thirteenth edition

Rypins' Medical Licensure Examinations

Edward D. Frohlich, M.D.

Vice President, Education and Research,
Alton Ochsner Medical Foundation;
Director, Division of Hypertensive Diseases,
Ochsner Clinic;
Professor of Medicine and Physiology,
Louisiana State University School of Medicine;
Adjunct Professor of Pharmacology and
Clinical Professor of Medicine,
Tulane University School of Medicine, New Orleans,
Louisiana

With the Collaboration of a Review Panel

thirteenth edition

Rypins'
Medical
Licensure
Examinations

topical summaries and questions

J. B. LIPPINCOTT COMPANY
Philadelphia • Toronto

The authors and publisher have exerted every effort to ensure that drug selection and dosage set forth in this text are in accord with current recommendations and practice at the time of publication. However, in view of ongoing research, changes in government regulations, and the constant flow of information relating to drug therapy and drug reactions, the reader is urged to check the package insert for each drug for any change in indications and dosage and for added warnings and precautions. This is particularly important when the recommended agent is a new or infrequently employed drug.

Thirteenth Edition

Copyright © 1981, by J. B. Lippincott Company.
Copyright © 1975, 1970, 1965, 1960, 1957 (edited by the late Arthur W. Wright, M.D.) by J. B. Lippincott Company.
Copyright 1952, 1947, 1945 (editions five to nine edited by the late Walter L. Bierring, M.D.) by J. B. Lippincott Company.
Copyright 1939, 1937, 1935, 1933 (editions one to four edited by the late Harold Rypins, M.D.) by J. B. Lippincott Company under the title MEDICAL STATE BOARD EXAMINATIONS.

6 5 4 3

Library of Congress Number 65–18856.

Printed in the United States of America

ISBN 0–397–52091–3

contents

editorial review panel

preface to the thirteenth edition

During the years that the thirteenth edition of RYPINS' will be available, we shall be celebrating the 50th anniversary of its availability to physicians who are preparing "for the ordeal of the licensing examination." This is indeed a remarkable achievement for any textbook; and the contemplation that three generations of physicians—grandparents, parents, and children—may have used this textbook to prepare for their same professional licensure provokes a thrilling sense of responsibility and satisfying reflections by the editor and contributors.

Initially, this textbook was prepared for those physicians planning to take State Board medical licensure examinations. It consisted of short treatises or summaries of nine major areas in medicine, each followed by typical questions from past examinations. This format has remained rather constant over the past twelve editions. With the thirteenth edition it remains the same although the number of areas have increased since the first edition to fourteen; however, the reviews are longer and the questions cover a wider range in proportion to the increasing knowledge in the respective fields.

I suspect that most experts, teachers, students, and specialists in preparing examinations would agree that all examinations have their faults. Nevertheless, licensing examinations remain the only means available for testing objectively the knowledge and competence of individuals to practice the art and science of medicine. As a result, the sophistication of examinations has increased and their scope and objectives have similarly expanded with the additional types of examinations: from the qualifying examination to National Board Examinations, and the several examinations that test the knowledge of practicing physicians worldwide. Each state jealously guards its right to determine which physician should be granted the privilege of practicing medicine within its borders; and, as a result, more than 50 jurisdictions have in the past prepared their own medical licensure examination. So great have been the differences in the kind and quality of these examinations, so low has been the rate of failure in some states and so high in others, that the interstate recognition of licenses has been found by some to be unsatisfactory. Indeed, because of the refusal of some states to accept the licenses of others, serious obstacles have been placed in the way of the interstate movement of physicians.

To resolve some of these difficulties, the Federation of State Medical Boards of the United States, after some years of study and research, developed a clinically oriented, reliable examination, the Federation Licensing Examination, that is offered to any State Board for its use as its own licensing examination. It is prepared by a committee of the Federation, in collaboration with the National Board of Medical Examiners. Known by the acronym FLEX (Federation Licensing EXamination), this examination is given in all participating states of the United States on the same three days, twice a year, in June and December. By far the largest number of graduates from American medical schools take another series of examinations, not identical to the FLEX, that are offered in three parts by the National Board of Medical Examiners (NBME): the first is given after the completion of the first two preclinical years in medical school; the second part, which focuses upon clinical medicine, is taken after the second two years; and part III, taken after at least six months of the first postgraduate training year, is an objective test of general clinical competence. With the Congress today considering health manpower legislation that may affect medical licensure, the use by all states of these high-quality examinations, prepared either under State Board auspices or by a nationally constituted medical licensure, may help forestall legislation of a Federal Licensing EXamination for graduates of American medical schools.

Nevertheless, the need for federal licensing examinations seems to have been mandated by the need to determine the competency of the knowledge of graduate physicians from foreign medical schools who are applying for the license to practice medicine in the United States. Over the years, two types of examinations have been developed for foreign medical graduates (FMG). The first of these, the ECFMG (Educational Commission for Foreign Medical Graduates), is a one-day test, in English, that consists of 300 well-chosen NBME multiple-choice questions, of which five out of every six come from the traditional clinical fields and the remaining question from basic medical sciences. Also included in the ECFMG examination is a one-hour test that is designed to assess the understanding of the English language. More recently, a second type of test has been introduced, the Visa Qualifying Examination (VQE) under mandate by a Congressional act in 1976. This law requires that all foreign medical graduates who are accepted for graduate training in the United States must pass the VQE before a visa can be issued to enter the United States. This examination is taken in three parts: the first in basic science, the second in clinical sciences, and the third in clinical and patient problems. Indeed, passing the VQE has been declared equivalent to passing parts I and II of the NBME. Still another area of medical licensure, of recent importance, is the requirement for relicensure by State medical boards of subspecialty organizations. Thus, examinations designed to determine medical knowledge and competence have undergone a tremendous growth in sophistication, number, and demands upon the professional physician.

We hope that this textbook will continue to be of value to all who are concerned with medical examinations—those who are preparing the examination; those who must prepare for medical licensure; those who must qualify for medical licensure (ECFMG); and those already licensed who are required to sit for relicensure examination. In addition, this textbook may also be of value to the medical educator planning for courses in continuing medical education, to the medical student who is interested in reviewing material for specific course examinations, and for the practicing physician interested in gaining a quick resumé of the present state of knowledge in some area of medical pedagogy. Indeed, this has been the text's aim over the past almost 50 years: to present, in a clear and concise manner, the most comprehensive and up-to-date knowledge of the various medical fields and to make the accompanying questions as pertinent and clinically oriented as possible. With respect to the questions that are appended to each chapter, it is suggested that the reader review not only the rhetorical questions; he should also consider the multiple-choice questions. These multiple-choice questions follow the style and format of the questions devised by the National Board of Medical Examiners and FLEX examinations. The answer key to the questions follows the listing of the questions.

As in previous editions, the textbook is divided into two parts. Part I, the basic medical sciences, contains sections on anatomy, physiology, biochemistry, microbiology and immunology, pathology, and pharmacology. Part II, the clinical sciences, includes chapters on surgery, internal medicine, obstetrics and gynecology, pediatrics, public health and community medicine, psychiatry, and the behavioral sciences. The introductory chapter on Medical Qualifying Examinations reviews the development of these examinations in greater detail than outlined above and points out the significance of each of the examinations, the testing procedures in all fields of medicine, and describes the examinations and the types of questions as well as the pitfalls that physicians preparing to sit for these examinations should anticipate.

With this thirteenth edition, the editorial responsibility for this textbook is assumed by its fourth editor. Editions one through four were edited by the late Harold Rypins, M.D.; editions five through nine, by the late Walter L. Bierring, M.D.; and editions ten through twelve, by the late Arthur W. Wright, M.D. I am especially grateful to the publisher, J. B. Lippincott Company, for selecting me to serve as the fourth editor, and I sincerely hope that this new edition measures up to the stature and achievement of the previous ones. Certainly, the former editors have provided a textbook of outstanding excellence and tradition to follow.

Several changes have been made in this book and should be acknowledged at this point. Dr. Calderon Howe has expanded the scope and responsibilities for the general microbiology chapter. Because of the burgeoning information in this field and the impact of the area of immunology in the practice of medicine, the chapter has been retitled General Microbiology and Immunology. Because of the untimely death of Dr. Wright, the immediately preceding editor of this book, we asked Dr. Jack Strong to author the Pathology chapter. Dr. Solomon Papper, a gifted teacher of Internal Medicine and known for his excellence in medical writing, has assumed the responsibility for that chapter. Drs. Gordon Deckert and Ronald Krug have revised the chapters in Psychiatry and Behavioral Sciences, each one taking senior authorship for his particular area of expertise in the areas in which they share outstanding competence. Each of these new authors has participated in and contributed importantly to medical education as well as to the formulation of medical examinations—State, National, and Specialty Board oriented. And, as already indicated, a major new feature of this volume is the addition of well-selected and pertinent multiple-choice questions (and their answers) at the end of each chapter.

Clearly, in this new task, the editor is especially grateful to those who have generously provided advice and assistance in preparation of this volume. To each and every one of these colleagues I offer my deep appreciation. I offer my never-ending thanks and gratefulness to my secretary, Mrs. Elizabeth Murray, for her unfailing and loyal support in preparing this manuscript. I also offer my gratitude to my institution, the Alton Ochsner Medical Foundation and Ochsner Clinic, for providing me the time and ambiance to pursue this academic challenge. I am most grateful to the staff of J. B. Lippincott Company, and particularly to Stuart Freeman for his advice. Above all, I offer my deep and grateful appreciation and love to my wife, Sherry, and my children, Margie, Bruce, and Lara, for their love and patience, and for their unquestioning understanding of the time and effort necessary to bring this manuscript to fruition.

EDWARD D. FROHLICH
New Orleans, Louisiana

preface to the first edition

This book is an expression of the writer's conviction that the average American medical graduate of today is well prepared for the practice of his profession and that consequently there is little basis for the obvious dread with which he approaches the ordeal of the licensing examination. It is based on fifteen years' experience as Secretary of the New York State Board of Medical Examiners, during which period he has had intimate contact not only with medical schools and boards of medical examiners throughout the country, but also with large numbers of candidates for the licensing examination.

After a critical survey of many thousands of questions actually used throughout the whole United States, a selection of typical questions has been made, and these immediately follow the review presented in each of the nine major medical subjects. By placing these questions at the end of the chapters the thought processes of the student are stimulated and his best interests more fully served than in the older forms of questions and answers.

It is the proper function of the state to submit to examination all candidates for the right to practice medicine, and the state medical licensing examination can, and in some instances does, serve as a valuable check upon the work of the medical schools. There should be, however, closer co-operation between licensing boards and medical schools. Medical faculties should recognize more clearly the function and intention of the licensing boards, and licensing boards should be more clearly aware of the progress which is being made in medical schools. It is evident that the examining boards are slowly realizing that medical schools are in better position than themselves to test the student's academic or encyclopedic knowledge of such subjects as anatomy, chemistry, and bacteriology; that such testing may be safely left in the hands of medical faculties; and that examining boards should limit themselves to inquiring into the ability of the medical graduate to apply such knowledge clinically.

As for the graduate's attitude toward the state licensing examination, his fear arises from failure to understand the point of view of the state examiners as well as from an ability to muster in due proportion the vast amount of material presented to him during his medical course.

Careful study of licensing examinations throughout the United States indicates a general agreement among examiners regarding the material essential for the candidate. It is this ground, and only this ground, that the present volume aims to cover.

Every effort has been made to treat as concisely as possible those portions of the medical curriculum generally selected for use by the various examining boards. Repetition and overlapping have been avoided. Where a subject such as rabies, for example, has been covered in the chapter on Preventive Medicine, it is not repeated under the consideration of the Filtrable Viruses in Bacteriology. The arrangement of the material emphasizes the relations of the whole and its parts. It is taken for granted that the student has been adequately trained in the medical sciences and there is no attempt to teach him anything new. The object is, not to cram his mind, rather, to assist him in selecting and rearranging his material intelligently and practically.

Deliberate omission has been made of nearly all technical procedures, such as physical diagnosis, blood-counting and blood-chemistry, basal metabolism, x-ray, or surgical technic. Technical procedures cannot be taught in books and the ability to employ them properly should be assumed in the modern graduate. For similar reasons there is no separate section on materia medica or prescription-writing. References to the use of therapeutic agents are included in the consideration of the disease for which they are indicated.

To the authors in the various fields of medicine from whose books and articles he has freely drawn, the author desires to express his appreciative thanks. His gratitude to Miss E. Marion Pilpel. Miss Florence S. Muffson, and particularly to his wife, Senta Jonas Rypins, for invaluable secretarial assistance, he is most happy to acknowledge.

HAROLD RYPINS
Albany, N.Y.

thirteenth edition

Rypins' Medical Licensure Examinations

1

Medical Qualifying Examinations

EDWARD D. FROHLICH, M.D.

Vice President, Education and Research, Alton Ochsner Medical
Foundation; Director, Division of Hypertensive Diseases, Ochsner Clinic;
Professor of Medicine and Physiology, Louisiana State University School
of Medicine; Adjunct Professor of Pharmacology and Clinical Professor
of Medicine, Tulane University School of Medicine, New Orleans,
Louisiana

The testing of professional competence before certifying for public responsibilities is an age-old practice. In China, for example, candidates for public service were required to submit to special examinations at least 3,000 years ago, and the tests were said to be not unlike those employed today. In the United States the practice developed slowly, first as a kind of contribution by the profession itself to public welfare; later as a responsibility of the state. In New York State the problem arose in the early 19th century as far as the practice of medicine is concerned. At that time, the Legislature found that attempts to control the practice of "physic and surgery" in unorganized fashion had been most unsatisfactory, since charlatans and quacks abounded, and passed "an act to incorporate Medical Societies for the purpose of regulating the practice of Physic and Surgery in this state." This law provided for the establishment of a medical society in each county and gave to the practicing physicians themselves, thus legally organized, the power to grant licenses to qualified applicants and to regulate the practice of medicine in their counties.

The methods of testing varied. In general, tests were clinical and practical, that is, they were limited to questions or discussions concerning the diagnosis and the treatment of diseases, for the candidates were chiefly those who had received their training as apprentices to practicing physicians. Not until nearly mid-century did the number of physicians who had had their education and training in medical schools predominate. Soon thereafter the states themselves began to assume the responsibilities of licensure and, consequently, for establishing formal testing procedures. With this development, Boards of Examiners, or similar bodies, were appointed to examine officially all applicants for fitness to practice the medical profession. Today, all 50 states, as well as the District of Columbia and the Commonwealth of Puerto Rico, have official medical licensing agencies.

The usual means of measuring knowledge is the for-

1

mal written examination, and it has an important place in all educational programs. "Examination," the late President Eliot of Harvard once stated, "is the most difficult of the educational arts and its influence on both students and teachers may be very great." Indeed, intelligently and thoughtfully prepared examinations can be made a most valuable educational exercise in any course of study. They not only force the student to review and stimulate him to keep up with his work, but they also may serve to test the quality of teaching if the examination is well designed and the results are interpreted carefully.

How effective are formal written examinations in testing professional competence? Perhaps not as effective as they are in an educational program. Nevertheless, they are the only practical means of assessing the competence of large numbers of applicants for professional licensure. Although this practice is not ideal and does not test for such essential attributes as ethical and moral standards, carefully designed tests do play a definite role in separating the qualified practitioner from the unqualified and, in doing so, protect the public from the charlatan and the incompetent.

Examinations for licensure, however, have not always kept pace with the remarkable advances in medical knowledge and the resultant changes in methods of training for the practice of medicine. For this reason, many of the examination methods employed in former years have become inadequate. Thus, the purpose of the licensing examination is not so much to test the candidate's general knowledge in such individual subjects as anatomy, pathology, medicine, and surgery as to determine his or her ability to apply this knowledge to the diagnosis and treatment of disease and to determine the candidate's general fitness to practice the art and the science of medicine. In the past, unfortunately, most licensing examinations failed miserably in this last category.

The existence of separate licensing boards in all the states, the District of Columbia and the Commonwealth of Puerto Rico, each setting its own type of qualifying examination for licensure, has led to great variation in the kind and quality of the examinations, has worked against unity of procedures and standards and has made difficult the movement of physicians from one licensing jurisdiction to another. Recently, however, as will be described in more detail later, through the efforts of the Federation of State Medical Boards of the United States, a high quality examination—the Federation Licensing Examination (FLEX) —prepared by a special Federation committee for administration twice a year, has been offered to any state medical board that wishes to use the examination as its own licensing test. A measure of its success is shown

by the fact that its use by nearly all states had been achieved by 1973.

Another confusing element in the licensing procedure has been added by the establishment in a number of states of separate boards of examiners in the basic sciences. These tests are designed to be given to candidates for admission to all branches of the healing professions, not only medicine but such other areas as chiropractic and neuropathy. In these jurisdictions certification by the basic science boards is required before admission to the specific professional examination is granted.

In most instances the members of these boards are teachers of such subjects as general chemistry, physics, biology, and anatomy. The tests are therefore not specifically prepared for physicians who have had intensive training in the basic medical sciences that form an integral part of medical education. The purpose of this examination is to determine whether the candidate has had adequate training in the several fundamental sciences considered to be essential for admission to the licensing examination of the particular healing art the applicant wishes to practice. At best these tests are elementary when compared with the comprehensive training in the basic medical sciences given in schools of medicine. The consequent repetition, in part at least, of an examination in basic sciences by the medical licensing boards in these states has complicated still further the licensing of physicians. Fortunately, the number of these basic science boards is diminishing, and the time appears not far off when they will be done away with.

All in all, then, with all their defects and deficiencies, examinations are essential to the licensing procedure. They form not only an integral part of any well-planned program of education but are also, when well constructed, the only generally satisfactory method of determining the professional competence and fitness to practice of large numbers of candidates. They constitute a dependable measure of coordinated thinking as well as a test of knowledge not to be gained in any other way. Examinations are therefore here to stay, and the objective of all boards of medical licensure must be to administer examinations that are as fair, comprehensive and valid tests of fundamental knowledge and clinical competence as it is possible to make.

TYPES OF EXAMINATIONS

The Essay Examination

Until recently many state boards of medical examiners employed the so-called essay examination, but this type is no longer generally used in licensing tests. In this test a limited number of questions is asked, and the candidate answers each one in a short composition or dissertation. The essay examination emphasizes description, definition, explanation and discussion. Symptoms, signs, abnormalities in function, pathologic changes, etiology and the diagnosis and treatment of disease conditions are described, and discussed by the candidate, sometimes at considerable length.

The advantages of the essay test are that it gives the candidate an opportunity to consider thoughtfully each of a limited number of problems posed, to reveal his ability to organize his answer, to demonstrate his skill at description and to present evidence of his general scholarship, his writing ability, penmanship, spelling, composition and neatness of execution. All of these qualities are desirable accomplishments, but not all of them are the particular attributes that define a physician's competence to practice medicine.

Among the disadvantages are the relatively long time it takes to grade essay answers, the difficulty the examiner has of being uniformly fair in grading answers to the same question on different papers and the frequent quandary the examiner finds himself in when, because of poor penmanship or a lack of knowledge of English on the part of the candidate, he cannot interpret an answer. The grading of essay examinations is therefore slow, subject to considerable subjective variation in evaluation of answers, and occupies an excessive amount of an examiner's time.

Finally, in view of the continued rapid expansion of medical knowledge in every field, it is now recognized that a limited number of essay questions does not permit as adequate testing of the candidate's general knowledge as is desired. Occasionally, therefore, oral or practical tests have been used to supplement the written test. With the additional information that such tests provide, the examining boards feel more secure in certifying a candidate for licensure. The great difficulty with this type of individual test, however, is that it cannot be given within a reasonable time, nor can adequate numbers of examiners be provided when great numbers of candidates must be examined. At present, if given at all, these individual tests are limited to those states where the number of candidates is small.

The Objective or Multiple-Choice Examination

In recent years more and more State Boards of Examiners have been turning to the objective or multiple-choice examination. In this type of test each question is so prepared that the candidate is faced with a problem, the correct answer to which is included in the question and must be selected and indicated on the answer sheet by making a mark in the appropriate place. The characteristic feature of these tests is that the candidate answers the questions by blackening, with a special pencil on the answer sheet, the space he believes to indicate the correct answer. Although this is considered a written examination, no actual writing of sentences is required. This kind of test has two important advantages: A great many more questions covering a much wider range of subjects can be asked in a given time than is possible in the essay examination, and the answers can be graded more objectively and with greater speed and accuracy than in any other type of examination. Thus, the number of questions that can be asked in an allotted period can be increased from 8 or 10, or at most 12, in an essay test to 100, 150, or even more, in the objective test, thereby effectively broadening the scope of the examination.

At first the objective or multiple-choice examination met with considerable disapproval on the candidate's part because the technique was so new and different, and on the examiners' part because the construction of valid, unambiguous, and reliable questions proved to be so difficult (far more difficult, in fact, than the preparation of essay questions). But with the passage of time the objective examination has come into its own as a valid, comprehensive and dependable test of a candidate's knowledge and, when applied effectively, of his competence and ability. Moreover, this type of examination seems to be the most searching, valid and comprehensive type of test to administer to large groups of candidates.

Many different forms of objective, multiple-choice questions have been devised to test not only medical knowledge but also the subtler qualities of discrimination, judgment and reasoning. Certain types of questions may test an individual's recognition of the similarity or the dissimilarity of diseases, drugs, physiologic or pathologic processes. Other questions test judgment as to cause and effect or the lack of causal relationships. Case histories are used to simulate the experience of a physician confronted with a diagnostic problem; a series of questions then tests the individual's understanding of related aspects of the case, such as associated laboratory findings, treatment, complications, and prognosis. In this type of examination each question has only one correct response among a number of possible choices—most often one correct response out of five choices, although the ratio may be somewhat less or considerably more.

The preparation of objective or multiple choice examinations is extremely difficult, for the work of the examiners, instead of consisting of the time-consuming and usually tiresome reading and grading of essay-type answers, shifts to the preparation of the many questions included in the tests. Because generally the objective is to construct questions with only one correct answer, the preparation of an examination is best done by a group, usually an examination construction committee. The members of each group or committee should be skilled in one basic or clinical science discipline. Usually each member prepares questions in advance of a committee meeting, at which each question will be subjected to a critical review. Doubtful items are revised, modified, or discarded and new items may be developed. All items not approved unanimously are discarded. An examination prepared in this way, which is the method used by the National Board of Medical Examiners, contains only material that has been thoroughly worked over and agreed upon as appropriate, free from ambiguity and representative not only of important aspects of the subject but also of high standards of education.

The Scoring of Multiple-Choice Examinations. When objective multiple-choice examinations are used, the examinations are usually scored by electronic machines. To the casual observer, this machine scoring may look like a highly mysterious business. The answer sheets are loaded into the machine, a button is pressed, and the machine reads the sheets, matches the answers against an answer key and punches the examinee's score into the automated machine data card. A manual check is also made to avoid the possibility of any technical error. Furthermore, these machines are not robots making their own decisions; they perform only in the way that they are programmed to perform. The responsible examiners determine whether an individual should pass or fail.

A grade of 75 has been established as the passing score for the examinations of the National Board. But it does not follow that it is necessary to respond correctly to 75 per cent of the items in order to obtain this grade. Indeed, the scoring procedure is such that usually a score of about 50 to 60 per cent of the questions answered correctly results in a passing grade of 75. In arriving at the passing score, the distribution curve of all those taking an examination is given consideration.

Examinations of the multiple-choice type have certain advantages over the time-honored essay tests. Although essay tests may probe more deeply into a limited number of subjects, multiple-choice examinations sample a much greater breadth of medical knowledge. Because the answer sheets can be scored by machine, the grading can be accomplished rapidly, accurately and impartially. With this type of examination it becomes possible to determine the level of difficulty of each test and to maintain comparability of examination scores from test to test and from year to year

for any single subject. Moreover, of even greater long-range significance is the facility with which the total test and the individual questions can be subjected to thorough and rapid statistical analysis, thus providing a sound basis for comparative studies and the continuing improvement in the quality of the test itself.

THE NATIONAL BOARD OF MEDICAL EXAMINERS

In the years following the issuance of the Flexner Report on the medical schools of the nation [Flexner, A.: Medical Education in the United States and Canada. Bulletin no. 4, Carnegie Foundation for the Advancement of Teaching, New York, 1910] it became evident that not only medical school programs, but also the licensing examinations of the various states, needed upgrading. One physician who took seriously the licensing examination matter was Dr. W. L. Rodman of Philadelphia, who, in 1915, founded the National Board of Medical Examiners. This Board, a voluntary and unofficial examining agency, was organized "to prepare and to administer qualifying examinations of such high quality that legal agencies governing the practice of medicine within each state" could, at their discretion, "grant a license without further examination to those candidates" who had passed the National Board examinations and had become Diplomates of the Board. The membership of the National Board of Medical Examiners has grown in strength and importance over the years and now includes representatives from the faculties of leading American medical schools and from the Association of American Medical Colleges, the American Medical Association, the Federation of State Medical Boards of the United States, the American Hospital Association, and various Federal medical services.

The National Board, however, is in no sense a licensing agency, and the last interest this board could have would be the responsibility of licensing physicians on a national basis. It is the function of each individual state to determine who shall practice within its borders and to set the standards of medical practice in accordance with its own rules and regulations. As its name implies, the National Board is an examining board, and currently all but a few states are willing to issue licenses to practice medicine within their borders to holders of the National Board Diploma; a few states do so with minor additional requirements. In a majority of states the National Board Diploma is accepted for full licensure. In New York State, for example, in 1973 approximately 37 per cent of all physicians licensed were licensed on the basis of their National

Board qualifications. It goes without saying that the reader preparing for licensure in a specific state should communicate directly with that state's Board of Medical Examiners to learn the requirements of that state.

Eligibility to take the National Board examinations is currently limited to candidates who are regularly enrolled as students in, or are graduates of, any approved medical school in the United States or Canada. Graduates of foreign medical schools are not admitted, although, before they may serve as interns or residents in any United States hospital, they must take and pass a qualifying examination, usually one given by the Educational Council for Foreign Medical Graduates—the so-called ECFMG examination—which itself is prepared for the Educational Council by the National Board of Medical Examiners. Recently there has been some modification of this requirement for United States citizens who, having completed their premedical education in the United States, have gone to a foreign country for their medical training and wish to return to this country to practice. More will be said about the ECFMG examination later in this chapter.

The examination of the National Board of Medical Examiners has from the outset been given in three parts, Part I in the basic medical sciences, Part II in the clinical sciences and Part III as a practical examination involving clinical and patient problems. Over the years, however, the examinations have not been static but have been changed in form and content to keep abreast of medical progress and changes in medical education. The examinations are prepared by special committees, one for each major basic science and clinical science field. These committees are selected with great care, and their members (usually six per committee) come from medical school faculties and the staffs of teaching hospitals all over the United States and Canada. Thus, the preparation of the examinations has been in the hands of leaders in the medical profession throughout the country, and the examinations themselves have reflected the progress and change occurring in the various fields of medicine and in science generally.

From carefully prepared essay tests in the various basic and clinical sciences the Board some years ago turned to the more efficient and valid objective or multiple-choice tests in the different subjects. The Board also decided to change from the Part III practical examinations given at the bedside in hospital centers throughout the country to a new, unique objective test of clinical competence that is taken by all candidates. This has resulted in more universally uniform and valid testing of a physician's fitness to practice, effectively eliminating the lack of uniformity that characterized the bedside examinations carried out in many

different centers. The National Board has not only kept constantly abreast of progress in medicine and medical education but has actually been a leader in bringing about progressive change, especially in the quality of examination procedures.

Today the Part I and Part II examinations are set up and scored as total comprehensive objective tests in the basic sciences and clinical sciences, respectively. The format of each part is changed since it is no longer subject oriented, that is, separated into sections specifically labeled Anatomy, Pathology, Medicine, Surgery, and so forth. Subject labels are therefore missing, and in each part questions from the different fields are intermixed or scrambled so that the subject origin of any individual question is not immediately apparent, although it is known in the National Board office. Therefore, if necessary, individual subject grades can be extracted.

Part I is a 2-day written test that includes questions in anatomy, biochemistry, microbiology, pathology, pharmacology, physiology and a recently added discipline, behavioral sciences. Each subject contributes to the examination a large number of questions designed to test not only knowledge of the subject itself but also "the subtler qualities of discrimination, judgment, and reasoning." Questions in such fields as molecular biology, cell biology and genetics are included, as are questions to test the "candidate's recognition of the similarity or dissimilarity of diseases, drugs, and physiologic, behavioral, or pathologic processes." Problems are presented in narrative, tabular or graphic form, followed by questions designed to assess the candidate's knowledge and comprehension of the situation described.

Part II is also a 2-day written test that includes questions in internal medicine, obstetrics and gynecology, pediatrics, preventive medicine and public health, psychiatry and surgery. The questions, like those in Part I, cover a broad spectrum of knowledge in each of the clinical fields. In addition to individual questions, clinical problems are presented in the form of case histories, charts, roentgenograms, photographs of gross and microscopic pathologic specimens, laboratory data, and the like, and the candidate must answer questions concerning the interpretation of the data presented and their relation to the clinical problems. The questions are "designed to explore the extent of the candidate's knowledge of clinical situations and to test his ability to bring information from many different clinical and basic science areas to bear upon these situations."

The examinations of both Part I and Part II are scored as a whole, certification being given on the basis of performance on the entire part, without reference to disciplinary breakdown. The grade for the part is derived from the total number of questions answered correctly, rather than from an average of the grades in the component basic science or clinical science subjects. A candidate who fails will be required to repeat the entire part. Nevertheless, as noted above, in spite of the interdisciplinary character of the examinations, all of the traditional disciplines are represented in the test, and separate grades for each subject can be extracted and reported separately to students, to state examining boards or to those medical schools that request them for their own educational and academic purposes.

This type of interdisciplinary examination and the method of scoring the entire test as a unit have definite advantages, especially in view of the changing character of the curricula in modern medical schools. The old type of rigid, almost standardized, curriculum, with its emphasis on specific subjects and specified numbers of hours in each, has been replaced by a more liberal, open-ended kind of curriculum, permitting emphasis in one or more fields and corresponding deemphasis in others. The result has been rather wide variations in the totality of education in different medical schools. Thus, the scoring of these tests as a whole permits accommodation to this variability in the curricula of different schools. Within the total score, weakness in one subject that has received relatively little emphasis in a given school may be balanced by strength in other subjects.

The rationale for this type of comprehensive examination as replacement for the traditional department-oriented examination in the basic sciences and the clinical sciences is given in The National Board Examiner:

The student, as he confronts these examinations, must abandon the idea of "thinking like a physiologist" in answering a question labeled "physiology" or "thinking like a surgeon" in answering a question labeled "surgery." The one question may have been written by a biochemist or a pharmacologist; the other question may have beeen written by an internist or a pediatrician. The pattern of these examinations will direct the student to thinking more broadly of the basic sciences in Part I and to thinking of patients and their problems in Part II.

Until a few years ago the Part I examination could not be taken until the work of the second year in medical school had been completed, and the Part II test was given only to the student who had completed the major part of the fourth year. Now a student, if he feels he is ready, may be admitted to any regularly scheduled Part I or Part II examination during any year of his medical course without prerequisite completion of specified courses or chronologic periods of study. Thus, emphasis is placed upon acquisition of knowledge and competence rather than completion of predetermined periods.

A candidate is eligible for Part III after he has passed Parts I and II, has received the M.D. degree from an approved medical school in the United States or Canada and, subsequent to the receipt of the M.D. degree, has served at least 6 months in an approved hospital internship or residency. Under certain circumstances, consideration may be given to other types of graduate training provided they meet with the approval of the National Board. After passing the Part III examination the candidate will receive his Diploma as of the date of the satisfactory completion of his internship or residency. If a candidate has completed his approved hospital training prior to completion of Part III, he will receive certification as of the date of the successful completion of Part III.

The Part III examination, as noted above, is an objective test of general clinical competence. It occupies one full day and is divided into two sections, the first of which is a multiple-choice examination that relates to the interpretation of clinical data presented primarily in pictorial form such as pictures of patients, gross and microscopic lesions, electrocardiograms, charts, and graphs. The second section, entitled Patient Management Problems, utilizes a programmed-testing technique (answer by erasure to uncover information or results of actions) designed to measure the candidate's clinical judgment in the management of patients. This technique simulates clinical situations in which the physician is faced with the problems of management presented in a sequential programmed pattern. A set of some four to six problems is related to each of a series of patients. In the scoring of this section, candidates are given credit for correct choices; they are penalized for errors of commission (selection of procedures that are unnecessary or are contraindicated) and for errors of omission (failure to select indicated procedures).

All parts of the National Board examinations are given in a great many centers, usually in medical schools, in nearly every large city in the United States, as well as in a few cities in Canada, in Puerto Rico and in the Canal Zone. In some cities, such as New York, Chicago and Baltimore, the examination may be given in more than one center.

The examinations of the National Board have become recognized as the most comprehensive test of knowledge of the medical sciences and their clinical application produced in this country. Approaching them in comprehensiveness and quality are the examinations, developed in close association with the National Board by a committee of the Federation of State Medical Boards of the United States, given twice a year under the auspices of the Federation in any state wishing to use them. These are known as the Federation Licensing Examinations or by the acronym FLEX. More will be said about these examinations later.

For years the National Board examinations have served as an index of the medical education of the period and have strongly influenced higher educational standards in each of the medical sciences. The Diploma of the National Board is accepted by 47 state licensing authorities, the District of Columbia and the Commonwealth of Puerto Rico in lieu of the examination usually required for licensure and is recognized in the American Medical Directory by the letters DNB following the name of the physician holding National Board certification.

The National Board of Medical Examiners has been a leader in developing new and more reliable techniques of testing, not only for knowledge in all medical fields but also for clinical competence and fitness to practice. In recent years, too, a number of medical schools, several specialty certifying boards, professional medical societies organized to encourage their members to keep abreast of progress in medicine and other professional qualifying agencies have called upon the National Board's professional staff for advice or for the actual preparation of tests to be employed in evaluating medical knowledge, effectiveness of teaching and professional competence in some medical fields. In all cases, advantage has been taken of the validity and effectiveness of the objective, multiple-choice type of examination, a technique the National Board has played an important role in bringing to its present state of perfection and discriminatory effectiveness.

THE ECFMG EXAMINATION

There have been three important developments in the field of medical qualifying examinations in recent years. The first was brought about as a result of the problems created by the ever increasing numbers of foreign-educated physicians, particularly from non-English speaking countries, who were coming to the United States for further education and training, many of whom decided to remain in this country to practice. After a 2-year study by a committee representing the American Hospital Association, the American Medical Association, the Association of American Medical Colleges and the Federation of State Medical Boards of the United States, with the unofficial cooperation of the US Department of State, the Educational Council for Foreign Medical Graduates (ECFMG) was created. The purpose of the Council is to develop and administer an evaluation procedure or qualifying examination, now called the ECFMG Examination, that will effectively ascertain the fitness of foreign medical graduates to serve as interns and residents in hospitals in the United States. Also included for those who come from countries where English is not the spoken language is a 1-hour examination designed to assess comprehension of English vocabulary and language structure.

It was only natural that the Council should turn to the National Board of Medical Examiners for advice and help. The result was that the examinations, given twice each year, were, and continue to be, prepared and scored by the National Board. Indeed, so close became the association between these two organizations because of this relationship, that the home office of the Council, formerly in Evanston, Illinois, was moved to Philadelphia, Pennsylvania, where it is now located. This is the same city in which the home office of the National Board is located.

The Council on Medical Education of the American Medical Association has adopted rules providing that no approved hospital in the United States can now employ as interns or residents any foreign-educated physicians who do not hold the ECFMG Certificate unless they already have a valid state license. In spite of some criticism (most of it unwarranted) of the Council as well as its sponsoring agencies in the first few years, the Council, after giving more than 315,000 examinations in more than 175 centers in this country and in over 85 foreign countries, has fully justified its existence. Indeed, at the present time practically every state that will accept foreign-educated physicians for licensure requires that all these applicants hold the ECFMG Certificate before being admitted to the licensing examination in that state.

The Council semiannually issues the *ECFMG Information Booklet** in which are set forth the requirements for ECFMG certification, and several pages are devoted to describing the examination itself. It is stated that this is primarily a comprehensive clinical examination. Although only about one tenth of the 360 questions come specifically from the basic sciences of anatomy, biochemistry, microbiology, pathology, pharmacology and physiology, many of the questions in the clinical fields require up-to-date knowledge of the basic sciences. Stress is laid on the various clinical fields in the following order: medicine, surgery, obstetrics and gynecology and pediatrics.

* Copies can be obtained by writing to the Educational Council for Foreign Medical Graduates, 3624 Market Street, Philadelphia, Pennsylvania 19104.

THE FEDERATION LICENSING EXAMINATION (FLEX)

The second significant achievement in the development of qualifying examinations was the introduction, in 1968, of the first Federation Licensing Examination (FLEX), prepared under the direction of the Examination Institute Committee of the Federation of State Medical Boards of the United States, Inc. Beginning in 1957, the Federation's Examination Institute Committee had held annual conferences designed to study examination procedures in the various states with the end in view of improving their quality and keeping them abreast of the continuing progress in medical education. As a result, there is general agreement to justify the continuation of this committee on a permanent basis.

At the present time this committee is charged: to provide state medical boards with high quality, uniform, and valid examinations for purposes of evaluating clinical competence and qualification for licensure; to place licensure in a definite relation to modern medical education by updating state board examination procedures and providing flexibility; to establish uniform levels of examinations among the states; to create a rational basis for interstate endorsement; and to provide a basis for the management of the foreign medical graduate problem.

Following publication of their first complete report, in 1961, the Examination Institute Committee continued to hold special conferences and symposia at each annual Federation meeting, and to press forward in its efforts to develop an examination of high quality that would be acceptable to the various state medical boards. At first, it was believed that the Federation itself could set up an examination center, staffed by a medical director and a specialist in examination construction and preparation, that would be in competition with other examination centers, particularly the National Board of Medical Examiners, which had been functioning for more than 50 years. Since the cost was found to be prohibitive, the Examination Institute Committee consulted with the staff of the National Board of Medical Examiners, and the Federation Licensing Examination came into being. Thus, in 1967, the Federation of State Medical Boards gave the new examination its unanimous approval at its annual meeting; and in June, 1968, candidates for licensure in six states took the first FLEX examinations. Since then, all but two states have accepted the FLEX examination as their own official licensing examination.

The Federation Licensing Examination (FLEX) is a uniform, valid and reliable licensing examination, planned and prepared by FLEX Test Committees composed of Federation members and designed for use by any state medical licensing board. It is a 3 day examination given simultaneously by participating medical boards in the name of their own states twice a year, in June and December.

The arrangement with the National Board calls for making pools of already tested and validated objective questions in the six major basic medical science disciplines and the six major clinical fields available to the Test Committees composed of Federation members who represent the state medical boards that have decided to use the FLEX examination. From this collection of questions two subcommittees—one for the basic sciences and one for the clinical sciences—prepare the licensing examinations in these two fields. A third subcommittee selects the questions or problems to be given in the test of clinical competence.

This latter test is relatively new in licensing examinations in spite of the fact that such competence is the most essential requirement of a physician. A few state boards had attempted to solve the problem by requiring oral or practical tests in addition to the standard written tests, but for those boards that had a large number of applicants for licensure, individual tests of this kind were out of the question. The National Board of Medical Examiners had developed an ideal and unique practical test that had been used for some years with great success. This, the Federation's FLEX Committee (now called the FLEX Board) felt, met every need, and it was decided to add this practical test to those in the basic and clinical sciences. However, because of the many changes in the curricula of medical schools in this country, it was held that individual tests in anatomy, physiology, surgery, etc., were becoming outmoded. A comprehensive interdisciplinary examination that covered all basic medical science fields in one test and the clinical sciences in another was established. Questions in all of the important areas would be included in these tests; they would be "scrambled" without regard to discipline, but with all fields adequately represented. It was decided that about 90 questions each in anatomy, biochemistry, microbiology, pathology, pharmacology and physiology would be mixed together in the basic sciences test, and about the same number of questions each in internal medicine, obstetrics and gynecology, pediatrics, preventive medicine and public health, psychiatry, and surgery would be mixed together in the clinical sciences test.

In each examination, the origin of the individual questions is known in the central office. Therefore, in spite of the scrambled character of the questions in the actual examination, it is possible to extract specific grades in each individual subject if these are needed. The FLEX Board felt, however, that each basic science and clinical science examination should be considered as a unit, with a single grade to be given for each entire test.

The examination in the basic sciences, given on the first day, is divided into three sections, A, B, and C, each lasting about 2½ hours, in which time some 180 questions must be answered, making a total of approximately 540 questions for the day. The clinical sciences examination, given on the second day, is presented in the same way.

On the third day the examination designed to test clinical competence is given. This test is divided into two sections that resemble in all details the two sections of Part III of the National Board examination. In the first section clinical material is presented in the form of pictures of patients or specimens, roentgenograms, electrocardiograms and graphic or tabulated material about which searching questions are asked. In the second section a distinctive technique described as programmed testing is employed, the object being to assess the candidate's judgment in the sequential management of patients in a manner similar to that which he would experience in relation to his own patients as he studied their disease processes or injuries, evaluated his findings and planned his treatment. A single overall grade is given to this entire part.

Because there will be many physicians who graduated from several to many years before appearing for this examination, the FLEX Board decided to provide, in addition to a single grade for each of the three parts (and of course, separate grades in each of the basic and clinical science subjects for those boards that might want them) a single overall grade for the entire examination, a grade that would give greater weight to the clinical, rather than the basic science, portion of the test. This is the so-called FLEX weighted average. This average is developed by emphasizing the importance of the clinical parts of the examination, inasmuch as a weight of 1 is given to the basic sciences grade, a weight of 2 to the clinical sciences grade and a weight of 3 to the clinical competence grade. How this weighted average is to be used will depend on the decision of each state medical board giving the FLEX examination. The FLEX Board recommends that a weighted average of 75 be the accepted passing grade.

Thus, there are now two important medical examinations, those given by the National Board of Medical Examiners and those given under the auspices of the Federation of State Medical Boards of the United States. These two examinations do not conflict since their purposes are not exactly the same. The National Board examinations are designed to test the knowledge of students as they are learning medicine in medical schools today; these tests are focused on the student of today and the physician of tomorrow. The FLEX examination is designed to assess fundamental knowledge and, more especially, the clinical competence of the physician of today. A dual examination system has thus emerged, each examination important in its own right, each with a different objective and each aimed at its own clearly defined target.

THE VISA QUALIFYING EXAMINATION (VQE)

Until 1976, all foreign medical graduates desiring to undergo postgraduate medical training in the United States were required to take the ECFMG examination before being certified by the ECFMG to be accepted by an accredited US hospital training program. But in 1976, and again in 1977, the United States Congress enacted amendments to the Immigration and Naturalization Act (INA) that require all foreign medical graduates who desire to enter the United States for postgraduate training (or to practice medicine) to pass the new Visa Qualifying Examination (VQE). Thus, passing this examination is required for eligibility for ECFMG certification based on VQE in order to obtain a visa to enter the United States. At this time this examination is not required for American citizens who are graduates of foreign medical schools, although it is possible that at some time in the future these individuals may be required to pass the VQE examination— not to be issued a visa to enter the United States but to obtain ECFMG certification for eligibility for postgraduate medical training.

The VQE is taken in two parts, the first in the basic sciences and the second in the clinical sciences; and they are very similar to the National Board examinations. Because of this extremely close similarity of the VQE and the National Boards (both, in fact, devote 50 per cent of the two parts to the basic sciences), a passing score on the VQE has been declared equivalent (by the ECFMG and the visa granting agency) to a passing score of Parts I and II of the National Board Examinations, providing the candidate also demonstrates competence in oral and written English. In 1977 there was a 75 per cent failure rate of the basic sciences (day 1) part of the VQE, an extremely high rate, particularly in comparison to the ECFMG examination (which has a much lower percentage of questions in the basic sciences area). Perhaps the candidates for examinations taking the VQE had thought that the VQE and ECFMG examinations were identical; clearly they are not, although both may provide ECFMG certification. The VQE (or its equivalent, as determined by the Secretary of Health and Human Resources) is a requirement for the immigration of physicians to the United States.

FIVE POINTS TO REMEMBER

In order for the candidate to maximize chances for passing these examinations, a few commonsense strategies or guidelines should be kept in mind.

First, it is imperative to thoroughly prepare for the examination. Know well the types of questions to be presented, the pedagogic areas of particular weakness, and devote more preparatory study time to these weak areas. Do not use too much time restudying areas in which there is a feeling of great confidence and do not leave unexplored those areas in which there is less confidence. Finally, be well rested before the test, and, if possible, avoid traveling to the city of testing just that morning or late the evening before.

Second, know well the format of the examination and the instructions before becoming immersed in the challenge at hand. This information can be obtained from many published texts and brochures or directly from the testing service (e.g., ECFMG and VQE from 3624 Market Street, Philadelphia, Pennsylvania 19104, USA; cable: EDCOUNCIL; telephone: (215) 386-5900). In addition, the many available texts and self-assessment types of examinations are valuable for practice.

Third, know well the overall time allotted for the examination and its components and the scope of the test to be faced. These may be learned by a rapid review of the examination itself. Then, proceed with the test at a careful, deliberate, and steady pace without spending inordinate time on any single question. For example, certain questions such as the "one best answer" (questions 1 to 3 of "Examples of Questions" below) probably should be allotted one to one and one-half minutes each. The "matching" type of questions (numbers 4 to 18) should be allotted similar time. The multiple "true-false" type should be given about a minute and a half. Thus, each question of the five-component questions should be allotted approximately 20 seconds. With respect to the "recall" type of question, there is great need for logical judgment, for the candidate to infer an answer from the presentation of the data, and to discard illogical answers from the multiplicity of the choices. Further, the candidate should be aware that those questions containing the word "always" or "never" are unlikely to be wise choices; questions with words such as "may" and "could" are wiser selections.

Fourth, it follows that if a question is particularly disturbing, the candidate should note appropriately the question (put a mark on the question sheet) and return to this point later. Don't compromise yourself by so concentrating on a likely "loser" that several "winners" are eliminated because of inadequate time. One way to save this time on a particular "stickler" is to play your initial choice; your chances of a correct answer are always best with your first impression. If there is no initial choice, reread the question.

Fifth, allow adequate time to review answers, to return to the questions that were unanswered and "flagged" for later attention, and check every *n*th (e.g., 20th) question to make certain that the answers are appropriate and that you did not inadvertently skip a question in the booklet or answer on the sheet (this can happen easily under these stressful circumstances).

There is nothing magical about these points. They are simple and just make sense. If the candidate prepared himself well and follows the preceding commonsense points, the chances are he will not return for a second go-round.

EXAMPLES OF QUESTIONS

The following questions are presented as a guide to the physician preparing for the above examinations. They offer the variety of types of multiple-choice questions that have been devised to provide objectivity in testing a large area of subject material that demands depth in knowledge and comprehension.

OBJECTIVE-MULTIPLE CHOICE TYPE

Completion Type

The so-called completion type item is the most common. Items of this type usually are placed together at the beginning of the test, as follows, with these directions:

Directions. *Each of the following questions or incomplete statements is followed by five suggested answers or completions. Select the one that is best in each case and blacken the corresponding space on the answer sheet.*

The following item illustrates this type, although obviously this question is rather easy.

Question 1:

To which one of the following systems of the body does the heart belong?

(a) The digestive system
(b) The central nervous system

(c) The circulatory system
(d) The endocrine system
(e) The musculoskeletal system

The correct answer, of course, is (c). To make this question somewhat more difficult and avoid naming the correct system among the choice, the circulatory system can be omitted and an alternative choice, "None of the above,"substituted for it. Then the question will appear as:

Question 2:

To which of the following systems of the body does the heart belong?

(a) The digestive system
(b) The central nervous system
(c) The endocrine system
(d) The musculoskeletal system
(e) None of the above

The fifth choice (e), now becomes the correct response. In this manner the candidate is made to think of the various systems of the body and must know the right answer without its being suggested to him as one of the possibilities. In these examinations the choice "None of the above" will appear and sometimes will be a correct and sometimes an incorrect response.

Another variant of the completion type of item is in the negative form, where all but one of the choices are applicable, and the candidate is asked to mark the one that does not apply. The following is an example:

Question 3:

All of the following are associated with prerenal azotemia EXCEPT

(a) Shock
(b) Dehydration
(c) Pernicious vomiting
(d) Gastrointestinal hemorrhage
(e) Multiple myeloma

The correct answer is (e).

Association and Relatedness Items

Items of a somewhat different nature may be used effectively, as, for example, in determining the candidate's knowledge of the action and the use of closely related drugs or the distinguishing features of similar diseases. There follow specific directions for items of this type with a group of items taken from a pharmacol-

ogy test and another group from a medicine test. As illustrated in this group of items, the candidate must have well-organized information about a number of related drugs and is required to demonstrate considerable understanding of the differential use of these drugs.

Directions. Each group of questions below consists of five lettered headings followed by a list of numbered words or phrases. For each numbered word or phrase, select the one heading that is related most closely to it.

Questions 4–9:

(a) Quinidine
(b) Theophylline
(c) Amyl nitrite
(d) Glyceryl trinitrate
(e) Papaverine

4. Relaxes smooth muscle of the arterial system; causes fall in arterial pressure; commonly administered in tablets sublingually *Answer:* (d).
5. An opium alkaloid; direct vasodilator action; used in instances of coronary occlusion and peripheral vascular disease. *Answer:* (e)
6. Commonly effective in relieving symptoms of bronchial asthma *Answer:* (b)
7. The best for quick treatment of cyanide poisoning *Answer:* (c)
8. Increases the contractile force of the heart and is diuretic *Answer:* (b)
9. May be used in auricular fibrillation *Answer:* (a)

Questions 10–17:

(a) Coarctation of the aorta
(b) Patent ductus arteriosus
(c) Tetralogy of Fallot
(d) Aortic vascular ring
(e) Tricuspid atresia

10. Benefited by systemic pulmonary artery anastomosis *Answer:* (c)
11. Most common type of congenital cyanotic heart disease *Answer:* (c)
12. Corrected surgically by resection and end-to-end anastomosis *Answer:* (a)
13. Possible cause of dysphagia in infants and children *Answer:* (d)
14. Wide pulse pressure *Answer:* (b)
15. Associated frequently with atrial septal defects *Answer:* (e)
16. A continuous murmur *Answer:* (b)

17. Hypertension in the arms and hypotension in the legs *Answer:* (a)

A further elaboration of association and relatedness items is considerably more searching and calls for a discriminatory understanding of a number of similar but distinguishable factors. For example, the following question reveals considerable information about the candidate's knowledge of the causes of hypoglycemia and the related functional disturbances: four of the five situations in the numbered list below are common to one of the three functional disturbances designated by letters. The candidate is instructed to select one situation that is the exception and the functional disturbance common to the remaining four.

Question 18:

(a) Clinically significant hypoglycemia
(b) Clinically significant hyperglycemia
(c) Clinically significant glycosuria

(1) Overdose of insulin
(2) Functional tumor of islet cells
(3) Renal glycosuria
(4) Hypopituitarism
(5) von Gierke's disease

If the candidate selects (a) and (3), the correct answer, he demonstrates that he knows that (1), (2), (4) and (5) may produce clinically significant hypoglycemia; that (3) does not; and that no combination of four of the five conditions is associated with hyperglycemia or glycosuria. In other words, the possession of both positive and negative information is probed. Specific directions for handling this form of discriminatory question read as follows:

Directions. There are two responses to be made to each of the following questions. There are three lettered categories; four of the five numbered items are related in some way to one of these categories. (1) On the answer sheet blacken the space under the letter of the category in which these four items belong. (2) Then blacken the space under the number of the item that does not belong in the same category with the other four.

Items of this type may be used to determine knowledge of disease symptomatology, laboratory findings or therapeutic procedures, as shown by the following:

Questions 19–21:

19.
(a) Multiple neurofibromatosis (von Recklinghausen's disease)

(b) Hemangioblastomas of the central nervous system
(c) Multiple sclerosis

(1) Neurofibromas of the skin
(2) Meningeal fibromas
(3) Congenital angiomas of the eye
(4) Lipomas of subcutaneous tissue
(5) Cystic disease of the pancreas

Answer: 1. (a)
    2. (5)

20.
(a) Contraindications to saddleblock anesthesia
(b) Contraindications to continuous caudal analgesia
(c) Contraindications to local anesthesia

(1) Deformity of the sacrum
(2) Cutaneous infections
(3) Perforated dura
(4) Decreased perineal resistance
(5) Prodromal labor

Answer: 1. (b)
    2. (4)

21.
(a) Eosinophilia of diagnostic significance
(b) Plasmacytosis of diagnostic significance
(c) Lymphoctyosis of diagnostic significance

(1) Trichinosis
(2) Multiple myeloma
(3) Löffler's syndrome
(4) Hodgkin's disease
(5) Schistosomiasis

Answer: 1. (a)
    2. (2)

Another variant of the association and relatedness type of question is demonstrated by the following example from a test in public health and preventive medicine:

Directions. Each set of lettered headings below is followed by a list of words or phrases. For each word or phrase blacken the space on the answer sheet under

A if the word or the phrase is associated with (a) *only*
B if the word or the phrase is associated with (b) *only*
C if the word or the phrase is associated with *both* (a) and (b)

D if the word or the phrase is associated with *neither*
(a) *nor* (b)

Questions 22–26:

(a) Maternal hygiene program
(b) School-health program
(c) Both
(d) Neither

22. Periodic physical examination *Answer:* C—
(a & b)
23. Audiometer test *Answer:* B
24. Nutritional guidance *Answer:* C—(a & b)
25. Serologic test for syphilis *Answer:* A
26. Immunization against rubella *Answer:* B

Quantitative Values and Comparisons

In general, questions in this category will call for an understanding of quantitative values rather than rote memory of the quantities themselves. The test committees have agreed that these examinations should contain a minimum of questions calling for the memorizing of absolute quantitative amounts. Actual figures will be found only where the details of the information are considered to be of such importance that they should be a part of the working knowledge that a practicing physician should have in mind without recourse to a reference book. Knowledge of the comparative significance of quantitative values may be called for by items such as the following:

Directions. The following paired statements describe two entities that are to be compared in a quantitative sense. On the answer sheet blacken the space under

A if (a) is *greater than* (b)
B if (b) is *greater than* (a)
C if the two are *equal or very nearly equal*

Questions 27–31:

27.
(a) The usual therapeutic dose of epinephrine
(b) The usual therapeutic dose of ephedrine *Answer:* B
28.
(a) The inflammability of nitrous oxide-ether mixtures *Answer:* A
(b) The inflammability of chloroform-air mixtures
29.
(a) The susceptibility of premature infants to rickets *Answer:* A
(b) The susceptibility of full-term infants to rickets
30.
(a) Life expectancy with glioblastoma of the occipital lobe
(b) Life expectancy with glioblastoma of the frontal lobe *Answer:* C
31.
(a) The amount of glycogen in the cells of Henle's loop in a diabetic *Answer:* A
(b) The amount of glycogen in the cells of Henle's loop in a nondiabetic

Directions. Each of the following pairs of phrases describes conditions or quantities that may or may not be related. On the answer sheet blacken the space under

A if increase in the first is accompanied by increase in the second or if decrease in the first is accompanied by decrease in the second
B if increase in the first is accompanied by decrease in the second or if decrease in the first is accompanied by increase in the second
C if changes in the second are independent of changes in the first

Questions 32–34:

32.
(1) Urine volume
(2) Urine specific gravity *Answer:* B
33.
(1) Plasma protein concentration
(2) Colloid osmotic pressure of plasma *Answer:* A
34.
(1) Cerebrospinal fluid pressure
(2) Intraocular pressure *Answer:* C

Cause and Effect

A type of item that is especially applicable to some of the more elusive aspects of medicine and calls for an understanding of cause and effect is illustrated in the following type of questions:

Directions. Each of the following sentences consists of two main parts: a statement and a reason for that statement. On the answer sheet blacken the space under

A if the statement and the proposed reason are *both true* and are *related* as cause and effect
B if the statement and the proposed reason are *both true* but are *not related* as cause and effect
C if the statement is *true* but the proposed reason is *false*

D if the statement is false but the proposed reason is *an accepted fact or principle*

E if the statement and the proposed reason are *both false*

Directions Summarized:

A = True True and related
B = True True and NOT related
C = True False
D = False True
E = False False

In situations that may be presented by this type of item, the right answer may sometimes be arrived at through good reasoning from an appreciation of the basic principles involved. The sample items are as follows:

Questions 35–39:

35. Herpes simplex usually is regarded as an autogenous infection BECAUSE patients given fever therapy frequently develop herpes. *Answer:* A

36. Cow's milk is preferable to breast milk in infant feeding BECAUSE cow's milk has a higher content of calcium. *Answer:* D

37. The corpus luteum of menstruation becomes the corpus luteum of pregnancy BECAUSE progesterone inhibits the activity of the anterior portion of the pituitary gland. *Answer:* B

38. The sinoauricular node serves as the pacemaker BECAUSE after its removal the heart fails to beat. *Answer:* C

39. A higher titer of antibody against the H antigen of the typhoid bacillus is a good index of immunity to typhoid BECAUSE any antibody to an organism can protect against disease caused by that organism. *Answer:* E

Question 40:

A modification of the true-false type of question that calls for careful thought and discrimination is the "multiple true-false" variety. In this question a list of numbered items follows a statement for which several possible answers are given and the candidate is required to select the appropriate response from a list of answers designated by letters:

40. Live virus is used in immunization against:
    1. influenza
    2. poliomyelitis
    3. cholera
    4. smallpox

Answers:
A. only 1, 2 and 3 are correct
B. only 1 and 3 are correct
C. only 2 and 4 are correct
D. only 4 is correct
E. all are correct

Structure and Function

Diagrams, charts, electrocardiograms, roentgenograms or photomicrographs may be used to elicit knowledge of structure, function, the course of a clinical situation or a statistical tabulation. Questions then may be asked in relation to designated elements of the same.

Case Histories

The most characteristic situation that confronts the practicing physician can be simulated by a case history followed by a series of questions concerning diagnosis, signs and symptoms, laboratory determinations, treatment and prognosis. In answering these questions, much depends on arriving at the proper diagnosis, for, if an incorrect diagnosis is made, related symptoms, laboratory data and treatment also will be wrong. These case history questions are set up purposely to place such emphasis on the correct diagnosis comparable with the experience of actual practice.

Directions. *This section of the test consists of several case histories, each followed by a series of questions. Study each history, select the best answer to each question following it, and blacken the space under the corresponding letter on the answer sheet.*

The patient is a 21-year-old white man with a complaint of malaise, cough and fever. The present illness had its onset 10 days prior to admission with malaise and a nonproductive cough, followed in 24 hours by a temperature varying from 100 to 101 that persisted up to the time of admission. On about the fourth day of illness the cough became more severe, producing scant amounts of white viscid sputum. Three days prior to admission, paroxysms of coughing began, followed sometimes by vomiting. Chilly sensations were noted but no frank shaking chills. Anterior parasternal pain on coughing has been present since the fifth day of illness.

On physical examination the temperature is 101; the pulse rate 110; the respiratory rate 32; and the blood pressure 108 systolic, 60 diastolic. The patient is well developed and well nourished, appears to be acutely but not chronically ill, and is dyspneic but not cyanotic.

Positive physical findings are limited to the chest and are as follows:

Vocal and tactile fremitus and resonance are within normal limits. In the left axilla a few fine rales are heard, and the bronchial quality of the sounds is increased, although the intensity is normal.

Blood findings are reported as follows:

White blood count 3,400 (polymorphonuclears 30%, lymphocytes 62%, monocytes 5%, eosinophils 3%).

Roentgenogram of the chest reveals an increase in the density of the perihilar markings with ill-defined areas of patchy, soft, increased radiodensity at both bases and in the left upper lung field.

Questions 41–45:

41. Which one of the following is the most likely diagnosis?
    (a) Tuberculosis
    (b) Pneumococcal pneumonia
    (c) Primary atypical pneumonia *Answer:* (c)
    (d) Coccidioidomycosis
    (e) Bronchopneumonia

42. Which one of the following is the most likely additional physical finding?
    (a) Splenomegaly
    (b) Signs of meningeal irritation
    (c) Pleural friction rub
    (d) Frequent changes in distribution of chest findings *Answer:* (d)
    (e) Signs of frank lobar consolidation

43. Which one of the following laboratory findings is consistent with the diagnosis?
    (a) Elevation and further increase of cold agglutinins *Answer:* (a)
    (b) Positive blood culture
    (c) Marked leukocytosis with the beginning of recovery
    (d) Positive sputum examination
    (e) Positive skin test

44. Which one of the following is the therapy that should be given?
    (a) Bed rest and streptomycin
    (b) Bed rest and penicillin
    (c) Streptomycin and paraaminosalicylic acid
    (d) Bed rest and Aureomycin *Answer:* (d)
    (e) Psychotherapy and physical rehabilitation

45. Which one of the following is the probable outcome of this disease in this patient if untreated?
    (a) The fever will subside spontaneously by crisis
    (b) Recovery will be gradual, with relapse not unexpected. *Answer:* (b)
    (c) Empyema will develop

    (d) Residual fibrosis will appear with healing
    (e) Lung cavitation will not be unexpected

Objective examinations permit a large number of questions to be asked, for 150 to 180 in each subject can be answered in a 2½-hour period. Because the answer sheets are scorable by machine, the grading can be accomplished rapidly, accurately and impartially. It is completely unbiased and percentile, since the human element is not a factor. Of long-range significance is the facility with which the total test and individual questions can be subjected to thorough and rapid statistical analyses, thus providing a sound basis for comparative studies of medical school teaching and for continuing improvement in the quality of the test itself. Furthermore, multiple-choice written examinations have certain advantages of real benefit to the candidate, to the medical school and, ultimately, to state boards of medical examiners.

REVIEW QUESTIONS

Following are examples of review questions. In those relating to the basic sciences in particular, an attempt has been made, in most of them at least, not merely to call for information based on recollection of past study but rather to relate the questions to practical clinical or patient problems.

Questions in the Basic Sciences

Describe or diagram the conduction pathways of the heart. Indicate the sites of pathology or disturbances in the presence of:

(a) paroxysmal tachycardia
(b) Adams-Stokes syndrome
(c) heart block after myocardial infarction

Diagram the anatomy encountered in doing a tracheotomy.

What neurologic structures are found at the cerebellopontine angle, both within and outside of the brain, where pathology might be reflected in clinical symptoms?

A patient has sustained fractures of the lower left ribs posteriorly. What subjacent structures might be injured? What studies should be performed to determine the extent of the injury?

Diagram a cross section of the spinal cord at the level of L2, indicating major tracts. Indicate the blood supply to the cord at this level.

Name five congenital defects that may be detected at birth and give their embryologic derivation.

Diagram the abdominal aorta with its major

branches. Indicate site of occlusion for Leriche syndrome.

Describe the embryologic development of the pituitary gland. Diagram its relationship to surrounding structures.

Diagram the relationship of the pancreas to the duodenum with its duct system. Describe its embryology.

Diagram the tracheobronchial tree, showing the major lung segments. Where will a foreign body aspirated into the tracheobronchial tree most frequently lodge?

Discuss the role of progesterone in pregnancy.

What is intermittent claudication? What is its cause?

What is meant by the specific dynamic action of food (SDA)? What is the significance of SDA in prescribing a diet for an obese patient?

Describe briefly the functions of the hypothalamus.

Define *each* of the following:

(a) conditioned reflex
(b) jaundice
(c) orthopnea
(d) emphysema
(e) tidal air
(f) heartburn

Name and discuss the factors responsible for the tonic activity of the respiratory center.

Explain why pulmonary edema develops first in dependent parts of the lungs.

Discuss the role of bile in fat digestion.

What is the origin of bilirubin found in the serum?

In a patient with jaundice and a mild anemia, what five *biochemical* determinations would, in your opinion, be most effective in the differential diagnosis? Explain your choices.

Define a vitamin.

Under what circumstances can hypervitaminosis develop? List the clinical and biochemical manifestations of any hypervitaminosis.

The following proteins may be found in human serum. Define four of the six listed below, list the methods by which they may be detected and explain their clinical significance: (a) cryoglobulin, (b) myeloma protein, (c) siderophilin (transferrin), (d) macroglobulin, (e) cold agglutinin, (f) haptoglobin.

Define a *buffer system*. Give an example of a buffer system important in clinical medicine and explain the operation of the system in (a) metabolic acidosis and (b) respiratory alkalosis.

What are the clinical manifestations of hypokalemia? What electrocardiographic changes are frequently associated with hypokalemia? List three clinical states in which hypokalemia is a common finding.

Define four of the following: (a) methemoglobin, (b) thyroglobulin, (c) respiratory quotient, (d) Pasteur effect, (e) nitrogen balance, (f) intrinsic factor.

In advising a community hospital that is about to establish a clinical diagnostic radioisotope laboratory, what radioactive chemical compounds would you recommend? List the compounds (*not* just elements) and give at least *one* use for *each*.

Name three microorganisms sensitive to penicillin and three resistant to penicillin as it is administered in clinical practice.

Define the terms *anamnestic response* and *booster effect*. How are these principles applied to artificial immunization?

List three infections in which disease is caused primarily by the toxin of the infecting microorganism.

Name a vaccine in which the immunizing principle is a modified toxin.

Describe two laboratory tests for the diagnosis of syphilis. How may these tests be modified by antiluetic therapy?

Name two microorganisms that may induce cavitating disease of the lung. Describe briefly the morphology and the staining characteristics of each.

What streptococcus is associated with "streptococcal" sore throat?

What distinguishes this microorganism on blood agar culture?

What are three possible sequelae of untreated streptococcal pharyngitis?

Name three bacteria that are frequency associated with meningitis.

For each of the three types of meningitis, list an antimicrobial drug that is effective in its treatment.

What is the etiologic significance of a pneumococcus in the throat culture of an adult patient with pharyngitis? In the sputum of a patient with pneumonia? In the nasopharynx of a child with otitis media?

List three cultural or biochemical characteristics of pneumococcus.

What is Sabin's vaccine? Are its antigenic constituents living or dead? Name one constituent of the vaccine in addition to those that are intended for immunization. Does the vaccine prevent infection?

Classify the etiologic agent of "Asiatic influenza."

Which antimicrobial agents are effective in the treatment of uncomplicated influenza?

What is the most frequent cause of death in influenza?

Name two microorganisms frequently implicated in the fatal termination of influenza.

Describe three characteristics by which viruses differ from bacteria.

Identify three diseases caused by rickettsia.

What are selective media? Give the name of one

such medium and its purpose. Of what value is penicillinase in diagnostic bacteriology?

Name two diseases that may be prevented or modified by the parenternal injection of antibody.

Name two diseases in which antibody must be used for optimal treatment.

What is the significance of:

(a) an elevated serum ASO (antistreptolysin O) titer?
(b) an elevated serum heterophile antibody titer?
(c) an elevated cold agglutinin titer in the serum?

Compare infectious hepatitis and serum hepatitis with respect to:

(a) etiologic agent
(b) epidemiology
(c) incubation period

Indicate for *each* of the following organisms whether it is sensitive or resistant in vitro to (a) penicillin and (b) tetracycline: *Streptococcus pyogenes, Neisseria gonorrhoeae, Neisseria meningitidis, Klebsiella pneumoniae, Hemophilus influenzae, Brucella abortus.*

Name three vaccines that contain living and three that contain dead infectious agents, listing also the microorganisms they contain. How would you test for the efficacy of immunization with any one of these agents (without exposing your patient to disease)?

List three gram-positive and three gram-negative bacteria. For *each* organism listed, give a brief description of its morphology.

Cite two laboratory characteristics of the staphylococci that are most commonly pathogenic for man. What is the drug of choice for treating most staphylococcal infections acquired outside the hospital?

Name three diseases of man caused by spirochetes. What are the names of the etiologic agents of these diseases?

Briefly discuss the most common gross pathology of an adenocarcinoma of the right hemicolon and contrast it with that most often seen in the descending colon. Correlate these gross findings with the usual initial symptom complex of each.

Which of the following is the most frequent site of carcinoma of the colon: (a) the cecum, (b) the splenic flexure, (c) the sigmoid, (d) the rectum?

Which of the following figures most nearly represents the percentage of carcinoma of the colon and the rectum that are detectable by digital rectal examination: (a) 10 per cent, (b) 2 per cent, (c) 20 per cent, (d) 50 per cent?

A 55-year-old woman is admitted to the hospital with complaints of tiredness, weakness, progressive enlargement of the abdomen and continuous mild generalized abdominal discomfort for "some time." No further reliable history is obtainable. Physical examination reveals a middle-aged woman with obvious recent wasting. Blood pressure 130/80; pulse 80 per minute and regular; temperature 97°F. The *only* other significant physical finding is an enlarged, tense abdomen exhibiting shifting dullness and fluid wave. (A routine urinalysis has revealed no significant abnormality, nor has an electrocardiogram.)

In the absence of other significant physical findings, what two conditions would you consider most probable in your provisional diagnosis?

What one simple and practical procedure, utilizing the clinical laboratory, would best aid in the differential diagnosis between the two?

Indicate the characteristic clinical laboratory findings elicited by this procedure for *each* of the two conditions that you have mentioned.

Very briefly discuss cancer of the lip under the following headings: (a) sex incidence, (b) location, (c) gross pathology, (d) microscopic pathology, (e) spread, (f) prognosis.

In cases of pernicious anemia, name:

(a) the fundamental defect involved in the pathogenesis.
(b) three laboratory findings indispensable to a diagnosis of pernicious anemia.
(c) three accessory laboratory findings that confirm the diagnosis.

The following phrases are descriptive of characteristics of certain neoplasms. In *each* case name a neoplasm to which the phrase might correctly pertain:

(a) a tumor that has a high mortality but rarely, if ever, metastasizes
(b) a serotonin-secreting tumor that may produce spells of flushing of the skin
(c) an invasive tumor of the skin that rarely, if ever, metastasizes
(d) a neoplasm that may be mistaken for eczema
(e) a malignant neoplasm originating from the placenta
(f) a neoplasm associated with intermittent episodes of hypertension

A man, age 55, has had a recent myocardial infarction. Anticoagulant therapy is ordered.

What drug should be used for rapid anticoagulant effect, and what laboratory procedure should be used to check the result?

What drug should be used for long-term anticoagulant effect, and what laboratory test should be used for its control? Give the normal values for this test and the range of values optimal for the patient receiving anticoagulant therapy.

Discuss briefly the pathology of bronchogenic carcinoma, indicating usual sites of primary origin, histologic types and method of spread.

List five common sites of metastasis of bronchogenic carcinoma, arranging them in order of frequency.

Following overindulgence in food and alcohol, a man, age 30, develops sudden severe epigastric pain with moderate rigidity and tenderness of the upper abdomen. There are nausea, vomiting, cyanosis, abdominal distention, rapid pulse and shock.

Indicate two conditions that should be considered and laboratory findings that would aid in the differential diagnosis.

Describe clinical features that should suggest that a skin lesion is a malignant melanoma.

Describe briefly the histopathology of malignant melanoma.

Indicate method of spread and prognosis.

Name three diseases that can be transmitted by blood or blood products from donor to recipient.

What precautions should be taken to prevent such transmission?

Questions in the Clinical Sciences

A patient is admitted to a hospital unconscious immediately following an automobile accident. The neurologic examination is normal. Consciousness is not regained. Two hours later respirations are irregular, the left pupil is a little dilated and the right arm is tonic. In another hour the right side of the face begins to twitch. The right arm is spastic, and the left pupil is fully dilated. Respirations are very irregular and slow. (Consider unmentioned phenomena to be normal.)

Write the letters *a* and *b* on your answer paper. After *each* letter write the *number* preceding the word or the expression that best completes the statement.

  (a) At this time the diagnosis is:
    1. depressed skull fracture
    2. intracranial hematoma
    3. subdural hematoma
    4. epidural hematoma
  (b) The immediate procedure should be:
    1. lumbar puncture
    2. neurologic consultation
    3. electroencephalogram
    4. angiogram
    5. temporal trephine

Outline the procedure to be followed in the evaluation of a severe injury of the pelvis.

What basic information must you have to order and manage intelligently a patient's fluid intake for the few days following a major abdominal surgical procedure during which oral fluids cannot be taken in adequate amounts?

Following a cholecystectomy for gallstones but with no previous history of jaundice, a patient drains bile from the incision. This drainage gradually becomes less and finally ceases after 2 weeks. Concomitantly, the patient becomes jaundiced and develops periodic attacks of chills and fever. The stools become somewhat lighter in color but are not clay colored.

What conditions would you consider in the differential diagnosis?

What laboratory tests or diagnostic procedures, if any, would definitely confirm your diagnosis?

Should this patient be operated upon?

If operation is indicated, when should it be performed?

List the procedures you might employ if necessary to arrive at the diagnosis of a lesion of the lung that has been noted on an anteroposterior chest x-ray film.

What means would you use to manage the problem presented by the elderly frail, weak individual who has great difficulty in getting rid of copious mucoid tracheobronchial secretions in the immediate postoperative period?

A 65-year-old man with chronic bronchitis and emphysema has a combined abdominal-perineal resection of the rectum and the sigmoid colon for carcinoma. During the immediate postoperative period he is being treated with an indwelling urethral catheter and an indwelling nasogastric tube. By the fourth postoperative day the patient's temperature has gradually risen since operation to 103° by rectum.

What significance, if any, is the amount of fever?

What should be done in an attempt to explain it?

Peptic ulcers of the duodenum are treated surgically by a variety of procedures. Indicate the rational basis for the treatment of his lesion by

  (a) vagotomy with pyloroplasty
  (b) subtotal gastric resection
  (c) gastroenterostomy

Outline your management of a patient presenting himself with a history of painless hematuria lasting for 1 day, 1 week ago.

Given a patient with severe hypertension, list some of the changes in the fundus of the eye that you would likely encounter in doing an ophthalmoscopic examination.

A 55-year-old woman with atrial fibrillation due to rheumatic heart disease experiences a sudden severe pain in the left leg. When she is seen at the hospital

4 hours later the pain is still present. The leg is cooler than the right from the knee down, and the skin is blanched. The toes can be moved, but sensation in the lower leg is decreased. Pulsation can be felt over the left common femoral artery at the level of Poupart's ligament on the left, but none below this level.

What is the clinical diagnosis?

At what specific point is the lesion most likely located?

What recommendations for management do you make?

A 32-year-old white man is found to have hypertension of 190 mm. Hg systolic and 100 mm. Hg diastolic on routine examination. What are the possible causes of this, and what clinical and laboratory findings would help in identifying these causes?

A 28-year-old Puerto Rican woman, the mother of children 6 and 8 years of age, complains of weakness, slight fever, anorexia and hemoptysis. How should this situation be managed from the diagnostic and therapeutic standpoints? What is the most likely diagnosis, and what are the implications with respect to this patient's family?

Discuss the management of *each* of the following clinical situations:

(a) congestive failure in a child with acute rheumatic pancarditis
(b) paroxysmal ventricular tachycardia
(c) premature ventricular beats in a patient with acute myocardial infarction

A 3-year-old child has a generalized convulsive seizure and is rushed to you in the emergency room of a hospital. Tabulate the more common causes and give the clinical and laboratory findings of *each* cause mentioned.

Indicate briefly the clinical significance of *each* of the following:

(a) Bence Jones protein in the urine
(b) a positive heterophil agglutination test
(c) a high blood alkaline phosphatase
(d) a high blood acid phosphatase
(e) a positive porphobilinogen in the urine

A moderately obese middle-aged female presents herself complaining of recurrent belching and a sense of a lump and burning in the substernal area. These symptoms occur especially when she stoops over or after a heavy meal, and when she goes to bed at night. Discuss differential diagnosis and treatment.

Outline the clinical and laboratory differential diagnosis of hematuria in an elderly male.

A middle-aged female patient with rheumatoid arthritis has been under long-term treatment with steroids. She now requires operation for acute appendicitis. What are the implications of the prior steroid therapy in such a situation, and how would you manage the medical aspects of the case?

Tabulate briefly the major indications and contraindications for use of each of the following:

(a) oral hypoglycemic agents
(b) nitrogen mustard
(c) parenteral iron preparations
(d) intravenous aminophylline
(e) intravenous ACTH

A young adult man has anorexia, vomiting and mild nausea for a few days and then notes dark urine and light stool. Discuss clinical and laboratory differential diagnosis and therapy.

Name one subjective complaint and one objective indication for estrogenic hormone in the management of the woman after her menopause.

A 9-year-old girl experiences prolonged vaginal bleeding. Examination reveals breast and vulvar development and a 6 by 9 cm. tumor in the pelvis. What would you suspect?

What two complaints warrant a suspicion of gonococcal infection in the female? Indicate two procedures, either of which would confirm the diagnosis.

A 60-year-old nulliparous woman, 9 years postmenopausal, reports serous to bloody vaginal discharge on several occasions in the past month.

Indicate two probabilities.

How would you establish the diagnosis?

What two possibly predisposing factors would you consider when suspecting vaginitis is due to Monilia?

What would confirm that diagnosis?

What treatment would you prescribe?

A patient, gravida I, with uterus approximately term size, states that she cannot be more than 30 weeks pregnant. What three possibilities would you consider?

The child survived delivery by section when profuse antepartum bleeding was due to placenta previa. Name three possible causes if menstruation fails to occur by the sixth month postpartum.

What two observations noted during labor warrant a suspicion that defibrination of maternal blood may occur?

How can you determine if this is occurring?

If undetected, what could be the result?

Name three laboratory procedures that might be indicated repeatedly during the prenatal care of a normal patient.

Name three disadvantages inherent in "deep" general anesthesia for delivery at term.

List the activities of the US Public Health Service.

What health hazards may be encountered in a boys' summer camp?

What voluntary agencies are active in the field of cardiovascular disease, and what are some of their activities?

What immunizations should be recommended for travelers to the Middle East and Africa?

What is meant by *each* of the following terms: (a) crude death rate, (b) standardized death rate, (c) infant mortality rate, (d) birth rate?

What services are offered by local health departments to the practicing physician?

Discuss health hazards in industry, and outline methods of preventing them.

Discuss health facilities provided by unions.

Part 1

Basic Medical Sciences

2

Anatomy

J. ROBERT TROYER, PH.D.

Professor and Chairman of Anatomy, Temple University
School of Medicine

NEAL E. PRATT, R.P.T., PH.D.

Professor of Anatomy, Temple University School of Medicine

THE BACK—HISTOLOGY OF BASIC TISSUES

VERTEBRAL COLUMN

Individual Vertebrae

Typical Vertebra. The component parts of the vertebral column are basically similar in construction. The two major portions are the anterior body and the posterior vertebral or neural arch. The body is in the form of a flattened cylinder that serves as the major weight-bearing portion of the vertebra. The vertebral arch consists of a series of continuous projections and prominences that form (together with the posterior aspect of the body) the vertebral foramen. The paired pedicles project posteriorly from the posterolateral aspect of the upper half of each body, and the laminae project posteromedially (to join in the midline) from the posterior extents of the pedicles. The transverse processes extend laterally from the arch; the single spinous process is directed posteriorly in the midline. The superior and inferior articular processes arise from the vertebral arch at about the junction of the pedicle and lamina. Each articular process contains an articular facet.

Regional Variation. The size of the vertebral bodies steadily increases from above downward to accommodate the increasing superincumbent weight. The delicate cervical vertebrae are distinguished by a bifid spine, foramina in the transverse processes that transmit the vertebral arteries, and prominent upward flares of the superolateral aspects of the body. Thoracic vertebrae have articular facets or costal fovea (with which the ribs form synovial joints) on the posterolateral aspects of the bodies and the anterior aspects of the tips of the transverse processes, and very long spinous processes that are directed obliquely inferiorly so that they overlap the next lower vertebra. Lumbar vertebrae have very large heavy bodies and short strong spinous processes that are directed posteriorly. Their laminae are about half as high (superoinferiorly) as their bodies, and hence an interlaminar space exists between lumbar vertebrae.

Connections Between Adjacent Vertebrae

Joints. The vertebral arches are connected by the intervertebral or zygapophyseal articulations. These are synovial joints between the superior articular facets of the vertebra below and the inferior articular facets of the vertebra above. A thin joint capsule permits a limited amount of gliding motion between the articular surfaces. The orientation or plane of the joint space is a major determinant of the direction of motion that occurs between adjacent vertebrae.

The bodies are united (and separated) by a fibrocartilaginous intervertebral disk. This is a cartilaginous joint and as such permits limited motion. The disk is composed of a gelatinous core (nucleus pulposus) which is surrounded by a strong distensible envelope (anulus fibrosus) and separated from each vertebral body by a hyaline cartilage plate. Thus, the disk has all the physical properties of a closed fluid-elastic system, i.e., any pressure is delivered equally and undiminished to all parts of the container, which in this case are the anulus fibrosus and the cartilaginous plates.

Ligaments. The ligaments of the vertebral column can be grouped into those that interconnect adjacent vertebrae and those that extend virtually the entire length of the vertebral column. The segmental ligaments include the ligamentum flavum, which connects the laminae, and the interspinous, supraspinous and intertransverse ligaments, whose locations are self-explanatory. Two ligaments extend from the atlas to the sacrum. The anterior longitudinal ligament reinforces the anterior and anterolateral aspects of the vertebral bodies and intervertebral disks. The posterior longitudinal ligament attaches to the posterior aspects of the bodies and disks and is therefore within the vertebral canal. This ligament supports the posterior aspect of the disk in the midline but adds little support posterolaterally.

These ligaments are strong and tight and act to support the vertebral column as well as restrict motion. Spinal extension is limited by only the anterior longitudinal ligament while the rest of the above-named ligaments limit flexion. Side-bending is limited by the intertransverse ligaments.

Vertebral Column as a Whole

Normal and Abnormal Curves. The anteroposterior curves of the vertebral column are compensatory adjustments that attempt to position the superincumbent weight above the next lower segment of support. Normally each junctional area (lumbo-sacral, thoraco-lumbar, cervico-thoracic, occipito-cervical) is directly above the center of gravity of the body as a whole, and as a result little or no muscular activity is necessary to hold the spine upright during quiet standing. These curves are such that the lumbar and cervical regions present posterior concavities while the thoracic and sacral regions present posterior convexities. No lateral curvature normally exists. An exaggerated lumbar curve is called *lordosis,* an exaggerated thoracic curve *kyphosis.* Any lateral curve is *scoliosis.*

Motion of Vertebral Column. Most motion of the vertebral column is the sum of the relatively small amount of actual motion that occurs between most pairs of adjacent vertebrae. Although the intervertebral disk is easily distorted in any direction, and thus permits motion in any direction, its thickness does regulate the extent of motion. In addition, motion is limited by the tension of the vertebral column ligaments. The direction of motion is limited to a large degree by the orientation of the plane of the zygapophyseal joint. In the cervical region the disks are relatively thick, and the joint spaces are oriented between the coronal and horizontal planes, being closer to the horizontal plane. As a result, flexion, extension, lateral bending and rotation are permitted. Flexion and extension are especially free between the occipital bone and the atlas, and rotation is very free between the atlas and axis. Motion in the thoracic region is greatly limited by the anatomy of the thoracic vertebrae and disks, as well as the stability of the rib cage. Lumbar disks are very thick, and the joint planes are almost sagittally and coronally oriented. Flexion and extension are free while lateral bending is slight in this region.

Integrity of the Vertebral Column. The static support of the normally aligned vertebral column is provided primarily by the ligaments discussed above. As soon as motion occurs the muscles become important in controlling the overall posture, but the relationship between adjacent vertebrae is still maintained by the ligaments. Bony support is a factor at only certain areas. The thoracic region is of course greatly reinforced by the thoracic cage, and as a result vertebral dislocations seldom occur there. At other levels the only possible bony support is derived from the articular facets that form the zygapophyseal joints, and this support is dependent upon the orientation of the joint space. In the cervical region these joint spaces are nearly horizontal. As a result there is no bony block that prevents one vertebra from sliding forward with respect to an adjoining vertebra. It follows that cervical dislocation can occur with only soft tissue damage (no fracture). On the other hand, the planes of the lumbar zygapophyseal joints are vertically oriented (the upper ones in the sagittal plane and the lower ones in the coronal plane), and the inferior articular facets overlap the next lower vertebra. Any tendency toward dislocation is resisted by interlocking of the articular surfaces, and fracture usually accompanies dislocation.

The lower lumbar region (especially the lumbosacral junction) requires special attention. The body of L5 is sitting on the anteriorly inclined superior aspect of the sacrum, and there is a natural tendency for this vertebra to slide (dislocate) anteriorly. This tendency is resisted by the zygapophyseal joints between L5 and the sacrum. Occasionally there is bony discontinuity of the lamina between the superior and inferior articular facets, a condition called spondylolysis. This means that the bony support normally provided by the zygapophyseal joint is lost, and anterior sliding is predisposed. If the body does slide anteriorly it is called spondylolisthesis.

Intervertebral Foramen

Normal Anatomy of the Intervertebral Foramen. The basic boundaries of this foramen are the same throughout the vertebral column. The superior and inferior aspects are the pedicles of the respective vertebrae. The anterior boundary consists of the intervertebral disk and portions of the adjacent vertebral bodies. Posteriorly the superior and inferior articular facets form the zygapophyseal joint. The specific anatomy of the foramen differs somewhat from region to region. Most pathologic change occurs in the more mobile cervical and lumbar regions, and this description will be limited to those areas.

Pathology Involving the Intervertebral Foramen. In the cervical region the foramen is small, the intervertebral disk forms most of the anterior wall, and the relatively large spinal nerve practically fills the opening. Protrusion or rupture of the disk into the foramen will impinge on the nerve in the foramen; i.e., rupture of the disk between cervical vertebrae 5 and 6 will involve spinal nerve C6. In addition, the size of the cervical intervertebral foramen can be reduced by inflammation of the zygapophyseal joint (arthritis) and by bony projections from the vertebral bodies. These bony spurs usually result from disk degeneration, which in turn causes irritation to "Luschka's joints" on the lateral aspects of the vertebral bodies. In the lumbar region the disk forms the lower half of the anterior wall of the foramen, and the upper vertebral body, the upper half. The opening is very large, and the relatively small spinal nerve exits in the upper part of the foramen opposite the vertebral body. Rupture of the disk at this level does not affect the spinal nerve in the same foramen but rather the spinal nerve that is descending in the anterolateral aspect of the vertebral canal (across the posterolateral aspect of the disk) to gain the next lower intervertebral foramen. Thus a rupture of the disk between lumbar vertebrae 4 and 5 will usually impinge on spinal nerve L5.

Microscopic Structure of the Connective and Supportive Tissues

The adult connective and supportive tissues are connective tissue proper, cartilage and bone. Connective tissue proper is further classified into loose irregular (areolar) connective tissue and dense regular and irregular connective tissues. These tissues contain cells and a preponderance of intercellular fibers and ground substance.

Loose Irregular Connective Tissue. Loose connective tissue is found in the superficial and deep fascia and as the stroma of most organs. It is generally considered as the packing material of the body. Loose connective tissue contains most of the cell types and all of the fiber types found in the other connective tissues. The most common cell types are the fibroblast, macrophage, adipose cell, mast cell, plasma cell and wandering cells from the blood. Fibroblasts contain the organelles that permit them to produce all of the fiber types and the intercellular material. In their production of these proteinaceous substances, messenger RNA, ribosomal RNA and transfer RNA are produced in the nucleus and pass to the cytoplasm. Amino acids that have been taken into the fibroblast attach to specific transfer RNA and are translated on the messenger RNA in the region of the ribosomes of the rough endoplasmic reticulum (RER). The polypeptides produced pass through the cisternae of the RER to the region of the Golgi complex where they are packaged into membrane-bound macromolecules that attach to the cell surface before discharge from the fibroblast. The Golgi complex also is responsible for adding the carbohydrate components to the glycosaminoglycans (mucopolysaccharides) of the ground substance. Macrophages are part of the reticuloendothelial system (mononuclear phagocyte system). They possess large lysosomes containing digestive enzymes, which are necessary for the digestion of phagocytized particles. Mast cells occur mostly along blood vessels and contain granules that represent the heparin and histamine produced by these cells. Plasma cells are part of the immune system in that they produce circulating antibodies. They are extremely basophilic because of their extensive rough endoplasmic reticulum. Adipose cells are found in varying quantities. When they predominate the tissue is called adipose tissue.

Collagenous, reticular and elastic fibers are irregularly distributed in loose connective tissue. Collagenous fibers are usually found in bundles of fibers and provide strength to the tissue. Each fiber is made up of fibrils. These are composed of staggered monomers of tropocollagen giving a 640 Å periodicity to most normal collagen in the body. Reticular fibers are smaller, more delicate fibers that form the basic framework of reticular connective tissue. Elastic fibers branch and provide elasticity and suppleness to connective tissue.

Ground substance is the gelatinous material that fills most of the space between the cells and fibers. It is composed of mucopolysaccharide and protein and its properties are important in determining the permeability and consistency of the connective tissue.

Dense Connective Tissue. Dense irregular connective tissue is found in the dermis, periosteum, perichondrium and capsules of some organs. All of the fiber types are present, but collagenous fibers predominate. Dense regular connective tissue occurs as aponeuroses, ligaments and tendons. In most ligaments and tendons collagenous fibers are most prevalent and are oriented parallel to each other; fibroblasts are the only cell type present. In the ligamenta flava, elastic fibers dominate and they are considered elastic ligaments.

Cartilage. Cartilage is composed of chondrocytes embedded in an intercellular substance consisting of fibers and an amorphous firm ground substance. Three types of cartilage (hyaline, elastic and fibrous) are distinguished on the basis of the amount of ground substance and the relative abundance of collagenous and elastic fibers.

Hyaline cartilage is found as costal cartilages, articular cartilages and cartilages of the nose, larynx, trachea and bronchi. The intercellular matrix consists primarily of collagenous fibers and a ground substance rich in chondromucoprotein, a copolymer of a protein and chondroitin sulfates. Chondrocytes occupy lacunae. During the growth period of the cartilage these cells existed as chondroblasts, and they produced the intercellular matrix. Cartilage grows interstitially by the mitoses of cells in the center of the cartilage mass. It also grows appositionally by the formation of chondroblasts from undifferentiated cells in the cellular layer of the perichondrium. Unlike the fibrous layer of the perichondrium, the cellular layer and the cartilage are avascular so they receive nutriments and oxygen through diffusion from blood vessels in the fibrous layer of the perichondrium. Articular cartilages receive nutriments by diffusion from blood vessels in the marrow and from the synovial fluid. With old age, there is a decrease of acid mucopolysaccharides, an increase in noncollagenous proteins, and calcification may occur because of degenerative changes in the cartilage cells.

Elastic cartilage is found in the pinna of the ear, auditory tube, epiglottis, and the corniculate and cuneiform cartilages. Elastic fibers predominate and thus provide greater flexibility. Calcification of this type of cartilage is rare.

Fibrous cartilage occurs in the anchorage of tendons and ligaments, in intervertebral disks, in the symphysis pubis and in some interarticular disks and ligaments.

Chondrocytes occur singly or in rows between large bundles of collagenous fibers. Compared with hyaline cartilage, only small amounts of hyaline matrix surround the chondrocytes of fibrous cartilage.

Bone. Bone tissue consists of osteocytes and an intercellular matrix that contains organic and inorganic components. The organic matrix consists of dense collagenous fibers and an osseomucoid substance containing chondroitin sulfate. The inorganic component is responsible for the rigidity of bone and is composed chiefly of calcium phosphate and calcium carbonate with small amounts of magnesium, fluoride, hydroxide and sulfate. Electron microscopic studies show that these minerals are deposited in an orderly fashion on the surface of and within the collagenous fibrils in their interband areas. In the basic organization of bone tissue, osteocytes lie in lacunae and extend protoplasmic processes into small canaliculi in the intercellular matrix. The protoplasmic processes of adjacent osteocytes are in contact with one another and gap junctions are present. The matrix is organized into adjacent layers or lamellae. The number and arrangement of lamellae differ between compact and cancellous bone.

Compact bone contains haversian systems (osteons), interstitial lamellae and circumferential lamellae. Haversian systems consist of extensively branching haversian canals that are oriented chiefly longitudinally in long bones. Each canal contains blood vessels and osteogenic cells and is surrounded by 8 to 15 concentric lamellae and osteocytes. The collagenous fibers in adjacent lamellae run at right angles to each other and spiral around the canal. Nutriments from blood vessels in the haversian canals pass through canaliculi and lacunae to reach all osteocytes in the system. Interstitial lamellae occur between haversian systems and represent the remains of parts of haversian and circumferential lamellae. Outer and inner circumferential lamellae occur under the periosteum and endosteum respectively. Volkmann's canals enter through the outer circumferential lamellae and carry blood vessels and nerves which are continuous with those of the haversian canals and the periosteum. Sharpey's fibers are coarse perforating fibers that anchor the periosteum to the outer circumferential lamellae.

Bones are supplied by a loop of blood vessels that enter from the periosteal region, penetrate the cortical bone, and enter the medulla before returning to the periphery of the bone. Long bones are specifically supplied by arteries which pass to the marrow through diaphyseal, metaphyseal and epiphyseal arteries. In the marrow cavity, some arteries end in sinusoids, and others branch and enter the haversian canals where they supply fenestrated capillaries. The marrow sinusoids drain to veins that leave through nutrient canals.

The capillaries of the haversian canals drain to veins that pass centrifugally to the periosteum and adjacent muscles.

Bone undergoes extensive remodeling, and haversian systems may break down or be resorbed in order that calcium can be made available to other parts of the body. Bone resorption occurs by osteocytic osteolysis or by osteoclastic activity. In *osteocytic osteolysis,* osteocytes resorb bone that lies immediately around the lacunae. In *osteoclastic activity,* large multinucleated osteoclasts arise from osteoprogenitor cells and abut against an osseous surface. Here, their extensive ruffled surfaces and proteolytic enzyme secretions seem to be involved in the resorption of more extensive portions of bone. In this way, portions of old haversian systems are resorbed, or longitudinal depressions are formed on the periosteal and endosteal surfaces of the bone. If new haversian systems are to be laid down in the gutters or tubes that remain after the resorptive process is complete, osteoblasts differentiate from the osteogenic cells of the enlarged haversian canal or periosteum and begin to lay down lamellae at the periphery of the space. Successive new concentric lamellae are laid down inside this initial lamella.

Cancellous bone differs from compact bone in that the lamellae are organized into trabeculae or spicules. Few haversian systems are present, and all osteocytes are generally closer to the blood supply than in compact bone.

Bone Development

Development of Vertebrae and Ribs. At the end of the second postfertilization week the primitive streak gives rise to cells that migrate laterally between the ectoderm and entoderm, forming the intraembryonic mesoderm. At appoximately the same time the notochord arises from a cranial midline migration from the primitive node. As development progresses, the intraembryonic mesoderm adjacent to the notochord thickens into longitudinal masses called the paraxial mesoderm. From the 21st to 30th days, the paraxial mesoderm differentiates into 42 to 44 paired segments called somites. This craniocaudal development of somites gives rise to four occipital, eight cervical, twelve thoracic, five lumbar, five sacral and eight to ten coccygeal somites. The somite further differentiates so that three distinct cellular regions are apparent. The ventromedial region, sclerotome, eventually gives rise to supportive skeletal structures (e.g., vertebrae and ribs); the dorsomedial part, myotome, forms the skeletal muscles; and the dorsolateral portion, dermatome, gives rise to the dermis of the skin and subcutaneous tissue.

During the fourth week the sclerotomic mesenchymal mass of each somite begins to migrate toward the midline to become aggregated about the notochord. In this migration, cells of the caudal half of each somite shift caudally to meet the cranially migrating cranial half of adjacent sclerotomes. From each of these joined masses, mesenchymal processes grow dorsally around the neural tube to form the neural arches of the vertebrae and also give rise to rib primordia. Since a vertebra develops from parts of two adjacent sclerotomes the original intersegmental arteries will come to pass across the middle of the vertebral bodies. The segmental spinal nerves to the myotomes will come to lie at the level of the intervertebral disks and the myotomes. The notochord degenerates in the region of the vertebral bodies but persists in the center of the intervertebral disk as the nucleus pulposus. In the cervical region, the migration of sclerotome accounts for the formation of seven cervical vertebrae from eight somites. This is due to the cranial half of the first sclerotome becoming part of the occipital bone while the caudal half of the eighth sclerotome becomes part of the first thoracic vertebra. Thus, the first cervical nerve passes between the occipital bone and first cervical vertebra while the eighth cervical nerve emerges between the seventh cervical and first thoracic vertebrae.

At 7 weeks separate chondrification centers develop in the bodies and the lateral half of each neural arch, and these subsequently fuse together. Later, ossification centers develop in the vertebral bodies, in each half of the neural arch and in each rib. These remain as separate centers throughout fetal life. The rib primordia give rise to ribs in the thoracic region, transverse processes in the lumbar region, parts of the transverse processes in the cervical region, and the alae of the sacrum. Excessive growth of the rib primordia can lead to cervical and lumbar ribs. In spondylolisthesis there is usually a defect in the formation of the pedicles due to nonunion of ossification centers. In this condition the spine, laminae and inferior articular processes of the affected lower lumbar vertebra stay in place, while the body migrates anteriorly with respect to the vertebra below it. In spina bifida conditions there is failure of the neural arches to unite properly in the formation of the spinous process.

The Microscopic Development of Bone. There are two basic patterns of bone formation: intramembranous and endochondral. In both of these types of bone formation, the process of forming bone tissue and the histologic structure of the bone formed are identical. The major difference between these two types of development is the environment within which bone tissue is laid down.

Intramembranous bone formation occurs in flat bones of the skull and face. In this type of development mesenchymal cells differentiate into osteoblasts in a region where mesenchymal cells have produced a fine-fibered vascular membrane. The osteoblasts lay down lamellae of collagenous fibers and ground substance in the form of a meshwork of trabeculae within the membrane. Some osteoblasts become entrapped as osteocytes in this osteoid tissue. When organic osteoid tissue becomes impregnated with inorganic salts it is called osseous tissue. Some intertrabecular spaces become marrow cavities when their mesenchyme differentiates into reticular connective tissue and blood-forming cells. Others become haversian canals as concentric lamellae are formed. At the periphery of the entire developing bone (e.g., outer and inner surfaces of skull bones) the bone becomes quite compact in its development. This is accomplished by a mesenchymal condensation around the bone that differentiates into a periosteum, the inner cells of which become osteoblasts and lay down compact bone. Thus the bone takes on an appearance of outer and inner tables of compact bone, between which is the diploe of spongy trabecular bone. Osteoclasts are associated with bone resorption, which takes place chiefly on the inner surfaces of the tables and trabeculae. The membranous junction between two developing flat bones is eventually ossified as a suture.

Endochondral bone formation is characterized by a cartilage model of the bone preceding bone histogenesis. In the formation of the cartilage model of a long bone, the oldest cartilage is found in the center of the shaft (diaphyseal) region. Cells in this region hypertrophy, produce phosphatase and bring about calcification of the surrounding cartilaginous matrix. The result of this calcification is inhibition of diffusion of nutrient materials to the chondrocytes, and they die or they may become osteoprogenitor cells. While the cartilage in the center of the shaft is calcifying, the chondrogenic layer of the perichondrium is becoming increasingly vascularized. In this new environment, the undifferentiated mesenchymal cells of the chondrogenic layer start to differentiate into osteoblasts, which lay down a bony collar around the shaft of the cartilage model. The perichondrium is now a periosteum. Osteogenic tissue and blood vessels from this osteogenic layer of the periosteum pass between the trabeculae of the bony collar and penetrate into the degenerating calcified cartilage. This periosteal bud of tissue is instrumental in resorption of some of the smaller calcified cartilage spicules between lacunae, and in the laying down of bone on remnants of the calcified cartilage. The center of the shaft now consists of osteogenic tissue and bony trabeculae that contain remnant cores of calcified cartilage. This area in the diaphysis is called the primary ossification center.

Since the newer cartilage lies toward the epiphyses, the metaphyses demonstrate the following developmental gradient as the diaphysis is approached: (1) a layer of tissue where cells are not dividing (zone of resting cartilage), (2) a layer where chondrocytes are dividing mitotically and interstitially in an axial orientation (zone of multiplication), (3) a layer where cells are enlarging (zone of cellular hypertrophy and maturation), and (4) a layer where the intercellular material is calcifying and cells are dying (zones of calcification). The shaft grows in length by the multiplication of cartilage cells at the zones of multiplication in each metaphyseal region and by osseous tissue being laid down on the remnants of calcified cartilage in the zone of calcification. This process also brings about an increase in length of the primary marrow cavity. An increase in width of the marrow cavity takes place by resorption of bone on the inner surface of the periosteal bony collar. Since this resorption is not as rapid as the appositional laying down of bone on the outer surface of the bony collar, the compact bone of the shaft increases in width.

Secondary ossification centers develop later in fetal life, or after birth, in the epiphyses. These are usually characterized by hypertrophy of chondrocytes and calcification of cartilage in the centers of the epiphyses where the older cartilage cells exist. Vascular and osteogenic buds of tissue enter the area from the metaphyseal region. A thin layer of dense bone is laid down on the surfaces of the epiphyses where a periosteum is present. On articular surfaces, no periosteum or perichondrium exists, and hyaline cartilage is retained as a covering to the underlying epiphyseal bone.

MUSCLES OF THE BACK

Superficial Muscles of the Back

These muscles are found superficial to the thoracolumbar fascia. They represent most of the extrinsic muscles of the shoulder in that they interconnect the axial and appendicular portions of the skeleton, specifically extending from the vertebral column or rib cage to the scapula, clavicle, or humerus. Functionally, they are concerned with motion of the shoulder girdle and humerus. Innervation is supplied mainly by branches of the brachial plexus. The trapezius is innervated by the accessory (11th cranial) nerve and controls the position of the shoulder statically as well as during virtually any motion, especially when the arm is abducted or flexed. The latissimus dorsi is the major extendor of the humerus and shoulder depressor (as in crutch walking), and is innervated by the thoracodorsal nerve. A plane of three muscles underlying the trapezius connects the vertebral column and scapula. The levator scapulae and rhomboids are innervated by the dorsal scapular nerve and direct branches of the cervical plexus. The serratus anterior extends from the medial border of the scapula to the anterolateral thoracic wall. It functions to hold the ventral surface of the scapula against the thorax and, working with the trapezius, is important in shoulder abduction and flexion. The long thoracic nerve innervates this mucle.

Deep Muscles of the Back

The deep muscles of the back, or the erector spinae, are deep to the thoracolumbar fascia and occupy the vertically oriented furrow formed between the spinous processes of the vertebrae and the angles of the ribs. These muscles extend from the occipital bone to the sacrum, and although they can be divided anatomically into many specific parts the entire mass functions as a unit. They are innervated segmentally by branches of the dorsal rami of spinal nerves. Bilateral contraction of these muscles produces extension of the vertebral column; unilateral contraction causes side-bending and rotation.

Microscopic Structure of Muscle Tissue

There are three types of muscle tissue: smooth, skeletal and cardiac. All three types are comprised of muscle cells (fibers) that contain myofibrils possessing contractile filaments of actin and myosin.

Smooth Muscle. Smooth muscle cells are spindle shaped and are organized chiefly into sheets or bands of smooth muscle tissue. This tissue is found in blood vessels and other tubular visceral structures. Smooth muscle cells contain both actin and myosin filaments, but the actin filaments predominate. The filaments are not organized into patterns that give cross striations as in cardiac and skeletal muscle. Filaments course obliquely in the cells and attach to the plasma membrane. Electron microscopy shows the plasma membrane as a "typical" trilaminar membrane. In specific regions where smooth muscle cells appose each other, leaving only narrow 20 Å intercellular gaps, specialized zones of contact occur which are known as nexuses or "gap" junctions. These junctions probably facilitate the transmission of impulses for contraction. In other intercellular regions a glycoprotein coat and a small amount of collagenous and reticular fibers are found.

Skeletal Muscle. Skeletal muscle fibers are characterized by their peripherally located nuclei and their striated myofibrils. The cross striations are due to the organization and distribution of actin and myosin filaments. These striations are organized within each muscle fiber into fundamental contractile units called sarcomeres, which are joined end to end at the Z lines. The striations in a sarcomere consist of an A band bordered toward the Z lines by I bands. The mid-region of the A band contains a variable light H band that is bisected by an M line. The light I band contains

actin filaments. These filaments interdigitate and are cross bridged in the A band with myosin filaments, forming a hexagonal pattern of one myosin filament surrounded by six actin filaments. In the contraction of a muscle fiber a chemical reaction takes place in the region of the cross bridges, causing the actin filaments of the I band to move deeper into the A band, thus resulting in a shortening of the I bands.

Each skeletal muscle fiber is invested with a sarcolemma (plasmalemma) that extends into the fiber as numerous small transverse T tubules. These tubules ring the myofibrils at the A-I junction and are bordered on each side by terminal cisternae of the sarcoplasmic (endoplasmic) reticulum. This arrangement of one T tubule with two terminal cisternae is called a triad. In excitation-contraction coupling, acetylcholine released from the motor end-plate causes depolarization of the muscle membrane, which is propagated to the T tubule-sarcoplasmic reticulum junction. This brings about release of calcium from the terminal cisternae of the sarcoplasmic reticulum, catalyzing the chemical reaction between the actin and myosin filaments in the region of the cross bridges. In this process, the troponin protein of the actin, which normally prevents activation of myosin ATP, may undergo a steric conformational change, thus permitting a ratchetlike attachment and release of the heavy meromyosin with successive actin binding sites. The actin molecules then slide into the A band.

Cardiac Muscle. Cardiac muscle contains striations and myofibrils that are similar to those of skeletal muscle. It differs from skeletal muscle in several major ways. Cardiac muscle fibers branch and contain centrally located nuclei and large numbers of mitochondria. Individual cardiac muscle cells are attached to each other at their ends by intercalated disks. These disks contain several types of membrane junctional complexes, the most important of which is the gap junction. This junction electrically couples one cell to its neighbor so that electrical depolarization is propagated through the heart by cell-to-cell contacts rather than by nerve innervation to each cell. The sarcoplasmic reticulum-T tubule system is arranged differently in cardiac muscle than in skeletal muscle. In cardiac muscle each T tubule enters at the Z line and forms a diad with only one terminal cisterna of sarcoplasmic reticulum.

Development of Skeletal Muscles

Histogenesis of Skeletal Muscle. Skeletal muscle cells develop from mesenchyme that arises from the myotomes of somites or from branchial arches. Stellate mesenchymal cells differentiate into elongate multinucleate myotubes containing peripherally located myofibrils and centrally located nuclei. Later in development, myofibrils will increase in size and number and the nuclei will migrate peripherally. In the limited regeneration of muscle, new fibers can be formed from satellite cells that lie between the skeletal muscle cell and its basement membrane.

Morphogenesis of the Skeletal Musculature. Myotomes divide into dorsal epaxial and ventral hypaxial condensations of mesenchyme. Dorsal and ventral rami develop from the segmental spinal nerves and innervate the epaxial and hypaxial portions respectively. The epaxial masses give rise to the deep muscles of the back. The hypaxial masses develop into anterior and lateral body wall muscles of the cervical and thoracolumbar regions. Muscles of the extremities and those that attach the limbs to the trunk may arise from local somatic lateral mesoderm but are innervated by the ventral rami of spinal nerves. Subsequent migrations of segmental myoblasts, trailing their respective nerves, lead to the formation of complex nerve fiber plexuses from successive spinal cord levels. In addition to migration, five other basic processes occur in the establishment of muscles: (1) fusions of portions of successive myotomes (e.g., erector spinae), (2) change from the original cephalocaudal direction of the fibers (e.g., transversus abdominus), (3) longitudinal splitting of a myotomic mass to form more than one muscle (e.g., rhomboideus major and minor), (4) tangential splitting (e.g., intercostals), and (5) degeneration of parts or all of a myotome with conversion of the degenerated part to connective tissue (e.g., serratus posterior inferior and superior).

SPINAL CORD AND SPINAL NERVES

Gross Anatomy of Spinal Cord and Spinal Nerves

Basic Organization. The nervous system is composed of the central and peripheral nervous systems. The central nervous system is enclosed within the cranial vault and vertebral canal and consists respectively of the brain and spinal cord. The peripheral nervous system is outside the bony encasement and is composed of peripheral nerves, which are branches of the cranial and spinal nerves. The autonomic nervous system is anatomically a portion of both the central and peripheral nervous systems, but the usual definition is a functional one that includes the motor side of the system controlling blood vessels, glands and viscera, and thus can be called the general visceral efferent system.

The spinal cord is a long cylindrical structure whose hollow core is called the central canal and is a portion of the ventricular system. The central canal is surrounded by the gray matter (cell bodies and terminal arborizations), which is in turn surrounded by the white matter (long ascending and descending cell processes). The cord is segmented, each segment corresponding to a specific portion of the body wall (including extremities) that it innervates. The diameter of the cord decreases from top to bottom with the exceptions of the low cervical and the lumbosacral regions whose enlargements reflect the upper and lower extremities respectively. The spinal cord terminates inferiorly at the inferior aspect of the first lumbar vertebra. This termination is in the form of an inverted cone and is thus called the conus medullaris. Vertical lines of nerve rootlets attach to the anterolateral and posterolateral aspects of the cord. The rootlets from a single segment converge and form anterior and posterior roots. The two roots join in the intervertebral foramen to form the spinal nerve. After exiting from the intervertebral foramen the spinal nerve divides into ventral and dorsal rami whose muscular and cutaneous branches supply the body wall structures.

Both the brain and spinal cord are surrounded by three membranes that have both trophic and protective functions. For the most part the meninges of brain and cord are similar. The differences are outlined later in this chapter. The innermost, the pia mater, is a thin membrane that conforms very closely to the contours of the spinal cord and is firmly attached to the neural tissue. The vessels that supply the central nervous system are found in this membrane. The denticulate ligament is a series of pial extensions that project laterally and attach to the outermost covering, the dura mater. These ligaments serve to stabilize the spinal cord. The intermediate arachnoid is a thin filmy membrane attached to the pia by numerous trabeculae. The area between the arachnoid and pia is the subarachnoid space, which is filled with cerebrospinal fluid. This fluid holds the arachnoid tightly against the outer dura mater, and since the arachnoid and dura are not firmly attached the subdural space is in reality only a potential space. Together the pia and arachnoid are the soft coverings of the spinal cord called the leptomeninges. The dura mater is a strong thin membrane, the pachymeninx. It is separated from the bones and ligaments of the vertebral canal by the epidural space in which the epidural fat and internal venous plexus are found. The dura, as well as the pia and arachnoid, extends laterally at the level of each spinal nerve and becomes continuous with the connective tissue covering of the nerves. Inferiorly the dural sac terminates at the second sacral vertebra. Since the arachnoid is so closely held against the inner aspect of the dura the dural sac and subarachnoid space can be considered the same in extent.

Relationship of Spinal Cord to Vertebral Column. The spinal cord extends from the foramen magnum to the lower border of the first lumbar vertebra. This means that only the very uppermost cervical cord segments are opposite the vertebra of the same name. Upper thoracic cord segments are one vertebral level higher than their correspondingly named vertebra, while the lumbar, sacral and coccygeal cord segments lie opposite the last two thoracic and first lumbar vertebrae. Since each spinal nerve exits through its original intervertebral foramen, only the highest cervical spinal nerves are horizontally oriented, while each next lower spinal nerve is more obliquely oriented as it travels farther to its intervertebral foramen. As a result of this incongruity between spinal cord and vertebral column, the symptoms resulting from a spinal cord lesion do not usually correspond to the vertebral level of the lesion. For example a lesion at vertebral level T12 could logically be accompanied by symptoms that correspond to cord segments L3 and below. In the interval between the end of the spinal cord and the dural sac the subarachnoid space contains only the dorsal and ventral roots, which form the cauda equina. This area is the region of choice for spinal tap as there is minimal risk to neural structures when a needle is inserted into the subarachnoid space. In addition the interlaminar space between lumbar vertebrae allows easy access.

Microscopic Structure of Spinal Nerves and the Spinal Cord

Spinal Nerves.   The basic cell type of nerve tissue is the neuron. Each neuron consists of a nerve cell body (perikaryon) and one or more nerve processes (fibers). The cell body of a typical neuron contains a nucleus, Nissl material of rough endoplasmic reticulum, free ribosomes, Golgi apparatus, mitochondria, neurotubules, neurofilaments and pigment inclusions. The cell processes of neurons occur as axons and dendrites. Dendrites contain most of the components of the cell body except the nucleus and Golgi apparatus, whereas axons contain the major structures found in dendrites except for the Nissl material. At the synaptic ends of axons, the presynaptic process contains vesicles from which are elaborated excitatory or inhibitory substances. The functional dendrites of some neurons, such as the sensory pseudounipolar neurons of spinal nerves are structurally the same as axons. Unmyelinated fibers in peripheral nerves lie in grooves on the surface of neurolemma (Schwann) cells and are incompletely invested by the plasmalemma of these cells. Myelinated peripheral neurons are invested by numerous "jellyroll" layers of Schwann cell plasma membrane that constitute a myelin sheath. The Schwann cell cytoplasm and nucleus lie peripheral to the myelin sheath. There are many Schwann cells along each myelinated fiber. In the junctional areas between adjacent Schwann cells there is a lack of myelin. These junctional areas along the myelinated process constitute the nodes of Ranvier.

Spinal nerves have an outer epineurial connective tissue investment and an inner more cellular perineurial covering that extends internally to surround nerve bundles. The cells of the perineurium form an epithelioid sheath wherein the cells are joined by occluding junctions and the layers of cells are separated by basal lamina material. This perineurial layer seems to be an effective barrier against material entering or leaving the nerve. A loose endoneurial connective tissue separates nerve processes and lies next to the basement membranes of the Schwann cells.

Spinal nerves contain the processes of neurons whose cell bodies are located in sensory dorsal root ganglia (pseudounipolar neurons), sympathetic ganglia (multipolar neurons), and in the gray matter of the spinal cord (multipolar neurons). Each spinal nerve contains myelinated and unmyelinated fibers which are invested by Schwann cells. In the ganglia, each cell body is surrounded by supportive satellite cells.

Spinal nerves contain neurons representing four functional components: (1) general somatic efferent fibers to skeletal muscles, (2) general visceral efferent fibers to smooth and cardiac muscle and glands, (3) general somatic afferent fibers from the skin, muscle and tendon spindles, and joints and, (4) general visceral afferent fibers from viscera.

Spinal Cord.   The spinal cord consists of a central canal lined with ependymal cells and bounded by central gray matter and peripheral white matter. The H-shaped gray matter has anterior, posterior and lateral horns. It consists of groups of nerve cell bodies (nuclei, cell columns), axons, dendrites and glial cells that form a meshwork called neuropil. An architectural lamination permits classification of the gray matter into nine Rexed's layers.

The anterior horn of gray matter contains the cell bodies of alpha and gamma motor neurons whose axons innervate extrafusal and intrafusal skeletal muscle fibers respectively. These nerve cell bodies constitute the general somatic efferent (GSE) cell column and are grouped into nuclei that supply axons to specific regions; e.g., those most medial in the anterior horn go to the more axial musculature while those most lateral innervate the extremities and the lateral muscles of the trunk. The alpha motor neurons are in Rexed's layer IX, the gamma motor neurons are in layer VII, and mostly commissural neurons occupy layer VIII. Preganglionic sympathetic neurons at thoracic and L1 and L2 levels are located in the intermediolateral cell column. This general visceral efferent (GVE) cell column is in Rexed's layer VII. Preganglionic parasympathetic cell bodies are scattered in layer VII of cord levels S2–S4. Axons of preganglionic autonomics leave the cord by the ventral root and become part of the spinal nerve. Sympathetic preganglionics leave the nerve via the white rami communicantes and enter the sympathetic chain ganglia or become components of splanchnic nerves. They will synapse with postganglionic sympathetic neurons in the sympathetic chain or prevertebral ganglia. Unmyelinated postganglionic axons reentering the spinal nerve constitute the gray rami communicantes. Sacral parasympathetic preganglionics form pelvic nerves, which terminate on ganglia near, or in, the organs innervated.

The posterior horn of gray matter consists of several nuclear groups that constitute the general somatic afferent (GSA) cell column. Most prominent of these nuclei are the substantia gelatinosa in Rexed's layer II, the nucleus proprius mostly in layer IV, and nucleus dorsalis of Clarke in layer VII. These nuclei are "nuclei of termination" for incoming somatic afferents in the dorsal roots. Pain and temperature first-order afferent neurons terminate on second-order neuron cell bodies in the substantia gelatinosa, nucleus proprius and deeper layers of the posterior horn. Axons of these second-order neurons transmit impulses contralaterally through the anterior white commissure and ascend in the lateral funiculus as the lateral spinothalamic tract. This tract synapses on third-order neurons in the ventral posterolateral (VPL) nucleus of the thalamus. Axons of VPL cells pass to the postcentral gyrus of the parietal lobe and to an area of parietal cortex immediately above the lateral fissure. Sensory information from intrafusal fibers of neuromuscular spindles and tendon spindles is transmitted via IA and IB myelinated first-order neurons respectively. These synapse on cells of the nucleus dorsalis at cord levels C8 to L3. Axons of these second-order neurons pass ipsilaterally to the cerebellum as the posterior spinocerebellar tract. 1A and 1B neurons entering the cervical cord above C8 ascend in the posterior white column to the medulla where they synapse on the accessory cuneate nucleus. Incoming fibers for crude (light) touch synapse in cells of the posterior horn. Most of the axons of these second-order neurons cross in the anterior white commissure and ascend in the anterior funiculus as the anterior spinothalamic tract. This tract synapses in the same nucleus of the thalamus and the impulses are probably relayed to the cortex in the same manner as in the pain and temperature pathways. Visceral sensation (GVA) is probably received by nuclei of termination in the lateral portion of the posterior horn. Its transmission to higher centers is probably through multisynaptic ascending paths in the funiculus proprius lying adjacent to the gray matter. Collaterals

from incoming neurons of the dorsal root enter the gray matter and synapse on internuncials and alpha motor neurons for reflex purposes. Those ending directly on alpha motor neurons are part of the monosynaptic stretch reflex. Terminals of association neurons interconnecting different segmental levels, as well as terminals of descending axons from suprasegmental levels, end on internuncials that synapse with gamma and alpha motor neurons.

The white matter is organized into posterior, lateral and white funiculi. Each funiculus contains both ascending and descending pathways. In the posterior funiculus (posterior white column) the most prominent pathway is that concerned with two-point touch, vibratory sense and stereognosis. Axons of this pathway in the posterior white column arise from cell bodies in the dorsal root ganglia, enter the cord in the medial bundle of the dorsal root and ascend to the medulla where they synapse on second-order neurons in the nuclei gracilis and cuneatus. Those axons entering dorsal roots below the T6 level constitute fasciculus gracilis and terminate in nucleus gracilis; those above T6 are in fasciculus cuneatus and terminate in nucleus cuneatus. Axons of the second-order neurons from the nuclei gracilis and cuneatus cross the midline as internal arcuate fibers and ascend as the medial lemniscus to the VPL nucleus of the thalamus where they synapse with third-order neurons whose axons go to the postcentral gyrus.

The most clinically prominent tracts of the lateral funiculus are the posterior spinocerebellar tract, the lateral spinothalamic tract, the lateral corticospinal tract and the lateral reticulospinal tract. The posterior spinocerebellar tract is peripherally located beneath the posterolateral fasciculus at all levels of the spinal cord above L4. It arises from cell bodies in Clarke's nucleus at the C8 to L3 levels and conveys spindle information to the cerebellum. The lateral spinothalamic tract is located ventrolaterally in the lateral funiculus and just deep to the anterior spinocerebellar tract. As previously mentioned, the lateral spinothalamic tract arises from cell bodies in the contralateral dorsal horn and ascends to the VPL nucleus of the thalamus. It represents the axons of second-order neurons of the pain and temperature pathway. The lateral corticospinal tract is located just medial to the posterior spinocerebellar tract in the more dorsal half of the lateral funiculus. This tract arises from pyramidal cells in the precentral gyrus and premotor area (areas 4 and 6) and postcentral (areas 3, 1, 2) gyrus. From these gyri, axons descend in the brain stem, cross in the pyramidal decussation and descend in the contralateral lateral funiculus before terminating on internuncial neurons, which, in turn, synapse on alpha and gamma motor neurons. The lateral corticospinal tract constitutes the upper motor neurons of the pyramidal motor system. It is involved primarily in fine voluntary movements involving chiefly the more distal phylogenetically "newer" musculature, and it is facilitory to the antagonists of the antigravity muscles. The lateral reticulospinal tract arises from large cells in the medial reticular formation of the medulla. Axons from these cells descend ipsilaterally in the lateral funiculus and are somewhat interspersed with axons of the lateral corticospinal tract. Stimulation of cells of the lateral reticulospinal tract inhibits alpha and gamma neurons innervating antigravity muscles (i.e., extensors of the lower extremity and flexors of the upper extremity). Other pathways are found in the lateral funiculus. These are the rubrospinal pathway from the red nucleus, the spinotectal pathway to the superior colliculus of the mesencephalon, spinoreticular fibers to the brain stem reticular formation and interconnections between the spinal cord and inferior olivary nucleus.

In the anterior funiculus, the anterior spinothalamic tract, anterior corticospinal tract, vestibulospinal tract, medial reticulospinal tract and medial longitudinal fasciculus (MLF) are most prominent. The anterior spinothalamic tract is located just anterior to the ventral horn. Its origin, destination and crude touch role were described previously. The anterior corticospinal tract has a similar origin and path to that of the lateral corticospinal tract, but it differs in that it is located near the anterior median fissure and its axons have not crossed in the pyramidal decussation. These axons will cross, however, at the level where they terminate on internuncials that synapse with gamma and alpha motor neurons, supplying the more proximal musculature. The vestibulospinal tract is interspersed with the anterior spinothalamic tract. It arises from cells in the lateral vestibular nucleus and descends ipsilaterally to end on internuncials that synapse with gamma and alpha motor neurons supplying antigravity muscles. Stimulation of this pathway results in facilitation of extensors of the lower extremity and of flexors of the upper extremity. The medial reticulospinal tract arises from nuclei in the medial portion of the pontine reticular formation. It descends ipsilaterally, lies lateral to the anterior corticospinal tract in the anterior funiculus and is involved in facilitation of antigravity muscles. The MLF lies in the most dorsal portion of the anterior funiculus next to the anterior median fissure. This composite tract contains axons arising from the mesencephalic tectum, vestibular nuclei and the reticular formation of the brain stem.

The spinal cord is supplied by descending branches from vertebral arteries and from radicular branches of segmental arteries. From these vessels paired poste-

rior spinal arteries arise that descend dorsal to the posterior funiculus, while a single midline anterior spinal artery arises from the paired anterior spinal arterial branches of the vertebral. An arterial vasocorona plexus, lying in the pia adjacent to the lateral funiculus, interconnects the anterior and posterior radicular branches. The posterior spinal arteries supply the posterior funiculus, dorsal part of the dorsal horn of gray matter and the posterolateral fasciculus. Sulcal branches of the anterior spinal artery supply all other parts of the spinal cord except the most peripheral portion of the lateral funiculus supplied by the arterial vasocorona. Spinal veins have a distribution that is generally similar to arteries. Sulcal and posterior veins empty into anteromedial, anterolateral, posteromedial and posterolateral veins. These drain, in turn, to radicular veins that enter the epidural venous plexus.

Development of the Spinal Cord and Spinal Nerves

The central nervous system appears early in the third embryonic week of development as a thickened neural (medullary) plate of ectoderm. This plate is elongate, wider cephalically than caudally, and is located rostral to the primitive node of Hensen. It is continuous laterally with ectoderm that will give rise to the epidermis of the skin. With further development the lateral edges of the plate elevate to form neural folds that close the neural groove into a neural tube. The closure begins at the fourth somite and progresses cephalically and caudally, with the anterior and posterior neuropores closing by the 25th day. Ectoderm arising at the junction of neural ectoderm with general surface ectoderm becomes segmentally arranged as a neural crest of material lying dorsolateral to the neural tube. The cephalic enlargement of the neural tube differentiates into the brain and gives rise to motor components of cranial nerves. The caudal part becomes the spinal cord and also gives rise to the ventral roots of spinal nerves. Neural crest gives rise to sensory neurons comprising the dorsal root ganglia and sensory cranial nerve ganglia, postganglionic autonomic ganglia of cranial and spinal nerves, Schwann cells, satellite cells, parenchyma of the adrenal medulla, pigment cells and cartilage cells.

Histogenesis of the Spinal Cord. The early neural tube consists of a neuroepithelium that differentiates into neuroblasts and spongioblasts (glioblasts). Neuroblasts differentiate into neurons whose cell bodies are localized into a mantle layer and whose axons contribute to a more peripheral marginal layer. Some of these axons ascend or descend in the marginal layer and become the association fibers of the tracts of the white matter. Others leave the white matter and become motor (efferent) nerve fibers of the ventral roots and spinal nerves. Spongioblasts lining the central canal differentiate into ependymal cells while others migrate into the marginal and mantle layers and become astrocytes and oligodendroglia. Oligodendroglia wrap nerve fibers in a jellyroll manner, thus, giving rise to myelin in the CNS. Microglia arise from cells that have invaded the developing spinal cord from the surrounding mesoderm.

The lateral walls of the neural tube are separated into dorsal alar plates and ventral basal plates by a longitudinally running sulcus limitans. The thin roof plate is obliterated in the fusions accompanying the formation of the posterior median septum; the floor plate remains as the anterior white and gray commissures. The mantle layer of the alar plate develops into the posterior horn of gray matter that contains the nuclei of termination for GSA and GVA neurons. Neurons of the posterior horn are internuncial, commissural and association neurons. The mantle layer of the basal plate becomes the anterior horn and lateral horn of gray matter. Neuroblasts of the anterior horn give rise to gamma and alpha GSE neurons whose axons leave the cord in the ventral root and innervate intrafusal and extrafusal skeletal muscle fibers respectively. Neuroblasts of the lateral horn give rise to preganglionic sympathetic neurons of the intermediolateral cell column at thoracic and L1-L3 levels. Preganglionic parasympathetic neurons arise in a similar position at S2-S4 levels.

Histogenesis of Spinal Nerves. General somatic afferent and general visceral afferent neurons arise from neural crest material, and their cell bodies are located in dorsal root ganglia. Axons of the sensory cells terminate in the posterior horn or, as in the case of the GSA discriminatory touch pathway, ascend in the posterior white column as the fasciculus gracilis and fasciculus cuneatus. General somatic efferent and preganglionic visceral efferent axons in spinal nerves arise from neuroblasts of the mantle layer as previously described. Postganglionic autonomic neurons differentiate from neural crest. Their cell bodies are aggregated into sympathetic and parasympathetic ganglia. Postganglionic axons are unmyelinated; those that traverse the spinal nerve enter it through the gray communicating rami. The myelin of all myelinated fibers in spinal nerves develop from neural crest material by the wrapping of differentiating Schwann cells around axons.

Nerve Degeneration and Regeneration. Injury to a nerve fiber leads to degeneration of the axon and myelin in the entire portion distal to the lesion (wallerian degeneration) and also for a distance of one to two internodes in the proximal stump of the fiber (retrograde degeneration). If injured neurons are components of ascending sensory pathways in the CNS, the sensory loss will be reflected as an anesthesia, hypesthesia, atonia, or hypotonia below the lesion. The degeneration, however, will be primarily in the entire distal stump above the lesion. When injured neurons are components of descending motor pathways then the loss may be expressed as paresis, paralysis of movement or atrophy. Both the motor functional deficit and degeneration of the distal stump are below the lesion.

In degeneration of myelinated peripheral nerves, myelin in the distal stump and in the region of damage will retract from the nodes, break up into segments and will be phagocytized by Schwann cells. Most myelin has degenerated by 3 weeks after the injury, but some may remain for up to 3 months. The axon of the distal stump swells, fragments and is phagocytized by the Schwann cells. Schwann cells of the distal stump, and for one to two internodes in the proximal stump, increase in size, divide and form longitudinal bands. These bands of Büngner move into the center of the nerve fiber as the myelin and axon degenerate, thus leaving a neurolemmal tubular space between the Schwann cells and their basement membrane. If the damage to the neuron is near the cell body the whole neuron will degenerate. If the injury is farther away the cell will not die but the cell body will swell, chromatolysis occurs, and the nucleus moves eccentrically to a position opposite the axon hillock. Chromatolysis is due to dispersion of rough endoplasmic reticulum and ribosomes and is not accompanied by loss of RNA.

In regeneration of the peripheral nerve, Nissl material starts to reappear around the nucleus in the third week, the nucleus returns to its original position, and turgescence subsides. Schwann cells bridge the area of the cut, and the swelling axon tip splits into fine fibers that enter neurolemmal tubes. Of the new fibers that enter each tube, the one that is usually first to reach the nerve ending will be moved deeply into gutters on the surface of the Schwann cells while the others degenerate. If the regenerating neuron is to become myelinated, the Schwann cells will wrap it with their plasmalemma. If it is to remain unmyelinated, it will be incompletely invested in the Schwann cell gutters.

Degeneration and regeneration processes of the central nervous system are similar to those in peripheral nerves, but regeneration is seldom as complete or successful. Since Schwann cells are absent, oligodendroglia perform similar functions but have more limited capacities. Vascular and neuroglial elements respond more to trauma. Microglia and astrocytes proliferate and extend into the cut area and compete with poor neurolemmal tube formation in the damaged area. Thus, regenerating fibers in the CNS pass into poor neurolemmal tubes if they are not first blocked by extensive scar tissue formation.

THE UPPER EXTREMITY

Bones and Joints of the Upper Extremity

The bones of the upper limb include the clavicle and scapula, which form the shoulder (pectoral) girdle, the humerus of the arm, the radius and ulna of the forearm and the carpals, metacarpals and phalanges of the hand.

Clavicle and Sternoclavicular and Acromioclavicular Articulations.

The clavicle through its articulations is the only bony connection between the upper extremity and the axial skeleton. As such, it keeps the limb away from the body and thereby allows for a large range of motion. Proximally directed force through the upper limb frequently causes clavicular fracture. These fractures are usually in the middle third of the bone because of its doubly curved shape, and they are also easily diagnosed by palpation because of the clavicle's completely subcutaneous location.

The medial end of the clavicle articulates with the superolateral aspect of the manubrium at the sternoclavicular joint. The bones are separated by an intraarticular disk, and thus two synovial cavities exist. The bones are held in position by the articular capsule and sternoclavicular, interclavicular and costoclavicular ligaments.

The lateral end of the clavicle articulates with the acromion at the acromioclavicular joint. The synovial space is enclosed by a capsule, but the major supports for this joint are the coracoclavicular ligaments (conoid and trapezoid ligaments), which extend between the clavicle and the coracoid process.

Humerus.

The humerus articulates with the scapula proximally and with the radius and ulna distally. The head forms a nearly hemispheric articular surface covered with articular cartilage. A constricted anatomic neck marks the attachment of the capsule of the shoulder joint. Lateral to the head is the greater tuberosity, on which are inserted the supraspinatus, infraspinatus and teres minor. The lesser tuberosity lies anteriorly below the head and receives the subscapularis. Between these tuberosities is the intertubercular groove lodging the tendon of the long head of the biceps. Immediately below the tuberosities is the tapering surgical neck, so named because of the frequency of fracture in that area. The spiral groove curves around the posterolateral aspect of the midshaft of the humerus, passing inferior to the laterally placed deltoid tuberosity.

The lower end of the humerus presents the trochlea medially and the rounded capitulum laterally. The trochlea articulates with the trochlear notch of the ulna and the capitulum with the radial head. Above the trochlea anteriorly the coronoid fossa receives the coronoid process of the ulna when the elbow is flexed.

Above the trochlea posteriorly the olecranon fossa is occupied by the olecranon process of the ulna when the elbow is extended. There is a small lateral and a larger medial epicondyle.

Shoulder Joint.

The shoulder joint is a loose ball and socket joint formed by the articulation of the head of the humerus with the glenoid fossa of the scapula. In this joint maximal mobility is available at the expense of stability. The very loose articular capsule is redundant inferiorly when the joint is in the anatomic position. The glenoid cavity is deepened to a small degree by the glenoid labrum, a dense fibrocartilaginous wedge that attaches to the periphery of the glenoid fossa. The capsule extends from the rim of the glenoid fossa and the labrum to the anatomic neck of the humerus. It is reinforced anteriorly by the variable glenohumeral ligaments and by the coracohumeral ligament. The tendon of the long head of the biceps brachii ascends through the intertubercular groove and then passes across the superior aspect of the humeral head (between the fibrous and synovial portions of the capsule) to attach to the supraglenoid tubercle.

The major supports of this joint are the muscles of the rotator (musculotendinous) cuff: the subscapularis, supraspinatus, infraspinatus and teres minor muscles. These muscles reinforce the anterior, superior and posterior aspects of the joint. The inferior aspect is virtually unsupported and contributory to the common anterior humeral dislocations.

Motion at the shoulder joint is very free and occurs around an infinite number of axes. Although shoulder joint motion is a major factor in allowing the hand to assume innumerable locations and positions, proper function of the entire shoulder complex is absolutely necessary. Scapular motion as well as motion of the clavicle accompanies virtually every position change of the arm, and a loss of scapular, sternoclavicular, acromioclavicular or glenohumeral range of motion will reduce the range of the entire upper limb. Scapular motion is controlled primarily by the trapezius and serratus anterior muscles. The motions listed below refer strictly to the shoulder joint, and the muscles that follow are the prime movers at that joint:

Flexion: anterior deltoid, pectoralis major, (especially the clavicular portion) coracobrachialis

Extension: latissimus dorsi, posterior deltoid, teres major

Abduction: middle deltoid, supraspinatus

Adduction: latissimus dorsi, pectoralis major (sternal portion)

Medial rotation: pectoralis minor, latissimus dorsi, anterior deltoid, subscapularis

Lateral rotation: posterior deltoid, teres minor, infraspinatus

Suprahumeral Space. This is not a space in any sense but rather an area that is packed with structures of various types. It is between the head of the humerus and the arch formed by the acromion, coracoid and the intervening coracoacromial ligament. The major structures involved are the superior portion of the capsule of the shoulder joint, the tendon and part of the supraspinatus muscle, the subdeltoid (subacromial) bursa, and the tendon of the long head of the biceps brachii muscle. During virtually every movement of the upper limb there is humeral motion and the structures in this space are compressed between the head of the humerus and the coracoacromial arch. This compression is especially necessary during flexion and abduction. Inflammation of any of these tissues results in loss of range of motion of the shoulder area.

Radius, Ulna and Their Articulations. The radius is the lateral bone of the forearm. It has a small head proximally that is flat and round, and an expanded distal extremity which is the major forearm contribution to the wrist joint. The ulnar notch is on the medial aspect of the expanded distal portion, and the lateral palpable radial styloid is the most distal bony prominence of the forearm. The radial (bicipital) tuberosity is on the ventral proximal aspect of the radius.

The ulna is large proximally but narrows distally into the small round (but flat) head with the ulnar styloid extending past the head medially. The proximal portion has the deep ventrally directed trochlear notch. The proximal lip of this notch extends well beyond the humerus and is the point of the elbow or the olecranon. The distal lipe of the notch is the coronoid process. The lateral aspect of the proximal ulna is indented to form the radial notch.

The ulna and radius are united through synovial joints both proximally and distally, with the interosseous membrane interconnecting the two shafts between these synovial joints. The proximal joint is between the radial head and the radial notch of the ulna; the distal joint is between the ulnar head and the ulnar notch of the radius. The proximal joint is stabilized primarily by the annular ligament of the radius, which attaches to the edges of the radial notch of the ulna and surrounds the head of the radius. The distal joint is reinforced primarily by an intra-articular disk that extends from the distal medial radius to the ulnar styloid. The proximal joint shares an articular capsule with the elbow joint; the distal joint shares one with the wrist.

Pronation and supination occur between the two bones of the forearm at the proximal and distal radioulnar joints. When the hand is supinated the two bones are parallel. When the hand is pronated the radius is wrapped around the ulna. Pronation is produced primarily by the pronator teres and pronator quadratus; supination by the biceps brachii and the supinator.

Elbow Joint. The elbow joint is formed between the trochlea of the humerus and the trochlear notch of the ulna medially, and between the capitulum of the humerus and the head of the radius laterally. The motion permitted at this joint—flexion and extension—is essentially determined by the part of the joint between the humerus and ulna. A common joint capsule encloses the two portions of the elbow joint as well as the proximal radioulnar joint. The capsule is thickened medially to form the ulnar collateral ligament and laterally to form the radial collateral ligament. The major flexors at the elbow are the brachialis, biceps brachii, and brachioradialis. The major extensor is the triceps brachii.

Bones of the Hand. The bones of the hand include the 8 carpal bones, 5 metacarpals and 14 phalanges. The bones of the carpus are arranged in two rows. From lateral to medial, the proximal row consists of the scaphoid, the lunate, the triquetrum and the pisiform bones. The distal row is composed of the trapezium, the trapezoid, the capitate and the hamate bones. Each of the digits is composed of three phalanges except the thumb, which has only two. The phalanges are named by their position, i.e., proximal, middle, and distal.

Wrist Joint and Joints of the Hand. The proximal articular surface of the wrist or radiocarpal joint is formed by the distal aspect of the radius and the medially-placed intra-articular disk which interconnects the ulnar styloid and the distomedial aspect of the radius. The distal articular surface is formed primarily by the scaphoid and lunate, with a small contribution from the triquetrum. The wrist joint has its own synovial cavity, which is separated from the distal radioulnar joint by the articular disk. The midcarpal articulation, which also has a separate joint cavity, is found between the two rows of carpal bones. The capsules of both joints are reinforced by collateral as well as dorsal and palmar ligaments. The motions that occur in the area of the wrist are contributed to by movement at both the radiocarpal and midcarpal joints. These motions and their major motors are:

Flexion: flexor carpi radialis, flexor carpi ulnaris
Extension: extensor carpi radialis longus, extensor carpi radialis brevis, extensor carpi ulnaris
Abduction or radial deviation: extensor carpi radialis longus, flexor carpi radialis, abductor pollicis longus
Adduction or ulnar deviation: flexor carpi ulnaris, extensor carpi ulnaris

The carpometacarpal (CM) articulations of the four medial digits allow essentially no motion, even though they are synovial joints. The carpometacarpal joint of the thumb is between the base of the first metacarpal and the trapezium. The shapes of these joint surfaces permit flexion, extension, abduction, adduction and, hence, circumduction. Rotation of the thumb is essential to opposition. Rotation occurs primarily at this joint and is provided by the action of the opponens pollicis.

The metacarpophalangeal (MP) joints are synovial in type and permit flexion, extension, abduction, adduction and circumduction. Abduction and adduction are free only in extension as the collateral ligaments become taut in flexion and thereby virtually eliminate any side-to-side movement. Abduction and adduction are very limited at the MP joint of the thumb. The interphalangeal (IP) joints are all synovial articulations that permit only flexion and extension.

The muscles producing motion in the hand are:

MP flexion (not thumb): lumbricals, dorsal and ventral interossei, flexor digitorum profundus, flexor digitorum superficialis

MP extension (not thumb): extensor digitorum

Digital abduction: dorsal interossei

Digital adduction: ventral interossei

Proximal IP extension: lumbricals, dorsal and ventral interossei

Distal IP extension: lumbrical, dorsal and ventral interossei

Proximal IP flexion: flexor digitorum superficialis, flexor digitorum profundus

Distal IP flexion: flexor digitorum profundus

NOTE: The combination of MP flexion and IP extention is a functional position that is used in many activities requiring infinite control and gradation. These motions are the combined functions of the lumbricals and the interossei muscles.

Thumb flexion: flexor pollicis longus and brevis

Thumb extension: extensor pollicis longus and brevis

Thumb abduction: abductor pollicis longus and brevis

Thumb adduction: adductor pollicis

Opposition of the thumb: opponens pollicis, abductor pollicis brevis and flexor pollicis brevis

Compartmentation of the Upper Extremity

Arm.   The arm is divided into anterior and posterior compartments by the medial and lateral intermuscular septa, which extend from the investing brachial fascia to the humerus. The muscles in the anterior compartment are the biceps brachii, brachialis, and coracobrachialis. These muscles are innervated by the musculocutaneous nerve and produce flexion at the elbow and supination of the forearm. Only the triceps brachii is found in the posterior compartment. This elbow extensor is innervated by the radial nerve.

Forearm.   The forearm is separated into anterior and posterior compartments by the medial and lateral intermuscular septa which extend from the antebrachial fascia to the ulna and radius respectively and by the interosseous membrane which interconnects the radius and ulna. The muscles in the anterior compartment originate from the medial humeral epicondyle and the ventral aspects of the radius and ulna and function to pronate the forearm and flex the wrist and fingers. The pronator teres, flexor carpi radialis, palmaris longus, flexor digitorum superficialis, flexor pollicis longus, pronator quadratus, and the lateral half of the flexor digitorum profundus (to digits 2 and 3) are innervated by the median nerve. The flexor carpi ulnaris and medial half of the flexor digitorum profundus (to digits 4 and 5) are innervated by the ulnar nerve. The muscles in the posterior compartment originate from the lateral humeral epicondyle and the dorsal aspects of the radius and ulna. These muscles are all innervated by the radial nerve, and they function to supinate the forearm and extend the wrist and digits at the MP joints. These muscles are the brachioradialis, extensor carpi radialis longus, extensor carpi radialis brevis, extensor digitorum, extensor digiti minimi, extensor carpi ulnaris, supinator, abductor pollicis longus, extensor pollicis brevis, extensor pollicis longus and extensor indicis.

Hand.   The ventral aspect of the hand is separated into thenar, hypothenar and central compartments. The antebrachial fascia continues into the hand and attaches along the first and fifth metacarpals. In the central region of the palm this fascia is greatly thickened to form the palmar aponeurosis. From the lateral border of this aponeurosis the thenar intermuscular septum extends into the palm and attaches to the first metacarpal. This septum together with the investing fascia around the lateral aspect of the palm delimits the thenar compartment, which contains the abductor pollicis brevis, flexor pollicis brevis and opponens pollicis muscles. These muscles are innervated by the recurrent or thenar branch of the median nerve. The hypothenar intermuscular septum extends between the medial extent of the palmar aponeurosis and the fifth metacarpal and with the investing fascia on the medial aspect of the palm defines the hypothenar compartment. This compartment contains the abductor digiti minimi, flexor digiti minimi brevis and opponens digiti minimi, all of which are innervated by the deep branch of the ulnar nerve. The central compartment is deep to the palmar aponeurosis in the center of the palm. It is bounded by the aponeurosis, the thenar and hypothenar intermuscular septa and a layer of fascia that extends between the first and fifth metacarpals deep in the palm. Only four small muscles are found here, the lumbricals. The two lateral lumbricals are innervated by the median nerve; the two medial ones, by the ulnar nerve. The long flexor tendons to the digits pass through this compartment. This compartment also contains the superficial palmar arterial arch, which is between the palmar aponeurosis and the long flexor tendons. The cutaneous branches of the median and ulnar nerves are distributed with the branches of the superficial arterial arch. The adductor interosseous compartment is essentially between the metacarpals. It is bounded dorsally by the dorsal interosseous fascia and ventrally by the adductor interosseous fascia. This space contains the dorsal and ventral interossei and the adductor pollicis, all of which are innervated by the deep branch of the ulnar nerve.

Bursae and Spaces. The radial and ulnar bursae are synovial tendon sheaths that surround the long flexor tendons of the digits. They both start proximal to the wrist, pass through the carpal tunnel with the tendons and extend either partially or completely through the palm and into the fingers. The radial bursa is associated only with the tendon of the flexor pollicis longus. The ulnar bursa surrounds all four tendons of both the flexor digitorum superficialis and profundus muscles. That part of this bursa associated with the little finger usually extends through the palm and into the digit while the others terminate at midpalmar levels. Thus, the synovial portions of the digital tendon sheaths of the index, middle, and ring fingers are not continuous with the ulnar bursa, per se.

A pair of potential spaces (really fascial planes) exists at the approximate level of the ventral adductor interosseous fascia, i.e., in the plane just deep to the long digital flexor tendons in the central compartment. This plane is divided into a medial midpalmar space and a lateral thenar space by a septum that extends from the palmar aponeurosis to the third metacarpal. As indicated above, these are only potential spaces but can become actual spaces when filled with blood, inflammatory material, etc.

Nerves of the Upper Extremity

Brachial Plexus. Most of the muscles of the upper extremity are supplied by branches of the brachial plexus. The plexus is formed by the ventral rami of spinal nerves C5, 6, 7, 8 and T1. Ventral rami of C5 and 6 unite to form the superior trunk, C7 continues as the middle trunk, and the inferior trunk is formed by the union of C8 and T1. The three trunks split into anterior and posterior divisions. This separation into divisions determines the basic innervation pattern for the extremity; i.e., the nerves formed from the ante-

rior divisions innervate the muscles in the anterior compartments, and those from posterior divisions innervate posterior compartment muscles. The lateral cord is formed from the anterior divisions of the superior and middle trunks, and the anterior division of the inferior trunk continues as the medial cord. The posterior divisions of all three trunks unite to form the posterior cord. The cords of the plexus receive their names from their relationships with the second part of the axillary artery. The terminal peripheral nerves are formed in the axilla from the cords. The median nerve (C6–T1) is formed by contributions from both the medial and lateral cords. The remainder of the medial cord forms the ulnar nerve (C7–T1), and the termination of the lateral cord is the musculocutaneous nerve (C5–7). The posterior cord gives rise to the radial (C5–8) and axillary nerves (C5, 6).

Branches from the plexus proper are called collateral branches, and they supply most of the extrinsic and intrinsic muscles of the shoulder. (Extrinsic muscles extend from the axial skeleton to the scapula, clavicle or humerus; intrinsic muscles connect the scapula or clavicle with the humerus.) The branches from the ventral rami are the dorsal scapular nerve (C5), which supplies both rhomboids and part of the levator scapulae, and the long thoracic nerve (C5–7) to the serratus anterior. From the superior trunk arise the nerve to the subclavius (C5) and the suprascapular nerve (C5), which innervates the supraspinatus and infraspinatus muscles. The medial (C8, T1) and lateral (C5–7) pectoral nerves branch from the medial and lateral cords respectively. The medial pectoral nerve innervates the pectoralis major and minor; the lateral, only the major. The three subscapular nerves branch from the posterior cord. The upper and lower subscapular nerves (C5, 6) innervate the subscapularis and teres major muscles. The thoracodorsal nerve (middle subscapular) (C7, 8) innervates the latissimus dorsi muscle.

Median Nerve. The median nerve passes through the arm in the medial neurovascular bundle, which is located where the medial intermuscular septum joins the brachial fascia. In the distal part of the arm it inclines laterally and passes through the cubital fossa just medial to the brachial artery. The median nerve enters the forearm by passing through the pronator teres muscle and descends in the forearm between the superficial and deep grounds of muscles. At the wrist the median nerve is between the tendons of the flexor carpi radialis and the palmaris longus. It enters the hand by going through the carpal tunnel. Just distal to the deep part of the flexor retinaculum (transverse carpal ligament) the nerve branches into the thenar or recurrent branch to the muscles in the thenar compartment, and the common and proper digital branches, which supply the skin on the ventral aspect of the lateral three and a half digits and some of the corresponding part of the palm. The lateral midpalmar skin is supplied by the palmar branch of the median nerve. This branch arises proximal to the wrist and does not pass through the carpal tunnel.

Musculocutaneous Nerve. From its origin in the axilla this nerve inclines laterally, going first through the coracobrachialis muscle and then between the biceps brachii and the brachialis. It enters the subcutaneous tissue in the distal lateral arm, after which it continues into the forearm as the lateral antebrachial cutaneous. It supplies the skin of the lateral aspect of the forearm.

Ulnar Nerve. The ulnar nerve passes through the proximal half of the arm in the medial neurovascular bundle. It inclines posteriorly in the distal half of the arm, enters the posterior compartment and then passes behind the medial epicondyle of the humerus to enter the forearm. The nerve passes through the forearm under cover of the flexor carpi ulnaris, and at the wrist it is deep to the tendon of the same muscle. It enters the hand by passing superficial to the deep part of the flexor retinaculum and lateral to the pisiform. Just distal to the pisiform it divides into deep and superficial branches. The superficial branch splits into common and proper digital nerves which innervate the palmar skin of the medial one and a half digits and corresponding part of the palm. The deep branch passes through the hypothenar compartment and then sweeps laterally across the palm deep to the long flexor tendons. It innervates the interossei as it crosses the palm and terminates in the adductor pollicis. The ulnar nerve also innervates the dorsal skin of the medial one and a half digits. This is accomplished by the dorsal cutaneous branch, which arises proximal to the wrist.

Radial Nerve. The radial nerve descends in the posterior compartment of the arm by curving obliquely around the posterior aspect of the midshaft of the humerus in the spiral groove. In the distal third of the arm it enters the anterior compartment by piercing the lateral intermuscular septum and is positioned between the brachioradialis and the brachialis muscles. Just proximal to the elbow and deep to the brachioradialis it divides into superficial and deep branches. The superficial branch descends in the forearm under cover of the brachioradialis. It enters the subcutaneous tissue in the distal forearm and is cutaneous to the dorsal surface of the lateral three and a half digits and corresponding part of the dorsal hand. The deep branch enters the posterior compartment of the forearm by wrapping around the neck of the radius in the substance of the supinator muscle. It then branches into its many muscular branches and continues through

the forearm as the posterior interosseous nerve, which terminates at the level of the wrist.

Axillary Nerve. The axillary nerve passes antero-inferior to the shoulder joint (where it is occasionally stretched in an anterior shoulder dislocation) and then horizontally around the posterior aspect of the surgical neck of the humerus. It then enters the under surface of the deltoid muscle.

Lesions Involving the Main Peripheral Nerves of the Upper Extremity

Radial Nerve. When the radial nerve is interrupted in the axilla, the following symptoms are apparent:

1. Extension of the elbow and wrist are lost, and wrist drop results.
2. Extension of the thumb is lost; abduction is weakened.
3. Extension of the metacarpophalangeal joints of the index, middle, ring, and little fingers is lost.
4. Grasp is weakened, due to inability to extend and stabilize the wrist.
5. Supination of the forearm is weakened.
6. Radial and ulnar deviation of the wrist are weakened.
7. Sensation is lost on the dorsolateral aspect of the hand, forearm, and arm.

A radial nerve lesion at the level of the elbow would differ primarily in that elbow extension would be unaffected, and the severity of other symptoms would be reduced. Sensory loss would be limited to the dorsolateral hand.

Median Nerve. Paralysis of the median nerve at the wrist (as it passes through the carpal tunnel, resulting in a carpal tunnel syndrome) produces the following problems:

1. Flexion of the thumb is weakened.
2. Opposition of the thumb is lost, resulting in a derotated and adducted thumb (simian hand).
3. Flexion of the MP joints of the middle and index fingers is weakened, resulting in a slight clawing of these fingers.
4. Sensation is lost on the palmar surface of the lateral three and a half fingers and the corresponding portion of the distal palm.

Paralysis of the median nerve proximal to the elbow or in the axilla causes additional difficulties:

5. Flexion of the IP joints of the index and middle fingers is lost, resulting in extension deformity, especially of the index finger.
6. Flexion of the PIP joints of the little and ring fingers is lost, resulting in slight clawing of those two fingers. (The combination of 5 and 6 produces a benediction attitude of the hand.)

7. Flexion of the distal joint of the thumb is lost.
8. Pronation of the forearm is lost.
9. Flexion of the wrist is weakened.
10. Sensation is lost on the palmar surface of the lateral three and a half fingers and the entire lateral palm.

Ulnar Nerve. Paralysis of the ulnar nerve at the wrist results in these difficulties:

1. Abduction and adduction of the fingers are lost.
2. Flexion of the MP joints and extension of the IP joints are weakened in the index and middle fingers and virtually lost in the ring and little fingers. As a result, clawing is severe in the little and ring fingers, and moderate in the middle and index fingers.
3. Adduction of the thumb is virtually lost.
4. Opposition of the little finger is lost.
5. Opposition of the thumb is somewhat difficult.
6. Palmar sensation of the medial one and a half digits and the corresponding portion of the palm is lost.

Paralysis of the ulnar nerve proximal to the elbow results in these additional problems:

7. Flexion of the DIP joints of the little and ring fingers is lost.
8. Flexion of the wrist is weakened and is accompanied by radial deviation.
9. Sensation of the dorsal and palmar aspects of the medial one and a half digits and corresponding portions of the hand is lost.

Combined Median–Ulnar Nerves. Interruption of both the median and ulnar nerves at the wrist results in:

1. Flexion of the MP joints and extension of the IP joints is lost; there is severe clawing of all four fingers.
2. Digital abduction and adduction are lost.
3. Thumb and little finger opposition are lost, hence a simian hand.
4. Sensation on the entire ventral surface of the hand is lost.

Blockage or lesion of the median and ulnar nerves proximal to the elbow causes the following additional difficulties:

5. Flexion of all joints distal to the elbow is lost.
6. Pronation of the forearm is lost.

Axillary Nerve. Paralysis of the axillary nerve as it leaves the posterior cord results in:

1. Virtual loss of useful shoulder joint abduction. Only a few degrees of abduction remain.

2. Weakened shoulder flexion.
3. Loss of sensation on the proximal lateral arm.

Musculocutaneous Nerve. Paralysis of the musculocutaneous nerve at its origin results in:

1. Very weakened elbow flexion
2. Weakened supination of the forearm
3. Loss of sensation on the lateral forearm.

Blood Supply of the Upper Extremity

Arteries. The blood supply of the upper limb is provided by the *subclavian artery,* which becomes the *axillary artery* as it crosses the first rib. The first part of the axillary artery extends from the first rib to the pectoralis minor muscle, the second part is deep to the muscle, and the third part extends between the pectoralis minor and the lower border of the teres major muscle. The first part of the artery has the superior thoracic branch to the upper chest wall. The second part of the artery has the thoracoacromial trunk which has branches to the acromial, deltoid, pectoral and clavicular regions, and the lateral thoracic branch which descends along the anterolateral chest wall. The third part has branches to the scapular and proximal humeral regions and to the latissimus dorsi. These are the subscapular branch, which bifurcates into the circumflex scapular and thoracodorsal arteries, and the anterior and posterior humeral circumflex arteries, which arise at the level of the surgical neck of the humerus. The circumflex scapular artery forms potential anastomoses posterior to the scapula with branches of the subclavian artery. The posterior humeral circumflex artery accompanies the axillary nerve as it passes around the posterior aspect of the proximal humerus.

The *brachial artery* is the continuation of the axillary artery. It passes through the arm in the medial neurovascular bundle. It inclines laterally in the distal half of the arm and crosses the elbow by passing through the cubital fossa. In the cubital fossa it is medial to the tendon of the biceps brachii muscle and lateral to the median nerve (between these two structures), and separated from the more superficial median cubital vein by the bicipital aponeurosis. It divides into the radial and ulnar arteries just opposite the radial head. Its largest branch is the deep brachial artery, which arises in the axilla and spirals around the humerus with the radial nerve.

The *ulnar artery* passes through the medial aspect of the forearm deep to the flexor carpi ulnaris muscle, and at the wrist it is just lateral to that muscle's tendon. It enters the hand by passing superficial to the deep part of the flexor retinaculum and lateral to the pisiform. Its largest branch is the common interosseous artery, which arises high in the forearm and gives rise to the anterior and posterior interosseous arteries.

The *radial artery* descends through the lateral part of the forearm under cover of the brachioradialis muscle. At the level of the radial styloid it inclines dorsally and enters the dorsum of the hand by passing through the anatomic snuff box. (The anatomic snuff box is bordered by the tendons of the abductor pollicis longus and extensor pollicis brevis laterally and the tendon of the extensor pollicis longus medially.) At the wrist a radial pulse can be obtained somewhat proximally just lateral to the tendon of the flexor carpi radialis.

The course of the ulnar artery in the hand is similar to that of the ulnar nerve in that it has a superficial and a deep branch. The superficial branch gives rise to the *superficial palmar arch*. This arch is at the level of the palmar border of the extended thumb between the palmar aponeurosis and the long flexor tendons. The arch is completed by the superficial palmar branch of the radial artery, which branches proximal to the wrist and passes superficially through the thenar muscles. The arch has common digital branches to the fingers and a proper digital branch to the thumb. The radial artery passes through the snuff box and then between (passing dorsal to ventral) the first and second metacarpals. This course brings it into the deep part of the lateral palm where it gives rise to the *deep palmar arterial arch*. This arch is completed by the deep branch of the ulnar artery, and it accompanies the deep ulnar nerve. This arch is proximal to the superficial arch and deep to the long flexor tendons. The palmar metacarpal branches of the deep arch communicate with branches of the superficial arch and the dorsal carpal arterial network.

Veins. The veins of the upper extremity consist of two sets: The deep veins accompany the arteries and communicate frequently with the superficial veins, which ramify in the subcutaneous tissue.

The *basilic vein* arises on the ulnar side of the back of the hand and extends along the ulnar side of the forearm to the elbow. It crosses the anteromedial aspect of the elbow, pierces the brachial fascia and empties into the brachial vein.

The *cephalic vein* begins at the radial side of the dorsal venous network and continues proximally through the lateral forearm and arm. At the shoulder it passes through the deltopectoral groove (separating the deltoid and pectoralis major muscles), after which it empties into the axillary vein.

The *median cubital vein* interconnects the cephalic and basilic systems superficial to the cubital fossa.

LOWER EXTREMITY

Bones and Joints of the Lower Extremity

Pelvis. The pelvis is composed of the two hip bones (os coxae) and the sacrum. The three bones are united at the two sacroiliac joints and the single symphysis pubis and thus form the pelvic ring.

The os coxae is made up of three bones that fuse early in life: the pubis, ischium, and ilium. The pubis is anteromedially located. It consists of a body (which forms the symphysis with the body of the opposite side) and posterolaterally directed superior and inferior rami. The superior pubic ramus unites with the ilium; the inferior, with the ischium. The palpable pubic tubercle springs from the anterior aspect of the body. The ischium is the posteroinferior portion of the hip bone. It has a heavy body, a palpable ischial tuberosity and an ischial spine. The tuberosity is the inferiormost aspect of the hip bone and the origin of the hamstring muscles. The ischial spine is projected posteromedially above the tuberosity, and it is palpable via rectal or vaginal examination. The ilium is the superiormost part of the os coxae. Its body is united with the ischium and the pubis. Its flattened superior part is a flat wing that flares superolaterally and has a thickened crest that terminates anteriorly and posteriorly in the anterior superior and posterior superior iliac spines respectively. The gluteal muscles attach to the lateral aspect of the iliac wing, and the iliacus muscle attaches medially. The posteromedial aspect of the iliac body presents the surface that articulates with the sacrum.

Inferiorly, portions of the three component bones surround the obturator foramen. Superior to the obturator foramen and on the lateral aspect of the os coxae the three component bones form the socket of the hip joint, the acetabulum. Posteriorly and inferiorly, the area between the ischial tuberosity and ischial spine is the lesser sciatic notch; the area between the ischial spine and the posterior inferior iliac spine is the greater sciatic notch.

The bones of the pelvis are involved in the formation of the walls of both the pelvic and abdominal cavities. The pelvic inlet separates the true pelvis below from the false pelvis (part of the abdominal cavity) above. The inlet is formed posteriorly by the sacral promontory, laterally by the arcuate line of the ilium and the iliopectineal line, and anteriorly by the superior aspects of the pubic body and symphysis.

Although there are many variations in pelvic architecture, the following classification has received general acceptance. It must be stressed that although the following discussion considers four categories of pelvic shape, in reality most pelves are mixtures of the various types. The gynecoid pelvis is regarded as the characteristic female pelvis. It is distinguished by an oval inlet with the transverse diameter exceeding the anteroposterior diameter. This pelvis is shallow with straight walls. The ischial spines are not prominent, and the subpubic arch is wide. It also has the appearance of being flattened from top to bottom, making it shorter and wider than the male pelvis. The android pelvis (male) has a heart-shaped inlet and is longer and heavier, and the angle of the subpubic arch is more acute. The anthropoid pelvis has an oval inlet with the long axis along the anteroposterior diameter. The platypelloid pelvis has a flattened oval inlet, which is caused by marked reduction in the anteroposterior diameter.

Femur. The femur is the largest and longest bone in the body. Proximally, the superomedially directed head is separated from the shaft by the neck, which joins the shaft at the trochanteric region. The head is slightly greater than a hemisphere and is covered with articular cartilage except in the region of the fovea. The angle between neck and shaft is greater than 90 degrees and generally greater in the female than in the male. The palpable greater trochanter is located superolaterally at this junctional area; the lesser is inferomedially. The long shaft inclines medially from above downward. The distal end of the femur has two separate condyles that are covered by articular cartilage. The articular surface comes together anteriorly to form a groove for the patella. An intercondylar fossa separates the condyles inferiorly and posteriorly. Each condyle is expanded superiorly to form an epicondyle.

Hip Joint. The acetabulum is a deep socket with the horseshoe-shaped articular surface oriented so that its open end is directed inferiorly. Therefore the articular surface is incomplete centrally and inferiorly. The head of the femur also has an area that is not covered by articular cartilage, the centrally located fovea. The bony congruency between the two surfaces is good. The head of the femur is actually gripped by the fibrocartilaginous acetabular labrum, which, in addition to deepening the socket, also reduces its diameter and thereby holds the femur in place. The labrum bridges the gap inferiorly between the two limbs of the horseshoe as the transverse acetabular ligament.

The capsule of the hip joint extends from the labrum and corresponding part of the os coxae across the joint and well down the femoral neck. Anteriorly it extends over the entire length of the neck and attaches to the area of the intertrochanteric line. Posteriorly it extends about two thirds of the way distally so that there is an extracapsular portion of the neck posteriorly. It is important to note that only the fibrous portion of the capsule is attached to the femur as just indicated. The synovial layer reflects on itself at these attachments and passes proximally along the neck to attach at the border of the articular surface of the head of the femur. Most of the blood vessels supplying the head and neck of the femur pass proximally along the neck of the femur deep to the synovial layer of the capsule. They are firmly held against the bone and vulnerable to laceration when the femoral neck is fractured. Again, it is important to note that the entire anterior aspect of the neck is intracapsular but only the medial two thirds is intracapsular posteriorly.

A major amount of support of the hip joint is provided by three extracapsular ligaments that blend with the fibrous portion of the joint capsule. The iliofemoral ligament (Y ligament of Bigelow) extends from the anterior aspect of the body of the ilium across the front of the hip joint to the lower part of the intertrochanteric line. This ligament becomes taut as the hip is extended and is a major stabilizing force of the hip joint. The ischiofemoral ligament curves around the superior aspect of the joint. In addition to tightening during hip extension it also forces the head of the femur into the acetabulum as the hip is extended. The pubofemoral ligament crosses the joint inferiorly. The fovea of the head of the femur and the nonarticular portion of the acetabulum are connected by the ligament of the head of the femur (ligamentum teres), an intra-articular ligament that conveys a small blood vessel to the head of the femur and offers virtually no joint support.

Although the number of potential motions that can occur at the hip joint is infinite, it is convenient to describe those that correspond to the cardinal planes of the body. These motions and their major motors are:

Flexion: psoas, iliacus, rectus femoris
Extension: biceps femoris, semitendinosus, semimembranosus, posterior portion of the adductor magnus, gluteus maximus
Abduction: gluteus medius, gluteus minimus
Adduction: adductor magnus, adductor longus, adductor brevis, adductor minimus, gracilis
Lateral rotation: gluteus maximus, obturator internus and externus, gemelli, quadratus femoris
Medial rotation: gluteus medius and gluteus minimus, tensor fasciae latae

It should be noted that, based on the position of the hip (flexion or extension), certain adductors may rotate the thigh either medially or laterally.

Tibia and Fibula. The *tibia* is the weightbearing bone of the leg and therefore is a major bone in the formation of both the ankle and knee joints. Superiorly it is expanded to form the flat tibial plateau, which is composed of the medial and lateral tibial condyles. These condyles are separated by the intercondylar area, which contains the intercondylar eminence. The anterior border of the shaft is subcutaneous throughout its length with an obvious protrusion superiorly where it begins as the tibial tuberosity. Inferiorly the tibia is expanded to form the articular surface for the ankle joint with the medialmost aspect extending distally as the medial malleolus.

The *fibula* is the lateral bone of the leg whose most apparent function is that of providing muscle attachments. This thin bone articulates with the tibia both proximally and distally. The interosseous membrane connects the two bones throughout most of their lengths. The inferior extent of the fibula is the lateral malleolus.

Knee Joint. The knee joint is formed between the rounded femoral condyles and the relatively flat tibial condyles (tibial plateau). The length of the articular surface (front to back) of the femoral condyles greatly exceeds that of the tibial condyles, and as a result most knee motion is a gliding of the femoral condyles on the tibial condyles. There is, however, some rocking motion between the two bones during the last few degrees of extension.

The poor congruency between the two sets of articular surfaces produces a dead space. This dead space is filled in part by the wedge-shaped disks or menisci. Each of these is somewhat C shaped and sits on the periphery of each tibial condyle and attaches centrally to the intercondylar area of the tibia. In addition to deepening the socket and increasing the congruency, the menisci are said to absorb shock that is transmitted from femur to tibia, and protect the capsule by keeping it from being pinched between the two bones. The lateral meniscus is almost a complete circle so that its central attachments are very close together. It is also loosely attached to the capsule, continuous with the meniscofemoral ligament and connected to the popliteus muscle. Thus, the lateral meniscus is relatively movable and this is presumably why it is seldom injured. The medial meniscus is relatively immovable and therefore very frequently injured as it is caught between the medial tibial and femoral condyles. It is immovable because it is C shaped and thus has wide central attachments, and it is attached very firmly to the capsule and the medial collateral ligament.

The fibrous and synovial portions of the joint capsule do not correspond to one another. The fibrous portion encloses the entire joint area and is made up of the quadriceps tendon, patella, and patellar ligament anteriorly, the patella retinacula anteromedially and anterolaterally, and the iliotibial tract (band) laterally.

Medially the tibial collateral ligament blends with the fibrous capsule. The synovial lining encloses the articular surfaces, but the intercondylar areas are outside the joint space (but within the fibrous capsule). The volume of the joint space is largest when the knee is slightly flexed (approximately 15 degrees), and thus patients whose knees are effused will usually be most comfortable with their knees in that position.

The major ligamentous support of the knee is provided by the collateral and cruciate ligaments. The lateral (fibular) collateral ligament extends between the lateral femoral epicondyle and the head of the fibula and restricts medial displacement of the leg on the thigh. This ropelike structure is easily palpable and separated from the joint capsule. The medial (tibial) collateral ligament is a strong broad band that connects the medial femoral epicondyle and the medial tibial condyle and restricts lateral displacement of the leg on the thigh. It is palpable as a thickening in the joint space medially. The collateral ligaments are taut when the knee is extended but loosen somewhat when the knee is flexed, thus permitting rotation in that position. The cruciate ligaments occupy the intercondylar area and give the knee anteroposterior stabilization. From its anterior tibial attachment the anterior cruciate ligament passes posteriorly, superiorly and laterally to attach to the medial aspect of the lateral femoral condyle. It protects against posterior dislocation of the femur on the tibia. The posterior cruciate extends from its posterior tibial attachment anteriorly, superiorly and medially to attach to the lateral aspect of the medial femoral condyle. It protects against anterior dislocation of the femur on the tibia. Although the cruciate ligaments are most tense in full flexion (posterior) and extension (anterior), portions of both are tense throughout the range of motion. And even though all of these ligaments are strong and reinforce the knee joint, the major stabilization of this joint is provided by the muscles (mainly quadriceps and hamstrings) that cross the joint.

The motions that occur at the knee and the major muscles that cause them are:

Extension: quadriceps femoris
Flexion: biceps femoris, semitendinosus, semimembranosus, gastrocnemius
Medial rotation: semimembranosus, semitendinosus, sartorius, popliteus
Lateral rotation: biceps femoris

Bones of the Foot. The bones of the foot are the tarsals, metatarsals, and phalanges. The seven tarsal bones are arranged in two rows with one bone between the rows. Proximally the talus sits on the calcaneus, and distally the bones (medial to lateral) are the medial, intermediate, and lateral cuneiforms and the cuboid. The navicular is essentially between the cuneiforms and the talus. The talus is the highest bone in the foot and it receives all of the superincumbent weight from the leg. The metatarsals and phalanges are similar in number and position to the metacarpals and phalanges of the hand.

The bones of the foot are arranged to provide flexibility and stability, i.e., they must perform the weight-bearing function while providing for a soft landing and forceful takeoff. These requirements are met by the presence of several arches that are arranged so that weight hits the floor at the calcaneal tuberosity posteriorly and at the heads of the metatarsals anteriorly. The most important arch is the medial longitudinal arch, which consists of the calcaneus, talus, navicular, three cuneiforms and the three medial metatarsals. The lateral longitudinal arch is made up of the calcaneus, cuboid and two lateral metatarsals. A transverse arch exists at the level of the distal row of tarsals and bases of the metatarsals. The major static support of these arches (primarily the medial longitudinal arch) is provided by ligaments, which are the very important plantar calcaneonavicular (spring) ligament, the long plantar ligament and the ligament-like plantar aponeurosis. Dynamic support is added by the intrinsic muscles of the foot. Three extrinsic muscles of the foot, the tibialis anterior and posterior and the peroneus longus, may provide additional dynamic support.

Ankle Joint. The ankle joint is formed above by the tibia and fibula and below by the trochlea of the talus. The trochlea is a tin-can-shaped process with its long axis oriented from side to side and its articular surface located on both its rounded upper aspect and flat ends. The tibia articulates with the superior aspect and medial end (via the medial malleous) of the talus; the lateral malleolus, with the lateral end. The talus glides around in the mortise formed by the tibia and fibula. The anterior aspect of the trochlea is wider than the posterior. As a result, in dorsiflexion the widest portion of the trochlea is wedged between the malleoli (good bony stability). In plantar flexion this support is lost. Thus, most sprains occur when the ankle is plantar flexed. The distal tibia and fibula are lashed together by anterior and posterior tibiofibular ligaments. The major ligaments supporting the ankle joint are the medial (deltoid) and lateral collateral ligaments. The deltoid ligament is a broad band that connects the medial malleolus with the talus, navicular and calcaneus. The lateral collateral ligament is composed of three distinct bands: the anterior and posterior talofibular ligaments and the calcaneofibular ligament. The anterior talofibular ligament is the most commonly injured ligament, accompanying the frequent plantar flexion-inversion sprain of the ankle.

The motions of the ankle and their major motors are:

Plantar flexion: gastrocnemius, soleus, tibialis posterior

Dorsiflexion: tibialis anterior

Subtalar and Transverse Tarsal Joints. Although the motions of the foot (other than toe motion) are the sum totals of the individual amounts of motion that occur at each intertarsal joint, there are two areas (called functional joints) where most of this motion does occur. These functional joints are the subtalar and transverse tarsal (midtarsal) joints. The motions of the foot are inversion, which is a combination of adduction and supination, and eversion, which is a combination of abduction and pronation. The subtalar joint is under the talus between the talus and the calcaneus. The two sets of articular surfaces are separated by a strong interosseous ligament. The orientation of these joint spaces is an inclined plane that is directed anteriorly, medially and inferiorly. The transverse tarsal joint consists of two joints that extend transversely across the foot. The medial articulation is between the talus and the navicular, the lateral between the calcaneus and the cuboid.

The motors of these foot motions are:

Inversion: tibialis anterior, tibialis posterior, flexor hallucis longus, flexor digitorum longus

Eversion: peroneus longus and brevis

Compartmentation of the Lower Extremity

Hip Region. Although there are no compartments around the hip as they exist in the rest of the lower extremity, the muscles in this region can be placed in logical groups. The gluteal muscles are the lateral and posterolateral muscles of the hip. The gluteus maximus is innervated by the inferior gluteal nerve, and the gluteus medius and minimus and the tensor fascia lata are supplied by the superior gluteal nerve. Deep to the gluteus maximus there is a group of muscles called the short external rotators of the thigh. These muscles are innervated by direct branches of the lumbosacral plexus and consist of the piriformis, obturator internus, superior and inferior gemelli and the quadratus femoris. Anteriorly the iliacus and psoas major come together to form the iliopsoas as they leave the abdominal cavity and enter the thigh. These hip flexors are innervated by direct branches of the lumbar plexus.

Thigh. The investing fascia of the thigh is the fascia lata. It is dramatically thickened laterally as the iliotibial tract or band. Two intermuscular septa extend from this investing fascia to attach to the femur. Thus, these medial and lateral intermuscular septa separate the thigh into anterior and posterior compartments.

The anterior compartment is actually anterolateral and the posterior compartment posteromedial. The muscles in the anterior compartment are innervated by the femoral nerve and consist of the sartorius and the four components of the quadriceps femoris—the rectus femoris, vastus medialis, vastus intermedius and vastus lateralis. The posterior compartment has two groups of muscles—the medial femoral or adductors and the posterior femoral or hamstrings. The medial femoral muscles are mostly innervated by the obturator nerve and consist of the adductor longus, adductor brevis, adductor magnus, pectineus, gracilis and obturator externus. The hamstrings are primarily innervated by the tibial portion of the sciatic nerve and consist of the biceps femoris, semitendinosus and semimembranosus.

Femoral Triangle. The femoral triangle is not a compartment per se, but it is an important area in that critical structures are found there. The triangle is defined by the inguinal ligament above, the sartorius muscle laterally, and the medial border of the adductor longus muscle medially. The floor is formed by the adductor longus, pectineus and iliopsoas muscles. The superficial and deep inguinal lymph nodes are found respectively superficially and deep to the investing fascia in this area. In addition to receiving superficial lymphatics from the lower extremity, the superficial nodes drain the lower abdominal wall, buttock, perineum, and lower portion of the anal canal and vagina. From lateral to medial the following structures descend through the triangle: the femoral nerve, the femoral artery and the femoral vein. The femoral artery is midway between the anterior superior spine of the ilium and the pubic tubercle. The femoral sheath is an extension of transversalis fascia that forms a sleeve around the femoral vessels as they enter the thigh. The area just medial to the vein is within the sheath and is called the femoral canal, the usual path of a femoral hernia. After leaving the triangle the femoral vessels pass through the thigh just deep to the sartorius muscle, an area called the adductor canal.

Popliteal Fossa. The popliteal fossa is a deep diamond-shaped area behind the knee. It is bounded superomedially by the tendons of the semitendinosus and semimembranosus muscles, superolaterally by the tendon of the biceps femoris and inferiorly by the heads of the gastrocnemius muscle. Its floor is the posterior (supracondylar) portion of the distal femur. The popliteal vessels pass vertically through this fossa with the artery closest to the bone and thereby vulnerable to laceration when this part of the femur is fractured. The tibial nerve passes through the middle of this fossa superficially, and the common peroneal nerve follows the tendon of the biceps femoris muscle. This space is packed with loose connective tissue.

Leg. The leg has anterior, lateral and posterior compartments. The major partition consists of the subcutaneous tibia, the interosseous membrane, the fibula and the posterior intermuscular septum, which separates the posteromedially situated posterior compartment from an anterolateral region. This anterolateral area is subdivided into anterior and lateral compartments by the anterior intermuscular septum. The anterior compartment contains the tibialis anterior, extensor hallucis longus, extensor digitorum longus and peroneus tertius muscles, all of which are innervated by the deep peroneal nerve. These muscles dorsiflex the ankle, invert the foot and extend the toes. The lateral compartment muscles are primarily everters of the foot. The two muscles in this compartment—the peroneus longus and brevis—are innervated by the superficial peroneal nerve. All posterior compartment muscles are innervated by the tibial nerve and function to plantar flex the ankle, invert the foot and flex the toes. The posterior compartment muscles are the gastrocnemius, soleus and plantaris superficially, and the deep group consisting of the flexor hallucis longus, flexor digitorum longus, tibialis posterior and popliteus.

Foot. The compartmentation of the foot is similar to that of the hand. The compartments of the great and little toes are completed by medial and lateral intermuscular septa that extend from the investing fascia to the first and fifth metatarsals respectively. The central compartment is deep to the plantar aponeurosis, between the medial and lateral intermuscular septa and superficial to the plantar adductor–interosseous fascia. The adductor–interosseous compartment is that area dorsal to the plantar adductor–interosseous fascia and between the metatarsals.

The compartment of the great toe contains the abductor hallucis and the flexor hallucis brevis muscles, both of which are innervated by the medial plantar nerve. The compartment of the small toe has the abductor digiti minimi and the flexor digiti minimi, and these muscles are innervated by the lateral plantar nerves. The muscles of the central compartment are the flexor digitorum brevis (medial plantar nerve) and the quadratus plantae (lateral plantar nerve). The lumbrical muscles arise from the tendons of the flexor digitorum longus as they pass through the central compartment. They are innervated by both the medial and lateral plantar nerves. All of the interossei and the adductor hallucis are in the adductor–interosseous compartment, and all are innervated by the deep branch of the lateral plantar nerve.

Nerves of the Lower Extremity

Lumbosacral Plexus. Branches of the lumbosacral plexus supply most of the lower extremity. The lumbar plexus is formed in the substance of the psoas major muscle from the ventral rami of L1 through L4. All of L1 and part of L2 give rise to cutaneous nerves that supply the lower abdominal wall, the anterior part of the perineum and the proximal portion of the lower limb. The rest of the plexus forms major nerves of the lower extremity. The sacral plexus (L4 through S4) is formed in the pelvis on the ventral aspect of the piriformis muscle. The combined contribution of L4 and L5 is the lumbosacral trunk, which enters the pelvis by passing just lateral to the sacral promontory. The lumbosacral plexus is not subjected to the stretching injuries as the brachial plexus because of the more limited motion of the hip joint. In addition it is deeply positioned and therefore well protected.

Femoral Nerve.   The femoral nerve (L2–4) emerges from the lateral aspect of the psoas major muscle and enters the thigh by passing deep to the inguinal ligament. Upon entering the femoral triangle it immediately branches into its many muscular branches. Its terminal branch, the cutaneous saphenous nerve, continues through the thigh in the adductor canal. It enters the subcutaneous tissue in the distal thigh and supplies the skin on the medial aspect of the leg and foot.

Obturator Nerve.   This nerve (L2–4) emerges from the medial aspect of the psoas major muscle just above the pelvic brim. It then enters the pelvic cavity and passes anteriorly and ventrally toward the obturator canal, through which it enters the medial aspect of the thigh. It ends there by dividing into its terminal muscular and cutaneous branches.

Gluteal Nerves.   The superior gluteal nerve (L4–S1) arises in the pelvis but immediately exits by passing above the piriformis muscle through the greater sciatic notch. It passes anteriorly between the gluteus medius and minimus muscles and terminates by supplying the tensor fasciae latae muscle. The inferior gluteal nerve (L5–S2) also arises in the pelvis and exits immediately by passing below the piriformis and through the greater sciatic notch directly into the substance of the gluteus maximus muscle.

Sciatic Nerve.   The sciatic nerve is the largest nerve in the body. It consists of the tibial and common peroneal nerves, which are enclosed in a common connective tissue sheath. The sacral plexus essentially terminates as the sciatic nerve. This nerve leaves the pelvis by passing below the piriformis (usually) and through the greater sciatic notch. It descends through the middle of the thigh between the medial and lateral hamstring muscles. It commonly divides into the common peroneal and tibial nerves in the distal thigh as it enters the popliteal fossa.

The *common peroneal nerve* passes superficially through the popliteal fossa just medial to the biceps femoris muscle and its tendon. It passes superficial to the lateral femoral condyle and then wraps around the lateral aspect of the neck of the fibula. The nerve divides into its terminal branches, the superficial and deep peroneal nerves, as it passes the neck of the fibula. The *superficial peroneal nerve* enters the lateral compartment of the leg where it descends to innervate the skin on the dorsum of the foot. The *deep peroneal nerve* passes through the lateral compartment into the anterior compartment. It descends through this compartment and enters the dorsum of the foot where it supplies the extensor digitorum brevis and the extensor hallucis brevis muscles. It has a very small cutaneous distribution to the web space between the great and second toes.

The *tibial nerve* descends superficially through the center of the popliteal fossa. It enters the posterior compartment of the leg by passing between, and then deep to, the two heads of the gastrocnemius muscle. It descends through the leg between the superficial and deep groups of muscles and enters the foot by passing behind the medial malleolus. As it enters the foot it divides into the medial and lateral plantar nerves. The medial plantar nerve is homologous with the median nerve of the hand. It enters the compartment of the great toe and divides into muscular branches and cutaneous branches (plantar digital nerves) that supply the skin on the plantar surface of the medial three and a half toes and corresponding part of the ball of the foot. The lateral plantar nerve is similar in course and distribution to the ulnar nerve in the hand. It passes diagonally across the plantar aspect of the foot by going between the flexor digitorum brevis and quadratus plantae muscles in the central compartment. It then terminates by dividing into superficial and deep branches. The superficial branch has muscular branches and is cutaneous to the plantar aspect of the lateral one and one-half toes and corresponding part of the sole in that area. The deep branch dives deeply and passes medially across the foot deep to long flexor tendons and terminates by supplying the adductor hallucis.

Peripheral Nerve Lesions in the Lower Extremity

In man the lower limb is used almost exclusively as a means of locomotion. The muscles are concerned with both weight bearing and forward propulsion of the entire body. In analyzing peripheral nerve lesions it is only reasonable to evaluate the disturbances in the normal gait pattern that are caused by nerve damage.

Superior Gluteal Nerve.   The abductors of the hip maintain the coronal balance at this joint during the stance phase of gait; i.e., when an individual is standing on one foot the hip abductors on the weight-bearing side prevent dropping of the pelvis to the opposite side (hip adduction). A patient with a superior gluteal nerve injury will exhibit a positive Trendelenburg sign during the stance phase of gait or when asked to stand on one foot; i.e., his pelvis will drop to the non-weight-bearing side, and he will shift his trunk laterally to the weight-bearing-side so as to bring the center of gravity over the supporting limb.

Inferior Gluteal Nerve. At heel-strike there is a tendency for the trunk to bend forward, i.e., hip flexion. This is counteracted by the gluteus maximus. If this nerve is totally severed the patient will compensate by throwing the trunk backward at heel strike and thus preventing the line of gravity from getting anterior to the hip joint.

Femoral Nerve. At heel-strike and continuing through the first part of the stance phase the quadriceps muscles maintain knee extension and thus support the body weight. With a loss of quadriceps function the patient must lock the knee and keep the line of gravity well in front of the joint. As a result this patient will whip his leg into extension by forceful thigh flexion followed by a rapid halt of this flexion (via the gluteus maximus), which snaps the knee into extension by pendulum action. As soon as the knee is extended he plants the heel on the floor, extends his hip (to hold the knee extension) and flexes his trunk (to get the line of gravity ahead of the knee joint). He then vaults over a rigidly extended knee.

Deep Peroneal Nerve. During gait the anterior compartment muscles of the leg shorten the length of the limb during the swing phase by dorsiflexing the ankle, and they prevent plantar flexion (foot-slap) at heel-strike. When a patient with a deep peroneal nerve lesion takes a step he must lift his leg high so that the plantar flexed foot can clear the ground (steppage gait). At heel-strike the ball of the foot hits the ground with a loud slap.

Tibial Nerve. The forward momentum for locomotion is provided by the foot pushing down and back against the ground (plantar flexion). When this action is missing unilaterally there is a noticeable lag in forward motion at the point of push off of the involved side.

Blood Supply of the Lower Limb

Arteries. Most of the lower extremity is supplied by the *femoral artery.* The gluteal region receives the *superior* and *inferior gluteal arteries* from the internal iliac, and the obturator artery (also a branch of the internal iliac) supplies a portion of the medial thigh. The femoral artery is the continuation of the internal iliac artery where it enters the thigh by going deep to the inguinal ligament. It descends through the femo-

ral triangle and adductor canal to the point where it passes through the adductor hiatus into the popliteal fossa where it becomes the popliteal artery. A femoral pulse is taken about midway between the anterior superior spine of the ilium and the pubic tubercle. The largest branch of the femoral is the *deep femoral artery,* which arises in the femoral triangle and descends just medial to the femur. The *medial and lateral circumflex arteries* arise from the deep femoral soon after it arises. The deep femoral also has perforating branches that pass into the posterior compartment of the thigh.

The *popliteal artery* passes through the deepest portion of the popliteal fossa, where it has several genicular branches. When a popliteal pulse is taken the artery must be compressed against the femur. This is done with the knee relaxed so as to relax the contents of the popliteal fossa, and then the contents of the fossa must be compressed at least several centimeters. The artery terminates by dividing into the anterior and posterior tibial arteries as it enters the posterior compartment of the leg.

The *anterior tibial artery* immediately enters the anterior compartment of the leg by passing above the superior margin of the interosseous membrane. It descends through the anterior compartment and enters the foot by crossing the anterior aspect of the ankle; there it becomes the *dorsalis pedis artery.* On the dorsum of the foot—where the pulse is best taken—the artery is between the tendons of the extensor hallucis longus and the extensor digitorum longus. The dorsalis pedis artery terminates as many branches, which supply the dorsum of the foot. One of these branches, the deep plantar branch, passes into the plantar aspect of the foot by going between the first and second metatarsals and there helps form the *plantar arterial arch.*

The *posterior tibial artery* descends through the deep portion of the posterior compartment of the leg. It inclines medially as it descends and enters the foot behind the medial malleolus where a posterior tibial pulse can be taken. It terminates as it passes around the medial malleolus by dividing into *medial and lateral plantar arteries.* It has a large peroneal branch high in the posterior compartment. The *peroneal artery* descends in the lateral part of the posterior compartment and terminates around the ankle.

The *medial and lateral plantar arteries* correspond in course and distribution to the medial and lateral plantar nerves. There is only one arterial arch in the foot, and it corresponds to the deep arch of the hand. It is formed by the deep branch of the lateral plantar artery and the deep plantar branch of the dorsalis pedis artery.

Veins. The veins of the lower extremity consist of deep and superficial veins. The deep veins correspond rather closely to the pattern of the arteries. The two saphenous veins are the main superficial veins. The *greater saphenous vein* begins on the dorsomedial aspect of the foot and ascends along the anteromedial aspect of the leg and thigh. It terminates by passing through the saphenous opening of the fascia lata and emptying into the femoral vein. The greater saphenous vein passes just anterior to the medial malleolus, where it is commonly secured for venous cutdown. The *lesser saphenous vein* begins as a network on the dorsolateral aspect of the foot. It ascends behind the lateral malleolus and through the middle of the calf. It terminates by emptying into the popliteal vein in the popliteal fossa.

HEAD AND NECK

Superficial Structures of the Head and Neck

Major Surface Landmarks and Regions. The anterolateral aspect of the neck is divided into anterior and posterior triangles by the prominent sternocleido-mastoid muscle. The anterior triangle is in front of this muscle and extends to the inferior margin of the mandible and midline. Behind the sternocleidomastoid the posterior triangle is also delimited by the superior border of the trapezius muscle and the middle third of the clavicle. The face can be divided into several areas that include the orbit, nose, forehead, temporal region, maxillary region and mandibular region. It is convenient to start with the well-defined orbit, which is protected and delimited by the prominent supraorbital and infraorbital margins, which meet laterally. Extending posteriorly at the level of the infraorbital margin, the zygomatic arch separates the temporal region above from the mandibular or lower jaw region below. The mandibular region extends inferiorly and then anteromedially to join the same region of the opposite side. The maxillary or upper jaw region is inferior to the infraorbital margin and lateral to the nose. The posterior part of the head is the occipital region.

Microscopic Structure of the Skin and Scalp. The skin consists of an outer epidermis of stratified squamous keratinized epithelium and an underlying dermis of dense irregularly arranged fibroelastic connective tissue. Beneath the dermis is a subcutaneous layer of loose connective tissue. The epidermis varies in structure and thickness, depending on the region of the body. On the palmar surface of the hand and on the soles of the feet the epidermis consists of four layers. These are, from the dermis to the surface, the stratum germinativum, stratum granulosum, stratum lucidum and stratum corneum.

The stratum germinativum is further divisible into a stratum basale and stratum spinosum. Epidermal cells in both of these layers are capable of mitoses. Cells of the stratum spinosum (prickle cells) are joined at numerous desmosomes (macula adherens) where many tonofilaments seem to converge toward the plasma membrane. Desmosomes are dense bodies where plasma membranes of adjacent cells appear thickened because of a dense layer on their cytoplasmic surfaces. A thin intermediate lamina occurs in the intercellular space at a desmosome. Tonofilaments will give rise to the fibrous protein keratin. Melanin granules are found in the deeper cells of the stratum germinativum in caucasians and in more of the deeper layers in colored races. Melanin is produced in melanocytes, which arise from neural crest. The melanin granules are distributed to the epidermal cells. The color of the skin is dependent on the amount of melanin, carotene and the vascularity of the skin.

The stratum granulosum represents cells that are older and further differentiated in the keratinization process than those of the deeper layers. Keratohyalin granules predominate and will give rise to a matrix of keratohyalin protein that will be prevalent in the more keratinized outer layers. The stratum lucidum contains flattened translucent cells that have lost their organelles. Cells of the stratum corneum also have lost their organelles and contain soft keratin, which consists of tightly packed filaments embedded in an amorphous matrix.

The dermis is divisible into papillary and reticular layers. The papillary layer is immediately underneath the epidermis and contains dense fine collagenous fibers, blood vessels and free and encapsulated (e.g., Meissner's tactile corpuscles) nerve endings. The reticular layer contains coarser bundles of collagenous fibers. Smooth muscle can be found in this layer in the nipple and scrotum. Hair follicles, sebaceous glands and the ducts of sweat glands are located in the reticular layer. The secretory portions of simple tubular sweat glands, the roots of hairs and pacinian corpuscles (deep pressure receptors) are constituents of the subcutaneous layer. Extensive accumulations of fat in this layer determine it as the panniculus adiposus.

Secretory portions of sweat glands consist of a high cuboidal epithelium invested by contractile myoepithelial cells. Since no part of the cell is lost in the secretory process, it is classified as a merocrine type of secretion. The ducts are stratified cuboidal, except for the intra-epidermal portion, which is lined by the epidermal epithelium.

Sebaceous glands have short ducts that empty into hair follicles, except for those in the labia minora and glans penis where they open directly to the surface. The secretory portion of the sebaceous gland is stratified cuboidal; the lumen is generally filled with rounded cells containing numerous fat droplets. The secretion of sebum involves the holocrine discharge of sebaceous cells. New cells proliferate and differentiate from more basal regions of the gland.

Hairs are most prevalent in the scalp and are lacking in such areas as the palms of the hands and soles of the feet. Each hair consists of a root and a shaft. The root is enclosed by a tubular hair follicle that consists of an inner cuticle and epithelial root sheath, both derived from epidermis, and an outer connective tissue root sheath that corresponds to the dermis. At its lower end the follicle and root expand into a hair bulb, which is indented by a connective tissue hair papilla. The hair, consisting of an inner medulla, a cortex and outer cuticle, grows upward from the differentiation of matrix cells in the hair bulb. Pigment in the cortical layer and air in the cortex and medulla determine the color of the skin. Arrectores pilorum of smooth muscle run in the obtuse angle between the follicle and epidermis, and they enclose sebaceous glands. Contraction causes erection of the hair and dimpling of the skin (goose flesh) at the smooth muscle attachment in the dermis. In the scalp and face, skeletal muscles are found in the superficial fascia.

Organization of the Blood Vessels to the Head and Neck. The common carotid arteries supply most of the head and neck structures outside the cranial cavity (as well as being a major source inside). On the right the vessel is one of the main terminal branches of the brachiocephalic trunk, while on the left it is a direct branch from the arch of the aorta. In a plane deep to the sternocleidomastoid muscle each artery extends along a line that passes behind the sternoclavicular joint and through the midpoint between the angle of the mandible and the mastoid process. It terminates by dividing into the internal and external carotids between the levels of the hyoid bone and the thyroid cartilage prominence (laryngeal prominence or Adam's Apple), where the carotid body and sinus can be palpated. The *internal carotid* has no branches and passes directly toward the carotid canal through which it enters the cranial cavity.

The *external carotid* artery ascends to the neck of the mandible where it divides into its terminal branches: the maxillary artery, which passes deep to the neck of the mandible into the infratemporal fossa, and the superficial temporal artery, which ascends into the temporal region to supply that region and the anterior part of the scalp. Six other branches commonly arise from this artery. The superior thyroid artery supplies primarily the thyroid gland and larynx. The lingual artery passes deeply toward the tongue. The facial artery crosses the inferior margin of the mandible just

anterior to the angle (where a facial pulse can be taken). From this point it follows a tortuous course obliquely across the face toward the angle between the nose and medial aspect of the eye. It supplies the superficial structures of the face as it winds superficial and deep to them. The ascending pharyngeal artery supplies the pharyngeal and palatal regions. The occipital and posterior auricular branches supply primarily the superficial regions designated in their names.

The *jugular system of veins* drains most of the head and neck. The main vessel is the internal jugular vein, which begins at the base of the skull where it receives most of the venous blood from the cranial cavity. It descends through the neck in company with the carotid arteries and terminates by joining the subclavian vein to form the brachiocephalic vein. As it descends through the neck it receives tributaries that drain the head and neck other than the cranial cavity.

Cutaneous Nerves. The cutaneous innervation is easily defined if the head and neck are divided into three areas. Area 1 includes the entire face and the anterior part of the scalp, extending posteriorly to a line across the top of the head that connects the two external auditory meatuses (interauricular line). The skin of this area is innervated by the three divisions of the fifth cranial (trigeminal) nerve. The ophthalmic nerve innervates the bridge of the nose, upper eyelid and cornea, forehead and scalp. The maxillary division covers the lateral aspect of the nose, cheek and anterior temporal region. The mandibular innervation corresponds to the area overlying the mandible and the posterior temporal region. Area 2 includes the medial aspect of the posterior neck and the corresponding part of the occipital region, which extends anteriorly to the interauricular line. This area is supplied by cutaneous branches of the dorsal rami of cervical spinal nerves. The third area is the anterolateral neck, including the posterior triangle and extending laterally to the shoulder plus a strip of skin around the superior and posterior aspects of the ear. The cutaneous branches of the cervical plexuses (lesser occipital, great auricular, transverse cervical and supraclavicular nerves) innervate this region.

Facial Muscles. The muscles of facial expression are found essentially in the subcutaneous tissue of the face, neck (platysma), and scalp (epicranius). They function to move the skin and regulate the shape of the openings on the face. Many muscles are associated with the muscle surrounding the mouth (orbicularis oris) and those surrounding the eyes (orbicularis oculi). The buccinator muscle is deeply located in the cheek and represents the only muscle in that area. All of these muscles are innervated by the seventh cranial (facial) nerve.

Parotid Gland.   The largest of the salivary glands is located anteroinferior to the ear and extends inferiorly to the level of the angle of the mandible. It has a deep portion that extends posterior and then medial to the ramus of the mandible. The main trunk of the facial nerve enters the posterior aspect of the gland and divides into its main divisions within the substance of the gland. The parotid duct passes anteriorly around the masseter muscle and empties into the oral cavity just opposite the second upper molar.

Microscopic Structure of Major Salivary Glands.   The parenchyma of the parotid gland consists of serous acini and ducts. The acini are grouped into lobules and lobes by connective tissue septa. Pyramid-shaped cells with apical accumulations of zymogen granules and basal concentrations of rough endoplasmic reticulum line the small lumina of the serous acini. Myoepithelial cells lie between acinar cells and the basal lamina. The serous secretion of the acinar cells passes into intercalated ducts, which empty into striated ducts. Both of these ducts are intralobular ducts. Intercalated ducts have small lumina and are lined by simple cuboidal epithelium. Striated (salivary) ducts are larger and are lined by a simple columnar epithelium whose cells have extensive infoldings of the plasma membrane on their basal surfaces. These basal striations with their interposed mitochondria are like those in cells of the distal convoluted tubules of the kidney and perform similar functions in the reabsorption of sodium and water from the luminal fluid. After reabsorption, the secretion in the striated ducts passes successively to interlobular, interlobar and the main excretory (Stensen's) ducts. The simple columnar epithelial lining of the ducts gets taller as the main duct is approached. Stensen's duct is lined by pseudostratified columnar epithelium that contains some goblet cells. At the opening of the duct into the oral cavity, the epithelium will become stratified squamous nonkeratinized epithelium.

The submandibular gland is a mixed seromucous gland whose acini are preponderantly serous. Mucous alveoli are frequently capped by serous demilunes or have serous cells lining their terminal portions. The secretion from serous demilunes passes between mucous cells to reach the lumen. Mucous cells contain basally flattened nuclei, rough endoplasmic reticulum and apical membrane-bound mucigen droplets. The ducts of the submandibular gland are microscopically similar to those of the parotid, but salivary ducts are longer and more numerous. The main duct (Wharton's) opens into the mouth beneath the tongue. It contains longitudinal smooth muscle in its wall.

The sublingual gland is a mixed gland, but the mucous alveoli predominate. Salivary ducts and intercalated ducts are few in number. The main excretory ducts open into the mouth at the side of the frenulum and, like the main ducts of the parotid and submandibular gland, are lined by pseudostratified columnar epithelium.

Fascial Planes and Compartments of the Neck

Fascial Planes.   The superficial layer (investing layer) of cervical fascia encircles the neck and encloses the sternocleidomastoid and trapezius muscles. The prevertebral fascia surrounds the vertebral column and its associated muscles, the longus capitis and colli, the scalenes, and the deep muscles of the back in the cervical region. The visceral structures of the neck are enclosed in a sleeve of fascia called the pretracheal fascia anteriorly and laterally and the buccopharyngeal fascia (between the pharynx or esophagus and the vertebral column) posteriorly. The infrahyoid muscles have their own fascia, which is between the investing and pretracheal layers of cervical fascia. In the lateral part of the neck and deep to the plane of the sternocleidomastoid muscle, the several layers of cervical fascia meet and contribute to the formation of the vertically oriented carotid sheath.

Anterior Triangle.   Many surgical approaches to the viscera of the neck are made through this area, which is bounded by the midline, inferior margin of the mandible and the sternocleidomastoid muscle. The part of the anterior triangle above the digastric muscle is the submandibular triangle, and the area below the digastric is sometimes divided into the carotid triangle above the omohyoid muscle and muscular triangle below. The carotid sheath structures—the vagus nerve, the carotid artery and the internal jugular vein—pass vertically through this area, located deep to the sternocleidomastoid muscle. The cervical sympathetic chain is deep in the triangle on the anterolateral aspects of the cervical vertebrae. The lateral lobes of the thyroid gland are immediately adjacent to the lateral aspects of the trachea and lower larynx, while the isthmus of the thyroid crosses the midline in front of the upper rings of the trachea. The parathyroids are related to the posterior surface of the upper and lower aspects of the lateral lobes of the thyroid. The esophagus lies behind the trachea and larynx.

The submandibular triangle contains (1) the submandibular gland, (2) the facial artery, (3) the facial vein and (4) the mylohyoid vessels and nerves. Posteriorly is (5) the upper part of the external carotid artery. More deeply lie (6) the internal jugular vein, (7) the internal carotid artery and (8) the vagus nerve.

Posterior Triangle.   The posterior triangle is bounded by the superior border of the trapezius, the posterior border of the sternocleidomastoid and the middle third of the clavicle. This area is easily visualized by asking the patient to hunch his shoulder anteriorly and turn his head to the opposite side. Several major structures supplying the upper limb are accessible through this triangle.

The cutaneous branches of the cervical plexus enter the subcutaneous tissue after curving around the posterior middle third of the sternocleidomastoid muscle. The accessory nerve emerges from beneath the middle of the posterior border of the sternocleidomastoid, passes obliquely across the triangle and dives deep to the superior border of the trapezius about 3 cm. above its clavicular attachment. The inferior belly of the omohyoid muscle crosses the inferior aspect of the triangle a few centimeters above the clavicle.

The floor of the posterior triangle is muscular, consisting of the splenius capitis and cervicis, levator scapulae and the scalene muscles. The anterior and middle scalene muscles attach inferiorly on the first rib. These two muscles, together with a small portion of the first rib, form a narrow triangle (scalene triangle or scalene groove) through which the roots (ventral rami) of the brachial plexus and the subclavian artery enter the posterior triangle. Any of these structures can be compressed as they pass through this narrow opening. This neurovascular compression can be caused by muscle hypertrophy, the occurrence of a cervical rib, etc. Since the posterior border of the anterior scalene muscle corresponds to the lower part of the posterior border of the sternocleidomastoid muscle, the scalene groove is readily palpable. Therefore, the roots of the plexus are palpable as hard cords, and the subclavian pulse can be taken by compressing the subclavian artery against the first rib. In addition, the inferior deep cervical lymph nodes are associated with the anterior scalene. These anterior scalene nodes—the final sentinel nodes for the thoracic duct on the left and the right lymphatic duct on the right—are palpated in the same area.

Although only a portion of the subclavian artery is in the posterior triangle, it will be covered here. This artery is divided into three parts on the basis of its relationship to the anterior scalene muscle. The first part arises from the arch of the aorta on the left and the brachiocephalic trunk on the right. It passes superolaterally to the medial margin of the anterior scalene. The first part branches are the vertebral artery, which ascends deep to the anterior scalene to enter the transverse foramen of C6, the thyrocervical trunk, which has suprascapular, transverse cervical and inferior thyroid branches, and the internal thoracic artery, which descends deep to the costal cartilages just lateral to the sternum. The second part of the subclavian lies posterior to the anterior scalene. Its only branch is the costocervical trunk, which gives rise to the deep cervical and highest intercostal arteries. The third part extends from the lateral border of the anterior scalene to the first rib. The dorsal scapular artery may arise from this part.

Visceral Structures of the Neck

Larynx. The larynx is a tubular organ composed of nine cartilages which are connected by elastic membranes and synovial joints. It is lined by a mucosa that covers the vocal cords and is innervated by branches of the vagus nerve. The cartilages of the larynx are (1) epiglottis, (2) thyroid (Adam's apple), (3) cricoid, (4) two arytenoids, (5) two corniculates and (6) two cuneiforms.

The larynx opens above into the pharynx and continues inferiorly as the trachea. It is anterior to cervical vertebrae 4 through 6, and covered anteriorly by the infrahyoid muscles and laterally by the lobes of the thyroid gland and the inferior constrictor muscle of the pharynx.

The vocal apparatus (glottis) consists of the true vocal folds and the opening (rima glottidis) between the folds. The area above the true folds extending to the laryngeal additis (entrance) is the vestibule or supraglottic portion. The false vocal folds are above the true folds, and the area extending laterally between the true and false folds is the ventricle. The vocal fold (true vocal cord) contains the thin cranial edge of the conus elasticus. This free edge is the so-called vocal cord. The vocal fold is divided into anterior intramembranous and posterior intracartilaginous portions. The intramembranous portion stretches between the thyroid and arytenoid cartilages and is capable of tension change and vibration. The intracartilaginous portion is formed by the arytenoid cartilage. The numerous intrinsic muscles moving the laryngeal cartilages lie deep to the thyroid cartilage except the cricothyroid, which alone is innervated by the external branch of the superior laryngeal nerve, and which functions to tense the focal cords. The others are innervated by the inferior (recurrent) branch of the vagus. These include the posterior cricoarytenoid, which abducts the vocal cords, the transvere arytenoid and lateral cricoarytenoid, which adduct the vocal cords, and the thyroarytenoid and vocalis muscles, which relax the vocal cords. The internal branch of the superior laryngeal nerve is sensory to the supraglottic portion of the larynx and the adjacent part of the pharynx. The recurrent laryngeal nerve innervates the infraglottic mucosa of the larynx. The blood supply is provided by the superior and inferior thyroid arteries.

Pharynx. The pharynx extends from the base of the skull to the beginning of the esophagus. Posteriorly it is in contact with the upper six cervical vertebrae; laterally it is in relation with the internal and the common carotid arteries, the internal jugular vein, the sympathetic trunk, and the last four cranial nerves. Anteriorly it communicates with the nasal cavity above and the oral cavity below the palate, and inferiorly with the larynx and esophagus.

That portion of the pharynx above the soft palate is the *nasopharynx*. The auditory (eustachian) tube opens on the lateral wall of the nasopharynx. The projecting cartilage of the auditory tube produces a marked elevation (the torus tubarius) around the opening. The pharyngeal recess is a fossa behind the posterior lip of the torus. The pharyngeal tonsil ("adenoid") is found on the posterior wall of the nasopharynx. The *oral pharynx* is posterior to the oral cavity, limited above by the soft palate and below by the superior aspect of the epiglottis. The oral pharynx communicates with the oral cavity through the *fauces* (throat), which is below the soft palate and above the root of the tongue. Laterally the fauces are bounded by two muscular columns (pillars of the fauces) which are covered by mucosa: anteriorly the palatoglossal fold and posteriorly the palatopharyngeal fold. The lateral area between the folds is the tonsillar fossa which contains the palatine tonsil. The *laryngopharynx* extends from the superior edge of the epiglottis inferiorly to the lower border of the cricoid cartilage, essentially surrounding the larynx laterally and posteriorly. The vertical groove between the lateral aspect of the larynx and the pharyngeal wall is the piriform recess.

The muscles of the pharynx are the three constrictors and the stylopharyngeus, the latter passing downward between the superior and the middle constrictors. The constrictors overlap each other from below upward and surround the pharynx, and all three are inserted into a fibrous raphe in the posterior midline. Between muscles and mucous membrane is the pharyngobasilar fascia, which is especially strong above, where it is attached to the basilar process of the occipital bone and the petrous portion of the temporal bone. The inferior constrictor arises from the cricoid cartilage and the oblique line of the thyroid cartilage and encircles the pharynx. The middle constrictor arises from the greater and the lesser horns of the hyoid bone. The superior constrictor arises from the lower end and the hamulus of the medial pterygoid plate, the pterygomandibular ligament and the posterior end of the mylohyoid line on the inner surface of the mandible. The constrictor muscles are innervated by the tenth cranial nerve and the stylopharyngeus by the ninth cranial nerve. The ninth cranial nerve is also a major sensory nerve innervating the pharyngeal mucosa. As a result, the sensory limb of the gag reflex is the ninth cranial nerve and the motor limb the tenth cranial nerve.

Microscopic Structure of the Thyroid and Parathyroid Glands. The thyroid gland is invested by a thin capsule of connective tissue that projects into its substance and divides it imperfectly into lobes and lobules. The parenchyma consists of follicles that are closed epithelial sacs lined by simple cuboidal or simple columnar epithelium, the cells being low when the gland is underactive and taller when the gland is overactive. Follicles vary from 50 to 500μ in diameter, and the size of each follicle is somewhat dependent on the degree of distention by the stored colloid in the lumen of the follicle. In the production of thyroxine and triiodothyronine the follicular cells receive iodide and amino acids from extensively distributed fenestrated capillaries lying adjacent to the basement membrane. Through the mechanisms of a basally located rough endoplasmic reticulum and apically oriented Golgi apparatus, a glycoproteinaceous thyroglobulin is produced. This substance is discharged at the apical end of the cell into the follicular lumen where it is stored along with nucleoproteins and proteolytic enzymes as colloid. Under the influence of TSH, portions of thyroglobulin are taken into the apex of the follicular cell by pinocytosis, and the droplets are hydrolyzed by lysosomal activity into thyroxine and triiodothyronine. These substances are then secreted from the basal aspect of the cell into the surrounding capillaries. Parafollicular cells located between follicle cells and the basement membrane, and also found between follicles, differ structurally from follicle cells by being larger and lighter staining. They probably produce thyrocalcitonin.

A connective tissue capsule separates parathyroid glands from the thyroid gland. Fine connective tissue septa penetrate the parathyroid glands and divide the parenchyma into irregular cords of chief (principal cells) and oxyphil cells. Chief cells produce parathyroid hormone and are found in two functional states as light and dark chief cells. Dark chief cells contain membrane-bound argyrophilic secretory granules, a relatively large Golgi complex and large filementous mitochondria. Light cells have a smaller Golgi complex and few secretory granules. Oxyphilic cells are very acidophilic, are engorged with mitochondria and have a small nucleus, and do not appear until the end of the first decade of life. Their function is unknown.

Microscopic Structure of the Larynx and Trachea. As previously mentioned the tubular larynx is composed of nine cartilages connected by elastic membranes and intrinsic skeletal muscles. It is lined with a mucosa whose folds form the true and false vocal folds. The mucosa of the true vocal folds covers the vocal ligament (free margin of the conus elasticus) and vocalis muscle. The lining epithelium of the true vocal fold and of most of the epiglottis is stratified squamous nonkeratinized epithelium. Some taste buds may be found in the epiglottic epithelium. The rest of the lining is pseudostratified ciliated columnar epithelium that contains goblet cells and is underlain by a lamina propria containing mixed seromucous glands. There are no glands in the true vocal folds, but the surface is kept moist by the secretions that arise from numerous glands lining the ventricles. Lymphatic tissue in the ventricles may constitute the laryngeal tonsil. The thyroid, cricoid and most of the arytenoid cartilages are hyaline cartilage. The epiglottis, cuneiform, corniculate and tips of the arytenoid cartilages are elastic cartilage.

The trachea is a tubular structure whose wall, from the luminal surface outward, consists of a mucosa, submucosa and adventitia. The mucosa is similar to that of most of the larynx in that it is comprised of a pseudostratified ciliated columnar epithelium with goblet cells, the most prominent basement membrane in the body, and a lamina propria that contains many logitudinally directed elastic fibers. The indistinct submucosa contains seromucous glands that also extend between the C- and Y-shaped hyaline cartilage rings in the adventitial layer. The open interval of the C-shaped cartilages faces the esophagus and is bridged with fibroelastic tissue and a trachealis smooth muscle that runs circularly, attaching at the inner surface of each cartilage end.

Microscopic Structure of the Pharynx. The wall of the pharynx consists of a mucosa, muscularis and fibrosa. A submucosal layer exists only in the superior lateral region and near the junction with the esophagus. The epithelium of the nasopharynx is pseudostratified ciliated columnar epithelium with goblet cells; that of the oropharynx and laryngopharynx is stratified squamous nonkeratinized epithelium. The lamina propria contains many elastic fibers that constitute a dense elastic layer immediately adjacent to the muscularis. Mucous glands are found beneath the stratified squamous epithelium, whereas mixed glands occupy the lamina propria under the pseudostratified ciliated columnar epithelium. Aggregations of lymphatic nodules in the posterior nasopharyngeal mucosa constitute the pharyngeal tonsils (adenoids). The superior, middle and inferior constrictor muscles and the stylopharyngeus and salpingopharyngeus muscles constitute the skeletal muscle of the muscularis layer. The fibrosa layer is a tough fibroelastic layer that attaches the pharynx to surrounding structures.

Temporal and Infratemporal Regions

Osteology. The temporal fossa is superficial to those areas of the frontal, parietal, and squamous portions of the temporal and greater wing of the sphenoid bones that are bounded superiorly and posteriorly by the temporal lines. It extends inferiorly to the zygomatic arch and anteriorly to the frontal process of the zygomatic bone.

The infratemporal fossa is deep to the ramus of the mandible and the zygomatic arch. It is limited above by the infratemporal crest of the sphenoid, medially by the lateral pterygoid plate, anteriorly by the maxilla and inferiorly by the alveolar border of the maxilla. The infratemporal fossa is continuous medially with the pterygopalatine fossa via the pterygomaxillary fissure. It communicates with the middle cranial fossa by openings in its roof, the foramen ovale and foramen spinosum. Connections with the orbit are established through the inferior orbital fissure.

Temporomandibular Joint. The temporomandibular articulation is formed by the anterior portion of the mandibular fossa and the glenoid ridge (articular tubercle) of the temporal bone above and the condyle of the mandible below. The articular surfaces are covered by fibrocartilage and are separated by an articular disk. The strong joint capsule is reinforced by the sphenomandibular and stylomandibular ligaments. The condyle moves like a hinge on the articular disk while the disk glides forward toward the articular eminence. Consequently, when the mandible is depressed as in opening the mouth, the mandibular condyle slides anteriorly and inferiorly and thus out of the mandibular fossa.

Muscles of Mastication. The muscles of mastication are the masseter, temporalis and the medial and lateral pterygoids. They are found in the temporal and infratemporal fossae and superficial to the ramus of the mandible.

The masseter runs from the zygomatic arch to the outer surface of the ramus of the mandible, and is an elevator of the mandible. The temporalis muscle arises from the temporal fossa of the skull and inserts on the borders and the inner surface of the coronoid process. It elevates and retracts the mandible. The medial pterygoid arises from the inner surface of the lateral pterygoid plate and inserts on the angle and the inner surface of the ramus of the mandible. The lateral pterygoid arises from the zygomatic surface of the great wing of the sphenoid and the outer surface of the lateral pterygoid plate. It inserts in the depression in front of the neck of the mandible and the articular disk. Both pterygoid muscles (especially the lateral) cause deviation of the mandible to the opposite side and are thereby responsible for the grinding action of chewing. In addition, the medial pterygoid is an elevator and the lateral pterygoid is a protruder of the mandible. Mandibular depression is produced by the lateral pterygoid and floor of the mouth muscles. All muscles of mastication are innervated by the mandibular division of the trigeminal nerve.

Contents of the Infratemporal Fossa. In addition to certain muscles of mastication, the infratemporal fossa contains the proximal portion of the maxillary artery, the mandibular division of the trigeminal nerve and the pterygoid plexus of veins.

The *maxillary artery* is the larger of the two terminal branches of the external carotid. It arises in the substance of the parotid gland and enters the infratemporal fossa by passing deep to the ramus of the mandible. It passes obliquely through the fossa (either deep or superficial to the lateral pterygoid muscle) on its course to the pterygopalatine fossa via the pterygomaxillary fissure. While in the infratemporal fossa it gives off the anterior tympanic, deep auricular, middle meningeal, inferior alveolar, pterygoid, masseteric, buccal and deep temporal branches. The middle meningeal artery enters the middle cranial fossa through the foramen spinosum and is the major arterial supply to the cranial dura mater and the arachnoid.

The *mandibular nerve* enters the infratemporal fossa through the foramen ovale. The main trunk of this nerve is short (1 cm.) so that it branches high in the fossa. Among its branches are branches to the muscles of mastication and the mylohyoid, tensor tympani and tensor veli palatini, the buccal nerve to the cheek, the auriculotemporal nerve to the posterior temporal region, the lingual nerve to the oral cavity and the inferior alveolar nerve to the mandibular dentition and the skin covering the chin.

Parasympathetics are distributed in certain branches of this nerve. The otic ganglion is located medial to the main trunk of the nerve. The preganglionic input is from the lesser petrosal nerve, whose fibers exit the brainstem in cranial nerve IX. (Between cranial nerve IX and the lesser petrosal these fibers pass through the tympanic nerve and the tympanic plexus.) The postganglionic fibers from the otic ganglion are distributed with the auriculotemporal branch to the parotid gland. The chorda tympani branch of the seventh cranial nerve enters the fossa through the petrotympanic fissure and joins the lingual nerve high in the fossa. The lingual nerve transports these preganglionic fibers to the submandibular ganglion (located in the submandibular triangle) where they synapse and are then distributed to the submandibular, sublingual and lingual gland.

The *pterygoid plexus of veins* surrounds the pterygoid muscles. It receives blood from the face, nasal cavity, orbit, palate, cranial cavity, pharynx and infratemporal fossa. It drains into the maxillary vein, which joins the superficial temporal vein to form the retromandibular vein.

Pterygopalatine Fossa

Osteology. The pterygopalatine fossa is between the maxilla in front and the pterygoid portion of the sphenoid behind. Medially it is bounded by the perpendicular plate of the palatine bone. It communicates laterally with the infratemporal fossa via the pterygomaxillary fissure, medially with the nasal cavity via the sphenopalatine foramen, inferiorly with the oral cavity via the palatine canal and the greater and lesser palatine foramina, posterosuperiorly with the middle cranial fossa via the foramen rotundum, anterosuperiorly with the orbit via the inferior orbital fissure and posteromedially with the pharynx via the pharyngeal canal. The pterygoid canal is a canal through the pterygoid portion of the sphenoid that opens onto the posterior wall of the pterygopalatine fossa.

Contents of the Pterygopalatine Fossa. This fossa contains the terminal portion of the maxillary artery, the maxillary division of the trigeminal nerve and the pterygopalatine parasympathetic ganglion. The preganglionic parasympathetic fibers that synapse in this ganglion leave the brain stem in the facial nerve. From the facial nerve the course of these fibers is in the greater petrosal nerve, which passes into the middle cranial fossa via the hiatus of the facial canal and then out of the fossa via a small foramen. The greater petrosal nerve then joins the deep petrosal nerve (postganglionic sympathetic), and together they pass through the pterygoid canal as the nerve of the pterygoid canal. This nerve terminates in the ganglion, the parasympathetics synapsing and sympathetics merely passing through. Both fiber types are then distributed with branches of the maxillary nerve. The parasympathetic secretomotor fibers are thus distributed to the mucosa of the nasal cavity, palate, pharynx and paranasal sinuses and to the lacrimal gland. The fibers to the lacrimal gland pass in the infraorbital nerve, and its zygomatic branch, and a communicating branch from the zygomatic nerve to the lacrimal nerve before the latter carries them to the lacrimal gland.

The maxillary nerve continues as the infraorbital nerve, which passes into the floor of the orbit and eventually terminates on the face via the infraorbital foramen. The branches of the maxillary nerve and the proximal portion of the infraorbital nerve are: the palatine (greater and lesser) to the palate, the nasopalatine and lateral nasal branches to the nasal cavity, the pharyngeal nerve to the nasopharynx, the zygomatic nerve to the skin of the zygomatic region of the face, and the superior alveolar nerves to the maxillary sinus and dentition.

The branches of the pterygopalatine artery are: the posterior superior alveolar to the maxillary sinus and maxillary dentition, the infraorbital artery, the descending palatine artery to the palate, the pharyngeal artery and the sphenopalatine artery to the nasal cavity.

Oral Cavity

The mouth or oral cavity consists of a vestibule and the mouth proper. The vestibule of the mouth lies between the lips and cheeks superficially and the gums and teeth internally. It receives the parotid duct opposite the second upper molar tooth.

The mouth proper is bounded laterally and in front by the alveolar arches and the teeth; behind, it communicates with the pharynx through the fauces. It is roofed by the hard and the soft palates. The floor is composed of the tongue and the reflection of its mucous membrane to the gum lining the inner aspect of the mandible; the midline reflection is elevated into a fold called the frenulum linguae. On each side of this fold is the caruncula sublingualis containing the openings of the submandibular (Wharton's) ducts. Behind these are the openings of the ducts of the sublingual glands.

Lips and Cheeks. The lips are muscular folds covered externally by skin and internally by mucosa (mucous membrane). The upper lip extends to the nasolabial sulcus and contains a vertical midline groove, the philtrum. The mentolabial sulcus separates the lower lip from the skin. The lips receive their blood supply from labial branches of the facial artery. Their sensory nerve supply is by infraorbital branches of the trigeminal nerve to the upper lip and mental branches to the lower lip; the facial nerve supplies the orbicularis oris muscle. Microscopically the cutaneous surface consists of a thin skin, which possesses hairs, and sweat and sebaceous glands. The vestibular surface consists of stratified squamous nonkeratinized epithelium, lamina propria and a submucosa rich in mucous and mixed seromucous labial glands. The orbicularis oris muscle lies between the dermis and submucosal layers. The red area of the lip lies in the free margin of the lip at the junction between skin and mucosa. It is covered by nonkeratinized epithelium containing deeply indenting vascular papillae. No glands are present, and the epithelium is kept moist by licking of the lips.

The cheeks are similar in structure to the lips. Thick submucosal fibers tightly bind the mucosa to the buccinator muscle, thus reducing the chance of chewing on mucosal folds. Mixed buccal glands occupy the submucosa.

Tongue. The tongue is a muscular organ whose bilateral muscle masses are separated in the midline by a fibrous septum. Extrinsic muscles arise from the hyoid bone, styloid process, mandible and palate as the hyoglossus, styloglossus, genioglossus and palatoglossus respectively. Portions of the genioglossus function in protrusion of the tongue; the styloglossus and palatoglossus elevate the tongue, the hyoglossus depresses the sides and the styloglossus and other portions of the genioglossus serve in retraction of the tongue. Intrinsic muscles are oriented in vertical longitudinal and transverse bundles, and function to control the shape of the tongue. Both intrinsic and extrinsic muscles, with the exception of the palatoglossus, which is innervated by the vagus nerve, are innervated by the hypoglossal (twelfth) nerve. At its root the tongue is connected to the pharynx, palate and epiglottis; the vallecula and glossoepiglottic folds separate the root from the epiglottis.

The tongue is divisible into an anterior two thirds and a posterior one third by a V-shaped sulcus terminalis on the dorsum of the tongue. The apex of the V points posteriorly and ends in the foramen cecum, which marks the site of the embryonic thyroid diverticulum.

The mucosa over the anterior two thirds is characterized by filiform, fungiform and vallate papillae. Filiform papillae are the most numerous and uniformly distributed. They have a slender vascular core of connective tissue and are covered by a hyalinized, but not fully keratinized, epithelium. Fungiform papillae are knoblike projections that are larger and more scattered than the filiform papillae. Their epithelium is stratified squamous nonkeratinized and contains taste buds. Vallate papillae are the largest and least numerous of the papillae. They are oriented parallel to the sulcus terminalis and are 9 to 12 in number. Each papilla is surrounded by a trench into which underlying serous glands of von Ebner empty. The sides of the papillae and trench contain many taste buds, which extend intraepithelially from the basement membrane to the surface. Taste buds contain spindle-shaped neuroepithelial cells that receive sensory nerve endings. Anterior lingual glands are located near the tip of the tongue and are mixed seromucous glands.

The mucosa over the posterior one third of the tongue is stratified squamous nonkeratinized epithelium overlying connective tissue, lymphatic nodules and mucous glands. Aggregations of lymphatic nodules around single crypts constitute lingual tonsils.

The tongue and floor of the mouth receive their blood supply from branches of the lingual artery.

Branches of the lingual vein drain the tongue. The fifth, seventh, ninth, tenth and twelfth cranial nerves supply the tongue. The hypoglossal nerve (twelfth) supplies somatic efferent (SE) fibers to the skeletal muscles. Temperature, pain and touch receptors are supplied in the anterior two thirds of the tongue by general somatic afferent (GSA) fibers of the lingual nerve from the mandibular branch of the trigeminal nerve (fifth), while general visceral afferent (GVA) fibers of the glossopharyngeal (ninth) nerve subserve the same function in the posterior one third of the tongue. Taste buds in the anterior two-thirds are supplied by special visceral afferent (SVA) fibers of the facial nerve (seventh) via the chorda tympani and lingual nerves. Taste buds of the vallate papillae are supplied by SVA fibers of the glossopharyngeal nerve. Taste buds and general sensations near the epiglottis are supplied by the superior laryngeal branch of the vagus nerve.

Teeth. Teeth, gums and alveolar bone provide a wall between the vestibule and the mouth proper. There are 20 deciduous teeth and 32 permanent teeth equally distributed between the upper and lower jaws. Each tooth consists of a free crown, a root buried in an alveolus (socket) of the jaw and a neck between the crown and root at the gum margin. Dental pulp of connective tissue, vessels and nerves occupies a pulp chamber in the crown and root. The root is suspended in the alveolar bone by a periodontal membrane. The wall of the tooth consists of enamel, dentin and cementum. Enamel is the hardest structure in the body, and it covers the crown. It consists of radially arranged rodlike enamel prisms that were elaborated by ameloblasts before the tooth erupted. Ameloblasts developed from the enamel organ, which differentiated from a dental ledge of oral ectoderm. Each of the enamel prisms is invested by a prism sheath which is rich in organic matter. Adjacent prism sheaths are cemented together by interprismatic substance. Dentin lines the pulp chamber and lies internal to enamel in the crown and internal to cementum in the root. Dentin consists of a meshwork of collagen fibers oriented parallel to the surface of the tooth, and a calcified ground substance composed of glycosaminoglycans and mineral salts. This dentin matrix is permeated by radially arranged dentinal tubules containing dentinal fibers (of Tomes), which are processes of odontoblasts lining the pulp chamber. These cells are necessary for the production of the dentin matrix. Cementum is like a bony covering of the dentin; it is more acellular and avascular than bone, but lamellation and bone cells (cementocytes) are present. Cementocytes and odontoblasts arise from mesenchyme.

The sensory nerves to the maxillary teeth are branches of the maxillary division of the fifth nerve.

The posterior superior alveolar nerve supplies the molars, the middle superior alveolar innervates the bicuspids, and the anterior superior alveolar supplies the canine and incisor teeth. These branches and palatine branches of the maxillary nerve also supply the gums. The lower teeth are supplied by the inferior alveolar nerve from the mandibular branch of the trigeminal nerve. Blood supply is by way of the superior alveolar branches of the maxillary artery and the inferior alveolar artery.

Palate, Isthmus of the Fauces, and Palatine Tonsil. The palate forms the roof of the mouth and consists of a hard and soft palate. The hard palate consists of the palatine processes of the maxillae and the horizontal portions of the palatine bones. An incisive canal penetrates it anteromedially, and greater and lesser palatine foramina lie posterolaterally. The bony palate is covered by a mucoperiosteum that is much like that of the gums in that it consists of a stratified squamous epithelium that contains a cornified layer. An accumulation of fat is found anteriorly in the submucosa; mucous glands are plentiful in the submucosa of the posterior two thirds of the hard palate. Transverse corrugations of the mucosa in the anterior region and a median raphe also are characteristic features.

The soft palate is a muscular organ that extends posteriorly from the hard palate. It is lined on the nasopharyngeal side by pseudostratified ciliated columnar epithelium and on the oral side and free margin by stratified squamous nonkeratinized epithelium. The submucosa contains mucous glands on the oral side and mixed glands on the nasal side. Most of the skeletal muscles of the soft palate insert into the palatine aponeurosis, which is continuous with the pharyngobasilar fascia, or they are continuous with their opposite partner in the midline. The lowest or most anterior layer of muscle is the glossopalatine muscle. As indicated previously this muscle and the mucosa covering it constitute the anterior pillar of the fauces (glossopalatine arch). The most posterior layer of muscle is formed by the palatopharyngeus muscle, which with its mucosa constitutes the posterior pillar of the fauces (palatopharyngeal arch). The uvular muscles run from the hard palate to the tip of the uvula.

The two most important muscles are the levator veli palatini and the tensor veli palatini. The tensor veli palatini arises from the scaphoid fossa at the root of the pterygoid plate; its tendon passes around the hamulus and spreads just above the glossopalatine muscle and attaches to the palatine aponeurosis. The levator veli palatini arises from the under surface of the petrous bone behind the tensor and spreads out in the soft palate above the tensor. These two muscles elevate the soft palate.

All of the muscles of the soft palate except the tensor are supplied by the vagus nerve; the tensor veli palatini is supplied by branches of the fifth cranial nerve. The principal artery of the hard palate is the greater palatine branch of the maxillary artery. It enters through the greater palatine foramen and runs forward toward the incisive canal where it anastomoses with branches of the sphenopalatine artery. The soft palate is supplied by the lesser palatine artery, ascending palatine branches of the facial artery and branches of the ascending pharyngeal artery. Palatine veins are tributaries to the pterygoid plexus.

The isthmus of the fauces is the communication between the oral cavity proper and the oral pharynx. It is bounded above by the soft palate, below by the tongue and laterally by the glossopalatine arch.

The palatine tonsil is located between the anterior and posterior pillars. It bulges into this depression and is covered by a mucosal fold of the anterior pillar; there is a depressed supratonsillar fossa above the tonsil. The free surface of the tonsil, lined by stratified squamous nonkeratinized epithelium, dips into the underlying lymphatic nodular aggregation as 10 to 20 branching primary and secondary crypts. Lymphocytes from the underlying diffuse and nodular lymphatic tissue often heavily infiltrate the epithelium. The tonsils produce lymphocytes; the presence of plasma cells indicates that tonsils are involved in antigen-antibody reactions. The presence of many neutrophils is characteristic of tonsillar inflammation. Each tonsil is partially invested basally by a connective tissue capsule that sends septa around the aggregations of nodules that invest each crypt. Some mucous glands and the superior pharyngeal constrictor and styloglossus muscles lie peripheral to the capsule. Efferent lymphatic vessels penetrate the pharyngeal wall and pass to superior deep cervical nodes, especially the jugulodigastric node. The arterial supply to the palatine tonsil is by the ascending palatine branch of the facial artery, tonsillar branch of the facial artery, palatine branch of the ascending pharyngeal artery, dorsal lingual branch of the lingual artery and descending palatine branch of the maxillary artery. The nerves innervating the tonsil are branches of the maxillary division of the trigeminal nerve and the glossopharyngeal nerve.

Nasal Cavity and Paranasal Sinuses

Nasal Cavity. The nasal cavity extends from the base of the anterior cranial fossa to the roof of the mouth (palate) and is divided into right and left sides by the nasal septum. The septum is formed by the perpendicular plate of the ethmoid, the vomer and the septal cartilage. The nasal cavity is related superiorly to the anterior cranial fossa; laterally to the ethmoid air cells, maxillary sinus, and orbit; inferiorly to the oral cavity; and posterosuperiorly to the sphenoid sinus. It opens anteriorly on the face via the nares and is continuous posteriorly via the choanae with the nasopharynx. The superior, middle and inferior conchae divide the cavity into superior, middle and inferior meatuses. The area posterosuperior to the superior concha is the sphenoethmoidal recess.

The GSA fibers to the mucosa of the nasal cavity are from the anterior and posterior ethmoidal nerves (ophthalmic V), and the lateral nasal and nasopalatine nerves (maxillary V). The olfactory epithelium in the upper part of the nasal cavity is innervated by SVA fibers from the olfactory (first cranial) nerve. All parasympathetic (GVE) fibers are from the pterygopalatine ganglion and distributed by branches of the maxillary division of the trigeminal nerve. The blood supply to the nasal cavity is from three sources: the maxillary, ophthalmic and facial arteries. The anterosuperior portions of the lateral wall and septum are supplied by the anterior and posterior ethmoidal branches of the ophthalmic artery. Most of the lateral wall (posteroinferior portion) is supplied by the lateral nasal branches of the maxillary artery, and the same area of the septum is supplied by the sphenopalatine branch of the maxillary. The area around the external nares is supplied by the superior labial branches of the facial artery.

Paranasal Sinuses. The relationships of each of the sinuses as well as communications with the nasal cavity are covered below.

The maxillary sinus is related to the orbit above, the nasal cavity medially, the posterior maxillary teeth inferiorly, the infratemporal fossa posterolaterally and the cheek anterolaterally. The sinus empties into the middle meatus via the hiatus semilunaris and is best drained when lying on the opposite side. Since the opening is well above the inferior extent of the sinus, the top of the head should be lower than the lower jaw if complete drainage is accomplished.

The frontal sinus is in the frontal bone deep to the superciliary ridge. It is related anteriorly to the forehead, posteriorly to the anterior cranial fossa and inferiorly to the orbit, ethmoid air cells and the nasal cavity. It empties into the middle meatus and is best drained in the upright position.

The ethmoid air cells are interposed between the upper portion of the nasal cavity and the orbit. They are related superiorly to the anterior cranial fossa and inferiorly to the mastoid sinus. These sinuses drain into the superior and middle meatus. The locations of these openings are variable, and hence the optional drainage position varies between upright and lying on the opposite side.

The sphenoid sinus is in the body of the sphenoid

bone. It is deep to the sella turcica, the hypophysis and the optic nerve. It is bounded laterally by the cavernous sinus through which runs the internal carotid artery and cranial nerves III, IV, ophthalmic and maxillary V, and VI. The pterygoid canal is in the floor of the sinus. This sinus empties into the sphenoethmoidal recess. It drains best with the head flexed more than 90 degrees.

The secretomotor fibers to the mucosa of the paranasal sinuses are postganglionic parasympathetics from the pterygopalatine ganglion that are distributed primarily with branches of the maxillary nerve.

Orbital Region

Osteology. The orbital cavities are four-sided pyramids. The roof of each is formed by the orbital plate of the frontal bone and the lesser wing of the sphenoid. The floor is formed by the orbital surface of the maxilla, the orbital process of the zygoma and the orbital process of the palatine bone. The medial wall is formed by the nasal process of the maxilla, the lacrimal, the ethmoid and the sphenoid bones. The lateral wall is formed by the orbital process of the zygomatic bone and the greater wing of the sphenoid. The orbit is related superiorly to the frontal sinus and anterior cranial fossa, medially to the nasal cavity, ethmoid air cells and sphenoid sinus, inferiorly to the maxillary sinus, and laterally to the temporal fossa and the middle cranial fossa. The orbit communicates with the cranial cavity via the superior orbital fissure and the optic canal, with the infratemporal and pterygopalatine fossae via the inferior orbital fissure, and with the sphenoid sinuses and nasal cavity via the anterior and posterior ethmoidal foramina.

Contents of the Orbit. The contents of the orbit are enclosed in a tough conically shaped layer of fascia, the periorbita. The periorbita is only loosely attached to the walls of the orbit (in reality it is the periosteum of these bones), and it is continuous at the apex of the orbit through the optic canal and the superior orbital fissure with the periosteal layer of cranial dura. The meningeal layer of cranial dura enters the orbit through the optic canal where it forms a sleeve around the optic nerve, which passes to the bulb of the eye. At the back of the bulb the meningeal layer of dura blends with the sclera of the eyeball. As the arachnoid and pia also follow the optic nerve to the eyeball, the subarachnoid space surrounds the optic nerve and extends the same distance. Within the confines of the periorbita the extraocular structures are embedded in fat.

The extraocular eye muscles control the movements of the eyeball and the upper eyelid. The inferior oblique, levator palpebrae and superior, medial and inferior rectus muscles are innervated by the oculomotor (third) nerve. The lateral rectus is supplied by the abducens (sixth) nerve and the superior oblique by the trochlear (fourth) nerve.

The optic nerve enters the orbit through the optic canal and passes through the center of the orbital cone toward the eyeball. The oculomotor, trochlear, ophthalmic and abducens nerves enter via the superior orbital fissure. One of the terminal branches of the oculomotor nerve is the superior branch, which passes above the optic nerve and supplies the upper muscles. The inferior branch passes below the optic nerve and provides the motor root to the ciliary ganglion. The trochlear nerve is very small and passes superomedially to the superior oblique muscle. The ophthalmic nerve divides into the lacrimal nerve, which supplies the lacrimal gland, the frontal nerve, which terminates as the supratrochlear and supraorbital nerves, and the nasociliary nerve, which has ethmoidal and infratrochlear branches. The abducens nerve passes through the lateral part of the orbit to the lateral rectus.

The ciliary ganglion is a parasympathetic ganglion located in the posterior third of the orbit just lateral to the optic nerve. Preganglionic fibers reach this ganglion through the motor root of the oculomotor nerve and after synapsing reach the eyeball via the short ciliary nerves. These fibers innervate the sphincter pupillae and the ciliary muscle. Sensory (GSA) fibers to the eyeball are provided by the nasociliary branch of the ophthalmic nerve. These fibers reach the bulb via the long ciliary nerves, which are branches of the nasociliary. In addition, the nasociliary nerve provides a sensory root to the ciliary ganglion through which sensory fibers reach the bulb via the ganglion and the short ciliary nerves. Sympathetic fibers reach the bulb through either long or short ciliary nerves as well as with various arteries. The sympathetics innervate the dilator pupillae muscle and the superior tarsal muscle.

The ophthalmic artery arises from the internal carotid artery as the latter passes the optic nerve. The artery enters the orbit just inferior to the optic nerve in the optic canal. The central artery of the retina enters the optic nerve about halfway along the orbital course of the nerve. It travels to the retina within the substance of the nerve (with the central vein of the retina) and is therefore surrounded by the subarachnoid space and is vulnerable to any pressure changes in that system. Other major branches of the ophthalmic artery are the ciliary branches to the eyeball, the lacrimal artery and the ethmoidals. The superior and inferior ophthalmic veins drain primarily into the sinus cavernosus although there are communications with the pterygoid plexus and the veins of the face.

Eyelid. The upper and lower eyelids are movable folds that are separated by a palpebral fissure at their free margins. Each lid is covered by thin skin that is modified posteriorly into a mucous membrane called the palpebral conjunctiva. The palpebral conjunctiva consists of a lamina propria and stratified epithelium whose surface cells fluctuate in various regions between squamous and columnar. The palpebral conjunctiva is continuous with the bulbar conjunctiva at the fornix. The lamina propria of the palpebral conjunctiva is firmly attached to the tarsal plate of dense connective tissue that contains the sebaceous tarsal (meibomian) glands. The tarsal glands open onto the free border of the lid. In the upper lid the superior tarsal muscle and tendinous slips of the levator palpebrae superioris attach to the tarsal plate. Ptosis of the eye can occur in: (1) Horner's syndrome, in which there is damage to the sympathetic innervation of the involuntary superior tarsal muscle, or (2) oculomotor nerve damage, in which the innervation to the skeletal superior levator palpebrae muscle is conpromised. The tarsal plate is attached laterally to the zygomatic bone and medially to the frontal process of the maxilla by lateral and medial palpebral ligaments. Anterior to the tarsal plate is the palpebral portion of the orbiculus oculi muscle. A subcutaneous tissue, which seldom contains fat, lies between the skin and the orbicularis oculi muscle. Cilia (eyelashes) are large hairs arranged in two or three irregular rows on the free margins of the eyelids. Large sebaceous glands (Zeis) and large spiral sweat glands (Moll) are closely associated with the cilia.

Lacrimal Apparatus. The lacrimal apparatus consists of the lacrimal gland, lacrimal ducts, lacrimal sac and the nasolacrimal duct. The lacrimal gland is situated near the front of the lateral roof of the orbit. Its main ducts open onto the upper lateral half of the conjunctival fornix. Microscopically this gland resembles the parotid in that it is comprised of serous acini. Tears from the lacrimal gland move across the eyeball to the medial angle of the eye where it enters the lacrimal canaliculi. The canaliculi arise on the medial margins of the upper and lower lids at the lacrimal puncta on the lacrimal papillae. The lacrimal ducts carry the lacrimal secretion medially to the lacrimal sac, which is an upward expansion of the nasolacrimal duct. The nasolacrimal duct is lined by columnar epithelium and passes downward, backward and slightly laterally to enter the nasal cavity at the inferior meatus.

Eyeball. The eyeball consists of three layers: (1) an outer fibrous tunic composed of the sclera and cornea, (2) a vascular coat (uvea) of choroid, ciliary body and iris, and (3) the retina formed of pigment and nervous layers. The anterior chamber lies between the cornea anteriorly and the iris and pupil posteriorly; the posterior chamber lies between the iris anteriorly and the ciliary processes, zonular fibers and lens posteriorly. Both chambers possess aqueous humor, which is produced in the region of the ciliary processes and exits through the uveal meshwork and canal of Schlemm at the lateral iris angle of the anterior chamber. The canal of Schlemm drains into the anterior ciliary veins. The vitreous body occupies the space between the lens and the retina.

In embryonic development the optic nerve and retina developed as an evagination of the diencephalon, the pigment layer of the retina arising from the outer layer and the nervous layer arising from the inner layer of the optic cup formed by indentation of the optic vesicle. The lens developed from a lens vesicle that took origin from a thickened lens placode of general surface ectoderm. The outer epithelium of the cornea also developed from surface ectoderm. The other investing tunics of the eyeball developed from head mesenchyme, while the extrinsic eye muscles arose from head (eye) somites.

The *cornea* constitutes the anterior one sixth of the eye. Its front free surface is lined with stratified squamous nonkeratinized epithelium, and its posterior surface is lined with endothelium that is continuous with the spaces of the uveal meshwork. Underlying the endothelium is a prominent basement membrane called Descemet's membrane; below the anterior epithelium is a thin connective tissue membrane (Bowman's membrane). Between both membranes is the substantia propria comprising the bulk of the cornea. This layer consists of many lamellae of collagenous fibrils held together by a glycoprotein ground substance. The collagen fibrils of adjacent layers run perpendicular to each other and may interweave from layer to layer.

The *sclera* forms the posterior five sixths of the eye and is composed of dense fibrous connective tissue. Although continuous with the cornea, it is delimited from the cornea by internal and external scleral sulci. Nerve fibers of the optic nerve perforate it posteromedially at the optic disc, forming the lamina cribrosa. Extrinsic eye muscles insert into the sclera, and the loose outer scleral layer is continuous with the loose tissue of Tenon's space investing the eyeball. Ciliary vessels and nerves perforate the sclera around the entrance of the optic nerve; other emissaria, which transmit venae vorticosae from the choroid layer, occur midway between the sclerocorneal junction and the optic nerve.

The *choroid* layer consists of a vascular loose connective tissue; it is separated externally from the sclera by a potential perichoroidal space and firmly attached internally to the pigment layer of the retina. The vessel and capillary layers of the choroid are the most prominent layers. The capillary layer supplies the outer layers of the retina and is the only portion of the choroid not continued forward into the ciliary body.

The *ciliary body* is bounded posteriorly at the ora serrata by the retina and choroid; laterally by the sclera; medially by the posterior chamber, vitreous body and lens; and anteriorly by the iris. The posterior two thirds of the ciliary body is heavily pigmented and smooth on its inner surface, whereas the anterior one third bears radially arranged ciliary processes. The forward continuation of the choroid forms the ciliary muscle layer, vessel layer and lamina vitrea. The forward continuation of the retina gives rise to the outer pigment and inner ciliary epithelial layers and to the internal limiting membrane. The smooth muscle of the ciliary body is oriented in meridional, radial and circular directions. Its action is to relax the tension on the suspensory zonular ligaments, thus allowing the lens to become more convex. It is supplied by parasympathetic fibers of the oculomotor nerve. Preganglionic fibers arise in the Edinger-Westphal complex of the mesencephalon, course through the oculomotor nerve and short motor root of the ciliary ganglion and synapse with postganglionic cell bodies in the ciliary ganglion. Myelinated postganglionic nerves traverse the 12 short ciliary nerves and choroid layer to reach the ciliary body.

The vascular layer thickens in the ciliary processes, contains fenestrated capillaries and is covered by the pigment and ciliary epithelia. The ciliary epithelium, over the summits of the processes, is modified by basal infoldings of the plasmalemma for transport. This epithelium is involved in aqueous humour formation. Occluding junctions between ciliary epithelial cells may be a major site of a blood-aqueous barrier.

The *iris* is attached peripherally to the anterior end of the ciliary body. The anterior surface of the iris demonstrates an inner pupillary zone separated from an outer ciliary zone by a collarette (iris frill). The iris is lined anteriorly by a discontinuous layer of fibroblasts and melanocytes, and posteriorly by pigment epithelium. Underlying the anterior surface layer is an anterior border layer formed principally of chromatophores; deep to this is a vascular stromal layer containing the sphincter pupillae muscle. These layers are an anterior continuation of the uvea. The vascular stroma is bordered posteriorly by the pigment epithelium and the more deeply lying dilator pupillae muscle; these two layers are a forward continuation of the iris. The color of the iris depends on the thickness of the anterior border layer and on the pigmentation of its cells. If the layer is thick and heavily pigmented, the eyes are seen as brown; if the layer is small and little pigment is present, the light passes through the vascular stroma and is reflected off of the pigment epithelium

as blue. The arterial supply to the iris is by way of long ciliary and anterior ciliary arteries from the ophthalmic division of the internal carotid arteries. These vessels form a major arterial circle in the vessel layer of the attached margin of the iris. Radial branches from this circle pass toward the pupillary margin, forming a minor arterial circle. The sphincter pupillae and dilator pupillae arise from the pigment epithelium and thus are of neural ectodermal origin. The sphincter pupillae is innervated by parasympathetic fibers of the oculomotor nerve by a pathway that is similar to that for the ciliary muscle. The dilator pupillae muscle is supplied by postganglionic sympathetic fibers that arise from cell bodies in the superior cervical ganglion, follow the internal carotid artery to the cavernous plexus, pass through the nasociliary and its long ciliary branch and traverse the choroid to reach the iris. The preganglionic sympathetic neurons arise in the intermediolateral cell column of T1 and T2 spinal cord segments, and their axons traverse the ventral roots, white communicating rami and sympathetic trunk to attain the superior cervical ganglion.

The *retina* is divisible into ten layers: (1) pigment epithelium, (2) layer of rod and cone outer and inner segments, (3) external limiting membrane, (4) outer nuclear layer, (5) outer plexiform layer, (6) inner nuclear layer, (7) inner plexiform layer, (8) ganglion cell layer, (9) nerve fiber layer and (10) internal limiting membrane. The simple cuboidal cells of the pigment epithelium have melanin-containing cytoplasmic processes that interdigitate with the rod and cone outer segments. Layers 2 to 5 contain the rod and cone receptors of the light pathway. The outer segments of rods and cones contain numerous stacked membranous discs derived from the plasma membrane and containing visual pigments. The outer discs of the rods differ from cones in that they lose their plasma membrane continuity and are discharged from the cell. The outer segment of cones and rods is connected to the inner segment by a connecting stalk containing a cilium. The inner segment contains the protein-producing endoplasmic reticulum and Golgi complex necessary for the replacement of rod discs and the nurturing of cone discs. The cell bodies and nuclei of rods and cones constitute the outer nuclear layer. The axons (pedicles) of these cells pass into the outer plexiform layer where they synapse with dendrites of bipolar cells and processes of horizontal cells. Bipolar cells are the second-order neuron in the visual pathway. Their nuclei are in the inner nuclear layer, and their axons synapse with dendrites of the third-order neuron ganglion cells in the inner plexiform layer. The cell bodies of midget and diffuse ganglion cells constitute the ganglion cell layer, and their axons form the nerve fiber layer. By these arrangements of cells one cone may synapse with one bipolar cell, which in turn synapses with one midget ganglion cell, or several rods or cones may synapse with one bipolar cell, which synapses with a diffuse ganglion cell. Horizontal interconnections are accomplished between rods and cones by horizontal cells and between ganglion cells by amacrine cells. The outer and inner limiting membranes are formed by the ends of processes of supporting Müller's cells whose nuclei, like those of bipolar, horizontal and amacrine cells, are located in the inner nuclear layer.

All of the retinal layers external to the inner nuclear layer receive nourishment from choroid capillaries. The rest of the retina is supplied by capillaries derived from branches of the central retinal artery of the optic nerve. The retinal arteries enter at the optic disc and branch into superior and inferior nasal and superior and inferior temporal arteries, the larger branches of which run in the nerve fiber layer. The veins accompany the arteries. Diagnostically the arteries are bright red; the veins are wine colored. The arterial "reflex" from the bloodstream is broader and brighter than the venous "reflex." Choroidal vessels are pinker, flatter and more bandlike than the retinal vessels.

In examination of the fundus of the eyeball a macula lutea is seen in the visual axis about 2½ disc diameters to the temporal side of the optic disc. It is a darker oval area in the reddish retinal field. It is devoid of vessels, and in its center is a depressed area, the fovea centralis. The fovea is a site for acute central vision where cones predominate and most retinal layers have been "moved aside" for more immediate access of light rays to the cones.

The lens is a biconvex body whose posterior surface has a greater convexity. It consists of a capsule, anterior epithelium and lens substance. The capsule consists of basal and reticular laminae ensheathing the lens into which zonular fibers insert. The anterior epithelium contains simple cuboidal cells that become elongate at the equator of the lens where they give rise to new lens fibers. The lens substance consists of prismatic lens fibers that are meridionally arranged, with older fibers more centrally located than the newer ones. Desmosome junctions are present between the newer cells; sutures mark the junction of fibers in the central part of the lens.

Ear

Temporal Bone. The temporal bone houses the internal and middle ear cavities, contains a network of interconnected canals and participates in the formation of various cranial and extracranial fossae. It is composed of squamous, mastoid, petrous and tympanic parts. The squamous portion forms part of the mastoid process, external auditory meatus and the mandibular fossa and has the zygomatic process, which forms part of the zygomatic arch. It helps define the middle cranial fossa. The mastoid portion forms most of the mastoid process and part of the wall of the posterior cranial fossa. The tympanic part forms most of the external auditory meatus and all of the styloid process. The pyramid-shaped petrous portion protrudes anteromedially toward the dorsum sellae where it ends. The petrous ridge separates the anterior face from the posterior face. The anterior face forms the posterior portion of the floor of the middle cranial cavity. The posterior face is the anterolateral aspect of the posterior cranial fossa and contains the opening of the internal auditory meatus.

External Ear. The external ear is composed of the external cartilaginous portion, the pinna or auricle, and the external auditory meatus. The external auditory meatus is about 3 cm. in length, connects the auricle and the middle ear cavity and consists of a lateral cartilaginous and a medial osseous portion. In the infant the osseous meatus is merely a bony ring, which in the adults grows to a length of about 2 cm. It is narrowest at the isthmus about 0.5 cm. from the tympanic membrane. The entire external auditory meatus is S-shaped. The convexity of the outer cartilaginous portion is directed upward and posteriorly while that of the inner osseous portion is directed downward and anteriorly.

Middle Ear. The middle ear, or tympanic cavity, is generally shaped like a flat cigar box. Its long axis parallels the tympanic membrane so that it is obliquely oriented, sloping medially from above downward and from behind forward. The cavity is divided into three regions: the middle ear cavity proper at the level of the tympanic membrane, the attic, or epitympanum, above the membrane, and the hypotympanum below the membrane. The cavity communicates posterolaterally with the mastoid air cells via the attic and mastoid antrum, and anteromedially with the nasopharynx via the auditory tube.

The lateral wall is formed primarily by the tympanic membrane. This membrane is angularly concave with its apex—the umbo—directed medially. It is composed of a fibrous stratum covered laterally by skin and medially by mucous membrane. The greater part of the periphery of the membrane is a thickened fibrocartilaginous ring which attaches to the bony tympanic sulcus. Superiorly the sulcus and fibrous stratum are deficient, and thus the membrane is lax (pars flaccida). The rest of the membrane is called pars tensa.

The medial wall separates the middle ear from the inner ear and presents: (1) the promontory, which corresponds to the first turn of the cochlea, (2) the oval window, which contains the foot plate of the stapes and lies a little above and behind the promontory, (3) the round window below the oval window, (4) the pyramid containing the stapedius muscle and (5) the aqueductus fallopii, a slight ridge of bone lying along the upper and posterior parts of the inner wall and containing the facial nerve, which emerges at the stylomastoid foramen.

The roof is the tegmen tympani, a thin portion of the petrous temporal bone, which forms part of the floor of the middle cranial fossa. The floor is formed by the roof of the jugular foramen. The anterior wall is formed below by the roof of the carotid canal; above it is deficient where the auditory tube opens into the tympanic cavity. The posterior wall is formed inferiorly by the descending portion of the facial canal; superiorly the attic is in communication with the mastoid antrum.

The ossicles of the middle ear are the malleus, incus and stapes. The manubrium of the malleus attaches to the umbo of the tympanic membrane, the foot plate of the stapes fits into the oval window, and the incus interconnects the stapes and malleus. The chorda tympani nerve branches from the facial nerve and passes between the incus and malleus. The tympanic plexus is located on the promontory. It contains sympathetics (via the caroticotympanic branch of the internal carotid plexus), and sensory and parasympathetic fibers (both via the tympanic branch of the glossopharyngeal nerve).

The auditory (eustachian) tube is about 3.8 to 4 cm. in length, extending from the tympanum obliquely forward, downward and inward. Its first third is bony; the pharyngeal two thirds are cartilaginous.

The air cells of the mastoid process communicate with the middle ear by means of the antrum and the attic. Up to the age of 5 years there is usually only one cell, the antrum, after which the mastoid consists of a large number of cells communicating with one another and the antrum. This area is lined with a continuation of the mucous membrane of the tympanum.

Inner Ear or Labyrinth.   The inner ear is contained in the petrous portion of the temporal bone and consists of an osseous labyrinth containing a membranous labyrinth. Between the bony and membranous labyrinth is perilymph. Within the membranous labyrinth is endolymph.

The *osseous labyrinth* is a series of cavities in bone consisting of a central vestibule off of which are three semicircular canals posterolaterally and the cochlea anteromedially. The vestibule is separated from the middle ear cavity medially by a bony wall containing the fenestra ovalis. This oval window is closed by the foot plate of the stapes. In the posteromedial wall of the vestibule is the opening of the vestibular aqueduct,

which extends to the posterior wall of the petrous portion of the temporal bone. The three semicircular canals are oriented at right angles to each other. The anterior (superior) and posterior canals are vertically oriented; the lateral (horizontal) canal is horizontally positioned. The positioning of the semicircular canals is such that the anterior canal of one osseous labyrinth runs parallel to the posterior canal of the other side. The anterior canal runs transverse to the long axis of the petrous bone. Its anterior limb is dilated into an ampulla just before its entrance into the vestibule; the posterior limb joins the anterior limb of the posterior canal to enter the vestibule as a crus commune. The posterior canal runs parallel to the posterior wall of the petrous bone, and its posterior limb enters the vestibule just beyond the ampulla. Both limbs of the lateral canal enter the vestibule, and an ampulla is located on the anterior limb. The cochlea is conical, has two and one-half turns, and its apex is directed forward, outward and downward. Mesenchymal epithelium lines the periosteum of the osseous labyrinth.

The *membranous labyrinth* consists of an interconnected series of fibrous sacs lined by simple squamous epithelium. The epithelium is derived from an otic vesicle that developed from an otic placode of general surface ectoderm. With the exception of the vestibule, the membranous labyrinth conforms generally to the contour of the osseous labyrinth. The larger portion in the upper posterior part of the vestibule is the utricle; that in front of the utricle is the saccule. The utricle receives the openings of the membranous semicircular canals. The saccule communicates with the membranous cochlear duct by the ductus reuniens. A utriculosacculor duct interconnects the utricle and saccule and continues backward through the vestibular aqueduct as the endolymphatic duct. The latter duct terminates as an endolymphatic sac under the dura lining the posterior surface of the petrous portion of the temporal bone. There are six neuroepithelial receptor areas in each labyrinth: (1) macula utriculi, (2) macula sacculi, (3–5) one crista ampullaris in each ampulla and, (6) organ of Corti in the cochlear duct. The organ of Corti is supplied by the cochlear division of the eighth nerve; the maculae and cristae are innervated by the vestibular division.

The *cristae ampullares* are thickened ridges of epithelium and connective tissue placed transversely to the long axis of each semicircular canal. The epithelium of each crista consists of sustentacular cells and two configurations (types I and II) of neuroepithelial cells called hair cells. Each hair cell contains one kinocilium and many stereocilia that project into an overlying gelatinous mass called the cupula. In the horizontal canals the kinocilia are on the utricular side of the hair cells; in the superior (anterior) and posterior canals the kinocilia are located away from the utricle. Displacement of the stereocilia toward the kinocilia increases the rate of discharge from the hair cells, while movement in the opposite direction decreases the rate of discharge in the vestibular nerve. Thus, movement of endolymph toward the utricle in the ampullary end of the horizontal semicircular canal causes an increased rate of discharge in that crista. Thus, when an individual is first rotated while the lateral canals are in a horizontal position, the endolymph flow in the horizontal canal on the side of direction of rotation would be essentially ampullopetal, resulting in increased rate of discharge, while the endolymph in the other horizontal canal is ampullofugal, and there is a decreased rate of discharge. In postrotation the opposite occurs. If the head is positioned so that the horizontal canals are vertically oriented, and warm water is added to one ear, then convection currents produce an ampullopetal flow in that ear resulting in a rate of discharge that exceeds that from the unstimulated ear. The use of cold water produces an opposite direction of endolymph flow; thus, the results are opposite to those for warm water. Both the type I and type II hair cells are innervated by the dendritic terminals of bipolar cells of the vestibular ganglion. Some cells receive efferent neurons. The vestibular ganglion lies in the upper part of the outer end of the internal auditory meatus. Axons from the vestibular ganglion pass medially in the internal auditory canal as the vestibular portion of the vestibulocochlear nerve and enter the brain stem at the pons–medulla junction.

The *maculae* are similar to the cristae in that they are local thickenings of the membrane, they contain hair cells and sustentacular cells, and their hair cells penetrate a gelatinous membrane. The macular gelatinous membrane contains calcium carbonate crystals called otoliths (otoconia) and is called the otolithic membrane. The hair cells in various regions of the macula utriculi have their kinocilia placed on different sides so that the macula can detect linear acceleration and the position of the head in respect to gravitational forces. The macula of the saccule seems to respond to slow vibrational stimuli.

The *organ of Corti* is located on the basilar membrane of the membranous cochlear duct. The cochlear duct (scala media) is filled with endolymph, runs throughout most of the cochlea and is separated from the upper scala vestibuli by the vestibular membrane and from the lower scala tympani by the basilar membrane. The basilar membrane is suspended between the centrally located osseous spiral lamina of the modiolus and the peripherally located periosteal thickening called the spiral ligament. On the lateral wall of the cochlear duct is the stria vascularis. It is highly vascular, is lined with pseudostratified columnar epithelium and is involved in endolymph production. The organ of Corti is an arrangement of supportive and hair cells on the upper border of the basilar membrane. The neuroepithelial hair cells are arranged into inner and outer hair cells by their relationship to an inner tunnel (of Corti) formed by inner and outer pillar cells. The hair cells are supported by outer and inner phalangeal cells whose phalangeal processes form a firm reticular lamina at the peripheral surfaces of the hair cells. The microvillous hairs of the hair cells are in contact with the overlying gelatinous tectorial membrane, thus establishing a mechanism wherein movement of the basilar membrane will cause stimulation of hair cells by bending of the hairs. This mechanical stimulus is transduced into electrical energy by the hair cells and transmitted to the terminal dendritic endings of the special somatic afferent (SSA) cells of the spiral cochlear ganglion. Axons of these bipolar nerve cells pass into the axis of the modiolus, course upward into the internal acoustic meatus, become the cochlear portion of the vestibulocochlear nerve and synapse in the dorsal and ventral cochlear nuclei at the pons–medulla junction of the brain stem.

The blood supply of the labyrinth is by way of the internal auditory (labyrinthine) and stylomastoid arteries. The stylomastoid is a branch of the posterior auricular. The internal auditory arises from the basilar artery, or in common with the anterior inferior cerebellar artery, and traverses the internal acoustic meatus before branching into cochlear and vestibular branches. The veins accompany the arteries and drain as internal auditory veins into the superior petrosal or transverse sinuses.

Development of the Head and Neck

Development and Fate of the Branchial Arches. During the third and fourth weeks of development the embryo develops head and tail folds that result in the incorporation of the dorsal portions of the primitive yolk sac entoderm as foregut, midgut and hindgut. The rostral portion of the foregut (primitive pharynx) develops five lateral pairs of pharyngeal pouches; these and the floor of the pharynx give rise to the tongue, pharynx, thyroid gland, parathyroid glands and thymus gland. The more caudal portions of the foregut will develop into the esophagus, stomach, part of the duodenum, and the liver and pancreas.

While the pharyngeal pouches are forming internally, five pairs of branchial (pharyngeal) arches appear externally. These are numbered 1, 2, 3, 4, and 6. They are separated by branchial (pharyngeal) grooves, which are aligned with the pharyngeal pouches to form branchial (pharyngeal) membranes consisting of outer ectodermal and inner entodermal layers. Each groove is numbered according to the arch that lies rostral to it. Each branchial arch also is comprised of an outer ectodermal layer and an inner entodermal lining, but a vertical bar of mesoderm and a cranial nerve are interposed between the two layers.

The first arch is divisible into mandibular and maxillary arches. The surface ectoderm of these arches will become the epidermis of the upper and lower jaws, the epithelium of most of the oral cavity, the parenchyma of the major salivary glands, and the enamel of the teeth. The mandibular and maxillary divisions of the trigeminal nerve course in these arches and supply the skin of the face with sensory nerves (GSA) and the muscles of mastication with motor (SVE) nerves. The muscles developing from the first arch are the temporalis, masseter, medial and lateral pterygoids, mylohyoid, anterior belly of the digastric, tensor veli palatini and tensor tympani. Mesenchyme of the first arch develops into a transitory Meckel's cartilage before forming a mandible, malleus, incus and maxilla. The first branchial groove gives rise to the external acoustic meatus. The first branchial membrane develops into the tympanic membrane, and the first pharyngeal pouch presages part of the auditory (eustachian) tube and middle ear cavity.

The second (hyoid) arch grows back over arches 3 to 6 and will fuse with them, obliterating branchial gooves 3 to 6 and a transitory cervical sinus that was formed in this caudal growth. Improper obliteration of the cervical sinus can result in a cervical cyst. Cervical fistulas may remain if communications are retained externally and/or internally through the branchial membranes. Since the ectoderm of the second arch gives rise to the epidermis of much of the neck, the openings of external branchial fistulas occur in the neck along the anterior margin of the sternocleidomastoid muscle. Internal fistulas most often occur into the second and third pouches. Since the tonsil develops in the region of the second pouch, internal fistulas of the second pouch open into the tonsillar region. Mesenchyme of the second arch gives rise to the muscles of facial expression, the stapedius, posterior belly of the digastric and stylohyoid muscles. It also gives rise to the stapes, styloid process, stylohyoid ligament and lesser cornua of the hyoid bone. The facial nerve runs in the second arch and supplies SVE neurons to the muscles developing from this arch.

The third pharyngeal arch gives rise to the stylopharyngeus muscle supplied by the glossopharyngeal nerve and to the body and greater cornua of the hyoid bone. The entoderm of the dorsal part of the third pharyngeal pouch gives rise to parathyroid III, which will develop further into the parenchyma of the inferior parathyroid gland. The ventral part of the third pharyngeal pouch becomes the thymus gland.

The fourth and sixth arches give rise to the laryngeal cartilages and the pharyngeal, palatal and laryngeal muscles. All of these, except for the tensor veli palatini, are innervated by the vagus (and accessory?) nerve, the recurrent laryngeal branch passing through the sixth arch. The dorsal part of the fourth pharyngeal pouch gives rise to the superior parathyroid gland; the fate of the ventral part is not certain. The fifth (sixth) pharyngeal pouch gives rise to the ultimobranchial body, which may be implicated in the formation of the thyrocalcitonin-producing parafollicular cells of the thyroid gland.

Aortic arches arise from the aortic bulb and enter each branchial arch, where they run chiefly caudal to the cranial nerve of each arch. The first two aortic arches in the mandibular and hyoid arches disappear. The third aortic arch becomes a part of the internal carotid artery. The right fourth arch becomes part of the right subclavian artery, and the left fourth arch becomes the arch of the aorta. The proximal portions of both sixth aortic arches become parts of the pulmonary arteries; the left distal part becomes the ductus arteriosus. Since the recurrent laryngeal is caudal to the sixth aortic arch, retention of the ductus arteriosus as the ligamentum arteriosum accounts for the left recurrent laryngeal looping around the arch of the aorta caudal to the ligament, whereas the right loops higher around the subclavian artery.

The tongue develops from elevations in the floor of the primitive pharynx and by forward migration of developing muscle from occipital somites. The body of the tongue arises from two lateral swellings and a median tuberculum impar in the floor of the mandibular arch. The root of the tongue develops from a copula of mesenchyme of the second, third, and fourth arches. The epiglottic swelling also comes from mesenchyme of the fourth arch. The muscles of the tongue develop from occipital somites and are innervated by somatic efferent (SE) fibers of the hypoglossal nerve. Since the oral membrane, demarcating the ectodermally lined stomodeum from the entodermal primitive pharynx, existed just in front of the fauces, most of the epithelium of the body of the tongue arose from ectoderm while the root and foramen cecum area developed from entoderm. Thus, general sensation of the anterior two-thirds of the tongue is supplied by branches of the trigeminal nerve, whereas the posterior one-third is innervated by the glossopharyngeal nerve. The thyroid gland develops as an evagination from the floor of the pharynx at the level of the first pharyngeal pouch. It migrates caudally to the region of the larynx, leaving the foramen cecum as the site of original evagination and often leaving thyroglossal duct cysts along its migratory course. Thyroglossal duct cysts along its migratory course. Thyroglossal duct cysts can be found in the root of the tongue and in or behind the hyoid bone.

Development of the Face, Nasal Cavity and Oral Cavity. By the sixth week of embryonic development a frontal prominence overhangs the cephalic end of the stomodeum. It is bounded laterally by nasal pits surrounded by horseshoe-shaped elevations. The medial portion of the horseshoe-shaped elevation is the nasomedial process; the lateral portion is the nasolateral process. The nasolateral process is delimited from the maxillary process by the naso-optic (nasolacrimal) furrow. The developing oral cavity is bounded inferiorly by distal fusion of the mandibular processes of the first branchial arch. As the maxillary processes become more prominent they fuse with the nasomedial processes and push them toward the midline; this displaces the frontal prominence upward and leads to fusion of the nasomedial processes in the midline. The fused nasomedial processes (intermaxillary segment) give rise to the medial part of the upper lip, incisor teeth and associated upper jaw and the primary palate (median palatine process). The maxillary process gives rise to the rest of the upper lip, teeth and jaw and the palatine shelves forming the secondary palate. The lower lips, jaw and teeth are formed from the mandibular processes. The nasolacrimal duct is formed at the point of obliteration of the naso-optic furrow by fusion of the nasolateral and maxillary processes. Inability of these processes to fuse leads to an oblique facial cleft. The nasolateral processes give rise to the alae of the nose.

The nasal pits become deeper and break through the bucconasal membrane into the primitive oral cavity. Toward the end of the second embryonic month the palatine shelves (lateral palatine processes) of the maxillary processes grow medially and fuse with the primary palate, rostrally, and with each other and with the inferiorly growing nasal septum, caudally. The lateral palatine processes, thus give rise to a secondary palate which separates the nasal cavity above from the definitive oral cavity below. The caudal free borders of the palatine shelves project as the soft palate into the pharynx, dividing it into an upper nasopharynx and lower oropharynx. Incomplete degeneration of the bucconasal membrane can lead to choanal atresia. Failure of the palatine shelves to fuse in the midline, or to fuse with the primary palate, produce cleft palate. Such clefts can be divided into three groups: (1) those occurring between the palatine shelves and the primary palate (anterior, primary palate types), (2) those occur-

ring posterior to the incisive foramen at the point of fusion of the palatine shelves with each other (posterior, secondary palate types) and, (3) those involving defects in both the anterior and posterior palate (complete unilateral or bilateral types. The anterior and complete types may be associated with cleft lip if the nasomedial and maxillary processes fail to merge (fuse). Median cleft of the upper lip and jaw is due to the lack of fusion of the nasomedial processes with each other.

Development of the Hypophysis. The hypophysis arises from two sources: Rathke's pouch and the infundibulum. Rathke's pouch arises as an evagination of stomodeal ectoderm that pinches off from the stomodeum and migrates toward the diencephalon where it becomes adherent to the rostral surface of the infundibulum. The infundibulum develops as an outgrowth of neural ectoderm from the hypothalamus of the diencephalon. The infundibulum gives rise to the neurohypophysis, i.e., infundibular stalk and pars nervosa (infundibular process). Rathke's pouch develops into the adenohypophysis, i.e., the pars tuberalis, pars intermedia, pars distalis (anterior lobe) and the vestigial lumen.

Central Nervous System and Cranial Nerves

The structure and localization of the spinal cord and spinal nerves were covered previously in the section on the back.

Gross Brain Topography. The brain consists of three basic parts, the cerebral hemispheres (telencephalon), the brain stem and the cerebellum. The cerebral hemispheres and cerebullum cover much of the superior and lateral surface of the brain stem. From the cerebral hemispheres to the spinal cord the brain stem consists of: (1) the diencephalon, (2) the mesencephalon, (3) the metencephalon (pons) and (4) the myelencephalon (medulla). In relation to the skull the frontal and temporal lobes of the cerebral hemispheres lie in the anterior and middle cranial fossae respectively; the cerebellar hemispheres are in the posterior cranial fossa. The diencephalon, mesencephalon and pons rest on the superior surface and clivus of the body of the sphenoid bone, while the medulla occupies a groove on the basilar part of the occipital bone extending from the sphenoid to the foramen magnum. The brain is invested by dura, arachnoid and pia mater.

The dura serves as the periosteum of the skull and also reflects between the cerebral hemispheres in the longitudinal cerebral fissure as the falx cerebri. The falx is continuous posteriorly with another dural reflection, the tentorium cerebelli, lying in the transverse cerebral fissure between the occipital lobe of the telencephalon and the superior surface of the cerebellum. Important venous sinuses are found in the dura. The superior sagittal sinus in the attached margin of the falx cerebri drains to the transverse sinuses at the periphery of the tentorium cerebelli. These in turn drain to the internal jugular veins. An inferior sagittal sinus in the free margin of the falx cerebri and the great vein of Galen from the brain drain to the straight sinus running in the junction of the falx and tentorium. The straight sinus drains to the transverse sinus. An anterior group of sinuses includes the cavernous, intercavernous, superior and inferior petrosal sinuses and basilar plexus.

The arachnoid does not project into the sulci of the telencephalon, and it is separated from the pia by a subarachnoid space. This space is enlarged into subarachnoid cisterna at the cerebellum-medulla junction (cisterna magna), between the cerebral peduncles (interpeduncular cistern), superior and lateral to the midbrain (cisterna ambiens) and at several other areas. Arachnoid granulations, projecting into the superior sagittal sinus, serve as a mechanism for the flow of cerebrospinal fluid from the subarachnoid space into the venous system. The pia is vascular, and the underlying glial membrane blends with the walls of pial blood vessels as they penetrate the brain substance. After branching of blood vessels in the brain, the capillary endothelium, basement membrane and glial processes constitute a blood-brain barrier.

The *cerebral hemispheres* are interconnected by a corpus callosum and an anterior commissure of commissural fibers and by the lamina terminalis, which lies rostral to the third ventricle. Each cerebral hemisphere consists of an outer gray cortex (pallium), and underlying white matter, a deeply located nuclear mass called the basal ganglia, and a lateral ventricle. The cortex and its underlying white matter are thrown into a fairly consistent localization of gyri and sulci that make it possible to define frontal, parietal, temporal, occipital, insular and limbic lobes. The more rostral frontal lobe is separated from the parietal lobe by the central sulcus (of Rolando). In the frontal lobe the precentral gyrus (motor area) borders the central sulcus and is demarcated from the more rostral superior, middle and inferior frontal gyri by the precentral sulcus. On the basal surface the frontal lobe is comprised of an olfactory bulb and tract lying between the gyrus rectus and the orbital gyri. The parietal lobe consists of the more rostral postcentral gyrus (somesthetic area) and the posteriorly located superior and inferior parietal gyri. On the medial aspect the parietal and occipital lobes are divisible by the parieto-occipital sulcus; laterally the boundary is less precise. The lateral fissure (sulcus) helps to form an inferior boundary to the fron-

tal and parietal lobes. It terminates caudally where the inferior parietal gyrus caps it as the supramarginal gyrus. The rest of the inferior parietal gyrus abuts against the posterior extent of the superior temporal gyrus and is called the angular gyrus.

The lateral surface of the occipital lobe consists of lateral occipital gyri. The medial surface is divided by the calcarine fissure into a cuneus above and a lingual gyrus below. That portion of the cortex immediately bordering the calcarine fissure is the striate cortex. The lateral surface of the temporal lobe is comprised of superior, middle and inferior temporal gyri. The transverse temporal gyri (of Heschl) lies medial to the superior temporal gyrus in the floor of the lateral fissure. It is the primary receptive area for hearing. The insula lies deep in the lateral fissure and constitutes a cortical cover to the lenticular nucleus. On the basal surface of the temporal lobe the occipitotemporal gyrus and parahippocampal gyri lie medial to the inferior temporal gyri. The more medial parahippocampal gyrus ends rostrally as the uncus, is bounded laterally by the collateral fissure and medially by the hippocampal fissure and is continuous around the caudal end (splenium) of the corpus callosum with the cingulate gyrus. The rostral part of the parahippocampal gyrus, the uncus and the lateral olfactory stria and gyrus (which project from the olfactory trigone and tract), comprise the primary olfactory receptive area. The limbic lobe consists of the subcallosal, cingulate and parahippocampal gyri, as well as the dentate gyrus and hippocampus, which lie deep to the hippocampal fissure.

The *diencephalon* contains the third ventricle and is divisible into four parts: the roof or epithalamus, the dorsolaterally located thalamus, the floor and ventromedially oriented hypothalamus and the ventrolateral subthalamus. The diencephalon is bounded above by the transverse cerebral fissure. While this fissure extends caudally between the occipital lobe and cerebellum and is occupied by the tentorium cerebelli, rostrally it lies between the corpus callosum and fornix above and the epithalamus (tela choroidea, pineal body, habenula) and thalamus below. It extends laterally and ventrally as the choroid fissures adjacent to the choroid plexuses of the lateral and third ventricles respectively. Rostrally, the transverse cerebral fissure ends blindly where the choroid plexus of the third ventricle is continuous with that of the lateral ventricle in the interventricular foramen (of Monro). The diencephalon is bounded laterally by the internal capsule and the cerebral peduncles. Basally the surface shows anteroposteriorly the optic chiasm, infundibular stalk and pituitary gland and mammillary bodies.

The *mesencephalon* lies between the diencephalon

and pons. Its dorsal surface consists of two superior colliculi, two inferior colliculi, the brachia of these colliculi, which connect to the lateral and medial geniculate nuclei of the diencephalon respectively, and the emerging trochlear (fourth) nerve. Ventrally the mesencephalon demonstrates cerebral peduncles, interpeduncular fossa, and emerging oculomotor (third) nerves. An iter (cerebral aqueduct of Sylvius) connects the third ventricle of the diencephalon with the fourth ventricle in the pons.

The *pons* is bounded above by the attached cerebellum. The lateral surface is made up of the middle cerebellar peduncle with its emerging root of the trigeminal (fifth) nerve. Ventrally, the basis pontis forms a bridge between the middle cerebellar peduncles. On the superior aspect the superior medullary velum, superior cerebellar peduncles and cerebellum form the roof of the fourth ventricle. The tegmentum forms the floor of the ventricle and demonstrates a facial colliculus in the medial eminence located medial to the sulcus limitans.

The upper part of the *medulla* (open medulla) contains a portion of the fourth ventricle. A tela choroidea of pia and ependyma form the roof of this part of the fourth ventricle. The floor is divisible into a medial eminence and a more lateral vestibular area. At the junction of the pons and medulla the fourth ventricle is open laterally with the subarachnoid space through the foramen of Luschka. A midline opening, the foramen of Magendie, is located at the caudalmost tip of the tela choroidea. The dorsal surface of the more inferior closed part of the medulla represents an enlarged upward continuation of the fasciculus cuneatus and fasciculus gracilis of the spinal cord. These areas are referred to as the tuberculum cuneatum and tuberculum gracilis (clava). They lie caudal and lateral to the fourth ventricle.

The ventral surface of the medulla, from the midline laterally, consists of pyramids and pyramidal decussation, preolivary sulcus, olivary eminence and postolivary sulcus. The abducens (sixth) nerve exits at the pons-medulla junction in line with the hypoglossal (twelfth) nerve rootlets, which emerge from the preolivary sulcus. The cranial accessory (eleventh), vagus (tenth) and glossopharyngeal (ninth) nerves exit from the postolivary sulcus. The facial (seventh) and vestibulocochlear (eighth) nerves emerge below the lateral recess of the fourth ventricle at the pons-medulla junction. They are in close anatomic relationship to the inferior cerebellar peduncle (restiform body), which courses below the lateral recess in passing from the medulla to the cerebellum.

Blood Supply to the Brain. The brain is supplied by the vertebral and internal carotid arteries. The vertebral arteries enter the foramen magnum and give off posterior inferior cerebellar and anterior and posterior spinal arteries. The vertebral arteries unite at the pons-medulla junction to form the basilar artery. The basilar artery runs in the basilar sulcus of the pons and terminates at the level of the mesencephalon by branching into posterior cerebral arteries. The basilar gives off the anterior inferior cerebellar, labyrinthine, paramedian, short and long circumferential and superior cerebellar arteries. Branches of the vertebral and basilar arteries supply the cerebellum, mesencephalon, pons, medulla, medial portion of the occipital lobe and part of the temporal lobe and diencephalon.

The internal carotid artery courses through the cavernous sinus and emerges from the sinus medial to the anterior clinoid process. It gives off the ophthalmic artery to the eye; the posterior communicating artery to the posterior cerebral artery; and the anterior choroidal artery, which supplies the optic tract, choroid plexus of the lateral ventricle, basal ganglia, posterior part of the internal capsule and the hippocampus. Lateral to the optic chiasm the internal carotid bifurcates into the middle cerebral and anterior cerebral arteries. The anterior cerebral arteries, connected by an anterior communicating artery, supply the medial surface of the frontal and parietal lobes. The middle cerebral artery passes into the lateral fissure and supplies the insula, lateral surface of the cerebral hemisphere and part of the inferior surface of the temporal lobe. Basal ganglia and part of the internal capsule are supplied by the lenticulostriate branches of the middle cerebral artery. The internal carotid and vertebral arterial supplies are interconnected, forming the circle of Willis, which consists of the anterior communicating, anterior cerebral, posterior communicating and posterior cerebral arteries. Central branches from the circle of Willis supply the basilar portion of the brain stem and basal ganglia and give rise to the hypophyseal portal arterial system of the adenohypophysis.

Superficial and deep cerebral veins drain to the dural venous sinuses. The great cerebral vein (Galen) receives the internal cerebral veins and drains to the straight sinus. Superior, middle and inferior superficial veins drain to the superior sagittal or basal sinuses. The midbrain, pons and medulla drain by small veins into the sinuses at the base of the brain. The cerebellum is drained by superior and inferior cerebellar veins into adjacent dural venous sinuses.

Circulation of Cerebrospinal Fluid. Cerebrospinal fluid is formed by the choroid plexuses of the lateral, third and fourth ventricles. The circulation of the cerebrospinal fluid begins at the lateral ventricles. The fluid passes through the interventricular foramen (of Monro) to the third ventricle and thence through the iter into the fourth ventricle. It passes through the foramina of Luschka and Magendie into the subarachnoid space (cisterna magna) and diffuses into the superior longitudinal sinus through the arachnoid granulations. Internal hydrocephalus may result from blockage of the ventricular pathway and most commonly occurs in the iter. Hydrocephalus resulting from blockage of the subarachnoid space at the tentorial apertures affects all of the ventricles.

Development of the Brain. By the fourth week of embryonic development the neural tube of the cephalic region appears as three vesicles: the prosencephalon, mesencephalon and rhombencephalon. The prosencephalon enlarges into two lateral telencephalic hemispheres and a midline diencephalon by the fifth week. The mesencephalon does not subdivide further, but the rhombencephalon differentiates into a more cephalic metencephalon and a caudal myelencephalon. With the extensive growth of the brain at this period the brain flexes in its confined space. The cephalic flexure occurs between the mesencephalon and metencephalon, the pontine flexure at the metencephalon-myelencephalon junction and the cervical flexure at the junction of the myelencephalon and spinal cord.

In later development, the telencephalic hemispheres enlarge greatly, flex into C-shaped structures and fuse with the lateral wall of the diencephalon at a point that will be occupied later by the posterior limb of the internal capsule. The pontine flexure will become more pronounced and a metencephalic rhombic lip of alar plate material will grow dorsally and develop into the cerebellum. The mantle layers of both the cerebral hemispheres and cerebellum give rise to deep nuclei and migrate peripherally to form the cortical gray material. The deep nuclei of the cerebral hemispheres are the basal ganglia consisting of amygdaloid, caudate, lenticular (putamen and globus pallidus) and claustrum. The deep nuclei of the cerebellum are the dentate, emboliform, globose and fastigial.

In the brain stem, the differentiation of mantle and marginal layers does not result in as distinct a layering of gray and white matter as in the cerebral hemispheres, cerebellum and spinal cord. Individual nuclei and fiber tracts are identifiable, but in many areas nuclei and fibers are interspersed and constitute a reticular formation. In addition to this major organizational difference between the spinal cord and brain stem, the structure of the latter also differs from the cord as a result of: (1) the expansion and thinning out of the roof plate in those areas that develop ventricles, (2) the development of phylogenetically newer structures, (3) the acquisition of cell columns for three new functional components of cranial nerves and (4) the specialization and lack of segmentation that leads to cranial

nerves that do not all have the same functional components.

The cell columns of the brain stem develop from the mantle layer. Those developing from the basal plate are nuclei of origin for motor (efferent) neurons whose axons leave the brain stem in cranial nerves. Those developing from of the alar plate are nuclei of termination on which incoming sensory (afferent) axons will synapse; these nuclei of termination represent cell bodies of association and internuncial neurons. Seven functional components are formed, but no cranial nerve contains all seven. These functional components are: (1) somatic efferent (SE) to skeletal muscles of occipital and eye somite origin, (2) special visceral efferent (SVE) to skeletal muscles of branchial arch origin, (3) general visceral efferent (GVE) to postganglionic parasympathetic ganglia, (4) general visceral afferent (GVA) receiving sensory neurons from visceral structures, (5) special visceral afferent (SVA) receiving neurons from taste and olfactory receptors, (6) general somatic afferent (GSA) from exteroceptive neurons and (7) special somatic afferent (SSA) receiving neurons from the eye and ear.

The cell columns of the brain stem are more discontinuous in their cephalocaudal extent than those of the spinal cord, and their localization corresponds generally to the emergence of the cranial nerves. A notable exception to this is the GSA cell column, which continues upward from the dorsal horn of the spinal cord (as the spinal and chief nuclei of cranial nerve V) to the mid-pons level, receiving trigeminal nerve fibers throughout its extent. There are no cell columns for the olfactory and optic nerves. Thus, the cell columns are limited to the mesencephalon, pons and medulla. The cross-sectional localization of brain stem cell columns differs markedly from those of the spinal cord. Most of this difference is due to the development of the ventricles. It is recalled that in the spinal cord the gray matter is oriented vertically into a dorsal horn (alar plate) and ventral horn (basal plate) lying lateral to the central canal. With the expansion of the central canal into the ventricles of the brain, the roof plate becomes stretched out as the tela choroidea (ependyma plus pia), and the alar plate is displaced lateral to the basal plate. Consequently in the pons and medulla the nuclei of termination transmitting sensory input are located lateral to the nuclei of origin for motor output. The basic sequential localization from the midline laterally is SE, SVE, GVE, GVA, SVA, GSA, SSA. All of the nuclei of these columns in the pons and medulla lie in the floor of the fourth ventricle or near the central canal, with the exception of the SVE column, which migrates ventrolaterally into the reticular formation.

In the phylogenetic development of the central nervous system, the older systems dealing with crude sensibilities and gross axial movements are retained centrally, while the phylogenetically newer structures dealing with discriminatory sensation and with the regulation of finer and more discrete movements are added more ventrolaterally.

The complex topography of the diencephalon and telencephalon and their interrelationships are better appreciated through an understanding of their development. As the ventricles of the diencephalon and telencephalon form, the roof plate of each becomes attenuated as the tela choroidea. Vascularized portions of this pia and ependyma extend into the ventricles as the choroid plexuses of the third and lateral ventricles. These choroid plexuses are continuous with each other at the interventricular foramen. The diencephalon may arise entirely from the alar plate; the optic nerve and retina develop as an evagination of the diencephalon.

The lamina terminalis arises as the most rostral wall of the telencephalon. As the telencephalic hemispheres grow tremendously in size, they grow forward, then backward, circumscribing a C-shaped growth pattern terminating at the temporal pole. The forward growth leaves the lamina terminalis displaced posterior to the frontal pole; the anterior commissure and corpus callosum develop in the lamina terminalis.

The C-shaped growth pattern is reflected in the formation of the anterior horn, body and inferior horn of the lateral ventricle. The caudate nucleus follows this path with its head in the ventral-lateral floor of the anterior horn and its tail extending into the dorsal-lateral wall of the inferior horn of the lateral ventricle. The caudate nucleus ends near the amygdaloid nucleus located just rostral to the inferior horn of the lateral ventricle. These basal ganglia seem to grow around the lenticular nucleus, which is anchored at its point of fusion with the diencephalon. The internal capsule develops in this point of fusion. The insular cortex, anchored to the lenticular nucleus, is overgrown by the extensive peripheral growth of the C-shaped hemisphere. The C-shaped growth is also reflected by the fornix. This structure is a fiber pathway which extends from the hippocampal formation in the temporal lobe to the mammillary bodies in the hypothalamus; it forms the anterior boundary of the interventricular foramen in its route.

Internal Topography of the Brain Stem. The brain stem is an upward continuation of the spinal cord. As each of the higher brain-stem and cortical centers was added to the nervous system in its phylogenetic development, connections between each of the levels were established, older centers at each level were retained, and many parts were traversed by tracts inter-

connecting the cerebral cortex with the spinal cord. In addition to these pathways and centers, central connections with cranial nerves also can be localized at the various brain-stem levels.

Medulla. The lower part of the closed medulla is similar to the spinal cord in that it has a central canal, fasciculus gracilis, fasciculus cuneatus, lateral and anterior spinothalamic tracts, posterior and anterior spinocerebellar tracts, lateral reticulospinal tracts and anterior corticospinal tracts in essentially the same locations as in the spinal cord. The substantia gelatinosa and posterolateral fasciculus continue upward as the spinal nucleus and tract of cranial nerve V respectively. The major difference between the low medulla and spinal cord is that the lateral corticospinal tract is just forming by the decussation of fibers from the pyramids. At this and higher levels there will be more of an admixture of gray matter and fibers in that area that corresponds to the gray matter of the spinal cord.

At higher regions of the closed medulla the ascending axons of the posterior funiculus synapse on cell bodies in the nucleus gracilis and nucleus cuneatus. Since these nuclei are displaced at higher levels by the expanding fourth ventricle, axons from these nuclei arch ventrally around the central canal as the internal arcuate fibers and decussate to form the medial lemniscus. This bundle of ascending fibers represents the axons of second-order neurons for the stereognosis—two-point touch pathway that will traverse the medulla, pons and mesencephalon before synapsing in the ventral posterior lateral nucleus of the thalamus. In the medial lemniscus, fibers carrying impulses from sacral levels are localized just above the pyramid, while fibers representing cervical levels are located more dorsally just below the MLF.

The inferior olivary nucleus occupies the ventral part of the medulla lateral to the medial lemniscus and pyramids. The vestibulospinal tract runs dorsal to the inferior olivary nucleus. The spinothalamic and spinocerebellar tracts lie along the lateral margin of the medulla in the postolivary sulcus region.

The hypoglossal nucleus (SE) extends throughout most of the medulla and lies dorsal to the MLF. Lateral to it is the dorsal motor nucleus (GVE) of the vagus. Axons from the hypoglossal nucleus pass ventrally and exit in the preolivary sulcus. Axons from the dorsal motor nucleus course laterally and exit from the postolivary sulcus. General visceral afferent and SVA fibers, which enter the brain stem in the vagus nerve and at higher levels in the glossopharyngeal and facial nerves, descend in the fasciculus solitarius and terminate on the cells of the nucleus solitarius and dorsal sensory nucleus of the vagus lying adjacent to the fasciculus. In the closed medulla the fasciculus and nucleus solitarius lie dorsal to the dorsal motor nucleus of cranial nerve X, and at open-medulla levels they lie lateral to the motor nuclei.

In the open medulla the hypoglossal and vagal nuclei form prominences in the floor of the fourth ventricle medial to the sulcus limitans. The sensory nuclei, i.e., the nucleus solitarius (GVA and SVA), vestibular nuclei (SSA), and spinal nucleus of cranial nerve V (GSA), lie lateral to the sulcus limitans. At high-medulla levels the vestibular nuclei (SSA) lie dorsomedial to the spinal nucleus and form a vestibular area in the floor of the fourth ventricle lateral to the sulcus limitans. At the level of the lateral recess, cochlear nuclei (SSA) form the most lateral prominence in the floor of the fourth ventricle. The nucleus ambiguus (SVE) is located in the reticular formation halfway between the spinal nucleus of cranial nerve V and the inferior olivary nucleus. Axons from this nucleus loop dorsomedially before exiting laterally in the vagus, accessory and glossopharyngeal nerves. Lateral to the spinal tract of cranial nerve V is the inferior cerebellar peduncle. It consists of the posterior spinocerebellar tract, olivocerebellar fibers from the contralateral inferior olivary nucleus, cuneocerebellar fibers from the accessory cuneate nucleus and some other ascending and reticular connections. The reticular formation is divisible into medial and lateral groups of nuclei. The lateral groups are sensory in that they receive ascending sensory information. The lateral small-celled area is associated with respiratory responses and is where the pressor center is located. The medial gigantocellular nucleus gives rise to the lateral reticulospinal tract and is inhibitory to antigravity muscles. This and adjacent medial nuclei constitute centers involved in respiratory and depressor circulatory responses. An ascending reticular activating system of multisynaptic connections arises primarily from the medial nuclei of the reticular formation.

Pons. The pons is divisible into a dorsal tegmentum and a ventral phylogenetically newer basis pontis. The tegmentum is an upward continuation of the medulla. It differs from the medulla in that the inferior olivary nucleus disappears and a central tegmental tract is located in its place; the medial lemniscus is oriented horizontally in the basal part of the tegmentum; the spinothalamic tracts are located at the lateral tip of the medial lemniscus; the corticospinal tracts are in the basis pointis and not in pyramids and cell columns and pathways relating to cranial nerves V to VIII are present.

At the pons-medulla junction the inferior cerebellar peduncle passes ventral to the lateral recess of the fourth ventricle before entering the cerebellum. At this location dorsal and ventral cochlear nuclei lie dorso-laterally and ventrally, the spinal tract and nucleus of cranial nerve V are medial, and the vestibular nuclei are dorsomedial to the inferior cerebellar peduncle. The cochlear nuclei receive axons of the bipolar neurons of the spiral cochlear ganglion. Axons from the cochlear nuclei pass medially through the tegmentum to ascend contralaterally and ipsilaterally just lateral to the spinothalamic tracts as the lateral lemniscus. Some of the axons of this pathway synapse in the superior olivary nucleus and nucleus of the lateral lemniscus before terminating in the inferior colliculus. The superior olivary nucleus lies dorsal to the spinothalamic tracts in the ventrolateral tegmentum. The vestibular nuclei receive axons from bipolar neurons of the vestibular ganglion and from the cerebellum. They send axons to the cerebellum, to the center for lateral gaze, to the oculomotor nuclei and spinal cord via the MLF, and into the spinal cord as the lateral vestibulospinal tract.

The basis pontis contains the corticospinal (pyramidal) tract, cortiobulbar (corticonuclear) fibers to cranial nerve motor nuclei, and corticopontine fibers that terminate on pontine nuclei. Axons of the pontine nuclei cross the midline and pass laterally and dorsally into the cerebellum as the middle cerebellar peduncle.

In lower pontine levels the facial (SVE) nucleus occupies the ventrolateral tegmentum. Axons from this nucleus course dorsomedially and superiorly and loop around the abducens nucleus before passing ventrolaterally and inferiorly to exit at the pons-medulla junction. The loop (internal genu) of the facial nerve and the adjacent abducens nucleus form an abducens (facial) colliculus in the floor of the fourth ventricle. Axons from the abducens (SE) nucleus pass ventrally and inferiorly to exit at the pons-medulla junction. A parabducens group of cell bodies representing a center for lateral gaze lies inferior to the MLF in the pontine paramedian reticular formation (PPRF). Superior and inferior salivatory nuclei, containing the cell bodies of parasympathetic preganglionic nerves of the facial and glossopharyngeal nerves respectively, occupy the tegmentum but are not sharply localized.

At mid-pons levels, the trigeminal nerve penetrates the middle cerebellar peduncle and runs to the lateral tegmentum. General somatic afferent fibers of this nerve, whose cell bodies are located in the trigeminal ganglion, terminate in the principal (chief, main) sensory nucleus and spinal nucleus of cranial nerve V. The principal sensory nucleus is the upward continuation of the spinal nucleus and receives touch fibers. Axons from this nucleus cross and ascend in the ventral secondary tract of cranial nerve V, running adjacent to the medial lemniscus, and terminate in the ventral posterior medial (VPM) nucleus of the thalamus. Some axons from the principal sensory nucleus ascend uncrossed to the VPM nucleus as the dorsal secondary tract of cranial nerve V running lateral to the MLF. Some entering touch fibers of the trigeminal nerve bifurcate and send descending branches to the upper part of the spinal nucleus of cranial nerve V. Pain fibers enter in the trigeminal nerve, descend as the spinal tract of cranial nerve V and terminate on cell bodies of the spinal nucleus of cranial nerve V. Axons from the spinal nucleus of cranial nerve V cross the midline and ascend in the ventral secondary tract of cranial nerve V. The motor (SVE) nucleus of cranial nerve V lies medial to the chief sensory nucleus of cranial nerve V. Its axons emerge from the pons in the motor root (portio minor) of the trigeminal nerve. A mesencephalic nucleus of cranial nerve V of unipolar neurons extends into the mesencephalon from midpons levels. It lies next to the lateral portion of the central gray material and represents the first-order neurons of a proprioceptive pathway of the fifth nerve. Thus, these cells are unique in that they are sensory ganglion cells that did not end up in ganglia but were retained in the brain stem during development of the neural tube.

At upper pons levels, the fourth ventricle narrows as the isthmus region of the pons-mesencephalon junction is approached. The superior medullary velum and superior cerebellar peduncles form the roof and lateral walls of the pons. In the region of the isthmus, the superior cerebellar peduncles move ventrally into the tegmentum. The fibers of these peduncles will decussate in the tegmentum of the mesencephalon and will ascend to the red nucleus and ventral lateral nucleus of the thalamus.

The reticular formation of the pons is an upward continuation of that in the medulla. The caudal and oral pontine reticular nuclei give rise to the pontine (medial) reticulospinal tract, which is facilitory to antigravity muscles. The main ascending pathway of the reticular formation is the central tegmental tract.

Mesencephalon. The mesencephalon is divided at the level of the cerebral aqueduct into a dorsal tectum and into two ventral cerebral peduncles. The tectum consists of two superior colliculi and two inferior colliculi. Each cerebral peduncle is subdivided into a dorsal tegmentum and a ventral crus cerebri by the substantia nigra.

At the inferior colliculus level axons of the lateral lemniscus terminate in the inferior colliculus. Fibers from this relay nucleus of the hearing pathway pass laterally into the brachium of the inferior colliculus and synapse on cells of the medial geniculate body which, in turn, send axons to the transverse temporal gyrus (of Heschl). The mesencephalic nucleus and root

and the nucleus pigmentosus lie ventral to the inferior colliculi in the lateral extent of the central gray. In the dorsomedial limits of the tegmentum the trochlear nucleus nestles in the dorsal surface of the MLF. Below the MLF fibers of the superior cerebellar peduncle decussate before passing upward toward the red nucleus; the medial lemniscus, secondary tracts of cranial nerve V and spinothalamics lie ventral and lateral to this decussation. Axons from the trochlear nucleus course dorsally in the central gray, decussate in the superior medullary velum and exit below the inferior colliculi. The crus cerebri contains the corticopontine, corticobulbar and corticospinal pathways. Corticobulbar and corticospinal fibers occupy the middle third of the crus.

The most significant features of the superior colliculus levels are the superior colliculi, oculomotor nuclear complex and nerves, and the red nucleus. The superior colliculus receives optic fibers from the optic tract and occipital cortex via the brachium of the superior colliculus. This brachium runs between the lateral geniculate body and the superior colliculus just below the pulvinar of the thalamus. The oculomotor nuclear complex consists of the oculomotor (SE) and Edinger-Westphal (GVE) nuclei, which are located medial to the MLF. The oculomotor nerve passes ventrally to exit medial to the crus cerebri in the interpeduncular fossa. Somatic efferent axons innervate the medial rectus, superior and inferior recti and inferior oblique muscles. Preganglionic parasympathetic axons from the Edinger-Westphal nucleus run to the ciliary ganglion where they synapse on postganglionic neurons that innervate the sphincter pupillae and ciliary muscles. The red nucleus lies in the ventromedial tegmentum and is surrounded by dentatothalamic axons of the superior cerebellar peduncle that are going to the ventral lateral nucleus of the thalamus. Some axons of the superior cerebellar peduncle synapse on cells of the red nucleus. The red nucleus also receives corticorubral fibers. Major efferent paths from the red nucleus are the rubrothalamic to the ventral lateral thalamic nucleus and the rubrospinal, which is a crossed pathway to anterior horn cells innervating the antagonists of antigravity muscles.

The pretectal area at the junction with the diencephalon is considered part of the mesencephalon. Features of this area are the pretectal nuclei, posterior commissure and subcommissural organ. Pretectal nuclei lie rostral to the superior colliculi, receive optic tract axons via the brachium of the superior colliculi and send crossed and uncrossed axons to the Edinger-Westphal nucleus. The pretectal nuclei constitute the association limb of the pupillary light reflex. The crossing fibers of this reflex either pass through the posterior commissure, or decussate in the central gray below the cerebral aqueduct. The posterior commissure lies dorsal to the cerebral aqueduct at the level where it joins the third ventricle. The subcommissural organ is modified ependyma located beneath the posterior commissure. The columnar ciliated cells of this organ may secrete aldosterone and may serve as a volume receptor.

Diencephalon. The diencephalon consists of an epithalamus, thalamus, hypothalamus and subthalamus. The epithalamus is in the roof of the third ventricle and is composed of the tela choroidea, striae medullares, habenular trigones and pineal gland. The stria medullaris conveys fibers from the septal and preoptic area to the habenular nuclei. Axons from the habenular nuclei pass to the mesencephalon through the fasciculus retroflexus.

The thalamus is bounded laterally by the posterior limb of the internal capsule and medially by the third ventricle. It extends anteroposteriorly from the interventricular foramen to the pretectal area, and it lies above the hypothalamus and subthalamus. The thalamus is separated into medial, lateral and anterior nuclear groups by the internal medullary lamina. The medial group nuclei are the midline and dorsomedial nuclei. The midline nuclei make connections with the hypothalamus. The dorsomedial nucleus receives afferents from the amygdaloid nucleus, hypothalamus and temporal cortex and sends axons to the prefrontal cortex. Intralaminar nuclei receive spinothalamic fibers and reticulothalamics from the reticular activating system. The centromedian nucleus is an intralaminar nucleus that receives fibers from the motor cortex (area 4) and globus pallidus and sends axons to the putamen. The lateral group of thalamic nuclei are divisible into a ventral tier and a dorsal tier. The ventral tier consists of the ventral anterior, ventral lateral and ventral posterior (VPL and VPM) nuclei. All of these ventral tier nuclei are relay nuclei. The VPL nucleus receives the medial lemniscus and spinothalamics. The VPM receives secondary ascending trigeminal pathways. Axons from both nuclei pass into the posterior limb of the internal capsule and terminate in the great somesthetic area (postcentral gyrus, area 3, 1, 2), those from VPM terminating closer to the more ventral portion of the postcentral gyrus than those from the VPL. Some axons from the VPL and VPM nuclei terminate in somatic sensory area II located in the parietal lobe above the lateral fissure. The ventral lateral nucleus receives dentatothalamic fibers and pallidothalamic fibers. The latter fibers arise from cells in the medial aspect of the globus pallidus and pass through the fasciculus lenticularis to reach the prerubral field. From here they loop laterally over the zone incerta

to enter the thalamus via the thalamic fasciculus. The ventral anterior nucleus receives pallidothalamic fibers via this same pathway. The dorsal tier nuclei are the lateral dorsal, lateral posterior and pulvinar. These nuclei are association nuclei and have interconnections with the parietal cortex. The pulvinar receives fibers from the metathalamus (medial and lateral geniculate bodies) and sends axons to the parastriate (area 18) and peristriate (area 19) areas in the occipital cortex and also to the inferior parietal cortex. The anterior nucleus of the thalamus relays mammillothalamic impulses from the mammillary bodies to the cingulate gyrus.

The subthalamus lies ventral to the thalamus between the hypothalamus and posterior limb of the internal capsule. It consists of the subthalamic nucleus, zona incerta, fasciculus lenticularis, prerubral field (of Forel) and the fasciculus thalamicus. The subthalamic nucleus lies on the internal capsule and substantia nigra and is separated form the zona incerta above by the fasciculus lenticularis. It has interconnections with the globus pallidus. Lesions of this nucleus produce hemiballism contralaterally.

The hypothalamus consists of groups of nuclei in the floor of the third ventricle. The nuclei are divided into medial and lateral groups by the fornix as it passes through the hypothalamus on its way to the mammillary body. The lateral group includes the lateral and tuberal nuclei. The medial group is subdivided anatomically into three groups: (1) anterior group, which includes the preoptic, anterior, supraoptic and paraventricular nuclei; (2) middle group, containing the dorsomedial and ventromedial nuclei, and (3) posterior group of posterior and mammillary nuclei.

The hypothalamic nuclei can also be grouped on the basis of their functional connections into autonomic, neuroendocrine and olfactory groups. The anteromedial hypothalamic group of nuclei generally are concerned with parasympathetic regulation, whereas the posterolateral group is more involved in sympathetic regulation. Both nuclear groups receive ascending GVA, GSA, and SVA (taste) input from the reticular formation and send out descending central autonomics to preganglionic neurons via reticulospinal and reticuloreticular pathways. These regions also receive olfactory input from the amygdaloid and septal areas and have interconnections with the thalamus, prefrontal cortex and limbic lobe.

The neuroendocrine nuclei are the supraoptic and paraventricular group, which produce posterior pituitary hormones, and a hypophysiotrophic group, which produce adenohypophyseal releasing factors. Axons of supraoptic and paraventricular neurons carry neurosecretory material in membrane-bound vesicles through the infundibular stem to the pars nervosa where the axons terminate in close association with capillaries. The neurosecretory material from supraoptic and paraventricular nuclei represents the antidiuretic (vasopressin) hormone or its precursor; oxytocin is also produced by cells of these nuclei. Cells of the hypophysiotrophic area are in nuclei in the median eminence region. Axons from these cells terminate near, and empty releasing factors into, the capillaries of the hypophyseal portal system in the pituitary stalk. The releasing factors are carried to the pars distalis where they bring about the release of anterior pituitary hormones.

The mammillary, preoptic and lateral hypothalamic nuclei receive input from the olfactory cortex. These nuclei have reciprocal connections with the limbic lobe and also project to other hypothalamic and brain stem nuclei.

Summary of Cranial Nerves. The *first (olfactory) nerve* is comprised of the central processes of bipolar olfactory cells (SVA) whose cell bodies are located in the olfactory epithelium on the upper part of the nasal septum and the lateral nasal wall. These unmyelinated fibers (fila olfactoria) pass into the anterior cranial fossa through the lamina cribrosa of the ethmoid bone and enter the olfactory bulb. After synapse with the mitral cells of the bulb the impulses travel in the olfactory tract to the lateral olfactory stria and terminate in the pyriform lobe. The pyriform lobe is the cortical receptive area for olfaction; it consists of the lateral olfactory stria, the uncus (periamygdaloid area) and the anterior part of the parahippocampal gyrus.

The *second (optic) nerve* is formed by the central processes of the retinal ganglion cells (SSA), which converge at the optic papilla. After piercing the sclera, the optic nerve passes through the orbital fat, traverses the optic foramen and joins with its opposite fellow to form the optic chiasma. The visual pathway from retina to occipital cortex consists of four orders of neurons. The first-order neurons are the rods and cones. The second-order neurons are bipolar cells, and the third-order neurons are ganglion cells. Axons of the ganglion cells comprise the optic nerve, chiasm and tract and terminate in the lateral geniculate body. Those axons from the nasal half of the retina decussate in the optic chiasm; those from the temporal half of the retina remain uncrossed. Thus the optic tract consists of axons from the temporal half of the ipsilateral eye and the nasal half of the contralateral eye. The fourth-order neurons are located in the lateral geniculate nucleus. Axons of these cells pass into the sublenticular and retrolenticular portion of the internal capsule, loop over the roof of the inferior horn of the lateral ventricle and course posteriorly as the optic

radiations to the striate cortex (area 17) located above and below the calcarine fissure in the occipital lobe. This pathway is also referred to as the geniculocalcarine tract.

Lesions in the visual pathway give rise to deficits in the visual fields and some loss of visual reflexes. Since light rays from specific portions of the visual field project to opposite parts of the retinal fields, lesions in the nasal retinal field will result in loss of vision in the temporal visual field while damage to the upper retinal field will demonstrate blindness in the lower visual field. In recalling the topographic distribution of fibers in the pathway, it is readily apparent that: (1) lesions in front of the chiasma lead to blindness (anopsia), or partial blindness, on the side of the damaged optic nerve or retina; (2) midline lesions of the optic chiasm result in bitemporal heteronymous hemianopsia; and (3) lesions of the pathway posterior to the chiasm give homonymous hemianopsias (or quadrantic anopsias) to the side opposite to that of the lesion.

When light is shone into one eye, the ipsilateral pupil will constrict (direct response) and the contralateral pupil will constrict (consensual response). The afferent limb of this pupillary light reflex consists of rods and cones → bipolar cells → ganglion cells whose axons pass through the brachium of the superior colliculus to the pretectal area. The association limb is comprised of neurons of the pretectal nucleus that send axons ipsilaterally, and contralaterally (via the posterior commissure or central gray) to the Edinger-Westphal nucleus. The efferent limb of the pupillary light reflex involves innervation of the sphincter pupillae muscles by a pathway involving the preganglionic neurons of both Edinger-Westphal nuclei and oculomotor nerves, and the postganglionic neurons of both ciliary ganglia. Section of one optic nerve results in blindness in that eye and loss of direct and consensual pupillary light response when light is shone into the blind eye. When light is shone into the other eye the direct and consensual responses are intact. Damage to an oculomotor nerve results in loss of pupillary constriction in that eye regardless of which eye is stimulated.

When a person focuses on a near object after focusing on a far object three responses take place: (1) convergence of the eyes by contraction of the medial recti muscles, (2) pupillary constriction by contraction of the sphincter pupillae muscles and (3) rounding of the lens due to constriction of the ciliary muscle. This reflex is referred to as the near reflex (accommodation-convergence-pupillary reflex). There are two notable distinctions between this reflex and the pupillary light reflex: (1) the pathway involves cortical connections and (2) the efferent limb involves both somatic efferent and general visceral efferent parasympathetic components. The afferent limb involves rods and cones → bipolar cells → ganglion cells → lateral geniculate nucleus → area 17. The association limb consists of connections from area 17 → area 18 (parastriate) → area 19 (peristriate) and its corticomesencephalic axons to the oculomotor complex. The efferent limb involves the oculomotor and Edinger-Westphal nuclei, the oculomotor nerves and the ciliary ganglia and nerves.

In the reflexes involving the turning of the head and eyes in response to visual impulses, there are cortical connections that project to centers for vertical gaze in the midbrain reticular formation and lateral gaze in the pons tegmental reticular nuclei. The lateral conjugate gaze center and pathways will be discussed further in the section on the abducens nerve. The association limb for reflex turning of the head probably relays through the superior colliculus and tectospinal tract to anterior horn cells and spinal accessory neurons in the cervical cord.

The *third (oculomotor) nerve* contains both somatic efferent and general visceral efferent parasympathetic fibers. These fibers arise from the oculomotor (SE) and Edinger-Westphal (GVE) nuclei of the midbrain, run ventrally through the tegmentum and emerge on the medial aspect of the cerebral peduncles. The third nerve traverses the cavernous sinus and enters the orbital cavity through the superior orbital fissure. Preganglionic neurons terminate on postganglionic cells of the ciliary ganglion. Axons of the postganglionic cells run as short ciliary nerves and innervate the sphincter pupillae and ciliary muscles. Somatic efferent fibers supply the levator palpebrae superioris, the superior, inferior and medial recti and the inferior oblique muscles.

Damage to the oculomotor nerve results in several characteristic symptoms. Ptosis (drooping of the upper eyelid) occurs as a result of denervation of the levator palpebrae superioris; the pupil is dilated, since the dilator pupillae is unopposed by the sphincter pupillae; and the direct and consensual responses of the pupillary light reflex are lost. The ciliary muscle is paralyzed and accommodation is impaired. Denervation of the extrinsic muscles results in external strabismus due to unopposed action of the lateral rectus and superior oblique muscles.

The *fourth (trochlear) nerve* arises from the trochlear nucleus (SE) at the inferior colliculus levels. Axons of these cells pass dorsally around the cerebral aqueduct, decussate with fibers of the opposite side and emerge as the fourth nerve at the superior medullary velum. The fourth nerve passes ventrally around the brain stem, traverses the cisterna basalis and the cavernous sinus and enters the orbit through the superior

orbital fissure. It supplies the superior oblique muscle, which intorts the eye when abducted, and depresses the eye when adducted.

The *fifth (trigeminal) nerve* contains both general somatic afferent fibers and special visceral efferent fibers. The motor fibers arise from the motor nucleus of cranial nerve V in the pons and emerge laterally from the middle cerebral peduncle in the motor root of the trigeminal nerve. The motor root passes beneath the trigeminal ganglion, exists the skull through the foramen ovale and joins sensory fibers to form the mandibular nerve. Motor branches of the mandibular nerve innervate the muscles of mastication and tensor tympani and tensor veli palatini muscles. Sensory pseudounipolar neurons have their cell bodies located in the trigeminal ganglion. They distribute their functional dendrites over the ophthalmic, maxillary and mandibular nerves and send axons to the pons as the sensory root of cranial nerve V. Upon entering the pons, the fibers from pain and temperature receptors descend as the spinal tract of cranial nerve V to terminate in its spinal nucleus. Touch fibers end in the principal sensory nucleus and in the upper part of the spinal nucleus of the fifth nerve. Crossed secondary fibers for pain, temperature and touch ascend as the ventral secondary tract of the fifth nerve to the VPM nucleus. Some touch fibers ascend ipsilaterally in the dorsal secondary tract to the VPM nucleus. Third-order neurons of the VPM nucleus send axons to the postcentral gyrus.

The cell bodies of proprioceptive fibers are located in the mesencephalic nucleus of cranial nerve V. The location of pathways to the cerebral cortex and cerebellum from this nucleus has not been completely established.

The ophthalmic nerve passes from the semilunar ganglion in the wall of the cavernous sinus through the superior orbital fissure. In the superior orbital fissure it breaks up into three terminal branches: (1) the frontal nerve with supraorbital, frontal and supratrochlear branches, (2) the lacrimal nerve and (3) the nasociliary nerve.

The maxillary nerve arises from the anterior border of the trigeminal ganglion, traverses the wall of the cavernous sinus and passes into the pterygopalatine fossa through the foramen rotundum. From the pterygopalatine fossa the nerve enters the orbit through the inferior orbital fissure and becomes the infraorbital nerve. This nerve passes into the infraorbital canal, where it gives off superior alveolar nerves, and emerges at the infraorbital foramen to supply the face through inferior palpebral, external nasal and superior labial branches. Major branches in the pterygopalatine fossa are: (1) zygomatic nerve, which supplies the skin of the side of the forehead and cheek, and communicates postganglionic parasympathetic fibers from the pterygopalatine ganglion to the lacrimal nerve, and (2) pterygopalatine nerves, which supply the posterior superior nasal cavity, nasopharynx, palate, orbit and posterior upper teeth. A middle meningeal nerve arises from the maxillary nerve near its origin and passes with the middle meningeal artery to the dura mater.

The mandibular division supplies the muscles of mastication and is sensory to the lower teeth, gums, mandible, tongue, lower lip, lower part of the face, and the skin of the auricula and temporal region. Just outside the foramen ovale it gives off a meningeal branch, which enters the skull through the foramen spinosum, and a medial pterygoid nerve supplying the medial pterygoid muscle and otic ganglion. Beyond these branches, the mandibular nerve divides into anterior and posterior divisions. The anterior division gives off motor branches to the temporalis, masseter and lateral pterygoid muscles and gives off a sensory buccal branch to the mucous membrane and skin of the cheek. The posterior division is mainly sensory and has several major branches: (1) the auriculotemporal whose roots encircle the middle meningeal artery and carry sensory fibers to the temporal and ear regions as well as postganglionic parasympathetic fibers to the parotid gland from the otic ganglion, (2) the inferior alveolar supplying the mylohyoid muscle, lower teeth, lower lip and chin, (3) the lingual nerve supplying the mucosa of the anterior two thirds of the tongue with GSA exteroceptive fibers of the fifth nerve and with SVA taste fibers of the facial nerve, the latter entering the lingual nerve via the chorda tympani nerve.

Lesions of the trigeminal nerve result in exteroceptive deficits of pain, temperature and touch in the areas supplied by the damaged components. Lesions of the ophthalmic division result in loss of the afferent limb of the corneal blink reflex. Thus, damage to one ophthalmic nerve produces loss of the direct and consensual blink. If the efferent limb, mediated by the facial nerve, were damaged and the ophthalmic was intact then stimulation of the cornea would result in blink of only that eye that had an intact seventh nerve. Lesion to the mandibular nerves could result in deviation of the jaw to the affected side upon opening of the jaws.

The *sixth (abducens) nerve* leaves the brain at the posterior border of the pons, traverses the cavernous sinus, enters the orbit through the superior orbital fissure and innervates the lateral rectus muscle. This nerve arises from SE cell bodies in the floor of the fourth ventricle at the facial colliculus level of the pons. The abducens nucleus receives afferents from the ipsilateral lateral gaze center (parabducens nucleus, pon-

tine paramedian reticular formation) located near the abducens nucleus below the MLF. Other axons from the lateral gaze center cross the midline and ascend in the contralateral medial longitudinal fasciculus to reach cells of the oculomotor nucleus that innervate the contralateral medial rectus muscle. Thus, stimulation of neurons in the pontine paramedian reticular formation results in conjugate deviation of the eyes to the side stimulated, since the ipsilateral abducens and lateral rectus, and contralateral oculomotor and medial rectus are activated. The abducens and oculomotor nuclei also are supplied by fibers that course through the MLF from vestibular nuclei and superior colliculi.

Section of the abducens nerve may lead to medial deviation (strabismus) of the affected eye since the medial rectus is unopposed. There is diplopia and inability to turn the eye laterally. Lesion of the abducens nucleus area often involves both the abducens and lateral gaze center. In this type of lesion there is inability for both eyes to look laterally toward the side of the lesion, and there is a tendency for persistent conjugate deviation toward the opposite side.

The *seventh (facial) nerve* contains GSA, SVA (taste), GVA, SVE and GVE functional components. General somatic afferent fibers arise from receptors in a small area near the external ear, pass to pseudounipolar cell bodies in the geniculate ganglion and course into the pons at the pons-medulla junction to terminate in the spinal nucleus of cranial nerve V. Special visceral afferent fibers arise from taste buds in the anterior two thirds of the tongue and traverse the lingual nerve and chorda tympani to reach the geniculate ganglion. Axons of these cells enter the pons and descend in the fasciculus solitarius to end in the upper part of the solitary (gustatory) nucleus. General visceral afferents arise from the submandibular, sublingual, lacrimal, nasal and minor salivary glands. Their cell bodies are in the geniculate ganglion, and their axons terminate in the nucleus solitarius. General visceral efferent preganglionic parasympathetic neurons arise in the superior salivatory nucleus of the pons and are distributed to the (1) pterygopalatine ganglion by way of the greater superficial petrosal nerve, and (2) to the submandibular ganglion via the chorda tympani and lingual nerves. Postganglionic fibers from the pterygopalatine ganglion supply the lacrimal gland and the small glands of the pharynx, palate and nasal cavity. Postganglionics leaving the submandibular ganglion supply the submandibular, sublingual and minor oral salivary glands. Special visceral efferent neurons arise in the facial motor nucleus, form an internal genu around the abducens nucleus, emerge in the facial nerve at the pons-medulla junction and are distributed through numerous branches to the muscles of facial expression, the stapedius muscle, posterior belly of the digastric muscle and stylohyoid muscle.

The facial nerve leaves the pons as two roots: (1) the motor root and, (2) the nervus intermedius. The latter nerve contains taste and parasympathetic fibers. Both roots enter the internal acoustic meatus with the vestibulocochlear nerve. At the fundus of the meatus, the facial nerve enters the facial canal in the petrous portion of the temporal bone. Near the tympanic cavity it bends (external genu) posteriorly above the oval window and descends to exit at the stylomastoid foramen. The geniculate ganglion is located at the bend, and the greater superficial petrosal nerve branches from this region. The nerve to the stapedius muscle and chorda tympani arise from the nerve while it is in the facial canal. The chorda tympani courses through the bone, enters the posterior wall of the tympanum and passes anteriorly between the mucous membrane medially and the tympanic membrane and manubrium of the malleus laterally. It exits anteriorly from the tympanum, emerges from the skull and joins the lingual nerve. That portion of the facial nerve exiting from the stylomastoid foramen divides into posterior auricular, digastric, stylohyoid, temporal, zygomatic, buccal, mandibular and cervical branches.

Lesions of the facial nerve (such as in Bell's palsy) result in weakness to all of the facial muscles ipsilateral to the lesion. This is distinct from lesions of the upper motor neurons (corticobulbar tract), which bilaterally innervate that part of the facial nucleus supplying the upper facial muscles but only contralaterally supply cells to the lower face. Thus, in upper motor neuron lesions there is weakness to the contralateral lower face. Peripheral nerve lesions also may result in (1) loss of taste in the anterior two thirds of the tongue, (2) impaired lacrimation and, (3) hyperacusis due to loss of the dampening affect of the stapedius muscle.

The *eighth (vestibulocochlear) nerve* is a special somatic afferent nerve arising from receptors for hearing in the cochlear duct and arising from the maculae and cristae of the vestibular apparatus. It is comprised of the processes of bipolar cells whose cell bodies lie in the spiral cochlear ganglion and vestibular ganglion. Axons of these cells run in the internal acoustic meatus and enter the pons at the pons-medulla junction.

Cochlear fibers synapse in the dorsal and ventral cochlear nuclei. From these nuclei axons pass bilaterally, synapsing in the superior olivary nucleus, nucleus of the lateral lemniscus and inferior colliculus. From the inferior colliculus axons pass to the medial geniculate nucleus where impulses are relayed to the transverse temporal gyrus (of Heschl). Lesions of one nerve result in deafness to that ear. Unilateral lesions of the central pathway lead to a diminution in hearing due to the bilateral representation.

Entering vestibular fibers may pass directly to the flocculonodular lobe of the cerebellum or synapse on vestibular nuclei. The vestibular pathway to consciousness is not known. There are reflex connections from vestibular nuclei to the spinal cord (via the MLF and vestibulospinal tract), to the center for lateral conjugate gaze and to motor nuclei of the brain stem reticular formation. Some of these connections are better appreciated when the pathways involving reflex activities that accompany angular rotation of the head are considered. When the head is first rotated to the right the endolymph of both horizontal semicircular canals does not move initially as fast as the cristae ampullares. This gives a relative displacement of endolymph to the left although endolymph is actually moving to the right. After rotation the cristae stop moving, but there is continued brief movement of endolymph to the right in the direction of rotation. Since stimulation of cristae of the horizontal canal toward the utricle results in depolarization of the hair cells, an imbalance occurs during rotation and postrotation between the two canals. In postrotation to the right the left vestibular nerve is stimulated while the right vestibular nerve is being inhibited. This results in rapid alternating eye movements (nystagmus). The pathway for the slow component of nystagmus in postrotation to the right involves the left vestibular nerve, left vestibular nuclei, right lateral gaze center, right abducens nucleus and nerve, left MLF and oculomotor nucleus and nerve. In this pathway axons from vestibular nuclei may ascend in the MLF to reach the oculomotor nucleus and cross to the opposite abducens nucleus, or they may go to the opposite lateral gaze center, which in turn, makes connections with the abducens and oculomotor nuclei. Accompanying past-pointing and a tendency to fall to the right are mediated through connections of the left vestibular nucleus with the cerebellum and through connections of the left vestibulospinal tract with anterior horn cells of antigravity muscles. Nausea, increased salivation and vomiting are mediated through connections of the vestibular nuclei with such motor nuclei as the dorsal motor nucleus of cranial nerve X, the nucleus ambiguus, the salivatory nuclei and other reticular nuclei.

The *ninth (glossopharyngeal) nerve* contains GSA, SVA (taste), GVA, SVE and GVE functional components. General somatic afferent fibers arise from skin receptors in the posterior part of the external auditory meatus and auricula. These fibers are distributed in the auricular branch of the vagus. They pass to the glossopharyngeal near the jugular foramen and the pseudounipolar cell bodies of these GSA neurons are located in the superior ganglion in the jugular foramen. Axons of these cells enter the upper medulla, in the postolivary sulcus, and synapse on cells of the spinal nucleus of cranial nerve V.

Special visceral afferent fibers arise from taste buds in the posterior one third of the tongue. They pass through lingual branches and their cell bodies are in the inferior ganglion. Axons terminate in the solitary (gustatory) nucleus. General visceral afferent fibers arise in the mucosa and glands of the posterior tongue, fauces and pharynx. Their cell bodies are located in the inferior ganglion and their axons terminate in the solitary nucleus. The carotid sinus nerve of the glossopharyngeal conveys GVA fibers from the carotid sinus to the nucleus solitarius. Axons from this nucleus course to the dorsal motor nucleus of cranial nerve X, where they synapse on neurons whose fibers pass into the vagus nerve and constitute the efferent limb of the carotid sinus reflex.

Special visceral efferent fibers arise in the nucleus ambiguus and pass through the glossopharyngeal nerve to innervate the stylopharyngeus. General visceral efferent preganglionic parasympathetics have their cell bodies in the inferior salivatory nucleus. Axons of these neurons pass into the tympanic nerve. This nerve arises from the inferior ganglion, courses through the temporal bone, runs on the promontory and helps to form the tympanic plexus in the middle ear cavity. The preganglionics leave the plexus in the lesser superficial petrosal nerve and synapse on postganglionics in the otic ganglion. Postganglionic axons run in the auriculotemporal branch of the trigeminal nerve and are distributed to the parotid gland.

In the gag reflex, the afferent limb is by way of GVA fibers from the oropharynx to the association limb in nucleus solitarius. Axons of the latter nucleus are both crossed and uncrossed to the hypoglossal nucleus for tongue movements and to the nucleus ambiguus for pharynx, larynx and soft palate movements. Lesions of the glossopharyngeal can result in some loss of taste in the posterior third of the tongue and in a loss of the gag reflex when the affected side is stimulated.

The *tenth (vagus) nerve* contains the same five functional components as do the facial and glossopharyngeal nerves. The small general somatic afferent component travels from the external ear in the auricular branch of the vagus and has its cell bodies located in the superior (jugular) ganglion lying in the posterior part of the jugular foramen. Axons from this ganglion enter the medulla in the postolivary sulcus and end in the spinal nucleus of cranial nerve V. The special visceral afferent fibers arise from taste buds in the region of the epiglottis. SVA cell bodies are in the inferior

(nodose) ganglion, located inferior to the jugular foramen, and their axons terminate in the gustatory part of the nucleus solitarius. General visceral afferent fibers arise in the mucosa and walls of the intestine (as far as the splenic flexure), the stomach, esophagus, pharynx, larynx, trachea, lungs, heart, carotid body and kidney. Their cell bodies are located in the inferior ganglion, and their axons terminate in the nucleus solitarius.

Special visceral efferent nerves arise from the nucleus ambiguus and are distributed to the skeletal muscles of the pharynx, soft palate, larynx and esophagus. Pharyngeal branches supply the pharyngeal plexus that gives branches to the pharyngeal constrictor muscles and all of the palatine muscles except the tensor veli palatini. The external branch of the superior laryngeal nerve supplies the cricothyroideus and part of the inferior pharyngeal constrictor muscles. The internal branch of the superior laryngeal supplies sensory and parasympathetic secretomotor fibers to the larynx and epiglottis. All of the laryngeal muscles, except the cricothyroideus, are supplied by the recurrent (inferior) laryngeal nerve. The right recurrent arises in the root of the neck and arches under the subclavian. The left recurrent arises in the upper thorax, loops around the arch of the aorta just below the ligamentum arteriosum and ascends to the larynx.

The general visceral efferent fibers arise from the dorsal motor nucleus of cranial nerve X. These preganglionics are distributed through numerous branches of the vagus to terminal parasympathetic ganglia in or on the heart, larynx, trachea, lungs and digestive system from the pharynx to the splenic flexure. The terminal ganglia of most of the gastrointestinal tract are the myenteric and submucosal nerve ganglia and plexi. Postganglionic axons from terminal ganglia supply smooth and cardiac muscle and glands.

The peripheral branches of the vagus nerve are extensive. In the jugular fossa, the vagus gives off auricular and meningeal nerves. In the neck it gives off pharyngeal, superior laryngeal, right recurrent laryngeal and the superior cardiac nerves. In the thorax the vagus gives off the left recurrent, inferior cardiac, anterior and posterior bronchial, and esophageal nerves. The right and left vagus form an esophageal plexus around the esophagus from which most of the left vagus enters the abdomen as the anterior vagus; most of the right contributes to the posterior vagus. Vagal branches in the abdomen are the gastric, hepatic and celiac.

A unilateral lesion of the vagus nerve or its nuclei produces paresis of the ipsilateral vocal cord, resulting in abnormal phonation and hoarseness. In addition, the affected side of the soft palate is lower than the normal side. Upon phonation, the uvula points toward the normal side. Lesions of the vagus also demonstrate abnormal gag and swallowing reflexes since the vagus constitutes the efferent limbs of those reflexes.

The *eleventh (accessory) nerve* consists of two parts, a cranial and a spinal part. The cranial part arises in the nucleus ambiguus (SVE), exits from the postolivary sulcus of the medulla, passes through the jugular foramen and merges with the vagus near the inferior vagal ganglion. The spinal part arises from anterior horn cells of the upper five cervical segments. Axons of these cells pass laterally through the lateral funiculus, ascend between the dentate ligament and the dorsal roots and pass as a nerve trunk through the foramen magnum into the cranial cavity. This nerve trunk communicates with the cranial part of the accessory and the vagus and exists from the jugular foramen to distribute fibers to the sternocleidomastoid and trapezius muscles.

Lesions of the spinal accessory produce weakness in shoulder shrugging on the affected side, and the arm cannot be raised above the vertical plane because of paresis of the trapezius. In addition, there may be weakness in rotating the head and face to the opposite side.

The *twelfth (hypoglossal) nerve* is a somatic efferent nerve that arises from the hypoglossal nucleus and emerges from the preolivary sulcus of the medulla. It passes through the hypoglossal canal, loops ventrally and anteriorly above the hyoid bone and innervates the tongue musculature.

Unilateral lesions of the hypoglossal nerve or nucleus result in deviation of the tongue to the affected side upon protrusion. This is due to the action of the unopposed genioglossus of the normal side. There may be fasciculations and wasting on the affected side.

Major Ascending and Descending Pathways. The following outline is a summary of some of the major clinically significant ascending and descending pathways that course through the spinal cord and ascend to higher levels.

Ascending Pathways of the Spinal Cord
1. Pain and temperature pathway
   Neuron I; Cell bodies in dorsal root ganglion and axon in dorsal root
   Neuron II: Cell bodies in the substantia gelatinosa and nucleus proprius. Axons cross to the opposite side and ascend as the lateral spinothalamic tract.
   Neuron III: Cell bodies in the VPL nucleus of the thalamus. Axons ascend in the posterior limb of the internal capsule to the postcentral gyrus and to a region of the parietal lobe bordering the lateral fissure.

2. Two-point touch, stereognosis, vibratory sense pathway
   Neuron I: Cell bodies in dorsal root ganglion. Axons of dorsal root ascend in the posterior white column. Those entering below T6 ascend in the fasciculus gracilis; those entering above T6 ascend in fasciculus cuneatus.
   Neuron II: Cell bodies in nucleus gracilis and cuneatus. Axons cross and ascend as the medial lemniscus.
   Neuron III: Cell bodies in the VPL nucleus of the thalamus. Axons to the postcentral gyrus via the internal capsule.

3. Crude (light) touch pathway
   Neuron I: Cell bodies in the dorsal root ganglion. Axons of the dorsal root enter the dorsal horn.
   Neuron II: Cell bodies in the dorsal horn. Axons are mostly crossed and ascend as the anterior spinothalamic tract.
   Neuron III: In the VPL nucleus of the thalamus

4. Posterior spinocerebellar and cuneocerebellar pathways
   Neuron I: Dendrites arise in neuromuscular and tendon spindles as IA and IB fibers respectively. Cell bodies in the dorsal root ganglia. Axons enter via dorsal roots; those below L3 and above C8 ascend in the posterior white column. The rest will enter the nucleus dorsalis near the level of entry.
   Neuron II: Cell bodies in the nucleus dorsalis (Clarke's column) receive first-order neurons from below the C8 cord level. Axons of these cells ascend ipsilaterally as the posterior spinocerebellar tract to the cerebellum. Cell bodies in the accessory cuneate nucleus receive ascending first-order neurons from levels above C8. Axons from this nucleus form the cuneocerebellar tract, which becomes part of the inferior cerebellar peduncle.

Ascending Pathways Arising at Brain Stem Levels
1. Pain and temperature pathway
   Neuron I: Dendrites in the maxillary, mandibular and ophthalmic division of the trigeminal nerve. Cell bodies in the trigeminal ganglion. Axons enter the pons and descend as the spinal tract of cranial nerve V. Some first-order neurons from the posterior ear region are part of the facial, glossopharyngeal and vagus nerves. Their axons enter the spinal nucleus of cranial nerve V.
   Neuron II: Cell bodies in the spinal nucleus of cranial nerve V. Axons cross and ascend as the ventral ascending secondary tract of cranial nerve V.

Neuron III: Cell bodies in the VPM nucleus. Axons to the postcentral gyrus via the posterior limb of the internal capsule

2. Touch pathways

Neuron I: Cell bodies in the trigeminal ganglion. Axons to the principal sensory nucleus and to the upper part of the spinal nucleus of cranial nerve V.

Neuron II: Cell bodies in the principal sensory nucleus and spinal nucleus of cranial nerve V. Axons from both nuclei cross and ascend as the ventral secondary ascending tract of cranial nerve V. Some axons from the principal sensory nucleus of cranial nerve V ascend ipsilaterally as the dorsal secondary ascending tract of cranial nerve V.

Neuron III: Cell bodies in the VPM nucleus of the thalamus; axons go to the postcentral gyrus.

3. Hearing pathway

Neuron I: Bipolar cells in the organ of Corti and spiral cochlear ganglion; axons to the pons–medulla junction

Neuron II: Cell bodies in the dorsal and ventral cochlear nuclei; axons are both crossed and uncrossed and ascend as the lateral lemniscus to the inferior colliculus. There may be relays through the superior olivary nucleus, nucleus of the lateral lemniscus and nucleus of the trapeziod body in this ascent.

Neuron III: Cell bodies in the inferior colliculus. Axons pass into the brachium of the inferior colliculus.

Neuron IV: Cell bodies in the medial geniculate body. Axons pass in the sublenticular limb of the internal capsule to the transverse temporal gyrus of Heschl.

4. Visual pathway

Neuron I: Rods and cones

Neuron II: Bipolar cells of the retina

Neuron III: Cell bodies are the ganglion cell layer of the retina. Axons course as the optic nerve, optic chiasm and optic tract. Axons from the nasal half of the retina cross in the optic chiasm.

Neuron IV: Cell bodies in the lateral geniculate body. Axons pass in the sublenticular and retrolenticular limbs of the internal capsule and in the geniculocalcarine tract (optic radiations) to the calcarine striate cortex (area 17).

Descending Pathways of the Brain and Spinal Cord

1. Pyramidal system

a. Corticospinal tract

Upper motor neuron: Cell bodies are in the precentral gyrus (area 4) and in the postcentral gyrus and premotor cortex. Axons descend in the posterior limb of the internal capsule, the crus cerebri, basis pontis and pyramids. Most cross at the pyramidal decussation and descend in the lateral corticospinal tract. They synapse on internuncials at the level of the lower motor neuron innervated.

Lower motor neuron: Cell bodies in the anterior horn of the spinal cord as alpha motor neurons to extrafusal muscle fibers and as gamma efferent neurons to intrafusal muscle fibers. This pathway tonically facilitates the antagonists of antigravity muscles and phasically controls the distal muscles in fine movements.

b. Corticobulbar pathways

Upper motor neuron: Cell bodies located near the lateral fissure in the precentral and postcentral gyri and in the premotor cortex. Axons pass through the genu of the internal capsule and crus cerebri. Those to the oculomotor, trochlear, abducens, motor nucleus of cranial nerve V, nucleus ambiguus and hypoglossal nucleus are mostly crossed, but uncrossed fibers are present. Those to the part of the motor nucleus of cranial nerve VII that supplies the upper facial muscles also are crossed and uncrossed, while those axons to cells supplying the lower facial muscles are only crossed. Those axons terminating on that part of the hypoglossal nucleus supplying the genioglossus also are crossed.

Lower motor neuron: Cell bodies in the SE and SVE nuclei of cranial nerves III through VII and IX through XII.

2. Major extrapyramidal tracts

a. Vestibulospinal tract

Upper motor neuron: Cell bodies are located in the lateral vestibular nucleus. Axons of this tract are located in the anterior funiculus and end on internuncial neurons.

Lower motor neuron: Gamma and alpha motor neurons to antigravity muscles are facilitated.

b. Lateral reticulospinal tract

Upper motor neuron: Cell bodies are in the gigantocellular nucleus in the reticular formation of the medulla. Axons of this tract are in the lateral funiculus.

Lower motor neuron: Gamma and alpha motor neurons to antigravity muscles are inhibited.

c. Medial reticulospinal tract

Upper motor neuron: Cell bodies are in the

oral and caudal pontine reticular nuclei. Axons of this tract descend in the reticular formation of the brain stem and in the anterior funiculus.

Lower motor neuron: Gamma and alpha motor neurons of antigravity muscles are facilitated.

d. Rubrospinal tract

Upper motor neuron: Cell bodies are in the red nucleus. Axons cross in the ventral tegmental decussation and descend in the rubrospinal tract. This tract is located in the lateral reticular formation of the brain stem and in the lateral funiculus of the spinal cord. Axons end on internuncials.

Lower motor neuron: Gamma and alpha motor neurons innervating the antagonists of antigravity muscles are facilitated.

Somatic Motor Control Mechanisms. The somatic motor anterior horn cells of the spinal cord and the somatic efferent (nuclei 3, 4, 6 and 12) and special visceral efferent (nucleus ambiguus and motor nuclei of 5 and 7) neurons of the brain stem are regulated by afferent and association fibers from all levels of the CNS. Afferent and internuncial neurons innervating anterior horn cells within one level of the spinal cord constitute a segmental level of motor control. An example of this is the myotatic stretch reflex where IA fibers from the muscle spindle of a stretched muscle convey impulses monosynaptically at the level of entry of the dorsal root, with an alpha motor neuron supplying the extrafusal muscle fibers of that muscle.

Intersegmental connections of afferent and association neurons within the spinal cord constitute a mechanism for intersegmental regulation of motor activity. Such connections may involve collaterals from long ascending and descending pathways or shorter spinospinal fibers of the fasciculus proprius. An example of this is the pain withdrawal reflex wherein pain fibers are stimulated (such as in the placing of the hand on a hot stove). The impulse is carried to several levels of the cord via the fasciculus proprius in order that motor neurons involved in the body adjustment of withdrawal can be stimulated.

Suprasegmental control pathways involve connections of the spinal cord with higher centers of the CNS. This constellation of numerous suprasegmental connections can best be appreciated if they are divided into phylogenetically older and newer systems. Such a scheme can include older antigravity and vestibular regulation, the next oldest regulation of the more stereotyped grosser movements involving the more axial musculature and the newer fine discrete movements.

Antigravity and vestibular connections involve input from muscle spindles and the vestibular apparatus. These afferents make connections through the spinocerebellar tracts and vestibular nuclei with the cerebellum; the vestibular fibers end in the flocculonodular lobe, while spindle information is conveyed to vermal and paravermal areas of the anterior and posterior lobes of the cerebellum. Cerebellar efferents, through dentatorubral fibers of the superior cerebellar peduncle, synapse in the red nucleus with cells of the rubrospinal tract, which bring about the facilitation of antagonists of the antigravity muscles. Cerebellar efferents from the flocculonodular lobe arise from the fastigial nuclei and terminate in the lateral vestibular nuclei. Axons from the lateral nucleus constitute the lateral vestibulospinal tract, which is facilitory to antigravity muscles. The medial and lateral reticulospinal tracts receive input from all levels of the CNS and are facilitory and inhibitory, respectively, to the antigravity muscles.

The regulation of gross stereotyped movements involves the basal ganglia and their ascending connections with the cortex and their descending connections through the reticular formation. In these circuits the premotor cortex and centromedial nucleus of the thalamus receive ascending afferent input and relay this information to the caudate and putamen. The latter two nuclei send axons to the globus pallidus and probably have an inhibitory effect on it. The putamen and globus pallidus also receive input from the substantia nigra. The efferent outflow from the basal ganglia (lenticular nucleus) is from the globus pallidus to: (1) the motor and premotor cortex by way of the ventral anterior and ventral lateral nuclei of the thalamus, and (2) the motor neurons of the spinal cord and brain stem by way of the subthalamus, prerubral field, red nucleus and the reticulospinal, rubrospinal and reticuloreticular pathways. Pallidal efferents to the thalamic nuclei course through the internal capsule and then pass between the subthalamic nucleus and zona incerta in the fasciculus lenticularis to reach the prerubral field (of Forel). From the prerubral field, axons loop laterally toward the thalamus in the fasciculus thalamicus, or they descend in the reticular formation to contralateral motor nuclei. Other pallidal efferents loop around the internal capsule in the ansa lenticularis in their pathway to the thalamus.

Lesions of the basal ganglia, subthalamus and substantia nigra are associated with disturbances in involuntary movements (dyskinesias) and in muscle tone. Lesions of the subthalamic nucleus can lead to hemiballism on the opposite side due to release of the globus pallidus from the inhibitory control of the subthalamus. Parkinsonism (paralysis agitans) is characterized by a decrease of dopamine in the substantia nigra and neostriatum (caudate and putamen). The tremor at rest and rigidity of this disorder may be due to inability of the neostriatum to inhibit the globus pallidus. Lesions producing chorea and athetosis are probably in the striatum but are not as clearly localized as the other basal ganglia disorders.

The pathways involved in the initiation and performance of a fine coordinated movement involve: (1) input to the cortex, (2) a feedback loop between the cerebral cortex and the cerebellum, (2) corticospinal and corticobulbar pathways and (4) alpha and gamma motor neurons of the spinal cord and brain stem. In these pathways ascending exteroceptive input is relayed through the thalamus to the primary receptive areas of the cortex (areas 3, 1, 2; 41 and 42; 43; 17). Projections from the primary receptive areas go to unisensory association areas lying adjacent to the primary receptive areas. The specific sensation for each receptive area is "recognized" in each unisensory association area. Projections from the unisensory association areas congregate in multisensory association areas in the junctional area of the inferior parietal gyrus (areas 39 and 40), superior temporal gyrus and lateral occipital gyri. In this area gnosis from more than one sensation is utilized in the initiation and formulation of learned complex motor activity.

Axons from these parietal, occipital and temporal regions, as well as axons from the prefrontal cortical center for initiative and judgment and from premotor and motor regions, descend as corticopontine pathways to pontine nuclei. Frontopontine fibers descend through the anterior limb of the internal capsule and medial portion of the crus cerebri. The other corticopontine fibers descend in the posterior limb of the internal capsule and lateral part of the crus cerebri. After they synapse on cells of the pontine nuclei, axons of the latter cells carry impulses across the midline of the basis pontis and ascend to the cerebellar cortex in the middle cerebellar peduncle. These pontocerebellar fibers are mossy fibers that end in the granule cell layer. From here impulses spread through the molecular layer of the neocerebellar cortex of the posterior lobe and are transmitted to Purkinje cells. Axons of Purkinje cells pass to the dentate nucleus, where they synapse on cells whose fibers cross the midline in the decussation of the superior cerebellar peduncle and ascend to the ventral lateral nucleus of the thalamus. From the ventral lateral nucleus axons ascend to the motor cortex.

The ultimate descending pathway for fine discrete movements is by way of the corticospinal and corticobulbar tracts to anterior horn cells and brain stem SE and SVE neurons. Both of these pathways are crossed pathways, although many of the corticobulbar tracts have some uncrossed representation. In this complex pathway, which involves a double crossing of fibers in the cerebral cortex—cerebellar loop and a single crossing of the corticospinal tract, the cerebellum acts as a computer coordinating the activity of numerous neurons.

Lesions of the cerebellum may demonstrate deficits in motor activity. Neocerebellar lesions produce a lateral cerebellar syndrome where the symptoms are on the same side of the body as the involved cerebellar hemisphere. This syndrome demonstrates an asynergia of voluntary skilled activity characterized by hypotonia and postural fixation defects, especially of the limbs. Some clinical signs and abnormal reflexes of neocerebellar disease are: dysmetria, intention tremor, rebound phenomenon, disdiadochokinesis, explosive speech, and decomposition of movement. Flocculonodular syndrome is primarily a disorder of locomotion and equilibrium. This is characterized by the patient falling, or walking on a wide base or with a drunken gait.

Lesions of various portions of the cerebral cortex lead to deficits in motor activity. Immediately after partial or complete lesions of the precentral gyrus there is flaccid paralysis of the contralateral limbs and loss of superficial and deep reflexes, and hypotonus and exaggerated deep reflexes may occur. Lesions of Broca's area in the inferior frontal opercular and triangular areas of the dominant hemisphere may result in expressive aphasia. Sensory aphasias are more often associated with lesions of the posterior temporoparietal region. Ideomotor and ideational apraxias appear to be associated with lesions of the dominant parietal lobe in the region of the inferior parietal gyrus. Ablative lesions of the frontal eye fields in the posterior part of the middle frontal gyrus interfere with voluntary conjugate eye movements to the opposite side. Damage to the corticospinal tract in the spinal cord will give an ipsilateral upper motor neuron complex of symptoms within several weeks of the onset of the injury. This constellation of symptoms includes: (1) increased segmental muscle tone (hypertonus), especially in extensors of the lower extremity and in flexors of the upper extremity, (2) increased deep tendon reflexes (hyperreflexia), (3) absence of or diminished superficial reflexes and (4) presence of pathologic reflexes such as the Babinski reflex. Lesions of lower motor neurons produce flaccid paralysis or paresis, loss of deep and superficial reflexes and some atrophy.

Visceral Motor Control Mechanisms. The hypothalamus is the highest subcortical center for the regulation of visceral activity. It receives ascending information from the spinal and cranial nerves by way of the reticular formation. In addition to these spinoreticular and reticuloreticular pathways, the hypothalamus receives input from the thalamus, basal ganglia and cerebral cortex. Efferents from the hypothalamus descend to the brain stem and spinal cord and also terminate in the thalamus, cortex and hypophysis.

As previously indicated, hypothalamic nuclei are structurally divisible into medial and lateral groups by the columns of the fornix. The lateral group includes lateral and tuberal nuclei. The medial group is further subdivided into anterior, middle and posterior groups. The anterior group includes the preoptic, anterior, supraoptic, paraventricular and periventricular nuclei. The dorsomedial and ventromedial nuclei comprise the middle group; the posterior and mammillary nuclei make up the posterior group.

Functional classification of nuclei into autonomic and endocrine neurosecretory groups makes the hypothalamic regions easier to appreciate. An anteromedial group of nuclei involved in parasympathetic regulation includes the anterior, preoptic, dorsomedial and part of the posterior hypothalamus. A posterolateral group of preoptic, anterior, ventromedial, posterior, tuberal and lateral nuclei regulate sympathethc activity. Outflow from the hypothalamus to preganglionic parasympathetic and preganglionic sympathetic cells of the brain stem and spinal cord is by way of periventricular fibers that multisynaptically utilize the dorsal longitudinal fasciculus and reticuloreticular and reticulospinal pathways.

The endocrine neurosecretory nuclei are the supraoptic and paraventricular and the hypophysiotrophic area of nuclei. The supraoptic and paraventricular nuclei produce a neurosecretory material (NSM) that travels in the unmyelinated axons of these cells through the infundibular stem to the pars nervosa of the pituitary gland. The NSM in the supraoptic neurons represents the precursor of vasopressin (ADH), whereas that in paraventricular cells is the precursor of vasopressin and oxytocin. Neurosecretory material is probably transformed into the hormones in the pericapillary spaces adjacent to posterior pituitary capillaries. The hypophysiotrophic nuclei encompass a crescent-shaped region starting anteriorly as part of the paraventricular nucleus and then dipping ventrally and caudally to include the suprachiasmatic, retrochiasmatic, ventromedial and arcuate (part of periventricular) nuclei. It is recalled that axons from these nuclei terminate in the infundibular stem adjacent to capillary loops of the hypophyseal portal vascular system. Releasing factors produced in neurons of the hypophysiotrophic area pass into these capillary loops and are transported via venous trunks of the pituitary stalk and capillaries of the pars distalis to the chromophobes and chromophiles of the anterior pituitary.

Visceral motor activity is influenced by descending pathways from the olfactory cortex and the limbic system. Olfactohypothalamic fibers course from the pyriform cortex to the hypothalamus. Impulses from the amygdala course in a ventral path and also in the stria terminalis to reach the hypothalamus and septal nuclei. Basal olfactory regions and the septal area are connected through the hypothalamus with the mesencephalic reticular formation by way of the medial forebrain bundle. The septal region is also in communication with the mesencephalic reticular formation through a pathway that includes the stria medullaris, habenular nucleus, habenulopeduncular tract (fasciculus retroflexus), interpeduncular nucleus and tegmental nuclei.

The limbic cortex is phylogenetically "older" cortex that forms a ring around the corpus callosum and diencephalon. It includes the subcallosal area, cingulate gyrus, isthmus (retrosplenial area), parahippocampal gyrus and hippocampal formation (hippocampus and dentate gyrus). All of these regions are connected through an association bundle called the cingulum. Axons from the hippocampal formation pass as the fimbria and fornix to the mammillary bodies and septal region. The mammillary bodies are linked to the cingulate gyrus through the mammillothalamic tract and its relay through the anterior nucleus of the thalamus. The mammillotegmental tract is a descending pathway from the mammillary bodies to the reticular formation of the brain stem.

In addition to the interconnections of the hypothalamus with the phylogenetically older olfactory and limbic cortex, there are neocortical connections. An important circuit is that between the prefrontal cortex and the hypothalamus through a relay in the dorsomedial nucleus of the thalamus.

Lesions of the hypothalamus affect visceral activity. Damage to the lateral hypothalamic nucleus may abolish appetite and lead to weight loss, whereas lesions of the satiety center in the ventromedial nucleus may lead to obesity through excessive eating. Lesions of the supraoptic nuclei can lead to diabetes insipidus. Bilateral temporal lobe lesions involving the pyriform cortex, amygdala and hippocampal formation may produce disturbances in emotional behavior.

THORAX

The thorax is bounded posteriorly by the thoracic vertebrae and the ribs, laterally by the ribs and the intercostal spaces and anteriorly by the sternum, the costal cartilages and ribs. The sternal angle (of Louis) is formed by the junction of the manubrium and the body of the sternum. It marks the level of the second costal cartilages, the bifurcation of the trachea, and the lower aspect of the fourth thoracic vertebra.

Surface Markings

Lungs and Pleura. The boundaries of the lungs and pleura may be mapped on the surface of the body as follows: The apex of the pleura extends about 2.5 cm. above the medial third of the clavicle. Its border then passes medially behind the sternoclavicular joint and the two pleura meet in the midline behind the sternal angle. The medial edge passes inferiorly to about the seventh costal cartilage where it inclines laterally. The medial edge of the left pleura inclines laterally at the level of the fourth costal cartilage because of the heart. This indentation of the medial edge of the pleura on the left is the cardiac notch. In the midclavicular line (below the middle of the clavicle) the lower border is at the level of the eighth rib, and in the midaxillary line at the tenth rib. Posteriorly at the scapular line (vertebral border of the scapula) the level of the pleura corresponds to the twelfth rib. The surface projection of the superior aspect of the lung corresponds to that of the pleura. The lung does not extend quite as far medially as the pleura so that the costal and mediastinal layers of parietal pleura are adjacent, thus forming the costomediastinal recess. The inferior border of the lung inclines laterally at the sixth costal cartilage. At the midclavicular line it is at the level of the sixth rib, at the midaxillary line the eighth rib, and at the scapular line the tenth rib. The area of pleural cavity below the inferior margin of the lung, where the parietal layers of costal and diaphragmatic pleura are adjacent, is called the costodiaphragmatic recess. During deep inspiration the lung descends into this recess.

The interlobar fissures separating the lobes of the lungs can also be reflected on the surface. The oblique fissure of the left lung divides the superior lobe from the middle lobe; that of the right lung separates the inferior lobe below from the superior and medial lobes above. The oblique fissure is at the level of the fourth rib posteriorly (base of the spine of the scapula), the fifth rib in the midaxillary line, and the sixth rib in the midclavicular line. A horizontal fissure separates the superior lobe from the middle lobe of the right lung. This fissure is at the level of the fourth costal cartilage next to the sternum, and at the level of the fifth rib in the midaxillary line where it joins the oblique fissure.

Surface Projections of the Heart. The heart may be mapped on the anterior thoracic wall by lines connecting four points. Point 1 is at the level of the second left costal cartilage, 1 to 2 cm. lateral to the edge of the sternum. Point 2 lies 1 to 2 cm. lateral to the edge of the sternum at the level of the third costal cartilage on the right. Point 3 is located at the level of the right sixth costal cartilage, 1 to 2 cm. from the sternal margin. Point 4 lies 7 to 8 cm. from the midline in the left fifth intercostal space, and marks the location of the apex of the heart. The lower (diaphragmatic) border corresponds to a line drawn from the apex through the xiphisternal articulation to point 3. The right border is indicated by a slightly convex line running from the right third costal cartilage to the right lower border. It is formed by the right atrium below and the superior vena cava above. The left border is formed by the left ventricle and the left auricular appendage. It curves from the third left costal cartilage to the apex. The posterior surface or base of the heart is formed largely by the left atrium, and a portion of the right atrium. All of the great veins—pulmonary and venae cavae—enter this portion of the heart. Most of the anterior (sternocostal) surface of the heart is formed by the right ventricle, with smaller portions of the left ventricle to the left and the right atrium to the right. The inferior or diaphragmatic surface is formed predominantly by the left and right ventricles.

The pulmonary and aortic orifices lie opposite the upper and lower margins of the third costal cartilage along the left margin of the sternum. The aortic valve lies behind the left side of the sternum at the level of the third interspace. The pulmonary valve is located to the left of the third chondrosternal articulation. The right atrioventricular (tricuspid) valve is in the midsternal line at the level of the fifth intercostal space. The left atrioventricular (mitral) valve lies at the left fourth sternochondral articulation.

Surface Projections of the Major Vessels. The thoracic aorta may be mapped on the surface of the body as follows: The ascending aorta extends from the aortic orifice on the left sternal margin to a point on the right margin of the sternum at the upper border of the second costal cartilage. The arch of the aorta curves to the left and backward, and its upper convexity lies about 2 cm. below the suprasternal notch. The descending thoracic aorta extends from the left side of the lower border of the fourth thoracic vertebra to the aortic hiatus of the diaphragm located in front of the body of the twelfth thoracic vertebra. The branches arising from the aortic arch are the brachiocephalic trunk lying in the midline, the left common carotid a little to the left and the left subclavian still further to the left and on a more dorsal plane.

The right and the left brachiocephalic veins unite to form the superior vena cava behind the first right chondrosternal junction. The brachiocephalic artery divides, and the right brachiocephalic vein originates, behind the right sternoclavicular joint. The left common carotid and the left subclavian enter the neck, and the left brachiocephalic vein begins, behind the left sternoclavicular articulation.

Mediastinum

The mediastinum contains all the thoracic viscera except the lungs. It is located between the pleural cavities and between the sternum and vertebral column. It is divisible into superior, anterior, posterior and middle regions.

Superior Mediastinum. The superior mediastinum is that part of the mediastinum located above the sternal angle. It contains the aortic arch and its branches, the superior vena cava and its tributaries, the vagus, recurrent laryngeal and phrenic nerves, trachea, esophagus, thoracic duct, left highest intercostal vein, the remains of the thymus and some lymph nodes.

Anterior Mediastinum. The anterior mediastinum is the area in front of the pericardial cavity. It contains the thymus, internal thoracic vessels, lymph nodes and surrounding connective tissue.

Posterior Mediastinum. The posterior cavity behind the heart and the great vessels contains the thoracic aorta, esophagus, vagus nerves, thoracic duct, azygos and hemiazygos veins, lymph nodes, and sympathetic trunks.

Middle Mediastinum. The middle mediastinum contains the heart and the pericardium.

Heart

Gross Structure of the Heart. The heart is a four-chambered organ consisting of two ventricles and two atria. An interatrial septum separates the two atria; an interventricular septum lies between the left and right ventricles. Anterior and posterior sulci on the sternocostal and diaphragmatic surfaces of the heart mark the location of the interventricular septum. The coronary sulcus encircles the heart at the atrioventricular junction. It is occupied by portions of the coronary vessels that supply the heart.

The borders of the heart were discussed previously in the section on surface markings. The apex of the heart is part of the left ventricle, and it points downward and to the left. It is located deep to the left fifth intercostal space about 4 cm. below and 2 cm. medial to the left nipple, and it is overlapped by an extension of the pleura and lungs. The base of the heart faces upward, to the right and toward the back. It consists mainly of the left atrium, part of the right atrium and proximal parts of the great vessels. Its superior boundary is at the bifurcation of the pulmonary artery, and its inferior boundary is at the coronary sulcus. The left boundary of the base is at the oblique vein of the left atrium, and the right boundary is at the sulcus terminalis. The base is separated from the bodies of T5-8 vertebrae by the thoracic aorta, esophagus and thoracic duct. The sternocostal surface of the heart is occupied by the right atrium, right ventricle and a small part of the left ventricle. The diaphragmatic surface is comprised of the two ventricles.

The *right atrium* is larger than that on the left and is comprised of two parts: (a) a principal cavity (sinus venarum) and (b) an auricula. The smooth-surfaced sinus venarum is that part of the atrium between the ostia of the superior and inferior venae cavae and the right atrioventricular opening. The superior vena cava opens into the upper and posterior part of the sinus venarum; the inferior vena cava opens into the lowest part of the sinus venarum near the interatrial septum. The coronary sinus opens between the ostium of the inferior vena cava and the atrioventricular foramen. Rudimentary valves guard openings of the inferior vena cava and coronary sinus. Small openings (foramina venarum minimarum) in the atrial wall allow for direct passage of blood from thebesian veins into the right atrium. The auricula is rough surfaced because of muscular ridges (musculi pectinati). It is demarcated externally from the sinus venarum by the sulcus terminalis and internally by the crista terminalis.

The dorsal wall of the right atrium consists of the interatrial septum. The fossa ovalis, representing the embryonic foramen ovale, is an oval depression in the septal wall located above the openings of the coronary sinus and inferior vena cava. It is bounded above and at its sides by the limbus fossa ovalis representing the embryonic free margin of septum secundum.

The *right ventricle* is bounded on the right by the coronary sulcus and on the left by the anterior longitudinal sulcus. Its superior part, the conus arteriosus (infundibulum), is continuous with the pulmonary trunk. Inferiorly, its wall forms the acute margin of the heart. The right ventricle is about one-third the thickness of the left ventricle, but the capacity (85 ml.) of both ventricles is the same. The internal surface is quite irregular because of ridges of muscle called trabeculae carneae. Some of these project from the wall of the ventricle and insert through chordae tendineae on the apices, margins and ventricular surfaces of cusps of the right atrioventricular valve.

The right atrioventricular (tricuspid) valve surrounds the right atrioventricular orifice and projects into the ventricle as anterior (infundibular), posterior (marginal) and medial (septal) cusps. The anterior cusp is the largest, the posterior is the smallest. These leaflets are composed of strong fibrous tissue that is continuous at their bases with the anuli fibrosi of the fibrous skeleton separating the atria from the ventricles. The anterior papillary muscle arises from the anterior and septal walls and is attached to the anterior and posterior cusps by chordae tendineae. The moderator band may arise from the anterior papillary muscle and extend across the lumen of the right ventricle. The posterior papillary muscle arises from the posterior wall, and its chordae tendineae insert on the posterior and septal cusps.

The conus arteriosus has a smooth inner surface, and it is limited from the rest of the ventricle by a ridge of muscular tissue called the crista supraventricularis. At the summit of the conus is the orifice of the pulmonary trunk. The pulmonary valve consists of three cusps, anterior, right and left. Each cusp contains a sinus behind it and has its convexity directed toward the ventricle. Adjacent cusps attach at a common commissure. A thin marginal lunula portion of each cusp runs from each commissure to a thickened nodule in the central free margin of the cusp. When the valve is closed the lunulae and nodules of the cusps are in contact.

The *left atrium* consists of a principal cavity (sinus venarum) and an auricula. The sinus venarum receives the four pulmonary veins and has a smooth surface. The interatrial septum covering the fossa ovalis of the right atrium constitutes a valve of the foramen ovale. The left auricula is longer than that of the right atrium. It curves ventrally around the base of the pulmonary trunk, and it lies over the proximal portion of the left coronary artery.

The *left ventricle* is longer, more conical and thicker than that on the right. It contains the apex of the heart and is separated from the right ventricle by the muscular and membranous parts of the interventricular septum. It has two openings, the left atrioventricular (mitral), guarded by the mitral valve and the aortic, limited by the aortic valve. The left atrioventricular valve consists of a large anterior (aortic) and a smaller posterior cusp. Each cusp receives chordae tendineae from both the anterior and posterior papillary muscles. The aortic opening is anterior and to the right of the mitral valve. The portion of the ventricle below the aortic orifice is called the aortic vestibule. The aortic valve consists of three cusps, posterior, right and left. The cusps are similar in structure to those of the pulmonary valve, but they are bigger and stronger. The right and left coronary arteries take origin from the right and left aortic sinuses (of Valsalva) respectively.

The *skeleton of the heart* consists of a series of fibrous rings (anuli fibrosi) and fibrous trigones. Fibrous rings surround each atrioventricular orifice, the aortic opening and the pulmonary orifice. The cusps of each of the associated valves are attached to the rings. The membranous part of the interventricular septum also is continuous with the fibrous tissue of these anuli. At the junction of the atrioventricular rings with the aortic ring a right fibrous trigone is formed. A left fibrous trigone occurs between the aortic and left atrioventricular rings.

Microscopic Structure of the Heart. The heart wall consists of three layers: (1) an inner endocardial layer, (2) a middle myocardial layer and (3) an outer epicardial layer. The endocardium consists of endothelium and a subendothelial connective tissue layer of fine collagenous and elastic fibers and some smooth muscle fibers. The endocardium of the atria is thicker than that of the ventricles. A subendocardial layer of loose connective tissue and blood vessels binds the endocardium to the myocardium. This layer in the ventricles contains the specialized muscle fibers of the conduction system.

The myocardium consists of spiraling bundles of cardiac muscle that take origin from the anuli fibrosi. In the atria the myocardium is a thin layer of fibers with a simple arrangement. The muscle of the ventricles is more complex and consists of several layers. The ventricular bands of muscle originate from the fibrous anulus and course in a helical manner from right to left and toward the apex. Some of the more superficial fibers can be traced in a mantle covering both ventricles. Some intermediate fibers weave from ventricle to ventricle in the septum. The more numerous deeper fibers pass into either of the ventricular walls and end by piercing deeply and becoming the papillary muscles. The microscopic structure of cardiac muscle was reviewed with skeletal muscle tissue in the section on the back.

The epicardium consists of mesothelium and an underlying connective tissue layer. A subepicardial layer of loose connective tissue containing blood vessels, nerves and fat binds the epicardium to the myocardium. The epicardium is the visceral pericardium.

The atrioventricular valves consist of a core of dense connective tissue, which is continuous with the anuli fibrosi, and an outer layer of endocardium. The endocardium on the atrial surface of the valves is thicker than that on the ventricular side. Chordae tendineae are composed of dense regularly arranged connective tissue. The aortic and pulmonary semilunar valves resemble the atrioventricular valves, but they are much thinner.

Conduction System of the Heart. This system is composed of specialized cardiac muscle found in the sinoatrial node and in the atrioventricular node and bundle. The heart beat is initiated in the sinoatrial node (pacemaker of the heart) located in the right atrium in the upper part of the crista terminalis just to the left of the opening of the superior vena cava.

Cells of the sinoatrial node are slender and fusiform. From the sinoatrial node the cardiac impulse spreads throughout the atrial musculature to reach the atrioventricular (A-V) node lying in the subendocardium of the atrial septum directly above the opening of the coronary sinus. The A-V node has small irregularly arranged branching fibers that contain few myofibrils. Thereafter the impulse is conducted to the ventricles by passing through the specialized (Purkinje) tissue of the atrioventricular bundle (of His). This bundle consists of a crus commune and right and left bundle branches. The common bundle travels from the A-V node into the membranous part of the interventricular septum. It divides into right and left bundle branches that pass in the subendocardium along the muscular part of the septum and distribute to the ventricles.

The innervation of the heart is from both the parasympathetic and sympathetic divisions of the autonomic nervous system. Right and left thoracic cardiac branches from the vagus nerves arise from the recurrent laryngeal nerves and pass to the deep cardiac plexus where they synapse on postganglionic parasympathetic neurons. The vagus nerves also give rise to superior and inferior cervical cardiac nerves. The left inferior cervical cardiac nerve ends in the superficial cardiac plexus; all of the rest end in the deep plexus. Superior, middle and inferior cervical cardiac nerves arising from sympathetic ganglia also descend to cardiac plexi. The left superior cervical cardiac sympathetic nerve ends in the superficial cardiac plexus; the rest end in the deep plexus. The deep cardiac plexus also receives thoracic cardiac branches from the upper four thoracic vertebral ganglia. The coronary and pulmonary plexi and the right and left atria are supplied by branches from the superficial and deep plexi. The right vagal and sympathetic branches end chiefly in the region of the sinoatrial node while the left branches end chiefly in the region of the A-V node.

Heart rate and force of contraction appear to be controlled mainly through the inhibitory action of the vagus nerves. Reflex slowing of the heart results from stimulation of the carotid sinus and the special pressure end organs in the carotid body. Impulses ascend in the carotid branch of the glossopharyngeal nerve to the inferior ganglion, thence to the solitary nucleus and finally to the dorsal motor nucleus of the vagus in the medulla. Efferent cardioinhibitory impulses pass down the vagi to the cardiac plexus to synapse there with postganglionic fibers that terminate at the sinoatrial (S-A) node.

Cardiac pain impulses arise in free nerve endings, in the cardiac connective tissue and adventitia of the cardiac blood vessels. They then travel in visceral sensory fibers through the cardiac plexus, then the middle and the inferior cervical cardiac and thoracic cardiac nerves and pass to the sympathetic chain ganglia of the neck and the upper thorax. From the middle and the inferior cervical chain ganglia these fibers descend, without synapsing, in the chain to the upper thoracic ganglia. Here other pain pathways join them, having passed directly through the cardiac nerves from the upper four or five thoracic chain ganglia. All the pain fibers continue through the white rami communicantes of spinal nerves T1 and T5 and traverse the corresponding dorsal roots and their ganglia. Their cell bodies are located in the dorsal root ganglia, and the central fibers pass from these spinal ganglia to the upper thoracic cord segments.

Cardiac pain is referred to cutaneous areas that supply sensory impulses to the same segments of the cord that receive the cardiac sensation. Thus they involve mainly the region of C7 through T5 and lie predominantly on the left side. The C8 and T1 segments are responsible for referred pain along the medial side of the arm and the forearm.

Blood Vessels of the Heart. The arterial supply of the heart is by way of right and left coronary arteries. Venous drainage is chiefly through cardiac veins, which empty into the coronary sinus.

The *right coronary artery* originates from the right aortic sinus and courses ventrally between the pulmonary trunk and the right atrium. It descends in the right part of the A-V groove, passing onto the posteroinferior aspect of the heart. It terminates by dividing into two branches: the posterior interventricular artery, which passes toward the apex in the posterior I-V sulcus where it anastomoses with the anterior interventricular branch of the left coronary, and a short continuation of the main trunk which anastomoses with the circumflex branch of the left coronary. Its marginal branch passes along the lower border of the right ventricle.

The *left coronary artery,* which is usually larger than the right, originates from the left aortic sinus. It runs close behind and then to the left of the pulmonary trunk, branching into the circumflex and anterior interventricular arteries as it emerges from behind the pulmonary trunk. The circumflex artery passes to the left in the left A-V sulcus and anastomoses with the right coronary artery on the posteroinferior aspect of the heart. The anterior interventricular artery descends toward the apex in the anterior I-V sulcus and passes onto the diaphragmatic surface where it anastomoses with the posterior interventricular branch of the right coronary.

The *cardiac veins* largely accompany the coronary arteries and open into the coronary sinus and thence into the right atrium. The remainder of the drainage occurs by means of small veins (venae cordis minimae and anterior cardiac veins) that drain much of the anterior surface of the heart and terminate directly into the right atrium.

The *coronary sinus* runs in the posterior A-V groove and drains into the right atrium at the left of the mouth of the inferior vena cava. It receives: (1) the great cardiac vein, which runs in the anterior interventricular groove, (2) the middle cardiac vein, located in the posterior interventricular groove, and, (3) the small cardiac vein, which accompanies the marginal artery along the caudal border of the heart.

Pericardium

The pericardium consists of two parts, an outer fibrous layer and an inner serous layer that adheres to the inner surface of the fibrous pericardium and reflects onto the outer surface of the heart.

Fibrous Pericardium. This tough connective tissue membrane surrounds the entire heart. Posteriorly and superiorly it blends with the adventitia of the great vessels. Inferiorly, it blends with the central tendon of the diaphragm. The outer surface of the fibrous pericardium is variably adherent to its neighboring structures. The anterior surface delimits the anterior from the middle mediastinum. It is attached superiorly to the manubrium by a superior pericardiosternal ligament. Inferiorly, fibrous condensations represent an inferior pericardiosternal ligament coursing to the xiphoid process. In the area between these two ligamentous attachments, most of the anterior surface of the pericardium is separated from the thoracic wall by the lungs and pleural cavities. Only a small portion of the pericardium is intimately related to the lower left portion of the sternum and the medial ends of the fourth through the sixth costal cartilages. In this region no lungs or pleura intervene between the chest wall and fibrous pericardium. This small portion of the pericardium corresponds to the cardiac notch in the left lung and underlies the left fourth and fifth intercostal spaces. This relation permits needle entry to the pericardial cavity without traversing the pleural cavity. Posteriorly the outer surface of this fibrous sac delimits the middle from the posterior mediastinum. It is in contact posteriorly with the bronchi, esophagus and descending thoracic aorta. The lateral outer surfaces of the fibrous pericardium are in close contact with the adjacent parietal pleura. The phrenic nerve and the pericardiacophrenic vessels descend between these two adherent layers.

Serous Pericardium. This is a thin membrane comprised of mesothelium and an underlying connective tissue lamina. This membrane lines the pericardial cavity with a smooth glistening surface that facilitates cardiac movement. The serous pericardium, by its location, is divisible into two layers, parietal and visceral. The parietal layer lines the fibrous pericardium. At a point where the fibrous pericardium intimately invests the walls of the great vessels entering and leaving the heart, the parietal layer of the serous pericardium is reflected to form the visceral layer (epicardium) of the serous pericardium. These reflections are in the form of two tubular sheaths, one sheath for the aorta and pulmonary trunk (arterial mesocardium), and the other for the pulmonary veins and venae cavae (venous mesocardium). That portion of the pericardial cavity passing horizontally between the two tubular sheaths remains as the transverse pericardial sinus. The reflection of the visceral pleura over the veins forms an inverted U-shaped cul-de-sac dorsal to the heart that is referred to as the oblique pericardial sinus.

Major Vessels of the Thorax

The great vessels entering and leaving the heart are constituents of either the pulmonary or systemic vascular circuits. The pulmonary circulation is represented by the: (1) pulmonary trunk originating from the right ventricle and branching into left and right pulmonary arteries, and (2) four pulmonary veins returning blood from the lungs to the left atrium. The systemic circulation is represented by the aorta, which originates from the left ventricle, and the superior and inferior venae cavae, which return blood to the right atrium. Lymphatic drainage from the thorax is by way of the thoracic duct and right lymphatic duct.

Pulmonary Trunk. This vessel arises from the infundibulum of the right ventricle and ascends obliquely and dorsally to the level of the sternal end of the second left costal cartilage where it divides into the left and right pulmonary arteries. In its course it passes in front of and then to the left of the ascending aorta. Anteriorly the pulmonary trunk is separated from the sternal end of the second left intercostal space by the left lung, pleura and pericardium. At its origin it is related on the left to the left auricle and the left coronary artery, on the right to the right auricle and occasionally the right coronary artery.

Pulmonary Arteries. The right pulmonary artery is longer and wider than the left. It passes horizontally to the right and enters the hilus of the lung immediately below the upper lobe (eparterial) bronchus. In its course it passes dorsal to the ascending aorta, the superior vena cava and the superior right pulmonary vein and lies ventral to the esophagus, right bronchus and anterior pulmonary plexus. The left pulmonary artery passes laterally and posteriorly, in front of the left bronchus and descending aorta, to enter the root of the left lung. The ligamentum arteriosum connects the arch of the aorta above with the left pulmonary artery below. The superior left pulmonary vein lies at first ventral and then inferior to the left pulmonary artery.

Pulmonary Veins. These vessels emerge from each of the five lobes of the lung. Upon entering the lung root, however, those from the superior and middle lobes of the right lung unite. Thus, four terminal pulmonary veins course from the roots of the lungs to the left atrium. The superior right pulmonary vein passes dorsal to the superior vena cava, and the inferior right pulmonary vein runs behind the right atrium before both enter independently through the dorsal and left wall of the left atrium. The superior and inferior left pulmonary veins course anterior to the descending aorta and enter separately through the posterior wall of the left atrium near its left border. Fusion of the left pulmonary veins into a common trunk is not uncommon.

Aorta. This vessel is the main arterial trunk of the systemic circulation. It ascends from the left ventricle, arches to the left and dorsalward over the root of the left lung, descends within the thorax on the left side of the vertebral column and enters the abdominal cavity through the aortic hiatus of the diaphragm. Thus the parts of the aorta are the ascending aorta, the arch of the aorta and the thoracic and abdominal portions of the descending aorta.

The *ascending aorta* arises from the base of the left ventricle at the caudal level of the third left costal cartilage. It passes obliquely upward to the right to the level of the second right costal cartilage. The ascending aorta is related anteriorly at its commencement by the infundibulum of the right ventricle, the pulmonary trunk and the right auricle. More cranially, it is separated from the sternum by the pericardium, variable portions of the right pleura, ventral margin of the right lung, loose areolar tissue and the remains of the thymus. The coronary arteries arise from the ascending aorta.

The *arch of the aorta* lies in the superior mediastinum. It begins at the upper border of the second right sternocostal articulation. It curves cranially and dorsally to the left and then descends along the left side of the vertebral column to the level of the intervertebral disk between the fourth and fifth thoracic vertebrae where it is continuous with the descending aorta. In its course it passes at first ventral to the trachea and then runs to the left of this structure and the esophagus. Arising from the superior aspect of the aortic arch are three large vessels: the brachiocephalic artery (innominate), the left common carotid artery and the left subclavian artery.

The *brachiocephalic artery* is the first branch from the arch of the aorta. It arises behind the middle of the manubrium sterni and courses obliquely upward to end behind the upper part of the right sternoclavicular joint where it divides into the right subclavian and common carotid arteries.

The *left common carotid artery* arises from the arch of the aorta behind and immediately to the left of the brachiocephalic artery. Its thoracic portion extends up to the level of the left sternoclavicular joint. In its course it passes in front of the trachea, left recurrent laryngeal nerve, esophagus, thoracic duct and left subclavian artery.

The *left subclavian artery* arises from the arch of the aorta about 2.5 cm. distal to the left common carotid. It ascends almost vertically on the left side of the trachea to the root of the neck where it arches upward and laterally. It lies behind the left vagus nerve, left phrenic nerve, left superior cardiac sympathetic nerve and left brachiocephalic vein. It passes in front of the left lung, pleura, esophagus and thoracic duct.

The *thoracic portion of the descending aorta* lies in the posterior mediastinum. It extends downward from the upper border of the body of the fifth thoracic vertebra to the aortic opening in the diaphragm at the level of the lower border of the twelfth thoracic vertebra. It gives off branches that supply the walls and viscera of the thorax. The thoracic descending aorta is in relation posteriorly with the left pleura and lung, the vertebral column and the hemiazygous veins. Anteriorly, from above downward, it lies next to the root of the left lung, pericardium, esophagus and diaphragm. On its right side are the azygos vein and thoracic duct, while on the left side are the left lung and pleura.

Superior Vena Cava. This vessel returns blood to the right atrium from the upper half of the body. It arises from the junction of the right and left brachiocephalic veins at the level of the lower border of the first right costal cartilage and enters the right atrium at the level of the third right costal cartilage. The superior vena cava is related anteriorly to the first and second intercostal spaces, the second costal cartilage, and intervening portions of the right lung, pleura and ascending aorta. Posteriorly it is in relation to the right margin of the trachea, azygos vein, the right bronchus, right pulmonary artery and the superior right pulmonary vein. On its left side lie a portion of the brachiocephalic trunk and the ascending aorta, while on the right can be found the phrenic nerve and right pleura. The superior vena cava receives the azygos vein on its posterior surface at the level of the second costal cartilage. The azygos vein enters the thorax through the aortic hiatus in the diaphragm, passes along the right side of the vertebral column, receives the hemiazygos vein at the T9 level (and possibly the accessory hemiazygos vein at the T8 level) and arches anteriorly over the root of the lung before entering the superior vena cava.

The *brachiocephalic veins* are formed by the union of the internal jugular and subclavian veins on each side. The right brachiocephalic vein arises dorsal to the sternal end of the clavicle and passes almost vertically downward in front of the trachea and vagus nerve and behind the sternohyoid and sternothyroid muscles and right lungs and pleura. The left brachiocephalic vein is longer than the right. It courses obliquely downward and to the right from its origin deep to the medial end of the clavicle, and joins the right brachiocephalic vein at the lower border of the right first costal cartilage. The thoracic portion of each brachiocephalic vein receives an internal thoracic and, often, an inferior thyroid vein. In addition, the left receives the left highest intercostal vein.

Inferior Vena Cava. This vessel returns blood to the right atrium from the caudal half of the body. It enters the thorax by piercing the diaphragm between the middle and right leaflets of the central tendon. It ascends in a slightly anteromedial direction in the middle mediastinum and pierces the fibrous pericardium. The inferior vena cava is separated, in its extrapericardial course, from the right pleura and lung by the right phrenicopericardiac ligament. In its short intrapericardial course it is invested on its right and left sides with a reflection of the serous pericardium.

Thoracic Duct. The thoracic duct is the common trunk of all lymphatics of the body except those that drain to the right lymphatic duct from the upper right quadrant of the body. It originates in the cisterna chyli of the abdomen at the second lumbar vertebra, enters the thorax through the aortic hiatus of the diaphragm and ascends through the posterior mediastinum between the aorta and azygos vein, and posterior to the esophagus. At the level of the T5 vertebra it crosses the midline to the left side, enters the superior mediastinum and ascends between the esophagus and pleura to enter the venous system at the junction of the left subclavian and internal jugular veins. The thoracic duct drains the posterior intercostal lymph nodes and posterior mediastinal nodes.

Right Lymphatic Duct. This duct receives lymph from the right side of the head and neck through the right jugular trunk; from the right upper extremity by way of the right subclavian trunk; and from the right side of the thorax, right side of the heart, right lung and part of the convex surface of the liver through the right bronchomediastinal trunk.

Microscopic Structure of Vessels. Blood and lymphatic vessels generally consist of three tunics: tunica intima, tunica media and tunica adventitia. These tunics are most pronounced in the larger vessels and vary with the type and size of vessels as to their constituents. Capillary walls consists of an endothelium and surrounding connective tissue. The endothelium may be continuous and contain no pores, or it may be fenestrated with pores closed by a thin membrane. Either type of endothelium contains tight intercellular junctions. Fenestrated capillaries can be found in the kidney and endocrine organs. In larger arteries and veins the three tunics are more pronounced. The tunica intima consists of endothelium, subendothelial connective tissue with smooth muscle, and an internal elastic membrane. In larger arteries the internal elastic membrane is fenestrated, often doubled and highly developed. The tunica media is more pronounced in arteries than in veins. In medium-sized (muscular, distributing) arteries it contains mostly circularly arranged smooth muscle and some elastic fibers. In larger arteries (elastic, conducting) elastic lamellae predominate, but smooth muscle is present. The media of arterioles consists of several layers of circularly arranged smooth muscle. The adventitia of arteries is not as pronounced as the tunica media. It is comprised of elastic and collagenous fibers and, in larger vessels, vasa vasorum that supply the outer layers.

Veins have a poorly defined tunica media, but the tunica adventitia is well developed. In medium-sized veins this outer layer contains mostly collagenous fibers. In the adventitia of large veins are longitudinally running smooth muscle fibers. Venous valves are local foldings of the intima. Venules have relatively thinner walls than arteries of similar diameter.

Lymphatic vessels are microscopically similar to veins. Lymphatic capillaries appear as endothelium lined clefts in connective tissue and have very thin walls. The thoracic duct has a thick tunica media consisting of longitudinal and circular smooth muscle bundles. Its tunica intima is prominent, but the adventitia is poorly defined.

Development of the Heart and Major Vessels

The heart and major vessels arise from blood islands of hemangioblastic tissue that were derived from mesoderm. The heart begins to form in the third embryonic week. An embryonic and two extraembryonic (umbilical and vitelline) vascular circuits are completed by the end of the first month of development.

Early Development of the Heart and Vascular Circuits. Two endocardial tubes are formed deep to the epimyocardial thickening of splanchnic mesoderm by the coalescence of blood islands. These tubes run longitudinally and are deep to the horseshoe–shaped prospective pericardial cavity. With the lateral folding and forward growth of the embryo, the endocardial tubes are shifted ventrocaudally and fuse in the midline. The adjacent epimyocardium fuses in the midline around the fused endocardial tubes, forming a single hollow heart tube that is suspended in the primitive pericardial cavity by the dorsal mesocardium.

The coalescence of other blood islands in the embryo forms blood vessels that are in continuity with the heart tube. In the embryonic circulation, paired anterior and posterior cardinal veins drain the embryo cranial and caudal to the heart respectively and join to form the paired common cardinal veins (ducts of Cuvier). This vessel drains into the caudal extent of the endocardial tube at the sinus venosus. Blood leaves the cranial extent of the endocardial tube and is distributed into six paired aortic arches that pass dorsally around the foregut in the branchial arches to empty into the paired dorsal aortae. Blood then circulates through branches of the aortae to capillaries that are in continuity with tributaries of the cardinal veins.

Blood vessels developing in the placenta (chorion) are linked to the embryonic circuit to form an umbilical (allantoic, placental) circuit. In this circuit umbilical arteries arise from the aorta, pass through the body stalk and go to capillaries of the placenta. Oxygenated and nutritive blood returns by the left umbilical vein to the sinus venosus. The right umbilical vein disappears soon after it is developed.

The vitelline circuit involves vascular channels in the yolk sac. Vitelline (omphalomesenteric) arteries arise from the abdominal aorta and pass along the yolk stalk to capillaries in the yolk sac. Blood returns to the sinus venosus by vitelline (omphalomesenteric) veins.

After birth the umbilical arteries will remain, in part, as a portion of the internal iliac and superior vesical arteries and the lateral umbilical ligaments. The umbilical vein persists as the round ligament of the liver. Portions of the vitelline veins become the portal vein. The vitelline artery gives rise to the superior mesenteric artery.

Folding and Partitioning of the Heart. With fusion of the endocardial tubes, several dilations become apparent. These are, from cephalic to caudal, the bulbus cordis (truncus arteriosus plus the conus arteriosus), ventricle, atrium and sinus venosus. Arteries leave the cephalic end of the bulbus cordis from a swelling called the aortic bulb (aortic sac). Veins enter at the sinus venosus. With the loss of the dorsal mesocardium, except where the veins and arteries enter and leave, the heart begins to flex into an S-shaped structure. The first flexure occurs at the junction of the bulbus cordis and ventricle. The second flexure causes the sinus venosus and atrium to shift dorsally. The adjacent bulboventricular walls disappear, and this part of the bulbus and primitive ventricle become part of a common ventricular chamber. The atrium becomes sandwiched between the pharynx dorsally and the rest of the conus and truncus ventrally, causing the atrium to bulge laterally into right and left swellings. The sinus venosus becomes shifted to the right and eventually is incorporated into the primitive right atrial swelling. The pattern of blood flow is from veins to atrium, to ventricle, to conus, to truncus, to aortic bulb and then to aortic arches.

During the second month of development the heart is partitioned into four chambers (two atria and two ventricles), atrioventricular valves are formed, and the conus, truncus and aortic bulb are partitioned into ascending aorta and pulmonary trunk.

In *partitioning of the atrium* endocardial tissue from the dorsal and ventral walls fuses into an endocardial cushion that separates the atrioventricular communication into right and left atrioventricular canals. While this is taking place an endocardial septum primum grows toward the endocardial cushion from the dorsal wall of the atrium. Before fusing with the cushion, an ostium primum exists temporarily between the free margin of the septum primum and the cushion. This ostium will not disappear before an ostium secundum arises from the degeneration of septum primum cephalically. In the seventh week a septum secundum grows dorsocaudally to the right of septum primum and leaves a crescentic free area covered only by septum primum. The communication from the right to the left atrium through the crescentic opening and ostium secundum is the foramen ovale. The valve of the foramen ovale is part of septum primum. The interatrial septum thus arises from septum primum and septum secundum.

The sinus venarum of the right atrium is formed by the incorporation of the sinus venosus into the right atrium so that the developing great veins enter independently. The smooth-surfaced portion of the left atrium arises after the absorption of the common trunk of the pulmonary veins, thus leaving four pulmonary veins entering at the boundaries of this area.

In *partitioning of the ventricle* a muscular interventricular septum grows toward the endocardial cushion. Just caudal to the cushion an interventricular foramen remains for a short time before it is closed by endocardial tissue from the free margin of the interventricular septum, the endocardial cushion and the conal septum.

In *septation of the aortic bulb, truncus arteriosus and conus arteriosus* a ridge of endocardial tissue develops on opposite walls of each of these structures. These ridges fuse in the middle of the lumen to form a bulbar (aortic, conal, truncal) septum. This septum spirals about 180 degrees as it descends from the aortic bulb into the conus, thus establishing a pulmonary trunk that intertwines with the ascending aorta. Semilunar valves develop in these vessels as localized swellings of endocardial tissue. The conal septum eventually descends to help close the intraventricular septum.

In *development of atrioventricular valves,* subendocardial and endocardial tissues project into the ventricle just below the A-V canals. These bulges of tissue are excavated from the ventricular side and invaded by muscle. Eventually all of the muscle, except that remaining as papillary muscles, disappears, and three right cusps of the right A-V valve and two cusps of the left A-V valve remain as fibrous structures.

Development of Major Arterial Vessels. Six pairs of aortic arches develop cephalocaudally in branchial arches. They bridge from the ventral aortic roots to the dorsal aortae. Of the six pairs, the first, second, fifth and distal part of the right sixth disappear. The remaining aortic arches, ventral aortic roots and dorsal aortae give rise to major arteries. The internal carotid arteries develop from the third aortic arches and the dorsal aorta cephalic to the third arch. The common carotids arise from the ventral aortic roots feeding the third arches. The external carotids arise in a similar position to the ventral aortic roots lying cephalic to the third arch. The right subclavian artery arises from the right fourth arch, the seventh dorsal intersegmental artery and the intervening portion of the right dorsal aorta. The left subclavian artery arises from the left seventh dorsal intersegmental artery. The arch of the aorta develops from the left fourth aortic arch and some septation of the aortic bulb. The pulmonary arteries arise from the proximal portions of the sixth arches along with some new vascular buds. The ductus arteriosus, linking the pulmonary trunk with the aorta, is the distal portion of the left sixth arch. The brachiocephalic artery originates from the right ventral aortic root between the fourth and sixth arches. The right dorsal aorta caudal to the right seventh dorsal intersegmental arteries disappears down to the embryonic low thoracic region where the paired dorsal aortae had fused into one midline vessel.

Development of Major Venous Channels. The superior and inferior caval systems and the portal vein arise from early embryonic vessels.

The *superior vena cava* forms from the right common cardinal vein and a caudal portion of the right anterior cardinal vein up to the entrance of the left brachiocephalic (innominate) vein. The latter vessel arises from a thymicothyroid anastomosis of veins. The right brachiocephalic develops from the right anterior cardinal vein between this anastomotic venous attachment and the right seventh intersegmental vein (right subclavian). The left common cardinal vein and part of

the left horn of the sinus venosus become the coronary sinus that drains the heart wall into the right atrium.

The *inferior vena cava,* from heart to common iliacs, arises from (1) a small portion of the right vitelline vein, (2) a new vessel in the mesenteric fold of the degenerating mesonephros, (3) the right subcardinal vein and (4) a sacrocardinal vein joining the caudal extent of the posterior cardinal veins. The subcardinals and their anastomosis, which developed to drain the mesonephros, also give rise to the renal, gonadal and suprarenal veins.

The *azygos venous system* arises mostly from the supracardinal veins and their anastomosis. The most cephalic portion of the azygos vein is derived from the right posterior cardinal vein.

The *portal and hepatic veins* arise from the vitelline (omphalomesenteric) veins and their anastomoses.

Fetal Circulation. The circulation of the blood in the embryo results in the shunting of well-oxygenated blood from the placenta to the brain and the heart while relatively desaturated blood is supplied to the less essential structures.

Blood returns from the placenta via the umbilical vein, is shunted in the ductus venosus through the liver to the inferior vena cava and thence to the right atrium. There is relatively little mixing of oxygenated and deoxygenated blood in the right atrium because the valve overlying the orifice of the inferior vena cava directs the flow of oxygenated blood from that vessel through the foramen ovale into the left atrium, while the deoxygenated stream from the superior vena cava is directed through the tricuspid valve into the right ventricle. From the left atrium the oxygenated blood and a small amount of deoxygenated blood from the lungs passes into the left ventricle and thence into the ascending aorta from which it is supplied to the brain and the heart through the vertebral, the carotid and the coronary arteries.

Because the lungs of the fetus are inactive, most of the deoxygenated blood from the right ventricle is shunted by way of the ductus arteriosus from the pulmonary trunk into the descending aorta. This blood supplies the abdominal viscera and the inferior extremities and is carried to the placenta, for oxygenation, through the umbilical arteries arising from the aorta.

Circulatory Changes at Birth. When respiration begins, the lungs expand, resulting in increased blood flow through the pulmonary arteries and a pressure change in the left atrium. This pressure change brings the septum primum and the septum secundum together and causes functional closure of the foramen ovale. Simultaneously, active contraction of the muscular wall of the ductus arteriosus results in its functional closure. Several months later it will become ligamentous as the ligamentum arteriosum. The ductus venosus functionally closes and becomes the ligamentum venosum. The fate of the umbilical arteries and veins was described previously in the section on extraembryonic circuits.

Congenital Abnormalities of the Heart and Great Vessels

The complicated sequence of development of changes in the heart and the major arteries accounts for the many congenital abnormalities that alone or in combination may affect these structures.

Septal defects include patent foramen ovale (incidence of about ten per cent) and atrial or ventricular septal defects. An ostium secundum defect lies cranial in the atrial wall and is relatively easy to close surgically. An ostium primum defect lies directly above the atrioventricular boundary and is often associated with a defect in the membranous part of the interventricular septum.

Interventricular septal defects usually involve the membranous part of the interventricular septum and are due to improper formation of the conal septum. Rarely the septal defect is so large that the ventricles form a single cavity, giving a trilocular heart (cor triloculare biatriatum).

Congenital pulmonary stenosis may involve the trunk of the pulmonary artery and its valve or the infundibulum of the right ventricle. If this is combined with an interventricular septal defect, the compensatory hypertrophy of the right ventricle develops sufficiently high pressure to shunt blood through the defect into the left side of the heart; this mixing of blood results in the child's being cyanosed at birth.

Fallot's tetralogy is the most common congenital abnormality causing cyanosis. It is comprised of pulmonary stenosis, right ventricular hypertrophy, a septal defect and an overriding aorta, the orifice of which lies cranial to the septal defect and receives blood from both ventricles.

Transposition of the great vessels is due to improper spiraling of the bulbar septum in the formation of the great vessels. This results in either complete transposition, where the aorta is from the right ventricle and the pulmonary trunk is from the left ventricle, or in incomplete transposition where both vessels are reversed but both exit from the right ventricle.

Aortic stenosis is due to either bulbar septum displacement or localized improper growth in supravalvular, valvular or subvalvular regions of the aorta.

Patent ductus arteriosus is a relatively common developmental abnormality. If not corrected it causes progressive work hypertrophy of the left heart and pulmonary hypertension.

Aortic coarctation may be due to abnormal retention of the fetal isthmus or to incorporation of smooth muscle from the ductus into the wall of the aorta. The constriction may occur from the level of the left subclavian artery to the ductus arteriosus, the latter being widely patent and maintaining the circulation to the lower part of the body. In other cases the coarctation may involve only a short segment near the ligamentum arteriosum, and the circulation to the lower limb is maintained by collateral arteries around the scapula that anastomose with the intercostal arteries.

Dextrorotation of the heart is the most spectacular of the abnormalities. The heart and its emerging vessels lie as a mirror image to the normal anatomy. It may be associated with reversal of all the intra-abdominal organs.

Abnormal development of the aortic arches may result in the arch of the aorta lying on the right or actually being double. Rarely an abnormal right subclavian artery arises from the dorsal aorta and passes behind the esophagus and thus causes difficulty in swallowing (dysphagia lusoria). Double aorta is due to retention of the right dorsal aorta between the seventh dorsal intersegmental artery and the point of fusion of the aortae. If this portion remains and the right fourth aortic arch disappears, then the right subclavian arises from the dorsal aorta.

Trachea and Lungs

Gross Structure of the Trachea and Lungs. The trachea extends from the cricoid cartilage at the C6 vertebral level to the level of the upper border of T5, where it bifurcates into left and right bronchi. It is related posteriorly to the esophagus and anteriorly to the thyroid gland and vessels, the sternohyoid and sternothyroid muscles, the thymus, the manubrium sterni, the major arteries and veins and the deep cardiac plexus.

The right bronchus is shorter, wider and diverges from the midline less than the left bronchus. Each bronchus enters the hilus of the lung at the mediastinal surface along with the pulmonary and bronchial arteries and veins, lymphatic vessels and lymph nodes, and autonomic nerve fibers. The right bronchus divides into three lobar bronchi, the superior, middle and inferior. The left bronchus divides into a superior and inferior lobe bronchus. Each of the lobar bronchi in turn subdivides to supply bronchopulmonary segments. In the right lung these segments are (1) the apical, posterior and anterior of the superior lobe, (2) the medial and lateral of the middle lobe and (3) the superior, medial basal, lateral basal, anterior basal and posterior basal of the inferior lobe. In the left lung these bronchopulmonary segments are (1) the apical-posterior, anterior, superior and inferior of the superior lobe and (2) the superior, anteriormedial basal, lateral basal and posterior basal of the inferior lobe. The segmental bronchi further subdivide to smaller bronchi and bronchioles in the substance of the lung.

The lungs project laterally from the mediastinum and are invested by visceral pleura, which is continuous at the hilum with the parietal pleura. The pleural cavity lies between the visceral and parietal pleura, and it surrounds the lung. The pleura is a moist serous membrane, and under normal circumstances its surfaces do not adhere to one another. Costal, mediastinal and diaphragmatic subdivisions of the parietal pleura are recognized.

Each lung is conical in shape and has an apex and base; three borders, the inferior, posterior and anterior; and three surfaces, the costal, diaphragmatic (base) and mediastinal. The apex extends 2.5 to 4.0 cm. into the root of the neck, while the base rests on the convex surface of the diaphragm. The costal surface faces the ribs. The mediastinal surface is in contact with mediastinal pleura and bears a cardiac impression in the region facing the pericardium. The posterior border is in the concavity on either side of the vertebral column. The anterior border is sharp and projects into the costomediastinal recess, except on the left in the cardiac notch region where the pericardium is not overlapped anteriorly by the lung. The inferior border is sharp and projects into the costodiaphragmatic recess. The right lung is divided into superior, middle and inferior lobes by two interlobar fissures; the left lung is divided into superior and inferior lobes by one interlobar fissure. The surface projections of these fissures were described previously in the section on surface markings.

The *afferent and the efferent innervation* of the lung is derived from the anterior and the posterior pulmonary plexuses, which receive branches from the vagus and the thoracic sympathetic trunk. Stimulation of the vagi brings about constriction of bronchioles, while stimulation of the sympathetic fibers causes dilation. The visceral afferents transmit pain and reflex activity, and return to the central nervous system via both the vagal and sympathetic pathways.

Microscopic Structure of the Trachea and Lungs. The conducting portion of the respiratory system includes the nasal cavity, nasopharynx, laryngopharynx, trachea, bronchi and bronchioles down to and including the terminal bronchioles. These regions are characterized by (1) a mucosa of pseudostratified ciliated columnar epithelium with goblet cells and an underlying connective tissue containing mixed seromucous glands, and (2) usually a cartilaginous or bony support. The respiratory portion consists of respiratory bronchioles, alveolar ducts, alveolar sacs and alveoli. A respiratory bronchiole and its branches constitute a lobule. All respiratory portions contain alveoli in their walls.

The microscopic structure of the larynx and trachea was described in the section on the head and neck. The main bronchi and segmental bronchi are similar to the trachea. The smaller bronchi have cartilaginous plates instead of rings. In bronchioles the cartilage disappears, circular smooth muscle becomes more prominent, and the ciliated epithelium becomes simple columnar and simple cuboidal. Glands are no longer present in the terminal bronchioles.

Respiratory bronchioles have simple cuboidal epithelium except at those sites where alveoli are present. Alveolar ducts are completely lined by alveolar sacs and alveoli, and their lumina are marked by spiraling bundles of smooth muscle. Alveoli are separated from each other by interalveolar septa that contain an extensive capillary net, reticular and elastic fibers, blood cells and macrophages. The alveolus is lined by an extremely attenuated simple squamous epithelium. Blood in the capillaries is separated from the air in the alveoli by endothelial cells and their basal lamina and the simple squamous cells and their basal lamina. Alveolar (septal) cells bulge between the squamous cells into the alveolar lumen and produce surfactant. Alveolar phagocytes (dust cells) migrate into alveolar spaces and engulf debris.

Bronchial arteries, carrying nourishment to the lungs, course along the bronchi to the distal ends of the alveolar ducts. Venous return of this blood is mainly through pulmonary veins, but some blood returns via the bronchial veins to the azygos system. Pulmonary arteries branch and follow the air tubes to the capillary plexi in the alveoli. Oxygenated blood is returned through pulmonary veins that travel in the interlobular connective tissue septa.

Esophagus

Gross Structure of the Esophagus. The esophagus extends from the pharynx at the C6 level to the stomach. It passes in front of the bodies of the vertebrae in the superior and posterior mediastinum and penetrates the diaphragm at the esophageal hiatus. It is supplied by the vagal nerves and sympathetic fibers that form an esophageal plexus around the esophagus. In the lower esophagus anterior and posterior vagal trunks descend through the diaphragm to the stomach. Parasympathetic preganglionic fibers penetrate the wall and synapse on postganglionic neurons in the myenteric (Auerbach's) and submucosal (Meissner's) plexi.

Microscopic Structure of the Esophagus. The

esophagus demonstrates well the general microscopic plan of the gastrointestinal system. The wall consists of four layers: (1) mucosa, (2) submucosa, (3) muscularis externa and (4) adventitia or serosa. The mucosa consists of stratified squamous nonkeratinized epithelium, a lamina propria with some mucous glands at the upper and lower extents of the esophagus, and a well-developed muscularis mucosae of smooth muscle. The submucosa contains some mucous glands and the autonomic submucosal nerve plexus. The muscularis externa consists of an outer longitudinal and inner circular layer of muscle with the myenteric plexus sandwiched between the two layers. In the upper esophagus the muscle is skeletal; in the lower portion it is smooth muscle, and in the middle it is mixed. The adventitia is connective tissue that merges imperceptibly with that of the surrounding mediastinum. In the short abdominal portion of the esophagus, the outer layer is peritoneum and thus consists of mesothelium and underlying connective tissue and is called a serosa.

Development of the Trachea, Lungs, Esophagus and Diaphragm

An entodermal respiratory diverticulum develops from the floor of the foregut just caudal to the last pharyngeal pouch. The larynx, trachea and lungs develop from this diverticulum. The esophagus differentiates from the foregut caudal to this outgrowth. In the development of the larynx, the opening is constricted into a narrow T-shaped laryngotracheal orifice by underlying mesodermal arytenoid swellings. There is a transitory period when the opening is completely obliterated by an overgrowth of epithelium. Persistence of portions of this may lead to webs that obstruct the laryngeal opening.

All cartilage, muscle and connective tissue of the larynx, trachea and lungs arise from splanchnic mesoderm. The epithelium and glands develop from branching of the entodermal diverticulum. The main bronchi divide dichotomously through 17 generations of subdivisions by the end of the sixth month. An additional six divisions will occur by early childhood.

As the bronchial buds divide, the lung increases in size, and it bulges laterally into the embryonic coelom. The early coelom consists of a more ventral prospective pericardial cavity in continuity with a more dorsal pleural cavity, which is continuous caudally above the septum transversum with the prospective peritoneal cavity. Right and left pleuropericardial folds project from the lateral body wall and septum transversum, grow medially between the heart and lungs, and fuse with the primitive mediastinum. Thus these folds become part of the definitive mediastinum and separate the pleural from the pericardial cavities. Pleuroperito-

neal folds grow from the septum transversum at right angles to the pleuropericardial membranes. These folds invest the esophagus and, along with the septum transversum, contribute to the formation of the diaphragm. In addition the definitive diaphragm receives a major contribution of muscle in its development from the lateral body wall.

Tracheoesophageal fistulas may develop from improper separation of the respiratory diverticulum from the foregut, by improper formation of the esophagotracheal septum, or by secondary fusion of the esophagus with the trachea. In the most usual circumstance the upper part of the esophagus ends blindly, while a lower portion is connected to the trachea by a narrow canal. This may result from dorsal deviation of the esophagotracheal septum in its caudal growth.

Diaphragmatic hernias can arise from improper formation of either the septum transversum or the pleuroperitoneal folds.

Lymphatic Organs of the Thorax

Thymus. The thymus is larger in the infant than it is in the adult. It consists of two lateral lobes invested by a connective tissue capsule that sends septa into the gland and divides it into lobules. The gland lies in the anterior part of the superior mediastinum and it extends from the fourth costal cartilage to the lower border of the thyroid gland. It lies anterior to the great vessels and fibrous pericardium. Microscopically the thymus is divisible into a central medulla and an outer cortex. The reticular connective tissue meshwork contains lymphocytes (thymocytes) and differs from the other lymphatic tissues in that the reticular cells are derived from entoderm (of the third pharyngeal pouch). The cortex contains more lymphocytes and is less vacular than the medulla. Thymic (Hassall's) corpuscles in the medulla are concentric arrangements of flattened, and often hyalinized, cells. The corpuscles vary in size and occurrence and may be indicative of degeneration of reticular cells of the thymus.

Branches of the internal thoracic and thyroid arteries pass through thymic septa and enter the cortex-medulla junctional area as arterioles. Here, the arterioles give off direct branches to the medulla and also feed capillaries that loop into the cortex before draining into postcapillary venules of the medulla and cortex-medulla junction. Since macromolecules cannot pass through the capillary loops, the cortical lymphocytes seem to be protected from circulating antigens by a blood-thymus barrier. Large numbers of lymphocytes pass through the walls of the postcapillary venules and drain by way of thymic veins into the left brachiocephalic, inferior thyroid, and internal thoracic veins. The thymus is essential for the production of thymus-dependent (T) lymphocytes that are involved in cell-mediated immunologic responses and that also assist β lymphocytes in humoral responses.

Lymph Nodes of the Thorax. The lymphatic nodes of the thorax are divided into parietal and visceral groups. The parietal nodes include the sternal, intercostal and diaphragmatic nodes. The sternal nodes are located along the internal thoracic artery and receive afferents from the mammae, the deeper structures of the anterior thoracic wall and the upper surface of the liver. Their efferents pass as a trunk to the junction of the subclavian and internal jugular veins. The intercostal nodes occupy the posterior parts of the intercostal spaces. They receive afferents from the posterolateral chest area. Efferents from the lower intercostal nodes carry lymph to the cisterna chyli, while the upper nodes send efferents to the thoracic duct and right lymphatic duct. Diaphragmatic nodes located anteriorly drain toward the sternal nodes, whereas those in the middle and posteriorly drain to the posterior mediastinal nodes. Superficial lymphatic vessels of the thoracic wall ramify beneath the skin and converge toward the axillary nodes. Lymphatic vessels of the mammary glands drain toward the surface along the interlobular septa and empty into a plexus located deep to the areola. This plexus also receives lymph from the areola and skin over the gland. It drains in two trunks to the axillary lymph nodes. Some drainage from the medial portion of the gland goes to the sternal nodes, while some efferents pass to interpectoral glands deep to the pectoralis major muscle, and others pass inferiorly toward abdominal nodes.

The visceral lymph nodes consist of anterior and posterior mediastinal and tracheobronchial nodes. The anterior mediastinal nodes are located in front of the great vessels and receive afferents from the thymus, pericardium and sternal nodes. Their efferents unite with those of the tracheobronchial nodes to form the right and left bronchomediastinal nodes. The posterior mediastinal nodes lie behind the pericardium and along the espohagus and descending aorta. Their afferents come from the liver, esophagus and pericardium. Most efferents from these nodes go to the thoracic duct. The tracheobronchial nodes filter lymph from the trachea, bronchi, lungs and heart.

Microscopically, lymph nodes are bean shaped, possess a hilum and are surrounded by a capsule that sends trabeculae into a stroma of reticular tissue containing lymphocytes. Nodules of dense lymphatic tissue are located peripherally in the cortical region. If the node is in the "active" stage the nodules contain germinal centers that consist of medium-sized lymphocytes and larger undifferentiated lymphocytes. These areas produce small lymphocytes that are pushed peripherally in the nodule and then into surrounding lymphatic sinuses. Nodes receive lymph peripherally through afferent vessels that penetrate the capsule and drain into a subcapsular sinus. This sinus drains along cortical peritrabecular sinuses to medullary sinuses (which lie between trabeculae and medullary cords of lymphatic tissue) before exiting from the lymph node at the hilum through efferent lymphatic vessels. Reticular cells lining the sinuses perform a filtering function by phagocytizing dead cells and particulate matter.

Lymph nodes also play a role in the immune response. The β lymphocytes are found in the subcapsular cortical tissue, in germinal centers and in medullary cords. In bacterial infections, antigens pass to the β lymphocytes and trigger them to form blast cells that proliferate and differentiate into antibody-producing lymphocytes and plasma cells. The antibodies pass into efferent lymphatic vessels and are transported by the circulatory system to the site of infection. T lymphocytes are located in deep cortical (paracortical) areas known as the thymus dependent zone. This zone contains many postcapillary venules, whose cuboidal endothelium permits a recirculating pool of T lymphocytes, and some β lymphocytes, to enter the lymph node. It is thought that uncommitted lymphocytes from the thymus and bone marrow enter the lymph node through these venules and react with antigens from foreign cells. In this response, T lymphocytes in the deep cortex become blast cells, proliferate, and form small long-lived memory cells and short-lived effector (killer) cells which enter the circulation.

Muscles, Nerves and Vessels of the Thoracic Wall

Muscles. The major muscles are the external and internal intercostals, the subcostal, and the transversus thoracis. The intercostal muscles fill the intercostal spaces, the external sloping medially from above downward and the internal sloping laterally from above downward. Subcostal muscles are fasciculi of the internal intercostals which extend over two or more intercostal spaces near the angles of the ribs. The transversus thoracis muscle arises from the dorsal surface of the lower sternum and xiphoid process and extends upward and laterally to insert on the second to the sixth costal cartilages. In respiration the intercostals probably keep the intercostal spaces constant during the elevating action of the scalene and sternocleidomastoid muscles and the downward pull of the abdominal muscles.

Nerves. All of the above muscles are innervated by intercostal nerves which are the continuations of the ventral rami of thoracic spinal nerves. The intercostal nerves and vessels occupy the costal grooves, with the nerves inferior to the intercostal arteries and veins. Each intercostal nerve has two cutaneous branches: the lateral cultaneous nerve in the midaxillary line and the anterior or cutaneous nerve just lateral to the sternum. Near the origin of the intercostal nerves, postganglionic sympathetic nerves are received from the sympathetic chain ganglia by way of gray rami communicantes. White rami communicantes carry preganglionic fibers from the spinal cord and intercostal nerves to the sympathetic chain ganglia, which lie adjacent to the necks of the ribs.

Arteries and Veins. Posterior intercostal arteries arise from the aorta and, in the upper spaces, from the costocervical trunk of the subclavian artery. They divide into anterior and posterior branches. The anterior branch and its collateral branch supply most of the intercostal space and end by anastomosing with intercostal branches of the internal thoracic artery. The posterior branch of the posterior intercostal artery follows the dorsal ramus of the spinal nerve and divides into spinal branches supplying the spinal cord and into muscular branches supplying the back.

Circulating Blood

Blood cells (formed elements) constitute 45 per cent of the total volume of circulating blood; plasma comprises the remaining 55 per cent. Of the 45 per cent cell volume, erythrocytes (red blood corpuscles, RBCs) make up 44 per cent, and the remainder is composed of leukocytes (white blood cells). The plasma, minus its blood clotting factors, is called serum.

Plasma acts as a medium for metabolic substances and circulating cells. Like tissue fluid, its primary components are water, inorganic salts and a number of proteins. Albumin, the most abundant plasma protein, maintains the colloid blood pressure. Gamma globulins are also important since they include the circulating antibodies. Beta globulins transport lipids, hormones and metal ions. Prothrombin and fibrinogen are essential components of the clotting process. Chylomicrons are microscopic particles of fat that are especially prominent in the plasma after a fatty meal.

Erythrocytes, when mature, are anucleate biconcave discs approximately 8 μm. in diameter and 2 μm. thick. There are about 4.8 and 5.5 million erythrocytes per cubic millimeter of blood in the normal female and normal male, respectively. Erythrocytes lack the usual complement of organelles and they do not have the capacity for protein synthesis. Each RBC exists for about 120 days and it lacks the mechanism to reproduce itself. About one per cent of the erythrocytes possess some residual ribosomal material and, due to their stained appearance, are called reticulocytes; they are considered to be immature erythrocytes. The reticulocyte count provides a rough index of the rate of erythrocyte development.

Leukocytes are divisible into granular leukocytes and nongranular leukocytes. The granular leukocytes are further classified as eosinophils, basophils, and neutrophils on the basis of the affinity of their granules for different stains. The nongranular leukocytes are the lymphocytes and monocytes.

Neutrophils are about twice the size of erythrocytes and make up about 60 per cent to 70 per cent of the white blood cells. Their nuclei consist of three to five lobes that are interconnected by fine filaments of nuclear material. Two types of granules are present in the cytoplasm: the specific granules, which stain with neutral dyes, and nonspecific granules, which are azurophilic. Both types of granules contain hydrolytic enzymes that are used by the cell in the digestion of phagocytized materials.

Eosinophils are about the size of neutrophils, but constitute only one per cent to three per cent of the total leukocyte population. The nucleus is usually bilobed and the chromatin is dense. The eosinophilic granules are membrane-bound vesicles containing lysosomal enzymes.

Basophils are about the same size as the other granular leukocytes. They constitute only 0.5 per cent of the white blood cells. The nucleus is usually S-shaped, its chromatin is less dense than that of the other granular leukocytes, and some of the membrane-bound cytoplasmic granules seem to obfuscate the outline of the nucleus. The basophilic granules contain histamine and heparin.

Lymphocytes constitute 20 per cent to 35 per cent of the white blood cell population. Most of the mature lymphocytes are the size of erythrocytes, but larger cells traditionally called large and medium lymphocytes are occasionally seen in circulating blood. The small lymphocyte has a relatively large round or slightly indented nucleus of dense chromatin. The nucleus is surrounded by a thin rim of cytoplasm containing a few ribosomes and some nonspecific azurophilic granules. The small lymphocytes are further designated as T and B lymphocytes. T lymphocytes are cytotoxic cells of the cell-mediated response that "kill" foreign cells and sensitizing agents that enter the body. They also assist the B lymphocytes in their humoral response to such invasive organisms as bacteria and viruses.

Monocytes range from 9 to 20 μm, in diameter and make up three per cent to eight per cent of the circulating leukocytes. The nucleus is oval, kidney-shaped or horseshoe-shaped. The cytoplasm contains a few azurophilic granules, a Golgi complex, polyribosomes and some glycogen; it is more abundant than that of the lymphocytes. Monocytes give rise to macrophages when they pass into connective tissues.

Platelets (thrombocytes) are small, irregular disk-shaped structures that are 1 to 2 μm in diameter. They are basophilic fragments of megakaryocytes containing a variety of granules. There are 250,000 to 300,000 platelets in a cubic millimeter of blood. They have a natural tendency to cling to each other and to all wettable surfaces they contact when blood is shed. Platelets contain serotonin which helps to constrict small blood vessels during vascular injury. They also contain thromboplastin, a substance released by platelets and injured endothelial cells. Thromboplastin helps convert prothombin of the plasma to thrombin. The thrombin then converts plasma fibrinogen to fibrin which forms a network trapping blood cells and platelets. Thus, a blood clot, or thrombus, is formed.

Blood Cell Formation (Hemopoiesis)

The main hemopoietic tissue in the body is bone marrow. Since all of the erythrocytes, platelets and granular leukocytes are produced in bone marrow, these blood components are called the myeloid elements. The specific development of these elements is referred to as myelopoiesis. Although the monogranular elements are produced in both lymphatic tissues and bone marrow, they are referred to as lymphoid elements; their development is termed lymphopoiesis.

The first blood cells develop in the third embryonic week from yolk sac and body stalk mesoderm. During the second month of development hemopoietic sites arise in the liver, spleen and mesonephric kidneys. In later months of fetal development, bones are established and the bone marrow becomes the dominant hemopoietically active tissue. Red bone marrow consists of a reticular fiber meshwork which contains and supports reticular cells, myelopoietic (blood forming) cells, adipose cells and thin-walled sinusoids. The myelopoietic cells occur in many stages. Some are relatively undifferentiated stem cells from which all myeloid elements come. Some are mature erythrocytes, granular leukocytes and nongranular leukocytes which are about ready to leave the bone marrow through the sinusoids and veins. The majority of cells, however, are the numerous stages of differentiation that stem cells go through during erythropoiesis, granulopoiesis and thrombopoiesis.

Erythropoiesis is the formation of erythrocytes from stem cells. In this process pluripotent stem cells, which have the potential to give rise to any blood cell type, differentiate into proerythroblasts. The latter cells divide into basophilic erythroblasts which contain free polyribosomes, a condensed nucleus, and no nucleoli. Without nucleoli the cells cannot produce ribosomes. Thus, when they divide into smaller polychromatophilic erythroblasts, their basophilia disappears and their acidophilia increases due to accumulating hemoglobin. When these cells have acquired their full amount of hemoglobin and their nuclei become very small and concentrated they are called normoblasts (orthochromatic erythroblasts). When the nuclei are extruded they become erythrocytes. Erythropoietin, produced by the kidney, regulates proerythroblast formation. The maturation of erythrocytes is regulated by the extrinsic factor (vitamin B$_{12}$) and the instrinsic factor (a mucoprotein produced in the stomach).

Granulopoiesis is the formation of basophils, eosinophils and neutrophils from stem cells that differentiate through myeloblast, promyelocyte, myelocyte and metamyelocyte stages. The myeloblast has a large nucleus with several prominent nucleoi; its cytoplasm is basophilic. When these cells acquire azurophilic granules, they are called promyelocytes. As promyelocytes mature into myelocytes, their nuclei become more dense, nonspecific azurophilic granules increase in number, and specific granules make their appearance. If the latter are neutrophilic, then the cell is a neutrophilic myelocyte; if basophilic or eosinophilic granules are present, the cell is a basophilic myelocyte or eosinophilic myelocyte. All of the cells from myeloblast through myelocyte are capable of mitosis. This ceases when the myelocyte nucleus becomes dense and more deeply indented as a metamyelocyte is formed. During maturation of the metamyelocyte into a mature granulocyte, the nucleus becomes more deeply indented and then becomes lobated or S-shaped. As this takes place, certain juvenile forms of cells are detected. In neutrophil formation the horseshoe-shaped nucleus often designates the cell as a band 'or stab cell. Since the life span of granular leukocytes is considerably shorter (about 14 hours) than that of erythrocytes (120 days), there are more developmental forms of granular leukocytes in the marrow than there are of erythrocytes.

Thrombopoiesis is the formation of blood platelets from megakaryocytes. In this process, plasma membranes of megakaryocytes partition off cytoplasmic fragments which are released from the cell and pass into the blood stream as platelets. The megakaryocyte may then die and is replaced by a stem cell in the marrow. Megakaryocytes are very large cells with multilobed nuclei. Blood platelets live for only about 8 to 11 days.

Lymphopoiesis is the formation of lymphocytes from a stem cell. In this process a large stem cell differentiates into a large lymphocyte (lymphoblast) that further divides and matures into medium lymphocytes, and then small lymphocytes. The sites of these lymphopoietic changes are in the bone marrow and in the lymphatic tissues of the spleen, thymus, lymph nodes, tonsils, and mucous membranes of the body. The theory that the small lymphocyte is an end point of differentiation is questioned, for it appears that the small lymphocyte can be the stem cell for large lymphoblasts that produce other small lymphocytes and antibody-producing plasma cells. In the establishment of the immune system, stem cells are sent to the thymus and the mucous membrane of the gut. In the thymus the stem cells become T lymphocyte precursors which pass to other tissues and become small cytotoxic "killer" lymphocytes. In the mucous membrane of the gut the stem cells become lymphocytes which develop into antibody producing lymphocytes.

Monopoiesis is the formation of monocytes from stem cells. Monocytes seem to develop in the marrow from pluripotent stem cells. After a few days developing in the marrow, monocytes pass into the circulation for one or two days before entering the connective tissue and becoming macrophages.

Mammary Gland

The mammary glands are integumentary glands located from the level of the second to sixth or seventh rib on the anterior of the thorax. In fetal development they first appear as ectodermal thickenings along a milk line extending between the upper and lower extremities. As development proceeds, 15 to 20 ectodermal invaginations branch and hollow out to give rise to the 15 to 20 lobes of the mammary gland, which are arranged in a radial fashion deep to the nipple. Thus each lobe has a single excretory duct opening on the nipple. Each of these ducts diverges at the base of the nipple and increases in size to form an ampulla (lactiferous sinus). Deep to the ampulla the ducts branch into intralobular ducts. In the male and non-pregnant gland there are few ducts present, and the epithelium changes from stratified to simple cuboidal epithelium in proceeding from larger to smaller ducts. In the lactating gland the ducts have proliferated, and their terminal portions develop into secretory alveoli lined by a simple pyramidal epithelium invested by myoepithelial cells. The lining epithelium demonstrates both apocrine and merocrine types of secretion. The lobes of the gland are supported by a dense connective tissue sheath, between the interstices of which are large accumulations of fat. Suspensory ligaments (of Cooper) run through the gland, attaching the deep layer of the superficial fascia to the dermis. The areola is covered by a thin, delicate pigmented skin. Underlying glands (of Montgomery) open on its surface. Smooth

muscle fibers also lie deep to the nipple and areola.

The nerves to the mammary gland are the intercostals (second to sixth), via lateral and anterior cutaneous branches. Sympathetic fibers accompany these nerves or the vessels supplying the gland. The arteries are the second and third perforating branches of the internal and the two external mammary branches of the lateral thoracic artery. Additional twigs from the intercostal arteries may enter the deep surface of the gland.

Diaphragm

The diaphragm is a thin dome-shaped muscle consisting of a series of radial fibers that arise from the inner side of the thoracic outlet and insert into a central aponeurosis or tendon. On the right its dome reaches to the fifth rib; on the left, to the fifth interspace.

Its origin has three parts: (1) a small sternal part that attaches to the posterior aspect of the xiphoid process, (2) an extensive costal portion that attaches to the subcostal margin and (3) a lumbar portion. The lumbar portion consists of the right and left crura, which arise from the anterior aspects of the lumbar vertebra and are separated by the aortic hiatus (T12), through which pass the aorta and thoracic duct. The esophageal hiatus (T10) is anterior to the aortic hiatus; most anterior and to the right is the opening for the inferior vena cava (T8). The diaphragm is supplied by the phrenic nerves with its peripheral portion receiving sensory fibers from the intercostals. The action of the muscles is to draw the central tendon downward, thus increasing the thoracic volume and decreasing the pressure within the thoracic cavity.

The phrenic nerve arises from the anterior rami of C3–5 nerves. It decends over the cupula of the pleura, in front of the root of the lung and between the pericardium and pleura to reach the diaphragm. Referred pain from the diaphragm occurs in the shoulder because both structures are innervated by sensory fibers to the C4 level of the spinal cord.

ABDOMEN

Surface Anatomy

Regions. The regions of the abdomen may be indicated by two horizontal and two vertical lines. The right and the left lateral lines are drawn vertically on each side through a point midway between the anterior superior iliac spine and the anterior median line. The transpyloric plane is a horizontal line through a point halfway between the suprasternal notch and the upper border of the pubic symphysis; this plane is also midway between the xiphisternal joint and the umbilicus. The transtubercular plane is a lower horizontal line at the level of the top of the iliac crest. These four lines subdivide the abdomen into the following nine regions; in the center the epigastric, the umbilical and the pubic regions; on the sides the right and the left hypochondriac, lumbar and inguinal regions.

The abdomen may also be divided into four areas by a vertical line and a horizontal line that pass through the umbilicus. This division establishes right and left upper and lower quadrants.

The transpyloric plane is at the level of the pylorus, the body of the first lumbar vertebra, the tip of the ninth costal cartilage on each side and the gallbladder on the right side. The semilunar line is the lateral border of the sheath of the rectus abdominis muscle and is a slightly curved line extending from the tip of the ninth costal cartilage to the pubic tubercle. The linea alba is the vertical median line between the rectus abdominis muscles.

Stomach. The stomach varies considerably in size and position, but its cardiac and pyloric portions are relatively fixed. The cardiac orific is opposite the seventh costal cartilage about 2.5 cm. to the left of the xiphisternal joint. The pyloric orifice is on the transpyloric plane about 1.5 cm. to the right of the midline. The lesser curvature is indicated by a curved line that passes downward and to the right and connects these two points. The fundus reaches the fifth interspace in the left lateral line. The greater curvature may extend to the level of the umbilicus. The pregastric space (Traube) overlies the stomach, is semilunar in outline and is bounded by the lower edge of the left lung, the anterior border of the spleen, the left costal margin and the lower edge of the left lobe of the liver.

Small Intestine. The duodenum may be mapped by four continuous lines: (1) a transverse line from the pylorus to the junction of the transpyloric and the right lateral lines, (2) a descending line passing inferiorly to the lowest level of the subcostal margin (subcostal line at L3), (3) another transverse line passing from right to left and ending about 3.0 cm. to the left of the midline, and (4) an ascending line for one to two vertebral levels that terminates at the duodenojejunal flexure. The rest of the small intestine occupies a large amount of the abdominal cavity. The coils of the jejunum are predominantly in the upper left quadrant and those of the ileum in the lower right quandrant. The ileocolic junction is slightly below and medial to the intersection of the right lateral and transtubercular lines.

Large Intestine and Vermiform Appendix. The cecum lies in the right iliac and hypogastric regions. The middle of its lower border is the midpoint of a line from the right anterior superior iliac spine to the upper margin of the symphysis pubis. This point (McBurney's) is the location at which point tenderness can be elicited when the appendix is inflamed. The right colic flexure is on a level just below the transpyloric plane 2.5 cm. lateral to the right lateral line. The left colic flexure lies just above the transpyloric plane 2.5 cm. lateral to the left lateral line.

Liver. The upper border of the liver corresponds to a horizontal line passing just below the nipples. The inferior border of the liver rather closely parallels the right inferior costal margin which it leaves at the tip of the ninth costal cartilage, extending from this point across the subcostal angle to just below the left nipple.

Pancreas. The head of the pancreas occupies the curve of the duodenum and is bounded accordingly. The neck is in the midline at the transpyloric line. The body extends to the left and slightly superiorly, and the tail is in contact with the spleen.

Spleen. The spleen is situated posteriorly beneath the left ninth, tenth and eleventh ribs. The upper pole lies about 3 cm. lateral to the left tenth thoracic spine. The lower pole extends as far forward as the midaxillary line at the level of the eleventh rib.

Kidney. The kidneys are about 10 cm. long; about one third of the length of the kidney lies above the transpyloric plane, the left kidney being about 1 to 1.5 cm. higher. The upper pole is about 5 cm. from the midline; the lower pole, 7.5 cm. from the midline. Both kidneys extend above the level of the twelfth rib. The hilum is 5 cm. from the middle line at the level of L1. On the dorsal aspect of the body the position of the kidneys may be indicated by a parallelogram. Two vertical lines are drawn 2.5 cm. and 10 cm. from the midline, and the parallelogram is completed by two horizontal lines at the levels of the tips of the spinous processes of T11 and L3.

Ureter. The location of the ureter is indicated by a line from the hilum to the bifurcation of the common iliac artery where the ureter enters the pelvis. This vertical line is 3 to 4 cm. lateral to the midline and is anterior to the transverse processes of the lumbar vertebrae.

Abdominal Wall

Superficial Fascia. This fascia is composed of superficial and deep layers. The superficial or fatty layer is continuous with the superficial fascia of adjacent areas, e.g., thigh and perineum. The deep or fibrous layer attaches to the deep fascia of the thigh but continues into the perineum as the superficial perineal fascia. Thus, fluid collecting in the superficial perineal space will find its way into the abdominal wall (between the fibrous layer of the superficial fascia and the external abdominal oblique muscle) but not into the thigh.

Muscles. The interval between the inferior costal margin and the superior aspect of the pelvis (pubis, inguinal ligament, iliac crest) contains four major muscles, all of which are segmentally innervated by thoracic and lumbar nerves. The external abdominal oblique, internal abdominal oblique and transversus abdominis are lateral to the semilunar line; the rectus abdominis is medial. The most superficial muscle is the external oblique whose fibers are directed anteriorly, medially and inferiorly. The fibers of the internal oblique are perpendicular to those of the external oblique. The transversus abdominis fibers are transversely oriented. The aponeuroses of all three muscles extend medially, and together they form the rectus sheath. The rectus abdominis is the only vertically oriented muscle, and it extends between the superomedial aspect of the pubis and the medial aspect of the inferior costal margin and the xiphoid process. Its tendinous intersections account for the "ripples" seen on the surface of the abdomen.

Inguinal Region. The inferior aspect of the abdominal wall is composed primarily of the aponeuroses of the abdominal muscles. The inferior margin of the external oblique aponeurosis forms the inguinal ligament as it stretches between the anterior superior iliac spine and the pubic tubercle. This tough band is an attachment for some of the other abdominal muscles, and it helps form the inguinal canal.

The inguinal canal is an obliquely oriented pathway through the abdominal wall. It stretches between the superficial (external) and deep (internal) inguinal rings and is directed inferomedially just above the inguinal ligament. The superficial ring is a split in the external oblique aponeurosis just superolateral to the pubic tubercle. The medial and lateral edges of the ring are called the medial (superior) and lateral (inferior) crura. The deep ring is the beginning of a sleeve of transversalis fascia that extends along the spermatic cord. This ring is located about halfway between the anterior superior iliac spine and the pubic tubercle.

The walls of the inguinal canal are as follows: (1) floor: inguinal ligament, (2) anterior wall: external oblique aponeurosis, (3) posterior wall: medially the conjoined tendon (falx inguinalis), which is composed of the arching medial attachments of the internal oblique and the transversus abdominis, and laterally the transversalis fascia, (4) roof: conjoined tendon as it arches over the contents of the canal.

The spermatic cord consists of the vas deferens and its artery, the pampiniform plexus of veins, lymphatic, sympathetics, the ilioinguinal nerve, the nerve and artery to the cremasteric muscle and the testicular artery. Most of these structures are enclosed within the (1) internal spermatic fascia, which is derived from the transversalis fascia, (2) the cremasteric muscle and fascia, which are derived from the internal oblique, and (3) the external spermatic fascia, which is derived from the aponeurosis of the external oblique.

Inguinal hernias are either direct or indirect, based on the path of the herniating sac. The indirect hernia follows the course of the testis during development, i.e., it passes into the canal through the internal opening and then through the canal. After exiting through the superficial ring it usually passes into the scrotum. At surgery the neck of this type of hernia is found lateral to the inferior epigastric vessels, and the hernial sac is covered with peritoneum and the three fascial coverings of the spermatic cord. A direct hernia passes through Hesselbach's triangle, i.e., the triangular area defined by the lateral border of the rectus abdominis, the inferior epigastric vessels and the inguinal ligament. At surgery the neck of this type of hernial sac is medial to the inferior epigastric vessels and covered by a layer of peritoneum and transversalis fascia. Since this hernia will pass through the superficial ring it is also covered by the external spermatic fascia.

Contents of the Abdominal Cavity
Peritoneum and Mesenteries

The peritoneum is similar to the pleura in that it consists of a parietal layer that lines the abdominopelvic cavity and a visceral layer that is reflected over organs. It is also similar in that the peritoneal cavity contains nothing other than a small amount of lubricating fluid and in reality is a potential space. It differs from the pleura in that its visceral layer reflects in varying degrees over multiple organs. Some organs—jejunum and ileum—are almost completely covered by peritoneum and attached to the posterior body wall by a mesentery and thus are said to be (completely) peritonealized. Other organs (kidneys) are essentially outside the peritoneum and covered by peritoneum on only one side. These organs are extraperitoneal or, if located on the posterior body wall, retroperitoneal. Those organs, which are neither peritonealized nor extraperitoneal, but are somewhere in between, are partially peritonealized.

The peritoneal cavity is separated into greater and lesser (omental bursa) peritoneal sacs. The lesser sac is posterior to the stomach, lesser omentum and caudate lobe of the liver. The greater sac is the rest of the peritoneal cavity. The two areas are connected only through the epiploic foramen (of Winslow), which is small and admits two fingers. Its anterior border is the right free margin of the lesser peritoneal sac, which is formed by the hepatoduodenal ligament and contains: (1) the common bile duct, (2) the portal vein, (3) the proper hepatic artery and (4) lymphatics and nerves.

Within the peritoneal cavity there are areas where inflammatory material can accumulate and become sequestered. These areas are as follows: In the abdomen there are the subphrenic and subhepatic spaces, and the paravertebral gutters. The subphrenic spaces are found between the liver and the diaphragm, being separated into right and left portions by the coronary and falciform ligaments and lesser omentum. The subhepatic spaces are inferior to the visceral surface of the liver, the right being inferior to the right and caudate lobes of the liver and the left (omental bursa) inferior to the left and quadrate lobes. These subhepatic spaces are connected through the epiploic foramen. The paravertebral gutters are vertically oriented and on either side of the lumbar vertebral bodies. Each is subdivided into two gutters by the ascending and descending portions of the colon. Thus, each paravertebral gutter consists of a medial and a lateral paracolic gutter. Material in the paracolic gutters tends to move superiorly into the subphrenic and subhepatic spaces. In the pelvis of both the male and female there are pararectal fossae on either side of the rectum. In the male the rectovesical pouch is found between the rectum and the bladder. In the female the uterus and broad ligament divide that similar area into two pouches, the vesicouterine pouch anteriorly and the rectouterine pouch (of Douglas) posteriorly.

Folds and fossae of the peritoneum occur on the lower part of the anterior abdominal wall. These consist of the single median umbilical fold, and the medial and lateral umbilical folds. The median fold overlies the remains of the urachus; the medial folds are formed by the obliterated umbilical arteries and the lateral by the inferior epigastric vessels. The supravesical fossae are between the median and medial folds; the medial and lateral inguinal fossae are medial and lateral respectively to the lateral fold. Indirect hernias pass through the lateral inguinal fossa while direct hernias pass through either the supravesical or medial inguinal fossa.

The specific peritoneal relationships of each organ will be covered with the discussion of that organ.

Stomach. This organ extends from the cardiac opening of the esophagus to the pylorus. It consists of a fundus, a body and a pyloric portion, the latter made up of the pyloric antrum, canal and sphincter. Its right or upper border forms the lesser curvature, to which the lesser omentum attaches. The lower and left border forms the greater curvature and gives attachment to the greater omentum and gastrolienal liga-

ment. Posteriorly the stomach is in contact with the spleen, the splenic artery, the diaphragm, the left kidney and suprarenal, the pancreas and the transverse mesocolon; anteriorly it is in contact with the liver, the diaphragm and the abdominal wall. The blood supply to the stomach is provided by the three main branches of the celiac trunk: the common hepatic, left gastric and splenic arteries. Each has branches which pass along the greater and lesser curvatures of the stomach. Venous and lymphatic drainage parallels the arterial supply. The veins are tributaries of the portal vein, and the lymphatics all pass eventually to the celiac group of aortic lymph nodes.

Small Intestine. The duodenum is a somewhat C-shaped tube that surrounds the head of the pancreas. It is divided into four parts, most of which are retroperitoneal. The first part is short and ascends slightly from the gastroduodenal junction. It is related anteriorly to the gallbladder and liver and posteriorly to the portal vein, common bile duct, gastroduodenal artery and the inferior vena cava. The second part descends in the right medial paracolic gutter. Posteriorly it is related to the right kidney and suprarenal gland while anteriorly it is crossed by the transverse colon. The common bile duct and main pancreatic duct empty into it posteromedially. The third part passes from right to left in front of the vena cava, the body of the third lumbar vertebra and the aorta; it passes behind the superior mesenteric vessels. The fourth part is short and curves superiorly and then anteriorly at the duodenojejunal junction. It is suspended from the area of the right crus of the diaphragm by a peritoneal fold called the suspensory ligament of Treitz.

The mesenteric portion of the small intestine is divided into the proximal jejunum and distal ileum. The mesentery is a fan-shaped double layer of peritoneum continuous with the serosa of the jejunum and ileum and enclosing their vessels. The root of the mesentery is about 15 cm. long, and its attachment to the posterior body wall extends from the duodenojejunal junction obliquely down and to the right, crossing the third part of the duodenum, the inferior vena cava and the right ureter. The mesentery contains the intestinal and ileocolic branches of the superior mesenteric vessels as well as lymphatics and autonomics. The transition from jejunum to ileum is not abrupt, but certain differences do exist. The amount of mesenteric fat tends to increase from above downward, as does the number of arcades formed by the vessels in the mesentery. However, the blood supply to the jejunum is greater, so that its pink color is more intense than that of the ileum. The jejunum has a thicker wall as the plicae circulares are higher at that level.

Large Intestine.   This portion extends from the ileocecal valve to the anus. It is characterized by sacculations (haustra) which are caused by three longitudinal muscle bands (taenia) that converge at the appendix. Between the sacculations are the semilunar folds, and along the free surface are pouches containing fat (appendices epiploicae).

The cecum is a cul-de-sac of the colon below the entrance of the ileum. It is found in the right iliac fossa and is usually almost entirely enveloped in peritoneum. The ileocecal valve is formed by two liplike folds projecting into the medial aspect of the cecum.

The vermiform appendix is a blind tube that comes off the posteromedial aspect of the cecum about 2.5 cm. below the ileocecal valve. It is most commonly found behind the cecum (retrocecal) although it may be in a variety of positions including hanging into the pelvis. It has a slight valve and although variable is usually about 10 cm. in length. It has no true mesentery but is covered with a peritoneal fold and is supplied by an appendicular branch of the ileocolic artery.

The ascending colon is the continuation of the cecum that passes superiorly against the posterior body wall and the right kidney. Just below the right lobe of the liver it makes a sharp bend to the left. This bend is the right colic or hepatic flexure. The transverse colon extends between the hepatic and the splenic flexures and is suspended from the posterior abdominal wall by the transverse mesocolon. The attachment of the mesocolon crosses the second part of the duodenum and the pancreas and attaches to the greater curvature of the stomach. The transverse colon is related to the liver, gallbladder and stomach anteriorly, and to the spleen superiorly. The descending colon extends from the splenic flexure to the left iliac fossa, passing along the lateral aspect of the left kidney and posterior body wall before becoming the sigmoid colon. Both the ascending and descending portions of the colon are usually partially peritonealized and therefore fixed in place, as opposed to the mobile transverse colon.

Liver.   The anterior, superior and posterior surfaces of the liver are in the form of a dome that is related to the thoracic diaphragm. Through the diaphragm the liver is related to the lungs, pleura, heart, and pericardium. Its posteroinferior or visceral surface is related to the hepatic flexure of the colon, right kidney and suprarenal gland, gallbladder, duodenum, esophagus and stomach. The visceral surface has an H-shaped configuration in which the center bar of the H is the porta hepatis where the portal vein autonomics and hepatic artery enter and the common hepatic duct and lymphatics exit. The limb of the H extending anteriorly on the right contains the gallbladder; posteriorly on the right is the inferior vena cava; anteriorly on the

left is the ligamentum teres; and posteriorly on the left is the ligamentum venosum. That part of the liver between the two anterior limbs is the quadrate lobe; that portion between the two posterior limbs is the caudate lobe. Functionally the liver is separated into a large right lobe and a smaller left lobe which includes the quadrate and caudate lobes.

The liver is semienclosed within a complicated system of peritoneal foldings. The falciform ligament reflects from the anterior belly wall to the liver and contains the ligamentum teres in its inferior border. Anteriorly the falciform ligament reflects over the right and left lobes of the liver. On the superior and posterior aspects of the dome of the liver the two layers of this ligament initially diverge toward the sides of the liver and at the most lateral extent of this reflection each layer sharply turns medially and posteriorly and converges toward the other in the region of the ligamentum venosum. As the two layers of the falciform ligament diverge and then converge in the pattern just indicated they reflect onto the diaphragm. This crown-shaped pattern of peritoneal reflections between the posterosuperior surface of the liver and the under surface of the diaphragm is termed the coronary ligament. It surrounds the bare area of the liver, an area in which no peritoneum separates the liver and the diaphragm. The right and left extents of the coronary ligament are called the right and left triangular ligaments respectively. The lesser omentum extends from the visceral surface of the liver to the lesser curvature of the stomach. The free edge of the lesser omentum is formed as the peritoneum surrounds the portal vein, hepatic artery and common bile duct. This free edge extends between the first part of the duodenum and the porta hepatis and forms the anterior boundary of the epiploic foramen (of Winslow), which is the entrance to the lesser omental sac.

The portal system includes all of the veins that drain the blood from the abdominal part of the digestive tube (except for the lower part of the rectum) and from the spleen, the pancreas and the gallbladder. The portal vein is formed behind the neck of the pancreas by the union of the superior mesenteric and the splenic veins. It enters the porta of the liver and there, with the hepatic artery, divides into right and left lobar arteries, whose branches supply the liver lobules and eventually drain to the inferior vena cava by way of hepatic veins. At the porta hepatis the hepatic artery and the common bile duct are in front of the vein: the artery to the left, the duct to the right.

In portal obstruction there are several alternate routes that blood may take to get from the portal venous system into the systemic circulation without going through the liver. These potential communications are between (1) the superior rectal veins with the middle and inferior rectal veins, which are tributaries of the internal iliac and internal pudendal respectively, (2) esophageal branches of the left gastric with esophageal tributaries of the azygous systems of veins, (3) portal tributaries in the mesenteries with body wall (retroperitoneal) tributaries of the lumbar, renal, and phrenic veins, (4) portal tributaries in the liver with tributaries to the abdominal wall veins in the falciform ligament and (5) portal tributaries in the liver with phrenic veins across the bare area of the liver.

Gallbladder and Ducts. The bile passages include the gallbladder, the cystic duct, the hepatic duct and the common bile duct. The gallbladder is a pear-shaped viscus lying below the liver between the right and the quadrate lobes. It has a broad fundus, a body and a neck that narrows into the cystic duct. The body of the gallbladder is related superiorly to the liver, inferiorly to the transverse colon and posteriorly with the duodenum or pyloric end of the stomach. The fundus of the gallbladder is at the tip of the ninth costal cartilage.

The cystic duct unites with the hepatic duct to form the common bile duct. The common bile duct and the main pancreatic duct unite just proximal to the point at which they empty into the second part of the duodenum at the major duodenal papilla. This common opening is protected by the sphincter of Oddi.

Pancreas. This organ lies between the stomach and the posterior abdominal wall, from the duodenum to the spleen. It is completely retroperitoneal. It is divided into a head, lying within the concavity of the duodenum, a neck, which is constricted posteriorly by the portal vein, a triangular body, and a tail that rests upon the spleen. The secretions of the neck, body and tail portions of the pancreas are carried through the main pancreatic duct, through which they enter the duodenum. The accessory pancreatic duct of Santorini traverses the head of the pancreas and enters the duodenum 2 cm. above the major duodenal papilla.

The main arteries supplying the pancreas are the superior and the inferior pancreaticoduodenal and the splenic, the latter running behind the upper part of the body and the tail of the pancreas.

Spleen. This organ occupies the left hypochondrium and epigastrium under the ribs. Its parietal surface is in relation to the dome of the diaphragm. Its visceral surface is related to the stomach, left kidney, splenic flexure of the colon and the tail of the pancreas. It is completely peritonealized and connected by peritoneal reflections to the posterior body wall in the region of the left kidney by the lienorenal ligament and to the stomach by the gastrolienal ligament. Its blood supply is provided by the splenic artery.

Kidney. The kidneys are surrounded by perirenal fat and supported by the renal fascia. They extend from the last thoracic to the third lumbar vertebrae, the right being lower than the left. The kidneys are entirely retroperitoneal and are partially separated from the peritoneum by the duodenum on the right and the pancreas on the left.

The kidneys occupy the most dorsal position of all the abdominal organs. Each kidney lies against the diaphragm and the twelfth rib above and against the psoas major and the quadratus lumborum below. The anterior relationships of the left kidney are spleen, stomach, pancreas, left colic flexure and the small intestine. The anterior surface of the right kidney is related to the liver, second part of the duodenum, and the right colic flexure.

The renal hilus is directed anteromedially and is the concave aspect of the kidney. The renal artery enters the kidney through this area, while the renal vein and ureter exit at this site. The final collecting cistern for urine is the renal pelvis. The pelvis occupies a large percentage of the hilus and is usually at the level of the body of L1. The pelvis narrows rapidly to form the ureter, which conducts the urine to the bladder. The ureters are retroperitoneal and descend through the abdominal cavity almost vertically on the anterior aspect of the psoas major muscle. The right ureter is related anteriorly to the duodenum, vessels to the ascending colon, root of the mesentery and the testicular or ovarian vessels. The left ureter is related anteriorly to the left colic vessels, testicular or ovarian vessels and the sigmoid colon. At roentgenographic examination in which the ureters are filled with contrast medium they are seen to cross the transverse processes of the lumbar vertebrae. As ureters enter the pelvis they incline medially, and they usually cross the termination of the common iliac arteries (or their branches). Their pelvic course is inferomedial to the posterior aspect of the bladder. The ureters have three natural constrictions: at the junction of the renal pelvis and the ureter, where they cross the common iliac arteries, and as they pass through the wall of the bladder.

Each kidney is generally supplied by a single large renal artery that is a direct branch from the abdominal aorta. A common variation is two or three renal arteries on one or both sides.

Suprarenal Glands. The retroperitoneal suprarenal (adrenal) glands sit on the superior poles of each kidney. Both glands are related posteriorly to the diaphragm. The right suprarenal is related anteriorly to the liver and medially to the inferior vena cava. The anterior aspect of the left gland forms part of the posterior wall of the omental bursa and may be related to the splenic artery and the pancreas. Each gland receives a rich blood supply via branches from the renal and inferior phrenic arteries and from the aorta.

Blood Supply of the Abdomen

The abdominal aorta enters the abdomen through the aortic hiatus (T12) and extends to the lower portion of the fourth lumbar vertbral body where it terminates by dividing into the large common iliac arteries and into its true continuation, the rudimentary median sacral artery. It descends vertically along the anterior (or slightly to the left) aspect of the lumbar vertebral bodies.

Its branches are as follows:

Inferior Phrenic. A pair of arteries that arise just below the diaphragm or from the celiac trunk and distribute to the under surface of the diaphragm.

Celiac Trunk. The highest of the unpaired vessels, it arises at L1. A very short trunk, it passes anteriorly behind the peritoneum and above the pancreas and divides into its three branches, the left gastric, splenic and common hepatic. The left gastric passes to the left and distributes to the lesser curvature of the stomach and has esophageal and hepatic branches. The splenic passes to the left embedded in the upper surface of the pancreas. It forms part of the floor of the lesser omental sac. It supplies the pancreas and spleen and has the short gastric and left gastroepiploic branches to the greater curvature of the stomach. The common hepatic artery runs anterolaterally to the right toward the upper aspect of the first part of the duodenum. The gastroduodenal branch descends behind the duodenum and has anterior and posterior superior pancreaticoduodenal, and right gastroepiploic branches. The continuation of the common hepatic after the gastroduodenal branch is the proper hepatic artery. This artery passes to the right and ascends to the porta hepatis through the lesser omentum. The right gastric artery usually branches from the proper hepatic soon after its beginning, and the cystic artery branches where the proper hepatic passes the cystic duct.

Middle Suprarenal. Usually a single vessel that passes directly to the suprarenal gland

Superior Mesenteric. The branches of this vessel supply the gastrointestinal tract from the middle of the duodenum through the transverse colon. One of its branches, the inferior pancreaticoduodenal artery, divides into anterior and posterior branches that form the pancreaticoduodenal arcades with the anterior and posterior superior pancreaticoduodenal arteries. The other branches are the intestinal arteries, the ileocolic artery, the right colic artery and the middle colic artery.

Renal Artery. Arising at about the level of the second lumbar vertebra these two large arteries pass across the crura of the diaphragm and the psoas major muscles in their transverse course to the hila of the kidneys. The right is longer than the left, and it passes posterior to the inferior vena cava.

Testicular or Ovarian Arteries. These small arteries arise just inferior to the renal arteries. The retroperitoneal testicular arteries descend obliquely toward the deep inguinal ring where they become part of the spermatic cord. The ureteric branches arise as the testicular arteries cross the ureters. The abdominal course of the ovarian arteries is similar to that of the testiculars. As they reach the pelvic brim the ovarian arteries swing medially and pass through the suspensory ligament of the ovary to the ovary.

Inferior Mesenteric. Arising just below the third part of the duodenum, this artery passes obliquely downward and to the left, behind the peritoneum. Its left colic, sigmoid and superior rectal branches supply the left third of the transverse colon, the descending colon, the sigmoid colon and the upper portion of the rectum.

Lumbar Arteries. The four lumbar arteries supply primarily the body wall and those structures within the vertebral canal.

Common Iliac Arteries. The large terminal branches of the aorta, the common iliacs, arise slightly to the left of the midline in front of the body of the fourth lumbar vertebra. The common iliacs divide into the internal and external iliac arteries just lateral to the sacral promotory. Each internal iliac enters the pelvis to supply pelvic and perineal structures. The external iliac passes under the inguinal ligament where it becomes the femoral artery.

Middle Sacral Artery. The true caudal continuation and termination of the aorta, this vessel arises from the posterior aspect of the aorta just above its bifurcation. It passes inferiorly on the ventral aspect of the lumbar vertebrae, enters the pelvis and descends on the anterior surface of the sacrum and coccyx. It gives rise to parietal branches in its course.

Nerve Supply of the Abdomen

Body Wall. The skin of the abdominal wall is innervated by the anterior and lateral cutaneous branches of intercostal nerves seven through eleven (T7–11), the subcostal nerve (T12) and the iliohypogastric branch of the first lumbar nerve. The underlying muscles of the abdominal wall are innervated segmentally by muscular branches of the same nerves.

Viscera. Autonomic innervation of the viscera of the abdominal cavity is provided by sympathetic fibers from spinal cord segments T5 through L1 or 2 and parasympathetic fibers from the vagus nerve and spinal cord segments S2 through 4. These fibers generally are distributed in periarterial plexuses that are associated with the abdominal aorta and its branches. The continuous plexus found on the ventral aspect of the aorta and associated with the three large unpaired arteries is divided into the celiac, superior mesenteric and inferior mesenteric plexuses, with the intermesenteric plexus connecting the superior and inferior mesenterics and the inferior mesenteric plexus continuing inferiorly as the superior hypogastric plexus. Continuations of these plexuses follow various other branches of the aorta to their respective destinations and bear the names of the arteries, e.g., the renal plexus.

The *sympathetic* input into these plexuses is as follows:

Greater (T5–10), lesser (T10–12), and least (T12) splanchnic nerves into the celiac and superior mesenteric plexuses. These nerves arise in the thorax and enter the abdomen by passing through the crura of the diaphragm.

Lumbar splanchnics (from the lumbar sympathetic trunk) into the intermesenteric, inferior mesenteric and superior hypogastric plexuses. The fibers in the thoracic and lumbar splanchnic nerves are preganglionic. They synapse with postganglionic fibers in ganglia associated with the aortic plexuses. The largest and most demonstrable of these is the celiac ganglion.

The *parasympathetic* input into these plexuses is as follows:

Vagal fibers supply the organs of the abdomen and the gastrointestinal tract as far distally as the splenic flexure of the large intestine. The vagus nerves enter the abdomen with the esophagus as the anterior and posterior vagal trunks. The trunks distribute on the anterior and posterior aspects of the stomach and enter the celiac plexus.

The pelvic splanchnics (from spinal cord segments S2–4) provide direct retroperitoneal branches to the descending and sigmoid portions of the large intestine.

The fibers in both the vagus and pelvic splanchnic nerves are preganglionic. They synapse with postganglionic fibers either in or very near the organ innervated.

Afferent fibers from the abdominal viscera reach the central nervous system through both the vagus and splanchnic nerves. Those sensory fibers in the vagus are concerned with muscular and secretory reflexes. Most pain fibers are thought to be carried in the splanchnic nerves.

Microscopic Structure of Abdominal Organs

Gastrointestinal Tract. The general histologic plan of the gastrointestinal tract consists of an inner mucosa, a submucosa, muscularis externa and serosa layers. These were reviewed in the section on the esophagus. Different parts of the gastrointestinal tract retain the basic plan but differ as to their internal configuration of the mucosa, epithelial lining, type and extent of mucosal and submucosal glands and by their thickness and configuration of muscle.

The *stomach* is structurally modified for the production of hydrochloric acid and pepsin and for the mixing of food with these substances. In the empty stomach the mucosa is thrown into longitudinal folds called rugae. Throughout the stomach the simple columnar lining epithelium produces mucus and indents into the mucosa as gastric pits. One or more mucosal glands empty into the base of each pit. The length of glands and pits and the glandular cell types differ in the cardiac, body (fundus) and pyloric regions of the stomach. Gastric glands of the body and fundus are the most prevalent and contain the most diverse cell types. In this type of gland, chief cells are located mostly in the base (fundus), parietal cells are located in the neck and isthmus region, mucous neck cells are in the neck, and argentaffin cells are scattered.

Chief cells produce pepsin and are typical enzyme-secreting cells in that they contain much rough endoplasmic reticulum, a well-established Golgi apparatus and membrane-bound zymogen granules. In these cells, amino acids attached to transfer RNA are carried to ribosomal RNA of the rough endoplasmic reticulum (RER) where the pepsinogen code is translated from messenger RNA. The protein product passes into the cisterna of the RER and is carried to condensing vacuoles near the Golgi apparatus. In this region the membrane-bound pepsinogen granule is formed. The granule passes to the apical surface of the cell where the product is discharged when the membrane of the granule fuses with the plasma membrane and then opens to the lumen. Parietal cells produce HCl and may produce the intrinsic antipernicious anemia factor. They are rounded, or pyramidal, cells whose apices open to the lumen through an intercellular canal between adjacent chief cells. An extensive infolding of the surface membrane forms intracellular canaliculi into which microvilli project. Smooth endoplasmic reticulum and mitochondria are prevalent, and the cells are often binucleate. In the production of HCl, sodium chloride probably passes to the intracellular canaliculi were hydrogen ion, supplied by carbonic acid in the cell, is exchanged for sodium. Thus, HCl passes into the lumen of the gland while bicarbonate passes from the cell into the blood. Mucous neck cells produce mucus of a different nature than that of the surface epithelium. Argentaffin cells are sandwiched between the other gland cells and the basement membrane. Some of these produce serotonin while other types of these cells produce cholinesterase; both of these secretions are discharged into the blood stream.

Pyloric and cardiac glands contain only cells that are similar to the neck mucous cell. In the pyloric region the gastric pits are deep, and the glands are very tortuous and appear shorter.

The muscularis externa layer of the stomach contains three layers, an outer longitudinal, a middle circular and an inner oblique layer. The two inner layers are thickened as the pyloric sphincter muscle. The serosa is continuous with the two layers of the greater and lesser omentum.

The *small intestine* is structurally modified for the absorption of nutritive substances. The absorptive surface is large because of (1) mucosal and submucosal folds called plicae circulares, (2) mucosal projections called villi and (3) microvilli forming a striated border on the simple columnar lining epithelium. Mucus is secreted by goblet cells in the lining epithelium. These cells increase in number at progressively lower levels of the gastrointestinal tract where drier wastes are accumulating. Crypts of Lieberkühn are mucosal glands that are found throughout the intestine; they empty at the bases of the villi. Their cells replace the lining cells of the villi every 7 to 8 days and thus show mitoses and gradations of differentiation. Some of these gland cells probably produce secretin and cholecystokinin. Argentaffin cells and Paneth's cells are present in the crypts of Lieberkühn. In the upper part of the duodenum, Brunner's glands occupy the submucosa and empty into the crypts or at the bases of villi. Their cells are similar to those in the pyloric glands and produce an alkaline mucus—carbohydrate secretion. The lower ileum contains aggregations of lymphatic nodules called Peyer's patches. These are located opposite the mesentery attachment, chiefly in the mucosa. The muscularis externa consists of inner circular and outer longitudinal smooth muscle layers. Myenteric and submucosal nerve plexi containing autonomic postganglionic cell bodies are present throughout the intestine and stomach.

The absorption of fats, carbohydrates, proteins and water in the small intestine takes place through the simple columnar lining cells of the villi since the tight junctions (zonula occludens) of the junctional complexes (zonula occludens, zonula adherens, macula adherens) do not permit intercellular passage. Thus, carbohydrates, fats and proteins must be broken down in the lumen before absorption can take place. Some of this is accomplished by pancreatic enzymes and liver bile salts. Intestinal juices produced by crypt glands and the lining epithelium are also involved in the terminal hydrolytic digestion of carbohydrates and proteins. The active sites of much of this activity seem to be in the microvillus region near the glycoprotein "fuzz" coat. Substances absorbed through the surface epithelium pass to capillaries or the central lacteal of the villi for distribution in the portal vein or thoracic duct respectively.

The *large intestine* absorbs much water and produces mucus that lubricates the feces. No villi are present, and the crypts open directly on the surface. The lining epithelium is simple columnar with a striated border, and it contains many goblet cells. The outer longitudinal layer of the muscularis externa is thickened into three longitudinally running bands of smooth muscle (taenia coli).

The *appendix* is microscopically similar to the colon except that it is smaller, does not have taenia and possesses a prominent ring of lymphatic nodules that occupy most of the lamina propria and the submucosa.

The *anal canal* functions to retain and eliminate wastes. The colon-like mucosa of the upper portion forms longitudinal anal columns just above the horizontally oriented anal valves. Epithelium over the anal valves is stratified squamous nonkeratinized epithelium. It becomes keratinized about 2.5 cm. below the valves. The lamina propria contains large internal hemorrhoidal veins and circumanal glands. The inner circular layer of the muscularis becomes the internal anal sphincter. The outer longitudinal layer disappears and is replaced in position by skeletal muscle of the external anal sphincter.

Liver and Gallbladder. The liver is surrounded by a tough connective tissue capsule that penetrates it at the porta to produce many septa. These septa provide support for the parenchyma and divide it into lobules. Branches of the portal vein and hepatic artery further subdivide within the septa and supply the lobules. These vessels and bile ducts constitute portal triads (portal canals) at the junction of adjacent lobules.

The lobules consist of a central vein from which anastomosing hepatic plates of cells, usually one cell thick, radiate toward the periphery. Between the plates are hepatic sinusoids that connect the portal vein and hepatic artery peripherally with the central vein centrally. Blood drains from the central vein to sublobular veins and leaves the liver by way of the hepatic veins. The sinusoids are discontinuously lined by endothelial cells and phagocytic Kupffer cells of the reticuloendothelial system. The lining cells abut against microvilli of the hepatocytes, leaving a space (of Disse) between the base of the endothelial cell and the hepatocyte that is continuous with the sinusoids. This provides for efficient interchange between blood in the sinusoid and the hepatocyte. Bile canaliculi lie between adjacent cells in the hepatic plates and are expansions of the intercellular spaces between the cells. These canaliculi receive bile produced by the hepatocytes and conduct it peripherally into small ducts that open into the bile ducts of the portal triad. Bile is transported out of the liver in hepatic ducts; it them traverses the cystic duct and is stored and condensed in the gallbladder. Bile is discharged from the gallbladder through the cystic duct and common bile duct and empties at the sphincters of Oddi and Boyden into the duodenum. The epithelium lining the bile ducts grades from low cuboidal to high columnar with the increasing caliber of the ducts. Hepatocytes are polyhedral, with one or more large rounded nuclei. They contain a wide range of organelles that are consistent with the many and diverse functions these cells perform.

The *gallbladder* is lined by a mucous membrane that is thrown into folds. It possesses a simple columnar epithelium that has extensive basal infoldings that are characteristic of surfaces where water and ion reabsorption is taking place. A circularly arranged smooth muscle layer is present and is surrounded by a prominent connective tissue layer.

Pancreas. The pancreas is divided into lobules by connective tissue septa. The lobules are packed with serous acini consisting of enzyme-secreting pyramidal cells and centroacinar cells. The serous-secreting cells are similar in structure to the previously described chief cells of the stomach, but these cells produce proteases, nucleases, amylase, lipase and high concentrations of sodium bicarbonate. The acini are drained by intercalated ducts that pass successively to larger intralobular ducts, interlobular ducts and the main pancreatic duct (of Wirsung) or accessory duct. The larger ducts have simple columnar epithelium, goblet cells and mucous glands; the smaller ducts are lined with simple cuboidal epithelium.

Islets of Langerhans are heavily vascularized groups of cells scattered throughout the pancreas. There are several cell types present in the islets. The most common type is the beta cell. It contains alcohol-soluble granules and produces insulin. Absence or malfunction of these cells leads to diabetes mellitus. The other prominent cell type of the islets is the alpha cell. It has alcohol-preserved granules and produces glucagon, a hyperglycemic-glycogenolytic factor.

Spleen. The spleen is the largest lymphoid organ in the body, and it is specialized for filtering blood. The spleen consists of white pulp (splenic nodules) and red pulp. The white pulp is dense lymphatic tissue; the red pulp is looser and consists of lymphatic splenic cords of tissue and venous sinusoids. Arterial blood enters the spleen at the hilum in the splenic artery. Branches of this artery pass in connective tissue trabeculae that radiate from the capsule at the hilar region. These are trabecular (interlobular) arteries. At the ends of the trabeculae the adventitia of the arteries takes on the character of reticular tissue and becomes infiltrated with lymphocytes forming splenic nodules (white pulp). These arteries are eccentrically located in the nodules and are called central arteries. After numerous branchings these arterioles leave the white pulp and enter the reticular connective tissue of the red pulp that surrounds the splenic nodules. In the red pulp the pulp arterioles divide into sheathed arterioles that empty into sinusoids via terminal arterial capillaries or empty first into the pulp reticulum and then filter between the lining cells of the sinusoids. Many macrophages of the reticuloendothelial system line the outer walls of the sinusoids and phagocytize worn-out red blood cells. The venous sinuses empty into pulp veins that pass to trabecular veins before blood is emptied via the splenic vein. In addition to the filtering of blood, the spleen controls the blood volume by storing red blood cells and by periodically discharging the blood through the contraction of smooth muscle and the action of elastic fibers in the capsule and trabeculae. The spleen also produces lymphocytes, monocytes, plasma cells and antibodies. Most of the lymphocytes that leave the spleen are from the recirculating pool of lymphocytes; relatively few new lymphocytes are formed in the spleen. The spleen is involved in both the cell-mediated and humoral responses to antigens. In the secondary responses to antigens by memory cells, the spleen is one of the most active organs in antibody secretion.

Suprarenal (Adrenal) Glands. The suprarenal glands are divisible into two parts: a mesodermally derived cortex and a neural ectodermally derived medulla. A thick connective tissue capsule sends radially directed trabeculae of reticular fibers into the underlying cortex. The cortex consists of an outer zona glomerulosa, a middle zona fasciculata and an inner zona reticularis. Columnar cells of the zona glomerulosa are arranged in arches. They produce aldosterone. The zona fasciculata consists of cords of cells that radiate inward from the zona glomerulosa. These cords are two cells thick, contain cuboidal cells that are often binucleate and are separated from adjacent cords by fenestrated capillaries that radiate inward from the capsule. Fasciculata cells often contain much lipid and appear vacuolated. The zona reticularis consists of irregularly arranged cords of cells that may contain lipofuscin pigment. Fasciculata and reticularis cells are under the control of ACTH from the adenohypophysis; they produce glucocorticoids and some sex hormones. The most prominent organelle in adrenal cortical cells is an extensive smooth endoplasmic reticulum (SER), which is indicative of steroid-secreting cells.

The suprarenal medulla produces epinephrine and norepinephrine in its polyhedral basophilic cells. These cells receive terminations of preganglionic sympathetic nerve fibers, and each cell is located between a venule and a capillary. The cells exhibit the chromaffin reaction. The blood supply of the suprarenal gland is by branches of the suprarenal arteries that (1) go directly to the medulla and (2) go indirectly to the medulla through capsular arterioles and their radiating capillary plexuses that pass between the cortical cords of cells before reaching the medulla.

Kidney, Ureter and Bladder. The *kidney* is divisible into an outer cortex and an inner medulla. The medulla consists of renal pyramids, with the broad base of each pyramid facing the cortex, while the apex (renal papilla) opens into a minor calyx. The 10 to 16 minor calyces open into two or three major calyces, which in turn empty into the funnel-shaped renal pelvis at the hilus of the kidney. The cortex lies peripheral to the medulla and extends between the pyramids as renal columns. The cortex consists of medullary rays (pars radiata) and cortical labyrinths (pars convoluta). The medullary rays are parallel extensions of medullary tubules into the cortex. Each of these is surrounded by cortical labyrinth tissue of glomeruli and convoluted tubules that empty into the tubules of the medullary ray. A medullary ray and its associated cortical labyrinth constitute a lobule. A kidney lobe is a renal pyramid with its overlying cortex and renal columns.

The functional unit of the kidney is the uriniferous tubule, which consists of a nephron and collecting tubule. The nephron is comprised of the renal corpuscle (of glomerulus and Bowman's capsule), the proximal convoluted tubule; the thick descending limb, thin portion, and thick ascending limb of the loop of Henle; and the distal convoluted tubule. The glomerulus is a tuft of fenestrated capillaries fed by an afferent arteriole and drained by a smaller efferent arteriole. It is invested by podocytes of the visceral layer of Bowman's capsule. The podocytes have pedicles that interdigitate with those from adjacent podocytes and attach to the basal lamina of the capillary endothelium. Filtration slits 250 Å wide exist between pedicles and communicate with the lumen of Bowman's capsule. At the basal lamina surface these slits are connected by a thin slit membrane. The podocytes, basal lamina and fenestrated endothelium constitute the filtration barrier. Mesangial (stalk) cells in the glomerulus probably remove filtration residues from the basal lamina which is the main filter for large molecules. The parietal layer of Bowman's capsule consists of simple squamous epithelium.

The proximal convoluted tubule is the longest and widest portion of the nephron. It is comprised of a simple pyramidal epithelium possessing a brush border (microvilli) and indistinct lateral borders. The proximal convoluted tubule is located in the cortical labyrinth. It is continuous with, and histologically similar to, the thick descending limb of Henle's loop that courses in the medullary ray. Both the proximal and straight descending tubules resorb 85 per cent or more of the water and sodium chloride of the glomerular filtrate. Sodium is actively transported by the cells. Glucose and amino acids also are resorbed by the epithelium of these tubules. The thin portion of Henle's loop is comprised of simple squamous epithelium. This portion resorbs water but adds sodium to the luminal contents.

The thick ascending and distal convoluted tubules have a low cuboidal epithelium with scattered microvilli, distinct lateral borders and an extensive infolding of the basal plasma membrane. In these tubules sodium is actively transported out of the cells, and the filtrate becomes hypotonic and acidic. Where the distal tubule abuts against the afferent glomerular arteriole the epithelium is columnar and constitutes the macula densa. The muscle cells of the adjacent afferent glomerular arteriole are replaced by large pale juxtaglomerular cells containing granules. These cells, the macula densa and some interposed cells constitute the juxtaglomerular complex that is responsible for the production of renin.

The collecting tubules consist of pale, clear simple cuboidal epithelium with distinct lateral boundaries. These tubules join to form papillary ducts lined by simple columnar epithelium. Under the influence of aldosterone from the suprarenal cortex, the collecting tubules are induced to reabsorb sodium from the glomerular filtrate and thus reduce the amount of sodium eliminated in the urine. Under the influence of antidiuretic hormone from the neurohypophysis, the epithelium of the collecting tubules becomes more permeable to water, and the latter is passively removed from the urine.

Arterial blood is carried to the hilar region of the kidney by the renal artery. This artery branches into interlobar branches that give rise to arcuate arteries passing along the cortex-medulla junction. Interlobular arteries arise from the arcuate arteries and pass peripherally in the cortical labyrinths to give rise to afferent glomerular arterioles supplying the glomeruli. From the glomeruli, efferent arterioles supply the capillary plexi around the tubules. Capillaries of the medulla are supplied by arteriolae rectae from the efferent arterioles. Venous drainage is by venae rectae, interlobular, arcuate, interlobar and renal veins that accompany the arteries.

The *ureters* are lined with transitional epithelium.

External to the lamina propria is a muscularis layer consisting of inner longitudinal and outer circular smooth muscle layers. Near the bladder an additional outer longitudinal layer is added.

The *urinary bladder* is histologically similar to the lower part of the ureter in that it has a mucosa with transitional epithelium, a three-layered muscularis layer and an outer connective tissue layer.

Development of Abdominal Organs

The development of the urogenital system will be covered in the section on the pelvis and perineum.

Development of the Digestive System. The entodermal foregut gives rise to the pharynx, esophagus, stomach, liver, pancreas and part of the duodenum. The midgut gives rise to the rest of the small intestine, ascending colon and proximal two thirds of the transverse colon. The hindgut develops into the rest of the large intestine as far as the upper part of the anal canal. The lower part of the rectum and anal canal is established by the separation of the cloaca into a dorsal anorectal canal and ventral urogenital sinus by the urorectal septum.

The *stomach* appears in the fourth embryonic week as a dilation of the foregut. As it shifts caudally from its position above the septum transversum it rotates so that its original left surface faces anteriorly. In addition, its caudal extent shifts to the right.

The *intestines* develop from cephalic and caudal limbs of a gut loop that extends into the belly stalk. The cephalic limb extends from the stomach to the yolk stalk. It gives rise to all of the small intestine, except the last 60 to 95 cm. of the ileum. The caudal limb extends from the yolk stalk to the hindgut and it gives rise to the rest of the ileum and much of the large intestine. As the loop develops it rotates counterclockwise (in an AP view) around the omphalomesenteric (vitelline) artery, the latter becoming the superior mesenteric artery. This rotation places the transverse colon above the jejunum and ileum, anterior to the duodenum, and just below the stomach. By the tenth week the abdomen enlarges, and the gut loop reenters the abdomen. The cephalic limb enters first, crowding the descending colon to the left. Partial persistence of the yolk stalk may remain as a Meckel's diverticulum attached to the ileum 60 to 95 cm. from the ileocolic junction.

The *liver* arises in the fourth embryonic week as a ventral diverticulum of the foregut. This diverticulum grows through the ventral mesentery and into the caudal face of the septum transversum. The more proximal part of the hepatic diverticulum gives rise to the common bile duct, cystic duct, gallbladder and hepatic ducts. The more distal portions differentiate into the hepatic plates and the smaller bile ducts. Since the liver grows in the septum transversum and bulges from its caudal face, it is covered by peritoneum lining the septum transversum, except at the bare area of the liver where it abuts directly against the septum (diaphragm).

The *pancreas* forms from dorsal and ventral entodermal buds located at the level of the duodenum. The dorsal bud grows into the dorsal mesentry. The proximal portion of the ventral bud joins with the common bile duct, whereas the distal portion grows into the dorsal mesentery and fuses with the dorsal bud. The pancreatic duct (of Wirsung) develops from the ventral anlage and the distal part of the dorsal primordium. The proximal portion of the dorsal bud may give rise to the accessory duct (of Santorini).

Development of the Abdominal Mesenteries and Spleen. The abdominal mesenteries develop primarily from the embryonic dorsal mesentry. The ventral mesentery may give rise to the lesser omentum and the falciform ligament, although the latter probably forms from a "shearing" of peritoneum covering the body wall. Much of the dorsal mesogastrium suspending the stomach fuses with the dorsal body wall to form the dorsal lining of the lesser sac. The rest of the dorsal mesogastrium fuses with the embryonic transverse mesocolon to form the definitive mesentery of the transverse colon and then drapes over the small intestine to become the greater omentum. The spleen develops from mesoderm of the dorsal mesogastrium. The dorsal mesentery of the duodenum fuses with the dorsal body wall, making it and the pancreas secondarily retroperitoneal. The dorsal mesentery of the jejunum and ileum becomes the mesentery proper. The dorsal mesentery of the ascending and descending colon mostly fuses with the dorsal body wall.

PELVIS AND PERINEUM

Gross Boundaries of the Pelvis and Perineum

Pelvis. The osteology of the bones that form the pelvis and basic types of pelvic architecture are discussed previously in the section on the lower extremity. The discussion here will include a definition of the pelvic cavity and the various planes of the pelvis.

The pelvic cavity proper (minor or true pelvis) is below the pelvic inlet and above the pelvic diaphragm or pelvic floor. The inlet is defined by the sacral promontory, arcuate line of the ilium, pecten pubis and the upper aspect of the symphysis pubis. The area above this plane is the major or false pelvis and is part of the abdominal cavity. The floor of the pelvis is a muscular sling composed of the levator ani and coccygeus muscles. This trough-shaped sling is inclined from lateral to medial and from posterior to anterior. Its lateral attachment extends along a tendinous arch from the symphysis pubis to the ischial spine. The levator ani attaches to this arch and after descending toward the midline attaches to its fellow along a median raphe. The coccygeus fills the gap between the ischial spine and the sacrum and coccyx. The lateral wall of the pelvic cavity consists of the obturator internus and piriformis muscles and the corresponding portions of the hip bone.

The plane of the pelvic inlet is the plane of greatest dimensions. The distance between the sacral promontory and the uppermost aspect of the symphysis pubis is the anteroposterior diameter of the inlet or the conjugate vera (true conjugate). Not strictly part of the pelvic inlet but important obstetrically is the obstetric conjugate, the distance between the promontory and the most posterior aspect of the symphysis pubis. The diagonal conjugate can be measured via vaginal exam and is the distance between the promontory and the inferior aspect of the symphysis pubis. The transverse diameter of the inlet is the greatest distance between the arcuate lines.

The plane of the pelvic outlet is defined by the inferior aspect of the symphysis pubis, the ischiopubic rami, the ischial tuberosities, the sacrotuberous ligaments and the tip of the sacrum. The AP diameter extends from the inferior aspect of the symphysis pubis to the tip of the sacrum. The transverse diameter of the outlet is the distance between the inner edges of the ischial tuberosities.

The plane of the midpelvis is the plane of least dimensions. The AP diameter of this plane extends from the inferior aspect of the symphysis to the sacrum, at the level of the ischial spines. The transverse diameter of the midpelvis is the distance between the ischial spines, the smallest diameter of the pelvis.

Perineum. The perineum is best defined as the region of the pelvic outlet below the pelvic floor. It is a diamond-shaped area that is defined by the inferior aspect of the symphysis pubis anteriorly, the ischial tuberosities laterally and the coccyx posteriorly. An imaginary line between the two ischial tuberosities separates the perineum into two triangular areas; the anterior urogenital triangle and the posterior anal triangle. The roof of the perineum is the floor of the pelvis, i.e., the pelvic sling that is formed by the levator ani and coccygeus muscles.

In the urogenital triangle is the urogenital diaphragm, which is a horizontal musculofascial shelf that stretches between the ischiopubic rami. It is formed by superior and inferior layers of fascia that enclose the sphincter urethrae and deep transverse perineal muscles. In the male it contains the bulbourethral glands (Cowper's glands). This diaphragm is penetrated by the membraneous urethra in both sexes and the vagina in the female. The area between the superior and inferior fasciae of the urogenital diaphragm encloses the deep perineal space or pouch.

The superficial perineal space is inferior or superficial to the inferior fascia of the urogenital diaphragm. It is limited externally or superficially by the membranous (fibrous) layer of subcutaneous tissue (Scarpa's fascia) of the abdomen, which continues into the perineum (as Colles' fascia) and attaches to the posterior extent of the urogenital diaphragm. This limiting layer also attaches to the ischiopubic ramus and the fascia lata of the thigh so that urine from a ruptured urethra or blood from hemorrhage may extravasate up into the abdominal wall (but not into the thigh) from the superficial perineal space. In the male this space contains the crura of the corpora cavernosa and related ischiocavernosus muscles, the corpus spongiosum and bulb of the penis with the related bulbocavernosus muscle and the superficial transverse perineal muscle. In the female this space contains the crura of the clitoris and related ischiocavernosus muscles, the bulbus vestibuli and related bulbocavernosus muscle, the superficial transverse perineal muscle and the greater vestibular glands (Bartholin's glands). The urethral opening is 2.5 cm. posterior to the clitoris.

The ischiorectal fossa is the fat-filled wedge-shaped area that is inferolateral to the pelvic sling and medial to the lower portions of the obturator internus muscle and the os coxae. In the region of the anal triangle the floor is the subcutaneous tissue and skin. The posterior recess of this fossa extends posterolaterally under the inferior margin of the gluteus maximus muscle. The anterior recess extends into the urogenital triangle above the urogenital diaphragm. The pudendal (Alcock's) canal is a slit in the obturator internus fascia along the lateral wall of this fossa in the anal triangle. The internal pudendal vessels and the pudendal nerve traverse this canal as they pass anteriorly into the urogenital triangle. The inferior rectal arteries and nerves branch from the parent structures in the pudendal canal and pass through the ischiorectal fossa toward the rectum and anal canal.

The nerve supply to the perineum is provided primarily by the pudendal nerve (S2–4). Its branches are the inferior rectal, perineal and posterior scrotal (labial) nerves. These branches supply all of the muscles and most of the skin of the perineum. The skin of the anterior part of the perineum is supplied by the

anterior scrotal (labial) branches of the ilioinguinal nerve. Autonomics to the perineum are apparently distributed through the pudendal nerve.

Viscera of the Pelvis and Perineum

Gastrointestinal Tract. The *sigmoid colon* begins at the pelvic rim, descends to the left pelvic wall, traverses the pelvis from left to right and bends upon itself to join the rectum in the midline. It is supported by the sigmoid mesocolon. The sigmoid and its mesocolon are extremely variable in length, exceeding by far the variability in other parts of the gastrointestinal system.

The *rectum* is that portion of the bowel below the midsacral region where the sigmoid mesocolon ceases. The lowest part of the infraperitoneal portion presents a dilated ampulla. Anteriorly the upper two-thirds of the rectum is in contact with the coils of the ileum. In the male the lower third is related anteriorly to the trigone of the bladder, the seminal vesicles, the ductus deferens and the prostate. In the female the lower third is in contact anteriorly with the vagina and the cervix. Posteriorly it is related to the sacrum in both sexes.

The upper third of the rectum is covered anteriorly and laterally by peritoneum, the middle third only anteriorly and the lower third passes below the peritoneum.

The *anal canal,* which is sometimes called the second portion of the rectum, is 2.5 to 3.5 cm. in length. It turns dorsally, making a right angle as it passes through the pelvic floor to the anus, and is surrounded by internal and external sphincters.

The following structures can be palpated during a rectal examination in the normal male: the anorectal ring, anteriorly the prostate, posteriorly the coccyx and sacrum and laterally the ischiorectal fossa and the ischial spines. The normal female presents the same structures with the exception of anteriorly, where the perineal body and the cervix of the uterus are palpable.

Urinary System. The pelvic portion of the *ureter* passes in front of the sacroiliac joint and medial to the internal iliac artery. In the male it passes posterior and inferior to the ductus deferens. In the female it passes inferior to the uterine artery and lateral to the cervix of the uterus. The vesical portion runs obliquely downward and medially through the bladder about 20 to 25 mm. from its fellow.

The empty *bladder* is posterior to the pubic symphysis and totally within the pelvic cavity below the pelvic inlet. The fully distended bladder of the adult projects well into the abdominal cavity. The bladder is extraperitoneal with its superior and posterosuperior surfaces covered with peritoneum. Laterally it is related to the levator ani and the obturator internus muscles. In the male the bladder is related superiorly to coils of small intestine and the sigmoid colon, posteriorly to the rectovesical pouch, the rectum, the seminal vesicles and termination of the vas deferens and inferiorly to the prostate gland. In the female it is related superiorly to coils of small intestine and the body of the uterus, posteriorly to the vagina and supravaginal portion of the cervix and inferiorly to the pelvic fascia and the urogenital diaphragm.

The *male urethra* extends from the bladder to the glans penis, traversing (1) the prostate gland, (2) the urogenital diaphragm, and (3) the length of the corpus cavernosum urethrae. The prostatic portion contains the numerous small openings of the prostatic ducts and the crista urethralis, with the colliculus seminalis containing the openings of the ejaculatory ducts. As the urethra passes through the urogenital diaphragm it is somewhat narrowed and is surrounded by the sphincter. In the cavernous portion the urethra is dilated at the openings of the Cowper's glands and also terminally at the fossa navicularis.

The *female urethra* is short in that it passes through the urogenital diaphragm, where it is surrounded by the sphincter urethrae, and ends shortly thereafter.

Male Reproductive System. The testis and the epididymis lie in the scrotum and are separated from the opposite side by the scrotal septum. The epididymis lies along the posterior border of the testis. It is enlarged above to form a head and tapers to a body and small tail below. It is formed mainly by the greatly contorted duct of the epididymis, which empties into the beginning of the ductus deferens.

Each ductus deferens ascends at first slender and tortuous, but before reaching the level of the head of the epididymis it becomes straight and runs vertically cranialward to traverse the inguinal canal. At the internal abdominal ring it leaves the spermatic cord, passes downward and backward over the lateral surface of the bladder and medially to the ureter, penetrates the prostate gland and opens into the prostatic portion of the urethra through the ejaculatory duct. Just before it enters the prostate it is joined by the club-shaped seminal vesicles.

The prostate gland surrounds the urethra between the inferior surface of the bladder and the superior surface of the urogenital diaphragm. It is related anteriorly to the symphysis pubis, laterally to the levator ani muscles, inferiorly to the urogenital diaphragm and posteriorly to the rectum.

Female Reproductive System. The ovaries lie against the lateral pelvic walls just below the pelvic

inlet and posteroinferior to the lateral aspect of the uterine tubes. Each ovary is enclosed in a mesovarium, a posterior reflection of peritoneum from the broad ligament. The ovary is suspended from the lateral pelvic wall by the suspensory ligament of the ovary, through which the ovarian vessels, nerves and lymphatics pass to the gland. Each ovary is connected to the uterus just below the uterine tube by the ovarian ligament.

The uterus consists of the fundus, body and cervix. The cavity of the uterus is continuous superolaterally with the narrow lumen of the uterine tubes and inferiorly with the cavity of the vagina. The fundus is the superior domed portion that projects above the cavity of the body. The body is the major portion of the uterus, and the cervix is the inferior portion that projects into the vagina. The uterine cavity is largest within the body. It narrows abruptly at the body-cervix junction to form the internal os. The lumen of the cervix (cervical canal) is narrow and ends inferiorly as the narrow external os, which is readily palpated during a rectal examination. The normally positioned uterus rests on the posterosuperior aspect of the bladder so that the uterovesical pouch is usually empty. The rectouterine pouch (of Douglas) separates the uterus from the rectum posteriorly. Laterally the uterus is related to the broad ligament and the ureter; the latter passing just lateral to the supravaginal portion of the cervix and inferior to the uterine artery.

The uterine (fallopian) tubes extend laterally from the superolateral aspects of the uterus. Each tube consists of a narrow-lumened isthmus, a dilated and long ampulla and the terminal infundibulum, which is composed of numerous fingerlike fimbriae. The tubes curve posteriorly near the lateral pelvic walls, and here their fimbriae partially cover the ovaries. The uterine tubes are the most superior structures in the broad ligament.

The normal uterus is both anteflexed and anteverted. Anteflexion is a forward bend within the uterus itself at the level of the internal os. Anteversion is a forward bend of about 90 degrees at the junction of the uterus and the vagina. This places the uterus in approximately the horizontal plane with its anterior surface resting on the posterosuperior surface of the bladder. Malposition usually involves one of the following: (1) turning of the entire organ, retroversion (backward turning) or anteversion (forward turning); (2) bending of the body on the cervix, retroflexion (backward bending) or anteflexion (anterior bending); (3) a shift in the position of the entire organ, retrocession, anteposition, prolapse or procidentia, the latter being the extreme degree of prolapse in which the cervix extrudes from the introitus. This results from extreme relaxation of the pelvic floor, the urogenital diaphragm and the uterine ligaments.

The vagina extends from above the inferior extent of the cervix of the uterus to its external opening in the vestibule. From above downward it is inclined anteriorly as it passes through the pelvic floor and the urogenital diaphragm. The upper portion of the vagina, which surrounds the inferior part of the cervix, is divided into anterior, lateral and posterior fornices. The vagina is related anteriorly to the base of the bladder and the urethra; posteriorly through the very thin wall of the posterior fornix to the rectouterine pouch, rectum and anal canal; and laterally to the levator ani muscle and the ureter, which passes near the lateral fornix.

In a vaginal examination the urethra, bladder and symphysis pubis are palpable anteriorly; the rectum and rectouterine pouch posteriorly; the ovary, uterine tube, and lateral pelvic wall laterally; and the cervix in the apex of the vagina.

The vestibule is surrounded by the labia minora and receives the vagina, urethra and major and minor vestibular glands.

The broad ligament is a reflection of peritoneum that passes over the uterus and related structures from front to back and extends laterally to the lateral pelvic walls. As such it forms a curtain across the pelvis from side to side, which has an anterior and a posterior layer. Lateral to the uterus the highest structure in the broad ligament is the uterine tube; below and behind that is the ovarian ligament; and below and anterior is the round ligament. The mesovarium is the reflection of the posterior layer that suspends the ovarian ligament and ovary. That part of the broad ligament above the mesovarium that suspends the uterine tube is called the mesosalpinx. That part of the broad ligament below the mesovarium is the mesometrium. At the base of the broad ligament posteriorly the posterior layer of mesometrium is elevated over the underlying uterosacral ligament as the rectouterine fold. The extraperitoneal connective tissue found between the layers of the broad ligament is the parametrium. The parametrium in the base of the broad ligament is thickened and forms the cardinal ligaments.

Blood Supply to the Pelvis and Perineum

The blood supply to the pelvic viscera and to the perineum is provided by branches of the internal iliac artery. The umbilical artery gives rise to the artery of the ductus deferens and the superior vesical artery, which supplies the bladder. The inferior vesical artery also supplies the bladder and the prostate and seminal vesicles in the male. The uterine artery (homologue

to the artery of the ductus deferens) usually arises separately and passes medially to supply the uterus, uterine tube and upper part of the vagina. The vaginal artery supplies most of the vagina. The middle rectal artery supplies the middle portion of the rectum and anastomoses with the superior and inferior rectal arteries. The internal pudendal artery exits the pelvis through the greater sciatic foramen, passes around the ischial spine and then enters the perineum through the lesser sciatic foramen. It supplies the somatic and visceral structures of the perineum. Other branches of the internal iliac artery are the superior and inferior gluteal arteries, which supply the gluteal region; the iliolumbar and lateral sacral arteries, which supply the posterior body wall; and the obturator, which passes into the medial thigh.

Microscopic Structure of Pelvic Contents

Male Reproductive System. The *testis* is ovoid and surrounded by a thick connective tissue capsule, the tunica albuginea. This capsule penetrates the testis at the mediastinum and sends radiating septula into it, dividing the testis into lobules. Within the lobules are seminiferous tubules and a loose fibrous stroma. The stroma contains interstitial cells of Leydig, which are characterized by rod-shaped crystalloids (of Reinke), much smooth endoplasmic reticulum and mitochondria with tubular cristae. These cells produce testosterone and the SER and tubular cristae are characteristic of steroid-secreting cells. The seminiferous tubules consist of contorted loops that join by straight tubules with the rete testis. The convoluted portions in the viable male are lined by a germinal (seminiferous) epithelium resting on a basal lamina that is bounded by a specialized layer of connective tissue fibers, fibroblasts and smooth muscle. The seminiferous epithelium contains supportive Sertoli cells and sex cells in various stages of spermatogenesis. From the basal lamina toward the lumen are located spermatogonia, primary spermatocytes, secondary spermatocytes, spermatids and spermatozoa. A cross section of a tubule may show several of six stages of development, and the entire tubule does not contain cells that are all in the same stages of development. This is due to different timing in the proliferation and division of stem cells.

Spermatogonia are the only sex cells present until the time of puberty when two different types are present. These are the A or stem cell and the B or derivative cell. A cells may divide into two A cells or into two B cells. B cells grow and differentiate into the primary spermatocytes of the middle zone of the epithelium. The primary spermatocyte undergoes the reduction division of meiosis and gives rise to two secondary spermatocytes containing the haploid number (23) of chromosomes. Each secondary spermatocyte divides quickly into two spermatids. Spermatids occupy infoldings in the walls of Sertoli cells and undergo transformation into spermatozoa. In this process the nucleus condenses, an acrosome vesicle is formed by the Golgi complex, the acrosome vesicle collapses as a head cap over the nucleus, an axial filament (flagellum) grows from the proximal centriole, and mitochondria form a helix around the proximal flagellum of the middle piece. Most of the cytoplasm is cast off, leaving only a thin cytoplasmic investment to the head, neck, middle piece and tail of the spermatozoon. In the principal piece of the tail it forms a fibrous sheath that does not extend into the end piece of the tail.

Straight seminiferous tubules and *rete testis* are lined by simple cuboidal to columnar epithelium. These empty into 10 to 15 *efferent ductules* that are lined by alternating cuboidal and tall ciliated columnar epithelium. A basal layer of rounded cells is surrounded by a lamina propria and some circular smooth muscle fibers. The cilia of the efferent ductules move spermatozoa into the *ductus epididymidis*. This duct contains pseudostratified columnar epithelium containing long microvilli (stereocilia). The thick viscid secretion of this duct supplies nutritive substances to the sperm while they mature and become motile. This duct has a circular smooth muscle layer.

The *ductus deferens* has a mucosa that is similar to that of the ductus epididymidis. The muscular layer is highly developed into inner longitudinal, middle circular and outer longitudinal layers. This duct is invested in the spermatic cord by the cremasteric muscle and the pampiniform plexus of veins. The ductus deferens dilates into an ampulla before terminating as the short slender ejaculatory duct, which pierces the prostate and opens into the urethra at the urethral crest. The mucosa of these structures is folded and the epithelium is not as tall as in the rest of the ductus deferens. The supporting wall of the ejaculatory duct is made up of fibrous tissue. Muscular contraction of the ductus deferens and the ductus epididymidis propel the spermatozoa to the urethra during the ejaculatory process.

The *seminal vesicle* consists of a mucosa folded into a complex system of elevations, a prominent muscularis and an adventitia. The epithelium is low pseudostratified columnar epithelium, and it secretes a viscid alkaline fluid rich in fructose.

The *prostate* is an aggregation of 30 to 50 tubulosaccular glands. The glandular epithelium is simple cuboidal to columnar, and the cells have apical secretion granules that contribute to the formation of the faintly acid secretion that is rich in citric acid and acid phosphatase. The lumina may contain lamellated prostatic concretions (corpora amylacea). The stroma between the tubules contains smooth muscle fibers.

The *male urethra* has three parts, the prostatic, membranous and cavernous (penile) portions. The prostatic urethra is lined mostly with transitional epithelium. The membranous and penile portions are lined with pseudostratified and stratified columnar epithelium, except at the meatus where the epithelium is stratified squamous. The prostatic urethra has a crest on its posterior wall. The paired ejaculatory ducts and prostatic utricle open on this crest. The ducts of the prostatic gland open into the prostatic uretha. The membranous urethra is encircled by a sphincter of skeletal muscle fibers from the deep transverse perineal muscle. The cavernous urethra extends throughout the penis. It occupies the corpus spongiosum and receives the ducts of the bulbourethral glands and the branching mucous urethral glands (of Littre).

The *bulbourethral glands* (Cowper's) are variably tubular, alveolar or saccular mucous glands that are enclosed in the membranous urethral sphincter. Their ducts, containing mucous areas of epithelium, open into the cavernous urethra about 2.5 cm. in front of the urogenital diaphragm.

The *penis* consists of three cylinders of erectile tissue: two dorsal corpora cavernosa and one ventral corpus spongiosum. The latter terminates distally as the glans penis, and it contains the cavernous urethra. A dense fibrous tunica albuginea surrounds the cavernous bodies and separates the corpora from one another by an incomplete median (pectiniform) septum. The three corpora are enclosed in a common loose irregularly arranged connective tissue layer that underlies the investing skin. The skin folds over the glans as the prepuce. The skin of the glans adheres firmly to the erectile tissue since the loose connective tissue layer is lacking. The epithelium of the inner surface of the prepuce and that of the glans is stratified squamous and is characteristic of that lining a moist surface. It is continuous at the urethral orifice with the epithelium lining the urethra.

The erectile tissue of the corpora cavernosa consists of endothelium lined lacunae that are separated by fibrous trabeculae containing smooth muscle. The lacunae are large centrally but are narrow peripherally where they communicate with a venous plexus underlying the tunica albuginea. In the corpus spongiosum the arrangement is similar except for an elastic tunica albuginea, thinner trabeculae and uniform lacunae. The corpora are supplied by two branches of the penile artery: the dorsal artery and the deep arteries. The branches of the dorsal arteries supply capillaries of the trabeculae that drain through the lacunae to the venous plexus. The deep arteries are the chief vessels for filling the lacunae during erection. These vessels run in the cavernous bodies and give off trabecular branches that empty directly to the lacunae through helicine arteries. The latter vessels have a thick circular muscle layer and an intima with longitudinal thickened cushions. During erection the smooth muscle in the cavernous trabeculae and helicine arteries relaxes, and the lacunae are engorged with more blood than can be rapidly drained by the compressed peripheral lacunae. At the end of erection, smooth muscle contraction shuts off the blood supplied by helicine arteries and forces blood into the peripheral venous plexus.

Female Reproductive System. The *ovary* is an exocrine organ secreting secondary oocytes, and it is an endocrine organ producing estrogens and progesterone. It is divided into an outer cortex and inner medulla. The cortex basically consists of a rather cellular connective tissue stroma, ovarian follicles and a simple cuboidal surface epithelium (germinal epithelium). The medulla consists of loose connective tissue, blood vessels, lymphatics, nerves, some smooth muscle and a few vestigial tubular structures called rete ovarii.

Ovarian follicles consist of a developing ovum and an investment of follicle cells and connective tissue. Follicles originate in the embryo and undergo extensive changes during the childbearing years when they are under the influence of adenohypophyseal hormones. In the embryo, primordial sex cells develop into oogonia which differentiate into primary oocytes; the latter go through the prophase of the first meiotic division before they enter an arrested dictyotene stage. Each of these cells is surrounded by a simple layer of follicle cells from the germinal epithelium. Many of these embryonic primary follicles die, but about 70,000 survive in the cortex of the ovary until the time of puberty.

At puberty, hypothalamic nerve cells produce follicle-stimulating hormone-releasing factor (FSH-RF). This hormone stimulates FSH production by basophils of the anterior pituitary gland. Under the influence of FSH, some oocytes emerge from the arrested dictyotene stage and start to complete the first meiotic division. Coincident with this, follicle cells enlarge and proliferate to form a stratified cuboidal epithelial layer around the oocyte. As the follicle enlarges, spaces between follicle cells coalesce to form an antrum filled with liquor folliculi. The growing follicle is now called a vesicular follicle. As this follicle differentiates, the follicular cells around the antrum form a stratified epithelial membrana granulosa that sits on a prominent basal lamina. This in turn is surrounded by an inner richly vascular theca interna and an outer more fibrous theca externa. The cells of the theca interna are relatively large, contain much smooth endoplasmic reticulum and are implicated in the production of estrogens. The oocyte is surrounded by a protein–polysaccharide layer called the zona pellucida. Cytoplasmic processes of the oocyte and of the immediate surrounding follicle cells of the corona radiata are closely aligned in the substance of the zona pellucida. The combined oocyte, zona pellucida and corona radiata project into the antrum of the follicle as the cumulus oophorus.

The mature vesicular follicle occupies much of the thickness of the cortex, and it causes a bulge (stigma) on the surface of the ovary. Its primary oocyte completes the first meiotic division and becomes a secondary oocyte. The secondary oocyte is relatively metabolically inactive, but it possesses more extensive protein producing mechanisms than are found in the primary oocyte. It starts its second meiotic division and reaches the metaphase stage at about the time it is ovulated from the ovary along with the zona pellucida and corona radiata. Just prior to ovulation small amounts of progesterone are produced by the follicle, and more luteinizing hormone is produced by the adenohypophysis.

After ovulation a small amount of blood accumulates in the collapsed follicular remains, and a clot is formed in the antrum region. The granulosa and theca interna cells enlarge, accumulate lipid and become lutein cells of a corpus luteum. The granulosa lutein cells constitute the bulk of the corpus luteum and produce progesterone. The theca lutein cells are smaller, less in number, more deeply staining, found at the periphery and may produce estrogens. Lutein cells possess major characteristics of steroid-secreting cells in that they have relatively more smooth endoplasmic reticulum and have mitochondria containing "tubular" lamellae rather than cristae. After clot formation the thecal connective tissue penetrates into the developing corpus luteum and replaces the blood clot in the central core.

If the ovulated secondary oocyte is fertilized and implantation takes place the corpus luteum will survive for about 6 months before it starts to regress. If the secondary oocyte is not fertilized the corpus luteum will last for about 14 days. When a corpus luteum degenerates the lutein cells become swollen, then pyknotic, and a hyalinized scar of connective tissue replaces the dead lutein cells. This white scar is called the corpus albicans.

Usually only one follicle reaches maturity and is involved in ovulation during each cycle. The other maturing follicles are no longer supported by the waning levels of FSH after ovulation and they degenerate. In small follicles the oocyte degenerates and the stroma invades the follicle, leaving no trace of the follicle.

In larger follicles, cells of the theca interna enlarge, and the basement membrane becomes a distinct glassy membrane before coarser stromal fibers penetrate the degenerating follicle, giving it the appearance of a small corpus albicans.

The *uterine tube (oviduct, fallopian tube)* has four regions: infundibulum, ampulla, isthmus and interstitial (intramural) portion. The wall of each of these parts consists of a mucosa, muscularis and serosa. The mucosa of the trumpet-shaped infundibulum, and to a lesser extent that of the ampulla, is characterized by many elongate fimbriae. The epithelium of all parts of the uterine tube is simple columnar and is comprised of ciliated cells and peg-shaped secreting cells. The relative numbers of these cell types vary, depending on the estrogenic or progesteronic influences. The muscularis consists of inner circular and outer longitudinal smooth muscle layers. These layers get relatively thicker in passing from the infundibulum to the interstitial portion. The serosa is lined by mesothelium and is a continuation of the peritoneal covering of the broad ligament.

The *uterus* is comprised of a body, fundus and cervix. The body and fundus are histologically similar, and their walls consist of three layers: perimetrium (serosa), myometrium (muscularis) and endometrium (mucosa). The perimetrium is the serosal continuation of the broad ligament. The myometrium is composed of an inner layer of longitudinal smooth muscle, a thick middle layer of circular smooth muscle and large blood vessels, and an outer layer of longitudinal and circular smooth muscle. These smooth muscle cells undergo hyperplasia and hypertrophy during pregnancy. The basic constituents of the endometrium are simple columnar epithelium that is partly ciliated; a lamina propria stroma containing mesenchymelike cells, reticular fibers and varying amounts of leukocytes; simple tubular glands; and two sets of arteries. One set of arteries (basal arteries) supplies the glands and stroma of the deepest part of the lamina propria. The other set (coiled, spiral arteries) supplies the rest of the endometrium.

The endometrium is under the influence of ovarian progesterone and estrogen. It reflects this influence in the marked structural changes characteristic of the menstrual cycle. Four uterine stages of the cycle are recognized: menstrual, proliferative (follicular, estrogenic), secretory (luteal, progesteronic) and premenstrual (ischemic). The menstrual stage takes place from days 1 to 5 of the cycle. The proliferative occurs from days 5 to 14, the secretory from days 14 to 27, and the premenstrual from days 27 to 28. These are approximate times.

During the proliferative stage the endometrium

grows from a height of 0.5 mm. to 2 to 3 mm. In this process, epithelial cells of the gland remnants form a new epithelial lining and straight glands. The stroma develops from the deep (basal layer). Spiral arteries grow into this new functional layer. In the secretory stage, under the influence of estrogen and progesterone, the endometrium grows another 2 mm. in height. An increase in interstitial fluid in part of the functional layer divides it into an inner edematous spongy layer and an outer compact layer. The uterine glands grow, become corkscrew shaped and produce a glycogen-rich mucoid secretion. Coiled arteries elongate and empty into venous sinusoids by way of capillaries. The premenstrual stage is the result of a decrease of progesterone and estrogen production by the corpus luteum. In this stage the coiled arteries kink, there is a drop in the blood supply to the functional layer, the edema decreases and the glands begin to fragment. During the menstrual stage the functional layer becomes anemic and ischemic. Arteries and veins break down, and blood oozes into the uterine cavity through the degenerating glands and surface epithelium. The entire functional layer is sloughed off during this stage. The basal arteries are not affected, so the basal layer is retained.

The *placenta* consists of a maternal component (decidua basalis) and a fetal component (chorion frondosum). Since the embryo implants into the compacta layer of the endometrium, the decidua basalis is that portion of the functional layer that lies deep to the embryo. Glands and blood vessels of this layer empty into intervillous spaces. The stromal cells swell markedly, accumulate glycogen and are called decidual cells. The chorion frondosum consists of a chorionic plate off of which anchoring villi arise and attach to the endometrium. Free villi extend from the anchoring villi into the intervillous spaces. In the first third of pregnancy the villi have cores of fetal connective tissue containing fetal capillaries with nucleated red blood corpuscles. This core of tissue is covered by an inner cytotrophoblastic and an outer syncytial trophoblastic epithelial layer. Later in pregnancy, the fetal vessels contain nonnucleated red blood cells, the cytotrophoblast disappears, and the syncytial trophoblast is thin except for clumps of syncytial knots. An acidophilic fibrinoid material accumulates over the syncytial trophoblast in late pregnancy. The "placental barrier" in the late placenta consists of the syncytial trophoblast, the endothelium of the fetal vessels and the intervening basal laminae of these epithelia. In the first trimester, the cytotrophoblast is an added layer in this barrier. The cells of the cytotrophoblast produce the syncytial trophoblast. The syncytial trophoblast cells probably produce estrogen, progesterone, human chorionic gonadotropin (HCG), and human placental lactogen (HPL).

The *cervix* consists of a mucosa, muscularis and adventitia. It does not undergo the extensive cyclic changes of the endometrium, although some changes in structure are seen in pregnancy. The portio vaginalis of the cervix projects into the vagina. The mucosa of the cervix is thrown into folds (plicae palmatae). It consists of simple columnar epithelium with some cilia, extensive forked mucus secreting glands and a firm stroma that is rich in collagenous and elastic fibers. The epithelium changes to stratified squamous at the portio vaginalis. During pregnancy the cervical glands become larger and secrete a mucus plug that seals the cervical canal. At the time of parturition the lamina propria becomes more edematous, looser and cellular. The muscularis layers are similar to those in the uterine body and fundus except that there is no inner longitudinal muscular layer. The adventitia contains collagenous fibers that are continuous with surrounding structures.

The *vagina* also is comprised of a mucosa, muscularis and adventitia. The lining epithelium of the mucosa is stratified squamous nonkeratinized, but keratohyaline granules may be found in some of the cells. Under the influence of estrogen the epithelium accumulates glycogen, and many pyknotic surface cells appear. When estrogen levels are low a basal layer of cells is prominent. The lamina propria contains many elastic fibers and some large blood vessels. No glands are present. The muscularis consists of a thin inner circular layer and a thicker outer longitudinal layer of smooth muscle. A sphincter of skeletal muscle is found at the lower end of the vagina.

The *hymen* has the same structure as the vaginal mucosa. It is a thin fold at the opening of the vagina into the vestibule.

The *clitoris* corresponds to the dorsal penis in the male. It has two small cavernous bodies of erectile tissue that end in a rudimentary glans clitoridis. It is covered by stratified squamous epithelium. Specialized nerve endings, such as Meissner's and pacinian corpuscles, are located in the subepithelial stroma.

The *labia minora* flank the vestibule. They have a vascularized connective tissue core that is covered by stratified squamous epithelium possessing a thin keratinized layer. Sebaceous glands, not associated with hairs, are located in the stroma.

The *labia majora* are folds of skin that cover the labia minora. The inner surface is like that of the labia minora. The outer surface is covered by skin containing hairs, sweat glands and sebaceous glands. The interior of these folds contains much adipose tissue.

The *vestibule* is lined by partially keratinized stratified squamous epithelium. Minor vestibular glands, placed chiefly near the clitoris and opening of the urethra, secrete mucus. The longer major vestibular glands are analogous to the bulbourethral glands of the male. They are located in the lateral wall of the vestibule. Their ducts open close to the attachment of the hymen.

Development of the Urogenital System

The urinary and reproductive systems take origin from the urogenital sinus and the intermediate mesoderm.

Development of the Kidney and Ureter. Three pairs of embryonic kidneys develop in man. These are the pronephros, mesenephros and metanephros. The pronephros and mesonephros will degenerate, but their development is essential for the establishment of the metanephros, which becomes the definitive kidney.

The *pronephros* arises at the C3–T1 vertebral levels by the dorsal proliferation of cords of cells from the intermediate mesoderm. These cords become pronephric tubules. They grow caudally and link up with the other pronephric tubules, forming a common pronephric duct that extends caudally toward the cloaca. The pronephric kidney does not function, but the pronephric duct seems to be important for the normal formation of the mesonephric kidney.

The *mesonephros* develops by the formation of mesonephric tubules from the intermediate mesoderm of the C6–L3 vertebral levels. Unlike the pronephric tubules, these tubules do not communicate with the coelom but receive a capillary glomerulus from the aorta at their blind end. The proximal blind end forms a capsule around the glomerulus. The distal ends of the mesonephric tubules tap into the pronephric duct and contribute to its caudal growth. This enlarged duct taps into the cloaca, and its name is changed to the mesonephric (wolffian) duct. The extensive growth of the mesonephros produces a large urogenital ridge projecting from the dorsal body wall.

The *metanephros* arises from two sources: the ureteric bud (metanephric diverticulum) and the metanephrogenic intermediate mesoderm of the L4–S1 vertebral levels. The ureteric bud arises as a tubular outgrowth from the mesonephric duct near its entrance into the cloaca. It grows toward the intermediate mesoderm where its blind end becomes capped by metanephrogenic tissue. The ureteric bud elongates as the ureter, and its blind end enlarges as the renal pelvis and undergoes a series of branchings. These branchings give rise to the major and minor calyces and the collecting tubules. The metanephrogenic condensations capping the blind ends of the collecting tubules develop into nephrons. One end of the blind nephron forms a Bowman's capsule around a glomerulus of capillaries. The other end taps into the collecting tubule.

Development of the Urinary Bladder and Urethra. The urinary bladder and urethra develop from the entoderm of the urogenital sinus and allantois. In early development the allantois is a diverticulum of the cloaca. A urorectal septum of mesoderm arises between the allantois and hindgut, grows caudally and divides the cloaca into a dorsal rectum and ventral urogenital sinus. With this division, the mesonephric duct empties into the urogenital sinus. As the urogenital sinus and a small adjacent portion of the allantois enlarge to form the urinary bladder, portions of the mesonephric and metanephric (ureter) ducts are incorporated into the wall of the urogenital sinus. This results in the ureters entering the bladder and the mesonephric ducts entering more caudally into the less dilated portion of the urogenital sinus. This distal portion of the urogenital sinus will become the urethra of the male and the urethra, vestibule and part of the vagina of the female.

Development of the Reproductive System. Even though the sex of the embryo is determined at fertilization, the gonads, ducts and external genitalia pass through an indifferent stage of development in which male and female components have the same appearance. This stage lasts until about the sixth week of development.

In the *indifferent stage,* gonads form on the medial wall of the urogenital ridges. Starting in the third week, primordial sex cells migrate from the yolk sac to the urogenital ridge. By the sixth week the coelomic epithelium has proliferated and surrounded the primordial sex cells to form primitive gonadal (sex) cords in the underlying mesoderm of the gonad.

In the indifferent stage of genital duct formation, both mesonephric and müllerian (paramesonephric) ducts are present. The müllerian ducts arise as longitudinal invaginations of the coelomic epithelium on the lateral wall of the urogenital ridge. Cranially this duct remains open to the coelom. Caudally it opens through the dorsal wall of the urogenital sinus. In its craniocaudal course it lies at first lateral to the mesonephric duct, then passes anterior to it and finally fuses with the opposite müllerian duct medial to the mesonephric ducts. During this fusion the urogenital ridges of the two sides are brought together to form a genital cord (septum) between the developing bladder anteriorly and the rectum posteriorly.

In the indifferent stage of the development of the external genitalia, mesoderm invades the lateral walls of the external opening of the urogenital sinus producing elevations called urogenital (urethral) folds. These folds unite anterior to the urogenital opening as the genital tubercle. Labioscrotal swellings develop lateral to the urogenital folds.

In the *development of the male reproductive system* the gonadal cords become testis cords that differentiate into seminiferous tubules and rete testis. The primordial sex cells become spermatogonia, whereas ingrowing coelomic epithelial cells give rise to supportive (Sertoli) cells. Efferent ductules develop from adjacent mesonephric tubules. The developing testis leads to the degeneration of the müllerian duct and to the differentiation of the mesonephric duct into the ductus epididymidis, vas (ductus) deferens and ejaculatory duct. The seminal vesicle arises as an outgrowth of the mesonephric duct. The urogenital sinus gives rise to the urethra and the prostate, bulbourethral and urethral glands. The genital tubercle enlarges and carries with it inferiorly a urethral plate of entoderm. This plate is transformed into the penile (cavernous) urethra after the urogenital folds fuse ventrally. The urethral plate, urogenital folds and genital tubercle (phallus) give rise to the definitive penis. The scrotum is formed by the ventral fusion of the labioscrotal swellings. The testes descend late in gestation from their retroperitoneal abdominal location. They are "anchored" in the scrotum by the mesenchymally derived gubernaculum testis. The path of descent is indicated by the inguinal canal. This follows the embryonic pathway of the processus vaginalis evaginating from the peritoneum.

In the *development of the female reproductive system* the initial gonadal cords degenerate and a second series of ovarian cords develop from primordial sex cells and coelomic epithelium. This second set of cords splits into groups of follicles near the surface of the developing ovary. Each primitive ovarian follicle consists of a developing sex cell surrounded by a flattened layer of follicular cells. The sex cells complete the prophase of the first meiotic division and are in the arrested dictyotene stage by the time of birth. From the sixth month until parturition there is a tremendous rate of degeneration of primitive follicles, the number decreasing from about 6 million to about 400,000 or less.

The unfused portions of the müllerian ducts develop into the uterine tubes. The fused portion gives rise to the uterus and part of the vagina. The genital cord remains as the broad ligament of the uterus. The proper ligament of the ovary and the round ligament of the uterus probably arise from the mesoderm of the urogenital ridge caudal to the ovary. The mesonephric duct and tubules degenerate, but some tubules remain as the paroophoron and epoophoron. Where the fused müllerian ducts empty into the urogenital sinus, some entodermal tissue forms a vaginal plate that eventually hollows out as part of the vagina. The urogenital sinus caudal to the vaginal opening becomes enlarged as the vestibule.

In the female the genital tubercle remains relatively small as the clitoris. The urethral folds become the labia minora, and the labioscrotal swellings develop into the labia majora. The hymen probably forms from the entoderm of the vaginal plate.

Congenital Malformations of the Urogenital System.

Horseshoe kidney is usually due to fusion of the caudal ends of the two kidneys across the midline. This probably occurs as they are approximated in their cranial migration out of the pelvis over the umbilical arteries. *Bifid ureter* is usually the result of a premature division of the ureteric bud. When this occurs it may result in double pelvis or double kidney. *Exstrophy of the bladder* is caused by failure of mesoderm to invade the area anterior to the developing bladder. This results in improper development of the anterior abdominal wall and bladder. *Congenital hydrocoele* is a collection of fluid in a remnant of the processus vaginalis. In *hypospadias* the external meatus of the urethra is on the ventral surface of the penis. This may be caused by improper closure of the urogenital folds or by failure of the outer ectodermal cells to grow into the glans and join the penile urethra.

Improper fusion of the müllerian ducts leads to many different abnormalities of the uterus. These range from uterus didelphys with its two bodies and two cervices to uterus arcuatus in which there is a minor degree of imperfect fusion. *Double vagina* is due to incomplete canalization of the vaginal plate. This may be associated with uterus didelphys and uterus bicornis bicollis.

Pseudohermaphroditism is a condition in which the individual has either testes (male pseudohermaphrodite) or ovaries (female pseudohermaphrodite) but possesses external genitalia of the opposite sex. In testicular feminization the male duct system and external genitalia are not induced to develop. An immature female duct system and female external genitalia remain. In adrenogenital syndrome a genetic abnormality results in absence of the enzyme C-21-hydroxylase, which is necessary for the production of hydrocortisone. This leads to an excess of ACTH, which causes overproduction of adrenal androgens. In females the excessive androgen causes hypertrophy of the clitoris and fusion of the labia majora, thus producing female hermaphroditism. In males the overproduction may cause precocious secondary sexual characteristics.

Early Embryology and Development of the Placenta

Fertilization. At ovulation a secondary oocyte, zona pellucida and corona radiata are discharged from the ovary and drawn into the infundibulum of the uterine tube where a spermatozoan can penetrate the zona pellucida and secondary oocyte. The union of the spermatozoan and secondary oocyte in the process of fertilization brings about the following major physical consequences: (1) reactivation of the secondary oocyte, (2) completion of the second meiotic division with formation of the second polar body, (3) establishment of a zygote (fertilized ovum) with the diploid number

(46) of chromosomes and (4) establishment of the mitotic spindle for the first cleavage division.

Cleavage and Blastodermic Vesicle Formation. During cleavage a series of mitoses occur in the zygote that result in successive 2, 4, 8 and 16 cell stages. These divisions take place over a period of about 3 days as the developing conceptus passes down the uterine tube. At about the time the 16 cell morula reaches the uterine cavity, fluid penetrates between some of the cells and produces a cavity in the solid ball of cells. The conceptus is now called a blastodermic vesicle (blastocyst). It consists of an outer layer of cells called the trophoblast, a cavity of the blastodermic vesicle (blastocoele) and an inner cell mass. After 3 days in the uterine cavity, the zona pellucida degenerates, and the sticky trophoblastic cells adhere to the endometrium.

Establishment of Ectoderm, Entoderm and Mesoderm. In the eighth day of development the inner cell mass cavitates to form an ectodermally lined amniotic cavity. The ectoderm of the embryonic disk will eventually give rise to the neural tube, neural crest and epidermis. An inner entodermal layer of cells also differentiates from the inner cell mass. These cells proliferate to form the yolk sac. The dorsal portion of the yolk sac later will become incorporated into the embryo as the primitive gut. Embryonic mesoderm arises from an elongate mass of cells called the primitive streak. The mesodermal cells turn inward along the midline and move laterally, insinuating themselves between the ectoderm and entoderm. In its forward, caudal and lateral movement, the embryonic mesoderm eventually joins the extraembryonic mesoderm that arises from the trophoblast. The notochord arises as a midline forward growth of cells from the primitive (Hensen's) node. In the third week of development, the embryonic mesoderm will have differentiated into paraxial (somite, dorsal), intermediate and lateral mesoderm. The paraxial mesoderm will develop further into paired somites that eventually give rise to vertebrae, ribs, skeletal muscle and connective tissues. The intermediate mesoderm will differentiate into much of the urogenital system. The lateral mesoderm, like the extraembryonic mesoderm, splits to form a coelom. That lateral mesoderm adjacent to the ectoderm is somatic mesoderm, while that next to entoderm is splanchnic mesoderm. Somatic mesoderm later will give rise to body wall tissues. Splanchnic mesoderm further differentiates into the cardiovascular system, smooth muscle and connective tissues in the walls of most visceral structures, mesenteries and the spleen.

Development of the Placenta. After the attachment of the blastodermic vesicle to the uterus at about the sixth postfertilization day, the trophoblast proliferates rapidly, and the conceptus begins to implant into the compacta layer of the endometrium. It is completely embedded in the uterine stroma by the eleventh day. In the rapid proliferation of cytotrophoblastic cells, cytokinesis has not kept pace with nuclear division, and an outer syncytial trophoblast appears over the single inner layer of cytotrophoblast. The coalescence of lacunae formed in the syncytial trophoblast leads to the formation of primary stem villi. These are most extensive in the trophoblast that faces the deeper layers of the endometrium. It is in this region where most of the nutriments are being supplied to the trophoblast from invaded uterine glands and blood vessels. The primary stem villi consist of a core of cytotrophoblast surrounded by syncytial trophoblast. Later, mesoderm invades these villi, and they become secondary stem villi containing a core of connective tissue. By the end of the third week, blood vessels start to form in the secondary villi. With the vascularization of the trophoblast it is called the chorion. That part of the chorion that is the deepest in the uterine wall becomes the chorion frondosum portion of the placenta; the rest of it loses its villi and is called the chorion laeve. An anchoring villus and its free floating villi constitute a cotyledon. Septa of the cytotrophoblastic coating of the intervillous space project from the decidua and incompletely separate the cotyledons from each other. The functional layer of the endometrium deep to the chorion frondosum is the decidua basalis; that adjacent to the chorion laeve is the decidua capsularis; and the rest is the decidua parietalis. As the embryo enlarges the uterine cavity is obliterated, and the decidua capsularis and decidua parietalis fuse into a much compressed layer. After birth of the newborn, the decidual layers, placenta, chorion laeve and amnion will be discharged as the afterbirth.

QUESTIONS IN ANATOMY

Both review and multiple choice questions are presented in this section. The answers to the multiple choice questions are at the end of this chapter. The answers to the review questions are in the text.

REVIEW QUESTIONS

Contrast the five principal regions of the vertebral column, giving the characteristics of typical vertebrae and curvatures and the exact movements permitted in each region.

Draw the normal curves of the spine.

Describe a typical thoracic vertebra.

List the various factors that permit movement of the vertebral column. Why do lumbar dislocations usually involve fracture while cervical dislocations do not?

Why does a rupture of the disk between lumbar vertebrae 4 and 5 usually impinge on spinal nerve L5?

How do cartilage and bone differ in their vascularity and in the mode of their nutritional supply?

How do seven cervical vertebrae develop from eight pairs of cervical sclerotomes? What is the embryologic basis of spondylolisthesis? spina bifida?

Describe the major components of the growing epiphyseal disk. How does a long bone grow in length and width?

What are the major functions of the superficial muscles of the back? the deep muscles of the back? What is the innervation to these muscles?

Describe a sarcomere. Are actin and myosin found in both the A and I bands? What is the T tubular system. What are the functions of intercalated disks?

What motor functional components of nerves innervate skeletal muscle of branchial arch origin? skeletal muscle of somite origin? smooth muscle of splanchnic mesoderm origin?

Draw a cross section of the thoracic cord, indicating the principal ascending and descending tracts.

Describe the formation of a typical spinal nerve.

Describe the contents and extent of the cauda equina. What area is the region of choice for a spinal tap? Why?

Give the extent and the relationships of the spinal cord and its meninges. Into which space is an anesthetic injected through the inferior aperture of the sacral canal as in caudal analgesia?

List the functional components of a spinal nerve. Which of these is a component of the autonomic nervous system? Where are preganglionic and postganglionic autonomic neurons located?

Name the nuclei of termination for incoming GSA fibers of spinal nerves.

Where would chromatolysis take place in hemisection of the spinal cord at the T3 level? What would be the sensory loss from this lesion? What would be the motor loss?

What is the fate of neural crest material? What cells are responsible for the formation of myelin in the CNS? in the PNS?

Describe the events of degeneration and regeneration of a peripheral nerve.

What would be the functional loss if the sulcal arteries supplying the C7 level were thrombosed? What area of the cord is supplied by the posterior spinal arteries?

Name the one bony link between the upper extremity and the axial skeleton.

What is the major support of the acromioclavicular joint?

Where is the surgical neck of the humerus?

Describe the articular capsule of the shoulder joint; its attachment.

What are the major supports of the shoulder joint?

What motions occur at the shoulder joint?

What muscles cause each of the motions at the shoulder joint?

Name the structures found in the suprahumeral space. What is the importance of the suprahumeral space?

At what joints do pronation and supination occur?

Describe the articular surfaces that form the elbow joint? What motions occur at this joint? What muscles cause the motions?

Between what bones is the wrist joint formed? What motions occur at the wrist joint? What muscles cause each of these motions?

What motions are available at the four medial carpometacarpal joints? How do the motions of the CM joint of the thumb differ from those of the other four?

List the motions that can occur at the metacarpophalangeal joints and the major motors of each.

Contraction of the muscles in the anterior compartment of the arm causes what motions? in the posterior compartment?

What nerve innervates the muscles in the anterior compartment of the arm? in the posterior compartment?

The muscles in the anterior compartment of the forearm are innervated by what nerves? in the posterior compartment?

What motions are caused by contraction of the muscles in the anterior compartment of the forearm? in the posterior compartment?

Describe the compartmentalization of the ventral aspect of the hand. What nerve(s) innervate(s) the muscles of each compartment?

Describe the radial and ulnar bursae.

Describe the locations of the midpalmar and thenar spaces.

Describe the organization of the brachial plexus.

Name the collateral branches of each part of the plexus.

Specifically define the locations of the ulnar and median nerves at the wrist.

What physical problems result following an injury to the radial nerve? musculocutaneous nerve? ulnar nerve? median nerve?

Trace the course of the brachial artery through the arm, and the radial and ulnar arteries through the forearm and hand.

Where exactly are radial and ulnar pulses taken?

Which artery terminates as the major contributor to the superficial palmar arterial arch? deep palmar arterial arch?

Describe the location and courses of the cephalic and basilic veins. Where does each empty into the deep veins?

What three bones form the os coxae? Describe the location of the acetabulum, obturator foramen, ischial spine, ischial tuberosity, greater sciatic notch, lesser sciatic notch, iliac crest with its anterior and posterior superior spines and the pubic tubercle.

Compare the articular surfaces that form the hip joint with those that form the shoulder joint.

Compare the acetabular labrum with the glenoid labrum.

Define the extent of the articular capsule of the hip joint. What parts of the femoral neck are intracapsular and what parts are extracapsular?

Describe in general the blood supply to the femoral neck and head. What is unique about the courses of some of these vessels?

Describe the extracapsular ligaments of the hip joint. What are their functions?

What motions can occur at the hip joint? What are the muscles involved in each motion?

Describe the articular surfaces that form the knee joint.

What motions are available at the knee joint? What muscles cause these motions?

Describe the menisci. What are their functions?

Against what types of forces do the cruciate ligaments protect the knee? the collateral ligaments?

List the bones of the foot. Which of these form the medial longitudinal arch? the lateral longitudinal arch?

What ligament is the most important support of the longitudinal arches of the foot?

Describe the formation of the ankle joint.

What motions are available at the ankle joint? What muscles cause each of the motions?

What ligament is usually injured in an inversion-plantar flexion sprain?

At what joints do inversion and eversion occur primarily? These motions are produced by the contraction of what muscles?

Describe the location of the gluteal muscles; innervation; functions.

Name the muscles of the anterior compartment of the thigh; innervation; functions.

List the medial and posterior femoral muscles; innervation; functions.

Describe the femoral triangle. What structures pass through the triangle and what are their relationships?

Describe the popliteal fossa and the relationships of the structures within the triangle.

List the muscles found in each of the compartments of the leg; innervations; functions.

Describe the compartmentation of the foot. What nerves innervate the muscles in each compartment?

Fibers from which spinal cord segments are found in the lumbosacral plexus? Where is the lumbar portion of the plexus formed? the sacral portion?

Describe the courses of the medial and lateral plantar nerves and compare each with its homologous nerve in the hand.

Describe the limp that would accompany an injury of the superior gluteal, inferior gluteal, femoral, deep peroneal and tibial nerves.

Describe the course of the femoral artery through the thigh. How does it begin? Where exactly is it located in the femoral triangle?

At what point does the femoral become the popliteal artery? Where is the artery in the popliteal fossa? How can a popliteal pulse be taken?

Describe the courses of the main arterial trunks through the leg.

Compare the arterial supply of the foot with that of the hand.

Describe the exact location of the greater saphenous vein as it crosses the ankle joint.

Which nerves leave the anterior cranial fossa?

Which structures are found in the posterior cranial fossa? What are the important foramina of this region? Name the structures passing through each foramen.

Which structures pass through the foramen magnum?

Name the structures passing from the middle cranial fossa to the orbit through: (1) the optic foramen, (2) the superior orbital fissure, (3) the foramen rotundum, (4) the foramen ovale and (5) the foramen lacerum.

List the contents of the infratemporal fossa. Where does this fossa communicate with the cranial cavity?

Describe the important relationships of the mastoid air cells.

Describe the location and the extent of the pharynx, the parts into which it is usually divided, the structure of its walls and the location of its various openings.

Describe the site and boundaries of the opening of the eustachian tube into the pharynx.

Describe the temporomandibular joint. In which direction does this joint usually become dislocated?

What are the structures and the spaces found just external to each part of the bony wall of the orbit? Indicate where each is related to the orbital wall.

Describe the extraocular muscles and give their nerve supply.

Describe the relationships of the palatine tonsil. Which artery is most commonly in close relation to the palatine tonsil? State the course of this artery and its relationships to the tonsil.

Give the relations of the branches of the external carotid artery? the internal carotid artery?

Describe the layers of the scalp. What are its blood and nerve supply?

Describe the meninges of the brain. In what parts of the brain are ventricles and choroid plexuses located?

Trace the pathway of the cerebrospinal fluid from its origin in the choroid plexus of the lateral ventricle to the superior sagittal sinus. What happens if the iter is occluded? At what other sites is the flow likely to be obstructed?

What are the principal fissures and lobes of the cerebrum?

Describe the internal and external topography of the medulla. Which cell columns extend into the medulla from the spinal cord?

Which cranial nerves arise from the medulla?

From what nuclei of origin in the brain stem do preganglionic parasympathetic fibers arise? Where do these fibers synapse and what organs do they supply?

Give, in general, the distribution of the vagus nerve. What are its functional components?

Give the origin, course and distribution of the hypoglossal nerve.

What cranial nerves convey the afferent and efferent nerves (limbs) of the cough reflex? carotid sinus reflex? gag reflex? corneal blink reflex? pupillary light reflex? What are the nuclei of termination and origin of these reflexes?

What nerves supply general somatic afferent, special visceral afferent and somatic efferent fibers to the tongue? How is the tongue mucosa modified to carry out the functions of the tongue?

If the uvula points to the right on phonation, which nerve is most likely damaged?

What is the relation of the facial nerve to the middle ear? the jugular vein? Describe the bony and the membranous labyrinths. Describe the middle ear and the mastoid. What is the anatomic basis for paralysis of only the lower contralateral face in corticobulbar lesions compared to paralysis of the whole contralateral side in facial nerve lesions?

Why do unilateral lesions of the auditory pathway within the CNS rarely result in deafness?

Describe the possible pathway for postrotational nystagmus starting with stimulation of the hair cells in the crista of the lateral semicircular canal.

Give the location within the central nervous system of the nuclei that directly innervate the voluntary ocular muscles. Where do afferent fibers to these nuclei originate and in which tracts do they travel to reach the nuclei? What are the necessary nerve connections for lateral conjugate gaze?

If the right fifth nerve is damaged, will the left eye blink if the right cornea is stimulated? If the right facial nerve is damaged and the fifth nerve is intact, will any eye blink if the right cornea is stimulated?

Describe the orbit and its contents.

Describe the eyeball.

Describe the normal anatomy of the fundus of the eye as seen with the ophthalmoscope. How are the arteries and the veins differentiated from each other?

What is the vascular supply of the retina? What nutritive pathway is compromised in detachment of the retina?

Describe the autonomic innervation of the eyeball and eyelid. Ptosis can occur following injury to what two nerve pathways? What are the symptoms of Horner's syndrome, and where might a lesion be located that could lead to this?

Describe the circulation of aqueous humor. In what area might blockage of the pathway lead to glaucoma?

Trace the flow of tears from their origin to their arrival in the nasal cavity. Where are the tarsal glands located and what types of glands are these?

What is the nerve pathway involved in the near reflex (accommodation, convergence and pupillary reflex)?

Describe the optic nerve, its termination and point of emergence from the skull.

Outline the visual pathway. Trace light rays from a point in the upper right quadrant of the visual field to the retina; then trace the impulses from the rods and cones stimulated to the specific site in the occipital cortex where the impulses would be received.

Contrast the effects of the destruction of the right optic nerve and of the left optic tract on the retina and the field of vision.

Describe the olfactory nerve, including its origin, termination and exit from the skull.

Locate the lamina cribrosa.

Give the course and function of the pyramidal (corticospinal) tract. What is its relation to the cerebral motor cortex?

Describe the course of the medial lemniscus. Where do these fibers originate and terminate? What is the functional significance of this pathway?

Where are the primary receptive cortical areas for two-point touch, vision, hearing and olfaction? Which relay nuclei of the diencephalon send fibers to these areas?

Where would be a likely site for a lesion that would give contralateral paralysis to the extremities and trunk below the lesion and would also give paralysis of lateral gaze to the side of the lesion? Where would the lesion be if there was contralateral paralysis of the body, ipsilateral paralysis of medial gaze, ptosis and dilated pupil?

Which functional components or pathways make up the internal capsule of the brain? Where in this structure is each component found?

Describe the paralysis resulting from a destructive lesion that involves the posterior limb of the internal capsule.

Where do the principal afferents to the cerebellum originate? Describe the course that each follows to reach its termination in the cerebellum.

What is the major output of the cerebellum? Where do the efferent pathways from the neocerebellum go? Where do the efferent pathways from the flocculonodular lobe terminate? What is the function of the cerebellum?

What is the major outflow of the lenticular nucleus? What connections are made with the subthalamic nucleus and what is the effect of this nucleus on the globus pallidus?

Which structures receive their blood supply from the internal carotid artery?

What blood vessels comprise the arterial circle of Willis?

Which major ascending and descending pathways could be compromised if there was occlusion of the anterior spinal artery where it arises from the vertebral artery?

What deficits would occur if the posterior inferior cerebral artery were occluded?

Give the position, relationships, attachments, innervation and embryonic origin of the pituitary gland. Into what parts is the pituitary gland divided and what are the characteristics of the cells in the various parts? What is the functional significance of each of the cell types?

Describe the pathway of hypothalamic releasing factors from their production in the hypothalamus to their site of action on chromophils of the adenohypophysis. How does this pathway differ from the neurosecretory tracts that terminate in the neurohypophysis?

Which structures are most susceptible to injury when the pituitary gland undergoes enlargement? Where are these structures found in relation to the pituitary?

Describe the major efferent pathways of the hypothalamus. What is the relationship between the hypothalamus and autonomic nervous system? the limbic system?

What are the two main divisions of the autonomic nervous system? Discuss the origins of the two parts from the central nervous system. Where, in general, are the peripheral adrenergic and cholinergic fibers found within these two systems?

To which structures are the nerve fibers from the superior cervical ganglion distributed? What would be the results of destruction of this ganglion?

Describe the microscopic structure of the salivary glands. Where do their ducts open into the oral cavity?

Which of the major salivary glands are mixed seromucous glands? Both the pancreas and parotid can be affected in mumps. Compare the exocrine portions of these two glands. How are the cells of the striated (salivary) ducts of the parotid similar to the nephron?

What are the major contents of the anterior triangle of the neck? the posterior triangle? In which triangle of the neck could you palpate the anterior scalene nodes? the roots of the brachial plexus?

Describe the carotid sheath, its contents and its relation to the cervical sympathetic trunk.

Describe the cervical plexus and give the structures innervated by it.

Which anatomic structures are traversed in tracheotomy?

What comprises the true vocal fold? What nerves regulate the muscles of the larynx? What would be the motor and sensory loss if the superior laryngeal nerve were severed?

Give the gross and the microscopic structures of the thyroid gland and its important relations. What is its blood supply? Where may ectopic and accessory thyroids be found? Explain their location on the basis of the embryonic development of the thyroid.

Give the number, the position and the relationships of the parathyroid glands. Describe briefly the origin and the development of these glands.

Give the position, relationships and microscopic structure of the thymus. Explain the occasional inclusion of parathyroid tissue in the thymus. Compare the thymus gland at birth and at puberty.

If there is a complete branchial fistula at the second pharyngeal pouch and cleft, where will it open internally and externally?

Describe the development of the face. What is the embryologic basis for cleft lip? cleft palate? choanal artresia?

Outline the boundaries of the lungs and pleura on the chest wall.

Name the lobes and the fissures of each lung and explain how they can be mapped out on the chest wall.

Give the outline of the heart as projected on the surface of the anterior thoracic wall. Which structures of the heart form the boundaries described above? Which chambers lie directly beneath the anterior chest wall?

Locate the heart valves as projected onto the anterior chest wall. Which of these valves lie near the surface and which are placed more deeply? If sounds from the more deeply placed valves are projected in the direction of blood flow through these valves, where would be the areas of maximum audibility for each?

What are the boundaries of the mediastinum? Give the contents of the anterior, the middle and the posterior portions.

Give the positions and the relationships of the trachea in the thorax. At what level does it branch into the right and the left bronchi? In which of these bronchi is a foreign body most likely to lodge? Explain.

How many bronchopulmonary segments are there in each lung and lobe?

Describe the right pleural sac. Why does the lung collapse when an opening forms from the air passages of the lung into the pleural sac?

Describe the innervation of the lungs. Indicate the functional significance of the nerve fibers involved.

Describe the changes in the histology of the walls of the respiratory tract as one proceeds from the trachea to the alveoli. How far down the conducting pathways do cartilage, glands and ciliated epithelium extend?

Describe the lining epithelium of the alveoli. What structures constitute a blood-air barrier?

Give the location and microscopic structure of the valves of the heart. What are the functions of the chordae tendineae and the papillary muscles? How are these structures arranged to subserve their functions? Compare the right and the left atrioventricular orifices and their valves. Why is one valve larger than the other?

Contrast the right and left ventricles of the heart as to structure of the walls, volume of the cavities and valvular arrangements.

Describe the development of the interatrial septum. Where is the foramen ovale? What is the embryologic basis of the foramen ovale defect and the foramen primum defect? What embryologic structures contribute to the development of the membranous part of the interventricular septum?

Describe the arch of the aorta, including its important relationships.

Describe the fate of the 6 pairs of aortic arches. What is the developmental reason for a right subclavian artery arising from the arch of the aorta? How does transposition of the aorta and pulmonary artery arise?

What embryologic vessels are retained and which fail to form in the formation of double superior venae cavae? What postnatal structures arise from the left umbilical vein, vitelline veins, vitelline arteries and umbilical arteries?

Describe the blood supply to the heart.

Describe the efferent innervation to the heart, including the location of the cell bodies of the various neurons involved.

Give the anatomic arrangements that provide for reflex slowing of the heart on stimulation of the carotid sinus.

The stellate ganglion has been removed for the relief of anginal pain. What effects other than the relief of anginal pain may result? Explain the anatomic basis for each of these additional effects.

Describe in detail the anatomic arrangement of the structures in the heart responsible for the initiation and transmission of the heart beat.

Describe in detail the anatomic modifications in the heart and the resultant changes in the circulation of the blood in a normal infant following birth. What results if these normal changes do not take place? Explain.

Describe the composition, the extent and the attachments of the pericardial sac. Where can it be opened for drainage without going through the pleura?

Describe the diaphragm, including its origin, structure, attachments and orifices. Give the mechanism of its action. Where is referred pain from the diaphragm commonly experienced and how is this related to its innervation?

What are the roles in inspiration of the diaphragm, abdominal muscles, intercostal muscles and scalene muscles?

Contrast the gross and the histologic features of the esophagus and the trachea as related to the functions of each of these tubes.

What is a possible embryologic reason for tracheoesophageal fistula? for diaphragmatic hernia?

Where does the thoracic duct empty and what does it drain?

Describe the lymphatics of the thoracic cavity. What is the effect, if any, of blocking the thoracic duct at the point at which it empties into the venous system?

Describe the pathway of lymph through a lymphatic node. What is the function of the reticuloendothelial system? What is the function of a lymph node?

Compare the microscopic structure of the thymus with that of a lymph node. What is the gross relationship of the thymus to the great vessels?

Discuss the lymphatic drainage of the breast, mentioning all possible pathways and connections.

Describe the normal gross and microscopic structure of the mammary gland.

Describe the origin, the course and the termination of the splanchnic nerves. What is the functional nature of the various fibers running in these nerves, and where are the cell bodies of these fibers located? What would be the vascular effects in the abdomen on section of the splanchnic nerves?

Divide the abdomen into 9 surface regions and name them. What structures do the horizontal dividing lines represent?

Divide the abdomen into 4 regions.

Locate the stomach on the surface, including the cardiac orifice and the pyloric orifice.

On the surface locate the duodenum, the ileocolic junction, the cecum and the right and left colic flexures.

On the surface outline the liver and indicate the exact location of the gallbladder.

On the surface locate the pancreas, spleen, kidneys, and ureter.

What muscles form the anterior abdominal wall?

What abdominal muscle or its aponeurosis forms the superficial inguinal ring, the deep inguinal ring, and the floor, roof, anterior and posterior walls of the inguinal canal?

Differentiate between the pathway of a direct versus an indirect inguinal hernia.

Differentiate between organs that are retroperitoneal, partially peritonealized and "completely" peritonealized. Give specific examples of each.

Describe the location of the lesser peritoneal sac.

Name the three structures in the free edge of the lesser omentum.

Describe the parts of the stomach.

What are the four parts of the duodenum?

Where may the jejunum and ileum normally be located? How does the jejunum grossly differ from the ileum?

How does the large intestine grossly differ from the small intestine?

With what organs are the ascending, transverse and descending parts of the colon related?

With what organs is the liver related? Where is the gallbladder found with respect to the liver? With what organs is the gallbladder related?

Describe the bare area of the liver.

Describe the peritoneal relationships of the liver.

What is the relationship between the inferior vena cava and the liver?

Where are the caudate and quadrate lobes of the liver?

What organs are drained by the portal vein? What alternate pathways may blood take when the normal path for portal blood through the liver is obstructed?

Describe the bile duct system of the liver and gallbladder.

Describe the relationships of the pancreas. Into what does the main pancreatic duct empty?

Describe the peritoneal relationships of the spleen.

At what vertebral levels are the kidneys found?

What structures form the kidney bed? What structures are related to the anterior surfaces of each kidney?

Describe the course of the ureters. To what structures is each ureter related? At what locations are the ureters naturally constricted?

Describe the location and relationships of each suprarenal gland.

At what vertebral level does the aorta pass through the thoracic diaphragm? At what vertebral level does the abdominal aorta bifurcate? Where is the abdominal aorta with respect to the lumbar vertebrae?

Name the three large unpaired branches of the aorta and give the distribution of each.

What general areas are supplied by the common iliac arteries?

The sympathetic fibers that innervate the abdominal viscera originate from what spinal cord segments? Where do the synapses occur between the preganglionic and postganglionic sympathetic and parasympathetic fibers that supply the abdominal viscera?

What part of the gastrointestinal tract is supplied by the vagus nerve?

Describe the system of nerve plexuses along the ventral aspect of the aorta.

What nerves innervate the skin and muscle of the abdominal wall?

What are the major differences in character in the normal mucosa of the alimentary canal, beginning with the esophagus and terminating at the anus? What are the associated changes in function?

Describe the stomach. Give its relations and describe the microscopic structure of gastric glands. What cells produce HCl? pepsin? mucus? serotonin?

Describe the modifications of the small intestine for the function of absorption. What structures accentuate the absorptive surface area. Locate Brunner's glands. What do they produce?

How do you distinguish microscopically a coil of small intestine from colon?

Describe the histologic structure of the vermiform appendix.

What is the microscopic structure of the liver? Describe the circulation of the blood through the liver. Explain on an anatomic basis why certain ingested poisons cause damage initially to the periphery of the liver lobules. In case of portal obstruction, what collateral venous circulation might be established?

Give the contents of the portal areas (canals, triads).

How is the mucosa of the gallbladder structurally adapted to the functions it performs?

Describe the histologic structure of the pancreas. Give the functional significance of the various structures included. What are the most prominent ultrastructural characteristics of cells of the exocrine secretory units?

What is the microscopic structure of the spleen?

Describe the flow of blood through the spleen. Describe the position, relationships and peritoneal attachments of the spleen.

Describe the microscopic structure of the adrenal gland. What is the nerve and blood supply to the cortex and medulla? Locate the cell bodies of neurons that supply the cortex and medulla.

Describe the histologic structure of the kidney. What is the blood supply to the various components of the renal cortex and medulla? How are the different parts of the nephron structurally adapted to carry out their functions?

What constitutes the filtration barrier of the renal corpuscle?

What are the histologic features of the ureter and urinary bladder that permit them to readily accommodate large quantitites of water?

Describe the rotation of the gut. What are the fates of the cephalic and caudal limbs of the gut loop?

How does the lesser peritoneal sac develop? What embryologic structures contribute to the formation of the greater omentum? What is the fate of the vitelline (omphalomesenteric) artery?

Locate the following structures and give the embryologic significance of them: (1) ligamentum arteriosum, (2) ligamentum venosum, (3) round ligament of the liver, (4) Meckel's diverticulum, (5) lateral umbilical ligaments.

Compare the peritoneal arrangements of the various parts of the large intestine. Explain the manner in which a structure that in early development is suspended by peritoneum becomes secondarily retroperitoneal.

Describe the origin of the pancreas.

Compare the suprarenal medulla with a sympathetic ganglion as to its origin, structure and function. Describe the development of the suprarenal gland.

How does the bare area of the liver reflect the development of the liver in the caudal face of the septum transversum? From what embryonic germ layer do the epithelium and glands of most of the digestive system arise?

Differentiate the true from the false pelvis.

Define the pelvic inlet and the pelvic outlet.

What muscles form the pelvic diaphragm? Describe their lateral attachments.

Define the AP and transverse diameters of the pelvic inlet, pelvic outlet and midpelvis.

Define the boundaries of the urogenital and anal triangles.

Describe the boundaries of the ischiorectal fossa, including its anterior and posterior recesses and its contents.

What is the pudendal canal and what are its contents?

Describe the deep perineal space. What are its contents in the male and the female?

Define the superficial perineal space. What are its contents in the male and the female?

What nerves innervate the skin of the perineum?

What structures are palpable in the male and female via rectal examination?

Define the locaton of the urinary bladder and name the organs to which it is related in both the male and female.

Trace the course of the urethra in both the male and female.

To what structures is the prostate gland related?

Describe the course of the ductus deferens.

Describe the location of the ovaries.

How are the ovaries related to the uterine tubes?

Define the parts of the uterus.

How is the uterus related to the vagina?

What is the normal position of the uterus? To what structures is it related?

What structures are normally palpable via a vaginal examination?

How is the broad ligament related to the uterus?

What are the mesometrium, mesovarium, mesosalpinx, parametrium and the cardinal ligaments?

Name the visceral branches of the internal iliac artery and describe their general distributions.

Describe the origin, migration and fate of primordial sex cells in the formation of the indifferent stage of the gonad and in the formation of the testis and ovary.

Describe the histologic structure of the testis. Where and how does spermatogenesis take place?

Describe the histologic structure of the epithelium lining the rete testis, efferent ductules, ductus epididymidis and ductus deferens.

Describe the male urethra, its parts, their characteristics and relationships. Explain on an anatomic basis where in the course of the urethra difficulty might be experienced in passing a rigid catheter.

What ducts empty into the urethra, and what is the nature of the substances being delivered to the urethra?

Describe the histologic characteristics of the penis. What structures are adapted for the function of erection? Why is the urethra not completely compressed during erection?

What is the origin of the vesicular ovarian (graafian) follicle? What is ovulation? When does it occur in relation to the menstrual cycle? When does it occur in relation to oogenesis?

Describe the development and histology of the corpus luteum.

If fertilization and implantation do not take place, when during the menstrual cycle will the corpus luteum degenerate? What is a corpus albicans?

Describe the histologic structure of the uterine (fallopian) tube. What is the function of the ciliated epithelium?

Describe the histologic structure of the uterus. State the major endometrial changes that take place during the menstrual cycle and during pregnancy. What is the effect of estrogen on the uterus? of progesterone?

Describe the mucosa of the cervix. What changes take place in the cervix during the menstrual cycle? during pregnancy?

Describe the histology of the vagina. How does its epithelium change during the menstrual cycle.

Compare the histology of the clitoris and penis.

What are the fates of the mesonephric ducts, müllerian ducts and urogenital sinus in the male? in the female?

What is the difference in origin of the nephrons and collecting tubules?

What is the embryologic basis of double vagina? uterus didelphys? bipartite uterus?

What is the normal fate of the processus vaginalis in the male? What is hydrocoele?

What is the fate of the urethral folds and labioscrotal swellings in the male? in the female? What embryologic structures are involved in the formation of hypospadias? What causes, and what is the effect of, congenital adrenal hyperplasia?

What series of events immediately follows penetration of a secondary oocyte by a spermatozoon? Where does fertilization usually occur?

How long is the developing conceptus in the uterine tube? in the uterine cavity? On what postfertilization day does implantation occur?

Into what layers of the endometrium does the embryo implant?

Describe the development of the placenta. When are both cytotrophoblast and syncytial trophoblast present? When are nucleated red blood cells normally found?

Describe the histologic structure of the placenta. What is the chorion frondosum? What is a cotyledon? Where are decidual cells found?

Describe the placental barrier. Describe the flow of blood through the placenta.

What is the fate of the primitive streak and primitive (Hensen's) node?

What is the developmental relation of the allantois to the urinary bladder?

What is the fate of the primitive yolk sac? How are the respiratory and digestive systems related to the yolk sac?

What is the fate of the neural plate?

What is the fate of the sclerotome? myotome? intermediate mesoderm?

MULTIPLE CHOICE QUESTIONS

One-Answer Type

Select the *one* statement that most accurately completes the sentence or answers the question. Answers are at the end of this chapter.

1. In a cell with especially high energy (ATP) requirements, which of the following organelles would you expect to be most highly developed:
   (a) rough endoplasmic reticulum
   (b) mitochondria
   (c) centrioles
   (d) peroxisomes

2. Cells with large amounts of rough endoplasmic reticulum are most likely to:
   (a) produce steroids
   (b) line the lumen of blood vessels
   (c) produce structural proteins that remain in the cell
   (d) synthesize a proteinaceous secretory product

3. Regarding the nucleus:
   (a) chromosomes in areas of euchromatin are probably less functionally active than in areas of heterochromatin
   (b) the nucleolar membrane separates the nucleolus from the chromosomes
   (c) the nuclear envelope consists of two membranes, and is penetrated by pores to allow passage of material between the nucleus and the cytoplasm
   (d) chromosomes and the nuclear envelope are most prominent during the metaphase stage of mitosis

4. Assuming a person had received enough exposure of x-rays to the whole body to destroy cells as they attempt to divide, which one of the following functions would survive best?
   (a) hair growth
   (b) red blood corpuscle production
   (c) intestinal absorption of fat
   (d) cardiac contraction

5. Choose the correct statement regarding the free surface specializations of epithelial cells.
   (a) Cilia contain a core of nine peripheral and two central microfilaments
   (b) Microvilli contain a core of microfilaments
   (c) Microvilli insert into centrioles (basal bodies)
   (d) Stereocilia contain a core of microtubules that inserts into centrioles (basal bodies).

6. Which of the following is *not* used in classifying the various types of epithelia?
   (a) The number of layers of cells

(b) The shape of the cells at only the free surface

(c) The terminal specialization or modification at the free surface

(d) The relative amount of intercellular material to the cellular content

7. The specific intercellular junctional mechanism through which cells are electrically coupled is the:
   (a) desmosome
   (b) tight junction
   (c) zonula adherens
   (d) gap junction

8. Which of the following fibers or fibrils is most like collagen in its chemical composition?
   (a) Muscle fibers
   (b) Elastic fibers
   (c) Neurofibrils
   (d) Reticular fibers

9. Tendons are composed of:
   (a) dense irregularly arranged connective tissue
   (b) dense regularly arranged connective tissue
   (c) large elastic fibers with fibroblasts lying between the fibers
   (d) large collagenous fibers with fibroblasts lying in lacunae between the fibers

10. In which of the following organs would you be most likely to find elastic cartilage?
    (a) Lungs
    (b) Developing long bone
    (c) Larynx
    (d) Inner ear

11. The stiffness of cartilage is due primarily to the presence of:
    (a) chondroitin sulfate
    (b) collagen fibers
    (c) hyaluronic acid
    (d) the perichondrium

12. Bone remodelling normally:
    (a) involves removal of existing bone by osteoblasts
    (b) involves deposition of calcified cartilage on existing trabeculae of bone
    (c) can occur in response to mechanical stress and fluctuations in the blood calcium level
    (d) occurs during the "growing years," but ceases by the age of 50

13. Which statement is true for muscle tissue?
    (a) Cardiac and smooth muscle cells both branch and have central nuclei
    (b) Cardiac and smooth muscle tissue both possess gap junctions
    (c) Skeletal muscle satellite cells lie outside the basement membrane of the muscle and are really connective tissue cells

(d) Cardiac and smooth muscle tissue are each more vascular than skeletal muscle tissue

14. Neurons:
    (a) of the central nervous system have nissl material that extends into both dendrites and axons
    (b) of the central nervous system are invested by myelin produced by Schwann cells
    (c) and glial cells in the gray matter of the spinal cord make up a meshwork called neuropil
    (d) of sympathetic ganglia are unipolar or pseudounipolar

15. Which of the following is *not* produced by a neuron?
    (a) Antidiuretic hormone (ADH)
    (b) Luteinizing releasing hormone (LHRH)
    (d) Epinephrine
    (d) Calcitonin

16. Neuromuscular spindles:
    (a) contain both afferent and efferent nerve fibers
    (b) contain intrafusal fibers which are usually larger than extrafusal fibers
    (c) are located in the myenteric plexus of the intestine
    (d) regulate the state of contraction of cardiac muscle

17. Which of the following cells is morphologically closest to the earlier "blast" stage?
    (a) Promyelocyte
    (b) Platelet
    (c) Neutrophilic metamyelocyte
    (d) Reticulocyte

18. Which of the following cell types is most numerous in a normal blood smear?
    (a) Neutrophil
    (b) Eosinophil
    (c) Lymphocyte
    (d) Monocyte

19. Myelocytes:
    (a) have an indented nucleus
    (b) are incapable of division
    (c) have "specific" granules
    (d) arise from metamyelocytes

20. In the heart:
    (a) Purkinje fibers are modified nerve fibers constituting part of the cardiac conduction system
    (b) the endocardium of the atria is thicker than that of the ventricles
    (c) papillary muscles are involuntary smooth muscle tissue that insert into chordae tendinae

(d) the sinoatrial (SA) node is modified connective tissue of the cardiac skeleton

21. Afferent lymphatic vessels are found supplying:
    (a) Peyer's patches
    (b) the spleen
    (c) lymph nodes
    (d) the thymus

22. Which one of the following does *not* filter blood through its sinusoids?
    (a) Bone marrow
    (b) Spleen
    (c) Lymph node
    (d) Liver

23. Which of the following organs is least likely to demonstrate mucus-secreting cells or glands?
    (a) Vagina
    (b) Esophagus
    (c) Cervix
    (d) Colon

24. Which of the following is a component of the mucosa (mucous membrane)?
    (a) Enteroendocrine cells of the stomach
    (b) Hair follicle
    (c) Auerbach's myenteric nerve plexus
    (d) Sweat gland

25. Which of the following is *not* correct for the small intestine?
    (a) Monoglycerides and fatty acids diffuse through the absorptive cell plasma membrane
    (b) The nodules of Peyer's patches may extend into the submucosal layer
    (c) Chylomicrons are often found in the intercellular spaces between absorptive cells
    (d) The outer longitudinal layer of the muscularis externa is thickened into taenia coli

26. In the kidney:
    (a) as much as 80 percent of the amino acids and glucose of the ultrafiltrate are reabsorbed by the thin portion of the loop of Henle
    (b) renin, produced by the juxtaglomerular apparatus, acts directly on arterial smooth muscle to cause vasodilation
    (c) antidiuretic hormone causes the collecting tubules to become more permeable to water, thus concentrating the urine
    (d) interlobular arteries arise from arcuate arteries and pass into the cortex via the medullary rays

27. During the differentiation of a spermatid (spermiogenesis) the acrosome arises by accumulation of material in:
    (a) mitochondria

(b) the nucleus
(c) the Golgi complex
(d) the nuclear envelope

28. In the male reproductive system:
    (a) spermatozoa are stored and undergo maturation in the rete testis
    (b) the ductus deferens, seminal vesicle, and prostate all have smooth muscle in their walls
    (c) the seminal vesicle is the main source of acid phosphatase in the semen
    (d) the prostate gland is a site where spermatozoa are stored and become mature

29. In the female reproductive system:
    (a) uterine glands secrete a carbohydrate-rich substance and also are necessary for regeneration of the surface epithelium of the uterus during the menstrual cycle
    (b) the cytotrophoblast of the placenta is most prominent during the third trimester of pregnancy
    (c) theca externa cells of ovarian follicles secrete most of the ovarian estrogen
    (d) ovulation occurs at the time when progesterone has reached its highest level in the blood plasma

30. Which one of the following "structure–secretory product" combinations is correct?
    (a) Syncytiotrophoblast–progesterone and estrogen
    (b) Acidophils of the pars distalis–follicle stimulating hormone (FSH)
    (c) Beta cells of the islets of Langerhans–glucagon
    (d) Zona glomerulosa of the suprarenal–cortisone

31. Which of the following is characteristic of the 27th day of the menstrual cycle?
    (a) Stasis of blood in the basal straight arteries of the endometrium
    (b) constriction of the coiled spiral arteries
    (c) increased proliferation of the endometrium
    (d) increased edema of the functional spongy layer of the endometrium

32. Which one of the following organs possesses all of these characteristics: both an exocrine and endocrine organ; under the influence of hypophyseal hormones; has cells completing the second meiotic division?
    (a) Ovary
    (b) Liver
    (c) Testis
    (d) Pancreas

33. Which one of the following organs possesses

all of these characteristics: serous acini, intercalated ducts, striated ducts, no mucous alveoli?
(a) Sebaceous gland
(b) Pancreas
(c) Sublingual gland
(d) Parotid gland

34. Which one of the following organs possesses
all of these characteristics: stratified squamous
non-keratinized epithelium, serous and mucous
glands, skeletal muscle, special visceral afferent
nerve fibers?
(a) Esophagus
(b) Tongue
(c) Vagina
(d) Anal canal

35. Three sites where substances readily pass between the vascular system and a surface lining
epithelium are in the lung alveoli, renal corpuscles, and chorionic villi. Which one of the following is found in all three structures?
(a) Lining cells which secrete lipoidal or steroidal substances
(b) Macrophages
(c) Fenestrated endothelial cells
(d) Angiotensin producing cells

36. In the ear:
(a) endolymph fills the scala tympani and scala
vestibuli
(b) the organ of Corti contains hair cells, each
of which possesses one true cilium
(c) bipolar neurons in the spiral cochlear ganglion have a peripheral process which end
on hair cells, and central process which are
components of the cochlear nerve
(d) the stapes is located in the round window
of the scala tympani

37. In the eye:
(a) visual pigments are located in discs of the
outer segments of cells of the pigmented
layer of the retina
(b) accommodation (focusing on a near object)
involves the relaxation of ciliary smooth
muscle, resulting in release of tension on
the ciliary zonule and rounding of the lens
(c) the blind spot produced by the optic disc
is medial to the visual axis
(d) the pupil gets larger in response to parasympathetic nerve stimulation

38. Which of the following primary afferent or efferent fibers of medullary cranial nerves is paired
with an *incorrect* nucleus of termination or origin?
(a) General somatic afferent (GSA) fibers of
IX–nucleus solitarius

(b) Special visceral efferent (SVE) fibers of XI–
nucleus ambiguus
(c) General visceral efferent (GVE) fibers of X–
dorsal motor nucleus
(d) Special visceral afferent (SVA) fibers of IX–
gustatory nucleus

39. After a peripheral lesion of the abducens nerve
in the orbit, one might expect to find all of the
following *except:*
(a) chromatolysis in the facial colliculus of the
pons
(b) chromatolysis in the ipsilateral mesencephalic nucleus of the fifth cranial nerve
(c) degenerating fibers in the contralateral medial longitudinal fasciculus (MLF)
(d) paralysis of the lateral rectus muscle

40. Which one of the following structures is *not*
supplied by direct branches of the artery with
which it is matched?
(a) Spinal tract of the trigeminal nerve–posterior inferior cerebellar artery
(b) Medial lemniscus–anterior spinal artery
(c) Corticospinal tract–posterior cerebral artery
(d) Visual (striate) cortex–anterior cerebral artery

41. Bilateral injury to the facial nerves at their emergence from the pons-medulla junction could result in:
(a) hyperacusis because of impaired stapedius
muscle activity
(b) loss of taste from the posterior one-third
of the tongue
(c) loss of all flow of saliva
(d) ptosis in both eyes

42. After a right upper motor neuron lesion of the
facial nerve there is a:
(a) loss of the sense of taste on the right anterior
portion of the tongue
(b) loss of the corneal reflex on the right side
(c) loss of ability to wrinkle the forehead on
the left side
(d) paralysis of lower facial muscles on the left
side

43. If there is a destructive lesion of the crista ampullaris in the left horizontal semicircular canal
all of the following are likely to be present *except:*
(a) a tendency to fall to the left
(b) past pointing to the left
(c) a sense of the room rotating to the right
(d) nystagmus with a fast component to the
right

44. A tumor in the cerebellopontine angle could
result in all of the following *except:*

(a) deafness in the ipsilateral ear

(b) lateral strabismus ipsilaterally

(c) corneal reflex

(d) absence of normal vestibular responses

45. All of the following result in constriction of the left pupil, *except:*

(a) focusing the eye on a near object after focusing on a far object

(b) shining light in the right eye of a normal person

(c) shining light on only the nasal half of the retina of the right eye of a person whose optic chiasm has been totally destroyed

(d) shining light in the right eye of a person whose left optic nerve was destroyed

46. Which of the following eye movements and reflexes would be *least* affected by bilateral destruction of the parastriate (18) and peristriate (19) areas of the cerebral cortex?

(a) Smooth eye pursuit of a moving object

(b) The near (synkinetic, accommodation-convergence) reflex

(c) The pupillary light reflex

(d) Saccadic movements occurring in the shift of gaze from one object to another

47. Destruction of which of the following would *most likely* result in a deficit of memory for recent events?

(a) Cingulate gyrus

(b) Parietal lobe

(c) Anterior-medial region of the temporal lobe

(d) Medial dorsal nucleus of the thalamus

48. The intervertebral foramen is bounded:

(a) superiorly and inferiorly by the lamina of the involved vertebrae

(b) posteriorly by the zygopophyseal joint

(c) posteriorly by the posterior longitudinal ligament

(d) anteriorly by the intervertebral disc and the anterior longitudinal ligament.

49. The shoulder joint is least reinforced by muscles of the rotator cuff:

(a) anteriorly

(b) inferiorly

(c) posteriorly

(d) superiorly

50. The major origin of the superficial group of anterior forearm muscles is the:

(a) lateral epicondyle of the humerus

(b) proximal ventral aspects of the radius and ulna

(c) olecranon process of the humerus

(d) medial epicondyle of the humerus

51. Which of the following intrinsic thumb muscles is *not* found in the thenar compartment?

(a) Adductor pollicis

(b) Flexor pollicis brevis

(c) Abductor pollicis brevis

(d) Opponens pollicis

52. The muscles in the adductor-interosseous compartment of the hand are innervated by the:

(a) median nerve

(b) median and ulnar nerves

(c) radial nerve

(d) ulnar nerve

53. The anterior cruciate ligament of the knee:

(a) is most taut when the knee is flexed

(b) attaches to the anterior intercondylar region of the tibia

(c) protects against posterior dislocation of the tibia on the femur

(d) protects against anterior dislocation of the femur on the tibia

54. Palpable just medial to the patellar ligament in the interval between the femur and tibia is the:

(a) anterior cruciate ligament

(b) fibular collateral ligament

(c) tendon of the popliteus muscle

(d) medial meniscus

55. Due to bony support, the most stable position of the ankle joint is:

(a) dorsiflexion

(b) inversion

(c) plantar flexion

(d) eversion

56. The major blood supply to the posterior femoral muscles is provided by:

(a) the obturator artery

(b) the perforating branches of the deep femoral artery

(c) the medial and lateral femoral circumflex vessels

(d) the superior gluteal artery

57. On the dorsum of the foot the dorsalis pedis pulse can be taken:

(a) medial to the tendon of the tibialis anterior muscle

(b) between the tendons of the tibialis anterior and extensor hallucis longus muscles

(c) between the tendons of the extensor hallucis longus and extensor digitorum longus muscles

(d) between the tendons of the extensor digitorum longus and peroneus tertius muscles

58. The posterior tibial pulse is taken:

(a) posterior to the medial malleolus

(b) anterior to the medial malleolus

(c) posterior to the lateral malleolus

(d) between the calcaneal tendon and the lateral malleolus

59. Which of the following functions of the muscles of mastication is incorrect?
    (a) Masseter: elevation of the mandible
    (b) Medial pterygoid: elevation of the mandible
    (c) Temporalis: protrusion of the mandible
    (d) Lateral pterygoid: deviation of the mandible to the same side

60. The majority of the muscle of the pharyngeal wall is innervated by cranial nerve:
    (a) IX
    (b) X
    (c) XI
    (d) XII

61. The parasympathetic fibers that innervate the sphincter pupillae muscle *do not* pass through the:
    (a) short ciliary nerves
    (b) cranial nerve III
    (c) long ciliary nerves
    (d) cavernous sinus

62. Laceration of the facial nerve immediately distal to the geniculate ganglion would *not* cause:
    (a) an inability to close the ipsilateral eye
    (b) loss of taste on the anterior two-thirds of the tongue
    (c) loss of lacrimation
    (d) loss of submandibular salivation

63. The common carotid artery bifurcates:
    (a) at the level of the cricoid cartilage
    (b) between the levels of the cricoid and thyroid cartilage
    (c) between the thyroid cartilage prominence and the hyoid bone
    (d) superior to the level of the hyoid bone

64. A lesion of the most superficial nerve in the posterior triangle of the neck would logically result in:
    (a) difficulty swallowing
    (b) difficulty breathing
    (c) difficulty turning the head to the same side
    (d) difficulty elevating (hunching) the shoulder

65. The pleural cavities:
    (a) contain the lungs
    (b) communicate across the midline
    (c) are composed of inner parietal and outer visceral layers
    (d) surround the lungs

66. A penetrating wound that enters the right fourth intercostal space in the midclavicular line would initially enter the:

(a) superior lobe of the right lung

(b) right lung below the oblique fissure

(c) inferior lobe of the right lung

(d) middle lobe of the right lung

67. *Not* participating in the formation of Hasselbach's triangle is the:
    (a) falx inguinalis (conjoined tendon)
    (b) lateral border of the rectus abdominis.
    (c) inguinal ligament
    (d) inferior epigastric vessels

68. The inguinal ligament extends between the:
    (a) pubic tubercle and the anterior superior iliac spine
    (b) anterior superior and inferior iliac spines
    (c) greater trochanter of the femur and the pubic tubercle
    (d) ischial spine and pubic tubercle

69. The neck of an indirect hernia is found:
    (a) medial to the pubic tubercle
    (b) medial to the inferior epigastric vessels
    (c) lateral to the deep inguinal ring
    (d) lateral to the inferior epigastric vessels

70. The renal pelvis is directed:
    (a) anteromedially
    (b) posteromedially
    (c) anterolaterally
    (d) posterolaterally

71. The pelvic diaphragm slopes inferiorly from:
    (a) anterior to posterior
    (b) medial to lateral
    (c) posterior to anterior
    (d) the pubic symphysis to the sacral promontory

72. The superficial perineal space (pouch) is continuous with the:
    (a) subcutaneous area of the thigh
    (b) peritoneal cavity
    (c) ischiorectal fossa
    (d) fascial plane in the abdominal wall between the external abdominal oblique fascia and the membraneous layer of superficial fascia

Possibly More Than One Answer

For each of the following questions answer:

(a) if only 1, 2, and 3 are correct

(b) if only 1 and 3 are correct

(c) if only 2 and 4 are correct

(d) if only 4 is correct

(e) if all are correct

1. The Golgi apparatus is involved in which of the following?
   1. Concentrating secretory products.

2. Packaging secretory products in condensing vacuoles
3. Producing thyroglobulin
4. Adding the carbohydrate component to the glycosaminoglycans of ground substance

2. Which of the following cells is/are characterized by smooth endoplasmic reticulum?
   1. Cells of the zona fasciculata of the suprarenal gland
   2. Cardiac muscle cells
   3. Granulosa lutein cells
   4. Pancreatic acinar cells

3. Which of the following cells is/are considered to be quite phagocytic?
   1. Cells of Kupffer
   2. Fibroblasts
   3. Macrophages
   4. Plasma cells

4. Which of the following statements is/are correct regarding epithelia?
   1. Stratified squamous epithelium lines surfaces that are subject to abrasion.
   2. Transitional epithelium is well adapted for absorptive functions.
   3. All cells of pseudostratified columnar epithelium reach the basement membrane, but not all of them reach the luminal surface.
   4. Epithelial cells usually receive nutritive substances from capillaries located in the intercellular spaces of the epithelium.

5. The basement membrane consists of:
   1. large collagen bundles
   2. reticular fibers
   3. the plasma membrane of basal epithelial cells
   4. a basal lamina

6. Which of the following are found within the intercellular spaces between epidermal cells?
   1. Tonofilaments
   2. Nerve fibers
   3. Meissner's tactile corpuscles
   4. Melanocytes

7. Osteons (Haversian systems) contain:
   1. collagenous fibers that, in adjacent lamellae, run perpendicular to each other
   2. interstitial lamellae
   3. osteoprogenitor cells that occupy the osteon (Haversian) canal
   4. canaliculi through which blood is transported to the osteocytes

8. Which of the following are characteristics of both hyaline cartilage and bone?
   1. Avascular tissue
   2. Cells occupy lacunae
   3. Grows by both appositional and interstitial growth
   4. The intercellular matrix contains numerous collagenous fibers and a mucoidal ground substance

9. Cardiac muscle differs from adult skeletal muscle in that cardiac muscle possesses:
   1. intercalated discs
   2. branching fibers
   3. centrally located nuclei
   4. T tubules which are located at the Z line

10. During excitation-contraction coupling in skeletal muscle:
    1. calcium is released from the cisterna of the sarcoplasmic reticulum
    2. the interaction of actin and myosin is regulated, at least in part, by troponin and tropomyosin
    3. a wave of membrane depolarization is carried into the depths of the muscle fiber by the T tubules
    4. the A band shortens as a result of the interaction between thick and thin filaments

11. Glial (neuroglial) cells are components of which of the following?
    1. Pars nervosa
    2. Pars distalis of the hypophysis
    3. Pineal gland
    4. Adrenal (suprarenal) medulla

12. A drug that interferes with mitosis would be likely to directly affect the division of:
    1. metamyelocytes
    2. myelocytes
    3. normoblasts
    4. polychromatophilic erythroblasts

13. Lymphatic nodules are found in the:
    1. spleen
    2. lymph nodes
    3. ileum
    4. thymus

14. Which of the following statements about the respiratory system are true?
    1. Great alveolar (giant septal, pneumonocyte II) cells produce surfactant.
    2. Bronchioles possess elastic cartilage which allows for expansion of bronchioles at inspiration.
    3. Respiratory bronchioles possess smooth muscle and alveoli.
    4. The true vocal cords (folds) and the rest of the larynx are lined by pseudostratified columnar epithelium.

15. Which of the following organs possess submucosal glands?

1. Duodenum
2. Fundus of the stomach
3. Esophagus
4. Colon

16. In which cell is/are there normally only 23 chromosomes (although there may be a normal diploid amount of DNA)?
    1. Parietal cell of the stomach
    2. Secondary spermatocyte
    3. Zygote
    4. An oocyte just after it is discharged from the ovary at ovulation

17. Which of the following statements about the liver is correct?
    1. Discontinuities in the sinusoidal epithelium permit passage of some substances between the lumen of the sinusoid and the perisinusoidal space of Disse.
    2. In the classical liver lobule bile flows toward the periphery, whereas a mixture of arterial and venous blood flows toward the center of the lobule.
    3. Hepatocytes constitute the walls of bile canaliculi.
    4. Hepatocytes possess both smooth and rough endoplasmic reticulum.

18. Following the administration of radioactive glucose, which of the following structures or substances would be labeled?
    1. The fuzz (glycocalyx) covering the free surface of the intestinal lining cell
    2. Colloid in the thyroid follicle
    3. Hyaline cartilage matrix
    4. Hepatocytes

19. Which one of the endocrine tissues listed below is correctly matched with a mechanism that is involved in the regulation of the production and/or release of the hormone produced by that tissue?
    1. Parathyroid–low levels of calcium in the blood
    2. Adrenal medulla–stimulation of preganglionic sympathetic neurons
    3. Pars distalis of hypophysis–releasing hormones which reach the pars distalis from hypothalamic neurons via the hypophyseal portal system
    4. Corpus luteum–placenta formation

20. Which of the following "cell–secretory product" combinations is/are correct?
    1. Plasma cell–circulating antibodies
    2. Mast cell–heparin
    3. Fibroblast–collagen precursor
    4. Enteroendocrine cell–serotonin

21. Which of the following "cell–secretory product" combinations is/are correct?
    1. Chief cell of the stomach–pepsinogen
    2. Acidophil of the pars distalis–growth hormone
    3. Zona glomerulosal cell of the adrenal gland–mineralocorticoids
    4. Parietal cell of the stomach–hydrochloric acid

22. A simple cuboidal or columnar epithelium with extensive basal infoldings of the plasma membrane is characteristically found in:
    1. distal convoluted tubules of the kidney
    2. the lining epithelium of the small intestine
    3. striated ducts of the parotid gland
    4. the lining epithelium of the oral cavity

23. Which of the following statements about the kidney is/are correct?
    1. The macula densa is a region of the distal tubule which is closely associated with an afferent glomerular arteriole.
    2. Collecting tubules are located in both the medulla and the cortex.
    3. Proximal convoluted tubules have an extensive microvillous (brush) border.
    4. Adjacent pedicels in the glomerulus are separated by a slit that is bridged by a very thin slit membrane.

24. Which of the following cells are correctly paired to its secretory product?
    1. Basophils of hypophysis–FSH (follicle stimulating hormone)
    2. oxyphil cells–parathyroid hormone
    3. Acidophils of hypophysis–prolactin (luteotropic hormone)
    4. Chromaffin cell of adrenal–aldosterone

25. Which of the following are target cells or target organs for the hormone indicated?
    1. Seminal vesicle–luteinizing hormone (LH)
    2. Prostate gland–testosterone
    3. Leydig cells–testosterone
    4. Sertoli cells–follicle stimulating hormone (FSH)

26. Which of the following statements is/are correct for the testis?
    1. Some spermatogonia proliferate and remain as stem cells, while others differentiate into primary spermatocytes.
    2. The smooth endoplasmic reticulum of Leydig cells is essential for testosterone production.
    3. Sertoli cells help control passage of macromolecules to haploid cells.
    4. Secondary spermatocytes are usually plentiful, since they are relatively slow to divide into spermatids.

27. The luteal (secretory) phase of the menstrual cycle is characterized by:
    1. a coiling or sacculation of endometrial glands
    2. relatively high amounts of progesterone in the plasma
    3. the presence of a functional corpus luteum
    4. atresia of some ovarian follicles

28. In the membranous labyrinth of the ear:
    1. maculae are receptors for position sense
    2. otoconia are components of the cristae
    3. efferent nerves end on some of the hair cells
    4. perilymph flow during head rotation produces forces on sensory hairs which cause them to fire nerve impulses

29. Which of the following statements is/are correct for the eye?
    1. The inner nuclear layer of the retina contains the nuclei of bipolar cells, horizontal cells and amacrine cells.
    2. Aqueous humour passes, in sequence, through the posterior chamber, anterior chamber, trabecular meshwork (spaces of Fontana), canal of Schlemm, and veins.
    3. Light striking the retina (excluding the fovea centralis and the optic papilla) encounters in order: ganglion cells, bipolar cells, and rods and cones.
    4. The pathway of visual impulses in the retina is from rods and cones to bipolar cells, and from the latter to ganglion cells.

30. Bilateral destruction of the posterior white column at spinal cord segment C5 might include a *loss* of:
    1. two point discrimination in both legs
    2. vibratory sense in both hands
    3. ability to identify objects placed in a patient's hands when the patient's hands are out of sight
    4. appreciation of passive limb movements in the hands and feet

31. One month after ipsilateral destruction of the C3 through T3 dorsal root ganglia there would be ipsilateral:
    1. anesthesia of the upper extremity
    2. slight increase in deep tendon reflexes of the upper extremity
    3. some nerve fiber degeneration in the medulla
    4. a complete dermatomal loss of sensation in only segments C6 to T1

32. Two months after complete destruction of the lateral funiculus in spinal cord segments C5 and C6 there would probably be:
    1. ipsilateral hemiplegia
    2. ipsilateral hypertonus at lower levels

3. absence of ipsilateral superficial (cutaneous) abdominal reflexes
    4. ipsilateral exaggerated deep tendon reflexes

33. Two months after complete ipsilateral destruction of the ventral roots of the C5 through T1 spinal nerves, one would expect to find:
    1. exaggerated myotatic (stretch) reflexes in the ipsilateral upper limb
    2. flaccid paralysis of muscles in the ipsilateral upper limb
    3. loss of superficial (cutaneous) abdominal reflexes
    4. muscle atrophy in the ipsilateral upper limb

34. When an axon is damaged there is dispersal of nissl material in the cell body (perikaryon) of the damaged neuron which is called chromatolysis. If the facial nerve was sectioned at its emergence from the brain stem, in which of the following would chromatolysis be present?
    1. nucleus solitarius
    2. geniculate ganglion
    3. pterygopalatine ganglion
    4. superior salivatory nucleus

35. A high medulla lesion involving the spinal tract (root) and nucleus of the trigeminal nerve on one side would:
    1. produce some loss of sensation from the ipsilateral external auditory canal
    2. cause contralateral and ipsilateral loss of crude touch on the face
    3. produce some ipsilateral loss of pain on the anterior two-thirds of the tongue
    4. cause a diminished jaw jerk reflex

36. A tumor obliterating the right striate cortex above the calcarine fissure would result in:
    1. damage to cells which receive impulses from both retinae via the lateral geniculate nucleus
    2. left lower quadrantic anopsia
    3. a homonymous type of visual defect
    4. chromatolysis of ganglion cells in the temporal half of the retina of the right eye

37. Which of the following structures are components of the hearing pathway:
    1. superior olivary nucleus
    2. inferior colliculus
    3. medial geniculate body (nucleus)
    4. lateral lemniscus

38. Destruction of the entire right tegmentum at the level of the facial colliculus would result in:
    1. contralateral loss of pain and temperature in the trunk, extremities, and part of the face
    2. complete contralateral loss of two-point touch in the trunk, extremities, and face
    3. paralysis of conjugate lateral gaze to the right

4. positive Babinski reflex on the left

39. A lesion of the mesencephalic tegmentum which destroys the left oculomotor nerve, left medial lemniscus and left red nucleus and adjacent cerebellar efferents, could result in:
   1. intention tremor in the right upper extremity
   2. ptosis in the left eye
   3. loss of touch on the right side of the body
   4. loss of the consensual response in the pupillary light reflex when light is shone in the left eye

40. Which of the following "destroyed structure–signs and symptoms" combinations is/are correct?
   1. Destruction of the subthalamic nucleus–hemiballism
   2. Destruction of the left inferior parietal gyrus (area 39, angular gyrus)–apraxia
   3. Destruction of the postcentral gyrus–agnosia
   4. Destruction of the supraoptic nucleus–diabetes insipidus

41. Which of the following lesions would produce the signs and symptoms indicated?
   1. A hemisection of the cord produces a contralateral loss of pain and temperature and an ipsilateral loss of two-point touch below the level of the lesion.
   2. Lesion of the vagus nerve near its emergence from the brain stem produces chromatolysis in the dorsal motor neuclus of the vagus and the nucleus ambiguus.
   3. Lesion of the hypoglossal nerve results in deviation of the tongue to the side of the lesion upon protrusion.
   4. Lesion of the inferior cerebellar peduncle causes chromatolysis in the ipsilateral nucleus dorsalis (Clarke's nucleus).

42. The location of the spinal nerve in the intervertebral foramen:
   1. is at the level of the intervertebral disc in the cervical region
   2. is above the level of the intervertebral disc in the lumbar region
   3. is at the level of Luschka's joints in the lower cervical region
   4. is at the level of the intervertebral disc in the lumbar region

43. With respect to the support provided by the ligaments of the vertebral column:
   1. The anterior logitudinal ligament resists flexion of the vertebral column.
   2. The posterior longitudinal ligament resists flexion of the vertebral canal.
   3. The interspinous ligaments resist extension of the vertebral column

4. The ligamenta flava resist flexion of the vertebral column.

44. With respect to the location of the ligaments of the vertebral column:
   1. The ligamenta flava interconnect the lamina of adjacent lamina
   2. The anterior longitudinal ligament lines the anterior aspect of the vertebral column.
   3. The posterior longitudinal ligament attaches to the posterior aspects of the vertebral bodies.
   4. The anterior longitudinal ligament attaches to the pedicles of adjacent vertebrae.

45. The radial nerve:
   1. passes posteriorly around the surgical neck of the humerus
   2. passes ventral to the lateral aspect of the elbow joint
   3. passes medial to the biceps tendon in the cubital fossa
   4. passes around the neck of the radius

46. Which of the following is/are palpable in the anatomic snuff box?
   1. Scaphoid
   2. Median nerve
   3. Radial artery
   4. Pisiform

47. The integrity of which of the following nerves can be checked by testing the motions of the thumb?
   1. Median
   2. Ulnar
   3. Radial
   4. Musculocutaneous

48. The superficial palmar arterial arch:
   1. is deep to the long flexor tendons
   2. is superficial to the palmar aponeurosis
   3. is proximal to the deep part of the flexor retinaculum
   4. is at the same level (depth) as the common digital branches of the median nerve

49. MP flexion and IP extension of the index, middle, ring and little fingers are produced by the:
   1. ventral interossei
   2. lumbricals
   3. dorsal interossei
   4. flexor digitorum profundus

50. The ulnar nerve:
   1. passes posterior to the medial epicondyle of the humerus
   2. passes lateral to the pisiform
   3. is deep to the flexor carpi ulnaris muscle in the forearm
   4. passes superficial to the deep part of the flexor retinaculum

51. The median nerve:
    1. is formed from both the medial and lateral cords of the brachial plexus
    2. passes through the carpal tunnel
    3. is medial to the brachial artery in the cubital fossa
    4. is lateral to the tendon of the flexor carpi radialis muscle at the wrist
52. The musculocutaneous nerve:
    1. passes deep to the brachialis muscle
    2. passes through the coracobrachialis muscle
    3. is the continuation of the medial cord of the brachial plexus
    4. passes between the biceps and brachialis muscles
53. The capsule of the hip joint:
    1. encloses the entire femoral neck
    2. is reinforced by the iliofemoral, ischiofemoral and pubofemoral ligaments
    3. encloses the proximal two-thirds of the femoral neck anteriorly
    4. encloses the proximal two-thirds of the femoral neck posteriorly
54. The transverse tarsal (midtarsal) joint is formed between the:
    1. talus and navicular
    2. talus and calcaneus
    3. cuboid and calcaneus
    4. navicular and cuboid
55. The lateral collateral ligament of the ankle extends between the lateral malleolus and the:
    1. calcaneus
    2. navicular
    3. talus
    4. cuboid
56. The femoral nerve:
    1. passes deep to the inguinal ligament
    2. contains fibers from spinal cord segments L2, 3 and 4.
    3. innervates muscles which extend the knee
    4. is medial to the femoral artery in the femoral triangle
57. The common peroneal nerve:
    1. is the deepest structure in the popliteal fossa
    2. passes around the neck of the fibula
    3. innervates the major plantar flexors of the foot
    4. is the most lateral nerve in the popliteal fossa
58. The tibial nerve:
    1. innervates all of the intrinsic muscles of the plantar foot
    2. enters the foot by passing behind the medial malleolus
    3. passes through the median area of the popliteal fossa

    4. innervates the muscles in the posterior compartment of the leg
59. The anterior cranial fossa is related to the:
    1. orbit
    2. nasal cavity
    3. frontal sinus
    4. ethmoid air cells
60. The lateral portion of the middle cranial fossa is related to the:
    1. infratemporal fossa
    2. middle ear cavity
    3. cavernous sinus
    4. orbit
61. The phrenic nerve:
    1. contains fibers from spinal cord segments C3, 4 and 5
    2. passes posterior to the root of the lung
    3. provides the motor innervation to the skeletal muscle fibers of the respiratory diaphragm
    4. contributes fibers to the cardiac plexus
62. The pterygopalatine fossa communicates with the:
    1. middle cranial fossa via the foramen rotundum
    2. nasal cavity via the sphenopalatine foramen
    3. oral cavity via the palatine canal
    4. orbit via the inferior orbital fissure
63. Regarding the openings of the paranasal sinuses:
    1. The anterior ethmoid air cells drain into the superior meatus of the nasal cavity.
    2. The maxillary sinus drains into the middle meatus of the nasal cavity.
    3. The frontal sinus drains into the inferior meatus of the nasal cavity.
    4. The sphenoid sinus drains into the sphenoethmoidal recess of the nasal cavity.
64. With respect to the areas or parts of the larynx:
    1. The glottis includes the true vocal folds plus the rima glottidis.
    2. The ventricle is a laterally extending pouch between the true and false folds.
    3. The vestibule and supraglottic portion are the same.
    4. The additis is the laryngeal entrance (from the pharynx).
65. Which of the following muscle–function pairs is/are correct?
    1. Cricothyroid–relaxation of vocal cords
    2. Posterior cricoarytenoid–abduction of vocal cords
    3. Lateral cricoarytenoid–abduction of vocal cords
    4. Transverse arytenoid–adduction of vocal cords
66. Relative to the heart:

1. Its diaphragmatic surface is formed primarily by the right and left ventricles.
2. Its posterior surface is formed predominantly by the right atrium.
3. Its sternocostal surface is formed by portions of all four chambers of the heart.
4. Its right border is formed by the right ventricle.

67. With respect to the relationships of the duodenum:
    1. Its first part is related posteriorly to the portal vein and common bile duct.
    2. Its second part is related medially to the head of the pancreas.
    3. Its third part is crossed anteriorly by the superior mesenteric vessels.
    4. Its third part is related posteriorly to the transverse colon.
68. The stomach is related:
    1. posteriorly to the caudate lobe of the liver
    2. anteriorly to the respiratory diaphragm
    3. anteriorly to the splenic artery
    4. posteriorly to the pancreas
69. The vermiform appendix:
    1. usually arises from the large intestine just superior to the entrance of the ileum
    2. arises from the cecum at the termination of the taeniae coli
    3. typically hangs into the (true) pelvic cavity
    4. is usually retrocecal in position
70. The spleen:
    1. lies under ribs 9, 10 and 11 posteriorly
    2. is related to the left kidney posteriorly
    3. is related anteriorly to the stomach
    4. is related to the right colic flexure
71. Pelvic splanchnic nerves:
    1. contain preganglionic parasympathethic nerve fibers
    2. contain fibers that innervate the gastrointestinal tract from the splenic flexure distally
    3. contain fibers that arise from sacral spinal cord segments 2, 3 and 4.
    4. contain the same type of efferent fibers as the lumbar splanchnic nerves
72. The portal vein is formed:
    1. between the pancreas and the stomach
    2. by the union of the splenic and superior mesenteric veins
    3. by the junction of the superior and inferior mesenteric veins
    4. posterior to the pancreas
73. The pudendal nerve:
    1. arises from spinal cord segments S2, 3 and 4
    2. passes through the pudendal canal
    3. passes through the lesser sciatic foramen

4. passes through the greater sciatic foramen
74. The urogenital diaphragm:
    1. is found both anterior and posterior to the ischial tuberosities
    2. is oriented in the sagittal plane
    3. is perforated by the urethra and anal canal
    4. extends between the ischiopubic rami

ANSWERS TO MULTIPLE CHOICE QUESTIONS

Multiple Choice: One-answer Type

1. b	19. c	37. c	55. a
2. d	20. b	38. a	56. b
3. c	21. c	39. c	57. c
4. d	22. c	40. d	58. a
5. b	23. a	41. a	59. d
6. d	24. a	42. d	60. b
7. d	25. d	43. c	61. c
8. d	26. c	44. b	62. c
9. b	27. c	45. c	63. c
10. c	28. b	46. c	64. d
11. a	29. a	47. c	65. d
12. c	30. a	48. b	66. d
13. b	31. b	49. b	67. a
14. c	32. c	50. d	68. a
15. d	33. d	51. a	69. d
16. a	34. b	52. d	70. a
17. a	35. b	53. b	71. c
18. a	36. c	54. d	72. d

Multiple Choice: Possibly More Than One Answer

1. e	20. e	39. a	57. c
2. a	21. e	40. e	58. e
3. b	22. b	41. e	59. e
4. b	23. e	42. a	60. e
5. c	24. b	43. c	61. b
6. c	25. c	44. a	62. c
7. b	26. a	45. c	63. c
8. c	27. e	46. b	64. e
9. e	28. b	47. a	65. c
10. a	29. e	48. d	66. b
11. b	30. e	49. a	67. a
12. c	31. b	50. e	68. c
13. a	32. e	51. a	69. c
14. b	33. c	52. c	70. a
15. b	34. c	53. c	71. a
16. c	35. b	54. b	72. c
17. e	36. a	55. b	73. e
18. e	37. e	56. a	74. d
19. e	38. b		

3

Physiology

ARTHUR C. GUYTON, M.D.

Chairman and Professor, Department of Physiology and Biophysics,
University of Mississippi School of Medicine

Physiology is the study of function in living matter, and *human physiology* is specifically the study of function in the human being. This discipline attempts to answer such questions as: How do we live? How do we reproduce? How do we move about? How do we think? How do we see? And what are the basic physical and chemical principles upon which the intricate functions of the body are based?

BASIC ORGANIZATION OF THE BODY AND "HOMEOSTASIS"

The basic living unit of the body is the *cell,* of which there are about 100 trillion in the body. The cells are continually bathed in *extracellular fluid,* which is sometimes called the *internal environment* of the body. The constituents of this fluid are very exactly controlled, and, as long as they remain within normal range, each cell is capable of living as an individual unit and performing its respective tasks for the body. A very large portion of our discussion of human physiology will deal with this exact regulation of the constituents in the extracellular fluid; this is called *homeostasis,* which means simply *maintenance of constant conditions in the internal environment.*

Functional Systems of the Body

The body can be divided into several major functional systems, each one of which performs a particular task in maintaining homeostasis as follows:

The *cardiovascular system* keeps the fluids of the internal environment continually mixed. It does this by pumping blood through the vascular system. As the blood passes through the capillaries, a large portion of its fluid diffuses back and forth into the *interstitial fluid* that lies between the cells.

The *respiratory system* provides oxygen for the body and removes carbon dioxide.

The *gastrointestinal system* provides the foods needed for cellular energy and for synthesis of new cellular and extracellular structures.

The *kidneys* provide a means for eliminating waste products left over after the chemical reactions in the cells have taken place. Most important among these are large quantities of urea, uric acid, creatinine and nitrates. In addition to ridding the body of the unwanted end products of metabolism, the kidneys also regulate the concentrations of most of the extracellular fluid constituents including the concentrations of sodium, potassium, calcium, magnesium, chloride, bicarbonate and phosphate ions. They also help to control the blood volume and volume of the extracellular fluid.

The *nervous system* directs the activity of the muscular system, thereby providing locomotion. It also controls the functions of many internal organs through the *autonomic nervous system,* and it allows us to be intelligent beings so that we can attain the most advantageous conditions for our survival.

The *endocrine glands* provide another regulatory system. Hormones secreted by these glands control many of the metabolic functions of the cells, such as growth, rate of metabolism, special cellular activities associated with reproduction, absorption of bone, rate of glucose metabolism and rate of amino acid metabolism.

The *reproductive system* provides for formation of new beings like ourselves; even this can be considered a homeostatic function, for it generates new bodies in which still trillions of more cells can exist in a well-regulated internal environment.

FUNCTION OF THE CELL

Cell Structure.   The cell is composed of two major parts: the *nucleus* and the *cytoplasm.* Surrounding the nucleus is a *nuclear membrane,* which is highly permeable, and surrounding the cytoplasm is a *cellular membrane* that is also permeable but only to certain substances. Both the nucleus and the cytoplasm are filled with a highly viscous fluid containing very large quantities of dissolved *proteins, glucose, electrolytes* and many other substances. In addition there are many intracellular organelles, some of which we will discuss in the following paragraphs.

The most important structures of the nucleus are the 23 pairs of *chromosomes,* each of which is composed of many thousand nucleoprotein molecules that are the *genes* that regulate cellular function and reproduction.

The most conspicuous structures in the cytoplasm are the *mitochondria* and the *endoplasmic reticulum.* The mitochondria are usually elongated bodies sometimes larger than 1 micron in length and containing large quantities of oxidative and other enzymes that are responsible for supplying energy to the cells, as will be discussed below. The endoplasmic reticulum is a system of tubes that connects with the nuclear membrane and spreads throughout the entire cytoplasm. Attached to the outer surface of the reticulum are often many minute particles, the *ribosomes,* which are composed principally of *ribose nucleic acid* (RNA) and are intimately concerned with the synthesis of proteins in the cytoplasm.

Energy Release in the Cell—Function of the Mitochondria.   An adequate supply of energy must always be available to energize the chemical reactions of the cells. This is provided principally by the chemical reaction of oxygen with any one of three different types of foods: glucose derived from carbohydrates, fatty acids derived from fats, and amino acids derived from proteins. On entering the cell the food molecules are split into still smaller molecules that in turn enter the mitochondria where still other enzymes remove carbon dioxide and hydrogen atoms in a process called the *citric acid cycle.* Then an oxidative enzyme system causes progressive oxidation of the food. The end products of the oxidative reactions in the mitochondria are water and carbon dioxide, and the energy liberated is used by the mitochondria to synthesize still another substance, *adenosine triphosphate,* a very highly reactive chemical that can diffuse throughout the cell and provide almost instantaneous energy for any cellular process that requires it.

Lysosomes.   Another organelle found in great numbers in all cells of the body is the lysosome. This is a small spherical vesicle surrounded by a membrane and containing digestive enzymes. The enzymes are used by the cell for various digestive purposes. For instance, when bacteria or other substances are phagocytized by cells, digestive enzymes from the lysosomes digest the phagocytized particles. Also, when cells become damaged, enzymes from lysosomes can digest the damaged portions of the cells and remove these. Finally, when tissues are no longer used for their normal functions, they frequently undergo *atrophy.* Lysosomes in the cells cause this atrophy by digesting portions of the cellular mass.

Regulation of Protein Synthesis in the Cell by the Genes.   Proteins are the basis of almost all the functions that occur in the cells for two reasons: (1) all of the enzymes that catalyze the chemical reactions of the cells are proteins, and (2) most of the important physical structures of the cell contain *structural proteins.*

The genes control protein synthesis in the cell and in this way control cell function. Each gene is a double stranded helical molecule of *deoxyribose nucleic acid,* called DNA, and it is composed of multiple units of (a) the sugar deoxyribose, (b) phosphoric acid, and (c) four bases of different types (two purines, *adenine* and *guanine,* and two pyrimidines, *thymine* and *cytosine*). It is the bases in this molecule that control the type of protein synthesized. These bases are held together in the long helical molecule by the deoxyribose and the phosphoric acid. The sequence of bases is different for each type of gene, and it is this sequence that determines the properties of each individual gene.

The Genetic Code.   Each unit of three successive bases in the strand of the deoxyribose nucleic acid

(DNA) molecule is called a *code word,* and these code words control the amino acids in a protein to be formed in the cytoplasm. One code word might be composed of adenine, thymine, and guanine, while the next code word might have a sequence of cytosine, guanine and thymine. These two code words have entirely different meanings because their sequences of bases are different. The sequences of bases in the successive code words on the DNA molecule are known as the genetic code.

Ribose Nucleic Acid (RNA) and Its Role in the Formation of Protein in the Cytoplasm. The deoxyribose nucleic acid molecule that makes up the gene controls formation of a similar molecule called a *ribose nucleic acid* molecule (RNA). This molecule is composed of the sugar ribose, phosphoric acid and four different bases (the same bases as those found in DNA except that thymine is replaced by uracil). Thus, this molecule is very similar to that of the gene, and it too carries the genetic code. When the DNA molecule of the gene causes formation of the RNA molecule, it transfers its code to the RNA molecule by controlling the sequence of bases in the RNA molecule. This control of RNA formation by DNA is called *transcription* because the genetic code is "transcribed" onto the RNA by the DNA.

Three different types of RNA molecules are formed: (1) ribosomal RNA, (2) transfer RNA, and (3) messenger RNA. All three diffuse from the cell nucleus through the nuclear membrane into the cytoplasm, where each plays a specific role in the manufacture of protein.

Ribosomal RNA becomes a major constituent of the small particles called *ribosomes.* Almost all of the ribosomes in turn become attached to the outside surface of the endoplasmic reticulum. Protein molecules are manufactured inside or on the surface of these ribosomes.

There are 20 separate types of *transfer RNA molecules,* each one of which combines specifically with one of the respective amino acids and conducts this amino acid to the ribosome, where it is combined into a protein molecule.

Messenger RNA carries the genetic code that determines the sequence in which successive amino acids will be arranged in the protein molecule. Messenger RNA is a single-stranded, long molecule, having a succession of genetic code *codons* along its axis. These codons are mirror images of the code words in the gene DNA, and they also consist of three successive bases. One end of the RNA strand enters the ribosome, and the entire strand then threads its way through the ribosome in a little over a minute. As it passes through, the ribosome "reads" the genetic code and causes the proper succession of amino acids to bind

together by chemical bonds called *peptide linkages,* which will be discussed later in the chapter. Actually, the messenger RNA does not recognize the different types of amino acids but instead recognizes the different transfer RNA molecules. However, each transfer RNA molecule carries only one specific type of amino acid; one can well understand that it is that type of amino acid that will be incorporated into the protein.

To recapitulate, as the strand of messenger RNA passes through the ribosome, each one of its codons draws to it a specific transfer RNA that in turn delivers a specific amino acid. This amino acid then combines with the preceding amino acid, the sequence continuing to build until an entire protein molecule is formed. At this point a special codon appears that states the process is complete, and the protein is released into the cytoplasm. This control of amino acid sequencing by the RNA code during protein formation is called *translation.*

It is believed that there are about 100,000 different types of genes in the nucleus; thus one can well understand that a multitude of different types of proteins can also be formed in each cell. The character of each cell depends on the relative proportions of the types of proteins that are formed. In essence, then, the genes control the structure of the cell through the types of structural proteins formed, and the genes also control the functions of the cell mainly through the types of protein enzymes that are formed.

Differentiation of Cells. During the course of development of the human being from the fertilized ovum, the ovum divides again and again until trillions of cells are formed. However, the new cells gradually *differentiate* from each other, certain cells attaining one set of genetic characteristics while other cells attain other characteristics. This process of differentiation occurs as a result of inactivation of certain of the genes and activation of others during successive stages of cellular division. This results in widely different functions in different cells.

Cellular Reproduction. Most cells of the body, with the exception of mature red blood cells and neurons in the nervous system, are capable of reproducing other cells of their own type. Ordinarily, if sufficient nutrients are available, each cell grows larger and larger until at a certain point it automatically divides by the process of *mitosis* to form two new cells. Before mitosis occurs, all the genes in the nucleus, as well as the chromosomes carrying the genes, are themselves reproduced to create a completely new set of genes. During mitosis one set of genes enters one of the daughter cells while the other set enters the second daughter cell. Thus, not only are the physical characteristics of the two new cells alike, but they are still controlled by the same types of genes so that their functions will also be very similar. If, during the process of reproduction, one or more of the genes fails to be reproduced or becomes suppressed, then the two new cells will not be exactly alike, and the cells will become slightly *differentiated* from each other.

THE BODY FLUIDS

Total Body Water: Extracellular and Intracellular Fluid. Approximately 57 per cent of the adult body is water. In the normal adult, this amounts to a *total body water* of approximately 40 liters. This can be divided into two major compartments: the *extracellular fluid,* which has a volume of about 15 liters, and the *intracellular fluid,* which has a volume of about 25 liters. The extracellular fluid is continually mixing and is called the *internal environment* of the body. Because of this mixing, its constituents are relatively uniform in all parts of the body. Frequently, it is desirable to divide the extracellular fluid into two subcompartments: the *plasma,* which is part of the blood and amounts to approximately 3 liters, and the *interstitial fluid,* which lies between the tissue cells and amounts to approximately 12 liters.

Though the intracellular fluids are not identical in all the different cells, they are sufficiently similar so that it is usually reasonable to consider them together as one large compartment of homogeneous fluid.

Comparison of Extracellular and Intracellular Fluid. Both extracellular and intracellular fluid contain nutrients that are needed for function of the cells. These include *glucose, fatty substances, amino acids* and *oxygen.* Some of the food substances are present in higher concentrations in the intracellular fluid than in the extracellular fluid because of specific concentrating abilities of the cell membranes.

A major difference between the extracellular and the intracellular fluids is in the electrolytes. Extracellular fluid contains large quantities of *sodium* and *chloride ions* but only small quantities of potassium, magnesium and phosphate ions. On the other hand, intracellular fluid contains very large quantities of these latter ions, *potassium, magnesium* and *phosphate,* but very few sodium and chloride ions. Also extracellular fluid contains small quantities of calcium ions, but intracellular fluid contains almost none. These differences in the fluids cause a *membrane potential* to develop between the two sides of the membrane—negative on the inside and positive outside. Later in the chapter we shall see how this potential develops and the manner in which it changes during the transmission of nerve and muscle impulses.

The Fluid of the Blood. The fluid of the blood is actually a composite of about 2 liters intracellular fluid inside the blood cells and 3 liters extracellular fluid in the plasma.

The plasma is almost identical with the interstitial fluid except that it contains dissolved proteins in a concentration of about seven per cent in comparison with an average protein concentration in the interstitial fluid of two to three per cent.

Exchange of Fluid and Electrolytes Through the Cell Membrane

Structure of the Cell Membrane. The cell membrane is composed basically of a *lipid matrix* but it also contains many large protein molecules that protrude all the way through the membrane. The protein molecules cause discontinuities in the lipid matrix, thus creating many *minute pores* in the membrane.

Diffusion Through the Cell Membrane. Many substances pass through the cell membrane, back and forth between the extracellular and the intracellular fluids, by the process of *diffusion.* Diffusion means simply *random motion of molecules.* That is, all molecules in liquids and gases are continually moving among each other, bouncing first one way and then another. The substances that diffuse readily through the cell membrane include water soluble unionized molecules and some *negative* ions with molecular or ionic weights less than 100 and almost all lipid-soluble substances regardless of molecular weight. The water soluble molecules and ions, including *water itself, chloride ions, lactate ions* and *urea,* diffuse through the pores, while the lipid soluble substances, including *fats, carbon dioxide* and *oxygen,* first become dissolved in the lipid matrix of the membrane and then diffuse through this. Positive ions diffuse through the pores only very poorly, potassium diffusing more readily than the others.

The net amount of each substance that will diffuse through the cell membrane depends on the relative concentrations of the substances on the two sides of the membrane. If the concentration difference is very great, the net movement of the substance will also be very great from the area of high concentration toward the area of low concentration.

Facilitated Diffusion. Some substances needed by the cell have molecular or ionic sizes too large for them to go through the membrane pores, and they are also insoluble in the lipid matrix of the cell membrane. Many of these substances are transported by a process called *facilitated diffusion,* in which the substance combines chemically with a *carrier* in the cell membrane and is transported in combination with this carrier. The combined substance and carrier are soluble in the membrane. On the other side of the membrane the substance is released from the carrier.

The most important substance transmitted through cell membranes by the process of facilitated diffusion is *glucose*. *Insulin* greatly increases this facilitated transport of glucose.

Active Transport Through the Cell Membrane. *Active transport* is similar to facilitated diffusion in that the substance to be transported combines with a *carrier* that makes it soluble in the matrix of the membrane. The substance is released from the carrier on the opposite side of the membrane, as is also true of facilitated diffusion. However, active transport causes movement of the substance *in only one direction*. Also, it can transport the substance even when the concentration of the substance is greater on the side to which it is being transported than on the other side.

The most important active transport system in the body is that for active transport of sodium out of cells and potassium into cells, which is called the *sodium–potassium pump*. This pump causes the concentration of sodium inside the cells to become very low and its concentration in the extracellular fluids very high, while causing the intracellular potassium concentration to build up to a very high level. It is this sodium–potassium pump that maintains most of the ionic concentration differences between the intracellular and the extracellular fluids and therefore is extremely important for function of nerve and muscle fibers, as will be described later in the chapter.

Other active transport systems include amino acid transport to the interior of cells and transport of large numbers of ions such as sodium, potassium, hydrogen, calcium, magnesium and phosphate through the renal tubular and gastrointestinal epithelial membranes.

Osmotic Pressure and Osmotic Equilibria at the Cell Membrane

Osmosis. Water molecules pass through the cell membrane at least 100 times as easily as most dissolved substances in either the extracellular or the intracellular fluids. Because of this, any time an excess concentration of dissolved substances occurs on either side of the membrane, water is forced by *osmosis* through the membrane; this can be explained as follows:

The presence of dissolved substances in a water solution reduces the concentration of water molecules in the fluid. Therefore, if such a solution is placed on one side of the cell membrane while pure water is placed on the other side, more water molecules will diffuse from the pure water, which has a high water concentration, through the pores of the membrane than from the solution which has a lower water concentra-

tion. As a result, an excess of water molecules will pass continuously from the pure water into the solution; this is osmosis.

Osmotic Pressure. If pressure is applied across a membrane through which osmosis is occurring, but with the pressure applied in the direction opposite to the osmotic flow, the osmosis can be slowed or even stopped. The amount of pressure that is required to stop the osmosis is called the *osmotic pressure*.

The normal concentration of osmotically active substances in the body fluids is so great that if these fluids should be placed on one side of a cell membrane and pure water on the other side, the amount of *osmotic pressure* across the membrane would be approximately 5,400 mm. Hg, which is more than 50 times as great as the mean arterial pressure of the human being. Obviously, pure water never exists in the normal person on either side of the cell membrane, but occasionally the concentrations of the extracellular and the intracellular fluids do differ slightly. When this occurs, small amounts of osmotic pressure develop immediately across the membrane and cause water to move through the membrane, *diluting the concentrated fluid and concentrating the dilute fluid* until their concentrations become equal. Therefore, *except for a few seconds at a time the extracellular and the intracellular fluids remain continuously in osmotic equilibrium with each other.*

Isotonicity, Hypotonicity and Hypertonicity. A solution is said to be *isotonic* if no osmotic force develops across the cell membrane when a normal cell is placed in the solution.

A solution is said to be *hypotonic* if the concentration of osmotic substances in the solution is less than their concentration in the cell. An osmotic force develops immediately when the cell is exposed to the solution, causing water to flow by osmosis into the cell; within less than a minute the cell swells until it either bursts or its fluids become diluted sufficiently to equal the concentration of the hypotonic solution.

A solution is said to be *hypertonic* when it contains a higher concentration of osmotic substances than does the cell. In this case osmotic forces develop that cause water to flow out of the cell into the solution, thereby greatly concentrating the intracellular fluid and markedly shrinking the cell.

Fluid Therapy. When fluid is administered to a patient, it is generally injected into the bloodstream or is absorbed into the blood from the gastrointestinal tract, and it immediately becomes part of the extracellular fluid. If the fluid is isotonic, it will generally remain in the extracellular fluid. If it is hypotonic, large portions of the water in the fluid will pass by osmosis into the cells. If it is hypertonic, it will draw large portions of the intracellular water out of the cells, thereby shrinking the cells.

Dehydration means loss of water from the body. If pure water is lost, such as by evaporation from the respiratory tract or from the surfaces of the skin, this will concentrate both the extracellular and the intracellular fluids. However, if pure extracellular fluid, or fluid very similar to extracellular fluid, is lost from the body, as occasionally occurs in different types of kidney disease or when a person sweats profusely, the fluid loss at first will be mainly from the extracellular compartment without affecting the intracellular fluid.

Exchange of Fluids Through the Capillary Membranes

Diffusion Between the Plasma and the Interstitial Fluid. The capillaries are porous structures with several million pores (the diameters of which are about 10 times as large as cell membrane pores) to each square centimeter of capillary surface. As the blood flows through the capillaries, very large quantities of dissolved substances diffuse in both directions through these pores. In this way sodium, chloride, potassium, glucose and almost all other dissolved substances in the plasma continually mix with the interstitial fluid. The rate of diffusion is so great that even cells as far as 50 microns away from the capillaries can still receive adequate quantities of nutrients.

Capillary Pressure. The blood inside the capillaries is under a considerable amount of pressure, averaging about 17 mm. Hg. This tends to cause fluid to leak out the pores of the capillaries into the interstitial fluid. Fortunately, however, the *colloid osmotic pressure* of the plasma proteins, which will be discussed below, prevents this loss of fluid and thereby helps to maintain the blood volume at a normal value essentially all of the time.

Colloid Osmotic Pressure of the Proteins. In the above discussion of osmosis and osmotic pressure, it was pointed out that essentially all dissolved substances in the extracellular and the intracellular fluids cause osmotic effects at the cellular pores. However, capillary pores are far larger than cellular pores, so that only dissolved proteins are large enough that they fail to pass to any significant extent through these pores. Since osmotic pressure is proportional to the number of dissolved molecules that *fail to pass* through the membrane, and since the total number of dissolved protein molecules is relatively small, the osmotic pressure of the plasma that develops at the capillary membrane is only 28 mm. Hg, some 200 times less than the osmotic pressure that can occur at the cellular membrane. Therefore, to distinguish the osmotic pressure at the capillary membrane from that at the cellular membrane, the capillary osmotic pressure is called *oncotic pressure* or *colloid osmotic pressure,* because protein solutions appear to be colloidal suspensions. The osmotic pressure at the cell membranes is frequently called *total osmotic pressure.*

Starling's Equilibrium of the Capillaries. The capillary pressure tends to push fluid out of the capillaries, while the colloid osmotic pressure tends to move fluid in. Furthermore, the pressure in the tissue spaces outside the capillaries, the *interstitial fluid pressure,* can push fluid inward if it is positive, and the protein in the interstitial fluids can cause *tissue colloid osmotic pressure* on the outside of the capillaries, which tends to move fluid out of the capillaries. To determine whether or not fluid will actually move inward through the membrane or outward, one adds the inward forces and the outward forces and determines which are the greater. Often these two will be exactly equal, so that there is no net loss or gain in either blood or interstitial fluid volume. This balance between the inward and the outward forces is called Starling's *equilibrium of the capillaries,* and it can be stated mathematically as follows:

Capillary pressure + tissue colloid osmotic pressure = interstitial fluid pressure + plasma colloid pressure

The normal values for these different pressures are the following:

Capillary pressure, 17 mm. Hg
Tissue colloid osmotic pressure, 5 mm. Hg
Plasma colloid osmotic pressure, 28 mm. Hg
Interstitial fluid pressure, −6 mm. Hg

Note particularly that the normal interstitial fluid pressure is *negative* rather than positive, putting these values into the above equation:

$$17 + 5 = -6 + 28$$
$$\text{or}$$
$$22 = 22$$

Edema. The collection of excess interstitial fluid between the cells is known as edema. The normal negative interstitial fluid pressure keeps the cells pulled tightly together because fluid is continually osmotically absorbed into the capillaries and is also pumped away from the tissues through the lymphatics. However, on occasion the interstitial fluid pressure becomes positive, which causes the interstitial fluid now to push the cells apart and cause edema. Thus, abnormalities that cause the interstitial fluid pressure to rise from its negative value into a positive range will cause edema. These include (1) *increased capillary pressure,* which can result from obstruction of a vein, excess flow of blood from the arteries into the capillaries, excess blood volume, or failure of the heart to pump blood rapidly out of the veins into the arterial system; (2) *decreased plasma colloid osmotic pressure,* which can result from failure of the liver to produce sufficient quantities of plasma proteins, loss of large quantities of proteins into the urine in certain kidney diseases, or loss of large quantities of proteins through burned areas of the skin or other denuding lesions; (3) *increased capillary permeability,* with allows excessive leakage of fluids and plasma proteins through the membranes— a number of allergic, bacterial and toxic diseases, including especially anaphylaxis and *Clostridium nouyi* infection, cause this type of damage to the capillaries; and (4) *excessive quantities of proteins in the interstitial fluids,* which will draw fluid out of the plasma into the tissue spaces because of high tissue colloid osmotic pressure—this results most frequently from *lymphatic blockage,* which prevents the return of proteins from the interstitial spaces to the blood, as will be discussed in the section below.

Lymphatic System

The lymphatics are a system of accessory vessels that accompany the blood vessels to almost all parts of the body. Minute *lymphatic capillaries* like the blood capillaries are found in almost all tissues; these lead into progressively larger lymphatic channels that finally converge mainly on the *thoracic duct,* which passes upward through the chest and empties into the venous system at the juncture of the internal jugular and subclavian veins. The lymphatic capillaries are so permeable that bacteria, various types of debris in the interstitial fluids, and large protein molecules can enter the lymph with great ease.

Lymph. Lymph is actually interstitial fluid that flows out of the interstitial spaces into the lymphatic capillaries. Therefore, its constitutents are almost identical with those of the interstitial fluid. Most lymph from the peripheral tissues contains a concentration of approximately 2 g. per 100 ml. of protein, while that from the liver contains a concentration of about 6 g. per 100 ml., and that from the intestines about 4 g. per 100 ml. Since the liver produces far more lymph in proportion to its weight than any other tissue of the body, the thoracic lymph has a protein concentration of about 4 g. per 100 ml.

Control of Lymph Flow. Two major factors control the rate of lymph flow: (1) the interstitial fluid pressure, and (2) the rate at which the lymphatics pump. The greater the volume of fluid in the tissue spaces, the greater becomes the interstitial fluid pressure. This, in turn, promotes increased flow of fluid into the lymphatic capillaries through their large openings. Once in the lymphatic capillaries, the fluid is pumped by intermittent compression of the lymphatic vessels. The compression results either from contraction of the lymphatic walls or from external compression of the lymph vessels by contracting muscles, joint movement or any other effect that compresses the tissues. The lymphatics contain valves that allow flow to occur only toward the point where the lymph empties into the blood stream. Therefore, during each compression cycle of a lymphatic vessel, fluid is pumped progressively along the vessel toward the circulation.

Removal of Bacteria and Debris from the Tissues by the Lymphatic System—Filtration by the Lymph Nodes. Because of the very high degree of permeability of the lymphatic capillaries, bacteria and any other type of very small particulate matter in the tissues can pass into the lymph. However, the lymph passes through a series of *lymph nodes* on its way to the blood. In these nodes the bacteria and other debris are filtered out, then phagocytized by reticuloendothelial cells in the nodes and finally digested into amino acids, glucose, fatty acids and other small molecular substances before being released into the body fluids.

Removal of Protein From the Interstitial Fluid by the Lymphatic System. Because of their large molecular size, most proteins that leak out of the blood capillaries into the interstitial fluids cannot pass back into the capillaries. After these collect in the interstitial fluid and become progressively more and more concentrated, they finally flow into the lymphatic system and are returned to the bloodstream in this way. Approximately one half of all the protein in the blood leaks into the interstitial spaces each day, and were it not for its return by the lymph to the blood, the person would lose most of his plasma colloid osmotic pressure within a few hours and would no longer be able to maintain normal blood volume. Therefore, this removal of protein from the interstitial spaces is probably the single most important function of the lymphatic system.

Special Fluid Systems of the Body

Cerebrospinal Fluid System. The *ventricles* of the brain and the *subarachnoid spaces* around the brain are filled with *cerebrospinal fluid.* The brain and the spinal cord actually float in this fluid, and it cushions the nervous system against blows to the skull or the spine.

Approximately 750 ml. of cerebrospinal fluid are secreted each day by the *choroid plexuses* in the four ventricles of the brain. This fluid then flows from the ventricular system into the subarachnoid space surrounding the cerebellum, then upward around the entire brain to be absorbed through many minute *arachnoidal villi* into the venous blood of the dural sinuses.

If the flow of cerebrospinal fluid is blocked at any point along its course from the choroid plexuses to the arachnoidal granulations, the fluid volume in at least part of the cerebrospinal system increases, causing *hydrocephalus,* which means simply "water in the head." The excess fluid can be inside the ventricles, in the subarachnoid space around the brain or in both regions. Hydrocephalus can also result from excessive secretion of cerebrospinal fluid by the choroid plexus.

Ocular Fluid System. The fluid in the eyes keeps the eyeballs stretched, thereby maintaining normal dimensions between the optical elements. The fluid behind the lens is mainly a gelatinous mass called the *vitreous humor,* while the fluid lying to the side and in front of the lens is a freely flowing fluid called the *aqueous humor.* Aqueous humor is continually secreted by many *ciliary processes* on the surface of the *ciliary body* that surrounds the eye on all sides of the lens. It then flows anteriorly through the pupillary opening and is absorbed continually into the *canal of Schlemm,* which lies at the iridocorneal angle.

The pressure in the eyeball is regulated principally by the rate of fluid absorption into the canal of Schlemm. The pressure normally remains almost exactly 15 mm. Hg, but any disease that blocks normal absorption of fluid from the anterior chamber into the canal of Schlemm causes this pressure to rise. Excessive rise of pressure—to 25 to 80 mm. Hg—is called *glaucoma;* this can cause either slow or rapid development of blindness. The blindness results from compression of the blood vessels that supply the retina with nutrients.

Potential Fluid Spaces. A potential fluid space is one that normally contains little or no fluid but under abnormal conditions can accumulate very large quantities of fluid. These spaces include: the *intrapleural space,* the *pericardial space,* the *peritoneal cavity,* the *joint spaces* and the *bursae.* In general, the membranes lining these spaces are very highly permeable so that the spaces communicate freely with the surrounding interstitial fluid spaces. Ordinarily, the tendency for absorption of fluid from the spaces is greater than the rate of filtration of fluid into the spaces, and this keeps them almost completely empty except for a small amount of highly viscid fluid that lubricates the movement of the surfaces against each other. However, the same conditions that cause edema in the interstitial spaces can also cause fluid to collect in the potential spaces. These include (1) high capillary pressure, (2) low plasma colloid osmotic pressure, (3) increased capillary permeability, and (4) increased colloid osmotic pressure of the fluid in the space.

An especially important cause of large quantities of fluid in a potential space is *infection.* This causes large amounts of white blood cells and tissue debris to appear in the space, and these in turn occlude or partially occlude the lymphatic drainage from the space. As a result, large quantities of proteins collect, building up the colloid osmotic pressure to a point that excessive quantities of fluids are drawn into the spaces. Such an infected fluid is called an *exudate,* while fluid that collects simply because of abnormal capillary dynamics is called a *transudate.*

KIDNEYS

Formation of Urine by the Kidneys

Nephron. The functional unit of the kidney is the *nephron,* and there are approximately 2 million nephrons in the two kidneys. The nephron is composed of a tuft of capillaries called the *glomerulus,* a capsule around the glomerulus called *Bowman's capsule* and a series of *tubules* that lead from Bowman's capsule to the *renal pelvis.* Blood flows into each glomerulus through an *afferent arteriole* and leaves it through an *efferent arteriole,* finally flowing into a system of *peritubular capillaries* that surround the tubules.

Rate of Blood Flow Through the Kidneys. Approximately 1,200 ml. of blood flow through the two kidneys each minute, this representing 20 to 25 per cent of the total cardiac output.

Glomerular Filtration. The normal pressure in the glomerulus is probably about 60 mm. Hg, and the colloid osmotic pressure of the plasma proteins averages about 32 mm. Hg. (This is slightly greater than the colloid osmotic pressure in other capillaries of the body because excessively large quantities of fluid are filtered through the glomerular capillaries, thereby concentrating the proteins.) The pressure in Bowman's capsule on the outside of the capillaries is approximately 18 mm. Hg. The glomerular pressure tends to force fluid out of the capillaries, while the colloid osmotic pressure and the pressure in Bowman's capsule tend to keep fluid from leaving the glomerulus. Therefore, the net force, called the *filtration pressure,* is equal to *glomerular pressure* minus both *plasma colloid osmotic pressure* and *Bowman's capsule pressure.* The normal filtration pressure therefore, is 60 minus 32 minus 18, or 10 mm. Hg, but it can be greatly altered in several ways: (1) by *increasing the arterial pressure,* which concomitantly increases the glomerular pressure; (2) by *dilation of the afferent arterioles,* which allows increased flow of blood into the glomerulus; (3) by *constriction of the efferent arterioles,* which impedes outflow of blood from the glomerulus; or (4) by *decreasing plasma colloid osmotic pressure.*

The total rate of fluid outflow from all glomeruli of both kidneys is about 125 ml. per minute, and this is called the *glomerular filtration rate;* this rate varies directly in proportion with the filtration pressure.

The *glomerular filtrate* is an ultrafiltrate of plasma having a composition almost identical with that of plasma except for very little proteins (only 0.03 per cent), but containing all the other constituents of plasma.

The Renal Tubules and Tubular Reabsorption. The renal tubular system is divided into four separate portions: (1) the proximal tubules; (2) the loops of Henle; (3) the distal tubules; and (4) the collecting ducts. As the glomerular filtrate (approximately 125 ml. per minute) passes progressively down this tubular system, 124 ml. are normally reabsorbed into the blood so that only 1 ml. passes into the urine. About 65 per cent is absorbed in the proximal tubules, 14 per cent in the loops of Henle, 15 per cent in the distal tubules and 6 per cent in the collecting ducts. Thus, one sees that most of the reabsorption occurs in the early portion of the tubular system.

The proximal tubules function specifically to conserve many substances that are needed by the body. For instance, all of the glucose, amino acids, aceto-acetic acid and proteins that are present in the glomerular filtrate are completely reabsorbed in the proximal tubules. Also approximately 65 per cent of the sodium, potassium and other electrolytes are reabsorbed. On the other hand, the proximal tubules are relatively impermeable to the waste products of the body.

In the loops of Henle a small amount of additional water and most of the remaining sodium and other electrolytes are reabsorbed, leaving about 4 per cent of the electrolytes and 18 per cent of the water. This ability of the loops of Henle to reabsorb most of the electrolytes plays a very important role in the ability of the kidney to concentrate urine, as will be discussed later.

Reabsorption of fluid and dissolved substances in the distal tubules and collecting ducts is quite variable—here the kidney plays it major role in controlling concentrations of various substances in the body fluids. Thus, if the concentration of sodium is very high in the body fluids, very little sodium will be reabsorbed in the distal tubules, so that large amounts of sodium will be lost into the urine. This mechanism, as well as the control mechanisms for other electrolytes, will be discussed at greater length later.

The collecting ducts collect fluid from a large number of distal tubules and transport this fluid to the pelvis of the kidney, where it is emptied as urine. As the fluid passes through the collecting duct, about six sevenths of the remainder of the fluid and small amounts of electrolytes are reabsorbed.

As fluids pass through all of the tubules, the usual waste products of metabolism such a urea, creatinine, uric acid, phosphates and sulfates, are poorly reabsorbed in comparison with water and the different electrolytes. Therefore, their concentrations become progressively greater as the tubular fluid passes from the glomerulus toward the renal pelvis. In this way, the waste products pass on into the urine and are lost.

Active Reabsorption Versus Passive Reabsorption. Reabsorption of nutrients and of many of the electrolytes from the tubules occurs by *active reabsorption,* that is, they are moved forcibly through the tubular membrane by chemical processes, as was explained earlier for cellular membranes. On the other hand, some substances such as water and urea pass through the membrane only by the process of *diffusion,* which is called *passive reabsorption.*

The Clearance Concept. From the above discussion it can be seen that a large portion of the plasma that enters the kidneys, about one fifth of it, leaks through the glomeruli into the tubular system of the kidneys and is reabsorbed. However, during its passage through the tubules certain portions of the glomerular filtrate are entirely reabsorbed, while other portions are either not reabsorbed at all or are reabsorbed very poorly. A substance that is not reabsorbed at all never returns to the plasma and therefore is completely cleared from the plasma. For instance, creatinine is not reabsorbed at all, so that the entire 125 ml. of plasma that filters into the tubules each minute is cleared of creatinine, while most of the water is reabsorbed into the blood. Therefore, it is said that the *plasma clearance* of creatinine is 125 ml. per minute.

About 60 ml. of plasma is cleared of urea each minute. About 1 ml. is cleared of sodium, and not any is cleared of glucose. Thus, the kidney acts as a "plasma clearing organ," removing those substances from the plasma that are not needed by the body while at the same time conserving those substances that are still valuable to the body.

Regulation of Extracellular Fluid Constituents and Volume

Regulation of the Ratio of Interstitial Fluid Volume to Blood Volume. As has already been explained, the extracellular fluid can move with ease back and forth between the interstitial spaces and the blood. When there is excess blood volume, the forces for movement of fluid out of the blood become greater than those for moving fluid into the blood. Therefore, some of the plasma portion of the blood is automatically transferred to the interstitial spaces, until the Starling forces at the capillary membrane once again become equilibrated. Conversely, if there is too little blood volume in relation to interstitial fluid volume, then the Starling forces become overbalanced in the direction that causes fluid to move from the interstitium into the plasma. Thus, the *ratio* of blood volume to interstitial volume is determined by the balance of the Starling forces at the capillary membrane.

Regulation of Overall Extracellular Fluid Volume. When the extracellular fluid volume becomes too great, this generally causes an increase in both the blood volume and the extracellular fluid volume. Likewise, dehydration causes a decrease in both of these. There are two mechanisms for regulation of the overall extracellular fluid volume, and therefore also regulation of both the blood volume and the interstitial fluid volume. The mechanisms are:

A rapidly acting mechanism is the *volume reflex* that controls the extracellular fluid volume. This reflex results from stretch of the two atria of the heart, especially the left atrium, which causes nerve signals to go to the brain stem and these in turn to cause two effects: First, they cause *decreased sympathetic nervous signals to the kidneys,* which allows increased renal vascular filtration and increased loss of fluid into the urine. Second, they cause *decreased secretion of antidiuretic hormone* by the hypothalamic-pituitary system. As will be explained subsequently, lack of antidiuretic hormone allows the kidneys to excrete excessive amounts of water, further decreasing the volume of fluid in the body. Thus, the volume reflex provides a very rapidly acting mechanism for adjusting both the blood volume and the total extracellular fluid volume when these become too great. However, this reflex is believed to adapt in 24 to 48 hours so that it is not capable of controlling the blood volume and extracellular fluid volume for long periods of time, such as for days and weeks.

A *long term mechanism* for control of blood volume and extracellular fluid volume is based on the interrelationship between blood volume and arterial pressure. In the section on the circulation we will discuss this interrelationship. Briefly, a prolonged increase in blood volume causes an increase in arterial pressure. The increased pressure in turn increases the rate of excretion of water and electrolytes by the kidneys, which is called *pressure diuresis.* In this way, the blood volume and extracellular fluid volume are both decreased back toward the normal level. This mechanism for control of the blood volume is called the *kidney volume-pressure control mechanism.* It is an extremely powerful mechanism and controls the volume very exactly over a period of weeks, months, and years.

Regulation of Body Fluid Osmolality and Sodium Ion Concentration by the Antidiuretic Hormone System and by the Thirst Mechanism. The body has two mechanisms for controlling the overall concentration of osmotically active substances in the body fluids. One of these mechanisms is the hypothalamic-pituitary *antidiuretic hormone* system and the other is the thirst mechanism. When the total osmotic pressure of the extracellular fluid becomes too great, this activates both of these systems, causing (1) increased thirst and therefore increased intake of water, and (2) decreased excretion of water by the kidneys because of the antidiuretic hormone. Therefore, the quantity of water in the body increases, thus diluting the concentrated electrolytes. In this way, the total concentration of electrolytes is controlled within very narrow limits.

While controlling the total concentration of osmotic substances in the extracellular fluid, the same two mechanisms control the concentration of sodium. The reason for this is that between 90 and 95 per cent of the osmotic substances in the extracellular fluid are either sodium itself or other constituents that are so closely linked to sodium that their concentrations are determined by the quantity of sodium that is available. For instance, the sum of the chloride ions and the bicarbonate ions is determined directly by the amount of sodium that is available. Therefore, the sodium ion concentration and the total concentration of all osmotically active substances in the extracellular fluids change almost exactly in parallel with each other; at the same time that the osmolality of the extracellular fluids is controlled, so also is the sodium ion concentration controlled.

Now, let us describe how the hypothalamic-pituitary antidiuretic hormone system functions and also how the thirst mechanism operates. First, a special arrangement in the kidneys affords a mechanism by which at times water can be reabsorbed more readily even than the electrolytes. To effect this, the *loops of Henle* of the renal tubules extend downward into the *medullae* of the kidneys. From these tubules active reabsorption of sodium and chloride ions occurs rapidly and strongly, causing a very high concentration of sodium chloride in the interstitial fluids of the renal medulla. Then when the tubular fluid later passes through the *collecting ducts,* which also pass through the medullae, the osmotic pressure exerted by the highly concentrated medullary fluid causes rapid absorption of water from the ducts. This leaves a concentrated fluid to pass into the urine. This mechanism for concentrating the urine is called the *countercurrent mechanism.*

The second portion of the system for control of water reabsorption is the sodium *osmoreceptor system,* which is located at the base of the brain. A high concentration of osmotic substances, especially of sodium, in the extracellular fluids causes the neuronal cells in the supraoptic nucleus of the hypothalamus, called *osmoreceptors,* to shrink, and this excites these cells. Impulses are transmitted to the *posterior pituitary gland,* which in turn releases a hormone called *antidiuretic hormone.* The antidiuretic hormone then passes by way of the blood to the kidneys where it *increases the permeability of the collecting ducts,* greatly increasing the rate at which water is reabsorbed osmotically. Therefore, when antidiuretic hormone is present in excess, the urine becomes highly concentrated. Without this antidiuretic hormone, the collecting ducts are almost impermeable to water; therefore, the water is lost into the urine, and the urine becomes highly dilute.

Thus, by means of this system, excess concentration of the extracellular fluids automatically increases the secretion of antidiuretic hormone, and this causes large quantities of water to be reabsorbed, which corrects the overconcentration of the extracellular fluids. On the other hand, dilute extracellular fluid inhibits the osmoreceptor system and therefore causes excessive loss of water into the urine, again automatically readjusting the extracellular fluid concentration to normal.

Thirst is the conscious perception of need for water, and it is caused by dehydration of neuronal cells located in the *drinking center* of the anterolateral hypothalamus. Any factor that overly increases the extracellular fluid concentration, especially excess sodium, which in turn causes excess intracellular fluid concentration, excites the thirst mechanism and makes the person seek water, thereby helping to correct the dehydration.

Regulation of Potassium Ion Concentration— Role of Aldosterone. Aldosterone has a direct effect on the renal tubules, especially the distal tubules and the collecting ducts, to increase reabsorption of sodium into the blood and also to increase the secretion of potassium from the blood into the tubules. The increased reabsorption of sodium into the blood does not affect the blood concentration of sodium significantly because the hypothalamic-pituitary antidiuretic hormone mechanism and the thirst mechanism discussed above still control the sodium ion concentration very exactly despite the increased sodium reabsorption from the renal tubules. Other mechanisms for control of potassium ion concentration, besides the aldosterone mechanism, are not so powerful. Therefore, when excess aldosterone circulates in the blood, the increased secretion of potassium into the renal tubules and subsequent excretion in the urine causes marked reduction of potassium in the extracellular fluid. Conversely, in the absence of aldosterone, the extracellular fluid potassium ion concentration increases markedly.

Now, to complete the control mechanism for potassium ion concentration: When the potassium ion concentration rises to very high levels, this has a direct effect on the adrenal cortex to stimulate increased aldosterone secretion. The aldosterone then causes increased secretion of potassium into the urine and return of the potassium ion concentration back toward normal.

Regulation of Other Extracellular Fluid Electrolytes. Other extracellular fluid electrolytes that are regulated in similar ways include the calcium, magnesium, chloride, bicarbonate, and other ions. An increase in calcium ion concentration causes decreased parathyroid hormone concentration; and this in turn causes decreased calcium reabsorption by the renal tubules and increased loss of calcium into the urine. The chloride and bicarbonate ion concentrations are adjusted by the respiratory and renal mechanism for control of acid–base balance as will be explained in the following paragraphs.

Regulation of Acid–Base Balance

When one speaks of acid–base balance, one actually means regulation of the *hydrogen ion concentration* in the body fluids. The hydrogen ion concentration is normally expressed in terms of pH, which is the *logarithm of the reciprocal of the hydrogen ion concentration* according to the following formula:

$$pH = \log\left(\frac{1}{H+}\right)$$

Arterial blood has a normal pH of 7.4. A pH of 7.8 is considered to be highly alkaline while a pH of 7.0 is considered to be highly acidic.

Acid–Base Buffer Systems. One of the important means for regulation of acid–base balance is the chemical *acid–base buffer systems* present in all the body fluids. An acid–base buffer is simply a combination of substances that will react chemically with either acids or alkalies, when these are added to a solution, to keep them from markedly changing the hydrogen ion concentration in the solution.

One of the major buffer systems of the body fluids is the *proteins of the cells* and, to a lesser extent, the proteins of the plasma and the interstitial fluids. Another buffer system that is extremely important in acid-base regulation is the *bicarbonate system.* This is a mixture of carbonic acid and bicarbonate ions that exists everywhere in the body fluids. The greater the carbonic acid, the lower is the pH; the greater the bicarbonate ions, the higher is the pH. The following equation, called the *Henderson–Hasselbalch equation,* describes this relationship:

$$pH = 6.1 + \log \frac{HCO_3^-}{CO_2}$$

Respiratory Regulation of Hydrogen Ion Concentration. Rapid ventilation of the lungs decreases the concentration of carbon dioxide in the alveoli, which in turn allows carbon dioxide to diffuse very readily from the blood. When carbon dioxide leaves the blood, large portions of the carbonic acid in the body fluids immediately dissociate into water and carbon dioxide, thus reducing the concentration of carbonic acid and also of hydrogen ions. Conversely, the less the pulmonary ventilation the greater becomes the concentration of carbonic acid and the higher becomes the hydrogen ion concentration.

Not only can pulmonary ventilation alter the hydrogen ion concentration, but also the hydrogen ion concentration can in turn control the rate and depth of pulmonary ventilation in the following manner: When the hydrogen ion concentration becomes too great, this has a direct effect on the respiratory center in the brain stem to cause an increase in the rate of pulmonary ventilation. In turn, the increased ventilation reduces the carbonic acid concentration in the body fluids and therefore returns the hydrogen ion concentration back toward normal. Conversely, if the hydrogen ion concentration becomes too little, the respiratory center becomes inhibited, pulmonary ventilation becomes reduced, and the carbonic acid concentration in the body fluids rises, thereby bringing the hydrogen ion concentration once again back near to normal. This respiratory mechanism of acid–base regulation can return the hydrogen ion concentration about two-thirds of the way back to normal within a minute or so after some foreign acid or alkali has entered the body fluids, provided the quantity is not too great.

Regulation of Hydrogen Ion Concentration by the Kidneys. When the respiratory system fails to readjust the hydrogen ion concentration to normal, the kidneys are still capable of bringing it back to normal during the ensuing 12 to 24 hours. If the renal mechanism has plenty of time to function, it is many times as effective as either the buffers or the respiratory mechanism in readjusting the pH of the body fluids.

The kidneys readjust the hydrogen ion concentration in the following way: Hydrogen ions are continually being secreted by the tubular epithelium into the tubular fluid, the hydrogen ions representing a loss of acid from the extracellular fluids. On the other hand, bicarbonate ions are continually filtering from the blood into the tubules, and this represents a loss of alkali. In acidosis the rate of hydrogen ion secretion exceeds that of bicarbonate loss because the tubular epithelial cells respond to acidosis by increased hydrogen se-

cretion. This allows the body fluids to lose excess acid and therefore to correct the acidosis. On the other hand, in alkalosis the rate of hydrogen ion secretion becomes very low, allowing excess loss of alkali. As a result, the body fluids become progressively more acidic, returning once again to a normal hydrogen ion concentration.

BLOOD AND IMMUNITY

Blood Cells

Red Blood Cells and Their Function. The body contains about 25 trillion red cells in an average concentration of about 5,000,000 per cu. mm. of blood. The percentage of the total blood volume comprised of red blood cells is called the *hematocrit,* and this is normally about 40 per cent.

The principal function of the red blood cells is to transport oxygen from the lungs to the tissues, but a secondary function is to transport carbon dioxide from the tissues back to the lungs. The dynamics of these functions will be presented later in the section on respiration.

Regulation of Red Blood Cell Formation. The rate of red blood cell formation is controlled by the delivery of oxygen to the tissues. The general mechanism of this is the following: Tissue hypoxia causes the tissues, particularly the kidneys, to release a hormone called *erythropoietin,* which then flows in the blood to the bone marrow where it stimulates erythropoiesis. In highly athletic persons, whose tissues require large amounts of oxygen, the total red cell mass in the body is often 20 to 50 per cent above normal, and in persons residing at very high altitudes where oxygen is rare in the air the total red cell mass sometimes becomes as much as 80 to 100 per cent above normal.

When the red blood cells are once formed, they normally have an average life span in the circulatory system of about 120 days.

Nutritive Factors Affecting Red Blood Cell Formation. The process of red blood cell formation can be divided into two principal processes: (1) formation of the cell structure itself, and (2) formation of hemoglobin. The red cell is formed in the bone marrow by a series of divisions from the *hemocytoblast.* Two vitamins, *vitamin B$_{12}$* and *folic acid,* are necessary for normal formation of the cell structure. If either of these is missing, the cell membrane is likely to be so friable that the cells are rapidly destroyed in the circulatory system; also, the cell is likely to be too large or occasionally too small, and its shape may be globular, ovoid, or any other shape besides the normal biconcave disk. This abnormal formation of red blood cells is called *maturation failure*.

A primary nutritive factor necessary for formation of hemoglobin is *iron*. Iron is present in the diet in only very small quantities and even then is rather poorly absorbed from the gastrointestinal tract; therefore, many persons frequently fail to form sufficient quantities of hemoglobin to fill the red blood cells as they are being produced. This causes *hypochromic anemia* in which the number of cells may be normal but the amount of hemoglobin in each cell is far below normal.

White Blood Cells. The number of white cells in the blood is normally only 1/600 the number of red blood cells, about 8,000 per cu. mm. of blood, but they perform the very important function of protecting or helping to protect the body from invasion by infectious agents. The white cells consist of *neutrophils, eosinophils, basophils* and *platelets*, all formed in the bone marrow, and *lymphocytes* and *monocytes*, formed in the lymph nodes.

The *neutrophils* are the most numerous of the white blood cells, these representing about 60 per cent of the total number in the blood. They are highly motile, highly phagocytic and are attracted out of the blood into tissue areas where tissue destruction is occurring by a process called *chemotaxis*, attraction of the neutrophils by the destruction products from the damaged tissues. Once in the tissue area, the neutrophils phagocytize bacteria and small amounts of dead tissue debris.

The *monocytes* are much larger cells than the neutrophils, and large numbers of them normally wander through the tissues all of the time. They can phagocytize five to ten times as many bacteria and much larger particles of tissue debris than can the neutrophils. However, they are not attracted nearly so rapidly into areas of tissue destruction as the neutrophils. In general, soon after an infection begins the concentration of neutrophils becomes very high in the infected area; then several days later the concentration of monocytes becomes very high, the monocytes replacing most of the neutrophils.

The monocytes enter the tissues, and during the next few hours they swell manyfold and become *macrophages*. Almost all tissues of the body contain macrophages, but they are especially abundant in those tissues that are exposed to bacteria, such as the lung alveoli, the sinusoids of the liver, the sinusoids of the bone marrow, the sinusoids of the lymph nodes, and the subcutaneous tissue. This extensive *monocyte-macrophage system* is frequently also called the *reticuloendothelial system*.

When tissues become infected or inflamed, breakdown products from these tissues not only cause chemotaxis of neutrophils and monocytes into the infected or inflamed tissue area, but the breakdown products also cause (1) rapid release of already stored white blood cells from the bone marrow, and (2) increased formation of new white blood cells.

The *eosinophils* are similar to the neutrophils except that they are less chemotactic and less phagocytic. Large numbers of eosinophils appear in the blood in allergic conditions and also when the body is invaded by certain parasites. It is possible that the eosinophils help to detoxify toxins that are released by parasites or by allergic reactions.

The *basophils* are similar to or the same as *mast* cells, which are found in the pericapillary tissues and secrete large quantities of *heparin*. Basophils also secrete heparin while still in the blood. This substance in turn prevents blood coagulation in the normal circulatory system.

The *platelets* are only fragments of cells instead of whole cells. Like heparin, they, too, are important in the blood coagulation process, as will be discussed below.

Blood Coagulation

The Blood Clot. When a blood vessel ruptures, a blood clot develops within a few minutes to fill the rent and stop the bleeding—if the vessel is small enough. This process is caused by polymerization of plasma *fibrinogen* molecules into long *fibrin threads* that entrap large numbers of red blood cells, white blood cells, platelets and plasma to form a soft gelatinous mass, the blood clot. The fibrin threads gradually contract, expressing most of the plasma from the clot, which leaves a reasonably solid barrier in the opening of the blood vessel.

Bleeding Diatheses. Several abnormalities of the blood coagulation mechanism can cause persons to become excessive bleeders. In *hemophilia* the substance called *antihemophilic factor* is absent from the plasma. This substance is required for function of the intrinsic pathway of blood coagulation; because of its absence in hemophilia, the hemophiliac person is an excessive bleeder.

The normal number of platelets in the blood is about 300,000 per cu. mm. In *thrombocytopenia* this number is greatly reduced. Platelets have the ability to attach themselves to very minute rupture points in blood vessels and thereby close these holes even without causing actual blood coagulation. In thrombocytopenia this function is lost, and as a result the person develops many minute bleeding spots over his entire body, causing *petechial hemorrhages* throughout all his organs and beneath the skin.

Prothrombin deficiency or *Factor VII deficiency* (as

well as deficiency of some other blood coagulation factors) frequently results from liver disease because each of these substances is a protein formed by the liver. Also, the concentration of each of them becomes reduced when vitamin K is not available to be used by the chemical systems of the liver for formation of the two substances. In deficiency of either prothrombin or Factor VII, the rate of thrombin formation is greatly reduced, thus preventing or depressing coagulation and allowing excessive bleeding.

Immunity

Innate Immunity. Immunity means resistance of the body to invasion by bacteria, viruses or other infectious agents or toxins. Each person is born with a certain amount of *innate immunity* that results from several special mechanisms: (1) the reticuloendothelial system and the white blood cells, which have already been discussed, (2) resistance of the intact skin to invasion by microorganisms, (3) destruction of bacterial organisms by the digestive enzymes in the stomach, and (4) substances circulating in the blood.

Adaptive Immunity—The Immune Process. In addition to the natural immunity that normally exists in all persons, a person can develop *adaptive immunity* to many destructive agents to which he is not naturally immune. Most destructive agents, such as bacteria, viruses or toxins, are mostly composed of protein molecules. On entering the body, these proteins act as *antigens* and cause two types of immunity: one is called *humoral immunity* and the other *lymphocytic immunity*. In humoral immunity, large protein molecules called *immune antiglobulins* or *antibodies* are formed, and these in turn destroy the invading agent. In the case of lymphocytic immunity, *sensitized lymphocytes* are formed, and these too have the capability of attacking and destroying the invading agents.

Humoral Immunity. In humoral immunity, the antigens first enter the lymphoid tissue, especially the lymph nodes. There they cause plasma cells, which are derived from lymphocytes, to produce large quantities of *antibodies* specifically reactive for the type of protein that initiated their production. Once these antibodies have been formed and released into the body fluids, which usually requires about a week to several weeks, they then destroy the specific invader that had caused their formation and can also destroy any future invader of this same type.

Antibodies are large protein molecules, usually gamma globulins, that are capable of combining chemically with invading agents. The antibodies attach to the surfaces of bacteria or viruses, or they combine directly with toxins. They either destroy the invading

agent or make it more susceptible to phagocytosis by the reticuloendothelial system and by white blood cells. Or, in the case of toxins, the antibodies can simply neutralize these by combining chemically with them.

Lymphocytic Immunity. In early fetal development of the lymph nodes, no lymphocytes are present in the nodes. Instead, the early lymphocytes are formed and processed in special structures, one of which is the thymus gland. After processing, the lymphocytes are then released into the circulating blood and eventually become entrapped in the lymphoid tissue. Once in this tissue, some lymphocytes are converted into plasma cells that become part of the humoral immune process to form antibodies.

Others of the lymphocytes in the lymph nodes subserve a second type of adaptive immune process called *lymphocytic immunity*. That is, instead of forming antibodies to be released into the circulating blood, antibodies are formed that remain inside the lymphocytes or remain attached to their membranes, and the whole lymphocytes are released into the circulating blood. These cells, called *sensitized lymphocytes* or *committed lymphocytes,* can squeeze through the pores of the capillaries and are attracted to damaged tissue areas by the process of chemotaxis. Once there, the sensitized lymphocytes attach directly to the invading organism and destroy it. Digestive enzymes in the lymphocyte exude through the membrane to engulf the invader and to digest it.

Tolerance; Autoimmune Disease. The immune process of the *normal* human body does not develop antibodies or sensitized lymphocytes that can destroy the body's own tissues, despite the fact that the body tissues are to a great extent like bacteria in their chemical composition. This phenomenon is called *tolerance* to the body's own proteins and tissues. This probably results from destruction during fetal life of those primordial lymphocytes capable of forming antibodies or sensitized lymphocytes against the body proteins and tissues.

Under abnormal conditions, however, both antibodies and sensitized lymphocytes that can attack the body's own tissues do occasionally develop. This process is called *autoimmunity*. It occurs particularly in older age or after some disease causes destruction of body tissue with release of tissue antigens into the circulating body fluids. Once the immune process has caused production of antibodies or sensitized lymphocytes that can attack the body's own tissues, these will then react against specific tissues and cause serious debility. Examples of autoimmune disease include rheumatic heart disease, acute glomerulonephritis, myasthenia gravis and lupus erythematosus.

Allergy

There are at least three different types of allergy, two of which can occur under appropriate conditions in normal persons and one of which occurs only in persons who have specific allergic tendency.

Allergies That Occur in Normal Persons. Two types of allergy that occur in normal persons are *anaphylaxis* and *delayed reaction allergy.*

Anaphylaxis occurs in persons who are strongly immunized against a foreign antigen. When a subsequent dose of the same foreign antigen is injected directly into the circulatory system, an immune reaction occurs in direct contact with the blood and the tissues immediately surrounding the blood vessels. This reaction causes local cellular damage. One of the effects is release of large quantities of histamine from the cells, and this in turn causes extreme vascular vasodilatation and circulatory collapse. Often a person dies as a result.

Delayed-Reaction Allergy. Delayed-reaction allergy is caused by sensitized lymphocytes and not by antibodies. A typical example is the reaction to poison ivy. The toxin of poison ivy becomes deposited in the skin, and a small portion of it finds its way to the lymph nodes, which, over a period of several days to a week or so, form sensitized lymphocytes. These then are carried by the blood back to the original site of entry of the poison ivy toxin. Reaction of the lymphocytes with the toxin in direct association with the cells produces severe local tissue damage, which is the well-known rash and vesicles associated with poison ivy.

Allergy in the Allergic Person. Some persons, called *allergic persons,* tend to form a type of antibody called *reagin.* Reagins have a different protein structure from that of normal antibodies and are called IgE antibodies. Also, the reagins tend to attach themselves to tissue cells throughout the body. When the specific antigen that reacts with the reagin (called the *allergin*) enters the tissue it combines with the reagin. This combination, occurring in intimate association with tissue cells, causes cellular damage with release of histamine and proteolytic enzymes from the affected cells, especially from tissue mast cells. Severe local tissue damage can result. Types of allergies of this type are hay fever, asthma and urticaria.

Transfusion; Transplantation of Tissues

Transfusion of blood from one person to another or transplantation of tissues or organs is principally a problem of immunity; the new host may be already immune to the transfused blood or the transplanted tissues, or he may develop immunity to these after a few weeks' time, which then causes death of the cells in the transfusion or the transplant.

Transfusion Reaction. If the host is immune to transfused blood or becomes immune soon after the transfusion, a *transfusion reaction* is likely to result. This consists of an attack on the red blood cells by the recipient's antibodies. The antibodies attach themselves to the surfaces of the cells and make them *agglutinate with each other,* which means that the cells stick together in clumps. Occasionally the antibodies are powerful enough also to cause the cells to rupture. However, even if the cells do not rupture from this cause, the clumped cells become caught in the capillaries of the circulatory system and during the next few hours become ruptured because of progressive trauma or attack by white blood cells or by tissue macrophages. Thus, the final result in all transfusion reactions is rupture of the red cells with release of hemoglobin and other intracellular substances into the blood. Many of the intracellular components have toxic effects throughout the body, causing a febrile reaction and sometimes depressing the circulation into a shocklike state. In addition, much of the free hemoglobin in the blood filters through the glomerular membrane into the renal tubules; then water is reabsorbed from the tubules, allowing the homoglobin to become so concentrated that it precipitates. This eventually blocks many or most of the tubules of the kidneys and causes either oliguria or anuria. As a result, a person occasionally dies a week or so later of uremia rather than as the immediate result of the transfusion reaction.

A-B-O Blood Groups. The membranes of the red blood cells in about 60 per cent of all human beings contain one or both of two very important antigens, called *group A* or *group B agglutinogens,* that frequently cause transfusion reactions. The bloods of different persons are generally *typed* on the basis of the presence or the absence of these agglutinogens in the blood cells. Thus, the four major blood groups of humans are *group A,* which contains A agglutinogen; *group B,* which contains B agglutinogen; *group AB,* which contains both A and B agglutinogens; and *group O,* which contains neither.

When a person does not have either A or B agglutinogens in his blood, he almost always does have antibodies that will agglutinate cells containing the missing agglutinogen. Antibodies that agglutinate the A agglutinogen are called *alpha agglutinins,* while those that agglutinate B agglutinogen are called *beta agglutinins.* Thus, group A blood contains beta agglutinins, while group B blood contains alpha agglutinins; group AB blood contains neither of the agglutinins; and group O blood, both alpha and beta agglutinins. Therefore, mixing bloods of different types will often cause agglutination of at least some of the cells and can result in a transfusion reaction.

Rh Blood Types. The blood cells of about 85 per cent of all white persons and 95 per cent of Negroes also contain another antigen, called the *Rh antigen,* which exists in several slightly different forms. Those persons who have the Rh antigen are said to be *Rh positive* while those who do not have any Rh antigen are said to be *Rh negative.*

A transfusion reaction occasionally results when Rh-positive blood is transfused into an Rh-negative person. However, this will not occur unless the Rh-negative person has been exposed previously to Rh-positive blood because, contrary to the alpha and the beta agglutinins, Rh antibodies do not occur spontaneously in the blood. Yet, if the Rh-negative person has been exposed previously to Rh-positive blood he will have developed antibodies against the Rh factor, and a subsequent transfusion with Rh-positive blood can cause an equally severe transfusion reaction as one that occurs with the group A-B-O bloods.

The Rh factor occasionally causes transfusion reactions in fetuses during pregnancy in the following way: If the mother is Rh negative, and the baby inherits the Rh-positive trait from the father, some of the Rh-positive antigens can gradually diffuse through the placenta into the mother and cause her to develop Rh antibodies; these antibodies then diffuse back through the placenta into the baby and cause agglutination of the circulating red cells. This effect rarely occurs with the first Rh-positive baby but occurs much more frequently during subsequent pregnancies because immunity develops in the mother mainly immediately after birth of the baby in response to antigens entering her blood from degenerating products of the placental tissues. If the mother is given antiserum against the Rh factor immediately after delivery, most instances of immunization can be prevented. But without such preventive measures, this is a cause of death in a large number of newborn or unborn children. The clinical condition, when present, is called *erythroblastosis fetalis* because the fetus responds with an erythroblastic reaction to form more blood cells.

Other Blood Types. In addition to the A, B, O and Rh factors in red blood cells there are still many other protein antigens in the blood cells that can occasionally cause transfusion reactions. These include the *M, N, S, P, Kell, Lewis, Duffy* and *Lutheran* factors. However, the transfusion reactions caused by these factors are usually so mild or so rare that these factors are not considered as being important in blood transfusions, but they are all very important in forensic medicine for determining parentage of children.

Transplantation of Tissues. Almost exactly the same problems are experienced in the transplantation of tissues as in transfusion, for other cells of the body besides the red blood cells also contain antigens to which the host is either already immune or to which the host can develop immunity within a few weeks after transplantation. For this reason, successful transplantation of organs that contain living cells can usually be achieved for only a few weeks unless the recipient is treated with immunosuppressive drugs, or unless transplantation is from one identical twin to another, whose tissues contain exactly the same types of antigens. After several weeks the immune processes of the body destroy the transplant. Fortunately the use of immunosuppressive drugs now allows transplantation of kidneys, hearts and other organs. Also, procedures for "typing" the antigens in tissues have now been developed so that the antigens from donor to recipient can be partially matched, thus reducing the severity of the transplant rejection reactions.

NERVE AND MUSCLE

Function of the Nerve Fiber

The Membrane Potential. A membrane potential occurs across the membranes of all cells. In nerve and muscle cells this potential amounts to about 90 millivolts, with negativity inside the cell membrane and positivity outside. The development of this potential occurs as follows: Every cell membrane contains a sodium–potassium pump that pumps sodium to the outside of the cell and potassium to the inside. However, more sodium is pumped outward than potassium inward. Also, the membrane is relatively permeable to potassium, so that potassium can leak out of the cell with ease. Therefore, the net effect of this pump is principally to transport sodium outward. This active transport of sodium, which is a positively charged ion, to the outside of the membrane causes loss of positive charges from the inside of the membrane and gain of positive charges on the outside, thus creating negativity inside the membrane and positivity outside. The resulting membrane potential is the basis of all conduction of impulses by nerve and muscle fibers.

The Action Potential. The action potential is the *change in electrical potential* at the membrane when an impulse spreads over its surface. This is caused in the following way: Any factor that makes the membrane excessively permeable—such as passing an electrical current through it, pinching the nerve fiber, pricking it with a pin, crushing it, or applying a drug such as acetylcholine—will usually cause the membrane to become very permeable to sodium ions. As a result, the positive sodium ions now flow rapidly to the inside of the membrane. Therefore, the membrane potential suddenly becomes reversed with positivity on the inside and negativity on the outside. This state is called *depolarization.*

Once depolarization has occurred, the loss of the negative potential on the inside of the membrane slows up the movement of sodium ions to the interior of the cell, and for reasons not yet understood, this slowing allows the membrane to become once more less permeable to sodium and more permeable to potassium. As a result, few sodium ions are now able to pass to the inside, but large numbers of potassium ions, which are present inside the cell in high concentration, diffuse to the outside; since potassium ions are also positively charged, this once again causes a buildup of positive charges outside the membrane and loss of positive charges from the inside, reestablishing the normal membrane potential. This process is called *repolarization.*

The action potential can spread along a nerve or muscle fiber in the following way: Every time an action potential begins at any given point on the membrane, the normal positive charge on the outside of the membrane and the normal negative charge on the inside are lost, which causes an electrical current to flow to the adjacent area(s) of the membrane and to stimulate these areas as well. As a result, an action potential then occurs at each of these points, and the process is repeated again and again until the action potential has spread to both ends of the fiber.

In large nerve fibers, the repolarization process follows about 1/2,500 second after the depolarization process. Therefore, as many as 2,500 impulses can be transmitted along a large nerve fiber per minute. On the other hand, the process of repolarization is so slow in many smooth muscle fibers that not over one impulse in every few seconds can be transmitted.

The All-or-Nothing Law. A very important aspect of nerve function is that a stimulus usually causes a nerve fiber either to transmit a complete impulse (action potential) or, if the stimulus is too weak, none at all. This is called the *all-or-nothing law.* Furthermore, once an impulse begins, it travels in all directions over the fiber—either backward or forward and into all branches of the fiber—until each portion of the neuronal membrane has become depolarized.

Relationship of Nerve Metabolism to Action Potentials. It is the metabolic processes of the cell that cause active transport of sodium and potassium through the cell membrane. Therefore, if metabolism in the cell is blocked, ionic differences between the extracellular and the intracellular fluids cannot be maintained. However, nerve metabolism can be blocked for as long as several hours at a time without greatly affecting transmission of the impulse, for, once the ionic differences have been built up, impulse transmission is purely a physical phenomenon without involving the enzymatic metabolic processes of the cells. With each impulse that is transmitted, a small portion of the ions concentrated on the two sides of the membrane are lost to the opposite fluid compartment. During the ensuing few seconds or minutes, the metabolic processes of the membrane normally retransport these ions, thus restoring completely normal ionic differences. The more impulses transmitted by the nerve fiber, the greater the rate of metabolism required to maintain the appropriate ionic concentrations.

Summation of Nerve Impulses. Since nerve impulses are an all-or-nothing function, the means by which the nervous system transmits weak or strong signals is to "summate" many numbers of nerve impulses, that is, the greater the number of impulses transmitted the greater the effect at the other end of the nerve. There are two means by which summation can occur: One of these is *multiple fiber summation,* in which simultaneous impulses are transmitted over many parallel nerve fibers at the same time, and the other is *temporal summation,* in which large numbers of impulses are transmitted over the same fiber in rapid succession one after another. In either instance, the effect at the opposite end of the nerve is very much the same because the degree of reaction is dependent on the number of impulses arriving at the end of the nerve in a given period.

The Neuromuscular Junction

The *neuromuscular junction* is the point at which a motor nerve fiber connects with a muscle fiber. The mechanism for transmission of the impulse from the nerve fiber to the muscle fiber follows.

Release of Acetylcholine at the Neuromuscular Junction. The nerve ending, where it lies on the muscle fiber, branches like the limbs of a tree to form a broad structure called the *endplate.* The nerve terminals in this end plate synthesize and store a chemical called *acetylcholine.* When a nerve impulse reaches the end plate, small portions of the stored acetylcholine are released into the *synaptic gap* between the nerve terminals and the muscle membrane, and this is turn acts on the membrane of the muscle fiber to increase its permeability to sodium. Within another 1/500 second a protein enzyme called *cholinesterase* destroys the acetylocholine. Thus, the net result of a nerve impulse reaching the end plate is the release of a small *pulse* of acetylcholine that lasts just long enough to stimulate the muscle fiber.

The End Plate Potential. When the short pulse

of acetylcholine increases the permeability of the muscle membrane, sodium ions immediately begin to pour to the inside of the fiber, which causes the outside of the fiber in the immediate vicinity of the end plate to become negative and the inside positive. This change in potential is called the *end plate potential*. The end plate potential in turn causes ions to being flowing along the inside and outside surfaces of the muscle membrane, which creates an action potential that spreads over the entire muscle fiber as described above for nerve fibers.

Occasionally the amount of acetylcholine released by the end plate is not very great, and the end plate potential also is considerably less than normal. Below a certain threshold value, the end plate potential is not strong enough to initiate an action potential in the muscle fiber. As a result, the impulse fails to pass on into the muscle.

The "Amplification" Function of the Neuromuscular Junction.   One often asks why such a complicated mechanism as that at the neuromuscular junction is needed to transmit impulses from nerve fibers into muscle fibers. However, the electrical currents generated around nerve fibers are far too weak to initiate an action potential directly in muscle fibers, for the muscle fibers are very much larger than nerve fibers. Therefore, the nerve fibers release acetylcholine, which causes the muscle fiber to generate its own electrical stimulus, the *end plate potential,* that has many times the stimulatory ability of the nerve impulse itself. Thus, the neuromuscular junction "amplifies" the stimulus.

Function of Skeletal Muscle

The Basic Contractile Mechanism.   In all muscle fibers there are two major types of fibrillar filaments: *actin filaments* and *myosin filaments*. These have lengths of 2.05 and 1.60 microns respectively. They are arranged linearly in the muscle fiber so that the myosin filaments alternate with the actin filaments. The ends of the myosin filaments overlap the ends of the actin filaments, and each of these then overlaps the ends of the next set of alternate filaments. This sort of arrangement continues throughout the entire length of the muscle fiber, which in some instances is as long as half a meter. When an action potential passes over the muscle fiber membrane, the actin and myosin filaments attract each other, and their ends slide together like pistons, thus shortening the fiber. As soon as the action potential is over, the attractive forces between the myosin and actin filaments disappear so that the alternate sets of filaments then slide away from each other like pistons moving backward.

Though the myosin filaments are composed entirely of myosin molecules, the actin filament is composed

of long threads of *actin* and *tropomyosin* wrapped around each other in a helical manner. Also, attached periodically to the tropomyosin is a protein complex called *troponin*. The troponin and tropomyosin control muscle contraction, as explained in the following sections.

Initiation of Contraction.   Transmission of an action potential over the muscle fiber membrane causes the fiber to contract a few milliseconds later. The mechanism by which this occurs is believed to be the following: Minute tubules, called *transverse tubules* or T tubules, pass transversely all the way through each segment of the muscle fiber. The action potential, on reaching one of these tubules, also travels to the interior of the muscle fiber along the membranes of the tubules. Thus, electrical current is distributed to the inner substance of the muscle fiber as well as along its surface. The tubules make physical contact in the substance of the muscle fiber with many additional very fine tubules called *longitudinal tubules*. These are part of the endoplasmic reticulum and are collectively called the *sarcoplasmic reticulum;* they lie parallel to the myofibrils that cause muscle contraction. Also, they contain large amounts of calcium ions. When the action potential travels over the muscle cell membrane, electrical currents pass through the T tubules to the longitudinal tubules, and these currents cause small amounts of calcium ions to be released from the longitudinal tubules into the intracellular fluid surrounding the myosin and actin filaments of the myofibrils. The calcium ions then combine with the troponin complex, and in some way not understood this changes the physical relationship of the tropomyosin and actin molecules; the net result is exposure of active sites on the actin that attract the myosin filament, causing contraction of the muscle. Within another few milliseconds the calcium ions are actively transported back into the longitudinal tubules, which decreases the calcium ion concentration and thereby inactivates the myosin, allowing relaxation of the muscle.

The Ratchet Theory of Muscle Contraction.   The nature of the forces that cause the actin and myosin filaments to slide along each other during the contractile process is not entirely understood. However, one theory is the following: Each myosin filament has approximately 200 arms, called *cross bridges,* that extend anglewise to the sides. At the end of each cross bridge is a hinged *head* that makes contact with one of the actin filaments. The head can attach temporarily to an active site on the actin filament, and it can also rock back and forth where it is hinged to the cross bridge. It is believed that when the head attaches to the actin filament, its molecular configuration changes, causing it to bend in a forward direction. This pulls the actin filament forward, but the forward bending also causes the head to disattach from the actin filament and to bend back to its original position. Next, it attaches to another active site farther along the actin filament. And the head bends again and pulls the actin filament still another short distance. Thus, by a process of attachment, bending, disattachment, and so forth, the actin and myosin filament are pulled together, causing muscle contraction. The effect that initiates this contractile process is uncovering of the active sites on the actin filament, which occurs when calcium combines with the troponin complex as described above.

Energetics of Muscle Contraction. Contraction of the muscle requires energy. Each time a muscle fiber contracts, a certain amount of *adenosine triphosphate,* the energy-rich compound that is synthesized during the metabolism of food, is destroyed. It is believed that one molecule of adenosine triphosphate is degraded each time the head of a cross bridge bends to cause movement of the actin filament. The energy derived from this adenosine triphosphate is used to return the head back to its original "cocked" position. In this way the energy is stored in the cocked head, and it is this energy that provides the force exerted by the head to pull the actin filament forward.

The more times a muscle fiber contracts and the greater the load against which the muscle contracts, the greater is the quantity of adenosine triphosphate that is degraded. When the quantity of adenosine triphosphate in the cell falls even slightly below normal, the intracellular processes for splitting and oxidizing foods go into high gear to generate new adenosine triphosphate. During extreme muscle activity, the rate of metabolism in individual muscles sometimes rises to as high as 50 times the metabolic rate of the resting muscle.

Muscle Twitch and Muscle Tetanization. When a single impulse passes over the muscle fiber, the fiber contracts for a very short time, about 1/5 second in the soleus muscle, 1/15 second in the gastrocnemius muscle and 1/50 second in an ocular muscle. This single short contraction is called a *muscle twitch.* However, this type of contraction normally does not occur in the body; instead, smooth and more prolonged contractions usually occur. These result from many individual muscle twitches occurring so close together, one after another, that the muscle appears to be contracting in one long continuous contraction rather than in many individual twitches. This effect is called *tetanization.*

Different Strengths of Muscle Contraction. A skeletal muscle is composed of many muscle fibers connected in parallel with each other. The strength of contraction of the entire muscle can be either very slight or very strong. To cause a weak contraction, nerve impulses are transmitted to only a few muscle fibers at a time, while to cause a very strong contraction, essentially all of the muscle fibers are contracted simultaneously. As is true in summation of nerve impulses, there are two different methods by which the strength of muscle contraction summates: (1) *multiple fiber summation,* in which many parallel muscle fibers contract simultaneously, and (2) *temporal summation,* also frequently called *wave summation,* in which successive contractions of each muscle fiber occur so close together that they add to each other.

Function of Cardiac and Smooth Muscle

The basic contractile mechanism of both cardiac and smooth muscle is essentially the same as that of skeletal muscle except that in smooth muscle the actin and myosin filaments are not arranged in distinct alternate segments as is true in both skeletal and cardiac muscle. Nevertheless, an action potential traveling over the membrane causes contraction, presumably as a result of the influx of calcium ions that makes the actin and myosin filaments attract each other.

Rhythmic Contraction in Cardiac and Smooth Muscle. A distinguishing characteristic of both cardiac and smooth muscle is that they normally exhibit repetitive rhythmic contractions. These rhythmic contractions are caused by spontaneously occurring action potentials in the muscle fibers. Every time the membrane potential returns to the resting state, a new action potential begins because the membranes of these types of muscle are naturally very permeable to sodium ions, these ions leak into the muscle fiber, cause a change in the local membrane permeability, and initiate the action potential. This repeats itself over and over: repolarization, depolarization, repolarization, depolarization, and so forth.

The action potential of cardiac muscle lasts about 0.3 second and of smooth muscle from as little as 0.01 second in some types of smooth muscle to more than a second in others. Also, these two types of muscle contract for prolonged periods rather than the very short period that occurs in skeletal muscle.

Tone and Plasticity of Smooth Muscle. Another important distinguishing characteristic of smooth muscle is that it can contract continuously in addition to the rhythmic contractions. The continuous contraction is called *tone.* The degree of tone can change from time to time, becoming almost none or increasing to a truly strong contraction. The intermittent rhythmic contractions are then superimposed on the basic tone. Thus, in the gastrointestinal tract, tonic contraction maintains a basal amount of pressure in the lumen of the gut, while rhythmic contractions superimposed on this cause propulsion of food along the gastrointestinal tract.

Another property of smooth muscle not evidenced by skeletal and cardiac muscle is *plasticity*. This means simply that smooth muscle can be stretched or shortened, and it will still maintain a relatively constant amount of tension. This allows smooth muscle organs such as the urinary bladder to increase very greatly in volume without the internal pressure changing to a great extent.

HEART

Rhythmic Excitation of the Heart

Basic Rhythmicity of Different Types of Cardiac Muscle. The natural rate of rhythmic contraction of cardiac muscle varies in different parts of the heart. The muscle fibers in the *S-A node,* a small area of special cardiac muscle located in the posterior wall of the right atrium beneath the opening of the superior vena cava, have a natural rate of rhythmicity of about 72 times per minute. The natural rate of rhythmicity of atrial muscle—if it is separated from the S-A node—is 40 to 60 times per minute, and that of ventricular muscle when separated from the remainder of the heart is about 15 to 30 times per minute. It is this basic rhythmicity of cardiac muscle that causes the intermittent pumping action of the heart.

Pacemaker Function of the S-A Node. Obviously a heart would be of less functional value if all of its parts beat at their own natural rates of rhythm than if all parts beat in unison. Fortunately, the portions of the heart that have slow rhythmicity are excited at a fast rate by impulses coming from the S-A node. For this reason the S-A node is said to be the normal *pacemaker* of the heart.

The pacemaker function of the S-A node is accomplished in the following manner: Every time the muscle fibers of the S-A node contract, an impulse is transmitted to the atrial muscle and from there into the ventricular muscle. Thus, contraction of the S-A node causes contraction of the entire heart. Then, long before either the atria or the ventricles can recover enough to contract spontaneously, another excitatory impulse arrives from the S-A node. Therefore, the other parts of the heart are never allowed to contract at their normal rates of rhythm.

Conduction of the Impulse Through the Heart— The Purkinje System. Cardiac muscle fibers are arranged in a functional *syncytium*—that is, the fibers interconnect with each other so that even a single impulse in a single fiber will spread over the entire muscle mass. However, the impulse is also conducted by specifically modified cardiac muscle fibers called *Purkinje fibers*. These conduct the impulse at a velocity of approximately 2 m. per second, which is four to six times the velocity in normal cardiac muscle. This rapid conduction allows all portions of the ventricular muscle to contract almost at the same time rather than one part contracting long ahead of another part; this in turn allows more forceful compression of the blood by the heart than would otherwise be true.

The *Purkinje system* begins in the S-A node and passes through the atria by way of several *internodal pathways* to the *A-V node,* which lies in the posterior wall of the right atrium near the tricuspid valve. From the A-V node a large bundle of Purkinje fibers called the *A-V bundle* or the *bundle of His* passes into the ventricular septum. Then the bundle divides into *left* and *right bundle branches,* which spread respectively around the endocardial surfaces of the left and right ventricles.

The atria and the ventricles are separated from each other by fibrous tissue everywhere except where the A-V bundle passes into the ventricles. Therefore, in the normal heart the only pathway by which an impulse can travel from the atria to the ventricles is through the A-V bundle.

Another very important feature of the Purkinje system is the *junctional fibers* that occur in the A-V node. These fibers are very small and have an extremely slow velocity of impulse transmission, on the order of one-tenth the velocity of transmission in normal cardiac muscle. This slow velocity allows a prolonged delay of the impulse so that *the atria contract 0.1 to 0.2 second ahead of the ventricles.* This allows the atria to pump blood into the ventricles before the ventricles begin their pumping cycle.

Heart Block. Occasionally, some pathologic condition destroys or damages the A-V bundle or A-V node so that impulses can no longer pass between the atria and the ventricles. When this happens, the atria continue to beat at the normal rate of the S-A node, while the ventricles establish their own rate of rhythm. Usually the Purkinje fibers in the A-V bundle or in one of the bundle branches of the ventricles becomes the *ventricular pacemaker,* because these fibers have a higher rate of rhythm than the muscle fibers of the ventricles. The natural rate of rhythm of the ventricles after heart block can be as little as 15 beats per minute or as high as 50 beats per minute. This condition is called *heart block.* Obviously, in heart block, the atrial contractions are not coordinated with the ventricular contractions, which prevents the ventricles from becoming as well filled before contraction as in the normal heart. This loss of atrial function impairs maximum heart pumping about 30 per cent; however, a person with heart block can continue to live for many years because the normal heart has tremendous reserve capacity for pumping blood.

The Circus Movement—Flutter and Fibrillation. Occasionally an impulse in the heart continues all the way around the heart, and, on arriving back at the starting point, reexcites the heart muscle to cause still another impulse to go around the heart, this process continuing around and around the heart indefinitely. This is called a *circus movement.* In the normal heart it does not occur for two reasons: First, normal cardiac muscle has a very long *refractory period,* usually about 0.25 second, which means that the muscle fiber cannot be reexcited during this time. Second, the impulse in the normal heart travels so rapidly that it will pass over the entire heart in far less than 0.25 second and therefore disappears before the heart muscle becomes reexcitable.

In the abnormal heart, however, the circus movement can occur in the following conditions: (1) Occasionally the refractory period of the cardiac muscle becomes much less than 0.25 second. (2) Sometimes the Purkinje system becomes destroyed so that the impulse takes a far longer period to travel through the ventricles. (3) Occasionally either the atria or the ventricles become greatly dilated so that the length of the pathway around the heart is greatly increased; this increases the time required for the impulse to travel around the heart. (4) Many times the impulse does not travel directly around the heart but instead travels in a zigzag direction, which lengthens the pathway sometimes to as much as ten times the direct distance around the heart; this obviously greatly prolongs the time for transmission of the impulse and can easily result in reexcitation of the cardiac muscle.

In the atria a regular circus movement around and around the atria causes *atrial flutter,* whereas zigzag impulses cause *atrial fibrillation.* The zigzag impulses in fibrillation also divide into multiple impulses so that there may be as many as five to ten impulses traveling in different directions at the same time. As a result, the atria remain partially contracted all the time, but they never contract rhythmically to provide any pumping action.

Flutter does not occur in the ventricles, but *ventricular fibrillation,* with many impulses of the zigzag variety spreading in all directions at once, is a very common cause of ventricular failure and death. An electric shock to the ventricles and ischemia of the ventricular muscle as a result of coronary thrombosis are very common initiating causes of ventricular fibrillation.

The principles of electrocardiography obviously cannot be presented in this chapter, but the normal electrocardiogram can be related to the rhythmic excitation process in the heart. The normal electrocardiogram consists of a *P wave,* which is caused by passage of the depolarization process throughout the atria; a *QRS complex of waves,* which is caused by passage of the depolarization process through the ventricles; and a *T wave,* which is caused by repolarization of the ventricles.

The PQ Interval. Normally, depolarization begins in the atria approximately 0.16 second before it begins in the ventricles. Therefore, the length of time between the beginning of the P wave and the Q wave, called the PQ interval (or PR interval when the Q wave is absent), is normally 0.16 second. Abnormally slow conduction of the impulse through the A-V bundle, as occurs when the bundle becomes ischemic following coronary thrombosis or inflamed in the acute phase of rheumatic fever, prolongs the PQ interval sometimes to as much as 0.30 to 0.50 second. The progress of rheumatic inflammation in the heart can be assessed by following the changes in the PQ interval. As the disease becomes worse, the PQ interval often increases; as it becomes better, the PQ interval often decreases back toward normal.

Abnormal QRS Waves. Since the QRS wave represents passage of the depolarization process through the ventricles, any condition that causes abnormal impulse transmission will alter the shape, the voltage or the duration of the QRS complex. For instance, hypertrophy of one ventricle will, on the average, cause increased voltage and is likely to increase preponderantly the R or the S wave, depending on the electrocardiographic lead and the ventricle affected. Also, damage to any portion of the Purkinje system will delay transmission of the impulse through the heart and therefore will cause an abnormal shape to the QRS complex as well as prolongation of the complex.

Abnormal T Wave. The T wave represents repolarization of the ventricular muscle. Many diseases damage the ventricular muscle just enough that it becomes difficult for the muscle to reestablish normal membrane potentials after each heart beat. As a result, certain of the ventricular fibers may continue to emit electrical current far longer than usual, which causes a bizarre pattern to the T wave or sometimes even inversion of the wave. Thus, an abnormal T wave ordinarily means mild to severe damage to at least a portion of the ventricular muscle.

Elevated or Depressed S-T Segment—Current of Injury. In an occasional electrocardiogram the segment between the S and the T waves is displaced either above or below the major axis of the electrocardiogram. This is caused by failure of some of the cardiac muscle fibers to repolarize between each two heart beats. As a result, between heart beats these fibers continue to emit large quantities of electrical current, called *current of injury,* that causes an elevated or depressed S-T segment. Therefore, when an elevated or depressed S-T segment is observed, one can be certain that at least some portion of the ventricular muscle has been severely damaged. This occurs very frequently following acute heart attacks.

Abnormal Rhythms.   One of the most important uses of the electrocardiogram is to diagnose abnormal cardiac rhythms. For instance, in *heart block* the P waves are completely dissociated from the QRS and T waves. In atrial fibrillation no true P wave can be discerned at all, but in its place are many fine noise like waves continuing indefinitely in the electrocardiogram. Finally, in extrasystoles of the heart, occasional QRST waves appear in the record at points completely out of rhythm with the remaining portions of the electrocardiogram.

Pumping Action of the Heart

Function of the Atria.   The heart is actually a four chamber pump; the right side of the heart pumps blood into the pulmonary circulation, and the left side pumps blood into the systemic circulation. The atria are "primer" pumps that pump their blood into the ventricles immediately before ventricular contraction, in this way enhancing the amount of blood pumped by the ventricles. The atria are not supplied with valves to prevent back flow of blood into the veins, and their pumping force is relatively slight, but fortunately only a minute amount of force is required to move blood into the ventricles.

Even when the atria fail to pump satisfactorily, as in atrial fibrillation or in heart block, blood still flows into the ventricles because the blood in the veins simply builds up a little higher pressure and forces its way on through the atria even without the advantage of the atrial pump. For this reason persons with nonfunctional atria can nevertheless live almost normal lives as long as they do not attempt to exercise strenuously.

Mechanics of Ventricular Pumping.   The ventricles are very strong pumps that are provided with inflow and outflow valves. During relaxation of the ventricles, their internal pressures are very low, which allows blood from the atria to push the A-V valves open and to flow into the ventricles. Then when the ventricles contract the intraventricular pressures immediately cause the A-V valves to close and the pulmonary and the aortic valves to open, and force most of the ventricular blood into the pulmonary and the systemic arterial systems. After another 0.3 second the ventricles relax, and the intraventricular pressures fall almost immediately back to zero. In the meantime the pulmonary artery and the aorta have become distended with excess blood; a minute portion of this rushes backward toward the ventricles, catches the vanes of the outflow valves, the pulmonary and the aortic valves, and closes them. As a result, the pressures in the arteries remain high even during the period between ventricular contractions.

The period of cardiac contraction is called *systole,* and the period of relaxation is called *diastole.*

Frank-Starling Law of the Heart.   When increased quantities of blood flow into the heart from the veins and distend its chambers, the stretched cardiac muscle automatically contracts with increased force. This increased force in turn pumps the extra blood on through the heart into the arterial system. This is called the *Frank-Starling law of the heart,* and it obviously allows the heart to adjust its pumping capability automatically to the amount of blood that needs to be pumped. This mechanism allows the heart to pump as much as two to three times the normal amount of blood even without increasing the rate of heart beat.

Nervous Control of the Heart.   The pumping action of the heart can also be altered by nervous control. Two types of nerve fibers supply the heart: *parasympathetic fibers,* which are carried in the vagus nerves, and *sympathetic fibers,* which are carried in the sympathetic nervous system. Stimulation of the sympathetic nerves increases the heart rate and also enhances the strength of the heart beat. Conversely, stimulation of the parasympathetics decreases the heart rate. In a normal person, the pumping action of the heart is regulated by both of these sets of nerves. To increase the degree of pumping action, the sympathetic nervous system is stimulated, while at the same time the normal impulses transmitted by the parasympathetic fibers are inhibited; these effects cause increased rate (up to 200 beats per minute) and strength of heart beat, which greatly enhance the overall pumping action. Conversely, during periods of rest the sympathetics become inhibited, and the parasympathetics again transmit a moderate number of impulses to the heart so that the degree of activity of the heart lessens.

This nervous control of the heart is an additional mechanism to the law of the heart to allow increased pumping action when increased quantities of cardiac output are required. For instance, in exercise these two mechanisms operate together to increase the cardiac output from the normal value of 5 liters per minute to as much as 20 to 25 liters—and in well trained athletes occasionally to as high as 30 to 40 liters per minute.

CIRCULATION

Dynamics of Blood Flow Through the Circulation

"Circuit" Concept of the Circulation. One of the most commonly forgotten features of the circulation is that it is a *complete circuit,* the same blood flowing again and again through the same vessels. Because of this, any alteration in blood flow in any single part of the circuit alters the flow in other parts. For instance, strong constriction of the arteries in the systemic circulation might well reduce the total cardiac output, in which case the blood flow through the lungs would be decreased equally as much as the flow through the systemic circulation. Another important feature of the circuit concept is that sudden constriction of a blood vessel must always be accompanied by an opposite dilatation of another part of the circulation, because the blood volume cannot change rapidly, and blood itself is incompressible. For instance, strong constriction of the veins in the systemic circulation displaces large quantities of blood into the heart, dilating the heart and causing it to pump with increased force. This is one of the mechanisms by which the cardiac output is regulated.

Distribution of Blood in the Circulation. Approximately 80 per cent of all the blood in the circulation is in the systemic circulatory system, approximately 10 per cent in the lungs and 10 per cent in the heart. About three-fourths of the blood is in the veins, about one-sixth in the arteries, and one-twelfth in the arterioles and the capillaries. It can be seen then that, even though it is the capillary blood that supplies nutrients to the tissues and exchanges gases in the lungs, only a minute portion of the total blood volume is in the capillaries at any one time.

Blood Pressure. This is the outward force of the blood against each unit area of the vessel wall. It is normally expressed in *millimeters of mercury* (mm. Hg). That is, if a vessel connected to a mercury manometer causes the mercury level to rise to a level of 100 mm., then the blood pressure is said to be 100 mm. Hg.

Blood Flow. This is the rate of movement of blood along the vessels, and it is usually expressed in *milliliters per minute* or *liters per minute.*

Resistance to Blood Flow. The viscous nature of blood causes it to flow only with difficulty through very small vessels, and the difficulty experienced by the movement of blood is called *resistance to blood flow.* The different factors that affect resistance are: (1) *the longer the length of the vessel the greater becomes the resistance;* (2) as the diameter of the vessel changes, the resistance changes in inverse proportion to the *fourth power of the diameter;* and (3) the *resistance increases directly in proportion to the viscosity* of the blood, which in turn is determined principally by the concentration of red cells in the blood.

Since changes in vessel diameter cause changes in resistance inversely proportional to the fourth power of the diameter, it is immediately obvious that even a minute change in diameter changes the resistance tremendously. Very small vessels in the circulation have a tremendous amount of resistance, while very large vessels have so little resistance that it can be disregarded. Thus, the only portions of the circulation that offer any significant amounts of resistance are the *very small arteries,* the *arterioles,* the *capillaries* and the *venules,* while the major arteries and the major veins normally offer almost no resistance (except where the veins are compressed by adjacent structures).

Relationship of Pressure, Flow and Resistance. When a blood vessel has a high pressure at one end and a low pressure at the other end, the rate of flow will be directly proportional to the *difference* in pressure between the two ends of the vessel, and it will be inversely proportional to the resistance to blood flow along the vessel. Thus the following formula applies:

$$\text{Blood Flow} = \frac{\text{Pressure Difference}}{\text{Resistance}}$$

Systemic Circulation

Mean Pressures in the Systemic Circulation. The left ventricle normally pumps about 5 liters of blood into the aorta each minute, and the mean aortic pressure is about 100 mm. Hg. The resistance to blood flow through the major arteries is so slight that the mean arterial pressure even in arteries as small as 3 mm. in diameter is still almost exactly 100 mm. Hg. Then the arteries become extremely small and lead into the *arterioles* where the resistance to blood flow is the greatest of any part of the systemic circulation. As a result, the mean pressure at the juncture of the arterioles and the capillaries averages only approximately 30 mm. Hg. The *capillaries* also contribute a moderate amount of resistance, causing the mean arterial pressure to fall another 20 mm. Hg to a level of 10 mm. at the juncture of the capillaries and the veins. The resistance in the venous system is relatively slight, the pressure falling only 10 mm. in the entire system. The pressure is approximately zero where the blood empties into the right atrium.

Pulsations in the Systemic Arteries. Blood is pumped by the heart in pulses, each beat of the heart normally ejecting approximately 70 ml. of blood; this is called the *stroke volume output.* As a result, the arteries become greatly distended during cardiac systole, and during diastole the excess blood stored in the arterial tree "runs off" through the systemic vessels to the veins. Thus, the aortic pressure rises to its highest point during systole and falls to its lowest point at the end of diastole. The high point and the low point are called, respectively, the *systolic* and the *diastolic pressures.* In the normal adult, the systolic pressure is approximately 120 mm. Hg and the diastolic pressure 80 mm. Hg. This is usually written 120/80.

The pulsatile pressure in the aorta causes approximately equally as great pulsations in the other major arteries of the systemic circulation, but in the very small arteries the intensity of pulsation progressively diminishes until very little occurs in the capillaries.

Regulation of Local Blood Flow by the Arterioles. In addition to having very large amounts of resistance, the arterioles are also capable of changing their resistance hundreds of times by increasing or decreasing their diameters. The arteriolar wall has an extremely strong smooth muscular coat in relation to the size of the vessel, and several different nervous and humoral stimuli can cause the arterioles to constrict so intensely that this can completely block all blood flow, while other stimuli can cause the arterioles to relax so completely that sometimes as much as 20 times normal amounts of blood are allowed to flow.

Autoregulation of Blood Flow in Each Tissue. In most tissues, blood flow in each local tissue area is *autoregulated,* which means that *the tissue itself regulates its own blood flow.* This obviously is very beneficial to the tissue because it allows the rate of delivery of oxygen and nutrients to the tissue to parallel the rate of activity.

The precise means by which autoregulation of local blood flow occurs is yet unknown. Many physiologists believe that active tissues release vasodilator substances such as *adenosine, carbon dioxide* and *potassium ions* into the surrounding fluids and that these in turn act on the arterioles to cause them to dilate. However, other experiments indicate that this regulation might be caused very simply in the following manner: When the tissues become very active, they rapidly utilize the available oxygen in the tissue fluids. This tends to decrease the amount of oxygen available for use by the smooth muscle cells of the arteriolar walls and therefore tends to decrease their strength of contraction. As a result, the arterioles dilate and allow adequate quantities of oxygen once more to become available to the tissues.

Nervous Regulation of Blood Flow. In essentially all areas of the body the sympathetic nerves secrete norepinephrine, and this causes vasoconstriction. Therefore, increased sympathetic stimulation causes decreased blood flow while decreased stimulation causes increased flow.

In general, nervous regulation of blood flow is concerned principally with changes in blood flow in large areas of the body at the same time. For instance, when a person becomes greatly overheated, skin vessels over the entire body become nervously dilated (vasodilation) to cause heat loss. Second, when a person exercises very strongly, the blood flow through the abdominal organs and the skin is decreased, thereby shifting the flow to the muscles. Third, when a person stands up, most of the blood vessels of the body are reflexly constricted, especially the veins. This offsets the tendency of blood to "pool" in the lower part of the body and therefore allows plenty of blood still to flow back to the heart and keep the cardiac output normal instead of falling as would otherwise occur.

Storage Function of the Veins. A reserve quantity of blood is stored in the circulatory system, especially in the veins, to be used in times of stress. Certain areas of the veins that store very large quantities of blood are called *blood reservoirs.* In order of importance these are (1) the *sinuses of the liver,* (2) the *major veins of the abdomen,* (3) the *veins of the pulmonary system,* (4) the *venous sinuses of the spleen* (the *pulp of the spleen* also stores concentrated red blood cells), and (5) the *subcutaneous venous plexuses.*

As much as one fourth of the total blood volume can usually be removed from a person without dire consequences because reflex nervous signals cause the veins to constrict, and blood continues to flow around the circulation almost normally. An interesting effect of the nerve signals is contraction of the spleen, for, on contracting, the spleen releases not only stored blood from its venous sinuses but also moderate amounts of concentrated red blood cells from its pulp. Thus, the spleen acts not only as a usual blood reservoir but also as a *blood cell reservoir.*

Special Areas of the Systemic Circulation

Muscle Circulation. During strenuous exercise the blood flow through a muscle can increase as much as 20-fold. This increase is caused almost entirely by *local regulation* in the muscle itself, the increased activity of the muscle automatically causing arteriolar dilation as described above.

Coronary Circulation. Blood flow through the myocardium obeys essentially the same principles as blood flow through the skeletal muscles. In general, coronary flow is controlled almost entirely by *local regulation* in the heart itself. The rate of blood flows parallels very closely the rate of oxygen consumption by the heart muscle, and it is believed that *low oxygen concentration* in the interstitial fluids of the heart muscle is in some way involved in the autoregulatory process; this was also discussed above as a possible mechanism of autoregulation throughout most of the body. Many physiologists believe that the low oxygen causes the tissues to release adenosine, and the adenosine in turn dilates the local blood vessels.

Normal coronary blood flow is about four per cent of the resting cardiac output. When the heart works very hard, the coronary blood flow increases as much as three to four fold.

Skin Circulation. The skin circulation is specifically geared for *control of body temperature.* When the body temperature rises above normal, nerve signals, as will be described later in the chapter, cause the blood vessels of the skin to dilate. This allows rapid flow of warm blood into the skin and therefore promotes loss of increased quantities of heat to the surroundings. Conversely, when the internal temperature of the body becomes too low, the skin vessels constrict, the skin becomes cold, and very little heat is lost.

Cerebral Circulation. The blood flow through the brain amounts to about 700 to 800 ml. per minute, and this remains very constant under almost all physiologic conditions. In general, blood flow through the brain is controlled almost entirely by *autoregulation.* It is believed that autoregulation occurs in the brain mainly in response to the *release of carbon dioxide* from the brain tissue, the carbon dioxide dilating the blood vessels in proportion to the amount that is released. This allows adequate blood flow to maintain an almost exact carbon dioxide concentration at all times in the interstitial fluids of the brain. Since neuronal function is highly dependent on changes in pH, and pH in turn is highly dependent on changes in carbon dioxide, this regulatory mechanism aids in the maintenance of normal cerebral activity. Decreased blood pH or oxygen concentration will also increase brain blood flow when either of these effects is severe.

Portal Circulation. Blood flows from the gastrointestinal tract and from the spleen into the *portal veins* and from these *through the liver* before emptying into the systemic veins. The liver vessels offer reasonable amounts of resistance to blood flow, which gives the portal circulatory system special characteristics of its own. Ordinarily, the portal venous pressure is about 8 mm. Hg because of the resistance to flow through the liver. However, in liver disease, such as *liver cirrhosis,* this resistance can increase so greatly that the portal venous pressure sometimes rises to as high as 20 to 30 mm. Hg. This causes the portal capillary pressure also to rise to a very high value, causing large quantities of fluid to leak out of the capillaries into the peritoneal cavity. Fortunately, if the blood flow through the liver becomes obstructed slowly, anastomotic channels can develop between the portal and the systemic veins. These especially occur through the esophageal veins, through the hemorrhoidal veins of the rectum and through posterior veins of the abdominal wall. Occasionally the veins of the esophagus and the hemorrhoidal veins become so enlarged that they rupture and cause serious bleeding, often causing death in the case of esophageal bleeding.

Pulmonary Circulation

Pulmonary Hemodynamics. Since the circulatory system is a circuit, the same amount of blood must flow through the lungs as through the entire systemic circulation. However, the *resistance to blood flow* through the lungs is only about one-ninth that in the systemic circulation, and the pressures are correspondingly smaller. The *pulmonary arterial systolic pressure* averages 22 mm. Hg, and the *diastolic pressure* averages 8 mm. Hg. The *mean pulmonary arterial pressure* averages 13 mm. Hg, and the *left atrial pressure* averages 2 mm. Hg, giving a total pressure drop through the pulmonary circulation of only 11 mm. Hg. The *pulmonary capillary pressure* is approximately 6 to 8 mm. Hg, which is only a few millimeters greater than the left atrial pressure. This low capillary pressure is very important in keeping the alveoli dry, which will be discussed below.

Effect of Blood Flow on Pulmonary Resistance. During strenuous exercise, and in other states of physiologic stress, the cardiac output sometimes increases to as much as four to five times normal, and in doing so the blood flow through the lungs also increases by this amount. However, the pulmonary arterial pressure hardly rises for the following reason: As the flow increases, many normally closed pulmonary capillaries open up, and those that are already open dilate more than ever. As a result, the pulmonary resistance decreases almost as much as the flow increases. Therefore, the mean pulmonary arterial pressure usually rises from 13 mm. Hg to only 15 to 20 mm. Hg when the cardiac output increases to as much as three to four times normal.

Shift of Blood From the Systemic Circulation to the Pulmonary Circulation. Approximately 10 per cent of all the blood in the circulatory system is normally in the lungs, and about 80 per cent is in the systemic circulation, the remainder being in the heart. Thus, there is approximately an eightfold difference in the amount of blood normally in the systemic circulation and in the lungs. However, the amounts of blood in the two circulations can change considerably when one side of the heart fails. *If the right heart* *fails,* as much as 50 per cent of the pulmonary blood can be displaced into the systemic circulation. Conversely, *if the left heart fails,* then a large portion of the systemic blood can be displaced into the lungs, sometimes increasing the pulmonary blood volume to as much as 100 percent above normal.

Another cause of excessive shift of blood into the lungs is *intense sympathetic stimulation* of the circulation. This constricts mainly the systemic circulation without significantly constricting the pulmonary circulation because the sympathetic nerve supply to the pulmonary vessels is extremely sparse. As a result, large quantities of blood are forced into the right atrium and the lungs to increase cardiac output and sometimes causing severe acute pulmonary edema.

Capillary Dynamics in the Lungs—the Basis of Dry Alveoli.   The normal pulmonary capillary pressure is approximately 7 mm. Hg, while the normal colloid osmotic pressure of the plasma is 28 mm. Hg. Thus, the pressure tending to force fluid out of the pores of the capillaries is only 7 mm. Hg, while that tending to cause absorption of fluid into the capillaries is 28 mm. Hg. Therefore, there is a large excess of "absorption pressure" at the pulmonary membrane, which causes any fluid that enters the alveoli to be absorbed, thus keeping the alveoli dry.

Pulmonary Edema.   Whenever excess blood shifts into the lungs as a result of failure of the left heart to pump adequately or as a result of excessive constriction of the systemic circulation, all of the pressures throughout the lungs, including the capillary pressure, rise very high. *As long as the capillary pressure remains less than a critical level, usually about* 30 mm. Hg, *the alveoli of the lungs will remain dry,* but, just as soon as the capillary pressure rises even slightly above the colloid osmotic pressure, large quantities of fluid immediately begin to filter out of the capillaries into the interstitial fluid and in severe conditions also through the alveolar membranes into the alveoli. This condition is *pulmonary edema.* If the pulmonary capillary pressure rises acutely to about 50 mm. Hg, sufficient pulmonary edema can develop in 20 minutes to cause death, and if the pulmonary capillary pressure rises acutely to only 30 mm. Hg, sufficient pulmonary edema can still develop in 3 to 6 hours to cause death. However, in chronic conditions such as mitral stenosis, the pulmonary capillary pressure can remain as high as 40 mm. Hg for long periods of time without causing pulmonary edema, probably because very large lymphatic vessels develop in the lungs and provide extra drainage of fluid from the lung tissues.

Regulation of the Mean Systemic Arterial Pressure.   Among the most important of all the control systems of the entire body are those that regulate the mean arterial pressure. The normal mean arterial pressure under resting conditions is approximately 100 mm. Hg, which is the force that causes blood to flow through the systemic circulation. During strenuous exercise and during other types of physiologic stress, the mean pressure can rise to as high as 150 to 200 mm. Hg in the normal person. In hypertension, the pressure remains elevated indefinitely.

There are two basic mechanisms for regulating mean arterial pressure: (1) the renal mechanism, and (2) the cardiovascular nervous reflex mechanism.

Renal Mechanism for Regulation of Mean Arterial Pressure.   When the mean arterial pressure falls too low in the kidneys, gradually over a period of several days the kidneys cause a reaction in the circulatory system to raise the mean systemic arterial pressure. Conversely, if the mean arterial pressure rises too high in the renal arteries, the kidneys cause reverse effects on the circulation to lower the arterial pressure back to a normal level. For instance, if a person is bled a considerable amount so that his arterial pressure falls very low, the renal mechanism begins immediately to bring the arterial pressure back to normal. Conversely, if excess fluids are injected into the circulatory system, elevating the arterial pressure even slightly, the renal mechanism immediately begins to reduce the arterial pressure back toward normal once again.

Many different mechanisms have been suggested to explain the mechanism by which the kidneys might regulate mean arterial pressure. Two of these that have received the most attention are the *renin mechanism* and the *renal-body fluid volume feedback mechanism.*

In the *renin mechanism,* the kidney secretes the enzyme *renin* when arterial pressure falls below normal. The renin in turn reacts with plasma proteins to form a substance called *angiotensin I.* This substance in turn is converted, mainly in the lungs, to *angiotensin II* by a lung enzyme called *converting enzyme.* The angiotensin II then causes vasoconstriction throughout the body; this increases the total peripheral resistance and also elevates the arterial pressure back toward normal.

Angiotensin II also has two other effects that play important roles in long-term pressure regulation: (1) It has a direct effect on the kidneys to cause sodium and water retention in the body. (2) It causes increased aldosterone secretion, and this, too, causes sodium and water retention. The resulting increase in body fluid helps to raise the arterial pressure.

The most important *long-term* mechanism for regulation of arterial pressure is the *renal-body fluid volume feedback mechanism.* When the arterial pressure rises too high, the kidneys excrete greatly increased quantities of both water and salt. As a result, the extracellular fluid volume and the blood volume both decrease, and they continue to decrease until the arterial pressure falls back to normal. Conversely, when the arterial pressure falls too low, the kidneys stop excreting water and salt, and, over a period of hours to days, the person drinks enough water and eats enough salt to build his blood volume back up to normal, thus also returning the arterial pressure to normal.

This renal-body fluid volume mechanism for control of arterial pressure is slow to act, sometimes requiring several days or perhaps as long as a week or more to come to equilibrium. Therefore, it is not of major significance in acute control of arterial pressure. On the other hand, it is by far the most potent of all arterial pressure controllers for long-term control of arterial pressure. It is almost invariably involved in one way or another, either as a result of kidney damage or as a result of external factors altering kidney function, in the causation of hypertension.

Regulation of Mean Arterial Pressure by Cardiovascular Nervous Reflexes. Several different nervous reflexes help to regulate the mean arterial pressure. The three most important of these are (1) the baroreceptor reflex, (2) the reflex response of arterial pressure to carbon dioxide, and (3) the reflex response of arterial pressure to cerebral ischemia.

The *baroreceptor system* operates as follows: In the walls of the carotid arteries, of the aorta and to a less extent of some of the other major arteries of the upper part of the body are many small stretch receptors called *baroreceptors*. When the pressure becomes excessively high in these arteries, these receptors are stimulated, and impulses are transmitted to the brain to inhibit the sympathetic nervous system. As a result, the normal sympathetic impulses throughout the body are reduced, causing the strength of the heart beat to decrease along with a simultaneous decrease in resistance in the peripheral vessels, both of which reduce the arterial pressure back toward normal. Conversely, a fall in arterial pressure decreases the number of impulses transmitted by the baroreceptors; then these no longer inhibit the sympathetic nervous system so that it becomes very active, which causes the arterial pressure to increase back toward normal.

An increase in carbon dioxide in the blood automatically increases the mean arterial pressure by *exciting the neurons of the vasomotor center* in the brain stem, resulting in strong sympathetic stimulation throughout the body. This mechanism helps to ensure adequate arterial pressure during stressful conditions, for almost all types of physical stress to the body increase the basal level of metabolism and the production of carbon dioxide.

Cerebral ischemia—lack of adequate blood flow to the brain—also causes the arterial pressure to rise.

In ischemia the *vasomotor center* in the brain stem automatically becomes highly excited, probably because of failure of the blood to carry carbon dioxide out of the vasomotor center rapidly enough. As a result, strong sympathetic stimulation throughout the body immediately elevates the arterial pressure; this in turn increases the cerebral blood flow back toward normal and helps to relieve the ischemia.

Relative Importance of the Renal-Body Fluid Volume and the Nervous Mechanisms in Regulating Mean Systemic Arterial Pressure. The renal-body fluid volume mechanism for regulating mean arterial pressure is slow to act, but it is a very powerful mechanism when it does act, having the capability of controlling the blood pressure to an extremely exact level. The cardiovascular reflexes, on the other hand, are of major importance for rapid control of arterial pressure such as (1) raising the pressure when a person stands after having been in a lying position, (2) resisting a fall in arterial pressure when a person bleeds severely, or (3) increasing the arterial pressure in times of physical stress such as during strenuous exercise. However, the cardiovascular reflexes are probably not of great importance in regulating arterial pressure from week to week, month to month or year to year. This is principally the function of the kidneys.

Hypertension

Hypertension is a disease characterized by *excessively high mean systemic arterial pressure,* and a person is usually considered to be hypertensive if the arterial pressure is greater than 140/90 mm. Hg. Approximately one-fifth of all persons develop hypertension before death, and approximately one-tenth die as a result of some secondary effect of hypertension. Yet, despite this great incidence of hypertension in the population, its cause in most cases is yet unknown. This type of hypertension is called *essential hypertension.* In the remaining cases the cause is usually renal disease or a hormonal disease that affects one of the pressure regulatory systems. These types of hypertension can be described as follows:

Renal Hypertension. Any condition that reduces the ability of the kidneys to excrete water and salt will usually cause hypertension. Such conditions include pyelonephritis, glomerulonephritis, polycystic kidney disease, amyloidosis, arteriosclerotic renal vascular disease and many other types of renal disease.

The type of kidney debility most likely to decrease water and salt excretion is pretubular damage to the kidney, such as constriction of the arteries to the kidneys, constriction of the afferent arterioles or increased resistance to fluid filtration through the glomerular membrane. All of these factors decrease the ability of the kidneys to form glomerular filtrate, which in turn causes fluid and electrolyte retention and thereby increases the blood volume until the arterial pressure rises to a hypertensive level. Once the pressure has risen, normal amounts of glomerular filtrate are once again formed, and the excretory function of the kidneys returns entirely to normal unless there is some simultaneous damage to the tubules.

The amount of increase in blood volume required to cause renal hypertension is probably less than 4 per cent, which is generally an unmeasurable quantity. However, the acute arterial pressure control mechanisms, especially the baroreceptor mechanism, oppose rapid changes in arterial pressure caused by alterations in blood volume. Therefore, an increase in blood volume that elicits hypertension will not cause the arterial pressure to rise instantaneously but instead to rise slowly over days to weeks. Even when hypertension is associated with increased blood volume, the cardiac output normally rises only during the onset of the hypertension. The increase in output causes excess blood flow to the tissues, and the arterioles in the tissues then, as a result, automatically constrict, a process called autoregulation. The cardiac output returns to normal while the total peripheral resistance becomes very high.

Ischemia of the kidney can also increase the arterial pressure by causing excess formation of renin, the renin in turn causing formation of angiotensin II in the blood. The angiotensin constricts the arterioles and thereby increases the arterial pressure. This effect occurs especially in malignant hypertension, but not to a significant extent in the great majority of usual essential hypertensive patients. It also occurs in hypertension caused by unilateral renal arterial disease when the renal ischemia fails to be relieved by the high pressure.

Hormonal Hypertension. Oversecretion of certain of the hormones, especially the *adrenal medullary hormones* and the *adrenocortical hormones,* can cause hypertension. For instance, a tumor of the adrenal medulla called a *pheochromocytoma* occasionally secretes large quantities of *norepinephrine* and *epinephrine.* These two substances have almost exactly the same effect on the circulatory system as stimulation of the entire sympathetic nervous system, thereby elevating the arterial pressure. Occasionally, also, either a tumor of the adrenal cortex or hyperplastic adrenal cortices secrete excessive quantities of cortical hormones. Certain of these, especially *aldosterone,* cause the kidneys to reabsorb large amounts of sodium and water from the tubules. The sodium and the water, in turn, lead to increased blood volume, which elevates the arterial pressure.

Essential Hypertension. Now that we have considered the two major categories of known types of hypertension we need to examine for a moment the possible cause of essential hypertension. Thus far, neither of the above two types of hypertension has definitely been proved to be the same as the essential hypertension that afflicts most of the patients. However, recent studies in patients who developed hypertension slowly over many years showed progressive sclerosis of the renal glomeruli. This obviously could decrease filtration of fluid into the tubules and could result in elevated arterial pressure, as described in the previous few pages.

Another widely believed mechanism of essential hypertension is one in which the sympathetic nervous system is excessively active and causes hypertension by constricting the blood vessels throughout the body, including those of the kidneys to prevent an increase in fluid loss when the hypertension occurs.

Regulation of Cardiac Output

The normal cardiac output in the adult is approximately 5 liters per minute, but this often increases to about four to five times this value during strenuous exercise. In general, the cardiac output is regulated in proportion to the need for blood flow through all the tissues of the body. That is, each respective tissue controls its own blood flow by *autoregulation,* which was discussed earlier in the chapter, and the cardiac output is then regulated to supply the required blood flow. This regulation is effected in two different ways: (1) by changing the *pumping ability of the heart* and (2) by changing the rate of blood flow into the heart from the systemic vessels, which is called *venous return.*

Regulation of the Pumping Action of the Heart. Earlier in the chapter it was pointed out that there are two major means by which the pumping action of the heart is regulated. One of these is the *Frank–Starling law of the heart,* and the other is *nervous regulation.*

In general, it can be said that, as a result of the combination of the above two mechanisms, the heart *under normal physiologic conditions* always pumps all the blood that flows into it without any hesitation. Therefore, *in normal physiologic states it is not the pumping action of the heart that determines cardiac output, but it is the venous return to the heart that determines the output.*

Regulation of Venous Return. Venous return is regulated by three major factors: (1) the average pressure of all the blood in the systemic circulation, called the *mean systemic pressure,* (2) the *right atrial pressure,* and (3) the *resistance to flow of the blood* through the systemic vessels.

In the *normal* circulatory system, the *right atrial pressure* is *not* one of the significant factors regulating venous return because, as pointed out above, the heart normally pumps all of the blood that comes into it and therefore maintains a right atrial pressure that is essentially zero. For this reason, the other two factors, the mean systemic pressure and the resistance to blood flow through the vessels, are the major controllers of venous return.

The *mean systemic pressure* is the "algebraic" average of all the pressures in the systemic circulation, and this amounts to approximately 7 mm. Hg in the normal animal. It is this low because by far the major portion of the blood is in the veins where the pressure is low rather than in the arteries where the pressure is high. The factors that can increase the mean systemic pressure are *increased blood volume* and *sympathetic stimulation of the blood vessels to cause constriction.* Therefore, both of these increase the return of blood toward the heart. Sympathetic stimulation of the veins is particularly important because by far the major portion of the blood is stored in the veins. When the veins constrict, large quantities of blood are forced into the heart, thus distending the heart chambers and increasing the cardiac output.

When the *resistance to blood flow* decreases, blood can then flow from the systemic vessels toward the heart with greater than normal ease, thus increasing the venous return. This is one of the principal means by which venous return is regulated, for *when the tissues become active, their blood vessels automatically dilate. Consequently, the venous return becomes increased, the cardiac output increases, and an adequate amount of blood flow is automatically made available to the active tissues.*

Regulation of Venous Pressure. The venous pressure is regulated mainly by the same two factors that regulate cardiac output—the *ability of the heart to pump blood* and the *venous return to the heart.* Normally the heart is capable of pumping all of the blood that returns to it and therefore keeps the right atrial pressure at essentially zero. However, if the heart becomes weak, or if the venous return to the heart becomes so much greater than normal that the heart cannot pump it all, blood begins to dam up in the right atrium, and the right atrial pressure rises. This occurs to a marked extent in cardiac failure, which will be discussed below. Thus, it is the balance between pumping by the heart and venous return that determines the right atrial pressure.

The right atrial pressure in turn is a major determinant of peripheral venous pressure, because the greater the right atrial pressure, the greater must the peripheral venous pressure be to keep the blood flowing toward the heart. Ordinarily the right atrial pressure must rise to about 5 to 6 mm. Hg above normal before significant distention of the peripheral veins begins to occur.

The Venous Pump. In the standing position blood does not flow with ease uphill through the veins. However, the veins are provided with valves, and when the surrounding muscles intermittently contract and compress the veins, this effect acts as a pump to keep the blood flowing toward the heart. This mechanism is called the *venous pump.* However, if a person stands completely still so that his veins are not intermittently compressed, or if the valves in his veins have become destroyed, as occurs in varicose veins, then the venous pump is no longer effective. Under these conditions the weight of the blood in the veins makes the venous pressure in the foot of standing person as high as 75 to 90 mm. Hg.

Physiology of Heart Failure

Coronary Thrombosis and Coronary Sclerosis. The usual cause of heart failure is diminished coronary blood flow to the heart muscle, which causes ischemia of the muscle and heart weakness or even destruction of portions of the heart. The most common cause of coronary insufficiency is *coronary atherosclerosis,* which occurs in everyone in old age. This means, simply, fatty–fibrotic lesions of the coronary vessels, causing progressive, usually localized constriction. However, in a large number of persons another condition, *coronary thrombosis,* occurs acutely as a result of a blood clot in a coronary artery, resulting in the well-known "heart attack." Both coronary atherosclerosis and coronary thrombosis normally result from *atheromata,* which means infiltration of the coronary wall with cholesterol and other fatty substances. The deposits of cholesterol form nidi for the growth of fibrous tissue and thereby cause sclerosis, or occasionally the cholesterol protrudes through the intima into the lumen of the vessel and causes a blood clot to form, thereby occluding the vessel and resulting in a heart attack.

Low Cardiac Output Failure. The immediate effect of a heart attack is usually greatly diminished pumping ability of the heart itself, which causes blood to dam up in one or both atria and the cardiac output to fall below normal. A person can live with a cardiac output as low as about one-half normal for many hours, but, if it falls below this level, he usually will die.

Nervous Compensations in Heart Failure. Immediately after an acute heart attack, the fall in cardiac output and the resulting fall in systemic arterial pressure initiate intense cardiovascular reflexes that strongly excite the sympathetic nervous system. The sympathetic impulses in turn help in two ways to compensate for the diminished pumping ability of the heart: First, the strength of contraction of the nondamaged portion of the heart is increased. Second, the sympathetic impulses increase the vasomotor tone throughout the systemic circulation, which results in increased venous return of blood to the heart. As a result of these two effects, the cardiac output is often returned either to normal or almost to normal within a few minutes after a mild or even moderate heart attack, and the person will often experience nothing more than a transient period of fainting. In most severe heart attacks, however, the nervous compensations are unable to return the cardiac output to normal, but, nevertheless, do return the output part way toward normal and thereby help to prevent death of the patient.

Fluid Retention in Heart Failure. Immediately after an acute heart attack, the output of urine by the kidneys usually decreases very greatly for three reasons: (1) Sympathetic reflexes cause intense afferent arteriolar constriction in the kidneys, thereby greatly reducing the glomerular filtration rate. (2) The low cardiac output tends to reduce the arterial pressure, and this too reduces the glomerular filtration rate. (3) When the cardiac output falls very low, the kidneys secrete large amounts of renin, and large amounts of angiotensin II therefore are also formed. This in turn causes the kidneys to retain fluid by a direct effect of angiotensin on the kidneys and also indirectly by stimulating aldosterone secretion, which then also acts on the kidneys to reduce fluid excretion. Consequently, in severe acute cardiac failure a person may become completely *anuric,* while in milder degrees of acute failure, he usually becomes *oliguric.*

Obviously, the retention of fluid by the kidneys increases the total volume of extracellular fluid, most of which leaks out of the capillaries into the interstitial spaces and causes at times very serious *edema.* However, a small amount remains in the blood and increases the blood volume.

Value of Fluid Retention. Most physicians have long considered fluid retention in heart failure to be a detrimental factor. However, experiments in animals indicate that moderate degrees of fluid retention are beneficial to the patient because the increase in blood and interstitial fluid volumes promotes increased return of blood to the heart, primes the heart better than usual and therefore allows increased pumping. Beyond a certain degree of priming, though, the heart can become overstretched; then, further retention of fluid becomes detrimental to heart function. Also, excessive fluid retention can cause pulmonary edema and death.

Left Heart Failure Versus Right Heart Failure. Since the heart is actually two separate pumps, it is obvious that one side of the heart can fail independently of the other. More often the left heart fails because most coronary thromboses affect principally the left ventricle. However, right heart failure frequently occurs in patients who have pulmonary hypertension or in patients with certain types of congenital heart defects.

Most of the differences between left heart failure and right heart failure are obvious. Left heart failure causes excessive shift of fluid into the lungs with resulting pulmonary edema, while right heart failure causes excessive shift of blood into the systemic circulation.

In right heart failure, so little blood is available in the lungs to shift into the systemic system that only a small amount of *venous congestion* occurs immediately in the systemic circulation. Indeed, *peripheral edema* does not occur at all immediately after *acute* right heart failure but instead must await retention of fluid by the kidneys.

On the other hand, in acute left heart failure the shift of blood into the lungs can be tremendous, and such severe *pulmonary edema* often occurs within a matter of minutes that it kills the person. Yet, sometimes the pulmonary capillary pressure rises only a moderate amount immediately after the failure, not enough to cause significant edema. But during the ensuing few days, as the kidneys retain fluid, the pulmonary capillary pressure rises still higher, and severe pulmonary edema then develops, causing a respiratory death.

Physiology of Valvular Heart Disease

In the past, before present-day therapy, much valvular disease of the heart was caused by *rheumatic fever,* which leads to partial or total destruction of the valves. Damage occurs most frequently in the mitral valve, almost as frequently in the aortic valve, and only rarely in the tricuspid and the pulmonary valves. Sometimes the damaged vanes of the valves fail to close, which results in *regurgitation* or *insufficiency.* At other times fibrosis of the valves greatly reduces the size of the valvular opening, which is called *stenosis.* In either instance, the function of the affected ventricle is greatly compromised. Consequently, rheumatic valvular heart disease usually causes the left heart to become a very poor pump, while the right heart remains essentially normal. As discussed above, this condition often causes excessive damming of blood in the lungs, resulting in pulmonary edema and eventually a respiratory death.

A particular feature of valvular heart disease is the rapidity with which pulmonary edema sometimes occurs following exercise. In the resting state the pulmonary capillary pressure may remain slightly below the critical level at which pulmonary edema develops. But, when the person exercises, the venous return to the right heart becomes greatly increased, thus resulting in further shift of blood into the lungs, with rapid development of edema.

Physiology of Congenital Heart Abnormalities

In many congenital heart abnormalities an abnormal opening exists somewhere between the pulmonary and the systemic arterial systems that allows much of the blood to bypass either the lungs or the systemic circulation; the condition is called a *right-to-left shunt* when the lungs are bypassed. When the blood bypasses the systemic circulation, it is called a *left-to-right shunt.*

A typical *right-to-left shunt* occurs in *tetralogy of Fallot* in which the principal defects are (1) an interventricular septal defect, (2) shift of the aorta to the right, its opening usually lying directly over the septal defect so that blood can flow into it from either the right or the left ventricle, (3) a greatly constricted pulmonary artery so that little blood will flow into the pulmonary system, and (4) hypertrophy of the right ventricle. In this condition the right ventricle pumps only small quantities of blood into the lungs but large quantities directly into the aorta. Thus, most of the systemic blood returning to the heart bypasses the lungs and reenters the systemic circulation without becoming aerated. The distinguishing physiologic abnormality of a right-to-left shunt, therefore, is poor aeration of the blood, and the person's skin always remains *cyanotic.*

A typical *left-to-right shunt* is a *patent ductus arteriosus,* in which the ductus arteriosus, an important blood vessel between the aorta and the pulmonary artery in fetal life, remains patent after birth of the baby. Another typical left-to-right shunt is an *interventricular septal defect.* In both of these conditions blood flows from the high pressure aorta or left ventricle into the low pressure pulmonary artery or right ventricle. As a result, the blood pumped by the left heart is forced immediately back into the pulmonary arterial system and traverses the lungs a second time and sometimes a third time before finally being pumped through the systemic circulation. Obviously, the blood that does eventually get to the systemic circulation is usually well aerated. Yet, this abnormal flow of blood around and around through the lungs markedly increases the work load of the heart, and, as a consequence, the heart is likely to fail at an early age. Also, the excess flow through the lungs often leads to progressive fibrosis of the lungs so that pulmonary debility sometimes leads to an early death.

CIRCULATORY SHOCK

Circulatory shock is a condition in which the cardiac output is so greatly reduced that tissues throughout the body begin to deteriorate. Any circulatory abnormality that greatly reduces the cardiac output can cause circulatory shock. There are three major classifications of shock: (1) *cardiac shock,* (2) *hypovolemic shock,* and (3) *neurogenic shock.*

Cardiac Shock. This occurs most frequently in acute heart failure, in which the cardiac output often falls very low for many hours at a time. This was described above in the discussion of low cardiac output failure.

Hypovolemic Shock. This means shock resulting from greatly reduced blood volume, and this in turn can be caused by (1) blood loss, (2) plasma loss, or (3) dehydration. Obviously, hypovolemia causes shock by decreasing the venous return to the heart.

Neurogenic Shock. This is circulatory shock that results from sudden inhibition of the sympathetic nervous system throughout the body. This allows all of the systemic vessels to dilate and the blood to "pool" in the lower part of the body rather than returning to the heart. If a person with loss of sympathetic tone is kept in a standing position, this can actually kill him, but, if he is placed in a horizontal position, sufficient blood will usually still flow back to the heart to allow survival.

The Progressive Nature of Shock. One of the essential features of true circulatory shock is that it creates a vicious cycle that tends to make the shock itself worse. That is, the shock causes very poor blood flow to different tissues of the body, including the tissues of the heart and the vascular system; this causes deterioration of the heart and the vessels; the cardiac output falls still more; the tissues deteriorate more; and the vicious cycle recycles again and again. Unless the cardiovascular reflexes and other compensatory mechanisms in the body overcome this progressive tendency of shock or unless therapy is instituted, the progression continues until death.

The progressive nature of shock is often very apparent in cardiac shock, for in this condition the heart is already greatly damaged. The decreased cardiac output results in further diminished coronary blood flow that makes the heart even weaker, thus initiating a very rapid vicious cycle of cardiac deterioration. For this reason, therapy must be instituted immediately in most cases of cardiac shock to prevent death.

Irreversible Shock. Another distinguishing characteristic of shock is that, beyond a certain stage in the progressive deterioration, any amount of therapy becomes ineffective in preventing death of the patient.

This is called the *irreversible stage of shock*. Often different types of therapy, such as blood transfusion or administration of norepinephrine, will actually return the arterial pressure to normal or above normal. Yet, after another 10 to 30 minutes the pressure begins to fall again, and any amount of therapy fails to keep this from proceeding on to death. When the circulatory organs have deteriorated beyond a certain degree, even though temporary measures can return the blood pressure and cardiac output to normal for a few minutes, the tissues themselves cannot recover rapidly enough to prevent subsequent death.

Circulatory Arrest

During many surgical operations, the heart arrests or fibrillates; also, since the advent of cardiac surgery, the heart is often stopped purposely. Ordinarily a person's body can stand about 3 minutes of complete *circulatory arrest* without any permanent damage whatsoever, but beyond 3 minutes, blood clots begin to develop in many of the peripheral vessels. With adequate preliminary anticoagulation procedures, circulatory arrest can be continued in an animal for as long as 10 to 20 minutes without serious damage to the body. Without this preliminary treatment, such extensive blood coagulation usually occurs in the vessels of the brain that permanent cerebral damage or death almost always ensues if the circulation remains arrested longer than 5 to 8 minutes.

RESPIRATORY SYSTEM

Ventilation of the Lungs

Lungs and Thoracic Cage. No muscles are attached directly to the lungs to cause them to inflate and deflate. Instead, the lungs float freely in the *thoracic cage* and anytime the thoracic cage enlarges or contracts, simultaneous changes in lung volume must also occur. The space between the visceral pleura of the lungs and the parietal pleura of the thoracic cage is called the *intrapleural space*. Normally, continuous absorption of fluid by the visceral pleura keeps the space almost entirely empty except for a few milliliters of viscid material that provides lubrication for the moving lungs.

If ever the intrapleural space is opened to the atmosphere, the lungs immediately collapse because the lungs themselves are highly elastic. This elasticity results from (1) elastic fibers in the lung tissue that extend in all directions and (2) surface tension of the fluid lining the alveoli; the surface of the fluid tends to contract because of intermolecular attraction between the water molecules. This factor is about three times as potent in causing lung collapse as are the elastic fibers.

Surface-Active Substance (Surfactant) in the Alveoli. If the alveoli were lined with water, the surface tension would be so great along the walls of the alveoli that they would remain collapsed all of the time. Fortunately, a substance called *surface-active substance or surfactant* is secreted into the fluids of the alveoli by the respiratory epithelium. This substance acts to decrease the surface tension of the fluids, which allows normal expansion of the lungs. Some newborn babies fail to secrete adequate quantities of surfactant, and therefore cannot expand their lungs normally; this sometimes leads to death.

Lack of surfactant also causes the development of pulmonary edema, when excess surface tension in the alveoli creates a powerful force to pull fluid into the alveoli from the interstitium.

Expansion of the Lungs. The lungs can be expanded in two ways, either by increasing the length of the thoracic cage or by increasing its thickness. The *diaphragm* is the main muscle that increases the length of the thoracic cage; all the muscles of the thorax and the neck that pull the chest cage upward increase the chest thickness, because the ribs normally hang downward, but on being pulled upward extend almost straight forward.

The major muscles of expiration are the *abdominal* muscles. These contract around the abdominal viscera, forcing them upward against the diaphragm. Also, some of the abdominal muscles pull downward on the ribs, which reduces the anteroposterior diameter of the thorax.

Tidal Air and Minute Respiratory Volume. The amount of air taken in and expelled with each breath is called the *tidal air*. This is normally about 500 ml. The *minute respiratory volume* is the sum of all the tidal air breathed during a minute. Since the normal respiratory rate is around 12 breaths per minute, the normal minute respiratory volume is about 6,000 ml.

Vital Capacity and Maximum Rate of Pulmonary Ventilation. The maximum amount of air that a person can expire after initially taking the deepest possible breath is called the *vital capacity*. In a normal male this is about 4.5 liters, and in a normal female about 3.5 liters. Thus, the vital capacity is about eight times the normal tidal air, which illustrates that there is a tremendous amount of *pulmonary reserve*. This reserve is even further enhanced by the ability of a person to breathe far more rapidly than the normal 12 breaths per minute. When a person breathes as rapidly and as deeply as he can, he can sustain for long periods a minute respiratory volume as high as 120 liters per minute and for a short time as high as 175 liters per minute. Therefore, a person can breathe about 20 to

30 times as much air per minute under stressful conditions as he breathes normally.

Dead Space and Alveolar Ventilation. Each time a person breathes air into his respiratory system, part of the new air must be used to fill the passageways between the nose and the alveloi. Since this portion of the air does not come in contact with the pulmonary membranes that aerate the blood, it is called *dead space air.* The dead space of the normal respiratory system is about 150 ml. Thus, with each normal tidal volume of air, 150 out of the 500 ml. fails to reach the alveoli and therefore is not available to aerate the blood. That portion of the air that does reach the alveoli is called the *alveolar ventilatory air,* and it normally amounts to about 350 ml. with each breath. With a normal respiratory rate of 12 per minute this amounts to an *alveolar ventilation* of 4.2 liters per minute.

Functional Residual Capacity. At the end of each normal expiration, approximately 2,300 ml. of air still remain in the lungs; this is called the *functional residual capacity.* And, even after the most forceful possible expiration, about 1,200 ml. still remain, which is called the *residual volume.* The air that remains in the lungs from breath to breath has a very important function: It keeps aerating the blood in the pulmonary capillaries even during expiration. Therefore, it prevents extensive rise and fall of blood oxygen and carbon dioxide concentrations during the respiratory cycle.

With a normal alveolar ventilatory air of only 350 ml. per breath and a normal functional residual volume of 2,300 ml., only about one seventh of the air in the lungs is exchanged with the atmosphere in each breath. If some foreign gas is placed in the alveoli, normal respiration will remove only half of this gas in a period of 17 seconds. Thus, it is a very false notion that the air of the lungs is completely replaced with each breath.

Alveolar Air

Concentration of the Alveolar Gases. The *alveolar air* normally contains major amounts of four different gases: *nitrogen, oxygen, carbon dioxide* and *water vapor.* The relative concentrations of these are nitrogen, 74 per cent; oxygen, 14 per cent; carbon dioxide, 6 per cent; and water vapor, 6 per cent. Thus, the amount of oxygen in the alveolar air is only 14 per cent in comparison with approximately 20 per cent in normal air. This difference is caused mainly by rapid absorption of oxygen from the alveoli into the blood. Also, alveolar air contains approximately 6 per cent carbon dioxide, while normal air contains almost no carbon dioxide. This high concentration of carbon dioxide is caused by continual excretion of carbon dioxide from the blood into the alveoli.

Partial Pressures of the Alveolar Gases. In es-

sentially all respiratory studies one expresses gas concentrations not in terms of percentage but in *partial pressures.* The partial pressure of a gas is the amount of pressure exerted by that gas alone. For instance, if a flask contains pure oxygen, and the total pressure in the flask is equal to atmospheric pressure, 760 mm. Hg, then the partial pressure of the oxygen is also 760 mm. Hg. However, if this flask contains half oxygen and half nitrogen while the total pressure is 760 mm. Hg, then the partial pressure of the oxygen would be 380 mm. Hg, and the partial pressure of nitrogen would also be 380 mm. Hg.

Partial pressures are used to express the concentrations of gases because it is *pressure* that causes the gases to move by diffusion from one part of the body to another. For instance, if the partial pressure of oxygen (Po_2) is 105 mm. Hg in the alveoli and only 100 mm. Hg in the blood, then oxygen will diffuse from the alveoli into the blood. Conversely, if the pressure is greater in the blood than in the alveoli, oxygen will actually diffuse in the backward direction. Thus, the direction and the rate at which gases will diffuse depend on the *pressure difference,* the gases always moving from a high pressure area toward a low pressure area.

The normal partial pressures of the different gases in the alveoli are:

Oxygen, 104 mm. Hg
Carbon dioxide, 40 mm. Hg
Water vapor, 47 mm. Hg
Nitrogen, 569 mm. Hg

Transport of Oxygen and Carbon Dioxide to the Tissues

Diffusion of O_2 and CO_2 Through the Pulmonary Membrane. The normal Po_2 in the alveoli is approximately 104 mm. Hg, while the Po_2 of the venous blood entering the pulmonary capillaries is approximately 40 mm. Hg. This is a pressure difference of 64 mm. Hg, which causes large quantities of oxygen to diffuse through the pulmonary membrane into the blood. By the time the blood has passed through the pulmonary capillaries, it will have become almost completely saturated with oxygen. That is, the Po_2 in the blood will have risen to about 100 mm. Hg, almost equal to that in the alveoli.

Carbon dioxide diffuses through the pulmonary membrane in the opposite direction to the diffusion of oxygen. The pressure of carbon dioxide (Pco_2) in the venous blood flowing into the lungs is approximately 45 mm. Hg, while the Pco_2 in the alveoli is 40 mm. Hg. This is a pressure difference of 5 mm. that causes carbon dioxide to diffuse out of the blood into the alveoli. Carbon dioxide is far more soluble in the pulmonary membrane than is oxygen, which allows it to diffuse through the pulmonary membrane approximately 20 times as readily as oxygen. Therefore, by the time the blood has passed through the pulmonary capillaries, its P_{CO_2} will have fallen to almost exactly the P_{CO_2} in the alveoli, that is, to about 40 mm. Hg.

In summary, as blood passes through the pulmonary capillaries, the blood P_{O_2} and P_{CO_2} approach very nearly the alveolar P_{O_2} and P_{CO_2}.

Diffusing Capacity of the Lungs. The rate at which a gas will diffuse from the alveoli into the blood for each mm. Hg pressure difference is called the *diffusing capacity of the lungs* for that particular gas. The diffusing capacity of the lungs for oxygen when a person is at rest is approximately 22 ml. per mm. Hg per minute. The diffusing capacity for carbon dioxide is about 20 times this value or approximately 440 ml. per mm. Hg per minute.

Transport of Oxygen by the Blood Hemoglobin. Ninety-seven per cent of all the oxygen normally carried from the lungs to the tissues is carried in chemical combination with *hemoglobin* in the red blood cells. Hemoglobin has the peculiar property of combining with large quantities of oxygen when the P_{O_2} is high and then releasing this when the P_{O_2} falls. Therefore, when the blood passes through the lungs, where the P_{O_2} rises to 100 mm. Hg, the hemoglobin picks up large quantities of oxygen. Then as it passes through the tissue capillaries, where the P_{O_2} falls to about 40 mm. Hg, large quantities of oxygen are released, this oxygen then diffusing into the tissue cells.

An especially important function of hemoglobin is that it releases oxygen to the tissues at a fairly constant P_{O_2}, between 20 and 50 mm. Hg, regardless of very wide fluctuations in the P_{O_2} in the air, for the following reason: If the oxygen in the alveolar air rises even as high as 1,000 mm. Hg, still the hemoglobin will combine with almost exactly the same amount of oxygen as it combines with at the the normal alveolar P_{O_2} of 104 mm. Hg. Therefore, essentially the same amount of oxygen is carried by the hemoglobin to the tissues. Because of this property, hemoglobin is frequently called an *oxygen buffer*.

Diffusion of Oxygen into the Tissues. When arterial blood enters the tissue capillaries, its P_{O_2} is still approximately 100 mm. Hg. On the other hand, the cells are continually using oxygen for metabolism, which keeps the P_{O_2} of the interstitial fluid low about 30 to 40 mm. Hg. Thus, a pressure difference exists between the blood and the cells of about 60 to 70 mm. Hg. This immediately causes rapid diffusion of oxygen into the interstitial fluid. As the blood passes through the capillaries its P_{O_2} normally falls to about

40 mm. Hg before it enters the veins. During high metabolic activity of the tissues, the venous P_{O_2} may fall to as low as 15 to 20 mm. Hg.

Transport of CO_2 in the Blood. When oxygen is metabolized in the cells, large quantities of carbon dioxide are formed, causing the intracellular P_{CO_2} to rise to values perhaps as high as 50 mm. Hg. On the other hand, the P_{CO_2} of the arterial blood entering the capillaries is only 40 mm. Hg. This 10 mm. pressure difference makes the carbon dioxide diffuse rapidly into the blood, raising the blood P_{CO_2} to about 45 mm. Hg before the blood passes on into the veins.

The carbon dioxide in the blood, like oxygen, is also carried mainly in combination with various chemical substances. The largest proportion combines with water inside the red blood cells to form *carbonic acid*. This reaction is catalyzed by a protein enzyme in the red cells called *carbonic anhydrase*. Most of the carbonic acid immediately dissociates into *bicarbonate ions* and *hydrogen ions,* the hydrogen ions in turn combining with hemoglobin. An additional small portion of the carbon dioxide combines directly with hemoglobin to form *carbaminohemoglobin*. When the blood arrives in the lungs, where the P_{CO_2} of the alveolar air is lower than that of blood, these chemical reactions are rapidly reversed, and the carbon dioxide diffuses out of the blood into the alveoli.

Regulation of Respiration

Respiratory Rhythm. The continual respiratory rhythm is caused by intermittent nerve impulses originating in the *respiratory center,* which is located in the brain stem in the reticular substance of the *medulla* and the *pons.* This center has a basic oscillating mechanism that causes it to emit rhythmic impulses to the respiratory muscles. However, its degree of activity can be increased or decreased by changes in the chemical composition of the blood as described below and also by sensory signals from the lungs.

A special reflex that is important in helping to regulate the respiratory rhythm is the *Hering-Breuer reflex.* This reflex is initiated by nerve receptors that detect the degree of stretch of the lungs. As the lungs become inflated, the receptors send signals into the respiratory center to inhibit inspiration and to excite expiration. Obviously, this reflex prevents overinflation of the lungs.

Control of the Alveolar Ventilation by Carbon Dioxide. The rate of alveolar ventilation is normally about 4.2 liters per minute, but this can be increased up to higher than 150 liters per minute, or it can be decreased to zero. By far the most powerful stimulus for increasing both the rate and the depth of respiration, and therefore increasing the rate of alveolar ventilation, is carbon dioxide. When increased quantities of carbon dioxide are formed in the body cells and these collect in the body fluids, the ventilation sometimes increases to as high as ten times normal. This in turn blows off the extra quantity of carbon dioxide from the lungs.

Regulation of Alveolar Ventilation by Blood pH. Earlier in the chapter it was pointed out that an increase in hydrogen ion concentration (that is, a decrease in pH) stimulates the respiratory center and increases alveolar ventilation. This causes increased quantities of carbon dioxide to be blown off from the blood which in turn decreases the amount of blood carbonic acid. And, since carbonic acid is in constant equilibrium with hydrogen ions of the blood, the hydrogen ion concentration also decreases back toward normal.

Regulation of Alveolar Ventilation by Oxygen Lack. Lack of oxygen in the blood can also increase the rate of alveolar ventilation. However, unlike the effects of carbon dioxide and hydrogen ion concentration, oxygen lack does not directly stimulate the respiratory center. Instead, it excites special nerve receptors called *chemoreceptors* located in minute *carotid* and *aortic bodies* that lie, respectively, in the carotid bifurcations and along the aorta. Each of these bodies has a special artery that supplies abundant amounts of arterial blood to the chemoreceptors. When the arterial oxygen concentration falls, signals from the chemoreceptors are transmitted to the respiratory center where they cause an increase in alveolar ventilation.

The oxygen lack stimulus for increasing alveolar ventilation is a weak one compared with stimulation by carbon dioxide and low pH. Maximal increase in carbon dioxide can increase alveolar ventilation about tenfold; maximal increase in hydrogen ion concentration can increase it about fivefold; but maximal oxygen lack (under acute conditions) can increase alveolar ventilation only by about one and two thirds.

One often wonders why oxygen lack is such a poor stimulus of respiration in comparison with carbon dioxide and hydrogen ions. However, oxygen concentration in the tissues is regulated principally by the hemoglobin buffer mechanism discussed above, while carbon dioxide concentration is regulated almost entirely by alveolar ventilation, and hydrogen ion concentration is regulated to a major extent in this way as was discussed earlier. Therefore, there is less need for oxygen to control respiration than for carbon dioxide and hydrogen ion concentration to control it.

Regulation of Respiration in Exercise. In exercise, alveolar ventilation sometimes increases as much as 30-fold, which is even more than the increase that occurs as a result of maximal carbon dioxide or maximal hydrogen ion stimulation. The precise cause of the greatly increased respiration during exercise has not been determined, but it is believed to result from nerve signals transmitted during exercise from other centers of the brain that are simultaneously providing nervous drive for the exercise itself, and from sensory signals originating in the active muscles.

Physiology of Respiratory Disorders

Hypoxia. The term *hypoxia* means insufficient oxygen in the body fluids to support normal tissue metabolism. If we very rapidly review the mechanisms of oxygen transport to the tissues, we can readily understand the different possible causes of hypoxia: (1) too little oxygen in the inspired air, (2) obstruction of the respiratory passageways, (3) decreased diffusing capacity of the lungs caused by destruction of large portions of the lung or thickened pulmonary membranes, (4) too little blood flow to the tissues to carry adequate oxygen, (5) absence of or diminished blood flow through large portions of the lungs, (6) too little hemoglobin in the blood to carry oxygen to the tissues, (7) too few capillaries in a particular tissue area to allow adequate tissue oxygenation, and (8) too few oxidative enzymes in the cells for the oxygen to be used.

Oxygen Therapy in Hypoxia. In certain types of hypoxia administration of high concentrations of oxygen in the respiratory air can relieve the hypoxic condition. This is particularly true of *atmospheric hypoxia, obstructive hypoxia* and *hypoxia caused by diminished diffusing capacity* of the lungs, for, in all of these, an increase in the oxygen concentration increases the P_{O_2} in the alveoli and thereby promotes increased oxygen diffusion into the blood. In other types of hypoxia the problem is mainly diminished transport of oxygen to the tissues or diminished use of oxygen by the tissues. In these types of hypoxia, oxygen therapy may be of slight benefit but not nearly so much so as in the types mentioned above.

Aviation Physiology

Hypoxia at High Altitudes. The main problem in aviation physiology is a progressive decrease in P_{O_2} at higher and higher altitudes. A normal person often becomes lethargic and loses much mental alertness at about 12,000 to 15,000 feet. At 18,000 feet, a person can become so disoriented that judgement is lost; pilots may actually fly still higher rather than returning to a lower level to correct the hypoxic condition. And at about 23,000 feet an aviator will become comatose in 20 to 30 minutes. If pure oxygen is used rather than normal air, a pilot can ascend to an altitude of about 45,000 feet before becoming hypoxic, because the oxygen replaces the nitrogen that normally fills the major amount of space in the alveoli.

Acclimatization to Hypoxia. Though an aviator almost never remains at a high altitude long enough to become adjusted to the altitude, mountain climbers often become *acclimatized* sufficiently that they can live and work at altitudes many thousand feet higher than normal persons. Acclimatization results from three major physiologic changes:

1. The oxygen lack mechanism for control of pulmonary ventilation normally increases ventilation only about 65 per cent, but after a person remains at high altitudes for several days, this mechanism becomes progressively more effective and increases ventilation about 400 per cent instead of the normal 65 per cent, thus providing much greater amounts of oxygen for the alveoli.

2. When one stays at a high altitude for several weeks, the hypoxia causes greatly increased production of red blood cells by the mechanism explained earlier in the chapter, sometimes increasing the total red cell mass to as much as 80 to 100 per cent above normal. This obviously increases the ability of the blood to transport oxygen to the tissues.

3. Associated with the increased blood cell mass is an increase in both the number of blood vessels in the tissues and also their sizes so that increased quantities of blood can flow through the tissues, thus again increasing the available oxygen in the tissues.

Acceleratory Forces in Aviation. Another major problem in aviation is *centrifugal acceleration,* which means that a person tends to be displaced in one direction or another when the airplane turns to one side or up or down. Centrifugal acceleration is especially of importance when one comes out of a dive or when one goes through a tight turn. Sometimes the aviator is pressed downward against the seat of the airplane with a force many times the weight of his body. The normal weight of the body is said to be 1 gravity (g), but if the total force against the seat is two times body weight, then the acceleration is 2 g. A person can withstand up to about 4 g without harm, but 5 g or more for only 10 seconds usually causes *blackout* because of "centrifuging" the blood of the head down into the vessels of the legs and the abdomen.

Space Physiology

Survival in space is mainly an engineering problem, for the person will have to exist in a *pressurized chamber* or in a *pressurized suit* that contains an adequate supply of oxygen. Other problems have to do with *linear acceleration* or deceleration, *weightlessness, radiation hazards* and *provision of a complete life cycle.*

The problem of *linear acceleration* exists principally when the space ship leaves the earth, for the ship must be accelerated to the velocity required to escape the pull of earth's gravity. Approximately the highest degree of linear acceleration developed is about 10 g— that is, the body is pushed backward against the seat with a force about ten times its own weight. The human body can stand up to 10 g in a horizontal or reclining position though not in the upright position. Therefore, takeoff has to be accomplished with the body horizontal to the line of takeoff. Linear deceleration occurs during reentry, and the problems are the same. Reentry is accomplished in a backwards direction, with the person again in the reclining position.

Weightlessness occurs in space because both the space ship and the human are traveling through space at the same speed, both of them affected by the same forces so that nothing pulls the human toward the bottom, the top, or the sides of the space ship. He simply floats in the ship. This has not proved to be a severe physiologic problem, mainly an engineering one to provide means for keeping the body properly oriented in the ship. However, it does cause some decalcification of the bones and loss of fluid from the tissues of the lower body.

The *radiation hazard* of space travel is likely to prevent prolonged space travel in a zone 500 to 20,000 miles above the earth. The play of cosmic particles on the stratosphere at this height creates a very strong field of gamma rays.

By far the greatest problem of space survival is that of providing a continuous supply of oxygen, water and food for the traveler, particularly since interplanetary space travel may well require months to years. This is expected to be accomplished by installing a *complete life cycle* in the space ship. Algae or some other type of plant life will be used to convert carbon dioxide, with use of the sun's energy, into oxygen and food. In turn, the excreta from the human being will be used as nutrients for the plant life. Thus survival can continue indefinitely.

Deep-Sea Diving Physiology

Effects of High Gaseous Pressures on the Body. When a person descends deep under the sea, air must be pumped into the lungs with progressively more and more pressure so that the chest can withstand the pressure of the water on the outside; otherwise, the chest would collapse. At a depth of 10 meters, the pressure must be two times normal atmospheric pressure; at 20 meters, 3 atmospheres; at 30 meters, 4 atmospheres; and so forth.

When air is compressed into the lungs under more than about 8 to 10 atmospheres of pressure, both the oxygen and the nitrogen become toxic. *High pressures of oxygen cause mental disorientation,* presumably because of excessive usage of oxygen by certain of the neuronal cells. The person first becomes quite irritable, and this is often followed by *convulsions* and *coma.* Obviously, if such should occur at great depths, it would be disastrous.

High nitrogen pressures have an anesthetic effect, causing first a *lethargic state,* then a *somnolent state* and finally *total anesthesia.* The deepest sea depth that a person can stand while breathing pure air for more than an hour is about 300 feet, at which depth the pressure is 10 atmospheres. At this pressure the nitrogen narcosis effect approaches the somnolent level, and the oxygen effect approaches the convulsion level. For safety's sake, a person rarely works below 250 feet even for short periods of time when breathing compressed air. At very deep levels, the nitrogen and part of the oxygen, are replaced by helium which causes none of the narcotic or convulsive effects of nitrogen or oxygen.

Bubble Formation on Ascent—Decompression Sickness. Another major problem in deep-sea diving physiology is the tendency for divers to develop bubbles in their body fluids as they ascend from the depths. When the body is exposed to high pressure, the inert gases of the breathing mixture—such as nitrogen or helium—become dissolved in high concentrations in all the body fluids. Then, when the person is again exposed to low pressure, these gases must diffuse out of the tissue spaces into the blood and then through the lungs into the expired air. This "degassing" process sometimes requires as much as 6 or more hours, and, if the pressure around the body is decreased rapidly rather than slowly, these gases will simply form bubbles in the body fluids rather than diffusing out through the lungs. Therefore, it is essential that the diver ascend from depths slowly or that he be decompressed slowly over a long period in a decompression chamber.

The development of bubbles in the body fluids can cause serious damage in the tissues or can cause gas emboli in the circulating blood. Two of the most distressing effects are (1) air emboli in the pulmonary vessels, which causes the "chokes," and (2) disruption of nerve pathways in the nervous system, which causes serious pain or even paralysis. This condition is generally called *decompression sickness,* the *bends, caisson disease* or *diver's paralysis.*

CENTRAL NERVOUS SYSTEM

Basic Organization of the Central Nervous System

Control Functions of the Central Nervous System. The central nervous system is a rapidly acting control system for the body. Control of the different bodily functions depends basically upon (1) *sensory receptors* that apprise the nervous system of the conditions in the body, (2) *effector organs* that perform functions dictated by the nervous system, and (3) *integrative mechanisms* in the central nervous system to determine the effector responses to receptor signals.

Sensory Receptors. The sensory receptors include any type of nerve ending in the body that can be stimulated by some physical or chemical stimulus originating either outside or within the body. These receptors include (1) the *rods* and the *cones* of the eyes for detection of light; (2) the *cochlear nerve endings* of the ear for detection of sound; (3) the *taste endings* in the mouth for detection of taste; (4) the *olfactory endings* in the nose for detection of smell; (5) the *sensory nerve endings in the skin* for detection of touch, pain, warmth, cold, pressure and tickle; (6) *sensory endings deep in the body* for detection of deep pressure, position of the limbs, vibratory impulses, and so forth; (7) *stretch receptors in the walls of the arteries* for detection of arterial pressure; (8) *stretch receptors in the veins, the lungs and other visceral organs;* (9) *chemical receptors* in different portions of the brain, such as in the vasomotor center and the hypothalamus, as well as in outlying organs such as the carotid and the aortic bodies; and (10) a variety of other specialized receptors. Thus, we have a long list of different types of receptors that can detect almost any type of normal stimulus to the body.

Effector Organs. These include every organ that can be stimulated by nerve impulses. Perhaps the most important effector system is the *skeletal muscular system.* In addition, the *smooth muscle* of the body and the *glandular cells* are among the important effector organs. However, *all cells of the body* react to circulating hormones in the body fluids, some of which are secreted in response to nerve impulses. For instance, sympathetic stimulation causes the adrenal medulla to release large amounts of epinephrine and norepinephrine. These are transported throughout the entire body and increase the metabolism of every known type of cell. In this sense, then, every cell of the body is an effector organ, though some cells are far more important in the scheme of nervous control than are others.

Reflex Arc. One basic means by which the nervous system controls functions in the body is the *reflex arc,* in which a stimulus excites a receptor, appropriate impulses are transmitted into the central nervous system where various nervous reactions take place, and then appropriate effector impulses are transmitted to an effector organ to cause a reflex effect.

Some reflexes are very simple with the effect following the stimulus within a fraction of a second. An example of such a reflex is the withdrawal of the hand from a hot stove. Other reflexes act extremely slowly. For instance, a person may see something he might desire in a store window today but not initiate the effector responses to buy the object until many months later. Nevertheless, this, in a sense, is still a reflex that requires many months of storage of information before the final effect occurs.

Integrative Centers of the Nervous System. Those parts of the nervous system that put many different types of sensory signals together before causing a reaction or first store the information and later cause a reaction are called the *integrative centers* of the nervous system. For instance, even in the simple reflex that causes a person to withdraw his hand from a hot stove, the areas of the spinal cord that are concerned with this withdrawal reaction are known as the centers for integration of the withdrawal reflex. At a much higher level of complexity are the integrative centers of the *cerebral* cortex that have to do with *memory* and *thinking*. The *medulla* is the integrative center for most respiratory control, for most control of arterial pressure and for control of swallowing; the *motor area of the cerebral cortex, the cerebellum, the basal ganglia and large parts of the reticular substance of the brain stem* are major parts of the integrative centers for control of muscular movement.

Function of the Single Neuron

The sum of all the actions of the single neurons determines the overall function of the brain. Therefore, it is necessary to understand the functional abilities of single neurons in order to comprehend the manner in which these operate together to give the integrative functions of the nervous system.

The Synapse. The neurons of the nervous system are arranged so that each neuron stimulates other neurons, and these in turn stimulate still others until the functions of the nervous system are performed. The point of contact between successive neurons is called a *synapse,* and the terminal endings of the nerve filaments that synapse with the next neuron are called *presynaptic terminals, synaptic knobs, boutons* or simply *end feet.* Usually, there are several hundred to several thousand synaptic knobs on each neuron, these having originated from preceding neurons. Each synaptic knob secretes a particular hormone called a *transmitter substance* that may either *excite* the next neuron or may *inhibit* it. These hormones are called *excitatory* or *inhibitory transmitters.*

Function of a Transmitter Substance at a Synapse. Over thirty different types of transmitter substances have been described, and undoubtedly many more will yet be described. However, each synaptic knob can secrete only one transmitter. It is synthesized within the synaptic knob and stored in thousands of small *vesicles.* When an action potential spreads over the end of the nerve fiber, the deplorization of the synaptic knob causes migration of a few of the vesicles to the membrane surface of the knob, and these vesicles extrude their contents of transmitter substance into the *synaptic cleft* between the synaptic knob and the membrane of the succeeding neuron. The transmitter then combines with a *receptor* (a protein molecule) that is an integral part of the neuronal membrane. This opens a pore in the membrane and allows ions to move through the pore. The receptor may be either an *excitatory receptor* or an *inhibitory receptor.* If it is excitatory, it opens sodium pores and allows sodium ions to move selectively to the inside of the membrane, which partially depolarizes the neuron and therefore helps to stimulate it. In the case of the inhibitory receptor, the pores become permeable to chloride and potassium ions. Movement of these ions through the membrane *hyperpolarizes* the neuron (makes the inside of the membrane more negative), and this inhibits the neuron rather than exciting it.

Thus, whether a transmitter substance will be excitatory or inhibitory depends on the receptor substance as well as the transmitter. Some transmitters can be either excitatory or inhibitory, depending on the receptor substance with which it reacts. On the other hand, other transmitters are almost always either excitatory or inhibitory.

Excitatory Transmitters. An excitatory transmitter that is released by a large number of synaptic knobs in the central nervous system is *acetylcholine.* This stimulates the successive neuron in exactly the same way that it stimulates a muscle fiber at the neuromuscular junction, that is, by increasing the permeability of the neuronal membrane to sodium. The sodium leaks rapidly to the interior of the cell, causing a sudden change in electrical potential across the membrane. However, stimulation of a single excitatory synapse almost never causes the neuron to "fire," for the amount of excitatory transmitter secreted at one synapse will not cause sufficient depolorization of the membrane to initiate an action potential. Each type of neuron is different in the number of synapses that must fire on its membrane to cause excitation. Certain neurons might require only five simultaneous firings; others might require as many as 100 to 1000 synapses discharging simultaneously. Thus, certain neurons allow signals to pass very easily, while others allow passage only with great difficulty. In this way, incoming signals can be channeled in the proper direction through the neuronal circuits of the brain.

Other transmitter substances that often function as excitatory transmitters include norepinephrine, epinephrine, dopamine, glutamic acid, enkephalin, endorphin, and substance P. However, some of these also function as inhibitory transmitters in the presence of inhibitory receptor substances.

Inhibitory Transmitters. Many synaptic knobs secrete inhibitory transmitters rather than excitatory transmitter. In fact, there are far more inhibitory synapses in the central nervous system than most people realize, for function of large parts of the brain, including the cerebral cortex, the basal ganglia, the thalamus, and the cerebellum, depend almost as much on inhibition of neurons as upon excitation. It is probable that as many as a third or even more of the synapses are of the inhibitory type rather than of the excitatory type.

Two inhibitory hormones that are secreted at many synapses are *gamma aminobutyric acid (GABA)* and *glycine*. Other transmitters that serve as inhibitory transmitters (in the presence of inhibitory receptors) include norepinephrine, epinephrine, serotonin, and dopamine.

Excitability of the Neuron. Whether or not a neuron will be excited depends on three major factors: (1) the basic nature of the neuron itself, whether it tends to be an excitable type of neuron or a relatively dormant type, (2) the number of excitatory synapses firing in any given time, and (3) the number of inhibitory synapses firing at any given time. In certain parts of the brain highly excitable neurons perform rapid and easily elicited actions; in others, relatively dormant neurons respond only when tremendously strong signals reach them. Thus, the *integrative capabilities* of the neurons differ in different parts of the brain.

Functions of "Pools" of Neurons

Each part of the brain usually contains large numbers of similar types of neurons that lie close to each other and are interconnected by means of many fine nerve filaments. Each such group of neurons is called a *neuronal pool*. Different patterns of nerve filament interconnections exist in different pools, and the type of pattern in turn determines the manner in which the pool operates in the overall function of the brain. In general, three basic types of circuits occur in neuronal pools: (1) the *diverging circuit*, (2) the *converging* or *integrative circuit,* and (3) *repetitive firing circuits.*

Diverging Circuit. This circuit is the simplest of all that occur in the neuronal pools. It is simply a circuit in which the nerve fibers entering the pool divide many times so that a few impulses entering the pool cause a large number of impulses to leave the pool. This type of circuit is typified by the nervous control of muscular activity, for stimulation of a single large neuron in the *motor cortex* will often stimulate many *interneurons* in the spinal cord, and these in turn might then stimulate as many as 50 to 100 *anterior motor neurons,* which in turn stimulate thousands of muscle fibers.

Converging or Integrative Circuit. An *integrative circuit* is one that, after receiving incoming signals from several sources, determines the type of reaction that will occur. That is, impulses "converge" into the pool, some from inhibitory nerves, some from excitatory nerves, some from peripheral nerves and some from other parts of the brain. The different factors that enter into the response of the pool are (1) the basic excitability of the neurons in the pool, (2) the number of excitatory impulses entering the pool, (3) the number of inhibitory impulses entering the pool, (4) whether or not there might be some diverging circuits also in the pool, (5) the distribution of excitatory and inhibitory impulses to the different neurons, and so forth. From this list of possible factors that can affect the output from the neuronal pool, one can readily understand that basic differences in the anatomic organization of different neuronal pools can give thousands of different responses to incoming signals. For instance, the pool may be a *high threshold pool* into which many excitatory impulses must arrive before an effect will occur. It might be a *low threshold pool* into which only a few impulses must arrive before an effect will occur. The low threshold circuit is typified by the neuronal response that causes withdrawal of a limb when only a few *pain* receptors are stimulated, while the high threshold circuit is typified by failure to withdraw a hand when tremendous numbers of *touch* receptors are stimulated.

Repetitive Firing Circuits. Among the most important types of circuits in the nervous system are the *repetitive firing circuits.* In these, impulses entering a pool of neurons cause the pool to emit a series of impulses lasting long after the incoming signal is over. Three types of circuits can cause this: The first is a pool of neurons consisting of very excitable neurons that have a natural tendency to fire repetitively. The second is a *long chain of neurons* arranged one after another so that an incoming stimulus activates each one in succession. From each neuron of the chain a nerve fiber extends to some outlying neuron. Thus, this outlying neuron receives repetitive impulses from the successive neurons of the chain, but after all these have fired the repetitive firing from the output neuron ceases.

Third, probably a much more important type of repetitive firing circuit is the *reverberating circuit* in which an incoming impulse is passed along a succession of neurons until finally one of the neurons restimulates an earlier neuron in the succession. This causes the impulse to go around the circuit again and again. Every time around the circuit, collateral impulses are emitted into outgoing nerve fibers that spread to other parts of the nervous system. Theoretically, this type of circuit might continue to oscillate indefinitely, but more usually the oscillation ceases when some of the neurons in the circuit become too fatigued to continue. The continual respiratory rhythm represents a continually reverberating circuit, while the thought processes of the cerebral cortex probably represent circuits that reverberate for short periods until neurons in the circuit fatigue or are inhibited so that the thought ceases.

To summarize, the nervous system is actually made up of many neuronal pools, each one of which has specific circuit characteristics that allow it to emit a certain pattern of output impulses in response to incoming signals. By combining the functional characteristics of the many different pools in the nervous system one can achieve almost any type of integrative function in one portion of the nervous system or another.

The Process of Cerebration

Thoughts. The bases of *cerebration* are the individual thoughts, many of which occur directly as a result of incoming sensory impulses. For instance, the impulses from the eyes when a person is looking at a beautiful scene certainly generate a number of different thoughts.

The precise mechanisms of thoughts in the brain are not understood, but one of the suggestions is that a thought represents a pattern of impulses passing through particular neurons in the conscious portion of the brain. For instance, electrical stimulation of a minute point on the surface of the cerebral cortex will often cause a person to have a very distinct and very clear thought. Since the same thought sometimes persists over a long time, it is reasonable to believe that at least many thoughts are caused by reverberating circuits of neurons that involve either small areas of the brain or at times very large areas.

Memory. Memory simply means storage of information in the brain. The precise mechanism by which information is stored for long periods is not known, though it is believed to result from permanent facilitation of synapses. This means simply that excitation of a synapse repetitively over a time will cause that synapse to become more and more effective in stimulating the neuron. In other words, the fact that an impulse passes through a synapse once makes it easier for successive impulses to pass through the same synapse. Therefore, if a thought pattern is evoked over and over again by incoming sensory stimuli, then even-

tually the pathway for transmission of impulses through that particular thought channel becomes facilitated so that even the slightest stimulus entering this pathway at a later time can elicit the entire thought. For instance, such a facilitated thought pathway might develop in response to seeing the beautiful scene referred to above. Then a year later, some stray impulse from another part of the brain might enter this particular thought pathway and allow the person to see the scene again in his mind. This is believed to be the basis of memory.

The portion of the brain most concerned with memory seems to be the *cerebral cortex,* for all through this structure are located neuronal pools that can be facilitated by sensory or electrical impulses so that subsequent signals entering these pools will evoke specific reactions. Furthermore, the storage of information in the brain is mostly lost when the cortex is gone.

"Programming" of the Thoughts. Now that we have discussed the possible basis of thoughts and memory, we still need to develop some understanding of the manner in which these are used in the thinking process. Everyone is familiar with the fact that different thoughts usually occur in rapid succession, and that each succeeding thought usually has some association with the preceding thought. Many sequences of thoughts are initiated by incoming sensory signals, whether these are from the somesthetic sensory system, from the eyes, from the ears, and so forth. For instance, a sudden knife cut on the leg would elicit first a thought of pain, then another thought that localizes the cut on the body, this followed by integrative processes that make the person turn his eyes and head to look at the pained area, followed by visual input impulses that combine with the previous thoughts to determine the nature of the stimulus causing the pain, and, finally, a series of integrations that cause motor movements to remove the body from the painful object or to remove the painful object from the body. In this sequence of cerebration, the person must call forth memories from past experiences in order to understand why and how his leg is being pained, for, if he has never seen a knife before and is not familiar with its cutting capabilities, simply looking at the leg and seeing a knife against the skin will not explain the cause of the pain. In short, for cerebration to occur, the thoughts must be *programmed.* Some part of the brain must determine where the attention of the mind will be directed, whether it will be directed to the incoming sensory signals from the leg, to the movement of the head and the eyes, or to one of the memory circuits to call forth information. The nature of this programming system of the brain is still unclear. However, the anatomic locations of the *thalamus* and the *reticular sub-*

stance of the mesencephalon have made many neurophysiologists point to these two areas as possible programming centers. Also, stimulation of specific points in these two areas can cause specific patterns of reaction in other parts of the brain and cord.

THE SOMATIC SENSORY SYSTEM

The sensory portion of the nervous system is often subdivided into three different systems: the *exterioceptive system,* which transmits impulses from the skin, the *proprioceptive system,* which transmits impulses mainly from the muscles and joints relating to the momentary physical condition of the body, and the *visceral sensory system,* which transmits impulses from the viscera. The first two of these are frequently called the *somatic sensory system.*

Modalities of Sensation. It is common knowledge that many different types of sensations can be perceived from the skin, including *light touch, tickle, pressure, pain, cold* and *warmth.* These are called *modalities* of sensation. Proprioceptive modalities of sensation include *sense of position of the limbs, degree of tension in the muscle tendons, degree of stretch of the muscle fibers* and *deep pressure on different parts of the body.* In addition to these, other modalities that are not transmitted by the somatic sensory system are *sight, hearing, equilibrium, smell* and *taste.*

Sensory Receptors. Each modality of sensation is usually detected by a particular type of nerve ending. The most common nerve ending is the *free nerve ending,* which is nothing more than a filamentous end of a nerve usually interwoven with other filamentous nerve endings. This type of ending can detect *pain, crude touch, tickle, heavy pressure* and probably *warmth.* In addition to the free nerve endings, the skin contains a number of specialized endings that are adapted to respond to some specific type of physical stimulus. For instance, one of these endings, called a *Meissner's corpuscle,* responds specifically to light touch.

Sensory endings deep in the body that subserve the different proprioceptive sensations are the *joint receptors,* which detect degree of angulation of the joints; *pacinian corpuscles,* which detect very rapid changes in pressure; *Golgi tendon apparatuses,* which detect degree of tension in the tendons, and *muscle spindles,* which detect degree of stretch of the muscle fibers.

Pathways for Transmission of Somatic Sensations into the Central Nervous System. The impulses generated in the sensory receptors are transmitted first into the *spinal nerves* and then through the dorsal roots of the spinal nerves into the cord. In general, the *proprioceptive impulses* are transmitted by large *type A nerve fibers,* which can transmit at velocities as high as 100 m. per second. This rapid velocity is especially important when a person is moving rapidly, for he needs to know during each split second the position of all parts of his body.

On the other hand, many of the *aching type pain* impulses are transmitted by the very small *type C fibers,* which transmit impulses at velocities as low as 1 m. per second. Here, rapidity of response is not needed. On the other hand, *sharp pain* is transmitted by intermediate velocity fibers, which allows rapid response to stimuli that might be damaging to the tissues.

Once the sensory fibers enter the spinal cord, most of them terminate on *second order neurons* that then transmit impulses either to other areas of the cord or all the way to the brain. However, some sensory signals pass through several neurons in the spinal cord before ascending to the brain, and some sensory fibers pass all the way to the medulla where they end in the *cuneate* and the *gracile nuclei,* which in turn send second order nerve fibers to higher centers of the brain. Most of the second order nerve fibers terminate in the ventrobasal complex of the thalamus, and *third order neurons* pass from this area to the cerebral cortex, especially to the *somesthetic cortex* and the *somesthetic association cortex,* which lie behind the central sulcus of the brain.

It should be noted particularly that along the entire course of the sensory fibers from the cord to the cerebral cortex many collateral fibers spread in all directions. Especially abundant are (1) collateral fibers that spread in the cord itself, (2) collateral fibers that spread into the cerebellum and into all parts of the reticular substance of the brain stem, and (3) collaterals that spread from the sensory neurons of the thalamus to most other portions of the thalamus, the hypothalamus and other closely associated nuclei. Thus, the "trunk line" sensory system carries sensory signals into essentially all parts of the brain.

The Law of Specific Nerve Energies. If a sensory nerve fiber is stimulated by an electrical stimulus, a person will perceive only one particular modality of sensation. For instance, excitation of a pain fiber will cause pain, excitation of a warmth fiber will cause the sensation of warmth, and so forth. Thus, each type of sensory nerve fiber transmits only one modality of sensation, and this is called the *law of specific nerve energies.*

However, it is not the type of fiber that determines the modality of sensation transmitted, but, instead, *it is the point in the central nervous system to which the fiber connects* that determines the modality. For instance, pain fibers end in a slightly different point in the thalamus from the warmth fibers, and these in a different point from the cold fibers.

Since most modalities of sensation can still be perceived even when the cerebral cortex is removed, it is believed that the lower sensory centers in the *brain stem* and the *thalamus* can determine at least some of the different sensory modalities, especially pain, cold, warmth, and crude touch. On the other hand, a person cannot localize sensations in different parts of his body accurately when the sensory portions of the cerebral cortex have been destroyed. Therefore, *discrete localization* is principally a function of the *somesthetic cortex*, though the thalamus by itself is capable of crude localization to general areas of the body.

Pain

The Basic Pain Stimulus; Threshold for Pain Perception.   Pain fibers are stimulated any time a tissue is *being* damaged. However, once the damage is complete the pain sensation gradually disappears in a few minutes or sometimes even in a few seconds. Pain nerve endings can be stimulated by *mechanical trauma* to the tissues, *excess heat, excess cold, chemical damage,* certain types of *radiation damage,* such as the pain associated with sunburn, and even *lack of adequate blood flow* to a tissue area, which causes *ischemic pain.* Again it should be emphasized that pain occurs when damage is actively occurring, and it is not felt very long after the damage has been accomplished.

Threshold for Pain Perception and Reactivity to Pain.   Frequently, it is said that some people perceive pain far more easily than others. This is not true, for actual research on various degrees of injury in relation to the perception of pain shows that all persons begin to perceive pain at almost exactly the same degree of injury.

However, once the pain has been perceived, the degree of transmission of pain signals in the nervous system, as well as the *reactivity* of different persons to the pain, varies tremendously. The reactivity to pain is partly an inherited characteristic of certain races of people, but it is also greatly influenced by previous training.

Control of Pain by Central Nervous System Mechanisms.   The brain has the capability to control the sensitivity of pain pathways. It does this by sending *centrifugal* inhibitory signals from the brain to the spinal cord and brain stem to control pain signal transmission.

One of the controlling centers for pain is the *reticular nuclei* extending from the area of the third ventricle in the hypothalamus into the central gray region around the aqueduct of Sylvius in the mesencephalon. These two areas can be stimulated by *enkephalins* and *endorphins,* which are morphinelike substances. Also, one or both of them are found in these areas of the brain. Therefore, they are believed to be an intrinsic brain opiate system for pain control.

Visceral Sensation

Visceral Pain and Referred Pain.   Essentially all internal organs of the body are supplied with pain nerve endings, but these are usually far more sparse than in the skin. Therefore, in general, sharp pain is much less likely to occur from the viscera than is the generalized aching or burning type of pain. The different types of stimuli that are particularly prone to cause visceral pain are (1) overdistention of a hollow viscus, (2) spasm of the smooth muscle of a viscus, (3) too little blood flow to the viscus, and (4) chemical damage such as that produced by spillage of acid gastric juice into the peritoneal cavity through a ruptured peptic ulcer. It is especially interesting that most deep tissues of the body, including even the organs of the abdomen, are relatively insensitive to a sharp knife cut, indicating that there are insufficient pain endings in any minute area to cause pain. Therefore, visceral pain usually occurs only on stimulation of pain endings over a wide area. However, this is not true in the periosteum, in the walls of the arteries, in the parietal pleura and in the parietal peritoneum, for these areas are almost equally as susceptible to pain as the skin.

Pain in a visceral organ is not always felt directly over the organ itself but may be referred to a distant area of the body. For instance, pain originating in the heart is often felt in one or both arms. This is called *referred pain.* Referred pain usually results from neuronal connections between the visceral pain fibers and the somatic pain pathways in the cord, the visceral impulses exciting the somatic pathways and the person feeling the pain in some nonvisceral part of his body.

Other Visceral Sensations.   There are few other types of visceral sensation besides pain that reach the conscious portions of the brain. However, many visceral sensations, such as stretch of arterial walls, stretch of the lungs, stretch of the gut, and so forth are of particular importance in reflex control of the specific organs. These reflexes and their initiating receptors are discussed at different points in this chapter in relation to the different organic systems.

Cord Reflexes

Many central nervous system functions occur locally in the spinal cord without the aid of the brain. Especially, the cord integrates many specific reflexes that help to control muscle movements.

The Stretch Reflex.   The simplest cord reflex, called the *stretch reflex,* is initiated by the *muscle spin-*

dles. These receptors continually send impulses into the spinal cord to excite the *anterior motoneurons;* these in turn transmit impulses back to the respective muscle. This continual flow of impulses helps to maintain a certain amount of basal tone in the muscle.

The stretch reflex is elicited by stretching the muscle. In its simplest form, the stretch reflex involves only two neurons, the neuron from the muscle spindle to the anterior motoneuron and the anterior motoneuron back to the muscle. Stretch of the muscle spindles increases the number of impulses transmitted by the spindles, and this increases the number of impulses transmitted by the anterior motoneurons back to the muscle. Therefore, muscle stretch enhances the contractile tension in the muscle. This tension in turn tends to shorten the muscle back to its initial length. Thus, the stretch reflex opposes changes in muscle length.

The stretch reflex has both a dynamic and a static component, called respectively the *dynamic stretch reflex* and the *static stretch reflex.* The dynamic effect occurs only when the muscle is stretched rapidly; this causes extreme feedback contraction of the muscle to oppose the sudden stretch. The static stretch reflex is much weaker than the dynamic reflex, but it maintains muscle contraction for minutes or hours when the muscle remains stretched beyond its normal length.

The muscle spindles themselves are provided with excitory nerve fibers from the spinal cord called *gamma efferent fibers,* and these in turn are controlled by signals from the reticular substance of the brain stem. Impulses transmitted through the gamma fibers can increase the degree of activity of the muscle spindle and therefore can also increase the intensity of either the dynamic stretch reflex or the static reflex. In this way, signals from the brain stem can alter the overall reactivity of the muscels.

The Withdrawal Response. *Withdrawal reflexes* can function in each part of the body to pull that part away from any painful object. For instance, if the hand is placed on a hot stove, impulses are transmitted from the pain receptors to the cord and immediately back to the flexor muscles of the arm to withdraw the hand. Because it is the flexor muscles that are involved in this instance, this particular withdrawal reflex is called a *flexor reflex.*

Part of the withdrawal response involves impulses transmitted to the opposite side of the body to extend the opposite limb, thereby pushing the whole body away from the vicinity of the painful object. This extensor effect is called the *crossed extensor reflex.*

The withdrawal response is different for each part of the body. For instance, a painful stimulus applied to the lower back will cause forward arching of the back, or if the right deltoid region of the shoulder becomes pained, the whole upper body shifts to the left and the shoulder drops. Even in persons with the spinal cord transected in the neck, most of these withdrawal reflexes can still occur in a crude fashion, though the human being has additional reflexes that go all the way to the brain and back that aid in the withdrawal response.

The Positive Supportive Reflex. Pressure on the bottoms of the feet causes the extensor muscles of the legs to tighten, which helps the legs to support the weight of the body against gravity. This reflex is integrated entirely in the few segments of the spinal cord that control the activity of each respective limb.

Walking Reflexes. Even walking movements can be performed by the limbs of a lower animal whose spinal cord has been transected. If the transection is placed in the thorax, the hind limbs can "walk" but without coordination with the movements of the fore-limbs. However, if the cord is transected in the neck, rhythmic to-and-fro coordinated walking movements among all four limbs often occur. Occasionally, trotting movements also occur and, very rarely, galloping movements.

Thus, the basic patterns for walking and other movements of locomotion are also integrated in the spinal cord. The nerve fiber tracts that coordinate the functions of the superior and the inferior segments of the cord are the *propriospinal fiber pathways* that lie near the gray matter and account for approximately one half of all the fiber tracts in the cord.

Functions of the Brain Stem

Support of the Body Against Gravity. Even though the spinal cord is capable of providing the positive supportive reflex that *helps* to support the body against gravity and also of supplying walking reflexes, the human body still cannot stand and certainly cannot walk without the aid of higher central nervous system centers. As animalhood has progressed from lower phylogenetic types to the higher types, more and more of the control systems have gradually shifted from the cord toward the brain. As stated above, a lower animal, such as an opossum, can still walk quite well with his hind limbs even when its spinal cord is transected in the thorax. In the dog, basic walking movements can occur in the hind limbs with the thoracic cord transected, but these cannot be coordinated sufficiently to provide functional walking. In the human being, even these walking reflexes are crude when the cord is cut.

Located in the brain stem are a number of centers that help the limbs support the body against gravity. These transmit impulses especially to the extensor muscles, tightening the muscles of the trunk, the buttocks, the thighs and the lower legs to allow the body to stand in an upright position. Therefore, it is frequently said that the brain stem supplies the nervous energy required for supporting the body against gravity. It is principally the *vestibular nuclei* and the *reticular nuclei of the mesencephalon and the pons* that are responsible for this function.

Maintenance of Equilibrium—Function of the Vestibular Apparatus. Closely associated with the support of the body against gravity is the maintenance of equilibrium. The vestibular and reticular nuclei of the brain stem can vary the degree of tension in the different extensor muscles in proportion to the need for maintenance of equilibrium. To do this these nuclei in turn are controlled by the *vestibular apparatuses* located on the two sides of the head in close association with the ears.

The vestibular apparatuses contain two types of receptor organs: One of these is the maculae of the utricle and saccule, which contain large numbers of small calcium crystals called *otoliths* that lie on "hairs" projecting from sensory receptor cells called *hair cells*. Leaning of the head to one side or forward or backward causes these otoliths to fall toward the direction of leaning, thus bending the hairs and resulting in signals transmitted into the brain and informing the brain of the position of the head in relation to the direction of gravitational pull.

The second receptor system of the vestibular apparatus is the *semicircular canals*. These are filled with fluid so that any time the head rotates in any plane, inertia of the fluid causes it to move through one or more of the canals and thereby to stimulate hair cells located in the *ampullae* of the semicircular canals. Thus, rotating movements of the head are also made known to the nervous system.

From the vestibular apparatus signals are transmitted to the *vestibular nuclei* in the medulla, to the *reticular nuclei* and into the *flocculonodular* lobes of the cerebellum. From the flocculonodular lobes the signals are also transmitted back into the reticular nuclei of the brain stem. After appropriate integration, the final necessary signals are emitted from the reticular and vestibular nuclei to cause shifts in tension of the different postural muscles, thereby causing the person's body to remain in a constantly upright position in relation to the pull of gravity.

Visceral Functions of the Brain Stem. Earlier in this chapter it was noted that the brain stem contains centers for respiratory control and vasomotor control. Also located in the brain stem are nerve centers for regulation of swallowing, secretion by the gastrointestinal glands, motor movements of the gastrointestinal tract and emptying of the urinary bladder—all functions that are discussed at further length elsewhere in the chapter. Thus, the brain stem controls many subconscious visceral functions in addition to providing subconscious support of the body against gravity and maintenance of equilibrium.

Integration of Sensory and Motor Functions in the Cerebral Cortex

Primary Sensory Areas of the Cortex. Signals from each type of sensory receptor are transmitted to a specific area of the cerebral cortex. For instance, the somesthetic sensations are relayed by the *thalamus* directly to the *somesthetic cortex*. Visual sensations are relayed from the optic tract by the *lateral geniculate bodies* directly to the *visual cortex* in the *calcarine fissure* area of the occipital lobes. Auditory impulses from the auditory nerves are relayed by the *medial geniculate bodies* to the *auditory cortex* in the central portion of the *superior temporal gyri*. Taste impulses are relayed through the *nuclei of the tractus solitarius* and the *thalamus* to a small area of the cerebral cortex deep in the fissure of Sylvius, and olfactory sensations are relayed mainly to the *uncus,* the *amygdala* (a subcortical mass of neurons in the anterior temporal lobe) and the *pyriform area.*

In the visual system each minute area of the retina is connected directly to a minute area of the visual cortex. In the somesthetic sensory system each point on the surface of the body connects with a specific point in the somesthetic cortex so that stimulation of a finger, for instance, will excite only a minute area of the cortex. In the auditory cortex certain sound frequencies stimulate the anterior portion of the auditory cortex, while others stimulate the posterior auditory cortex.

In general, therefore, the types of information transmitted into the cerebral cortex by the different sensory systems are (1) the locations in the body from which the signals are arriving, (2) the types of receptors detecting the sensations, and (3) the intensities of the sensory stimuli. Once this information has entered the primary sensory areas, signals are relayed to other portions of the brain where the different types of information began to be assembled into usable thoughts.

Sensory Association Areas. Located immediately adjacent to the primary sensory areas are the *sensory association areas,* which receive direct communications from the primary sensory areas. In the sensory association areas many memories of past sensory experiences are stored, and here the new information arriving from the primary sensory areas is compared with information that has been stored from the past. In this way the significance of the new sensory signals is determined. For instance, when a person hears a word, he will not know that it is a word unless memory of that word has been stored in the auditory association areas. Likewise, when a person sees an airplane, the primary visual cortex is unable to determine the nature of the object, but, on transmission of appropriate information into the visual association areas, the person becomes aware that he is seeing an object that he has seen before and classifies it as an airplane. Similar functions are performed by somesthetic, taste and smell association areas.

Gnostic Function of the Brain. Brain surgeons have found that destruction of the posterior part of the *superior temporal lobe,* an area called *Wernicke's area,* in the left hemisphere of the right-handed person will destroy one's ability to put together information from the different sensory association areas and thereby determine the overall meaning. For this reason, this region of the brain has been called the *gnostic center,* which means simply the "knowing center." This area is well located for this purpose because it lies at the juncture of the temporal, the parietal and the occipital lobes in very close association with most of the sensory areas of the cortex.

Ideomotor Function of the Brain. Once all the information from the different sensory association areas has been integrated into a distinct conscious meaning, the brain then decides what type of physical reaction should occur—from no reaction at all to very violent reaction. This is called the ideomotor function of the brain. Again, in neurosurgical patients it has been found that damage of Wernicke's area will cause a person to lose ideomotor ability.

After all sensory information is put together, appropriate signals are then sent to the motor portion of the brain, which in turn causes muscular movements.

The Motor Pathways

Primary Motor Cortex. A strip of the cortex averaging about 2 cm. in width and lying immediately in front of the central sulcus of the brain is called the *primary motor cortex.* Stimulation of discrete points in the primary motor cortex will cause contraction of discrete muscles in the body. For instance, stimulation of the primary motor cortex at a point on top of the brain where it dips into the longitudinal fissure will cause contraction of a leg muscle on the opposite side of the body, while stimulation of the primary motor cortex where it begins to dip into the fissure of Sylvius will contract a muscle somewhere on the opposite side of the face.

Pyramidal System and Pyramidal Tracts. In the primary motor cortex of each hemisphere are some 30,000 large neuronal cells called *pyramidal* or *Betz cells.* Fibers from these cells pass downward through the *pyramidal tracts* all the way into the spinal cord. There they synapse with *interneurons located in the gray matter* of the cord. The interneurons also receive many nerve endings from (1) sensory nerve fibers entering the spinal cord through the spinal nerves, (2) propriospinal fibers originating in other segments of the cord, and (3) other nerve fibers from the brain. The interneurons, after integrating the signals from all these sources, in turn transmit impulses to the *anterior motoneurons* located in the anterior gray matter of the cord. These neurons receive additional impulses directly from (1) proprioceptive nerve fibers from the spinal nerves, (2) a few nuclei in the brain stem, and (3) other segments of the spinal cord. After integrating these signals, the anterior motoneurons in turn send impulses through the peripheral nerves to all the skeletal muscles of the body. This entire system for transmission of impulses from the motor cortex to the muscles is called the *pyramidal system.*

Stimulation of a discrete point in the motor cortex causes a discrete muscle to contract.

Premotor Cortex. Located anterior to the motor cortex is still another strip averaging about 2.5 cm in width called the *premotor cortex.* Stimulation of a discrete point in the premotor cortex usually does not cause contraction of a discrete muscle but, instead, causes a "pattern" of contraction. That is, it might cause the whole arm to rise upward, or it might cause the whole hand to flex forward, or stimulation of still another point might cause the thumb and the forefinger to move back and forth toward each other rhythmically as if cutting with scissors.

There is reason to believe that different patterns of movements can be learned and stored in the premotor cortex and that essentially all movements of the body consist of *sequences* of such learned movements. For instance, if a person should wish to throw a baseball, he would stimulate one minute portion of the premotor cortex to grip the ball, then another to pull the arm backward and upward, then another to sling the arm foward and, finally, still another to allow him to release the grip on the ball at the appropriate time. It is believed that the ideomotor function of the cortex controls the sequence of patterns of movement. Probably not more than a few hundred different patterns of movement are stored in the normal premotor cortex. However, of the thousands to millions of different combinations into which these patterns of movement can be organized, even this few number of movements allows almost any type of activity.

Extrapyramidal Pathways. To cause many of the actual muscle movements, the premotor cortex transmits signals into the motor cortex, which in turn controls the actions of the discrete muscles. However, some *gross* patterns of movement, such as those involving the trunk of the body, are transmitted through the *extrapyramidal system,* the nerve tracts of which pass first to lower centers of the brain and then from these through additional pathways to the spinal cord. For instance, one major extrapyramidal pathway is from the motor and premotor cortex to the *reticular substance* of the brain stem and from there through the *reticulospinal tracts* to the *spinal cord.* Another extrapyramidal pathway is from the motor and premotor cortex to the *basal ganglia,* to the *brain stem* and then to the *cord.*

Function of the Basal Ganglia

The *basal ganglia* are aggregates of neuronal cells that lie to the sides of the thalamus. They have very extensive neuronal connections with the premotor and the motor portions of the cortex, with the thalamus and with the nuclei of the lower brain stem. Unfortunately, little is known about the basic neurophysiology of these structures, though from a clinical point of view they are known to have four particular functions:

1. They operate in association with the premotor and the motor cortex to help *control most of the patterns of movements.* Damage to certain areas of the basal ganglia will cause abnormal and often continuous movements such as *choreiform movements, writhing movements,* and so forth.

2. The basal ganglia help to *control the basal degree of activity of the entire motor system.* Damage to certain areas of the basal ganglia can cause portions of the motor system to become greatly overexcitable, resulting in intense tonic contraction of either localized portions of the body or of the whole body. This results in a state of *rigidity.*

3. The basal ganglia operate in conjunction with the nuclei of the brain stem to *damp the antagonistic movements of the postural muscles.* For instance, if a trunk *extensor* muscle should attempt to extend the back, this would immediately elicit certain proprioceptive reflexes that would make trunk *flexor* muscles tend to contract. This in turn would tend to make the *extensor* muscles contract again, and, as a result, a continuous state of oscillation would develop. However, this effect is normally *damped* by some of the lower basal ganglia so that antagonistic postural movements throughout the body are normally very smooth rather than tremorous. But in patients who have *Parkinson's disease,* which results from damage to the *substantia nigra,* one of the lower basal ganglia, a continuous tremor exists between the antagonistic pairs of muscles either in the entire body or in certain affected areas.

4. Recent studies show that when a person performs voluntary muscle activity the basal ganglia become activated before the cerebral cortex. Therefore, it is believed that the volitional drive to incite muscle activity originates in the middle regions of the brain rather than in the cerebral cortex. A scheme that has been suggested is that the reticular substance of the mesencephalon, and perhaps portions of the thalamus, initiates the original signal and that this then spreads to the basal ganglia, cerebral cortex, and cerebellum all at the same time. Then coordinate activity in all these areas at the same time provides the motor signals to contract discrete muscles during the course of an overall pattern of muscle activity.

Function of the Cerebellum

The cerebellum receives collateral signals from the pyramidal and the extrapyramidal fibers whenever they are stimulated by the basal ganglia, the primary motor cortex and the premotor cortex, and it also receives impulses from proprioceptor nerves originating in all peripheral parts of the body. Thus, every time a motor movement is instituted by the brain, the cerebellum receives direct information of the *projected* movement from the cerebrum and receives information from the peripheral parts of the body telling it whether the movement has been accomplished and how much so. Putting these different types of information together, the cerebellum helps the motor system to stop the movements when the mission has been accomplished. To do this, the cerebellum performs two basic functions: First, it performs a *predictive function.* From the proprioceptor impulses it can tell how rapidly a part of the body is moving and from this can predict when the part will get to a desired position. As it approaches the appropriate point, impulses are transmitted from the cerebellum through the thalamus to the motor cortex and basal ganglia, there initiating the motor signals that stop the movement.

A second function of the cerebellum closely associated with the predictive function is its *damping function.* By starting to stop the movement of a limb before it gets to the desired point, the momentum of the limb will not carry it beyond its intended position. However, if the cerebellum has been destroyed, the momentum will carry the limb beyond the position. Then the other areas of the brain attempt to bring it back again to the desired position, but again the limb overshoots, and this continues several times until the intended movement is finally accomplished. Thus, in cerebellar damage, tremors occur that are very similar to those that result from basal ganglia damage. However, there is one particular difference: the basal ganglia tremor continues almost all the time when the person is awake, while the cerebellar tremor occurs only during movements associated with specific voluntary motor acts such as intentional movement of the hand from one point to another.

Failure of the predictive and the damping functions of the cerebellum causes a person to walk with *ataxic movements,* causes hand movements to be jerky if they are performed rapidly, and even causes speech to become *dysarthric,* which means that some sounds are overemphasized or held too long while other sounds are underemphasized to such an extent that the words are frequently unintelligible. It should be emphasized, though, that a person without a cerebellum can still perform most functions, even with precision, if he performs them very, very slowly. Therefore, the cerebellum is a system for helping to control very rapid motor movements while they are actually occurring, keeping them precise despite rapidity of movement.

Autonomic Nervous System

Sympathetic Nervous System. The motor impulses from the central nervous system to the visceral portions of the body are transmitted differently from those to the skeletal muscles. These pass through two different divisions of the *autonomic nervous system* called the *sympathetic* and the *parasympathetic systems.*

The sympathetic nervous system originates in neurons located in the *lateral horns* of the gray matter in the spinal cord between the first thoracic segment and the second lumbar segment. Nerve fibers pass by way of the anterior spinal roots first into the spinal nerves and then immediately into the *sympathetic chain.* From here, fiber pathways are transmitted to all portions of the body, especially to the different visceral organs.

Most sympathetic nerve endings secrete a hormone called *norepinephrine* that excites most of the visceral structures but inhibits a few. In general, it excites the heart and most of the blood vessels of the body, causing increased force of cardiac contraction and increased total peripheral resistance, with a resultant rise in arterial pressure. It inhibits the activity of the gastrointestinal tract, thereby slowing peristalsis, and it inhibits the urinary bladder, dilates the pupil of the eye, excites the liver to cause release of glucose and increases the rate of metabolism of essentially all cells of the body.

Secretion of Epinephrine and Norepinephrine by the Adrenal Medullae. Sympathetic nerves control the rate of secretion of both epinephrine and norepinephrine by the adrenal medullae, the central portions of the two adrenal glands. These hormones are carried by the blood and cause essentially the same effects in most parts of the body as those caused by direct sympathetic stimulation in each respective part. Furthermore, these hormones reach some cells that have no sympathetic nerve supply. They especially increase the rate of metabolism in all cells of the body.

The adrenal medullae represent a second means by which the central nervous system can cause sympathetic effects throughout the body. When sympathetic nerves to some organs have been destroyed, these hormones can still elicit the usual sympathetic functions when the overall sympathetic nervous system is excited.

Parasympathetic System. The parasympathetic fibers pass mainly through the vagus nerves, though a few fibers pass through several of the other cranial nerves and through the anterior roots of the sacral segments of the spinal cord. Parasympathetic fibers do not spread so extensively through the body as do sympathetic fibers, but they do innervate essentially all of the thoracic and abdominal organs, as well as the pupillary sphincter and ciliary muscles of the eye and the salivary glands.

The parasympathetic nerve endings secrete *acetylcholine,* which, like norepinephrine, stimulates some organs and inhibits others. In general, it inhibits the heart and those blood vessels that have parasympathetic innervation, but it excites the ciliary and the pupillary sphincter muscles of the eye, the glandular and motor functions of the gastrointestinal tract, the urinary bladder and the gallbladder.

Control of the Autonomic Nerves by the Central Nervous System. The activities of the sympathetic and the parasympathetic nerves are controlled in four different levels in the central nervous system: (1) in the cord, (2) in the brain stem, (3) in the hypothalamus, and (4) in the cortex. The *autonomic cord reflexes* have to do principally with local reactions in discrete parts of the body. For instance, excess filling of the rectum causes a parasympathetic reflex from the sacral cord that promotes emptying of the rectum. Visceral pain from the small intestine causes reflex sympathetic inhibition of the entire gastrointestinal tract, and excess heat to a skin area causes reflex sympathetic vasodilation of the localized blood vessels, which helps to reduce the local skin temperature.

In the *brain stem* such factors as *blood pressure, swallowing, vomiting, salivary secretion, stomach* and *pancreatic secretion* and, to a certain extent, *emptying of the urinary bladder* are all controlled. These different functions are discussed in relation to different systems of the body at other points in the chapter.

The autonomic centers of the *hypothalamus* control such functions as *body temperature, degree of overall excitability* of the body and various responses of the viscera to emotions. To perform these functions the hypothalamus transmits impulses into the lower brain stem and thence either into the vagus nerves or down into the spinal cord to stimulate the spinal autonomic centers.

Centers in the cerebral cortex can elicit almost any type of autonomic response. These responses are often of an emotional nature, such as fainting caused by widespread vasodilation through the body. Also, some are associated with muscular exercise, such as a rise in blood pressure and vasodilation in the muscles. The responses caused by the cerebral cortex are transmitted mainly through the autonomic centers in the hypothalamus and the lower brain stem.

EYE

Optics of the Eye

Function of the Eye as a Camera—the Lens System. The eye is constructed very much like a camera. The *retina* is analogous to the film in a camera, the *cornea* and the *lens* of the eye are analogous to the lens system of a camera, and the *pupil* is analogous to the diaphragm of a camera.

Light rays on entering the eye are refracted—that is, they are bent—at four different surfaces: (1) the anterior surface of the cornea, (2) the posterior surface of the cornea, (3) the anterior surface of the lens, and (4) the posterior surface of the lens. It is this bending of the light rays that allows an image of the scene in front of the eyes to be focused on the retina in exactly the same way that an image is focused by the lens system of a camera on the film. The image is upside down and reversed to the opposite side from the orientation of the object in front of the eyes.

Mechanism of Focusing. For a clear image to be formed on the retina, the surfaces of the cornea and of the lens of the eye must have the appropriate degrees of curvature in relation to the distance of the retina behind the lens system. That is, the image must be focused on the retina. The eye can change the curvature of the lens in the following way: Attached around the periphery of the lens are approximately 70 ligaments that pull continually to the side, keeping the lens normally in a flattened shape. The lens itself is a very elastic structure so that when these ligaments are loosened, it assumes a round, globular shape. When an object comes close to the eye, increased curvature of the lens is required to focus a clear image on the retina. To do this a muscle called the *ciliary muscle* is tightened. This muscle is a circular sphincter extending all the way around the peripheral attachments of the ligaments, and on contraction the ligaments are loosened. This automatically allows the lens to change from its normal flattened shape to a globular shape, thereby assuming far greater curvature and allowing adequate focusing of the images of nearby objects.

Yet, the tension on the lens ligaments must be controlled very exactly, or the lens might become too round for adequate focusing. This is controlled by the cerebral cortex. If the image is in poor focus, the visual image in the brain also is indistinct, and appropriate impulses are transmitted back through the third cranial nerve to the ciliary muscle to adjust the degree of contraction.

The diameter of the pupil is controlled by a nervous reflex originating in the retina called the *light reflex*. Impulses caused by strong light on the retina are transmitted along the optic nerve and the optic tract into the *pretectal nuclei* of the midbrain, from there to the *visceral nucleus of the third nerve* and then back to the pupillary constrictor to decrease the pupillary aperture. Conversely, in darkness, lack of light signals from the retina reverses the reflex and causes the diameter of the pupil to increase.

Another importance of the pupil is that it alters the *depth of focus* of the eye. When the image on the retina is not in exact focus, the light rays passing through the peripheral edges of the lens will be much more out of focus than those passing through the very center of the lens. However, as the pupillary diameter becomes smaller, the light rays entering the peripheral edges of the eye are blocked and do not reach the retina. Therefore, by constricting the size of the pupil, which occurs in bright light, a person whose lens is not in exact focus will still have fairly clear vision.

Function of the Retina

Rods and Cones. The light sensitive receptors of the retina are millions of minute cells called *rods* and *cones.* The rods distinguish only the white and the black aspects of an image while the cones are capable of distinguishing its colors as well.

In general, from 50 to 400 rods are connected to a single optic nerve fiber while, in the central portion of the retina, a single cone is connected to a single optic nerve fiber. As a result, minute points of light on the retina can be localized to very discrete positions by the cones but can be localized far less acutely by the rods. Thus, very acute and clear vision of objects is mediated by the cones, while only a diffuse type of vision is mediated by the rods. The central portion of the retina, called the *fovea centralis,* has only cones, which allows this portion to have very sharp vision, while the peripheral areas, which contain progressively more and more rods, have progressively more diffuse vision.

Rhodopsin–Retinene Cycle. For a person to see an image, the light energy entering the eye must be changed into nerve impulses. In the rods this is accomplished by means of a chemical system called the *rhodopsin–retinene cycle.* Large quantities of the light-sensitive substance *rhodopsin,* also known as *visual purple,* are present in the rods. When light impinges on these, a small portion of the rhodopsin is transformed immediately into another substance called *lumi-rhodopsin,* which is a very unstable compound and lasts in the rods for only a fraction of a second. Instead, it degenerates through a series of chemical steps to form two substances called *retinene* and scotopsin (a protein). But, during the split second while the rhodopsin is being degraded, the rod becomes excited, sending nerve impulses from the retina into the optic nerve.

The retinene and scotopsin are gradually recombined by the metabolic processes of the rod to re-form rhodopsin, thereby continually supplying the rod with new rhodopsin.

Retinene is derived from vitamin A; therefore, when a person has a very serious deficiency of vitamin A in his diet, his retina is likely to become relatively insensitive to light, causing the condition known as *night blindness.*

Dark and Light Adaptation. The retina is capable of adapting its sensitivity so that the eye can see almost equally as well in both very bright light and moderate darkness. This retinal adaptation is a far more powerful mechanism than the pupillary adaptation discussed above, though it requires several minutes to several hours to develop fully each time the person changes to a new level of light intensity. The mechanism of dark and light adaptation is the following:

When a person remains in very bright light for a long time, extremely large quantities of rhodopsin are split into retinene and scotopsin; this reduces the quantity of rhodopsin in the rods and therefore makes them become insensitive to light, which is called *light adaptation.* Conversely, when a person spends a long time in darkness, only very small amounts of rhodopsin are split while the metabolic systems of the rods are continually building more and more rhodopsin. Consequently, rhodopsin collects in very high concentrations after a while and greatly increases the sensitivity of the retina; this is called *dark adaptation.*

One might wonder why it is important for the sensitivity of the retina to change. However, it must be remembered that to see an image clearly there must be dark areas in the image as well as light areas. If the retina should remain highly sensitive all of the time and a person should then go out into the bright sunlight, all portions of the image would be so bright that everything would appear white without any dark areas.

Color Vision. The cones of the eye function in very much the same way as the rods except that the light sensitive chemicals are slightly different from rhodopsin. These chemicals still utilize retinene as the basis for light sensitivity, but the retinene combines with a *photopsin* rather than with scotopsin. Each photopsin, like scotopsin, is a protein, but slightly different from other photopsins. The nature of this protein determines the color sensitivity of the light sensitive chemical. There are three major groups of cones that respond especially intensely to certain colors of light. These cones are classified as *blue* cones, *green* cones and *red* cones.

The eye determines the color of an object by the *relative intensities* of stimulation of the different types of cones. For instance, yellow is a color having a wavelength midway between green and red. Therefore, it stimulates the green and the red cones about equally, which gives one the sensation of seeing the color yellow. Orange has a wavelength somewhat closer to that of red light than of green light. Therefore, it stimulates the red cones about twice as much as it does the green cones, giving the sensation of orange. Finally, pure red light stimulates the red cones very strongly while stimulating the green and blue cones only weakly. This gives the sensation of red. The same principles hold true for the different shades of color between green, blue, and yellow.

Transmission of Impulses from the Retina to the Cerebral Cortex. Each point of the retina is represented by a discrete point in the visual cortex located in the calcarine fissure area of the occipital cortex. Therefore, every time a spot of light hits a particular area of the retina, a corresponding area is stimulated in the visual cortex. From here second order and third order impulses pass to the visual association and gnostic areas of the brain as described earlier in the chapter.

In addition to transmitting the light and the dark spots of the image to the brain, the retina also sends surges of extra impulses into the brain when the intensity of light on the retina increases or decreases or when some object moves across the surface of the retina. The function of these impulses seems to be to call one's attention either to moving objects or to rapid changes in light intensities.

The retina, the visual transmission pathways, and the visual cortex also respond especially strongly to contrast points in the visual pattern. For instance, at borders between light and dark areas, the visual cortex is very strongly stimulated.

EAR

Transmissions of Sound from the Tympanum to the Cochlea. Sound is caused by compression waves that travel through the air at a velocity of about $\frac{1}{5}$ mile per second. As each compression wave strikes the *tympanum,* it is forced inward, and between compressions the tympanum moves outward. The center of the tympanum is connected to the *ossicular system,* which consists of a series of bony levers that transmit the sound vibrations into the *cochlea* at the *oval window.* The tympanum and the ossicular system function as a sound "transformer," for the tympanum itself has a surface area some 20 times the surface area of the oval window, giving a total increase in force of the sound vibrations against the oval window of about 20-fold.

Resonance in the Cochlea—Determination of Pitch. The cochlea is composed of two major fluid chambers, the *scala vestibuli* and the *scala tympani,* which lie side by side in a coil and are separated by the *basilar membrane.* Inward movement of the stapes against the oval window pushes the fluid in the scala vestibuli, and this in turn causes the basilar membrane to push the fluid in the scala tympani. Finally, the fluid in the scala tympani pushes outward against the *round window.* Thus, every time the stapes moves inward, the round window bulges outward into the middle ear.

Low frequency sound causes the stapes to move back and forth very slowly, which allows the pressure waves to travel far up into the scala vestibuli before maximum bulging of the basilar membrane into the scala tympani occurs. On the other hand, high frequency sound waves cause very rapid vibration of the stapes, and the waves travel only a short distance into the scala vestibuli before maximum bulging occurs. In this way a form of resonance occurs in the cochlea, with low frequency waves causing maximum back-and-forth vibration of the basilar membrane near the far tip of the cochlea and high frequency sound causing vibration of the basilar membrane near the base of the cochlea, that is, close to the oval and round windows. The brain determines the pitch of the sound mainly from the portion of the basilar membrane that vibrates—high pitch near the base of the cochlea and low pitch near the apex.

Stimulation of the Hair Cells—Determination of Loudness. Located on the surface of the basilar membrane are many *hair cells* similar to those in the vestibular apparatus discussed earlier. When the basilar membrane vibrates, these cells are stimuated—the more forceful the vibration the greater the frequency of stimulation. And the loudness of the sound is determined by this frequency of impulses transmitted from the hair cells into the brain.

Transmission of Auditory Impulses into the Brain. Approximately 25,000 nerve fibers are attached to the hair cells of the cochlear apparatus. The auditory signals in the auditory nerves go first to the *cochlear nuclei* located in the brain stem; from here they pass upward to the *medial geniculate body* and then to the *auditory cortex* in the superior temporal gyrus. The spatial orientation of the nerve fibers is maintained all the way from the basilar membrane to the auditory cortex so that one sound frequency excites one area of the auditory cortex while another sound frequency excites another area. The meanings of the auditory signals are then interpreted in the *auditory association areas* immediately adjacent to the primary auditory cortex.

CHEMICAL SENSES

Taste

Taste Buds and the Primary Sensations of Taste. Located on the surfaces of the tongue, especially on the circumvallate papillae, which lie in a V line on the posterior part of the tongue, and also in small numbers on the lateral walls of the pharynx, are many small nerve receptors called *taste buds.* These have a hollow cavity that communicates through a small *pore* with the mouth. Lining the cavity are sensory taste receptor cells, and taste "hairs" protrude from the ends of these cells into the cavity. Certain types of chemicals that diffuse through the taste pores can excite the hairs of the taste cells.

Four different types of taste buds are known to exist, each of these responding principally to (1) saltiness, (2) sweetness, (3) sourness, and (4) bitterness. The first three of these taste sensations help the person to select the quality of food that he eats and in some instances even makes him desire certain substances such as salt that may be deficient in his body. The last of the taste sensations, bitterness, is principally for protection, because most of the naturally occurring poisons among plant foods elicit a bitter taste that normally will cause an animal to reject the food.

Transmission of Taste Impulses into the Brain. Most of the taste impulses are transmitted by way of the *chorda tympani* into the *seventh nerve* and then into the brain stem; the remainder are transmitted through the *ninth nerve* into the brain stem. The impulses pass mainly to the *nucleus of the tractus solitarius,* then to the *thalamus,* and finally to the *primary taste cortex,* which lies immediately posterior to the central sulcus of the brain deep in the fissure of Sylvius.

Smell

The Olfactory Epithelium and Its Stimulation. Located in the superiormost part of each nostril is a small area having a surface of about 2 sq. cm. called the *olfactory epithelium.* This contains large numbers of *olfactory cells* that send *cilialike* processes into the mucus lining the nose. Almost any chemical substance that can diffuse through the mucus and then into these cilia will stimulate one or more of the olfactory cells. Since the cilia themselves have lipid membranes, lipid-soluble substances stimulate the cells much more readily than non-lipid-soluble substances. The precise types of chemicals that stimulate different olfactory cells are not known, for it has been very difficult to study by either subjective or objective means the olfactory stimulus from a single olfactory cell. It is believed that there might be seven or more primary sensations of smell and that the many hundreds of different smells to which we are accustomed are actually combinations of these primary sensations.

Transmission of Olfactory Impulses into the Brain. From the olfactory cells signals are transmitted through the *olfactory tract* into the *midline nuclei* of the brain that lie superior and anterior to the hypothalamus, and into the *pyriform cortex* and *amygdala*. The midline nuclei control the crude functions of smell, such as eliciting salivation or licking the lips. The pyriform cortex and amygdala deal with olfactory conditioned reflexes that determine appetite or the more social responses to food.

GASTROINTESTINAL TRACT

Motor Movements of the Gastrointestinal Tract

Propulsive Movements. There are two general types of movements in the gastrointestinal tract: the *propulsive movements* that propel food forward along the tract and the *mixing movements* that keep mixing the intestinal contents.

The principal propulsive movement is *peristalsis,* which occurs in all smooth muscle tubes. That is, stimulus of a single section of the gut causes a constrictive ring to move forward along the gut, pushing any material in the gut ahead of the constriction. A nerve plexus in the wall of the gut called the *myenteric plexus* helps to control the peristalsis, keeping the peristaltic movements oriented principally in the analward direction along the gut rather than in the upward direction, and also strengthening the peristalsis.

In the lower end of the stomach and in the small intestine the propulsive movements are relatively strong, so that ingested food moves all the way to the large intestine within 3 to 10 hours. However, the propulsive movements in the large intestine are strong only for a few minutes out of each day. As a result, the intestinal contents remain for many hours in the large intestine, allowing reabsorption of most of the electrolytes and water before expulsion of the feces.

Swallowing is a special type of propulsive movement.

When food is pushed into the back of the mouth by the tongue, nerve receptors on the sides of the pharynx elicit an automatic swallowing process. Signals are transmitted from these receptors to the brain stem, integrated there and then transmitted back to the pharynx and upper esophagus. A peristaltic wave begins in the pharyngeal constrictors, the glottis closes so that food cannot pass into the trachea, the constrictor muscle at the opening of the esophagus relaxes so that the food will enter the esophagus, and then the peristaltic wave proceeds downward along the upper esophagus, all of this controlled directly by nerve impulses from the brain stem. On reaching the lower half of the esophagus, the natural peristaltic process of the gastrointestinal tract takes over and propels the food the rest of the way to the stomach.

The Mixing Movements. *Chyme.* Special movements promote mixing of the food with intestinal secretions. In the stomach these are mainly peristaltic waves that are not strong enough to propel the food through the pylorus but are strong enough to keep mixing the food with the secretions. The mixture of food and secretions that results is called *chyme*.

In the small intestine, intermittent constrictive rings occur as often as several times a minute, dividing the intestine into segments. Then the constrictions relax and others occur at other points. In this way the chyme is chopped again and again into small aliquots. These movements are called *segmenting contractions*. In the large intestine similar segmenting contractions called *haustrations* occur; these slowly roll the fecal matter over and over, allowing almost complete absorption of the water and electrolytes.

Secretion in the Gastrointestinal Tract

Secretion of Saliva. Saliva is secreted principally by the *parotid,* the *submaxillary* and the *sublingual glands.* Their secretion is controlled by the *salivatory nuclei* in the brain stem, and these in turn can be stimulated either by nerve impulses from the mouth when food is eaten or by psychic stimuli from the cerebral cortex.

Secretion in the Stomach. Stomach secretion occurs in response to either nervous stimuli or hormonal stimuli. About half of the secretion is caused by vagal impulses transmitted from the *dorsal motor nuclei of the vagi* in the brain stem. These in turn are caused by (1) impulses from the cerebrum initiated by the thought of food or the smell of food, (2) impulses from the mouth during the chewing process, and (3) impulses from the stomach when food is actually in the stomach; this last is the stimulus that causes at least half of all the stomach secretion.

The hormonal mechanism operates in the following

way: Certain types of food, especially those that have a high degree of taste, extract a hormone called *gastrin* from the mucosa of the stomach antrum. This hormone then passes by way of the blood stream to the *gastric glands* of the stomach body and fundus to cause secretion of a very highly acid gastric juice.

Secretion by the Pancreas. The pancreas, like the stomach, is also stimulated by both nervous and hormonal stimuli. The same factors that cause nervous impulses to the stomach also cause impulses to the pancreas and thereby promote secretion of digestive enzymes.

Stimulation of the pancreas by hormonal mechanisms occurs as follows: The chyme, on entering the small intestine, extracts two different hormones from the intestinal mucosa, *secretin* and *cholecystokinin,* and these are carried in the blood to the pancreatic acini. Secretin causes the pancreas to secrete large amounts of highly alkaline solution, and cholecystokinin causes the pancreatic cells to release large quantities of digestive enzymes. Secretin is released from the intestinal mucosa mainly in response to acid emptied from the stomach into the duodenum, and the alkaline pancreatic secretion in turn neutralizes the acid. The cholecystokinin is released mainly in response to the presence of protein and fats in the chyme, and the secreted enzymes in turn help to digest the proteins and fats.

Secretion in the Small Intestine. Almost all of the secretion in the small intestine is caused by local stimulation of the intestinal glands. This results from either mechanical stimulation of the mucosa by the chyme or distention of the gut, both of which elicit very rapid flow of intestinal juices mainly by way of *intramural nervous reflexes* in the *submucosal* and *myenteric plexuses.*

Secretion of Mucus. Mucus is secreted in all parts of the gastrointestinal tract, from the salivary glands all the way to the mucosal glands of the large intestine. Mucus is an excellent lubricant and is also very resistant to chemical destruction either by the intestinal juices or by different types of foods. Therefore, it provides excellent protection for the mucosa of the gastrointestinal tract.

Digestion in the Small Intestinal Tract

The chemical processes of digestion are all processes of *hydrolysis* of the different foods. This means that the food molecule splits into two smaller molecules, and at the same time a hydrogen atom from a water molecule combines at the point of splitting with one of the food products while the remaining hydroxyl radical from the water combines with the other food product. The carbohydrates are hydrolyzed into *monosaccharides,* the fats into *glycerol* and *fatty acids* and the proteins into *amino acids.* Hydrolysis of the different types of foods is catalyzed by different types of enzymes called the *digestive enzymes.*

Digestion of *carbohydrates* is begun by *salivary amylase* secreted in the saliva, and their digestion is carried still much further by *pancreatic amylase* secreted in the pancreatic juice. After the action of these two, the carbohydrates will have been split principally into *disaccharides.* Then four enzymes in the epithelial cells of the small intestinal mucosa, *sucrase, maltase, isomaltase* and *lactase,* split the disaccharides into *monosaccharides,* principally *glucose, fructose* and *galactose.*

The *fats* are split into *glycerol* and *fatty acid molecules* by *lipases* secreted mainly in the pancreatic juice but to a very slight extent in other digestive secretions.

Protein digestion begins in the stomach under the influence of *pepsin* and *hydrochloric* acid. Then it continues under the influence of *trypsin* and *chymotrypsin* secreted by the pancreas. At this point, the proteins will have been digested into large *polypeptides.* Then several different *peptidases* secreted in the pancreatic juice or found in the intestinal epithelial cells split the polypeptides into *amino acids.*

Absorption From the Gastrointestinal Tract

Active Absorption. Certain substances can be *actively absorbed* from the gastrointestinal tract. This means that the molecules are transported through the intestinal mucosa by a chemical process that greatly enhances the rate of absorption. This active absorption is very similar to that which occurs in the urinary tubules, which was explained earlier in the chapter. Substances that can be actively absorbed are most *monosaccharides*—especially glucose, fructose, and galactose—the *amino acids, sodium ions* and several *other ions.*

Passive Absorption. Passive absorption means absorption of substances simply by diffusion through the membrane. When substances in the chyme are actively absorbed, such as glucose, the amount of osmotically active substances increases in the intestinal wall interstitial fluids, while the amount decreases in the chyme. As a result, tremendous quantities of water are osmotically absorbed from the gut. Also, when positively charged ions such as sodium ions are actively absorbed, a positive charge builds up on the vascular side of the membrane, and this pulls negatively charged substances such as chloride ions through the membrane. The most important substances passively absorbed are water, chloride ions and fats.

Portal and Lymphatic Routes of Absorption.

Almost all of the water-soluble substances are absorbed directly into the blood capillaries of the villi, and they then pass with the portal blood through the liver into the general circulatory system. This is called the portal route of absorption, and the substances absorbed in this way are (1) most of the water and electrolytes, (2) the carbohydrates, and (3) the proteins.

Fatty acids are not absorbed into the blood of the villi but, instead, while passing through the epithelium of the villus, recombine with glycerol to form neutral fat. This then passes into the lymphatics and is transmitted upward along the thoracic duct in the form of *chylomicrons* to be emptied into the veins of the neck.

Gastrointestinal Disorders

Peptic Ulcer. The digestive enzymes in the stomach juice can digest the mucosa of the stomach itself or of the duodenum, if ever the secretions penetrate through the mucous cell coat of the mucosa. Ordinarily, especially large quantities of mucus are secreted by the entire mucosal surface of the stomach and duodenum. Furthermore, the acidity of the stomach secretions is immediately neutralized by alkaline pancreatic juice when the secretions enter the duodenum. However, the protective barrier against the stomach juice sometimes loses some of its effectiveness. For instance, continued sympathetic stimulation reduces the secretion of mucus by the glands of Brunner in the upper duodenum and therefore predisposes to the development of a duodenal ulcer. Also, some persons have been shown to secrete five or more times as much stomach juice as the normal person during the interdigestive period between meals, the normal person usually secreting only a few milliliters during the whole night. Obviously, the excess acid in the stomach juice is difficult to neutralize in the absence of food in the stomach to combine with much of the acid; therefore, this is perhaps the most common cause of peptic ulcer. Worry and anxiety commonly increase this interdigestive secretion.

Diarrhea and Constipation. Almost any irritation of the gastrointestinal mucosa greatly increases the local rate of secretion of intestinal juices and also the intensity of peristalsis. This causes a "washout" phenomenon, the material in the irritated area flowing rapidly toward the anus. Thus, the most common cause of *diarrhea* is mucosal irritation, often due to *bacterial infection* but sometimes to *irritative foods*.

Diarrhea can also result from *excessive activity of the parasympathetic nervous system*, because parasympathetic stimulation increases the secretory and pro-pulsive activities of the GI tract throughout its entire extent but especially so of the latter half of the large intestine. This, too, results in rapid "washout" of the gut.

Exactly the opposite effects can cause *constipation*. *Sympathetic stimulation*, for instance, decreases the activity of the gastrointestinal tract throughout its entire extent and can result in serious constipation. Also, *spasm* of the gut at some point in *the descending colon or the sigmoid* is a common cause of constipation, for spasm of even a small area in this region can prevent adequate emptying of the large intestine even though colon activity elsewhere may be completely normal. Such spasm is often caused by *local irritation.*

Achalasia and Megacolon. Two gastrointestinal disorders have been shown to be caused by either lack of or dysfunction of the myenteric plexus in the intestinal wall. One of these is *achalasia,* which results from neuronal dysfunction at the lower end of the esophagus, and the other is *megacolon,* which results from lack of or deranged myenteric plexus in the sigmoid. In either instance, the propulsive movements through the affected area are either greatly inhibited or blocked. In achalasia the food piles up in the esophagus, sometimes causing an extreme enlargement of the esophagus called *megaesophagus*. In the case of megacolon, the failure of feces to pass through the sigmoid causes progressive dilatation of the colon, sometimes resulting in bowel movements as infrequently as once a month.

METABOLISM AND ENERGY

Metabolism of Carbohydrates and Synthesis of Adenosine Triphosphate

Glucose as the "Common Denominator" in Carbohydrate Metabolism. The digestive products of essentially all carbohydrates are *glucose, fructose* and *galactose*. Much of the fructose is converted to glucose as it is absorbed by the intestinal epithelium, and the galactose, after being absorbed, is transmitted by the portal blood mainly to the liver where it is almost immediately converted into glucose. Then this glucose eventually passes back out of the liver cells into the blood to join the glucose that is absorbed directly from the gastrointestinal tract. Therefore, it is in the form of glucose that essentially all carbohydrates are made available to the cells to be metabolized.

Storage of Glycogen in the Liver. Large quantities of glucose, either that converted from fructose and galactose or that directly absorbed from the gastrointestinal tract, can be stored in the liver cells in the form of *glycogen granules*, glycogen being a polymer of glucose. Special enzymes in the liver cells cause the polymerization of glucose into glycogen. Then when the glucose level in the blood falls too low, the glycogen is split by still other enzymes back into glucose, which then passes into the blood to be utilized elsewhere in the body. In this way extra glucose is removed from the blood when the blood glucose concentration is too high and then is returned when the blood glucose falls too low. Thus, the liver provides a *blood glucose-buffering function.*

Entry of Glucose into the Cells—Effect of Insulin. The pores of the cell membranes are almost completely impermeable to glucose. Fortunately, glucose is *transported* through the membrane by a facilitated diffusion carrier mechanism, as was discussed in the early part of the chapter. The activity of this carrier mechanism for glucose transport is controlled by the amount of *insulin* secreted by the pancreas. Large amounts of insulin increase the rate of glucose transport to about 15 times the rate when no insulin is available. When the pancreas fails to secrete insulin, very little glucose can enter most cells, but when excess insulin is secreted, glucose enters the cells so rapidly that the blood glucose level falls very low.

Glycolysis and Synthesis of Adenosine Triphosphate. After entry into the cells, glucose can be polymerized into glycogen and stored temporarily as glycogen granules, or it can be used immediately to provide energy for cellular functions. The initial process for providing energy is principally *glycolysis,* which means splitting each molecule of glucose to form *pyruvic acid.* This occurs by a series of chemical reactions involving several stages of *phosphorylation* and several *transformations* all catalyzed by protein enzymes in the cells.

During the different stages of glycolysis, a net of two molecules of *adenosine triphosphate* are synthesized for every molecule of glucose converted into pyruvic acid. In this way a small portion (about three per cent) of the energy stored in the glucose molecule is transferred to adenosine triphosphate molecules, which in turn are very highly reactive and can provide immediate energy to other functional systems of the cells as it is needed.

Citric Acid Cycle and the Release of Carbon Dioxide and Hydrogen from Pyruvic Acid. The two molecules of pyruvic acid formed from glucose in the glycolysis process contain about nine tenths of the energy that was originally in the glucose molecule. To make this available to the cell, each molecule of pyruvic acid is first split into carbon dioxide and hydrogen. This occurs principally by means of a series of chemical reactions called by various names: the *Krebs cycle,* the *tricarboxylic acid cycle* or the *citric acid cycle.*

The pyruvic acid is first decarboxylated to form *acetyl coenzyme A,* and this immediately combines with *oxaloacetic acid* to form *citric acid.* Then the citric acid is progressively decomposed, liberating carbon dioxide and hydrogen atoms. The carbon dioxide diffuses out of the cells and is blown off by the lungs into the expired air. However, the hydrogen atoms are then made available to react with oxygen, a process that provides tremendous amounts of energy to the cell as will be disscussed below. After the carbon dioxide and hydrogen atoms have been removed, the residue of the citric acid molecule is a new molecule of oxaloacetic acid that can be used over and over again in the citric acid cycle.

All the chemical reactions in the citric acid cycle are catalyzed by another series of enzymes called *decarboxylases* (which remove the carbon dioxide) and *dehydrogenases* (which remove the hydrogen atoms).

Oxidation of Hydrogen and Synthesis of More Adenosine Triphosphate. Most of the hydrogen that is released during the breakdown of pyruvic acid combines with nicotinamide adenine dinucleotide and from this is rapidly passed to another substance, a *flavoprotein.* Then the hydrogen leaves the flavoprotein to become hydrogen ions, and the electrons removed from the hydrogen atoms are passed rapidly through a series of *electron carriers,* including cytochrome B, cytochrome C, cytochrome A, and cytochrome oxidase, and finally to the dissolved oxygen in the fluids of the cell to convert the oxygen into hydroxyl ions. The presence of both hydrogen and hydroxyl ions in the same fluid allows immediate combination of the two to form water. The water in turn diffuses out of the cell and eventually is excreted by the kidneys or evaporates from the body.

The important feature about this oxidation of hydrogen is not the formation of water but, instead, the use of energy from the hydrogen and oxygen atoms for synthesis of *adenosine triphosphate* (ATP). Thirty-six molecules of adenosine triphosphate are formed for each molecule of glucose oxidized, 18 times as many molecules as are formed by the process of glycolysis. Therefore, it is this final oxidation of pyruvic acid that is the main source of energy for the cells.

Role of the Mitochondria in the Citric Acid Cycle and in "Oxidative Phosphorylation." The overall process by which hydrogen ions are oxidized and the released energy is used to generate adenosine triphosphate is called *oxidative phosphorylation.* This entire process occurs inside the mitochondria. It begins with transport of acetyl coenzyme A, which is formed from pyruvic acid, through the double wall of the mitochondrion into the mitochondrial cavity. It is here that the chemical reactions of the citric acid cycle occur and hydrogen atoms are released. The exact manner in which the hydrogen atoms are then utilized to cause the formation of adenosine triphosphate is not clear. However, experiments suggest the following mechanism: The first step is ionization of the hydrogen atoms and passage of the electrons removed during the ionization process through the electron carrier system. The electron carriers are large protein molecules that are integral parts of the inner wall of the mitochondrion. As the electrons pass from one carrier to the next, they give up energy, and the energy is used to pump hydrogen ions from the central cavity of the mitochondrion into the space between the two mitochondrial walls. This creates a high concentration of hydrogen ions in this space. Then the large hydrogen ion gradient across the inner wall of the mitochondrion causes the hydrogen ions to leak back through the wall toward the central cavity. As they do so, they interact with still other large protein molecules that are also integral parts of the wall. These molecules are ATPase enzymes that are capable of catalyzing adenosine triphosphate synthesis and are called *ATP synthetase*. They utilize energy from the moving hydrogen ions to cause conversion of adenosine diphosphate plus a phosphate radical into ATP. Thus, in this roundabout way, the tremendous energy that had been present in the glucose molecule is finally used to form ATP, which itself stores a large portion of this energy and uses it later to catalyze almost all intracellular reactions.

Functions of Adenosine Triphosphate. Adenosine triphosphate is a highly labile compound, the formula for which is the following:

At each point where the last two phosphate radicals attach (indicated by the curving bonds, called "high energy phosphate bonds") about 8,000 calories of energy are available in each mole of adenosine triphosphate. These two phosphate radicals can split away with great ease and can transfer this energy to other chemical processes in the cells. Thus, adenosine triphosphate is almost an explosive compound that is ready to act immediately. As it is used up, more adenosine triphosphate is formed by the processes described above.

Some of the specific functions of adenosine triphosphate are (1) to provide the immediate energy needed for contraction of muscle cells, (2) to provide the en-

ergy needed to pump sodium out of nerve and muscle cells so that action potentials can be transmitted along the membranes, (3) to provide the energy needed to synthesize new proteins by the ribosomes in the cytoplasm, and (4) to provide the energy needed for synthesis and secretion of almost all substances formed by the glands. These are only a few of the functions of adenosine triphosphate, for, actually, without adenosine triphosphate almost no chemical reactions can occur in cells.

Metabolism of Fats

Transport of Fats in the Plasma—the Lipoproteins. Most fatty substances are not soluble in the body fluids. Therefore, most of the fatty substances in the blood are in the form of minute suspended particles, only a fraction of a micron in size, called *lipoproteins*. The fatty substances in the lipoproteins are loosely bound with varying amounts of protein. The proteins in turn, being miscible with water, increase the suspension stability of the lipoproteins in the plasma and prevent excessive adherence of them to each other or to the endothelium.

A very small amount of fatty acids, about 10 mg. per 100 ml., is present in the plasma *in combination with the albumin of the plasma proteins*. These are called *free fatty acids*. Despite this very small concentration, this fatty acid is transferred extremely rapidly back and forth with the tissue fats, as much as one half of it transferring every 2 to 3 minutes. Such rapid mobility makes this the *principal means of transport* of most of the fat from one area of the body to another.

Chylomicrons. After absorption of fatty acids from the small intestine, these acids immediately recombine in the intestinal epithelial cells with glycerol to form minute particles of neutral fat that then aggregate to form minute fat globules called *chylomicrons*. These pass through the intestinal lymphatics and the thoracic duct to empty into the blood. Within an hour or so after a meal has been completely absorbed most of the chylomicrons will have been removed from the circulating blood, some of them being absorbed by the liver cells and a very large portion being split by an enzyme, *lipoprotein lipase*, into fatty acids that are either metabolized for energy or are resynthesized into fat by the *fat cells* and stored.

Fat Depots. All the fat cells of the body are known collectively as *fat depots*. Fat can remain stored in the fat cells for hours, days or months. When the amount of circulating fatty acid falls very low in the blood during the interdigestive period between meals, the stored fat is split by *tissue lipoprotein lipase* into fatty acid and then transported in the blood to other cells of the body where it may be needed.

Use of Fat for Energy—Synthesis of Adenosine Triphosphate. Fat is used by the body to provide energy in almost identically the same way that carbohydrates are used. The chemical processes for deriving energy from fats include the following stages: (1) The neutral fat is split inside the fat cells into *glycerol* and *fatty acids.* The glycerol, having a chemical composition very similar to that of certain glucose breakdown products, can easily be oxidized to energize the formation of adenosine triphosphate molecules. (2) The fatty acid molecules are partially oxidized mainly in the liver cells by a process called *beta carbon oxidation,* which causes the fatty acid to split and form many *acetyl coenzyme A molecules.* These in turn enter the mitochondria where they are decomposed by the citric acid cycle and then completely oxidized by the oxidative phosphorylation process to synthesize large numbers of adenosine triphosphate molecules in exactly the same way that the acetyl coenzyme A derived from pyruvic acid is used for the same purpose. Thus, fats provide energy in nearly the same manner as carbohydrates except that the initial stage for splitting carbohydrates is mainly the *glycolysis* mechanism while the initial stage for splitting fats is principally an *oxidation* mechanism.

A large share of all fatty acid degradation begins in the liver, but only a small portion of the acetyl coenzyme A formed in the liver cells can be used for energy in the liver itself. Instead, this is transported away from the liver by the blood in the form of *acetoacetic acid,* a condensation product of two molecules of acetyl coenzyme A. This in turn is absorbed by the other cells of the body where it is split again into acetyl coenzyme A, then enters the citric acid cycle and is used for energy.

Phospholipids. All cells of the body synthesize *phospholipids,* which are chemical substances derived mainly from fat and have certain of the physical and chemical characteristics of fats, but most of these are synthesized in the liver or intestinal epithelial cells. The phospholipids are used by the cells to form part of the cellular membrane, different intracellular membranes and other intracellular structures. One of the most important features of all cellular life is the different compartments into which each cell is divided by lipid membranes. The physical characteristics of the phospholipids and other fatty substances in these membranes make it possible for them to separate the cytoplasm from the extracellular fluid, the nucleoplasm from the cytoplasm, the fluids of the mitochondria from the cytoplasm, and so forth.

Cholesterol. Another substance derived from fats is *cholesterol;* it, too, has many physical and chemical characteristics similar to those of fat. Like phospholip-

ids, cholesterol is synthesized by all cells of the body and is used along with phospholipids and neutral fat in composing the different membranous structures of cells. An especially large amount of cholesterol is formed by the liver, and about 80 per cent of this is then used by the liver to synthesize bile acids that are secreted with the bile into the small intestine. These in turn promote emulsification of fats in the gastrointestinal tract so that they can be digested, and they also promote fat absorption. Also, cholesterol is used by the sex glands and the adrenal cortex for synthesis of different steroid hormones.

Atherosclerosis. Unfortunately, large quantities of cholesterol are occasionally either synthesized by the walls of the arteries or are deposited there from the blood. As a result, large *plaques* of cholesterol frequently develop in the arterial walls and protrude through the intima into the flowing arterial blood. This disease is called *atherosclerosis.* Blood clots often develop on the protruding cholesterol plaques, the clot at times becoming large enough to occlude completely the lumen of the vessel. This is the cause of most acute coronary occlusions that bring about heart attacks.

The rate at which cholesterol is deposited in the walls of the arteries is directly proportional to the intake of calories in the diet, especially when this is above the daily requirements for energy. Atherosclerosis also seems to be more severe when most of the intake of calories is in the form of highly saturated fats rather than in the form of unsaturated fats, proteins and carbohydrates. Certain persons are genetically inclined to very severe atherosclerosis.

Metabolism of Proteins

Transport and Storage of Amino Acids. The amino acids, which are the end products of protein digestion in the gastrointestinal tract, are absorbed into the portal blood and then are disseminated into all parts of the body. Small amounts of the amino acids diffuse into the liver cells and are temporarily stored there, though this is of minor importance in comparison with the storage of glucose and fat by the liver. By far the greater portion of the amono acids is rapidly absorbed directly into all the cells of the body.

Cellular Synthesis of Proteins. Once inside the cells, most amino acids are rapidly synthesized into proteins. This process is controlled by *messenger ribonucleic acid molecules* that act as *templates* for the formation of the protein molecules. This overall mechanism was described at the beginning of this chapter in the discussion of cellular physiology.

Essential Amino Acids. The usual proteins of the body contain 20 different amino acids, and these are available in almost all protein foods that are eaten.

However, an occasional protein of the diet has a deficiency of one or more of the usual amino acids. Often one of the available amino acids can be converted into the missing one, but 10 of the 20 amino acids cannot be formed this way and must be present in the diet in order for the cells to synthesize their normal complements of proteins. These 10 amino acids are called *essential amino acids.*

Synthesis of Other Substances from Amino Acids. Many special chemical substances needed in the cells are synthesized from amino acids. For instance, many of the hormones are either modified amino acids or small polypeptides, including *thyroxine, epinephrine, parathyroid hormone, posterior pituitary hormones* and *insulin.* In addition, such important substances as *adenosine triphosphate* and *creatine phosphate* derive parts of their structures from proteins.

Catabolism of Proteins in the Cells. *Catabolism* of proteins means splitting of the proteins back into amino acids. A small concentration of amino acids, about 30 mg. per 100 ml., is always maintained in the plasma and interstitial fluid. When this amount decreases, amino acids begin to diffuse out of the cells, and this causes the proteins of the cells to begin to be catabolized into amino acids. This catabolism is catalyzed by intracellular enzymes called *cathepsins,* which are digestive enzymes released from *lysosomes* in the cells. In this way a small concentration of amino acids is always maintained in the body fluids. Then, if a particular cell becomes damaged or for some other reason needs an immediate source of amino acids to repair its structural and enzyme systems, the amino acids are available. Thus, amino acids can be mobilized from one part of the body to another by this process—to wherever the need is momentarily greatest. Amino acid mobilization is greatly accelerated by *glucocorticoid hormones.*

Deamination of Amino Acids and Their Use for Energy. If a person eats more protein than the amount needed to maintain adequate protein stores in the cells, all the excess amino acids are degraded and then used for energy as carbohydrates and fats are used. The first stage in this process is *deamination,* which means removal of the amino radical from the amino acid. This is accomplished by a specific enzyme system in the liver cells. The amino radical is then synthesized into *urea,* which is excreted through the kidneys into the urine.

Many of the resultant deaminated amino acids are similar to pyruvic acid and can enter the citric acid cycle either directly or after a few stages of minor alterations. In this way, the amino acids become oxidized in very much the same way as carbohydrates and fats, and large quantities of adenosine triphosphate are formed to be used as an energy source everywhere in the cells.

Nutrition

The Energy Equivalent of Foods—Calories. In the above sections it has been noted that carbohydrates, fats and proteins can all supply energy to the cells. Energy is generally expressed in terms of Calories (spelled with a capital C), which are equivalent to kilocalories. However, the different types of food are not equal in their capabilities for supplying energy. One g. of carbohydrate or 1 g. of protein supplies 4.1 Calories of energy to the body, while 1 g. of fat supplies 9.3 Calories of energy. Therefore, it is evident that over twice as much carbohydrate or protein must be eaten to provide the same amount of energy as a specified quantity of fat.

Energy Requirements. A normal adult requires about 1,600 Calories of energy each day simply to exist even without sitting up or walking around. To provide the energy needed for sitting, another 200 to 400 Calories is required; and for walking a moderate amount, still another 500 Calories. The total daily energy requirement for the average person adds up to about 2,500 Calories. This is called the *metabolic rate* of the body. For performing very heavy physical labor this can occasionally be as great as 6,000 to 7,000 Calories per day.

Basal Metabolic Rate. The *basal metabolic rate* is the metabolic rate of an awake person whose body is as inactive as possible. To attain the *basal state* a person must have had essentially no exercise for the past 8 to 10 hours, no food for the past 12 hours, and he must have quiet conditions and normal room temperature. The normal basal metabolic rate of the young male adult is about 40 Calories per sq. m. of body surface area per hour or a total of about 70 Calories per hour for the whole body.

Daily Protein Requirement. About 30 g. of amino acids are degraded each day and used by the body mainly for synthesizing various necessary intracellular substances. Even when a person is starving, this degradation of amino acids continues. Therefore, simply to maintain normal protein stores of the body, about 30 g. of proteins are needed in the diet per day. And, if these proteins do not contain the correct *ratios* of amino acids, or if they are not utilized completely by the body, still larger amounts of protein are required.

Obesity. Obesity means simply the storage of excess amounts of fat in the body. When more energy foods are ingested than are utilized each day, the extra amount is stored in the form of fat. Even excess carbohydrates and proteins are converted into fat and then stored. Thus, obesity actually develops from a greater intake of energy each day than utilization of energy. Unfortunately, certain people have far more insatiable appetites than others, which causes them to continue eating far beyond their energy needs. Sometimes this results from abnormal function of the feeding centers in the hypothalamus.

Starvation. In starvation, the stored energy substances in the body are utilized very rapidly. Sufficient *glycogen* is stored in the liver and muscle cells to provide significant amounts of energy for about ½ to 1 day. Beyond that, almost all the energy made available to the body at first comes from the stored fat, this sometimes lasting for as long as 3 to 8 weeks. However, during the entire process of starvation a small amount of body protein is continually degraded and used for energy as well, and when the fat stores begin to run out, tremendous amounts of protein then begin to be used for energy. When this happens, the functional state of the cells quickly deteriorates, and death soon follows. However, it is fortunate that most of the proteins are spared until the last.

Functions of the Vitamins. Vitamins are substances ingested in the food in only minute quantities but that play key roles in the metabolic systems of the body. The functions of some of the important vitamins are the following:

Vitamin A is used to synthesize rhodopsin, which was discussed earlier as a necessary chemical for vision. It also aids in the normal growth of cells, especially epithelial cells.

Thiamine operates as part of a *cocarboxylase* for removal of carbon dioxide from foods being used by the cells.

Niacin functions in the body in the forms of *nicotinamide adenine dinucleotide (NAD)* and *micotinamide adenine dinucleotide phosphate (NADP)*. These act as hydrogen acceptors when hydrogen is removed from the foods; therefore, they are important in the oxidation of food.

Riboflavin is used to form flavoprotein, which is also a hydrogen carrier in the oxidation of foodstuffs.

Vitamin B₁₂ and *folic acid* were discussed earlier in the chapter as substances needed for the maturation of red blood cells in the bone marrow.

Pantothenic acid is a precursor of *coenzyme A,* which is needed for acetylation of many substances in the body. It is especially needed for the formation of acetyl coenzyme A prior to oxidation of both glucose and fatty acids.

Pyridoxine is used as a coenzyme in many reactions involving amino acid metabolism, one of which acts to transfer amino radicals from one substance to another, and another of which causes deamination.

Ascorbic acid (vitamin C) is a strong *reducing compound* that probably acts in several metabolic processes in which electrons are exchanged with oxidative chemicals. Though the precise nature of these specific chemical reactions is not known, the major physiologic function of ascorbic acid is to maintain normal intercellular substances, including normal collagen fibers and normal intercellular cement substance between the cells.

Vitamin D is needed for absorption of calcium from the gastrointestinal tract.

Vitamin K, which was discussed in connection with blood coagulation, is needed in the synthetic processes of the liver for formation of prothrombin, Factor VII, and several other factors that are utilized in blood coagulation.

Regulation of Body Temperature

Body temperature is controlled by the balance between the *rate of heat production* in the body and the *rate of heat loss.* If the rate at which heat is produced is greater than the rate at which it is lost, the body temperature will rise. On the other hand, if the rate of loss is greater, then the body temperature will fall.

Heat Production and Its Control. All the metabolic processes of the body produce heat as a byproduct, for almost all the energy in the food eventually becomes heat after it has performed its other functions. Thus, in the average person at least 2,000 Calories of heat are formed each day. Therefore, the rate of heat production is controlled by the metabolic rate of the body.

Under basal conditions it is mainly the internal organs—the brain, the heart, the kidneys, the gastrointestinal tract and especially the liver—that produce most of the heat. However, when a person uses his muscles for various activities, these produce tremendous amounts of heat. During extreme muscular activity the total heat production of the body can increase temporarily to as much as 15 times normal, over 90 per cent of the heat than coming from the muscles.

Heat Loss. Normally, the most important means by which the skin loses heat to the surroundings is by *radiation;* that is, heat waves, a type of electromagnetic radiation, are transmitted from the surface of the body to surrounding objects. A large portion of the heat is also lost by *conduction* to the surrounding air and then *convection* of the heated air away from the body. Finally, when a person sweats, very large amounts of heat are consumed to cause *evaporation* of the water in the sweat.

The skin is supplied with an abundant vasculature, but the amount of blood that flows through these vessels is controlled very exactly by the sympathetic nervous system so that when the body becomes overly heated blood flow will be tremendous, and when the body is underheated blood flow will be negligible. Rapid flow of blood heats the skin, allowing large amounts of heat to be lost to the surroundings. Also, sympathetic stimuli to the sweat glands increase sweat production and consequently greatly increase the evaporative loss of heat. Slow blood flow prevents heat loss because the skin temperature falls rapidly to approach that of the surroundings.

Regulation of Body Temperature by the Hypothalamus. Portions of the hypothalamus are sensitive to changes in body temperature, so that whenever the blood becomes too hot or too cold, appropriate readjustments in the rates of heat production and heat loss return the body temperature to normal.

Located in the *preoptic area* of the anterior hypothalamus is a small region called the *heat center.* When this becomes too cold, signals are transmitted into the posterior hypothalamus, and this causes three effects: (1) *it reduces the rate of heat loss* by constricting the blood vessels to the skin; (2) it transmits signals through the brain stem and spinal cord to stimulate the skeletal muscles throughout the body; this in turn increases muscle tone and causes *shivering,* which increases the muscle metabolic rate, sometimes *increasing heat production* as much as 300 per cent; and (3) it *increases heat production by causing release of epinephrine* which has a small effect to increase the rate of metabolism of all cells in the body, sometimes increasing heat production as much as 20 to 40 per cent. As a result of all these effects, the body temperature rises back toward normal.

When the preoptic area becomes too hot, this same temperature system functions in exactly the opposite manner. It *decreases heat production* by reducing the tone of the skeletal muscles throughout the body and reducing the sympathetic release of epinephrine. More important, however, it *increases the rate of heat loss* in two ways: (1) lack of sympathetic vasoconstriction allows the blood vessels of the skin to become greatly dilated; the skin temperature rises, and increased amounts of heat are lost to the surroundings; and (2) stimulation of a sweat center also in the preoptic area of the anterior hypothalamus causes sweating over the entire body, with resultant evaporative loss of heat.

In summary, if the preoptic area of the anterior hypothalamus becomes too hot, heat production is decreased while heat loss is increased, and the body temperature falls back toward normal. Conversely, if the anterior hypothalamus becomes too cold, heat production is increased, while heat loss is decreased so that the body temperature now rises toward normal.

Effect of Skin Temperature Signals on Body Temperature Regulation. Not only do signals from the preoptic area of the hypothalamus play an important role in body temperature regulation, but temperature signals from the skin do also. When the skin becomes too warm, nerve impulses are transmitted from the skin warm receptors all the way to the preoptic area of the hypothalamus to increase sweating, and this obviously increases body heat loss. Conversely, when the skin becomes too cold, signals from the skin cold receptors are transmitted to the posterior hypothalamus where they activate shivering, which in turn helps to increase the body temperature back toward normal. Therefore, body temperature control is vested in an integrated mechanism in which the hypothalamus is the central integrator, but reacts to signals both from the preoptic area and from the skin.

Local reflexes from the skin to the spinal cord and then back to the skin to control the degree of local sweating and local vasodilatation or constriction also play a minor role in temperature control.

ENDOCRINE GLANDS

The endocrine glands secrete *hormones* that control many of the body's functions. Hormones function in three major ways: (1) by controlling transport of substances through cell membranes, (2) by controlling the activity of specific cellular genes, which in turn determine the formation of specific enzymes and other cellular factors, and (3) by controlling directly some metabolic systems of cells.

Some hormones perform their functions by first activating an *intracellular hormonal mediator* called a *second messenger* that then performs the specific intracellular function. The most important of the second messengers is *cyclic adenosine monophosphate.* To activate this intracellular mediator, the general hormone first binds with a receptor on the surface of the membrane of the target cell. This receptor in turn activates the enzyme *adenylcyclase* in the membrane, and this in turn causes formation of cyclic AMP inside the cell. And, finally, the cyclic AMP performs a specific function within the cell such as causing an increase of enzymes, alteration of cell permeability or modification of chemical reactions within the cytoplasm.

Pituitary Hormones

The pituitary gland secretes hormones that regulate a wide variety of functions in the body. This gland is divided into two major divisions: the *anterior pituitary gland* and the *posterior pituitary gland.* At least six well-known hormones are secreted by the anterior pituitary gland—*growth hormone, thyroid stimulating hormone, adrenocorticotropic hormone, prolactin* and two *gonadotropic hormones*—while two well-known posterior pituitary hormones are secreted—*antidiuretic hormone,* also called *vasopressin,* and *oxytocic hormone.*

Control of Pituitary Hormone Secretion by Hypothalamic Hormones. When the anterior pituitary gland is separated from the hypothalamus, secretion of most of its hormones, with the exception of prolactin, decreases to very small amounts. This occurs because secretion by the anterior pituitary gland is controlled mainly by hormones formed in the hypothalamus and then conducted to the pituitary through the hypothalamic-hypophyseal portal system. This system consists of small veins that carry blood (and hormones) from capillaries in the lower hypothalamus to the venous sinuses of the anterior pituitary gland. Here, the hormones from the hypothalamus act directly on the anterior pituitary cells to control secretion of the pituitary hormones. Most of the hormones from the hypothalamus have a positive effect on the anterior pituitary cells, causing release of the pituitary hormones, but some of them have a negative effect, inhibiting release.

The important hypothalamic hormones that control the function of the anterior pituitary gland are the following:

Growth hormone-releasing hormone that causes release of *growth hormone*

Corticotropin-releasing hormone that causes release of *adrenocorticotropic hormone*

Thyrotropin-releasing hormone that causes the release of *thyroid-stimulating hormone*

Luteinizing hormone-releasing hormone that causes release of the two gonadotropins, *luteinizing hormones* and *follicle-stimulating hormone*

Prolactin inhibitory hormone that inhibits the release of *prolactin* (in the absence of this hormone, the rate of prolactin secretion increases to about three times normal)

Growth Hormone. Growth hormone causes growth of the body. It is secreted by the anterior pituitary gland throughout life, not merely while a person is growing. It causes enlargement and proliferation of cells in all parts of the body, resulting in progressive growth of the body stature until adolescence. At this time the epiphyses of the long bones unite with the shafts of the bones so that further increase in height of the body cannot occur. However, certain of the "membranous" bones and soft tissues, such as the bones of the nose and certain bones of the skull, as well as the tissues of some of the internal organs, still continue to grow.

The precise mechanism by which growth hormone exerts its effects on the cells is not clear. However, it is known to act on the liver to cause formation of several small protein substances called *somatomedin.* It is this substance that in turn causes growth of the bones and perhaps also causes many of the other effects of growth hormone.

Growth hormone also promotes transport of some amino acids through cell membranes, thereby making more of these available to the cells. In addition, it (1) activates the RNA translation process to cause increased formation of proteins by the ribosomes, (2) increases the rate of DNA transcription to increase the amount of messenger RNA, (3) increases the replication of DNA which causes increased reproduction of the cells themselves, and (4) decreases the rate of breakdown of proteins in the cells. Thus, growth hormone has a potent effect to enhance all aspects of protein synthesis and storage in the cells of the body. It is resumably this effect that is most important in promoting growth.

After adolescence, growth hormone continues to be secreted at about two-thirds the preadolescent rate. Though most growth in the body stops at this time, primarily because the growth potential of the long bones ceases when the epiphyses unite with the shafts, the other metabolic effects of growth hormones continue. Growth hormone also affects carbohydrate metabolism, though not nearly as much as protein metabolism. It increases the blood sugar and decreases the rate of metabolism of carbohydrates by the cells. Growth hormone affects fat metabolism as well. It increases the rate of breakdown of fats into fatty acids and increases their use for energy by all the cells.

Growth hormone secretion is controlled by *growth hormone-releasing hormone* that is secreted in the hypothalamus and transported to the anterior pituitary gland *through the hypothalamic-hypophyseal portal system.* When nutritional debility causes hypoglycemia or decreases the body's protein stores, the secretion of growth hormone-releasing hormone and therefore also the rate of growth hormone secretion are increased. Also, other types of physical stress or mental stress can increase the rate of growth hormone secretion under some conditions.

Thyroid-Stimulating Hormone. Thyroid-stimulating hormone stimulates the thyroid glandular cells in many ways: (1) it increases the rate of synthesis of thyroglobulin, (2) it increases the rate of uptake of iodide ions from the blood by the glandular cells, and (3) it activates all the chemical processes that cause thyroxine production and release by the thyroid gland. Therefore, indirectly, thyroid-stimulating hormone increases the overall rate of metabolism of the body, for, as will be discussed later, this is the principal effect of thyroxine.

The degree of activation of the anterior pituitary gland to secrete thyroid–stimulating hormone is controlled principally by a negative feedback effect of thyroxine on the hypothalamus. When the thyroxine concentration is high, this decreases the rate of secretion of *thyrotropin-releasing hormone* by the hypothalamus and also decreases the activity of the anterior pituitary glandular cells to produce thyroxine. Therefore, when excess thyroxine is already present in the blood, this feedback effect turns off further production.

Adrenocorticotropic Hormone. Adrenocorticotropic hormone strongly stimulates *cortisol* production by the adrenal cortex, and it stimulates the production of other adrenocortical hormones to a much less extent. Cortisol in turn has many different metabolic effects in the body, including especially degradation of proteins in the tissues, release of amino acids into the circulating blood, conversion of many of these amino acids into glucose (the process of gluconeogenesis), and decreasing utilization of glucose by tissue cells. These effects will be discussed later in relation to the adrenal hormones.

The secretion of adrenocorticotropic hormone by the anterior pituitary is controlled mainly by *corticotropin-releasing hormone* from the hypothalamus. The rate of secretion of this hormone, in turn, is strongly stimulated by stressful states such as disease, trauma to the body, and even emotional excitement. Also, when excessive quantities of cortisol are present in the blood, the depressant effect on the hypothalamus and anterior pituitary cells results in a decrease the rate of secretion of adrenocorticotropic hormone, thus providing a negative feedback mechanism for controlling the concentration of cortisol in the blood.

The Gonadotropic Hormones. The anterior pituitary gland secretes two hormones called *gonadotropic hormones* that regulate many male and female sexual functions. These are *follicle-stimulating hormone* and *luteinizing hormone*. The rates of secretion of these hormones are controlled mainly by *luteinizing hormone-releasing hormone* from the hypothalamus. However, feedback effects from the sex hormones also help to control their rates of secretion. The gonadotropic hormones will be discussed in more detail later in the chapter in relation to the male and female functions.

Prolactin. Prolactin plays an important role in the development of the breasts during pregnancy and also in promoting milk secretion by the breasts after birth of the baby. These functions will be discussed in more detail in relation to milk production.

The secretion of prolactin is controlled mainly by *prolactin inhibitory hormone* from the hypothalamus. Prolactin secretion increases about 10-fold during pregnancy. Its rate of secretion is also increased by suckling of the nipples by the baby; this in turn causes production of more milk.

Posterior Pituitary Hormones. Two different hormones are secreted by the posterior pituitary gland. The first of these is *antidiuretic* hormone, which was discussed earlier in relation to water reabsorption from the renal tubules. Briefly, when the body fluids become excessively concentrated, neuronal cells in or near the supraoptic nucleus of the hypothalamus, called *osmoreceptors,* cause antidiuretic hormone to the released from the posterior pituitary gland. On reaching the kidney, this hormone enhances the rate of water reabsorption from the renal tubules and tends to correct the overconcentration of the body fluids.

Antidiuretic hormone also constricts the arterioles and causes the arterial pressure to rise, for which reason it is sometimes called *vasopressin.* Finally, this hormone can also cause contraction of many other smooth muscle structures throughout the body.

The second posterior pituitary hormone, *oxytocin,* causes contraction especially of the uterus but to a less extent of some of the other smooth muscle structures of the body. Oxytocin is released by the posterior pituitary gland in increased amounts during parturition, and it may play a significant role in initiating birth of the baby. Oxytocin also plays a role in lactation in the following way: Sucking on the breast initiates nerve impulses that pass all the way from the nipple to the hypothalamus, which then sends signals to the posterior pituitary gland to cause release of oxytocin. The oxytocin in turn stimulates *myoepithelial cells* that constrict the alveoli of the breast in a manner that makes the milk flow into the ducts. This is called *milk ejection* or *milk letdown.*

Adrenocortical Hormones

The adrenal cortex secretes three different types of steroid hormones that are chemically similar to each other but physiologically widely different. These are: (1) the *mineralocorticoids,* which are represented principally by *aldosterone,* (2) the *glucocorticoids,* which are represented mainly by *cortisol,* and (3) the *androgens.*

Mineralocorticoids—Aldosterone. The mineralocorticoids have significant effects on electrolyte balance in the body. Several such hromones are secreted by the adrenal cortex, but probably 95 per cent or more of the total mineralocorticoid activity is due to *aldosterone.*

Aldosterone was discussed earlier in this chapter in relation to reabsorption of sodium from the renal tubules and tubular secretion of potassium. Briefly, aldosterone enhances sodium transport from the tubules into the peritubular fluids, and at the same time enhances potassium transport from the peritubular fluids into the tubules. Therefore, aldosterone causes conservation of sodium in the body and excretion of potassium in the urine.

Aldosterone also causes increased reabsorption of choloride ions and water from the tubules in the following ways: When sodium is reabsorbed, this immediately creates a positive charge on the outside of the renal tubules that pulls the negative chloride ions through the membrane. When increased amounts of sodium and chloride are reabsorbed, the osmotic concentration of the tubular fluid decreases, while the osmotic concentration of the peritubular fluids increases. As a result, large quantities of water are absorbed by osmosis into the extracellular fluid, and the total extracellular fluid volume increases.

The important factors for control of aldosterone secretion are: (1) An increase in potassium ion concentration has an especially powerful effect to cause increased aldosterone secretion. This provides a negative feedback system for controlling the extracellular fluid potassium ion concentration because the aldosterone then promotes excretion of the excess potassium from the extracellular fluid into the urine. (2) Angiotensin also can strongly stimulate the secretion of aldosterone. This controls the total extracellular fluid volume in the following way: When the extracellular fluid volume decreases, the arterial pressure also tends to decrease. This then causes the kidney to form renin and angiotensin as was explained earlier in the chapter. The angiotensin stimulates aldosterone secretion, which in turn causes absorption of sodium, chloride, and water, thus increasing the extracellular fluid volume back toward normal. (3) Decreased sodium ion concentration in the extracellular fluid also stimulates aldosterone secretion. This may occur because decreased sodium also stimulates angiotensin formation. (4) Adrenocorticotropic hormone has a slight effect to increase aldosterone secretion.

Glucocorticoids—Cortisol. Several different *glucocorticoids* are secreted by the adrenal cortex, but almost all of the glucocorticoid activity is caused by *cortisol,* also called *hydrocortisone.* Glucocorticoids affect the metabolism of glucose, proteins and fats.

Cortisol decreases glucose uptake into cells and also decreases the rate of utilization of glucose by the cells. In addition, it increases the rate of *gluconeogenesis* in the liver cells, which converts amino acids into glucose that is then emptied into the blood. Thus, several different effects cause the blood concentration of glucose to increase.

Cortisol also causes degradation of proteins and decreases protein synthesis in most tissues of the body. This causes amino acids to be released from the cells and therefore increases their concentration in the blood. The liver, however, is different from the other tissues because cortisol increases amino acid uptake by liver cells. There they are used to synthesize increased quantities of plasma proteins, to provide metabolic energy for the liver, and to be converted into glucose by the process of gluconeogenesis as noted above.

Cortisol causes increased use of fat for energy. This results mainly from an effect of cortisol to activate *hormone sensitive lipase* in the fat cells that causes splitting of the fat and release of fatty acids into the circulating blood.

In an animal that does not secrete cortisol, the body's tissues are very susceptible to cellular destructive processes. However, stress of almost any type—such as trauma, surgical operations, disease, mental stresses, and so forth—causes increased secretion of cortisol. This cortisol in turn seems to be essential for repair of damaged tissues. However, the manner in which cortisol stimulates tissue repair still is not understood. Perhaps it is the increase in availability of amino acids and glucose in the blood induced by cortisol that is mainly responsible for this effect.

Cortisol can also suppress inflammation. One of the most important mechanisms of this is that cortisol stabilizes the cellular lysosomes, preventing them from rupturing and releasing their digestive enzymes, histamine, bradykinin, and other factors that promote the inflammation process. Cortisol also decreases the permeability of capillary membranes, which minimizes edema formation during inflammation.

Androgens. The androgens are steroid hormones that cause masculinizing effects in the body. Though the most important androgen is testosterone secreted by the testis, the adrenal cortex also secretes several androgenic hormones. These are normally of minor importance, but, when an adrenal tumor develops or when the adrenal glands become hyperplastic and secrete excess quantities of hormones, the amounts of androgens secreted occasionally become great enough to cause even a child or an adult female to take on adult masculine characteristics, including growth of a beard, change of the voice to a bass quality and increased muscular strenght.

Thyroid Hormones

Formation and Release of Thyroxine. The thyroid gland is composed of follicles lined with glandular cells. These cells secrete a very large glycoprotein called *thyroglobulin* to the inside of the follicle. They also absorb iodide ions from the circulating blood and secrete these in an oxidized form into the follicles along with the thyroglobulin. This oxidized iodine combines with tyrosine amino acid molecules that are integral parts of the large thyroglobulin molecule. In this manner, large quantities of *thyroxine* (and much smaller quantities of *triiodothyronine*) are formed within the thyroglobulin molecule, and the thyroglobulin is then stored in the thyroid follicles for an average of about 6 weeks. As thyroid hormones are needed in the circulating blood, some of the thyroglobulin is reabsorbed back into the glandular cells by the process of *pinocytosis*. Then the thyroglobulin is digested by *proteases* released from lysosomes, thus releasing thyroxine and triiodothyronine into the blood.

The rate of formation of the thyroid hormones, and especially their rate of release from thyroglobulin, is controlled by *thyroid stimulating hormone* from the anterior pituitary gland, as was discussed earlier.

Once the thyroid hormones have been released into the blood, they combine with several different plasma proteins. Then during the next week they are slowly released from the blood into the tissue cells.

Effect of Thyroxine on the Cells. Thyroxine increases the rate of activity and metabolism of almost all cells in the body. It also increases the breakdown of all cellular foodstuffs and the rate of heat release from the cells.

Unfortunately, the exact manner in which thyroxine performs its functions in the cells is still unknown. However, it does increase the rate of synthesis of proteins in most cells and especially the rate of synthesis of many different enzymes that in turn are the basis for the increased metabolic activities of the cells. It also increases the sizes and numbers of mitochondria in the cells, and these in turn increase the rate of production of ATP, which might be another factor that promotes enhanced cellular metabolism.

Hyperthyroidism. An excess of thyroxine secretion above that needed for normal function of the body is called hyperthyroidism. Briefly, this causes excessive activity of essentially all the functional systems of the body including (1) greatly increased rate of metabolism throughout the body, (2) increased heart rate and increased cardiac output, (3) increased gastrointestinal secretion and gastrointestinal motility, (4) increased activity of the nervous system, sometimes causing a fine tremor of all the muscles, (5) increased respiratory rate, (6) often abnormal glandular secretion by the other endocrine glands, and (7) severe loss of weight in extreme cases.

Hypothyroidism. The opposite of hyperthyroidism is hypothyroidism; it results from too little secretion of thyroxine. It causes greatly inhibited activity of almost all the functional systems, including (1) a decrease in metabolic rate to as low as 40 per cent below normal, (2) sometimes such lethargy that the person sleeps 14 to 16 hours per day and even when awake has difficulty cerebrating, and (3) collection of a mucinous fluid in the tissue spaces between the cells, creating an edematous state called *myxedema*.

Pancreatic Hormones—Insulin and Glucagon

The pancreas secretes two different hormones, *insulin* and *glucagon,* the first of which is of extreme importance to normal function of the body. Insulin is a small protein, molecular weight about 6000, formed by the *beta cells* of the *islets of Langerhans*. Glucagon likewise is a small protein, molecular weight about 3500, formed by the *alpha cells* of the islets of Langerhans.

The Metabolic Role of Insulin. Insulin is often called the "storage hormone" because its secretion is greatly increased immediately after a meal, and it causes cellular storage of all of the different foodstuffs including carbohydrate, fat, and protein.

Effect of Insulin on Carbohydrate Metabolism. Insulin has an especially large effect to cause glucose storage following a meal. Approximately 60 per cent of this is stored in the liver, and about 15 per cent is stored in the muscles, while most of the remainder is used for energy. The mechanism by which insulin promotes glucose storage in the liver is quite different from the mechanism in muscle. In the liver, glucose diffuses through the cell membrane with ease but is trapped in the hepatic cells by being converted first into *glucose phosphate* and then into *glycogen*. Insulin promotes this effect by greatly increasing the activities of two liver enzymes, *glucokinase* and *glycogen synthetase*. In muscle and most other cells of the body (besides the liver and the brain) insulin increases the permeability of the cell membranes to glucose. In the presence of large amounts of insulin, the membrane of resting muscle is about 15 times as permeable to glucose as it is when there is no insulin. Insulin also moderately increases the activity of the enzymes in these cells both for storing glucose in the form of glycogen and also for increased metabolic usage of the glucose.

Insulin has no measurable effect on transport of glucose into the brain cells. Instead, the rate of glucose diffusion into these cells is directly proportional to blood glucose concentration.

The insulin system plays the most important role of all the hormones in maintaining a normal blood glucose concentration. The large amounts of insulin secreted after each meal prevent the glucose concentration from rising too high by causing storage of almost all of the absorbed glucose in the liver. Then, between meals, in the absence of insulin, most of this glucose returns to the blood because of a continual breakdown of glycogen in the liver when insulin is not present.

It is especially important that the blood glucose concentration be regulated in this manner because it assures a relatively unvarying rate of delivery of glucose to the brain. Unfortunately, the brain cells are special in that they cannot utilize fats and proteins for energy. Therefore, the regulation of blood glucose concentration—which is performed principally by the action of insulin—helps to maintain a steady rate of neuronal activity.

Effect of Insulin on Fat Metabolism. Insulin has both direct and indirect effects on fat metabolism. The direct effect is to decrease the rate of fatty acid release from fat tissues into the body fluids. The mechanism of this is mainly intense depression of *hormone sensitive lipase* by insulin which prevents the hydrolysis of triglycerides in the fat tissue and therefore prevents fatty acid release. Conversely, when there is little insulin, this enzyme becomes excessively active and causes large quantities of fatty acids to be released into the tissue fluid. In this way, fatty acids become mobilized and are utilized for energy in place of glucose that cannot be utilized in most tissues of the body without insulin.

The indirect effect of insulin on fat metabolism occurs secondarily to insulin induced changes in carbohydrate metabolism. Insulin has the same effect on fat cells that it has on muscle cells to cause increased glucose transport into the fat cells. This causes some increase in formation of fatty acids in these cells and then storage of these in the form of triglycerides. However, the most important effect is that the glucose inside the fat cells is used to form the *glycerol portion* of the stored triglycerides. In addition to this small amount of fat synthesized entirely in the fat cells, much larger quantities of fatty acids are synthesized in the liver when there is excess blood glucose and insulin. These fatty acids are then transported to the fat cells where they too are stored as triglycerides.

When large quantities of fatty acids are released from the fat cells in the absence of insulin, many of these are transported to the liver where they form excessive quantities of (1) stored fat in the liver, (2) cholesterol, phospholipids, and triglycerides that are then released into the blood, and (3) acetoacetic acid that is also released into the blood. In prolonged periods of no insulin secretion, the acetoacetic acid can become so great that it causes severe acidosis.

Effect of Insulin on Growth and Protein Metabolism. Insulin is absolutely essential for growth. Even growth hormone will not cause a significant amount of growth in an animal in the absence of insulin. Insulin probably has this effect because it increases the formation of protein in cells. It does this by promoting active transport of amino acids through the cell membrane to the interior of the cell, by increasing the number of functional ribosomes for forming proteins, and by increasing the activity of the DNA–RNA system that controls protein formation.

Control of Insulin Secretion. The rate of secretion of insulin by the pancreas is controlled mainly by the concentration of glucose in the circulating blood but also by the concentration of amino acids as well. At high concentrations of these, large quantities of insulin are secreted, and the insulin in turn promotes storage of both glucose and amino acids in the body cells. At low concentrations, the rate of insulin secretion decreases, and both glucose and amino acids are then transported out of the cells.

Diabetes Mellitus. Failure of the pancreas to secrete sufficient amounts of insulin results in *diabetes*. In this disease, the metabolism of all the basic foodstuffs is altered. The basic effect on glucose is to prevent its uptake by essentially all cells of the body besides those of the brain. As a result, blood glucose concentration rises very high, while cellular utilization of glucose falls lower and lower. Fat utilization rises higher and higher to make up the difference. Four principal sequelae often result from these basic effects:

First, the very high blood glucose concentration causes far more glucose to filter into the renal tubules than can be reabsorbed. Because this unabsorbed glucose creates osmotic pressure in the tubules, it also prevents reabsorption of much of the tubular water, thereby promoting very rapid diuresis with loss of large quantities of extracellular fluid into the urine and resulting *dehydration*.

The second effect, which can be even more detrimental than the first, results from the increased utilization of fats for energy. This causes the liver to release acetoacetic acid into the plasma far more rapidly than it can be taken up and oxidized by the tissue cells. As a result, the patient develops severe *acidosis*, which, in association with the dehydration, causes *diabetic coma*. This leads rapidly to death unless the condition is treated immediately with large amounts of insulin.

A third effect is to cause, over a prolonged period of time, depletion of the body's proteins. Also, failure to utilize glucose for energy leads to decreased storage of fat as well. Therefore, a person with severe untreated diabetes suffers rapid loss of weight and often death within a few weeks without treatment.

Fourth, also over a long period of time, the excess fat utilization in the liver causes very large amounts of cholesterol in the circulating blood and also increased deposition of cholesterol in the arterial walls. This leads to severe *arteriosclerosis* and other *vascular lesions*.

Glucagon. Glucagon has the opposite effect on

blood glucose to that of insulin, sometimes causing it to double in as little as 20 minutes. It causes this effect by increasing the rate of breakdown of glycogen in the liver cells. Over a longer period of time, it also causes marked increase in gluconeogenesis, which is the process by which amino acids are converted into glucose. The mechanism by which glucagon causes release from the liver cells is believed to be the following: Glucagon activates *adenylcyclase* in the liver cell membranes. This in turn causes formation of cyclic AMP in the cells, which then activates *phosphorylase,* the enzyme that causes glycogen to split into glucose molecules.

When the blood concentration of glucose falls below normal, the pancreas secretes large amounts of glucagon. The blood glucose raising effect of glucagon then obviously helps to correct the hypoglycemia. Therefore, glucagon is also important for control of blood glucose concentration, though probably not nearly so important as insulin.

Parathyroid Hormone and Physiology of Bone

Formation of Bone. Before the function of parathyroid hormone can be explained, we must first discuss the basic physiology of bone and its relation to calcium and phosphate in the extracellular fluids. Bone is formed by *osteoblasts,* which line the outer surfaces of all bones and are also present inside most of the bone cavities. The osteoblasts secrete a very strong *protein matrix,* comprised mainly of collagen fibers, which gives the bone its toughness. This matrix has the special property of causing phosphate ions to combine with calcium ions, precipitating a complicated salt of calcium and phosphate called *hydroxyapatite* in the protein matrix to make it extremely hard. The extreme strength of the collagen fibers gives the bone tremendous tensile strength, while the hardness of the bone salt gives it tremendous compressive strength.

When calcium is not available is large quantities in the body fluids, bone is poorly formed. Calcium is difficult to absorb from the gastrointestinal tract, and when it fails to be absorbed, phosphate is also poorly absorbed because the two substances form insoluble compounds in the gut. However, *vitamin D* greatly increases calcium absorption, which in turn allows increased phosphate absorption. Therefore, lack of vitamin D decreases the amount of available calcium and phosphate for bone formation and can result in such poor mineralization of the bones that they no longer resist compressive forces. This is the disease known as *rickets.* Before vitamin D can increase calcium absorption by the gastrointestinal tract, it must be converted from its natural form into the substance

1,25-dihydroxycholecalciferol. The first stage of this conversion occurs in the liver and a second stage in the kidney; the second stage requires the presence of parathyroid hormone. Therefore severe liver disease, kidney disease, or lack of parathyroid hormone can lead to diminished calcium absorption by the intestinal tract.

Absorption of Bone. Bone is also continually absorbed by large numbers of *osteoclasts* present in the bone cavities. This absorption of bone has two major functions: (1) In all bones the protein matrix gradually becomes aged and loses its toughness, thus allowing the bone to become brittle. The absorptive process removes the aging bone, which is continually replaced by new bone formed by the osteoblasts. (2) Absorption of bone provides a means by which calcium ions can be made available rapidly to the extracellular fluids.

Function of Parathyroid Hormone. Parathyroid hormone is principally concerned with the regulation of calcium ion concentration in the body fluids. It does this to a great extent by regulating the activity of the osteoclasts—the greater the parathyroid secretion, the greater becomes the number of osteoclasts and the greater their rates of activity, thereby markedly accelerating the absorption of bone. In this way, parathyroid hormone in tremendous quantities can increase the calcium ion concentration in the extracellular fluid as much as 50 per cent in as little as 4 hours. Another means by which parathyroid hormone increases calcium ion concentration in the extracellular fluid is to promote increased absorption of calcium ions from both the gastrointestinal tract and the renal tubules. At least part of the increased absorption from the intestine results from the effect of parathyroid hormone to activate vitamin D as explained earlier.

Large quantities of phosphate are also released into the blood by the absorption of bone. However, parathyroid hormone also accelerates the rate of phosphate excretion by the kidneys so that extracellular phosphate concentration, in contradistinction to the calcium concentration, usually does not rise but may actually fall when parathyroid hormone is administered.

This regulation of calcium ions by parathyroid hormone is extremely important because almost all of the excitable tissues of the body, including nerves, muscle fibers, the heart and all smooth muscle organs, depend upon a well-regulated calcium ion concentration for normal function. For instance, a low calcium ion concentration causes such extreme decreases of irritability in the peripheral nerves that they begin to emit impulses spontaneously, these causing a state of continual muscular contraction called *tetany.* Also, greatly decreased calcium ion concentration reduces the contractility of the cardiac muscle. Parathyroid hormone secretion is the principal method by which normal calcium ion concentration is maintained in the body fluids at all times, and the bones act as a large reservoir of calcium to be used for this purpose.

Regulation of Parathyroid Hormone Secretion. Whenever the calcium ion concentration in the body fluids falls too low, this causes proliferation of and increased secretion by the parathyroid cells. Among the conditions that increase the output of parathyroid hormone are: (1) low calcium ion concentration in rickets, (2) low calcium ion concentration in osteomalacia (adult rickets), (3) lactation, in which large amounts of calcium are secreted in the milk, and (4) low calcium diet.

Calcitonin and Its Role in Regulation of Calcium Ion Concentration. A relatively recently discovered hormone called *calcitonin* causes, when injected into an animal, rapid deposition of calcium in the bones and therefore rapid decrease in calcium ion concentration in the body fluids. This hormone is secreted by special cells in the thyroid gland in the human. Its rate of secretion increases when the calcium ion concentration rises above normal. Therefore, it functions in exactly the opposite manner to parathyroid hormone, returning the calcium ion concentration back toward normal when this concentration rises too high. Furthermore, it responds much more rapidly than does parathyroid hormone. However, the quantitative role of calcitonin in calcium ion regulation is far less than that of parathyroid hormone. Also, it is doubtful whether its effects can continue for more than a few hours to a few days.

Reproductive Functions of the Male

Spermatogenesis. The basic reproductive function of the male is the formation of *sperm* by the *testes.* The *seminiferous tubules* of the testes contain a basal layer of *germinal epithelium,* the cells of which divide through several stages and gradually form the sperm. During formation, essentially all of the cytoplasm is lost from the cell, and the cell membrane elongates in one direction to form a tail. Also, at one stage of division, the 23 pairs of chromosomes split into two sets of unpaired chromosomes, one of these sets going to one sperm and the other to the second sperm. One pair of chromosomes, called the *XY pair,* is known as the sex pair. After separation of the chromosomal pairs in the process of sperm formation, half of the sperm carry X chromosomes and the other half Y chromosomes. The X chromosome causes a female child to be formed, while the Y chromosome causes a male child to be formed. Thus, the sex of the offspring is determined by the type of sperm that fertilizes the

ovum. Furthermore, this division of the chromosomes allows only half of the genes of the father to be inherited by the child, while the other half come from the mother.

In addition to germinal cells, the seminiferous tubules contain large *Sertoli cells* from which the developing sperm obtain nutrient substances during their development.

Testosterone. Large quantities of testosterone are formed by the *interstitial cells* of the testes located between the seminiferous tubules. This testosterone has a local effect in the testes on the production of sperm by the seminiferous tubules, and without it spermatogenesis cannot occur. However, in addition to its effects on spermatogenesis, it also causes development of the sexual and secondary sexual characteristics of the male, including (1) development of the penis when the fetus is developing, (2) descent of the testes into the scrotum during intrauterine life, (3) development of the enlarged musculature of the male, (4) increase in the thickness of the skin, (5) bass quality of the male voice, (6) growth of a beard on the face and of hair on many other areas of the body, and (7) baldness in those male individuals who are genetically predisposed to this.

Regulation of Testicular Function by the Anterior Pituitary Gland. At least two *gonadotropic hormones* secreted by the pituitary gland help to control spermatogenesis and testosterone secretion by the testes. During childhood, essentially no gonadotropic hormones are secreted by the anterior pituitary gland, but at puberty both *follicle stimulating hormone* and *luteinizing hormone* begin to be secreted, the follicle stimulating hormone promoting division of the germinal cells to initiate spermatogenesis, while luteinizing hormone stimulates the interstitial cells to produce testosterone. The testosterone in turn is required for proper development of the sperm and for their maturation. The testes continue to produce both sperm and testosterone from puberty until death, though beyond approximately the 40th year of life the rates of production gradually decline.

Regulation of Gonadotropic Hormone Secretion—Role of Luteinizing Hormone Releasing Hormone. The rate of secretion of gonadotropic hormones by the anterior pituitary gland is controlled mainly by *luteinizing hormone releasing hormone,* a hormone formed in the hypothalamus and transported to the anterior pituitary gland through the hypothalamic-hypophyseal portal system. This hormone causes both luteinizing hormone and follicle stimulating hormone to be released from the anterior pituitary gland.

Testosterone secreted by the testes inhibits the formation of luteinizing hormone releasing hormone by the hypothalamus, thus providing a negative feedback mechanism for control of testosterone secretion. A substance called *inhibin* is secreted by the seminiferous tubules; this has an effect on the anterior pituitary gland to diminish the rate of secretion of follicle stimulating hormone, thus providing a feedback mechanism for controlling the formation of sperm.

During childhood, the rate of secretion of luteinizing hormone releasing hormone is very low because the hypothalamus is extremely sensitive to the inhibitory effects of even minute amounts of circulating testosterone. However, at approximately the age of 12, the hypothalamus loses most of this inhibitory sensitivity, and large amounts of luteinizing hormone releasing hormone then begin to be secreted, and the sex life of the male begins. This is the period of puberty.

Storage of Sperm and Ejaculation. After sperm are formed in the seminiferous tubules, they then pass into the *epidydimis* where they must remain for approximately a day while they mature within this new environment. From there, they pass into the *vas deferens* and the *ampulla* where they are stored. During coitus, sexual stimulation transmits impulses to the spinal cord, which cause reflex (parasympathetic mediated) erection of the penis. Then, at the height of sexual stimulation, rhythmic peristalsis begins in the epidydimis and spreads up the vas deferens, into the ampulla and seminal vasicles, and finally through the prostate gland. This expels the semen into the posterior urethra. Then, rhythmical contractions of the bulbocavernosus muscle cause rhythmic compression of the urethra, and about 3 ml. of *semen* is expelled. This process is called *ejaculation* (sympathetic mediated).

The *ejaculate* is composed of a mixture of (1) sperm from the *testes,* (2) a highly mucid and nutritive fluid from the *seminal vesicles,* and (3) a highly alkaline fluid from the *prostate gland.* The alkalinity of the prostate fluid causes the sperm to become immediately *motile* because of movement of the sperm tail, traveling at a velocity as much as 1 to 4 mm. per minute, which allows the sperm to pass upward through the *uterus* and the *fallopian tubes* to fertilize the ovum.

Failure of the male to ejaculate more than 60 to 80 million sperm in each ejaculate usually results in *sterility.* This may be caused by the lack of sufficient *hyaluronidase,* and various proteolytic enzymes that are secreted by the sperm. These enzymes dissolve the mucous plug of the cervix and possibly also help to break granulosal cells away from the surface of the ovum, thereby allowing a sperm to penetrate the ovum.

Reproductive Functions of the Female

Ovarian Cycle and Oogenesis. Oogenesis means the formation of ova. The newborn female child has approximately two million *primordial ova* in her two ovaries. Many of these degenerate during childhood so that only about 300,000 remain at puberty. At that time, under the stimulation of gonadotropic hormones from the anterior pituitary gland, a rhythmic monthly sexual cycle begins. At the beginning of each month, cells surrounding a few of the ova, the *granulosal* and the *thecal cells,* begin to proliferate, and these secrete large quantities of *estrogens,* one of the female sex hormones. Fluid is also secreted, forming cavities around the ova called *follicles.* After approximately 14 days of growth, one of the growing follicles breaks open and expels its ovum into the abdominal cavity. Then, all the other growing follicles begin to degenerate within a few hours, a process called artesia. Presumably, this results from some type of inhibiting hormonal action on the ovaries after ovulation occurs. Nevertheless, the result is the release of one single ovum each month at approximately the 14th day of the female sexual cycle.

Immediately after the ovum has been expelled, the granulosal cells undergo rapid fatty changes and considerable swelling, a process called *luteinization,* and they begin to secrete large amounts of *progesterone* in addition to *estrogens.* This modified mass of cells, now called a *corpus luteum,* persists for approximately another 14 days, at the end of which time it degenerates. Then a new set of follicles begins to develop, and at the end of another 14 days another ovum is expelled into the abdominal cavity, the cycle continuing on and on.

At about the same time that the ovum is expelled from the follicle, its nucleus divides two times in rapid succession. During one of these divisions, the pairs of chromosomes separate, and half of them are expelled from the ovum, leaving only 23 unpaired chromosomes in the final *mature ovum,* which is then ready for fertilization.

Effects of Estrogens and Progesterone on the Endometrium. The estrogens and the progesterone secreted by the ovaries have very important effects on the uterine *endometrium,* preparing it for implantation of a fertilized ovum. The estrogens secreted during the first half of the monthly ovarian cycle cause very rapid proliferation of the endometrial stroma and glandular cells. Then during the second half of the ovarian cycle progesterone causes both the stromal and the glandular cells to enlarge and the glandular cells to begin secreting a serous fluid while the stromal cells store large quantities of protein and glycogen in preparation for supplying nutrition to the developing ovum.

Menstruation. When the corpus luteum degenerates at the end of the ovarian cycle, almost no estrogens or progesterone are then secreted by the ovaries for the next few days. Lack of the normal stimulatory effect of these hormones causes the endometrial cells to lose their stimulus for increased activity. As one of the results, the blood vessels to the endometrium become spastic, which causes very rapid necrosis of most of the endometrium, the dead tissue sloughing away and being expelled through the vagina along with about 50 ml. of blood and much more serous exudate. This process, called *menstruation,* normally lasts about 4 days. By the end of menstruation, new follicles that have begun to develop in the ovary are beginning to secrete estrogens once again, and under the influence of these the endometrium begins a new cycle of development.

Effects of Estrogens and Progesterone on Other Tissues. In addition to the effects of estrogens and progesterone on the endometrium, these hormones, particularly estrogens, have a number of other effects throughout the body. Estrogens cause proliferation and enlargement of the smooth muscle cells in the uterus, increasing the uterine size after puberty to about double the childhood size. Estrogens also cause proliferation of the glandular cells of the breast and cause deposition of fat in the breast tissues, thus giving the characteristic growth of the female breasts. They cause fat deposition on the hips and in other points peculiar to the female. They cause very rapid growth of the bones immediately after puberty but also promote early uniting of the epiphyses with the shafts of the long bones so that the final height of the female, despite her rapid growth immediately after puberty, is less than it otherwise would have been. Finally, they cause broadening of the pelvic outlet of the female and enlargement of the external genitalia.

Progesterone has very much the same effect on the breasts that it has on the uterine endometrium, causing the glandular cells to increase in size and to develop secretory granules in their cells. In addition, it causes accumulation of fluid and electrolytes in the breast tissue, making them swell during the latter half of each monthly sexual cycle.

Regulation of the Female Sexual Cycle by the Hypothalamus and Anterior Pituitary Gland. Until the female is approximately 12 years of age, the anterior pituitary gland secretes no gonadotropic hormones, as is also true in the male. This is believed to result from exquisite sensitivity of the hypothalamus to inhibition by even the minutest amounts of estrogen and progesterone secreted by the ovaries. However, at this age, the age of puberty, the hypothalamus loses this inhibitory sensitivity and begins to secrete luteinizing hormone releasing hormone, in the same manner that occurs in the male. This hormone in turn stimulates the secretion of both luteinizing hormone and

follicle stimulating hormone by the anterior pituitary gland. It is the follicle stimulating hormone that causes initial growth of the ovarian follicles during the first few days of the monthly ovarian cycle. Then this hormone, aided by luteinizing hormone as well, causes the thecal cells, and possibly also the granulosal cells, to secrete estrogens plus large quantities of fluid into the developing follicles.

At about the 13th day of the ovarian cycle, an especially large amount of luteinizing hormone is secreted by the anterior pituitary gland, which is called the *luteinizing hormone surge.* The excess luteinizing hormone, in some way not completely understood, causes ovulation 16 to 24 hours later. The luteinizing hormone also causes the granulosal cells to change into *lutein cells* which in the aggregate become the *corpus luteum.* Luteinizing hormone also stimulates the corpus luteum to produce large quantities of both progesterone and estrogen during the latter half of the female sexual cycle. Then, when the corpus luteum degenerates at the end of the cycle, the resulting lack of progesterone and estrogen production leads to menstruation as described above.

It is not clear exactly how the successive changes in secretion of follicle stimulating hormone, luteinizing hormone, estrogen, and progesterone during the female sexual cycle are controlled. However, it is known that estrogen in particular, and progesterone to a less extent, normally cause feedback inhibition of luteinizing hormone releasing hormone secretion by the hypothalamus. Therefore, during the latter part of the ovarian cycle, when large amounts of progesterone and estrogen are secreted by the corpus luteum, secretion of both follicle stimulating hormone and luteinizing hormone by the anterior pituitary gland becomes diminished. This in turn leads to degeneration of the corpus luteum and cessation of production of the large quantities of progesterone and estrogen. Lacking the feedback inhibition from these two hormones, the hypothalamus and the pituitary gland become active once again, and the rates of secretion of follicle stimulating hormone and luteinizing hormone rise once more, thus beginning a new cycle.

However, it is still difficult to understand what causes the midmonthly luteinizing hormone surge, but it is believed to occur in the following way: Experiments have shown that when large quantities of estrogen circulate in the blood (but in the absence of progesterone) for several days, this has exactly the opposite effect on the hypothalamus and anterior pituitary gland from its normal inhibiting effect. That is, it causes a positive feedback effect instead of negative feedback and actually stimulates the production of more luteinizing hormone releasing hormone, which in turn leads to massive production of luteinizing hormone (and lesser amounts of follicle stimulating hormone as well) by the anterior pituitary gland. And this leads to ovulation, followed by development of the corpus luteum and the subsequent events described above. Thus, the cycle begins again.

Menopause. At 40 to 55 years of age essentially all of the ova in the ovaries have been used up, a few expelled into the abdominal cavity by ovulation and vast numbers degenerated in situ in the ovaries. Therefore, no follicles or any corpus luteum can develop in the ovaries to secrete either estrogens or progesterone. The anterior pituitary gland continues to secrete large quantities of gonadotropic hormones, but since no estrogen or progesterone can be secreted to inhibit the hypothalamus or the pituitary, no monthly sexual cycle occurs thereafter. Loss of the female sex hormones sometimes causes rather drastic psychic and psychosomatic effects, resulting often in depressive states, hallucinatory states, and "hot flashes" of the skin. This period in the life of the female is called the *menopause*.

Physiology of Pregnancy

Fertilization and Implantation. After coitus, millions of motile sperm make their way upward through the uterus and fallopian tubes. These sperm are capable of living in the genital tract of the female for as long as 72 hours but are very fertile for only about 24 hours. If during this time an ovum is expelled from the ovary, or, if an ovum has been expelled up to 24 hours prior to coitus, then a sperm can cause fertilization. In the process of fertilization, the head of the sperm combines with the nucleus of the ovum. Since each of these contains 23 unpaired chromosomes, the combination restores the normal cellular complement of *23 pairs* of chromosomes. This allows the ovum to begin a process of division, the first division occurring approximately 30 hours after fertilization. Subsequent divisions then take place at a rate of about once every 18 to 24 hours.

The ovum usually passes shortly before fertilization into one of the two fallopian tubes, the *fimbriated ends* of which lie in approximation to the ovaries. Gradually, the cilia that line the fallopian tube and beat toward the uterus move the dividing ovum downward along the tube to reach the uterus in about 3 days.

The dividing ovum develops an outer layer of *trophoblast cells;* these are capable of phagocytizing nutrient materials from the secretions of the fallopian tube and the uterus, thus making these secretions available to the developing mass of cells. The trophoblast cells also secrete *proteolytic enzymes* that allow the developing mass of cells to eat its way into the endometrium and thereby *implant* itself.

Function of Chorionic Gonadotropin in Pregnancy. When the corpus luteum degenerates at the end of the *normal* monthly cycle, the endometrium of the uterus sloughs away, and menstruation occurs. However, when the ovum becomes fertilized, it is important that the endometrium remain intact in order for the early developing fetus to implant and grow. Fortunately, the trophoblast cells secrete a hormone called *chorionic gonadotropin* that has almost identically the same effects on the corpus luteum as luteinizing hormone from the pituitary gland. Therefore, this hormone keeps the corpus luteum from degenerating and keeps it secreting large quantities of estrogens and progesterone; as a result, menstruation does not occur. Instead, the endometrium actually grows thicker and is gradually phagocytized by the growing fetal tissues, in this way providing the major portion of the nutrition for the fetus during approximately the first 8 to 12 weeks of pregnancy.

After the first 3 to 4 months of pregnancy, the placenta begins to secrete large quantities of estrogens and progesterone. From then on the corpus luteum is not needed.

Function of the Placenta. During the early weeks of pregnancy, the trophoblast cells and other fetal tissues gradually develop the placenta. This organ contains several very large chambers filled with mother's blood, and into these project millions of small villi containing blood capillaries from the fetus. Trophoblast cells cover the surfaces of the villi, and these actively absorb many nutrients from the mother's blood and transport them into the fetal blood during the first few weeks of pregnancy. However, this time by far the greater proportion of the necessary nutrients is absorbed *passively* from the mother's blood into the fetal blood. That is, the concentrations of the nutrients are greater in the mother's blood than in the fetal blood, and as a result they simply *diffuse* through the placental membrane into the fetal blood. Conversely, excretory substances such as urea, uric acid and phosphates accumulate in high concentrations in the fetal blood and then diffuse backward through the placental membrane into the mother's blood, then to be excreted by the mother's kidneys.

Hormones Secreted by the Placenta. In addition to secreting chorionic gonadotropin, which was discussed above, the placenta also secretes several other important hormones, especially estrogens and progesterone. After approximately the third month, the rate of secretion of chorionic gonadotropin becomes very little, and the corpus luteum begins to degenerate. Therefore, from that time onward the estrogens and progesterone from the placenta are essential for the maintenance of pregnancy. Toward the end of pregnancy, the rate of secretion of estrogens is as much as 100 times that during the normal ovarian cycle, and the rate of secretion of progesterone is about ten times as great. The estrogens and the progesterone also are essential for growth of the fetus. The progesterone secreted by the placenta is formed from cholesterol derived from the mother's blood. However, secretion of estrogens by the placenta requires a double stage process. The first stage is the formation of large quantities of androgens by greatly enlarged adrenal cortices in the fetus. These androgens are then converted by the placenta into several different types of estrogens, including estradiol, the most potent of all the estrogens.

The placenta also produces large quantities of another hormone called *human chorionic somatomammotropin*. This hormone has several important effects: First, it promotes growth of the fetus. Second, it causes increased use of fatty acids by the mother for energy and decreased use of glucose; this makes the excess glucose of the mother available for use by the fetus, an important effect because the fetus is especially geared for utilization of glucose. Third, human chorionic somatomammotropin also aids in the growth and development of the breasts during pregnancy, thus preparing the breasts for lactation following birth of the baby.

Growth of the Fetus.   During the first few weeks of pregnancy the fetus grows hardly at all, though the surrounding fetal membranes, especially the placenta, develop very rapidly. After 4 weeks, however, the length of the fetus increases approximately directly in proportion to the time of gestation, and the weight increases with the cube of the time. Thus, at 6 months the length is approximately six-ninths the final length, but the weight is still only one-fourth the final weight. It can be seen, then, that by far the greatest growth in weight of the fetus occurs in the last 3 months, and during this time, pregnancy makes many demands on the mother for nutritive substances needed by the baby, including especially proteins, vitamins, large amounts of calcium for the bones and iron for the red blood cells.

Parturition.   When the fetus is fully formed, approximately 9 months after fertilization, the uterus suddenly becomes far more excitable than usual, labor begins, and the baby is expelled. This is called *parturition.* The precise factors that initiate parturition have never been determined, but it seems that it results from a combination of several different factors that progressively increase the excitability of the uterine musculature as follows: (1) Near term the placenta begins to secrete a progressively higher ratio of estrogens to progesterone. Since estrogens normally excite uterine activity while progesterone inhibits it, this change in ratio increases the excitability of the uterine musculature. (2) The fetus itself increases in size, which stretches the uterine musculature, thus also increasing its excitability. (3) The head of the fetus presses downward against the cervical opening of the uterus and begins to stretch the cervix; this, too, seems to increase the excitability of the uterus. (4) The posterior pituitary gland begins to secrete increased quantities of oxytocic hormone, and at the same time the sensitivity of the uterine musculature to oxytocin increases greatly, both of which together further increase the excitability of the uterine musculature. As a result of the combination of all of these factors, the rhythmic contractions of the uterus become stronger and stronger. Finally, they become strong enough to begin pushing the baby into the birth canal. This in turn stretches the cervix very rapidly, which causes a still greater increase in the excitability of the uterus itself, making the uterus contract still harder. Also, sensory signals from the cervix to the hypothalamus cause progressively increasing secretion of oxytocin that in turn excites the uterus still more. Thus a cycle is set up as follows: strong uterine contraction, stretching of the cervix, stimulation of still stronger uterine contraction caused by this stretch, still more stretch of the cervix and so forth until the baby is expelled.

Changes in the Baby Immediately upon Birth. Prior to birth, the baby receives its nutrition and oxygen through the placenta. Normally the first function performed by the newborn baby is rapid expansion of its lungs to aerate its own blood, thereby allowing it to lead an independent existence. A baby can usually go as long as 4 to 6 minutes without breathing before damage occurs. However, beyond this time many neuronal cells of the brain are likely to be destroyed.

In the fetus, blood bypasses the lungs by two routes: (1) It flows from the right atrium through the *foramen ovale* directly into the left atrium. (2) Most of the blood that does not take this route is pumped by the right ventricle into the pulmonary artery and then through the *ductus arteriosus* directly into the aorta rather than through the lungs. However, birth of the baby changes these directions of blood flow in the following ways: (1) Loss of blood flow through the placenta after birth greatly increases the total peripheral resistance in the baby's systemic circulatory system. (2) Expansion of the lungs also expands the pulmonary blood vessels and in this way greatly reduces the resistance to blood flow through the pulmonary circulation. As a result, the ratio of resistance in the systemic circulation to resistance in the pulmonary circulation increases several fold, allowing much easier flow of blood through the lungs, but considerably more difficult flow through the systemic circulation. Because of this, the pulmonary arterial pressure falls, while the systemic arterial pressure rises so that blood now begins to flow backward from the aorta through the ductus arteriosus rather than forward. This brings arterialized blood, containing a high oxygen concentration, into contact with the ductus, and the oxygen constricts the ductus causing *functional closure* within a few hours. Then fibrous tissue grows into the ductus walls and causes *permanent closure* in one to two months in most babies.

Also, immediately after birth, the increased resistance in the systemic circulation increases the load on the left heart and therefore increases the left atrial pressure. At the same time the decreased resistance in the lungs decreases the right atrial pressure. This higher pressure in the left atrium than in the right atrium closes a valvelike structure over the foramen ovale, preventing further flow through this route. Thus, these two changes in the circulatory system now provide normal blood flow through the lungs.

Lactation

All during pregnancy large quantities of estrogens and progesterone are secreted either by the corpus luteum or the placenta. The estrogens cause proliferation of the glandular tissues of the breasts, and the progesterone causes development of the alveoli as well as storage of nutrient materials in the glandular cells. Other hormones that also help to promote breast development during pregnancy include prolactin and growth hormone from the mother's anterior pituitary gland, insulin from her pancreas, glucocorticoids from her adrenal glands, and human chorionic somatomammotropin from the placenta. However, the progesterone and estrogens also inhibit actual milk production despite their effect on breast proliferation. Therefore, before birth of the baby the mother does not secrete milk. Loss of the placenta from the mother's body when the baby is born removes the secretion of progesterone and estrogens so that the breasts are now no longer inhibited; within 24 to 48 hours milk begins to flow.

During pregnancy, the mother's anterior pituitary gland produces increasing quantities of *prolactin*, increasing to about 10 times the normal rate of secretion. This hormone is especially required to cause final development of the breasts and also to cause them to secrete milk. After birth of the baby, continued removal of milk from the breasts causes the anterior pituitary gland to continue producing large quantities of prolactin, and this in turn stimulates the breasts to continue producing milk. When milk is no longer removed from the breasts, the anterior pituitary gland stops producing prolactin, and milk production ceases within a few days.

Oxytocin secreted by the posterior pituitary gland is also important for lactation, causing milk ejection from the breast alveoli, which was discussed earlier in relation to the posterior pituitary hormones.

QUESTIONS IN PHYSIOLOGY

GENERAL

What is meant by homeostasis?

What are the differences between extracellular and intracellular fluids?

What is meant by the internal environment of the body?

List the functional systems of the body and describe the manner in which each helps to provide homeostasis.

THE CELL

Describe the parts of the cell.

What is the function of the chromosomes and the genes in the cells?

Describe the principal mechanism by which energy is released in the cell, and give the function of the mitochondria.

How do the genes regulate protein synthesis by the cell?

What are the functions of codons?

Describe the functions of the special types of cells throughout the body.

How does cellular reproduction come about?

BODY FLUIDS

How are the body fluids distributed between the extracellular and the intracellular compartments, and how does the blood fit into these two compartments of fluid?

What is the difference between the ionic composition of extracellular fluid and intracellular fluid?

Describe the structure of the cell membrane.

Explain the mechanism of diffusion through the cell membrane, and list the common substances that normally pass through the membrane in this manner.

What is meant by active transport through the cell membrane? Give the mechanism of active transport.

What is the significance of the sodium pump?

Explain the mechanism of osmosis through the cell membrane, and explain how osmotic pressure can develop across a semipermeable membrane.

What is meant by isotonicity, hypotonicity and hypertonicity?

Explain how different types of intravenous fluids

are partitioned between the extracellular and the intracellular fluids when administered intravenously.

What are the functional differences between the capillary membrane and the cellular membrane?

What is the difference between colloid osmotic pressure at the capillary membrane and total osmotic pressure at the cellular membrane?

Explain the law of the capillaries. How do capillary pressure, tissue pressure and tissue colloid osmotic pressure enter into the law of the capillaries?

Outline the abnormalities in capillary dynamics that can cause interstitial fluid edema.

How is lymph formed?

List the functions of the lymphatic system.

What part does the lymphatic system play in the control of tissue fluid protein concentration?

Trace the flow of fluid in the cerebrospinal fluid system.

Describe the mechanisms of formation and absorption of fluid in the eye. How is the pressure in the eye regulated?

What is meant by a potential fluid space, and under what conditions can transudates appear in the potential fluid spaces?

KIDNEYS

Describe the nephron, and give the hemodynamics of blood flow through the kidneys.

Describe the mechanism by which glomerular filtrate is formed in a nephron.

Explain how solutes are reabsorbed from the tubules, and explain the difference between absorption by diffusion and by active absorption.

Explain the clearance concept in relation to the formation of urine.

How is sodium ion concentration in the extracellular fluids regulated?

How are the concentrations of chloride and potassium ions regulated in the extracellular fluids?

Explain the role of aldosterone in the control of body fluid electrolytes.

Explain the mechanism of the osmoreceptor system and its importance in the regulation of total concentration of solutes in the extracellular fluids.

How does the thirst mechanism enter into the regulation of electrolyte concentration in the body fluids?

Explain the chemical mechanism of an acid-base buffer.

How does the respiratory system regulate hydrogen ion concentration?

What are the different mechanisms by which the kidneys help to regulate hydrogen ion concentration?

BLOOD AND IMMUNITY

What are the normal concentrations of red and white cells in the blood, and what is meant by the hematocrit?

How is the concentration of the red cells in the blood regulated?

What are the nutritive factors that are necessary for red blood cell formation?

Give the basic functions of the different types of white blood cells.

Describe the mechanisms by which blood coagulation occurs. What is the importance of thromboplastin, and what is its origin?

What is the significance of prothrombin, fibrinogen, accelerator globulin, calcium ions and platelets in blood coagulation?

Explain the cause of bleeding in hemophilia, in thrombocytopenia and in prothrombin deficiency.

What factors in the body provide a certain degree of innate immunity?

Explain the mechanism of the immune process by which a person develops adaptive immunity.

Explain the difference in function of antibodies and sensitized lymphocytes in the process of immunity.

What is meant by immunologic tolerance?

What is the basic cause of autoimmune disease?

What is the significance of IgE antibodies in allergy?

How does histamine enter into allergic reactions?

Describe the effects of a transfusion reaction.

What is meant by the A-B-O blood groups, and how can mismatching of these groups cause transfusion reactions?

How do the Rh blood types differ from the A-B-O blood groups in causing transfusion reactions?

Explain the problems of transplantation of tissues from one person to another.

NERVE AND MUSCLE

How does a membrane potential develop across the nerve membrane?

Explain the mechanism of the action potential. How does an action potential spread along a nerve membrane?

What is meant by the all-or-nothing law?

If oxidative metabolism in the nerve suddenly stops, can the nerve continue to transmit nerve impulses?

Describe the mechanism by which an impulse is transmitted through a neuromuscular junction.

Explain the "amplification" function of the neuromuscular junction.

Describe the ultramicroscopic structure of a skeletal muscle fiber and explain the mechanism of contraction.

How is contraction initiated in a skeletal muscle fiber?

Explain the mechanism of muscle tetanization.

Explain the mechanisms by which different strengths of muscle contraction can be achieved.

How does smooth muscle differ from skeletal and cardiac muscle?

How does cardiac muscle differ from smooth and skeletal muscle?

Explain the significance of tone and plasticity of smooth muscle.

HEART

Explain the basic mechanisms for control of rhythmicity in the heart and explain the "pacemaker" function of the S-A node.

Trace the conduction of the cardiac impulse through the heart.

What is the significance of the junctional fibers in the Purkinje system?

What is meant by heart block and how does it come about?

Explain the circus movement in the heart, and describe the mechanisms of flutter and fibrillation.

What is the significance of the P-Q interval in the electrocardiogram?

What types of conditions can cause abnormal QRS waves in the electrocardiogram?

What conditions can cause abnormal T waves in the electrocardiogram?

How does a "current of injury" affect the electrocardiogram?

What is the function of the atria in the pumping action of the heart?

Explain the mechanisms of pumping by the ventricles.

Give the Frank-Starling law of the heart, and explain its significance.

Describe the nervous control of the heart.

What is the difference between sympathetic and parasympathetic control?

CIRCULATION

Explain the "circuit" concept of the circulation.

Outline the distribution of blood in the different segments of the circulation.

Give the formula relating blood flow to blood pressure and resistance.

What are the factors that determine the resistance of a blood vessel?

What are the mean pressures in the different parts of the systemic circulation?

How is blood flow regulated in local tissue areas by the arterioles?

Explain the possible mechanisms of autoregulation of blood flow.

What are the blood reservoirs, and what is their significance?

Under what conditions is nervous regulation of blood flow important in the systemic circulation?

How is blood flow in the skeletal muscles regulated?

How is blood flow through the skin regulated to control body heat?

What is the relationship of carbon dioxide to the regulation of cerebral blood flow?

What is the relationship of the portal circulatory system to ascites?

List the mean pressures in the different parts of the pulmonary circulation.

How does increasing the blood flow through the lungs affect the resistance to blood flow in the pulmonary circulation?

Under what conditions do large quantities of blood shift from the pulmonary circulation to the systemic circulation and vice versa?

Explain why the pulmonary alveoli normally remain empty of fluid.

Under what conditions will pulmonary edema develop?

Describe the renal-body fluid volume mechanism for regulation of mean arterial pressure.

Describe the renin-angiotensin mechanism for control of arterial pressure.

How do the different cardiovascular reflexes enter into the regulation of mean arterial pressure?

Give the mechanism of the baroreceptor reflex control of arterial pressure.

What conditions of the kidneys can cause renal hypertension?

What is meant by neurogenic hypertension, and how can it develop?

List the different types of hormonal hypertension.

Discuss the possible basic mechanisms of essential hypertension.

What are the factors that are of importance in the regulation of cardiac output?

How can the pumping action of the heart be increased or decreased in different conditions?

What are the factors that regulate venous return?

What is the significance of the mean systemic filling pressure, and how does sympathetic stimulation affect venous return?

How is venous pressure regulated?

Explain the mechanism of the venous pump.

What is meant by low cardiac output failure?

How can the nervous system compensate for mild degrees of cardiac failure?

Under what conditions can fluid retention be of

value, and under what conditions can it be of harm in heart failure?

What conditions can cause left heart failure, and what conditions can cause right heart failure? Also, what are the differences that occur in the circulation in these two types of failure?

Describe the dynamics of the circulation in aortic stenosis, aortic regurgitation, mitral stenosis and mitral regurgitation.

What is meant by a right-to-left shunt, and how does this affect the circulation?

What are the dynamics of cardiac shock?

What are the significant differences between hypovolemic shock and neurogenic shock?

Explain why circulatory shock is progressive in nature.

Under what conditions does circulatory shock become irreversible?

How long can a person stand circulatory arrest, and what is the significance of coagulation in the circulation in circulatory arrest?

RESPIRATORY SYSTEM

Define and give the values for tidal air, minute respiratory volume, vital capacity, maximum rate of pulmonary ventilation, alveolar ventilation per minute, dead space and functional residual capacity.

What is the importance of the functional residual capacity?

List the concentrations and the partial pressures of the different gases in the alveoli.

Why is it important that gases utilized by the respiratory system be expressed in terms of partial pressure?

Why does carbon dioxide diffuse through the pulmonary membrane far more rapidly than does oxygen?

Define the "diffusing capacity" of the lungs and give its value for oxygen.

Explain the mechanism by which hemoglobin transports oxygen in the blood.

Give the different mechanisms by which carbon dioxide is transported in the blood.

What causes the continual respiratory rhythm?

How do carbon dioxide, blood pH and oxygen lack increase pulmonary ventilation?

List the different causes of hypoxia.

In what hypoxic conditions is oxygen therapy particularly valuable?

How does pneumonia affect the respiratory system?

How does emphysema affect the respiratory system?

How does atelectasis affect the respiratory system?

How high can an aviator ascend without developing coma from hypoxia?

What are the mechanisms by which a person becomes acclimatized to hypoxia?

What is meant by an acceleratory force of 5 g, and approximately how much centrifugal acceleratory force can an aviator stand?

What are the particular physiologic problems involved in space travel?

What are the toxic effects of high oxygen pressure and high nitrogen pressure on the body?

What is decompression sickness, and what is its cause in deep sea diving?

CENTRAL NERVOUS SYSTEM

List the different types of sensory receptors.

List the different types of effector organs.

Describe the basic mechanism of the reflex arc.

What is meant by the integrative centers of the nervous system?

Describe the synapse and its functions.

What is meant by the excitatory transmitter, and under what conditions will it excite a neuron?

What is meant by the inhibitory transmitter, and how does it function at the synapse?

What factors determine the excitability of the neuron?

Explain how an amplifying circuit in a neuronal pool works.

Explain the mechanism and the significance of a converging or an integrative circuit in a neuronal pool.

Give the types of repetitive firing circuits in a neuronal pool. What are the specific characteristics of each?

Describe a possible mechanism by which thoughts occur in the central nervous system.

Describe a possible mechanism of memory.

What is meant by programming of thoughts?

What is meant by modality of sensation? List the different modalities.

What determines the modality of sensation that will be felt when a nerve fiber is electrically stimulated?

Trace the pathways for transmission of different types of somatic sensations into the central nervous system.

What is meant by the law of specific nerve energies?

What is the basic stimulus necessary to cause pain?

Distinguish between the threshold for pain perception and reactivity to pain.

What types of stimuli can cause visceral pain?

Explain the mechanism of referred pain.

How is pain intensity controlled by the central nervous system?

Describe the stretch reflex, and give its functions.

What are the functions of the gamma efferent fibers?

Describe the withdrawal response and explain its relationship to the flexor reflex and the crossed extensor reflex.

Describe the positive supportive reflex and explain its importance.

How are walking reflexes integrated in the spinal cord?

Explain the function of the brain stem in the support of the body against gravity.

What is the difference between the functions of the macula of the utricle and the semicircular canals in equilibrium?

List the different visceral functions of the brain stem?

List the locations of the primary sensory areas of the cerebral cortex.

What is meant by sensory association areas, and what are the functions of the somatic, the auditory and the visual sensory association areas?

What is meant by the gnostic function of the brain?

What is the ideomotor function of the brain?

Trace the pyramidal system from the motor cortex to the spinal cord.

What is the function of the premotor cortex in the control of muscular movements?

Trace the extrapyramidal pathways from the cerebral cortex to the spinal cord.

List the functions of the basal ganglia in the control of muscular movements.

How does the cerebellum damp the movements of the body?

Why does cerebellar dysfunction frequently cause ataxic movements?

What are the hormones secreted by the sympathetic and the parasympathetic nerve endings?

How does the central nervous system control the autonomic nerves?

EYE

What are the four refractive surfaces of the eye?

Explain the mechanism by which the eye focuses images on the retina.

What is the relationship of the pupil to the depth of focus on the eye?

Give the mechanism of the pupillary light reflex.

Distinguish between the functions of the rods and the cones.

Explain how the rhodopsin-retinene cycle of the rods operates.

Explain the mechanism of dark and light adaptation.

Explain the method by which the eye distinguishes different colors.

Trace the transmission of nerve impulses from the retina to the cerebral cortex.

EAR

Explain the mechanics of sound transmission from the tympanum to the cochlea.

How does resonance occur in the cochlea?

Explain the mechanism by which the cochlea determines the pitch of a sound.

Explain how the cochlea determines the loudness of a sound.

Trace the transmission of auditory impulses into the brain.

CHEMICAL SENSES

What are the four different types of taste buds?

Trace the transmission of taste impulses into the brain.

What types of substances can stimulate the olfactory cells?

Trace the transmission of olfactory impulses into the brain.

GASTROINTESTINAL TRACT

What are the two major types of movements in the gastrointestinal tract?

Explain the mechanism of peristalsis and its control.

Describe the mechanism of swallowing.

Explain how the intestinal contents are mixed in the stomach, in the small intestine and in the large intestine.

Describe the mechanisms by which gastric secretions are controlled.

Explain how pancreatic secretion is controlled.

What is the major mechanism by which small-intestinal secretion is controlled?

What is the importance of mucus secretion throughout the gastrointestinal tract?

Explain the mechanisms of digestion of carbohydrates, fats and proteins in the gastrointestinal tract.

What substances are actively absorbed from the gastrointestinal tract?

What substances are absorbed by diffusion?

What substances are absorbed into the portal blood, and what substances are absorbed into the lymphatic system from the gastrointestinal tract?

What abnormal conditions can cause peptic ulceration?

What abnormal conditions can cause diarrhea and constipation?

What is the basic abnormality of achylasia or mega-colon?

METABOLISM AND ENERGY

Explain why glucose is called the common denominator in carbohydrate metabolism.

What is the importance of glycogen storage in the liver?

How is glucose transported in the cells, and how does insulin affect this transport?

What is meant by glucolysis, and what is meant by the citric acid cycle?

What are the significance and the functions of adenosine triphosphate in the metabolic scheme?

Describe the mechanisms by which adenosine triphosphate can be formed in the cells.

How are fats transported in the plasma?

What are chylomicrons, and how are they removed from the blood?

What are fat depots?

How can fat be utilized to synthesize adenosine triphosphate?

What are the functions of phospholipids and cholesterol in the body?

Discuss what is known about the cause of atherosclerosis.

How are amino acids transported, and how are they stored in the body?

What is meant by an essential amino acid?

Under what conditions does catabolism of proteins occur in the cells?

Why must deamination of amino acids occur before these can be used for energy?

Explain the energy equivalent of foods and give the energy equivalents for carbohydrates, fats and proteins.

What are the daily energy requirements of the body under different physiologic conditions?

What is meant by the basal metabolic rate?

What is the cause of obesity?

What types of stored foods are utilized by the body in starvation?

Give the functions of vitamin A, thiamine, niacin, riboflavin, vitamin B_{12}, folic acid, pantothenic acid, pyridoxine, ascorbic acid, vitamin D and vitamin K.

What are the mechanisms by which heat is produced in the body?

What are the mechanisms by which heat is lost from the body?

Explain the hypothalamic mechanism for automatic control of body temperature.

ENDOCRINE GLANDS

Explain how cyclic AMP acts as an intracellular hormonal "second messenger."

List the six significant anterior pituitary hormones.

Explain the control of anterior pituitary hormone secretion by the hormones.

List the functions of growth hormone.

How does growth hormone promote tissue growth?

How does thyroid-stimulating hormone affect the thyroid gland?

How does adrenocorticotropin affect the adrenal cortices?

How is the secretion of adrenocorticotropin by the anterior pituitary gland controlled?

What are the two posterior pituitary hormones, and what are their functions?

How do mineralocorticoids function in the body?

What is the function of the glucocorticoids, and how is their secretion regulated?

What are the adrenal androgens, and under what conditions are they important?

What are the basic effects of thyroxine on the cells?

List the physiologic abnormalities in hyperthyroidism.

List the physiologic abnormalities in hypothyroidism.

What portions of the pancreas secrete insulin and glucagon?

What are the basic functions of insulin?

How does insulin affect the overall aspects of carbohydrate metabolism?

How does insulin affect the overall aspects of fat and protein metabolism.

What physiologic abnormalities result from diabetes mellitus?

What are the significant functions of glucagon?

Outline the principal steps in the formation of bone.

Under what conditions are bones absorbed in the body?

Explain how parathyroid hormone regulates calcium ion concentration in the extracellular fluids.

Describe the function of calcitonin.

What factors can cause increased secretion of parathyroid hormone?

Describe the formation of sperm in the testes.

What are the physiologic functions of testosterone?

Describe the secretion of testosterone and the regulation of testicular function by the anterior pituitary gland.

Explain the process of ejaculation.

Explain maturation of the ovum.

Describe the events in the ovarian cycle during the female sexual month.

How do estrogens and progesterone affect the endometrium?

Explain the cause of menstruation.

What are the effects of estrogens and progesterone on the tissues of the body other than the sex organs?

Explain the regulation of the female sexual cycle by the hypothalamus and the anterior pituitary gland.

How does the ovum become fertilized and later implanted in the uterus?

Why is chorionic gonadotropin necessary for the continuation of pregnancy?

Describe the nutritive functions of the placenta.

Outline the schedule of growth of the fetus during gestation.

Explain the mechanism of parturition.

Describe specifically the changes that occur in the baby's respiration and in its circulation immediately after birth.

List the factors that cause growth of the mother's breasts and then milk secretion following birth of the baby.

What is the function of oxytocin in lactation?

MULTIPLE CHOICE QUESTIONS

Choose the *best* answer. Answers are at the end of this chapter.

1. What is the probable structure of pores in the cell membrane?
   (a) A cylindrical hole through the membrane
   (b) A protein molecule entrapped in the membrane
   (c) A phosolipid molecule entrapped in the membrane
   (d) A large polysaccharide molecule entrapped in the membrane
   (e) A slit in the membrane

2. The ribosomes are formed by:
   (a) the Golgi apparatus
   (b) the endoplasmic reticulum
   (c) the lysosomes
   (d) the mitochondria
   (e) the nucleolus in the nucleus

3. Cardiac muscle:
   (a) has a velocity of conduction of action potentials of .3 to .5 meters per second
   (b) never contracts for more than .12 second
   (c) is not influenced by norepinephrine
   (d) has a longer duration of contraction during tachycardia
   (e) all of the above

4. During the middle of diastole:
   (a) the second heart sound is heard
   (b) the mitral valve is closed
   (c) aortic pressure is falling
   (d) all of the above

5. During the middle of systole:
   (a) the pulmonic valve is open
   (b) the QRS complex is occurring
   (c) ventricular volume is increasing
   (d) all of the above

6. An irregular, rapid heart rate with normal QRS complexes and no P waves suggests:
   (a) sinus arrhythmia
   (b) second degree heart block
   (c) paroxysmal tachycardia with a ventricular pacemaker
   (d) atrial fibrillation

7. The delay between the P wave and the Q wave in the normal electrocardiogram is primarily caused by:
   (a) a slow transmission through the A-V node and junctional fibers
   (b) delay at the internodal pathways
   (c) circus movement
   (d) the slow rate of conduction in atrial heart muscle

8. A stronger than normal heart might be observed during:
   (a) sympathetic stimulation
   (b) myocardial ischemia
   (c) Stokes-Adams syndrome
   (d) atrial fibrillation

9. The Purkinje fibers:
   (a) are myelinated axons
   (b) have a conduction velocity of about five times that seen in heart muscle
   (c) have action potentials about a tenth as long as those in heart muscle
   (d) all of the above

10. The heart is predisposed to ventricular fibrillation:
    (a) when action potentials follow a short, but circular pathway
    (b) during sinus bradycardia
    (c) if conduction velocity through the myocardium is decreased
    (d) all of the above

11. Which of the following statements is *incorrect*?
    (a) Blood flow velocity in the capillaries is greater than in the large veins.
    (b) Total surface area of the capillaries is much greater than in the large veins.
    (c) Reduced oxygen tension in the tissues would tend to relax precapillary sphincters.
    (d) Increased sympathetic nerve stimulation would tend to constrict the small arterioles.

12. Which of the following changes would tend to cause accumulation of fluid (edema) in the tissues?
    (a) Increased precapillary vascular resistance
    (b) Decreased postcapillary vascular resistance
    (c) Increased plasma colloid osmotic pressure
    (d) Increased venous pressure

13. Which of the following changes would probably occur as a result of a two-fold increase in the net filtration of fluid into the tissues?
    (a) A marked increase in lymph flow rate
    (b) approximately a two-fold increase in interstitial fluid volume
    (c) a decrease in interstitial fluid colloid osmotic pressure
    (d) (a) and (b)
    (e) (a) and (c)

14. Vitamin B_{12} is essential for what aspect of blood cell reproduction?
    (a) Formation of hemoglobin
    (b) Extrusion of the nucleus from the normoblasts
    (c) Formation of DNA
    (d) Activation of erythropoietin
    (e) Promotion of iron absorption from the intestinal tract

15. What type of cells found in lymph nodes phagocytizes unwanted particles in the lymph?
    (a) Neutrophils
    (b) Lymphocytes
    (c) Plasma cells
    (d) Microphages
    (e) Macrophages

16. In a person with type O blood, what type or types of agglutinins does he have in his plasma?
    (a) None
    (b) Alpha
    (c) Beta
    (d) Alpha and beta

17. In most instances of erythroblastosis fetalis:
    (a) the mother is Rh positive, the father Rh negative, and the baby Rh negative
    (b) the mother is Rh negative, the father Rh positive, and the baby Rh negative
    (c) the mother is Rh negative, the father Rh negative, and the baby Rh negative
    (d) the mother is Rh positive, the father Rh positive, and the baby Rh positive
    (e) the mother is Rh negative, the father Rh positive, and the baby Rh positive

18. Contraction of which of the following muscles is most important for causing forceful expiration?
    (a) Internal intercostals
    (b) Diaphragm
    (c) External intercostals
    (d) Sternocleidomastoids
    (e) Abdominals

19. The major cause of the hyperpnea of muscular exercise is:
    (a) stimulation of the respiratory center by the cerebral cortex and the joint proprioceptors
    (b) hypercapnia
    (c) hypoxemia
    (d) alkalosis
    (e) peripheral chemoreceptors

20. Which of the following factors has no direct stimulatory effect on the medullary respiratory center?
    (a) Changes in arterial PCO_2
    (b) Changes in arterial pH
    (c) Changes in arterial PO_2
    (d) Changes in the nervous output from the joint proprioceptors

21. In which of the following diseases would you expect to find an increase in thickness of the respiratory membrane?
    (a) Emphysema
    (b) Asthma
    (c) Pulmonary artery thrombosis
    (d) Skeletal abnormalities of the chest
    (e) Pulmonary edema

22. Which of the following would *not* be expected to cause hypoxia?
    (a) Hypoventilation
    (b) Abnormal ventilation to perfusion ratio
    (c) Hyperpnea
    (d) Diminished diffusing capacity for O_2
    (e) Excessive blood flow through venous to arterial shunts

23. The peripheral vasculature under the least control of the sympathetic nervous system is the:
    (a) arteries
    (b) arterioles
    (c) capillaries
    (d) venules
    (e) veins

24. Baroreceptor impulses:
    (a) inhibit the vagal center
    (b) increase in number with decreased carotid arterial pressure
    (c) result in increased heart rate
    (d) excite the sympathetic vasoconstrictor center
    (e) none of the above

25. Which of the following changes would tend to *decrease* glomerular filtration rate?
    (a) Increased afferent arteriolar resistance
    (b) Increased glomerular capillary filtration coefficient

(c) Decreased hydrostatic pressure in Bowman's capsule

(d) Decreased plasma colloid osmotic pressure

26. The bicarbonate buffer system is important in regulating extracellular fluid H^+ concentration because:
    (a) the concentrations of CO_2 and HCO_3^- in the extracellular fluid are relatively high
    (b) the pK of the bicarbonate buffer system is very close to the pH of the extracellular fluid
    (c) the two elements of the bicarbonate buffer systems (CO_2 and HCO_3^-) are regulated by renal and respiratory mechanisms
    (d) (a) and (c)
    (e) (b) and (c)

27. Which of the following statements is *incorrect?*
    (a) Countercurrent flow in the vasa recta minimizes solute loss from the medulla of the kidney
    (b) There is a net movement of water out of the descending loop of Henle
    (c) The thick ascending loop of Henle is highly permeable to water
    (d) Blood flow through the vasa recta is very low, compared to blood flow through peritubular capillaries of coritical nephrons

28. Vasodilation of the *efferent* arterioles of the kidney *tends to:*
    (a) increase renal blood flow
    (b) decrease glomerular filtration rate
    (c) decrease peritubular capillary colloid osmotic pressure
    (d) decrease glomerular capillary hydrostatic pressure
    (e) all of the above

29. Which of the following changes would *not* occur, under *steady-state conditions* in a normal person as a result of a 50 per cent decrease in sodium intake?
    (a) Increased plasma concentration of angiotensin II
    (b) Increased plasma aldosterone concentration
    (c) Approximately a 50 per cent decrease in sodium excretion
    (d) A large (greater than 10 per cent) decrease in plasma sodium concentration

30. For which of the following substances would you expect the renal clearance to be the *lowest,* under normal conditions?
    (a) Urea
    (b) Creatinine
    (c) Sodium
    (d) Glucose
    (e) Water

31. Which of the following changes would *not* occur as a result of dehydration (loss of water, but not solute)?
    (a) Increased secretion of antidiuretic hormone
    (b) Increased plasma sodium concentration
    (c) Decreased permeability of the collecting ducts to water
    (d) Increased solute concentration in the renal medulla

32. If a person has a tidal volume of 411 ml., a physiological dead space volume of 100 ml., and a respiratory minute ventilation of 3600 ml./min., what is his alveolar ventilation?
    (a) 3600 ml./min.
    (b) 3000 ml./min.
    (c) 2700 ml./min.
    (d) 1500 ml./min.
    (e) 900 ml./min.

33. The major factor regulating alveolar ventilation during rest is:
    (a) arterial PO_2
    (b) arterial PCO_2
    (c) arterial pH
    (d) nervous output from the joint proprioceptors
    (e) none of the above

34. Which one of the following effects in the heart would *not* be a result of increased vagal nerve activity?
    (a) Acetylcholine release at the nerve endings
    (b) Decreased S-T interval
    (c) bradycardia
    (d) Hyperpolarization of the S-A node

35. Increased venous return leads to increased cardiac output by way of the Frank-Starling mechanism. Which one of the following would *not* happen?
    (a) Increased end diastolic sarcomere length
    (b) Increased myocardial tension during systole
    (c) Increased stroke volume
    (d) Decreased end diastolic volume

36. Just before atrial depolarization and contraction:
    (a) the heart is completely polarized
    (b) a period of diastasis occurs
    (c) the pulmonic valve is closed
    (d) left ventricular pressure is less than 20 mm. Hg
    (e) all of the above

37. A possible cause of sinus bradycardia is:
    (a) complete heart block
    (b) decreased sympathetic outflow
    (c) atropine
    (d) decreased vagal outflow
    (e) all of the above

38. Secretory granules in secretory cells are mainly formed by which intracellular organ?
    (a) Mitochondria
    (b) Golgi complex
    (c) Endoplasmic reticulum
    (d) Lysosomes
    (e) Microtubules

39. What is the maximum concentration of hemoglobin normally found in red blood cells?
    (a) 5 per cent
    (b) 10 per cent
    (c) 16 per cent
    (d) 20 per cent
    (e) 34 per cent

40. When infection occurs in a tissue, what type of white blood cell is first attracted from the blood into the tissue by the process of chemotaxis?
    (a) Neutrophils
    (b) Monocytes
    (c) Eosinophils
    (d) Basophils
    (e) Plasma cells

41. What is the first important event in hemostatis following severe tissue injury?
    (a) Blood coagulation
    (b) Formation of a platelet plug
    (c) Vascular spasm
    (d) Formation of thromboplastin
    (e) Formation of prothrombin activator

42. If a nerve membrane of a large A nerve fiber is not able to pump sodium and potassium ions through the membrane but otherwise it is in the normal resting state, approximately how many nerve impulses can be transmitted by the nerve fiber before it cannot transmit any more impulses?
    (a) one
    (b) About 10
    (c) About 5000
    (d) Usually 50,000 or more

43. Skeletal muscle contraction is excited when the intracellular concentration of which ion rises above 10^{-5} moles per liter in the sarcoplasm of the muscle cells?
    (a) Na
    (b) K
    (c) Mg
    (d) Ca
    (e) Cl

44. With normal cardiac function, a 10 mm. Hg change in which of the following pressures would have the greatest effect on cardiac output?
    (a) Pressure in the carotid arteries
    (b) Pressure in the renal artery
    (c) Aortic pressure
    (d) right atrial pressure
    (e) Pulmonary artery pressure

45. Following acute failure of the left ventricle of the heart in man, pulmonary edema generally begins to appear when left atrial pressure approaches:
    (a) 7 mm. Hg
    (b) 15 mm. Hg
    (c) 20 mm. Hg
    (d) 30 mm. Hg
    (e) 50 mm. Hg

46. The factors that cause arterial pressure to recover from moderate degrees of hemorrhagic shock include:
    (a) formation of angiotensin
    (b) baroreceptor reflexes
    (c) absorption of fluid from interstitial spaces of the body
    (d) release of vasopressin
    (e) all of the above

47. When a normal person suddenly changes from recumbent to standing posture:
    (a) blood pressure falls dramatically
    (b) renin secretion is suppressed
    (c) blood pools in the jugular vein
    (d) heart rate increases

48. The partial pressure of water vapor in the lungs:
    (a) increases with hyperventilation
    (b) is relatively constant with changes in altitude
    (c) is proportional to the CO_2 concentration
    (d) becomes negative when barometric pressure falls below 47 mm. Hg

49. What type of ions is probably most important in causing release of transmitter vesicles at nerve endings?
    (a) Sodium ions
    (b) Potassium ions
    (c) Magnesium ions
    (d) Calcium ions
    (e) Chloride ions

50. The type of nerve fiber that has a conduction velocity of approximately 1 meter per second is:
    (a) type A alpha
    (b) type A beta
    (c) type A gamma
    (d) type A delta
    (e) type C

51. Kinesthetic sensations are detected mainly by what type of receptors?
    (a) Muscle spindles
    (b) Golgi tendon apparati
    (c) Skin receptors
    (d) Joint receptors

52. The Betz cells of the primary motor cotrex are located in which layer of the cortex?
    (a) Layer II
    (b) Layer III
    (c) Layer IV
    (d) Layer V
    (e) Layer VI

53. Which primary cortical sensory area is located in the middle of the superior temporal gyrus?
    (a) Vision
    (b) Hearing
    (c) Somatic sensation
    (d) Taste
    (e) Smell

54. Damaging what area of the brain is likely to cause anterograde amnesia?
    (a) Prefrontal cortex
    (b) Occipital cortex
    (c) The amygdala
    (d) The hippocampus
    (e) The thalamus

55. When a person wishes to speak a certain thought, where does the thought originate?
    (a) In Broca's area
    (b) In the posterior part of the temporal cortex
    (c) In the supramarginal gyrus
    (d) In the facial region of the motor cortex
    (e) In the prefrontal cortex

56. In what layer of the retina is a large store of vitamin A found?
    (a) The choroid
    (b) The pigment layer
    (c) The outer nuclear layer
    (d) The outer plexiform layer
    (e) The inner nuclear layer

57. Which type of cone is it that has a peak absorbancy at a light wavelength of 430 millimicrons?
    (a) Red cones
    (b) Green cones
    (c) Blue cones

58. The red cones and the green cones are stimulated approximately equally. What color will the person see?
    (a) Red
    (b) Yellow
    (c) Green
    (d) Purple
    (e) Blue

59. The type of taste that is most sensitive to minute concentrations of the substance to be tasted is:
    (a) The sour taste
    (b) The salty taste
    (c) The sweet taste
    (d) The bitter taste

60. What hormone causes contraction of the gall bladder?
    (a) Secretin
    (b) Gastrin
    (c) Villikinin
    (d) Cholecystokinin
    (e) Bradykinin

61. What of the following enzymes requires an acid pH of approximately 2.0 to function optimally?
    (a) Trypsin
    (b) Chymotrypsin
    (c) Pepsin
    (d) Pancreatic lipase
    (e) Parotid amylase

62. What is the usual cause of megacolon (also called Hirschsprung's disease)?
    (a) Infection in the colon
    (b) Excessive parasympathetic stimulation
    (c) Excessive sympathetic stimulation
    (d) Congenital absence of the myenteric plexus in the sigmoid

63. Approximately what porportion of the bile salts is normally reabsorbed and then resecreted by the liver?
    (a) 5 per cent
    (b) 15 per cent
    (c) 40 per cent
    (d) 70 per cent
    (e) 95 per cent

64. What substance in gallstones causes them to be sometimes x-ray opaque?
    (a) Bile salts
    (b) Bilirubin
    (c) Cholesterol
    (d) Calcium
    (e) Phospholipids

65. At normal room temperature most body heat loss is by:
    (a) convention
    (b) direct conduction
    (c) radiation
    (d) sweating

66. The hormone responsible for increased body temperature after ovulation is:
    (a) luteinizing hormone
    (b) progesterone
    (c) increased estrogen
    (d) androgens

67. Secretion of estriol during pregnancy:
    (a) is dependent on both a viable fetus and a functioning placenta
    (b) is largely produced by the maternal ovaries
    (c) is not dependent on a viable fetus

(d) is lower than the secretion rate of estriol in the nonpregnant female

68. In the female rat, selective neutralization of folli-cle-stimulating hormone with anti-FSH antibodies:
    (a) increases estrogen and progesterone secretion by the corpus luteum
    (b) prevents early uniting of the epiphyses
    (c) prevents early follicular growth
    (d) suppresses the secretion of hypothalamic releasing factors

69. Toxemia of pregnancy:
    (a) is caused by abnormal hormone production
    (b) is associated with retention of salt and water
    (c) is associated with hypotension
    (d) always results in eclampsia

70. In the female rat, selective neutralization of estrogen with antiestrogen antibodies just prior to midcycle:
    (a) prevents menstruation
    (b) prolongs the female sexual cycle
    (c) inhibits ovulation
    (d) prevents the preovulatory surge of gonadotropins

71. What probably causes stimulation of the thermal receptors?
    (a) Change in the membrane structure caused by heat or cold
    (b) Change in the metabolic rate of the nerve ending
    (c) Change in the viscosity of the fluid surrounding the neuron
    (d) Change in the concentration of sodium ions outside the neuron caused by changes in temperature
    (e) Changes in the concentration of potassium ions outside the neuron caused by changes in temperature

72. The energy levels in two different sounds differ from each other by 10,000 times; how much difference is this in decibels?
    (a) 10,000
    (b) 4
    (c) 40
    (d) 20
    (e) 80

73. Which theory probably explains long-term memory the best?
    (a) The theory that it causes actual physical or chemical changes at the synapses
    (b) The theory that there is change in RNA inside the soma of the neuron
    (c) The theory that the glial cells around the neuron change

(d) The theory that the ionic composition of the neurons change
(e) The theory that the electrical potential of the neuron changes

74. Which of the basal ganglia plays the greatest role in initiating and regulating gross intentional movements of the body?
    (a) The substantia nigra
    (b) The globus pallidus
    (c) The subthalamic nucleus
    (d) The claustrum
    (e) The striate body

75. What part of the lower regions of the brain probably plays the most significant role in directing one's attention to one particular type of brain activity?
    (a) The thalamus
    (b) The hypothalamus
    (c) The mesencephalon
    (d) The pons
    (e) The septal region of the limbic system

76. Motor aphasia results from damage to:
    (a) the general interpretative area
    (b) Broca's area
    (c) the angular gyrus area
    (d) the superior temporal cortex
    (e) the prefrontal area

77. Very light stimulation of the primary sensory cortex is most likely to cause:
    (a) movement of an area of the body to which the sensory cortex is connected
    (b) pain in the area of representation
    (c) a feeling that someone has touched the area of representation
    (d) a mild electric, tingling feeling in the area of representation
    (e) a hot feeling in the area of representation

78. Amino acids are transported in the blood mainly in the form of:
    (a) plasma proteins
    (b) lipoproteins
    (c) in combination with a carbohydrate carrier
    (d) in combination with a phospholipid carrier
    (e) amino acids themselves

79. If the baroreceptor reflexes are fully functional when upright posture is assumed:
    (a) the blood vessels of the arms will become vasodilated
    (b) arterial pressure in the foot will be maintained at 120/80 mm. Hg
    (c) bradycardia will occur
    (d) cerebral blood flow will not change appreciably

80. Menstruation is caused by the:
    (a) surge of LH just prior to midcycle
    (b) failure of the corpus luteum to involute
    (c) sudden reduction of progesterone and estrogen at the end of the ovarian cycle
    (d) excessive secretion of estrogen and progesterone at the end of the ovarian cycle

81. The onset of puberty in the male is caused by:
    (a) the sudden "ripening" of the testicles with secretion of large quantities of testosterone
    (b) spontaneous secretion of FSH and LH by anterior pituitary gland at the age of 12
    (c) an aging process of the hypothalamic sexual control centers
    (d) a sudden sharp decrease in hypothalamic sensitivity to testosterone

82. Oxygen debt:
    (a) is impossible to incur when breathing pure oxygen
    (b) can never occur in a healthy individual
    (c) is often evidenced by an increase in lactic concentration in the blood
    (d) is caused by lack of anaerobic metabolism

83. If a person whose normal core body temperature is 98.6 is placed in a tub of water that is 98 F, and the person is breathing air that is 98 F and 100 per cent humidified:
    (a) the person's core temperature will rise
    (b) the person's core temperature will fall to 98 F.
    (c) shivering is likely
    (d) sweating will occur and maintain constant body temperature

84. The most important factor that tends to collapse the lungs (the recoil tendency) is the:
    (a) elastic fiber in the lungs
    (b) intrapleural fluid pressure
    (c) total intrapleural pressure
    (d) surface tension of the alveolar fluid
    (e) tension in the intercostal muscles

85. Oxygen therapy has significant value in all the following types of hypoxia *except:*
    (a) atmospheric hypoxia
    (b) hypoventilation hypoxia
    (c) hypoxia due to pulmonary edema
    (d) hypoxia due to decreased hemoglobin in the blood
    (e) histotoxic hypoxia due to cyanide poisoning

86. The blood vessels of the systemic circulation that are responsible for most of the resistance to blood flow in the circulation are the:
    (a) aorta and large arteries
    (b) arterioles
    (c) capillaries
    (d) venules
    (e) venae cavae and large veins

87. After drinking a large amount of *hypotonic* fluid and after absorption of the fluid from the gut into the blood, which of the following changes would you expect?
    (a) Increased secretion of antidiuretic hormone
    (b) A decrease in distal tubular permeability to water
    (c) A marked decrease in glomerular filtration rate
    (d) A marked increase in sodium excretion

88. If one loses a large quantity of saliva externally, which of the following ions would be lost in the greatest amount in relation to its concentration in plasma?
    (a) Sodium
    (b) Chloride
    (c) Potassium

89. The hormone generally considered to be the major stimulus for enzyme secretion by the pancreas is:
    (a) cholecystokinin
    (b) secretin
    (c) trypsin
    (d) gastrin

90. Failure to absorb bile salts in the distal ileum causes:
    (a) constipation
    (b) no effect
    (c) diarrhea

91. The absence of lactase in the intestine would cause failure to digest completely:
    (a) steak
    (b) beer
    (c) milk
    (d) table sugar

92. A large greasy smelly stool usually indicates failure of digestion of:
    (a) carbohydrates
    (b) fats
    (c) proteins
    (d) peptones

93. Sudden exposure of an unacclimatized subject to 25,000 feet would produce after 10 minutes?
    (a) improved night vision
    (b) falling pH
    (c) helium bubbles in the blood
    (d) coma
    (e) all of the above

94. The maximum number of ribosomes that a messenger RNA molecule can be attached to at any one time is:
    (a) zero

(b) one
(c) two
(d) more than two

95. Which of the following is correct about the energy required to cause diffusion through a cell membrane?
    (a) No energy is required
    (b) The energy that causes the diffusion comes from chemical reactions in the cell membrane
    (c) Energy for diffusion is required only when a net rate of diffusion must occur against a concentration gradient
    (d) The energy that causes the diffusion comes from the kinetic energy of the particles of the solution

96. The sodium concentration in extracellular fluid is progressively decreased. What happens to the degree of postivity of the plateau in the monophasic cardiac action potential?
    (a) It increases
    (b) It decreases
    (c) Essentially no change

97. When energy is derived from creatine phosphate to cause muscle contraction, what is the first step in this transfer of energy?
    (a) The creatine phosphate transfers its energy to the cross bridges to cause them to become cocked
    (b) The creatine phosphate causes the power stroke of the cross bridges
    (c) The creatine phosphate transfers its energy to the actin filament
    (d) The creatine phosphate transfers its energy to the myosin filament
    (e) The energy of the creatine phosphate is used to convert ADP into ATP

98. What provides most of the energy that is used to maintain a normal resting membrane potential of about 70 millivolts inside the neuronal soma?
    (a) The potassium pump
    (b) The chloride pump
    (c) The sodium pump
    (d) The calcium pump
    (e) Diffusion of chloride ions

99. When temporal summation occurs at the neuronal soma, which of the following will cause the greatest degree of summation?
    (a) Fiber stimulus frequency of 1,000 impulses per second
    (b) Fiber stimulus frequency of 100 impulses per second
    (c) Fiber stimulus frequency of 10 impulses per second
    (d) Fiber stimulus frequency of 1 impulse per second

100. To what part of the brain do most of the signals from the Golgi tendon apparati and muscle spindles go?
    (a) The somesthetic cortex
    (b) The thalamus
    (c) The basal ganglia
    (d) The motor cortex
    (e) The cerebellum

101. In what part of the central nervous system do the signals probably originate to provide most of the support of the body against gravity?
    (a) The bulboreticular facilitatory area
    (b) The basal ganglia
    (c) The motor cortex
    (d) The cerebellum
    (e) The spinal cord

102. Where are the centers located for causing such gross sterotype body movements as rotational movements of the head, raising movements of the head and body, flexing movements of the head and body, and turning movements of the body?
    (a) Motor cortex
    (b) Cerebellum
    (c) Amygdala
    (d) Mesencephalon

103. Damage to which area of the cerebral cortex is likely to cause the greatest degree of loss of intellectual capabilities in a right-handed person?
    (a) The frontal lobes
    (b) The left somesthetic sensory and sensory association areas
    (c) The right somesthetic sensory and sensory association areas
    (d) The left posterior superior temporal gyrus
    (e) The right posterior temporal and angular gyrus regions

104. What determines whether norepinephrine circulating in the body fluids will be excitatory or inhibitory in a particular organ?
    (a) The nature of the receptor in the cells of the organ
    (b) The intensity of nerve stimulation of the organ
    (c) The chemical changes that occur in the norepinephrine before it excites the cells
    (d) The position on the cells where norepinephrine is secreted by the nerve endings

105. When rhodopsin is decomposed by light energy, what happens to change the membrane potential of the rod?
    (a) The activity of the sodium pump is increased
    (b) Membrane permeability in the outer segment is increased
    (c) The membrane permeability for potassium greatly increases

(d) Membrane permeability for sodium ions in the outer segment is decreased

(e) The activity of the postassium pump is increased

106. Integration of temperature information by the nervous system occurs mainly in the:
(a) Spinal cord
(b) Hypothalamus
(c) Amygdala
(d) Peripheral receptors

107. The arterial pulse pressure in the femoral artery is normally:
(a) Less than the pulse pressure in the upper aorta
(b) Less than 20 mm. Hg
(c) Greater than the pulse pressure in the upper aorta
(d) Equal to the pulse pressure in the upper aorta
(e) None of the above

108. Macrophages are the mature form of:
(a) Neutrophils
(b) Eosinophils
(c) Basophils
(d) Monocytes
(e) Lymphocytes

109. Hemophilia is most commonly caused by deficiency of which of the following clotting factors?
(a) Platelet factor 3
(b) Factor V
(c) Thromboplastin
(d) Factor VIII
(e) Factor XII

110. The troponin-tropomyosin complex is believed to play what role in the muscle contractile process?
(a) It provides the major amount of elastic tension during the contractile process
(b) It is believed that in the resting state it covers or in some other way inactivates the active sites on the actin strands of the actin helix
(c) Combination of this complex with myosin excites the activity of the "power stroke"
(d) Combination of potassium with the troponin portion of this complex is believed to trigger muscle contraction

111. The endoplasmic reticulum has which of the following functions?
(a) Formation of glucose by the granular portion of the reticulum
(b) Formation of proteins by the granular portion of the reticulum
(c) Digestion of proteins by all portions of the reticulum
(d) Transport of protein molecules in some cases from one part of the cell to another part

112. What portion of the cell membrane acts as a barrier to limit the movement of water and water-soluble substances through the membrane?
(a) The lipid portion
(b) The protein portion
(c) The mucopolysaccharide portion
(d) The pores
(e) The membrane enzymes

113. The concentration of sodium on the first side of a membrane is two times as great as on the second side of the membrane. This concentration is now increased to five times as great on the first side as on the second side. How many times does the net rate of sodium diffusion through the membrane increase?
(a) five times
(b) four times
(c) 2.5 times
(d) two times
(e) 1.25 times

114. A solution contains 1 gram-mole of magnesium sulfate per liter. Assuming full ionization of this compound, calculate the osmotic pressure of the solution (1 mosmole/liter concentration is equivalent to 19.3 mm. Hg osmotic pressure).
(a) 19.3 mm. Hg
(b) 38.6 mm. Hg
(c) 19,300 mm. Hg
(d) 38,600 mm. Hg
(e) 57,900 mm. Hg

115. In a self-excitable tissue such as the sinoatrial node of the heart where the rhythm of the heart is generated, what causes the pause between successive action potentials?
(a) Prolonged increased permeability of the sodium channels during this period
(b) Prolonged excess permeability of the potassium channels during this period
(c) Increased leakage of calcium ions to the interior of the fiber during this period
(d) Excessive gating potential on the potassium channels during this period of time
(e) Excessive gating potential on the sodium channels at this time

116. Which of the following cortical layers is stimulated most by the diffuse thalamocortical system?
(a) Layer 2
(b) Layer 3
(c) Layer 4
(d) Layer 5
(e) Layer 6

117. If the connections are cut between the cortex and the thalamus, which one of the following types of brain waves can still be recorded in the cortex?

(a) alpha waves
(b) beta waves
(c) theta waves
(d) delta waves

118. Almost all of the cerebral cortex has direct two-way communication with which one of the following subcortical structures?
(a) Cerebellum
(b) Thalamus
(c) Hypothalamus
(d) Bulboreticular facilitory area
(e) Putamen

119. Under resting conditions the ganglion cells of the retina discharge at approximately what rate?
(a) one per second
(b) five per second
(c) 25 per second
(d) 125 per second
(e) 1250 per second

120. Stimulation of the hair cells in the cochlea is caused by:
(a) compression of the hair cells by the sound waves
(b) vibration of the hair cells by the sound waves
(c) movement of the hair cells back and forth so that the hairs are bent by fluid or the tectorial membrane
(d) the electrical current generated by potential differences between the endolymph and the perilymph
(e) nerve stimuli originating from the cochlea nerve

121. What of the following statements is *not* true about brain waves?
(a) The brain wave of petit mal epilepsy is a spike and dome pattern.
(b) Grand mal epilepsy is characterized by high frequency high voltage waves.
(c) Psychomotor epilepsy is characterized by lower than normal frequency waves.
(d) Deep sleep is characterized by alpha waves.

122. Which of the following statements is true?
(a) The transmitter secreted at the endings of the sympathetic preganglionic neurons is norepinephrine.
(b) The transmitter secreted at the endings of the preganglionic neurons of the parasympathetic neurons is epinephrine.
(c) The transmitter secreted at the postganglionic neuron endings of the parasympathetic neurons is atropine.
(d) The transmitter secreted at most postganglionic neuron endings of the sympathetic nervous system is norepinephrine.

123. Which of the following is *not* important in dark adaptation?
(a) Conversion of retinene into rhodopsin
(b) Conversion of vitamin A into retinene
(c) The pupillary reflex
(d) Conversion of retinene into lumirhodopsin

124. Two basic types of electrical waves in smooth muscle of the gastrointestinal tract are:
(a) fast waves and spikes
(b) short and long spikes
(c) slow waves and spikes
(d) slow waves and fast waves

125. The usual stimulus of peristalsis is:
(a) distention
(b) sympathetic stimulation
(c) acid chyme
(d) alkaline chyme

126. The principal function of the gastroesophageal spincter is:
(a) to allow stomach acid into the esophagus
(b) to maintain food in the esophagus for digestion
(c) to prevent reflux of stomach contents
(d) nonexistent

127. Hydrochloric acid is secreted by the:
(a) Paneth cells
(b) goblet cells
(c) chief cells
(d) parietal cells

128. The three phases of gastric secretion are:
(a) first, second, and third
(b) cephalic, gastric, and intestinal
(c) ptylin, gastrin, secretion
(d) gastric, intestinal colonic

129. A transmitter substance is applied to the surface of a neuron, and this causes the pores to open up with greatly increased permeability to chloride ions and potassium ions but no increase in permeability to sodium ions. However, the potential across the cell membrane does not change when the pores open up. What happens to the excitability of the neuron?
(a) The neuron is facilitated
(b) The neuron is inhibited
(c) There is no change in degree of facilitation or inhibition
(d) The neuron is facilitated but there is a long latent period for development of the excitation
(e) The neuron is inhibited but there is a long latent period for development of the inhibition

130. What is the most important deficit that occurs

when the somesthetic association area is removed?
(a) Loss of tactile sensation
(b) Loss of thermal sensation
(c) Loss of pain sensation
(d) Loss of three dimensional conception of the body
(e) Loss of ability to localize sensations on the surface of the body

131. The portion of the vestibular system that is most important for preventing a person from suddenly falling if he makes a sudden turn while moving forward is the:
(a) saccule
(b) utricle
(c) cochlea duct
(d) otoconia
(e) semicircular canals

132. Where is motor activity probably initiated in the brain?
(a) Motor cortex
(b) Premotor cortex
(c) Basal ganglia
(d) Cerebellum
(e) The mesencephalon and thalamus

133. Braxton-Hicks contractions:
(a) is a positive feedback system
(b) is another term for labor contractions
(c) occur during most of the months of pregnancy
(d) result in hypoxia of the fetus

ANSWERS TO MULTIPLE CHOICE QUESTIONS

1. b	35. d	68. c	101. a
2. e	36. e	69. b	102. d
3. a	37. b	70. c	103. d
4. c	38. b	71. b	104. a
5. a	39. e	72. c	105. d
6. d	40. a	73. a	106. b
7. a	41. c	74. e	107. c
8. a	42. d	75. a	108. d
9. b	43. d	76. b	109. d
10. c	44. d	77. d	110. b
11. a	45. d	78. e	111. d
12. d	46. e	79. d	112. a
13. e	47. d	80. c	113. b
14. c	48. b	81. d	114. d
15. e	49. d	82. c	115. b
16. d	50. e	83. a	116. a
17. e	51. d	84. d	117. d
18. e	52. d	85. e	118. b
19. a	53. b	86. b	119. b
20. c	54. d	87. b	120. c
21. e	55. b	88. c	121. d
22. c	56. b	89. a	122. d
23. c	57. c	90. c	123. d
24. e	58. b	91. c	124. c
25. a	59. d	92. b	125. a
26. e	60. d	93. d	126. c
27. c	61. c	94. d	127. d
28. e	62. d	95. d	128. b
29. d	63. e	96. b	129. b
30. d	64. d	97. e	130. d
31. c	65. c	98. c	131. e
32. c	66. b	99. a	132. e
33. b	67. a	100. e	133. c
34. b			

4

Biochemistry

ALFRED E. WILHELMI, D. PHIL.

Charles Howard Candler Professor of Biochemistry, Emeritus, Emory University

COMPOSITION OF LIVING TISSUES

The elements comprising the major organic constituents of the body are C, H, O, N, P and S. These organic constituents are of two classes: very large molecules, which may be classed as elements of storage, structure or function, and small molecules, which are (a) the constituents of the macromolecules, (b) derivatives of these constituents with special functions (e.g., coenzymes, vitamins) and (c) sources of energy, through fermentation or oxidation. The inorganic elements are also of two classes: (1) monovalent and divalent ions, which are major constituents of the body fluids Na^+, K^+, Cl^-, HCO_3^-, Ca^{2+}, Mg^{2+}, HPO_4^{2-}, $H_2PO_4^-$, and (2) trace elements Fe, Cu, Mn, Zn, I, Co, Mo, Si, V, F.

The most abundant single compound in the body is *water*—65 to 70 per cent of the lean body mass, or 55 per cent of the whole body weight. The water is distributed between extracellular and intracellular compartments, and the extracellular compartment is divided into a stationary component, the interstitial fluid, and the continuously moving blood plasma. Soluble and diffusible substances are rapidly and efficiently distributed throughout the system.

The principal *solid constituents* of the body are *proteins* (19 per cent of the total body weight); *lipids* (19 per cent); *ash,* mainly calcium and phosphorus in the skeleton (5 per cent); and 2 per cent of *other organic substances, including the carbohydrates.*

The Cell

The unit of organization and of metabolic operations in the body is the cell. Cells exhibit great variety of form and function, but they all have structural and functional components in common. Every cell is bounded by a plasma membrane, which is an active guardian of the internal environment of the cell, excluding certain materials, allowing some to pass and expending energy to facilitate the transport of others. The fabric of the membrane is a bimolecular layer of lipid, mainly of phosphoglyceride molecules presenting their polar ends to the surfaces of the membrane and their hydrocarbon tails toward one another, to the interior. This fabric is partly or completely penetrated by a variety of proteins, many of them enzymes. Each surface of the plasma membrane therefore presents a different pattern of protein and of metabolic activity to the aqueous environment of the exterior and the interior of the cell.

The plasma membrane is neither passive nor static. Both its lipid and its protein constituents are constantly being replaced, although at different rates, and its metabolic activities, with respect to receptor sites and specific enzymatic activities, may alter in response to change in metabolic needs and the environment of the cell.

The endoplasmic reticulum is an internal membranous system of the cell, forming channels or vesicles, and connected to the outer nuclear membrane and possibly to the plasma membrane. The membrane is composed of lipoprotein and is the locus of many specific enzymatic activities. Certain regions, the "rough" endoplasmic reticulum, are covered with ribosomes, which are the sites of protein synthesis. The "smooth" endoplasmic reticulum is the site of steroid synthesis, of polysaccharide synthesis and of a variety of specialized metabolic reactions, many of them involving the direct addition of oxygen in hydroxylations. In the differential centrifugation of cell homogenates the disintegrated endoplasmic reticulum is found as small vesicles, microsomes, which retain many of their specific enzymatic activities.

Another internal membranous structure communicating with both the endoplasmic reticulum and the plasma membrane is the Golgi apparatus. It is a site of synthesis of heteropolysaccharides and the place where many proteins, transferred from the ribosomes, acquire their carbohydrate moieties. This is a more important function of the Golgi apparatus than was once thought, since it now appears that the glycoproteins, containing covalently bound carbohydrate, may be the largest class of all proteins.

Every nucleated cell contains its own digestive apparatus in the form of lysosomes, small vesicles (0.5 to 3μ in diameter) bounded by a simple membrane and containing a great array of acid hydrolases capable in the aggregate of reducing all of the compound molecules in the cell to their simplest constituents. They are clearly involved in the processes of pinocytosis and phagocytosis, and they play a part in the internal cellular housekeeping by means of which the constituents of macromolecules are salvaged for reuse, and in the processes by which, in fasting, protein is mobilized for gluconeogenesis. The lysosomes release their contents when cells die and undergo autolysis.

The largest organelles other than the nucleus are the mitochondria. These small particles (0.5 by 3μ) appearing in a variety of shapes, are enclosed by a double membrane. The outer membrane resembles that of the endoplasmic reticulum. The inner membrane is a far more elaborate structure, richer in lipid, more rigid, and more selective in its permeability than the outer membrane. The inner membrane is thrown into folds, or cristae, projecting inward toward the matrix of the mitochondria, and the inner surface of the cristae carries on slender stalks numerous spherical particles. Embedded in these particles are the enzymes of the respiratory chain. The mitochondria are the sites of oxidative energy production in cells. The matrix, enclosed by the inner membrane, contains the enzyme systems for the oxidation of fatty acids, the pyruvate oxidation system, and the tricarboxylic acid cycle. The inner membrane contains the elements of the final common pathway, the respiratory chain. The principal products of mitochondrial oxidations are carbon dioxide, water, and adenosine triphosphate (ATP), the main form in which energy is conserved and utilized in the cell. The number of mitochondria in a cell depends upon its size and the intensity of its oxidative metabolism. In all cells they account for nearly all of the oxygen utilized, but they carry out many other processes that differ in their detail in different cells. For example, the mitochondria of liver cells carry out the initial steps of urea synthesis. These reactions do not take place in other cells.

The largest organelle of a cell is the nucleus, a dense structure large enough to be seen in the light microscope. The nucleus is also surrounded by a double membrane. There is evidence to suggest that the outer membrane may be continuous with the endoplasmic reticulum. The double membrane has numerous "pores" where the structure is thin, permitting free exchange of materials with the cytoplasm. The principal constituents of the nucleus are the nucleoproteins. With the exception of a small quantity in the mitochondria, the DNA of the cell is in the nucleus, distributed as small dense nucleoprotein particles called chromatin. RNA is thought to be synthesized in a denser region of the nucleus called the nucleolus. The nucleus contains the enzymes required for the replication of DNA, at the time of cell division, and for the transcription of DNA into the various forms of RNA required for the synthesis of protein. In the nucleus the genetic information in DNA is stored and reproduced as required, and it is transmitted, through RNA, to the rest of the cell, in the form of a characteristic pattern of functional and structural proteins.

The internal membranes and organelles of the cell are bathed in the cytosol, which provides a means of communication between them. In addition, the cytosol contains enzymes and enzyme systems not firmly associated with any structure: the enzymes of glycolysis, glycogenesis and glycogenolysis, of fatty acid synthesis, of amino-acyl-tRNA synthesis and many others.

The cell, with its many internal membranes and organelles, is itself a little organism. The chemical changes supporting its life are not random but are highly structured. It is this that makes possible the large degree of cellular self-regulation, efficiency and economy.

CHEMISTRY OF PROTEINS AND NUCLEIC ACIDS

Proteins

The principal nitrogen-containing compounds of plant and animal tissues are the proteins. Their essential nature is illustrated in their role as biologic catalysts, the enzymes, but they act also as constituents of membranes, as prominent components of connective tissues, bone matrix, cartilage, hair, horn, claws, nails; as hormones, antigens and antibodies; as osmotic regulators; and as both specific and general carriers, not only of the respiratory gases but also of a host of simpler organic compounds and many inorganic ions. Their elementary composition is simple: C = 50 to 55 per cent; H = 6.0 to 7.3 per cent; O = 19 to 24 per cent; N = 13 to 19 per cent; S = 0 to 4 per cent. Many other elements are associated with proteins in more or less firm combination, but only iodine is found as a constituent of an α-amino acid in a derived protein, thyroglobulin.

Proteins are polymers of α-amino acids. They owe their infinite variety and individuality to differences in the kind, number and order of the 20 amino acids occurring naturally in proteins and to the presence of nonprotein constituents: carbohydrate, lipid, nucleic acid, metals and a wide array of complex organic substances, serving, like the heme of hemoglobin, some special function, sometimes covalently bound to the protein, sometimes in a looser, reversible association with it.

The range of sizes of proteins is enormous, from tiny proteins such as insulin (M_r about 6,000) to large aggregates having masses of millions of daltons.* The structure common to them all is the peptide bond, formed by loss of water between the carboxyl group of one α-amino acid and the α-amino group of another. This yields a repeating backbone structure as follows:

$$\cdots N - \underset{\underset{R_1}{|}}{\overset{\overset{H}{|}}{C}} - \overset{\overset{O}{\|}}{C} - \underset{}{\overset{\overset{H}{|}}{N}} - \underset{\underset{R_2}{|}}{\overset{\overset{H}{|}}{C}} - \overset{\overset{O}{\|}}{C} \cdots$$

* Molecular weight (M_r) is the *ratio* of the sum of the atomic weights of the atoms in a molecule to $\frac{1}{12}$ of the weight of the atom of ^{12}C. It is a termless number. The *dalton* is a measure of the *mass* of a particle as a multiple of $\frac{1}{12}$ of the mass of ^{12}C. It is usefully applied to large heterogeneous particles, such as ribosomes, or to polymers of indefinite size (e.g., glycogen).

Compounds formed in this way are peptides. Proteins, containing many such bonds, are polypeptides. They may consist of a single chain or of two or more identical or different chains. The distinction between large polypeptides (e.g., ACTH, 39 amino acids, M_r about 4,500) and small proteins is somewhat arbitrary. The simplest peptide, containing two amino acids, is a dipeptide. One containing five amino acids is a pentapeptide; one containing 20 is a dodecapeptide, and so on.

Proteins differ radically in shape as well as size. The soluble globular proteins are formed by folding of the polypeptide chains to form a more or less tight ball, such as one might make rolling up a bit of string between thumb and forefinger. The fibrous proteins (usually insoluble, like collagen or the keratin of hair) are formed of long chains of monomers in side-by-side and end-to-end array or, like F actin, one of the contractile proteins, are formed by the string-of-beads alignment of many globular subunits. The association of large polypeptides with one another, or the aggregation of different subunits, is an important property of proteins. Hemoglobin, for example, is a globular protein composed of two pairs of subunits, and some fundamental properties of the molecule arise from interactions among the nonidentical subunits. The activity of certain enzymes is regulated by the reversible association of their subunits.

Proteins can be hydrolyzed by heating in mineral acid or alkali or by treatment with a mixture of proteolytic enzymes. Complete hydrolysis yields a mixture of simple crystalline compounds, the α-amino acids. With the exception of the simplest amino acid, glycine (α-aminoacetic acid), all of the α-amino acids contain at least one asymmetric center at the α-carbon, are optically active and are all of the L-series (related to L-glyceraldehyde). The complete amino acid analysis of proteins is now achieved with as little as 2 mg. of sample by automated methods using ion-exchange chromatography. The amino acid tryptophan, which is destroyed by acid hydrolysis, is estimated separately in the intact protein, and cysteine, which is often partly destroyed, is oxidized to cysteic acid before hydrolysis.

The 20 amino acids found in proteins fall into several classes. The largest includes the monoamino-monocarboxylic acids. These are subdivided as follows:

1. Aliphatic amino acids: glycine, alanine, valine, leucine, isoleucine
2. Hydroxy amino acids: serine, threonine
3. Sulfur-containing amino acids: methionine, cysteine (disulfide form: cystine)
4. Aromatic amino acids: phenylalanine, tyrosine, tryptophan

5. A single imino acid, proline, in which the α-nitrogen is part of a five-membered ring

In addition, there are two dicarboxylic acids and their amides:

6. Aspartic acid and asparagine; glutamic acid and glutamine.

Finally, there are three basic amino acids:

7. Lysine, containing an ϵ-amino group
8. Arginine, containing a strongly basic guanido group
9. Histidine, containing the imidazole group

The structures of the amino acids are shown in Table 4-1. Two *derived* amino acids are found in collagen and a few other related structural proteins: 4-hydroxyproline or 3-hydroxyproline, and 5-hydroxylysine. The iodinated amino acids, monoiodotyrosine and diiodotyrosine, 3,5,3',5'-tetraiodothyronine (thyroxine) and 3,5,3'-triiodothyronine, are found in thyroglobulin, synthesized in the thyroid gland. The amino acid, β-alanine, $H_2NCH_2CH_2COOH$, is a constituent of the vitamin, pantothenic acid, and of the naturally occurring peptides carnosine (β-alanyl histidine) and anserine (β-alanyl-N_1-methyl histidine). Ornithine, the next lower homologue of lysine, $H_2N-CH_2-CH_2CH_2-CH(NH_2)COOH$, is a component of the urea-synthesizing cycle, together with citrulline, $H_2N-CO-NH-CH_2-CH_2-CH_2-CH(NH_2)COOH$. γ-Aminobutyric acid (GABA), $H_2N-CH_2-CH_2-CH_2-COOH$, derived by decarboxylation of glutamic acid, is an important intermediate of amino acid metabolism in brain and spinal cord, where it may act as a neuroregulator.

With the exception of the leucines and tyrosine, the amino acids are all easily soluble in water. They are both weak acids and weak bases and are effective buffers in the regions of the pKa of the carboxyl and the amino groups (about pH 2.4 and pH 9.8 respectively). In the physiologic range of pH, however, the amino acids, with the exception of histidine, are not effective buffers. In neutral solutions they exist as zwitterions: $^+H_3N-CH(R)-COO^-$. Addition of sufficient acid suppresses the dissociation of the carboxyl group, generating the cation:

$$^+H_3N-CH(R)-COOH.$$

The addition of alkali titrates the amino group, yielding the anion:

$$H_2N-CH(R)-COO^-$$

Although the α-amino and carboxyl groups are involved in the peptide bond of proteins their behavior as electrolytes is a model for the behavior of proteins as polyelectrolytes. The free carboxyl groups in proteins are the γ- and β-carboxyls of glutamic and aspartic acid and the carboxyl of the terminal amino acid of the polypeptide chain. The free basic groups of proteins are the NH_2-terminal amino group, the ϵ-amino group of lysine, the guanido group of arginine and the imidazole nitrogen of histidine. The titration behavior of these groups is quite like that of the carboxyl and the amino group of the model amino acid described above: addition of acid suppresses the ionization of the carboxyl groups; addition of base suppresses ionization of the basic groups. The amino acid above, with its single cation and anion, is neutral in neutral solution: It is isoelectric and will not migrate in an electric field.

Proteins, as polyelectrolytes, have numerous cationic and anionic groups. If there is a predominance of dicarboxylic amino acids, the protein is acidic, and it has a net negative charge in neutral solutions; if basic amino acids are present in excess, the protein is basic and will have a net positive charge in neutral solution. The difference between negative and positive charges can be brought to zero by titrating the protein in the appropriate direction; e.g., by adding acid to a neutral solution of an acidic protein, the ionization of the carboxyl groups is gradually suppressed, and a pH is reached at which the excess of negative charge is removed: The protein is then at its isoelectric point (zero net charge), and it will not migrate in an electric field. Table 4-2 lists the pK values of the ionizing groups of proteins. Like the amino acids, proteins are in general poor buffers in the physiologic range of pH, since only the imidazole nitrogen of histidine has a pK near pH 7.4, and relatively few proteins have a high content of histidine. Some of the properties of proteins as polyelectrolytes will be considered below.

The amino acids have the characteristic properties of amines and carboxylic acids. In addition, they have reactions characteristic of any other special group in the molecule, the phenolic hydroxyl of tyrosine, for example, or the sulfhydryl of cysteine. The reactions of these groups are also given by the proteins that contain these amino acids.

The method most commonly used to estimate α-amino acids quantitatively is the reaction with ninhydrin (triketohydrindene hydrate), yielding a blue color, CO_2, ammonia and an aldehyde containing one less carbon atom than the amino acid. Since ammonia and other amino compounds give a color with ninhydrin, only the measurement of evolved CO_2 is specific for α-amino acids. With suitable precautions, however, ninhydrin can be used in the colorimetric measurement of amino acids. Proline and the hydroxyprolines give a yellow color with ninhydrin. A variety of color reactions are available for the detection and estimation

TABLE 4-1. The Amino Acids: General Formula:
$$^+H_3N-\underset{\underset{R}{|}}{\overset{\overset{COO^-}{|}}{C}}-H$$

Name	Abbreviation	R
1. Glycine	Gly	$H-$
Alanine	Ala	$-CH_3$
Valine	Val	$CH_3-\underset{\underset{CH_3}{\|}}{CH}-$
Leucine	Leu	$CH_3-\underset{\underset{CH_3}{\|}}{CH}-CH_2-$
Isoleucine	Ile	$CH_3CH_2\underset{\underset{CH_3}{\|}}{CH}-$
2. Serine	Ser	$HO-CH_2-$
Threonine	Thr	$CH_3-\underset{\underset{OH}{\|}}{\overset{\overset{H}{\|}}{C}}-$
3. Cysteine	Cys	$HS-CH_2-$
Methionine	Met	$CH_3-S-CH_2CH_2-$
4. Phenylalanine	Phe	$-CH_2-$
Tyrosine	Tyr	$HO-$ $-CH_2-$
Tryptophan	Trp	$-CH_2-$
5. Proline	Pro	COOH
6. Aspartic acid	Asp	$^-OOC-CH_2-$
Asparagine	Asn	$H_2N-CO-CH_2-$
Glutamic acid	Glu	$^-OOC-CH_2CH_2-$
Glutamine	Gln	$H_2N-CO-CH_2-CH_2-$
7. Lysine	Lys	$^+H_3N-CH_2-CH_2-CH_2-CH_2-$
8. Arginine	Arg	$^+H_3N-\underset{\underset{NH}{\|}}{C}-NH-CH_2-CH_2-CH_2-$
9. Histidine	His	$-CH_2-$

TABLE 4-2. pK Values for Acidic and Basic Groups in Proteins

Protein	pKa at 25 C.
α-carboxyl (terminal)	3.0–3.2
β-carboxyl (aspartic)	3.0–4.7
γ-carboxyl (glutamic)	4.4
Imidazole (histidine)	5.6–7.0
α-amino (terminal)	7.6–8.4
ϵ-amino (lysine)	9.4–10.6
Guanidinium (arginine)	11.6–12.6
Phenolic hydroxyl (tyrosine)	9.8–10.4
Sulfhydryl (cysteine)	8–9

of individual amino acids. The aromatic amino acids tyrosine and tryptophan have absorption spectra with maxima at 275 to 280 nm. Their presence accounts for the ultraviolet absorption maximum of proteins at about 280 nm., which is often used for the measurement of the amount of protein in a solution.

The reactions of amino acids of greatest importance are those that make it possible to form peptide bonds. Technical developments in recent years have made the synthesis of oligopeptides relatively easy and practical and have made scarce materials much more readily available (examples: L-pyroglutamyl-L-histidyl-L-proline amide, the tripeptide thyrotropin-releasing factor of the hypothalamus; oxytocin, vasopressin and a variety of analogues; the C-terminal pentapeptide amide of gastrin: glycyl-L-tryptophanyl-L-methionyl-L-aspartyl-L-phenylalanine amide).

The biologically active synthetic peptides provide evidence that the amino acids are linked in proteins mainly by peptide bonds. In addition the peptide bonds of specific synthetic peptides are cleaved by proteolytic enzymes that cleave similar linkages in proteins. When proteins are hydrolyzed by acid or enzymes, free amino and free carboxyl groups appear in equal numbers. Intact proteins have very little free amino nitrogen, but this appears in abundance during hydrolysis. Polypeptides and proteins also give the biuret reaction, the development of a violet color with copper sulfate in strongly alkaline solution. This is dependent on the backbone structure, just sufficient in a tripeptide:

$$-\overset{|}{\underset{|}{C}}-CO-NH-\overset{|}{\underset{|}{C}}-CO-NH-\overset{|}{\underset{|}{C}}-$$

Finally, the evidence of the process of biosynthesis of proteins (presented later in this chapter) indicates that the peptide bond is the only type of linkage between amino acids in the primary structure of a protein.

The sulfhydryl group of a specific cysteine residue in a protein may play an essential part in its biologic activity. Very often the cysteine residues of proteins

are joined by oxidation to the disulfide. When this occurs in the same polypeptide chain a loop is formed; when it occurs between cysteine residues in different chains, they are linked covalently by the -S-S-bond. In both instances the structure of the protein is stabilized and made more rigid. In mature collagen, elastin and the "hard clot" of fibrin, intermolecular covalent bonds are formed by oxidation and condensation of lysine and hydroxylysine side chains. These linkages increase the stability and depress the solubility of the proteins in which they occur.

The carbonyl oxygen and the amide nitrogen of the peptide bonds of proteins make an important contribution to their structure and stability by the formation of hydrogen bonds:

$$\begin{array}{ccc} & R & \\ & | & \\ -C-C-N- \\ \| & | & | \\ O & H & H \\ \cdot & & \cdot \\ \cdot & & \cdot \\ \cdot & & \cdot \\ H & & O \\ | & H & \| \\ -N-C-C- \\ & | & \\ & R & \end{array}$$

The electron of the amide hydrogen is shared with the oxygen. Individually such noncovalent bonds are weak, but in a large protein molecule the formation of many such bonds helps to maintain a stable conformation.

In the folding of the polypeptide chains to form a protein, most of the ionizing groups appear on the surface of the molecule, in contact with the aqueous medium. Ionic bonds (salt linkages) between such groups are infrequent, and because they are subject to the effect of changes in the hydrogen ion concentration of the medium they do not make an important contribution to the stability of the protein. They do, however, help to determine the conformation of the protein and, as in hemoglobin, play a part in holding the subunits of the protein together and in the conformational changes accompanying oxygenation and deoxygenation. Occasionally an ionic bond between the -COO$^-$ of a dicarboxylic acid and -NH$_3^+$ of lysine in the interior of the molecule makes an important contribution to the structure.

Just as the hydrophilic ionizing groups of a protein tend to appear at its surface, so do the hydrophobic hydrocarbon side chains in the polypeptide tend to seek one another out in the interior, coming into apposition and displacing water from between them. This process of hydrophobic bonding is important not only for stabilizing the structure of the nonaqueous interior of a globular protein, but also in the association of subunits of a molecule and in the aggregation of many molecules to form, for example, fibers, as in collagen or in hair. The amino acids involved in hydrophobic bonding are the aromatics, phenylalanine, tyrosine and tryptophan, and the neutral amino acids, methionine, valine, leucine, isoleucine, alanine and glycine.

After the amino acid composition and the molecular weight of a polypeptide or a protein have been determined, the next most important step is to determine the primary structure, the amino acid sequence. The carboxyl-terminal amino acid may be determined by treatment of the protein with the enzyme carboxypeptidase. The amino-terminal amino acid may be determined by treatment of the protein with fluorodinitrobenzene, which reacts with the free amino group to form the dinitrophenyl derivative:

$$C_6H_3(NO_2)_2F + H_2N\text{-}R\cdots$$
$$= C_6H_3(NO_2)_2NH\text{-}R\cdots + HF$$

After acid hydrolysis of the protein, the yellow dinitrophenyl amino acid can be separated and identified by paper chromatography.

Another method, devised by Edman, uses phenylisothiocyanate, which reacts with the free amino group to form a phenylthiocarbamyl derivative. Under acid conditions the phenylthiohydantoin of the NH_2-terminal residue is formed, leaving behind the polypeptide containing one less amino acid. The phenylthiohydantoin can be identified in one or more ways. This procedure can be repeated many times in some instances, yielding the amino acid sequence directly. The process is limited by nonspecific cleavage of acid-sensitive peptide bonds.

A large polypeptide or a protein can be hydrolyzed at specific points by treatment with a proteolytic enzyme of high specificity. Trypsin, for example, cleaves polypeptides at the carboxyl side of arginyl and lysyl residues. After tryptic hydrolysis, the resulting mixture of peptides can be separated and purified by electrophoresis and chromatography, and the amino acid composition and sequence of each peptide can be determined. The amino- and carboxyl-terminal peptides can be readily identified, but the order of the remaining peptides must be established by degrading the protein by a different method, providing a set of overlapping peptides. This is done by using an enzyme of different specificity or by cleaving the polypeptide at a specific point by means of a chemical reagent that acts upon a specific amino acid. Cyanogen bromide, for example, attacks methionyl residues to cleave them at the car-

boxyl side, removing the sulfur, and converting the methionine to homoserine. By a combination of systematic degradation and analysis with careful bookkeeping the entire amino acid sequence of a protein may be determined. If the protein has one or more nonidentical subunits, these must be separated so that the sequence of the individual polypeptides can be determined. If disulfide bonds are present, these are reduced and alkylated in order to facilitate the sequence analysis.

It is thought that the conformation of a polypeptide or protein is determined essentially by its amino acid sequence. This is illustrated convincingly by an experiment with the small globular soluble enzyme ribonuclease (M_r 11,000). In the presence of 6 M guanidine HCl and the reducing agent thioethanol, the four disulfide bonds of the enzyme are opened, and the molecule unfolds to form an unstructured linear polypeptide. If the reagents are slowly removed by dialysis at pH 7 and room temperature, the molecule recovers its original configuration spontaneously and at the same time completely regains its biologic activity. The experiment demonstrates that the biologic activity of the protein depends upon its three-dimensional configuration, but that this depends in turn upon the primary structure—the nature and order of the constituent amino acids.

Present knowledge of the three-dimensional structure of proteins is derived mainly from x-ray diffraction analysis of a number of crystalline proteins and of certain fibrous proteins such as hair keratin, silk fibroin and collagen. One of the characteristic arrangements of amino acids in proteins discovered by these studies is the α-helix. L-Amino acids of certain kinds in polypeptides arrange themselves in a right-handed helix of 3.7 residues per turn; the shape of the helix is maintained by hydrogen bonds between adjacent turns. Peptide bonds involving the amino acid proline are unable to accommodate to this pattern, and the helical structure is interrupted in the vicinity of prolyl residues. At such points the polypeptide chain may take a turn, or fold back upon itself. The hair protein keratin has predominantly an α-helical structure. Adjacent polypeptide strands, in bundles of three or seven, are bonded together by disulfide bonds. The structure is strong and because the helices can unwind to an extended configuration, hair protein can be stretched to nearly twice its length before it breaks. Polypeptide chains in a linear, or extended, β-configuration, may align themselves adjacent to one another, strongly hydrogen bonded, in the structure known as the "pleated sheet." The adjacent chains may run parallel or antiparallel. Such a structure is found in silk fibroin, but it may occur also in globular proteins.

The amino acid sequence of a protein is defined as

the primary structure. Secondary structure refers to sectors of α-helix, pleated sheet, β-configuration or the regions of intrachain disulfide bonds. Tertiary structure comprises the conformation of the entire folded polypeptide. For proteins comprised of two or more subunits, identical or not, the compact array of the subunits is referred to as the quaternary structure.

When the original (native) conformation of a protein is altered, it is said to be denatured. This may be caused by heat, by acid or alkali, by high concentrations of urea or of guanidinium hydrochloride, by detergents, by organic solvents and by mechanical agitation. The most sensitive indicator of denaturation is loss of biologic activity, but most of the other indices of protein conformation—solubility, optical rotation, ability to crystallize, absorption spectrum—also change. Native proteins, often resistant to attack by proteolytic enzymes, are readily digested after denaturation. Denaturation itself, however, does not involve cleavage of peptide bonds. In some instances, as in the experiment with ribonuclease described above, denaturation is reversible.

Many of the properties of proteins are functions of their total charge, or their net charge. Proteins with many ionizing groups attract water molecules, are strongly hydrophilic and very soluble, like serum albumin. At zero net charge, the solubility of proteins is minimal, and they are most readily precipitated by high concentrations of salts such as ammonium sulfate or sodium sulfate. At a pH above the isoelectric point, proteins have a net negative charge and combine readily with heavy metals (Zn, Ba, Ag, Cu, Hg), forming insoluble salts. At acid pH proteins combine with acid anions (tungstate, trichloroacetate, picrate, perchlorate) to form insoluble salts. Similarly, they combine with basic or acid dyes. These properties are exploited in the separation of proteins by ion exchange or in devising a long-acting form of a biologically active protein (e.g., by the combination of the acidic protein insulin with the basic proteins globin or protamine to form a poorly soluble salt). A mixture of proteins in solution may be separated by applying a potential difference across the solution. The proteins migrate in the electrical field at different rates according to their net charge. The process is called electrophoresis. It can be carried out in buffer solution permeating a solid support such as starch gel, paper or polyacrylamide gel. The proteins are located by staining them with a dye and determined quantitatively by measuring the intensity of the color. This method is used in the analysis of serum or plasma proteins for diagnostic purposes.

Proteins are classified according to three systems: by structure, as globular or fibrous, by solubility and by composition. Most of the soluble proteins belong to the globular class. The classes by solubility are (1) albumins: soluble in water, precipitated by saturation with $(NH_4)_2SO_4$; (2) globulins: insoluble in water, soluble in dilute neutral salt solutions or in dilute acid or alkali, precipitated by half-saturation with $(NH_4)_2SO_4$; (3) albuminoids (scleroproteins): insoluble in water and dilute neutral salt solutions; (4) histones: soluble in water, dilute acid and alkali; insoluble in dilute ammonia; (5) protamines: soluble in water, dilute acid and alkali, and ammonia.

The classes by composition are defined in terms of constituents other than amino acids. (a) Simple proteins contain only amino acids. (b) Glycoproteins contain carbohydrate. (c) Nucleoproteins contain nucleic acids. (d) Metalloproteins contain metal ions. (e) Lipoproteins contain lipids (usually of more than one type). (f) Chromoproteins contain a colored prosthetic group. The special substituent of the conjugated proteins (classes b to f) may or may not be covalently bound to the protein moiety. When the binding is noncovalent, the complete protein is called the holoprotein; the protein free of its substituent is the apoprotein.

Nucleic Acids

In addition to the proteins, the other class of nitrogenous high molecular weight constituents of cells is the nucleic acids. These compounds are of two types, named, according to one of their distinguishing features, deoxyribonucleic acid (DNA) and ribonucleic acid (RNA). DNA is found mainly in the nucleus of cells, and in quite small amounts in the mitochondria. The molecules are enormous, their mass exceeding 2×10^9 daltons. RNA is found in the nucleus, but mainly in the cytoplasm. There are three main functional types of RNA: (1) soluble or transfer, tRNA, M_r about 28,000; (2) messenger, mRNA, M_r about 10^6; and ribosomal, rRNA, M_r, 0.5 to 1×10^6. On hydrolysis both DNA and RNA yield equimolar amounts of a nitrogenous base, a pentose and inorganic phosphate. In RNA the pentose is ribose; in DNA 2-deoxyribose. A peculiarity of DNA, related to the presence of the deoxypentose, is that it is not sensitive to alkaline hydrolysis, whereas RNA is. Both RNA and DNA contain the purine bases adenine (A) and guanine (G) and the pyrimidine base cytosine (C). RNA however, contains uracil (U), and DNA contains thymine (5-methyl uracil) (T). These bases are illustrated in Figure 4-1. The fundamental unit of structure of the nucleic acids is the *nucleotide*, consisting of base + pentose + phosphate. The pentose is linked to a nitrogen of the base by its 1′ carbon. Phosphate is esterified to the pentose in the 5′ position. The combination of base + pentose is a *nucleoside*. The nucleotide can be described as a

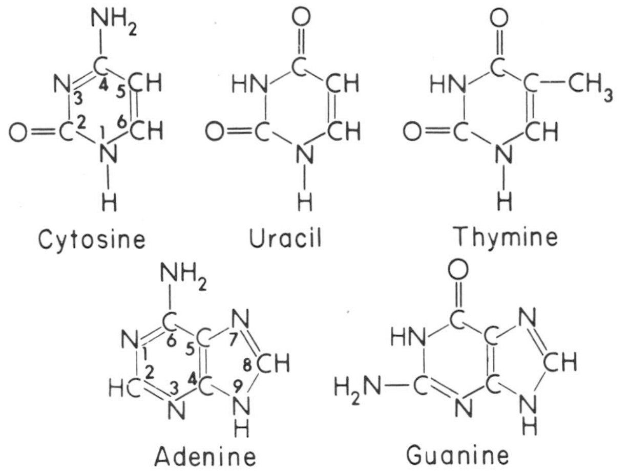

Fig. 4-1. The pyrimidine and purine bases.

nucleoside monophosphate, or named as an acid. Thus, for adenine, the nucleoside is adenosine (or deoxyadenosine); the nucleotide is adenylic acid (or deoxyadenylic acid) or adenosine 5'-monophosphate (AMP) (deoxyadenosine 5'-monophosphate (dAMP). Both RNA and DNA are linear polymers. The individual nucleotides are joined by phosphodiester linkages between the pentoses, from the 5' position of one of the 3' position of the next one. A model oligonucleotide might be:

phosphate-pentose-adenine
phosphate-pentose-uracil
phosphate-pentose-adenine
phosphate-pentose-cytosine

A shorthand for this tetranucleotide is pApUpApC, where the capital letters represent the nucleoside and lower case p the phosphate. It is conventionally written with the 5'-terminal at the left and the 3'-terminal at the right. The corresponding deoxyoligonucleotide is written: pdApdTpdApdC.

A significant regularity of the composition of DNA from many sources, discovered by Chargaff, is that the concentration of adenine always equals that of thymine, and the concentration of guanine always equals that of cytosine (A = T; G = C), although, in different DNAs, the ratio A + T/G + C could vary widely. This fundamental observation, combined with the regularities of structure of DNA revealed by x-ray diffraction analysis, led to the concept of the double helical structure, in which adenine in one strand is paired by hydrogen bonding to thymine in the other, and likewise guanine with cytosine. The two strands run anti-parallel:

$$5' \cdots \text{pdApdCpdTpdA} \cdots 3'$$
$$3' \cdots \text{dTpdCpdApdTp} \cdots 5'$$

In this array the hydrogen-bonded bases lie in planes and stack closely to form a linear molecule in which the backbone is formed by the phosphate-linked deoxyribose molecules. The stacking forces between the bases are as important as the hydrogen bonds between them in conferring stability on the molecule. These forces are disrupted by heating, so that DNA, like protein, can be denatured. The transformation from ordered helix to random coil is attended by an abrupt increase in absorption of light at 260 nm., due to lessened interaction between the unstacked bases. The melting temperature (Tm) at which this occurs increases with increasing proportions of G + C in the DNA, because these two bases are held by three hydrogen bonds, rather than two, as between A and T, and it is a useful rough measure of the base composition of a DNA. If the solution is cooled slowly the disordered DNA can reform an intact helix.

In animal cells, DNA is associated with polyamines and basic proteins of the class of histones. The deoxyribonucleoproteins are soluble in 1 M salt solution and insoluble in 0.15 M NaCl. The precipitated nucleoprotein is extremely viscous and sticky, and like the DNA it contains (25 to 50 percent of the dry weight) it has a very high molecular weight. The component proteins are bound to the DNA by salt linkages between the phosphate and the side chains of the basic amino acids, and are easily separated from the DNA by extraction with dilute acid. The histones are small proteins (M_r 12,000 to 20,000) and are distinguished by their high content of arginine and lysine, the absence of tryptophan, and, except for one subclass, the absence of cysteine or cystine. The histones are a heterogeneous group of molecules, distinguished from one another by their relative content of arginine and lysine. The amino acid side chains are frequently modified by N-methylation of lysine and arginine, by O-phosphorylation of serine and by N-acetylation of lysine. The histones are thought to play a part in the regulation of transcription of DNA and possibly in protecting it. In mature spermatozoa the histones present in the deoxyribonucleoprotein during development are displaced by a group of even more basic small proteins, the protamines. In the DNA-protamine complex, the ratio of arginine to phosphate is 1, and the charges are completely neutralized. The role of the protamines is unknown.

Transfer RNA forms an activated complex with a specific amino acid, which it transfers to the site of polypeptide synthesis on the ribosome. A number of tRNAs have been sequenced. The molecule contains from 75 to 90 nucleotides. Base pairing gives it roughly a cloverleaf shape. At the 3' end, the sequence characteristic of all tRNAs is $\cdots$ pCpCpA. The aminoacyl group attaches to the 3'-hydroxyl of the terminal adenosine. A distinctive feature of tRNA is the occurrence of many modified bases as minor components. The most frequent type of modification is the methylation of one or more of the bases. A very common altered base is pseudouridine, in which the ribose is attached by carbon to carbon linkage between the 1-carbon of the sugar and the 5-carbon of uracil. These alterations all take place after the polynucleotide has been synthesized. The methylated bases cannot be hydrogen bonded, and they may therefore play a part in determining the characteristic conformation of the tRNAs. About 10 to 20 per cent of the cellular RNA is tRNA.

Messenger RNA forms a single strand of length varying with the message. It carries the information required for the synthesis of a polypeptide from DNA to the site of protein synthesis in the ribosome. About 2 per cent of the cellular RNA is mRNA.

About 80 per cent of the cellular RNA is in the ribosomes, the particles on which protein synthesis takes place. Ribosomal RNA is heterogeneous, and the functions of each type have not been established.

DNA and RNA are so important that all cells have retained the capability of synthesizing the component mononucleotides. Nucleic acids can be completely hydrolyzed in the intestine. Ribose, deoxyribose, phosphate and adenine can be absorbed and utilized in nucleic acid synthesis. The other bases are catabolized. Guanine is deaminated, oxidized to uric acid and excreted. The nitrogen of the pyrimidine bases is ultimately excreted as urea.

Adenosine
triphosphate

In addition to their role as constituents of RNA, the adenine, guanine, cytidine and uridine nucleotides, as free compounds, have other important functions. The most important of these is the mediation of energy transfer between energy-producing and energy-using systems, mainly carried out by adenosine monophosphate, diphosphate and triphosphate (AMP, ADP, ATP). Guanosine diphosphate and triphosphate play a similar part in some reactions. AMP is also a constit-

uent of a number of coenzymes (e.g., nicotinamide adenine dinucleotide; coenzyme A). The nucleoside phosphates function also as vehicles of group transfer: amino-acyl-adenylates as the activated intermediates in the formation of amino-acyl-tRNA in protein synthesis; uridine diphosphoglucose in glucosyl transfer; cytidine diphosphocholine in the synthesis of phospholipids. Cyclic 3′,5′-adenosine monophosphate (cAMP), cyclic GMP, and cyclic CMP, play important parts as "second messengers," relaying signals initiated by hormones at the cell surface to the interior of the cell.

ENZYMES

All of the chemical reactions in the body take place at constant, relatively low temperature, and most of these would be infinitely slow unless they were catalyzed. A major function of proteins is to serve as enzymes, the biologic catalysts synthesized in living cells. The characteristics of a differentiated cell are determined not only by its structural proteins but also by the nature, variety and amounts of its constituent enzymes and by their ordering into enzyme systems. Over 1,500 enzymes are known, and many of these have been isolated in crystalline form and studied in detail. All enzymes have proved to be proteins.

The general properties of enzymes are those of the proteins. Enzymes range in molecular weight from about 12,000 to well over a million. They can be inactivated by heating, by exposure to strong acid and alkali, by treatment with organic solvents, by high concentrations of denaturing agents such as urea or guanidine hydrochloride and in some cases by exposure to cold or by mechanical agitation. They are highly diverse in structure. Some are simple proteins, consisting only of amino acids in a single polypeptide chain. Some are made up of two or more polypeptides, which may or may not be identical. Many enzymes require an additional heat-stable component, or cofactor, for activity. In some cases these are metal ions (Mg^{2+}, Zn^{2+}, Cu^{2+}) or an anion such as Cl^- (an absolute requirement of salivary and pancreatic amylase). In other cases the cofactor is a complex organic molecule such as the iron-containing porphyrins of the cytochromes, peroxidase, and catalase. When cofactors are firmly bound to the enzyme, or linked covalently to it, they are called prosthetic groups. In many cases the association of cofactor and enzyme is easily reversible. Such cofactors are called coenzymes, and they often serve a large group of enzymes having similar functions. For example, many oxidation-reduction enzymes of the class of dehydrogenases are served by the coenzyme nicotinamide adenine dinucleotide (NAD^+), which acts as an electron acceptor. The complete system, enzyme + coenzyme, is called a holoenzyme; the protein alone is called the apoenzyme. In each case it is the protein that determines the kind of reaction catalyzed and the particular substrate or substrates acted upon. Certain of the digestive enzymes are secreted as proenzymes, which are activated only when they reach their site of action. The active gastric proteinase pepsin, for example, is produced from pepsinogen by the action of HCl in the stomach, and then autocatalytically. The activation involves cleaving a single peptide bond of pepsinogen, releasing a blocking peptide and permitting the residual pepsin to assume a configuration appropriate for its activity.

As catalysts, enzymes affect the rate at which a thermodynamically possible reaction reaches equilibrium without affecting either the equilibrium or the net energy change of the reaction. Like other catalysts, the enzyme is unchanged by the reaction, although it participates intimately in it. In any chemical reaction the net energy change may be large or small, but the reaction proceeds at a rate determined by the rate at which a certain proportion of the population of molecules reaches a higher level of energy known as the transition state. The extra energy required to attain the transition state is the activation energy. Enzymes, like other catalysts, have the effect of lowering the activation energy of the reactions they catalyze, making it possible for many more molecules to reach the transition state per unit of time. Their extraordinary efficiency in doing this may be related to the ability of enzymes to impose a definite spatial orientation upon their substrates. The turnover number—the number of moles of substrate converted per mole of enzyme per minute—is a measure of catalytic efficiency. For β-galactosidase it is 12,500; for carbonic anhydrase (catalyzing the hydration of CO_2 to H_2CO_3) it is 36,000,000, the greatest of any known enzyme.

The rates of enzymatic reactions vary with temperature, pH, enzyme concentration and substrate concentration. As in ordinary chemical reactions, the rate of an enzyme-catalyzed reaction doubles for every 10 C. rise in temperature up to about 45 to 60 C. when the thermal lability of proteins begins to take effect, and the enzyme is rapidly inactivated. In addition to being affected unfavorably by extremes of acid and alkali, enzymes are affected by pH within the physiologic range of hydrogen ion concentrations. In general, the activity of an enzyme is maximal at a given pH, falling fairly symmetrically to low levels on either side of this optimum. In the study of enzymes, or in their determination, the use of buffers to control the pH is essential. In the body the close regulation of the pH of the intracellular and extracellular fluid maintains an appropriate milieu for enzyme action. In the stomach the secretion of HCl secures an optimum pH (around 2) for the proteolytic enzyme pepsin, while the alkaline secretions of the small intestine and pancreas assure a neutral or mildly alkaline medium in which the pancreatic and intestinal enzymes work best.

At a favorable constant temperature and optimum pH the rate of an enzyme-catalyzed reaction is directly proportional to the concentration of enzyme. When, however, one varies the concentration of substrate (enzyme, pH and temperature constant) it is seen that at first the rate increases rapidly in proportion to the substrate concentration, then more slowly and finally not at all: the enzyme appears to be saturated with substrate. Michaelis and Menten interpreted these observations to mean that there was a combination of enzyme and substrate, as follows:

$$E + S \rightleftharpoons ES \rightarrow E + P$$

where E is the free enzyme, S is the substrate, ES an enzyme-substrate complex, and P the product, and from this with certain simple assumptions they were able to derive a kinetic equation that fitted their experimental data relating the observed velocity of the reaction (v) to the substrate concentration [S]:

$$v = \frac{V_{max} [S]}{K_m + [S]}$$

where V_{max} is the maximum velocity and K_m (moles per liter) is a constant derived from three rate constants, for the formation and breakdown of ES from E and S, and its breakdown into E and P. The curve relating v to [S] is a rectangular hyperbola. From the kinetic equation, K_m equals the substrate concentration at which the reaction reaches half its maximal velocity, that is, at which half of the enzyme molecules are occupied by substrate. K_m is a characteristic of the enzyme. The lower the value, the more readily enzyme and substrate interact. Michaelis constants range between 10^{-2} and 10^{-8} moles per liter.

A distinguishing characteristic of enzymes is their specificity. Urease, for example, has absolute specificity for the hydrolysis of urea to ammonia and CO_2. No substituted urea is affected by the enzyme. Many enzymes are specific for only one optical isomer, α-glycosides, for example, as opposed to β-glycosides. There may be specificity for a geometric isomer. Fumarate hydratase converts fumarate to malate but does not react with maleate, the cis-isomer of fumarate. Enzymes are usually specific for the type of reaction catalyzed. Some enzymes have very broad specificity, acting on compounds with a common structural feature. Alkaline phosphatase catalyzes the hydrolysis of a variety of monoesters of phosphoric acid. The rates are different for different substrates, reflecting differences in the accommodation of the substrates at the catalytic center or the active site of the enzyme.

Some compounds resemble natural substrates closely enough to combine with enzymes at the active site, forming an inactive ES-complex. These compounds are competitive inhibitors of the enzyme. They can be displaced from the enzyme by increasing the concentration of substrate. The classic example is the inhibition of succinic dehydrogenase by malonic acid ($HOOC \cdot CH_2 \cdot COOH$), a homologue of succinic acid ($HOOC \cdot CH_2CH_2 \cdot COOH$). The total amount of active enzyme is not reduced by the inhibitor, so V_{max} is unchanged, but a higher concentration of substrate is required to reach half-maximal velocity, that is, K_m is increased. Many drugs may act by competitive inhibition of enzymes. Sulfanilamide (para-aminobenzenesulfonamide) inhibits the utilization of para-aminobenzoic acid by bacteria for the synthesis of folic acid and arrests their growth.

Many enzyme poisons react with functional groups of the protein that are essential for activity. They cannot be displaced by substrate. The inhibition is therefore noncompetitive. K_m is unchanged, but the total amount of active enzyme is reduced, and V_{max} is lowered. When the functional group is altered or destroyed, the inhibition is irreversible. For example, an enzyme requiring free sulfhydryl ($-SH$) for activity is irreversibly inhibited by monoiodoacetic acid (ICH_2COOH), which reacts with ($-SH$) to form the carboxymethyl derivative ($-SCH_2COOH$). The nerve poison, diisopropylphosphofluoridate, alkylates the serine hydroxyl at the active site of many esterases, including acetylcholinesterase, which is essential for the orderly transmission of nerve impulses.

Enzymes catalyzing the same reaction in different cells, or in different parts of the same cell, i.e., mitochondria and cytosol, often occur in multiple forms, called isoenzymes or isozymes. Lactic dehydrogenase occurs in five electrophoretically distinguishable forms. The enzyme is made up of four subunits of two types, H (for heart) and M (for muscle), and may occur as H_4, H_3M, H_2M_2, HM_3 or M_4. The heart enzyme (H_4) is found in tissues that are capable of sustained aerobic activity; the muscle enzyme (M_4) occurs where there is intense intermittent activity. The heart enzyme is inhibited by low concentrations of pyruvate ($K_m = 8.9 \times 10^{-5}$), while the muscle enzyme is much less sensitive ($K_m = 3.2 \times 10^{-3}$). The identification of a particular isozyme in the plasma of a patient can help to establish the locus of damaged tissue and, from the quantity of isozyme present, the severity of the injury.

Intracellular enzymes seldom act alone but are components of multienzyme systems involved in the orderly breakdown or biosynthesis of metabolites. The sequence of reactions is controlled at certain points by enzymes that are subject to regulation either by the product of the sequence of reactions or by changes in the concentration of substances such as ATP, ADP or inorganic phosphate that reflect changing requirements for energy in the cell. Regulatory or *allosteric* enzymes are usually large molecules containing several subunits. In addition to the substrate-binding site they contain specific binding sites, the allosteric (other) space or site, for one or more modulators or effectors. An effector may be positive, increasing activity by increasing V_{max} or decreasing K_m, or negative, acting by decreasing V_{max} or increasing K_m. In some regulatory enzymes the substrate itself acts as an allosteric effector. In such enzymes the relation between velocity of reaction and substrate concentration is not hyperbolic but sigmoid. At low substrate concentration the reaction rate is initially low, but as substrate binds to the allosteric site, the conformation of the enzyme changes, and a rapid increase in rate occurs with a small additional increment in substrate concentration (Fig. 4-2). such a cooperative effect is also seen in hemoglobin: the addition of the first oxygen molecule causes an intramolecular change such that rapid addition of more oxygen takes place during a relatively small increase in Po_2 (Fig. 4-9).

The numerous chemical reactions and the great variety of substrates involved in living systems have made the naming and classification of enzymes a difficult and still unfinished task. Some enzymes are still known by the trivial names given to them by their discoverers: pepsin and trypsin, the gastric and pancreatic proteinases. Some are named after the substrate upon which they act: urease; lipase. These names give no clue to the nature of the reaction catalyzed. More recently, enzymes have been named by the class of reaction catalyzed: esterase; dehydrogenase. The name is made more complete by adding the name of the substrate or class of substrate: cholinesterase; phosphomonoesterase; alcohol dehydrogenase. The International Enzyme Commission in 1964 proposed a new classification of enzymes in six major categories, each with many subgroups: (1) *oxidoreductases;* (2) *transferases;* (3) *hydrolases;* (4) *lyases;* (5) *isomerases;* (6) *ligases.*

The *oxidoreductases* include all the enzymes involved in hydrogen and electron transfer. Among these are the dehydrogenases using NAD^+ or $NADP^+$ as coenzymes (lactic or malic dehydrogenase); oxidases in which oxygen is the acceptor, forming hydrogen peroxide (xanthine oxidase; D-amino acid oxidase); oxygenases, catalyzing reactions in which oxygen is partly

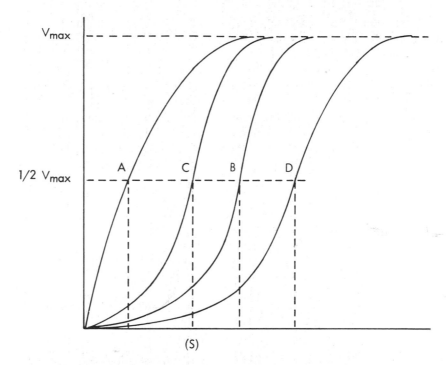

Fig. 4-2. Relation between velocity of reaction and substrate concentration in some regulatory enzymes. A = hyperbolic (Michaelis–Menten) kinetics; B = allosteric kinetics; C = action of positive effector; D = action of negative effector.

incorporated into the substrate (phenylalanine hydroxylase); peroxidases and catalases, which catalyze the decomposition of hydrogen peroxide.

Transferases catalyze transfer of groups such as one-carbon groups (methyl-, hydroxymethyl-, formyl-transferases, usually involving tetrahydrofolic acid as carrier coenzyme). This group includes enzymes catalyzing phosphate transfer (ATP: creatine phosphotransferase; creatine kinase; creatine phosphokinase) (CPK). The amino-transferases (transaminases) also fall into this category.

The *hydrolases* act by introducing the elements of water at a specific bond of the substrate. This division includes the carbohydrases, the proteases, the nucleases, the amidases and amidinases, the purine deaminases and the esterases. The important carbohydrases are the polysaccharidases (α- and β-amylases, hyaluronidases, sulfomucases), the α-glucosidases (maltase), the β-glucosidases (emulsin) and sucrases (invertase). Peptide linkages are hydrolyzed by the proteases, which are divided into two groups: (1) the endopeptidases (pepsin, trypsin, chymotrypsin, rennin and cathepsins) that act on peptide linkages in the interior of a peptide chain; and (2) exopeptidases (carboxypeptidases, aminopolypeptidases, prolinases, dipeptidases) that act on a terminal peptide linkage. Carboxypeptidase requires a free carboxyl group to remove the carboxyl-terminal amino acid; aminopeptidases split the peptide bond involving the NH_2-terminal residue. Dipeptidases hydrolyze only dipeptides. The amidases include urease, asparaginase, glutaminase (arginase is an amidinase). Histidase and urocanase are imidazolases that occur in the liver. Adenase and guanase are the important purine deaminases. The nucleases include polynucleotidases, nucleotidases and nucleosidases. The esterases include the carboxylesterases (simple esterases and specific esterases such as acetylcholinesterase, cholesterolesterase, cholinesterase) sulfatases and phosphatases.

Lyases catalyze reactions involving the addition of groups to substances containing double bonds, or the nonhydrolytic removal of groups from substrates to yield products with double bonds. Examples are: aldolase: 3-phosphoglyceraldehyde + dihydroxyacetone phosphate $\rightleftarrows$ fructose-1, 6, diphosphate (formation and cleavage of a C-C bond); fumarate hydratase: fumaric acid + H_2O $\rightleftarrows$ malic acid (formation and cleavage of a C-O bond); histidine decarboxylase: histidine $\rightleftarrows$ histamine + CO_2 (cleavage of a C-C bond).

Isomerases catalyze the conversion of a compound to its isomer. An example is phosphohexose isomerase: glucose-6-phosphate $\rightleftarrows$ fructose-6-phosphate. This category also includes the epimerases, converting compounds to an isomer with altered configuration around one carbon atom. Example: uridinediphosphoglucose 4-epimerase, which catalyzes the important reaction UDP-glucose $\rightleftharpoons$ UDP-galactose.

Ligases catalyze the joining of two molecules coupled with the breaking of a pyrophosphate bond. ATP or a comparable nucleoside triphosphate is involved in the reaction. Examples: formation of aminoacyl-transfer RNA in protein synthesis: L-amino acid + tRNA + ATP $\rightleftharpoons$ L-aminoacyl-tRNA + AMP + PP_i (L-amino acid: tRNA ligase (AMP), or aminoacyl-tRNA synthase); formation of acetyl CoA: acetic acid + HS-CoA + ATP $\rightleftharpoons$ acetyl-CoA + AMP + PP_i (acetate: CoA-SH ligase (AMP), familiar name, acetic thiokinase). Reactions of this class are made essentially irreversible by hydrolysis of the inorganic pyrophosphate by a pyrophosphatase.

An increase in the amount of some intracellular enzymes in the plasma is a sign of disease or damage to an organ. For many years it has been known that an increase in acid phosphatase in the blood is seen in carcinoma of the prostate, an increase in alkaline phosphatase is observed in bone or liver disease, and an increase in amylase is found in pancreatic disease. More recently it has been found that increases in glutamic-oxaloacetic transaminase, in glutamic-pyruvic transaminase and in lactic dehydrogenase all occur in liver and heart disease. Damage to voluntary muscle or to the heart muscle, or to brain, is accompanied by an increase in creatine phosphokinase. The assay of these enzymes in blood is an aid to diagnosis, and in some instances, as has been noted above, the determination of characteristic isozymes may be an aid to differential diagnosis. Many genetic disorders are characterized by absence or deficiency of specific enzymes, for example, glucose 6-phosphate dehydrogenase or glutathione reductase in red cells, attending primaquine sensitivity in certain individuals.

A number of important coenzymes are derivatives of the water-soluble vitamins. Niacin is a constituent of nicotinamide-adenine dinucleotide (NAD^+), which acts as an electron and hydrogen acceptor for a large group of dehydrogenases. The related coenzyme of another group of dehydrogenases, nicotinamide adenine dinucleotide phosphate ($NADP^+$) has an additional molecule of phosphoric acid esterified to the 2′ position of the ribose of the adenylic acid moiety of the dinucleotide. Riboflavin appears both as the ribitol 5′-phosphate ester, flavin mononucleotide (FMN), and in pyrophosphate linkage with adenylic acid as flavin adenine dinucleotide (FAD). Both forms of the coenzyme act as hydrogen acceptors, serving different sets of dehydrogenases or acting as essential intermediates in a respiratory chain.

The coenzyme functions of thiamine, biotin, pyri-

doxine, folic acid and vitamin B_{12} are noted in the section on vitamins.

ENERGY EXCHANGE AND PRODUCTION

Living organisms are enclaves of order open to an environment continually tending to disorder. Organisms are maintained by constant expenditure of energy derived from the foodstuffs by processes that are, in the long run, oxidative. All of the life processes of growth, reproduction, repair, maintenance and chemical, electrical and mechanical work are supported by chemical reactions that, taking the entire system, animal + input + output, proceed with a net loss of free energy, that is, of the component of the total energy that is available for useful work. Thus, although an organism may maintain constancy of composition, internal order and total internal energy for a large part of a lifetime, it does so at the continuous expense of its environment.

The quantitative aspects of the energy exchanges of the whole organism and of the energy of individual chemical reactions are important to an understanding of bioenergetics in man. The former involves appreciation of the total energy cost of operations; the latter involves appreciation of the free energy of chemical reactions, the fraction of the total energy available for work.

Overall Energy Exchange. In adult individuals in a steady state of body composition the sum of all the processes of energy production and utilization appears as heat. This is produced at the expense of the foodstuffs. It has been demonstrated that the oxidation of carbohydrate and lipid in the body yields the same amount of heat as their oxidation in a bomb calorimeter. For proteins, the values do not agree, because oxidation of the nitrogen in the body is not complete; it appears mainly as urea, which still has a considerable energy content. In studies of energy metabolism in man, the unit of energy is the *kilocalorie* (kcal.): the amount of heat required to raise the temperature of 1,000 g. of water from 15 to 16 C. The caloric value of the foodstuffs varies somewhat with each individual constituent. Average values are, for carbohydrate, lipid, and protein, respectively, 4.1, 9.3, and 4.1 kcal. per g. These are often conveniently rounded off to 4, 9, and 4 (Table 4-3).

The ratio of carbon dioxide produced to oxygen consumed in the utilization of each individual foodstuff is the *respiratory quotient* (RQ). For carbohydrates the RQ is 1.0, for example:

$$C_6H_{12}O_6(\text{glucose}) + 6O_2 \rightarrow 6CO_2 + 6H_2O$$
$$6CO_2/6O_2 = 1.0$$

TABLE 4-3. Caloric, O_2, and CO_2 Equivalents of Carbohydrate, Fat and Protein

	Carbohydrate	Fat	Protein
Kilocalories per gram	3.7–4.3	9.5	4.3
Liter CO_2 per gram	0.75–0.83	1.43	0.78
Liters O_2 per gram	0.75–0.83	2.03	0.97
Respiratory quotient	1.0	0.707	0.801
Kilocalories per liter O_2	5.0	4.7	4.5

For lipid, the average RQ is 0.7; the generally saturated hydrocarbon chains of the lipids require more oxygen per mole of CO_2 produced than do the oxygen-rich carbohydrates. The average RQ for protein is 0.8. Over any period, the RQ is the resultant of many processes involving all the foodstuffs. It is sometimes useful to calculate the nonprotein RQ. This is done by measuring the nitrogen excretion over a time in which O_2 consumption and CO_2 production are being measured. The protein consumed during the interval is estimated by multiplying grams of N excreted by 6.25 (based on an average protein N content of 16 per cent). The amounts of O_2 used and CO_2 produced in consuming the estimated amount of protein utilized are computed and subtracted from the total O_2 used and CO_2 produced. The remainders represent the contributions from carbohydrate and lipid, and the ratio, CO_2/O_2, reflects the proportions of the two foodstuffs in the metabolic mixture being oxidized. At a nonprotein RQ of 1.0, only carbohydrate is being oxidized; at RQ 0.7, only lipid. Midway between, at RQ 0.85, one half of the oxygen is being consumed in burning fat. For each value of the nonprotein RQ, the calories produced per liter of oxygen consumed can be computed from the relative contributions of the two substrates. In the estimation of basal metabolic rates by the measurement of oxygen consumption for short intervals, it is assumed that the nonprotein RQ is 0.82. The corresponding caloric equivalent of the oxygen consumed (60 per cent by fat, 40 per cent by carbohydrate) is 4.825 kcal. per liter.

The energy required and produced by an individual may be divided into two components, a variable one related to physical activity and work and a more constant component related to the resting needs of the body: the *basal metabolic rate (BMR)*. This is measured in the waking but resting and relaxed state, in a quiet room, some hours after the last meal (in the postabsorptive period) and at a comfortable room temperature, to avoid any extra metabolic work required for cooling and heating. Oxygen consumption is measured with a respirometer, usually for several 10-minute intervals. From this an estimate of BMR is obtained in kcal. per hour. From the height and weight of the

subject an estimate of the body surface area, in square meters, is computed, and the results are expressed in terms of kcal. per square meter per hour. For a single species in a fairly narrow range of sizes of subjects, the metabolic rate correlates well with the body surface area. When a great range of animals, from shrew to elephant, is studied it is found that the metabolic rate is more exactly a function of the three-quarters power of the body weight. The metabolic rate varies with age and sex. It is higher in children (at 6 years, 50 to 53 kcal. per sq. m. per hr.), falls to a plateau (42 to 37 kcal. per sq. m. per hr.) between the ages of 20 and 50 and declines slowly thereafter. The rate in males at any age is higher by 3 to 5 kcal. per sq. m. per hr. The BMR is low at birth and accelerates during the first 1½ years. Variations from the normal BMR may occur in a number of pathologic conditions, for example, in hyperthyroidism, when it may be much increased, or hypothyroidism, when it is severely depressed. Measurement of BMR may still be a useful diagnostic procedure, although in many instances, for example, in thyroid disease, it has been supplanted by other more precise and convenient methods of evaluating thyroid status. The concept is important for the insight it yields into the magnitude of the energy exchange required to support the bodily processes at rest.

The total metabolism of an individual varies with occupation and other pursuits. For sedentary workers, the additional energy required may be no more than one-half the basal requirement; a steelworker or a lumberjack may require 6,000 to 8,000 kcal. per day, three to four times the basal requirement.

The rate of heat production of an individual is not primarily regulated by the rate of heat loss, although the BMR may be increased in consequence of increased activity during continued exposure to cold. The rate of heat production is most strictly governed by the rate of energy utilization. Any acceleration of an energy-using process, such as muscular activity, is attended by an increase in the rate of the processes of utilization of substrate to furnish the energy for the increased activity. The ingestion and assimilation of food are themselves attended by an increase in oxygen consumption and heat production. This so-called *specific dynamic effect of foodstuffs* is related to the costs of handling: digestion, transport, storage, transformation, catabolism. It is largest when the individual foodstuffs are fed singly: 5 per cent for carbohydrate; 13 per cent for fat; as much as 30 per cent for protein or even individual amino acids, but it is not additive: the extra heat production induced by an average balanced meal is only about 10 per cent. The large specific dynamic effect of protein when it is fed by itself may be attributed to two factors: the energy cost of urea synthesis and excretion and the extra oxygen consumed in converting the α-keto acids to a useful form. For example, only three carbon atoms of arginine, proline, ornithine, glutamine and glutamic acid are available for gluconeogenesis; the remainder is oxidized away and the energy is lost as heat.

Free Energy. At the level of individual chemical reactions in the body, events take place at nearly constant pressure, volume and temperature. The system cannot act as a heat engine, and biologically useful work is not accomplished by changes in volume or pressure. Although living organisms are open systems, it is useful to an understanding of the energetics of biochemical processes to look upon them as if they were taking place in the ideal, isolated, closed, reversible system of thermodynamics. In a system of this kind, the addition of a certain amount of heat (energy) results either in work being done or in an increase in the heat content, the *enthalpy* (H) of the system. The amount of useful work that can be done is, however, limited by the tendency of all systems to come to equilibrium or to arrive, by whatever pathway, at a less ordered state. The *entropy* (S) of the system tends to increase, and a measure of this increase in disorder or randomness is given by the term $T\Delta S$, where T is the absolute temperature. The amount of the total change in energy of a chemical reaction that is available for doing useful work, the free energy (ΔG), is given by the expression:

$$\Delta G = \Delta H - T\Delta S$$

Consider a chemical reaction under way toward equilibrium:

$$A \rightleftharpoons B$$

If ΔG is negative the reaction is exergonic and will proceed spontaneously to the right. If ΔG is positive, the reaction is endergonic and will proceed spontaneously to the left. At equilibrium, no work can be done; ΔG is zero. Similarly, the reaction is exothermic if ΔH is negative: it will give off heat; and it is endothermic if ΔH is positive: it will take up heat. The

reaction is isothermic if ΔH is zero. In a series of reactions proceeding in steps:

$$\begin{matrix} (1) & (2) & (3) \\ W \rightleftharpoons X \rightleftharpoons Y \rightleftharpoons Z \end{matrix}$$

the overall reaction, $W \rightleftharpoons Z$, will go forward if the *net* change in free energy ($\Delta G_1 + \Delta G_2 + \Delta G_3$) is negative, even if ΔG_2, for example, were zero or positive. This principle is seen to operate in the many steps of a number of metabolic processes. A common intermediate is shared at each step, and endergonic steps may be made to go forward if they are suitably coupled to one or more exergonic reactions.

The reference value for computing changes in free energy is the standard free energy, $\Delta G°$, usually calculated at 25 C. and 1 atm. For solutions, the standard state is defined as a concentration of 1 mole per liter. For water, the standard state is the pure liquid; it may be taken to apply also to the dilute solutions encountered in physiologic systems. Changes in free energy are expressed as calories per mole.

For reactions such as:

$$aA + bB \rightleftharpoons cC + dD$$

it can be shown that

$$\Delta G = \Delta G° + RT \ln \frac{[C]^c[D]^d}{[A]^a[B]^b}$$

where R is the gas constant (1.987 calories per mole · degree), T is the absolute temperature, and ln signifies the natural logarithm. Since at equilibrium $\Delta G = 0$, then

$$\Delta G° = -RT \ln \frac{[C_{eq}]^c[D_{eq}]^d}{[A_{eq}]^a[B_{eq}]^b} = -RT \ln K_{eq}$$

The standard free energy of a reaction may thus be determined from the equilibrium constant (Table 4-4). Once this has been done, it is possible to compute the free energy change ΔG, for a reaction under any conditions of temperature and concentration of the reactants. Very often ΔG, computed for physiologic concentrations of the reactants, is larger than $\Delta G°$.

TABLE 4-4. Relationship Between the Equilibrium Constant and the Standard Free Energy at 25C

K_{eq}	G°,cal.
1,000.0	−4089
100.0	−2726
10.0	−1363
1.0	0
0.1	+1363

The change in free energy involved in effecting changes in the concentration of a molecule or ion may be determined from the equation:

$$\Delta G = RT \ln C_2/C_1$$

where C_1 is the initial and C_2 is the final concentration. For values of the ratio greater than 1, concentration is taking place, ΔG is positive, and work must be done. The system must be coupled to a reaction expending free energy; for example, the hydrolysis of ATP is coupled to the removal of Na^+ from the intracellular to the extracellular fluid.

In oxygen-dependent organisms such as man, the oxidation of substrates is essential for the liberation of energy for doing work. The most common type of oxidative reaction is catalyzed by the dehydrogenase enzymes and is represented by

$$SH_2 \rightleftarrows S + 2H^+ + 2e$$

where S is any substrate molecule. The reaction is completed by the reduction of a specialized acceptor, a coenzyme:

$$Co + 2H^+ + 2e \rightleftarrows CoH_2$$

and the entire oxidation-reduction reaction is represented by

$$SH_2 + Co \rightleftarrows S + CoH_2$$

Oxidation (loss of electrons) of one component of the system must always be coupled to reduction (gain of electrons) of another component. The flow of electrons from S to Co can be thought of as generating a voltage, a potential difference proportional to the energy driving the reaction. For the systematic study of oxidation-reduction reactions, a reference half-reaction is required. This is provided by the hydrogen electrode, obtained by bubbling hydrogen gas at 25 C. and 1 atm. through a solution containing H^+ ions at 1 M concentration. Its potential is arbitrarily defined as zero volts. The reaction is:

$$2H^+ + 2e \rightleftarrows H_2(gas). \quad E_0 = 0.0 \text{ volts}$$

For convenience in dealing with biologic oxidations a secondary standard has been defined by bubbling hydrogen gas at 30 C. and 1 atm. through a solution of H^+ ions at a pH of 7 (10^{-7} M). The potential of this half cell is, with reference to the primary hydrogen electrode, $E'_0 = -0.42$ volts. The reaction is

$$2H^+ + 2e \rightleftarrows H_2(gas) \text{ (pH = 7.0) (30 C.)}$$

For comparison, the reduction of oxygen to water:

$$1/2 \; O_2 + 2H^+ + 2e \rightarrow H_2O \text{ (pH 7.0; 30 C.)}$$

has $E'_0 = 0.815$ volts. When two half reactions are combined, the half reaction with the more positive potential is the oxidizing agent. For example, if the oxygen and hydrogen half reactions are coupled, the values for E'_0 predict that oxygen will be reduced and hydrogen oxidized. The free energy change for such a reaction is given by the equation

$$\Delta G° = -nF(E'_0) + \frac{RT}{nF} \ln \frac{[\text{oxidant}]}{[\text{reductant}]}$$

or, when the ratio of concentration of oxidant to reductant is 1,

$$\Delta G° = -nF(E'_0)$$

where n is the number of electrons transferred, F is the caloric equivalent of the Faraday, 23,058 calories per volt, and E'_0 is the potential difference between the two half reactions (that is, for this example, the *span* between -0.42 volts and 0.815 volts, or 1.235 volts). For the oxidation of hydrogen to water, then,

$$\Delta G° = -2 \times 23,058 \times 1.235$$
$$= -56,953 \text{ calories}$$

Biological Oxidation and Energy Production. Many of the steps of oxidation of substrates in the cell are catalyzed by dehydrogenases assisted by the coenzyme nicotinamide adenine dinucleotide (NAD^+). The reduction potential of the half-reaction

$$NAD^+ + 2H^+ + 2e \rightleftarrows NADH + H^+$$

is -0.32 volts. The free energy of the reaction

$$NADH + H^+ + 1/2 \; O_2 \rightleftarrows NAD^+ + H_2O$$

which has a span of 1.14 volts, is 52,572 calories. Such a large release of free energy does not take place all at once. There is instead a coupled series of oxidation-reduction reactions, at some points of which the fall in potential, while still small, is large enough to allow for the synthesis of a compound, ATP, that provides, in a generalized and useful form, energy for a very large part of all the energy-requiring processes of the cell.

The coenzymes serving the dehydrogenases of the cell are devices for converging the output of large numbers of individual oxidative steps upon a few mediators, NAD^+, $NADP^+$, flavin mononucleotide (FMN) and flavin-adenine dinucleotide (FAD). In many cases, reduced $NADP^+$ mainly serves the reductive steps of many biosynthetic reactions (fatty acid synthesis, for example) in which the potential energy of a hydrogen pair of the precursor is invested in the product. NAD^+ and the flavoproteins are directed toward a final common pathway, the respiratory chain, that provides for their rapid and efficient reoxidation, and that also is closely coupled to the process by which ATP is formed from ADP and P_i The locus of the respiratory chain is the inner membrane of the mitochondria. The input to the chain is provided entirely by reduced NAD^+ and reduced flavoproteins.

Reduced NAD^+ is linked to the respiratory chain by a flavoprotein, the NADH-cytochrome b reductase, that acts as a specific reoxidizing agent for the NAD^+-linked dehydrogenases. A second point of entry into the respiratory chain is provided by succinate dehydrogenase, a flavoprotein that can also act as a cytochrome b reductase. The hydrogen of these two reduced flavoproteins is passed to coenzyme Q (ubiquinone):

$$H_3C \overset{O}{\underset{O}{\bigcirc}} CH_3 (R) \quad \overset{2H}{\rightleftharpoons} \quad H_3C \overset{OH}{\underset{OH}{\bigcirc}} CH_3 (R)$$

where (R) is an isoprenoid side chain of $n = 10$ units ($-CH_2-CH=C(CH_3)-CH_2-)_n$ in mammalian cells. In the reoxidation of ubiquinone electrons are transferred to cytochrome b and hydrogen ions are liberated:

$$2CytbFe^{3+} + CoQH_2 \rightleftharpoons 2CytbFe^{2+} + CoQ + 2H^+$$

This can be done in steps, through the semiquinone, to accommodate the 1-electron requirement of the cytochromes, which operate by the alternate reduction and oxidation of iron. The hydrogen ions set free in the reoxidation of coenzyme Q combine later with oxygen activated by cytochrome oxidase to complete the oxidation of substrate hydrogen to water.

The four main cytochromes, in the order of their increasing reduction potential, b, c, a, and a_3 (cytochrome oxidase) form the electron-transporting components of the respiratory chain. They are iron porphyrin proteins in which the porphyrin is covalently bound to the protein. Cytochrome c is the best known of these compounds, because it is readily extractable from mitochondria. The others are firmly bound to the lipid matrix. Cytochrome a_3 is the only one capable of reacting with molecular oxygen.

Each of the steps of the respiratory chain, from substrate to oxygen, takes place with a fall in reduction potential, that is, in free energy. In the pathway, substrate $\rightarrow NAD^+ \rightarrow FAD \rightarrow CoQ \rightarrow Cyt\ b \rightarrow Cyt\ C \rightarrow Cyt\ a \rightarrow Cyt\ a_3 \rightarrow 1/2\ O_2$, there are three sites at which the fall in potential is large enough to allow for the capture of the energy: between NAD^+ and FAD, between cytochromes b and c and between cytochromes a and a_3. The conservation of energy at these sites involves the synthesis of ATP from ADP and P_i, an endergonic reaction: $\Delta G° = + 7,300$ calories. For each pair of hydrogen atoms entering the pathway

from NADH 3 moles of ATP are synthesized and an atom of oxygen is consumed; the P/O ratio is 3. A total of $3 \times 7,300$ calories or 21,900 calories is conserved from the available free energy of 52,572 calories for an efficiency of 42 per cent.

The synthesis of ATP is intimately connected with the passage of electrons; the processes of oxidation and phosphorylation are closely coupled. This can be understood by considering events in a fresh preparation of mitochondria. Oxygen is plentiful, but the rate of O_2 consumption is low. If substrate is added, O_2 consumption hardly changes. If ADP is added, O_2 consumption increases smartly until all the ADP is converted to ATP. Addition of more ADP increases the O_2 consumption until the concentration of substrate becomes limiting. If ADP and substrate are then added in excess, the O_2 consumption increases until all the oxygen is used. The concentrations of substrate and of oxygen are clearly important, but the critical regulator of the system is ADP. As the ratio ATP/ADP increases, the rate of respiration slows. Oxygen consumption is coupled to need, since the acceleration of processes utilizing ATP automatically increases the concentration of ADP and the rate of respiration. The ratio ATP/ADP also plays a part in regulating the flow of substrate, so this need is met at the same time.

The respiratory pathway can be inhibited at several sites. Amytal and other barbiturates act on transfers from FAD to CoQ. Antimycin A inhibits electron transfer from cytochrome b to cytochrome c. Cytochrome a_3 is inhibited by cyanide and carbon monoxide. The quantity of a_3 in the body is extremely small, and its affinity for cyanide is high, which explains why cyanide is so deadly a poison. Some inhibitors, including certain antibiotics such as aureomycin, valinomycin and oligomycin, act at all three sites by inhibiting phosphorylation.

The tight couple between oxidation and phosphorylation is loosened or destroyed by a number of natural or synthetic agents, the bile pigment bilirubin, free fatty acids, thyroxine, all in fairly high concentrations, 2,4-dinitrophenol and dicumarol. They are all lipid soluble, and they are thought to act by altering the permeability of the inner mitochondrial membrane. The effect of an uncoupling agent is to allow oxidation to proceed unrestrained, with no or reduced yield of ATP.

Mechanism of Oxidative Phosphorylation: The Chemiosmotic Hypothesis. Respiration in mitochondria does not appear to be coupled to the generation of a phosphorylated compound comparable to 3-phosphoglyceryl-1-phosphate, formed in glycolysis, which can transfer a phosphoryl group to ADP, making ATP. No firm evidence for such a process in mitochondria has been obtained. Recently it has been proposed that the elements of the respiratory chain may be oriented in the inner mitochondrial membrane in such a way that the passage of electrons is coupled to the secretion of protons (H^+) into the space between the inner and outer mitochondrial membranes. Since the inner membrane is impermeable to protons, this creates both a pH gradient and an electrochemical gradient between the mitochondrial matrix and the inter-membranous space. The projections on the cristae of the inner membrane, facing the matrix, are comprised of a group of proteins that a) together form a reversible Ca^{2+}, Mg^{2+}-dependent ATPase, and b) make a channel through the inner membrane. The return of protons through the channel, down the potential gradient, furnishes the driving force for the synthesis of ATP from ADP and P_i. The protons may arise from two sources: 1) the reduction of Coenzyme Q, as noted above, and 2) changes in the dissociation of ionizable groups in proteins of the electron transport chain as they are alternately reduced and reoxidized, rather like the Bohr effect in hemoglobin. It is not certain whether two or four protons are secreted per electron pair at each energy realizing step. Newly formed ATP is not released from the enzyme unless ADP is also present; the flow of protons and electrons is thus controlled by the supply of ADP. Uncoupling agents are lipid soluble, and destroy the membrane barrier to protons, discharging the potential difference. Oxidation thus continues without phosphorylation. The chemiosmotic hypothesis, very simply described here, is not yet fully worked out, but it embraces the widest range of phenomena associated with energy production in mitochondria.

ATP and Other "High-Energy" Compounds. Ninety per cent or more of the oxygen utilization of most cells takes place in the mitochondria. A significant fraction of the potential energy of the controlled, stepwise oxidation is realized as ATP. The pyrophosphate bonds of the nucleoside triphosphate are relatively stable at physiologic pH and temperature, but the reactions

$$ATP + H_2O \rightarrow ADP + P_i, \text{ and}$$
$$ADP + H_2O \rightarrow AMP + P_i$$

are exergonic: $\Delta G°$ for both is -7.3 kcal. It is customary to describe ATP and ADP as containing "high-energy" phosphate bonds. Thus, when ATP is coupled to an endergonic reaction such as the synthesis of glucose-6-phosphate, the energy is thought of as being provided by the conversion of the high-energy phosphate bond of ATP to the lower energy phosphate ester bond. Another way of looking at ATP, derived

from the work of Daniel Atkinson, may yield greater insight into its function and significance:

For a $\Delta G°$ of -7.3 kcal./mole, the ratio (ATP)/(ADP)(P_i) at equilibrium is about $4 \times 10^{-6} M^{-1}$. If the concentration of inorganic phosphate in the cell is $10^{-2} M$, the ratio (ATP)/(ADP) is about 10^{-8}. In an actively respiring cell the ratio (ATP)/(ADP)(P_i) is actually about 500. It differs from the equilibrium ratio by about 10^8. This means that for any reaction coupled to ATP the equilibrium concentration ratio will be about 10^8 times as large as it would be when the uncoupled reaction is at equilibrium. For example, if the K_{eq} for the reaction $A \rightarrow C$ is 10^{-4}, and the concentration of A is $10^{-5} M$, the conversion could occur, uncoupled, only at concentrations of C less than $10^{-9} M$. If the reaction is coupled ($A + ATP \rightarrow C + ADP + P_i$) it can take place at any concentration of C up to 0.1M.

From this point of view, the objective of mitochondrial respiration is to maintain the ratio (ATP)/(ADP) at about 10^8 times the equilibrium ratio. This provides the driving force for nearly all biochemical processes, since any useful reaction may be made thermodynamically favorable by coupling it to the utilization of a suitable number of ATP equivalents.

These considerations apply to all the nucleoside and deoxynucleoside di- and triphosphates, and to a select group of compounds that may also be maintained at concentrations far from their equilibrium values: 1) acid anhydrides such as acetyl phosphate or phosphoglycerylphosphate; 2) enol-phosphates such as phosphoenolpyruvate; guanidinium phosphates such as phosphocreatine; acylthioesters such as acetyl CoA. The free energy of hydrolysis of these compounds lies in the range 9 to 15 kcal. Their utilization is coupled to the synthesis of ATP and to other biosynthetic reactions, as will be seen below.

Other Oxidative Reactions in the Cell. A limited group of aerobic dehydrogenases, many of them flavoproteins, react directly with molecular oxygen, producing hydrogen peroxide:

$$SH_2 + FP \rightarrow S + FPH_2 + O_2 \rightarrow H_2O_2 + FP$$

The peroxide is usually promptly decomposed by the widely distributed heme protein, catalase:

$$2 H_2O_2 \rightarrow 2 H_2O + O_2$$

Catalase may also act as a peroxidase:

$$SH_2 + H_2O_2 \rightarrow 2 H_2O + S$$

Catalase is found, along with numerous aerobic dehydrogenases, in small particles called peroxisomes, in liver and other tissues.

Oxygenases catalyze the incorporation of oxygen into a substrate molecule. Dioxygenases (example tryptophan pyrrolase) catalyze the incorporation of both atoms of oxygen. Monooxygenases catalyze the incorporation of only one atom of oxygen into their substrates. The other atom is reduced to water. A source of reducing equivalents is required. Some steroid hydroxylations are carried out in this way:

$$St\text{-}H + O_2 + NADPH + H^+ \rightarrow$$
$$St\text{-}OH + H_2O + NADP^+$$

Other steroid hydroxylations, and the hydroxylation of many drugs in liver, are carried out by a mixed function oxygenase involving Cytochrome P450, so called because the absorption spectrum is the presence of carbon monoxide exhibits an unusual band at 450 nm. Reducing equivalents are provided by NADH or NADPH. Electron transport is mediated by a flavoprotein, cytochrome P450 reductase, sometimes assisted by a small iron-sulfur-containing protein (in the adrenal cortex, called adrenodoxin). The action may be summarized as follows (AH is a drug or steroid substrate):

$$P450Fe^{3+} + AH \rightarrow P450Fe^{3+}AH + e^- \rightarrow$$
$$P450Fe^{2+}AH + O_2 \rightarrow P450Fe^{2+}AHO_2 + e^- \rightarrow$$
$$\rightarrow P450Fe^{2+}AHO_2^- \rightarrow P450Fe^{2+}O^- + AOH \rightarrow$$
$$P450Fe^{3+} + O^{2-} + 2H^+ \rightarrow H_2O$$

The hydroxylated substrate dissociates readily from the complex, oxygen is further reduced, and water is formed with the protons arising from the reoxidation of the flavoprotein. There are numerous cytochromes P450. Those in liver are inducible, increasing manyfold in response to the administration of some drugs, such as phenobarbital.

Oxidases catalyze the removal of hydrogen from their substrates, but use only oxygen as their hydrogen acceptor. In some instances the product is water, but monoamine oxidase, for example, yields hydrogen peroxide. All enzymes of this class contain copper.

Reactions involving oxygen directly are important, but play no part in energy production. They account for only a few percent of the oxygen utilization of an organism. The numerous reactions of this kind, however, are thought to lead frequently to the formation of the superoxide radical:

$$EnzH_2 + O_2 \rightarrow EnzH + H^+ + O_2^-$$

Superoxide is a vigorous oxidizing agent. Its persistence could be damaging, and it is thought to be responsible for the toxicity of oxygen. A widely distributed enzyme, superoxide dismutase, holds superoxide in check by converting it to oxygen and hydrogen peroxide:

$$O_2^- + O_2^- \rightarrow H_2O_2 + O_2$$

The dismutase of mitochondria requires Mn^{2+}, like that in bacteria, but the cytosolic enzyme requires Cu^{2+} and Zn^{2+} in one of each of its two subunits.

The reader will note the frequent occurrence of metals—Fe, Cu, Mn, Mg—in reactions of oxidation, reduction, and group transfer. This underlines the importance of mineral constituents in the diet.

CHEMISTRY AND METABOLISM OF CARBOHYDRATES

Chemistry

The carbohydrates are a numerous and heterogeneous group of compounds that may be defined as polyhydroxy aldehydes and ketones and their derivatives. They are classified as monosaccharides, oligosaccharides (2 to 10 monosaccharide units) and polysaccharides, macromolecules, sometimes of indefinite sizes (polydisperse), with masses of thousands to millions of daltons. The primary product of photosynthesis is carbohydrate; it is the first representative of the captive energy of sunlight upon which the entire biosphere depends. In the human diet it is a major source of energy, and it is strictly required for certain critical life processes in the central nervous system, voluntary muscles, the red cell and the retina.

Monosaccharides. The simplest carbohydrates are the three-carbon compounds (trioses) glyceraldehyde and dihydroxyacetone:

L-glyceraldehyde   D-glyceraldehyde

dihydroxyacetone

The aldotriose has an asymmetric carbon atom. A D- and an L- series of higher homologues is generated by the successive addition of HCOH groups. At each step a new asymmetric center is added. A comparable series begins with the ketotetrose. For both aldosugars and ketosugars the D series is defined by convention as having the configuration around the carbon atom adjacent to the primary alcohol identical to that of D-glyceraldehyde. Monosaccharides occurring in na-

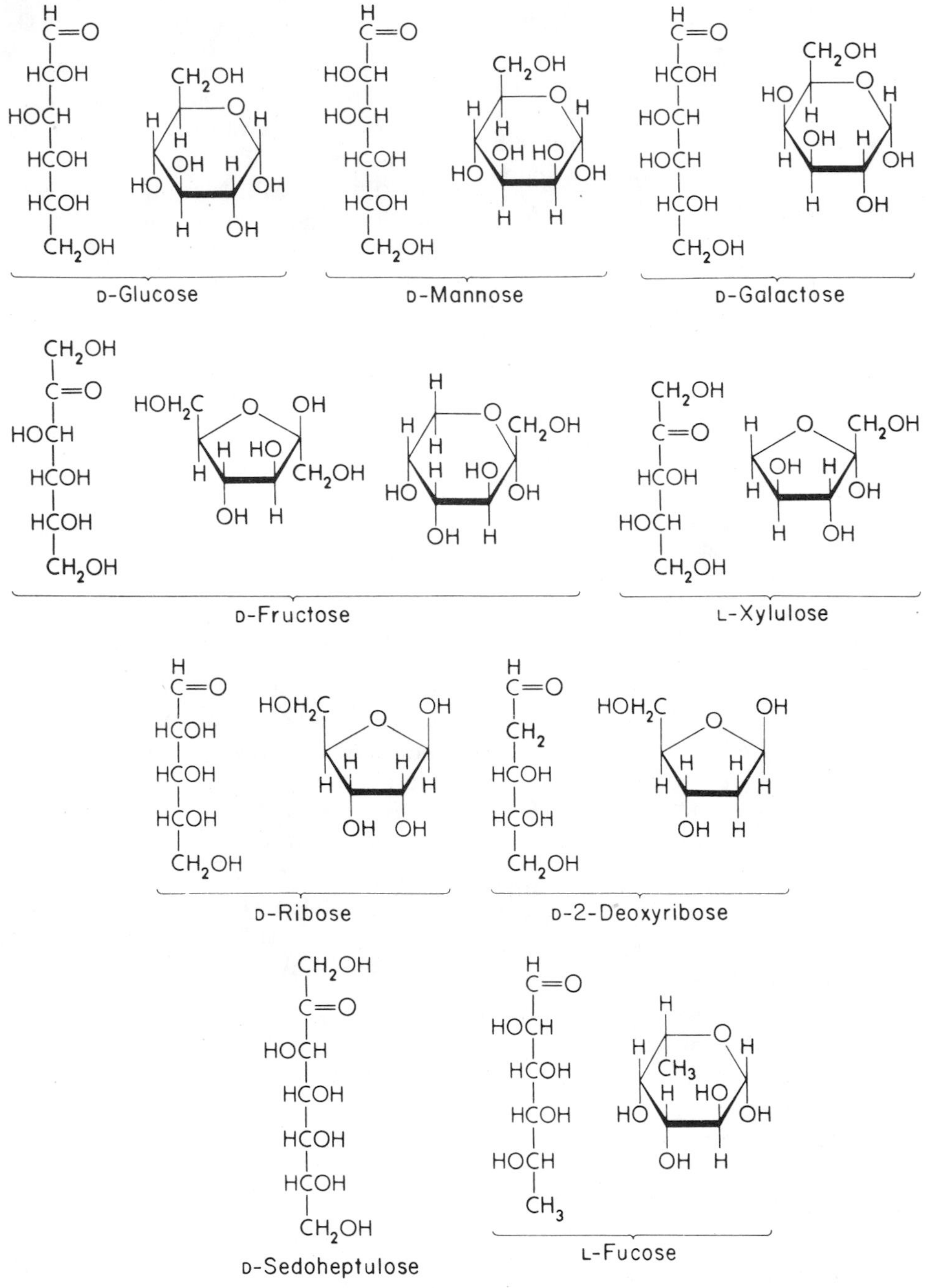

Fig. 4-3. Principal monosaccharides in animal metabolism.

ture have from three to seven carbon atoms. The number of possible isomers is 2^n, where n is the number of asymmetric centers. All of the isomers do not occur in nature. The monosaccharides of principal interest in animal metabolism, in addition to the trioses noted above, are the aldotetrose D-erythrose; the aldopentoses D-ribose, its derivative D-2-deoxyribose, and D-xylose; the ketopentoses D-ribulose and D-xylulose (insertion of -ul- between the stem of the name and

the class suffix -ose denotes a ketosugar); the three aldohexoses D-glucose, D-galactose and D-mannose; the ketohexose D-fructose and the seven-carbon D-sedoheptulose; and D-fucose, a frequent member of the oligosaccharide chains of glycoproteins. The structures of some of these are shown in Figure 4-3. They are all colorless crystalline compounds highly soluble in water and insoluble in organic solvents.

Three- and four-carbon monosaccharides have a lin-

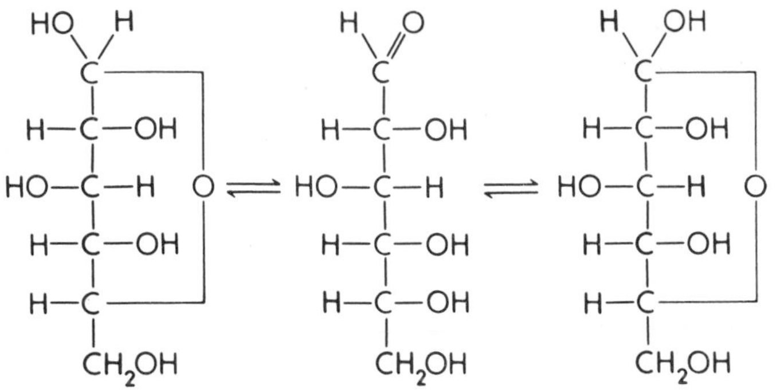

Fig. 4-4. Mutarotation of glucose isomers.

ear structure, and their properties as aldehydes and ketones are readily expressed. Keto- and aldo- pentoses and hexoses react sluggishly. This is accounted for by the intramolecular formation of a hemiacetal or a hemiketal, produced by condensation of the carbonyl group with an alcohol group, yielding a five- or six-membered ring containing oxygen. The six- and five-membered rings are related to the compounds pyran and furan respectively, and monosaccharides in this form are designated pyranose and furanose respectively. The carbon originally carrying the carbonyl oxygen is known as the anomeric carbon. It is a new asymmetric center, yielding isomers designated α and β. The anomers are in equilibrium with each other and with a minute amount of the free aldehyde or ketone. The optical rotation of a solution of β-D-glucose will change, over a period of hours, in a direction indicating that the α-isomer is forming. The equilibration of the two isomers in this way is called *mutarotation* (Fig. 4-4).

The properties of the sugars are still better accounted for by the formulation of Haworth, in which the ring is represented as projecting at a right angle to the plane of the paper, the substituents projecting above and below the plane of the ring. (Fig. 4-3). Galactose and mannose differ from glucose in the configuration round one carbon atom: they are *epimers*.

The chemical properties of the monosaccharides are those of both alcohols and aldehydes or ketones. They can form esters with other organic acids, with sulfuric acid and (a most important group) with phosphoric acid. At the anomeric carbon they can react with another alcohol (including other monosaccharides) to form full acetals or ketals, called glycosides. This is

the reaction by which the oligosaccharides and polysaccharides are constructed. Glycosides may also be formed with phenolic hydroxyl groups, with carboxylic acids or with phosphoric acid (glucose 1-phosphate is an ester glycoside). The pentoses of the nucleotides are N-glycosides, formed by loss of water between the hemiacetal hydroxyl and an -NH group of the constituent base. Because of the asymmetry at the anomeric carbon, glycosides have either the α or the β configuration. They form distinct compounds and are hydrolyzed only by enzymes specific for one optical isomer. The noncarbohydrate constituent of a glycoside is called the aglycone.

Aldoses and ketoses can react with phenylhydrazine to form hydrazones and osazones, crystalline derivaties useful in identifying individual sugars and establishing structural relationships. The simpler carbohydrates, including some disaccharides, are reducing sugars, reacting with cupric ion in hot alkaline solution to produce cuprous oxide, a reaction used in both the qualitative and the quantitative analysis of the sugars. Reduction of the aldehyde or ketone group forms the sugar alcohols. Reduction of glucose yields sorbitol; fructose gives rise to both sorbitol and mannitol. Ribitol (from ribose) is the carbohydrate moiety of riboflavin; glycerol (from glyceraldehyde or dihydroxyacetone) is the alcohol of neutral fats (triacylglycerols). Uronic acids are formed by oxidation of the terminal primary alcohol of an aldohexose to a carboxylic acid. Glucuronic and galacturonic acid are constituents of polysaccharides and, combined as glycosides with a variety of compounds, such as the steroids or bile pigments, make them soluble and facilitate their excretion. Oxidation of the aldehyde yields the aldonic acids, and oxidation at both C-1 and C-6 of the aldoses yields saccharic acids, useful mainly in the preparation and identification of carbohydrates.

The pentose ribose is important because it is the constituent sugar of many free nucleotides (ATP, NAD^+, etc.) and of the ribonucleic acids. Its 2-deoxy derivative is present in DNA. The 5-phosphate esters of the epimeric ketopentoses ribulose and xylulose are intermediates in the reactions of the direct oxidation pathway of glucose.

Amino sugars are formed from each of the three important aldohexoses by replacement of the 2-hydroxyl group with an amino group. Glucosamine (chitosamine) is found in chitin, the polysaccharide of insect cuticle, in glycolipids and in a number of heteropolysaccharides. Galactosamine (chondrosamine) is also found in glycolipids and mucopolysaccharides. Both amino sugars are most frequently found as the N-acetyl derivative. Mannosamine is found condensed with pyruvic acid to form neuraminic acid. N-acetyl neuraminic acid is one of a group of N- and O-acyl derivatives of neuraminic acids called sialic acids. They are constituents of complex glycolipids (gangliosides) and are present in many heteropolysaccharides, mucoproteins and glycoproteins.

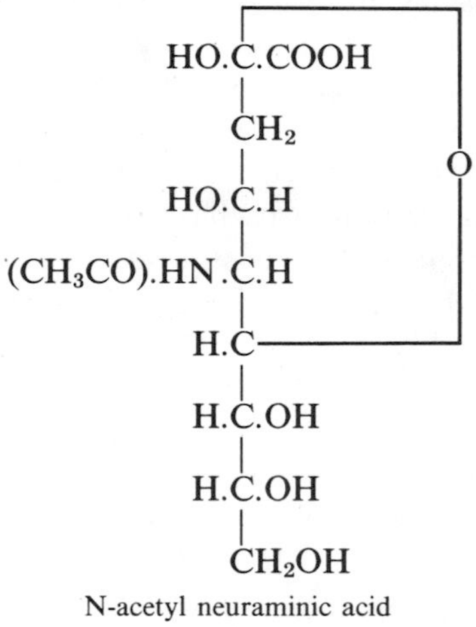

N-acetyl neuraminic acid

Oligosaccharides. Only three disaccharides are of interest for mammalian metabolism, maltose, lactose and sucrose. Maltose is a glycoside containing two glucose units in α-1,4 linkage. It is a product of digestion of starch and glycogen by amylases. Since the

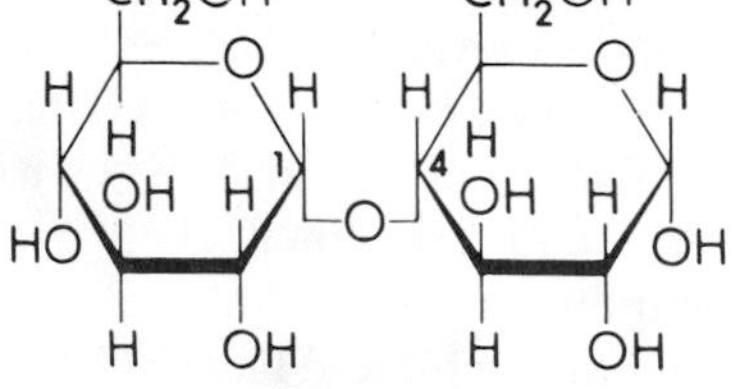

Maltose

anomeric carbon of one of the glucose units is free, maltose is a reducing sugar and exhibits other reactions characteristic of the carbonyl carbon (formation of an osazone, etc.). The same is true of lactose, a galactoside containing glucose in β-1,4 linkage. Lactose is the sugar of milk and is the carbohydrate of the infant diet. The third disaccharide of interest is sucrose. It

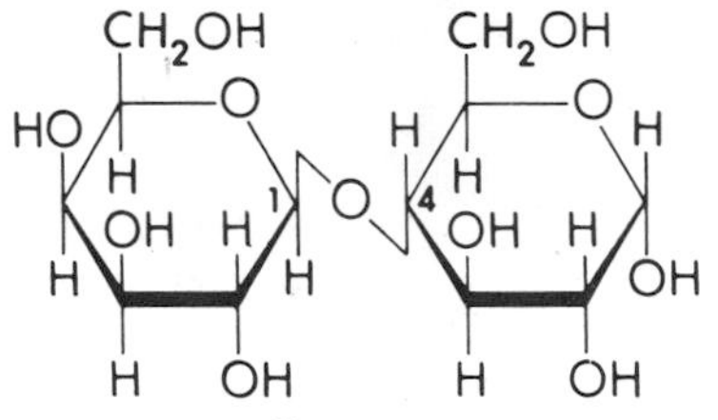

Lactose

yields glucose and fructose on hydrolysis but is not a reducing sugar because the two molecules are linked by loss of water between the two anomeric carbon atoms, C-1 of glucose and C-2 of fructose. Sucrose, derived from sugar cane and beet, is probably the most widely used of the simpler sugars. It is digestible but not metabolizable: injected sucrose is recovered completely in the urine. The disaccharide is dextrorotatory. The mixture of glucose and fructose formed on hydrolysis is levorotatory, and for this reason is called invert sugar. The enzymes catalyzing the hydrolysis are called invertases.

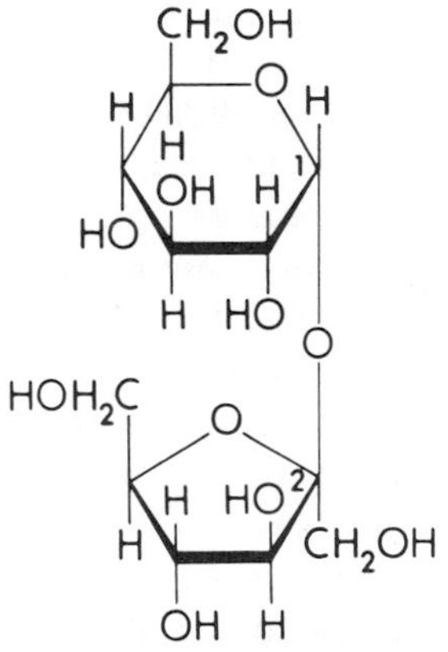

Sucrose

Polysaccharides. Homopolysaccharides are polymers containing many identical monosaccharide units bound in glycosidic linkage. Cellulose, starch and glycogen are homoglucans, composed entirely of glucose. Cellulose is the principal structural component of many plants. It is a linear polymer of glucose units joined in β-1,4 glycosidic linkage. The long slender molecules aggregate to form strong fibers. Cotton is nearly pure cellulose. In wood the cellulose fibers are cemented together with lignin. Cellulose is not digestible by man. The starches are storage forms of carbo-

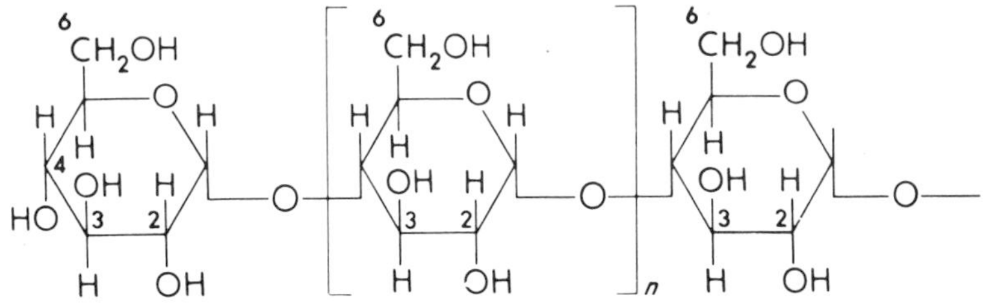

Fig. 4-5. Amylose-type chain.

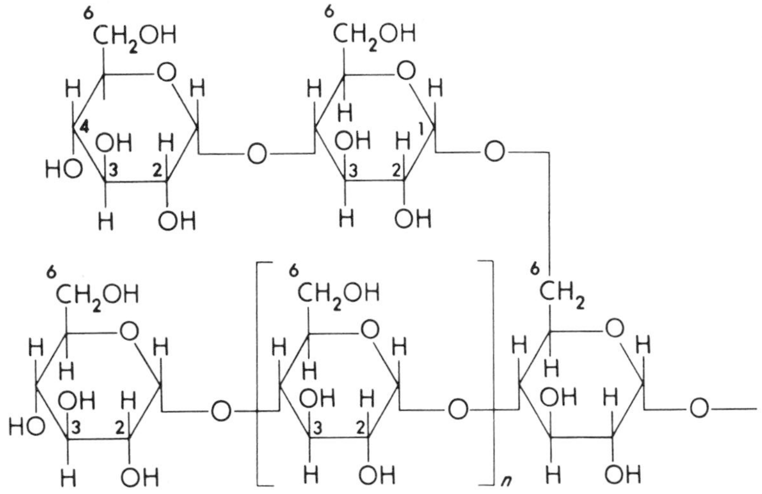

Fig. 4-6. Amylopectin-type chain.

hydrate in plants. Two components are present (Figs. 4–5 and 4–6). Amylose (20 to 30 per cent of most starches) is made up of 250 to 300 glucose units in α-1,4 glucosidic linkage. The molecule is coiled in a helix rather than in the extended configuration of cellulose. Because of this it gives an intense blue color with iodine; the atoms can slip inside the helix, and in the somewhat hydrophobic interior they absorb light strongly. The degradation of amylose by α-amylase (α-1,4 glucan 4-glucanohydrolase) occurs by a random attack on interior glycosidic linkages, yielding a mixture of glucose and maltose. The β-amylases (α-1,4 glucan maltohydrolases) of bacteria and plants are exo-amylases attacking only from the nonreducing ends of the chains to set free maltose.

The second component, amylopectin, is a branched polysaccharide, the branches being formed by the occurrence at intervals of glucose in α-1,6 glucosidic linkage with a glucose forming part of a chain joined together in α,1,4 glucosidic linkage. A new chain of glucose units in α-1,4 linkage grows from the branch. The molecule branches repeatedly to form a treelike structure. In amylopectins the average interval between branches is 24 to 30 glucose units. The chains of amy-

lopectin are coiled loosely like those of amylose. The compound gives a purple color with iodine. The molecules of amylopectin are polydisperse, ranging in mass from 50,000 to several million daltons. Enzymatic attack by α-amylase on interior linkages results in rapid degradation of the molecule to smaller units (dextrins) and finally to glucose, maltose and isomaltose (α-1,6 glucosidoglucose). The β-amylases attack only the outer tier of branches, liberating maltose and leaving over half the molecule intact as a β-amylase limit dextrin. The comparable animal storage form of glucose is glycogen. The molecule is constructed like amylopectin, but branching is far more frequent, with only 8 to 12 glucose units per nonreducing end group. Glycogen is also polydisperse, the particles ranging in mass from 250,000 to 100×10^6 daltons. Because of the shorter intervals between branches, glycogen gives a reddish color with iodine. Its degradation by the amylases is like that of amylopectin. Glycogen is stable to hot alkali. It is isolated from tissues by digestion with hot KOH, followed by precipitation of the glycogen with ethanol.

A group of glucose homopolysaccharides of special interest are the dextrans of bacterial origin. These contain glucose in α-1,6 linkage and are infrequently branched. Partly degraded dextrans, suitably purified and graded for molecular size (70,000 to 100,000 daltons), are nicely soluble and are useful as plasma volume expanders. They are nontoxic and are slowly metabolized.

Inulin is a homopolysaccharide of fructose, in β-2,1 bond, M_r about 10,000, found in the Jerusalem artichoke and related plants. It is not metabolized by animals or man, does not penetrate into cells and is not reabsorbed by the kidney. It has been used to measure extracellular space and glomerular filtration rate.

The homopolysaccharide chitin, found in the shells of crustaceans, molds and insects, is, next to cellulose, the most abundant polysaccharide. It is a linear polymer of N-acetyl-glucosamine in β-1,4 linkage, analogous to cellulose. Its aggregated fibers make a tough and durable integument.

The heteropolysaccharides are large molecules yielding more than one constituent monosaccharide on hydrolysis. They are a numerous and diverse group of animal and plant compounds. Among these, the acid mucopolysaccharides are of greatest interest. Their distinguishing characteristic is that they are composed of repeating units of a uronic acid, usually in β-1,3 glycosidic linkage with an N-acetylated amino sugar. These disaccharide units are linked by β-1,4, linkages between the amino sugar and the uronic acid. Hyaluronic acid is composed in this way of glucuronic acid and N-acetylglucosamine. A polydisperse macromolecule of 10^5 to 10^7 daltons, it forms highly viscous solutions. It is a component of synovial fluid, of the vitreous humor and of Wharton's jelly, which is most often used in its isolation.

Hyaluronic acid, like other mucopolysaccharides, is often associated with small amounts of protein. The polysaccharide is attacked by an enzyme, hyaluronidase, which first depolymerizes the macromolecule and then cleaves it into tetrasaccharides. At the site of attack the normal barrier to the movement of particles and macromolecules through the connective tissue is destroyed. For this reason, hyaluronidase is called the spreading factor.

The disaccharide unit of chondroitin is also composed of glucuronic acid and N-acetylglucosamine. It is associated in cartilage with two more abundant derivatives, chondroitin-4-sulfate and -6-sulfate, in which N-acetylglucosamine is esterified with sulfate. Dermatan sulfate (formerly chondroitin sulfate B) contains the unusual monosaccharide L-iduronic acid (the 5-epimer of glucuronic acid) in α-1,3 linkage with N-acetylgalactosamine 4-sulfate. The disaccharide units are linked by β-1,4 linkages.

A related sulfated polysaccharide is heparin, in which the repeating unit is a hexasaccharide containing 2,6-disulfoglucosamine, 2-sulfoiduronic acid and glucuronic acid in the proportions 3:2:1. Heparin is polydisperse, occurring in small molecules (M_r = 3,000 to 11,000) and as macromolecules (up to 10^6 daltons). It is found in abundance in mast cells and basophilic leucocytes, but it may also be synthesized on demand in other tissues. The anticoagulant activity of heparin preparations may be due to only a small fraction of the molecules. The effectiveness of heparin in preventing thrombosis may be due to absorption of these linear anionic polyelectrolytes onto blood vessel walls, imparting a negative charge to them. Heparin affects the activity of many enzymes. It displaces lipoprotein lipase from cell surfaces, helping to initiate hydrolysis of the triacylglycerols of chylomicrons and very low density lipoproteins. Appreciation of the wide variety of effects of heparin on many processes has given it new importance.

Heteropolysaccharides and oligosaccharides linked covalently to proteins and lipids are of very common occurrence. Examples are the mucin of saliva and the mucoproteins found among the α-globulins of plasma, as well as the numerous glycoproteins of cell membranes.

Metabolism of Carbohydrates

The digestion of carbohydrates is accomplished mainly in the small intestine. Saliva contains an α-amylase (α-1,4-glucan 4-glucano-hydrolase) capable of hydrolyzing the homopolysaccharides of starches, and glycogen. It is inactivated by acid, and the extent of digestion of the polysaccharides in the stomach is limited by the acid gastric juice permeating successive layers of swallowed food. Proteolysis in the stomach sets free the cell contents, making their contained carbohydrates more accessible to the action of the pancreatic enzymes.

The α-amylase secreted by the pancreas is identical to the salivary amylase. Its pH optimum is 7, and it has a strict requirement for Cl^-. By its action, amylose is hydrolyzed to glucose and maltose, amylopectin and glycogen to glucose, maltose, and small branched oligosaccharides containing glucose in α-1,6 linkage, which can be split by an α-1,6 glucosidase. Enzymes capable of hydrolyzing the disaccharides maltose, lactose and sucrose are found in the brush border of the intestinal epithelial cells. The monosaccharides glucose, galactose and fructose are the main products of carbohydrate digestion that enter the bloodstream. There are no digestive enzymes in man capable of hydrolyzing polysaccharides such as cellulose. Undigested vegetable fibers therefore provide no nutrient but add bulk to the feces and may facilitate their elimination.

Monosaccharides are absorbed from the intestine at different rates, the order being galactose > glucose > fructose > mannose > xylose > arabinose. Galactose and glucose are absorbed against a concentration gradient by a process of active transport that is dependent on the presence of sodium ion in the intestinal lumen. No metabolic energy is required; the movement of Na^+ into a region of lower concentration in the cytosol of the epithelial cells is coupled in an as yet unknown way with the carriage of glucose and galactose from a region of low concentration in the intestinal lumen into the cells and through the serosal side into the blood. The system is saturable, and the actively absorbed sugars (including the nonmetabolizable sugars 3-0-methylglucose, 6-deoxyglucose and 6-deoxygalactose) apparently compete for a common carrier. Phlorhizin is a potent inhibitor of sugar transport, and ouabain, which inhibits the active transport of $Na+$ from the serosal side of the epithelial cells into the plasma, also blocks the active transport of glucose. The more slowly absorbed monosaccharides leave the intestine more rapidly than can be accounted for by simple diffusion but are not concentrated against a concentration gradient. The absorption of sugars through the large surface of the small intestine is highly efficient; very little normally escapes.

The metabolism of glucose in all tissues begins with its esterification with phosphate:

$$glucose + ATP \xrightarrow{Mg^{2+}} glucose\ 6\text{-phosphate} + ADP$$

This reaction is catalyzed in most tissues by a *hexokinase* of broad specificity, capable of acting upon mannose, fructose, and galactose as well. Hexokinase is inhibited by the product, glucose-6-phosphate, but one of its substrates, $Mg^{2+}\ ATP^{4-}$, is a positive effector, favoring the reaction at physiological concentrations of glucose-6-phosphate in the cell. The Km of most hexokinases is low, 1 to 10 μM. Glucose is therefore readily esterified as it enters the cell. Liver contains a specific *glucokinase* which is not product inhibited. Its Km is 20 mM, and it acts best when the portal vein glucose concentration is high, for example, during a meal.

A major pathway of glucose utilization in all tissues is the process of breakdown into the three-carbon product, pyruvic acid, which is oxidized further to carbon dioxide and water, but which, in most tissues in the absence of oxygen, can be reduced to lactic acid. The anaerobic conversion of glucose to 2 moles of lactic acid is called *glycolysis*. This pathway is particularly well developed in voluntary muscle, serving the useful purpose of providing energy for the synthesis of ATP at a time when the oxygen supply to the working mus-cle is insufficient to meet the demand for energy. The process begins with glucose-6-phosphate, derived from blood glucose or, by way of glucose-1-phosphate, from glycogen. The enzyme phosphoglucose isomerase converts the glucose ester to fructose-6-phosphate. The next step is the formation of fructose 1,6-diphosphate by the enzyme phosphofructokinase (PFK):

$$fructose\text{-}6\text{-phosphate} + Mg^{2+}ATP^{4-}$$
$$\rightarrow fructose\ 1,6\text{-diphosphate} + Mg^{2+}ADP^{3-}$$

This reaction, essentially irreversible, is the "committed" step of glycolysis. PFK is a closely regulated enzyme. Its activity is increased by increases in the concentration of ADP, AMP and inorganic phosphate. It is inhibited by ATP, citrate and 2,3-diphosphoglycerate (in liver and red cell). Thus it may be seen that when ATP utilization is high, PFK activity is increased; at high ATP concentration, the activity is depressed. The enzyme is also inhibited by increased concentrations of free fatty acid, so that when this substrate is readily available, glucose utilization is depressed.

Fructose diphosphate is cleaved between carbons 3 and 4 by the enzyme aldolase to yield 3-phosphoglyceraldehyde and its isomer dihydroxyacetone phosphate. These isomers, like glucose 6-phosphate and fructose 6-phosphate, are interconvertible through the action of triose phosphate isomerase. By this means both triose phosphates are capable of undergoing the further reactions of glycolysis.

Up to this point, if one has started with glucose, 2 moles of ATP have been utilized. In the subsequent steps this "debt" is repaid, and a net yield of 2 additional moles of ATP is achieved. The first of these steps involves the oxidation of 3-phosphoglyceraldehyde to 1,3-diphosphoglyceric acid by the enzyme 3-phosphoglyceraldehyde dehydrogenase: inorganic phosphate is taken up and a mixed anhydride of phosphoglyceric acid and phosphoric acid is formed. A large fraction of the chemical potential energy of the oxidation is conserved by this device, and in the next step, catalyzed by phosphoglycerate kinase, ATP is formed:

$$1,3\text{-diphosphoglycerate} + Mg^{2+}ADP^{3-}$$
$$\rightleftharpoons 3\text{-phosphoglycerate} + mg^{2+}ATP^{4-}$$

The oxidation of phosphoglyceraldehyde to phosphoglycerate, an energy-yielding reaction, is coupled to the uptake of inorganic phosphate and the synthesis of ATP. Since 2 moles of triose phosphate are available for oxidation, 2 moles of ATP can be generated. In the reaction, the coenzyme NAD^+ is reduced. As will presently be seen, the essence of this and other fermentations is the means chosen to reoxidize NADH.

$$\begin{array}{c}
HC\!=\!O \\
| \\
HCOH \\
| \\
H_2COPO_3H_2
\end{array}
\; + NAD^+ + P_i \rightleftharpoons
\begin{array}{c}
O \\
\parallel \\
C\!-\!O \sim PO_3H_2 \\
| \\
HCOH \\
| \\
H_2COPO_3H_2
\end{array}
\; + NADH + H^+$$

Oxidation of phosphoglyceraldehyde

The enzyme phosphoglyceromutase next catalyzes the conversion of 3-phosphoglycerate to 2-phosphoglycerate, and the latter compound is dehydrated by the enzyme enolase to yield phosphoenolpyruvate:

$$\begin{array}{c}
COOH \\
| \\
HC\!-\!OPO_3H_2 \\
| \\
H_2C\!-\!OH
\end{array}
\;\overset{Mg^{2+}}{\rightleftharpoons}\;
\begin{array}{c}
COOH \\
| \\
C\!-\!O \sim PO_3H_2 \\
\parallel \\
CH_2
\end{array}
\; + H_2O$$

A large fraction of the potential energy of the dehydration of glycerate to pyruvate is conserved by the formation of the phosphate ester of the enol-tautomer of pyruvate. ATP can be synthesized by the transfer of the phosphate to ADP, catalyzed by the enzyme pyruvate kinase. This step is essentially irreversible. Pyruvate kinase is, like PFK, closely regulated. The behavior of the enzymes in muscle and liver is quite different. In muscle, high concentrations of ATP are inhibitory. In the liver as well, the enzyme is inhibited by ATP and alanine, but a high concentration of fructose 1,6-diphosphate can override the inhibition. The liver enzyme is also inhibited by long-chain fatty acids and by acetyl CoA. Thus under conditions in which lipid substrate is available, and in which gluconeogenesis from amino acids may be occurring, the breakdown of phosphoenolpyruvate is firmly restrained. Since 2 moles of phosphoenolpyruvate are formed, 2 moles of ATP may be synthesized. The gross yield of the transformation, glucose → 2 pyruvate, is 4 moles of ATP; the net yield is 2, or if one has started with glycogen, 3.

In the absence of oxygen the reduced coenzyme must be reoxidized by other means. This is accomplished by the reduction of pyruvate by lactate dehydrogenase:

$$CH_3COCOOH + NADH + H^+ \rightleftharpoons$$
$$CH_3CHOHCOOH + NAD^+$$

Glycolysis can continue until the accumulation of acid results in a fall in pH unfavorable to continued action of the glycolytic enzymes. The isozymes of lactate dehydrogenase were mentioned earlier in this chapter.

The process of fermentation of glucose in many microorganisms follows the identical pathway to pyruvate as it occurs in animal tissues, but a different choice of hydrogen acceptor is made, and the product is the neutral compound ethanol. Pyruvate is decarboxylated by the enzyme carboxylase, thiamine pyrophosphate (co-carboxylase) acting as coenzyme, and the resulting acetaldehyde is reduced to ethanol:

$$CH_3COCOOH \rightarrow CH_3CHO + CO_2$$
$$NADH + H^+ + CH_3CHO \rightleftharpoons CH_3CH_2OH + NAD^+$$

These are the terminal steps of the alcoholic fermentation of yeast.

Lactic acid is a metabolic dead end. When the supply of oxygen is adequate, lactate need not be produced, since NADH can be reoxidized by other means. Lactate that may have accumulated can only be reoxidized to pyruvate.

Cytosolic NADH has no direct access to mitochondria. It is reoxidized by a rather elaborate "shuttle" involving cytosolic and mitochondrial malate dehydrogenases and glutamate-oxaloacetate (OAA) transaminases. The scheme is as follows:

T_1 is a device in the mitochondrial membrane permitting exchange of glutamate (Glu) for aspartate (Asp). T_2 is a similar device permitting exchange of α-ketoglutarate (KGA) for malate. Imagine that in the cytosol the concentration of NADH rises. Then (since the equilibrium favors malate):

$$NADH + H^+ + OAA \rightleftharpoons malate + NAD^+ \text{ (cytosol)}$$

Malate enters the mitochondria in exchange for KGA, and is there reoxidized to OAA, producing mitochondrial NADH, now in touch with the respiratory chain. The reactants of the transaminases ($K_{eq} = 1$), linked in easy balance by T_1, are essentially in equilibrium. The system therefore responds sensitively to the reduction of OAA in the cytosol.

The Pyruvate Oxidation System. Pyruvate is oxidatively decarboxylated by a highly organized enzyme system located in the mitochondrial matrix. In the

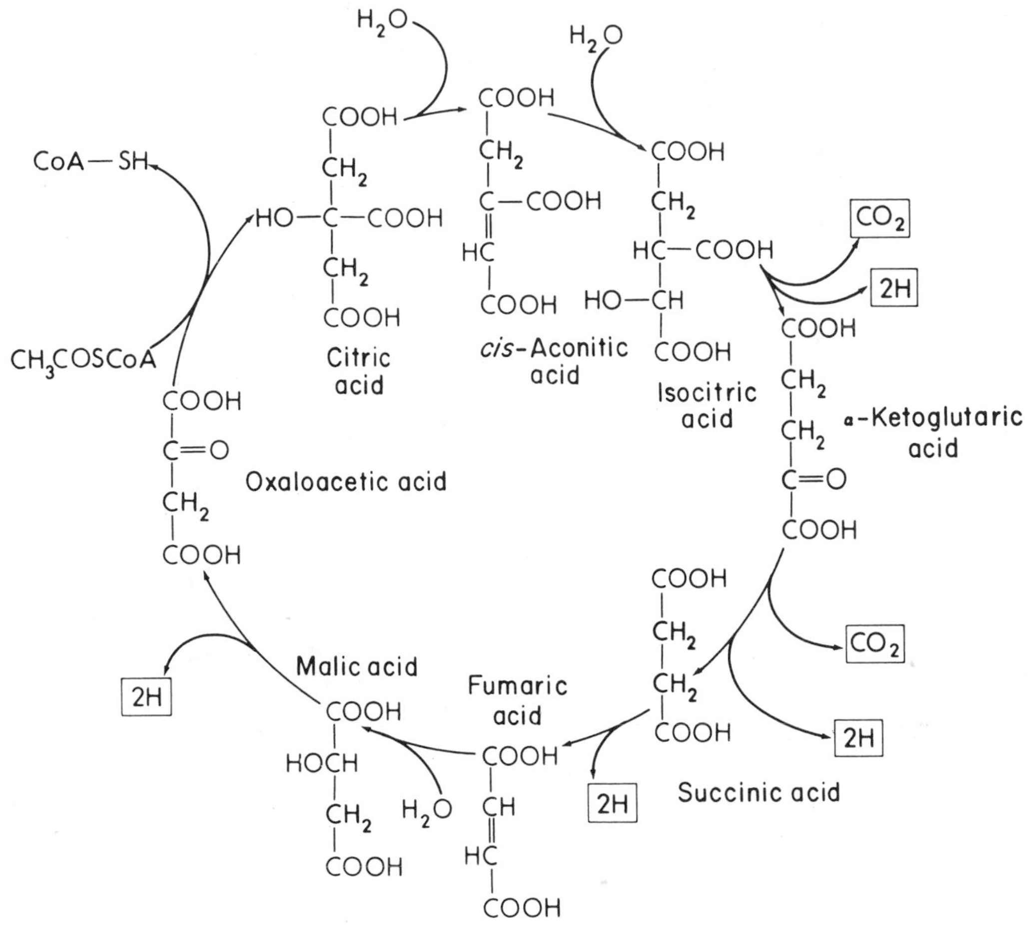

Fig. 4-7. Tricarboxylic acid cycle.

first step pyruvate is decarboxylated by pyruvate dehydrogenase, yielding CO_2 and α-hydroxyethyl-thiamine pyrophosphate. "Active acetaldehyde" is transferred by the same enzyme to the prosthetic group, lipoamide, of the enzyme lipoyl transacetylase. In this transfer, the disulfide of lipoamide is reduced, acetaldehyde is oxidized to "active acetyl" and bound as a thioester:

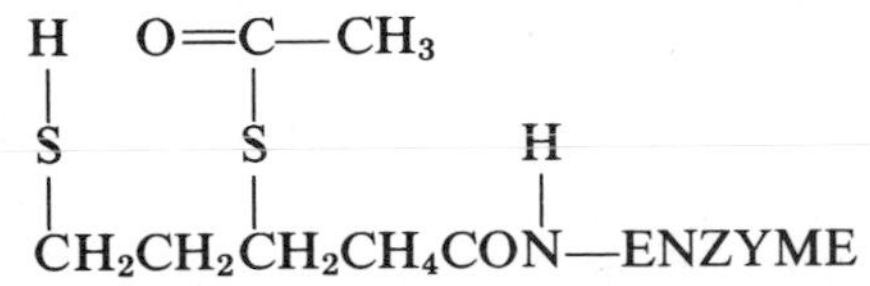

$$\begin{array}{c} H \quad O=C-CH_3 \\ | \qquad | \qquad\qquad H \\ S \qquad S \qquad\quad | \\ CH_2CH_2CH_2CH_4CON-ENZYME \end{array}$$

The acetyl group is then transferred to coenzyme A, forming acetyl-SCoA, leaving lipoamide in the disulf-hydryl form. The reduced coenzyme is reoxidized by a flavoprotein, dihydrolipoyl dehydrogenase. The reduced flavoprotein is in turn reoxidized by NAD^+. The overall reaction is described by the equation:

$$CH_3COCOOH + HSCoA + NAD^+ \rightarrow$$
$$CH_3CO\text{-}SCoA + CO_2 + NADH + H^+$$

The pyruvate oxidation system is arrayed in particles of about 9×10^6 daltons, containing many replicas of the constituent enzymes. The system is closely regulated. Pyruvate dehydrogenase is activated by fructose diphosphate. It is product inhibited, by both NADH and acetyl-SCoA. ATP affects it by means of a pyruvate dehydrogenase kinase, also present in the particle; phosphorylation of the enzyme at a specific site inhibits its action on pyruvate. The kinase is also activated by NADH and acetyl-SCoA. The inhibition is relieved by a phosphatase, also present in the particle.

The Citric Acid Cycle. Acetyl-SCoA is oxidized in the mitochondria by means of the citric (tricarboxylic) acid cycle (Fig. 4-7). Citrate synthetase catalyzes the condensation of acetyl-SCoA with oxaloacetate to yield citrate and HSCoA. The reaction is essentially irreversible. Aconitase catalyzes the conversion of citrate to cis-aconitate and isocitrate. Isocitrate is oxidatively decarboxylated to α-ketoglutarate and CO_2 by the NAD^+-requiring isocitrate dehydrogenase. The enzyme has an absolute requirement for Mg^{2+} and is strongly activated by ADP. The oxidative decarboxylation of α-ketoglutarate is carried out by a particle analogous to the pyruvate oxidation system. Succinate semialdehyde is formed on thiamine pyrophosphate, and with the intermediate aid of lipoamide this is oxidized to succinyl-SCoA. NAD^+ is reduced in the reoxidation of the lipoamide. These oxidative decarboxylations account for the carbons of acetyl SCoA as CO_2.

The energy of succinyl-SCoA is conserved by the action of succinate thiokinase:

$$\text{succinyl-SCoA} + \text{GDP} + P_i \rightleftharpoons \text{succinate} + \text{GTP} + \text{HSCoA}$$

GTP may be utilized directly, or its terminal phosphate may be transferred to ADP.

Succinate is next oxidized to fumarate by a flavoprotein, succinate dehydrogenase. Fumarate is hydrated to malate, and oxaloacetate is regenerated by oxidation of malate by the NAD^+-requiring malate dehydrogenase.

The four oxidations of the citric acid cycle furnish substrate hydrogen to the respiratory chain. The rate of operation of the cycle is governed by the concentration of substrates and of cofactors. Citrate synthetase is inhibited by NADH and succinyl-SCoA. Isocitrate dehydrogenase is activated by its substrate, ADP, and AMP, and inhibited by NADH and ATP. α-ketoglutarate dehydrogenase is inhibited by NADH and succinyl-SCoA. In general, when the demand for energy is high the rates of production and oxidation of acetyl-SCoA are high. When the ratios, $NADH/NAD^+$ and ATP/ADP increase, the rate of operation of the cycle decreases.

Characteristics of the Tricarboxylic Acid Cycle: Anaplerosis.

The tricarboxylic acid cycle provides an ingenious solution to the problem of oxidizing a small two-carbon compound to CO_2 and water by combining it with a four-carbon keto acid to form a six-carbon intermediate that is oxidatively decarboxylated to yield first a five- and then a four-carbon dicarboxylic acid. Two further steps of oxidation regenerate the keto acid. The products of the cycle are 2 moles of CO_2, 3 moles of NADH, 1 mole of reduced flavoprotein and 1 mole of GTP. The oxidation of the four pairs of hydrogen atoms to water realizes a high proportion of the potential energy of acetate as ATP. The pathways of oxidation of carbohydrate, of fatty acids, and of most of the carbon of the amino acids converge upon the tricarboxylic acid cycle. It is the prime source of the potential energy that makes the mitochondrion the powerhouse of the cell.

The citric acid cycle is also a source of substrate for a variety of biosynthetic processes. Oxaloacetate

and α-ketoglutarate, for example, yield aspartate and glutamate by transamination. Decarboxylation of oxaloacetate yields pyruvate which, by transamination, yields alanine. Citrate, diffusing into the cytosol, is cleaved to oxaloacetate and acetyl-SCoA, furnishing substrate for fatty acid synthesis. The source of phosphoenolpyruvate for gluconeogenesis is oxaloacetate.

The concentration of intermediates of the cycle is maintained by a number of reactions, the most important of which is the reaction of CO_2 fixation catalyzed by the enzyme pyruvate carboxylase:

$$CH_3COCOOH + HCO_3^- + ATP \xrightarrow[\text{AcCoA}]{Mg^{2+}}$$

$$HOOCCH_2COCOOH + P_i + ADP$$

The enzyme contains covalently linked biotin as a cofactor for the fixation of CO_2, and it has an absolute requirement for acetyl-SCoA, without which CO_2 cannot be bound to the biotin. Reactions of this type, restoring the concentration of citric acid cycle intermediates, are called anaplerotic (filling up) reactions. In heart and voluntary muscle, pyruvate carboxylase is not present, but two types of anaplerotic reaction may take its place. One is by transamination between glutamate and pyruvate:

$$\text{pyruvate} + \text{glutamate} \rightleftharpoons \text{alanine} + \alpha\text{-ketoglutarate}.$$

The other is by the malic enzyme:

$$\text{pyruvate} + CO_2 + NADPH + H^+ \rightleftharpoons \text{L-malate} + NAD^+$$

Other functions of these enzymes are noted below

Energy Yield of Glycolysis and Oxidation of Glucose.

In glycolysis, 1 mole of glucose yields 2 moles of pyruvate, 2 moles (net) of ATP, and 2 moles of NADH, which can be reoxidized as described above. Reoxidation of the corresponding 2 moles of mitochondrial NADH yields 2×3 moles of ATP. The oxidative decarboxylation of 2 moles of pyruvate yields 2 moles of acetyl-SCoA and 2 moles of NADH, which on reoxidation yields 2×3 moles of ATP. The oxidation of 2 moles of acetyl-SCoA by the citric acid cycle yields directly 2 moles of GTP, 6 moles of NADH, and 2 moles of reduced flavoprotein. Reoxidation yields $6 \times 3 + 2 \times 2$ moles of ATP. The total, $2 + 6 + 6 + 2 + 18 + 4 = 38$ moles of ATP. If the free energy of hydrolysis of ATP is taken to be 7,300 calories per mole, then, of the 686,000 calories of potential energy in 1 mole of glucose, about 277,400 calories are conserved, with an apparent efficiency of about 40 per cent.

Under anaerobic conditions the reaction glucose $\rightarrow$

2 lactate, yielding only 2 moles of ATP (net), is vastly less efficient in terms of energy yield per mole of substrate utilized, but in voluntary muscle it offers the advantage for survival of rapid development of full power and acceleration independently of the immediate oxygen supply. In the red cell, glycolysis is the sole source of energy, supporting a complex of requirements, including the maintenance of the peculiar properties of the red cell membrane, for nearly its life span of 126 days.

The "Direct" Oxidation of Glucose. In tissues that are active sites of fatty acid or steroid synthesis—liver, adipose tissue, mammary gland, testis, adrenal cortex—a direct oxidation pathway for glucose 6-phosphate (the phosphogluconate pathway, hexose–monophosphate shunt, pentose–phosphate pathway) is usually well developed. Its functions are (1) to provide NADPH for use in biosynthesis, and (2) the synthesis and metabolism of pentoses.

1. The reactions producing NADPH are catalyzed by glucose 6-phosphate dehydrogenase:

glucose 6-phosphate + NADP$^+$ $\rightleftarrows$
6-phosphogluconate + NADPH + H$^+$

and a second oxidation catalyzed by 6-phosphogluconate dehydrogenase:

6-phosphogluconate + NADP$^+$ $\rightleftarrows$
ribulose 5-phosphate + CO$_2$ + NADPH + H$^+$

The NADPH is a source of hydrogen for the reductive steps of fatty acid and of steroid biosynthesis from acetyl CoA.

2. The ketopentose D-ribulose 5-phosphate is converted to D-ribose 5-phosphate by a phosphopentose isomerase, and to D-xylulose 5-phosphate by an epimerase:

D-Xylulose 5-P $\rightleftarrows$ D-Ribulose 5-P $\rightleftarrows$ D-Ribose 5-P

D-Xylulose 5-phosphate and D-ribose 5-phosphate are substrates for a transketolase, an enzyme requiring thiamine pyrophosphate, which transfers "active glycolaldehyde" from xylulose to ribose to form the seven-carbon ketose D-sedoheptulose 7-phosphate and D-glyceraldehyde 3-phosphate:

The enzyme transaldolase catalyzes the transfer of the dihydroxyacetone moiety of a ketose phosphate to C-1 of an aldose phosphate:

With D-sedoheptulose 7-phosphate and D-3-phosphoglyceraldehyde the products are D-fructose 6-phosphate and D-erythrose 4-phosphate.

Transketolase can catalyze the transfer of a two-carbon moiety from D-xylulose 5-phosphate to D-erythrose 4-phosphate, forming D-fructose 6-phosphate and D-3-phosphoglyceraldehyde.

These four sets of reactions, nonoxidative and reversible, can account for both the production and disposal of ribose and its relatives. Note that fructose

6-phosphate is formed in two of the reactions, as well as 3-phosphoglyceraldehyde, providing a reversible pathway from the pentoses to both hexose and triose. With a little ingenuity a "balance sheet" can be drafted in which 6 moles of glucose 6-phosphate can be oxidatively decarboxylated, with the production of 12 moles of $NADPH + H^+$, 6 moles of CO_2 and 5 moles of fructose 6-phosphate, which is of course readily convertible to glucose 6-phosphate. A "cycle" is thus established for the economical production of reducing equivalents by the oxidation of glucose 6-phosphate. An important point of control is the 6-phosphogluconate dehydrogenase. This enzyme is powerfully inhibited by NADPH, and the reactions do not go forward until NADPH begins to be utilized, and its concentration falls. Note that the production of ribose 5-phosphate is not dependent upon the oxidations.

Interconversions of the Hexoses. The reaction of fructose and mannose with hexokinase and ATP yields the respective 6-phosphate esters. Fructose 6-phosphate is an intermediate of glycolysis. Mannose 6-phosphate is convertible to fructose 6-phosphate by a phosphomannose isomerase similar to the phosphoglucose isomerase relating glucose 6-phosphate to fructose 6-phosphate. In liver, a fructokinase, with ATP, yields fructose 1-phosphate. This is broken down by a specific aldolase to dihydroxyacetone phosphate and glyceraldehyde. The glyceraldehyde, reduced to glycerol, is phosphorylated by glycerokinase with ATP, and the glycerophosphate can be used in lipid biosynthesis or reduced to dihydroxyacetone phosphate, entering the glycolytic pathway. Lack of fructokinase leads to an essentially benign fructosuria. Fructose intolerance caused by genetic lack of the specific aldolase is a serious disease, because the accumulation of fructose 1-phosphate causes inhibition of a variety of enzyme systems. Individuals lacking the aldolase must not receive fructose or sucrose. The old term "levulose" is occasionally used in packaging fructose and is not recognized as a synonym of fructose, with awkward consequences for the aldolase-deficient patient.

The first metabolic product of galactose is galactose 1-phosphate, produced with galactokinase and ATP. The next step is catalyzed by phosphogalactose uridyl transferase:

UDP-glucose + galactose 1-phosphate ⇌
  UDP-galactose + glucose 1-phosphate

Uridine diphosphate glucose epimerase catalyzes the reaction:

UDP-glucose ⇌ UDP-galactose

In this way galactose is brought into the metabolic pathway of glucose. In galactosemia of infants, phosphogalactose uridyl transferase is lacking, resulting in intolerance for lactose and galactose, failure of growth, and cataract formation. Galactosuria is symptomatic of the disorder. Once it is recognized, the consequences are avoided by rigorous exclusion of galactose from the diet. The formation of UDP-galactose from galactose 1-phosphate and UTP by UDP-galactose pyrophosphorylase is a pathway negligible in infant liver and not very significant in adults.

Glycogen Synthesis and Glycogenolysis. The distribution of glycogen in tissues and organs is not uniform. Many tissues, e.g., kidney, adrenal, brain, contain small quantities (0.05 to 0.1 per cent) that are constant except under anoxic conditions. More than half the glycogen in the body is found in voluntary muscle; the concentration in the fed state is 0.6 to 2.0 per cent. In fasting, the amount falls by about 20 per cent. In voluntary muscle, glycogen forms an emergency reserve of fuel in physical activity, providing energy through glycogenolysis and glycolysis before the rate of the blood flow and the oxygen supply are adjusted to the demands of muscular work, and perhaps also in supreme muscular effort. It is replenished during recovery at the expense of the blood sugar. Diaphragm and cardiac muscle contain lesser amounts of glycogen (0.3 to 0.6 per cent). The glycogen of the heart, unlike that of other tissues, increases in fasting. It decreases rapidly in the anoxic working heart, providing a small reserve against oxygen lack. The human liver after an overnight fast contains about 4.5 per cent of glycogen. Infusion of glucose at a rate of 1 g. per kg. per hr. does not increase it beyond six per cent. In a prolonged fast, liver glycogen may fall to one per cent or less. The store of glycogen is used mainly to support the blood glucose, allowing time for the process of gluconeogenesis to accelerate and for the factors restraining glucose utilization to come into play. The glycogen of both muscle and liver is not an inert store, but turns over constantly during phases of feeding and fasting, rest and activity.

Glycogenesis. The synthesis of glycogen begins with the conversion of glucose-6-phosphate to glucose-1-phosphate by phosphoglucomutase (glucose-1,6-diphosphate acting as coenzyme). The enzyme uridine diphosphate glucose pyrophosphorylase catalyzes the synthesis of uridine diphosphate glucose:

UTP + glucose-1-phosphate = UDP-glucose + PP_i.

The formation of UDPG is made essentially irreversible by the hydrolysis of inorganic pyrophosphate set free in the reaction. The enzyme glycogen synthase transfers the active glucosyl of UDPG to the nonreducing end of a branch of glycogen, forming an α-1,4 glucosidic linkage. Repeated transfers build up glycogen by extending the terminal branches. At intervals, the "branching enzyme," an amylo- (α-1,4 → α-1,6) transglucosylase, removes a six or seven-unit portion from the end of a branch and transfers it to form an α-1,6 linkage on a glucose residue near the new end of the branch. Both branches then continue to grow. The uridine diphosphate set free when the glucosyl unit is transferred from UDPG is resynthesized to UTP at the expense of ATP. The net cost of storing a mole of glucose as glycogen is equivalent to the hydrolysis of 2 moles of ATP to 2ADP and 2P_i, less than 6 per cent of the yield of ATP from the oxidation of a mole of glucose to CO_2 and water. Glycogen synthase is a regulated enzyme, existing in a fully active form (synthase I) and in a phosphorylated form (synthase D), dependent for its activity on the presence of glucose-6-phosphate. When there is a demand for glucose, the same protein kinase that activates phosphorylase kinase deactivates glycogen synthase. The dephosphorylation of the enzymes by the appropriate phosphatases activates the synthase, deactivates phosphorylase. In liver or muscle at rest glycogen synthase is mainly turned on and glycogen phosphorylase is mainly turned off, conditions favoring the maintenance of a steady state of the glycogen as well as an increase in the store when an excess of glucose is presented, e.g., during a meal.

Glycogen isolated from rat liver with gentle care always contains protein. Krisman has advanced the hypothesis that native glycogen is a glycoprotein. In *de novo* synthesis of glycogen, the protein is the primer upon which an *initiator glycogen synthase*, with UDPG as substrate, attaches a number of oligosaccharide (α-1,4,-glucan) chains sufficiently long to permit glycogen synthase and branching enzyme to build the new macromolecule.

Glycogenolysis. The breakdown of glycogen in liver and muscle is catalyzed by an enzyme quite different from the hydrolytic digestive enzymes, a glycogen phosphorylase, which cleaves a glucose unit from the nonreducing end of a branch of glycogen:

$$(\text{glucose})_n + H_3PO_4 \rightleftarrows (\text{glucose})_{n-1}$$
$$+ \text{glucose-1-phosphate}$$

The enzyme acts only on α-1,4 glycosidic linkages, and it stops four residues away from a branching point. "Debranching" enzyme, an amylo (α-1,4-α-1,4) glucosyl transferase, transfers the trisaccharide attached to the glucose residue in α-1,6 linkage to another chain, and the glucose residue thus exposed is hydrolyzed by an amylo-α-1,6 glucosidase. Phosphorylase then acts until the next branch point is approached. In phosphorolysis, the energy of the α-1,4 glycosidic bond is conserved in glucose-1-phosphate. This compound is readily transformed to glucose-6-phosphate by the enzyme phosphoglucomutase, and the glucose unit of glycogen is ready to enter the glycolytic or other pathways. *In liver, kidney, and the epithelium of small intestine* a specific glucose-6-phosphatase hydrolyzes the ester, delivering free glucose to the bloodstream. This enzyme is not present in muscle.

Muscle glycogen phosphorylase, comprising about 5 per cent of the soluble muscle protein, is composed of identical subunits (M_r-100,000) and is present as dimers and tetramers. Each subunit contains a molecule of pyridoxal phosphate, acting as a structural component and essential for activity. The inactive form, phosphorylase *b*, may be activated by binding of one AMP to each subunit, or by conversion to the tetramer, phosphorylase *a*, by the phosphorylation of a specific serine residue in each subunit at the expense of ATP. The activation of phosphorylase *b* by AMP is opposed by ATP, which binds at the same site and acts as an inhibitor, and by glucose-6-phosphate. In muscle at rest, almost all the phosphorylase is present in the *b* form, and the breakdown of glycogen is extremely slow. Although the enzyme is reversible, synthesis does not occur by this route because the concentration of glucose-1-phosphate is too low and that of inorganic phosphate is too high, with no means for its removal. When the muscle is stimulated, glycogen breakdown accelerates remarkably, owing to the very rapid conversion of phosphorylase *b* to *a* by the specific enzyme, phosphorylase kinase. When contraction is initiated by a nerve impulse, Ca^{2+} is released and the kinase, which is absolutely dependent upon the concentration of Ca^{2+}, is activated. When stimulation of the nerve stops, phosphorylase kinase is deactivated by the rapid withdrawal of Ca^{2+}, followed by inactivation of phosphorylase *a* by a specific phosphatase.

An alternative activation of the kinase occurs in response to epinephrine. The hormone, arriving at receptors in the muscle membrane, activates an enzyme, adenylate cyclase, which converts ATP into cyclic 3',5'-AMP. This compound activates a protein kinase, which, in its turn, phosphorylates phosphorylase kinase at the expense of ATP. The phosphorylated form of phosphorylase kinase is active at the low Ca^{2+} concentration of resting muscle. It converts phosphorylase *b* to phosphorylase *a* at the expense of ATP, leading to rapid acceleration of glycogen breakdown. Each step involves an amplification of the preceding step, and the entire process occurs in a very short time. The system is self closing. When epinephrine is removed or destroyed, adenylate cyclase becomes inactive, cyclic 3',5'-AMP is hydrolyzed by a phosphodiesterase, protein kinase is dephosphorylated by a phosphoprotein phosphatase, and phosphorylase *a* is converted to phosphorylase *b* by a specific phosphatase.

In the liver, glycogenolysis is more directly dependent upon activation of phosphorylase kinase through the sequence of reactions beginning with adenylate cyclase. In liver, adenylate cyclase is activated mainly by glucagon, which induces maximal activation of adenylate cyclase at much lower concentration than is necessary for activation by epinephrine. Since the secretion of glucagon varies inversely with the rise and fall of blood glucose, the hormone may be regarded as exerting a tonic fine control of glycogenolysis, whereas the effect of epinephrine may be that of demand in an emergency.

The protein kinase that activates phosphorylase kinase also phosphorylates glycogen synthase, inhibiting glycogen synthesis. The two systems are therefore in reciprocal relationship in respect to control of their activity. The enzymes immediately related to glycogen—phosphorylase, glycogen synthase, branching and debranching enzyme and the specific phosphatases and kinases—are closely associated with the glycogen particles in the cell, another circumstance allowing for rapid and close control of glycogen synthesis and breakdown.

Since muscle lacks glucose 6-phosphatase, the breakdown of glycogen in muscle cannot lead directly to restoring blood glucose. (The small proportion of glucose units set free by hydrolysis of the branch points is very likely rapidly phosphorylated inside the cell.) Lactate and pyruvate formed by glycogenolysis and glycolysis readily leave the muscle and pass via the blood to the liver, where they may be resynthesized to glucose. This in turn can reappear as blood sugar and serve to replenish the muscle glycogen. Some of the lactate and pyruvate is taken up by other tissues (e.g., heart, kidney) and oxidized there.

Disorders of Glycogen Metabolism. One or another of the complex of enzymes governing the synthesis and breakdown of glycogen may be absent or defective. In rare instances liver glycogen synthase is absent, so that storage of glycogen cannot occur. The enzyme defect in von Gierke's disease is peripheral to the glycogen complex of enzymes but leads to glycogen accumulation in liver, kidney and intestine. Glucose-6-phosphatase is absent. Glycogen can form, but, since glucose cannot be released, glycogenolysis cannot occur. Both liver and muscle glycogen phosphorylase may be absent, independently. In the absence of muscle phosphofructokinase, both glycogen and hexose monophosphate accumulate, and no energy can be realized from glucose. Deficiency of branching enzyme leads to an amylopectin-like glycogen with very long inner and outer chains. In amylo-1,6-glucosidase deficiency,

the outer chains are missing or very short; there is no real substrate for phosphorylase. In Pompe's disease, all tissues seem to be affected by generalized glycogenosis. The disorder is attributed to a deficiency of α-1,4 glucosidase, an enzyme, possibly associated with lysosomes, that it is assumed would have the effect of breaking very large glycogen molecules into smaller ones, leading to increase in new end groups, i.e., in effective substrate concentration. In disorders of liver glycogen storage, delivery of glucose to the blood is slow or impossible, and the tendency to hypoglycemia and ketosis is marked. The reflex discharge of epinephrine is without effect on the blood sugar, although blood lactate and pyruvate increase. Growth is poor, and an afflicted infant does not thrive. Defects in muscle glycogen storage are attended by muscular weakness and inability to initiate muscular work, underlining the importance of glycogen as a substrate for glycolysis in the anaerobic phase of vigorous muscular activity.

Gluconeogenesis. A 70 kg. man in the fed state may have six per cent of glycogen in his 1800 g. liver, or 108 g. In 35 kg. of muscle, at 0.7 per cent glycogen, he has 235 g. of glycogen. The total store of 343 g., equivalent to about 1400 kcal., would barely support his daily energy needs in a sedentary occupation. During an overnight fast about 20 per cent of muscle glycogen (47 g., 193 kcal.) disappears. Liver glycogen is now about 4.5 per cent; 27 g. (111 kcal. equivalent) has disappeared in support of the blood sugar, which has decreased from the postabsorptive level of 100 mg. per dl. (14 g. in 14 liters of extracellular water) to about 60 mg. per dl. (8.4 g. total in extracellular water). After a week's fast, liver glycogen will have fallen to about one per cent. For many days of continued fasting there is no significant change in blood sugar or liver and muscle glycogen. Experiments in animals have shown that if the liver is removed or sequestered, the blood sugar falls. It falls more rapidly if the kidneys are also removed. In fasting man the liver and kidneys are the sources of the blood glucose. They are synthesizing glucose from non-carbohydrate precursors.

The substrates for gluconeogenesis are pyruvate and lactate (from muscle, red cells, renal medulla, retina, and bone marrow), glycerol (from triacylglycerols), and amino acids (from tissue protein). The conservation of glucose derived from these limited sources for meeting essential needs is secured by making fatty acids nearly the exclusive source of energy during the fast.

The increased oxidation of fatty acids in liver and kidney has additional consequences. (1) It helps to maintain a high ratio of ATP to ADP, furnishing energy for gluconeogenesis. (2) It provides reducing equivalents which, exported from the mitochondria as malate, yield both NADH and oxaloacetate needed in the cytosol. (3) Increased concentration of fatty acid in the cytosol and of acetyl-SCoA in the mitochondria further satisfy the conditions for inhibiting phosphofructokinase, pyruvate kinase, and pyruvate dehydrogenase, and for activating pyruvate carboxylase and fructose-1,6-diphosphate-1-phosphatase. In addition, glucagon, activating adenylate cyclase to increase the concentration of cAMP, promotes the inhibitory phosphorylation of pyruvate dehydrogenase, the activation of phosphorylase, the inhibition of glycogen synthase, and an increase in glucose-6-phosphatase, for which glucocorticoids are permissive.

The steps of glycolysis can now be reversed. A steady supply of phosphoenolpyruvate (PEP) is provided by the action of phosphoenolpyruvate carboxykinase:

$$oxaloacetate + GTP \rightarrow PEP + GDP + CO_2$$

The amount of this kinase and of pyruvate carboxylase is increased in fasting. Their synthesis is dependent upon the action of adrenal glucocorticoids. From PEP to phosphoglycerate are easy, reversible steps. ATP and NADH promote the reduction of phosphoglycerate to phosphoglyceraldehyde and the formation of dihydroxyacetone phosphate. The equilibrium of the aldolase reaction favors fructose-1,6-diphosphate. The activated 1-phosphatase leads to the hexose phosphates and glucose. Since the action of glucokinase is suppressed, there is only net output of glucose.

The energy requirement of gluconeogenesis from lactate may be reckoned from the equation:

$$2 \text{ lactate} + 6 \text{ ATP} \rightarrow \text{glucose} + 6 \text{ ADP} + 6 \text{ P}_i$$

Note that lactate furnishes its own reducing equivalents. For pyruvate, used directly or derived from glucogenic amino acids, the equation is:

$$2 \text{ pyruvate} + 6 \text{ ATP} + 2 \text{ NADH} + 2 \text{ H}^+$$
$$\rightarrow \text{glucose} + 6 \text{ ADP} + 6 \text{ P}_i + 2 \text{ NAD}^+$$

The equivalent energy cost is 12 ATP per mole of glucose. Glycerol pays its own way. It is phosphorylated by glycerokinase:

$$2 \text{ glycerol} + 2 \text{ ATP} \rightarrow 2\alpha\text{-phosphoglycerol} + 2\text{ADP}$$

The product is oxidized:

$$2 \text{ } \alpha\text{-phosphoglycerol} + 2 \text{ NAD}^+$$
$$\rightleftharpoons 2 \text{ dihydroxyacetone phosphate}$$
$$+ 2 \text{ NADH} + 2 \text{ H}^+$$

The overall reaction is:

$$2 \text{ glycerol} + 2 \text{ ATP} + 2 \text{ NAD}^+$$
$$\rightarrow \text{glucose} + 2 \text{ ADP} + 2 \text{ P}_i$$
$$+ 2 \text{ NADH} + 2 \text{ H}^+$$

for a net equivalent yield of 4 ATP.

In man in the postabsorptive state, as liver glycogen is decreasing, the processes of glucogenesis are already getting underway. The most striking signs of this are a rise in plasma alanine, a marked increase in the output of alanine from muscle and a corresponding increase in the uptake of alanine by the liver. The amount of alanine leaving the muscle is greatly in excess of that present in the muscle protein, and it is concluded that alanine is formed by transamination, especially from the branched chain amino acids (Leu, Ileu, Val), to pyruvate derived from glycogen or blood glucose. Early in fasting plasma alanine accounts for about one-half the splanchnic extraction of amino acids. Glucose derived from alanine in the liver may be used again to form alanine in muscle. There is thus an *alanine cycle,* which appears to be a device for transferring the nitrogen of the branched-chain amino acids from muscle to liver. The corresponding keto-acids are oxidized in the muscle. In the traffic of amino acids from the muscle, glutamine is also conspicuous. It is utilized by the gut, but mainly by the kidney, since in addition to being glucogenic it is a source of urinary ammonia. As fasting is prolonged, the rate of carbohydrate utilization by muscle falls, and the alanine output is diminished. The plasma alanine falls, and the supply of alanine becomes rate limiting for hepatic glucogenesis. By this time, the processes leading to conservation of body protein and carbohydrate are in full swing, fat mobilization has accelerated, and the body is obtaining more than 90 per cent of its energy from the oxidation of fat.

It is important to realize that about one-half of the glucose formed per day in fasting man is derived from pyruvate and lactate produced by tissues *obliged* to use glucose (e.g., red cells and others already noted). The remainder, coming from amino acids and glycerol, and mostly required by the brain, must be strictly rationed.

Regulation of the blood sugar. In the postabsorptive state in man the blood glucose lies in the range of 90 to 110 mg. per dl., and in fasting the concentration falls to 59 to 70 mg. per dl. Blood glucose is not constant but may normally swing between extremes of 50 to over 150 mg. per dl. in the course of a day's events, depending upon meals, physical activity and states of excitement. A number of devices operate to return the blood glucose to the characteristic concentrations noted above. Glucose is removed from the blood by all tissues. Replenishing the carbohydrate supply by a meal leads to storage of glucose as glycogen in liver, muscle and in adipose tissue, conversion of excess glucose into fatty acids in liver and adipose tissue and increased oxidation. These events are reflected in the rise and subsequent fall of the blood glucose, and in a rise of the RQ toward 1.0, indicative of increased utilization of glucose. Assimilation of glucose by the liver is a function mainly of the blood glucose concentration and the status of the liver enzymes. At concentrations of glucose exceeding 100 mg. per dl. the liver extracts glucose from the blood. This capability of the liver is a function of the duration of fasting and of diet. The activity of hepatic glucokinase falls during a fast or during dietary regimens low in carbohydrate. The activity increases quickly in response to a carbohydrate meal and may be considerably increased in response to diets high in carbohydrate or when most of the daily caloric requirement is taken at a single meal rich in carbohydrate. These events are to some degree independent of insulin, which can, however, diminish hepatic glucose output. It accelerates glycogen synthesis by increasing the amount of the active independent form of glycogen synthase, and promotes fatty acid synthesis from carbohydrate by means not yet clearly established. Assimilation of glucose by the intestine, the kidneys and the brain is independent of insulin and is a function of the concentration of glucose in the blood. The passage of glucose into voluntary muscle and adipose tissue requires insulin. It is the failure of these two large organs to assimilate glucose that accounts for the prolonged high blood glucose level of the diabetic subject after a meal. Some of the glucose intolerance is due to glucagon, which sustains a high hepatic output of glucose in insulin deficiency. In the normal subject an increase of plasma insulin in response to the rise in blood glucose during a meal insures the removal of glucose by the replenishment of muscle and adipose tissue glycogen, by glucose oxidation (reflected in a rise in RQ) and by conversion of glucose to fat.

After the assimilation of glucose from a meal is completed, continuing peripheral utilization results in a fall in blood glucose, usually below the preprandial level. Glucose begins to leave the liver, possibly because the fall in the blood sugar excites an increased output of glucagon, which, working through hepatic adenylate cyclase and cyclic AMP, causes acceleration of glycogenolysis and inhibition of glycogen synthesis. As the blood sugar falls, insulin secretion rate falls, and the rate of peripheral utilization of glucose diminishes. Even while hepatic glycogen is far from depleted, gluconeogenesis begins and accelerates. The supply of amino acid substrate for gluconeogenesis increases as peripheral tissue protein is mobilized under the influence of increased secretion of adrenocortical hormones. (In adrenalectomized or hypophysectomized animals, in which mobilization of protein for gluconeogenesis is slow, the rate of depletion of liver glycogen in fasting is much greater than normal.) Net lipolysis in adipose tissue increases, plasma glycerol and free fatty acids increase, and fat begins to make up an increasing fraction of the energy supply of the tissues. The blood sugar, over a period of hours, settles to the steady state typical of fasting, reflecting the balance between gluconeogenesis and continuing but limited glucose utilization.

In summary, the factors favoring disposal of glucose are (1) high plasma concentration of glucose, (2) the pattern of cellular enzymatic activity determined by dietary status and habit and (3) insulin. Factors favoring glucose mobilization are (1) low plasma glucose concentration, (2) glucagon and (3) the supply of substrate for gluconeogenesis. Factors limiting peripheral glucose utilization are (1) low plasma glucose concentration, (2) increased plasma free fatty acids and muscle tissue fatty acids and (3) increase in secretion of growth hormone.

In response to emergency the reflex discharge of epinephrine from the adrenal medulla leads to rapid glycogenolysis in liver and muscle, causing a brisk increase of blood glucose, lactate and pyruvate, and free fatty acids. Lactate and pyruvate are taken up by the liver and other tissues, oxidized in part, and in part converted to glucose. The free fatty acids disappear quickly as net lipolysis in adipose tissue slows in response to the rise in glucose. The blood glucose falls more slowly, in part because the epinephrine-induced glycogenolysis in muscle leads to a marked temporary increase in glucose-6-phosphate, and glucose assimilation is slow because muscle hexokinase is strongly product inhibited. It should be noted that stimulation by epinephrine is a *preparation* for activity. The stimulated resting muscle is well oxygenated (epinephrine is a peripheral vasodilator) and has a high ATP/ADP ratio, so that there is an effective restraint on phosphofructokinase. Hexose monophosphate accumulates. If the initial excitement is followed by physical activity then the consequent increase in the concentration of ADP, activating phosphofructokinase, finds an ample supply of substrate ready for glycolysis. Very shortly thereafter, glucose uptake is accelerated.

In addition to insulin, glucagon, the glucocorticoids, growth hormone and epinephrine, the thyroid hormone, through its effects on metabolic rate, influences the blood sugar. In hypothyroidism the depressed metabolic rate is reflected in a slowing of glucose absorption from the intestine, a decreased rate of utilization of glucose and low fasting blood sugar (due perhaps to a decreased rate of gluconeogenesis). In hyperthyroid states the rate of absorption of glucose is accelerated, but the rate of removal of glucose from the blood is also increased. In fasting, the liver glycogen is depleted much more quickly than normal, and since the hyperthyroid individual may be in marked negative nitrogen balance, there is much greater substrate for gluconeogenesis than usual, and the fasting blood sugar remains higher than normal. Enhanced sensitivity to catecholamines may be responsible in part for these phenomena.

In a normal individual, fasted overnight, the taking of 1 g. per kg. of glucose by mouth is followed by an increase in blood glucose from an initial 70 to 90 mg. per dl. to a maximum of 140 to 150 mg. per dl. in 1 hour, and a fall to or slightly below the initial concentration in 2 to 2½ hours. In the diabetic individual the initial blood glucose concentration may be high or in the normal range; it rises after oral intake of glucose to concentrations well over 150 mg. per dl., and the return to the initial level of blood glucose may be long delayed. Intolerance to glucose may also occur in individuals who have been on low carbohydrate diets. This quickly disappears with normal adaptation of the appropriate enzymes, so that a second glucose tolerance test is usually normal. The rate of disposal of glucose may be reduced in liver disease. Reduced glucose tolerance is also often seen in hyperactivity of the adrenal cortex and of the pituitary.

CHEMISTRY AND METABOLISM OF LIPIDS

Chemistry

The class of lipids is defined as those compounds in animal tissues that are soluble in organic solvents. This group of mainly hydrocarbon substances is heterogeneous. The simplest of the lipids are the fatty acids, monocarboxylic acids of the type $CH_3(CH_2)_nCOOH$, where n may be 0, 2, 4, 6, 8, etc., in steps of two carbons, from acetic acid, CH_3COOH, to acids of 24 to 40 carbon atoms. In animal fats, including those of man, palmitic acid (C-16) and stearic acid (C-18) are the members of greatest interest in this series of saturated fatty acids. In addition to these, a group of monounsaturated fatty acids is also important:

palmitoleic acid: $CH_3(CH_2)_5CH = CH(CH_2)_7COOH$

oleic acid: $CH_3(CH_2)_7CH = CH(CH_2)_7COOH$

These four saturated and unsaturated fatty acids, in human and most animal fats, make up more than 90 per cent of the component fatty acids. These acids are rarely found free in the tissues or the blood. In the cells, in the course of their metabolism, they are usually present as fatty acyl CoA derivatives. In the blood they are transported from depots to tissues bound to serum albumin as "free" or "unesterified"

fatty acids (FFA or UFA respectively). Binding to serum albumin is essential to the release of fatty acids from the depots and equally essential for their easy uptake into tissues.

The polyunsaturated fatty acids, linoleic (Δ9, 12 octadecadienoic acid):

$$CH_3(CH_2)_4CH = CHCH_2CH = CH(CH_2)_7COOH$$

linolenic (Δ9, 12, 15 octadecatrienoic acid):

$$CH_3CH_2CH = CHCH_2CH = CHCH_2CH$$
$$= CH(CH_2)_7COOH$$

and arachadonic (Δ5, 8, 11, 14 eicosatetraenoic acid):

$$CH_3(CH_2)_3CH_2CH = CHCH_2CH = CHCH_2CH$$
$$= CHCH_2CH = CH(CH_2)_3COOH$$

are of great interest because of their supposed effect of lowering plasma cholesterol and because they are precursors of the prostaglandins. These three acids are described as essential fatty acids, but linolenic and arachadonic acid can be synthesized from linoleic acid, which is the only truly essential fatty acid.

Fatty acids of four to ten carbon atoms, minor component acids in many fats, are prominent only in milk fats.

Only the lower members of the series, C-2 to C-8, have any appreciable solubility in water. The melting point increases regularly with increasing chain length; the higher fatty acids, C_{16} and greater, are solid at room temperature (20C.). Unsaturation lowers the melting point: oleic acid (Δ9, C-18) is liquid at 20C. These acids all share the reactions characteristic of the carboxyl group: they can form esters and salts. The salts with Na^+ and $K+$ are water soluble, and are called *soaps*. With divalent cations, Ca^{2+}, Mg^{2+}, etc., the salts are weakly ionized, insoluble, forming the curd characteristic of the reaction of soaps in hard waters. The unsaturated fatty acids have the reactions characteristic of the carbon-carbon double bond. (1) In the presence of an appropriate catalyst (Ni) they can add hydrogen. This is the reaction used to form solid cooking fats from vegetable oils. (2) Halogens (Br_2; I_2) are readily taken up at the double bond. The iodination of fats is used as a means of measuring their degree of unsaturation. (3) The double bond is subject to attack by oxygen or by ozone. The reaction leads to cleavage of the molecule, with the formation of fatty aldehydes. These have the unpleasant odors associated with the *rancidity* of fats. The fatty aldehydes are inhibitors of some enzymatic processes in cells. In the living organism these processes are suppressed by the action of antioxidants, e.g., the tocopherols (vitamin E).

The next important class of the lipids are esters of the polyhydric alcohol, glycerol, with fatty acids:

$$
\begin{array}{ll}
\text{H}_2\text{COH} & \text{R}_1\text{COOH} \\
| & \\
\text{HCOH} + \text{R}_2\text{COOH} \rightleftarrows \\
| & \\
\text{H}_2\text{COH} & \text{R}_3\text{COOH}
\end{array}
\qquad
\begin{array}{l}
\text{H}_2\text{COOCR}_1 \\
| \\
\text{HCOOCR}_2 + 3\text{H}_2\text{O} \\
| \\
\text{H}_2\text{COOCR}_3
\end{array}
$$

The triacylglycerols, or the *neutral fats,* comprise the principal combined form of the fatty acids in the body. They are the major constituents of the fat depots and are found in significant concentration in most tissues except the brain. The equation above suggests (R_1, R_2, R_3) that triglycerides are randomly composed of different fatty acids, and this is in fact the case. The component fatty acids in a neutral fat rarely form "pure" triglycerides, e.g., tristearin or tripalmitin. In some vegetable oils in which a single fatty acid, oleic, makes up more than 80 per cent of the whole, triolein must be a major component. The triglycerides comprise the storage form of the fatty acids in the body. These hydrocarbon acids are fuel, yielding about 9 kcal. per g. In an average adult male there may be 15 kg. of triacylglycerol. This could support his energy requirements (at 3,000 kcal. per day) for 45 days.

The neutral fats are insoluble in water. Their melting point is a function of their composition: the greater the degree of unsaturation of the constituent fatty acids, the lower the melting point. The reactions occurring at the double bond of unsaturated fatty acids can occur in the triglycerides as well: They can be hydrogenated, iodinated and attacked by oxygen. In addition, the triglycerides can be hydrolyzed, yielding glycerol and free fatty acids. This reaction, carried out in alkali, yields *soaps:*

$$
\begin{array}{l}
\text{H}_2\text{COOCR}_1 \\
| \\
\text{HCOOCR}_2 + 3\ \text{KOH} \rightarrow \\
| \\
\text{H}_2\text{COOCR}_3
\end{array}
\qquad
\begin{array}{ll}
\text{H}_2\text{COH} & \text{R}_1\text{COO}^-\text{K}^+ \\
| & \\
\text{HCOH} + \text{R}_2\text{COO}^-\text{K}^+ \\
| & \\
\text{H}_2\text{COH} & \text{R}_3\text{COO}^-\text{K}^+
\end{array}
$$

One measure of the character of a mixture of triglycerides (any fat) is the *saponification number:* the number of milligrams of KOH required to hydrolyze 1 g. of fat. For butter, this number is high, since the short-chain fatty acids predominate, and there will be more molecules per gram of fat. For beef fat (palmitic and stearic acid (C-16, C-18) predominating) the number is low, since there must be fewer molecules per gram of fat. The iodine number of a fat is also used to characterize it. This is the number of grams of iodine taken up by 100 g. of fat. The higher the number, the more double bonds, the greater the degree of unsaturation.

Esters of fatty acids with alcohols of 16 carbon atoms or more are called waxes. The cholesterol esters of blood and other tissues are waxes. Other examples are beeswax, sperm oil (mainly cetyl palmitate) and lanolin, or wool fat.

The next important class of lipids are the glycerophospholipids. They are composed of 1 mole of glycerol, 2 moles of fatty acid, one of which is usually unsaturated, 1 mole of phosphoric acid, and 1 mole of any of three nitrogenous bases: the amino acid serine ($\text{HOCH}_2\text{CHNH}_2\text{COOH}$), its product of decarboxylation, ethanolamine ($\text{HOCH}_2\text{CH}_2\text{NH}_2$) or the N-trimethyl derivative of ethanolamine, choline ($\text{HOCH}_2\text{CH}_2\text{N}^+(\text{CH}_3)_3$). Less frequently, inositol, the cyclic hexitol, replaces the base. The simplest glycerophospholipid is phosphatidic acid:

$$
\begin{array}{l}
\text{H}_2\text{COOCR}_1 \\
| \\
\text{HCOOCR}_2 \\
| \\
\text{H}_2\text{CO}-\text{PO}_3\text{H}_2
\end{array}
$$

If the phosphate is esterified with choline, the product is a lecithin, the most common type of glycerophospholipid:

$$
\begin{array}{l}
\text{H}_2\text{COOCR}_1 \\
| \\
\text{HCOOCR}_2 \\
\quad\quad\quad\ \ \text{O} \\
| \quad\quad\quad \| \\
\text{H}_2\text{CO}-\text{PO}-\text{CH}_2\text{CH}_2\text{N}^+(\text{CH}_3)_3 \\
| \\
\text{O}-
\end{array}
$$

The class of glycerophospholipids called cephalins contain ethanolamine or serine esterified to phosphate in the same manner as choline. The inositol-containing glycerophospholipids are important constituents of the lipids of brain. It is usual now to describe the various glycerophopholipids as derivatives of phosphatidic acid: phosphatidyl choline; phosphatidyl ethanolamine, etc. Phosphatidic acid is an intermediate in the synthesis of triglycerides: The phosphate is hydrolyzed off and the 1, 2-diacylglycerol reacts with a mole of fatty acyl-SCoA to form triacylglycerol and HSCoA.

The glycerophospholipids are distributed throughout the body as essential constituents of cell membranes, including the membranes of organelles such as mitochondria. They are constituents of the plasma lipoproteins, and in this respect they play a role in lipid transport. They are also prominent constituents of the myelin of brain and nerves. The presence of phosphate and a base in most of the glycerophospholipids confers both cationic and anionic properties upon them. They are appreciably soluble in water as well as in organic solvents, and this undoubtedly plays a part in their function in membranes. An enzyme, *phospholipase A,* found in certain snake venoms and in many tissues, hydrolyzes the fatty acid in the β position of lecithin to yield *lysolecithin,* a strong detergent. When this happens in the blood of a victim of snake bite, lysolecithin is released from the plasma lipoproteins and causes extensive hemolysis. A *lysophosphatidase,* present in many tissues as well as pancreas, removes the second fatty acid from lysolecithin. *Phosphatidase C* hydrolyzes the base, leaving phosphatidic acid. *Phosphatidase D* removes base and phosphate, leaving an α, β-diacylglycerol.

Plasmalogens resemble the glycerophospholipids but have on the α-carbon of the glycerol, a long-chain α, β-unsaturated ether, which on hydrolysis yields an aldehyde. Their function is unknown.

The *sphingolipids* are characterized by the presence of the base, *sphingosine:*

$$CH_3(CH_2)_{12}—CH$$
$$\|$$
$$CH—CH—CH—CH_2OH$$
$$|\quad\quad|$$
$$OH\quad NH_2$$

When a long-chain saturated fatty acid is present in amide linkage on the amino group, the resulting compound is a *ceramide:*

$$CH_3(CH_2)_{12}—CH$$
$$\|$$
$$CH—CH—CH—CH_2OH*$$
$$|\quad\quad|$$
$$OH\quad NH$$
$$|$$
$$RC=O$$

The addition of phosphoryl choline to the primary alcohol group (*) yields *sphingomyelins,* which together with glycerophospholipids, are important constituents of myelin. The presence of a hexose (most often galactose) in glycosidic linkage with the primary alcohol (*) of ceramide yields compounds called *cerebrosides.* The gangliosides are formed similarly, except that they contain more than 1 mole of carbohydrate: 1 mole of N-acetylgalactosamine and 1 mole at least of N-acetylneuraminic acid (sialic acid). These lipids, containing no phosphate, are also called *glycolipids.*

There is a large class of lipids built upon the repeating unit, isoprene:

$$CH_3$$
$$|$$
$$CH_2=C—CH=CH_2$$

This class of compounds is called *terpenes* and includes camphor, rubber, carotenes and vitamin A. A typical member of the class is β-carotene, a precursor of vitamin A.

The side chains of the tocopherols (vitamin E), of vitamin K, and of ubiquinone, Coenzyme Q, are built up of isoprene units.

Steroid is a generic name for a diverse group of condensed ring hydrocarbon compounds that are derivatives of cyclopentanoperhydrophenanthrene (sterane). The important animal steroids are cholesterol, the bile acids, vitamin D, the sex hormones and the adrenocortical hormones. The designation of the rings and the numbering system are best illustrated by the parent hydrocarbon of cholesterol, cholestane. The ring system is essentially planar and in all naturally

Cholestane

occurring steroids, rings B and C and C and D are attached *trans.* In consequence, the angular methyl groups at carbons 10 and 13 and the hydrogen atom at carbon 8 extend above the plane of the ring, and the hydrogen atoms at carbons 9 and 14 extend below the plane of the rings. Substitutents *cis* to the methyl group at carbon 10 (above the plane of the ring) are designated β; those extending below the plane of the ring are designated α.

Cholesterol, the sterol of all animal cells, has a 3-β-hydroxyl group and a double bond between carbons 5 and 6. It crystallizes from ether as waxy rhomboidal plates. It is readily soluble in organic solvents but insoluble in water. In the tissues and the blood, it occurs both as the free alcohol and esterified to fatty acids. It is an important constituent of membranes, and it is present in high concentration in nervous tissue. It serves as the precursor of the other steroids of the

β-carotene

body. Cholesterol gives rise to 7-dehydrocholesterol, having an additional double bond at carbon 7, which is converted to cholecalciferol, vitamin D_3, by the action of sunlight on the skin. The plant sterol, ergosterol, identical in ring structure to 7-dehydrocholesterol but

Cholesterol

having a double bond in the side chain at carbon 24 and an additional methyl substituent at carbon 24, is also converted by irradiation with ultraviolet light to ergocalciferol, vitamin D_2.

The bile acids are derived from cholesterol in the liver. The side chain is shortened to five carbon atoms, and the rings are saturated. The parent hydrocarbon is cholanic acid. Human bile contains mainly cholic acid,

Cholanic acid

3α, 7α, 12α-trihydroxycholanic acid, and chenodeoxycholic acid, 3α, 7α-dihydroxycholanic acid. These compounds are conjugated, through the carboxyl group, with the amino group of glycine ($NH_2 \cdot CH_2COOH$) or taurine ($NH_2 \cdot CH_2CH_2 \cdot SO_3H$). The bile acids and their salts are highly polar substances, lower surface tension, act as detergents and assist in emulsifying lipid in the intestine, and form molecular complexes with fatty acids, aiding in their absorption from the intestine.

The structures and relationships of the steroid hormones are dealt with in the section on hormones.

Metabolism of Lipid

Digestion of lipid occurs mainly in the small intestine. A gastric lipase with a pH optimum near neutrality may be significant in infants, but in the stomach, lipid is merely set free by the proteolytic rupture of cell membranes. In the small intestine, digestion is accomplished by the combined action of the bile and of lipases in the pancreatic juice. The bile acids, glycocholic and taurocholic acid, are ionized at the neutral or slightly acid pH of the duodenum and act as emulsifying agents, dispersing insoluble lipid into fine particles with an extended interface with the aqueous medium. Triacylglycerols are attacked by pancreatic

lipase which, in combination with a colipase, has a pH optimum of about 6. The action of lipase leads to a mixture of free fatty acids, glycerol, diacylglycerols and monoacylglycerols. The pancreas secretes a prophospholipase A, which is converted to phospholipase A by tryptic action. This enzyme sets free one fatty acid from phosphatidylcholine and other phosphatides, forming lysophosphatidyl compounds, which, like the monoacylglycerols, are strongly polar and contribute to the emulsification and dispersion of the lipids. Other enzymes (phosphodiesterase, phosphatase) assist in the hydrolysis of the phospholipids. A group of esterases of broad specificity hydrolyze esters of short chain fatty acids and of cholesterol. The bile acids and other detergents disperse the free fatty acids in the form of micelles, which can pass into the epithelial cells. The micelles provide a medium for the absorption of other lipids and of lipid-soluble substances such as the fat-soluble vitamins and their precursors. Hydrolysis of the lipids need not be complete. It is estimated that about 40 per cent of ingested triacylglycerols are absorbed as glycerol and free fatty acids, 3 to 10 per cent as intact triacylglycerols and the rest as diacylglycerols and mainly monoacylglycerols. The bile salts absorbed with the fatty acids and attendant lipids are returned to the liver via the bloodstream and are secreted again into the bile.

The water-soluble products of lipid digestion (glycerol; fatty acids of less than 12 carbon atoms, choline, etc.) are absorbed into the portal bloodstream and pass directly to the liver. Both neutral fat and phospholipids are reconstituted in the epithelial cells of the small intestine and passed into the lymph as lipoprotein particles called chylomicrons, about 1 μ in diameter (83 per cent triacylglycerol, 7 per cent phospholipid, 8 per cent free and esterified cholesterol, and 2 per cent protein). Triacylglycerols appear in the lymph even when the meal consists exclusively of free C-16 and C-18 fatty acids. The chylomicrons enter the blood through the thoracic duct. They are thus generally distributed to both adipose tissue and the liver.

Numerous factors affect the digestion and absorption of lipid. The three most important are the bile, the pancreatic secretion and the functional integrity of the intestinal mucosa. In the absence of bile, hydrolysis of lipid occurs extensively, but there is little or no absorption, and the feces contain large amounts of free fatty acids. The stools are bulky and clay colored because of the absence of bile pigment. When pancreatic secretion is defective, neither digestion nor absorption occurs, and the bulky stools contain unhydrolyzed lipid. In celiac disease in children and sprue in adults, biliary and pancreatic function may be intact, but absorption of lipid is incomplete because of defective metabolism of the epithelial cells. In all these instances steatorrhea leads to loss of essential lipid-soluble substances, the polyunsaturated fatty acids and the fat-soluble vitamins.

The lipids of the feces are made up normally of a small amount of unabsorbed dietary lipid, of lipid secreted by the intestine itself and of the lipids of the intestinal bacteria.

Blood Lipids and Lipid Transport. In normal man in the postabsorptive state, blood plasma contains about 500 mg. per dl. of total lipid. Of this, triacylglycerols comprise 160 mg. per dl., phosphoglycerols, 160 mg. per dl., and cholesterol, 180 mg. per dl. (about two-thirds as ester). Unesterified (free) fatty acid (about 0.3 mmoles per liter is present bound to albumin. All of the lipids of the plasma are present as constituents of lipoproteins. It is only in this way that the insoluble lipid substances are dispersed and dissolved in the aqueous phase of the plasma. The lipoproteins can be separated by ultracentrifugation and are classified according to their densities. Very low density lipoproteins (VLDL, density, 1.006 to 1.019) contain about 60 per cent triacylglycerol and 9 per cent protein. Low density and high density lipoproteins (LDL and HDL, respectively) contain only about 15 per cent triacylglycerol, much more free and esterified cholesterol 20 to 48 per cent, and more protein. The proportion of phospholipid in the lipoproteins is about twice in HDL (48 per cent) what it is in the others. The HDL, about three per cent of the plasma proteins, migrate electrophoretically with the α-globulins. The VLDL and LDL, about five per cent of the plasma proteins, migrate with the β-globulins. The lipoproteins are formed and secreted by the liver and intestine.

Isolation and characterization of the apoproteins of the lipoproteins has illuminated their functional relationships. Apo-A_1 and Apo-A_2 are the main proteins of the HDL. Apo-B is the main protein of the chylomicrons and of VLDL and LDL. Apo-C_1,C_2,C_3 are associated with HDL, VLDL, and chylomicrons, and exchange freely among them. Apo-E, "arginine-rich" protein, is found in HDL. Apo-C_1 is an activator of the lecithin : cholesterol acyl-transferase (LCAT) which plays a part in the collection of cholesterol from peripheral tissues by the HDL. Apo-C_2 is a potent activator of the lipoprotein lipase found in the wall of capillaries of heart, lung, and adipose tissue.

After a meal, chylomicrons appear in the plasma, rising to a maximum at the peak of absorption and disappearing as lipid is taken up by the peripheral tissues, mainly the adipose tissue, and the liver. There is a concomitant rise and fall of plasma lipoproteins, particularly the VLDL. The plasma nonesterified fatty acids, which may have doubled or tripled in concentra-

tion during the fasting period, decrease rapidly, since net synthesis of triacylglycerol in the adipose tissue is taking place.

As the lipid content of the plasma increases, the normally clear fluid becomes milky (lactescent) because of reflection of light by the particles of the chylomicrons and very low density lipoproteins. Clearing of the lipemic plasma is brought about by lipoprotein lipase, released from cell walls by heparin, activated by Apo-C_2, which specifically hydrolyzes the triacylglycerols of chylomicrons and VLDL. The glycerol goes to the liver where it may be used again. Adipose tissue cells lack glycerol kinase and cannot use glycerol. The fatty acids that are set free combine with plasma albumin and are readily taken up by the adipocytes where they are resynthesized to triacylglycerols.

The lipoprotein lipase associated with adipose tissue has a low affinity for its substrate and is sensitive to insulin, increasing in activity in the fed state, and rapidly losing activity in fasting, as the plasma insulin falls. The lipoprotein lipase of heart and other nonadipose tissues has a high affinity for its substrate and is more active in fasting than it is in the fed state. The two enzymes are therefore nicely adapted to their respective functions of storage and utilization of fatty acids. The 3-phosphoglycerol used for synthesis of triacylglycerols must be formed by reduction of dihydroxyacetone phosphate, derived from glucose. *The storage of neutral fat in adipose tissue therefore depends on the availability of glucose.*

It is now known that the LDL arise from the VLDL as the latter are stripped of neutral fat. The LDL thus become major carriers of cholesterol in the plasma. They are taken up by specific receptors located in crypts on the surface of, for example, fibroblasts and smooth muscle cells. The LDL are assimilated by endocytosis, fused with lysosomes, and destroyed. The protein is hydrolyzed, and cholesterol is set free. The free cholesterol inhibits the committed step in cholesterol synthesis, catalyzed by 3-hydroxy-3-methyl-glutaryl-SCoA reductase, and activates acyl-SCoA : cholesteryl-acyltransferase, which reesterifies the cholesterol. The LDL therefore deliver cholesterol to tissues that require it and help to regulate cholesterol synthesis in the same tissues. The genetic disorder, familial hypercholesterolemia, occurs in individuals homozygous for a defect resulting in the absence of specific LDL receptors.

In a healthy 70 kg. man, lipid makes up not less than 10 per cent of the body weight. It is present mainly as triacylglycerol, in adipose tissue located beneath the skin, in the abdominal cavity, in the intermuscular spaces and near or around certain organs such as the kidney. Although the liver plays an active role in lipid oxidation, biosynthesis and transport, it normally contains no more than four to five per cent of fat, not usually visible in the light microscope in sections stained for fat. The composition of the body fat is such that it is liquid at the temperature of the fat depot: subcutaneous fat therefore is more highly unsaturated than that surrounding the internal organs. The body fat also has a composition characteristic of the species, resulting from the nature of the diet, saturation or unsaturation of dietary fat, possibly selective utilization, and biosynthesis from carbohydrate. These processes may be overwhelmed by feeding large amounts of a particular fat, as in a peanut-fed hog, in which the fat becomes highly unsaturated, or in cattle in the finishing lots, in which a low fat, high carbohydrate diet of grains leads to biosynthesis of a "hard" relatively saturated fat. The body fat serves as insulation against cold and against mechanical shock and injury. It is also a major energy reserve. A man containing 15 kg. of stored triacylglycerol has an energy store of 141,000 kcal., which could support him through many days of fasting. An obese individual, with 80 kg. of triacylglycerol, has stored away 750,000 kcal. of excess energy. The adipose tissue is normally not a passive store. The daily cycle of feeding and fasting leads to frequent mobilization of fat from the depots and to its replenishment both by dietary fat and by biosynthesis from carbohydrate.

The activity of the adipose tissue is reflected in the behavior of the free fatty acids (FFA) of the plasma. In the postabsorptive state their concentration is low, about 0.3 mmoles per liter. During an overnight fast, the blood sugar falls, plasma insulin falls, and the rate of supply of glucose to the peripheral tissues decreases. A hormone-sensitive lipase in the adipocytes is activated by an increase in the secretion of glucagon, catecholamines, glucocorticoids, and growth hormone. The balance between triacylglycerol synthesis, which depends on the glucose supply, and lipolysis, shifts in favor of release of fatty acids and glycerol. The concentration of the plasma FFA increases to about 0.6 mmoles per liter. The turnover rate also increases to 139 mg. (0.54 mmoles) per min. About 30 per cent is oxidized at once, yielding 0.4 kcal. per min., or about 50 per cent of the non-protein calories required by a 70 kg. man at rest. After 3 days of a fast the plasma FFA plateau at about 1.6 mmoles per liter. The turnover rate increases with the concentration, and the oxidation of FFA is yielding over 90 per cent of the required calories. After a meal, blood glucose and plasma insulin increase, the net synthesis of triacylglycerols in the adipose tissue is reestablished, and the plasma FFA quickly fall.

Fatty Acid Oxidation. Most of the tissues of the body oxidize fatty acids as an important source of energy. The process takes place in mitochondria, but it is preceded by activation of the fatty acids in the cytosol to form the fatty acyl CoA derivative:

$$R\ (CH_2)_nCOOH + HSCoA + ATP \rightleftharpoons$$
$$R\ (CH_2)_n\ CO\text{-}SCoA + AMP + PP_i$$

The subsequent hydrolysis of inorganic pyrophosphate makes the reaction irreversible. The enzyme is acyl CoA synthase. The activated fatty acid cannot enter mitochondria directly; its entrance is mediated by carnitine, β-hydroxy, γ-trimethylamino-butyric acid,

$$(CH_3)_3{}^+NCH_2CHOHCH_2COOH$$

The enzyme palmitoyl CoA carnitine palmitoyl transferase catalyzes the formation of fatty acyl carnitine. This compound enters the mitochondrion, where a like transferase reverses the transfer and fatty acyl CoA is reconstituted.

The fatty acid then is oxidized by a repeated cycle of four enzymatic steps.

1. Dehydrogenation by the flavin enzyme, fatty acyl CoA dehydrogenase:

$$RCH_2CH_2CO\text{-}SCoA + E\text{-}FAD \rightleftharpoons$$
$$RCH = CHCO\text{-}SCoA + E\text{-}FADH_2$$

2. The 2,3-*trans*-unsaturated fatty acyl CoA is hydrated by enoyl CoA hydratase, forming L-3-hydroxyacyl CoA:

$$RCH = CHCOSCoA + H_2O \rightleftharpoons$$
$$RCHOH\text{-}CH_2COSCoA$$

3. L-3-hydroxyacyl CoA is dehydrogenated by the NAD^+-requiring enzyme L-3-hydroxy CoA dehydrogenase:

$$RCHOH\text{-}CH_2COSCoA + NAD^+ \rightleftharpoons$$
$$R\text{-}CO\text{-}CH_2COSCoA + NADH + H^+$$

4. The 3-ketoacyl CoA is cleaved by the enzyme β-ketothiolase to form acetyl CoA and the fatty acyl CoA two carbon atoms shorter:

$$RCOCH_2COSCoA + HSCoA \rightleftharpoons$$
$$RCOSCoA + CH_3COSCoA$$

Three sets of the four enzymes, with specificity respectively for long, intermediate, and shortchain fatty acids, are present in the mitochondria. In seven turns of the cycle, palmitoyl CoA is oxidized to 8 moles of acetyl CoA, with the formation of 7 moles of reduced flavoprotein and 7 moles of NADH. Reoxidation of the coenzymes yields, respectively, 14 and 21 moles of

ATP. Oxidation of acetyl CoA by the citric acid cycle yields $8 \times 12 = 96$ ATP. The balance sheet of the complete oxidation is:

$$CH_3(CH_2)_{14}CO\text{-}SCoA + 23\ O_2 + 131\ P_i + 131\ ADP \rightarrow CoA + 16\ CO_2 + 146\ H_2O + 131\ ATP$$

More than 40 per cent of the potential energy of palmitic acid is recovered in newly synthesized ATP, counting the initial investment of 2 equivalents of ATP in the activation step. The process of degradation of the fatty acid to acetyl CoA is known as β-oxidation. The same steps are used, reversibly, in mitochondria, to lengthen or shorten fatty acids by two carbon atoms.

Acetoacetate and β-hydroxybutyrate. The mobilization of FFA in fasting furnishes a readily utilizable substrate to all tissues not strictly dependent on carbohydrate. In addition, as fasting is prolonged, the liver produces increased amounts of two simple products of partial oxidation of fatty acids, acetoacetate and β-hydroxybutyrate. Acetoacetate, in some circumstances, decomposes to acetone and CO_2. This has led to all three metabolites being known, incorrectly, as ketone bodies.

The first step in the synthesis of acetoacetate is catalyzed by acetyl-SCoA acetyl transferase:

$$2\ CH_3CO\text{-}SCoA \rightleftharpoons CH_3COCH_2CO\text{-}SCoA + HSCoA$$

Acetoacetyl-SCoA is combined with another mole of acetyl-SCoA to yield 3-hydroxy,3-methyl-glutaryl-SCoA (HMG-SCoA):

$$\underset{\displaystyle OH}{\overset{\displaystyle CH_3}{HOOC\text{-}CH_2\text{-}\overset{|}{\underset{|}{C}}\text{—}CH_2CO\text{-}SCoA}}$$

HMG-SCoA is cleaved by a specific lyase, to acetoacetate and acetyl-SCoA.

Acetoacetate is reduced to β-hydroxybutyrate by an NAD^+-linked mitochondrial β-hydroxybutyrate dehydrogenase:

$$CH_3COCH_2COOH + NADH + H^+ \rightleftharpoons CH_3CHOHCH_2COOH + NAD^+$$

The free compounds are released to the blood. They are readily taken up by tissues such as muscle. β-Hydroxybutyrate is reoxidized to acetoacetate, and this is activated by the enzyme thiophorase and succinyl coenzyme A:

acetoacetate + succinyl CoA $\rightleftharpoons$

acetoacetyl CoA + succinate

Reaction of acetoacetyl CoA with thiolase and HSCoA

yields acetyl CoA for oxidation by the tricarboxylic acid cycle.

The rate of production of acetoacetate is inversely related to the amount of liver glycogen. In overnight fasting, the plasma ketone bodies may be only 0.1 mmoles per liter. In prolonged fasting, when the liver glycogen is depleted, the rate of ketone body production rises to about 1.1 mmoles per min., and it just slightly exceeds the rate of oxidation; the concentration in plasma may be about 7 mmoles per liter. In the steady state of a long fast the brain adapts to utilize β-hydroxybutyrate to cover more than half its energy expenditure, but it never loses its dependence on glucose. In normal man, as much as 120 to 130 g. of ketone bodies may be oxidized per day.

With the depletion of liver glycogen and an increased rate of gluconeogenesis the flow of carbon from the citric acid cycle toward glucose limits the capability of oxidizing acetyl-SCoA arising from the oxidation of fatty acids. The flow of fatty acid carbon is directed toward acetoacetate and β-hydroxybutyrate. In these circumstances carnitine (the means of access to the mitochondria) becomes rate limiting for the oxidation of fatty acids.

In diabetic ketoacidosis the rate of production of ketone bodies is, like that of long-fasting obese subjects, about 1.1 mmoles per min., but the rate of oxidation is severely depressed, to about 0.2 mmoles per min., and the plasma ketone bodies may rise to over 12 mmoles per liter. Acetoacetate and β-hydroxybutyrate are excreted in the urine, in amounts as much as 100 g. per day. Sodium required for their partial neutralization is lost in the urine. The resulting acidosis, complicated further by dehydration arising from the obligatory loss of water in the large volume of urine high in solutes (urea, glucose, ketone bodies), leads to coma and eventually to death.

Fatty Acid Synthesis. In the daily cycle of deposition and mobilization the fat stores are replenished both by dietary fat and by fatty acids synthesized from carbohydrate and amino acids. In man, lipogenesis takes place mainly in the liver, not simply by reversal of the steps of oxidation in the mitochondria but by means of a distinct enzyme system in the cytosol. The reactants are: acetyl SCoA, malonyl SCoA and, for both reductive steps in the synthesis, the coenzyme NADPH. Synthesis is accomplished upon a multienzyme particle catalyzing, in reverse order, each of the steps of β-oxidation, but not releasing the product until the new 16-carbon fatty acid is fully formed. The growing fatty acid is retained upon a small protein, the acyl carrier protein (ACP), combined with 4' phosphopantetheine:

$$ACP-O-\overset{\overset{\textstyle O}{\|}}{\underset{\underset{\textstyle OH}{|}}{P}}-O-CH_2-\overset{\overset{\textstyle CH_3}{|}}{\underset{\underset{\textstyle CH_3}{|}}{C}}-\overset{\overset{\textstyle OH}{|}}{\underset{\underset{\textstyle H}{|}}{C}}-\overset{\overset{\textstyle O}{\|}}{C}$$

$$HS-CH_2CH_2NH-OC-CH_2CH_2-NH$$

which is the CoA-like prosthetic group of the ACP.

Malonyl CoA is formed by the biotin enzyme, acetyl CoA carboxylase:

$$CH_3COSCoA + HCO_3^- + ATP \rightleftharpoons ADP$$
$$+ P_i + HOOCCH_2COSCoA$$

This is the rate-limiting step in fatty acid biosynthesis. The enzyme is activated by citrate or isocitrate. Their concentration in the cytosol increases in the presence of an abundant carbohydrate supply.

The steps of the biosynthesis are as follows:

1. Acetyl-SCoA + HSACP $\rightleftharpoons$ acetyl-SACP + HSCoA.
2. Acetyl-SACP + HS-Enz $\rightleftharpoons$ acetyl-S-Enz + HSACP.
3. Malonyl-SCoA + HSACP $\rightleftharpoons$ malonyl-SCAP + HSCoA.
4. Malonyl-SACP + acetyl-S-Enz $\rightleftharpoons$ acetoacetyl-SACP + HS-Enz + CO_2.
5. Acetoacetyl-SACP + NADPH + H^+ $\rightleftharpoons$ D-β-hydroxybutyryl-SACP + $NADP^+$.
6. D-β-hydroxybutyryl-SACP $\rightleftharpoons$ crotonyl-SACP + H_2O.
7. Crotonyl-SACP + NADPH + H^+ $\rightleftharpoons$ butyryl-SACP + $NADP^+$.

The cycle begins anew with:

8. Butyryl-SACP + malonyl-SACP $\rightleftharpoons$ β-keto-caproyl-SACP + CO_2 + HSACP. Seven turns of the cycle yield palmitoyl-SACP, which is released from the complex by a deacylase.

The acetyl SCoA required for the synthesis arises in the cytosol from citrate by the action of citrate lyase:

$$Citrate + ATP + HSCoA \rightarrow acetyl-SCoA$$
$$+ oxaloacetate + ADP + P_i$$

When the carbohydrate supply is abundant and the level of ATP is high, the action of isocitric dehydrogenase is restrained, citrate accumulates, diffuses from the mitochondria and supplies acetyl-SCoA for the synthesis. Oxaloacetate is reduced to malate, which returns to the mitochondria and re-enters the tricarboxylic acid cycle. Acetyl SCoA arising from oxidation of pyruvate is in this way transferred to the cytosol. NADPH is provided mainly by the two oxidative steps of the phosphogluconate pathway.

Synthesis of triacylglycerols and phosphoglycerols.

The essential intermediate for the synthesis is L-glycerol-3-phosphate, formed either by reduction of dihydroxyacetone phosphate or by phosphorylation of glycerol by glycerokinase. The first step of triacylglycerol synthesis, and of the synthesis of some phospholipids, is the formation of phosphatidic acid:

$$2 \text{ Acyl-SCoA} + \text{L-3-phosphoglycerol} \rightarrow$$
$$\text{L-phosphatidic acid} + 2HSCoA$$

The phosphatidic acid next loses its phosphate by hydrolysis, and the resulting L-1,2-diacylglycerol reacts with a third molecule of acyl-SCoA to form the triacylglycerol and HSCoA.

Phosphatidylethanolamine is synthesized by the reaction of a 1,2-diacylglycerol with the activated intermediate, cytidine diphosphoethanolamine:

$$\text{CDP-ethanolamine} + \text{L-1,2-diacylglycerol} \rightarrow$$
$$\text{phosphatidylethanolamine} + \text{CMP}$$

Phosphatidylcholine is formed from phosphatidylethanolamine by transfer of methyl groups from S-adenosylmethionine. Dietary choline is also utilized directly. After phosphorylation by a kinase and ATP, the phosphocholine reacts with cytidine triphosphate to form cytidine diphosphocholine, and the activated phosphocholine group is transferred to a 1,2-diacylglycerol to form phosphatidyl choline.

The phospholipids are essential constituents of the membranes, internal and external, of all cells. In this role they are not static structural components but turn over at varying rates, rapid in some cells (e.g., kidney cortex), much more slowly in others. This continuing breakdown and resynthesis is entirely local. The plasma phospholipids arise in the liver and are taken up again by the liver, evidently playing some essential part in the production and secretion of the plasma lipoproteins and in the balance of traffic in lipids between the liver and the peripheral tissues. In this process the lecithins (phosphatidylcholine) play a critical part. In the absence of a dietary source of methyl groups (that is, on a diet low in protein of poor quality) and of dietary choline, animals develop a fatty liver, accumulating up to 30 or 40 per cent of triglyceride, far in excess of the normal accumulation seen even in the starving animal. The condition is relieved by choline, or by protein of high quality containing enough methionine to provide methyl groups sufficient to support the synthesis of needed choline. The effect of choline or methionine on dietary fatty liver is called a *lipotropic* action. Fatty livers occur in other circumstances, on high cholesterol diets, or in diabetes, when the catabolism of fat is very intense and the liver is in effect presented with a continuous excess of substrate, and in injury to the liver by poisons such as alcohol, carbon tetrachloride or white phosphorus. The injured liver cells appear to lose quite early their capacity for synthesizing and secreting lipoproteins. Triglyceride accumulates as a first consequence of the injury, which may be followed by the disorganization of other cellular processes. The fatty liver of choline deficiency has not been satisfactorily explained. It is possible that this too might reflect a failure of some aspect of the synthesis and secretion of the lipoproteins.

The *sphingolipids* (sphingomyelins; cerebrosides; gangliosides) are actively and continuously synthesized in the tissues in which they are found, especially in the nervous system. They are normally degraded to ceramide by a variety of hydrolases, and the net concentration remains constant. Nine instances are now known of a hereditary deficiency of one or another specific hydrolase. One or more of the sphingolipids accumulates, especially in nervous tissue, giving rise to neurologic disturbances that develop in early infancy and soon lead to death. In Niemann-Pick disease, sphingomyelin accumulates in brain, spleen, liver and kidney, in the absence of a sphingomyelinase that normally cleaves the compound to sphingosine and phosphocholine. In Tay-Sachs disease, absence of hexoseaminidase A leads to accumulation of the ganglioside galactosyl, N-acetyl galactosyl, glucosyl ceramide in brain and spleen. In Gaucher's disease, absence of β-glucosidase results in glucosylceramide accumulation in brain and in reticuloendothelial cells of liver, spleen and bone marrow. Most of these deficiencies can be detected during fetal life by enzyme assay of cells obtained from samples of the amniotic fluid.

Cholesterol. The sterol characteristic of animal tissues originates both in the diet and by synthesis in the body. Cholesterol is easily absorbed during normal digestion. The usual daily dietary intake is 0.2 to 0.3 g. The liver synthesizes about 1.0 to 1.5 g. per day, and about 0.5 g. is made in adrenal cortex, testis, skin, intestine and in the smooth muscle of arterial walls. This endogenous production may be partly suppressed by dietary cholesterol. In man, this effect does not seem to be substantial.

The serum cholesterol varies widely, from 150 to 250 mg. per dl. About two-thirds of serum cholesterol is esterified. A plasma enzyme, phosphatidyl choline : cholesterol acyl transferase, catalyzes transfer of an unsaturated fatty acid from the 2-position of phosphatidyl choline to the 3-hydroxyl of cholesterol. All of the plasma lipoproteins contain cholesterol, but the principal carriers are the LDL, and the HDL. Recent work suggests that the HDL may be critically important in collecting cholesterol and transporting it to the liver for disposal. Plasma cholesterol is not much affected by varying the cholesterol intake but may be lowered considerably (along with the plasma lipids in general) by limiting the intake of animal fats and increasing the proportion of more highly unsaturated fats in the diet. In atherosclerosis the lesions in the walls of the blood vessels accumulate cholesterol and other lipids, and it is thought that the occurrence and progress of atherosclerosis are correlated with conditions in which there are sustained high concentrations of blood cholesterol: diets rich in animal fat; diabetes; lipoid nephrosis; hypothyroidism.

The biosynthesis of cholesterol in liver and other tissues begins with acetyl-SCoA. The critical intermediate is 3-hydroxy, 3-methyl glutaryl-SCoA, and the committed step of the synthesis (feedback inhibited by cholesterol) is the reduction of HMG-SCoA to mevalonic acid:

$$HOCH_2 - CH_2 - \overset{\overset{\displaystyle OH}{|}}{\underset{\underset{\displaystyle CH_3}{|}}{C}} - CH_2COOH$$

Six 5-carbon units derived from mevalonic acid condense to form cholesterol. An important intermediate in the process is the linear hydrocarbon squalene, which folds to form the four condensed rings of the first true steroid in the synthetic pathway, lanosterol.

Direct loss of cholesterol from the body may occur by secretion into the small intestine and into the bile. A major route of utilization occurs by conversion of cholesterol into the bile acids, their conjugation with taurine or glycine, and their secretion in the bile. They are in part reabsorbed, in an enterohepatic circulation that also involves cholesterol, organic iodine-containing compounds, bile pigments and a variety of other difficulty soluble substances. Portions of all of these are not reabsorbed but pass on into the large bowel to be excreted in the feces. The concentration of bile acids in the liver exerts a feedback control upon the conversion of cholesterol to bile acids. If the level of cholesterol increases in turn, it moderates its own synthesis by acting upon HMG-SCoA reductase.

NITROGEN METABOLISM

The cooking of foods usually denatures the proteins, making them more susceptible to attack by the enzymes of the gastrointestinal tract. This attack begins in the stomach. The chief cells of the gastric glands secrete the proenzyme pepsinogen, which in the presence of gastric HCl undergoes partial hydrolysis to yield the active proteolytic enzyme, pepsin. This in turn acts on pepsinogen: the process of activation is autocatalytic. The active enzyme ($M_r = 33,000$) is an acidic protein, with an isoelectric point of about pH 1 and an optimum pH of 2 to 3. Pepsin is an endopeptidase, attacking interior linkages of the polypeptide chain. Its specificity is directed mainly to attack upon the aromatic amino acids, phenylalanine, tyrosine and tryptophan, hydrolyzing the bond involving the carboxyl group. It acts somewhat less readily upon bonds involving the carboxyl group of leucine and the acidic amino acids. Since food spends only a limited time in the stomach, peptic digestion proceeds mainly to the stage of large polypeptides. In the absence of sufficient HCl to maintain a pH of 2 to 3 in the stomach, for example, in the achlorhydria of pernicious anemia, peptic digestion cannot occur.

The array of proteolytic enzymes secreted by the pancreas is fully capable of carrying out the entire process of protein digestion. Trypsinogen is converted to trypsin by hydrolysis of the NH_2-terminal hexapeptide Val-(Asp)$_4$-Lys by the enzyme enterokinase, secreted by the intestinal cells. Trypsin is in turn responsible for the activation of the chymotrypsinogens and of procarboxypeptidase A and B. Trypsin hydrolyzes bonds involving the carboxyl groups of lysine and arginine. The chymotrypsins, like pepsin, hydrolyze bonds involving the carboxyl groups of the aromatic amino acids. Carboxypeptidase A, an exopeptidase, hydrolyzes aromatic or aliphatic amino acids at the carboxyl end of polypeptide chains. Carboxypeptidase B releases only carboxyl-terminal arginine or lysine residues. These two enzymes together carry on the further degradation of the peptides set free by both trypsin and chymotrypsin. The result of the combined actions of the pancreatic enzymes on proteins and polypeptides is a host of small peptides and some free amino acids.

The terminal stages of protein digestion probably take place in the cells of the intestinal mucosa, which are rich in peptidases. Among the more important of these are the aminopolypeptidases, enzymes of broad specificity capable of setting free amino acids successively from the amino-terminal end of the polypeptide chain. In addition there is a variety of dipeptidases. These enzymes complete the breakdown of proteins to free amino acids.

The absorption of amino acids from the intestinal lumen is normally rapid and complete. The process requires energy, and it involves a number of transport systems with specificities for different amino acids. The mechanisms of the active transport are not finally established. There is in adults no absorption of intact protein or even of large polypeptides. If the pancreatic enzymes are lacking, digestion of protein is incomplete, and much undigested protein is found in the feces.

The amino acids, and possibly a few simple peptides, enter the portal blood and pass to the liver and other tissues. They are quickly removed from the plasma. Liver, kidney and intestinal mucosa are most active in this respect, other tissues less so, in proportion to the magnitude and rate of protein turnover in the different organs.

The amino acids are (1) incorporated into newly synthesized protein after mixing with the "pool" of free amino acids in the extracellular fluid and the tissues; (2) utilized as precursors of other amino acids and of nonprotein nitrogenous constituents of various tissues; and (3) deaminated or transaminated, after which the carbon skeletons may be used for gluconeogenesis or for replenishing the intermediates of the tricarboxylic acid cycle, for fatty acid synthesis or for oxidation and energy production. The nitrogen may be used in the synthesis of other amino acids, or it may be excreted as urea or as ammonium salts.

In human adults in good health, a steady state of the body composition is maintained, and as much nitrogen is excreted in urine and feces as is taken in the food: the individual is in nitrogen balance. In infants and growing children there is steady gain of body substance, with net retention of nitrogen: positive N balance. Net loss of body nitrogen—negative N balance—is seen (1) in fasting; (2) during insufficient intake of food, especially of carbohydrate; (3) when the diet is lacking in one or more of the essential amino acids; (4) in conditions of stress or after injury; (5) in debilitating illness; (6) in insulin deficiency; (7) in a number of vitamin deficiencies affecting intermediary metabolism.

The normal condition of nitrogen balance is not static; there is a continuing interchange of dietary and body nitrogen such that in any 24 hour period only about one half of the nitrogen in the urine is derived from dietary protein. This does not reveal the whole extent of the continuing processes of protein synthesis and degradation in the body. From studies with labeled amino acids it is estimated that in man about 0.8 g N per kg. per day is incorporated into newly synthesized protein. For a 70 kg. adult in nitrogen balance, about $70 \times 0.8 \times 6.25 = 350$ g. of protein are synthesized and degraded per day. The dietary intake of proteins (35 to 100 g. per day) provides only a fraction of the amino acids involved in the daily turnover of protein.

Not all of the body proteins take part equally in the continuing metabolism of protein. The collagen of some tendons, and the matrix of parts of bones and teeth, may last an individual lifetime without replacement. In other types of connective tissue, and in basement membranes of cells, the rates of repair and replacement of collagen and elastin may be significant. In the liver there is a continuous process of synthesis and export of the plasma proteins, but there is also a diurnal waxing and waning of the concentration of specific proteins as the rhythms of feeding and fasting, of plethora and scarcity, require alterations in the complement of enzymes needed for specific tasks such as glycogen synthesis, accelerated delivery of glucose to the blood or gluconeogenesis. Other tissues share in lesser degree the dynamic response of the liver to changing conditions. In every tissue it is the enzymes, as the tools of adaptation, that take part most extensively in the turnover of protein. It is not known how the body sums up all of the individual acts of protein synthesis and breakdown to achieve nitrogen balance.

Protein Synthesis. The process begins in the nucleus, where the information is stored in DNA as a sequence of deoxyribonucleotides. In response to appropriate signals, a portion of DNA is exposed, the helix is unwound, and a complementary copy of one strand of the DNA is made under the influence of a DNA-dependent RNA synthetase. The required substrates for this process are the complete mixture of the ribonucleotide triphosphates, ATP, GTP, UTP and CTP. The products are inorganic pyrophosphate and a polyribonucleotide, a messenger RNA comprising (1) a sequence of nucleotides that facilitates the initial association of mRNA with the ribosomes; (2) a sequence of bases, which, as triplets (codons), can be translated into the amino acid sequence of the protein to be synthesized; (3) a sequence of bases containing at least one triplet that denotes the end of the message. The synthesis of mRNA (in fact, of *any* RNA) in the nucleus in this way is known as *transcription*.

The process of *translation* takes place in the rough endoplasmic reticulum of the cells. It involves the ribosomes (a kind of biochemical machine tool), messenger RNA and an appropriate array of activated amino acids. These are synthesized by a group of 20 amino-acyl-tRNA synthases, each of them specific for one of the amino acids. These are cytoplasmic enzymes, which carry out the following reactions:

1. Amino acid + ATP + enzyme $\rightleftharpoons$ amino-acyl-adenylate-enzyme + pyrophosphate.
2. Amino-acyl-adenylate-enzyme + tRNA $\rightarrow$ amino-acyl-tRNA + enzyme + AMP.

The first reaction is made virtually irreversible by the hydrolysis of the inorganic pyrophosphate by a pyrophosphatase. The activated amino acid is attached to the 3' position of the ribose in the terminal adenylate residue at the 3' end of the tRNA. Each tRNA carries a sequence of three bases (an anticodon) that is complementary to the base sequence in mRNA (the codon) corresponding to that amino acid. For example, the

codon for methionine is AUG. The anticodon for methionyl tRNA should be CAU, and the two will pair in anti-parallel fashion as follows: tRNA: 3' - UAC - 5'; mRNA: 5' - AUG - 3'. In this way, each activated amino acid carried upon its specific tRNA finds its correct place on the messenger. This association exemplifies the process of translation of the message of the base sequence of mRNA into the amino acid sequence of the protein. The process is consummated upon the ribosome.

Ribosomes are tiny but complex structures containing several sizes of molecules of RNA and about 70 different proteins. In eukaryotic cells the ribosomes have a mass of about 4×10^6 daltons and a Svedberg number (related to their rate of sedimentation in the ultracentrifuge) of 80S. Ribosomes dissociate into a 60S particle, 2.7×10^6 daltons, and a 40S particle, 1.3×10^6 daltons.

The amino-terminal amino acid in polypeptide chain synthesis is always methionine. A special $tRNA^{Met}_F$ is used. (When methionine appears elsewhere in the polypeptide chain a different $tRNA^{Met}_M$ is required.) Protein synthesis starts when, (a) in the presence of three small protein initiation factors, and GTP, mRNA binds near its 5' end to the 40S subunit; (b) Met-$tRNA^{Met}_F$ binds to the 40S subunit, and to the appropriate initiating codon (AUG) of the mRNA, and (c) the 60S subunit attaches to complete the 80S ribosome, releasing the initiation factors, GDP and P_i. The next amino-acyl-tRNA, assisted by an elongation factor (EF-1), finds its place on the mRNA adjacent to the Met-tRNA. Another mole of GTP is hydrolyzed to GDP and Pi in this step. The place in the ribosome occupied by the Met-tRNA is called the P (for peptidyl) site; that adjacent to it (in the 3' direction of the mRNA) is called the A (for amino-acyl-tRNA) site. When the A site is occupied, the amino-acyl group at the P site is transferred by ribosomal peptidyl transferase to the amino group of the amino-acyl-tRNA at the A site. Since the transferred group is already activated, no further energy is required in the formation of the peptide bond. The P site is now occupied by the deacylated $tRNA^{Met}_F$. It is displaced in a reaction involving elongation factor (EF-2) and requiring the hydrolysis of GTP. At the same time the newly formed peptidyl-tRNA at the A site is translocated, still bonded to the mRNA, to the P site of the ribosome. The cycle of elongation can then be repeated with the next incoming amino-acyl-tRNA. The ribosome steadily works its way toward the 3' end of the mRNA, and the polypeptide chain of the protein grows on the ribosome.

In prokaryotes and in mitochondria the principle of operation of protein synthesis is the same, but there are differences in detail. The ribosomes are lighter (70S) and their constituent subunits are 30S and 50S. The initiating amino-acyl-tRNA is N-formylmethionyl-tRNA$^{Met}_F$. The methionine is N-formylated after the acyl-tRNA is synthesized. Formyltetrahydrofolic acid is the coenzyme. There are minor differences in detail in the number and kind of the initiating, elongating and terminating factors.

The synthesis of the protein is terminated when one of three codons (UAA, UAG, UGA) is reached at the end of the message. Since there is no amino-acyl-tRNA corresponding to these codons the A site remains unoccupied. In the presence of GTP and a release factor, the completed protein is released from the P site, the vacant tRNA is discharged, GTP is hydrolyzed and the ribosome dissociates, falling away from the messenger.

Each mRNA can accommodate a number of ribosomes at once, according to its length. These polyribosomes, strung on the mRNA like spaced beads on a string, synthesize many molecules of the protein simultaneously. The process continues for the lifetime of the mRNA. In bacterial cells, the turnover of messenger is very rapid; in mammalian cells, some mRNA has a relatively long life.

Some antibiotics act by inhibiting protein synthesis. Chloramphenicol inhibits ribosomal peptidyl transferase (cycloheximide also does this, but only in animal cells). Tetracycline prevents attachment of amino-acyl-tRNA to the ribosome. Puromycin, in both animal and bacterial cells, acts as a false amino-acyl-tRNA, accepts the peptidyl chain and terminates growth of the polypeptide.

Diphtheria toxin inactivates elongation factor 2 in animal cells by catalyzing the transfer of EF-2 to NAD$^+$, replacing the nicotinamide at its glycosidic linkage with the ribose with EF-2. The enzyme is one of the most potent toxins known, and its action dramatizes the importance of continuing protein synthesis in animal cells.

Several features of the process of protein synthesis may be emphasized:

1. The equivalent of four high energy phosphate bonds is required to synthesize a single peptide bond. This is in addition to the energy requirement for the synthesis and maintenance of tRNA, MRNA and the ribosomes, but since many more molecules of protein are synthesized than of the various RNA's, the principal energy cost may be laid to peptide bond synthesis. If a 70 kg. adult synthesizes 350 g. of protein per day, he incorporates 56 g. N or 4 g.-atoms N per day. This requires the expenditure of 16 moles of high energy phosphate. At a P/O ratio of 3, the oxygen used

will be 5.33 g.-atoms or 2.665 moles per day, or at 22.4 liters per mole, 59.74 liters O$_2$ per day. At an average RQ of 0.82 the caloric equivalent of oxygen is 4.825 kcal. per liter. The total energy expenditure for protein synthesis is 4.825 × 59.74 or 278 kcal. per day. This is 15 per cent of the 1800 kcal. required to support the basal metabolism of our subject. The high cost of synthesis of the peptide bond reflects the fact that this is an ordered process in which two particular amino acids are joined in a specified sequence.

2. The process yields the primary sequence of the protein, which, upon being set free, must adopt a conformation determined by that sequence. All other changes in the protein : iodination, glycosylation, phosphorylation, hydroxylation, carboxylation, are post-translational events.

3. The ribosomes are general tools for the synthesis of the polypeptide prescribed by any mRNA. Neither is necessarily species specific for the process.

4. Old or damaged proteins are not repaired but are replaced by total synthesis of new proteins. The process requires that the complete mixture of amino acids be available for activation. This explains why the absence of any essential amino acid results in negative N balance—the failure to maintain a net steady state of the body protein. It explains why restricted intake of a single essential amino acid—e.g., methionine—is rate limiting for growth and why a single large dose of an amino acid is nearly completely catabolized.

5. A sequence of three nucleotide bases in mRNA (a codon) specifies the position of an amino acid in a polypeptide. Since there are four bases (A;G;U;C) in RNA, there are $4^3 = 64$ possible codons. Three of these function as signals for termination, as noted above; the other 61 form the code words for the amino acids, as shown in Table 4-5, of the genetic code. The code is the same for all species. There is more than one codon for many of the amino acids; the code is degenerate. The first two bases of a codon are very specific; the same amino acid may be coded although the third base is different. A mutation may cause a base to change so that a terminator codon is generated; such a "nonense" codon causes premature chain termination and failure to synthesize a given protein. In other mutations, the sequence of a triplet may alter in such a way that a different amino acid is specified. This may alter the properties of the resulting protein, for example hemoglobin S, of sickle cell anemia, in which Glu at position 6 of the β-chains is replaced by Val. In many instances, mutations involving the third base of a codon lead to no change at all, since the code is degenerate. A different tRNA is not required for each codon. It is found that some tRNAs

TABLE 4-5. Genetic Code

First Position 5' end	Second position U	C	A	G	Third Position 3' end
U	Phe	Ser	Tyr	Cys	U
	Phe	Ser	Tyr	Cys	C
	Leu	Ser	Term*	Term	A
	Leu	Ser	Term	Trp	G
C	Leu	Pro	His	Arg	U
	Leu	Pro	His	Arg	C
	Leu	Pro	Gln	Arg	A
	Leu	Pro	Gln	Arg	G
A	Ile	Thr	Asn	Ser	U
	Ile	Thr	Asn	Ser	C
	Ile	Thr	Lys	Arg	A
	Met	Thr	Lys	Arg	G
G	Val	Ala	Asp	Gly	U
	Val	Ala	Asp	Gly	C
	Val	Ala	Asp	Gly	A
	Val	Ala	Asp	Gly	G

* Term = terminator codons

can recognize several codons belonging to a single amino acid.

6. The synthesis of protein can take place in all nucleated cells. In addition, mitochondria contain DNA that specifies some of their proteins. These proteins are synthesized within the mitochondria, using mitochondrial ribosomes, tRNAs and mRNAs, together with the appropriate enzymes and factors resembling those of prokaryotes, quite distinct from the components of the protein-synthesizing system of the cell.

Amino Acid Metabolism. The amino acids serve many purposes other than the synthesis of protein. Only ten amino acids are required for normal growth: Arg, His, Ile, Leu, Val, Thr, Lys, Met, Phe and Trp. In human adults, only the last eight are essential. All of the rest of the amino acids can be derived from these ten if they are furnished in sufficient amounts in a diet supplying enough calories from carbohydrate and fat and including the mineral elements and vitamins. If ^{15}N is fed to an animal as ammonium salt, glycine or any amino acid other than lysine, the isotope can eventually be found in the α-amino group of all the amino acids except lysine. Apart from the precursor, the isotope is found in greatest concentration in glutamate and aspartate, in the amidine nitrogens of arginine, and in urea. One of the processes by which this distribution of nitrogen takes place is transamination. The transaminases are a group of amino-transferases, requiring pyridoxal phosphate as coenzyme, that catalyze the transfer of α-amino nitrogen between an α-keto acid and an α-amino acid, one of which must

be a dicarboxylic acid. Thus, alanine may be synthesized from glutamate by the glutamate-pyruvate transaminase (GPT):

$$CH_3COCOOH + HOOCCH_2CH_2CHNH_2COOH \rightleftharpoons$$
$$CH_3CHNH_2COOH + HOOCCH_2CH_2COCOOH$$

Similarly, glutamate may be synthesized from aspartate and α-keto-glutarate by the glutamate-oxaloacetate transaminase (GOT). The equilibrium constant of these enzymes is near unity, the interchange requires little energy, and the reactions are easily reversible. Note that pyruvate is derived from glucose and that oxaloacetate and α-ketoglutarate are intermediates of the Krebs cycle. These two transaminases are most prominent in many tissues, but many others exist, making possible the passage of α-amino nitrogen from many amino acids into glutamate and aspartate. Glutamate may also be synthesized by the action of glutamate dehydrogenase on α-ketoglutarate and ammonia:

$$NH_4^+ + HOOCCH_2CH_2COCOOH + NADH$$
$$+ H^+ \rightleftharpoons HOOCCH_2CH_2CHNH_2COOH + NAD^+$$
$$+ H_2O$$

The amides of the two dicarboxylic acids, glutamine and asparagine, are formed from ammonia and the respective amino acid at the expense of ATP. A γ-glutamyl phosphate is the intermediate in one instance ($ADP + P_i$ are products); in the other, a Δ-aspartyl-adenylate is the intermediate. Ammonia exchanges with the adenylate, and the products are AMP and PP_i.

The glycolytic pathway is a source of the carbon of serine as well as that of alanine. The precursor is 3-phosphoglycerate. This may be oxidized, by an NAD-requiring enzyme, to 3-0-phosphohydroxypyruvate, which by transamination with glutamate, yields 3-0-phosphoserine. Hydrolysis by a phosphatase yields the free amino acid. By another route, 3-phosphoglycerate is transformed to 2-phosphoglycerate, which on hydrolysis yields glycerate. This is oxidized to hydroxypyruvate (NAD^+ is required), which is transaminated to yield serine.

Serine is a source of glycine. The hydroxymethyl group is transferred to tetrahydrofolic acid to form 5,10 methylene THF, glycine and water. Decarboxylation of serine yields ethanolamine: $H_2NCH_2CH_2OH$. This may be transaminated to yield glycolaldehyde, $HCOCH_2OH$, and this in turn is oxidized to glycolic acid and then to glyoxalic acid: $HCOCOOH$. Glycine can be formed by transamination.

Serine collaborates with methionine in the synthesis of cysteine. Methionine must first transfer its methyl group to a suitable acceptor, after activation of the methyl group. This is done by the formation, with ATP, of S-adenosyl-methionine, in which the sulfur is attached to the 5' carbon of the ribose. The activated methyl may be passed to guanidoacetic acid to form creatine, to norepinephrine to form epinephrine, to phosphatidylethanolamine to form phosphatidylcholine, or it may be used in the methylation of selected bases of rRNA and tRNA, or of DNA. The compound left after methyl transfer, S-adenosyl-L-homocysteine, is hydrolyzed to L-homocysteine and adenosine. An enzyme, cystathionine synthase, catalyzes the condensation of serine with homocysteine to form cystathionine:

$$\underset{\underset{\text{NH}_2}{|}}{\text{HOOC CHCH}_2\text{CH}_2\text{SCH}_2}\underset{\underset{\text{NH}_2}{|}}{\text{CHCOOH}}$$

which is hydrolyzed by cystathionase to form cysteine and homoserine. Both enzymes require pyridoxal phosphate. Methionine thus contributes only its sulfur in the synthesis of cysteine.

Several inborn errors of cysteine synthesis are recognized. In homocystinuria the defect is in cystathionine synthetase. In cystathionuria the cleavage enzyme, cystathionase, is defective. In cystinuria the defect is not in the synthesis of the amino acid but in the renal tubular transport of cystine, lysine, arginine and ornithine.

Proline and ornithine arise by way of the γ-semialdehyde of glutamate. Loss of water between the aldehyde and the α-amino group forms the five-membered ring; the double bond at the nitrogen is reduced by NADH. If the γ-semialdehyde transaminates with another molecule of glutamate, ornithine and α-ketoglutarate are formed:

$$\text{HOOCCHNH}_2\text{CH}_2\text{CH}_2\text{CHO}$$
$$+ \text{HOOCCHNH}_2\text{CH}_2\text{CH}_2\text{COOH} \rightleftarrows$$
$$\text{HOOCCHNH}_2\text{CH}_2\text{CH}_2\text{CH}_2\text{NH}_2$$
$$+ \text{HOOCCOCH}_2\text{CH}_2\text{COOH}$$

Phenylalanine is converted to tyrosine by the action of phenylalanine hydroxylase. The reaction is mediated by a folic acid-like coenzyme, tetrahydrobiopterin:

Phe + O_2 + H_4-biopterin → Tyr + H_2O + H_2-biopterin.
H_2biopterin + NADH + H^+ → H_4biopterin + NAD^+

In phenylketonuria the oxygenase is defective or lacking. The concentration of phenylalanine in plasma is high, and the amino acid and some of its metabolites—phenylpyruvate, phenyllactate, and phenylacetate—are found in large amounts in the urine. Severe mental retardation is associated with the defect, but this may be avoided if phenylketonuria is detected early in infant life, by restricting the dietary intake of phenylalanine. In these circumstances tyrosine becomes an essential amino acid and must be provided in adequate amounts.

The genetic defect is carried as an autosomal recessive in about two per cent of the population, and it has an incidence of about one in 10,000 births.

The question whether histidine is an essential amino acid for adults has not been settled. On diets free of histidine, adults remain in nitrogen balance for the relatively short period of observation. It is noticed, however, that the concentration of histidine in plasma falls by as much as 50 per cent in a short period of deprivation, suggesting that in a long-term experiment histidine would prove to be essential.

Certain of the amino acids are precursors of important constituents of the tissues. Creatine (methylguanidoacetic acid) is formed from glycine, arginine and methionine. Guanidoacetic acid is formed by transfer of the amidine group from arginine to glycine:

$$\underset{\underset{\text{}}{}}{\overset{\text{NH}}{\overset{\|}{\text{H}_2\text{N}-\text{C}}}}-\text{NH(CH}_2)_3\text{CHNH}_2\text{COOH}$$
$$+ \text{H}_2\text{N}-\text{CH}_2\text{COOH} \rightarrow$$
$$\overset{\text{NH}}{\overset{\|}{\text{H}_2\text{N}-\text{C}}}-\text{NHCH}_2\text{COOH}$$
$$+ \text{H}_2\text{N(CH}_2)_3\text{CHNH}_2\text{COOH}$$

This is the rate-limiting step. Transamidinase activity in liver decreases in fasting, and is suppressed by dietary creatine. Guanidoacetic acid, as noted above, is methylated at the expense of S-adenosylmethionine. About two per cent of the total body creatine is excreted in the urine each day as creatinine. The anhydride arises from phosphocreatine in muscle by loss of phosphate. The rate of the process is a function of the total creatine, which is in turn a function of the total mass of muscle. In adults the daily urinary creatinine is sufficiently constant to be a reliable measure of the completeness of 24 hour urine collections. Increase or decrease of the muscle mass is reflected in a rise or fall of the urinary creatinine. Rapid loss of muscle mass, and certain diseases of muscle, are characterized by failure to retain creatine, which appears as such in the urine. Of the total muscle creatine, 70 to 80 percent is present as phosphocreatine.

Glycine is utilized in the synthesis of heme, of purines, and of the tripeptide, glutathione: L-γ-glutamyl-L-cysteinyl-glycine.

The products of decarboxylation of a number of the α-amino acids are interesting and important. Most of the enzymes responsible for these reactions require pyridoxal phosphate as a coenzyme. An exception is the histidine decarboxylase of mast cells, which catalyzes the formation of histamine, a powerful vasodilator, liberated at sites of inflammation and more generally in traumatic shock, in anaphylaxis and in allergic reactions. Histamine is a potent excitor of gastric secretion of both pepsin and acid. Serotonin (5-

hydroxytryptamine) is a product of decarboxylation of 5-hydroxytryptophan. The amine is found in the central nervous system and is believed to function at certain sites as a neurotransmitter. Decarboxylation of glutamic acid yields γ-aminobutyric acid, found in high concentration in brain and spinal cord. It is thought to act as an inhibitory neurotransmitter. Decarboxylation of aspartic acid yields β-alanine ($H_2NCH_2CH_2COOH$). This reaction occurs in microorganisms, but in animals, β-alanine is derived from propionyl-SCoA by way of malonic semialdehyde: $CHOCH_2COOH$. Decarboxylation of ornithine yields putrescine: H_2N-$(CH_2)_4$-NH_2. This base reacts with a molecule of S-adenosylmethionine to form the polyamine, spermidine: $H_2N(CH_2)_4NH(CH_2)_3NH_2$. Reaction of the latter with a second molecule of S-adenosylmethionine yields spermine:

$$H_2N(CH_2)_3NH(CH_2)_4NH(CH_2)_3NH_2$$

Spermine and spermidine are essential for growth of some microorganisms, are found in high concentrations in sperm and may be important in the growth of tissues. The enzyme ornithine decarboxylase is increased in a variety of tissues by general or specific stimuli to growth. The functions of the polyamines are not known, but it is suspected that they may play a part in regulating RNA synthesis.

The sulfur of cysteine can be oxidized to cysteic acid, which, upon decarboxylation, yields taurine, $H_2NCH_2CH_2SO_3H$, a component of the bile acid, taurocholic acid.

Tryptophan, in addition to being a precursor of serotonin, can be a precursor of nicotinic acid, and in this respect has a vitamin-sparing action.

Tyrosine is a precursor of the thyroid hormones, of the catecholamines dihydroxyphenylethylamine (dopamine), norepinephrine and epinephrine, and of melanin.

In the catabolism of amino acids the nitrogen is removed by deamination or transamination. The nitrogen appears as urea: The carbon skeleton of the amino acids suffers a variety of fates. The many transaminases converge upon glutamate:

amino acid + α-ketoglutarate $\rightleftharpoons$ α-keto acid + glutamate.

Ammonia is set free by glutamate dehydrogenase:

H_2O + glutamate + NAD^+ $\rightleftharpoons$ α-ketoglutarate + NH_4
$\qquad\qquad\qquad\qquad\qquad$ + NADH + H^+

Glutamate and aspartate also equilibrate through the glutamate–oxaloacetate transaminase. By these steps the α-amino nitrogen of many amino acids is partitioned among glutamate, aspartate and ammonia. Oxidative deamination of individual amino acids other than glutamate is quantitatively less important than the system described above. The L-amino acid oxidases (flavoproteins) of liver and kidney have broad specificities but are sluggish enzymes.

Ammonia is disposed of in two ways. In the tissues it is converted to glutamine for transport to the liver and the kidneys. In the liver it is converted to urea—neutral, highly soluble, and nontoxic. Ammonium ion is extremely toxic. Normally, it is quickly and almost completely removed from the blood. Ammonia produced in digestion enters the portal blood and is efficiently cleared by the liver. This organ is exclusively the site of urea synthesis.

The simple reaction

$$CO_2 + 2NH_3 \rightarrow CO(NH_2)_2 + H_2O$$

requires energy and is accomplished by a cyclic process in the liver that is at the same time a pathway of arginine synthesis.

The first step is the formation of carbamyl phosphate:

$$CO_2 + NH_4^+ + 2ATP \rightarrow H_2N\text{-}CO\text{-}OPO_3H_2 + 2ADP + P_i$$

The enzyme, carbamyl phosphate synthase, is located in the mitochondria and requires acetylglutamate as a cofactor. The reaction is essentially irreversible. Carbamyl phosphate is transferred to ornithine by another mitochondrial enzyme, ornithine transcarbamylase, to form citrulline:

$$H_2N(CH_2)_3CHNH_2COOH + H_2N\text{-}CO\text{-}OPO_3H_2 \rightarrow$$
$$H_2N\text{-}CO\text{-}NH\text{-}(CH_2)_3CHNH_2COOH + P_i$$

The second molecule of ammonia is provided by aspartate, which, in an ATP-requiring reaction catalyzed by argininosuccinate synthase in the cytoplasm, condenses with citrulline to form argininosuccinate:

$$H_2N\text{—}CO\text{—}NH\text{—}(CH_2)_3CHNH_2COOH$$
$$+$$
$$HOOCCHNH_2CH_2COOH + ATP$$
$$\downarrow$$
$$H_2N\text{—}C\text{—}NH\text{—}(CH_2)_3CHNH_2COOH$$
$$\underset{|}{\overset{\parallel}{N}}$$
$$HOOCCH\text{—}CH_2COOH + AMP + PP_i + H_2O$$

The cytoplasmic enzyme, argininosuccinase, decomposes the condensation product to arginine:

$$H_2N\text{-}C(=NH)NH(CH_2)_3CHNH_2COOH$$

and fumarate: $HOOCCH=CHCOOH$. The enzyme arginase completes the cycle:

$$\text{arginine} + H_2O \rightarrow \text{ornithine} + CO(NH_2)_2$$

Urea synthesis requires the equivalent of 4 moles of ATP per mole of nitrogen. The cost is less than five per cent of the caloric value of the corresponding amount of protein catabolized.

The carbon skeletons of the amino acids are economically disposed of by oxidation or by transformation to carbohydrate, acetoacetate or fatty acids, depending on the circumstances. Most of the amino acids can provide carbon for gluconeogenesis. Arginine, ornithine, proline, histidine, glutamine, through glutamate, lead to α-ketoglutarate and the tricarboxylic acid cycle. Alanine, serine, glycine and cystine lead to pyruvate and thence either to acetyl-SCoA or, over oxaloacetate and phosphoenolpyruvate, to glucose. Asparagine and aspartate lead to oxaloacetate. The decomposition of phenylalanine and tyrosine produces both fumarate and acetoacetate and that of tryptophan yields alanine and acetoacetate. Valine, isoleucine, methionine and threonine are degraded by reactions leading to propionyl-SCoA, methyl malonyl-SCoA and succinyl-SCoA. Only leucine and lysine are unequivocally ketogenic, giving rise to acetoacetate or acetyl-SCoA, which allow of no net transfer of carbon to carbohydrate in their oxidation by the tricarboxylic acid cycle.

The branched-chain amino acids leucine, isoleucine and valine share common first steps in their catabolism. The α-keto acids are formed by transamination with α-ketoglutarate, and these are in turn oxidatively decarboxylated by a dehydrogenase complex involving NAD^+, a flavoprotein, thiamine pyrophosphate, lipoic acid and coenzyme A, which acts in principle like the similar systems that oxidatively decarboxylate pyruvate and α-ketoglutarate. The acyl-SCoA derivative at this step is different for the three amino acids and, as noted above, yields a different ultimate product. The enzyme complex catalyzing the decarboxylation of the branched-chain amino acids is defective in maple syrup urine disease, in which the keto acids, excreted in significant amounts, impart their characteristic odor to the urine.

Proteins and amino acids do not normally serve as a large source of energy to the organism. An adult in nitrogen balance with an intake of 70 g. of protein per day derives from it only 280 kcal. (less the cost of handling the protein) or about 10 per cent of the total basal plus activity expenditure of energy. In fasting, the amino acids become important as a source of glucose, or by their oxidation in place of glucose, but the major energy source in fasting is triglyceride. Only in protein-calorie insufficiency of long duration does the body draw upon its protein (mainly the large mass of muscle protein) as a principal energy source.

Synthesis and Metabolism of Purines and Pyrimidines.   The body has retained the capability of total synthesis of purines and pyrimidines. In the synthesis of the purine nucleus, the first step is the formation of 5-phosphoribosylamine from glutamine and 5-phospho-α-D-ribosyl-1-pyrophosphate (PRPP) (Fig. 4-8). The reaction is catalyzed by PRPP amidotransferase. This is a regulated step. Accumulation of any of the purine nucleotides results in feedback inhibition of the enzyme. From the phosphoribosylamine (N9), the purine nucleotide is constructed by the successive addition of glycine (C4,5;N7) formate (C8); the amide N of glutamine (N3); CO_2(C6); the α-amino N of aspartate (N1); and formate (C2).

The primary product, inosine monophosphate (IMP) is aminated at C6 to form adenosine monophosphate (AMP), or oxidized at C6 to yield xanthosine monophosphate (XMP), which is aminated at C2 to form guanosine monophosphate (GMP). The synthesis of IMP requires ATP at several steps. The formation of AMP from IMP requires GTP; the formation of GMP from XMP requires ATP, so that the respective levels of GTP and ATP may control the synthesis of AMP or GMP from IMP. The nucleoside triphosphates are formed from ATP by nucleoside mono- and diphosphate kinases.

Degradation of AMP involves first the loss of the 5'-phosphate, then the deamination of adenosine to

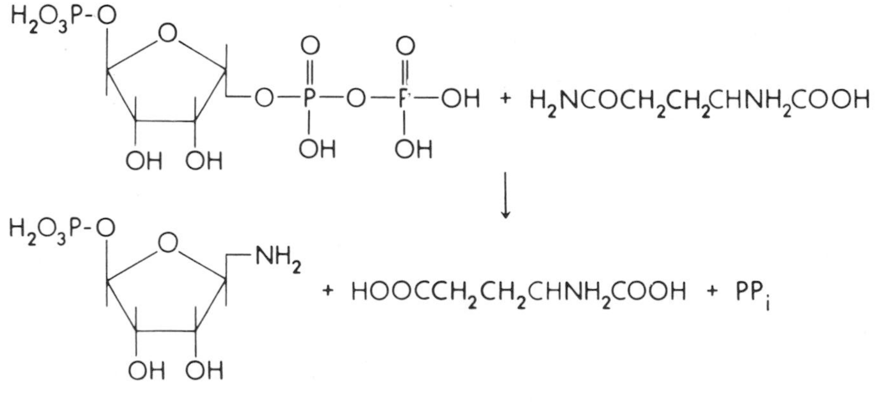

Fig. 4-8. Synthesis of purine ribotide, first step.

form inosine, followed by hydrolysis of the ribose to form hypoxanthine. Guanine is deaminated to form xanthine. Hypoxanthine and xanthine are oxidized to uric acid, which is the end product of purine catabolism in man. Hypoxanthine and guanine take part in what was first called a salvage pathway but what may be the main route of synthesis of IMP and GMP in nonhepatic tissues from the free bases or nucleosides synthesized in the liver. The enzyme is hypoxanthine-guanine phosphoribosyl transferase (PRT), and the reaction is:

$$\text{hypoxanthine} + \text{PRPP} \rightarrow \text{IMP} + \text{PP}_i$$
$$\text{(guanine)} \qquad\qquad \text{(GMP)}$$

This enzyme is absent in the Lesch-Nyhan syndrome, in which there is great overproduction of purines. This disease is linked to the X chromosome and is found in males only. It is characterized by early onset, aggressive behavior, self-mutilation, mental retardation, excretion of uric acid three to six times normal, renal stones and renal failure. If the concentrations of IMP and GMP are normally maintained in part by the action of PRT, a defect in the enzyme would allow their concentration to fall and remove the feedback restraint from the PRPP amidotransferase. It is also possible that lack of PRT reduces the utilization of PRPP, and that a rise in PRPP concentration might increase the formation of 5-phosphoribosylamine. Gout is another disease in which overproduction of purines occurs. It is thought that in some cases the feedback-sensitive enzyme PRPP-amidotransferase might be altered in such a way that it is less sensitive to IMP and GMP so that the operating level of production of the purine nucleotides would be higher than normal. Some patients, however, may have a partial deficiency of PRT, with moderate overproduction of purines giving the gouty symptoms without the other serious abnormalities of the Lesch-Nyhan syndrome.

The biosynthesis of pyrimidines begins with the synthesis of carbamyl phosphate. The synthase is a cytoplasmic enzyme. Glutamine is the source of the nitrogen:

$$CO_2 + 2ATP + H_2O + \text{glutamine} \rightarrow$$
$$\text{carbamylphosphate} + 2ADP + P_i + \text{glutamate}$$

This is a regulated step; the enzyme is feedback inhibited by UTP. The next step in the synthesis of the pyrimidine ring is the condensation of aspartate with carbamyl phosphate by aspartate transcarbamylase. The product, carbamylaspartate:

$$HOOC—CH—CH_2—COOH$$
$$| $$
$$HN—CO—NH_2$$

loses water to form a six-membered ring and is oxidized by orotate dehydrogenase (NAD$^+$) to orotate. This

Orotate

reacts with PRPP and orotidylate pyrophosphorylase to form orotidylate and PP$_i$, and the product is decarboxylated to form uridine monophosphate (UMP). UTP is formed from UMP at the expense of ATP. Cytidine triphosphate is formed from UTP by amination at the 4-carbon by transfer of the amide group of glutamine. The energy for the transfer is derived by the breakdown of ATP to ADP and P$_i$.

The deoxyribonucleotides are derived by the reduction of the ribose in the ribonucleoside diphosphates, UDP, CDP, ADP, GDP. The reductase utilizes as coenzyme a small protein, thioredoxin, which acts as a hydrogen donor, by the oxidation of a pair of proximal -SH groups to -S-S-. Thioredoxin is reduced by an NADPH$^+$-requiring reductase.

Thymidylic acid, the deoxyribonucleotide exclusive to DNA, is synthesized by methylation of dUMP which, in animal cells, may be formed by deamination of dCMP. The methylating agent is 5,10-methylene tetrahydrofolate, which is oxidized to dihydrofolate. This is reduced to THF by DHF-reductase, requiring NADPH. The compounds methotrexate and aminopterin are folic acid analogues that are potent inhibitors of DHF reductase and are effective agents in cancer chemotherapy because, by interfering with the formation of the THF coenzymes, they slow down nucleic acid synthesis in all rapidly growing cells.

In the degradation of the pyrimidines the nucleotides are first hydrolyzed to the free bases, and these are decomposed to ammonia, carbon dioxide and malonate (or, from thymine, methylmalonate). All of the breakdown products are easily disposed of.

DNA: Replication and Transcription. During cell division in man, the DNA is densely packed, in association with an array of small basic proteins, the histones, together with some non-histone, acidic protein, into 23 pairs of chromosomes. At other times, the complex of nucleoprotein, called chromatin, is dispersed through the nucleus. In this "resting" interval, DNA may be replicated in preparation for division. The mode of replication is semiconservative: each of the complementary strands of DNA gives rise to *its* complement during replication, and the two new molecules each contain one daughter strand. This is shown as follows. If *Escherichia coli* are grown in the presence of $^{15}NH_4Cl$, the purine and pyrimidine bases of DNA acquire the heavy isotope. If the labeled cells are transferred to new medium containing $^{14}NH_4Cl$, the DNA isolated after one generation has a density, on gradient centrifugation, midway between that of "^{15}N" DNA from the parent generation and "^{14}N" DNA from a control culture. All of the molecules contain one light and one heavy strand. In the next generation, half of the new DNA molecules are "light"; the other half, "medium."

DNA serves as its own template for replication. Several DNA polymerases take part in the action, some generating portions of the new strands, others putting the pieces together to form the continuous complementary daughter strand. All four deoxyribonucleoside triphosphates must be present. The two strands of DNA unwind, and synthesis of the new strands proceeds simultaneously. Initiation of synthesis occurs at each of several sites of attachment of a template of RNA about ten nucleotides in length. The complementary new chain of DNA ($A = T$; $G = C$) grows from the 3' end of this primer, in the direction, 5' to 3'. As sections about 100 nucleotides long are completed, the RNA initiator is displaced and the gap is filled by the appropriate deoxyribonucleotide. In this manner the antiparallel strands of DNA are both copied, in sections synthesized in the 5' to 3' direction for which the DNA polymerases are specific.

Transcription of DNA is catalyzed by several DNA-dependent RNA polymerases, each of which may be responsible for the different sets of genes. A single strand of RNA is synthesized as the complement of one of the two strands of DNA. All four nucleotide triphosphates (ATP, UTP, GTP, CTP) must be present. Synthesis is initiated by the attachment of RNA polymerase to a promoter site on the DNA with the aid of an initiation factor, sigma. The RNA grows in the direction, 5' to 3', from the 3' end of the section of DNA being transcribed. The sigma factor is released. Another small protein, rho factor, recognizes the specific termination site on the DNA and facilitates release of the RNA and of the enzyme.

Ribosomal RNA (rRNA) is produced in the nucleolus. In animal cells there are thousands of copies of the genes for rRNA, but it is not known how this large reserve is regulated. It is probably related to the control of the synthesis of the ribosomal proteins. Nucleolar rRNA is synthesized as a large molecule (45S) from which the 5.8S, 18S and 28S components of the ribosomes are derived. In the processing of the 45S precursor, the portions that become parts of the 60S and 40S ribosomal subunits are heavily methylated on both the ribose and the bases. The two subunits self assemble with their complement of ribosomal proteins.

Transfer RNA (tRNA) is synthesized first as part of a large precursor molecule that is partly degraded and modified in the nucleus, and folded, by base pairing, into the characteristic shape of these adapter molecules. In the cytoplasm, the modifications are completed, and the activating sequence, C-C-A, is added to the 3' end. More than 50 tRNAs have been isolated and sequenced. The mode of regulation of their synthesis is not known.

Messenger RNA (mRNA) is synthesized in the nucleus as a component of a precursor molecule many times as large as the eventual message. The precursor molecules turn over rapidly, and only a small fraction of the total RNA leaves the nucleus as mRNA. Many mammalian RNAs contain, at the 5' end, a "cap" structure—7-methylguanosine triphosphate—and, at the 3' end, a tail of polyadenylic acid comprising as many as 200 nucleotides. A recently discovered peculiarity of the genes for eukaryotic mRNAs is that the complete message is not all of one piece, but is interspersed with two or more "silent" sections. The transcribed RNA must therefore be cleaved, and the proper message coding for the protein or its precursor reassembled before the completed mRNA is released.

The regulation of transcription of genes in animal cells is not yet well understood, but it is thought that it may follow in some respects the model derived from studies on microorganisms such as *Escherichia coli*. A sector of DNA containing the information for one or more proteins (related, as in an enzyme sequence) is called an operon. The genes coding for protein in this region are called structural genes. Adjacent to the operon is an operator site, of about 20 base pairs, and beyond it a promoter site to which the DNA-dependent RNA polymerase can attach. Next to this is a repressor gene, which is coded for the synthesis of a repressor protein specific only for the adjacent operator site. When the repressor is in situ the polymerase cannot move along the DNA. If the repressor is removed by an appropriate agent, usually a small molecule, transcription can take place: the operon is "derepressed." The classical example is lactose in *E. coli*. It derepresses the Lac-operon, permitting the synthesis of a polycistronic mRNA coded for the synthesis of the enzymes required for the utilization of lactose by the cell. This can take place because, in the absence of usable carbon, the concentration of cAMP, normally kept low in the presence of substrate, increases. cAMP combines with a small protein, the catabolite gene activator, and the combination binds at the promoter site to permit initiation of transcription.

A number of variations can be played upon the theme of repression–derepression. End product inhibition, for example, is brought about when the end product of an enzyme sequence, accumulating in sufficient amount, combines as a corepressor with the repressor protein to activate it and block further transcription of the DNA operon coded for the enzyme sequence.

BLOOD

The blood (eight per cent of body weight) is the circulating tissue, consisting of the formed elements, the red and the white cells and the platelets, and the liquid medium, the plasma. Normally the cells comprise 45 per cent of the volume (hematocrit reading) in males, slightly less (41 per cent) in females. The average specific gravity of normal blood varies from 1.055 to 1.060; of the plasma, from 1.024 to 1.028. Its viscosity is about 4.5 times that of water. The osmotic pressure of human blood is equivalent to that of a 0.9 per cent sodium chloride solution (physiologic saline). The functions of the blood are (1) transport, of O_2 and CO_2, nutrients, metabolic products, and water; (2) communication and regulation, by the distribution of hormones and other chemical signals, and of heat; (3) defense, against infection by the circulation of leukocytes and antibodies, against wounding by the system of coagulation and against large fluctuations of hydrogen ion concentration by an efficient buffer system.

The Red Cell. The normal red blood cell contains about 65 per cent water and 35 per cent solids. Its distinctive feature is that it contains a 34 per cent solution of hemoglobin packed into a biconcave disk from 6 to 9 mμ in diameter and about 1 mμ thick in the center, increasing to 2 to 2.5 mμ at the periphery. There are about 5 million red cells per cubic millimeter of blood. By this device, 14 to 16 g. of hemoglobin per 100 ml. of blood are easily moved about without a very large increase in viscosity. The primary function of the red cell is the transport of oxygen and carbon dioxide.

The mature red cell has no nucleus. An increased rate of red cell formation is indicated by the presence of a higher proportion than normal of reticulocytes, red cells that have not quite lost all remnants of the nucleus, DNA and RNA, and of mitochondria. Some reticulocytes are normally present, since there is daily turnover of about 20 ml. of red cells, just under one per cent of the total. The lifetime of the red cells is about 126 days. Glycine labeled with ^{15}N is incorporated bodily into heme. The concentration of the isotope in heme rises quickly to a maximum during 2 days of feeding glycine, then falls, between days 119 and 133, while the concentration of isotope in the bile pigment rises abruptly during the same period.

As in other cells, the principal cation of the red cell is potassium, with smaller amounts of sodium and magnesium. The anions are chloride, bicarbonate, inorganic phosphate, 2,3-diphosphoglycerate and smaller amounts of other phosphate esters, nucleotides such as ATP, and hemoglobin. Chloride, bicarbonate, hydrogen ion and inorganic phosphate move freely across the red cell membrane. The concentration of glucose within the red cell is maintained at the same level as that of the plasma by a process of active transport. A continuing supply of energy, derived mainly from glycolysis and the hexosemonophosphate oxidation pathway, is required to maintain the internal composition of the red cell. There is a small rate of consumption of oxygen, due mainly to the autooxidation of some hemoglobin to methemoglobin. This process results in the production of a superoxide radical O_2^-, which is scavenged by the reaction, $2O_2^- + 2H^+ = O_2 + H_2O_2$, catalyzed by superoxide dismutase (the copper-containing enzyme once called erythrocuprein). The hemeprotein, catalase, in the red cell completes the protective reaction by decomposing the hydrogen peroxide.

Further protection against hydrogen peroxide is afforded by reduced glutathione, which together with the enzyme glutathione peroxidase, decomposes H_2O_2. Glutathione is maintained in the reduced state by glutathione reductase, utilizing NADPH derived from the actions of glucose 6-phosphate dehydrogenase and 6-phosphogluconate dehydrogenase. This system of enzymes is related to the phenomenon of primaquine sensitivity. In susceptible individuals a wide array of agents, including the antimalarial drug primaquine, induces extensive hemolysis due to hypersensitivity to peroxides because of a low concentration of reduced glutathione. This is most often ascribable to a deficiency in glucose 6-phosphate dehydrogenase (insufficient generation of NADPH), but it can also be due to deficiency in glutathione reductase, 6-phosphogluconate dehydrogenase or the enzymes catalyzing glutathione synthesis. The latter are ATP dependent, and defects in the enzymes of the glycolytic pathway that limit the supply of ATP may also limit the supply of reduced glutathione.

The glycolytic system of the red cell produces lactate and ATP from glucose as usual, but it is modified by the addition of two enzymes. (1) Diphosphoglyceromutase catalyzes the essentially irreversible reaction:

phosphoglyceryl phosphate →

2,3-diphosphoglycerate

The transfer of the acyl phosphate (normally transferred to ADP) to the 2-ester position occurs with a large fall in free energy. (2) Phosphoglycerate phosphatase catalyzes the hydrolysis of 2,3-diphosphoglycerate at the 2 position, yielding inorganic phosphate and the normal glycolytic intermediate, 3-phosphoglyceric acid. This little metabolic cycle maintains and regulates the concentration of 2,3-diphosphoglycerate in the red cell. Diphosphoglycerate binds to hemoglobin strongly but to oxyhemoglobin very slightly. The binding to Hb (mole for mole) ties the β-chains firmly together and facilitates the unloading of oxygen by diminishing the affinity of hemoglobin for oxygen. Diphosphoglycerate is mainly responsible for the sigmoid shape of the oxygen dissociation curve of hemoglobin and for the effective delivery of oxygen at the partial pressures of the gas in the peripheral tissues. Inborn errors involving defects of enzymes of the glycolytic system in the red cell have been recognized in a number of instances. The lifetime of the cell is reduced, probably because of limitations of the supply of energy required to maintain the integrity of the cell membrane. The result is a hemolytic anemia.

Hemoglobin. The red ferro-heme protein hemoglobin, M_r about 65,000, is a molecule composed of four polypeptide subunits each containing a heme. It is a member of a family of iron-porphyrin proteins that includes myoglobin, the cytochromes and the enzymes peroxidase and catalase. The iron-porphyrin prosthetic group is responsible for the color.

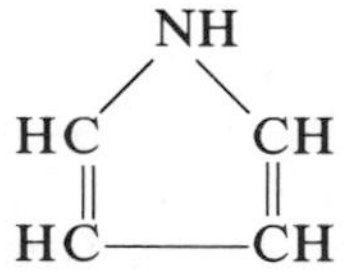

Pyrrole

The parent compound of the numerous family of metalloporphyrins is the cyclic tetrapyrrole, porphin, composed of four pyrrole rings joined to one another

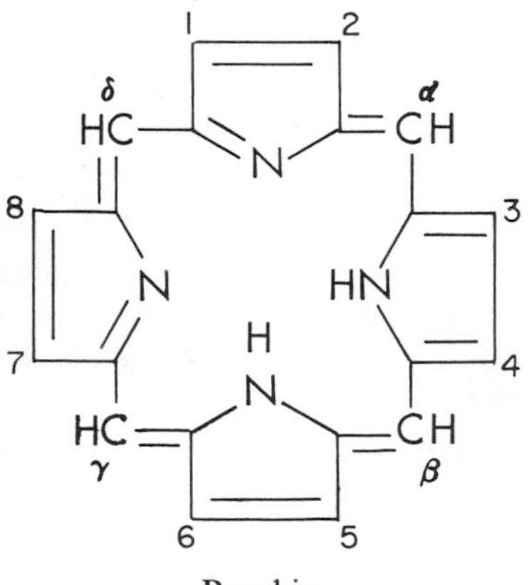

Porphin

by methenyl bridges. The numbering of the carbon atoms of the porphin ring is shown in the structural formula. The porphyrins differ from one another in the substituents to the carbon atoms numbered 1 to 8 in porphin. The porphyrin of hemoglobin is protoporphyrin IX (type III). There is a methyl group at positions, 1,3,5 and 8, vinyl groups on carbons 2 and 4 and propionic acid groups at positions 6 and 7. The capability of synthesizing porphyrins is nearly universal in living organisms. The first step is the synthesis of delta-amino-levulinic acid from glycine and succi-

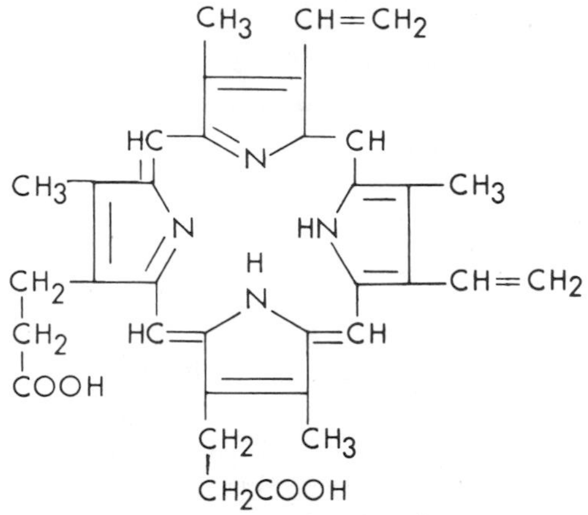

Protoporphyrin IX

nyl-SCoA by the pyridoxal phosphate-requiring enzyme delta-aminolevulinate synthase (the rate-limiting enzyme in the synthesis, controlled by feedback of heme):

$$H_2N\text{-}CH_2\text{-}COOH + HOOC\text{-}CH_2CH_2CO\text{-}S\text{-}CoA$$
$$= HOOC\text{-}CH_2CH_2CO\text{-}CH_2\text{-}NH_2 + CO_2 + HS\text{-}CoA.$$

The enzyme delta-aminolevulinate dehydrase catalyzes the condensation of 2 moles of delta-aminolevulinate to form porphobilinogen:

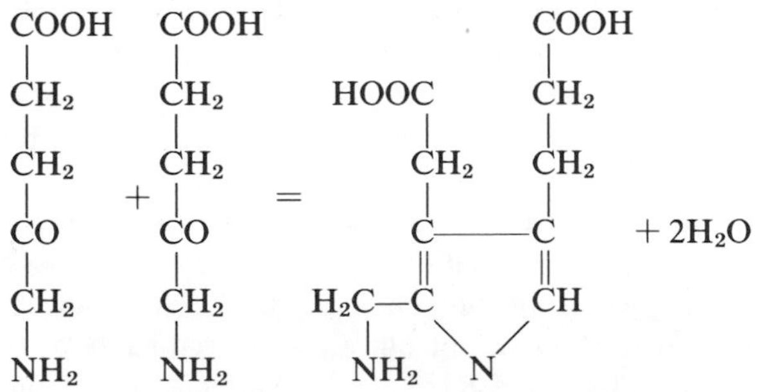

Protoporphyrin is synthesized by the condensation of 4 moles of porphobilinogen accompanied by deamination and appropriate modifications of the side chains. The iron is introduced last, by the enzyme heme synthase, to form ferroprotoporphyrin, or heme. The iron displaces the hydrogen atoms on two of the pyrrole rings and forms coordinate bonds with the other two tertiary nitrogens. In the red cell the rate of synthesis of protoporphyrin is normally nicely balanced against the rate of synthesis of the globin, so that neither is at any time in excess of the other. This balance is disturbed in the hereditary erythropoietic porphyrias, in which excess porphyrins accumulate in normoblasts and erythrocytes, are deposited in tissues, causing skin photosensitivity, and are excreted in urine and feces. Other types of hereditary porphyria, of hepatic origin, are not accompanied by sensitivity to light, and are characterized by excretion of large amounts of delta-aminolevulinic acid and porphobilinogen in the urine, as well as of increased amounts of porphyrins in urine and feces. Porphyrinurias, characterized by increased excretion of coproporphyrins, may be acquired as a result of exposure to toxic agents, in consequence of liver disease, and in leukemia, pernicious anemia, hemolytic anemias and a variety of other disorders.

The hemoglobins of different species all contain heme. The differences in their properties are due to differences in the amino acid sequence of the protein, globin. The heme is readily dissociated by treatment of hemoglobin with acids or bases. Free heme is easily oxidized to hemin, which crystallizes readily. This property is exploited in a simple method for the detection of blood. Oxidation of the iron of hemoglobin, forming ferriprotoporphyrins, yields methemoglobin.

The normal human hemoglobins are composed of two pairs of four polypeptide subunits, α, together with β, γ or δ. Adult hemoglobin (HbA) has the composition α_2^A, β_2^A; normal fetal hemoglobin (HbF) is designated α_2^A, γ_2^F. About two to three per cent of normal adult hemoglobin is present as α_2^A, δ_2^A. Abnormalities may arise from limited ability to synthesize α subunits (α-thalassemia) or β subunits (β-thalassemia). In the former case hemoglobins of the type β_4^A and γ_4^F are found; in the latter there are abnormal quantities of $\alpha_2\delta_2$ or $\alpha_2\gamma_2$. Individuals homozygous for these defects do not survive for long.

A small amount of HbA is glycosylated by a nonenzymatic reaction between glucose-6-phosphate and the NH_2-terminal valyl residues of the β-chains (HbA$_{Ic}$). The quantity varies with the mean concentration of blood glucose, and it has been suggested that this may be used as an indicator of the effectiveness of long term regulation of the blood sugar in diabetic subjects.

Numerous instances are now known of amino acid substitutions in the hemoglobin of individuals, occurring as a result of mutations. One of the best known examples is sickle cell anemia, in which the glutamic acid at position 6 of the β subunits of hemoglobin is replaced by valine. The altered charge of the molecule (HbS) makes it easy to recognize, since it migrates electrophoretically at a different rate from normal hemoglobin. This change in the molecule also leads to a marked change in the solubility of the deoxy form

of HbS; it tends to crystallize, distorting the cell into the sickle shape, in which it is fragile, hemolyzing in the capillaries. The rate of red cell destruction is high, leading to the anemia. Individuals homozygous for the trait have severe anemia, are seriously ill and lead a short and painful life. Individuals heterozygous for the trait have a microcytic anemia, and their red cells are inhospitable to the malaria parasite. In malarial regions their chances of survival are greater than those of individuals with HbA. This may also be true of individuals heterozygous for the thalassemias.

The complete amino acid sequences of the α, β and γ chains of hemoglobin are known. By x-ray diffraction analysis the conformation of all four chains in the molecule, both in the deoxygenated and in the oxygenated state, is now known, providing a great deal of information in molecular terms about the properties of hemoglobin. The α chains (141 residues) are similar in sequence and conformation to the β chains (146 residues), and they both closely resemble the single chain of myoglobin, the reserve oxygen carrier of muscle. Both chains are compactly folded, and the two pairs fit closely together, held by ionic and hydrogen bonds and by hydrophobic interactions. The hemes are tucked into pockets that provide a strongly hydrophobic environment. The iron is coordinated with two histidine residues at opposite sides of the pocket; in oxyhemoglobin one of these coordinate bonds of the iron is occupied by O_2. It is the hydrophobic environment of the heme that allows the combination of ferrous iron with oxygen to take place without oxidizing the iron. This is the essential condition for the carriage of oxygen by hemoglobin.

Carriage of Oxygen. The transport of oxygen in the blood is accomplished by the reversible combination of oxygen with hemoglobin. This takes place along gradients of partial pressure of O_2 maintained on the one hand by the continuing movements of respiration, aerating the lungs, and on the other hand by the continual but varying oxidative processes in the peripheral tissues. The partial pressure of O_2 in the alveolar space in the lungs is maintained at or near 100 mm. Hg; that in the venous blood entering the lung may be 50 mm. Hg or less. Oxygen diffuses into the red cell and combines with hemoglobin. The blood leaves the lung with the hemoglobin about 96 per cent saturated, at a partial pressure of O_2 of about 100 mm. Hg (95 during exercise). At the lower partial pressure of O_2 in the peripheral tissues, hemoglobin surrenders its oxygen. The extent of unsaturation is related to the intensity of the local oxygen-using processes. A very small amount of oxygen is carried in solution (0.3 ml. per 100 ml. blood). In blood containing 15 g. of hemoglobin per 100 ml., 1.34 ml. of O_2 can be carried per

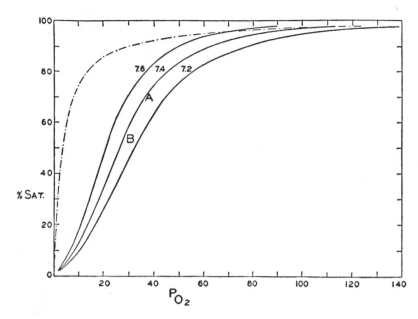

Fig. 4-9. Normal oxygen dissociation curves of the system hemoglobin, O_2, oxyhemoglobin at several pH values. Also a representative curve for myoglobin (dashed curve) whose molecular weight is about one-fourth that of hemoglobin. (Clark, W.: Topics in Physical Chemistry, p. 208. Baltimore, Williams and Wilkins, 1948).

gram of hemoglobin, or at full saturation, 20.1 ml. O_2 per 100 ml.

The curve describing the relation between partial pressure of oxygen and per cent saturation of hemoglobin has a sigmoid shape (Fig. 4-9). The significance of this relationship is that hemoglobin readily gives up an appreciable portion of its oxygen at still moderate partial pressure of oxygen such as might be encountered in resting tissues, and that it is nearly completely saturated at partial pressures of oxygen well below the partial pressure in the lungs. By contrast, the oxygen saturation curve of myoglobin, a heme protein similar to a subunit of hemoglobin, which combines with only 1 mole of oxygen, is a rectangular hyperbola. It is very nearly completely saturated at a partial pressure of O_2 of 40 mm. Hg, and it is still nearly 60 per cent saturated at a partial pressure of O_2 of 10 mm. Hg. The dissociation of oxygen is also affected by pH. At an increased partial pressure of carbon dioxide (decrease in pH), oxygen dissociates more readily; if the system becomes more alkaline, oxygen dissociates less readily, at any P_{O_2}. This effect, known as the Bohr effect, has the physiologic significance that in the tissues, where carbon dioxide is being generated, the P_{CO_2} is high, pH falls, and O_2 dissociates more completely at any given P_{O_2}. In the lungs carbon dioxide diffuses out, P_{CO_2} is less, pH increases, and the uptake of O_2 is facilitated. This property of hemoglobin is expressed in the equation:

$$HHb + O_2 \rightleftarrows HbO_2^- + H^+$$

This equation says (1) that the oxygenation of hemoglobin increases with the concentration of oxygen (P_{O_2}); (2) that oxyhemoglobin is a stronger acid than hemoglobin (H^+ dissociates); (3) that increasing the hydrogen ion concentration will push the reaction to the left (favor dissociation of O_2); (4) that the net anionic ($-$) charge on oxyhemoglobin is greater than that on hemoglobin. (At the pH of the red cell interior, alkaline to the isoelectric point of hemoglobin, the protein always has a net negative charge). The binding of 1 mole of O_2 to hemoglobin results in the release of 0.7 equivalents of H^+.

The oxygenation of hemoglobin is accompanied by marked changes in the conformation of the molecule. The tight packing of the two pairs of chains is relaxed by dissolution of the ionic bonds holding the α chains to one another and to the β chains. The binding of diphosphoglycerate to the β chains is decreased, allowing them greater freedom of motion. The pockets holding the heme in the β chains, too narrow to receive oxygen at first, increase in width. The pockets holding the heme in the α chains are wide enough at all times but access to one of them is limited by the tight packing to the corresponding beta chain. The shape of the dissociation curve is interpreted to mean that the entry of the first oxygen molecule, although slow, initiates the conformational changes that facilitate access of oxygen to the other heme groups. The Bohr effect is attributed to changes in the pKa of some of the ionizing groups involved in the disrupted salt bridges, especially those that link the α and the β chains together. These phenomena are determined by the interactions of the two pairs of different chains. In abnormal hemoglobins of the type $\beta_4{}^A$ no cooperative effects are seen, and the oxygen dissociation curve is a rectangular hyperbola like that of myoglobin.

Carriage of Carbon Dioxide. The transport of carbon dioxide in the blood is accomplished mainly through the actions of two red cell proteins, hemoglobin and the zinc-containing enzyme carbonic anhydrase. About 27 per cent of the total carbon dioxide is carried on hemoglobin as carbamino acid formed by the reaction of carbon dioxide with undissociated amino groups:

$$R\text{-}NH_2 + CO_2 \rightleftarrows RNHCOOH = RNHCOO^- + H^+$$

Hemoglobin has a greater capacity for carbamino-CO_2 formation than oxyhemoglobin. The difference is increased by the greater partial pressure of CO_2 and the increased acidity of venous blood. The plasma proteins make no significant contribution to carbon dioxide transport in this form.

Carbon dioxide dissolves in the plasma water and diffuses into the red cell. In any aqueous system CO_2 can react with water to form carbonic acid:

$$CO_2 + H_2O \rightleftarrows H_2CO_3 \rightleftarrows H^+ + HCO_3{}^-$$

The uncatalyzed hydration of carbon dioxide is very slow and is negligible in the plasma. In the red cell, carbonic anhydrase, present in large excess, brings this reaction almost instantly to equilibrium. The ionization of carbonic acid is fast and complete. What happens to the hydrogen and the bicarbonate ions?

One must imagine arterial blood at P_{O_2} of 100 mm. Hg (96 per cent HbO_2) and a P_{CO_2} of 40 mm. Hg arriving at the capillary bed of resting muscle, where the P_{O_2} is 36 mm. Hg and the P_{CO_2} is 50 mm. Hg. Oxygen diffuses into the muscle along its pressure gradient. There is a slight increase of dissolved CO_2, and CO_2 diffuses into plasma and red cell along its gradient. Some CO_2 reacts with hemoglobin to form carbamino CO_2. Most of it is rapidly hydrated in the red cell to form carbonic acid, which ionizes. Now at this time the reaction

$$HHb + O_2 \rightleftarrows HbO_2{}^- + H^+$$

is shifting to the left as O_2 leaves the cell: Hemoglobin must take up H^+ ion. Consequently, most of the H^+ ions generated by the dissociation of carbonic acid in the red cell are accommodated on hemoglobin with no change in pH. This phenomenon is known as the isohydric shift, or the isohydric transport of CO_2. If CO_2 enters and is hydrated in excess of about 0.7 mole per mole of O_2 leaving, the additional hydrogen ions are buffered by hemoglobin, which is unusually rich in histidine, the only amino acid that can act effectively as a buffer in the physiologic pH range.

There is a rapid increase in the concentration of bicarbonate ion in the red cell. The equilibrium between cells and plasma is restored by the diffusion of bicarbonate ions into the plasma. Electrical balance is preserved by the diffusion of chloride ions from the plasma to the red cells. This so-called chloride shift occurs because the decrease in the net anionic charge of the large indiffusible anion hemoglobin requires a change in the distribution of diffusible ions between the cells and the plasma. The working rule derives from the Gibbs–Donnan equilibrium, by which the distribution of diffusible ions between cells and plasma is determined by the degree of ionization of hemoglobin:

$$r = \frac{[Cl^-]c}{[Cl^-]p} = \frac{[HCO_3{}^-]c}{[HCO_3{}^-]p} = \frac{[H^+]p}{[H^+]c} = \frac{1 - [Hb^-]c}{2[A^-]p}$$

The value of r is less than 1. A fall in the net anionic charge on hemoglobin brings the value of r nearer to 1, and chloride must move from plasma to cells. The sum of bicarbonate and chloride in the red cell is increased, and this increase in effective osmotic pressure within the cells is adjusted by the entrance of water. The increase in red cell volume is reflected in the higher value of the hematocrit for venous than for arterial blood (48 per cent as opposed to 45 per cent).

At the lungs the reactions occurring in the tissues are reversed. The formation of oxyhemoglobin creates a stronger acid than carbonic acid, which is decomposed; CO_2 escapes into the alveoli. The following equation sums up the succession of chemical events:

$$O_2 + HHb + HCO_3{}^- \rightleftarrows HbO_2{}^- + H_2O + CO_2$$

Increase in P_{O_2} drives the reactions to the right; increase in P_{CO_2} drives them to the left. The speed and the easy reversibility of the reactions are assured by the presence of carbonic anhydrase in the red cell. The quantitative aspects of CO_2 transport are summarized in Table 4-6. Note that most of the bicarbonate, generated in the red cell, is carried in the plasma, that the plasma proteins play a negligible role in buffering the carbonic acid and that the pH change is minimal (2.1 nanomoles of H^+ per liter).

Blood as a Buffer. The system, plasma + red cells, is, in addition to its role in gas transport, the effective buffer system of the blood. Hemoglobin, the protein present in the highest concentration in the

TABLE 4-6. CO_2 Transport*

	Arterial (mM.)	Venous (mM.)	Difference (mM.)
Total CO_2 in 1 liter of blood	21.53	23.21	1.68
Plasma (600 ml.)			
Total CO_2	15.94	16.99	1.05
As dissolved CO_2	0.71	0.80	0.09
As bicarbonate ions	15.23	16.19	0.96
Chloride ions	59.59	58.72	−0.87
Net negative charges on plasma proteins	7.89	7.80	−0.09
pH	7.455	7.429	−0.026
Red cells (400 ml.)			
Net negative charges on hemoglobin	22.60	21.15	−1.45
Carbamino-CO_2 ions	0.97	1.42	+0.45
Bicarbonate ions	4.28	4.41	+0.13
Chloride ions	18.11	18.98	+0.87

* The data are for 1 liter of normal human blood containing 8.93 mM. of hemoglobin and having a hematocrit of 40 per cent.

blood, is, unlike the plasma proteins, an effective buffer in the physiologic pH range. The location of carbonic anhydrase in great excess in the red cell makes the system sensitive and responsive to the gain or loss of acid by the blood. In the reaction:

$$P_{CO_2} = CO_{2(dissolved)} + H_2O = H_2CO_3 = H^+ + HCO_3^-$$

it may be seen that $[H^+]$ is governed by the partial pressure of carbon dioxide (P_{CO_2}). If a sample of plasma is titrated by equilibrating it with increasing P_{CO_2}, it is observed that its buffer capacity, the amount of acid required to change the pH by one unit, is 5.4 mmoles per liter. If a sample of whole blood is similarly titrated, it is found that the buffer capacity of the plasma equilibrated in this way, the "true" plasma, is 21.6 mmoles per liter per pH unit. The difference reflects the buffering power of hemoglobin. This property is independent of the state of oxygenation. It is a function of the concentration of hemoglobin. The buffer capacity of true plasma is therefore decreased in anemia.

Carbonic acid is not by itself a suitable buffer acid for physiologic conditions, but the system, dissolved carbon dioxide, carbonic acid, bicarbonate described in the equation above, in which the gas may be regarded as the acid component, behaves like a weak acid with an apparent pK (pK') of 6.1. The Henderson-Hasselbalch equation for this system is:

$$pH = 6.1 + \log \frac{[HCO_3^-]}{[CO_{2(dis)} + H_2CO_3]}$$

It is not possible to determine the quantities in the ratio directly, but the pH and the [total CO_2] can be determined. From this $[HCO_3^-]$ can be computed by the equation:

$$pH = 6.1 + \log \frac{[HCO_3^-]}{[Total\ CO_2] - [HCO_3^-]}$$

and a value for $[CO_{2(dis)} + H_2CO_3]$ is obtained from the computed value for the denominator of the equation. Since the amount of H_2CO_3 is always very small, the denominator can now be written $[CO_{2(dis)}]$. The concentration of CO_2 in plasma is given by the Bunsen solubility coefficient, 0.51 ml. CO_2 (at STP) per ml. of plasma at 38 C. and 1 atm. pressure of CO_2. From the molar volume of CO_2 (22.26 liters) it can be calculated that the amount of CO_2 dissolved in 1,000 ml. of plasma is:

$$\frac{0.51 \times 1,000}{760 \times 22.26} = 0.0301\ mmoles/mm.\ Hg$$

partial pressure of CO_2

The equation relating pH to [total CO_2] and P_{CO_2} can now be written:

$$pH = 6.1 + \log \frac{[total\ CO_2] = 0.0301 P_{CO_2}}{0.0301 P_{CO_2}}$$

In a resting subject total CO_2 is 25.3 mmoles per liter and P_{CO_2} is 40 mm. Hg; the value of the ratio is

$$\frac{25.3 - 1.2}{1.2} = 20$$

and the pH is 7.4.

The fact that one of the components of this buffer system is a gas makes possible rapid adjustment of pH by alteration of the rate and depth of respiration. If the breath is held, CO_2 accumulates, P_{CO_2} increases, and the pH of the blood falls. *Respiratory acidosis* may thus be induced by conditions such as pulmonary edema and emphysema that interfere with diffusion of CO_2 and its escape from the lungs, or by conditions such as narcosis that slow or suppress respiration. When the condition is sustained, the first line of defense of the blood pH is compromised, and the kidney must be relied upon for compensation of the acidosis by excretion of a more acid urine.

Increasing the rate and depth of the respiration removes CO_2 from the lungs more rapidly than it enters them, Pco_2 falls, and the pH of the blood increases. *Respiratory alkalosis* may thus be induced by hysterical excitement, by crying in infants and children, by some infections affecting the central nervous system and by drugs such as salicylates. It may lead to the convulsions of tetany, since the rise in blood pH increases the calcium-binding capacity of the plasma proteins, and the fall in $[Ca^{2+}]$ may precipitate an attack. The kidney compensates for sustained respiratory alkalosis by excreting a more alkaline urine.

An entry of acid into the blood, for example, an increase of blood lactic acid in exercise, induces *metabolic acidosis*. Bicarbonate is decomposed, Pco_2 increases, and the blood pH falls. The increase in Pco_2 and in $[H^+]$ stimulates the respiratory center, CO_2 is removed more rapidly from the lungs, and the pH returns toward normal: the metabolic acidosis is nearly completely compensated. As the lactate is removed from the blood by the liver, heart and kidney, more CO_2 can be retained as bicarbonate, Pco_2 falls, and the rate of respiration returns to normal as the pH increases. In extreme conditions the accumulation of metabolic acids in the blood diminishes the CO_2-carrying capacity beyond the point at which the Pco_2 can be reduced any further by hyperventilation. Compensation is no longer possible, and the blood pH falls. The classical example is the ketoacidosis of unregulated diabetes mellitus, in which the increased concentrations of acetoacetate and β-hydroxybutyrate in the blood, coupled with the loss of sodium as the partially neutralized ketoacids are excreted in the urine, lead to severe uncompensated metabolic acidosis.

During digestion the gastric glands secrete HCl. The hydrogen ions are derived by concentration from the plasma. The blood pH rises, Pco_2 falls, and in response the respiratory rate slows. There is a state of *metabolic alkalosis* (the so-called alkaline tide of the first phase of digestion), which is partially compensated by the lungs. In severe vomiting, with loss of HCl and other electrolytes and water, the metabolic alkalosis is more extreme and serious.

The buffering power of hemoglobin, the strategic location of carbonic anhydrase in the red cell and the consequent quickness of response of the CO_2/bicarbonate system, coupled to the pH-sensitive respiratory center and the lungs, provide the first line of defense of the hydrogen ion concentration of the blood and body fluids. In the long term, however, excess acid and alkali are dealt with by the kidney, which is ultimately responsible for acid-base, electrolyte and water balance in the body.

Fate of Red Cells: Bile Pigments. Aged red cells are destroyed by macrophages in liver, spleen and bone marrow. The α-methene bridge of heme is cleaved to give the iron-pyrrole-protein choleglobin. This is split into verdohemochrome and globin. The protein is degraded to amino acids, which are further catabolized or reused. Verdohemochrome is converted to bilirubin, giving up its iron in the process. The iron returns to the iron stores for reuse. Bilirubin bound to plasma albumin goes to the liver, where it is conjugated to glucuronic acid, and excreted in the bile. In the intestine the conjugate is hydrolyzed and bilirubin is converted, by successive reductions, to the colorless urobilinogen and stercobilinogen. The latter appears in the feces, reoxidized to the brown pigment stercobilin. Urobilinogen is reabsorbed and excreted in the urine, reoxidized to the pigment urobilin. About 250 mg. of bile pigment appears in the feces, and 1 to 2 mg. in the urine of normal individuals each day.

Jaundice, characterized by yellow skin and conjuctiva, occurs when there is a sustained large increase in the concentration of bile pigments in the plasma. A great increase in destruction of red cells, exceeding the capacity of the liver to remove the resulting bile pigment, causes hemolytic jaundice. The pigment is mainly bilirubin tightly bound to serum albumin and giving the indirect van den Bergh test (development of a color with diazotized sulfanilic acid after addition of alcohol to the serum). In hepatitis or cirrhosis, the liver fails to conjugate and secrete bilirubin. The indirect van den Bergh test reveals high concentrations of bilirubin in the serum, but the excretion of bile pigment in feces and urine is low. In obstruction of the bile duct, bilirubin is at first conjugated normally but the conjugates accumulate in the plasma, yielding, with diazotized sulfanilic acid, an immediate color (direct van den Bergh test). Longstanding obstruction causes liver damage. Both albumin-bound and conjugated bilirubin appear in serum. Little or no bile pigment appears in the feces, but urinary excretion of bilirubin is high.

The biochemistry of leukocytes and platelets is a specialized topic and will not be dealt with here.

Blood Plasma. The blood plasma contains 90 per cent water, about 7 per cent proteins, 0.9 per cent inorganic salts, and about 2 per cent of a wide variety of organic solutes of low molecular weight. The number and variety of the constitutents, including the individual proteins, is enormous. The fluid obtained after blood is allowed to clot, the blood serum, differs from plasma mainly in lacking the proteins associated with clotting. In the analysis of blood, the choice of serum or plasma depends upon the nature of the substance to be measured. In many instances, analyses are made upon protein-free filtrates of whole blood; the method of deproteinization also may depend on the analysis to be made. Table 4-7 presents normal values for a large number of the constituents of blood plasma or serum that are of clinical interest. Continuing improvements in analytic technology constantly increase the variety, sensitivity, specificity and ease of performance of methods. An example is the current development of numerous applications of the principle of radioimmunoassay.

Plasma Proteins. The plasma proteins are separable by chemical methods into two classes: globulins (precipitable at half saturation with ammonium sulfate) and albumins (precipitable at full saturation with ammonium sulfate). By electrophoresis the proteins are separated into albumin, α-1, α-2, β and γ globulins, and fibrinogen, which are present as 55, 5, 9, 13, 11 and 7 per cent of the total respectively. Direct determinations of this kind are of diagnostic value, since they reveal which class of protein is present in abnormally great or small proportion. The total protein of normal human plasma may range from 6 to 8 g. per dl.

Albumin (M_r 69,000, isoelectric point pH 4.7) has a very high proportion of ionizing groups and is extremely soluble in neutral solution. Because it is the smallest of the plasma proteins, and is present in the highest concentration, albumin exerts about 80 per cent of the total osmotic effect of the plasma proteins. It is therefore of major importance in regulating the distribution of water and nonprotein solutes between the plasma and the extracellular space. Because of its numerous polar groups it is a powerfully hydrophilic protein; this contributes to the osmotic effectiveness of the molecule. Again, probably because of its highly polar character, albumin improves the solubility of many substances in plasma by binding them. In this way it transports unesterified fatty acids, bilirubin and a great variety of other difficultly soluble compounds. In addition, albumin binds anions and cations; about half the plasma calcium is bound to albumin. The binding is noncovalent, reversible and dependent on the concentration of the unbound molecule or ion.

The α-1 globulins are high-density lipoproteins and glycoproteins. α-2 globulins include the very low density lipoproteins, the copper-transport protein, ceruloplasmin, prothrombin (see below), haptoglobin, which combines with hemoglobin set free by hemolysis, and glycoproteins.

The principal beta globulins are the low-density lipoproteins, the iron-transport protein, transferrin, and plasminogen.

The gamma globulins are the class of proteins that migrate most slowly in electrophoresis. They comprise the immunoglobulins (Ig) or antibodies. The three major classes of gamma globulins are IgG (80 per cent of total Ig; M_r 150,000); IgA (13 per cent of Ig; M_r 160,000); IgM (7 per cent of Ig; M_r 750,000). A typical IgG molecule consists of two symmetrical halves joined together by two disulfide bonds. Each half consists of a heavy chain (420 amino acids) joined by a disulfide bond to a light chain (214 amino acids). The unique specificity of each IgG molecule appears to be related to the fact that the primary sequence of the first 107 amino acids from the amino-terminal end of both the heavy and the light chains is different for each antibody. The remainder of the sequence of the light chains and the heavy chains is identical for every IgG molecule. Two types of light chains are common to every class of Ig, but each class has its own heavy chain. Some immunoglobulins (IgM) consist of multiples of the common dimeric structure. In newborn mammals, including man, the ability to synthesize antibodies has not yet developed. Passive immunity is conferred by the passage of maternal antibodies across the placenta. In rare instances there is a hereditary inability to synthesize gamma globulins (agammaglobulinemia). When the initial passive immunity has lapsed, during the first year of life, such individuals are at great risk from infections.

Fibrinogen (M_r 330,000) is a very long slender molecule that migrates between the beta and the gamma globulins in electrophoresis of plasma. Its concentration is about 0.3 g. per ml. It is the essential substrate of the final activated enzyme in the clotting process.

Most of the plasma proteins are made in the liver. The immunoglobulins are made by the plasma cells of the reticuloendothelial system. The plasma proteins undergo continuous breakdown and renewal at rates characteristic of each. Maintenance of the steady state of their concentration in plasma is therefore critically dependent upon the quality and quantity of the dietary protein, upon vitamins and minerals, and upon the caloric intake.

Coagulation of Blood. The clotting of blood is a chemical device to seal breaks in the cardiovascular system. The device is stable, capable of rapid initiation and acceleration, and self closing. These objectives are achieved by a system of catalysts and cofactors, in blood and tissue, leading to the conversion of fibrinogen to fibrin, which polymerizes to form the clot. The *essential* process is summarized in two equations:

$$\text{prothrombin} \xrightarrow{\text{Ca}^{2+};\ \text{thromboplastin}} \text{thrombin}$$

$$\text{fibrinogen} \xrightarrow{\text{thrombin}} \text{fibrin}$$

Calcium ion is essential; anything that removes or sequestrates Ca^{2+} prevents clotting (e.g., oxalate, fluoride, citrate, ethylenediaminetetraacetate, or removal of Ca^{2+} by ion exchange). "Thromboplastin" is an inclusive term for several other essential components of the system.

Injury to the surface of blood vessels initiates the *intrinsic* pathway of clotting; injury to tissues sets free tissue thromboplastin, initiating the shorter and more rapid *extrinsic* pathway. The clotting factors of these pathways form a system of serine proteases, with specificities resembling those of trypsin, present in plasma as inactive precursors, or zymogens.

At the site of injury to a blood vessel, with exposure of subendothelial collagen to blood, temporary local excess of the prostaglandin thromboxane A_2 causes platelets to adhere to collagen, become sticky and extrude their contents. Serotonin, norepinephrine and histamine are released, causing local vasoconstriction. ADP accelerates the aggregation of platelets to form the primary hemostatic plug, the nucleus of the eventual fibrin clot. The plug of platelets contracts, because of shortening of an actomyosin-like platelet protein, thrombosthenin. The disruption of platelets sets free thromboplastin and a mixture of phosphatidyl serines and phosphatidyl ethanolamines containing polyunsaturated fatty acids, which facilitate steps of the clotting process. If the injury is slight, the platelet plug alone may be sufficient to effect closure and initiate repair.

The intrinsic pathway is also initiated at a site of injury of a vessel wall. Contact with the injured surface activates the Hageman factor (Factor XII). The process is accelerated by the conversion of prokallikrein to kallikrein.

Factor XIIa in turn activates Factor XI (plasma thromboplastin antecedent), and Factor XIa in its turn activates Christmas Factor, Factor IX, a step requiring calcium. Factor IXa activates the antihemophilic globulin, Factor VIII (not itself an enzyme), and then the complex formed by Factor IXa, VIIIa, Ca^{2+}, and the phosphoglycerides (PG) mentioned above, converts Factor X (Stuart factor) to its active form. Factor Xa activates Factor V (proaccelerin, also not an enzyme), and then the complex of Factors Xa, V', Ca^{2+}, and PG convert prothrombin (Factor II) to thrombin.

The extrinsic pathway involves activation of Factor VII (proconvertin) by means at present ill defined, and later by Factors Xa and thrombin itself, which also activate Factor V. The complex, Factor VIIa, tissue factor, Ca^{2+}, and PG then can activate Factor X. The pathways converge at Factor Xa and the activation of prothrombin, as above.

Phosphoglyceride surfaces play a critical part in these processes. First, by drawing the participants together, PG concentrates them by a factor of as much as 10^4, tending to overwhelm the natural inhibitors of clotting. Second, the lipid surface provided by disrupted platelets or damaged cells, assures that the accelerated reactions will occur at, and only at, the site of injury. Third, the concentrating function of PG greatly accelerates the reactions. The following data on the relative rates of thrombin formation from bovine prothrombin are instructive:

1) Factor Xa, Ca^{2+}		1
2) " " " , PG		50
3) " " " , Factor V'		350
4) " " " , Factor V', PG		19000

It is probable that the activation of Factor X, involving a similar organization, is also enormously accelerated. The binding of Factors IXa, Xa, VIIa and prothrombin to PG depends on their calcium-binding capabilities. This they owe to the post-translational, vitamin K-dependent formation of γ-carboxy-glutamyl residues near the NH_2-terminal ends of these molecules.

By a limited proteolytic attack on fibrinogen (Factor I) thrombin cleaves a small peptide from each of the two α-chains and the two β-chains. The resulting fibrin monomer rapidly aggregates to form fibrils, strands, and the meshwork of the clot, entrapping red and white cells in the process. The clot is hardened by the action of a transaminase, fibrinase, derived from fibrin-stabilizing Factor XIII from platelets and in plasma by the action of thrombin. In the presence of Ca^{2+} the enzyme catalyzes the crosslinking of fibrin by exchanging the amide group of glutamine residues in one molecule for the ϵ-amino group of lysine residues in another, setting free ammonia in the process. The cross-linked fibrin is highly insoluble.

Fibrin adsorbs thrombin, so that as the clot is formed it also removes the last active factor in the chain, tending to limit the reaction to the site of injury.

Each active factor leads to the formation of a greater quantity of the next one, so that the cascade of reactions has a large amplifier effect: The clotting of 250 mg. of fibrinogen in 100 ml. of blood may be initiated by a small fraction of a milligram of active Hageman factor (XII). Most of these factors have been recognized by their absence in certain individuals with disorders of the clotting process. Classical hemophilia (type A) is due to the synthesis of an ineffective form of

TABLE 4-7. Composition of Human Blood

This table considers only components important in clinical medicine. Values are expressed as mg. per 100 ml.(dl.) unless otherwise indicated. When a single value is given it is understood to be a mean value. The medium upon which the analysis is carried out is indicated thus: (B) = whole blood; (P) = plasma; (S) = serum.

Component		Normal Range	Pathologic Deviations
Total serum protein	(S)	6.4–7.7 g.	Low in nephrosis with marked decrease in albumin; high in dehydration
Albumin*	(S)	3.9–4.9 g.	Low in starvation; lack of formation by the liver; loss of protein in the urine
Globulin	(S)	2.3–3.5 g.	Increased in chronic infections, multiple myeloma and liver disease
Fibrinogen	(P)	0.2–0.4 g.	High in infectious diseases; decrease may be present after gross bleeding in obstetric cases; also low in severe hepatic disorders
Hemoglobin	(B)		High in polycythemia
Male		14–17 g.	
Female		12–16 g.	Low in anemia
% of Total hemoglobin			
Hemoglobin-A		90–95%	
Hemoglobin-A$_2$		2–2.5%	
Hemoglobin-F (adult)		0.5%	
Methemoglobin	(B)	0.2–0.3 g.	Increased on exposure to certain organic chemicals and nitrites; cyanosis at 10–20%; anoxia at about 30%
Nonprotein N, NPN	(B)	15–35	High in nephritis, eclampsia, metallic poisoning; normal in nephrosis
Urea nitrogen, BUN	(B)	8–18	High in kidney failure and urinary obstruction, acute glomerulonephritis, mercury poisoning, dehydration; low in acute hepatic insufficiency, severe hepatic failure; often low in pregnancy; low or normal in nephrosis
Creatinine	(S)	0.5–1.2	Increased in nephritis
Creatine	(S)	0.16–0.4	
Uric acid	(S)	2–6	High in gout, eclampsia, nephritis, arthritis
α-amino acid nitrogen	(S)	3.5–5.5	Low in nephrosis (during crisis); high in severe liver disease
Ammonia	(B)	0.04–0.07	High in liver disease; high in newborn
Glucose	(B)		
reducing substance		80–120	High in diabetes mellitus
"true"		60–100	
Calcium	(S)	9–11 4.5–5.5 mEq./L.	Low in infantile tetany, severe nephritis, parathyroidectomy, deficient absorption of vitamin D; lower when serum protein is low; high following excessive doses of vitamin D and in hyperparathyroidism.
Phosphorus, inorganic	(S)	3–4 (adults) 4–7 (children)	Increased in chronic nephritis, hypothyroidism and rickets
Phosphorus, lipid	(S)	6–11	Increases in liver disease, hypothyroidism
Phosphatase, alkaline (Bodansky)	(P)	1–4 units (adults) 5–14 (children)	High in rickets, Paget's disease, cancer of bone, liver disease, hyperthyroidism Low in genetic disorder: hypophosphatasia
Phosphatase, acid	(P)	0–1 units	High in cancer of prostate
Cholesterol, total	(S)	150–280	High in diabetes, lipoid nephrosis, hypothyroidism, severe nephritis, atherosclerosis
Cholesterol ester	(S)	110–200	Low in liver disease
Bilirubin, total	(S)	0.2–1.5	High in red blood cell destruction, liver disease, hemolytic anemia. First month of life values are greater in normal infant— up to 12 mg. at 3 to 5 days; even higher in premature infant
1-Minute bilirubin		0.05–0.25	
Acetone	(S)	0.3–2.0	High in diabetes, starvation
Lipids, total	(P)	500–820	

* Values based on precipitation of globulins with a Na_2SO_4-Na_2SO_3 mixture (20.8% Na_2SO_4 + 7% Na_2SO_3). This mixture gives a partition that agrees closely with results obtained by electrophoresis.

TABLE 4-7. Composition of Human Blood (*Continued*)

Component		Normal Range	Pathologic Deviations
Chlorides	(S)	98–100 mEq./L.	High in nephritis, congestive heart failure, dehydration, prostatic obstruction, eclampsia, anemia; low in diabetes, fever and pneumonia
Sodium	(S)	139–146 mEq./L.	Low in diabetic acidosis, alkali deficit; decreased on administration of excessive fluid
Potassium	(S)	4.1–5.6 mEq./L.	High in pneumonia and acute infections; may be decreased in treatment of diabetes and restoration of plasma volume and in diarrhea and vomiting
Magnesium	(S)	1.1–2.2 mEq./L.	Decreased in severe diarrhea, tetany, acute uremia; increased in chronic nephritis and liver disease
Sulfates as SO_4— (inorganic)	(S)	2.5–5.0	
Iron	(B)	46–55	
Iron	(S)	0.05–0.18	Low in anemias with iron deficiency, hemorrhage; elevated in hemochromatosis and thalassemia
Iron-combining capacity	(S)	0.3–0.45	
Total cations Na, K, Ca, Mg	(S)	142–150 mEq./L.	Low in diabetic acidosis, alkali deficit
CO_2 content	(S)	24.5–33.5 mEq./L.	Low in primary alkali deficit, severe protracted diarrhea, administration of ammonia salts; high in hypoventilation
CO_2 combining power	(S)	20.0–30 mEq./L.	
Serum protein cation–binding power	(S)	15.5–18.0 mEq./L.	
CO_2 tension (Pco_2) (arterial)		35–45 mm.	
pH(at 38 C.)		7.30–7.45	High in uncompensated alkalosis; low in uncompensated acidosis
Lactic acid	(B)	6–16	
Oxygen content, arterial	(B)	15–22 vol. %	
Oxygen content, venous	(B)	11–16 vol. %	
Oxygen capacity	(B)	16–24 vol. %	
Oxygen tension		85–100 mm. Hg	
Osmolality	(P)	270–290 mOsm./L. plasma water	
Protein-bound iodine (PBI)	(S)	4–8.0 µg	High in hyperthyroidism; low in cretinism, hypothyroidism
Water	(B)	79–81 g.	
	(S)	91–92 g.	
Transaminases:			
Glutamic-oxalo-acetic (SGOT)	(S)	5–40 units	(Karmen units) Increased within 24 hours after myocardial infarction; falls to normal by 6th or 7th day
Glutamic-pyruvic (SGPT)	(S)	5–35 units	(Karmen units) Much higher values, and more prolonged, in infectious hepatitis and other hepatic diseases
Lactate dehydrogenase	(S)	90–200 IU/liter	
Amylase	(S)	60–180 units	(Somogyi) Increased in pancreatitis, mumps
Lipase	(S)	0.2–1.5 units/ml.	Elevated in acute pancreatitis, mumps
Ascorbic acid	(P)	0.4–1.5	Low in severe vitamin C deficiency
Copper	(S)	0.08–235	Decreased in anemia, Wilson's disease
Zinc	(S)	0.100–0.140	

Factor VIII. Hemophilia B is due to the absence of Christmas factor (IX), and hemophilia C is due to the absence of Factor XI (plasma thromboplastin antecedent). In congenital parahemophilia the accelerator globulin (V), proaccelerin, is missing.

The lysis of clots is brought about by a proteolytic enzyme, plasmin (fibrinolysin), which is synthesized in the kidney as the inactive precursor, plasminogen. Active plasmin is formed by tissue factors, by the enzyme urokinase, present in blood and urine, and by a number of unphysiologic agents (chloroform; streptokinase). It is a trypsin-like enzyme that breaks down insoluble fibrin to small soluble peptides.

CEREBROSPINAL FLUID

Cerebrospinal fluid is a clear colorless fluid of low viscosity. Unlike lymph and plasma, it does not coagulate. It is secreted by the choroid plexus into the subarachnoid space of the brain and spinal cord and the ventricles of the brain, and it returns to the blood in the lumbar region. The normal pressure is between 100 and 200 mm. of water. The total amount of fluid in the adult is between 100 and 150 ml., and, since it is renewed several times a day, from 5 to 10 ml. can be withdrawn at a time with no ill effects. The protein concentration is low, from 15 to 45 mg. per dl., about 80 per cent albumin, the rest globulin. The pH and the bicarbonate concentration are the same as in normal serum. The glucose concentration in normal spinal fluid is lower than that in plasma: between 45 and 80 mg. per dl. The concentration of non-protein nitrogenous constituents is, in mg. per dl., total NPN, 12.5 to 30; amino acids, 1.5 to 3.0; creatinine, 0.45 to 1.5; urea nitrogen, 6 to 15; uric acid, 0.4 to 2.8. Plasma lipids are absent.

The spinal fluid is in osmotic equilibrium with the plasma, but the concentrations of individual electrolytes differ. Chloride is high: 118 to 130 mEq. per liter. Sodium is about 140 mEq. per liter, as it is in plasma. The concentrations of other cations (in mEq. per liter) are: calcium, 2.43; magnesium, 2.4; potassium, 2.2. The inorganic phosphorus is low in spinal fluid, 1.25 to 2.0 mg. per dl. in adults, 1.5 to 3.5 mg. per dl. in children.

In many diseases there is a significant and characteristic increase in the concentration of protein, most frequently of globulin, in the cerebrospinal fluid. The Pandy test, in which a drop of spinal fluid added to 1 ml. of ten per cent phenol produces immediately a bluish-white cloud of precipitated globulin, is a standard qualitative test. Lange's colloidal gold reagent may be used in a semi-quantitative test for characteristic increases in cerebrospinal fluid protein.

LYMPH

The chemical composition of lymph is qualitatively similar to that of plasma. The concentration of protein is much lower (from 0.3 to 6 per cent) and variable. Lymph from gut and liver is high in protein; that from skin and muscle contains much less. The proteins are identical to the plasma proteins, but the ratio of albumin to globulin is higher: 3:1 to 5:1. Lymph contains fibrinogen, prothrombin and leukocytes, and coagulates slowly, forming a softer clot than does plasma. The concentrations of nonprotein nitrogen, urea, inorganic phosphorus, chlorides, amino acids, creatinine and calcium are about the same as in blood plasma. Lymph is derived from the interstitial fluid, which permeates the tissues, supplying nutrients and receiving waste products and secretions from the cells. The composition of lymph therefore depends both on the rate of irrigation of a tissue and on local metabolic activity. The composition of thoracic duct lymph varies significantly during digestion and absorption of a meal, since lymph flowing from the gut to the thoracic duct is the main vehicle for the transport of fat to the blood. The total volume of lymph returned to the blood per day is 1 to 2 liters.

MILK

Milk is the normal secretion of the mammary gland. Human milk differs markedly from cow's milk in a number of ways. A comparison of average compositions of the two milks is given in Table 4-8.

The protein and mineral content of human milk are much lower than those of cow's milk, while the lactose in human milk is much higher. For infant feeding, cow's milk generally is diluted with water and fortified with sucrose, to approximate the protein mineral, and carbohydrate content of human milk. No single food has so many nutritional virtues as milk.

The milk proteins are casein, lactalbumin and lactoglobulin. They are of very high quality, containing all the essential amino acids in ideal proportions. Milk supplements the cereal proteins, for it supplies the lysine and the tryptophan that are lacking in cereals. Fresh milk does not coagulate on boiling, but a surface film is formed that contains casein and calcium salts. The pH of fresh milk is between 6.6 and 7.0. When unsterilized milk is allowed to stand, organisms in the

TABLE 4-8. Relative Composition of Cow's and Human Milk

	Water %	Protein %	Lactose %	Fat %	Ash %	Calories per 100 g.
Cow's milk	87	3.5	4.8	3.9	0.7	65
Human milk	87	1.5	7.2	3.6	0.2	67

milk grow and produce lactic acid from lactose, and the pH may become low enough to coagulate the casein (pH 4.7). Casein may also be clotted by pepsin, chymotrypsin and by rennin, an enzyme from the fourth stomach of the suckling calf. The protein of cow's milk is 80 per cent casein, whereas the casein in human milk is only 40 per cent of the total protein. The distribution of the amino acids in the protein and the percentage distribution of the mineral elements in the ash are quite similar in the two types of milk. The sulfur of milk is almost entirely in the form of the sulfur-containing amino acids in the protein. Many enzymes are present in milk (lactoperoxidase, catalase, lipase, xanthine oxidase, aldolase). The phosphatase content of cow's milk is the basis of a test for adequate pasteurization. Human milk is particularly rich in amylase. Casein and lactoglobulin are synthesized only in the mammary gland, and only during lactation. Milk contains immunoglobulins similar to those of serum.

Lactose is the sole carbohydrate of milk. It is less sweet than other sugars. It favors the growth of acid-producing bacteria and thus helps to prevent intestinal putrefaction. It likewise favors the absorption of calcium and phosphorus. Lactose is synthesized in the mammary gland from glucose and UDP-galactose. It is found only in female mammals, and only during lactation. The enzyme galactosyltransferase normally transfers galactose from UDP-galactose to N-acetylglucosamine. The product (lactosamine) is a common constituent of the carbohydrate present in many glycoproteins, and the enzyme is found in nearly all tissues. Under the influence of prolactin the mammary gland synthesizes a new protein, alpha lactalbumin, which combines with the galactosyltransferase, greatly reduces its Km for glucose, and makes possible the reaction:

$$\text{UDP-galactose} + \text{glucose} \rightarrow \text{lactose} + \text{UDP}$$

The enzyme is membrane bound, in the Golgi apparatus. "Lactose synthase" is a remarkable instance of the facultative adaptation of a common enzyme to a special purpose by the formation of a complex with a positive effector protein.

Fat of milk is more variable than any other constituent. The fat in cow's milk contains all the even-carbon fatty acids from C4 to C20. There are qualitative differ-

ences in the fat of human and cow's milk. Both contain mainly oleic, palmitic, and stearic acids, but human milk contains more oleic acid and only small amounts of the volatile short chain fatty acids. Whole milk contains from 9 to 17 mg. of cholesterol per 100 ml. Skimmed milk contains only 4 mg. of the sterol per liter.

There is no adequate substitute for milk in meeting the calcium requirements. Milk is also a good source of riboflavin. It contains a liberal amount of vitamins A, B_{12} and thiamine. Most milk sold today is fortified with vitamin D. Milk is low in iron, copper, and ascorbic acid.

Colostrum, the fluid obtained from the mammary gland the first few days after parturition, differs markedly from ordinary milk. Human colostrum has a higher concentration of protein, immune globulin, β-carotene, riboflavin, niacinamide and other vitamins. Colostrum has less fat and lactose than milk.

URINE

About 1,200 ml. of blood flow through the two kidneys per minute. Plasma is filtered in the glomeruli, yielding a nearly protein-free filtrate, about 125 ml. per minute in an adult male, slightly less in the female. The rate of filtration is proportional to the net filtration pressure [blood pressure − (colloid osmotic pressure of the plasma proteins + hydrostatic pressure of the glomerular filtrate)] and to the rate of blood flow through the kidneys. Of the total volume of filtrate formed each day (about 180 liters) more than 99 per cent is normally reabsorbed. In this process the plasma is cleared of waste materials, of excess of water or electrolyte and of excess acid or base. About 85 per cent of the glomerular filtrate is reabsorbed in the proximal convoluted tubule. Glucose is completely recovered, and about 75 per cent of the filtered Na^+ ion is actively reabsorbed. Water and Cl^- ion passively follow the Na^+ ion, along with a small fraction of the urea present in the filtrate. An essentially isotonic solution is reabsorbed; the filtrate is very little concentrated at this stage. Waste materials such as sulfate and creatinine are not reabsorbed at all and are completely cleared from the blood. In the loop of Henle another 15 per cent of the sodium is reabsorbed, with only 5 per cent of the water, and the filtrate reaching the distal tubules is hypotonic. In the distal and collecting tubules the remainder of the Na^+ is reabsorbed, and water is reabsorbed in the presence of the antidiuretic hormone (ADH); otherwise these sections of the nephron are essentially impermeable to water, and a dilute urine is secreted.

The active reabsorption of sodium is accomplished in part by exchange for K^+ and H^+ ions. The H^+ ions are dealt with in three ways: (1) Filtered HPO_4^{2-} is converted to $H_2PO_4^-$. (2) Ammonia formed from glutamine is converted to ammonium ion:

$$L\text{-glutamine} + H_2O = L\text{-glutamate} + NH_3.$$
$$NH_3 + H^+ = NH_4^+$$

This device can spare Na^+ otherwise required for the partial neutralization of the anions of filtered acid. (3) The H^+ ions can react with filtered HCO_3^- to form H_2CO_3, which is decomposed to H_2O and CO_2. The CO_2, absorbed into the tubule cells, which are rich in carbonic anhydrase, is rehydrated to H_2CO_3, which dissociates into H^+ and HCO_3^-. The anion is returned to the blood, and the H^+ can cycle again in exchange for Na^+. The average daily diet yields about 70 mEq. of excess acid (H^+). About half of this is excreted by the conversion of HPO_4^{2-} to $H_2PO_4^-$ in the urine, and the other half is excreted as ammonium ion. Filtered bicarbonate is completely returned to the plasma at concentrations below 26 to 27 mmole per liter, and by means of the exchanges described above, the concentration of $NaHCO_3$ in plasma is restored to normal. When plasma bicarbonate is low, the concentration is restored by the hydration of metabolic CO_2 in the tubule cells, the dissociation of the resulting carbonic acid, exchange of H^+ for Na^+ and secretion of Na^+ with the bicarbonate counterion into the plasma. When sodium intake is restricted, aldosterone, operating in the distal tubule, facilitates reabsorption so that recovery of filtered Na^+ is essentially complete. Even when the intake is restricted, there is unavoidably some daily loss of potassium because of the way in which the management of Na^+ and H^+ is carried out. The reabsorption of water under the influence of ADH is governed by the secretion of the hormone in response to changes in total plasma volume and osmolality. The concentration of solute in the urine may vary correspondingly from 50 to 1,400 milliosmoles per liter in the course of regulation of the plasma osmolarity at about 310 milliosmoles per liter.

The rate of urine secretion is quite variable, as is also the concentration of the solid constituents with each voiding. It is customary to consider the composition of the 24 hour output as giving more information than that of the output over shorter periods.

The adult secretes from 1,000 to 1,500 ml. of urine in a 24 hour period, the day volume being from two to four times as much as the night volume. The latter is more concentrated. The child excretes from three to four times as much as the adult per kg. body weight. Under normal conditions the volume is determined primarily by the amount of fluid ingested. The specific gravity of urine varies between 1.015 and 1.025, but in unusual circumstances it may be as low as 1.003 and as high as 1.045. Urine normally is clear, pale straw to deep brown in color and has an aromatic odor. Depending on the diet, the pH may vary from 5.5 to 5.7; under extreme conditions the pH may be as low as 4.5, or, in uncompensated alkalosis, as high as that of the blood (7.8 to 8.0).

Protein. About 75 mg. of protein is excreted normally in 24 hours, an amount too small to be detected by ordinary chemical tests. The protein found in proteinuria is mainly albumin, but always with some globulin. Urine also may contain mucin, which can be distinguished and removed by acidifying with strong acetic acid and filtering. An abnormal protein, the Bence Jones protein, may be present in urine of patients who have multiple myeloma. Bence Jones proteins have been identified as the light chains of immunoglobulins, arising from unbalanced synthesis of IgG, IgA or IgM in rapidly proliferating lymphoid cells. Light chains produced in excess of heavy chains are excreted in the urine.

Sugar. Glucose is a so-called threshold substance, appearing in the urine when the blood glucose rises to about 170 mg. per dl. Glucose in the glomerular filtrate at a lower concentration is reabsorbed entirely.

Pentoses may be present in the urine after large amounts of cherries, grapes, plums or other foods rich in pentoses are eaten. Pentosuria also occurs as a hereditary condition in which L-xylulose is excreted independently of the nature of the diet. There is congenital lack of the enzyme, L-xylulose dehydrogenase, required for the metabolism of this pentose. It is a harmless disorder, but care must be taken that it not be mistaken for glucosuria.

Acetone Bodies. Acetoacetate, β-hydroxybutyrate and acetone are normal products of oxidation of fatty acids, and are not excreted in the urine unless their concentration in blood exceeds about 20 mg. per dl. Their presence in urine is therefore indicative of intense fatty acid metabolism such as may occur in fasting or in diabetic ketosis.

Porphyrins. Coproporphyrin and uroporphyrin are present in small amounts in normal urine. *Porphyrinuria,* symptomatic of many diseases, is characterized by moderate increases in urinary coproporphyrin. *Porphyrias* may be congenital or acquired. They are characterized by excretion of large amounts, several hundred mg. per day, of both uroporphyrin and coproporphyrin.

Nonprotein Nitrogen Constituents of Urine. With a mixed diet the total nitrogen of urine per 24 hours may be between 8 and 18 g., depending on the amount of protein ingested. Urea is the principal end-product of protein (amino acid) metabolism in man. With a high protein diet it may represent 90 per cent of the total urinary nitrogen, while with a low protein diet it may be only 60 per cent of the total. The excretion of urea may be decreased in certain liver diseases in which the capacity to produce urea is decreased, in severe acidosis and in advanced nephritis. Ammonia nitrogen represents ordinarily from 2.5 to 5.0 per cent of the total urinary nitrogen. It is present in urine as ammonium salts. The amount is increased greatly in diabetic acidosis and decreased greatly in nephritis. Urinary ammonia may be increased greatly owing to hydrolysis of urea by bacteria in the bladder or in other parts of the urinary tract. Urine standing exposed to air becomes very alkaline, because of the conversion of urea to ammonia by bacteria. Creatinine, the anhydride of creatine, is excreted in the urine in amounts of 1 to 2 g. per 24 hr., depending somewhat on the creatinine in the diet, which is excreted unchanged, and mainly on the total muscle mass (i.e., the total body creatine). Daily urinary creatinine is therefore roughly constant for a given individual adult, and is independent of exercise and of nitrogen intake. Creatine is found more commonly in the urine of women than in that of men. It is a regular constituent of the urine of children (from 10 to 51 mg. per day). Starving adults and patients with certain muscular dystrophies excrete creatine in the urine.

The total amino acid excretion in urine per 24 hours is about 1.5 g., of which more than half is in peptide or other combinations from which it is liberated by acid hydrolysis. About 0.4 to 1.0 g. of uric acid is excreted in 24 hours in the urine. The excretion is quite variable. It is increased by exercise and diets rich in purine foods. The strength of uric acid (pKa = 5.7) is such that part of the uric acid in normal urine is excreted as urate and part as free uric acid.

The nature and origin of urinary calculi are discussed in the chapter on Pathology.

BILE

Bile plays an important role in digestion. It is secreted continuously (about 500 to 700 ml. per day) by liver cells and is stored in the gallbladder. The outflow into the intestine is intermittent; the contraction of the gallbladder is stimulated by free fatty acids, protein, bile salts in the intestine and also by the hormone cholecystokinin, which originates in the intestinal mucosa. Bladder bile is green to yellowish brown, bitter to taste and more concentrated than hepatic duct bile. Bile is alkaline in reaction (pH 7.1 to 7.7) and contains bile acids, pigments, cholesterol, inorganic salts, fats and fatty acids. In the gallbladder, part of the bicarbonate ions may be reabsorbed.

The bile salts, sodium glycocholate and sodium taurocholate, aid in protein and fat digestion and in fatty acid absorption. The chief pigments of bile, bilirubin and biliverdin (a mild oxidation product of bilirubin) are derived from the breakdown of hemoglobin. In the bile pigments, the pyrrole groups are in open-chain formation. In the intestine, bile pigments are reduced to urobilinogen, which is partly excreted in the urine and partly reabsorbed, carried to the liver and reconverted to bile pigment. Part of the bile pigments are reduced by bacteria to a brown pigment, stercobilin, that gives the characteristic brown color to feces.

The functions of the bile are: (1) to promote absorption of fats, fat-soluble vitamins and calcium, (2) to activate lipase, (3) to diminish putrefaction in the large intestine, (4) to stimulate peristalsis, (5) to provide a reservoir of alkali to help neutralize the acid chyme from the stomach and (6) to serve as an excretory channel for cholesterol, lecithin, poisonous toxins, bile pigments and certain inorganic wastes. Metal ions, such as copper and zinc, are removed from the blood by the liver and excreted in the bile.

Biliary calculi (gallstones) may be almost pure cholesterol. Other types contain calcium salts, and most types contain varying amounts of bile pigment. Formation of the stones is associated with conditions in which stasis, infection or both exist in the gallbladder. Other factors may enter into their formation.

MUSCLE

The property of motion of living cells is most clearly illustrated by striated voluntary and cardiac muscle and by smooth muscle, but the molecular device of the contractile protein is employed by many cells for a variety of tasks such as the moving apart of the chromosomes during cell division or the extrusion of the contents of blood platelets. The energetics and molecular dynamics of contraction are best understood in voluntary striated muscle, which will be the subject of this brief account.

The principal constituents of mammalian skeletal

TABLE 4-9. Partial Composition of Mammalian Skeletal Muscle

Component	g./100 g. Wet Weight
Total solids	20.0–28.0
Water	72.0–80.0
Total protein	16.5–20.9
Creatine + creatinine	0.27–0.58
Carnitine	0.19–0.30
Glycogen	0.7–2.0
Inorganic constituents	1.0–1.5
Potassium	0.39
Phosphorus	0.20
Magnesium	0.02
Sodium	0.07
Chloride	0.05
Calcium*	0.006

* The low concentration of calcium is not insignificant. In terms of muscle water, it is 7.4 to 8.4 mg. per dl., and locally it may be much higher.

muscle are listed in Table 4-9. About 90 per cent of the total protein of muscle is accounted for by four proteins that are directly concerned with contraction: myosin; actin; tropomyosin; and troponin T, C and I. The remainder of the protein makes up the cell membranes and the enzymes required for glycolysis, respiration and the other metabolic activities of the cell. In voluntary muscle the glycolytic system is particularly prominent, since the organ is usefully adapted to delivering full power for a limited time in the absence of oxygen.

The cells of voluntary muscle are multinucleated, have many mitochondria and may be up to 40 mm. in length and 10 to 100μ in diameter. Each muscle fiber is composed of a number of fibrils, 1 to 2μ in diameter. It is the complex structure of the myofibrils that accounts for the striations of the fiber. Under polarized light a muscle fiber exhibits alternating light and dark bands. The I (for isotropic) bands have uniform optical properties, while the A (for anisotropic) bands change appearance with change in the plane of the polarized light in which they are observed. Each light I band is bisected by a thin dense transverse line, the Z line, running right through the fiber. Midway in each dark A band is a light region, the H band, bisected by a faint transverse line, the M line, running right through the fiber. The interval between two Z lines is the sarcomere, the operating subunit of the myofibril. Sarcomeres are about 2.3μ in length, but they are shorter and more numerous, the faster the muscle.

Looked at still more closely, the band pattern of the sarcomeres is seen to be determined by an orderly array of thin and thick filaments running longitudinally in the myofibril. The thin filaments are attached at the Z line, extend across the I band and partly overlap the thick filaments, which extend throughout the A band. The thick filaments are seen to have, except in the pale H band region, numerous small processes that do not quite touch the thin filaments. In cross section, the myofibril presents a hexagonal array of thin and thick filaments such that every thin filament is surrounded by thick filaments and vice versa.

The thin filaments are mainly composed of the fibrous protein, F actin, formed by the action of ATP on the globular protein monomer, G actin (M_r 46,000):

$$n \text{ G actin} + n \text{ ATP} = F \text{ actin(ADP)} + (P_i)n$$

The molecules of G actin, like a doubled string of beads, form the long helix of F actin. The diameter of the polymer is nearly the diameter of a thin filament, 50 Å. The protein tropomyosin B, also a long slender double helical molecule, lies in the grooves of the helix of F actin, covering about 7 monomer units. At intervals of about 400 Å a molecule of the protein troponin is bound to the terminus of tropomyosin. One subunit of the troponin (T) binds to tropomyosin; one subunit (I) inhibits the Mg^{2+}-activated ATP-ase of actomyosin; one subunit (C) binds Ca^{2+} strongly and overrides the inhibition when it does. In the absence of calcium ion, troponin affects the long helix of tropomyosin, so that it does not quite lie in the grooves of the helix of the F actin, interfering with the close approach of myosin to actin. This is the resting condition; the muscle is soft, flexible and extensible.

The thick filaments are composed of the major protein of the contractile system, myosin. The molecule, M_r about 470,000, is about 1,600 Å long. It is separable by tryptic hydrolysis into a tail, L meromyosin, consisting of two polypeptide chains in α-helical configuration, wound about one another in a double helix, and a head, H-meromyosin, comprised of two tightly folded globular pieces, set at an angle to the tail, so that the whole molecule somewhat resembles a golf club. The head-pieces are associated with two light chains of about 20,000 daltons. These can be phosphorylated by a specific myosin light chain kinase requiring calmodulin and calcium ion for its activity. The head-pieces contain sites for combining with actin and a catalytic site binding ATP. The thick filaments, about 100 Å in diameter, are bundles of myosin molecules arranged in a staggered array so that the angled heads appear at many points on the surface of the filament except at the center, the H band, where only L meromyosin is present. The thick filaments are polarized, with the protruding heads of the myosin extending toward each Z line, and overlapping the thin filaments, but not quite touching them in the resting state. The thin and

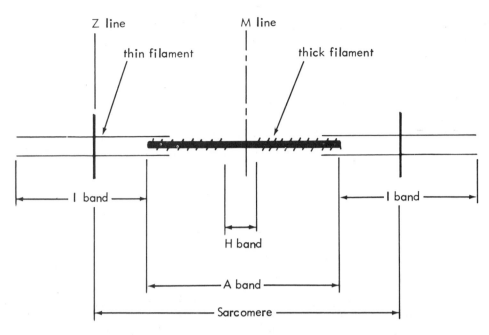

Fig. 4-10. Filaments of muscle in the resting condition.

thick filaments easily slide by one another as the resting muscle is stretched (Fig. 4-10).

In milliseconds after a stimulus a muscle becomes stiff and inextensible, develops tension and, if allowed, will shorten and lift a load, doing work. Each sarcomere is activated, and it can be seen that as the muscle shortens, the I bands nearly disappear, without any notable change in the width of the A bands. The thin filaments move into the A band region, increasing their degree of interdigitation with the thick filaments. The rapid activation is a function of the membrane investing the muscle fibers, the sarcolemma, and interpenetrating them to form the sarcoplasmic reticulum. The nerve impulse to the muscle depolarizes this membrane, which is swept by a wave of potential change of about 60 mv. The membrane becomes permeable to Ca^{2+} ions, which gain access to troponin C.

The binding of Ca^{2+} by troponin C results in a change in the configuration of tropomyosin. It lies more deeply in the grooves of F actin, and this allows contact to take place between the subunits of F actin and the angled heads of myosin. The actomyosin complex formed in this way is a potent ATP-ase. ATP bound to the myosin head is hydrolyzed to ADP and Pi, and a configurational change occurs, altering the angle of the head and drawing the attached F actin more deeply between the thick filaments. When ADP on the myosin head is displaced by ATP, contact with F actin is broken and the head assumes its resting angle, but it can at once engage again with F actin, hydrolyzing the ATP and shifting the thin filament another step further. Each thin filament is engaged

simultaneously by the heads of several thick filaments, which in turn are engaged with surrounding thin filaments. The latter, anchored to the Z lines, are drawn as far as possible into the A region, and the sarcomere shortens.

When the stimulus passes, Ca^{2+} is actively withdrawn by the sarcoplasmic membrane, the myosin heads load with ATP and remain disengaged, because by the action of troponin I and of tropomyosin, an active actomyosin complex can no longer be formed. The muscle becomes soft and extensible and returns to rest length if it is lightly loaded, as it usually is, in situ.

In smooth muscle and non-muscle cells utilizing actomyosin, phosphorylation of the myosin light chains is essential for the combination of myosin with actin. An increase of $[Ca^{2+}]$ to $10^{-5}M$ activates myosin light chain kinase. The phosphorylated myosin combines with actin and contraction occurs. When the $[Ca^{2+}]$ falls to $10^{-7}M$, contraction continues until a phosphatase dephosphorylates the myosin light chains. Actomyosin dissociates and relaxation occurs. In skeletal and cardiac muscle, phosphorylation of the myosin light chains is not required for the combination of myosin with actin, but it increases the rate of that process.

If the supply of ATP fails, the myosin heads cannot disengage from F actin, and the muscle remains short and inextensible, in rigor. When this is due merely to fatigue it is relieved by rest, during which ATP is replenished. The slow passing of rigor post mortem may be due to the hydrolysis of ADP bound to F actin, with reversion of the linear polymer to G actin monomers and dissolution of the thin filaments.

The immediate source of energy for contraction, for doing work and for relaxation is ATP. The supply is maintained by three back-up devices. Minor support is provided by the enzyme myokinase, which catalyzes the reaction

$$2ADP = ATP + AMP.$$

Of greater importance is phosphocreatine (PC) which, through the action of creatine phosphokinase (CPK) transfers phosphate to ADP:

$$PC + ADP \rightleftharpoons ATP + \text{creatine}$$

Four isozymes of CPK are known; a special one, representing 40 per cent of the total CPK activity, is bound to the inner membrane of the mitochondria, close to the ADP–ATP translocase. Another isozyme (MM) is bound to the muscle fibrils and the sarcoplasmic reticulum (20 per cent of the activity). It is thought that ATP may be compartmentalized in the muscle cell, and that PC may serve not merely as a store but also for intracellular energy transport. A critical observation in support of this hypothesis is that when CPK is inhibited by fluorodinitrobenzine, only a small fraction of the total ATP is utilized before the muscle fails to respond to further stimulation.

Resynthesis of PC and ATP is provided by glycolysis, which comes into play at the onset of muscular activity, before the blood flow and the oxygen supply are adjusted to the needs of work. Recall that the protein kinase of muscle that activates glycogen phosphorylase is itself activated by Ca^{2+}; the onset of contraction is coupled with the provision of substrate for glycolysis. The resynthesis of ATP by anaerobic glycolysis can continue until the accumulation of lactic acid reaches a point—about 250 mg. per 100 g. of muscle—at which the buffer capacity of muscle is exceeded. The fall in pH results in abrupt cutoff, most probably of phosphofructokinase, which is exquisitely sensitive to change in pH, and glycolysis is inhibited.

Finally the maintenance and restoration of the supply of ATP and PC during continued activity is accomplished by oxidative phosphorylation. With an adequate blood and oxygen supply a muscle can work at moderate rate almost indefinitely. Carbohydrate is an obligatory substrate for muscle only during anaerobiosis. Fat is an equally good fuel for oxidative muscular exercise. It may in fact be a preferred substrate. The rate of energy utilization of active muscle may be 50 times its resting rate. This capability is reflected in the presence of a large number of mitochondria in intimate contact with the myofibrils, and in a rich capillary bed, providing for minimal distances of diffusion of oxygen during full activity.

CONNECTIVE TISSUE

Connective tissue is found everywhere in the body, in and around blood vessels, in the renal pelvis, ureters and urethra, in ligaments and tendons, in cartilage, in the matrix of bones and teeth, as a component of the intercellular substance of organs, lining the body cavities and the organs they contain, investing the muscles and underlying the skin. The characteristics and composition of connective tissue vary with the proportions of the two principal proteins present and with the amount of glycoprotein, embedded in a heteropolysaccharide ground substance of which the main constituent is in many instances hyaluronic acid. The constituents of connective tissue are synthesized and secreted by fibroblasts, macrophages, mast cells and other cells of the reticuloendothelial system, which also have housekeeping functions of removal of debris, renewal and repair.

The insoluble fibrous proteins of connective tissue are collagen and elastin. Collagen comprises from 25 to 30 per cent of the total body protein in an adult. It is synthesized in fibroblasts as procollagen, a molecule comprising three polypeptide chains, each forming a left helix quite different from the usual α-helix of proteins, and each chain having a small globular domain at the amino and carboxyl ends. These domains assist in the twisting of the three chains round one another in a slow right helix to form a thread, and they may inhibit aggregation of the procollagen monomers. They contain all of the cystine found in procollagen. The central helical portion of procollagen is distinguished by its content of three derived amino acids, 3- and 4-hydroxyproline and 5-hydroxylysine, formed by the action of specific oxygenases on certain prolyl and lysyl sidechains of procollagen during or just after synthesis. The carboxy- and amino-terminal propeptides of procollagen are removed by enzymatic scission as the collagen (tropocollagen) thus set free is secreted. Collagen monomer is now a molecule of 300,000 daltons, a triple helix about 15 Å in diameter and 3,000 Å long. The composition is extraordinary: 25 to 33 per cent glycine; 21 per cent proline, 11 per cent alanine; no cystine. Short non-helical domains at each end of the molecule contain most of the polar amino acids. A small amount of carbohydrate is present in the helical portion. In the extracellular fluid collagen monomers aggregate side by side and head to tail to form fibrils, fibers, strands and cables. The ends of adjacent molecules are offset about a quarter length, which results in regular electron-dense bands across the fibers, spaced 640 to 700 Å apart. Different collagens differ in the makeup of the three polypeptide chains forming the monomer; several are known, each differing in amino acid composition and sequence. A fair portion of the collagen of young animals is soluble in dilute acid, yielding collagen monomers. As the animal grows older, the collagen matures, becoming less soluble by virtue of progressive cross-linking within and between molecules. The sidechains of some lysine and hydroxylysine residues are oxidized to aldehyde by an amine oxidase, a Cu-containing enzyme. The aldehyde groups may condense with one another in an aldol condensation, or they may react with ε-amino groups of other lysine and hydroxylysine molecules to form a variety of firm covalent cross-links. If the amine oxidase is inhibited or is hereditarily deficient, collagen structure is weak and skeletal development is defective. The disorder, lathyrism, is induced experimentally by feeding peas *(Lathyrus odoratus)* or the active principle, β-aminopropionitrile. The oxygenases responsible for the hydroxylation of prolyl and lysyl residues of procollagen require O_2, Fe^{2+}, α-ketoglutarate and ascorbic acid. Succinate, CO_2 and H^+ are products of the reaction. If the oxygenases are inhibited, formation of procollagen is defective; there is delayed secretion of a non-functional molecule. This may account for some of the characteristic lesions of scurvy.

Collagen heated in dilute acid is converted to the soluble derived protein, gelatin. It is useful as a food supplement but is an incomplete protein, lacking tryptophan and cysteine. Once secreted, collagen is, in many sites in the body, enduring and inert metabolically, but in bone it is subject to breakdown and reconstruction as the bone is remodeled.

Elastin is characteristically more prominent than collagen in structures such as the walls of large arteries or ligamentum nuchae. It is an important component of the connective tissue of skin. Elastic connective tissue tends to be yellow; collagenous tissue, white. Heat denaturation of elastin does not yield gelatin. Elastin is an exceedingly insoluble protein of unusual composition: glycine, 27 per cent; alanine, 20 per cent; valine, 10 per cent; proline and hydroxyproline, 10 per cent. The molecule is highly cross-linked by reactions between lysyl side chains like those occurring in collagen, but somewhat more complicated. The native protein has elastic properties superior to those of rubber, but the molecular structure accounting for this is at present unknown. In lathyrism or in the presence of inhibitors of amine oxidase, or in pyridoxine or copper deficiency, the cross-linking of elastin is defective, with consequent serious weakness of such tissues as aorta.

The ground substance of connective tissue is comprised of a variety of heteropolysaccharides, mucopolysaccharides usually found in combination with protein. These are: hyaluronic acid, chondroitin and the chondroitin sulfates, keratosulfates and heparin. These molecules form part of the intercellular substance. They are highly hydrophilic and are capable of binding an-ions such as Na^+ and Ca^{2+}. They assist in maintaining the state of hydration of tissues, and they may play a part in the orientation of the collagen matrix of bone and teeth and in determining the direction and interlacing of collagen in other sites. The mucopolysaccharides are, with the exception of some chondroitin sulfates, metabolically active, undergoing constant breakdown and renewal. Their proportions in different tissues change with age. The turnover of these compounds may require an appreciable fraction of the supply of carbohydrate, but an accurate estimate is not available.

BRAIN AND NERVE

The brain and spinal cord and their dependent and related structures comprise an organization of more than 10^{10} cells. In life, the activity of large aggregates of these cells is incessant. About 20 per cent of the oxygen consumption of an individual at rest is used by the brain, which is 2 per cent of the body weight. The usual substrate is glucose, but in the fetus and the newborn, and in prolonged starvation, the brain adapts to use acetoacetate or β-hydroxybutyrate to cover about one-half its energy requirement. Glucose is nonetheless indispensable, since if in any circumstances the blood glucose falls to low levels, the function of the nervous system is impaired. If the condition is not quickly corrected, convulsions, coma and death follow. The utilization of glucose occurs mainly by the glycolytic pathway to pyruvate, and then over acetyl-S CoA to the tricarboxylic acid cycle. A remarkably high proportion of glucose carbon finds its way into amino acids in the brain. Very little carbohydrate is stored in brain or nerve. The glycogen content is about 0.1 per cent, a negligible reserve against hypoxia. Indeed, a brief period of oxygen lack causes unconsciousness and may cause irreparable damage.

The metabolism of amino acids in the brain centers around glutamate and aspartate, the two amino acids most immediately related to the TCA cycle. About 75 per cent of the free amino acids of the brain are accounted for by glutamate, glutamine, γ-aminobutyrate, aspartate and N-acetylaspartate. The brain, like the liver, can synthesize oxaloacetate from CO_2 and pyruvate, and it can therefore maintain and replenish the supply of intermediates of the TCA cycle and, by amination and transamination, the supply of the amino acids related to it. This may be functionally significant, for example, if brain ammonia increases in consequence of a rise in the level of blood ammonia. This may be dealt with by acceleration of the pathway, CO_2 + pyruvate → oxaloacetate → α-ketoglutarate → glutamate → glutamine, a process by which 2 moles of ammonia are sequestered. Protein synthesis in brain and nerve is very active during growth and development, less active but still significant in adult brain. The possibility that the synthesis of protein or polypeptides, as representatives of information, may be related to memory is being investigated. The synthesis of RNA in brain is an active, continuing process related to the intensity of nervous activity. It is astonishing to discover that the brain is dependent for its pyrimidines and purines on a supply of uridine and of guanine and hypoxanthine from the blood. The latter are utilized by means of the guanine-hypoxanthine phosphoribosyl transferase, the enzyme of the salvage pathway. It will be recalled that absence or deficiency of this enzyme causes severe behavioral and neuronal disorder (the Lesch-Nyhan syndrome). A role for RNA in the function of memory has also been adumbrated, but no convincing evidence in support of the proposition has been brought forward.

The brain is capable of synthesizing fatty acids. Although a large fraction of the brain lipids turns over very slowly, the phospholipids containing choline and inositol turn over rapidly. The lipid storage diseases, resulting from defects in the enzymes that break down the sphingolipids, have been mentioned previously.

Nervous tissue has a high content of water, 75 to 80 per cent. Of the solids, 38 to 40 per cent is protein; 51 to 54 per cent is lipid, mostly compound lipid. There is about 10 per cent of cholesterol, mostly unesterified. The lipids are to a large degree associated with protein, as lipoprotein (water soluble) or as proteolipid (soluble in chloroform-methanol). The structure forming the white matter of brain and nerve is myelin, 40 per cent water, 70 to 80 per cent lipid, and 20 to 30 per cent protein. Most of this is present as a proteolipid. About 30 per cent of the protein of myelin is a basic protein (isoelectric point 10.6) that, when injected into animals (rabbit, monkey, guinea pig), produces an allergic encephalomyelitis. Two short polypeptide sequences of this small encephalitogenic basic protein have been shown to be active in susceptible species. The disorder is being studied as a possible useful model of human demyelinating diseases.

The business of nerves is to establish and maintain connections with other nerves and effector organs and to transmit impulses. The establishment and maintenance of connections is a function of growth and development; it is most vigorous early in life, but it continues as part of the processes of interneuronal communication in the brain supporting the activities of habit, memory and thought. It is related to the vigor of the biosynthetic processes already mentioned. The transmission of impulses occurs in two stages, electrical, involving the cell body and the axon, and chemical, at the synapse. The electrical component exploits the characteristic of all cell membranes of maintaining a high internal concentration of K^+, and a low Na^+ concentration, against a high external concentration of Na^+ and a low concentration of K^+, with a resulting resting membrane potential of 60 to 75 mv. between the interior of the axon and the extracellular medium. Stimulation of the nerve causes depolarization of the membrane. Na^+ enters, K^+ leaves, the sign of the resting potential reverses, the ion flux destabilizes the adjacent membrane, and the impulse progresses as a wave of negativity sweeping down the fiber. Behind it, the membrane is restored to the resting state assisted by the action of the Na^+, K^+-dependent ATP-ase (very high in nerve membrane), extruding Na^+ and recapturing K^+. The impulse may be propagated great distances (meters in a large animal) without decrement. It is a metabolic phenomenon, not a physical one, dependent upon oxygen and the supply of energy. A current hypothesis is that the initiation and propagation of the nerve impulse is due to the progressive release, all along the axon, of bound acetylcholine. The liberated amine reacts with an acceptor protein, setting free in turn its bound Ca^{2+} ions, which act upon the membrane, altering its permeability. The current generated by the movement of K^+ and Na^+ ions across the membrane releases more bound acetylcholine, and the impulse progresses down the axon. The local reaction is closed by hydrolysis of acetylcholine by a specific acetylcholinesterase. When this happens, the receptor protein binds Ca^{2+} again, and the properties of the membrane are restored. Acetylcholine is resynthesized from choline and acetyl-SCoA by choline acetylase and is stored in bound form.

In cholinergic nerves the same process supports the second stage of transmission of the impulse at the synapse. Here acetylcholine acts as the neurotransmitter, diffusing to the sensitive site of the effector cell (e.g., a muscle end-plate) and depolarizing its membrane, eliciting the characteristic response of the cell by means of the propagated new impulse. The reaction is closed by the action of cholinesterase at the effector cell site. Acetylcholine, resynthesized, is stored in vesicles at the nerve ending. Acetylcholinesterase is inhibited by a number of compounds: other quaternary amines; prostigmine, physostigmine, and alkylating agents such as di-isopropylphosphofluoridate and its relatives, the so-called nerve gases.

The neurotransmitter of the adrenergic nerves in the sympathetic nervous system and several parts of the brain is the catecholamine, norepinephrine, also produced along with its methylated derivative epinephrine, in the adrenal medulla. A precursor, dopamine (dihydroxyphenylethylamine) also acts as a neurotransmitter, affecting the basal ganglia. Its concentration in the caudate nucleus is low in Parkinson's disease. Administration of large amounts of its precursor, dopa (dihydroxyphenylalanine) can relieve the symptoms of that disease. Another amine, serotonin, 5-hydroxytryptamine, is associated with cells in the hypothalamus and brain stem. Although the neuronal amines tend to be conserved by recapture into storage sites, they can be inactivated by amine oxidase. Their action is prolonged by inhibitors of the oxidase such as amphetamine.

In recent years, a host of small and large molecules, including polypeptide hormones normally secreted by the hypothalamus, the pituitary, and the gastrointestinal tract, have been found widespread in the brain. At present their origin and function are unknown, but they are the objects of excited scrutiny. Among the more interesting of these are the opioid pentapeptides, methionine and leucine enkephalin:

$$\text{Tyr-Gly-Gly-Phe-Met (or -Leu)}$$

which bind specifically to morphine receptors in the brain, and, like β-endorphin from the pituitary appear to be natural opiates.

THE HORMONES

The hormones comprise a system of chemical regulators elaborated in specific organs, complementary to the nervous system, communicating with their targets by means of the blood plasma and the extracellular fluid, serving the organism as a whole and supplementing the autoregulatory devices operating in the cells. In general, hormones do not initiate new processes, but affect the rate of operation of existing systems. The most striking instance of this is the action of the thyroid hormone on the metabolic rate. In the absence of the hormone the myriad reactions of metabolism take place, but slowly. The thyroid hormone permits acceleration of the reactions to a new steady state. At puberty the hormones of the reproductive system effect a kind of metamorphosis. It appears that they do indeed affect the nucleus of their target cells, unmasking different sectors of DNA and provoking the synthesis of mRNAs that serve to establish an altered array of enzymes in support of the new task of the adult cells of the reproductive system and of the body as a whole. In this instance the hormones appear as another of the numerous devices regulating gene expression.

The secretion of hormones is regulated in a number of ways. A direct signal may be transmitted to an endocrine organ by a change in the concentration of a metabolite in the plasma. A rise in blood sugar, for example, elicits secretion of insulin by the β-cells of the islet tissue of the pancreas. A fall in serum $[Ca^{2+}]$ is a signal for increased output of parathyroid hormone. Increase of glucose utilization lowers the blood sugar and turns off the signal to the pancreas. Mobilization of Ca^{2+} from the bones increases serum $[Ca^{2+}]$ and shuts off the secretion of parathormone. The blood-borne signal may be physical rather than chemical. Infusion of a hypertonic solution of NaCl increases the effective osmotic pressure of the plasma. This excites osmoreceptor cells in the hypothalamus to emit signals leading to the sensation of thirst and also to the increased secretion of the antidiuretic hormone (ADH; vasopressin), which increases the retention of water by the kidney. At the same time the chemical signal of increased plasma $[Na^+]$ acts directly on the adrenal cortex to suppress aldosterone secretion and thus facilitate the renal secretion of sodium. The two signals act together until the plasma $[Na^+]$ and osmolarity are restored to normal.

A stimulus to hormone output may be mediated by the nervous system. The adrenal medulla is provoked to discharge epinephrine by anger, fear or anxiety as well as by hypoglycemia. The action is short lived because of the rapid metabolic inactivation of the catecholamines, so the signal must be repeated frequently or sustained.

A gland such as the adrenal cortex is both nourished and stimulated by a tropic hormone, the adrenocorticotropic hormone (ACTH) of the adenohypophysis. A portion of the output of the glucocorticoids from the adrenal cortex feeds back upon the source of the stimulus to the secretion of ACTH, the hypothalamic neurosecretory cells that produce corticotropin-releasing hormone (CRH). The rate of delivery of CRH to the anterior pituitary is slowed, the output of ACTH is depressed, and the activity of the adrenal cortex is diminished. Feedback systems of this kind often oscillate in short cycles of stimulus and suppression. They are always "on" and are responsive within the brief span of a cycle to overriding stimulus or inhibition. Thus the severe hypoglycemia that leads to discharge of epinephrine, glycogenolysis and increase of blood sugar and blood lactate as well as of plasma free fatty acids for the short term of need, also elicits discharge of CRF and ACTH, increased output of glucocorticoids, mobilization of protein, accelerated gluconeogenesis and preparation of the organism for the long term of effort and stress.

Other modes of regulation of hormonal activity are more subtle, a function of the state of the target cells, which may be affected by the presence of local modulators such as one of the prostaglandins, making them sometimes more, sometimes less sensitive to the action of a hormone. In other instances, the cells of a target organ may, upon long exposure to increased concentrations of a hormone, become less sensitive to its effects by altering the pattern and the number of binding sites for that hormone in the plasma membrane.

Except for the steroid hormones and the thyroid hormone, which find their target in the nuclei of the cells that they affect, most of the polypeptide hormones, and the catecholamines act by attaching to specific binding sites in the plasma membrane of cells of their target organs. Their effect is amplified by the activation of an enzyme, adenylate cyclase, that catalyzes the transformation of ATP into cyclic $3', 5'$-AMP (cAMP), the so-called second messenger. This effector in turn activates other systems in the cell, differing in different target cells, and eliciting a response characteristic of the hormone. The specificity of the response lies in the receptor site and in the systems responsive to cAMP. For example, ACTH activates adenylate cyclase in cells of the adrenal cortex, and cAMP activates enzymes leading to cortisol production and secretion, but ACTH has no effect in liver. Epinephrine and glucagon activate adenylate cyclase in liver, leading to glycogenolysis, but have no action on the adrenal cortex. Epinephrine, but not glucagon, activates adenylate cyclase in muscle. This example of the action of the second messenger was described in detail earlier in this chapter.

A hormone may exert some of its effects by inhibiting production of cAMP. Thus insulin, which inhibits lipolysis in adipocytes, does so at least in part by inhibiting adenylate cyclase. Since cAMP is continuously hydrolyzed to AMP by a phosphodiesterase, its concentration quickly falls and adipocyte lipase returns to inactive status. The adenylate cyclase/cAMP system is very widespread, and it may have counterparts employing other nucleotides such as GTP to form $3',5'$-cGMP, which could be an activator of systems other than those influenced by cAMP.

Although the list of hormones thought to activate adenylate cyclase (or inhibit it) at their receptor sites is very long, it cannot yet be said that the release or restraint of cAMP accounts satisfactorily for all the actions of a given hormone. cAMP may be one rather noticeable component of a complex response initiated by a hormone at its specific receptor site in the plasma membrane and reverberating through the target cell.

Another form of second messenger is encountered in somatomedin (once known as sulfation factor), which is made, possibly in the liver, under the influence of growth hormone, disappears slowly from the plasma in its absence and reappears when growth hormone is injected. The response has not been shown to be dose related. Somatomedin affects primarily the skeleton, stimulating chondrogenesis and osteogenesis; its stimulation of synthesis of chondroitin sulfate accounts for the name, sulfation factor. Some investigators think that somatomedin may account for all of the protein anabolic effects of growth hormone, but the evidence in support of this idea is poor. Somatomedin may, however, be representative of a wider group of accessory hormone-dependent factors supporting aspects of a complex process such as growth.

The Adenohypophysis

The anterior pituitary secretes six hormones: growth hormone (GH) or somatotropin (STH), prolactin (Prl), adrenocorticotropic hormone (ACTH), thyrotropic or thyroid-stimulating hormone (TSH), luteinizing hormone (LH) and follicle-stimulating hormone (FSH). The last three of these are glycoproteins of molecular weight about 30,000. Each is composed of two subunits of nearly equal size. The α-subunit is common to them all; the β-subunit in each instance confers the specific biologic activity. The β-subunits are immunologically distinct and make possible the specific radioimmunoassay of each of these closely related glycoproteins. TSH nourishes and stimulates the thyroid gland, promoting the synthesis and release of T_4 and T_3. Prolonged stimulation of the thyroid by TSH, as in iodine lack, leads to hypertrophy and hyperplasia (simple goiter). LH stimulates ovulation, the development of the corpus luteum and secretion of progesterone. FSH brings about maturation of the ovum and, with LH, secretion of estrogen by both ovary and follicle. In males, LH stimulates the interstitial cells of the testis to secrete testosterone. In combination with FSH it supports the germinal epithelium and the maturation of sperm.

Prolactin is a simple protein of molecular weight about 25,000. The amino acid sequence of the sheep hormone is known. Doubt about the existence of a distinct prolactin in humans and in nonhuman primates has been resolved by the isolation and characterization of human prolactin. Its resemblance to sheep prolactin is greater than its resemblance to human growth hormone, and it is immunochemically distinct from human growth hormone. A principal function of prolactin is the stimulation of milk production and secretion. In some animals, the hormone is luteotropic, prolonging the life of the corpus luteum, but it is probably not so in man.

Growth hormone is also a simple protein. It is now recognized that the growth hormones of mammals, possibly of all vertebrates, are uniform in size (M_r about 22,000) and similar in amino acid composition. Growth hormone of humans and of nonhuman primates is active in man and lower animals, but the GH of other mammals is not active in man. Human

GH is immunologically distinct from the other growth hormones, and this forms the basis for its specific radio-immunoassay. Human and other primate GH also has prolactin activity. GH is essential for continued symmetrical growth of the body in young animals. In non-growing adults in a steady state of body composition, GH supports the protein-anabolic side of the balanced processes of protein synthesis and degradation that constitute the continuing metabolism of nitrogen. GH assists in conserving body nitrogen in fasting. It is an effective mobilizer of fat, and it assists in the economizing of carbohydrate by suppressing its utilization in the fasting animal. An exaggeration of these effects is seen in the induction of diabetes ("metahypophyseal diabetes") by the chronic administration of large doses of growth hormone to dogs. Acromegaly in man, in consequence of a GH-secreting tumor, is frequently accompanied by diabetes.

ACTH is found in plasma as a polypeptide of 39 amino acid residues (4.5K ACTH) and as a glycopeptide (13K ACTH), larger because of a single oligosaccharide attached to an asparagine residue near the carboxyl end of the peptide. The sequence of the first 13 residues of ACTH from the NH$_2$-terminal end is identical to that of α-MSH, one form of melanocyte-stimulating hormone. In α-MSH, the NH$_2$-terminal serine is N-acetylated, and the carboxyl-terminal valine is amidated. ACTH has about one per cent of the melanocyte-stimulating activity of α-MSH. ACTH stimulates the synthesis and secretion of the glucocorticoid hormones, maintains the adrenal cortex, and, in excess, causes enlargement of the gland.

Study of the biosynthesis of ACTH reveals that it is produced as a glycoprotein prohormone of molecular weight 31,000, that is a precursor of *several* biologically active polypeptides. The 31K prohormone is thought first to be cleaved to yield 23K ACTH and "11.7K endorphin," a molecule similar to the presumed hormone, β-lipotropin, so-called because it induces mobilization of fatty acids from adipose tissue. The 23K ACTH is thought first to be cleaved to an NH$_2$-terminal peptide of unknown function, and 13K and 4.5K ACTH, which are secreted. The β-lipotropin-like 11.7K endorphin gives rise on further cleavage to β-MSH (in man, a peptide of 22 amino acid residues, which may be the only form of human MSH), and 3.5K endorphin, comprising the 30 carboxyl-terminal residues of the 31K precursor. β-endorphin is a natural opiate, about 30 times as active as morphine, mole for mole, that can combine specifically with opiate receptors in the brain.

MSH causes dispersion of the pigments of melanocytes, darkening the skin, and also stimulates synthesis of melanin. Thus it is easier to see from the composition of the common prohormone, why, in adrenal insufficiency, when feedback inhibition of ACTH secretion by glucocorticoids is lacking, *both* ACTH and MSH are present in excess in the plasma, each contributing to the darkening of the skin and mucous membranes characteristic of the disorder in man.

An antagonist of MSH, melatonin, N-acetyl-5-methoxytryptamine, is found in the pineal gland. Melatonin also exerts inhibitory effects on the reproductive system in both young and adult animals, apparently by inhibiting the release or the action of the hypothalamic gonadotropin-releasing hormone.

The Neurohypophysis

The hormones of the neurohypophysis are stored in combination with the carrier protein, neurophysin. Both are nonapeptides:

Cys-Tyr-Phe-Gln-Asn-Cys-Pro-Arg-Gly-NH$_2$

is vasopressin (ADH). It resembles oxytocin:

Cys-Tyr-Ile-Gln-Asn-Cys-Pro-Leu-Gly-NH$_2$

Both have been isolated, identified, and synthesized. Vasopressin functions as an antidiuretic agent, regulating water reabsorption by the kidney. In its absence there is diabetes insipidus, characterized by the excretion of very large volumes of dilute urine. The secretion of vasopressin is regulated by plasma osmotic pressure, blood volume and blood pressure. Ingestion of a large volume of water is followed by diuresis. A hemorrhage, reducing blood volume and pressure, is a powerful stimulus of vasopressin secretion, causing water retention and even occasionally a pressor effect. Oxytocin, which affects the contraction of the pregnant uterus, plays a role in parturition. In the lactating female, oxytocin assists in the expression of milk from the mammary gland. It is secreted in response to the act of suckling. The close chemical resemblance of the two compounds endows each with some activity characteristic of the other.

The posterior lobe hormones are secreted in association with two proteins of molecular weight about 10,000 called neurophysins—oxytocin with neurophysin I, vasopressin with neurophysin II. The association is a loose one, partly ionic and partly noncovalent, and the peptides are easily set free from their respective neurophysin when they are secreted from the posterior lobe.

Regulation of Pituitary Secretion

The secretion of the adenohypophyseal hormones is controlled by polypeptide neurohormones elaborated in cells of the hypothalamus and reaching the pituitary by a venous portal system. There are both releasing and inhibiting hormones. So far, three such agents have been isolated, identified, and synthesized. Thyrotropin-releasing hormone (TRH), the simplest of these, is a tripeptide, L-pyroglutamyl, L-histidyl-L-proline-amide. A decapeptide, pGlu-His-Trp-Ser-Tyr-Gly-Leu-Arg-Pro-Gly-NH$_2$, is a releasing hormone (LH/FSH-RH) for both LH and FSH. The secretion of GH is inhibited by a tetradecapeptide H-Ala-Gly-Cys-Lys-Asn-Phe-Phe-Trp-Lys-Thr-Phe-Thr-Ser-Cys-OH, named somatostatin. These agents are effective in vivo in nanogram amounts and in vitro in picogram amounts. With TRH, it has been shown that the feedback inhibition of TSH secretion by thyroid hormone is due to stimulation of the synthesis of a protein that blocks the action of TRH on the TSH-secreting cell. The feedback is therefore effective at the pituitary rather than the hypothalamus. Evidence for other releasing factors is physiologic, based on the effects of interrupting the hypothalamicohypophyseal portal venous system by stalk section, by ablation of selected hypothalamic nuclei, by stimulation of discrete centers through fine implanted electrodes and by pituitary transplantation. The isolation and identification of releasing (and possibly release-inhibiting hormones) for each of the adenohypophyseal hormones will be accomplished in the next decade. Their importance is indicated by evidence that in a significant number of instances of growth hormone deficiency, for example, the defect lies not in the pituitary but in the hypothalamus. If the releasing hormones all prove to be simple peptides, then their synthesis and therapeutic application will be far easier than supplying the anterior pituitary hormones themselves.

The Steroid Hormones

The steroid hormones are derivatives of cholesterol. They are products of the adrenal cortex, the testis, the ovary and corpus luteum, and the placenta. A great variety of these compounds are known, but the major active principles are relatively few. In man, the hormones of the adrenal cortex are corticosterone, cortisol (17α-hydroxycorticosterone) and aldosterone; that of the testis is testosterone; and the hormones of the ovary and corpus luteum are, respectively, estradiol and progesterone. During pregnancy the placenta, in addition to secreting a gonadotropin with the activities of LH and FSH, produces both estrogen and progesterone.

The biosynthesis of the steroid hormones is illustrated in Figure 4-11. The side chain of cholesterol (I) is first shortened by a "desmolase" to yield the 21-carbon derivative, pregnenolone (II). This compound is converted by a 17α-hydroxylase to a 17α-hydroxypregnenolone (III). Compounds II and III give rise to progesterone (IV) and 17α-hydroxyprogesterone (V) by the action of the steroid 3β-ol dehydrogenase and of an isomerase shifting the double bond from the Δ5 position characteristic of cholesterol to the Δ4 position characteristic of the adrenal steroids and the androgens. Both IV and V are converted by a 21-hydroxylase to deoxycorticosterone (VI) and 17α-hydroxydeoxycorticosterone (VII) respectively. These compounds, with marked mineralocorticoid activity, are normally not produced in significant amounts. An 11β-hydroxylase converts VI to corticosterone (VIII) and VII to 17α-hydroxycorticosterone (IX; cortisol). Aldosterone (X) is produced by the action of an 18-hydroxylase on VIII, followed by the oxidation of the 18-hydroxyl group to an aldehyde, by an 18-hydroxy-dehydrogenase.

In the testis, 17α-hydroxypregnenolone (III) loses its side chain to become dehydroepiandrosterone (XI). The action of the steroid 3β-ol dehydrogenase and isomerase converts this to the Δ4, 3 ketone, androstenedione (XII). Reduction of the 17-ketone leads to testosterone (XIII). Inspection of the figure will suggest alternative pathways to the reader.

In the ovary, the precursor of estradiol (XIV) is testosterone, through the intermediate compounds 19-hydroxy- and 19-aldo-testosterone. The oxidative removal of the 19-substituent and the reduction of the 3-ketone to a hydroxyl lead to the aromatization of the A ring and formation of the phenolic estrogen.

The formation of progesterone in the corpus luteum and the placenta follows the pathway outlined above.

The metabolism of the steroid hormones has several characteristic features. The liver is the site of formation of most of the metabolites. Cortisol, corticosterone and aldosterone are converted to their tetrahydro-derivatives by reduction of the 3-ketone and saturation of the Δ4 double bond in the A ring. These derivatives are conjugated (at C-21) in the liver and excreted mainly as glucosiduronidates. There may be, to a small extent, oxidation of the 20-ketone to a secondary alcohol. About 5 to 10 per cent of the secreted 21-C adrenal steroids lose their side chain and are excreted as 11-oxy-17-ketosteroids. The two principal metabolites of testosterone, 5α-androsterone and 5β-androsterone (etiocholanolone) also arise by reduction of the 3-ketone and saturation of the A ring. Both compounds are oxidized at C-17, and are therefore 17-ketosteroids. They are excreted as glucosiduronidates and sulfates. Estradiol is converted to the 17-keto derivative, estrone, and also to the 16-hydroxy derivative, estriol. All three compounds appear in the urine, as glucosiduronidates and sulfates. The principal metabolite of progesterone, pregnane-3α,20α-diol, also arises by

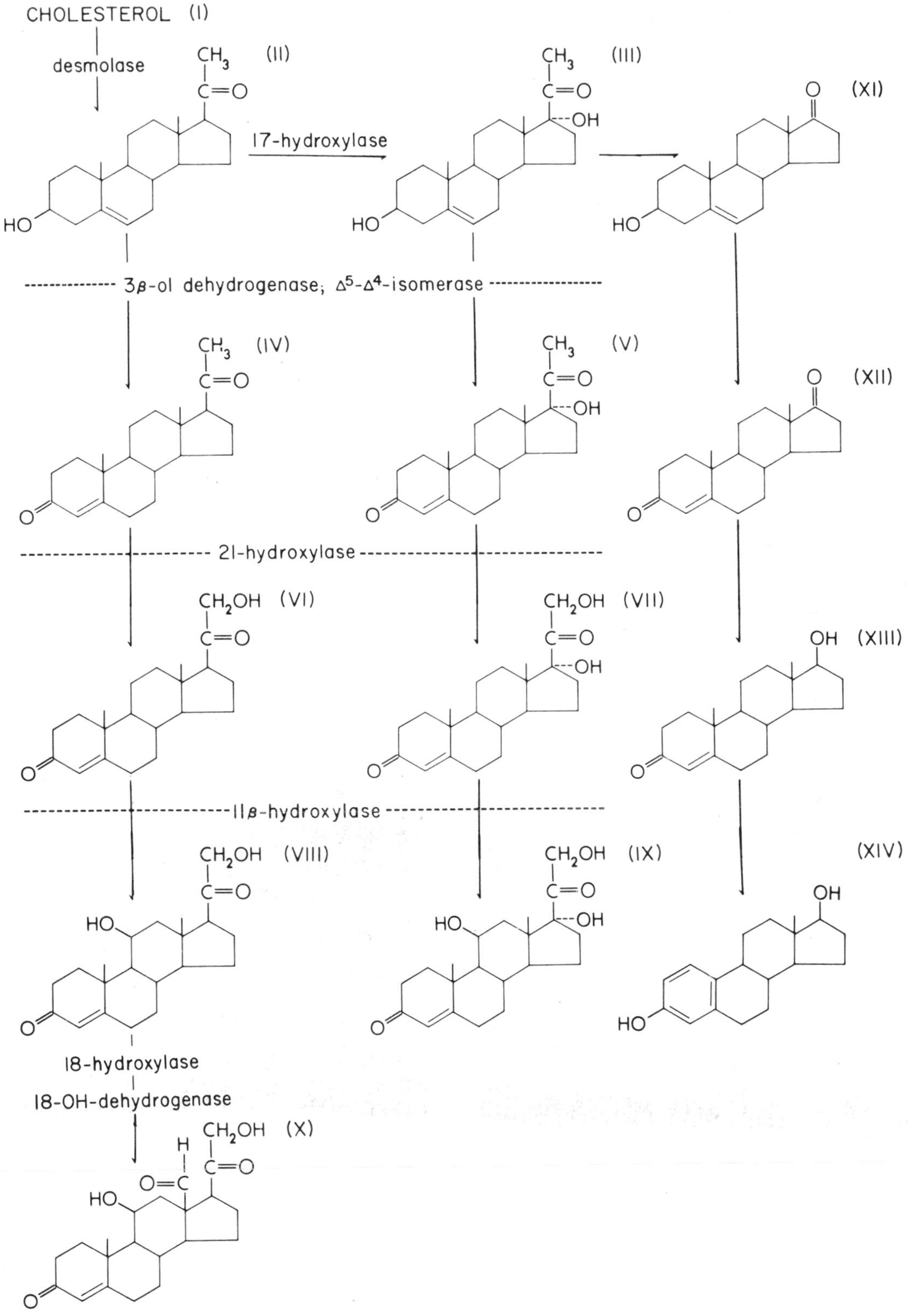

Fig. 4-11. Biosynthesis of steroid hormones.

reduction of the 3-ketone and saturation of the A ring. It is excreted as the 3-glucosiduronidate or the 3-sulfate.

The quantitative relations among these compounds are of interest. The adrenal cortex daily produces (in man) 10 to 30 mg. of cortisol, 2 to 4 mg. of corticosterone and 0.3 to 0.4 mg. of aldosterone. The testis secretes 4 to 9 mg. of testosterone per day. In the female, urinary neutral 17-ketosteroids (derived entirely from the adrenal cortex) amount to 4 to 17 mg per day; in the male, they are greater by the amount arising from the testis: 6 to 28 mg. per day. The production of estrogens and of progesterone is more difficult to determine, since the rates of secretion vary with the stage of the cycle. It is estimated that the secretion rate of estradiol may range from 200 to 1500 μg. per day and for progesterone, in the luteal phase of the cycle, from 2 to 25 mg. per day.

Mode of Action of the Steroid Hormones. Recent studies have formed the basis for a general model of the action of steroid hormones upon their target cells. These water-insoluble molecules are carried in the plasma mainly bound to proteins (e.g., *transcortin,* a small globulin that binds adrenocortical hormones). At the target, the lipophilic steroid penetrates the cell membrane and is bound to specific receptors in the cytosol. In this form, by one or more stages, the steroid gains access to the nucleus, where there are specific receptors for the steroid/cytosolic complex. These events initiate the activation of DNA and the synthesis of RNA in amounts and kinds appropriate to the nature of the steroid hormone and the special character of the target cell. Many details remain to be worked out, and it is not yet clear whether this model, accounting for the action of steroid hormones entirely by their ability to regulate gene expression, is sufficient to account for all of their actions.

The Testis

Testosterone, the male hormone, originates in the interstitial cells of the testis. Its production is regulated by the luteinizing (interstitial cell stimulating) hormone of the anterior pituitary, and the output of the tropic hormone is in turn modified by the action of testosterone upon the rate of secretion of LH-RH from the hypothalamus. Dihydrotestosterone, formed by the action of a 5α-reductase, is the active form of the hormone in the prostate, and perhaps in other target tissues. The male hormone is essential for spermatogenesis and is necessary for the growth and maintenance of the accessory sexual organs: penis and scrotum, prostate, seminal vesicles, and other glands of the reproductive tract. Testosterone, in conjunction with FSH, is necessary for growth and function of the testis.

The secondary male characteristics—shape of the skeleton, musculature, hair pattern, voice and behavior—depend upon testosterone. The hormone is responsible for the closure of the epiphyses of the long bones, so that it at first accelerates growth and later limits height. Testosterone and other androgens are powerful protein anabolic agents. Testosterone (or an orally more effective androgen, 17α-methyltestosterone) has been used to improve growth in prepubertal boys and to promote nitrogen retention in debilitating diseases. Much effort has been put into the search for derivatives of testosterone in which the protein anabolic effect is favored over the androgenic actions, with only limited success. The most promising derivatives are 19-nortestosterone, lacking the angular methyl group at carbon 10, and its 17α-ethyl derivative.

Testosterone is metabolized by saturation of the $\Delta 4$ double bond, reduction of the 3-ketone to hydroxyl and oxidation of the 17-hydroxyl to a ketone. The two main urinary metabolites are 5α-androsterone and its 5β-isomer, etiocholanolone. These metabolites are produced mainly in the liver, where they are conjugated to glucuronic acid or to sulfate. Many other minor derivatives of the androgens are known.

The Ovary

The principal female sex hormone is 17β-estradiol. It is found in the ovary and in the urine along with the 17-keto derivative, estrone, and the 16-hydroxy derivative, estriol, the least active of the three. During pregnancy the placenta is also a source of estrogens. These phenolic steroids are derived from testosterone. All three estrogens are excreted as conjugates with sulfate or glucuronic acid. The site of their inactivation is the liver. Although a variety of metabolites of estradiol have been found, the 2-hydroxy and the 16-hydroxy derivatives are quantitatively most important.

The estrogens are responsible for the development and maintenance of the secondary sex characteristics of the female: the pattern of body hair, the shape of the skeleton, the voice and the nature of the skin. Estrogens play a critical role in the development of the mammary gland and in the proliferation of the gland during pregnancy, prior to lactation. They support the development of the uterus, the vagina and the glands associated with these organs. During the ovarian cycle the estrogens initiate proliferation of the uterine endometrium and of the vaginal epithelium and augment secretion of the cervical glands. Like the androgens in the male, the estrogens in the female hasten the rate of closure of the epiphyses of the long bones.

After ovulation the corpus luteum takes on the function of a second hormone-producing site within the ovary, secreting progesterone. In the latter half of the ovarian cycle progesterone acts on the uterine endometrium, partially prepared by estradiol, to stimulate the development of the uterine glands and the secretory activity required for implantation of the fertilized ovum. Its continued production is essential to the maintenance of pregnancy. The hormone has effects on salt and water retention similar to those of the mineralocorticoids. This action may play a part in keeping the uterine muscle in a quiescent state, relatively insensitive to stimulation by oxytocin. Progesterone plays a part with estrogen in mammary gland development, but it inhibits the final stages of preparation for the secretion of milk. The precipitate fall in progesterone output at parturition allows the biosynthesis of the components of milk to proceed.

Progesterone, like other related steroids, is metabolized by saturation of the A ring and reduction of the 3-ketone. The 20-ketone is also reduced, and the chief metabolite of progesterone, formed mainly in the liver, is pregnane-3α, 20α-diol. It is excreted as the glucosiduronidate or the sulfate.

Like estradiol, progesterone is not very active by mouth. A number of derivatives of both hormones have been devised for oral administration. Of these, the synthetic estrogen diethylstilbestrol is probably the best known. One of the most effective oral progestins, ten times as active as progesterone is 17α-ethynyl--(. . . C$\equiv$CH)19-nortestosterone.

Relaxin. The corpus luteum also produces a polypeptide hormone, relaxin, a substance that softens the ligaments of the symphysis pubis in guinea pigs and mice. The effect is dose related and is the basis of the bioassay. The hormone is a small molecule, molecular weight 6,000, containing two polypeptide chains joined by disulfide bonds. It is analogous in structure to insulin, but is a basic, rather than an acidic protein. Histidine, proline, and tyrosine are absent, but by introducing a tyrosyl residue at the NH_2-terminal end, a site for iodination is established and radioimmunoassay is made possible. By this means the rise and fall of relaxin in the serum of pregnant women has been followed. Its function in man has not been established.

The Placenta. In addition to producing estradiol and progesterone, the placenta secretes two polypeptide hormones in abundance. Human chorionic gonadotropin (hCG) appears in blood and urine early, about a week after the first missed period. Its detection is a test for pregnancy. The hormone is a glycoprotein closely related to TSH, LH, and FSH, but the β-subunit of hCG has an additional 23 amino acids at its carboxyl end. Antisera to this terminal polypeptide react *only* with hCG. By this means it has been found that hCG in minute amounts is present in the pituitary, blood, and urine of men and non-pregnant women.

The hormone has the activities of both LH and FSH, and it serves to maintain the corpus luteum of pregnancy.

The other polypeptide hormone of the placenta is a protein of 191 amino acid residues, highly homologous with hGH, but having only feeble growth-promoting activity and marked prolactin activity. This human placental lactogen (hPL) or chorionic somatomammotropin (hCS) appears in the blood early in pregnancy, rises to a high plateau by the third trimester, and disappears after delivery of the placenta. The function of hCS is not firmly established.

The Adrenal Cortex and Medulla

Two types of hormonal activity are associated with the adrenal cortex: (1) regulation of electrolyte metabolism (Na^+ and K^+), a primary function of the mineralocorticoids; (2) regulatory actions on carbohydrate, protein and lipid metabolism, a primary function of the glucocorticoids. The glucocorticoids have some effects on electrolytes, but the mineralocorticoids have no other metabolic effects, at the concentrations at which they act effectively in the control of Na^+ and K^+. In man, the important mineralocorticoid is aldosterone, the principal glucocorticoids are cortisol and corticosterone. Aldosterone production is located in the outermost layer of the adrenal cortex, the glomerulosa. The glucocorticoids are produced in the cells of the fasciculata and the reticularis. These cells atrophy after hypophysectomy, but the secretory activity of the glomerulosa is only moderately affected. For this reason hypophysectomy is not a fatal operation, but adrenalectomy is.

In adrenal insufficiency the kidney loses its ability to retain sodium and to excrete potassium. Loss of sodium chloride in the urine is accompanied by loss of water. In addition, the fall in extracellular NaCl results in osmotic movement of water into the tissues. In consequence there is hemoconcentration, decreased cardiac output and fall in blood pressure. There is progressive renal failure, leading to retention of urea. Ultimately there is circulatory collapse and death. The action of the heart is affected by the increase in plasma K^+ concentration, and the heart may stop in diastole.

If the intake of potassium is restricted and plentiful sodium chloride is provided, the consequences of mineral imbalance can be avoided. The partial correction of adrenal insufficiency in this way makes clear the effects of deprivation of the glucocorticoids. In fasting there is rapid depletion of the store of liver glycogen, and an early fall of the blood sugar to hypoglycemic levels. The urinary nitrogen is less than normal, and there is evidence of deficient protein mobilization and gluconeogenesis. There is a great increase in sensitivity to insulin, most probably because of diminished gluconeogenesis. The fasting rise in plasma free fatty acids is slower than normal but the RQ falls as usual, giving no indication of excessive fasting carbohydrate utilization. The capacity for muscular work is very much reduced, and sensitivity to stress is greatly increased. The individual is much more susceptible to infection and the processes of inflammation are intensified. The ability to excrete a water load is much impaired. In the absence of maintenance with extra NaCl these metabolic defects are compounded by the electrolyte imbalance. There is loss of appetite, weight loss, gastrointestinal distress, anemia and a general sense of overall weakness and depression.

The secretion of glucocorticoids is regulated by feedback upon the hypothalamus. Cortisol or corticosterone affects the output of corticotropin-releasing hormone, which in turn controls the output of ACTH by the anterior pituitary. In adrenal cortical insufficiency, the absence of the 11-oxycorticoids in plasma leads to continuous unrestrained output of ACTH and MSH. The pigmentation of the skin and mucous membranes seen in adrenal insufficiency in man have been mentioned before.

The regulation of aldosterone production is complex. The glomerulosa is responsive directly to a fall in plasma Na^+ concentration or to a rise in plasma K^+. ACTH itself has a minor effect. The kidney, responding to a fall in blood volume or blood pressure, acts to reverse these changes by increasing its output of renin. This enzyme acts upon an α-2 globulin, angiotensinogen, to produce the decapeptide angiotensin I, which is attacked by a second enzyme to produce the octapeptide angiotensin II, Asp-Arg-Val-Tyr-Ile-His-Pro-Phe. This powerful pressor substance stimulates the release of aldosterone, increasing Na^+ retention and helping to retore the blood volume.

In adrenal insufficiency the injection of aldosterone leads quickly to reversal of the changes in electrolyte and water metabolism. Sodium and water are retained, potassium is excreted, and the distribution of fluid between the intracellular and extracellular compartments is restored to normal. There is no repair of the metabolic defects, but in the absence of stress or injury life is maintained. In primary aldosteronism, due to a tumor of the glomerulosa, there is weakness and headache associated with mild hypertension, increased renal loss of potassium, hypokalemia and a moderate increase in plasma Na^+. Excessive amounts of aldosterone and its metabolites are found in the urine. Removal of the tumor results in disappearance of the weakness and hypertension and restoration of normal plasma $[Na^+]$ and $[K^+]$. Secondary aldosteronism is seen in many patients with edema due to various causes. It is not certain why this occurs.

Cortisol and corticosterone can reverse all the effects of adrenalectomy or adrenal insufficiency. Injection of these hormones leads to increase in blood sugar and liver glycogen, increase in protein mobilization and nitrogen excretion, reduction in insulin sensitivity, involution of lymphoid tissue and suppression of the inflammatory response, restoration of muscular strength and endurance and of resistance to stress of all kinds, and, in some instances, to marked euphoria. These effects are exaggerated when excessive amounts of glucocorticoids are produced by tumors of the adrenal cortex or in response to ACTH-producing tumors in the pituitary or occasionally in extrahypophyseal sites. The resulting syndrome, Cushing's syndrome, is characterized by a moon face, hirsutism in the female, thin and fragile skin, thin arms and legs, a heavy, obese torso and, because of continuing loss of body protein and muscle mass, general physical weakness. There is a tendency to osteoporosis, possibly due to deficient maintenance of the protein matrix upon which calcification occurs.

Individuals with hereditary deficiencies of one or more of the enzymes required for the synthesis of cortisol have been recognized. Perhaps the best known of these are the deficiencies of 21-hydroxylase and 11β-hydroxylase. In both instances, 11-oxycorticoids cannot be formed, there is no feedback regulation of ACTH output, and adrenal hyperplasia occurs. The enzymatic block leads to greater use of the pathways leading to androgen production, resulting in masculinization in the female and precocious puberty in the male. When 11β-hydroxylase is absent there is also hypertension, resulting from excessive accumulation of the mineralocorticoid intermediates 11-deoxycorticosterone (DOC) and its 17α-hydroxy derivative (compound S). Treatment with cortisol or an active synthetic glucocorticoid restores the feedback, represses the excessive androgen output and protects the patient, who is otherwise deficient in glucocorticoids.

The adrenal glands are a composite endocrine organ, the medulla deriving from the nervous system, and the cortex deriving from the embryonic mesoderm. The products of the two parts are very different chemically, but they are in part related functionally through the reactions of the organism to stress.

The *adrenal medulla* secretes two hormones, the catecholamines, epinephrine (E) and norepinephrine (N), lacking the N-methyl group. The ratio N/E differs from species to species; in man 10 to 30 per cent is N. The hormones are derived from phenylalanine, as follows: Phe → Tyr (phenylalanine hydroxylase); Tyr

HO—[benzene ring]—$\overset{\text{H}}{\underset{\text{OH}}{\text{C}}}$—$CH_2$—$NH \bullet CH_3$

HO—

Epinephrine

→ dihydroxyphenylalanine (dopa) in the rate limiting step (tyrosine hydroxylase); dopa to dopamine (aromatic L-amino acid decarboxylase, requiring pyridoxal phosphate); dopamine → norepinephrine (dopamine β-hydroxylase); epinephrine by methylation, using S-adenosylmethionine (phenylethanolamine N-methyl transferase, regulated by product inhibition). Normal concentrations in plasma are, for E, 0.06 μg. per liter; N,. 0.03 μg. per liter. In 24 hour urine, E, 10 to 15 μg.; N, 30 to 50 μg. Both hormones are metabolized mainly by two enzymatic changes: 3–0 methylation (O-methyl transferase) and deamination (monoamine-oxidase). The principal urinary metabolite is 3-methoxy, 4-hydroxymandelic acid.

The hormones are secreted in response to emergency (preparation for fight or flight), to emotion (fear, anger) and to hypoglycemia, reflexly, through the central nervous system. The metabolic effects of E are: glycogenolysis in liver and muscle, with increase in blood sugar and lactate; increase in O_2 consumption and heat production and acute increase in plasma nonesterified fatty acids (also the only metabolic effect of N). In addition, E causes increase in heart rate, cardiac output and systolic blood pressure; dilates blood vessels of heart, voluntary muscles and viscera, causing fall in peripheral resistance; dilates bronchial musculature; relaxes the muscles of the intestine, but contracts the pyloric and ileocaecal sphincters. N acts mainly as a peripheral vasoconstrictor, increasing peripheral resistance and both systolic and diastolic blood pressure. The metabolic effects of E and N are mediated by their action upon the adenylate cyclase system of their target cells.

Tumors of the chromaffin tissue of the medulla itself or of outlying rests (pheochromocytomas) have effects that depend on the proportions of the two hormones secreted by the tumor: increased basal metabolic rate, hyperglycemia, glycosuria, with persistent or intermittent hypertension, or paroxysmal hypertension. Concentrations of the hormones and their metabolites are greatly increased in both plasma and urine.

The Pancreas. The islets of Langerhans of the pancreas make and secrete insulin from the beta (B) cells, glucagon from the alpha (A) cells, and somatostatin from the delta (D) cells.

The tetradecapeptide *somatostatin* is also found in numerous cells of the gastrointestinal tract. It inhibits the secretion of *both* insulin and glucagon, just as it does that of GH in the pituitary. The situation of the D cells, relative to the A and B cells of the islets, suggests that somatostatin may normally moderate their responses. Its actions, and the control of its secretion, are not yet fully explained.

Glucagon, a polypeptide of 29 amino acids, the "hyperglycemic-glycogenolytic factor," is secreted in response to a fall in blood sugar. Its main site of action is the liver, where it stimulates adenylate cyclase, leading to activation of phosphorylase and rapid glycogenolysis. Glucagon also stimulates lipolysis, fatty acid oxidation, and ketogenesis, and it promotes gluconeogenesis from amino acids. In adipose tissue, glucagon stimulates lipolysis and release of fatty acids. Unlike epinephrine, it does not stimulate glycogenolysis in muscle. Recent evidence suggests that the secretion of insulin and glucagon is "on" continuously, the action of the one moderating the opposing action of the other, under resting conditions. It has been suggested that the severity of some cases of diabetes may be due to the unopposed action of glucagon released by A cells that have escaped from the inhibitory effect of high blood glucose.

Insulin is a small protein (M_r about 6,000) comprised of 51 amino acids, arranged in an A chain of 21 residues joined through a pair of disulfide bonds to a B chain of 30 residues. The A chain also contains an intrachain disulfide bond. If any of these disulfide bonds is cleaved, activity is lost. The hormone is synthesized as a larger molecule of 81 residues, proinsulin, a single polypeptide chain, starting with the A chain at the amino-terminal end and ending in the B chain. The final step in the synthesis of insulin occurs at its storage, by enzymatic scission of the C peptide of 30 residues connecting the two chains. Insulin is stored as such, along with C peptide, in the secretory granules of the β cell. The rate of secretion of insulin rises and falls with rise and fall of the blood glucose. Glucose also acts as a stimulus to insulin synthesis. Insulin is released in response to a protein meal or to intravenous administration of large doses of arginine or leucine. Glucagon also stimulates insulin release, by increasing the concentration of cyclic AMP in the β cells. The oral hypoglycemic agents such as the sulfonylureas stimulate insulin release, possibly by inhibiting the phosphodiesterase that destroys cAMP.

The action of insulin is rapid and of short duration. Its property as an acidic protein is exploited by combining it with basic proteins, protamine or globin, to form neutral, insoluble complexes from which insulin is slowly released from the site of injection. Insulin acts to increase glucose utilization by the tissues, particularly muscle and adipose tissue. Its action is reflected in a fall in blood sugar, an increased oxidation rate of glucose (rise in RQ), increases in liver, muscle and adipose tissue glycogen and an increase in fatty acid synthesis from carbohydrate. The release of fatty acids from adipose tissue is suppressed, plasma free fatty acids fall, and ketogenesis subsides as hepatic fatty acid oxidation falls. Insulin increases amino acid transport into muscle and stimulates protein synthesis in both muscle and liver. Insulin is essential for growth and for the maintenance of nitrogen balance in adults. In its absence growth hormone cannot exert its normal effect but instead acts as a diabetogenic agent, worsening the effects of insulin lack.

Diabetes mellitus results from insulin lack or deficiency. Glucose utilization by peripheral tissues is impaired, blood glucose rises to high levels, and glucose appears in the urine, even in fasting. The capacity to maintain a steady state of protein in the tissues is lost, and negative nitrogen balance obtains, with wasting of tissues. There is accelerated gluconeogenesis from the lost protein, with concomitant urinary loss of the glucose and increased excretion of urea. Maintenance of a steady state of stored neutral fat is lost, there is unbalanced lipolysis and excessive mobilization of free fatty acids. The liver is flooded with this substrate, which is stored in part as neutral fat and oxidized in large amounts to acetyl-SCoA. The production of ketone bodies is greatly increased, often in excess of the rate of utilization, leading to ketonemia, ketonuria and diabetic acidosis. The excretion of large amounts of glucose, urea and ketone bodies results in a large urine volume. In addition, acetoacetic and beta-hydroxybutyric acids are moderately strong acids and are excreted in part as sodium salts. The loss of electrolyte leads to acidosis, and the large fluid loss leads to dehydration. In severe acidosis, depression of the central nervous system leads to coma. Vigorous treatment with insulin brings about reversal of these changes.

The foregoing description is of a "worst case" of an insulin-dependent individual producing no insulin at all. The invention of the radioimmunoassay for insulin in serum showed at once that many diabetics have circulating insulin that, for reasons yet unknown, is relatively ineffective. Such individuals, described as "maturity-onset" diabetics, are often obese, and their disease can be controlled by reduction in weight through diet and exercise.

The Thyroid

The thyroid gland produces a polypeptide hormone regulating serum calcium (calcitonin; thyrocalcitonin) and two iodine-containing hormones that are amino

acids, thyroxine (3,5,3',5'-tetraiodothyronine (T_4) and 3,5,3'-triiodothyronine (T_3). The modes of synthesis and secretion of the latter hormones are unique. The thyroid gland actively concentrates iodide from the plasma, oxidizes it to iodine and iodinates tyrosine residues in situ in a large protein, thyroglobulin, synthesized in the gland. Monoiodotyrosyl and diiodotyrosyl residues, formed in this way, undergo an enzyme-controlled coupling reaction leading to the formation of triiodothyronine and tetraiodothyronine as constituents of thyroglobulin, which is stored as colloid in the acini of the gland. The hormones are set free upon an appropriate stimulus by thyrotropic hormone (TSH) by proteolysis of the thyroglobulin. The free T_3 and T_4, enter the bloodstream and are carried to their targets bound to protein, mainly by a specific thyroxine-binding globulin (TBG). Only the unbound hormone (about 0.1 per cent) is active. The binding of T_3 and T_4 to the serum proteins provides a physiologic "buffer," a circulating reserve of the hormones. In pregnancy T_4 and T_3 are increased, but the TBG is increased as well, and the amount of free T_4 is not abnormally high. T_4 and T_3 can now be estimated separately and conveniently by radioimmunoassay.

The trapping of iodide by the thyroid is inhibited by thiocyanate and perchlorate. Other antithyroid drugs, the thioureas, aminothiazoles and mercaptoimidazoles, appear to block the formation of iodine and of the iodotyrosines. These substances are all goitrogens. T_3 and T_4 are not produced, the serum concentration falls, and this is a signal to the hypothalamus to increase the secretion of thyrotropin-releasing hormone (TRH). The pituitary increases its output of TSH, and, under prolonged stimulation, the thyroid gland undergoes hypertrophy, hyperplasia and hypervascularization. Goiter is also seen in response to an insufficient dietary intake of iodine. In regions deficient in iodine, goiter is endemic, but its occurrence can be prevented by adding a small amount of iodide to table salt.

The thyroid hormones regulate the metabolic rate. In their absence the rates of O_2 consumption and heat production are low. In addition the hormones are critically important in the development and maturation of the brain, the skeleton and perhaps other systems as well. In their absence in the infant mental development is defective; the condition is known as cretinism, and it can be cured by giving T_3 or T_4 if it is discovered soon enough. Growth is impaired in hypothyroidism, possibly because thyroid hormone is essential for the production and secretion of growth hormone by the pituitary. T_4 has no effect on growth of the hypophysectomized animal, but growth hormone can stimulate growth in the thyroidectomized animal. Metabolism of the thyroid hormones involves loss of iodine. The iodide may be lost in the urine, it may leave the body by way of the intestine, or it may be trapped in the thyroid and recycled. The iodothyronines and other organic iodides are secreted in the bile, and there may be minor enterohepatic secretion and reabsorption.

The actions of the thyroid hormone at its target cells are unusual. T_3 is lipophilic, and penetrates the plasma membrane easily. There are, however, specific receptors for T_3 on the plasma membrane, to which it binds. In this respect T_3 behaves like the polypeptide hormones and the catecholamines. T_3 entering the cytosol is bound to numerous specific receptors. Unlike those for the steroid hormones, the T_3 receptors are not vehicles for entry into the nucleus; T_3 attaches directly to receptors in the nuclear chromatin. By this means it may exert the effects on gene expression accounting for its long-term influence on maturation and development. Finally, T_3 also is bound to specific receptors on the inner membrane of the mitochondria, and it can be shown to stimulate oxygen uptake and ATP turnover. This action may account for the fast calorigenic action of the thyroid hormone. The large reservoir of cytosolic receptors, in equilibrium with a minute amount of T_3, may serve as both a buffer and an intracellular store, accounting in part for the long period of development of thyroid insufficiency.

Calcitonin is a polypeptide (M_r 4,500) containing 32 amino acids. Human calcitonin has been sequenced and synthesized. The main site of action of the hormone is on bone, inhibiting bone resorption and increasing calcium deposition. Its effect is to lower serum calcium, and it is therefore an antagonist of the parathyroid hormone. Its secretion rate is directly proportional to the concentration of serum calcium, and its duration of action is brief. Calcitonin is formed in the clear cells of the thyroid gland, which are derived from the ultimobranchial body. In the fowl, which has an ultimobranchial body, calcitonin is found there, rather than in the thyroid gland.

Parathyroid Glands

Parathyroid hormone (PTH) is a polypeptide (M_r 9,500) of 84 amino acid residues. The amino-terminal sequence of 30 residues has all the activities of PTH but is less potent. The hormone acts on small intestine, kidney and bone. In the gut, it promotes absorption of Ca^{2+} and P_i, but only in the presence of vitamin D. In kidney, PTH increases tubular reabsorption of Ca^{2+}, Mg^{2+}, decreases the reabsorption of P_i. In bone it (1) inhibits collagen synthesis; (2) enhances osteolysis, both osteocytic and osteoclastic; (3) increases rate of maturation of both osteoclasts and osteoblasts; (4) causes release of Ca^{2+} and acidic mucopolysaccharide from bone matrix; (5) increases accumulation of lactate and isocitrate; and (6) increases collagen breakdown. The effect of these actions is to increase serum $[Ca^{2+}]$ and to cause phosphaturia. PTH acts by binding to bone cell plasma membrane, activating adenylate cyclase; cyclic AMP enhances entry of Ca^{2+} into bone cells, stimulating them to osteoclastic activity. The secretion of PTH is regulated by the serum $[Ca^{2+}]$, increasing as it falls, decreasing as it rises. The size and activity of the glands are inversely related to the dietary intake of calcium. In hypoparathyroidism, serum $[Ca^{2+}]$ falls, $[P_i]$ rises. In young animals, tetany and convulsions may occur leading to death. Hyperparathyroidism, resulting from a tumor or hyperplasia of the glands, leads to *osteitis fibrosa cystica,* due to resorption of bone. Serum $[Ca^{2+}]$ is increased, $[P_i]$ decreased, and renal excretion of Ca^{2+} is greatly increased, leading often to the formation of urinary calculi. Hyperparathyroidism may arise secondary to chronic renal insufficiency. Retention of P_i depresses serum $[Ca^{2+}]$, and this in turn stimulates PTH production.

PTH, by helping to maintain a low concentration of P_i in the renal cortex, facilitates the action of the enzyme responsible for the l-hydroxylation of 25-hydroxycholecalciferol and thus promotes the synthesis of the active form of vitamin D_3, which is in turn required for the action of PTH on the gut and on bone.

Prostaglandins

The prostaglandins (PG) are a group of unsaturated C-20 hydrocarbon acids, first discovered in human semen but now known to be synthesized in nearly all tissues. They are derivatives of linoleic acid and, more immediately, arachidonic acid. The pathway of synthesis is outlined in Figure 4-12. No store of PG exists, but biosynthesis is easily provoked when a tissue is even lightly traumatized. The rate-limiting step is the activation of phospholipase A to release arachidonic acid from phospholipid in the cell membrane. A lipo-

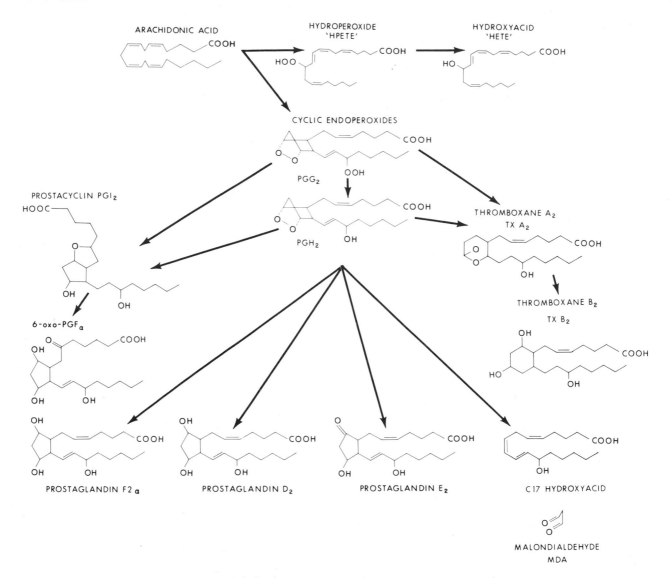

Fig. 4-12. Metabolic pathway of arachidonic acid. Reproduced with permission from Moncada, S., and Vane, J. R.: Mode of action of aspirin-like drugs. In Stollerman, G. H. et al. (eds.): Advances in Internal Medicine, Vol. 24. Copyright © 1979 by Year Book Medical Publishers, Inc., Chicago.

oxygenase catalyzes the formation of the unstable hydroperoxide ("HPETE"), leading to the hydroxyacid ("HETE"). The function of these compounds is unknown. A cyclo-oxygenase catalyzes the formation of cyclic endoperoxides (PGG_2; PGH_2), leading to the production of the short-lived prostacyclin (PGI_2) and thromboxane (Tx_2), and of the somewhat more stable $PGF_2\alpha$, PGD_2, and PGE_2. (The subscript number denotes the number of double bonds.) $PGF_2\alpha$ is a venoconstrictor and a bronchoconstrictor; PGE_2 has the opposite effects. Both compounds stimulate contraction of uterine and gastrointestinal smooth muscle. Many analogues of these compounds have been syn-thesized, but their therapeutic application has so far been limited (see Chapter 7). Greater interest now attaches to prostacyclin and thromboxane A_2 because of their effects on platelet aggregation and thrombus formation. At physiological pH and temperature PGI_2 disappears, and the nearly inactive 6-oxo-$PGF_1\alpha$ is formed, in 2 to 3 minutes, and TxA_2 is converted, in about 30 seconds, to the inactive TxB_2. For this reason these substances were missed in early studies of the prostaglandins.

Prostaglandin synthesis in blood platelets is stimulated when they adhere to damaged vascular epithelium or to collagen, begin to aggregate, and release their contents. In platelets, the intermediate endoperoxides are converted mainly to TxA_2, which is a potent stimulator of aggregation and a powerful vasoconstrictor. This process is fortified by a similar emphasis on synthesis and release of TxA_2 in the deeper layers of the damaged vessel wall. Formation of a hemostatic plug is initiated, the cascade of reactions leading to coagulation is stimulated, and a thrombus forms.

Platelets do not adhere to healthy vascular endothelium. It is found that the cells of the intima synthesize mainly prostacyclin, and that they may in addition produce PGI_2 from endoperoxides released from platelets coming into contact with the vessel wall. Finally it is observed that many cells in the lung produce PGI_2 in abundance, and that despite its short life a significant concentration (in the order of ng. per ml.) is maintained in the plasma. Prostacyclin stimulates platelet adenylate cyclase and increases the concentration of cyclic AMP in the platelet. This in some way prevents platelets from adhering to healthy epithelial cells. At sites of minor inury, and at much lower concentrations of PGI_2, platelets may adhere, but aggregation is prevented, and the adhering platelets may take part in repair of the vascular epithelium. It is noted that PGI_2 may even disperse clumps of platelets that have already aggregated. Platelet endoperoxides and TxA_2 inhibit adenylate cyclase. It appears, therefore, that platelet activity may be regulated by changes in the balance between PGI_2 and TxA_2 and PG endoperoxides in the platelets and the local environment.

Aspirin, which in a single small dose (0.3g.) prolongs bleeding time, inhibits platelet cyclo-oxygenase irreversibly by acetylating the enzyme at its active site, and thus inhibits *all* PG synthesis for the lifetime of that cohort of platelets (9 to 13 days). It is thus a rather blunt instrument. A selective inhibitor of TxA_2 synthesis should provide a better solution to the control of thrombus formation both in vivo and in vitro.

Gastrointestinal Hormones

The events of digestion are regulated in part by stimuli arising from the foodstuffs themselves, and the signals are mediated by both nervous and chemical means. Three polypeptide hormones are produced by cells of the gastrointestinal mucosa: gastrin, cholecystokinin (pancreozymin) and secretin. Gastrin, a heptadecapeptide amide, is produced in the mucosa of the pylorus and the antrum in response to HCl and to soluble agents in foods. It stimulates secretion of HCl by the parietal cells of the stomach. The terminal pentapeptide amide is as active as the entire molecule. The other two hormones are secreted by the duodenal mucosa in response to the presence of HCl and large polypeptides arising from peptic digestion of proteins.

Cholecystokinin, a polypeptide amide of 33 amino acids, stimulates the secretion of enzymes by the pancreas and elicits contraction of the gallbladder. The terminal pentapeptide amide is identical to that of gastrin. Each hormone has all the actions of the other, but they differ in relative potency. Secretin, a polypeptide amide of 27 residues, elicits a copious alkaline secretion, low in enzyme activity, from the pancreas. It is secreted in response to HCl in the first part of the duodenum. It inhibits the production of gastrin. The combined action of secretin and cholecystokinin elicits an enzyme-rich alkaline secretion of the pancreas sufficient to neutralize the gastric contents and to carry forward the processes of digestion of the major foodstuffs. Secretin and glucagon have a high degree of similarity in amino acid sequence, suggesting that the two polypeptide hormones, differing and not overlapping in function, may have arisen long ago by gene duplication and subsequent mutations.

The three gastrointestinal hormones described above are established members of what may in time be a numerous family. Some candidates are: enteroglucagon, affecting motility of the ileum; gastric inhibitory polypeptide (GIP); vasoactive intestinal peptide (VIP), of uncertain function; and motilin, stimulating gastric motility.

NUTRITION

The essential requirements of the organism for growth, development, maintenance and activity are oxygen; water; energy-yielding substrate, mainly carbohydrate and fat; protein, primarily for replacement of indispensable nitrogen-containing compounds; vitamins and minerals.

The requirement for oxygen and the processes of respiration have already been discussed.

Water

About 70 per cent of the lean body mass is made up of water, which is divided into an intracellular compartment (50 per cent) and an extracellular compartment (20 per cent) including the blood plasma (5 per cent) and the interstitial fluid (15 per cent). The daily losses of water average, for a 70 kg. man, about 2,600 ml.: in the expired air, 840 ml.; urine, 1,200 ml.; stool, 200 ml.; visible and invisible perspiration, 360 ml. The amount of each and the total vary with intake, temperature and humidity, physical activity and state of health. The sources of water are: from oxidation of substrates, about 300 ml. per day. Water in the food, a small and variable amount, and beverages, make up the required 2,300 ml. The clearance of wastes by the kidney imposes an obligatory requirement for solvent water, since the concentrating ability of the kidneys is limited. This requirement, plus the unavoidable losses through lungs and skin, must be met. If fluid intake is inadequate, water is supplied from the body fluids, leading to dehydration. Rapid loss of body weight is indicative of dehydration; a change of as much as 12 per cent indicates that the process is dangerously advanced.

The daily gains and losses of water amount to only about six per cent of the total body water, but the internal traffic of the body fluids is very much greater. About 180 liters of glomerular filtrate are formed each day; all but about 1,200 ml. are normally returned to the blood. In diabetes insipidus the urine volume may be five to ten times normal, with concomitant dehydration and thirst. The 200 ml. of water lost in the feces are the remainder of a large aggregate volume of secretions in the alimentary canal: 500 to 1,500 ml. of saliva; 1,000 to 2,500 ml. of gastric juice; 100 to 400 ml. of bile; over 1,000 ml. of pancreatic juice; and 700 to 3,000 ml. of intestinal fluids; in sum, from one to three times the plasma volume. It is easy to see why dehydration (and disturbance of electrolyte and acid–base balance) can occur quickly in persistent vomiting or diarrhea. This is particularly true in infants. Their water content is near 80 per cent; in a 10 kg. infant the total body water is 8 liters, and the extracellular volume is only 1.6 liters. Vomiting or diarrhea can swiftly dehydrate such an infant. Since the gastrointestinal secretions are isotonic with the blood plasma, the loss is borne by the extracellular fluid.

The regulation of water balance is managed by the central nervous system and the kidney. Water loss increases the osmolarity of the extracellular fluid. This is detected by osmoreceptors in the brain, eliciting sensations of thirst and secretion of antidiuretic hormone. Water is taken, and retained, until the osmolarity of the body fluids falls to normal, and the stimulus to the osmoreceptors is relieved. By some more subtle means not fully understood, an increase in extracellular volume is also detected, and both water and salt are excreted until the normal volume is restored. This has been discussed briefly in the section on the adrenal cortex.

The distribution of water among the body compartments is governed by several factors. As between the blood plasma and the extracellular fluid, the critical factors are the plasma proteins, which do not readily cross the capillary membrane and therefore exert an osmotic effect, tending to retain water, and the opposing hydrostatic effect of the blood pressure. These two opposing effects are normally nearly in balance. The distribution of water between the intracellular and extracellular compartments is determined essentially by the peculiarities of the plasma membrane of the tissue cells. The main intracellular cation is K^+, which as it slowly leaks away, is recaptured and retained by the cell. The dominant extracellular cation is Na^+. It slowly leaks into cells, but a low steady state intracellular concentration is maintained by pumping sodium out, in exchange for potassium. The motive power for this process is the Na^+, K^+-dependent ATP-ase of the plasma membrane. The effective separation of K^+ and Na^+ in the two compartments means that alterations in the solute concentration in either compartment are adjusted by a corresponding osmotic movement of water. If water is lost without salt, the Na^+ concentration in the extracellular compartments rises, and water will move osmotically from the intracellular compartment. Simple dehydration is therefore shared out over the whole of the body water. Loss of salt without water, as in adrenal cortical deficiency, lowers the concentration of Na^+, and water moves osmotically into the intracellular space. A gain or loss of isotonic fluid affects only the extracellular fluid volume. These relationships are discussed further in the chapter on Physiology.

Carbohydrate and Fat

Factors affecting the requirement for energy-yielding substrates have been discussed in relation to energy production and utilization. The proportions of carbohydrate and fat supplying energy may vary widely in different diets with no ill effects. There are no "essential" carbohydrates that the body cannot synthesize, but carbohydrate in the diet is important because it "spares" protein that must otherwise be used for gluconeogenesis. Glucose is an essential carbohydrate in a special sense: (1) it is exclusively the substrate for the red cell; (2) even when, after prolonged fasting, the brain adapts to utilize acetoacetate and β-hydroxybutyrate glucose is still required by the brain; (3) only glucose can be used by the anaerobic energy-yielding process of glycolysis. Dietary and body protein will, if necessary, be used to meet these requirements for glucose. The dietary sources of carbohydrate are potatoes, rice and cereal grains. In the average diet, 50 per cent or more of the calories are provided by carbohydrate, in the amount of 250 to 500 g. per day, but more is often taken.

Fat, mainly in the form of triacylglycerol, is an efficient fuel and energy store in the body, since it yields per unit weight more than twice the energy of carbohydrate and protein. There appears to be only one essential fatty acid, linoleic acid. All the rest, in fact nearly all of the compound lipids, can be synthesized in the body. In an affluent country such as the United

States, more than 20 to 25 per cent of the daily calories may be derived from fat in meats, milk and other dairy products and from vegetable oils. In any diet, about one per cent of the calories should be present as linoleic acid or equivalent polyunsaturated acid. Since only the glycerol moiety of the lipids is a source of glucose, fat is an inefficient source of carbohydrate, and by itself it cannot exert a protein-sparing action. Since cholesterol is a prominent constituent of atherosclerotic lesions, it is thought prudent to limit the dietary intake of the sterol. This does not itself result in a reduction of the plasma cholesterol, but in combination with increased intake of polyunsaturated fatty acids, substantial reductions in plasma cholesterol may occur. Thus, many nutritionists recommend careful restriction in the intake of animal fats and cholesterol together with an increase in the use of vegetable oils. In the absence of better knowledge of the origins of vascular disease this is a discreet policy.

The body is an energy-saving system. Excess calories ingested as carbohydrate, fat or protein are stored as fat. This is an inescapable rule, underlying overweight and obesity. Weight is lost when the caloric intake is restricted and energy production is increased by moderate exercise. The important considerations in dealing with obesity are education and motivation. When the caloric intake is restricted, it is important to provide protein of good quality and the necessary vitamins and minerals.

Protein

Vigorous young men, exercising daily, with a total requirement of 3,000 kcal. per day, remain in nitrogen balance and in excellent health on a daily intake of 0.5 g. per kg. body weight of protein of good quality. For a 70 kg. man, this is 35 g. of protein per day, 140 kcal., about five per cent of the daily caloric intake. The requirement for protein is not large. The significant phrase is "protein of good quality." The protein of milk and eggs is representative of such high quality protein. (1) It contains all of the essential amino acids. (2) The distribution of the amino acids approximates the average composition of the body protein. (3) It is easily and completely digested and absorbed and efficiently utilized in the growing animal: The ratio, gain in body N/N ingested, is highest for such protein. Most proteins fall short of this ideal, especially the vegetable proteins, since they have quite different proportions of the amino acids than the animal proteins and are often deficient or lacking in one or more of the essential amino acids. A mixture of animal and vegetable sources of protein is therefore recommended for the average diet, and the daily requirement is set at 1 g. per kg. to assure an adequate intake of the essential amino acids and of the amino acids, such as cysteine and tyrosine, that can spare essential amino acids such as methionine and phenylalanine. For infants and growing children, adolescents and pregnant women, the recommended intake is 2 g. per kg. Taking the world as a whole, in the present day, it is doubtful that these requirements for protein nutrition are satisfied for the great majority of mankind.

Protein is utilized most efficiently when it is a constituent of a balanced meal containing both carbohydrate and fat; the calorie-providing foodstuffs spare amino acids for their proper function as substrates for protein synthesis. It should be appreciated that in addition the meal must contain the appropriate minerals, especially the cations Na^+, K^+, Mg^{2+}. A patient receiving a well-balanced mixture of amino acids, carbohydrate and lipid by intravenous hyperalimentation does not retain nitrogen well if any of the important cations is missing from the mixture.

Vitamins

The vitamins are accessory food factors not synthesized by the body but required in small amounts for maintenance of normal function. They are not related chemically but are classified as fat soluble (A, D, E, K) and water soluble (C and the B complex). Most of the vitamins, especially those of the B complex, have been identified as constituents of coenzymes, and one vitamin (D_3) is now perfectly well qualified to be regarded as a hormone.

The Fat-Soluble Vitamins. Vitamins A, D, E and K are the fat-soluble vitamins. They and their precursors in the diet depend for their absorption on the normal absorption of lipids. If this is disturbed, the fat-soluble vitamins are lost along with the lipids in the fatty stools, and deficiencies of these vitamins may complicate the disturbances due to faulty digestion and absorption of lipids.

Retinol

Vitamin A (retinol) occurs in cod liver oil, halibut liver oil, milk fat, egg yolk and liver. Yellow vegetables and fruits (carrots, sweet potatoes, apricots, cantaloupe) and leafy green vegetables (spinach, greens) contain pigments (α, β, and γ-carotene and cryptoxanthin) that can be converted to vitamin A in the intestinal epithelium. The symmetric β-carotene (see p. 263) is oxidized by a dioxygenase to 2 moles of vitamin A aldehyde (retinal). This is reduced to retinol, the alcohol is esterified to palmitate, and the ester is carried by chylomicra to the liver, where it is stored. Retinol is transported in plasma by a specific retinol-binding globulin. Vitamin A aldehyde (retinal) is the active form of the vitamin in vision.

In adults the store of retinyl ester in the liver defers the onset of deficiency symptoms for many months. The first sign of deficiency is night blindness. In infants and children there is no reserve of the vitamin, and the profound effects of deficiency are readily apparent. There is failure of growth, both of the skeleton and of the soft tissues, and keratinizing metaplasia of all epithelial tissues. In the eyes this leads to xerophthalmia and blindness. Increased susceptibility to infection is common. Male animals become sterile because of atrophy of the germinal epithelium, and female animals do not bear normal young.

The best defined action of the vitamin is its role in vision. In the retina, the visual pigment rhodopsin (visual purple) is formed by combination of the protein opsin with 11-*cis*-retinal. Absorption of light by rhodopsin causes isomerization of 11-*cis*- to all-*trans*-retinal; this event triggers the nerve impulse. All-*trans*-retinal dissociates from opsin. It is slowly reconverted to 11-*cis*-retinal by light, but the conversion is achieved more rapidly by reduction of retinal to retinol, followed by enzymatic isomerization to the 11-*cis*-form and reoxidation to 11-*cis*-retinal. This part of the visual cycle may take place mainly in the liver. Retinal is essential for the prevention of night-blindness, and it is required for the preservation of the rods, since in prolonged severe deficiency of retinal (retinoic acid being provided to prevent deficiency in other respects) the rods degenerate.

Many effects of vitamin A are mediated by retinoic acid. Recent work has shown that a derivative, retinyl phosphate, may play a part in glycoprotein synthesis, reacting with guanosine diphosphate mannose to form mannosyl-retinyl phosphate (MRP). MRP is used in turn to transfer mannose to specific sites on the proteins being glycosylated. It has been shown, in support of this proposed function, that rat serum α-1-macroglobulin exhibits defective glycosylation in vitamin A deficient animals.

Pure vitamin A alcohol forms pale yellow crystals, is unsaponifiable, fairly heat stable but easily destroyed by oxidation. Its loss in foods by oxidation may be prevented by vitamin E. One international unit of the vitamin is defined as the activity of 0.6 μg. of β-carotene. Recommended daily allowance of the vitamin for adults is 5,000 I.U. Very large excesses of the vitamin (500,000 I.U. per day over long periods) are toxic.

Vitamin D, the antirachitic factor, is produced by irradiation of the plant sterol, ergosterol, with ultra-violet light. The product (ergocalciferol, viosterol, vitamin D_2) forms white odorless crystals, soluble in fat solvents and stable to heat, acids, alkalies and most oxidizing agents. Vitamin D_3 (cholecalciferol, the natural form in animals) is formed from 7-dehydrocholesterol by the action of sunlight on the skin (Fig. 4-13). It is found in high concentration in fish liver oils. Vitamins D_2 and D_3 are essentially equipotent in humans. Cholecalciferol is oxidized to 25-(OH)-D_3 in the liver, in a reaction that is strongly product inhibited, providing a safeguard against overproduction. The 25-(OH)-D_3 is further oxidized in the kidney to 1,25-(OH)$_2D_3$, the active form, which exerts its effects without the time lag seen after giving D_2 and D_3 to experimental animals. The reaction in kidney is enhanced by parathyroid hormone and is inhibited by high serum calcium and by a high concentration of phosphate in renal cortical cells. It may be seen that vitamin D is a true vitamin only in the absence of sunlight. The active agent, 1,25-(OH)$_2D_3$, can also be regarded as a hormone.

In vitamin D deficiency, calcium is poorly absorbed from the intestine, and both calcium and phosphate are lost in the feces. Serum inorganic phosphate is decreased, but calcium may be normal. In the absence of vitamin D and of an adequate supply of calcium and phosphate, the matrix of growing bone is poorly calcified. The bones remain soft and are easily distorted. The condition is known as rickets.

1,25-(OH)$_2D_3$ increases absorption of calcium from the small intestine by stimulating the formation of a specific calcium-binding protein in the brush border of the intestinal epithelial cells, facilitating transport of calcium into the bloodstream. Parathyroid hormone also stimulates this process, but only in the presence of the active vitamin. 1,25-(OH)$_2D_3$ mobilizes calcium from bone, and, acting with parathyroid hormone, may assist in the regulation of the serum calcium. In addition to increasing the supply of calcium by improving its absorption from the gut, 1,25-(OH)$_2D_3$ acts in some way to improve the rate of calcification of the bone matrix. The healing of rickets is greater and faster than one would expect merely from the improved supply of calcium and phosphate. The vitamin may act together with calcitonin, which increases the deposition of bone salt. Vitamin D-resistant rickets and the resistance to the vitamin in chronic uremia may be due to failure of the kidney to make the required active form.

The international unit of the vitamin is the activity of 0.05 μg. of D_2. The recommended daily allowance is 400 I.U. Most foods are poor sources of the vitamin, and the natural source for growing children is by the action of sunlight on the skin. This is now supple-

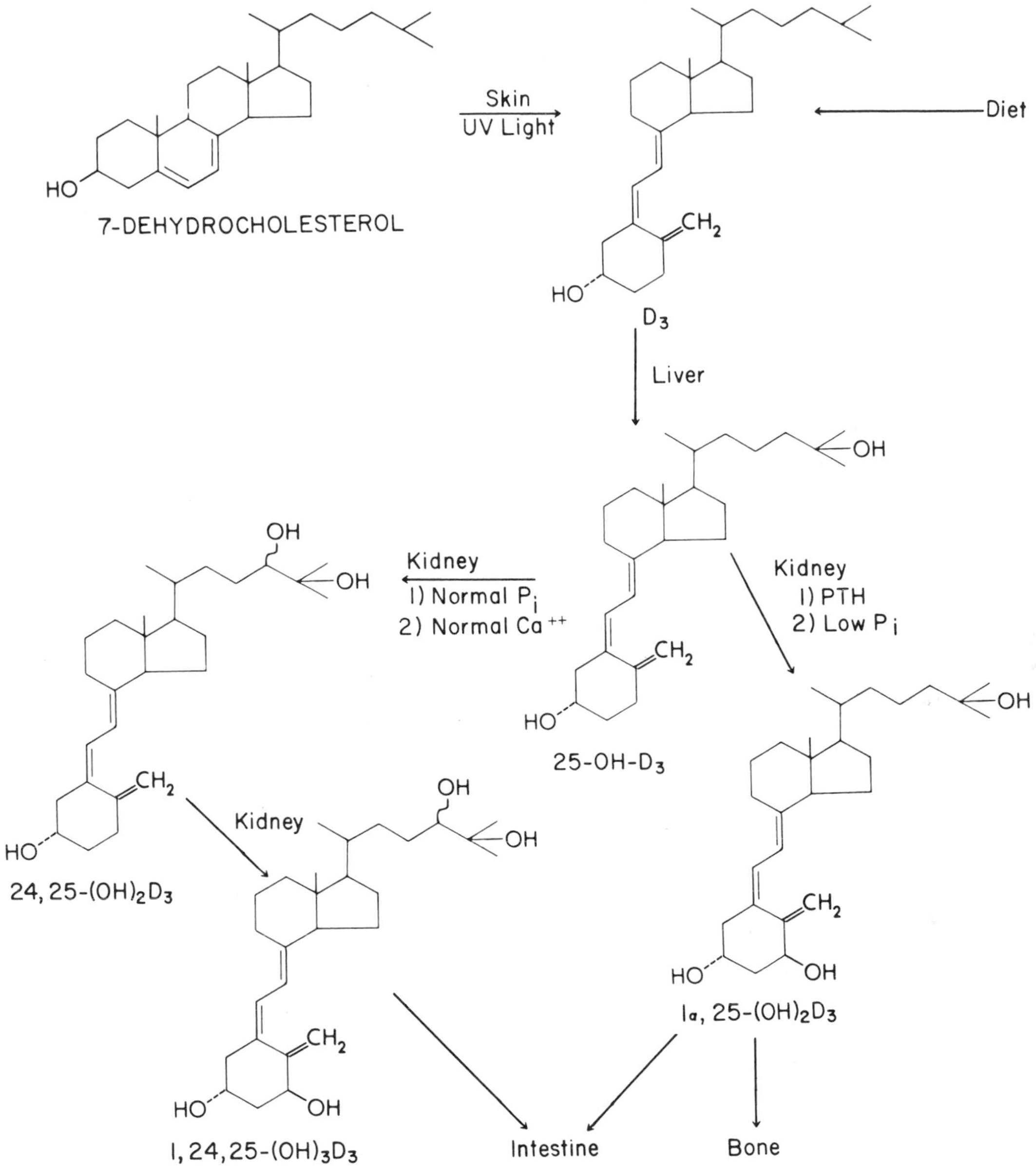

Fig. 4-13. Vitamin D_3 as a prohormone; schematic summary of the origin of vitamin D_3 and its various biologically active metabolites. (Holrick, M. F., and DeLuca, H. F.: Am. Rev. Med., *25:*349, 1974).

mented by fortification of milk with vitamin D, either by adding ergocalciferol or by ultraviolet irradiation. A continuous supply of the vitamin is necessary. Storage in the body is limited, and there is some loss both in the urine and in the feces (through excretion in the bile) and perhaps some complete destruction of the vitamin by unknown pathways.

Vitamin D taken in excess (more than 4,000 I.U. per day for many days) is toxic. Large amounts of bone salt are mobilized, and the bones become easily liable to multiple fractures. Serum calcium and inor-

ganic phosphate are high, and there may be metastatic calcification of soft tissues. Renal calculi may form, leading to disturbances of renal function.

Vitamin E is found in wheat germ oil, green leafy vegetables, nuts, legumes, liver and egg yolk. From these sources, seven complex alcohols, known as tocopherols, have been isolated. Of these α-tocopherol has the widest distribution and the greatest biologic activity. The tocopherols are viscous oils, soluble in fat solvents, stable to heat in the absence of oxygen. They are strong antioxidants and are unstable to oxyα-Tocopherol

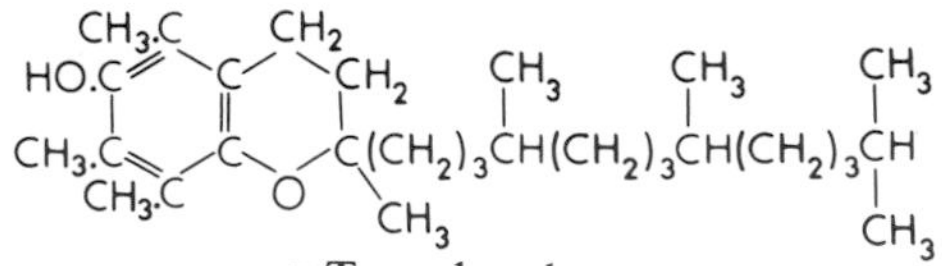

gen, ultraviolet light and rancid fats. In natural foods, they inhibit development of rancidity and oxidative destruction of vitamin A.

Vitamin E deficiency in the rat leads to failure of reproduction—in the female because of early fetal death and in the male because of immobility of spermatozoa and degeneration of the germinal epithelium. In advanced deficiency the rat develops muscular dystrophy. In rabbits and guinea pigs, E deficiency leads very quickly to muscular dystrophy, with progressive paralysis. Similar effects are seen in calves, lambs and ducklings on an E-deficient diet. The effects of E deficiency seen in various animal species are numerous and diverse, but they may all be related to the antioxidant properties of the vitamin and its protective effects on unsaturated lipids. The work on animals leads to the assumption that vitamin E is essential for man, but the vitamin is so widespread that deficiency in man is rare. The requirement for the vitamin may be increased with increasing dietary intake of polyunsaturated fatty acids. A sign of vitamin E deficiency is reduction of the normal resistance of red cells to hemolysis by oxidizing agents such as peroxide or dialuric acid. This was noted in one human subject suspected of E deficiency because of cirrhosis and faulty lipid absorption from the intestine.

Vitamin K, which prevents hemorrhagic disease in chicks fed a synthetic ration, has been isolated from alfalfa (K_1) and fish meal (K_2). The compounds are derivatives of naphthoquinone containing a long hydrocarbon side chain. Menadione (2-methyl, 1,4,-naphthoquinone) is as active as the natural compounds, on a molar basis, and is used therapeutically. Vitamin

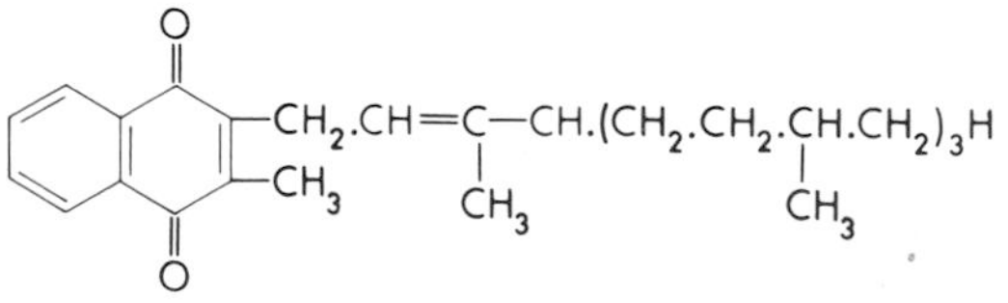

K compounds are easily destroyed by oxidizing agents, alcoholic alkali, strong acid and light. The natural sources for man are green vegetables, tomatoes, soybean oil and bran. These sources are supplemented by K produced by intestinal bacteria. Deficiency in man arises from severe disturbances of lipid digestion and absorption. Newborn infants, before an intestinal flora has been established, may show signs of K defi-

ciency. Treatment of the mother with K before birth can prevent the disorder (hemorrhagic disease of the newborn).

Vitamin K is essential for the synthesis in the liver of the clotting factors prothrombin, proconvertin, Christmas factor and Stuart factor (factors II, VII, IX, and X, respectively). In the absence of K these proteins are synthesized and secreted by the liver, but they are ineffectual, lacking the capability of binding Ca^{2+} and therefore unable to associate with the phospholipid required for their activity. In the liver, K mediates the transfer of CO_2 to prothrombin to form, on the first ten residues of glutamic acid nearest the NH_2-terminal end of the polypeptide chain, carboxyglutamic acid:

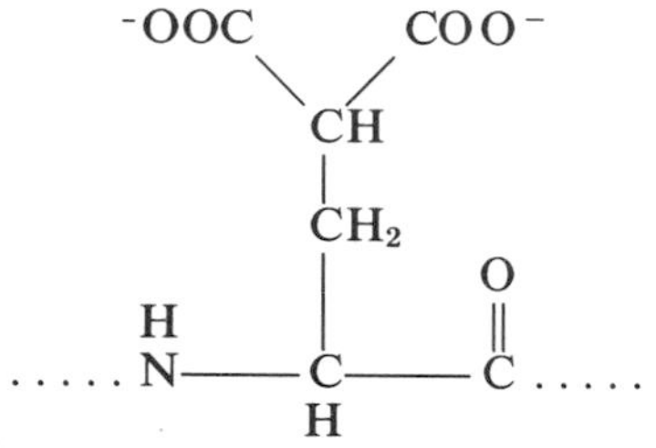

The reaction requires the presence of oxygen, and ATP is utilized. The details are as yet unknown. A similar post-translational modification of factors VII, IX, and X, mediated by K, establishes their calcium-binding activity. Dicoumarol owes its anticoagulant activity to its ability to inhibit this action of vitamin K.

The Water-Soluble Vitamins. The vitamins of the B complex, ascorbic acid and choline constitute the water-soluble vitamins. Most of them form part of the essential apparatus of the enzyme systems of plant and animal cells, and with a good mixed diet, well prepared to avoid losses by cooking, they should be present in amounts sufficient to prevent deficiency.

Thiamine Hydrochloride is a white crystalline substance that possesses a nutlike, salty taste and a yeastlike odor. It is stable in the dry form and in acid

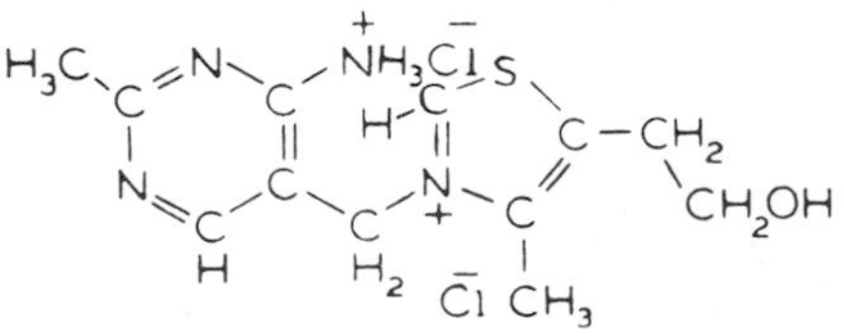

solution. Heating in neutral or mildly alkaline solution rapidly inactivates it. Mild oxidants easily convert it to thiochrome, the blue fluorescence of which is used in the quantitative determination of the vitamin. Thiamine is found free in fairly high concentration in the outer layers of the cereal grains, in peas and beans, in yeast, in animal tissues, especially pork, and (in low concentration) in milk. Wheat flour is a poor source of thiamine, which is lost in the milling, but white bread made with enriched wheat flour is now an important dietary source of the vitamin. Much of the vitamin in vegetable foods may be lost by prolonged cooking in excessive amounts of water. Thiamine is not stored, and a constant supply is required. The recommended daily allowance is 0.5 mg. per 1,000 kcal. of diet. The need varies with state of physical activity, food intake and composition of the diet. Protein and lipid spare thiamine; carbohydrate increases the requirement.

Thiamine deficiency in man takes the form of dry or wet beriberi, and it is seen most often in the Far East, where polished rice is a major component of the diet. There is loss of appetite, rapid loss of weight, muscle wasting and weakness, enlargement of the heart, peripheral neuritis, emotional disturbances and mental confusion. In wet beriberi there is, in addition, generalized edema. These disorders are rapidly and dramatically reversed by administration of the vitamin. Except in certain cases of chronic alcoholism, thiamine deficiency is not seen in Western countries, but widespread mild or marginal deficiency may exist. There is at present no simple satisfactory laboratory test for thiamine deficiency. The normal concentration of the vitamin in whole blood is about 7 μg. per dl., most of it is in the red cells. A small amount (50 to 250 μg.) may appear in the urine daily at normal levels of intake.

The active form of the vitamin is thiamine pyrophosphate (TPP) formed by direct transfer of pyrophosphate from ATP. TPP acts as a coenzyme in the decarboxylation of pyruvate and α-ketoglutarate, in the transketolase reaction of the pentose phosphate shunt pathway and in the oxidative decarboxylation of the branched-chain keto acids derived from leucine, isoleucine and valine. The critical importance of thiamine is apparent from these functions.

Riboflavin (7,8 dimethyl-10-(1'-D-ribityl)-isoalloxazine) is a bitter-tasting orange-yellow pigment that dissolves sparingly in water to give a greenish yellow fluorescence that can be used in the simplest method of measuring the vitamin. Riboflavin is stable to dry heat and in acid solution, stable to mild oxidation and is sensitive to ultraviolet light, yielding lumichrome, which has an intense blue fluorescence, in acid solution and lumiflavin, a yellow pigment, in alkaline solution. Riboflavin is generally distributed in plant and animal tissues, but there are few particularly rich sources: milk, eggs, green leafy vegetables, liver, yeast and wheat germ.

Uncomplicated riboflavin deficiency in man is rare. It usually occurs in other deficiency diseases (pellagra;

beriberi). The symptoms are like those of other deficiency states: magenta-colored tongue, fissures at the corners of the mouth, dermatitis, corneal vascularization. The importance of the vitamin for normal growth and reproduction is indicated from studies in experimental animals. The vitamin is not stored. The daily requirement is estimated to be 0.4 to 0.6 mg. for young children, rising to 1 to 2 mg. for older children and adults. The normal concentration of riboflavin in whole blood is 20 μg. per dl. It is mostly in the erythrocytes, which may provide the most sensitive measure of deficiency. The need for the vitamin may best be correlated with growth and protein synthesis.

Riboflavin-5'-monophosphate (somewhat loosely called flavin mononucleotide, FMN), and flavin-adenine dinucleotide (FAD), formed by joining FMN in pyrophosphate linkage to adenylic acid, are found as prosthetic groups of a large array of oxidases, oxygenases and dehydrogenases, in which they act, reversibly, as hydrogen and electron donors and acceptors. FMN and FAD are usually firmly bound, indeed often covalently linked, to their respective apoenzymes. A number of forms of FMN and FAD are known, in which there are substitutions in the isoalloxazine ring system. These may serve different functions. A specific riboflavin-binding protein has been found, in the gamma globulin fraction, in plasma.

Niacin (nicotinic acid; pyridine-3-carboxylic acid) is the pellagra-preventing factor. It occurs as the free acid, but in animal tissues it is found as the acid amide (nicotinamide) serving as a constituent of two pyridine nucleotides. The food sources of niacin are liver, meat, whole-grain cereals and fish; it is added as a supplement to white flour. The essential amino acid tryptophan can be converted to niacin in the body. The need for the vitamin is diminished with diets rich in sources of tryptophan (eggs and milk). It is estimated that 60 mg. of tryptophan are equivalent to 1 mg. of niacin. In pellagra the niacin deficiency is complicated by deficiencies of other B vitamins and especially by a diet low in protein or unbalanced in its constituent amino acids. There is failure of growth, loss of appetite, severe gastrointestinal disturbances, dermatitis in areas of skin exposed to sunlight, and dementia. Treatment of pellagra requires not only niacin but also a diet adequate in the other B vitamins and in protein.

Niacin functions as a constituent of the coenzymes nicotinamide-adenine dinucleotide (NAD^+) and nicotinamide-adenine dinucleotide phosphate ($NADP^+$). The two coenzymes serve two separate systems of dehydrogenases, acting as hydrogen and electron acceptors and donors, NAD^+ mainly in systems concerned with energy production (e.g., 3-phosphoglyceraldehyde dehydrogenase; lactic dehydrogenase), $NADP^+$ in systems concerned with energy storage (glucose 6-phosphate dehydrogenase; both of the reductive steps in fatty acid synthesis). The symptoms of niacin deficiency are not well correlated with the known metabolic functions of the coenzymes.

The major urinary metabolite of niacin is N^1-methylnicotinamide, formed from nicotinamide in the liver. The vitamin is not stored, and a constant supply is required. The requirement is a complex function of the status of the individual and the nature of the diet, especially the amount and quality of the protein. The recommended daily allowances are 5 to 15 mg. for infants and children, 15 to 20 for adolescents and adults of both sexes.

Vitamin B_6 (pyridoxine; pyridoxal; pyridoxamine) is a pyridine derivative found in three forms in nature, all equally effective in animals and man. The natural sources of the vitamin are yeast, liver, kidney, meat,

milk, legumes, green vegetables and whole-grain cereals. The active form of the vitamin is pyridoxal phosphate, which acts as a coenzyme in many reactions involving amino acids: transamination, decarboxylation, dehydration/deamination; in the synthesis of δ-amino-levulinic acid from glycine and succinyl CoA; and as an essential structural constituent of glycogen phosphorylase. The main urinary metabolite of the vitamin is 4-pyridoxic acid.

B_6-deficient rats fail to grow and develop a scaly, edematous dermatitis on tail, ears, paws and mouth (acrodynia). This may be due to a deficiency of polyunsaturated fatty acids, which causes a similar dermatitis, without the edema. B_6-deficient rats develop a hypochromic anemia and suffer demyelination of the spinal cord and peripheral nerves. They become extremely sensitive to noise, convulsing readily. A naturally occurring deficiency state has not been seen in adult humans, but symptoms (nausea, vomiting, anorexia, dermatitis) are readily elicited by administration of the analogue deoxypyridoxine, or of isonicotinoylhydrazide (isoniazid). Deoxypyridoxine phosphate competes with pyridoxal phosphate for its place on the enzymes that it serves. Isoniazid forms a hydrazone of pyridoxal and pyridoxal phosphate, which is excreted in the urine. Human subjects receiving deoxypyridoxine excrete oxalic acid and large amounts of kynurenine and xanthurenic acid, indicating a disturbance in the metabolism of tryptophan. Convulsions have been seen in children receiving a commercial baby food deficient in pyridoxine and in children with a hereditary defect who require large amounts (2 to 10 mg. per day) of pyridoxine.

The requirement for pyridoxine is a function of age, activity and the level of protein intake. It is increased with high protein diets. There may be some synthesis of the vitamin by intestinal bacteria. The recommended daily allowances range from 0.2 to 1.2 mg. in infants and children to 1.4 to 2.5 mg. in adolescents and adults of both sexes, and in pregnant and lactating women.

Pantothenic acid (pantoyl-β-alanine) is a constituent of coenzyme A and of the prosthetic group of the

acyl carrier protein concerned in fatty acid synthesis. The richest sources of the vitamin are meat, milk, yeast, liver and eggs. It is an essential factor in all animals that have been studied, but it has not been established as essential for man. In the rat, pantothenic acid deficiency causes a diminished rate of growth, poor reproduction and adrenal cortical hypofunction due to hemorrhagic necrosis. Coenzyme A plays an essential role in the oxidation of pyruvate, α-ketoglutarate and the fatty acids, and in the biosynthesis of the fatty acids, cholesterol and the porphyrins. A recommended daily allowance for the vitamin is 5 to 10 mg.

Biotin was first recognized as a growth factor for yeast, and it was later established that it is identical to a factor required for growth and respiration by *Rhizobium* and to the factor in yeast and liver that protects rats from the consequences of eating large amounts of raw egg white. In most animals and in man biotin deficiency can be induced only by sterilizing the intestinal tract with an antibiotic. The effect of raw egg white is due to the presence of a protein, avidin, that binds tightly to biotin and prevents its absorption. In normal animals and in man, the intestinal bacteria are adequate sources of the vitamin. Beef liver, yeast and eggs are rich food sources. Probably as little as 10 μg. per day are required by humans.

Biotin is the coenzyme, covalently bound as a prosthetic group in amide linkage with the ϵ-amino group of a specific lysine residue in the molecule, of a number of enzymes involved in the fixation of carbon dioxide. These include pyruvate carboxylase, acetyl-SCoA carboxylase, methylmalonyl transcarboxylase, and propionyl-SCoA carboxylase, In biotin deficiency, as might be expected, the incorporation of carbon dioxide into oxaloacetate is reduced, and fatty acid biosynthesis is impaired, but in addition there are reductions in urea synthesis, purine synthesis and tryptophan catabolism that are difficult to explain, since no biotin-containing enzymes are known to be involved.

Folic acid (folacin; pteroylglutamic acid) contains glutamic acid, p-aminobenzoic acid, and a pterin (2-amino-4-hydroxy-6-methyl pteridine). The compound shown is the pteroylglutamic acid of liver. Folic acid is also found in many organisms and tissues as a polyglutamyl derivative, containing three to seven residues in γ-glutamyl linkage. These are hydrolyzed enzymatically to the active monoglutamyl compound. The meta-

bolically active form of folic acid is the 5,6,7,8 tetrahydrofolic acid (THF). It is the coenzyme of a group of enzymes involved in "one-carbon" metabolism, acting as acceptor and donor of "active" formyl, formaldehyde, formimino, methoxy and methyl

groups. It is essential for the synthesis of purines and of thymine and is required, along with pyridoxal phosphate, in the synthesis of serine from glycine. It can act as a source of methyl groups in the synthesis of choline from ethanolamine.

In folic acid deficiency there is growth failure, anemia and leukopenia. The vitamin is effective in treating sprue and the megaloblastic anemias of some infants and pregnant women. These disorders may arise from a defect in the absorption of folic acid or from inability to convert the polyglutamates to the active form, since dietary insufficiency is rare because of the wide distribution of the vitamin, and since folic acid may be synthesized by the intestinal bacteria. The richest food sources are liver, kidney, yeast, meat and green leafy vegetables. The recommended daily allowance is 400 μg., but the requirement is much less, nearer 50 μg.

Since folic acid is essential for the synthesis of purines and of thymine, and therefore of DNA, and since folic acid deficiency causes leukopenia, a number of antimetabolites have been studied for their possible beneficial effect in leukemia. Aminopterin (4-aminopteroyl-glutamic acid) and its 9-methyl derivative have produced temporary remissions of acute leukemia in children. The drug is extremely potent: In a concentration of $1:10^6$ in the diet, aminopterin kills rats or mice in less than a week.

Vitamin B$_{12}$ (antipernicious anemia factor; Castle's extrinsic factor) is not synthesized by animals or higher plants but is exclusively of microbial origin, including the microbial flora of the intestine in man and other animals. The richest dietary sources of the vitamin are liver and kidney, but the amounts of B$_{12}$ in most foods are very low (1 to 5 μg. per 100 g.). It is probably entirely absent from higher plants. Symptoms of deficiency of the vitamin have been observed in individuals eating a strict vegetarian diet; otherwise a true deficiency of B₁₂ is rare. In pernicious anemia the defect is in the production of a gastric mucoprotein (intrinsic factor) that combines mole for mole with the vitamin and facilitates its absorption from the ileum. If enough B₁₂ is given orally (200 to 300 μg. per day) pernicious anemia can be prevented or cured even in the absence of intrinsic factor. The requirement for the vitamin in man is not known exactly, but may be about 0.6 to 1.2 μg. per day.

Vitamin B₁₂ is isolated as a red crystalline compound containing cobalt and phosphate. It is stable to heating in neutral or mildly acid solution but is rapidly destroyed above pH 9. One of the common coenzyme forms of B₁₂ is shown. The central structure is composed of four condensed pyrrole rings, as in the porphyrins, but in this "corrin" ring system two of the pyrroles are attached directly rather than through a methene bridge. As the vitamin is isolated, the central cobalt atom is attached covalently to cyanide (cyanocobalamin). In the coenzyme form the cyanide is replaced by a deoxyadenosine moiety, attached covalently to the cobalt through the 5'-carbon of deoxyribose. Also attached covalently to the cobalt is a 5,6-dimethylbenzimidazole riboside connected through phosphate and aminopropanol to a side chain on ring IV of the tetrapyrrole nucleus.

The vitamin B₁₂ coenzymes are concerned in the interconversion of glutamate and β-methylaspartate and in the analogous interconversion of methylmalonyl SCoA and succinyl SCoA. B₁₂ also participates in the methylation of homocysteine to methionine and of deoxyuridine monosphosphate to deoxythymidine monophosphate. It is this latter function that may relate the coenzyme function of B₁₂ to the macrocytic anemia characteristic of its deficiency, but all the phenomena of B₁₂ deficiency cannot yet be accounted for in terms of known metabolic reactions.

Lipoic acid (thioctic acid) is often classified with the water-soluble B complex. It is required by some microorganisms, but there is no evidence that it is required by man. In its functional form (lipoamide) it is bound covalently through its carboxyl group to the ε-amino nitrogen of a specific lysine residue in the enzyme lipoate acetyl transferase. It functions as a coenzyme in the oxidative decarboxylation of pyruvate and α-ketoglutarate, accepting "active aldehyde"

from thiamine pyrophosphate, assisting in its conversion to the activated acid (thioester) and in its transfer to form the active acyl-coenzyme A derivative. In this process the disulfide of the lipoamide is reduced to disulfhydryl. The dihydrolipoamide is reoxidized to the disulfide by the flavoprotein dihydrolipoyl dehydrogenase.

Ascorbic acid (vitamin C) cannot be synthesized by man and other primates or by the guinea pig. Other animals and many plants can synthesize ascorbic acid from glucose. The compound, which occurs as a γ-lactone, is readily and reversibly oxidized to dehydroascorbic acid. Ascorbic acid is an effective reducing agent in mildly acid solution. Its ability to reduce quantitatively the dye 2,6-dichlorophenolindophenol to its colorless form is the basis of a widely used, very sensitive analytic method. Vitamin C is found in highest concentrations in citrus fruits, berries, melons, tomatoes, green pepper, raw cabbage and leafy green vegetables. The concentration in potatoes is low, but when potatoes are a large component of the diet, they can be a major source of vitamin C. Because it is easily oxidized, losses of ascorbic acid in storage, processing and cooking of food are large and variable.

Ascorbic acid is found in varying amounts in all tissues and body fluids. The amount in adrenal cortex (about 400 mg. per 100 g.) is greater than in any other tissue. High concentrations are also found in the corpus luteum. In the adrenal, ACTH and in the corpus luteum, LH causes a marked fall in ascorbic acid that is proportional to the dose, providing a basis for the bioassay of these two hormones. The role of ascorbic acid in steroidogenesis in these organs is unknown. In human subjects with an intake of 75 to 100 mg. per day of vitamin C the concentration of ascorbic acid in serum is 1 to 1.4 mg. per dl. At higher concentrations in blood, vitamin C is readily excreted in the urine. With diets free of the vitamin, the concentration in blood falls very slowly, and 3 to 4 months are required before deficiency symptoms appear.

Deficiency of vitamin C leads to scurvy. The disorder is characterized by a breakdown or disorganization of tissues of mesenchymal origin: bone, dentine, cartilage, connective tissue and intercellular substance. In adults, the gums become sore; the teeth loosen and may fall out; subcutaneous hemorrhages and edema occur because of increased capillary fragility; there is joint pain, anemia and loss of appetite. Wound healing is slow, and the scars of old wounds may break down. In children, in addition, growth and development are impaired. The developing teeth and skeleton are particularly affected. Most of these defects are attributable to poor formation of collagen and intercellular substance. The anemia may be related to inability to use stored iron and to effects on the metabolism of folic acid.

Although the relationship between ascorbic acid and dehydroascorbic acid suggests a role in oxidation-reduction reactions, no reaction is known in which the vitamin plays a direct role as coenzyme. Yet its presence is required in a number of biologic oxidations: in the hydroxylation of proline and lysine in collagen biosynthesis and in the hydroxylation of γ-butyrobetaine to carnitine. An obligatory role for ascorbic acid in the oxidation of certain aromatic acids, ρ-hydroxyphenylpyruvic acid, ρ-hydroxyphenylacetic acid and tryptamine is not certainly established. Vitamin C facilitates removal of the iron from ferritin and may play a part in making stored iron available.

The requirement for Vitamin C is a subject of long and occasionally heated discussion. There is no doubt that a daily intake of 70 to 100 mg. per day is more than sufficient to avoid scurvy and to assure well-being. The requirement may be substantially greater in infections and fever, and larger intakes (up to 1 g. or more per day) have been recommended for the prevention of colds and for improved resistance to other stresses. The whole question is being re-examined experimentally, but it is too soon to form a judgement.

Inositol is a carbocyclic hexitol, found in wide distribution among microorganisms, plants and animals. Of

the nine possible stereoisomers, only one, *myo*-inositol, is biologically active. No human requirement for inositol has been shown. It has been found that for the successful culture of numerous strains of human cells, inositol is required in the medium. Phosphatidylinositol is found as one of the constituent phospholipids of many tissues. The free compound is found in high concentration in mammalian cardiac muscle and in shark skeletal muscle. In plants it is often esterified to phosphate. Phytic acid, inositol hexaphosphate, found in cereal grains, can be rachitogenic in large amounts in the diet, since it forms an insoluble salt with calcium. It may also interfere with the absorption of iron and zinc.

Choline, N-trimethylethanolamine, is normally present in large amounts in the diet and can in any case be synthesized by animals receiving adequate amounts of protein. It is formed by the decarboxylation of serine to ethanolamine, which is methylated at the expense of methionine. Lecithin, phosphatidyl choline, is widely distributed in all tissues and is a prominent constituent in many membranes. Acetylcholine is an essential neurotransmitter. In rats and certain other animals on diets low in protein, choline is required to prevent the development of fatty liver. It is not clear how directly this may be related to the synthesis of phosphatidyl choline. In young rats shortly after weaning, choline deficiency leads to the development of hemorrhagic kidneys. The lesions are cured by choline or by a diet high in methionine. The need for choline may be related to the rapid synthesis of phosphoglycerides in the kidneys of these young animals. Choline is oxidized in the body to betaine (N-trimethylglycine), an active methyl donor. Methyl groups are lost successively, first by direct transfer, and then by oxidation and transfer of the "one-carbon" (formyl) fragment to tetrahydrofolic acid. The reactions proceed from dimethylglycine, to sarcosine, and finally to glycine. Choline makes an important contribution to the one-carbon pool, and this may explain some of the consequences of choline deficiency in animals on diets low in protein. Rich food sources of choline are egg yolk, brain, kidney, liver, sweetbreads and yeast. It may be regarded more as a useful nutrient than as a vitamin.

Minerals

Minerals may be defined as those chemical elements that remain largely in the ash when the substance is ignited at a high temperature. These elements exist in the body both in inorganic and organic combination. Four chemical elements compose about 96 per cent of the body weight (oxygen, 65 per cent, carbon, 18 per cent, hydrogen, 10 per cent and nitrogen, 3 per cent). The remaining four per cent is made up of the elements usually called minerals, which include calcium, phosphorus, potassium, sodium, sulfur, chlorine, magnesium, iron and the so-called trace elements iodine, copper, manganese, zinc, fluorine, cobalt, silicon, molybdenum, tin, nickel, chromium, selenium and vanadium.

The normal adult is in a steady state with respect to minerals, the intake being equal to the amounts excreted. Minerals are lost by various routes, namely, the kidney, the bowel and the skin. About one-fourth of the solid matter of urine and one tenth of the solid matter of feces is mineral. In growth, pregnancy and lactation, positive balances in some minerals should exist to allow for the building of tissue. The quantitatively important inorganic cations of tissues and body fluids are Na^+, K^+, Ca^{2+} and Mg^{2+}; and the inorganic anions are Cl^-, HCO_3^-, $H_2PO_4^-$, HPO_4^{2-} and SO_4^{2-}.

Calcium is the most abundant mineral element in the body, about 99 per cent of this mineral occurring in the bones and the teeth. However, the remaining one per cent in the body fluids is of great importance. The level in the blood serum remains very constant (9 to 11 mg. per dl.); about half of this is protein bound. The degree of ionization of the calcium, usually about 60 per cent, depends upon the protein and the pH of the plasma. Its presence in proper proportions with sodium, potassium and magnesium is necessary in the fluids surrounding the tissues for their proper function. Calcium is an essential element in blood coagulation, in the normal response to stimulation of nerves, in the activation of some enzymes, in muscular contraction, and in mediating the responses of many kinds of cells to various stimuli.

Calcium-binding proteins play a critical part in many of the actions of calcium (for example, troponin C). A ubiquitous member of this class, *calmodulin,* has recently been discovered and studied intensively. Calmodulin is a small heat-stable acidic protein (16,700 daltons) remarkably conserved in amino acid sequence and structure in many species, capable of combining with four atoms of Ca^{2+}/mole. It is activated by a rising concentration of calcium, takes up the ion, changes conformation, and combines with a dependent enzyme, activating it:

$$Calmodulin + Ca^{2+} \leftrightharpoons Calmodulin\text{-}Ca^{2+}$$
$$Calmodulin\text{-}Ca^{2+} + Enzyme(inactive) \leftrightharpoons Calmodulin\text{-}Ca^{2+}\text{-}Enzyme(active)$$

Calmodulin-dependent enzymes include 3',5'-cyclic nucleotide phosphodiesterase, adenylate cyclase, the myosin light chain kinase required for contraction of myosin of smooth muscle and non-muscle cells, and phosphorylase kinase, in which it is present, tightly bound, as the delta subunit.

In the maintenance of calcium balance it is necessary to consider the absolute levels of calcium and phosphorus (Ca/P ratio) of food, amount of fat, phytic acid, iron, oxalates, protein and vitamin D in the diet and the pH of the intestine. These factors all have a bearing on proper calcium absorption. Dietary calcium is absorbed into the blood from the small intestine. It is removed from the blood for the bones and teeth during growth and also to a less extent at all ages. During periods of low calcium intake it is withdrawn from the bones to maintain the normal blood calcium level. The more easily mobilized calcium is present in the trabeculae; the calcium of the teeth, dentine, and enamel is more stable. Deficiency of calcium in the diet may lead to generalized rarefaction and demineralization of bone (osteomalacia); vitamin D deficiency is almost always present. Insufficient intake of calcium and phosphorus may also cause rickets in children. Calcium is excreted in the urine and the feces. Normally the amount of calcium excreted in urine is small. The fecal calcium consists of unabsorbed calcium and also calcium that has been secreted into the intestinal tract with the digestive juices and not reabsorbed. The absorption of calcium is dependent upon vitamin D; this vitamin, together with the parathyroid hormone and calcitonin, regulates the concentration of calcium in the blood and body fluids.

Phosphorus constitutes about one fourth of the body minerals, approximately 90 per cent being combined with calcium in bone and teeth. Organic phosphates are numerous, ubiquitous and essential to many metabolic processes. The inorganic phosphates of the body fluids form an important buffer system in the neutrality regulation of the body. This is of particular importance and utility in the intracellular fluid and in the urine, where phosphate is used in the conservation of sodium and the excretion of hydrogen ions.

About 70 per cent of the phosphate in food is normally absorbed from the small intestine. Intestinal phosphatases liberate phosphate from organic combinations. Phosphates are widely distributed in food, and when protein and calcium requirements are satisfied by a mixed diet there is no danger of a phosphorus deficit. Absorption of phosphates is decreased by substances that tend to form insoluble phosphate salts (excess calcium, strontium, magnesium, aluminum, barium and thallium, for example). Phosphates are excreted in the urine and the feces, the proportion varying considerably. With a balanced diet the urinary phosphorus constitutes 60 per cent of the total excretion. All of the blood plasma inorganic phosphate is diffusible and filterable through the glomeruli. Most of the phosphate of the glomerular filtrate is reabsorbed; the clearance is always below the inulin clearance. Vitamin D increases and parathyroid hormone decreases reabsorption of phosphate by the renal tubules. Fecal phosphate represents unabsorbed phosphate and that secreted into the intestine. Under normal conditions the fecal phosphorus is about 30 per cent of the amount in the diet. The normal concentrations of inorganic phosphorus in the blood plasma of the adult is between 3 and 4 mg. per dl.; it is slightly higher in infants and children: 4 to 5 mg. per dl. Plasma inorganic phosphate is present mainly as the ions HPO_4^{2-} and $H_2PO_4^-$ in the ratio 4/1. A very small amount is present as inorganic pyrophosphate.

Magnesium is widely distributed in both plant and animal tissue. It is the essential metallic element in chlorophyll. There are about 25 g. of magnesium in the adult body; about 70 per cent is in the bones. It is primarily an intracellular ion. Magnesium is present in most foods in sufficient amounts to prevent a nutritional deficiency. It is absorbed from the intestine, but the absorption is usually incomplete; its absorption is influenced by the same factors that influence calcium absorption. It is excreted in both the urine and the feces; the latter includes nonabsorbed magnesium from the diet. The blood plasma contains 1.5 to 3 mg. per dl., 80 per cent of which is ionized and diffusible; the remainder is bound to protein. The red blood cells contain a slightly higher concentration of the element (4 mg. per dl. of cells). Low levels of magnesium in the blood plasma will produce tetany similar to that observed in hypocalcemia. Excess plasma magnesium decreases muscle and nerve irritability; an extremely high level will bring about anesthesia.

Return to consciousness can be obtained quickly by intravenous administration of calcium. Magnesium is essential for many enzymic reactions; it is an activator for the phosphate-transferring enzymes. It also activates pyruvate carboxylase, the condensing enzyme of the citric acid cycle, leucine aminopeptidase, the conversion of G actin to F actin in muscle, the synthesis of glutamine, and the methylation of guanidoacetic acid

Sodium is found mostly as an ion in the extracellular fluid. It does not readily cross cell membranes. It is therefore important in the maintenance of the normal osmotic relationships between the intracellular and extracellular fluids. It is absorbed readily, and the body content is kept within narrow limits by the kidney. Sodium is lost in the feces and from the skin. Sodium in the blood is kept at a relatively constant level. There is some evidence to support the opinion that excess salt consumption is a factor in the etiology of human hypertension. Dietary sodium restriction is used in the treatment of hypertension and congestive heart failure. The major pathway for the excretion of sodium is by the kidney. On diets low in sodium the urinary excretion of the ion falls to a very low level; about 99.5 per cent of the sodium filtered at the glomerulus is reabsorbed. With the average diet, the excretion of sodium in the urine amounts to 4 or 5 g. per day.

Potassium occurs mainly in the intracellular fluid.

Of the approximately 4,000 mEq. of potassium in the adult human body only about 70 mEq. are in the extracellular fluid. Potassium ions influence the contractility of muscle and affect the excitability of nerves. Potassium is widely distributed and plentiful in foods, efficiently absorbed from the intestine and readily excreted by the normal kidney. Under ordinary circumstances the 2 to 4 g. present in the normal diet are more than enough to meet the daily requirements. The plasma concentration of this element must be maintained within narrow limits. If the concentration of plasma potassium reaches values above 10 mEq. per liter the heart may stop in diastole. Hyperkalemia may occur in the terminal stages of nephritis and in Addison's disease. The "artificial kidney" or proper ion-exchange resins may be lifesaving in certain conditions of hyperkalemia. Potassium deficiencies may occur after long-continued administration of parenteral fluids consisting of sodium chloride and glucose, after loss of digestive juices (diarrhea), in acidosis and in a period of negative nitrogen balance. In many cases of potassium deficiency a state of alkalosis develops. The hypokalemia and alkalosis are more severe if dietary sodium is increased. This occurs because of the renal mechanism of exchange of Na^+ for K^+ or H^+. In the absence of potassium, excess hydrogen ion is exchanged, and more bicarbonate is returned to the plasma. Deficits in body potassium may exist even though the blood plasma concentration is within normal limits. About 1 to 3 g. of potassium are excreted in the urine per day with a normal diet. In complete absence of potassium in the diet the kidney allows from 30 to 60 mEq. to escape daily in the urine. Conservation of potassium by renal tubules appears to require the presence of chloride. It has been shown that potassium chloride is more effective than alkaline salts of potassium in relieving potassium deficiency. A number of enzymes have been found to be dependent on potassium ions. During the synthesis of glycogen potassium migrates into the cells, and during glycogenolysis it is released. Less than ten per cent of the ingested potassium is excreted in the feces.

Chlorine is associated with potassium and sodium. The chloride ion readily crosses cell membranes and is found both within cells and in the extracellular fluid. It is an important element for the regulation of acid-base balance, and it helps to maintain the osmotic pressure relationships between the intracellular and extracellular fluids. Chloride is the principal anion in gastric juice, and it is an activator of salivary amylase. On the average about 90 per cent of ingested chloride is excreted in the urine, 4 per cent in perspiration and 1 per cent in feces.

Fluorine is a normal constituent of bone and teeth

and it functions in their development. It has been observed that in regions where the water contains 1 part per million or more of fluoride, the incidence of caries in the population is very low. For this reason it is recommended that drinking water contain 1 part per million of fluoride. There have been, and still are, vigorous objections to this practice as a public health measure for the control of dental caries. If excess fluoride is present in water, mottling occurs, especially in the permanent teeth of children at the time of eruption. Excess fluoride is excreted readily by the kidneys and sweat glands. Trace amounts of fluorine salts are present in most foods. Recent studies with highly refined methods have shown that fluorine may be essential for normal growth and development of both skeleton and soft tissues. The distribution of fluorides is such that there is very little likelihood of a deficiency occurring during normal growth.

Sulfur, as a constituent of the amino acids methionine, cysteine and cystine, is furnished almost entirely by dietary protein. It is metabolized to sulfate, which is in turn used in the formation of certain mucopolysaccharides (e.g., heparin) and in the esterification of a variety of phenols, including the estrogenic steroids, to facilitate their excretion in the urine. The sulfur of the vitamins biotin, thiamine and pantothenic acid, as well as that of methionine, represents the essential dietary requirement of this element.

Iron is a constituent of hemoglobin and of important enzymes such as catalase, peroxidase, the cytochromes and cytochrome oxidase, and the oxygen-carrying heme protein of muscle, myoglobin. The human body contains from 4 to 5 g. of iron; 2 to 3 g. in hemoglobin, 1 to 1.5 g. stored as ferritin and hemosiderin and the rest in myoglobin, respiratory enzymes and blood plasma. The body uses its iron supply efficiently. The iron that is released daily (20 mg.) by the breakdown of erythrocytes is used again in the formation of new hemoglobin.

Iron in plasma (about 100 μg. per dl.) is carried mainly as ferric iron by a specific iron-binding protein, transferrin, which can bind two atoms of Fe^{3+} per mole and is normally about 30 per cent saturated. Because nearly all the iron in plasma is protein bound, almost none is excreted by the kidney. A little iron is lost in the bile, and by the desquamation of cells of the gastrointestinal mucosa. The loss is only 1 to 2 mg. per day. There is no effective route of excretion of excess iron.

Iron in the food is converted in part into salts in the course of digestion, and ferric iron is reduced to some extent to the ferrous state by various agents in the food (e.g., ascorbic acid or glutathione). Acid conditions in the small intestine favor the absorption of iron; alkaline conditions, excess phosphate, oxalate, and phytates decrease the absorption of iron. Normally only about ten per cent of the dietary iron is absorbed.

Because iron is not readily excreted, its absorption from the gut is guarded. The passage of soluble iron through the intestinal cells into the plasma is thought to be mediated by a carrier system in which a protein resembling transferrin plays a part. When the carrier is loaded, it provokes the synthesis of a colorless protein, apoferritin, which combines with excess carrier iron in the form of ferric hydroxide to make the red iron storage protein ferritin. When iron is needed, the carrier system delivers it rapidly to the plasma. The concentration of carrier iron does not rise, and the synthesis of apoferritin and ferritin is not stimulated. It is not clear what signal directs the delivery of carrier iron to the plasma. It is thought by some that the intestinal store of ferritin iron may be drawn upon in case of need. Others think that it is not a ready store, and is lost when epithelial cells are desquamated.

Stores of ferritin are also found in the liver, spleen, and bone marrow. These play an active role in surrendering iron in time of need. Excess iron, which may accumulate after vigorous parenteral administration, large-scale destruction of red cells, or repeated transfusions, is found in many cells as dense particles of hemosiderin, thought to be made of many molecules of ferritin, with additional iron. These deposits may damage the cells in which they are laid down.

The requirement for iron varies with age, sex, and state of health. In adult males, the daily loss of 1 to 2 mg. is easily replaced, but in females of reproductive age the usual diet is barely adequate to cover the additional loss of iron in the menses, or the extra need imposed by pregnancy and lactation. Iron deficiency develops slowly. The stores are depleted, serum iron falls, transferrin may be only 12 per cent saturated, intestinal absorption of iron increases. Anemia is a late manifestation of iron deficiency. It has been reported that an early signal of a draft upon the iron stores is a change in concentration of serum *ferritin*. Minute amounts are present: in males, 123 μg. per liter, in females 56 μg per liter; in iron deficiency, as little as 12 μg. per liter. Ferritin in serum is estimated by radioimmunoassay. The early detection of iron deficiency in this way may prove immensely useful.

Copper is a component of the enzyme polyphenol oxidase (tyrosinase), which is necessary for melanin pigment formation. It is part of, or essential for, the action of uricase, the cytochromes and many oxidases. It is required for hemoglobin synthesis. In the blood, copper appears to be distributed fairly equally between cells and plasma. Essentially all of the copper of the red cell is bound to the protein erythrocuprein. About 95 per cent of the copper in the blood plasma is present in a copper protein, an α-2 globulin called ceruloplasmin, and the rest is loosely bound to albumin. Ceruloplasmin has a molecular weight of 151,000, has 0.34 per cent of copper and contains hexosamine, hexose and neuraminic acid. Its physiologic function is unknown, but it probably regulates the utilization of copper by releasing it to various tissues as needed, meanwhile maintaining a very low concentration of free copper in the body fluids. In a rare familial disorder of copper metabolism known as hepatolenticular degeneration (Wilson's disease) the concentration of ceruloplasmin is greatly reduced. The copper content of liver and brain is greatly increased, leading to severe liver damage and neurologic defects. About 2 mg. of copper is present in the average daily intake. It is poorly absorbed from the upper portion of the small intestine. Copper is stored in the liver as a protein-copper complex. It is excreted in the bile. Excessive amounts of copper are very toxic.

Copper is essential for the normal absorption and utilization of iron, and it is required in the reactions of cross-linking of the lysine side chains in elastin upon which the properties of that important protein depend. A deficiency of copper may be seen in infants receiving only milk, who exhibit a microcytic, normochromic anemia apparently due to poor absorption and utilization of iron. A fatal outcome of copper deficiency is not, however, avoided by correcting the deficiency of iron.

Iodine is a component of the thyroid hormone. Most of the iodine in the adult body is found in the thyroid gland. The concentration in thyroid tissue is about 2500 times as great as that in any other tissue. In absence of sufficient iodine the gland increases its secretory activity and becomes enlarged (simple or endemic goiter). Iodine (iodide) is absorbed from the small intestine. In the blood it is present as inorganic iodide and protein-bound iodine. It is taken up by the thyroid gland as iodide, concentrated and oxidized to iodine and incorporated into thyroglobulin.

The normal iodine content of the thyroid gland is about 40 mg. per 100 g. The distribution of iodine in foods varies markedly with soils and waters over the world. Seafoods and vegetables grown on iodine-rich soils are good sources of the element. Iodized common salt containing 0.01 per cent potassium iodide is highly recommended for use in regions in which goiter is endemic. The adult requirement is 0.15 to 0.30 mg. per day. Increased amounts are needed during puberty, pregnancy and lactation.

Zinc is present in many enzymes, including carbonic anhydrase, carboxypeptidase and alcohol dehydrogenase. It is essential for the proper growth and development of young animals. It is widely distributed in foods of both plant and animal origin. Although it is poorly absorbed from the intestine (most of the zinc is excreted in the feces), the requirement, 15 to 20 mg. per day, is easily met except when the diet is very high in cereals. Phytic acid prevents the absorption of zinc as well as of calcium and magnesium. Zinc deficiency in man causes poor growth and hypogonadism. In the rare autosomal recessive disorder, acrodermatitis enteropathica, there is a defect in the absorption of zinc, possibly due to chelation of the ion by unabsorbed oligopeptides. The disorder may be overcome by giving large doses of zinc, up to 150 mg. per day, by mouth. The value of treating other dermatoses with zinc is being studied. In long-term intravenous feeding, a zinc supplement may be necessary to maintain serum zinc at the normal concentration of 110 to 125 μg. per dl. A human adult may contain 2 to 3 g. of zinc. It is present in all tissues, in amounts varying from 10 mg. per g. wet weight to as much as 860 mg. per g. in normal prostate.

Manganese is found in all animal and plant tissue. It is considered an indispensable trace element because it is an activator of arginase, phosphatases, cholinesterase and many other enzymes of metabolic importance. In cells, it tends to be concentrated in the mitochondria, which may indicate its importance in aerobic energy production. The manganese ion can be substituted for magnesium in the activation of some enzymes. No deficiency syndrome has been detected in the human. The average American intake of manganese is about 6 to 8 mg. per day. It is poorly absorbed and is excreted mostly in the feces (only traces are found in the urine).

Cobalt is an essential component of vitamin B_{12}. It is found in many common foods, readily absorbed from the intestine and excreted in the urine. The requirement for the element is small, and very little is retained. Cobalt may be used for the formation of vitamin B_{12} by the rumen bacteria of cattle and sheep. No other requirement for cobalt in man is known. Parenterally administered cobalt salts induce polycythemia that is not connected with vitamin B_{12}. The mechanism of this effect is unknown.

Molybdenum is part of the structure of two flavoprotein enzymes: xanthine oxidase and aldehydeoxidase. Therefore it is considered an essential trace element. Molybdenum is present in legumes and cereals; liver, kidney and spleen contain fair amounts. No deficiency caused by molybdenum has been recognized. The human requirement for this element is not known.

Silicon, next to oxygen the most abundant of the elements, is present in minute amounts in most plant and animal tissues. It is now known that silicon deficiency in young animals causes poor growth and defects in skeletal development. The element is apparently essential for the formation and composition of mucopolysaccharides required as nuclei for the initiation of calcification. It is an integral component of the chondroitin-sulfate-protein complexes and of the mature collagen of connective tissue and articular cartilage. It is apparently exceedingly important for the structural integrity of connective tissue. Interest in silicon in the past has been mainly in the role of silica in silicosis; it has hitherto been regarded as an environmental contaminant rather than as an essential nutrient.

Selenium, a notably toxic element, has in the past been associated with diseases of cattle and sheep reared in districts where the soil is rich in selenium. In minute amounts it is an essential dietary factor affording protection against massive liver necrosis in rats on diets poor in sulfur-containing amino acids and high in fats or carbohydrates. Its action is enhanced by vitamin E, although their functions do not seem to be related. The manifestations of selenium deficiency vary widely in different species. Selenium is a constituent of the enzyme glutathione peroxidase, and it may therefore be important for normal metabolism of the red cell. It has also been found in a cytochrome b_5-like heme protein (M_r about 10,000) in extracts of heart and voluntary muscle of selenium-deficient lambs injected with selenium.

Chromium, in the trivalent form, is thought to facilitate glucose utilization. In chromium III deficiency the glucose tolerance of rats is significantly reduced, although there is no insulin deficiency.

Tin, nearly ubiquitous in foods and animal tissues, and long thought to be an environmental contaminant, has been shown to be essential for normal growth and development in the rat.

Vanadium is likewise essential for normal growth and development in the rat.

Nickel, an element of biologic interest because of its wide occurrence in plant and animal tissues, has now been shown to be required for normal organization and function of the liver in rats and chicks.

In summary, the important points about the mineral elements required for normal growth, development and function are (1) without exception, taken in excess, they are toxic; (2) it is difficult to become deficient in any of them except calcium, iodine and iron; (3) knowledge of their requirements in man at every stage of life is still incomplete; (4) for the trace elements, a concentration of 1 part per billion (as a requirement)

is still several trillion atoms per gram or several thousand per cell.

QUESTIONS IN BIOCHEMISTRY

REVIEW QUESTIONS

What are the principal constituents and the structural characteristics of the plasma membrane of cells?

A reaction, A $\rightleftarrows$ B has an equilibrium constant of 1.0 at 25 C. Another reaction, B $\rightleftarrows$ C has a K_{eq} of 0.01 at 25 C. If the two reactions are coupled, will A go appreciably to C?

What is $\Delta G°$ for the reaction A $\rightleftarrows$ B ($K_{eq} = 1.0$)?

Is the second reaction, B $\rightleftarrows$ C, exergonic or endergonic?

The concentration of H^+ ions in plasma is $4 \times 10^{-8}M$ and that in gastric juice is $2 \times 10^{-2}M$. Using the relation $\Delta G = 2.303RT \log C_2/C_1$ compute the energy required to move 1 mole of HCl from plasma to gastric juice at 37C. Is this process exergonic or endergonic?

What effect would a powerful inhibitor of carbonic anhydrase have (a) upon CO_2 transport in blood; (b) on renal regulation of pH?

Define an isoenzyme, and give an example of the clinical value of determining isoenzymes in blood.

In the hereditary disorders known as the lipidoses, what class of lipids is affected?

Describe the biochemical basis of the value of methotrexate and aminopterin in the chemotherapy of leukemia.

The brain has a very active turnover of RNA. How does it make the nucleotides required for RNA synthesis?

Phosphofructokinase (PFK) is a regulated enzyme. What is meant by that term? At what points in metabolic pathways are regulated enzymes usually found? Of the following, which are negative and which are positive effectors of PFK? ATP; P_i; citric acid; AMP; ADP; fatty acids.

What is the importance of Ca^{2+} in muscle?

The concentration of Ca^{2+} in muscle is about 1 mg. per 100 g. wet weight. How does the concentration of Ca^{2+} in muscle water (assuming uniform distribution) compare with the concentration of calcium in plasma?

Fluoride ion (0.001 M) inhibits the enzyme enolase. What sources of energy for muscular contraction are interdicted by this poison, and what sources are still available (a) during anaerobiosis; (b) in the presence of oxygen?

Under what circumstances would you expect to find a constraint upon the action of isocitric dehydrogenase in liver? What important biosynthetic process would be favored?

An enzyme such as the transaminases requires pyridoxal phosphate as coenzyme. What would be the effect on an individual's requirement for vitamin B_6 if, because of a mutation, the equilibrium constant for the reaction:

apoenzyme + pyridoxal phosphate $\rightleftharpoons$ holoenzyme

changed from 10^6 to 10^2?

In the reaction scheme:

$$A \rightleftharpoons B \rightleftharpoons C \rightleftharpoons D \rightleftharpoons E \rightleftharpoons F \rightleftharpoons G$$
$$\Updownarrow$$
$$H$$

at which step would you expect the pathway leading to G to be regulated?

Both ATP and GTP are required in protein synthesis. Describe the respective processes in which they take part.

Suppose that an amino acid was altered chemically after it had been incorporated into its proper tRNA. Would the altered aminoacyl-tRNA be utilized? Why?

An enzyme is found to have broad specificity for a certain group of phosphate esters. Its Km for ester A is 10^{-7}; its Km for ester B is 10^{-3}. If A and B are present together at a concentration of 10^{-5} M, which will be utilized more rapidly?

What is the source of hydrogen for the reductive step of fatty acid biosynthesis?

Name two important oxidative enzymes supporting fatty acid biosynthesis.

If an inhibitor of lactic dehydrogenase is present, what becomes the limiting factor in anaerobic glycolysis?

An individual producing urine of maximal acidity (pH 4.5) is excreting an organic acid of pK = 4.5. What is the degree of neutralization of the acid in the urine being secreted? What cations are available for this?

An individual in a state of partially compensated metabolic acidosis has a plasma [Total CO_2] of 15 mM. per liter. If his blood pH is 7.34, you would expect the pCO_2 to be (normal; higher than normal; lower than normal).

What is the reasonable basis for classifying 1,25,-dihydroxycholecalciferol as a hormone?

Thiamine deficiency is readily associated with a defect in the utilization of pyruvate. Why should one also think of a possible defect in the metabolism of the branched-chain amino acids and in the pentose phosphate pathway?

On a diet entirely free of stearic acid an individual will nevertheless deposit this C-18 saturated fatty acid as a constituent of his depot fat. How is this done, and where does it take place?

In an in vitro experiment with normal mitochondria a substrate is found to yield a P/O ratio of 2. Name a likely substrate. Suggest a likely coenzyme for its oxidation.

List three ways in which the kidney accomplishes the excretion of hydrogen ions.

Name a divalent cation indispensable in blood coagulation.

Which one of the following proteins is not made in the liver? albumin; very low density lipoprotein; IgG; fibrinogen.

What is the significance of the appearance in urine of a high concentration of small peptides containing hydroxyproline?

The hydrolysis of a peptide bond has a $\Delta G°$ of about -500 calories per mole at pH 7. What is the significance of the requirement of 4 ATP for the biosynthesis of a peptide bond in a protein?

What advantage is gained for a liver or a muscle cell in employing an enzyme such as glycogen phosphorylase rather than amylase, as the digestive tract does?

Outline a nonoxidative pathway for the production of ribose from glucose.

In what two important biosyntheses is phosphoribosylpyrophosphate involved?

Show how galactose, fructose or mannose can arise from glucose in the human organism.

Where does the enzymatic defect lie in galactosemia?

A female infant exhibits signs of masculinization of the genitalia, hypertension and a very marked increase in urinary 17-ketosteroids, together with a negligible output of tetrahydrocortisol. What biochemical lesion is most likely present?

What are the two sources of nitrogen in the hepatic biosynthesis of urea?

Name two kinds of reaction of activation of substrates or groups involving nucleoside triphosphates other than ATP.

A man encounters a bull unexpectedly in a field. He runs 50 yards, climbs a 6-foot fence and escapes the bull. For some minutes he breathes fast and deeply and has a high pulse rate. Account for all the phenomena in biochemical terms, indicating what your findings would be on analysis of blood samples taken (1) immediately after the escape and (b) 20 minutes later.

Account in biochemical terms for the fact that rigor sets in most quickly following a violent death immediately after extreme physical effort.

What tentative conclusions would you draw from a laboratory report indicating that a sample of a patient's blood showed increased creatine phosphokinase, glutamic-oxaloacetic transaminase and H_4 isozyme of lactic dehydrogenase?

What is the significance of the term "closely coupled oxidative phosphorylation? With what cell organelle do you associate this process?

Name the two anterior pituitary hormones that are simple proteins.

Describe three modes of regulation of an enzymatic pathway.

What physical signal controls the secretion rate of antidiuretic hormone?

Such a signal cannot be expected in hemorrhage, yet there is a powerful stimulus to the secretion of ADH. Why?

Which of the plasma proteins is most effective in determining the osmotic pressure of the plasma? Why?

What would be the consequences of a biochemical lesion involving loss of the enzyme in liver that cleaves argininosuccinate? Would this necessarily be an incapacitating lesion?

In general terms, what are the conditions promoting, or inhibiting, the operation of the tricarboxylic acid cycle?

What is the component of the respiratory pathway that acts as a "transformer" from the hydrogen-transfer sector to the electron-transfer sector of the pathway?

In fasting man, what plasma amino acids show the greatest increase in concentration and leave muscle in the greatest amount?

What is ceramide? Name two classes of compound based on it as a constituent.

Give an example of an inducible enzyme and summarize the current idea of the mechanism of induction.

In the reaction, fumarate $\rightleftharpoons$ malate, maleic acid, the geometric isomer of fumarate, acts as a competitive inhibitor. What is meant by that term? What effect does a competitive inhibitor of an enzyme have on V_{max}? on K_m?

A high intracellular concentration of fatty acids has a powerful negative effect on phosphofructokinase. Explain what part this might play in the phenomenon of "starvation diabetes."

Describe the process by which the triacylglycerol of chylomicra becomes triacylglycerol in the adipose tissue cell.

What would be the consequences of a serious reduction in plasma albumin on the mobilization of fat in the fasting organism?

What is the effect of a marked degree of anemia on the buffer capacity of true plasma?

Name two phosphatases indispensable for the delivery of newly formed glucose to the blood by the liver of the fasting subject.

How can muscle glycogen be a source of blood glucose?

Define the processes of transcription and translation as they are applied to protein biosynthesis.

What critical role does methionine play in protein synthesis in both prokaryotes and eukaryotes?

What are the precursors of the prostaglandins?

Discuss the proposition: Lactose is a disaccharide unique to the postpartum female mammal.

In an enzyme system, what is meant by control by product inhibition? Give an example.

How can the product of an enzyme system regulate not just the activity but the total amount of the enzymes of the system?

In mitochondria, which is the more selective of the two investing membranes? With which membrane is the respiratory pathway associated?

What is the distinguishing functional characteristic of the rough endoplasmic reticulum?

What are the consequences of a defect in the production of blood platelets?

What factor or factors are critical for platelet aggregation?

An increase in the dietary polyunsaturated fatty acids might require an increase in the intake of what vitamin?

Identify opsin by nature and function. With what vitamin derivative is it associated?

Among the following, identify the basic peptides; the neutral peptides; the acidic peptides:

1. Phe-Ser-Tyr-Leu-Leu-Pro-Gly
2. Glu-Glu-Glu
3. Ala-Pro-Gly-Ser-Met-Lys-Phe
4. Arg-Arg-Glu-Phe-Ser-Pro-NH$_2$
5. Gly-Glu-Pro-Gly-HOPro-Leu-Gly-Lys-Pro

From what important protein might peptide (5) above be derived?

A patient with glycogen storage disease is discovered to have muscle glycogen with very short outer chains. What is the nature of the defect?

What is the activated form of glucose that takes part in glycogen synthesis?

What is the distinction between glycogen synthase I and D?

Define phosphatidic acid. Of what lipids can it be a precursor?

What are the acidic ionizing groups of proteins? At what pH are they essentially completely dissociated? Do they buffer effectively at pH 7.4?

In the reaction, glucose 6-phosphate $\rightleftharpoons$ glucose 1-phosphate, equilibrium is attained at 94 per cent G

6-P, 6 per cent G 1-P. In which direction is the reaction exergonic?

In general, what is the pH optimum of the enzymes contained in lysosomes? What is the function of lysosomes?

3-Hydroxy-3-methylglutarylCoA is the precursor of what two important substances in lipid metabolism?

How is acetoacetate taken up and utilized by muscle?

Why is the storage of fat in adipose tissue dependent upon the ability of the tissue to take up glucose?

What is the sole metabolic effect of norepinephrine?

What is required for the occurrence of polyribosomes?

Of the plasma lipoproteins, which are the main transporters of triacylglycerols?

What is the function of 2,3-diphosphoglycerate in the red cells?

What is meant by the statement that choline is a lipotropic substance?

If a substrate, on combination with an enzyme, increases its K_m, is it acting as a positive or a negative effector?

Can the normal substrate of an enzyme be itself an allosteric effector?

What is meant by the cooperative effect in the association of oxygen and hemoglobin?

How many atoms of oxygen must be used to provide the energy for the synthesis of 1 mole of urea?

What is a carbohydrate chemically? What general chemical and physical properties distinguish a sugar from a polysaccharide?

Write the pyranose-ring structure of glucose and indicate which carbon atoms are asymmetric.

Explain briefly what basis is used for classifying the monosaccharides into the D series and the L series.

Write the Haworth cyclic-type formula for glucose and galactose. At what numbered carbon atom does the arrangement of the H and OH differ? Why do these sugars form different osazones?

Why does sucrose not have reducing properties?

Name a compound among the carbohydrates that fits the specifications in each of the following groups: (a) a ketohexose, (b) a disaccharide that will *not* undergo mutarotation, (c) a sugar containing an amino group attached to the number 2 carbon atom of the hexose.

Give the hydrolysis products of each of the following disaccharides: lactose, maltose and sucrose.

What is a glycoside? Distinguish between glycoside and glucoside.

Glucose and mannose are epimers. Explain why.

Ribose and ribulose are isomers. How do they differ structurally?

What is starch? Name and discuss the properties of the two components that make up starch. What reducing sugar is produced by the action of salivary amylase on boiled starch?

What is glycogen? What color does a dilute solution of iodine give with glycogen? amylopectin?

Compare the properties and the structure of starch, glycogen and cellulose.

Name the polyglucoside that consists mostly of 1,6-glucoside chains with occasional 1,4-glucoside branches. What useful application does it have?

What are the general structural characteristics of the uronic acids? Why do they have reducing properties? Name two uronic acids and state where they occur in nature.

What is the difference between an aldonic and a saccharic acid?

Name the end-product of the acid hydrolysis of glycogen.

What is the difference between a homopolysaccharide and a heteropolysaccharide? Give an example of each group.

Name the major classes of lipids.

What is the chemical composition of a fat?

Distinguish between a fat and a wax.

Distinguish between a simple and a mixed triglyceride.

What is saponification of a fat? What conclusions can be drawn from the saponification number of a fat?

How does the iodine number of lard compare with that of linseed oil?

Discuss the factors that make a fat rancid.

To what class of chemical compounds does glycerol belong?

What is a phospholipid?

What products are obtained on complete hydrolysis of lecithins?

How is lysolecithin produced? Name an important property of this substance.

How do cephalins differ from the lecithins?

What type of chemical compound is sphingosine?

Name the hydrolysis products of the cerebrosides. Name two important cerebrosides.

What is the structural feature common to all the steroids?

Write the structural formula for cholesterol, indicating the numbering of the carbon atoms.

Why is 7-dehydrocholesterol an important compound?

In what forms is cholesterol present in the blood?

Name the four groups of steroid hormones. Which steroid hormones have no side chain attached to carbon 17?

What steroid hormones are derivatives of pregnane?

What are the structural features of the adrenocortical hormones?

What is the influence of the presence of an oxygen atom on carbon 11 of an adrenocortical steroid on the physiological effects of the compound?

What changes accompany overproduction of aldosterone?

Name the principal bile acids. From what compound are they produced in the liver? To what substances are these compounds conjugated?

What is another name for sialic acid?

What is the difference in ring A in estrone as compared to ring A in androsterone?

What chemical elements are found in protein? What units are used to build up the complex protein molecule?

Outline the generally accepted classification of proteins.

What properties distinguish an albumin from a globulin?

Nutritionally, what is a complete protein? Name the essential amino acids. What types of food are particularly good sources of these amino acids?

Discuss the modern concepts of the structure of the protein molecule.

Discuss the changes that occur when a native protein is denatured.

Classify the α-amino acids that are found in proteins.

Describe two color tests for the detection of protein.

Into what class of proteins do we place nucleoproteins?

Where do nucleoproteins occur in the animal body?

What units make up the structure of nucleic acid? Discuss the two types of nucleic acid that have been isolated.

Give the structural formulas for purine and pyrimidine; for the two purine bases with their common names.

Name the principal pyrimidines that occur in nucleic acid. Which one occurs only in ribonucleic acid? Which one occurs only in deoxyribonucleic acid?

What are the components of a nucleotide and how are they linked together? How are the nucleotides linked together in nucleic acid?

What is a nucleoside? Name the nucleosides obtained from nucleotides of ribonucleic acid.

Show the chemical relationship of hypoxanthine, xanthine and uric acid.

A protein is in a solution at pH greater than its isoelectric point. To what pole will the protein migrate on passage of an electric current through the solution?

At what pH in relation to the isoelectric point would a protein bind heavy metals?

In what native protein do we find hydroxylysine?

What types of protein are highly resistant to proteolytic enzymes?

2,6,8-Trioxypurine is known by what common name?

What amino acid contains a disulfide?

What is the important function of deoxyribonucleic acid in the cell nuclei?

Name the types of ribonucleic acids and give their function.

List the vitamins that are insoluble in water but soluble in fat solvents.

Under what conditions in the intestine would the absorption of vitamin A be decreased?

What is the chemical relation of vitamin A to β-carotene? Compare the two with respect to their occurrence in nature.

What symptoms have been observed and associated with a vitamin A deficiency?

Why is carotene often called provitamin A?

Under what conditions can vitamin A and carotene be destroyed?

What are the sources of vitamin D_2 and vitamin D_3?

Since natural foods are poor sources of vitamin D, how can the needs of children for this vitamin be provided?

What are the known functions of vitamin D? When vitamin D is given to a rachitic infant, the amount of inorganic phosphorus in the urine is reduced. How is this change brought about by the vitamin?

What symptoms are observed with an overdosage of vitamin D?

What vitamin is concerned with the synthesis of prothrombin in the liver?

What fat-soluble vitamin protects against the destruction of vitamin A by oxidation?

Under what conditions is vitamin K deficiency observed clinically? How is menadione related to this vitamin?

What are good sources of the tocopherols?

Name the important members of the B complex of vitamins. Designate those that are components of one or more coenzymes. Name those that have antianemic properties.

What is the function of the pyrophosphoric acid ester of thiamine?

What factors increase the normal human requirements for thiamine?

Discuss the deficiency symptoms that may be present with a lack of thiamine.

What needs of the human increase the daily requirement for riboflavin?

What foods are the best sources of riboflavin?

Describe the two coenzymes in which niacinamide functions as a component. What acute condition is cured by niacin?

Discuss the relation of niacin and tryptophan in the treatment and prevention of pellagra. Explain why milk, relatively low in niacin, helps the patient with this deficiency condition.

Discuss the foods of animal and plant origin that are good sources of niacin.

Discuss an important function of pyridoxal phosphate.

What are the best food sources of vitamin B_6?

Discuss the importance of the coenzyme in which pantothenic acid is one of the components.

What are the functions of biotin?

What clinical conditions are relieved by the administration of folic acid? What enzyme is required for the hydrolysis of the pteroylglutamic acid isolated from yeast? What are the hydrolysis products?

What unusual chemical element is present in vitamin B_{12}? What is needed for the proper absorption of this vitamin from the intestine?

Discuss probable roles of vitamin C in the body. What organ contains the highest concentration of this vitamin? Discuss the requirements and the best food sources to supply the needs of the body.

Where in the body is β-carotene converted to vitamin A?

To which class of proteins does keratin belong?

Where is keratin formed in the human body?

Name the three principal solids in the organic matrix of cartilage.

What is collagen? Where does it occur? How is gelatin obtained from collagen?

Which albuminoid is predominant in yellow connective tissue?

What is the role of phosphoric acid in the contraction of muscle?

Give the values for the composition of muscle (water, protein, lipid, ash and carbohydrate).

Distinguish between myosin and actomyosin.

Distinguish between G actin and F actin.

What types of lipids are present in nervous tissue?

What is the function of acetylcholine? What is the action of acetylcholinesterase on acetylcholine? Where does cholinesterase occur in the body?

What is the function of secretin? What is the function of cholecystokinin?

What is the relation of proinsulin to insulin?

What type of compound is glucagon?

Tabulate the hormones secreted by the thyroid gland. What are their effects on tissue metabolism?

What is thyroglobulin?

What is the function of the parathyroid hormone? What symptoms can be relieved by administration of this hormone?

What is the function of calcitonin?

Discuss the hormones secreted by the adrenal medulla.

Discuss the nature and the properties of the adrenocorticotropic hormone (ACTH). Give the principal physiologic and chemical effects observed on administration of this hormone.

List the hormones that have been isolated from the anterior lobe of the pituitary gland. State their functions.

Differentiate the physiologic effects of oxytocin and vasopressin.

What are the principal functions of blood?

Discuss in detail the chemistry of hemoglobin. What is heme? What is hemin? What use is made of the hemin test?

What is the valence of iron in carbon monoxide hemoglobin? in hemin? in methemoglobin?

Which chemical substances act on hemoglobin to give methemoglobin? What is the percentage of iron in hemoglobin?

What is the source of the bile pigments? What happens to the iron when the red blood cell is disintegrated in the liver? What is the relationship of biliverdin to bilirubin?

Describe in a general way the chemical composition of blood plasma. How does the composition of blood plasma differ from that of serum?

Outline the steps in the coagulation of blood.

What is the function of the liver in the coagulation of blood?

Contrast the effects of heparin and vitamin K on the processes involved in the coagulation of blood.

Discuss the proteins that are present in blood serum. How do we characterize the lipoproteins?

Name the compounds that contribute to the synthesis of porphobilinogen.

What type of protein is transferrin?

What is the normal range for serum calcium? What factors would lower the serum calcium?

Compare the normal concentration of inorganic phosphorus in the serum of a child with that in the adult.

Under what clinical conditions do we observe a high blood cholesterol?

Discuss a representative curve that would be obtained from the glucose tolerance test on a person showing no abnormality in the metabolism of glucose.

Comment briefly on the following blood constituents: uric acid, fibrinogen, serum amylase, carbonic anhydrase, plasma bicarbonate, alkaline phosphatase and serum transaminase.

Give a number (in mg. per dl.) falling within the normal range for the following blood serum constituents: urea nitrogen; creatinine; calcium; total cholesterol; albumin (in g. per dl.) and protein-bound iodine (in ug. per dl.).

What are considered to be the ranges of hemoglobin concentration in the blood of normal adult men and women?

Define these terms: enzyme, apoenzyme, coenzyme, substrate, antienzyme, kinase, proenzyme and endoenzyme. Name three proenzymes secreted into the alimentary tract.

Discuss the stereochemical specificity of enzymes.

Name the divisions in which enzymes can be broadly classified.

Describe briefly the occurrence of one enzyme of each of the following classes: 1) hydrolase; 2) oxidase.

Name the enzymes (common names), their substrates and their hydrolysis products of the following classes: an amidase, and a deaminase.

Name two enzymes that are known to contain copper.

Distinguish between the action of catalase and peroxidases.

What is the importance of superoxide dismutase?

Name three proteolytic enzymes and state their function.

State important factors that influence enzyme action.

Hexokinase is a transferring enzyme. Which substance is transferred in the reaction catalyzed by the enzyme?

What is the function of salivary amylase? What inorganic anion acts as an activator?

What is pepsinogen?

What enzymes are secreted by the pancreas?

Discuss the part that bile plays in the digestion of food. What is the pH of bile?

Name the bile salts. What is the function of the bile salts?

What is the origin of urobilinogen? stercobilin? urobilin?

What metal ions are removed from the blood by the liver and excreted in the bile?

What is the principal constituent of most biliary calculi?

Which digestive enzymes in the alimentary tract participate in the hydrolysis of starch?

To what extent does the absence of bile from the intestinal tract influence digestion and absorption? By what changes in physical appearance and chemical composition of the feces would such an absence of bile be manifested?

What may be determined from a chemical analysis of gastric juice?

Discuss the absorption of the products of digestion.

Discuss the mechanisms of fat absorption. By what path is the major part of neutral fat able to reach the blood?

How are the amino acids absorbed? What happens to the rate of absorption of glucose, fructose and galactose when phosphorylation is prevented? How can this be accomplished?

Discuss the mechanisms by which the content of glucose in the blood of a healthy individual is maintained at an approximately constant level.

The enzymes hexokinase, phosphoglucomutase, phosphatase, cocarboxylase and phosphorylase are concerned in carbohydrate metabolism. Explain briefly the role of each.

In what organs in the body do we find a store of glycogen?

Define gluconeogenesis; glycogenolysis; glycolysis.

Write the structural formulas for glucose 1-phosphate and fructose 1,6-diphosphate. Name the enzyme and the compound with which fructose 6-phosphate reacts to form the diphosphate.

Why is the conversion of glycogen to glucose limited to the liver and the kidney?

Discuss the breakdown of glycogen to lactic acid in muscle. What is the fate of this lactic acid?

Discuss some hormonal influences on the blood sugar level.

Define the terms: exergonic reaction; endergonic reaction. Which type of reaction is the phosphorylation of glucose?

Under what conditions does glycosuria occur?

What is the reaction catalyzed by aldolase?

What is the end product of glycolysis?

What are the steps in the oxidation of pyruvate? How is citric acid formed? What happens to the citric acid? What products are liberated and what product is consumed in the cycle?

Discuss the conversion of galactose 1-phosphate to glucose 1-phosphate.

Discuss the dynamic state of lipids in the fat depots.

Outline the steps in the oxidation of fatty acids in the body.

Describe the conditions under which ketone bodies are formed in excess. Define "ketosis." What produces ketonuria? What amino acids are ketogenic?

Discuss the absorption and the metabolism of cholesterol. What foods are relatively high in cholesterol? How much cholesterol can be synthesized in a day by the normal adult?

What are the end-products of the oxidation of fat in the body?

Proteins are needed for the regulation of many vital body functions. Name four such functions.

What is the principal nitrogenous end-product of protein metabolism in man?

How is urea synthesized in the body from the ammonia formed by deamination of the amino acids? In what organ does this occur? How is the metabolism of urea affected by severe hepatic disease? Outline the steps in the urea cycle. What happens in animals that lack arginase?

Define and illustrate transamination. What amino acids are very active in transamination?

What is the fate of amino acids absorbed from the intestine? How may these acids enter the citric acid cycle? Define deamination; nitrogen equilibrium. What is meant by negative nitrogen balance? positive nitrogen balance? Under what conditions do we see these states in clinical medicine?

Name three compounds that occur in the body for which glycine is needed for synthesis.

What amino acids may be used in the body for the synthesis of purines?

What are the hydrolysis products of arginine?

In what proteins do we find hydroxylysine?

What amino acids contain sulfur? Name three important compounds in the body whose methyl group may be obtained from methionine. Describe the mechanism whereby methylation from methionine is accomplished.

What metabolic disorder is caused by the inability of an infant to convert phenylalanine into tyrosine? Outline the steps in the normal metabolism of tyrosine.

What is the relation of tryptophan to serotonin?

Where does creatine occur in the body? What amino acids are used in the synthesis of creatine? What is the relation of creatine to creatinine?

Write the structural formula of uric acid. What compound is formed from adenine in the presence of adenase? From guanine in the presence of guanase? What enzyme is required for the oxidation of these compounds to uric acid?

Discuss the normal metabolism of the pyrimidines. What substances are used by the body for the synthesis of purines and pyrimidines?

About 1.5 per cent of the body is calcium. Discuss the distribution of calcium in the body.

Name the important cations and anions that occur in body fluids. Discuss the distribution of these elements in the blood plasma, in the erythrocytes and in the intracellular fluids.

List the factors that influence the absorption of calcium from the intestine.

Discuss clinical conditions associated with a deficiency of calcium in the diet.

What is the source of fecal calcium? What hormones regulate the blood serum calcium? What are the sources of calcium if the level is below normal?

Almost all the calcium and the phosphorus is found in bone and teeth. Name three other important functions of calcium. Name three other functions of phosphorus. Which factors affect the utilization of these minerals?

Discuss the absorption of phosphorus from the intestine. What influence do vitamin D and the parathyroid hormone have on the reabsorption of phosphate by the renal tubule?

Discuss the distribution of magnesium in the various compartments of the body.

Discuss the needs for sodium chloride in the body fluids.

Discuss the seriousness of hyperpotassemia. Under what clinical conditions may potassium deficiency be present?

Since there is no effective route for the excretion of excess iron, discuss the manner in which the body is guarded against absorption of excessive amounts of iron. What is ferritin? What is hemosiderin?

Discuss the needs of the body for copper. What is ceruloplasmin?

In what form is iodine present in the blood? What foods are good sources of iodine?

Enumerate four trace elements and give one site in the body where they occur or are used.

What are the daily requirements of the body for water? Name the various ways that the body may lose water, giving the approximate amounts lost in each case.

Enumerate the common clinical conditions in which abnormal losses of water are important factors.

Give the caloric values of 1 g. of carbohydrate; 1 g. of fat; 1 g. of protein.

Define or explain: respiratory quotient; specific dynamic action of food; direct calorimetry; indirect calorimetry.

What factors affect the total heat production of an individual?

Describe the conditions and the factors to be considered in the determination of the basal metabolism. Define basal metabolic rate.

What is assumed in the commonly used clinical procedure for the determination of basal metabolic rate that allows us to neglect the measurement of the amount of carbon dioxide produced during the period and measure only the oxygen consumed?

Under what clinical conditions is the basal metabolic rate subnormal?

Outline the principal chemical changes that occur in the venous blood when it comes into equilibrium with the alveolar air in the lung. Why is there a small change in the volume of the erythrocyte?

How is oxygen transported in the blood to the tissue?

In what forms is carbon dioxide carried in the blood? Explain two ways in which hemoglobin aids in its transport.

What factors cause an increase in the rate and the depth of respiration? What factors cause a decrease?

Define or explain: chloride shift; carbon dioxide tension of blood; isohydric carbon dioxide transport; carbaminohemoglobin; Bohr effect.

What is the importance of carbonic anhydrase in the erythrocyte?

Define or explain: acidosis, alkalosis, alkali reserve.

When does metabolic alkalosis occur? What conditions induce respiratory acidosis?

When there is metabolic acidosis or metabolic alkalosis, determination of the total carbon dioxide content of plasma or serum is usually sufficient to tell the clinician the acid-base condition of the patient. With respiratory acidosis or respiratory alkalosis, it is necessary to determine the blood pH as well as the total carbon dioxide content. Explain why.

What changes would you expect in the urinary pH under the following conditions: (a) after persistent vomiting; (b) after vigorous overbreathing; (c) after eating a very high protein diet; (d) after eating a low protein diet and large amounts of orange juice; and (e) after taking sodium bicarbonate?

How does the kidney help in the acid-base regulation of the body?

What is the origin of the ammonia excreted in the urine. What factors increase ammonia production?

Summarize the factors that work toward keeping the blood pH within such narrow limits.

In severe liver disease, blood urea falls and blood amino acids rise. Explain.

Describe and explain the van den Bergh tests for bilirubin in blood serum.

Discuss the composition of cerebrospinal fluid, comparing the concentration of the constituents with their concentration in blood plasma. What is the concentration of protein in normal fluid? Describe the Pandy test.

How does the protein concentration in lymph vary with the site of origin of the fluid? Compare its protein concentration with that of blood plasma.

In a 24 hour urine specimen name (a) the principal nitrogen-containing compound that is present and (b) the organic compound containing nitrogen that is excreted in constant amounts from day to day. Discuss the sources of uric acid in the urine.

Discuss the origin and the significance of acetone bodies in the urine.

Compare the composition of cow's milk and human milk in regard to the concentrations of water, protein, lactose, fat and ash.

Pasteurized cow's milk is deficient in what vitamins and minerals?

Milk contains all required amino acids in adequate amounts. Although it contains little niacin (or niacinamide) no deficiency of this vitamin occurs in those using large amounts of milk with insufficient amounts of other protein of high biologic value. Explain how this is possible.

What is colostrum? Compare its chemical and physical properties with those of milk.

What is considered a safe protein allowance per kilogram of body weight for an adult man or woman? Should this allowance be increased with muscular activity? Why is it recommended that animal protein should supply half of the total protein intake?

Why should the adolescent girl require more protein, calcium, iron, ascorbic acid and total calories than a mature woman?

What classes of individuals require special consideration in reference to their vitamin D intake?

Why are fats required in the diet? In what foods do we find significant amounts of polyunsaturated fatty acids?

How do we obtain adequate amounts of sulfur in the diet? How can we make sure that the iodine intake is adequate?

What groups of foods should be considered with the patient in planning an adequate diet?

MULTIPLE CHOICE QUESTIONS

Answers to multiple choice questions are found at the end of this chapter. There is one best answer to the following questions.

1. A drug of some value in studying prostaglandins is:
   (a) phenobarbital
   (b) aspirin
   (c) caffeine
   (d) morphine
   (e) phenolphthalein
2. The following values for a group of serum electrolytes fall within the normal range EXCEPT (values in Meq/liter):
   (a) $Na^+ = 100$
   (b) $HCO_3^- = 25$
   (c) $Cl^- = 110$
   (d) $K^+ = 4$
   (e) $Ca^{2+} = 5$

3. In the absence of dietary copper, there is a deficiency of plasma:
   (a) haptoglobin
   (b) ceruloplasmin
   (c) thyroxine-binding globulin
   (d) transferrin
   (e) prothrombin
4. A plasma albumin concentration of less than 2 g. per liter would affect specifically the transport of:
   (a) glucose
   (b) iron
   (c) bilirubin
   (d) creatine
   (e) cholesterol
5. An enzyme of importance in maintaining hemoglobin iron in the ferrous state is:
   (a) glucokinase
   (b) glutathione reductase
   (c) enolase
   (d) aldolase
   (e) phosphoglyceraldehyde dehydrogenase

In the following questions, answer:
(a) if 1, 2, and 3 are correct;
(b) if 1 and 3 are correct;
(c) if 2 and 4 are correct;
(d) if 4 only is correct;
(e) if all are correct.

6. The tricarboxylic acid cycle requires:
   (1) an activated substrate
   (2) NAD^+
   (3) a flavoprotein
   (4) GDP

7. The fatty acid oxidation system requires:
   (1) FAD
   (2) NAD^+
   (3) HSCoA
   (4) an activated substrate
8. Immediate precursors of ATP in glycolysis include:
   (1) fructose-6-phosphate
   (2) phosphoenolpyruvate
   (3) 3-phosphoglycerate
   (4) phosphoglycerylphosphate
9. Ionizing groups of proteins include:
   (1) terminal carboxyl
   (2) serine hydroxyl
   (3) γ-carboxyl of glutamate
   (4) asparagine amide

Match the appropriate hormone to the following chemical signals in the plasma:
10. aldosterone   (a) rise in glucose
11. testosterone   (b) fall in Na^+
12. glucagon   (c) rise in Ca^{2+}
13. insulin   (d) moderate fall in glucose
14. calcitonin   (e) rise in luteinizing hormone

ANSWERS TO MULTIPLE CHOICE QUESTIONS

1. (b)	**5.** (b)	**9.** (b)	**13.** (a)
2. (a)	**6.** (e)	**10.** (b)	**14.** (c)
3. (b)	**7.** (e)	**11.** (e)	
4. (c)	**8.** (c)	**12.** (d)	

5

General Microbiology and Immunology

CALDERON HOWE, M.D.*

Professor and Head, Department of Microbiology and Immunology,
Louisiana State University Medical Center, New Orleans, Louisiana

THE MICROORGANISMS

Microorganisms (not including viruses) are found in the heterogeneous group first designated as the Kingdom Protista by Haeckel in 1866. This included all unicellular or coenocytic organisms and some primitive algae and fungi, any single cell of which is undifferented, i.e., can reproduce the entire species autonomously and asexually: bacteria, protozoa, some fungi and all blue-green algae, the last being of no known medical importance. Viruses are now included, though they were unknown before 1892 when tobacco mosaic virus was discovered by Iwanowski.

Bacteria and the medically negligible blue-green algae are together often called lower protists. They constitute a separate kingdom at one time called Monera;

* With the invaluable collaboration of the following members of the Basic Sciences Faculty: Bettie M. Catchings, Ph.D., Jane E. Deas, Ph.D., Michael L. Murray, Ph.D., Richard J. O'Callaghan, Ph.D., and Lawrence A. Wilson, Ph.D.

more recently, Procaryotae. They are distinguished from *all other forms of life* by their *procaryotic structure,* i.e., their nuclear material *(nucleoid)* is not enclosed in a nuclear membrane; the cytoplasm contains chiefly ribosomes and certain membrane-associated structures called mesosomes suggestive of primitive endoplasmic reticulum. They are generally spoken of as procaryotes. The cells of all other organisms, including humans, are said to be eucaryotic, i.e., their nucleus is enclosed in a perforate nuclear membrane, and the cytoplasm contains numerous organelles, including ribosomes (protein synthesis); mitochondria (mediate energy transfer); chloroplasts (photosynthesis in green plants); endoplasmic reticulum (energy transfer and other enzymic functions); lysosomes; Golgi bodies; microtubules. Eucaryotic protists are often called higher protists. Unlike viruses, *all* protists contain both DNA and RNA. Viruses may contain either, never both.

As between the two groups of procaryotes, all blue-green algae are photosynthetic and contain chlorophyll

a. No bacteria of any kind contain chlorophyll a. Therefore all bacteria may be succinctly defined as procaryotes without chlorophyll a. Bacteria have traditionally been assigned to the plant kingdom as fission fungi (Class Schizomycetes) and are still often so called.

Classification of Bacteria (Procaryotes)

At present the classification of bacteria has no phylogenetic basis and is therefore entirely artificial and arbitrary. So-called classifications are at present chiefly keys for identification. Bacteria are still classified primarily on the basis of morphology, secondarily on various physiologic properties such as pigment, spore formation, staining reactions, motility and enzyme equipment (e.g., aerobic or anaerobic, proteolytic, fermentative). Immunologic properties (antigenic structure) and susceptibility to highly specific phages are also used in differentiation and identification.

All medically significant species of bacteria are chemosynthetic and heterotrophic (chemoorganotrophs; see Bacterial Metabolism) having diameters typically <5 μm. (usually 1 to 2 μm., and less in *Rickettsia* and *Chlamydia*). Unlike viruses, all except rickettsia and chlamydia and two or three other species of pathogenic bacteria, e.g., syphilis spirochetes and leprosy bacilli, are cultivable in *inanimate* media. Viruses, rickettsia and chlamydia can multiply only in living cells (cell and tissue cultures, etc.). All bacteria have cell walls of peptidoglycan or murein that contain muramic acid, a substance unique to the procaryotes. Medically significant bacteria occur in six orders as follows:

1. **Order Pseudomonadales:** Family Pseudomonadaceae: gram-negative rods (one genus, *Spirillum,* is helical but *not flexible;* see Spirochetes); grow in simple peptone media at 10° to 40° C; generally motile with *polar* flagella; strictly aerobic. Some produce blue pyocyanin, yellow fluorescent pigment or both. Representatives: *Pseudomonas aeruginosa, P. pseudomallei*

2. **Order Eubacteriales:** ("true bacteria"): gram-positive or gram-negative rods or cocci, no helical forms; motile species have *peritrichous* flagella; aerobic, facultative or strict anaerobes; only two genera (*Clostridium* and *Bacillus*) produce heat-resistant endospores; must grow at 37 C in peptone or meat infusion media; some also require blood, yeast extract or serum. This order contains most of the pathogenic bacteria. Representatives: *Salmonella typhi* and *related Enterobacteriaceae, Streptococcus pyogenes, Staphylococcus aureus, Clostridium tetani, Bacillus anthracis, Neisseria gonorrhoeae*

3. **Order Actinomycetales:** branching, rod-like or filamentous cells; no motile pathogens; generally gram-positive; some species are acid-fast. Representatives: *Mycobacterium tuberculosis, M. leprae, Actinomyces israeli, Nocardia* sp.

4. **Order Spirochaetales:** helical; *flexible;* motile without flagella; generally gram-negative, but preferentially observed with darkfield microscope; contain a central, fibrillar, elastic structure (axial filament) around which the tubular cell is wound. Representatives: *Treponema pallidum, Leptospira icterohaemorrhagiae, Borrelia recurrentis*

5. **Order Mycoplasmatales:** *no cell wall,* therefore osmotically fragile and extremely pleomorphic; complex developmental cycle involves extremely minute "minimal reproductive units" <0.2μm. and filtrable; the smallest known living units capable of independent multiplication in inanimate media; nonmotile, though some have flagella; no heat-resistant endospores; colonies on special "enriched media" extremely minute, typically with fried egg appearance (except Eaton agent); aerobic or facultative; parasitic species are rich in lipids and require media with serum and steroids. Representatives: *Mycoplasma pneumoniae (Eaton agent), Ureaplasma, M. hominis*

6. **Order Rickettsiales:** bacteria that lack important enzyme systems characteristic of other bacteria, hence their *obligate intracellular parasitism* and extremely minute size: diameters are around 0.3μm.; no heat-resistant endospores; none is cultivable in or on inanimate media, but all are cultivable in cell and tissue cultures, and most in viable chick embryos; procaryotic, bacteria-like cell structure

   a. Family Rickettsiaceae: lack several synthetic enzyme systems but *can synthesize ATP;* multiply by binary fission like other bacteria; have distinct cell walls with muramic acid; morphologically are distinct rods, cocci or filaments. Representatives: *Rickettsia prowazeki, Coxiella burneti*

   b. Family Chlamydiaceae: formerly thought to be viruses: lack many synthetic enzymes; unlike all other bacteria, *cannot synthesize ATP;* complex intracellular mode of multiplication; cell walls are layered and, like bacteria, contain muramic acid; morphology spheroidal. Representatives: *Chlamydia trachomatis, C. psittaci*

Classification of Protozoa, Fungi and Helminths (Eucaryotes)

In addition to bacteria, other groups containing pathogenic microorganisms may be listed as follows:

A. Phylum Protozoa: unicellular animals; rarely cultivable on artificial media; five groups differentiated by type of motility:

1. Superclass Sarcodina (move with pseudopodia): *Entamoeba histolytica;* enteric and tissue parasites
2. Subphylum Ciliophora (move with cilia): *Balantidium coli;* enteric
3. Superclass Mastigophora (move with flagella): arthropod-borne: *Leishmania, Trypanosoma;* blood and tissues; *Trichomonas,* chiefly genitalia.
4. Subphylum Sporozoa (ameboid movement in some trophozoites): alternating sexual and asexual multiplication in different hosts, e.g., man and mosquito in *Plasmodium* (malaria parasites): blood and tissues
5. Class Toxoplasmea: (gliding and flexing motility) asexual multiplication by binary fission, endogony or sporogony, or both; trophozoites in cysts or pseudocysts. *Toxoplasma gondii, Pneumocystis carinii, Sarcocystis lindemanni*

B. Division Eumycetes = Mycophyta = Mycota; Subdivision Eumycotina (true fungi): eucaryotic cellular structure; may be branching and filamentous or yeast-like, or both; not photosynthetic; chemoorganotrophic; cultivable on inanimate media, e.g., Saboraud's agar; pathogens are mainly Fungi Imperfecti or Deuteromycetes.

1. Superficial infections (tineas, athlete's foot, onychomycosis, etc.) due to dermatophytes: *Trichophyton* spp; *Microsporum* spp; *Epidermophyton*
2. Deep or systemic infections (histoplasmosis, coccidioidomycosis, blastomycosis, etc.) due to yeast-like or dimorphic fungi

C. Multicellular Microorganisms (eucaryotic cell structure; contain DNA and RNA) *Helminths* (parasitic worms); adult helminths are not microscopic, but many of their developmental, infective and diagnostically important forms are.

1. Phylum Platyhelminthes (flatworms)
   a. Class Trematoda—flukes: nonsegmented; digenetic (alternate sexual and asexual generations in different hosts); sexual stage in man; bilaterally symmetrical; dorsoventrally compressed; hermaphroditic except dioecious (♀ and ♂) schistosomes (blood flukes); e.g., liver flukes, lung flukes
   b. Class Cestoidea—tapeworms: hermaphroditic; consist of enlarged scolex ("head") with suckers (and hooks, depending on species) for attachment to intestinal mucosa; narrow "neck" produces, by budding, successive flat segments; these form the ribbon-like strobilia or chain of from three to several thousand hermaphroditic proglottids, e.g., beef tapeworms

2. Phylum Nematoda—roundworms: nonsegmented; long, slender, cylindrical; dioecious
   a. Intestinal parasites: typically no intermediate hosts; eggs, larvae or both mature in intestine, on skin, in or on soil; e.g., pinworms, hookworms, ascaris
   b. Blood and tissue parasites (intermediate hosts necessary)
      (1) *Trichinella spiralis* (pork worm)
      (2) Filaria worms (various species and insect vectors)

D. Noncellular Infective Agents—Viruses: except for some pox viruses, are visible only with electron microscopes; obligate intracellular parasites; no intracellular multiplication; nonmotile; without metabolic mechanisms; without autonomous reproductive mechanisms; contain core of genetic and infective DNA *or* RNA, *never* both; associated with protein (capsid) in either cubic or either helical configuration, some have an outer, host-cell-derived, lipid-containing envelope; no muramic acid, which is unique to procaryotic cell walls.

MICROSCOPIC METHODS

The compound microscope commonly used in medical work consists of three principal lens groups: condenser (with iris diaphragm), objective and ocular or eyepiece; and a source of visible light. Light enters at the lowest part of the optical system and passes upward toward the eye through the object on the stage and the magnifying lenses. Immersion oil is placed between the object and the objective lens to prevent loss of light due to refraction and reflection at the several glass surfaces. An objective lens designed to operate in oil is called an *oil-immersion* objective.

The objective produces a real image magnified about 90 times. The ocular or eyepiece further enlarges it about 10 times, giving a final image about 900 times the size of the object (i.e., 10×90 or $900\times$).

The Electron Microscope

Because of the relatively long wavelength of visible light (about 500 nm. or 5000 Å), objects less than a certain distance (0.2 μm.) apart cannot be differentiated (or *resolved*). Thus, the *resolving power* of the common *(optical)* microscope is limited by the *nature of visible light;* images are fuzzy at magnifications beyond about 1,200. Electrons have a much *shorter wavelength* than ordinary light (about 0.5 nm. or 5 Å). Therefore, a microscope utilizing electron streams instead of visible light rays has a much greater *resolving power* and is capable of giving distinct images at magnifications of 100,000 or more.

Glass is opaque to electrons. However, electrons are deflected from their path by magnetic fields. Therefore, in the electron microscope, circular electromagnets take the place of glass lenses and are "focused" by varying the strength of the magnetic fields. Three major magnet-lens systems are used, each having a function analogous to its counterpart in an ordinary microscope. Since electrons travel well only in a vacuum, the entire instrument is arranged for evacuation. Because electron images are not directly visible to the eye, they are viewed on a fluorescent screen or are recorded on photographic plates. Like x-ray pictures, they are electron-shadowgraphs (electron micrographs). If photographic enlargements are made, final magnifications over $10^5\times$ are possible. Objects invisible with optical microscopes, such as viruses, become visible by this means.

Until recently, electron images have depended on passage of electrons *through* the object, degrees of contrast in the picture depending on differing degrees of electron density or opacity in the object.

The Scanning Electron Microscope

Striking topographic pictures giving the illusion of perspective or 3-D effect are now obtainable with the *scanning electron microscope* (SEM), which uses secondarily activated electrons (in a sense "reflected" from just beneath the surface of the opaque object) rather than transmitted electrons (TEM).

The surface of opaque objects is scanned by a focused beam or "probe" of electrons much as a TV camera scans a scene, with great depth of focus. The probing beam, being only about 5 to 10 nm. in diameter, penetrates into very narrow and deep crevices or reveals high prominences with great clarity. The scanning beam is synchronized with a TV projecting beam. Secondary electrons from the microprobing beam are collected and transmitted to the TV screen at magnifications that may be varied from less than 100× to 100,000× or more.

Other Optical Methods

Other optical methods are: (1) *phase microscopy,* in which light rays passing *through* the object, and those diffracted *around* it (and therefore out of wave-phase with the rays passing through the object) are integrated into a single image; (2) x-ray and (3) fluorescence microscopy.

In *fluorescence microscopy* the microorganisms are stained with a fluorescent dye. When excited by ultraviolet light (invisible), the dye emits light at visible wavelengths. Fluorescein yields a yellow-green color. The method is sometimes used to find tubercle bacilli in sputum, etc. The procedure is like the Ziehl-Neelsen acid-fast stain but substitutes fluorescent auramine O for the carbolfuchsin.

Darkfield Microscopy

By means of a darkfield condenser or a "stop," central rays of light (usually admitted) are prevented from passing upward through the object to the eye. Peripheral rays (usually eliminated) are refracted by the darkfield condenser to emerge so obliquely from the surface of the slide that they do not reach the eye when the field is devoid of any object. The field therefore appears dark (hence darkfield). When the oblique rays impinge on an object on the slide, e.g., a spirochete, dust, bacterium, they are reflected upward from the surface of the object of the eye through the lenses. The object is then seen brightly oublined by the rays reflected from its surface.

STAINING METHODS

Gram's Stain

1. Smear the material to be stained on a slide. Allow to dry in air.
2. Apply an appropriate solution of crystal violet. Allow to stain about 1 minute. Wash gently.
3. Apply Gram's or Lugol's iodine solution for 1 minute. Wash gently.
4. Apply 95 per cent ethyl alcohol or acetone or both until all but the thickest part of the smear are decolorized, or for not more than 10 to 15 sec. Wash.
5. Counterstain with safranine for 1 minute. Wash. Blot dry.
6. Examine naked smear with oil immersion.

Bacteria are differentiated by their ability to either hold or lose the violet-iodine combination in the presence of decolorizing agent. Those that hold the violet dye are called gram positive. Those that are decolorized and take the red counterstain are called gram negative. Many are intermediate and will appear gram positive or gram negative, depending on length of application of decolorizing agent, age of cells, kind of medium, pH, etc.

With respect to reaction toward Gram's stain, medically important bacteria may be listed as follows:

Gram-Positive Bacteria

All streptococci

All staphylococci

Pneumococci (*Streptococcus* [*Diplococcus*] *pneumoniae*)

Diphtheria bacillus (*Corynebacterium diphtheriae*) and diphtheroids

All acid-fast bacilli, such as *Mycobacterium tuberculosis*

All spore-forming anaerobes (genus *Clostridium*)

Bacillus anthracis

Listeria, Erysipelothrix, Actinomyces, Nocardia, Streptomyces, Coxiella

Gram-Negative Bacteria

Gennus *Neisseria*

The Enterobacteriaceae, including *Salmonella, Shigella,* the coliform group

The Hemophilus groups (*H. influenzae, H. vaginalis, H. ducreyi*)

Organisms of
  pertussis (*Bordetella pertussis*)
  plague (*Yersinia pestis*)
  cholera (*Vibrio cholerae*)

All species of *Pseudomonas*, e.g. *Pseudomonas aeruginosa*

Spirillum minus, Brucella sp., *Francisella* (Pasteurella) *tularensis, Bacteroides, Fusobacterium, Veillonella.*

Differences in reaction to the Gram stain reflect numerous profound differences in properties of the organisms, chiefly susceptibility to antibiotics affecting cell wall synthesis (see Table 5-1).

Acid-Fast Stain (Ziehl-Neelsen) and Kinyoun (Cold) Methods

Organisms of tuberculosis and leprosy, and several related saprophytic species of *Mycobacterium* such as the smegma bacillus, have the distinctive character called acid-fastness (AF), presumably due to the presence of lipids (wax-like mycolic acid) in the cell wall. They quickly absorb red carbolfuchsin dye when warmed, and hold the dye against acidified alcohol solution. In stained smears, all non-acid-fast bacteria, mucus, pus cells, etc., lose the carbolfuchsin when treated with acid alcohol and take a contrasting counterstain, e.g., methylene blue, yellow picric acid or brilliant green. The acid-fast stain is used as follows:

1. Smear as for Gram's stain.
2. Flood slide with carbolfuchsin, steam gently for 5 minutes over low flame, do not allow to dry, add more stain if necessary. Cool. Alternatively, carbolfuchsin containing phenol and alcohol (cool) may be used without heat.
3. Apply 90 per cent alcohol containing 3 to 5 per cent HCl until all but thickest parts of smear cease to give off color (about 1 to 3 minutes). Wash.
4. Counterstain 1 minute with methylene blue. Wash.

Tubercle bacilli are more strongly acid-fast than other members of the acid-fast group, and give a characteristic beaded appearance. Both Gram's stain and acid-fast stain depend on the integrity of the cell wall. Broken or disintegrated bacilli or their parts are neither gram positive nor acid-fast.

Fluorescent-Antibody Staining

Antibodies may be conjugated with fluorescent substances (e.g., fluorescein, rhodamine) without loss of specificity. They combine with their specific antigen in the usual way. The fluorescence of the antibody renders an (ordinarily) invisible antigen-antibody combination readily visible with the microscope using ultraviolet illumination. For example, in the direct method to determine the localization of a mass of specific viral protein, i.e., a specific antigen, in a frozen tissue section or acetone-fixed cell, the specimen is flooded with the specific fluorescent antibody. The excess fluorescent antibody is then washed away. On examining with ultraviolet light, the fluorescent-stained viral antigen, or any other antigen (e.g., bacterial) coated with fluorescent specific antibody, is easily seen.

In an "indirect" method, *nonfluorescent* specific antibodies (immune globulins) are applied to the specimen as above. The excess is washed away. The specific antigen-antibody combination is invisible but is easily made visible by flooding the slide with fluorescent antibody (made in another species) to *any immunoglobulin* of the species in which the primary unlabeled antibody was made. Since, in the smear under discussion, all globulin, *except* that held in the *specific* antigen-antibody combination, has been washed away, the fluorescent *antiglobulin* antibody will reveal the immunoglobulin remaining in the specific antigen-antibody combination.

Labeling for Electron Microscopy

Because fluorescent antibodies cast no electron shadows they are not visible in electron micrographs. For examination of antigen-antibody complexes, reactions, locations, etc., with the electron microscope, antibodies are conjugated with ferritin, an organic iron compound opaque to electrons. Ferritin-labeled antigen-antibody complexes are seen as minute black specks in electron micrographs. Antibody conjugated with peroxidase after union with antigen *in situ* is revealed by reaction with hydrogen peroxide and then benzidine, the reaction product being visible by either light or electron microscopy. Peroxidase-labeled and developed tissue preparations last indefinitely and can be fixed and permanently mounted, in contrast to preparations stained with fluorescent antibody that, because of rapid fluorochrome decay, cannot be fixed.

THE ANATOMY AND PHYSIOLOGY OF BACTERIA

The Bacterial Nucleus

This is more appropriately called a nucleoid. Unlike the chromosomes of eucaryotes it is not enclosed in a nuclear membrane and is more or less intermingled with the cytoplasm. It consists of a single, tenuous, circular thread of double-stranded deoxyribonucleic acid (DNA). The DNA is bound to a membrane and is held in a compact configuration by numerous noncovalent cross-links, composed of RNA and/or protein. In the cell it appears like a tangled skein of yarn. It constitutes the entire genome of the bacterial cell.

Disentangled, each of the two DNA strands is seen to be a long-chain polymer of deoxyribonucleotides, each nucleotide bearing either a purine base: guanine (G) or adenine (A), or a pyrimidine base: thymine (T) or cytosine (C). The nucleotides of each strand are held together lengthwise by strong, covalent, phosphodiester linkages between the sugars while the two strands themselves are held together by relatively weak hydrogen bonds between the bases:

$$
\begin{array}{ll}
\text{deoxyribose} & \text{deoxyribose} \\
\text{---phosphate ---} & \text{phosphate ---} \\
| & | \\
\text{purine (A or G)} & \text{pyrimidine (C or T)} \\
\|(|) & \|(|) \\
\text{pyrimidine (C or T)} & \text{purine (A or G)} \\
| & | \\
\text{deoxyribose} & \text{deoxyribose} \\
\text{---phosphate ---} & \text{phosphate ---}
\end{array}
$$

A always pairs with T; C with G. The whole structure is formed like a helical ladder, the sides being the firm phosphosugar polymers, the rungs are the separable purine-pyrimidine base pairs. The numbers, sequence and kinds of nucleotides and their pairing are fixed characters for each species and constitute its genetic code. The ends of the helix are connected, forming a twisted closed circle, an arrangement important in its replication. The twists in the circle are highly strained, as in a twisted rope. The resulting "supercoils" are released in a controlled manner, presumably facilitating revolution of the molecule about the helical axis during replication and recombination.

The contrast between procaryotic and eucaryotic chromosomes is not limited to physical arrangement of molecules, but extends to the organization of the genetic message. The DNA of procaryotes has few repeated sequences, most of the DNA is transcribed, and there are no intervening sequences within structural genes. Eucaryotic DNA contains many repeated sequences; some repeat millions of times. Much of the DNA has no transcript; portions of structural genes are separated from each other by intervening sequences.

The presence of intervening sequences in the genes of eucaryotes has many implications for the new science of genetic engineering. Eucaryotic DNA generally is not translated properly in procaryotic cells because of the inability of the procaryotic translation mechanism to deal with interruptions within structural genes.

Bacterial Cytoplasm

This consists of a fluid matrix or "cell sap" having various ions, wastes, enzymes, amino acids, vitamins, nucleotides, tRNA, etc., in solution. Because of the selective permeability of the cell membrane and the action of "one-way" permease enzymes in the cell envelope, many of these substances increase in concentration inside the cell sufficiently to raise the intracellular osmotic pressure to several atmospheres. When the cell (especially a gram-positive cell) is deprived of its strong wall of peptidoglycan or murein (as by lysozyme or growth in contact with penicillin, cephalothin, etc.), in a hypotonic solution the fragile cell membrane ruptures (see Table 5-2).

Particulate matter includes inert granules of stored food such as polymetaphosphates (volutin); lipids, principally as poly-betahydroxybutyric acid; starch-like granules, etc.

The largest portion of cytoplasmic particulate matter of the bacterial cell consists of ribosomes, minute granules of rRNA with some protein. Each 70s ribosome monomer consists of two subunits, 50s and 30s. Ribosomes function in the synthesis of proteins. With the assistance of tRNA anticodons to transfer amino acids, and mRNA codons to carry the genetic code of the nuclear DNA, the sequence of the amino acids in the polypeptides made by the ribosomes is determined. The 50s and 30s subunits of the ribosomes are the points of attachment of numerous antibiotics that interfere with protein synthesis (see Table 5-3).

Mesosomes (possibly primitive endoplasmic reticulum) appear to be saccular invaginations of the cytoplasmic membrane and to be associated, in contact with the nuclear material, with cell fission. Mesosomes are absent from mycoplasmas. There are no mitochondria, lysosomes, Golgi bodies, or other complex organelles that characterize eucaryotic cells.

Bacterial Flagella

Procaryotic flagella lack the enclosing membrane and patterned, internal, multifibrillar structure (9 + 2 pairs) characteristic of all eucaryotic flagella. Bacterial flagella are capable of rhythmic, wave-like motion and, among pathogenic species, are responsible for motility (except in spirochetes). Among the Enterobacteriaceae, flagellar protein confers species or type specificity on the cell. Flagellar antigens are called H (for Hauch, germ. film) antigens. In the genus *Salmonella* they vary in degree of specificity between phase I and phase II (see Table 5-4). H antigens may be removed by violent shaking or may be destroyed by heat, alcohol or acid.

O or somatic *(ohne Hauch)* antigens of gram-negative bacteria reside in the cell wall, which, in these organisms, consists of only about 10 per cent peptidoglycan. The remainder is mainly lipopolysaccharide-protein-phosphatide complexes, the molecular structures of which confer O antigenic specificity and the endotoxicity so characteristic of gram-negative cells.

Closely related species of bacteria, such as the many serotypes of *Salmonella,* may contain identical O antigens (see Table 5-5). (See also discussion of A, B, H, blood-group antigens under Immunohematology.) Thus, if a person is stimulated antigenically, either by injections of vaccine or by infection with any of the genus *Salmonella,* say *S. typhi,* the blood may contain O agglutinins for several other species of *Salmonella.* This is helpful in diagnosing salmonellosis retrospectively by serum agglutination titrations with any of several group-related (Table 5-5) species of *Salmonella* (Widal test). With *S. typhi,* it is customary to use both O and H (type) antigens.

O bacterial suspensions are prepared by treating the organisms with alcohol at 37 C. This destroys the flagellar antigens and leaves the somatic intact. The agglutinated cells then form fine granules. H antigens are prepared by treating the bacteria with 0.2 per cent formalin in saline. This stiffens the flagella and prevents the O antigens from bringing the bacilli close together; flocculent agglutination results.

Flagella of spirochetes are polar but, unlike the separate flagella of other bacteria, occur in bipolar bundles bent sharply back on the tubular cell, their ends meeting near the midlength. These bundles together form an end-to-end axial filament around which the helical cell is twined. Like other flagella they are attached in the cell wall by hooks and rings.

Pili or Fimbriae

These are typically straight, rigid, very tenuous hairs or spikes, visible only with the electron microscope, rooted in the cell membrane and projecting from all surfaces of gram-negative rods. There are several types of pili, varying in length, diameter and function. One function of the common types of pili is to cause the cells to adhere to each other, as in forming pellicles on the surface of broth cultures, and to other particles and surfaces. Pili cause marked hemagglutination of guinea pig erythrocytes.

F-type pili are found only on "male," donor, or F+ cells. These pili are larger, longer and less rigid and much less numerous than other types of pili and appear to serve as conjugation tubes during mating (see Conjugation). Being protein *(pilin),* pili can give marked antigenic specificity, which may cause confusion in H and O agglutination tests unless precautions are taken to eliminate them.

The Cytoplasmic Membrane

This is commonly of the three-layer, unit-membrane type: a double, inner, lipid leaflet between two outer layers of protein. It acts as a highly selective, semipermeable, osmotic barrier for the cell. In bacteria (except pathogenic mycoplasmas, which have no cell wall) sterols are not present, whereas they are present in pathogenic fungi in which they constitute points of attack by such fungicidal antibiotics as nystatin and amphotericin B (see Table 5-3).

Attached to the cell membrane are many ribosomes, and integrated with it are many enzymes of energy-mediating systems, with cytochromes and the associated oxidative phosphorylation (ATP-producing) systems.

Endospores

These are intracellular, minute, dehydrated, round or oval bodies, only one per cell, with thick, multilayered walls. They contain the essential cell contents in compact form. Endospores are highly resistant to heat, sunlight, radiation, drying, chemical disinfectants and other unfavorable influences. Under suitable conditions of moisture, nutrition and warmth, they germinate, much as seeds germinate, and grow into the vulnerable, vegetative form of the organism. Spores or conidia of eucaryotic fungi are only slightly thermostable.

The only known pathogenic organisms forming such highly heat- and disinfectant-resisting spores are species of the aerobic genus *Bacillus (B. anthracis)* and of the anaerobic genus *Clostridium,* including *C. tetani, C. perfringens, C. botulinum* and several species associated with *C. perfringens* in gas gangrene of dirty wounds.

Slimes and Capsules

Some species of bacteria produce more or less slimy outer coatings. When diffuse and soluble such coatings are called *slimes;* when more compact, gel-like and adherent they are called *capsules.* Capsules commonly consist of polysaccharides (e.g., capsules of pneumococci), polypeptide (e.g., *B. anthracis*), mucopolysaccharide (e.g., hyaluronic acid capsules of group A and C *Streptococcus pyogenes*), and other polymers. The capsular polysaccharides usually confer immunologic specificity, e.g., type specificity of pneumococci and meningococci. Capsules serve to protect the cell from dehydration and phagocytosis and thus contribute to virulence. They occur typically on cells in pathologic material or in smooth (S) type colonies.

Some very thin capsules are called *microcapsules, K antigens,* sheath antigens, etc. One of these is the Vi (virulence) antigen of typhoid bacilli. It prevents O agglutination by antibodies and tends to disappear after artificial cultivation.

The Cell Wall and Periplasmic Space

The procaryotic cell wall differs markedly from that of eucaryotic green plants and from that of eucaryotic fungi, which contain chitin. Typical animal cells have no true cell wall.

The cell walls of gram-positive bacteria consist wholly of relatively thick layers of *peptidoglycan* or *murein;* i.e., complex, cross-linked polymers of N-acetyl glucosamine and N-acetyl muramic acid (unique to procaryotic cells), linked to teichoic acids and some D-("unnatural") amino acids, often with diaminopimelic acid (DAP).

Externally associated with the gram-positive cell wall are certain proteins, some of which confer immunologic specificity on the cell, e.g., the M proteins of group A streptococci, e.g., *S. pyogenes.*

Gram-negative cells have a rather loosely attached outer membrane or layer with unit-type-membrane structure that contains the O (endotoxin) antigen and a relatively thin inner layer of lysozyme-soluble peptidoglycan that is in contact with the plasma membrane. The outer membrane acts as a nonselectively permeable molecular sieve.

Differences between envelope structures are associated with numerous differences between gram-positive and gram-negative species.

Deprived of the strong mucocomplex of their cell wall (e.g., by penicillin or mutation), gram-positive species become completely naked and osmotically fragile *protoplasts;* gram-negative species become *spheroplasts.* These are less osmotically fragile because they are partly protected by the lipopolysaccharide moiety of their cell walls, which is not affected by penicillin.

GENETIC TRANSFER IN BACTERIA

Three mechanisms for transfer of bacterial DNA from cell to cell are known: (a) conjugation, (b) transformation and (c) transduction.

Conjugation

Conjugation, the nearest approach to true sexuality in bacteria, depends on the presence of fertility genes that are often associated with extrachromosomal elements called plasmids, some of which confer ability to produce sexual organelles. Such plasmids, through the action of transfer genes, produce sex pili and mediate the intercellular transfer of DNA by the replicative processs. An autonomously replicating molecule (replicon) bearing genes for sexual organelles constitutes a self-transferable fertility factor. Furthermore, plasmids bearing transfer genes can transiently insert into other replicons, including the chromosome, and thus promote the transfer by conjugation of the entire genetic complex.

Recent rapid bacterial evolution has been mediated by plasmids and is attributable to their ability to transfer genetic information from cell to cell during conjugation. The importance of plasmids to medicine lies in the fact that they may contain genes for drug resistance and toxin production as well as the means for transferring these traits across interspecies barriers. Moreover, plasmid genes possess "transposon" activity, in that genetic information can be freely exchanged from plasmid to plasmid, or from plasmid to chromosome, within the same cell. The existence of such "genetic loose change" has aroused intense interest among researchers and practitioners interested in the containment of infectious diseases.

In this regard, the emergence of plasmid-born penicillinase genes among clinical isolates of *Hemophilus* and *Neisseria* has caused much concern for the future effectiveness of antibiotic therapy. The DNA responsible has been shown to be derived from enterobacteriaceae. Based on chronological order of acquired resistance, the information was carried, by plasmids, from the enterobacteriaceae into species of *Hemophilus.*

Transformation

In bacteria, this is the transfer of cell-free, genetic DNA from one cell to another by exposing the recipient cells, in vitro or in vivo, to contact with DNA derived from a different (but related through adequate base-pair homology of their DNAs) donor cell. This is exemplified by the transformation of pneumococcus serologic (capsular) types and can occur between other related species. Only fragments of DNA from the donor cell enter the recipient cell through the cell wall and membrane. The recipient cell must be in a competent state (i.e., R, or no interfering capsule, etc.) to receive the transforming DNA. Competence also depends on the presence of a particular surface protein. The transformation of fibroma virus to myxoma virus is a related phenomenon, though the mechanism of the transfer is different.

Do not confuse it with *malignant transformation* of animal cells due to prophage-like integration of oncogenic viruses with the cell chromosome. This results in heritable alterations of morphology, membrane composition and structure, associated with loss of contact inhibition of movement and cell multiplication; in changes in antigenic composition and in aneuploidy. All are associated with malignancy.

Transduction

Bacterial DNA mispackaged into phage particles may be transmitted to other cells by viral infection (transduction). Mispackaging of bacterial DNA sometimes occurs as a consequence of errors in the coupling of the processes of replication and packaging of viral DNA (generalized transduction). Excision of prophage DNA (see phage) from the bacterial chromosome is another source of transducing particles. During excision, the prophage may include within its own chromosome or replicon a few or many linked bacterial genes, sometimes in exchange for some of its own genes (specialized transduction).

Phage Conversion. This results when a temperate phage introduces certain specific genetic properties that are coded solely by phage genes, not by chromosomal genes; e.g., introduction of the property of toxigenicity into a cell of a nontoxigenic *Corynebacterium diphtheriae*. The nontoxigenic cell becomes toxigenic, but *only as long* as the converting prophage remains in the cell genome. "Curing" the converted cell of its phage (e.g., failure of the phage to be transmitted during cell fission) causes the cell to revert to nontoxigenicity. Phage conversion is not true genetic recombination, since the converting nucleic acid is not of bacterial origin.

Because the cell containing the converting prophage is in a lysogenic state, i.e., potentially lytic by induced prophage, such conversion is often called *lysogenic conversion*. All toxigenic strains of *C. diphtheriae* contain a prophage. Similar examples of phage-borne toxigenicity are found in other species, e.g., *Streptococcus pyogenes*.

VARIATION AND MUTATION

Phenotypic Changes

The distinguishing characteristics of any cell and its progeny are phenotypic (visible or demonstrable) expressions of the genetic makeup of the cell. Because the DNA molecule is remarkably stable, phenotypic characters remain quite constant under ordinary conditions of growth. However, while the genotype (entire sequence of nucleotides and genetic units in the chromosome) may remain unaltered the phenotypic manifestations of its messages via mRNA and tRNA and rRNA may be greatly altered by environmental circumstances such as pH, temperature, presence of certain ions or nutritional or toxic substances. Characters commonly altered by such influences are pigment, slime formation, sporulation, filamentous growth, and so on. Changes of this nature are variously called fluctuations, modifications, variations, etc. Characteristically they are nonheritable; each cell reverts to its original or unaltered state immediately on removal of the altering influence; the genotype has remained intact.

Induced Enzymes. A particular type of phenotypic variation is seen in inducible (or "adaptive") enzyme function. The genotype may code for production of certain enxymes such as β-galactosidase, penicillinase, or certain permeases, which are ordinarily suppressed by an intracellular repressor. In the presence of the specific substrate of the enzyme, or of a chemically related substance (e.g., β-galactose or lactose), the repressor is removed or inactivated, and the genetic potentiality is phenotypically expressed by fermentation of the lactose, destruction of penicillin or admission to the cell of the substrate of the particular permease involved. An important aspect of this is the development of bacteria, notably staphylococci, that, originally susceptible to penicillin, on contact with penicillin produce the enzyme penicillinase, thus becoming wholly resistant to penicillin (see Drug Resistance.) The induced change appears to be permanent though it is not a genetic change. *Inducibility* of an enzyme represents an inherited potentiality under repression; its *induction* is the result of removal of the repressor by an external stimulus.

Colony Variation

An important aspect of bacterial variation (formerly often called *dissociation*) is seen in the formation of different types of colony. Bacteria of any given species may form, on agar plates, variant colonies that have very different properties.

Smooth, or S, Type. These colonies are of pasty or butyrous consistency, smooth, moist looking, glistening, domed and circular, with even, regular margin. The cells in S colonies tend to be encapsulated and to occur singly; i.e., not in long chains or filaments.

Rough, or R, Type. These have a dull, dry, rough or granular surface and are rather flat, with a crenated, or indented, and irregular margin. R colonies are brittle or granular in consistency. Long chains of cells, especially of rod forms, or long filaments, tend to occur. These cells generally are not encapsulated.

Practically any culture of any organism may produce either R or S variant, depending in great part on environment. The activating mechanism may be alternating mutations and back-mutations. The S ⇌ R change often occurs as a result of environmental conditions such as presence of certain amino acids and reduced oxygen tension. Usually it is not a stable change.

The capsular substance of S type cells, usually carbohydrate, is *antigenically active* and highly *specific* and, in species like *Streptococcus pneumoniae, Haemophilus influenzae* and *Neisseria meningitidis,* is *associated with virulence.* Therefore, in selecting an organism for making an immunizing antigen or for immunologic studies in general, it is usually best to select a smooth, encapsulated strain of known virulence. In general, rough variants are of lesser virulence and lack capsules, antigenic activity and immunologic specificity. These relationships are especially well demonstrated in making pertussis and typhoid vaccines.

Mucoid and Dwarf Colonies. *Mucoid colonies* are mucoid in consistency and often are voluminous and semifluid, tending to flow across agar. They may contain gummy or slimy glucans, dextrans, or other polysaccharides, depending on species. *Dwarf colonies* are extremely minute, sometimes barely visible to the unaided eye. Organisms from any variant colony may produce colonies of other phases. The pathologic significance of the mucoid and the dwarf colonies is not clear.

Recombination

It is important to distinguish recombination, which involves rearrangement of sequences within one or more molecules of DNA, from simple reassortment of DNA molecules between cells, such as occurs with plasmid transfer.

The bacterial chromosome is not a fixed structure; any homologous sequences present within the genome will be foci of virtually constant recombinational activity. Indeed, it is possible that a few *E. coli* cells in fact contain identical genomes. A strikingly evident example of the consequences of recombination within homologous sequences is the phenomenon of phase variation. The antigenic specificity of the flagella of *Salmonella* alternates periodically between two states. It is now known that this antigenic alteration is due to recombination between homologous DNA sequences that bracket the flagellar structural genes. With each recombination event, the chromosomal sequence of the flagella genes is reversed: When the genes

are inserted into the genome in one orientation, the H_1 antigenic phase is expressed; when they are inserted in the other orientation, the H_2 phase is expressed. Many recombination events go undetected; it is nevertheless becoming apparent that the normal condition of the *E. coli* genome is one of dynamic flux.

It is interesting to note that the highly repetitive DNA of eucaryotes would probably be unstable to the point of chaos in the presence of such an indiscriminate and fiercely active recombination system.

Genotypic Changes

These are true genetic mutations; the actual chemical composition of the DNA molecule or genome is altered and if the change is not lethal, as often happens, the change is passed on to the progeny of the cell. Because of the stability of the DNA molecule most types of mutation are rare, ordinarily occurring at frequencies of from about 1 in 10^5 to 1 in 10^{11} unless the frequency is increased by certain mutagenic agents.

The smallest genetic unit, the presence, absence or alteration of which can result in a mutation, is a single nucleotide, a *muton*. The presence, or structure, or a single nucleotide or base pair may determine a heritable character and be a gene or recombinational unit or *recon*, but genes generally consist of many nucleotides. A gene, in current terminology, is any genetically functional segment of the chromosome.

Mutagenic agents may be chemical or physical. Among the most potent physical mutagens are ultraviolet and ionizing radiations. Ultraviolet, among other effects, tends especially to cause aberrant linkages (dimers) between pyrimidines: T to T, T to C or C to C. Ionizing radiations can cause destructive effects due to release of free radicals, or mutations due to deletion of nucleotides.

Several chemicals are active mutagens. Alkalating agents like N and S mustards affect guanine; all are changes that result in erroneous pairing of bases. Nitrosated amines are an important possible source of some base analogues, e.g., 5-bromouracil (enol form) can cause false pairing with G instead of A; AT is thus replaced by GC. Some dyes like acridine orange cause distortion of the secondary structure of the DNA helix, resulting in faulty replication or recombination.

Potentially lethal lesions occur repeatedly in the DNA of living organisms. Only the presence of error-free DNA repair systems prevents the loss of genetic fidelity. Bacteria continue to provide valuable insights into DNA repair mechanisms and mutagenesis. Bacteria also serve as a principal short-term screen for detection and analysis of environmental mutagens that are responsible for increasing the endogenous load of premutational lesions in mammalian DNA.

The most widely used test (Ames test) has been shown to have highly accurate predictive value for carcinogenic activity. Indeed, of 176 chemical carcinogens tested, 158 or 90 per cent were mutagenic. Conversely, of 108 "noncarcinogens," only 13 were mutagenic. These 13 negatives may reflect the relative lack of sensitivity of tests in animals.

Many mutagens and carcinogens are metabolized to active forms by enzymes present in mammalian cells. Cellular extracts containing these enzymes are often included in the test plate so that compounds requiring activation will not be missed.

As a point of reference, the condensate of the smoke from a single cigarette causes approximately 20,000 mutations when tested in the presence of cellular enzymes.

Auxotrophs

Among the many important mutant forms of microorganisms are "deficient" auxotrophs. *Auxotrophs* are mutants that have lost one or more synthetic properties characteristic of the original type ("wild type" or prototype) from which the auxotroph was derived.

Mutations that affect antigenic, metabolic, morphologic, and similar properties, that are the basis of diagnostic tests are also of obvious importance, as are changes in properties that alter virulence (toxigenicity, capsule formation, etc.). Possibly, epidemics may in part result from, or be affected by, genetic changes in virulence factors.

Resistance to chemotherapeutic drugs and dependence on antibiotics are particularly undesirable types of mutation; some are transmissible by certain episomes (R or RTF) during conjugation among certain gram-negative bacteria. (See Antibiotics.)

BACTERIAL METABOLISM; BIOENERGETICS

Metabolic Types

All living cells depend on extraneous sources of energy for growth, reproduction and self-synthesis. Those obtaining energy from the sun, e.g., green plants, blue-green algae and a few species of nonpathogenic bacteria, are said to be *photosynthetic*. All microorganisms of medical significance (except viruses) obtain energy from exothermic (exergonic) chemical reactions, i.e., oxidations; they are said to be *chemosynthetic*. Viruses obtain their energy from the cells they infect.

Some chemosynthetic bacteria of the soil, called *chemolithotrophs,* oxidize only inorganic substrates (e.g., $2NH_3 + 4O_2 \rightarrow 2HNO_3 + 2H_2O$) as sources of energy. They can use CO_2 as a sole source of carbon. Organisms capable of using CO_2 as a sole source of carbon

are often called *autotrophs*. All microorganisms of medical interest, including bacteria, protozoans and fungi, etc., are chemosynthetic but, unlike autotrophs or chemolithotrophs, can utilize only *organic* substrates as sources of energy *and* carbon, i.e., they are *chemoorganotrophic*. Organisms requiring organic sources of CO_2 are often called *heterotrophs*. Many of these also require CO_2. The various metabolic types may be listed as follows:

Photosynthetic
  Green plants
  Blue-green algae
  Some bacteria of no medical interest
Chemosynthetic
  Chemolithotrophs: oxidize inorganic substrates; use only inorganic N, S and C (are autotrophic with respect to C source) (of no medical interest.)
  Chemo-organotrophs: oxidize only organic substrates; use mainly organic sources of S, N and C (are heterotrophic with respect to C source); may also require CO_2.

Although all pathogenic microorganisms are chemoorganotrophs, some, e.g., certain enteric species, require only a single organic compound such as glucose if furnished with a complete mineral supplement. Others, like the strict anaerobes, streptococci, gonococci, etc., require numerous preformed complex substances: peptones, carbohydrates, amino acids, vitamins, etc. Bacteria cannot ingest solid particles of food, i.e., their nutrition is entirely by osmosis and diffusion of nutrients in solution. They are said to be *osmotrophic*.

Energy Metabolism of Bacteria

In all chemo-organotrophs, bacterial as well as human, the most generally used source of carbon and energy is glucose. The most common first stage in energy metabolism of glucose is glycolysis by the Embden-Meyerhof scheme. Among bacteria, other systems may also be used, depending on species: the pentose-phosphate pathway, which is thermodynamically less efficient than glycolysis, and the Entner-Doudoroff pathway, found especially in species of *Pseudomonas*. Some species of bacteria can also use numerous other sugars and organic compounds (e.g., phenol and petroleum) as sources of energy and carbon, depending on the enzymic ability of the organism to convert the sugar, etc., into a form such that at some point in the metabolic process it can enter the glycolytic or other pathway. These differences often have value in diagnostic microbiology.

Among bacteria, and depending on species, glucose may be used in one or two of three general types of exergonic reactions: (a) *aerobic respiration*, (b) *anaerobic respiration* and (c) *fermentation*. In all three the prime source of energy is enzymic (dehydrogenase) removal, from a substrate, of pairs of hydrogen atoms with liberation of their electrons ($H = H^+ + e^-$). Removal of electrons is oxidation and yields energy; acceptance of electrons is reduction. In cell metabolism, when hydrogen (e^-) is removed from a substrate by a dehydrogenase, it is transferred to an agent at a higher oxidative potential, commonly nicotinamide-adenine dinucleotide (NAD), which then becomes $NADH_2$. The functioning part of the dehydrogenase is "niacin," which can accept the hydrogen and yield it up. In order to continue to function, the $NADH_2$ must be reoxidized (i.e., 2H removed).

a. *In aerobic respiration* the $NADH_2$ becomes reoxidized by enzymically transferring the hydrogen to a second O–R system, usually the riboflavin (or flavoprotein) system. Here the electrons are diverted and transferred to a series of four or five enzymes called *cytochromes,* each of greater e^--accepting (oxidizing) potency than the one before it. The coenzymes of the cytochromes are much like heme in having an atom of iron chelated in a porphyrin ring, the iron being able to accept and transfer e^-. In aerobic respiration the final cytochrome of the series, in the presence of the enzyme oxidase and $2H^+$, transfers the $2e^-$ to $\frac{1}{2}O_2$, forming H_2O. The entire series of enzymes and reactions from flavin to, and including, oxidase is called a *respiratory chain.* Many bacteria are *restricted* to the use of O_2 as a final hydrogen (electron) acceptor; they are called strict or *obligate aerobes.*

b. Many *common organisms* (called *facultative*) are capable of respiration under anaerobic conditions as well as under aerobic conditions as above. In the absence of O_2 they can use, as an alternative, several readily reducible inorganic compounds like $NaNO_3$ (substances depending on species) as final hydrogen acceptor in place of O_2: $NaNO_3 + 2H \rightleftharpoons NaNO_2 + H_2O$. Nitrate reduction is a familiar "test" in laboratory microbiology. Nitrite (NO_2) is a toxic product. It is also mutagenic and possibly carcinogenic. Furthermore, it can react with endogenous cellular amines (particularly the ubiquitous compounds spermine and spermidine) to produce nitroso compounds of great mutagenic potency. Some species reduce the nitrite, which is toxic, to N or NH_3 in stepwise reactions.

c. *In fermentation* two (or more) parts of the same organic substrate molecule (or two similar organic molecules, e.g., the Stickland reaction between two amino acids: alanine + glycine → acetic acid + NH_3 + CO_2) serve as hydrogen (electron) donor and hydrogen (electron) acceptor, respectively, a thermodynamically inefficient mechanism since much less energy is released

than in either form of respiration as described above.

In aerobic and anaerobic respiration the pyruvate resulting from glycolysis (or alternate pathway) is first combined with acetyl-s-coenzyme A, with liberation of 2H, via NAD, to the respiratory chain. The pyruvate then undergoes the series of changes constituting the Krebs or citric acid or tricarboxylic acid cycle. The overall reaction in bacterial respiration (aerobic or anaerobic) is: $C_6H_{12}O_6 + 6O_2 \rightarrow 6CO_2 + 6H_2O$ (plus 34 ATP and 688 kcal., not all of which is available for cell synthesis and reproduction. Some is given off as heat or otherwise lost to entropy.

In fermentation the pyruvate undergoes various alterations different from those seen in aerobic respiration, depending on species. There is no respiratory chain of cytochromes; much of the energy is not used. Reoxidation of the $NADH_2$ produced by glycolysis is accomplished by the reduction of cellular metabolites (e.g., pyruvate) followed by excretion of the reduced product (e.g., lactate) from the cell. In this way, the $NADH_2$ is oxidized, but its reducing power is lost to that cell. Some lactic acid bacteria, for example, reduce all of the pyruvate to lactic acid; some produce mainly propionic acid; and others produce a variety of substances, some of which are distinctive: acetylmethyl carbinol (basis of the Voges-Proskauer reaction), ethyl alcohol, acetone, butryic acid, CO_2, and others. All of these products of fermentation contain much of the original energy of the glucose and can serve as energy sources for other species of bacteria and fungi.

Energy and Phosphorylation. The most important result of any form of energy metabolism for the cell is the phosphorylation of certain organic compounds that, because of the strained state of the phosphate ester bond, become high-energy compounds. Among these are adenosine triphosphate (ATP), guanosine triphosphate (GTP), acetyl phosphate, 1,3-diphosphoglyceric acid, and others. The high-energy ester bond on hydrolysis yields energy to the compound temporarily associated with the high-energy compound. ATP, ADP and AMP constitute a series of energy transfer compounds, each of the latter two absorbing energy on phosphorylation that is transferred to ATP and H_3PO_4. Together they constitute an almost universally used energy transfer system in the cell.

In the bacterial respiratory chain, energy from electrons passing along the chain of cytochromes is transferred to the cell at two or three specific points, forming, with inorganic phosphate, ATP from ADP (oxidative level phosphorylation). Two molecules of ATP are also formed (from ADP + H_3PO_4) during glycolysis, from hydrolysis of 1,3-phosphoglyceric acid to 3-phosphoglyceric acid (substrate level oxidative phosphorylation) and hydrolysis of phosphoenol pyruvic acid to pyruvic acid. This is almost the entire yield of energy in fermentation.

All forms of exothermic reaction in living cells are sometimes referred to collectively as *biooxidations.*

Three other types of bacteria, differing in respect to oxygen requirements, deserve mention: (a) the microaerophils; (b) the indifferent organisms; and (c) the obligate aerobes.

Microaerophils require somewhat lowered oxygen pressures, neither complete anaerobiosis nor full aerobiosis. Probably certain of their enzymes are sensitive to atmospheric oxygen tension. Some pathogens are microaerophils, e.g., *Leptospira, Brucella* when first isolated.

Indifferent species can grow in the presence of air but do not contain cytochrome or the citric-acid cycle enzymes. Such species grow better in the absence of free oxygen than aerobically. They have no metabolic pathway to oxygen from glucose. They neither need nor utilize free oxygen, though they can use it for metabolizing glycerol to H_2O_2, which kills them because they do not produce catalase. Neither are they "poisoned" by free oxygen, as are strict anaerobes. They are *indifferent* to it. Examples are *Streptococcus pyogenes* and *Lactobacillus species.*

Strict or **obligate anaerobes** not only cannot grow but cannot survive in the presence of free oxygen. They are obliged to live in the absence of air (anaerobically). Their metabolism is entirely fermentative. Their sensitivity to free oxygen may depend on certain enzymes or conenzymes that are poisoned by oxygen or must remain in a reduced condition. Typically they do not produce catalase, which decomposes the highly toxic H_2O_2 that is produced by them in contact with O_2. Examples of strict anaerobes are *Clostridium tetani,* certain hemolytic streptococci and *Bacteroides* species. Anaerobic enzyme systems function only at low O–R potentials, e.g., −0.3 volt.

Cultivation of Anaerobes

Cultural conditions suitable for strictly anaerobic bacteria are found in the bottom of tubes filled to a depth of at least 10 cm. with chopped animal tissue and covered with broth containing 1 per cent glucose and heated to drive off air (oxygen) shortly before use, or in any organic or tissue medium *from which free oxygen is excluded.* A plating medium for isolating pure cultures of strict anaerobes consists of meat–infusion glucose agar containing a strong reducing substance, such as cysteine or sodium thioglycollate. In a hermetically sealed "anaerobic jar" device, using chemicals in a plastic pack *(Gaspak),* combination of oxygen with hydrogen is catalyzed at room temperature without use of electricity or exterior source of hydrogen.

Saprophytes

Not all chemo-organotrophs are pathogens. Some are of great value in dairy and fermentation industries, production of antibiotics, and so on. Many are indispensable as scavengers. They are called *saprophytes* (Gr. decay-plants). They inhabit the soil, the oceans and swamps, the intestinal tract and the outer surfaces of the body, the genital tract, the mouth and the nose. They do not commonly invade *live* tissues or blood, but some can grow in dead tissues, as in dirty wounds, or in certain foods, and cause disease by secreting toxins. Examples of the latter are *Clostridium tetani,* the cause of tetanus; *C. perfringens,* the gas bacillus involved in gas gangrene; and *C. botulinum,* the cause of botulism. Thus we may have noninvasive but highly *pathogenic saprophytes.*

Parasitic microorganisms include all species capable of growth in or on live tissues or the bloodstream. Their pathogenic potentialities range from virtual commensalism or mutualism (e.g., most coliform species, *Staphylococcus epidermidis*) through opportunism (e.g., *Proteus* sp., *Pseudomonas aeruginosa*) to high-grade virulence (e.g., *Yersinia pestis, Neisseria gonorrhoeae*). The first two groups are *opportunists* or *secondary invaders;* the last two species are *primary pathogens.*

A DESCRIPTIVE CHECK LIST OF BACTERIA OF MAJOR IMPORTANCE IN MEDICAL MICROBIOLOGY

I. Rods
  A. **Non-spore-forming**
    1. Gram-negative
      a. Enteric bacteria:
         The enteric bacteria include many genera, some of them normal flora and others (*Salmonella* and *Shigella*), exogenous and regularly pathogenic. Enteric organisms are aerobic, ferment a variety of carbohydrates and possess complex antigenic structures. Because on Gram stain they all look more or less alike, their identification rests on biochemical reactions and antigenic analysis and on susceptibility to colicins (e.g., *Pseudomonas*). All have endotoxin (LPS); some secrete potent enterotoxins. As a group, these organisms are responsible for a

large number of nosocomial infections, and many of them are resistant to multiple antibiotics because of their acquisition of drug-resistance plasmids. Most of the enteric organisms are opportunistic pathogens, particularly of the genitourinary tract and central nervous system, in burn patients and in the compromised host. For all these reasons, careful antibiotic sensitivity testing is central to effective antibacterial chemotherapy.

The main "relatedness" groups of enteric bacteria are:

Escherichia coli, (Shigella)
Klebsiella, Enterobacter, *Serratia* group
Arizona-*Edwardsiella*-Citrobacter, *(Salmonella)* group
Proteus-Providence *(Providencia)* group, including *P. rettgeri* and *P. morganii*
Pseudomonas group, the only strict aerobe among the enteric bacteria, with wide distribution in soil, water, sewage and air.
Vibrio—*Vibrio cholerae* causes cholera (a surface infection) in humans by elaboration of cholera toxin, which is similar to the toxins elaborated by enteropathogenic *E. coli. Campylobacter* (previously *Vibrio*) *fetus* elaborates no toxin, but causes gastroenteritis in infants and children and, occasionally, invasive infections with bacteremia.

b. Respiratory pathogens:
Haemophilus influenzae (very tiny; nonmotile; pleomorphic; aerobic; requires vitamins, hemin [X factor] and NADP [V factor]; chocolate agar); infant tracheobronchitis, meningitis, conjunctivitis.
Bordetella pertussis (morphologically like *H. influenzae;* requires cystine, methionine, and nicotinic acid; Bordet-Gengou medium, best on first isolation; use of penicillin to make the medium selective; hemolytic, pearl-like colonies identify by FA) whooping cough; related species are *B. parapertussis* and motile *B. bronchiseptica* (these do not require blood media).
c. Genitourinary pathogen:
Haemophilus ducreyi (morphologically

like *H. influenzae;* very fastidious nutritionally; hemolytic) chancroid.
d. Blood and tissue pathogens:
Brucella: suis (hogs); *abortus* (cattle); *melitensis* (goats and sheep) [all may infect man]; (blood-infusion broth or special agar of liver infusion, tryptone, etc., with CO_2 at pH 6.8; very tiny; nonmotile; facultative with $NaNO_3$) brucellosis or undulant fever in man.
Yersinia, pestis, Francisella tularensis (small rods; require ordinary rich media except *F. tularensis,* which requires egg or cystein with blood and glucose; distinctive bipolar staining in blood; arthropod-borne).
Mima polymorpha and *Herellea vaginicola:* identity moot; now are species of *Acinetobacter* or *Moraxella,* q.v. (ubiquitous in and on human body; tiny diplococcobacilli often resembling *Neisseria;* aerobic; catalase +; oxidase − except *M. polymorpha* var. *oxidans*) possibly minor pathogens or secondary invaders in many pathologic situations, especially conjunctivitis.
Bacteroides fragilis and other species (*strict* anaerobes; blood agar; motile or nonmotile; inhabit mouth and intestines) opportunists in various suppurative situations such as appendicitis, lung abscess, surgical wounds.
Pseudomonas pseudomallei (similar to *P. aeruginosa* but yellow, honey-like growth) melioidosis.
Spirillum minus (small; short; 3 to 7 tight spirals; *not* flexible); rapid rotatory and progressive motion; well-developed *polar* flagella; never cultivated in vitro) ratbite fever or sodoku, common in Japan; rare in North America *(S. Minor).*
2. *Gram-positive–nonsporulating*
a. Gastrointestinal pathogens: none common in U.S.A.; bovine tuberculosis elsewhere
b. Respiratory pathogens:
Corynebacterium diphtheriae (methylene blue stain: clublike, beaded and barred forms; soluble exotoxin) A-P toxoid prophyl. vs diphtheria, DTP (Table 5-21).

Mycobacterium tuberculosis (acid-fast; niacin +; nonmotile; obligate aerobe slow growth on Lowenstein-Jensen egg yolk–glycerine–malachite green medium; *rapid* growth in Dubos' fluid medium with Tween 80; virulent strains form "cords"; isoniazid sensitive; colonies dry and friable; not to be confused with *M. smegmatis* and *M. phlei* and "atypical" or Runyon-group species, which grow rapidly; bovine type of tubercle bacilli is used in BCG); tuberculosis.

c. *Mycobacterium laprae* (morphologically like *M. tuberculosis*); obligate intracellular parasite; intracellular in "lepra cells"; not cultivable on lifeless media.

d. Blood and tissue pathogens:
Listeria monocytogenes (a motile diphtheroid; blood agar with increased CO_2; slow growth); animal reservoir, especially sheep; listeriosis is a zoonosis; clinically protean including amnionitis and meningitis.

Actinomyces israelii (branching, filamentous bacterium; strictly anaerobic; found only in man [bovine species is *A. bovis*]; gram-positive but not acid-fast; "sulfur granules" in masses of "ray fungus" in pus) actinomycosis, penicillin-sensitive.

Nocardia asteroides, etc. (branching forms that readily fragment to bacillus-like or coccoid segments; gram-positive; *N. asteroides* and some others acid-fast in exudates; strictly aerobic; some species form "sulfur-granules" in pus) Madura foot or systemic and pulmonary nocardiosis.

B. Endospore forming (special spore stains required)
Endospores resist 15 minutes or longer boiling at 100 C. and 1 hour or more of dry heat at 150 C.
1. Gram-negative: none of medical importance
2. Gram-positive:
a. Aerobic or facultative (sporulate only in contact with free oxygen)
*Bacillus anthracis** (grows well on blood-free media; spores contaminate pastures, hides, wool) pulmonary anthrax or woolsorters' disease; malignant pustule; septicemia, toxemia.

b. Anaerobic or microaerophilic. (Spores form and germinate only under anaerobic conditions)
Clostridium species (all inhabit soil, many occur in animal feces; cultivable in thioglycollate media etc.; all pathogens motile except *C. perfringens*)
C. tetani fecally contaminated wounds; soluble exotoxin affects motor nerve endings; alum-precipitated toxoid prophyl. vs tetanus DTP (Table 5-21).
C. perfringens "gas bacillus"; associated with *C. novyi, C. histolyticum, C. septicum* and *C. tetani* in fecally contaminated, deep wounds; exotoxins are various proteolytic and saccharolytic enzymes, collagenases, and gas gangrene.
C. botulinum ("snow-shoe" sporulation; grows in soil-contaminated, improperly heat-processed, canned foods, forming exotoxin that causes flaccid paralysis; toxin destroyed by 80 C. in 15 minutes) botulism (infant, endogenous).

II. COCCI
A. Diplococci
1. Gram-negative:
Neisseria species ("coffee-bean" morphology; aerobic with added CO_2; colonies indophenol-oxidase-positive)
N. gonorrhoeae (*requires* "chocolate agar"* [or equivalent, e.g., Thayer-Martin selective agar with CO_2; grows only at 35 to 37 C.; culture essential for diagnosis in females and chronic cases; typically inside polymorphonuclear leukocytes; oxidase-positive colonies must be identified biochemically; maltose negative) gonorrhea, ophthalmia neonatorum, endocarditis, septic arthritis, proctitis, pharyngitis, meningitis. Penicillinase-producing strains.
N. meningitidis (culturally and morphologically like *N. gonorrhoeae* but ferments maltose; in leukocytes in spinal fluid) *epidemic* meningitis.

---

* Distinguish between the general use of the term "bacillus" in reference to any rod-shaped organism and the generic use of the term *Bacillus* in reference to the genus of aerobic spore-formers, e.g., *Bacillus anthracis.*

* Meat-infusion agar containing 5 per cent blood and heated at 90 C. for 15 minutes.

N. catarrhalis, flava, sicca etc. (respiratory "saprophytes"; grow well on blood-free media at 25 C.; opaque or pigmented colonies) must be distinguished from pathogenic *Neisseria* and *Veillonella* in vagina.

2. *Gram-positive:*

Streptococcus pneumoniae (viridans i.e., green zone [alpha] hemolytic-type colonies on blood agar; lancet-shaped cocci paired in type-specific polysaccharide capsules; swelling reaction with type-specific serum; optochin-sensitive; inulin +) lobar pneumonia, meningitis, otitis.

S. pyogenes (β-hemolytic, i.e., clear zones in blood agar pour plates; cell wall polysaccharides determine Lancefield groups A–U; type specificity determined by M or T cell wall proteins) scarlet fever, puerperal sepsis, septicemia, septic sore throat, pyoderma. Nonsuppurative sequelae to group A only: rheumatic fever, glomerulonephritis. Group B—neonatal sepsis, meningitis.

S. mitis, S. salivarius, S. faecalis (α-hemolytic or viridans blood agar type; slow growth on blood agar plates) direct etiologic role in dental plaque formation and dental caries; hematogenous endocarditis.

Enterococcus group (includes *Streptococcus faecalis* and its varieties *zymogenes* and *liquefaciens, S. faecium* and *S. durans;* alpha or beta type; Lancefield group D; intestinal; wide temperature range and resistant to environment of intestines; occur in sewage; *S. faecalis* an index of fecal pollution analogous to *Escherichia coli*) urinary tract infections, endocarditis.

Staphylococcus species (irregular clusters, pairs and single cocci; facultative; catalase +; anaerobic use of glucose and pyruvate; grow well on blood-free media at 20 to 40 C.) bacteriophage typing.

S. aureus (golden pigment; most of the pathogenic strains produce coagulase, leukocidin, hemolysin and other tissue-damaging factors; also ferment mannitol, produce DNase, and liquefy gelatin; penicillin-resistance due to production of penicillinase) nosocomial, pyogenic infections, thermostable enterotoxin causes food poisoning, toxic shock, and "scalded skin" syndromes. (Differentiate: exotoxin, endotoxin, enterotoxin.)

S. epidermidis (S. albus) (no pigment; coagulase not produced; culturally like *S. aureus*) commensal skin organism, opportunistic endocarditis.

III. HELICAL, *flexible* bacteria

Treponema species (4 to 14 close, regular spirals; tubular cell wound around an axial filament composed of bundles of modified polar flagella; best seen in darkfield; rotatory and flexing motion; pathogenic species morphologically indistinguishable; antigenically closely related; not cultivable in artificial media; the anaerobically cultivable Reiter treponeme is antigenically similar to *T. pallidum* but not virulent; *T. genitalis, T. microdentium* and other saprophytes can be confused morphologically with *T. pallidum* in darkfield) *T. pallidum,* syphilis and bejel; *T. pertenue,* yaws; *T. carateum,* pinta. Numerous saprophytic strains are cultivable in vitro.

Borrelia species (longer, coarser, more open and irregular spirals than *Treponema;* vigorous lashing motion; stain readily; gram-negative; not cultivable in nonliving media).

Leptospira species (thinnest [<0.2μm.] and most tightly coiled [12 to 24 turns] of the spirochetes; hooked ends; unifibrillar axial filament; rapid rotatory and progressive motion; readily cultivable in media with serum; microaerophilic; blood and tissue parasites), zoonoses source of human infection, "aseptic" meningitis.

L. icterohemorrhagiae Weil's disease or hemorrhagic jaundice.

IV. BACTERIA WITHOUT CELL WALLS: MYCOPLASMA, PLEUROPNEUMONIA-LIKE ORGANISMS (PPLO)

These organisms lack the enzymes that synthesize cell walls, the entire cell (except rare flagella) being enclosed within the thin, pliable, typically bacterial, cell membrane. In general, lack of the strong cell wall leaves them osmotically fragile (i.e., subject to osmotic rupture) unless suspended in special PPLO medium of increased osmotic pressure (e.g., 20 per cent serum, 3 per cent sucrose, etc.). Colonies on agar begin growth just below the surface and spread on the surface forming a foamy-looking colony with a fried-egg appearance. As a result of their pliable cell membrane, mycoplasmas are highly pleomorphic, forming cocci, branched filaments, ringforms, etc. Some of the forms are so minute as to be filterable. Lack of cell wall makes mycoplasmas totally resistant to antibiotics that inhibit cell wall formation: penicillin, cephalosporins, etc. They are very sensitive to surfactant substances such as soaps and bile and to tetracyclines. Except for *Mycoplasma pneumoniae*, they are nonhemolytic.

Over 30 species of genus *Mycoplasma* are recognized. These require sterols for growth. Some are associated with a variety of pathologic processes of man and lower vertebrates: *M. hominis*, *M. gallisepticum*, *M. arthritidis*, *M. agalactiae*, *M. pneumoniae*. *Ureaplasma urealyticum* causes "nongonococcal" urethritis (NGU). Of a second genus, *Acholeplasma*, most are saprophytes or of doubtful pathogenicity. They do not require sterols for growth and are osmotically very fragile (e.g., *A. laidlawi*).

V. **Minute Bacteria**; Obligate intracellular parasites. All are real bacteria, nonmotile, nonsporing rods or cocci, 0.3–0.6 μm by 0.8–2.0 μm. Two Orders are now recognized: Rickettsiales and Chlamydiales.

Order I. *Rickettsiales*. Of three Families containing some seventeen genera, only two (Genus *Rickettsia* and Genus *Coxiella*) contain human pathogens of general importance though several are of veterinary importance.

Genus *Rickettsia* (not filterable; normally only arthropod-borne; can synthesize their own ATP) Typhus, Rocky Mountain spotted fever, etc.

Genus *Coxiella* (much like *Rickettsia* but filterable: raw milk, dust of barns and cattle yards, infected lochia, etc.; probably also several species of ticks) Q fever *(C. burneti)*

Order II. *Chlamydiales*. *Chlamydia trachomatis*: trachoma, inclusion conjunctivitis, infant pneumonia (perinatal), lymphogranuloma venereum (L). Nongonoccocal urethritis, salpingitis (D–K), well-defined glycogen-rich in-

clusions, sensitive to sulfonamide, tetracyclines.

C. Psittaci: Ornithosis (many species of mammals and birds), no glycogen in inclusions, insensitive to sulfonamide, sensitive to tetracyclines.

Bartonella bacilliformis: Oroya fever, verruga peruana.

STERILIZATION AND DISINFECTION

Sterilization

In relation to microbiology, sterilization means the destruction of all life. It is often incorrectly used interchangeably with disinfection, which means the destruction of *pathogenic* organisms. Thus, milk that is pasteurized (heated at 63 C. for 30 minutes and quickly cooled) is disinfected but is not sterile, since many common harmless organisms and spores resist this heating process.

Disinfection

A disinfectant is a substance that kills pathogenic microorganisms but is generally understood not to be sporicidal. A sporicidal disinfectant would also be a sterilizing agent, e.g., ethylene oxide, betapropiolactone.

Chemical disinfectants are indiscriminately poisonous. They may combine in cells with a variety of chemical groups, e.g., carboxyl, sulfhydryl and hydroxyl. They may act by (a) injuring cell membranes (especially lipid components), causing leakages, rupture or both, e.g., lipid solvents like ethyl or propyl alcohol or emulsifying agents like cationic detergents, (e.g., Zephiran) and other surfactants like phenolic compounds, (e.g., hexachlorophene, Lysol, Creolin); (b) chemically or physically altering enzymes and other proteins and DNA by breaking hydrogen and sulfide bonds and causing denaturation, coagulation, precipitation (e.g., phenolics, heavy metals like organic mercurials and $AgNO3$); (c) oxidizing cell components, e.g., $KMnO4$; chlorine free or loosely combined as chloramines ($CL_2 + H_2O = HOCl + H^+ + Cl^-$; HOCl a potent oxidizer); (d) toxic combinations, as with I in surfactant iodophors (e.g., *Wescodyne*) or alkylations as in the presence of ethylene oxide. In many instances the action of any agent is not clearly of one type or another but a combination of effects on different cell components. Factors that affect the action of any disinfectant are: kind, numbers and age of bacterial cells present, pH, temperature, time of exposure, concentration. In general, within limits, increase of any of the physical factors increases disinfectant action.

Sepsis; Antiseptic

Sepsis means the presence of pathogenic organisms growing in the tissues or blood. An antiseptic, strictly speaking, is a substance that combats sepsis but is generally thought of as a microbicidal or microbistatic substance applicable to exposed *living* tissues without undue damage to the tissues; e.g., as dilute alcohol, surfactant compounds of iodine (iodophors), *mild* tincture of iodine, and some organic mercurials. Antiseptics are not used internally. The terms antiseptic and disinfectant are often loosely used interchangeably.

Asepsis, strictly speaking, means absence of sepsis, but generally it is used to mean the absence of any living organisms. *Aseptic technique* is any procedure designed to eliminate live organisms and to keep them away. Modern surgical and microbiologic procedures are based on aseptic technique.

METHODS

Sterilization may be accomplished by (1) heat; (2) mechanical means such as filtration; (3) use of sporicidal chemicals, notably ethylene oxide and betapropiolactone. Less widely used are penetrating, ionizing radiations in dosages of 2.5 mrad, chiefly for sterilization of heat-labile drugs, surgical equipment, etc. Ultraviolet (about 260 nm.) has little power of penetration and is best used to control contamination by dust in air in enclosed spaces like meat warehouses.

Dry Heat

A. *Incineration.* Useful for bandages, paper dishes, sputum cups, etc.
B. *Oven Baking.* Useful for articles not containing water or that may be injured by steam. Applied usually to laboratory glassware and to materials not readily permeable by steam, such as petrolatum, mineral oil, sand, wooden articles and glass syringes. A temperature of 165 C. for at least 2 hours is necessary to kill all spores.

Moist Heat

A. *Boiling* (100 C. at sea level). Some bacterial spores can survive 90 minutes or more of boiling. Hepatitis viruses can survive at least 10 minutes of boiling and probably longer. Therefore, boiling is not satisfactory as a means of *sterilization* under ordinary circumstances. Boiling for 10 minutes is suitable for *disinfection* in situations from which (1) spores of pathogenic bacteria and (2) hepatitis viruses are known to be *absent.*

B. *Fractional or Intermittent Sterilization* (also called *tyndallization* after Tyndall, British physicist). This consists of the application of free steam at 100 C. for 10 to 30 minutes on 3 successive days, with incubation at about 23 C. between heatings. Vegetative (non-spore-containing) microorganisms and spores that have germinated are killed at each heating. Fractional sterilization is necessary only for solutions that are injured by temperatures higher than 100 C. It is not in common use.

C. *Autoclaving.* Steam, when compressed, is much hotter than free steam, and at 15 pounds pressure has a temperature of 121 C. An autoclave is a vessel that may be closed hermetically so as to exclude all air but retain steam under pressure. An ordinary household pressure cooker is a miniature autoclave capable of perfect sterilization.

In autoclaving, steam pressure of 15 to 20 pounds is usually applied from 10 to 30 minutes. All *air* must escape and all space filled with *steam.* Air does not reach the desired temperature. Also, since steam is depended on to bring about *hydrolysis* of bacteria and their spores, mixture with dry air reduces the effectiveness of the process. Autoclaving is generally used for culture media, saline solutions, etc., for surgical supplies, for solutions intended for intravenous injections, and for bandages, dressings, etc. Glassware is often autoclaved. Autoclaving is not used for oils, petrolatum, etc., which cannot absorb steam and therefore remain dry.

Sporicidal Vapors

A. *Formaldehyde* vapor is sometimes used to disinfect (sterilize?) interiors of rooms, ships, etc., but has the disadvantage of polymerizing (paraformaldehyde) on surfaces and being difficult to remove. In high concentration it is sporicidal. It is commonly used dissolved 37 per cent (weight) in water as Formalin or Formol for tissue fixation and embalming.

B. *Ethylene Oxide,* an alkylating agent, is used, diluted about 1:10 with CO_2 or other vapor to reduce toxicity and inflammability, inside autoclaves under conditions of controlled concentration (around 500 mg. per l. of air), pressure (around 10 lb.), temperature (around 130 F. or 55 C.) and relative humidity (around 40 per cent). It is effective but rather expensive and is useful mainly for objects that are damaged by ordinary methods of heat sterilization.

C. *Betapropiolactone,* liquid at room temperatures, forms a sporicidal vapor in concentrations around 1.5 mg. per l. of air at relative humidities around 80 per cent and temperatures around 25 C. It does not penetrate surgical packets, etc., very well. It is used principally as a substitute for formaldehyde, not for ethylene oxide. It has a tendency to polymerize.

Filtration

Fine-pored filters, long used for mechanical sterilization [e.g., cellulose mixed with asbestos (Seitz disks); sintered (fused) granular glass], have been supplanted by paper-thin membrane filters that depend chiefly on pore size (about 12 to 0.22 μm.) for mechanical sieve action, especially if the perforations in the filters have been made by regulated nuclear bombardment. Such filters also serve to collect microorganisms from fluids for microscopic examination or cultivation directly on the filter when placed on pads saturated with culture medium, often selective media.

MICROBISTASIS (BACTERIOSTASIS)

By this term is meant nonlethal inhibition of growth of microorganisms for hours, days or years, generally by interfering with certain enzyme functions. Microbistatic agents may be physical, e.g., refrigeration, freeze-drying, pickling brines or dehydration, or chemical, e.g., various aniline dyes in media, antibodies, antibiotics, sulfonamide drugs. In selective bacteriostasis in the diagnostic laboratory, such agents are used to inhibit growth of undesired contaminants in specimens such as feces or sputum and permit the desired species to grow. Microbistasis is an inexact term, since, if microorganisms are held "static" long enough, they eventually die, though they may survive for many years under some microbistatic conditions, such as freeze-drying.

Microbistasis is characteristically reversible, e.g., by chemical neutralization of the bacteriostatic agent (Hg + H$_2$S); mechanical removal (washing or dilution); cessation (warming of frozen cells); or rehydrating dried cells.

Surface Disinfection

By this is meant the application of solutions of microbicidal surfactant substances, such as saponated cresols, that are adsorbed on surfaces of floors, furniture, etc., exerting a prolonged disinfectant action. Hexachlorophene is such a substance. It is commonly com-

bined in hand soaps for surgical and hospital use. The cationic quaternary ammonium compounds such as Zephiran have similar properties.

ANTIBIOTICS

Antimicrobial agents used in the treatment of infectious diseases must have deleterious effects on the microorganism with little toxicity for host tissue. This difference in selective toxicity is expressed quantitatively as the therapeutic index. Selective toxicity is based on the binding of the drug to a microbial structure or protein that is either absent or significantly different from its counterpart in mammalian tissue. Metabolic pathways producing carbohydrate intermediates and energy are similar in microbial and mammalian cells and are not the usual targets for chemotherapeutic agents. The procaryotic ribosome is much smaller than its eucaryotic counterpart (70 s vs. 80s) and is a key target for antimicrobial agents. The peptidoglycan layer of the bacterial cell wall is unique to microorganisms and its synthesis is a prime target. Differences between eucaryotes and procaryotes with respect to cell membranes and nucleic acid synthesis, although subtle, are sufficiently distinctive to provide a basis for selective toxicity of chemotherapeutic agents.

Mode of Action of Cell Wall Inhibitors

The drugs that inhibit cell wall synthesis are listed in Table 5-1. The inhibition of peptidoglycan synthesis is usually a lethal event for a bacterium because the process of adding new material to the wall is coupled with autolytic digestion of the wall at the anticipated growth sites. In the absence of synthesis, the continuation of enzymatic digestion weakens the wall until osmotic pressure causes bursting of the cytoplasmic membrane. Cells can survive inhibition of cell wall synthesis if the autolytic enzymes are not functioning, as in nongrowing cells. They can survive also in spite of wall digestion if the osmotic pressure is not sufficient to force lysis, a condition occurring in hypertonic solutions (e.g., pus). These factors support the need for wound drainage concurrent with the institution of antimicrobial therapy.

The process of cell wall synthesis must be understood to appreciate the activity of various antimicrobials. The process includes a cytoplasmic component leading to the synthesis of a peptidoglycan subunit, secretion of this subunit through the cytoplasmic membrane into the periplasmic space, and finally enzymatic addition and cross-linking of the subunit to the growing portion of the peptidoglycan. Each of these three major sets

TABLE 5-1. Antimicrobial Agents That Inhibit Cell Wall Synthesis

Drug	Chemical Group	1° Site of Binding	Activity Blocked	Active On	Adverse Reactions	Sensitivity to β-Lactamases
Penicillin G	β-lactam ring	Periplasmic space (cross-linking enzyme)	Blocks peptidoglycan cross-linking (cidal)	Gram-positive, fastidious gram-negative	Hypersensitivity develops to all penicillins	Gram-positive and gram-negative
Penicillin V	β-lactam ring	Periplasmic space	Blocks peptidoglycan cross-linking	Gram-positive, fastidious gram-negative	Hypersensitivity develops to all penicillins	Gram-positive and gram-negative
Methicillin, Nafcillin, Oxacillin	β-lactam ring	Periplasmic space	Blocks peptidoglycan cross-linking	Staph and other gram-positive	Hypersensitivity develops to all penicillins	Resistant to penicillinase
Ampicillin	β-lactam ring	Periplasmic space	Blocks peptidoglycan cross-linking	Broad spectrum	Hypersensitivity develops to all penicillins	Sensitive to most
Carbenicillin	β-lactam ring	Periplasmic space	Blocks peptidoglycan cross-linking	Broad spectrum (Pseudomonas)	Hypersensitivity develops to all penicillins	Resistant to some gram-negative enzymes
Cephalothin	β-lactam ring	Periplasmic space	Blocks peptidoglycan cross-linking	Broad spectrum	Hypersensitivity to all cephalosporins	Sensitive to many gram-negative enzymes
Cefamandole, Cefoxitin	β-lactam ring	Periplasmic space	Blocks peptidoglycan cross-linking	Broad spectrum	Hypersensitivity to all cephalosporins	Resistant to most
Cycloserine	D-alanine analog	Cytoplasmic enzyme	Inhibits conversion of D-alanine to L-alanine for subunit synthesis	Gram-positive		
Bacitracin	Polypeptide	Cytoplasmic lipid	Inhibits subunit synthesis	Gram-positive	Limited to topical use	
Vancomycin		Cell membrane	Blocks secretion of cell wall subunit	Gram-positive		

of reactions is subject to selective interference by various antimicrobials. Synthesis of the subunit is blocked by cycloserine and bacitracin. Secretion through the membrane is blocked by vancomycin. Cross-linking of the subunit is blocked by penicillins, semisynthetic penicillins and cephalosporins.

No antimicrobial agent has effects on all types of microorganisms. There are whole classes or genera of organisms none of which are ever found sensitive to a particular drug. These organisms are considered to be inherently insensitive to that drug. On the other hand, most isolates of a given genus or species may be sensitive to a given drug, but occasional isolates are found not to be. These exceptions are generally designated as being resistant, that is, insusceptible to concentrations of drug that inhibit other strains of the same organism. Accordingly, the sensitivity of a group of microbes can generally be predicted because it is due to physiologic or structural traits common to all members of that group. Strains resistant to a given drug occur at rates that cannot always be predicted.

Careful *in vitro* susceptibility testing of each isolate is therefore required.

Problems of Insensitivity and Resistance Related to Antimicrobials Affecting Cell Wall Synthesis

Most gram-negative organisms are insensitive to clinically attainable levels of penicillin G and V. This insensitivity is determined by the impermeability of the lipopolysaccharide layer of the cell wall. Most gram-positive organisms and some of the fastidious gram-negative bacteria allow the penicillins to reach the periplasmic space and exert their lethal action. Some strains of these normally sensitive species resist penicillin because they lack certain proteins in the periplasmic space or because they produce penicillinase. Penicillinase cleaves the β-lactam ring of the penicillin molecule to form penicilloic acid, thereby completely eliminating the activity of the drug. The pencillinases of gram-positive organisms tend to be inducible exoenzymes, whereas the penicillinases of gram-negative organisms remain in the periplasmic space and can be constitutive. Each penicillinase has a range of substrates, most semisynthetic penicillins and cephalosporins being subject to digestion by penicillinases. Chemical substitutions that lead to the protection of the β-lactam ring are partial solutions to the chemotherapeutic problems posed by penicillinase. Nafcillin, methicillin and oxacillin are resistant to penicillinases common in *Staphylococcus aureus*. Carbenicillin resists some penicillinases of gram-negative rods. Some of the new cephalosporins, for example, cefoxitin and cefamandole, resist a wide variety of penicillinases.

The similarity between penicillins and cephalosporins includes their mechanisms of action but fortunately excludes to a large degree their haptenic properties. Penicillin, like almost all antimicrobial agents, following combination with host proteins, can induce hypersensitivity to the penicillin molecule. A person allergic to penicillin G produces an allergic reaction when exposed to semisynthetic penicillins (i.e., nafcillin, oxacillin, ampicillin). Fortunately, such hypersensitive individuals fail in most cases to react with cephalosporins. Atopic individuals however can become hypersensitive to cephalosporins as well as to any of the other drugs.

Vancomycin inhibits cell wall synthesis by blocking the secretion of peptidoglycan subunits into the periplasmic space. Vancomycin should be held in reserve as a valuable drug for use against gram-positive organisms resistant to penicillins and other antimicrobial agents.

Bacitracin and cycloserine, in the bacterial cytoplasm, inhibit cell wall synthesis by different mechanisms. Bacitracin limits the availability of a lipid carrier, the functions of which include binding of newly formed subunits to the internal surface of the cytoplasmic membrane. Cycloserine inhibits synthesis of subunits by blocking the enzymatic conversion of L-alanine to D-alanine.

Mode of Action of Drugs Affecting Synthesis of Nucleic Acids

During synthesis, DNA may be cleaved at specific points by endonucleases, which thus allow modifications to be introduced, provided that normal repair mechanisms can act to reconstitute the integrity of the molecule. If normal DNA repair mechanisms are blocked, the nicks caused by endonucleases are lethal to the microorganism.

The inhibitors of nucleic acids act either at the macromolecular level or on the synthesis of nucleic acid bases (Table 5-2).

Two drugs that function at the macromolecular level are *nalidixic acid* and *rifampicin*. Nalidixic acid exerts a bactericidal effect on gram-negative organisms by blocking one enzyme required for normal DNA synthesis. Nalidixic acid binds to the enzyme gyrase, the functions of which include the unwinding of tightly coiled regions of DNA during DNA synthesis. Gyrase-mediated unwinding of DNA is induced by cutting the DNA and allowing relaxation of supercoils and then repair of the nicks. Nalidixic acid binding to this bifunctional enzyme allows the DNA nicking to continue but inhibits repair of the nicks. The action of *rifampicin* requires its binding to DNA-dependent RNA polymerase of bacteria. This enzyme is composed of a core of four protein subunits plus a separate regulatory protein, sigma (σ). Synthesis of messenger RNA (mRNA) by this enzyme begins when the core binds to the promoter region of a bacterial operon. However, construction of the mRNA requires the binding of protein to the core portion of the enzyme. Rifampicin binds to the core portion of the enzyme, inhibiting the core–sigma interaction required for mRNA synthesis.

The synthesis of nucleic acid bases in bacteria requires the addition of single carbon units, a reaction mediated by folic acid. Folic acid is synthesized *de novo* in bacterial cells but not in eucaryotic cells, in which it is only consumed or enzymatically modified. Two important enzymatic reactions involved in the synthesis of bacterial folic acid are sensitive to chemotherapeutic agents. The conversion of para-aminobenzoic acid to dihydrofolic acid, a reaction mediated by dihydrofolic acid synthetase, is sensitive to competitive inhibition by "sulfa" drugs, e.g., sulfanilamide. These drugs do not affect the mammalian cell, which, because it lacks mechanisms for primary synthesis, has a nutritional requirement for dihydrofolic acid.

The second enzymatic reaction in folic acid synthesis that is sensitive to antimicrobial agents is the conversion of dihydrofolic acid to tetrahydrofolic acid. Dihydrofolic acid reductase mediates this reaction in both eucaryotic and bacterial cells. The drug trimethoprim binds about 10,000 times more avidly to the bacterial than to the mammalian enzyme because of differences in structure between the two species of protein. Bacteriostatic concentrations of the drug are therefore well tolerated by the eucaryotic cell. Both sulfonamides and trimethoprim effect a folic acid deficiency; but because they act at different stages in the pathway, a mixture of the two drugs generates a synergistic antibacterial effect. Griseofulvin is an analogue of the purine base, guanosine, and inhibits DNA synthesis by a mechanism that is not clear.

TABLE 5-2. Antimicrobial Agents Affecting Membrane or Nucleic Acid Synthesis

Name	Chemical Feature	Site of Binding	Activity Blocked	Range of Activity
Polymyxins, Gramicidin	Polypeptide ring	Cell membrane	Retention of cytoplasm	Gram-positive and gram-negative
Nystatin, Amphotericin	Polyene	Cell membrane	Retention of cytoplasm	Fungi
Sulfanilamide	PABA-analog	Cytoplasmic enzyme (dihydrofolic acid synthetase)	Purine and thymidine shortages block RNA and DNA synthesis	Broad
Trimethoprim	—	Cytoplasmic enzymes (dihydrofolic acid reductase)	Purine and thymidine shortages block RNA and DNA synthesis	Broad
Griseofulvin	Guanosine analog	Unknown	DNA replication	Fungi
Rifampicins	Semisynthetic Macrolide	Cytoplasmic enzyme (RNA polymerase)	Transcription of mRNA	Broad
Nalidixic acid	—	Cytoplasmic enzyme (gyrase)	Inhibits DNA unwinding needed for DNA synthesis	Gram-negative
Nitrofurantoin	—	Reduced by microorganisms and reacts with DNA	Integrity of DNA replication	Broad
Metronidazole	—	Reduced by microorganisms and reacts with DNA	Integrity of DNA replication	Anaerobes

Mode of Action of Drugs Directly Affecting Cell Membranes

Microbial cell membranes resemble those of eucaryotic cells in general organization and chemistry. This fact makes it likely that drugs designed to act directly on cell membrane structure would be unacceptably toxic. However, there are subtle differences that permit selective binding of certain antimicrobial agents (e.g., lack of sterols in bacterial membranes) (Table 5-2). Polymyxins and gramicidin bind to bacterial membranes and cause reorganization of phospholipids around the drug, thereby introducing sites of ionic leakage. Unlike many other bactericidal agents, the polymyxins exert an almost immediately lethal effect, in this respect resembling the action of detergents.

Nystatin (Mycostatin) and amphotericin interact in a detergent-like manner with the membrane of susceptible fungi. The toxicity of nystatin for host tissue limits its application to treatment of surface infections.

Mode of Action of Drugs Affecting Protein Synthesis

Protein synthesis in bacteria begins when the 30s portion of ribosomes, through the action of soluble initiation proteins, binds to mRNA (Table 5-4). The amino acids to be linked into a protein are each bound to species of transfer RNA (tRNA) that in turn recognize specific sequences in mRNA. The binding of tRNA, charged with amino acids, to the 30s portion of the ribosome–mRNA complex is the first stage of protein synthesis susceptible to antibiotic action. Drugs that bind to the 30s subunit and block tRNA recognition include aminoglycosides, spectinomycin, and tetracycline (Table 5-3).

The formation of peptide bonds requires both 30s and 50s portions of the ribosome. The actual formation of peptide bonds may be blocked by certain drugs, such as chloramphenicol, lincomycin and clindamycin, which bind to the 50s subunit.

In the normal process of protein synthesis, the ribosome moves relative to the mRNA (i.e., translocates), a reaction that requires soluble proteins and GTP for energy. Erythromycin blocks translocation by binding to proteins comprising the 50s subunit. Fusidic acid blocks translocation by binding to one of the soluble proteins (elongation factor G) involved in energizing the movement.

The consequences, to the bacterium, of inhibition of protein synthesis, vary depending upon the manner in which the process is inhibited. Inhibition by chlor-

TABLE 5-3. Antimicrobial Agents Blocking Protein Synthesis

Drug	Chemical	1° Site of Binding	Step Blocked	Range of Activity
Streptomycin, Neomycin, Kanamycin, Gentamicin, Tobramycin, Amikacin	Aminoglycoside	30s ribosomal subunit	Binding of tRNA to ribosome	Broad spectrum
Spectinomycin	Aminocyclitol	30s ribosomal subunit	Binding of tRNA to ribosome	Broad spectrum
Tetracycline	—	30s ribosomal subunit	Binding of tRNA to ribosome	Broad spectrum
Chloramphenicol	—	50s ribosomal subunit	Formation of peptide bond	Broad spectrum
Lincomycin	Macrolide	50s ribosomal subunit	Formation of peptide bond	Gram-positive
Clindamycin	Macrolide	50s ribosomal subunit	Formation of peptide bond	Broad (anaerobes) spectrum
Erythromycin	Macrolide	50s ribosomal subunit	Translocation of ribosome on mRNA	Broad spectrum
Fusidic acid	—	Cytoplasmic soluble protein (elongation factor)	Translocation of ribosome on mRNA	Gram-positive

amphenicol is completely reversible and is therefore only bacteriostatic. This implies that continuous protein synthesis *per se* is not absolutely required for bacterial survival. An antibiotic such as streptomycin binds irreversibly to the ribosome, thereby causing nearly complete inhibition of protein synthesis, and hence causing death of the bacterium. The killing effect is related to the production of "mis-sense" proteins, which are synthesized in the presence of the drug and which misfunction because of incorrect amino acid sequences caused by drug-induced alterations of the ribosome. Mis-sense proteins in the cell lead to changes in internal structures or enzymes, thus accounting for the death of the cell.

MAJOR MECHANISMS OF ANTIBIOTIC RESISTANCE

Changes in the structural or physiologic components of an organism that occur by mutation can result in resistance to antibiotics. Significant levels of resistance may occur after a single mutation or after a series of mutations. Antimicrobial drugs do not themselves induce mutation(s), but select out those organisms that have undergone mutation. This sequence is the most common mechanism of resistance to vancomycin, rifampicin, nalidixic acid, and polymyxins. Although resistance to other drugs can emerge as a result of

bacterial mutation, acquisition of specific plasmids more often accounts for observed changes in sensitivity to drugs (Table 5-4).

Resistance plasmids (R) govern their own replication and confer resistance on the bacterial host cell. Plasmids that in addition contain a set of transfer genes are called resistance transfer factors (RFT) because they mediate conjugation. R and RTF plasmids thus differ in size and in ability to initiate conjugation. One bacterium can accommodate a variety of plasmids, and it is not uncommon to encounter mixtures of R and RTF plasmids in a single organism. R plasmids, although unable to initiate conjugation, can be transferred by conjugation mediated by an RTF in the same organism. In the absence of an RTF, the R plasmid can be transferred only when the organism is infected with a bacteriophage capable of generalized transduction. Because RTF plasmids are not encountered in *Staphylococcus,* the transfer of R plasmids in this organism is dependent on phage. In enteric bacteria, hemophilus and a variety of other organisms, transfer of R plasmids occurs by either RTF-mediated conjugation or by transduction.

The resistance to antibiotics that is mediated by R and RTF plasmids is determined by a protein product of the plasmid. In the case of penicillins and cephalosporins, this protein has β-lactamase activity and destroys the antibiotic in the periplasmic space or outside

TABLE 5-4. Major Mechanisms of Specific Antibiotic Resistance

Drug	Mechanism of Resistance	Genetic Basis of Resistance
Penicillin	β-lactamase	Plasmid*
Ampicillin	β-lactamase	Plasmid*
Cephalothin	β-lactamase	Plasmid*
Methicillin	Impermeability	Plasmid
Vancomycin	Membrane alteration	Chromosome (mutation)
Sulfanilamide	Novel dihydrofolic acid synthetase	Plasmid*
Trimethoprim	Novel dihydrofolic acid synthetase	Plasmid
Rifampicin	Altered RNA polymerase	Chromosome (mutation)
Nalidixic acid	Altered gyrase enzyme	Chromosome (mutation
Polymixins	Altered membrane components	Chromosome (mutation)
Aminoglycosides	Antibiotic-modifying enzyme	Plasmid*
Spectinomycin	Antibiotic-modifying enzyme	Plasmid
Tetracycline	Permeability barrier	Plasmid*
Chloramphenicol	Antibiotic-modifying enzyme	Plasmid*
Lincomycin	Ribosome-modifying enzyme	Plasmid
Clindamycin	Ribosome-modifying enzyme	Plasmid
Erythromycin	Ribosome-modifying enzyme	Plasmid

* Resistance may be part of a transposon.

of the cell wall. Chloramphenicol, aminoglycosides and spectinomycin are inactivated because the plasmid protein in the periplasmic space mediates the enzymatic attachment of acetyl, phosphate or adenyl groups. Lincomycin, clindamycin and erythromycin are inactivated because the plasmid protein mediates the enzymatic methylation of an RNA molecule in the ribosome, methylation inhibiting the binding of drug to the ribosome. The plasmid product in some way reduces the uptake of tetracycline drug into the bacterium. In the case of folic acid inhibitors, the plasmid product is a pathway enzyme that is not competitively inhibited by the drug as is the chromosomally produced enzyme.

The single product of a plasmid in some cases reacts with a variety of compounds, that is, a given β-lactamase may destroy ampicillin, penicillin G and cephalothin, or a given aminoglycoside-modifying enzyme may react with kanamycin, gentamicin and tobramycin. Thus the expression of resistance to several related drugs is often mediated by one gene product of the plasmid. A single plasmid may contain multiple genes each mediating resistance(s). Because a bacterium can harbor numerous plasmids, the emergence of genetically complex and highly resistant strains is encountered in environments subject to the powerful selective pressure of multiple antibiotics (e.g., a hosptial).

One further complication introduced by R and RTF plasmids is that the plasmid gene responsible for resistance may comprise a transposon. A transposon is capable of "hopping" from the plasmid on which it entered a bacterium to another plasmid, to the chromosome, or even to the DNA of a phage that infects the same cell. Hopping of transposons accounts for the spread of resistance to organisms that are otherwise unable to support the replication of the plasmid originally harboring the resistance gene. This process accounts for the spread of β-lactamase genes from plasmids of enteric bacteria to species of *Hemophilus* and *Neisseria*.

METHODS FOR TESTING BACTERIAL SENSITIVITY TO ANTIBIOTICS

Because of occasional adverse side effects and increasing emergence of antibiotic-resistant organisms, chemotherapeutic agents must be used in critical fashion to safeguard their clinical efficacy. The purpose of testing an organism for sensitivity to several antibiotics is to allow the physician some latitude in the ultimate choice of therapy. This consideration may be important in avoiding undesirable complications attending the use of a particular drug in a given patient (e.g., allergy) and to offer a choice of potentially effective substitutes. The selection of drugs to be tested is based primarily on knowledge of the infection, that is, whether it is in the urinary tract, blood, localized pus or spinal fluid. In this connection, a carefully done Gram stain, particularly of pus, spinal fluid and unspun urine correctly collected, yields vital information about the initial choice of antibiotics that will then be confirmed or modified on the basis of results of sensitivity testing of the organism(s) in question.

The widely used Kirby-Bauer method is based on the inhibition of surface bacterial growth under standard conditions. Several colonies of the organism to be tested are inoculated into Todd-Hewitt broth and grown to a standard optical density. Inoculum from this culture is then spread across the surface of a nutrient agar plate in a manner that gives heavy confluent growth. Disks containing antibiotics are then placed on the agar. After incubation, the diameter of the zone of growth inhibition around each antibiotic disk is measured. Each organism is then scored as sensitive, intermediate or resistant, according to the size of the zone of inhibition, which is a direct function of the sensitivity of the organism to the antibiotic. However, other factors also affect the zone size (e.g., diffusion, stability and concentration of the drug, characteristics of the particular organism, size of inoculum) that collectively impose upper and lower limits within which variations in sensitivity among individual strains of a bacterial species can be judged. Infections due to organisms designated as sensitive to a given antibiotic are more likely to yield clinically to that antibiotic than are infections with strains designated as intermediate or resistant.

It is sometimes important to determine accurately the concentration of an antibiotic that must be achieved to inhibit a particular microorganism. For such determinations, the tube dilution method is employed in addition to the Kirby-Bauer method. In this procedure, an antibiotic is serially diluted in growth medium and inoculated with relatively small numbers (10^5/ml.) of a particular organism. The lowest concentration of antibiotic that prevents bacterial growth (turbidity) is the minimal inhibitory concentration (MIC).

For antibiotics that are bactericidal, the bactericidal endpoint can be determined by subculturing the tubes in which there is no turbidity and in which viable organisms from the inoculum may have survived. The bactericidal concentration is higher than the bacteriostatic. The MIC refers to the bacteriostatic endpoint. The minimal lethal concentration (MLC) refers to the bactericidal endpoint.

HISTORICAL NOTES

Francesco Redi (1668) demonstrated that maggots in meat came from eggs laid by flies and not from spontaneous generation as generally believed at that time.

Antonj van Leeuwenhoek (1672), Dutch merchant and amateur lens maker, was the first to see and de-scribe bacteria and protozoa. He called them all animalcules, or "little animals," and is often called the "father of bacteriology and protozoology."

Joblot (1718) and **Lazaro Spallanzani** (1765), studying putrefaction and fermentation (at that time thought to be spontaneous chemical changes), placed putrescible fluids, such as meat soup, urine, or hay infusion, in closed flasks, heated them, and observed that no putrefaction occurred as it did in similar flasks that afterward were opened and exposed to the air. This was explained on the basis that the cause of the spoilage was living beings (like Leeuwenhoek's animalcules) in the air. **John Turberville Needham** (1749) had obtained different results and opposed this view, stating that heating destroyed a "vital principle" in the fusions and that the "animalcules" seen in the spoiled material formed spontaneously as a result of a chemical reaction when air was admitted, and failed to form when air was withheld.

Edward Jenner, in 1798 and 1806, demonstrated that inoculation with active cow pox vesical material conferred immunity to smallpox. Recently published evidence (Vela, G. R., and Coomes, M., Amer. Soc. Microbiol. News., 1973, 39 [Nov.]: 735) indicates that Jenner's discovery and work were antedated in 1774 and 1805 by an intelligent farmer, Benjamin Jesty (1737–1816) of Yetminster, southern England.

Schultze (1836) and **Schwann** (1837) admitted air to heated infusions and showed that even then no animalcules developed if the air was passed through strong acid or alkali or through red-hot glass tubes. These experiments were criticized on the ground that the acid, the alkali and the heat destroyed a mysterious "vital principle" in the air.

Schröder and **von Dusch** (1854) admitted, to heated infusions, air that was not treated in any way but merely filtered through cotton wool. (The present use of cotton plugs in bacteriology probably had its origin in these experiments.) The infusions remained sterile, but the idea of spontaneous generation of "animalcules'" persisted.

Louis Pasteur (1822–1895), French chemist, interested in the cause of spoilage ("diseases") of beer and wines, entered the controversy concerning spontaneous generation and finally refuted the doctrine by heating infusions in flasks with long, down-twisted necks that excluded dust but were open to the air without any substance between the outer air and the infusion. Such flasks remained sterile until dust was put into them. Pasteur later became interested in the analogy between diseases of beer and wine and human disease and formulated anew the old idea that disease was caused by invasive microorganisms. His later works were chiefly in the field of immunology, and he discovered most of the basic facts of immunity and devised methods of immunizing against anthrax, rabies and other diseases. He is often called the "father of immunology."

Joseph Lister (1827–1912), English physician and scientist, contemporary with Pasteur and well acquainted with his ideas on dust in the air as a source of contaminating organisms, conceived the idea of using phenol solutions on surgical wounds to prevent sepsis and, later, of operating in an atmosphere filled with phenol-solution mist. This opened the door to antiseptic surgery and later to aseptic surgery. Lister is the "father of modern aseptic surgery."

Robert Koch (1843–1910), (Nobel Prize winner), German physician, interested in bacteria as the cause of disease, worked with anthrax and later became famous as the discoverer of the tubercle bacillus, the cholera vibrio and other organisms causing disease. Koch was very critical of his own results when claiming to have discovered the causative agent of a disease. He established four criteria (Koch's postulates) for judging an organism as a true etiologic agent. These were:

1. The organism should be constantly present in the pathologic condition.
2. It should be isolated in pure culture from the pathologic material.
3. When inoculated in pure culture into suitable animals it should reproduce the pathologic conditions.
4. It should be recovered in pure culture from the experimental animal.

In Koch's laboratory the idea of using solid media containing agar, in constant use today to isolate pure cultures of microorganisms, was first developed as were practical methods of staining and the Petri dish. During the decade from 1880 to 1890 pupils of Koch, using Koch's isolation methods, discovered most of the organisms causing common infectious diseases. Löffler, Pfeiffer, Neisser, Escherich, Eberth and others were in the group of bacteriologists who became famous by following Koch's methods.

John Tyndall, English physicist, from his experiments inferred the existence of heat-resistant "phases" (later called endospores) of bacteria. In 1878 he devised the method of intermittent heating, now called *Tyndallization,* to kill them.

Elie Metchnikoff (Nobel Prize winner), Russian scientist, pupil of Koch, in 1883 discovered phagocytosis.

H. C. J. Gram in 1884 devised his method for differential staining of bacteria.

Emil A. Von Behring (Nobel Prize winner), **Shibasa-**

buro **Kitasato** and **Albert Fränkel** in 1890 discovered the phenomena of active and passive immunization against diphtheria and tetanus.

Iwanowski, Russian scientist, demonstrated in 1892 the first noncultivable, nonvisible and filterable agent of disease—tobacco mosaic virus.

F. A. J. Löffler and **Paul Frosch** in 1898 discovered the agent of hoof-and-mouth disease, the first-described agent of a viral disease of lower animals. **Walter Reed,** and the U.S. Army Yellow Fever Commission at Havana, in 1899 confirmed the mosquito *(Aedes aegypti)* as vector and discovered the viral agent of yellow fever, first to be described as the cause of a viral disease of man.

Howard Taylor Ricketts in 1909 discovered rickettsiae as the cause of Rocky Mountain spotted fever.

Ross Harrison in 1907 developed methods for explantation and cultivation of tissues *in vitro.*

Peyton Rous in 1911 was the first to demonstrate the transmission of a malignant tumor (chicken sarcoma) by means of cell-free filtrate.

Frederick W. Twort (1915) and **Felix H. d'Herelle** (1917) were first to discover the bacterial viruses—bacteriophages.

Alexander Fleming (Nobel Prize winner, with Sir Howard W. Florey and E. B. Chain) discovered penicillin in 1929.

M. Heidelberger and **F. E. Kendall** in 1929 developed the quantitative precipitin reaction, which underlies the interpretation of most antigen/antibody reactions.

In 1931, **Max Theiler** (Nobel Prize winner) discovered a means of attenuating the virus of yellow fever, leading to the development of the 17D yellow fever vaccine.

A. Tiselius and **E. A. Kabat** in 1939 demonstrated that antibodies were contained in the γ-globulin fraction of serum.

A. H. Coons and his collaborators in 1942 developed the fluorescent antibody technique.

In 1944 **Selman A. Waksman** (Nobel Prize winner) discovered streptomycin.

O. T. Avery, C. M. McCleod and **M. McCarty,** in 1944, demonstrated that the genetic information responsible for transformation of pneumococci was embodied in nucleic acid and in no other biological macromolecular entity. This was the genesis of molecular biology and molecular genetics.

In 1949, **John F. Enders, T. H. Weller** and **F. C. Robbins** (Nobel Prize winners) cultivated the virus of poliomyelitis in non–neural tissue explants, making possible the development of poliomyelitis and other attenuated viral vaccines.

E. Chargaff in 1950 described the principle of base

pairing in DNA, a key to elucidating the structure of nucleic acids and the genetic code.

In 1953 **F. Lipman** and **H. Krebs** (Nobel Prize winners) contributed fundamental knowledge in the fields of energy metabolism and synthetic phenomena in living cells (Krebs cycle).

Wilton Earle and colleagues at the National Institutes of Health (1954) and **J. T. Syverton** and **W. F. Scherer** (1954) adapted continuous cell culture systems to virologic investigation.

J. Lederberg, G. Beadle and **E. Tatum** (Nobel Prize winners, 1958) made fundamental contributions to knowledge of molecular genetics.

Nobel Prize winners in the fields of immunologic unresponsiveness (clonal selection theory and mechanisms of induced tolerance) were **Sir F. M. Burnet** and **P. B. Medawar** in 1960.

In 1962, **F. H. C. Crick, J. D. Watson** and **M. H. F. Wilkins** received the Nobel Prize for elucidating the structure of DNA.

In 1965, **F. Jacob, A. Lwoff** and **J. Monod** received the Nobel Prize for their studies on bacterial and viral genetics.

Other Nobel Prize winners in related fields have been **M. W. Nirenberg, H. G. Khorana,** and **R. W. Holley,** 1968 (decipherment of the genetic code) and **S. E. Luria, M. Delbruck** and **A. D. Hershey** (microbial genetics) 1969.

BACTERIAL INFECTIONS

GRAM-NEGATIVE ENTERIC BACTERIA

The cell walls of these bacteria, like most other gram-negative bacteria, contain lipopolysaccharides that constitute heat-stable *endotoxins* and O antigens and contribute to their pathogenicity. For further details on pathology of infectious diseases see Chapter 6.

Salmonellosis

Any of several hundred serotypes or bioserotypes of *Salmonella* may cause gastroenteritis. On the basis of H and O antigens they are arranged in a system

TABLE 5-5. A Portion of the Kauffman-White Schema Showing Antigenic Content of Representative *Salmonellae*

Groups, Species, Serotypes and Bioserotypes	O Antigens	H Antigens Phase I	H Antigens Phase II
S. enteritidis			
Serogroup A			
bioserotype paratyphi A	1, 2, 12	a	—
serotype typhimurium	1, 4, 5, 12	i	1, 2
Serogroup B			
serotype paratyphi B	1, 4, 5, 12	b	1, 2
Serogroup C₁			
bioserotype paratyphi C	6, 7, (Vi)	c	1, 5
Serogroup D₁			
serotype enteritidis	1, 9, 12	g, m	—
S. typhi	9, 12 (Vi)	d	—
S. choleraesuis	6, 7	c	1, 5

called the *Kauffman-White schema* and divided into groups on the basis of O and H antigens. A few are shown in Table 5-5. While salmonellosis correctly means infection with any species of the genus, a distinction is made between *S. typhi* (typhoid fever) and infections by other *Salmonella* species. The latter are generally referred to as food infection or (improperly) food poisoning.

All typical strains grow well on common laboratory media without blood or serum, at 35 to 40 C. All are facultative. None produces urease and all decarboxylate lysine, arginine and (except *S. typhi*) ornithine. In the eighth edition of "Bergey's Manual," 1974, some 1700 named species or serotypes constitute the genus *Salmonella*. Serotypes and species that are of most medical importance retain their familiar names in this text.

Excepting typhoid fever, salmonellosis is commonly (but not invariably) localized in the intestinal tract, is mild or acute and self-limited. Occasional cases resemble typhoid fever, dysentery or even cholera, especially in debilitated patients. Neither species nor clinical picture is constant. *S. typhi, S. paratyphi A, S. paratyphi B* and *S. paratyphi C* are especially invasive.

SALMONELLOSIS

Typical Typhoid Fever	Typical Food Infection
Relatively long incubation	Incubation period commonly 24 to 48 hours
Early septicemia	Septicemia uncommon
Later enteritis with ulceration	Enteritis early; ulceration uncommon
Stool cultures positive later	Stool cultures positive early
Rose spots characteristic	Rose spots uncommon or rare
Persistent infection	Infection usually self-limited
Carrier state uncommon	Carrier state common
Fatality in untreated cases 10 per cent	Fatality uncommon

Meningitis, pneumonia, osteomyelitis, etc., may occur, especially in typhoid fever. Also in typhoid fever, intestinal perforation may occur at necrotic lymphatic areas (Peyer's patches) that are the site of initial localization of *S. typhi*. In typhoid fever, stubborn residual infection of the gallbladder sometimes develops, resulting in cholelithiasis and its complications, one of which is a persistent carrier state, usually curable by cholecystectomy, and especially dangerous in public food handlers ("Typhoid Mary").

S. typhimurium, S. choleraesuis, S. oranienburg and *S. enteritidis* are among species commonly involved in *Salmonella* infection through ingestion of contaminated food. They and others (not *S. typhi*, which is restricted to man) commonly infect a wide range of wild and domestic animals and poultry, which thus become reservoirs of infection of man via foods: raw meats of infected birds and animals, raw dairy products, raw eggs. All *Salmonella* species are transmitted in human feces (*S typhi* sometimes also in urine following pyelonephritis and cystitis), hence in sewage and in sewage- or feces-polluted water, food and dairy products; by coprophagic arthropods (flies, ants, roaches, etc.); fomites (pronounced *fómitēz*).

In typical *Salmonella* food *infection,* symptoms commonly begin *after* 10 hours following ingestion, i.e., long enough for bacterial multiplication to occur, in contrast with food *poisoning,* especially the common staphylococcal food poisoning, in which symptoms of intense gastroenteritis commonly begin *within* about 10 hours following ingestion, since the toxin is preformed and growth of staphylococci in the alimentary tract does not ordinarily occur.

Diagnosis. In food infection by *Salmonella* (except *S. typhi*) the organisms occur in the *stool* early during the enteritis and may be isolated and identified on appropriate media (Table 5-6). They usually do not invade the bloodstream.

In typhoid fever, on the contrary, the incubation period may be 2 to 3 weeks, symptoms delayed, and the bacilli appear in the *blood* (2 per cent bile infusion broth and plain infusion broth) during the first 10 days and in the stool or the urine only *after* the first week. They often persist in the stools up to 12 weeks, and in about 3 per cent of cases they persist more or less intermittently for years. In overt typhoid fever, splenomegaly and rose spots on the trunk are distinctive.

Serologic diagnosis of salmonellosis. Patients' sera are examined for antibodies against *Salmonella* using standard strains of *S. typhi* as antigen in titered agglutination tests. A significant (greater than 1:160) level or a rise (fourfold or greater) in titer with O antigen (*S. typhi* treated so that primarily the somatic antigens are exposed) denotes active infection. A significant rise

TABLE 5-6. Preliminary Identification of *Salmonella* and *Shigella*

1. Plate sample (blood culture, stool, etc.) on (a) S-S; desoxycholate; bismuth sulfite; EMB; and MacConkey agar. (Samples incubated previously for 18 hours in selective tetrathionate or selenite broth also are plated on the same media.) Incubate overnight at 37 C.
2. Pick suspicious lac⁻ colonies to:
   A. Triple-sugar-iron (TSI) agar slant. (Detects gas, acid and H₂S.) Additional differential information may be obtained by including lysine-iron-agar (LIA) and motility-ornithine decarboxylase and indol (MOI) agar.
      Salmonella: Acid and gas (*S. typhi,* no gas) in butt; alkaline slant; H₂S+; motile.
      Shigella: Acid butt, no gas; alkaline slant; H₂S−; nonmotile.
      Proteus Arizona group and Citrobacter or intermediates: often resemble *Salmonella* or *Shigella* (lac⁻).
   B. Urea medium. *Proteus* hydrolyzes urea in 4 hours or less. *Salmonella* and *Shigella* do not attack urea.
3. If organism gives a *Salmonella* or a *Shigella* type of reaction in above tests, try agglutination with polyvalent *Salmonella* or *Shigella* sera.
4. If positive, confirm biochemically and by definitive serologic tests with monospecific antisera to O and H antigens. This service is available through state departments of health.

in antibody to H antigen (*S. typhi* treated to preserve the flagellar antigens that will then be the primary reactants with antibody) was usually found to follow immunization with typhoid vaccine, which is little used nowadays. Antibodies to a surface (capsular) antigen (Vi) characteristic of some strains of *S. typhi* are thought to be associated with the presence of *S. typhi* in asymptomatic carriers.

Phage Types. Strains of *S. typhi* possessing Vi antigen and antigenically indistinguishable from one another can be further subdivided on the basis of differential sensitivity to bacteriophages. At least 50 phage types are known. This differentiation by phage typing is useful in epidemiologic studies; for example, in tracing possible different sources of infection during a supposedly single-source epidemic. Similar systems of phage typing have been developed for several other groups of bacteria: *Salmonella paratyphi A* and *S. paratyphi B; Shigella; Escherichia coli; Vibrio cholerae; Staphylococcus aureus.*

Prevention of salmonellosis as well as of other communicable diseases of the intestinal tract centers primarily around thorough cooking of foods containing animal products or eggs or liable to contamination by sewage or excreta of avian or mammalian carriers, including man. Human carriers should not serve as food handlers or nurses. Typhoid carriers are generally registered with, and supervised by, health departments.

Active immunization against typhoid is justified for persons in intimate continued household exposure to a documented typhoid carrier or for travelers to areas in which there is a recognized risk of exposure to typhoid because of poor sanitation practices. Adults and children over 10 years of age: 0.5 ml. subcutaneously on two occasions 4 weeks apart. Children younger than 10 years of age: 0.25 ml. subcutaneously on two occasions 4 weeks apart. Under conditions of continued or repeated exposure or for indications if more than 3 years after primary immunization, boosters (single dose subcutaneously as recommended above for each age group, or 0.1 ml. intracutaneously for all age groups) should be given. Only monovalent *Salmonella typhi* vaccine should be used; previous formulations of "TAB" vaccines (combining typhoid and "paratyphoid A and B" antigens) should not be used.

Shigellosis (Bacillary Dysentery)

Clinical dysentery may be caused by a variety of agents: certain protozoa, viruses, unripe apples, *Salmonella,* etc. Shiga, a Japanese scientist, in 1896 first isolated the bacterium now called *Shigella dysenteriae* during outbreaks of severe dysentery in Japan. Flexner later (ca. 1900) isolated a different species from cases of dysentery in the Philippines. Many varieties were afterward described elsewhere. The various strains were named according to names of discoverers or places where found.

The genus *Shigella* is now classified into four major groups, each with several numbered serotypes based on O antigens (not H antigens; why?):

Group A. *S. dysenteriae*
Group B. *S. flexneri*
Group C. *S. boydii*
Group D. *S. sonnei*

General properties of *Shigella* are as for *Salmonella typhi* except that *Shigella* is nonmotile; like *Salmonella typhi* produces no gas from glucose; and has other different enzymic properties (Table 5-6) and is much less durable in the outer world.

Multiplication of dysentery bacilli occurs in the mucosa and the lymph nodes of the lower ileum and colon, with ulceration and sometimes pseudomembrane formation. Acute gastroenteritis is common. Bacteremia is rare. Stools typically contain mucus, pus and blood. All of the gram-negative enteric bacilli possess lipopolysaccharide (endotoxin) in their cell walls. *Shigella dysenteriae* and *S. flexneri* produce antigenically similar toxins, the former in larger amounts than the latter. The enterotoxin is probably responsible for the watery, small-bowel diarrhea, often severe, that is characteristic of the first few days of shigellosis. *S. dysenteriae* infections cause higher fatality rates (20 per cent) than infections by other *Shigella* species and occur chiefly in epidemic form. They are rare in the United States. In this country *S. flexneri* and *S. sonnei* are the most common species. Infections due to them are widespread in carriers and occur in endemic and occasional cases as well as in epidemics. The fatality rate for these species is relatively low in adults; it is higher in infants.

Transmission of shigellosis is almost entirely fecal-oral: by soiled hands and by feces-contaminated foods and objects. Bacillary dysentery is less commonly water borne than typhoid fever, as these organisms do not survive long in water. However, numerous water-borne epidemics have occurred. Infected milk and milk substitutes for infants prepared by unrecognized carriers and not properly sterilized have caused dysentery in nurseries.

Control measures are much the same as for salmonellosis. *Shigella* has been found in monkeys and, rarely, in dogs. There is a distinct correlation between unsanitary living conditions and feces-borne diseases. Prevalence of such diseases is related inversely to availability of clean water for domestic purposes. Vaccines have not been satisfactory in preventing shigellosis.

Laboratory Diagnosis. Blood cultures are rarely positive. Stool cultures are made as in the salmonelloses. They should be made *early* in the disease, with *freshly* passed specimens, and *repeatedly* if negative. Stools in bacillary dysentery are distinctly purulent; those in amebic dysentery much less so. Dysentery agglutinins appear late (in from 12 to 14 days) in patients and often are of low titer or absent. A polyvalent serum may be used to identify the organism isolated from the patient as belonging to the genus *Shigella;* specific sera determine the species and the serotype. Fermentation and other tests also are useful.

Because of widespread resistance to multiple antibiotics among strains of *Shigella,* isolates should be tested *in vitro* for susceptibility to ampicillin and tetracycline, the two drugs of choice for treatment of infections due to sensitive strains. Infections due to resistant strains are treated with trimethoprim plus sulfamethoxazole.

Infections Due to Colon Bacilli (Escherichia) and Other Intestinal Gram-Negative Bacteria

Escherichia coli normally inhabits the intestinal canal in enormous numbers and is sometimes found as an opportunist in various pathologic conditions of the genitourinary tract, often chronic in nature: pyelitis, pyonephrosis, cystitis, appendicitis, postoperative peritonitis and neonatal meningitis. The majority of strains causing meningitis carry the K_1 capsular antigen, which is related to the polysaccharide antigen of group B *Neisseria meningitidis.* Generalized infections can arise, which are frequently fatal because many of the strains are antibiotic resistant. Often associated with *E. coli* and, like it, often introduced by surgery or urologic instrumentation or as opportunistic or nosocomial infections are *Proteus species* and *Pseudomonas aeruginosa,* both of which pose particular problems in resistance to antibiotics.

Certain strains of *E. coli* are etiologic agents in bacterial infant diarrhea, especially in children's institutions, and in some adult cases. The strains implicated in diarrhea are commonly designated as enteropathogenic because they produce either a heat-labile toxin (LT) or a heat-stable toxin (ST), both of which are the expression of plasmids. LT appears to act in a manner similar to that of cholera toxin in stimulating the production of adenosine 3':5'-cyclic monophosphate (cAMP) in small-bowel epithelial cells. The mechanism of action of ST remains obscure. Certain enteroinvasive strains have been recognized that cause true dysentery (diarrhea with blood and pus) in contrast to the cholera-like clinical picture caused by enterotoxin. This character is probably also plasmid controlled. Serogrouping of *E. coli* outbreaks is of value only as an epidemiologic tool in investigation of outbreaks and not as a routine analysis of nonepidemic isolates. Travelers' diarrhea, frequently due to toxigenic *E. coli,* may be prevented (but not treated) by administration of doxycycline (100 mg./day).

Klebsiella pneumoniae, species of *Enterobacter,* and *Serratia* are all closely related Enterobacteriaceae (Tribe Klebsielleae), all having the same sort of endotoxin in their cell walls. Any may be found in the same sorts of opportunistic infections as *E. coli.* All grow on the same sorts of media at 25 to 40 C. and can be differentiated by various biochemical reactions. The capsules of *K. pneumoniae* are polysaccharides and serve as the basis for serologic identification. Some serotypes cross-react with *S. pneumoniae.* Besides being a frequent cause of nosocomial infection, *K. pneumoniae* is one of the few gram-negative bacilli that can cause primary lobar pneumonia, particularly in compromised patients in whom the upper lobes are usually involved and, the infection being necrotizing, cavitation may occur. Therapy is sometimes successful with a combination of an aminoglycoside with a cephalosporin. Prevalence of multiply resistant strains in a hospital environment is directly related to the unregulated use of antibiotics.

Asiatic Cholera

The principal agents of cholera are *Vibrio cholerae* and *V. El Tor. V. cholerae* resembles *Salmonella typhi* in many respects but is curved like a comma. Whereas all motile Enterobacteriaceae have *peritrichous* flagella, the flagella of *V. cholerae* are *polar* (Pseudomonadales). *V. cholerae* differs from *S. typhi* also in being proteolytic and in growing well in alkaline (pH 9) media with blood and egg (Dieudonne's medium). *V. cholerae*

resembles *S. typhi* in being an intestinal pathogen restricted to man, surviving for long periods in polluted water, and in modes of transmission. Also like *S. typhi,* it contains heat-stable O antigens and lipopolysaccharide endotoxin and a heat-labile flagellar antigen.

Antigenic groupings (I to VI) are based on at least three type-specific O antigens: A, B and C. The Inaba group is designated AC; Ogawa group, AB; Hikojima group, ABC. The Inaba and Ogawa antigenic types are included in vaccines. For diagnosis an O-group serum with Inaba and Ogawa immunoglobulins is sufficient since all *V. cholerae* and El Tor vibrios are agglutinated by these.

V. El Tor causes endemic and epidemic cholera-like disease (El Tor cholera), generally with lower death rates than in *V. cholerae* outbreaks. It is of importance in Malaysia and adjacent lands. Both *V. cholerae* and *V. El Tor* agglutinate with cholera serum of O group I (A). All may be variants of a common stock. Cholera vibrios also share O antigens with *Brucella,* so that persons who have received cholera vaccine may show significant levels of serum agglutinins for *Br. abortus,* the standard test antigen (see below). The El Tor vibrio produces hemolysin (Greig positive) and its cultures agglutinate chick erythrocytes. Unlike *V. cholerae,* it kills chick embryos and resists polymyxin.

There are saprophytic species of vibrios and some that are pathogenic for lower animals: *V. metschnikovi* (pigeons); *V. proteus; V. fetus* (sheep, cattle, goats, sometimes man).

In *V. cholera,* multiplication of the vibrios is entirely in the gut, the endotoxin producing intense gastritis and nausea and irritation of the bowel, chiefly the ileum. The exotoxin produced by *Vibrio* is the prototypic enterotoxin, which causes fluid secretion through the activation of tissue adenylcyclase to increase intestinal cAMP concentration. Similar LTs are produced by *E. coli* and all are coded for by transmissible plasmids. Ingestion of contaminated water leads to the penetration of the mucous layer and colonization of the lining epithelium of the small intestine by the vibrios. The epithelium remains intact, but it passes immense quantities of watery fluid, turbid with mucus ("rice-water" stools), with resulting dehydration, hemoconcentration, electrolyte imbalance, toxemia and shock. Administration of fluids and electrolytes is of critical importance and dramatic effectiveness in therapy. Without treatment, mortality in *V. cholerae* outbreaks may range from 5 to 75 per cent.

Epidemic cholera is largely water borne, but sporadic cases may be transmitted by any raw foods contaminated with feces or vomitus of patients or of temporary carriers. *Chronic* carriers of *V. cholerae* seem to be rare, but convalescent carriers and mild, ambulatory cases seem to be common. The disease is at present absent from the Western hemisphere but is endemic and epidemic in India and mainland Southeast Asia. Isolated outbreaks in Louisiana have been associated with ingestion of raw oysters taken from contaminated coastal waters.

Control measures are basically as in other enteric bacterial disease. Rigid inspection and control of travelers from endemic and epidemic areas are important in preventing the international spread of cholera.

Vaccines are required for U.S. travelers to the epidemic or endemic areas. Modern cholera vaccine consists of killed *V. cholerae* suspensions, 10^8 cells per ml., half Inaba, half Ogawa. Studies and experience in the Orient indicate the desirability of including El Tor vibrios. Protection begins about 10 days after vaccination and lasts only about 6 months. It is not very solid and should be reinforced by booster doses each 6 months. The vaccine also evokes antibodies that agglutinate *Brucella* organisms. Toxoid derived from the "permeability factor" or exotoxin is currently under field trial.

Laboratory Diagnosis. Liquid (rice water) stools of patients may be examined microscopically for typical vibrios, blood, mucus and pus. Cultivation of stools or suspect water in selective (pH 9.0) alkaline peptone water often yields prolific growth of the vibrios in a surface pellicle after 6 to 8 hours at 37 C. This pellicle may be examined microscopically and used to inoculate plates of a special thiosulfate-citrate-bile-salts medium containing 1:200,000 KTe for selectivity, for isolation of colonies, also for a rapid, preliminary, slide agglutination test. Colonies resemble those of *Shigella*. Final identification depends on morphology, cultural properties and serologic tests.

Neither serum nor chemotherapy is of recognized value in cholera.

Vibrio parahemolyticus. This vibrio, an inhabitant of saline, estuarine, coastal waters is very similar to *V. cholerae*. It is the cause of a severe form of gastroenteritis associated especially with eating insufficiently cooked or raw crustaceae or shellfish. It differs from *V. cholerae* in requiring 3 to 7 per cent of NaCl in culture media, growth at 43 C., ability to metabolize chitin and positive Greig reaction. It is transmitted in stools of patients and by sewage-contaminated foods, waters, etc.

PATHOGENIC, GRAM-POSITIVE, PYOGENIC COCCI (STREPTOCOCCI, PEPTOSTREPTOCOCCI, STAPHYLOCOCCI, PEPTOCOCCI).

Hemolytic Types

For convenience three subdivisions of streptococci may be made on the basis of types of hemolytic zones produced around colonies on sheep or rabbit blood agar plates incubated *aerobically* at 37 C., as follows:

Hemolytic:

1. Beta type ("Strep hemolyticus," beta hemolytic strep," etc.). With one or two exceptions, these comprise the *pyogenic group* of streptococci. They form a clear, colorless, zone of hemolysis, devoid of intact erythrocytes around small colonies.
2. Alpha type ("Strep viridans," "green strep"). These form a greenish zone of *intact erythrocytes* around small colonies, with varying degrees of hemolysis at the periphery. The group includes *S. mitis, S. mutans S. salivarius, S. bovis, S. thermophilus, S. faecium, S. pneumoniae* and others.

Nonhemolytic:

3. Gamma type ("indifferent strep," "nonhemolytic strep"). These produce no visible change in the blood around their colonies. The group includes *S. lactis,* some of the Enterococcus group: *S. faecalis, S. liquefaciens,* etc. (Table 5-7).

Serologic Subdivisions of Streptococci

Lancefield subdivided the *beta-type* hemolytic streptococci into immunologic groups on the basis of cell-wall polysaccharide antigens. Grouping is done with highly specific antisera as a precipitin reaction or with counterimmunoelectrophoresis (CIE), using streptococcal extracts, as a coagglutination reaction with antibody-coated staphylococcal cells (protein A) or latex particles, or by ultraviolet light microscopy with fluorescein-labeled antibody (Table 5-7). The Lancefield groups are lettered A to U, and with a few exceptions, are beta hemolytic.

Lancefield Groups. Group A includes the classic *Streptococcus pyogenes* from human sources. *S. pyogenes* is the principal human pathogen, causing scarlet fever, septic sore throat, erysipelas, puerperal sepsis, empyema, meningitis. Group A strains are sensitive to bacitracin; most other beta-hemolytic streptococci are resistant. All group A strains are sensitive to penicillin, the drug of choice for therapy and/or prophylaxis of acute rheumatic fever.

Group B strains are a frequent cause of neonatal infections (especially type 3) and are distinguished from all others in (a) producing double-zone ("hot-cold") beta hemolysis, (b) hydrolyzing sodium hippurate, and (c) positive CAMP test. These are mainly *S. agalactiae* strains.

Group D streptococci include enterococci *(S. faecalis)* and are found in miscellaneous human infections such as arthritis, sinusitis, endocarditis, and cystitis, probably as opportunistic invaders. Group D streptococci, although usually indifferently hemolytic (γ), may be viridans or, less frequently beta hemolytic. All group D streptococci grow on bile-esculin (B-E) agar with a positive reaction; only enterococci grow in broth containing 6.5 per cent NaCl.

Other groups, through K, Q, and T, occur in lower animals or in dairy products. A few alpha-type and gamma-type (e.g., *S. lactis*) streptococci contain Lancefield group N antigens.

The determination of the Lancefield group of a beta-hemolytic streptococcus is of diagnostic and prognostic value as well as an index to epidemiology and therapy.

A further subdivision of *group A streptococci* is made into over 50 numbered serologic types on the basis of precipitin tests with type-specific soluble *protein* antigens (M proteins) in these streptococci. M proteins are essential to virulence. The M types of group A streptococci are related to certain clinical conditions; for example, types 1, 3, 4, 6, 12 and 25 have been found to predominate in certain epidemics in which acute hemorrhagic nephritis was a prominent complication of acute pharyngitis. Type 2 and a few higher serotypes (49, 55, 57, 59, 60, 61) have been reported as the cause of pyoderma-associated acute glomerulonephritis (AGN). This fact accounts for the sporadic occurrence and geographic localization of AGN in contrast to the relatively constant seasonal incidence of ARF without evident geographic localization in temperate climates. There is little or no cross immunity between M types. Therefore, repeated group A streptococcal infections may occur in the same individual, each caused by a different M type of streptococcus.

Other cell-wall fractions of group A streptococci include acid- and heat-labile but trypsin-resistant T proteins. These can be used as antigens to prepare specific antisera that differentiate some 45 T-agglutinin types. T-agglutination typing is useful in epidemiologic studies on group-A *Streptococcus* infection, especially when M antigens are ill-defined.

Fibrinolysin or *streptokinase* is a protein elaborated by streptococci of groups A, C and G, that activates a serum enzyme, plasmin, able to digest supposedly protective, retaining, fibrin clots that may be formed around infected lesions. *Antifibrinolysin* or *antistreptokinase* appears in the blood of patients recovering from infections with streptococci of these groups and, if increasing in titer, is of diagnostic value.

Beta-type streptococci of group A also produce at least two kinds of soluble hemolysin: S and O. *Streptolysin O* is readily oxidized and appears, in blood agar plates, only around *sub-surface* colonies unless *anaerobically* incubated. *Streptolysin S* is sensitive to heat, acid, or both, but *not* to oxygen. A significant increase in titer of antisteptolysin O or of other antienzymes (streptozyme test) during beta-hemolytic streptococcal infection, especially respiratory infections, is of diagnostic significance in relation to the subsequent emergence of acute rheumatic fever (ARF). *Streptolysin S* is not antigenic.

Capsules and Hyaluronidase. Group A streptococci, especially M types 4 and 22, form protective capsules of hyaluronic acid, a slimy polysaccharide. These capsules may be hydrolyzed by *hyaluronidase*, produced in varying amounts by the streptococci themselves. Although this may offset the antiphagocytic effect of the capsules, it can also digest the ground substance of the connective tissues and has therefore been regarded by some as a spreading factor, permitting invasion of the tissues by the streptococci.

Streptodornase is an enzyme found in cultures of beta-type streptococci that digests deoxyribonucleic acid (hence strepto-*dorn*ase). Much of the slimy, fibrinous exudate in empyema, etc., consists of fibrin and DNA from lysed leukocytes. Streptokinase and streptodornase have clinical use in chemical debridement of such highly viscous exudates. Antibodies to hyaluronidase and/or to deoxyribonuclease B have the same significance as ASO. In the absence of a significant elevation in one or more of these antienzymes (titer greater than 1/100) a diagnosis of ARF is most unlikely. In streptococcal pyoderma, little or no ASO response may occur, but anti-DNase titers rise.

Infections by Streptococci

Scarlet Fever and Septic Sore Throat. Many strains of *S. pyogenes* (group A) produce an exotoxin (erythrogenic or scarlet-fever toxin) that, when absorbed by the susceptible host, produces the nausea, chills, fever and rash of scarlet fever.

Like the toxin of *Corynebacterium diphtheriae*, erythrogenic toxin is produced only by lysogenic streptococci *(lysogenic conversion)*.

Scarlet fever and septic sore throat are two manifestations of the same infection. In both, a septic sore throat is present. Persons susceptible to the erythrogenic toxin also develop a rash and are said to have scarlet fever. Persons insusceptible to the toxin, that is, with antitoxic immunity, have no rash, and such cases are diagnosed as septic sore throat. Reinfections and septic sore throat without rash, due to different M types of toxigenic streptococci are possible.

Transmission of streptococcal infections is as for respiratory infections in general: oronasopharyngeal secretions and contact.

For diagnostic cultures swabbings from nose or throat are streaked on blood agar, and undercut, or better, emulsified in broth that is then used to inoculate blood agar pour plates to obtain subsurface colonies. Beta-type hemolytic colonies found after 24 hours at 35 C. are fished to blood broth and incubated. Pure cultures may be subjected to appropriate differential tests shown in Table 5-7.

TABLE 5-7. Properties of Streptococci Most Frequently Isolated from Clinical Specimens (aerobic)

Lancefield Serogroup (Species)*	Group-specific Cell Wall Polysaccharide	Usual Type of Hemolysis (sheep blood)	Growth at 37 C.	10 C.	45 C.	Fermentation of Trehalose	Sorbitol	Inulin	Hippurate Hydrolysis	Sensitivity to Bacitracin†	Optochin	BE‡	Tolerance to 6.5% NaCl	Diseases
A (S. pyogenes)	Rhamnose-GNac	β	+	−	−	+	−	−	−	+			−	Pharyngitis, tonsillitis, otitis, pyoderma, systemic infections, nonsuppurative sequelae: ARF, AGN
B (S. agalactiae)	Rhamnose-GNH₂	β(α γ)§	+	−	−	+	−		+	−(+)	−	−		Ascending amnionitis, neonatal sepsis, pneumonia, meningitis
C (S. equi, equisimilis, dysgalactiae)	Rhamnose-Gal-Nac	β	+	−	−	−	−		−	−	−			Mild URI, puerperal sepsis, endocarditis
D (S. fecalis, bovis, equinus)	Glycerol-teichoic acid-D-ala-glu	Enterococcus (S. fecalis, faecium, durans): α β γ							v	−	−	+	+	UTI, endocarditis (Enterococci: penicillin resistant)
		Nonenterococcus (S. bovis, equinus): α γ							−	−	−	+	−	
F (S. milleri, anginosus, minutus, MG)								−		−				Respiratory infections, pneumonia
G (S. canis)								+		+				Puerperal, skin, wound infections
VIRIDANS		α									−	−(+)	−	Dental caries, endocarditis
S. salivarius (K)			+	−	+									
S. mitis			+	−	+									
S. mutans			+	−	+									
S. sanguis (H)		(β)	+	−	−									
S. pneumoniae (84 serotypes)		α									+	−	−	Pneumonia, septicemia, meningitis, endocarditis, otitis

* Representative species named.
† 5–10% of group B and C–G are bacitracin sensitive.
‡ Growth and hydrolysis of esculin on bile–esculin (BE) agar.
§ CAMP test positive.

AGN = acute glomerulonephritis.
ARF = acute rheumatic fever.
URI = upper respiratory infection.
UTI = urinary tract infection.
v = variable.

In severe cases septicemia may develop, and blood cultures (10 ml. of blood in 150 ml. of tryptose broth) are of utmost importance as a guide to treatment.

Acute rhematic fever is a nonsuppurative sequel to group A streptococcal infection only (acute pharyngitis and tonsillitis and inapparent infection). There is a relatively constant level of incidence up to 3% following all untreated cases regardless of the serotype. The pathogenesis of ARF is based on the cumulative immune response (IR) to group specific (?protoplast membrane) antigens stimulated by successive streptococcal infections with different serotypes and is signalled by elevated or persistently rising antibody titers to streptococcal enzymes. The group specific antibody cross-reacts with sarcolemma of cardiac muscle. This cross-reaction, with other as yet unknown factors, underlies the tissue-damaging lesions of ARF. Patients with a history of ARF are about 10 times more at risk of recurrence of ARF with each successive acute group A streptococcal infection than are persons without known previous history of streptococcal infection. ARF can be effectively *prevented* by prompt and adequate penicillin *treatment* of acute streptococcal pharyngitis.

Other Streptococcal Infections. Beta-type hemolytic streptococci of any Lancefield group, but especially groups A, C and G, may cause various nonepidemic infections, such as otitis media, empyema, sore throat, erysipelas and meningitis. Puerperal sepsis may be transmitted to parturient women by carriers of beta-type hemolytic streptococci, which are common, and by unsterile hands, instruments, gloves, dressings, dust.

Group B streptococci *(Streptococcus agalactiae)* are found in 25% of normal vaginas and from this source may cause severe and often fatal infection in infants in the first two months of life, particularly subtype III. Maternal antibody to group B streptococci protects infants at risk from ascending infection by B streptococci. About 5 per cent of the group B strains are nonhemolytic and may therefore be missed. Up to 30 per cent of the strains may be bacitracin sensitive and thus may be mistaken for group A streptococci. Definitive identification is made by fluorescent antibody techniques and by the CAMP test. Penicillin and related antibiotics are effective in the treatment of these infections in which early diagnosis is life-saving.

Alpha-hemolytic (viridans) streptococci fall into several serogroups and some are untypeable. *S. mutans,* by virtue of its capacity to produce high-molecular weight dextran, is a prime cause of dental plaque formation that, if unchecked, leads directly to dental caries. *S. mitis* and *S. sanguis* are the viridans streptococci most commonly causing endocarditis. All viridans streptococci are universally found in the normal oropharynx and from this site may gain transient entrance into the blood following minor trauma to the supporting periodontal tissues. In patients with damaged endocardial surfaces (healed rheumatic fever, congenital deformities, prostheses), these otherwise noninvasive bacteria of low intrinsic virulence are the primary cause of endocarditis initiated at the site of endocardial discontinuity or denudation. In the same way, group D streptococci account for up to 10 per cent of endocardial infections. If endocarditis is suspected, a persistent effort should be made *prior to therapy* to recover organisms from the blood. To this end, bidaily cultures should be made until at least three separate blood samples yield the same organisms, for which the minimal inhibitory concentrations of penicillin and streptomycin should be determined. Upon primary isolation, most group D and many viridans streptococci are relatively resistant to penicillin *in vitro* but still yield clinically to adequate dosage of combined antibiotics, usually penicillin and streptomycin with the adjunctive administration of probenecid.

Streptococcus pneumoniae, distinguished from viridans streptococci by sensitivity to optochin, is the most common cause of lobar pneumonia and a frequent cause of meningitis. There are 84 serotypes determined by the capsular swelling reaction with type-specific rabbit antisera. The capuslar polysaccharide is antiphagocytic (i.e., the chief virulence factor) and is also the protective antigen. A vaccine is now available that is composed of purified capsular polysaccharide from each of the 14 serotypes that account for over 90 per cent of infections. It is effective in preventing pneumococcal pneumonia in selective high-risk population groups with any of the types in the vaccine (e.g., patients compromised by kyphoscoliosis, diabetes, cellular immunodeficiencies, sickle cell disease, splenectomy). Most strains of *S. pneumoniae* are sensitive to penicillin at levels easily achieved in the blood. Recently, penicillin-resistant strains of *S. pneumoniae* have appeared. Respiratory infection with *S. pneumoniae* is not highly contagious. In contrast to lobar pneumonia, which almost always yields to appropriate antibiotic treatment, pneumococcal meningitis carries a high mortality despite what appears to be adequate treatment. Counterimmunoelectrophoresis is an important aid in diagnosis of meningial infection when viable organisms cannot be recovered in cultures of the spinal fluid.

Peptostreptococci

Gram-positive, chain-forming cocci of a related family, Peptococcaceae, similar in general characters to genus *Streptococcus* but strictly anaerobic, are grouped in the genus *Peptostreptococcus.* These cocci attack proteins and carbohydrates and are often found in grassy, foul-smelling lesions of various organs, frequently associated with other anaerobic bacteria. They may be primary pathogens, and are also important as secondary invaders. Peptostreptococci are generally sensitive to penicillin.

Staphylococci

Staphylococcal Infections

Staphylococci cause numerous types of suppurative inflammatory conditions in any or every part of the body. They commonly form abscesses and furuncles of the skin and produce a number of metabolites of varying degrees of toxicity. Most pathogenic strains produce β-type hemolysis (but not α type) on blood-agar plates. Staphylococci grow vigorously on media like those used for streptococci but are somewhat less fastidious as to temperature (15 to 40 C.) and requirements for blood or serum, though they also require organic N and glucose. Like streptococci, they are facultative anaerobes. Blood agar with mannitol, 7 per cent NaCl, and tellurite is a useful selective medium.

Staphylococci differ from streptococci in producing catalase, having cytochrome systems, and in producing, at 25 C., large opaque, white, cream-colored or butter-yellow colonies. *S. aureus* tends to produce more yellow pigment than *S. epidermidis,* especially in pus. Resistance of staphylococci to penicillin is transmissible by plasmids that code for penicillinase. Most strains of *S. aureus* pathogenic for man are characterized by the production of the enzyme coagulase *(bound or free),* which induces clotting of citrated or oxalated human or rabbit plasma. Other characters often associated with (but not necessarily the cause of) pathogenicity of *S. aureus* are: (a) fermentation of mannitol; (b) elaboration of acid phosphatase, β-lactamase (penicillinase), protease, hyaluronidase, lysozyme, catalase, deoxyribonuclease; (c) protein A (in cell wall), which binds to Fc portion of immunoglobulins; (d) several hemolysins or toxins, including exfoliatin (which causes the "scalded skin syndrome") and enterotoxins (causing acute gastroenteritis and possibly "toxic shock syndrome"). The cell-wall teichoic acid is polyribitol in *Staphylococcus aureus* and polyglycerol in *Staphylococcus epidermidis.* Cell-wall, cross-linked peptidoglycan (PG) is synthesized in successive stages: (1) production of N-acetyl muramyl pentapeptide, (2) assembly of linear PG strands, and (3) cross-linking of polymerized strands with pentaglycine bridges. Several antibiotics inhibit growth by competing with enzymes at different stages (e.g., transpeptidation) of cell wall synthesis.

S. epidermidis and nonpathogenic micrococci are ubiquitous on the human skin and rarely have any combination of any of these characteristics. *S. aureus* is markedly resistant to phagocytosis; *S. epidermidis* is not. Infections by *S. epidermidis* are typically superficial and rarely severe. *S. aureus* produces proteolytic enzymes that may cause necrosis and destruction of tissues. Excessive allergy develops in certain individuals with prolonged *S. aureus* infections, e.g., chronic furunculosis. Desensitization using *autogenous vaccines* has been recommended in the past, but has been largely discredited. Cell-mediated immune responses to recurrent staphylococcal infection probably account for the occasionally accentuated inflammatory reaction characteristic of recrudescent staphylococcal infections (recurrent furmeulosis).

Phage Types and Antibiotic Resistance

By means of phage typing (with 22 phages) it is possible to trace sources of antibiotic-resistant and coagulase-producing strains of staphylococci. Phage types of *S. aureus,* for example 42B/52/81 or 53/VA4, may occur in outbreaks and be traceable by phage typing to a certain patient or hospital-personnel carrier of that type. *Staphylococcus aureus* of phage type 80/81/52 was at one time responsible for widespread nosocomial infections. These strains were highly resistant to penicillin, caused highly invasive infection and persisted in carriers among hospital personnel. Their prevalence has presently declined. Staphylococcus phages have been divided into four lytic groups: (I, II, III, IV). Epidemic strains of staphylococci are generally lysed by phages of groups I, II, and III; enterotoxic strains, by phages of groups III and IV.

Antibiotic Resistance

Antibiotic-resistant strains of *S. aureus* are still common and are found in carriers among hospital personnel, who then become the principal potential sources of nosocomial infection.

Food Poisoning

Some strains of coagulase-positive staphylococci produce a thermostable exotoxin (enterotoxin) that, when ingested, causes acute staphylococcal food poisoning or gastroenteritis. There are at least five antigenic types of staphylococcal enterotoxin (A to E).

Heat-stable enterotoxin is preformed in contaminated food that has been allowed to stand at 22 to 38 C. (room or incubating temperature) for some hours. A wide variety of foods is suitable for growth of staphylococci.

Contamination of foods, resulting in staphylococcal food poisoning, often is traced to food handlers who have abscesses or boils on hands or arms or in the nose, etc. Foods exposed openly in shops and cafeterias may be infected by coughing and sneezing workers or customers. Most communities have laws against such exposure and require refrigeration of cream-filled pastries.

Intoxication is characterized primarily by the sudden onset of nausea and vomiting after a short incubation period (2–6 hours) and is unaccompanied by fever. Dehydration may be severe and even life-threatening, particularly in infants and elderly or debilitated patients. True enterocolitis (bloody diarrhea, necrotizing lesions of small and/or large bowel) as contrasted with acute upper gastroenterointoxication may be caused by antibiotic-resistant strains that colonize the colon, overgrowing the normal flora and producing enterotoxin *in situ*. Another soluble exotoxin (exofoliatin) produced particularly by phage type 71 causes the scalded skin syndrome, bullous impetigo, and scarlatiniform rash.

Toxic Shock Syndrome

Toxic shock syndrome (TSS) has recently been recognized as a distinct entity occurring in women who use tampons during normal menstrual flow. With few exceptions, *Staphylococcus* has been recovered from vaginal cultures from these patients whose symptoms include sudden onset, nausea, vomiting, shock, and later an exfoliative dermatitis not unlike that seen in scalded skin syndrome. TSS probably results from systemic intoxication with staphylococcal toxin.

GRAM-NEGATIVE COCCI

Infections Due to Neisseria

This genus, found only in man, is named for Neisser, first to recognize (in 1879) the causative agent for gonorrhea.

Gonorrhea

Although no demonstrable *exo*toxins are produced, the organisms contain endotoxin and are highly pyogenic. Gaining entrance to suitable tissues such as glandular or mucosal surfaces of the genitalia, especially those covered by columnar epithelium, they produce an intense inflammatory exudate. Usually within less than 10 (1 to 31) days of infection there is a rapid formation of thick, mucopurulent exudate from the posterior urethra of males and from the cervix. Invasion of neighboring tissues (e.g., prostate and fallopian tubes) often occurs and uncommonly there is bacteremia with arthritis and endocarditis. The gonococci in an infected mother may gain entrance to the conjunctival sac of the infant during birth, causing severe ophthalmia *(ophthalmia neonatorum)*. Gonococcal ophthalmia of adults may occur as a result of autoinfection. Gonococci may be found in the urethra, prostate, Bartholin's glands, cervix, vagina, rectum, pharynx (*Veillonella* and nonpatholgenic respiratory *Neisseria* may confuse), in septicemia, in cutaneous lesions, and are a leading cause of septic arthritis.

In diagnosis of gonorrhea, positive gram-stained smears are useful in fresh, clinically typical disease when exposure within 10 days is established.

Detection of "gram-negative intracellular diplococci" resembling *N. gonorrheae* is good presumptive evidence (which should be fortified by culture on Thayer-Martin agar in a candle jar) of infection in the male and is sufficient to warrant prompt treatment. In the female the presence of saprophytic gram-negative diplococci *(Neisseria, Veillonella, Herellea)* may make the interpretation of smears difficult, and reliance must be placed on endocervical culture. Causes of nongonococcal urethritis (NGU) must be kept in mind, especially chlamydiae and ureaplasma, in cases of "treatment failure." It should be kept in mind that *N. gonorrheae* can cause meningitis and that disseminated gonococcemia is not unusual. Secondary manifestations include arthritis and acute endocarditis. *N. gonorrheae* is also the occasional cause of tracheitis and pneumonitis and may be found in the posterior nasophraynx. Conversely, *N. meningitidis* can be found in the genital tract and cause essentially all of the same syndromes as *N. gonorrheae*. The control of gonorrheal infection depends on case detection, reporting and prompt therapy. Gonorrhea continues to increase in prevalence, especially among teenagers, in company with syphilis and chlamydial infections. Neisserial ophthalmia neonatorum may be prevented by the instillation (mandatory in most states) of 1 per cent silver nitrate solution. Penicillin resistance among isolated strains of *N. gonorrheae* poses the most serious problem in therapy. Penicillinase-producing strains of *N. gonorrhea* (PPNG) have been reported.

Fluorescent antibody staining is useful for microscopic diagnosis. Examination should also be made for *Candida albicans* and *Trichomonas vaginalis*. For initial isolation of any pathogenic neisseria, swabs of the endocervix taken through a speculum or freshly expressed urethral exudate from the man or sediment of spinal fluid are immediately plated on warmed chocolate or Thayer-Martin agar and incubated in a candle jar. Oxidase-positive colonies appearing in 18 to 24 hours are subcultured and inoculated into semisolid agar containing differential sugars (glucose, maltose and sucrose). *N. gonorrheae* ferments only dextrose, *N. meningitidis,* dextrose and maltose and common commensal organisms, all three or none. Definitive identification can be made with fluorescent antibody on smears of purified cultures.

Organisms of small colony types (T1, T2) typical of fresh isolates from patients possess pili that mediate initial attachment to cells and have inherent antiphagocytic (virulence) properties. Pili constitute the protective antigen of gonococci. Strains may be typed for epidemiologic purposes by ability to grow on defined media lacking certain nutrients ("auxotyping"). Arginine-, hypoxanthine-, and uracil-requiring strains are usually penicillin sensitive but are resistant to the bactericidal effect of normal serum and cause asymptomatic urethritis in men and the bacteremia–arthritis syndrome. More than 30 auxotypes have been defined. All gonococci and pneumococci produce proteases that inactivate IgA at mucosal surfaces. Conjugally transferable plasmids coding for penicillinase are present in many random clinical isolates.

Meningococcal Meningitis

Meningococci closely resemble gonococci not only culturally and biologically but in producing similar infections. Unlike gonococci, meningococci most commonly infect the upper respiratory tract, often causing, initially, catarrhal rhinitis. Transmission is mainly by *fresh* droplets of oronasal secretions of patients and carriers; meningococci are very sensitive to environmental temperatures and to drying. Invasion of the bloodstream from the nasopharynx frequently follows, often with extensive purpura, particularly when meningococcal infection assumes epidemic proportions. Invasion of the meninges appears to follow bacteremia only occasionally. Thus, relatively few overt cases of meningitis may develop although the carrier rate may be 50 per cent or more. Blood cultures usually are positive early in meningococcal meningitis. Limited, chronic or overwhelming meningococcemia may occur, with adrenal damage and Waterhouse-Friedrichsen syndrome. Chronic meningococcemia is a syndrome that should suggest itself as a possible cause of unexplained recurrent generalized petechial hemorrhages.

Meningococci are separable by agglutination tests into 9 serogroups. Capsular polysaccharides have been purified from types A, B, C, X and Y; only A and C are suitable for human vaccines. After 6 months of age and during the first 12 years, the incidence of meningococcal infection, particularly meningococcal meningitis, is inversely proportional to the meningococcidal activity of the serum. Maximum incidence of meningitis occurs from the 6 to the 24th month. The stimulus for the natural cumulative acquistion of antibody is the presence in the oropharynx of nontypeable *Neisseria* and other species of bacteria with cross-reactive antigens.

Primary isolation is made on chocolate agar. Pathogenic *Neisseria* can be identified by differential sugar fermentation and/or fluorescent antibody. Cerebrospinal fluid that contains polymorphonuclear leukocytes and low sugar levels but from which no organisms are recovered should be analyzed, along with urine samples, by counterimmunoelectrophoresis (CIE) for meningococcoal, pneumococcal and *H. influenzae* capsular polysaccharides. Group B meningococcus is currently the prevalent type in the United States.

Treatment and Control. Penicillin G is the drug of choice, given initially intravenuously. In patients with pencillin allergies chloramphenicol is used. Intimate medical and household family contacts should be carefully watched for early signs and not be given chemoprophylaxis. Compromised patients at risk can be immunized with commercially available A and C vaccines. Because B strains are sulfadiazine sensitive, this drug can be used for prophylaxis in well-indicated situations. There has been an increase in infections due to Y strains.

Infections Due to Brucella

Brucellosis (Undulant Fever)

Undulant fever in man may be caused by any species of the genus *Brucella: B. abortus, B. melitensis* or *B. suis,* or variants of these. Brucella species are distinguishable by agglutination tests with adsorbed, monovalent serum and by special biochemical tests (Table 5-8). Some species *(B. canis, B. ovis, B. neotomae)* are restricted to other animals.

The species names refer to origin or special affinities for respective animal hosts, e.g., *B. abortus*—cattle; *B. melitensis*—from Malta (Melita is the ancient name for Malta); the principal vector is infected goat's milk; *Br. suis*—swine. Cross infections by any of the organisms can occur between various animal species, but *B. suis* is largely restricted to swine and *B. melitensis* to goats. Any may infect man. All of the organisms are highly endotoxic and typically, but not obligately, intracellular parasites. No exotoxin is formed. Usual portals of entry are through the gastrointestinal tract and cuts and abrasions of skin and possibly via inhalation or through unbroken skin or mucosal surfaces such as the conjunctivae. The organisms invade the bloodstream and localize in lymph nodes, liver, spleen, glandular tissues and elsewhere. They multiply inside macrophages and can persist there. They can produce mastitis, orchitis, etc. Unpasteurized milk from infection udders of cattle, goats, etc., is highly infectious.

TABLE 5-8. Properties of *Brucella*

Organism	Principal Animal Host	Duration of H$_2$S Production (days)	Rate of Urease Production	Growth on Agar with Fuchsin	Growth on Agar with Thionine
B. abortus	Cattle	2–4	±	+	−
B. suis	Swine	4–8	++	−	+
B. melitensis	Goats	±1–2	±	+	+

In farm animals, especially those pregnant for the first time (i.e., not immune), fetus, placenta, membranes, etc., contain large numbers of the bacilli, due to high concentrations of erythritol, a growth stimulant. Due to acute placentitis, abortion results, especially in cows, mares, ewes and sows, but rarely in women. In man the disease is rarely fatal but often is prolonged and debilitating, with relapses and muscle pains, sweating, chills and many ill-defined symptoms referable to the nervous system, the gastrointestinal tract, etc. Prolonged latent infection of the reticuloendothelial cells may occur with development of allergic complications and neurologic symptoms. A prolonged and variable antibody response characterizes most infections and is detectable by agglutination with *Brucella abortus* antigen, which cross-reacts broadly with other strains. Agglutinins may be present concomitantly with or in the absence or circulating *Brucella* organisms and thus probably have little to do with localization or host control of infection.

B. suis and *B. melitensis* are most virulent for man and can infect cattle. Most severe human cases in the United States are due to these varieties. *B. abortus* infections are more common in cattle and human beings, usually less severe in man; many unrecognized human *B. abortus* infections doubtless occur. Raw milk, lochia and carcasses of infected cattle, swine, goats and some other animals are highly infectious, and brucellosis is found most commonly among men engaged in handling these materials: breeders, veterinarians, abattoir employees. Person-to-person transmission is rare. The organisms occur in feces and urine and may survive for considerable periods in infected dairy products.

Control of Brucellosis. Handling of animal products and products of abortions should be avoided, or rubber gloves should be used. Only pasteurized dairy products should be used. Farm animals should be vaccinated (attenuated live *B. abortus* strain 19, occasionally causing accidental infection in veterinarians and farm personnel) especially females before first pregnancy (does not prevent infection but reduces abortion rate), and infected animals should be eliminated.

Diagnosis. Skin tests with extracts of *Brucella* (brucellergin) are no longer recommended for diagnostic use. Primary diagnosis must be made by repeated cultures of the blood, of exudates or liver biopsy along with serial serum agglutination tests.

Cultures of blood, especially of blood *clots,* are most valuable and conclusive in diagnosis. Incubation of special *Brucella*-broth medium, with daily subcultures to agar plates, should continue for at least a month at 35 C. in an atmosphere with about 10 per cent CO$_2$. Brucella will grow reluctantly on solid media, e.g., plates of liver infusion, tryptose or trypticase-soy agar at pH 6.8. In Castaneda's method, a layer of agar in a flat-sided flask is bathed periodically with inoculated broth in the same bottle by daily laying the flask on its side for an hour or so.

Isolation of *Brucella* from contaminated materials such as milk or feces is accomplished by adding, to one of the above media, selectively inhibitory agents: crystal violet plus polymyxin B, penicillin, cycloheximide. The last is included to control saprophytic fungi.

Serum agglutinins may appear about 2 weeks after onset of acute brucellosis but are not always demonstrable, even in severe cases. Titers may range from 1:50 to 1:20,000. Titers below about 1:160 are of doubtful significance. Extensive prozones (blocking antibodies) appear in brucellosis; accordingly, dilutions of patient's serum should be carried out to at least 1:2,560 in all tests. As in any serologic diagnosis, a *rise* in titer between two samples taken 5 to 10 days apart is of greater significance than any single titer. Agglutinin tests with milk whey of infected cattle usually are positive.

Positive Brucella agglutination in man can occur as a result of previous tularemia or vaccination against cholera. For antibiotic therapy, combinations of streptomycin with broad-spectrum antibiotics, especially the tetracyclines, are recommended. Relapses are frequent because the organisms persist intracellularly.

Infections Due to Bordetella

Pertussis and Related Diseases

The etiologic agent of pertussis (whooping cough) is *Bordetella pertussis.* Clinical conditions much like

TABLE 5-9. Some Differential Properties of *Haemophilus* and *Bordetella*

Organism	Production of		Growth Factors Req.		Motility	Brown Color in Peptone Agar	Urease Produced	Colonies on Blood Agar	Fermentation of Glucose
	Indole	NaNO$_2$	X*	V†					
H. influenzae	±	+	+	+	−	−		Small, "dewdrop"	+
H. ducreyii	−	−	+	−	−	−		Small, gray, hemolytic	
H. parainfluenzae	−	−	−	+	−	−			
B. bronchiseptica	−	+	−	−	+	−	+	Large, white	−
B. pertussis	−	−	{ niacin, cysteine	−	−	−	−	Tiny, pearl-like‡	−
B. parapertussis	−	−	{ methionine	−	−	+	+	Resemble *B. pertussis*	−

* Hemin.

† Coenzyme I or nicotinamide-adenine-dinucleotide (NAD). Responsible for "satellite phenomenon" when cocultured near colonies of *S. aureus.*

‡ Hemolytic.

classic pertussis but usually milder, may be produced by *B. parapertussis* and, rarely in man, *B. bronchiseptica*. These organisms are readily differentiated by laboratory procedures (Table 5-9). All are related immunologically. All are easily killed by heat, standard disinfectants and sunlight.

In pertussis the organisms enter the upper respiratory tract. After a "sniffly" catarrhal period, obstructive edema with more or less anoxia occurs. Interstitial pneumonia may develop, with secondary invasion by other respiratory pathogens. The pertussis bacilli characteristically localize in the cilia of the bronchial epithelium and may mechanically immobilze or paralyze them. The mucous membrane of the respiratory tract becomes hyperesthetic. There is probably damage to superficial layers by both endotoxin and exotoxin, or other biologically active substances elaborated by the organisms (lymphocytosis-stimulating and histamine-sensitizing factors). The familiar strangling and coughing attacks may be related to this and may be partly central in origin. Excessive coughing and difficulty in inspiration lead to anoxia, which in infants and young children may trigger convulsions. Large numbers of the organisms are found in the viscid, mucoid material, probably produced, at least in part, by the "rough" phases of the organisms, and coughed up during the first 2 to 3 weeks of the disease. They disappear after the fourth week. Carriers are unknown or very rare. Bacteremia does not occur.

As in most diseases of the upper respiratory tract, transmission is by droplets of saliva and respiratory mucus.

Control. Infected children should be isolated from susceptibles for 5 weeks after onset. Susceptible children should be isolated for 3 weeks after last exposure unless seen by physician or school nurse daily. Young children never should come into contact with infective cases, as postpertussis pneumonia is a frequent cause of mortality in children under 5.

Three *rough* variants or phases 2, 3, 4 of low virulence and antigenicity, occur in cultures (S → R) and are not associated with human disease. Vaccines are made of killed *B. pertussis* of the encapsulated *smooth* (S) type (phase 1), alum-precipitated and usually mixed with alum-precipitated diphtheria and tetanus toxoids (DTP). Presently accepted schedules call for routine immunization of normal infants and children by subcutaneous inoculation with DTP at 2, 4, 6, and 15 months of age, with boosters at 4 to 6 years. Adult type D and P toxoids (Td) should be used after 6 years of age.

Laboratory Diagnosis. Plates of Bordet-Gengou medium (improved formulas contain penicillin and cycloheximide to inhibit gram-positive respiratory organisms and saprophytic fungi) may be inoculated with a pernasal swab. The organism is found only in the respiratory secretions and not in blood or organs. The plates are incubated at 35 C. for at least 6 days, being examined frequently for minute, pearly, hemolytic colonies. Mild pertussis-like diseases are sometimes due to *B. parapertussis* or to *B. bronchiseptica*. Colonies are fished to "chocolate" blood agar slants for serologic and cultural verification (Table 5-9). Fluorescent antibody stains of smears of respiratory secretions are useful as are adjunctive diagnostic procedure. Blood lymphocytosis is a frequent and diagnostic sign in the acute "whooping" stage. Antimicrobials have no effect on the clinical course during the paroxysmal stage. Erythromycin eliminates *B. pertussis* from patients within a few days. Corticosteroids may favorably influence severe pertussis.

Infections Due to Haemophilus

Haemophilus Infections

Included in the hemophilic group are *H. ducreyi; H. aegyptius; H. influenzae;* and *H. parainfluenzae* (endocarditis) (Table 5-9). *H. aeqyptius,* a cause of acute contagious conjunctivitis, is a biotype of *H. influenzae.*

Haemophilus influenzae, a common resident of the normal upper respiratory tract, does *not* cause influenza but was formerly thought to do so, hence its species name. It causes several other diseases, among them conjunctivitis (pink-eye), meningitis (especially in children), especially in infants, a severe obstructive epiglotitis or tracheolaryngitis with septicemia. Invasions of sinuses and bronchopneumonia are not uncommon. Several types of *H. influenzae* (a, b, c, d, e and f) are distinguished by the specificity of antiphagocytic capsular polysaccharides in a manner analogous to type specificity of pneumococci and are similarly demonstrable by capsular swelling with type-specific antisera. Capsular polysaccharide can be detected in cerebrospinal fluid and urine by CIE. *H. influenzae* infections are generally due to type b (capsule has polyribitol phosphate). Blood cultures in infusion broth, and sputum cultures on "chocolate" agar plates usually are positive in acute epiglotitis and laryngotracheobronchitis; blood and spinal fluid cultures, in meningitis. Broad-spectrum antibiotics, especially ampicillin, are the drugs of choice. The appearance of ampicillin-resistant strains of *H. influenzae* b requires substitution of other drugs such as chloramphenicol.

Chancroid

Chancroid (soft chancre) is an acute, inflammatory, localized and self-limited necrotizing disease, due to

Haemophilus ducreyi, occurring on or near the genitalia. It begins as a small pustule, which soon ruptures, leaving an irregular, painful ulcer with undermined edges and a necrotic, erosive, soft base (soft chancre) that spreads rapidly. Like syphilis it usually produces buboes, but, unlike syphilis, these buboes are soft, painful and often suppurate. Chancroid also differs from syphilitic chancre in the absence of induration and in its violent inflammatory nature. Chancroidlike lesions are sometimes due to (or involve) *Herpesvirus hominis* type 2 and must be differentiated from syphilitic lesions.

Haemophilus ducreyi is *typically* seen within leukocytes, *sometimes* in small clusters ("schools of fish") in direct smears, and morphologically resembles *H. influenzae. H. ducreyi* resembles *H. influenzae* also in being very fragile and susceptible to environmental conditions (Table 5-9).

Diagnosis is based largely on clinical findings and history of exposure. Smears of the exudate in the chancroid or, better, in pus aspirated from closed buboes, may demonstrate the organisms. Rich (25 per cent) rabbit-blood infusion agar (3 per cent) in an atmosphere with 10 per cent CO_2 is essential to growth in initial isolation, which is not often successful.

Transmission is typically by coitus, *rarely* by fomites. The infection is autoinoculable and transmissible by pus and exudates. Although broad-spectrum antibiotics are effective in treatment, use of antibiotics in any venereal disease entails danger of masking syphilis. For this reason, oral sulfisoxazole is considered the treatment of choice.

Infections Due to Yersinia and Francisella

Plague-like Diseases

This term includes bubonic plague, due to *Yersinia pestis;* tularemia, due to *Francisella tularensis;* and hemorrhagic septicemia, due to *Pasteurella multocida.*

All of the above are primarily *zoonoses* (animal diseases transmissible to man) and are fundamentally alike in pathogenesis. All are, in varying degrees, generalized, homorrhagic and septicemic, with localization in various organs and tissues and in lymph nodes that become suppurative, painful buboes. In each disease the organisms occur in pathologic exudates (respiratory, ulcers, draining buboes, etc.).

P. multocida infection is neither common nor serious in man but is highly fatal in animals.

Bubonic Plague and Tularemia. In the advanced, septicemic stage, these diseases are transmissible to man by the bites of arthropods: *Yersinia pestis* by rat fleas (*Xenopsylla cheopis* and others) and by arthropod parasites of ground squirrels and other rodents of forest and prairie (*sylvatic* and *campestral* plague respectively). *Francisella tularensis* is transmitted by deer flies *(Chrysops discalis)* and various ticks (*Dermacentor variabilis, D. andersoni,* etc.). Man-to-man transmission may also occur via man-biting fleas, *Pulex irritans.* In either disease an infectious pustule develops at the site of the bite. Local buboes develop (hence, "bubonic" plague); in many cases septicemia follows. Tularemia is also transmitted to man by his handling of carcasses of infected animals, notably wild rabbits, resulting in rabbit fever in hunters, market men, housewives, etc. Lakes and streams contaminated from decaying infected animal carcasses may also be a source of infection by ingestion or inhalation.

In bubonic plague, fatality may range from 50 to 80 per cent in untreated cases; much less with early treatment. The less common septicemic (hemorrhagic plague with marked terminal cyanosis—black death) and pneumonic forms, untreated, are almost invariably fatal.

In pneumonic plague, which not infrequently develops from severe bubonic cases, respiratory secretions are high infectious, and, as in other infectious respiratory diseases, are impossible to control under ordinary conditions of life.

Tularemia is often very severe, prolonged and debilitating though rarely fatal if treated early with streptomycin and other broad-spectrum antibiotics. Fatality may range to 5 per cent if untreated. Pulmonary tularemia is especially serious.

Prevention. Rat flea-borne bubonic plague is prevented by measures that diminish contact between man and rats (live or dead) and rat fleas. Elimination of open garbage dumps and rat-proofing of buildings are important measures. Dusting rat runways with insecticides to control the fleas, and antirat-poisoning campaigns are often effective. *Pneumonic* plague is controlled only by *prompt* diagnosis, *immediate* and *rigid* segregation of patients and *expert* communicable-disease nursing. Streptomycin is the drug of choice for tularemia. Uncomplicated bubonic plague responds to streptomycin, tetracycline, chloramphenicol or sulfadiazine if treatment is begun early. Streptomycin or tetracyclines are preferred for septicemic plague. A living attenuated vaccine is recommended under special circumstances involving high risk of exposure (e.g., laboratory workers). Chemoprophylaxis of plague contacts (i.e., close household contacts) with either tetracycline or sulfadiazine is recommended.

Recovery from both tularemia and bubonic plague confers high-grade, durable immunity, evidenced by sustained levels of agglutinins, which are cross-reactive with *Fr. tularensis* and *V. cholerae.*

In *diagnosis,* pathologic material stained with Wayson's stain (methylene blue and carbol fuchsin) reveals the organisms as ovoid rods. *Yersinia pestis* is distinguished by having well-maked bipolar staining, most of the cells resembling a closed safety pin. The other species show this character to a lesser degree. The polar granules tend to disappear in cultures.

Yersinia pestis grows well on any media, is motile and produces an exotoxin and soluble protein antigen (fraction 1) that is antiphagocytic. The lipopolysaccharides of both *Francisella* and *Yersinia* contribute to clinical manifestations of disease. *Yersinia* exhibit capsules and bipolar staining and can be reaidly identified with fluorescent antibody. *Francisella tularensis* is difficult to recover on primary isolation, for which blood glucose cysteine agar or other media containing sufficient SH compounds are required; the organism is identified by specific agglutination or by fluorescent antibody. Phagocytized by polymorphonuclear leukocytes, *Y. pestis* is killed; in monocytes it survives, multiplies, forms capsules and gains virulence.

ACTINOMYCETES AND RELATED ORGANISMS

Infections Due to Corynebacterium

Diphtheria

Corynebacterium diphtheriae, the cause of diphtheria, occurs on the oropharyngeal mucosa, and in overt disease it may spread to larynx, trachea, bronchi, nares and lips. Strictly aerobic, it is not invasive during life but grows superficially, exuding diphtheria toxin *if it is lysogenic* with a specific bacteriophage (prophage-β), a classic example of lysogenic conversion.

At the sites of primary infection in the mucosa of the respiratory tract or on the skin, diphtherial toxin causes intense irritation and an acute inflammatory response. The toxin is absorbed into the lymphatics and blood and thereby disseminated to distant sites. The consequent disease depends on obstruction of the air passage, due to local swelling and pseudomembrane formation, plus systemic poisoning. Death may result from the local obstruction unless tracheotomy and intubation are performed. The toxin causes severe myocardial degeneration; the adrenals also are markedly affected. The toxin may cause acute nephritis as well as various transitory nerve damages resulting in aphonia, peripheral neuritis and paresis.

Transmission is as in other respiratory diseases; milk-borne outbreaks, once common, are now rare as a result of pasteurization of milk. Patients with overt diphtheria should be isolated until two or three successive daily negative throat cultures are obtained. If antibiotic therapy or chemotherapy has been employed, negative cultures are of no significance until 1 week after the last dose of the drug.

The *Shick test* consists of an *intra*cutaneous injection of 1/50 of a guinea-pig M.L.D. of active diphtheria toxin. (One M.L.D. of diphtheria toxin is the least amount necessary to kill a 250-gram guinea pig in 4 to 5 days.) If the blood serum has less than about 0.01 unit of antitoxin per ml., a positive reaction appears in 24 to 36 hours, consisting of a slight infiltration of the skin, surrounded by a red areola 1 to 5 cm. in diameter and is caused by the direct dermonecrotic action of the toxin. It is not a hypersensitivity reaction. The reaction persists for at least 5 days. False or pseudoreactions due to allergy to diphtherial protein fade before 5 days as a rule.

A negative reaction indicates that sufficient antitoxin is present to protect from severe diphtheria. It is unnecessary to give prophylactic antitoxin or toxoid to persons showing such reactions.

The *Moloney test* is a test for allergy to diphtherial antigen. In a person allergic to diphtherial protein, intradermal injection of 0.1 ml. of 1:100 *fluid* toxoid may cause a type IV allergic reaction. Persons reacting severely should not be immunized because about 80 per cent of such reactors already have antitoxic immunity.

Laboratory Diagnosis. On slants of Löffler's coagulated-serum medium or Pai's coagulated-egg medium the organism grows readily at 35 C. when inoculated with swabbings from local lesions. Stained with alkaline methylene blue, *C. diphtheriae* has a very distinctive beaded, barred, club-, spindle-, and dumbbell-shaped morphology readily recognized by the experienced bacteriologist. *C. diphtheriae* is readily isolated by streaking throat swabs on blood agar containing about 0.04 per cent of potassium tellurite as a selective agent. Suspicious black colonies are fished to slants for pure culture study, including determinations of type and toxigenicity or freshly prepared Tinsdale (tellurite) agar. *C. diphtheriae* grows in black colonies surrounded by a brown "halo." Staphylococci and commensal *Corynebacteria* (diphtheroids) produce similar black colonies, but without halos. *Listeria monocytogenes* may be misdiagnosed as a "hemolytic diphtheroid."

Suspected diphtheriae-like organism should be tested for toxigenicity by *immunodiffusion* (in-vitro toxigenicity test). A simple form of the latter consists of embedding, in special serum-agar medium in a Petri dish, a strip of filter paper saturated with diphtheria antitoxin. After the agar hardens, the suspected culture is heavily streaked linearly across the agar surface at right angles to the paper. A precipitin reaction, visible as a white line in the agar, develops where toxin diffusing from virulent cultures meets antitoxin diffusing from the paper strip.

Physiologic Types. Several physiologic types of

C. diphtheriae are recognized: gravis, mitis, intermedius; these type-distinctions have no relation to clinical severity of diphtheria. All types form the same toxin.

The xerosis organism *(C. xerosis)* and *C. pseudodiphtheriticum* (Hofmann's bacillus)—so-called diphtheroids, common harmless saprophytes of the throat—are distinguished by their morphology and fermentation reactions (*C. xerosis* attacks both glucose and sucrose; *C. pseudodiphtheriticum* attacks neither).

Diphtheria antitoxin is produced commercially by the subcutaneous injection of horses with diphtheria toxin or toxoid or both until the serum contains about 1,200 units of antitoxin per ml. This is concentrated by standard methods of serum fractionation and is "despeciated" by peptic digestion, which reduces its antigenicity by removing most of the Fc portion of the immunoglobulin. The final immunoglobulin product contains 20,000 units per ml.

Since, to be effective, antitoxin of any sort (tetanus, botulism, etc.) must be given before the specific toxin is bound to the tissues (particularly myocardial and neural tissues), and since antitoxin, if injected subcutaneously, is absorbed slowly, proper serum therapy requires: (a) early diagnosis, (b) early injection of antitoxin intramuscularly and (c) sufficient antitoxin. A skin test for sensitivity to horse serum should be made before injection of *any* equine product, especially if there is any history of allergy, asthma, previous injection of horse serum, etc. Epinephrine should be readily available. Antibiotics (penicillin or erythromycin) are given to eliminate organisms from the upper respiratory tract and terminate the carrier state. Tonsillectomy and adenoidectomy are recommended for the chronic intractable carrier.

Immunization. Recommended schedules for normal infants and children call for DPT at 2 to 3 months of age, followed by two boosters respectively at 2-month intervals and again at 15 months. Boosters are also given at 4 to 6 years and subsequently if needed, the latter with adult type toxoid (Td).

Chemotherapy is of no specific benefit against diphtheria toxin. However, chemotherapeutic drugs in diphtheria help to prevent complications due to other bacteria. The value of chemotherapy in curing the carrier state is debatable.

Infections Due to Mycobacteria

Tuberculosis

Mycobacterium tuberculosis, var. *hominis,* is the principal pathogen of the genus and the etiologic agent of human tuberculosis. Many of the unusual characteristics of the organism are attributable to the extraordinarily high lipid content of the cell and cell wall, for example, resistance to staining, acid-fastness, slow growth rate, resistance to the action of antibodies plus complement, virulence, and resistance to the action of physical and chemical agents.

A primary infection that follows the inhalation of airborne tubercle bacilli induces in the patient a cell-mediated immune response, detectable by the intradermal tuberculin skin test, and an allergic hypersensitivity to tuberculoproteins. Delayed or tuberculin-type allergy is directly referable to intracellular persistence of tubercle bacilli and greatly affects the course of the disease in either reinfection or reactivation type seen in adults. Resistance to reinfection, which is usually endogenous, depends on the capacity of the host to contain the organism by the same cell-mediated mechanisms that produce the inflammatory response in delayed dermal hypersensitivity, that is, T lymphocytes and lymphokines such as MIF and MAF.

Consequences of infection depend upon the immune status of the host, size of the inoculating dose and virulence of the bacilli. Progressive tuberculosis is a chronic granulomatous process that may eventually involve multiple organ systems.

Specimens collected for smear and culture include 24-hour sputa, gastric washings (especially desirable for infants, for some adults who swallow their sputum, and for sputum-negative individuals with minimal activity), 24-hour urines, cerebrospinal fluid and other appropriate materials. Microscopic examination of direct smears stained with either the Kinyoun acid-fast or the immunofluorescent techniques may not reveal any acid-fast bacilli. Sediments of specimens concentrated by centrifugation following digestion using one of several standard techniques provide better material from which to isolate tubercle bacilli. Cultures are an absolute necessity for speciation of mycobacteria because identification cannot be accomplished using only microscopic morphology. Growth on solid media such as coagulated egg proteins, (e.g., Lowenstein-Jensen medium) or oleic acid–albumin (e.g., Dubos–Middlebrook medium) permits observations regarding colonial morphology, thermal tolerance and growth rate and also provides organisms for various biochemical tests, for example, niacin production, nitrate reduction, Tween-80 hydrolysis, catalase activity; for virulence tests, e.g., serpentine cord formation or presence of cord factor, neutral red binding, guinea pig inoculation; and drug-susceptibility assays (Table 5-10).

M. tuberculosis grows best at 37 C. and requires 2 to 4 weeks to produce typical, dry, crumbly, cornmeal-like colonies. The organism is niacin positive, reduces nitrate to nitrite, does not hydrolyse Tween-80, is negative for catalase activity after heating at 68 C.

TABLE 5-10. Differential Properties of *Mycobacterium* Species of Recognized Pathogenicity for Man

Species and Groupings	Niacin	NO$_3$ Reduced	Growth on 5% NaCl	Tween 80 Hydroly.	Cata-lase	Resistant to Isoniazid	Pathogenic for		
							G. Pig	Rabbit	Mice
Mycobacterium tuberculosis	+	+	–	–	+	–	+	–	±
M. bovis	+ or –	–	–	–	+	–	+	+	±
Group I—photochromogens (lemon yellow)*									
M. kansasii	±	+	–	+	+	+	–	–	±
M. marinum (ulcerans?)	–	–	–	+	+	+	–	–	+
Group II—scotochromogens (yellow to dark red)†									
M. scrofulaceum	–	–	–	–	+	+	–	–	±
Group III—no pigments in light									
M. intracellulare (Battey)	–	–	–	–	+	+	–	–	–
Group IV—rapid growers; some scotochromogens									
M. fortuitum—no pigments	–	+	+	v	+	+	–	–	–
M. abscessus—no pigments	–	–	–	–	+	+	–	–	±
M. borstelensis—no pigments	±	–	–	–	+	+	–	–	±

* Produce pigments upon exposure to light.
† Produce pigments in darkness.
v = variable.

for 20 minutes, produces cord factor (serpentine cords), binds neutral red dye and is virulent for guinea pigs.

Antigens used in the tuberculin skin test are standardized based on milligrams of tuberculoprotein and expressed as tuberculin units (TU), old tuberculin (OT) or purified protein derivative (PPD). The greatest value of the tuberculin skin test is in the detection of those individuals whose reactions have converted from negative to positive. Equivocal reactions may be seen in patients infected with a mycobacterial species other than *M. tuberculosis*, in which instances, species-specific antigens may be used to aid in the differentiation process. Antituberculous drugs are prescribed for converters with clinical symptoms and may be prescribed for prophylaxis for asymptomatic converters. The latter should be distinguished by their age and the chronology of their responses to PPD-testing from persons who show a "booster" response and who may therefore be presumed to have longstanding infection and should not be treated.

A vaccine (BCG, bacille of Calmette and Guérin), prepared from an attenuated strain of *M. bovis*, is available for prophylactic immunization. The vaccine should be administered only to those who are nonreactive to tuberculin. Although the vaccine is widely used in Europe and other countries, its use in the United States is restricted to certain high-risk groups, such as young children in a household in which there is an open case of tuberculosis, because immunization vitiates the usefulness of the tuberculin test. BCG should not be given to anyone with a positive tuberculin (PPD) skin test.

Many BCG vaccines are available, all derived from the original strain, but varying widely in immunogenicity, efficacy, and reactogenicity. Lasting protection cannot be assured by vaccination. Therefore tuberculosis must be included in the differential diagnosis even in vaccinees.

Treatment usually consists of a combination of drugs (at least two) to increase therapeutic effectiveness and to minimize the emergence of drug-resistant mutants. When the patient's bacterial population is thought to be particularly large, three drugs are frequently used during the early phase of therapy, for instance when there are extensive infiltrates or cavitary lesions and thus bacilli can be found on direct smears of unconcentrated sputum.

Isoniazid (INH), ethambutol, rifampin and streptomycin are generally considered first line drugs. The most frequently used regimen in the United States is a combination of the first two. Prevention of infection secondary to open cases is effectively achieved by isoniazid, especially if the tuberculin test is negative, indicating maximal susceptibility, or in cases in which

tuberculin tests have converted recently from negative to positive. In the latter instance, whether or not roentgenographic evidence of tuberculosis is present, INH is indicated to prevent progression of active disease.

Other mycobacterial species, although less pathogenic for man than *M. tuberculosis*, are capable of causing human tuberculous disease and therefore present diagnostic and therapeutic problems. *M. bovis* causes bovine tuberculosis and at one time was a leading cause of human tuberculosis. *M. avium*, the cause of avian tuberculosis, has been isolated from human pulmonary lesions. *M. ulcerans* is the etiologic agent of chronic cutaneous tuberculosis. Species classified in the Runyon groups I -IV, sometimes called the "atypical mycobacteria", cause both pulmonary disease and chronic cutaneous lesions. Identification of these less virulent mycobacterial species is necessary because many of them exhibit responses to chemotherapeutic drugs which are different from those of *M. tuberculosis*. The close antigenic relationships that exist among the mycobacteria make immunologic differentiation difficult or impossible. Identification therefore depends upon accurate observations regarding colonial morphology, nutritional and environmental influences on growth and growth rate, and precise performance of the variety of biochemical tests described in other literature (Table 5-10).

Leprosy

Mycobacterium leprae, the etiologic agent of human leprosy, is unique among the bacteria in that it has never been cultured either on lifeless media or in tissue explants. A generation time of 20 to 30 days has been obtained from serial passages in mouse foot pads. Lesion distribution suggests a diminished ability to multiply in body areas where temperatures exceed 30 C. In tissues, the acid-fast organism closely resembles *M. tuberculosis*. Athymic ("nude") mice offer a good host cell medium for propagation of *Mycobacterium leprae*. The nine-banded armadillo has been shown to develop a chronic infection in which *M. leprae* multiples to high numbers and with little harm to the animal.

M. leprae is probably as communicable as *M. tuberculosis*. However, the portal of entry, method of spread, genesis of lesions and manner of dissemination are still unclear. Children are infected more readily than adults. Disease usually occurs in individuals who live in endemic areas, e.g., Africa, Asia, Pacific islands, and certain areas of the United States and who have a history of long and close contacts with leprosy patients. The usually prolonged incubation period varies from several months to 30 years. Regardless of the portal of entry and incubation period, the bacilli eventually find their way to the mucous membranes, skin and peripheral nerves, giving rise to cutaneous lesions and peripheral anesthesias.

The tuberculoid or mild form and the lepromatous or progressive form are the two recognized types of leprosy. Tuberculoid leprosy lesions are usually localized and confined to the skin, mucous membranes and area nerves. Histologically, they resemble tubercles and are comprised of epithelioid cells, lymphocytes and plasma cells; there is usually no caseation, and organisms are rare. In contrast, lepromatous leprosy lesions appear as cutaneous nodules called lepromas that occur principally on the face and extremities, but may involve the liver, spleen, bone marrow, viscera and other areas. Histologically, the lepromas are composed of lymphocytes, plasma cells, and lipid-laden macrophages and giant cells (called lepra cells) containing numerous bacilli arranged in bundles or globular masses (globi).

The status of the patient's cellular immune system and the ability to mount a competent cell-mediated immune response determines to a large degree the type of leprosy that will develop. Tuberculoid leprosy is seen in the more resistant patients whereas lepromatous leprosy is seen in patients with T-lymphocyte defects.

Patients with tuberculoid leprosy react positively to intradermal injections of lepromin, an antigen derived from homogenized leprous tissue, and to tuberculin. Lepromatous leprosy patients give a negative response to lepromin, indicating a defect in the cell-mediated immune responses. Normal individuals, persons immunized with BCG and tuberculosis patients also give a positive reaction to lepromin, indicating cross-reactivity with tuberculoproteins and tissue antigens. The only real value of the lepromin test rests in its ability to identify anergic leprosy patients.

Excepting injuries stemming from peripheral anesthesias, complications of leprosy appear to have an immunologic origin, e.g., erythema nodosum, erythema necroticans and others.

Sulfone drugs are most effective in treatment, especially dapsone (DDS, 4'-4'-diamino-diphenylsulfone). Rifampin kills *M. leprae* and shows promise as a useful drug. Clofazimine has been shown to suppress the erythema nodosum reaction. Thalidomide has shown promise experimentally.

Infections Due to Actinomyces and Nocardia

Actinomyces and *Nocardia* species, the chief etiologic agents of these infectious diseases, are gram-positive bacilli that grow slowly producing, delicate, branching filaments that tend to fragment into bacillary elements. These organisms and the infections they cause are usu-

ally grouped and studied with the fungi for the reasons stated previously and because they cause chronic infections characterized by suppuration and abscess and granuloma formation. The two genera are classified into separate families, Actinomycetaceae and Nocardiaceae, respectively, based on oxygen requirements, catabolic activities and cell wall composition. *Actinomyces* species are anaerobic, ferment carbohydrates, are non-acid-fast, and their cell walls do not contain diaminopimelic acid (DAP). *Nocardia* species are aerobic, produce acid from carbohydrates oxidatively, are partially acid-fast and contain meso-DAP and nocardiomycolic acid in their cell walls.

Among the *Actinomyces* species, *Actinomyces israelii* and *Actinomyces bovis* are the principal etiologic agents of actinomycosis, the former in humans, the latter in cattle. Differentiation of the two species is dependent upon biochemical tests such as nitrate reduction, starch hydrolysis, carbohydrate fermentations; upon serologic tests such as immunofluorescent tests (FA) and immunodiffusion tests (ID); upon the appearance of micro- and macrocolonies; and upon microscopic morphology.

The disease is seen more frequently in cattle than in man. The organisms are indigenous in man and probably in cattle, initiating infection following oral tissue trauma. Bovine infections, called "lumpy jaw," usually involve the mandible with the formation of tumefactions, abscesses, fistulas and sinus tracts, producing soft-tissue and bone destruction and marked cicatrization. The disease is chronic, spreading to contiguous tissues rather than involving blood and lymph vessels. The animal's general health is not affected unless mastication or breathing is impaired.

Human actinomycosis occurs as cervicofacial, abdominal and thoracic infections. Similar to the bovine counterpart in its initiation and clinical picture, the cervicofacial type is the most common and has the best prognosis. Abdominal actinomycosis is thought to arise from swallowing *A. israelii* bacilli or from abdominal trauma and may occur concurrently with or in the absence of a preexisting cervicofacial infection. Abdominal disease often involves the appendix with spread to nearby tissues. Symptoms are referable to the organ systems involved. Thoracic actinomycosis is thought to arise as an extension through the neck from a cervicofacial infection or as an extension through the diaphragm from an abdominal hepatic infection or as a primary infection initiated by aspirating organisms present in the mouth. Symptoms are those of a subacute pulmonary infection, often resembling tuberculosis. Disseminated infections may occur, and death may supervene as a result of secondary bacterial infections. Rarely are pure cultures of *Actino-*

myces israelii (or *Actinomyces bovis*) obtained from lesions or exudates.

In the purulent discharges from the sinus tracts are minute yellow-white granules, often called "sulfur granules." The granules, crushed under a coverslip and examined microscopically, are composed of tangled, branching filaments with peripheral ends radially arranged and clubbed. After washing to remove contaminants, the granules should be cultured in a broth medium containing a reducing agent or on blood agar and incubated anaerobically at 37 C. Examination of cultures for microcolonies at 48 hours and macrocolonies at 14 days facilitate identification.

Penicillin, the drug of choice, is administered intravenously in doses that vary from 3 to 20 million units per day, depending upon the severity of the disease. Energetic surgical intervention to incise and drain lesions and to excise lesions and devitalized tissues is a highly recommended procedure. Other drugs used for therapy are tetracycline, chloramphenicol, streptomycin and sulfadiazine. Antibiotic therapy should be continued for 12 to 18 months following surgical procedures.

Nocardiosis is an acute or chronic disease usually caused by *Nocardia asteroides*. It most often begins as a primary pulmonary infection characterized by suppuration, less frequently by granuloma formation. Bacilli are hematogenously disseminated to subcutaneous tissues and other organs, particularly the central nervous system where they produce multiple abscesses in the brain and meninges. Delicate, branching filaments that are gram-positive and acid-fast are seen in sputum, infected tissues and exudates from abscesses. Granules are not produced.

Nocardiosis is a term usually reserved for primary pulmonary infections or systemic infections resulting from dissemination from a pulmonary locus. Other infections caused by the *Nocardia* are mycetoma, a localized, chronic process characterized by the development of tumefactions, abscesses, fistulas and sinus tracts, and the lymphocutaneous syndrome characterized by the progression of abscesses along a lymphatic channel, producing a clinical picture similar to that seen in lymphocutaneous sporotrichosis. Granules, composed of fine, radially arranged, branching, acid-fast, filaments with or without terminal clubbing, are produced and found in exudates from mycetoma lesions. Granule morphology facilitates a presumptive diagnosis by permitting differentation between bacterial and fungal etiology. Mycetoma is usually caused by *Nocardia brasiliensis* or *Nocardia caviae*. *N. brasiliensis* is the usual etiologic agent of the lymphocutaneous syndrome. All are soil saprobes, initiating infections following inhalation or traumatic cutaneous implantation of the bacilli.

Sputum from nocardiosis patients and deep-tissue biopsies (preferred because fewer contaminants are present) or granules (processed as are actinomycosis granules) from mycetoma patients are cultured on Sabouraud's dextrose or blood agar without added antibiotics and incubated aerobically and anaerobically at 22 and 37 C. All three species produce similar colonies that appear as dry, brittle, orange or yellow, cauliflower-like or cerebriform growths that are often covered with a short-napped mycelium. Speciation of the nocardiae is based on biochemical reactions, principally casein, tyrosine, and xanthine hydrolysis and oxidative acid production from carbohydrates.

Sulfadiazine, the drug of choice for nocardiosis, is administered in doses of 3 to 10 grams/day to achieve a blood level of 9 to 20 mg./100 ml. (depending upon the severity of the infection) for 3 to 6 months. Sulfamethoxazole is also effective. Therapy for mycetoma depends upon the etiologic agent; bacterial or actinomycotic mycetoma responds to antibiotic or antibacterial drugs whereas eumycotic mycetoma is extremely refractory to antibiotics or antimycotic drugs. Early actinomycotic mycetoma lesions (before bone involvement) respond to sulfadiazine. More advanced cases respond to high doses of penicillin. Surgical intervention to drain abscesses and remove devitalized tissues augments healing.

PATHOGENIC AEROBIC AND ANAEROBIC RODS

Improved techniques with prereduced media and apparatus for initial isolation and for identification of strictly anaerobic bacteria of many types have shed much light on the variety, occurrence and properties of these organisms. Their rigid anaerobic requirements appear to depend on (a) lack of cytochrome respiratory chains but presence of flavoprotein enzymes that transfer hydrogen to free oxygen, forming H_2O_2, a very toxic product; (b) failure of strict anaerobes to form peroxidase or catalase to destroy the H_2O_2. Typical aerobes produce catalse.

Prominent among the strict anaerobes are (1) endospore-forming rods, *Clostridium tetani* (tetanus); *C. perfringens* (gas gangrene and food poisoning); *C. botulinum* (food poisoning—botulism); (2) various species of gram-negative, non-spore-forming pleomorphic rods, represented by *Bacteroides fragilis,* and *Fusobacterium necrophorum;* (3) *Peptostreptococcus.* Species of *Peptostreptococcus* often acquire the ability to grow aerobically after several transfers in the laboratory.

On initial isolation all require strictly anaerobic conditions and rich organic media like cooked chopped meat. Generally they are associated (commonly together) with foul smelling, necrotizing, mixed infections. The nonsporing anaerobes account for over half the clinical infections in this class. In most of them, one or more penicillin-resistant, gram-negative anaerobes (*Bacteroides, Fusobacteria*) are involved, occasionally with anaerobic cocci (*Peptostreptococci, Peptococci*). The oral cavity and gastrointestinal tract are the sources of metastatic endogenous infections (brain abscess, pulmonary ("putrid lung" abscess, endocarditis).

Infections Due to Clostridia

Tetanus

Clostridium tetani, the cause of tetanus or lockjaw, has the general properties of the genus (Table 5-11). It is not invasive but grows well in dead tissue; there it can produce its soluble exotoxin. It normally inhabits superficial layers of the soil, especially of cultivated and manured fields, because of its regular presence in the feces of domestic and wild animals and sometimes of man. The spores of *C. tetani* resist dry heat at 150 C. for 1 hour, autoclaving at 121 C. for 5 to 10 minutes and 5 per cent phenol for 12 to 15 hours. Protected from sunlight (ultraviolet light), the dried spores remain viable for many years. Toxin interferes with neuromuscular transmission by inhibiting release of acetylcholine from nerve terminals in muscle. Muscle spasms are due to interference, by the toxin, with spinal cord synaptic reflexes, leading to inhibition of antagonists (strychnine-like action). Secondary disturbances of autonomic functions occur.

Tetanus Toxin. The fraction of the toxin responsible for tetany is called *tetanospasmin*. This has marked affinity for nervous tissue and reaches the CNS (spinal cord) via the blood and lymphatics, especially those associated with nervous trunks.

Tetanus bacilli or spores are doubtless frequently introduced into wounds. The nature of the wound determines whether the bacilli can proliferate. Deep (anaerobic), soil-contaminated wounds in which there has been considerable tissue destruction are especially likely to supply these conditions.

Tetanus neonatorum occurs especially when filthy conditions surround parturition. Infection of the umbilical stump by feces and soil containing *C. tetani* spores is the most common cause.

In the acute form of tetanus the incubation time ranges from 3 to 14 days; in the chronic form the incubation period may exceed a month.

In treatment, prompt surgical debridement of wounds is essential. Tetanus immune globulin (TIg, human) is available and should be given to individuals who have sustained tetanus-prone injuries and who have no known history of immunization with toxoid.

Prevention of tetanus is based primarily on prompt surgical opening, cleansing and disinfecting of wounds. A preliminary dose of 1,000 units of tetanus immune globulin (human [TIG]) is given when conditions are unfavorable to the patient. Equine or bovine antitoxic serums should no longer be used. A dose of tetanus toxoid should also be given at the time of tetanus-prone wounds sustained by individuals with a known history of primary immunization. Basic primary immunity is achieved by routine immunization of infants with DPT (diphtheria and tetanus toxoids combined with pertussis vaccine) at 2, 4, and 6 months of age. Boosters are given at 18 months and at 4 to 6 years. Adult type toxoids (Td) should be used after 6 years of age (Table 5-21).

Diagnostis is primary clinical. Gram-stained smears from an infected wound may reveal the presence of the organism (also anaerobic streptococci, *C. perfringens* of gas gangrene, etc.).

Gas Gangrene (Clostridial Myositis)

Gas gangrene may occur when deep (anaerobic), contused wounds are contaminated with soil that contains spores of one of more of several species of clostridia. Devitalized tissue provides an environment with reduced redox potential that favors the germination and multiplication of anaerobic bacteria. *Clostridium perfringens,* the principal agent in gas gangrene, inhabits the mammalian intestine and female genital tract, and soil and is nearly always accompanied in infected wounds by one or more other soil clostridia that act synergistically with *C. perfringens: C. putrificum, C. histolyticum, C. novyi, C. fallax, C. septicum* and others; the bacteriology is rather variable and heterogeneous. *C. tetani* is also commonly present. As in tetanus, whether or not gas gangrene develops depends on the nature of the wound and the virulence of the bacteria present. Approximately 30 species of *Clostridium* can be isolated from human infections. Taxonomic differentiation, usually impractical for the routine diagnostic laboratory, is based on morphologic and cultural characteristics and on gas–liquid chromatography to identify fermentation products.

Clinical manifestations of clostridial infections are highly varied. Clostridial food poisoning ranks second or third on the list of common forms, usually involves ingestion of meat contaminated with *C. perfringens;* and has an attack rate of 50 to 70 per cent. Diarrheal

TABLE 5-11. Differential Properties of *Clostridium* Species

Clostridium:	Distinctive Morphology	Motile	Capsules	Spores	Proteo-lytic*	Fermentation of Glu-cose	Fermentation of Su-crose	Fermentation of Lac-tose	Diseases
C. botulinum	Sporulating rods have snow-shoe form	+	−	Oval, subterminal	+	+	−	−	Botulism
C. perfringens	Short, thick rods; minute spores (rare)	−	+	Oval, subterminal	+	+	+	+	Myonecrosis, suppuration, cellulitis, septicemia,
C. septicum	Like C. botulinum	+	−	Oval, subterminal	+	+	−	+	enterocolitis,
C. novyi	Like C. botulinum	+	−	Oval, subterminal	+	±	−	−	food poisoning
C. histolyticum	Like C. botulinum	+	−	Oval, subterminal	+	−	−	−	
C. tetani	Sporulating rods resemble drumstick	+	−	Terminal, spherical	+	−	−	−	Tetanus

* All liquefy gelatin, an incomplete protein, but only *C. histolyticum* digests complete proteins *in vitro* and in wounds.

disease is caused by heat-labile protein enterotoxin associated with the spore coat that is released as the ingested vegetative cells are lysed in the intestine. Maximum activity occurs in the ileum. The toxin inhibits glucose transport and causes protein loss into the intestinal lumen. Diagnosis is made by isolation of toxigenic *Clostridium perfringens* from food and/or feces of afflicted patients. Enteritis necrotans is caused by ingestion of meat contaminated with *Clostridium perfringens* type C, the β toxin of which is the cause of an acute ulcerative process, restricted to the small intestine in which the mucosa is denuded and sloughed. It is accompanied by acute abdominal pain, bloody diarrhea, vomiting, shock and a high incidence of peritonitis by direct extension; it is frequently fatal. A somewhat similar process has been recognized as occurring in association with prolonged broad-spectrum antibiotic therapy, most often clindamycin, in the presence of which *Clostridium difficile,* a member of the normal flora, overgrows to produce a potent necrotizing toxin, which is heat labile and acid sensitive. Vancomycin is effective in suppressing *C. difficile. Clostridium perfringens* and *Clostridium ramosum* together represent almost half of the total isolates from clostridial infections of soft tissue, which can occur in almost any region of the body and in which devitalization of tissue and polymicrobial contamination promote anaerobic conditions. These include intra- and abdominal sepsis, carcinoma, empyema and pelvic, brain, pulmonary, prostatic and perianal abscesses. Localized infection of the skin and subcutaneous tissue occurs, particularly in compromised patients such as diabetics and heroin addicts (suppurative myositis), and may develop into diffuse spreading cellulitis and fasciitis, with widespread gas formation, toxemia, shock, renal failure, intravascular hemolysis, ending in death. *C. perfringens, ramosum* and *septicum* may be recovered in blood cultures. In contrast to the foregoing, clostridial myonecrosis (gas gangrene) is a process in which muscle destruction is prominent, in association with crepitance and systemic toxemia, and usually follows trauma or a surgical procedure (e.g., elective colon resection, biliary tract surgery). Gram-stained watery discharges show myriads of gram-positive rods and relatively few inflammatory cells. Blood cultures frequently yield *Clostridia. C. perfringens* accounts for 80 per cent of cases, the remaining being attributable to *C. novyi, septicum* and *bifermentans.* Diagnosis rests on the characteristic appearance of affected muscle, which initially is pale, edematous, and devitalized, progressing inward to frank gangrene. The same condition may occur in the absence of evident trauma (nontraumatic myonecrosis) and is occasionally associated with silent colonic carcinoma. Septic abortion and less frequently normal delivery may be complicated by uterine myonecrosis, usually signalled by jaundice, massive intravenous hemolysis (due to the α toxin, lecithinase) and renal failure with hemoglobinuria, and hypotension. Uncomplicated clostridial bacteremia may occur in the absence of clear-cut localizing signs of infection. Central to treatment is adequate debridement, along with judiciously selected antimicrobial therapy, particularly of suppurative infections in which broad-spectrum antibiotics can serve to suppress aerobic as well as anaerobic bacteria in this invariably polymicrobial infection (aerobes: aminoglycosides such as gentamicin, tobramycin, amikacin; anaerobes: clindamycin, chloramphenicol, metronidazole, cefoxitin). Penicillin G is maximally effective against *C. perfringens.* The use of pentavalent clostridial antitoxin is controversial and should be limited to those patients clearly exhibiting toxemia (hemoglobinemia, disseminated intravascular coagulation, shock, renal failure). The decision to use it must be weighed against the hazards of serum sickness or anaphylactic shock. Skin tests should precede the administration of antitoxin (horse serum). Exchange erythrocyte transfusion to remove damaged erythrocytes has adjunctive therapeutic value. Hyperbaric oxygen, also a controversial topic, has its proponents. Substantial risks are involved and the number of centers with hyperbaric chambers is limited. It cannot replace other modalities of therapy focused on containing and obliterating the source of infection according to good surgical principles.

Botulism (Food Poisoning)

Botulism was first described in cases of poisoning by meat sausage (*botulus* is Latin for sausage). *C. botulinum* may grow in sausages, hams and canned foods of any sort not too dry, and not too acid (limiting pH 4.5) for growth, that are (1) contaminated with soil or marine sediment (E spores); (2) anaerobically packed; and (3) heat processed at a temperature inadequate to kill spores of *C. botulinum,* which are highly resistant to heat and drying. In storage at room temperatures the spores germinate and the growing bacilli form the potent exotoxin. Under commercial canning conditions in the United States botulism is uncommon.

The ability of organisms to produce toxin is probably dependent on lysogenization with specific bacteriophage, as with diphtherial and streptococcal erythrogenic toxins. Toxins type A, B, and E affect man most commonly; types C and D affect cattle and avian species. The toxins are polypeptides with a molecular weight of about 150,000 daltons, which interfere with neurotransmission by preventing the release of acetylcholine at peripheral cholinergic synapses. The heat-labile toxin is inactivated by boiling for 10 minutes or by heating to 80 C. for 30 minutes and by ultraviolet light.

Botulism presents as an afebrile neurologic disorder, characterized by symmetric descending weakness or paralysis (diplopia, photophobia, fixed pupils, dysphonia, dysarthria, dysphagia, respiratory muscle weakness), diminished salivation, oropharyngial desiccation, ileus, and urinary retention. Any or all of these signs and symptoms may occur beginning 6 hours to 8 days after ingestion of toxin-containing food. Specific diagnosis rests on a demonstration of toxin in the blood or in the stool and/or food, in which Clostridium botulinium may also be found (mouse bioassay for toxin). Death is from respiratory failure. Polyvalent antitoxin (horse serum) preceded by a skin test is recommended, 1 vial intravenously, 1 intramusculary. Expectant supportive care is essential, particularly respiratory care, and may be life saving, because intoxication is self-limited. Contaminated wounds have been reported as a primary source of botulin. Infantile botulism (the hypotonic or "floppy" infant) and sudden infant death syndrome (SIDS) are both caused by botulin (types A and B) emanating from organisms that colonize the gastrointestinal tract from some unknown source.

Infections Due to Bacillus

Anthrax

Anthrax, due to *Bacillus anthracis,* a strict aerobe, is primarily a disease of domestic herbivora grazing on spore-infested pastures. It is contracted by man usually via skin abrasions, mainly from (1) tissues or body fluids of infected animals; (2) handling spore-contaminated hides or wool from infected animals or fertilizer made from infected bone meal. Spores sometimes occur in dust on sheep's wool or other animal hair, and inhalation of the infectious dust produces a dangerous pneumonic form of anthrax sometimes called woolsorters' disease. Gastrointestinal anthrax, highly fatal, may also occur. Infection of the face through improperly sterilized shaving brushes and analogous accidents have occurred. A skin lesion (malignant pustule) is most typical.

Most species of *Bacillus* are harmless, motile, ubiquitous saprophytes of the soil and environment. *B. anthracis* is distinctive, being highly pathogenic, nonmotile and nonhemolytic. A hemolytic, harmless species closely similar to *B. anthracis* is *B. cereus.* Most species of *Bacillus* are more or less strict aerobes or facultative and readily cultivable on simple peptone media or blood agar at 25 to 40 C. Oval spores occur near the middle of anthrax bacilli without swelling the rod. Anthrax spores are long lived and unusually resistant to heat and chemicals. In infected tissues *B. anthracis* forms a large polypeptide capsule that is antiphagocytic and therefore associated with virulence, illustrative of a general phenomenon in bacterial infection.

In *cutaneous anthrax,* the most common form, the characteristic ulcer appears within about 24 hours after infection, teeming with bacilli. Its center soon changes into a black, central necrosis with an angry, markedly edematous areola, spreading eschar ("malignant pustule") and painful local lymphadenopathy. With severe local reactions, especially around the head and neck, toxemia may occur ("malignant edema"). Anthrax in any form, but especially pulmonary and gastrointestinal forms with toxemia, is accompanied by bacteremia and may be the source of hematogenous meningitis. Penicillin is the drug of choice in therapy. Cortisone is indicated in cases of malignant edema. Penicillin-allergic patients can be successfully treated with erythromycin, tetracycline or chloramphenicol.

A potent and complex protein exotoxin consisting of three distinct factors was first discovered in tissues and exudates of infected animals and was later demonstrated in cultures rich in serum and bicarbonate ions, which also increase capsule production. Virulence of *B. anthracis* depends on production of both capsules and toxin. Infection evokes antibodies against both. Artificial immunity is evoked by the use of AP antigenic fraction of the toxin and is especially valuable among the heavily exposed. Occasional nontoxigenic, encapsulated variants occur.

Control. Careful incineration or *deep* burial of dead animals, their exudates, contaminated straw, etc., is necessary. Animal autopsies should not be performed on farms, as all body fluids and tissues are highly infectious, and *exposure to air* induces anthrax organisms to sporulate. Legislation requires disinfection of hides, wool, bone meal fertilizer, and brush bristles in commercial use. During an outbreak, animals should be immunized with a nonencapsulated spore vaccine. A "protective antigen" (PA) vaccine is available for people who are at particular risk.

Diagnosis. Gram-stained smears of pustule exudate, body fluids, tissues or blood show the characteristic, encapsulated rods. Cultures of these materials should also be made, leading to conclusive diagnosis by animal inoculation (mice are highly susceptible) and serologic and biochemical tests.

SPIROCHETAL DISEASES

The order Spirochaetales (spirochetes) includes spiral, *flexible* bacteria (contrast with *rigid Spirillum*). Although procaryons, the spirochetes are structurally the most complex of bacteria, consisting of three principal parts: (a) an outer envelope or periplast probably containing murein, on which marked susceptibility of some species to penicillin presumably depends; (b) the cell proper, an elongated cylindrical tube with cytoplasmic membrane; (c) a fibrillar, axial filament arising, like flagella (and, seemingly like them, contractile), from basal granules at one end of the tubular cell and gathered into a bundle constituting an axial filament around which the cell is wound helically. In general, spirochetes are not readily stained and are commonly examined in the living state in moist material by means of the darkfield microscope. (See also Fluorescent Antibody-Staining Technique.)

The order contains numerous saprophytes, but only three genera are of medical importance (see p. 1).

All pathogenic spirochetes are quite fragile and readily killed by drying, heat, and disinfectants. However, they can survive for years at − 76 C.

Syphilis

Treponema pallidum, the cause of syphilis, is from 4 to 20 μm. in length and 0.2 μm in diameter. The cytoplasm is surrounded by a trilaminar cytoplasmic membrane, a delicate inner mucopeptide layer (periplast) and an outer lipoprotein membrane containing lipopolysaccharides. Three fibriles are inserted into the tapered ends of the cell. The organism has 4 to 14 coils and differs from *Borrelia* (see below) in the tightness and regularity of its coils. Its distinctive movements consist of occasional rotation about the long axis, slow to-and-fro gliding and occasional sedate bending.

For diagnostic darkfield examination fluid should be taken from a cleanly scraped chancre or, better, punctured bubo and should contain as little blood and solid material as possible. Dried smears, negatively stained with India ink, nigrosin or other stains in lieu of darkfield for diagnosis can lead to error because distinctive motility permits some degree of differentiation from saprophytic treponemes of the genitalia.

Spirochetes are demonstrated in tissues by the silver impregnation method of Levaditi or Fontana. *Treponema pallidum* has never been cultivated in a virulent state on artificial media though several readily cultured nonpathogenic strains (notably the Reiter strain) morphologically identical with, and antigenically very closely similar to, *T. pallidum,* are well known.

Demonstrable immunity appears in 2 to 4 weeks after appearance of the primary lesion (chancre) when standard serologic tests [SST or STS] become positive. Specific antitreponemal tests also become positive.

Primary (2 to 6 weeks) and secondary stages (4

weeks to 4 months) subside with developing specific resistance. Years later, tertiary gummatous lesions of arteries, CNS, bones, viscera, etc., with intense cytologic response and necrosis, probably related to allergy, develop. Transplacental transmission leads to congenital syphilis. A healthy neonate of a syphilitic mother may have syphilitic IgG globulins in its blood since IgG molecules pass the placenta. Syphilitic IgM cannot pass the placenta and appears in the neonate only as a result of active fetal syphilitic infection.

If effective antispirochetal therapy (e.g., penicillin) is instituted *early* in the disease, i.e., before immunity has developed, *reinfection* can occur. High-grade immunity develops in 2 to 6 weeks. *Relapse* may occur if the early therapy is not totally effective.

Transmission is by sexual contact (vaginal or oral) or, rarely (0.01 per cent) by contact with *fresh* exudates from any open lesions at any stage; direct blood transfusion, or insufficiently aged (less than 4 days) blood-bank blood can transmit during any septicemic stage. Freshly infected needles, syringes, etc., can also transmit the disease to nonimmune persons.

Diagnostic procedures include:

1. *Darkfield examination* of material from open lesions at any stage. A single negative darkfield is not conclusive.

2. *Standardized serologic tests* (SST) or serologic tests for syphilis (STS) depend on the presence in serum of immunoglobulins (IgM or IgG) reactive with a lipoidal antigen derived from bovine tissues (cardiolipin). This antibody (referred to as reagin or reaginic antibody) results from the interaction of the host with *T. pallidum* and has nothing to do with IgE, also fortuitously referred to as reagin or reaginic antibody associated with atopic allergy. Syphilitic reaginic antibody is distinct from antibody to *T. pallidum* and is measured by flocculation with cardiolipin-cholesterol-lecithin antigen in the Veneral Disease Research Laboratory (VDRL) or Rapid Plasma Reagin (RPR) tests.

3. *Tests for specific antitreponemal antibody.* These antibodies are evoked by, and are *specific* for, *Treponema pallidum* and persist during even chronic, clinically minimal, stages when SSTs are negative. They are detected with the fluorescent treponemal antibody adsorption (FTA-ABS) test, which utilizes the principle of the indirect or "sandwich" fluorescent antibody staining procedure (p. 100). Patient's sera and known positive and negative control sera (clear and unhemolyzed) are inactivated at 56 C. for 30 minutes and adsorbed with material (sorbent) from Reiter

treponemes to remove antibody to commensal spirochetes that cross-react with *T. pallidum*. Fixed smears of *T. pallidum* grown in rabbit testis (Nicholas strain) are used as the antigen substrate. The stained slides serve as permanent records. A positive nontreponemal reaginic test may occur in many conditions other than syphilis, from which they must be distinguished by a negative specific test for treponemal antibody (FTA-ABS). "Biological false positive" reaginic antibody tests occur frequently in infectious mononucleosis, malaria, granulomatous disease of many etiologies, some viral and chlamydial infections, dysgammaglobulinemias and autoimmune diseases such as rheumatoid arthritis and systemic lupus erythematosus.

Yaws, Pinta, Bejel

These nonvenereal, tropical treponematoses are caused by *Treponema pertenue, T. carateum* and *T. pallidum,* respectively. Bejel is endemic (nonvenereal) syphilis. As with venereal syphilis, all of these diseases are characterized by self-limited primary and secondary lesions, a latent period apparently disease-free and late lesions that are frequently destructive, particularly of bone and skin. All give at some stage positive VDRL or RPR tests and/or treponemal antibody (FTA-ABS) tests. In yaws the distinctive frambesia (raspberry-like) lesion is diagnostic. All three may be diagnosed by darkfield examination, the organisms being morphologically indistinguishable from one another. These diseases respond dramatically to penicillin. Unlike syphilis, they are commonly transmitted by fomites (pronounced fómĭtēz) and nonvenereal contact as between mother and child; in addition yaws is transmitted (probably mechanically) by small flies, notably *Hippelates* species.

A single injection of long-acting penicillin G is effective in the treatment of all of these treponematoses.

Leptospirosis

Leptospirosis is infection by any of approximately 150 sorotypes of a single species *(Leptospira interrogans)* (Gr. *leptos* = thin). Morphologically and culturally the pathogenic species or types are distinguishable from one another, but as a genus leptospires are distinguished by properties listed on page 351. There are numerous free-living saprophytic species, often collectively spoken of as *L. biflexa*. These are commonly found in wet, decomposing materials, domestic drain pipes, etc. They differ markedly from pathogenic species in resistance to azaguanine, conditions in contaminated cultures, sewage and the like, and in growth at 5 to 15 C.

Pathogens grow well only at about 30 to 37 C. and, like *Treponema pallidum,* are extremely sensitive to surface-tension reducers (detergents, bile, soap, etc.) and to acid (e.g., acid urine or water). Bacterial contaminants in cultures are usually lethal to them. Leptospires traverse ordinary bacteriostatic filters. The various pathogenic species or serotypes can be differentiated from each other only by using highly specific, adsorbed, agglutinating sera. They survive (grow?) in urine-polluted water if not too acid or too heavily contaminated.

Zoonoses. Leptospirosis is primarily a disease of wild and domestic animals and is readily transmissible to man by water contaminated by infected *urine* of rats, dogs, cats, cattle and man, (in these species the organisms colonize the renal tubules, sometimes for life); by infected carcasses of animals in rivers, lakes and swimming holes; by urine-polluted bilge or mine water; by infected birds in poultry-dressing establishments, etc. Thus, leptospirosis is a good example of the zoonoses: infectious diseases of animals communicable to man. Person-to-person transmission occurs rarely. Leptospires enter the blood mainly via abrasions in the skin, possibly via intact skin, and probably via the oral mucosa during ingestion of contaminated foods, water, etc. Neither endotoxins nor exotoxins have been demonstrated.

In severe cases of Weil's disease (icteric leptospirosis) there is much damage to liver and kidneys. Hemorrhages into stomach, intestines and skin are common, and jaundice is marked. Temperature is high. The organisms appear in the blood during the initial febrile period, later in the urine and tissues. Mortality varies and may be, at times, fairly high. Many cases are mild and anicteric (subclinical).

Infections by leptospires may involve meninges, eyes, lungs, etc., with protean symptomatology. Meningitis and iridocyclitis without jaundice often occur.

Prevention. Avoidance of rat-infested quarters; water or food susceptible to urinary pollution by man or lower animals; handling infected animals; exposure of the body, as by swimming in streams or ponds, to water susceptible to pollution by urine or infected carcasses, and control of rat breeding will prevent leptospirosis. Vaccination of domestic livestock and pets with killed leptospires is widely practiced.

Vaccines made of suspensions of killed leptospires are good antigens but must be so broadly polyvalent as to be generally impracticable, and they do not prevent renal colonization. Recovery confers immunity.

Diagnosis often can be made immediately by darkfield examination of fresh urine (*not* blood because of paucity of leptospires and confusion with inert fibrils in blood). Blood or urine cultures in peptone-mineral media with 10 per cent serum often yield leptospires. Inoculation of first-week blood or urine into young hamsters or guinea pigs often yields the infecting leptospira. Live leptospires are also demonstrable by all three methods in emulsions of kidney and liver of infected animals. About 50 per cent of wild rats in some garbage dumps have been shown with darkfield to harbor *L. icterohaemorrhagiae.* Agglutination and bacteriolytic (agglutination-lysis) tests and complement-fixation tests with convalescent serum, using mixed antigenic types of leptospires, are usually positive to high titers.

Treatment. Mild cases are self-limited. Tetracycline is recommended for severe Weil's disease.

Relapsing Fever (Borreliosis)

Various closely related spirochetes, serotypes of the genus *Borrelia,* cause relapsing fevers (do not confuse with undulant fever due to *Brucella* sp.). Borrelias resemble treponemes in many respects. They are best observed with a darkfield apparatus in febrile blood of patients or of diagnostically infected white rats that quickly develop marked borrelemias. Blood film stained with Giemsa's stain also reveal them. Borreliosis is an arthropod-borne disease.

Transmission in south-central Europe, India, Asia and North Africa and other areas where pediculosis occurs is by body lice *(Pediculus humanus)* crushed on bite wounds, and in these geographical areas is due principally to *Borrelia recurrentis,* for which man is the only host. In South Africa, the Balkans, eastern Mediterranean regions, South and Central America and the western United States other closely similar species, notably *B. duttoni,* are transmitted in the bites, joint (coxal) fluids and feces (depending on involved species) of various *Ornithodoros* ticks. The tick-borne disease is a true zoonosis, since there are animal reservoirs, principally wild rodents, but also monkeys, armadillos, opossums, etc. Man is only accidentally infected. The spirochetes are also transmissible transplacentally, causing fatal infection of the fetus. In *Ornithodorus* ticks, borrelias are transmitted transovarially; not so in lice.

The organisms multiply in the bloodstream, probably also in tissues. After an initial acute, febrile attack with headache, chills and splenomegaly, the fever ends by crisis in 1 to 2 weeks. After about 5 days immunity develops, and readily visible agglutination (rosette forms) of the spirochetes occurs in the bloodstream. The organisms persist in certain tissues and apparently become resistant to the antibodies, presumably by appearance of antigenically distinct mutants, and again invade the bloodstream after 1 to 3 weeks, causing a febrile relapse followed again by agglutination. This may recur two to ten times before true convalescence begins, each relapse being a little less severe than the preceding one.

Prevention depends on anti-louse measures where lice are the vectors; elsewhere, anti-tick measures, chiefly avoidance of tick-infested rodents in caves, deserted camps, use of insect repellents, and so on. Antibiotic therapy (tetracycline or erythromycin) is effective. If given during a febrile attack, Jarisch–Herxheimer-like reactions may occur.

Class Mollicutes = (Lat.*mollis*-pliable; *cutis*-skin)

Order Mycoplasmatales

Genus Mycoplasma

Mycoplasma mycoides, the first of this group to be discovered (1898), was found in bovine pleuropneumonia. Later, similar forms, called pleuropneumonia-like organisms (PPLO), were found in cases of mastitis in sheep and goats, and in rodents, often associated with arthritis and lesions of eyes and ears. Most mycoplasmas are inhabitants of the normal upper respiratory and genitourinary tracts. Strains *(Ureaplasma urealyticum)* characterized by producing very tiny colonies) (T strains) cause nongonococcal urethritis (NGU).

Mycoplasma pneumoniae (Eaton agent), the first mycoplasma proven to be a cause of human disease, causes an interstitial pneumonia called "primary atypical pneumonia" that is transmitted like other respiratory diseases. The mortality rate is low. It was for years thought to be due to a virus, especially after it was shown by Eaton and associates, in 1944, to be filterable. Not until 1962 was an Eaton agent cultivated on artificial medium and is now called *Mycoplasma penumoniae.*

Mycoplasma pneumoniae is a significant cause of respiratory infection (pneumonia) in temperate climates and may occur in periodic epidemics, most frequently affecting school-age children and young adults. Spread is by respiratory droplet and close contact. Illness is increasingly severe wtih increasing age. The primary target of the organism is the respiratory epithelium, in which normal ciliary motion is interrupted. It is primarily a surface infection. Recovery is due to local accumulation of IgG and IgA antibody. Treatment with tetracyclines or erythromycin is effective; penicillin is contraindicated.

The organism may be cultivated on blood and serum media with yeast extract; it also may be cultivated in avian embryos and in tissue cultures with penicillin, polymyxin B and thallium acetate as antibacterial agents. Colonies on agar differ from those of most other mycoplasma in being domed and granular. *M. pneumoniae* colonies produce β-type hemolysis on blood-agar plates and hemadsorption of erythrocytes of various species. The organisms are best identified by serologic methods, including the aerobic, tetrazolium-reduction-inhibition (TRI) test and by fluorescent antibody-staining techniques. Primary atypical pneumonia is also indicated by the appearance in the serum of *cold agglutinins* (agglutination of human O erythrocytes at 4 C., eluted at 37 C.) due to IgM with cross-reactive specificity for erythrocyte glycophorin and *M. pneumoniae.*

Ureaplasma urealyticum (11 serotypes previously called T or "tiny" mycoplasma because of colonial size) and *M. hominis* (7 serotypes) colonize the genital tract and have been implicated in inflammatory disease and its consequences in the female internal genitalia. Antibody to both organisms is detected with increasing frequency in relation to increasing age. Infection is venereally transmitted. *U. urealyticum* is an important cause of nongonoccal urethritis (NGU) and infection of the male adnexa and salpingitis. Diagnosis is based on cultivation of mycoplasma on specially enriched media and on biochemical speciation by metabolic inhibition with specific antibody. Serologic responses to this organisms are irregular so that serodiagnosis is not feasible as a routine measure in acute infection. Tetracycline is the drug of choice in treatment.

L Forms of Bacteria. Many common gram-positive bacteria, cultivated in the presence of penicillin in media with *increased osmotic pressure* (e.g., 3 per cent sucrose), grow without their cell wall and are therefore called *protoplasts;* in many respects they are much like PPLO. Gram-negative bacteria retain the lipoprotein portions of their cell wall in the presence of penicillin and are therefore not wholly naked and are called *spheroplasts.* These cell-wall-less or cell-wall-defective forms are called L forms (from the Lister Institute, where they were first described) of the particular bacterium involved. Removed from the *osmotically protective* medium they undergo plasmoptysis, i.e., they are "osmotically fragile." With the removal of penicillin they revert to true bacteria. PPLO also not uncommonly revert to well-known species of bacteria, and vice versa. It is suggested that *nonreverting PPLO* are genetically stabilized bacterial L form mutants with decreased osmotic fragility. The possible development of L forms of pathogens in vivo, especially during penicillin therapy, with establishment of latent and *antibiotic-resistant* infections, is of obvious importance clinically.

A number of other species of PPLO, also bacterial L forms, are of importance in diagnostic work with viruses, since they can contaminate tissues used as sources of cell cultures for diagnostic virology as well as animal sera used in cell culture media.

Streptobacillus moniliformis is a bacterial species, bacillary and streptobacillary in form, that produces minute PPLO called L_1 bodies, that revert in turn to *S. moniliformis*. Both forms may occur in the same culture. *Streptobacillus maniliformis* is related to one form of rat-bite fever and to Haverhill fever.

MINUTE BACTERIA

This Order is named for Howard T. Ricketts, who died of typhus fever, a rickettsial disease, in 1910, while investigating the causative agent.

Family Rickettsiaceae

Genus Rickettsia

Morphologically, rickettsias are very like minute cocci and rods, the later often containing bipolar granules of unknown significance. The organisms can grow in tissue cell cultures but are commonly propagated in cells of the yolk sac of embryonated hens' eggs. Machiavello's stain, is commonly used. In spite of their minute size rickettsias do not pass through bacteria-retaining filters (but see *Coxiella* of Q fever, the exception). Their cell structure is procaryotic, and their cell walls contain muramic acid, a substance found only in bacteria. They are obligate intracellular parasites. Rickettsias contain a potent endotoxin but produce no exotoxin. Cellular subtances are antigenic and species specific, except the antigen that is shared with *Proteus* (see Weil-Felix reaction).

Habitat. Most rickettsias are primarily parasites of insects and only secondarily of animals. They are transmitted from insects to man, and from man to man, by the bites of insects or by being rubbed into scratches and cuts when infected insects are crushed on the skin or deposit feces there.

Antibiotic Susceptibility. Rickettsias possess bacterium-like, though limited, enzyme systems, including those of the Krebs cycle and those necessary to the synthesis of ATP, cell wall and some proteins. Hence rickettsias are susceptible to enzyme-inhibiting chemotherapeutic drugs, especially the tetracyclines and chloramphenicol. Relapses occur during therapy because the organisms are chiefly intracellular.

Vaccines. Rickettsias grow in the yolk-sac membranes of eggs, as mentioned above, at 32 C. They are separated from this material by differential centrifugation. After inactivation with formaldehyde they are used for making vaccines (e.g., Cox-type typhus vaccine) and as antigen in serologic studies. Before injection of any egg-derived product, including several virus

TABLE 5-12. Rickettsial Diseases

Diseases	Rickettsias	Scrotal Reaction	Common Vector	Weil-Felix Reaction Proteus OX 19	OX 2	OX K
Rocky Mountain spotted fever	*R. rickettsii*	++++	Dog tick *(Dermacentor variabilis)* Rabbit tick *(D. andersoni)*	+++	++	—
Murine (endemic) typhus	*R. mooseri*	++	Rat flea *(Xenopsylla cheopis)* (lice?)	+++	+	—
Classic (epidemic) typhus	*R. prowazeki*	+	Body louse *(Pediculus corporis)*	++++	+	—
Brill's disease (recrudescent typhus) (Brill-Zinsser disease)	*R. prowazeki*		Original infection	v*	v*	—
Tsutsugamushi (Japanese or Oriental river or swamp fever; scrub typhus)	*R. orientalis*	—	Harvest (field) mite *(Trombicula akamushi)*	—	—	++++
Q fever	*Coxiella burneti*	—	Dust, ticks, improperly pasteurized milk	—	—	—
Rickettsialpox	*R. akari*	—	Mouse mite *(Allodermanyssus sanguineus)*	—	—	—

* v = variable.

vaccines, e.g., yellow fever, inquiry should be made concerning allergy to eggs; fatal reactions have occurred. Vaccine is used mainly against louse-borne or epidemic typhus and in persons at high risk from murine typhus.

Laboratory diagnosis of rickettsial disease is done most conveniently and reliably by agglutination tests using purified yolk sac antigens. These can reveal group-specific antibodies. Rabbit, mouse or guinea-pig inoculation, followed by records of febrile response; examination of sections of tissues; and serologic tests are valuable but hazardous procedures. The intensity of the effect of rickettsias on the scrotum of guinea pigs is a valuable diagnostic datum (Table 5-12).

The *Weil-Felix test* depends on agglutination of *Proteus vulgaris* (variety OX-19, OX-2 or OX-K) by the serum of patients with certain rickettsial infections. *Proteus* has no etiologic relationship with rickettsial diseases but shares an O antigen with certain rickettsias. Nonspecific misleading reactions are obtained with the serum of patients having *Proteus* infection or borelliosis but no rickettsial infection. (See Table 5-12).

Diseases Due to Rickettsias. Three main groups of diseases due to Rickettsia species are recognized: (1) the *Rocky Mountain spotted fever* group; (2) the *typhus* group; and (3) the *tsutsugamushi* (oriental swamp or scrub or river fever) group. Diseases of the first group are mainly tick borne. The ticks maintain infection transovarially and by copulation and among a varied mammalian reservoir by biting; man is an incidental host. The typhus group includes European or "classic" or epidemic typhus and Brill's disease (recrudescent typhus); man-to-louse-to-man cycle; the lice die of the infection. Also in this group is rat flea–borne murine or endemic typhus. Diseases of the third group are larval-mite borne. Q fever and its causative organisms differ from all of the above in clinical respects and vectors.

Another rickettsial disease, rickettsialpox, occurs, so far as is known, only in restricted areas of some cities of the eastern seaboard of the U.S., Korea, and Russia. It is transmitted by mites that infest house mice and therefore is a household disease.

Clinically, all rickettsial diseases (except Q fever, which resembles influenza, and rickettsialpox, which resembles chickenpox) have certain cardinal features in common: stupor and other neurologic signs, rash, and invasion of reticuloendothelial cells by the rickettsias. Usually there are both clinical and pathologic diagnostic differences between these rickettsioses, such as chronology, intensity and distribution of the rash, development of eschar at site of arthropod bite, etc.

In nature, epidemic typhus occurs only in man, the other rickettsioses being primarily zoonoses (i.e., enzootic in lower animals, occurring only secondarily in man). The rickettsias of typhus and tsutsugamushi fevers remain in the cytoplasm of infected cells, while those of Rocky Mountain spotted fever and of rickettsialpox also invade the nucleus. In severe Rocky Mountain spotted fever the smooth muscles of peripheral vascular walls are destroyed. In rickettsialpox and tsutsugamushi there is a definite ulcer or eschar at the site of the infecting bite. Rickettsialpox is distinguished by its poxlike vesicles. Tsutsugamushi, Rocky Mountain spotted fever and epidemic typhus are generally more severe than murine typhus or rickettsialpox.

Brill-Zinsser disease is epidemic or classic typhus, occurring as sporadic cases in the total absence of body lice, as a relatively mild *recrudescence* of latent infection years after the initial attack. In the febrile stage the disease is transmissible by body lice. Apparently the rickettsias can remain viable but quiescent in the tissues for many years after initial infection. Occasionally, this disease appears in the United States, especially in immigrants from central Europe, Asia Minor and Eastern Mediterranean areas.

Genus Coxiella

This genus contains only one species, *Coxiella burneti,* named for H. L. Cox and F. M. Burnet, simultaneous discoverers. It is immunologically distinct from other rickettsias. *C. burneti* causes Q fever (Q for "query") first observed and named by Derrick in Australia. *C. burneti,* has most of the properties of *Rickettsia* but differs in being (1) filterable; (2) quite resistant to environmental conditions such as drying, diffuse sunlight, disinfectants, heating at 62 C. for 30 minutes; (3) mode of transmission: improperly pasteurized contaminated milk; dust, from barns housing infected sheep, cattle, goats, rodents; tissues and parturition fluids, etc., from infectious animals; several species of ticks.

In *Q fever* the respiratory tract is most commonly affected. There is no rash. The disease clinically resembles influenza, often with interstitial pneumonitis. Mortality is low or nil. Q fever appears to be disseminated widely, especially among persons in the animal industries. The organisms may be isolated from the blood by animal inoculation. Diagnosis also may be made by serologic methods but *not* by the Weil-Felix test. Milk can be made safe only by pasteurization for 30 minutes at a temperature of 63 C. (145 F.). Tetracycline and chloramphenicol are the drugs of choice in treatment.

ORDER CHLAMYDIALES

Family Chlamydiaceae

Genus Chlamydia

The various species of Chlamydia are all very similar and are probably host-modified mutants of one parent stock. They have been called Bedsonia, for Sir Thomas Bedson who, with Bland, first described the psittacosis organism. Formerly classified with viruses, the chlamydias, like *Rickettsia* and *Coxiella,* are bacteria modified to obligate intracellular parasitism by lack of certain protein-synthetic and oxidative-enzyme systems. Chlamydias are distinctive in lacking enzymes that synthesize ATP; they must use host-derived energy.

They are not arthropod-borne. They exhibit a complex developmental cycle involving initial and elementary bodies.

The genus is divided into two main groups. Group A *(Chlamydia trachomatis)* includes (1) the TRIC agents, of which ocular types cause trachoma and genital types cause inclusion conjunctivitis, and (2) the agent of lymphogranuloma venereum (LGV). Group B includes the agents of psittacosis and ornithosis.

In trachoma (ocular *types* A, B, C) intracellular inclusions in infected cells are discrete and rather dense, staining brown with iodine because of glycogen content. Their occurrence is prevented by sulfadiazine and cycloserine. The trachoma organisms are demonstrable culturally (egg yolk or tissue culture) or microscopically (Giemsa or fluorescent antibody) in epithelial cells scraped from tarsal plates.

In inclusion conjunctivitis (group A, genital *types* D, E, F) the organisms, closely resembling *types* A, B and C, occur in the eyes of newborn infants and are usually derived from the mother's genital tract. They are coitally transmissible and common among the sexually promiscuous. Infections of ears, nose and genitalia may also occur in neonates. Trachoma in neonates is rare. In adults the organisms are an important cause of nongonococcal penicillin-resistant urethritis (NGU). *C. trachomatis* is also a major cause of pelvic inflammatory disease and a distinctive form of neonatal interstitial pneumonia.

The chlamydias in lymphogranuloma venereum differ from the foregoing in being lethal for mice on intracerebral inoculation and in being less infective for the eyes of lower primates. In human females and homosexual males they commonly cause ramifying, destructive, painful rectal disease. The LGV organisms are related to TRIC types E and D. Chlamydial infections tend to become chronic or latent and relapsing.

Group B organisms *(C. psittaci)* cause psittacosis, or parrot fever, named for the psittacine birds that are its natural hosts and carriers. Ornithosis, contracted from a variety of other species of birds, is due to the same, or virtually identical, organisms. These chlamydias are transmitted in dried dust containing feces and respiratory secretions of sick birds. Psittacosis (or ornithosis) in man occurs as a primary interstitial pneumonia that must be distinguished from influenza, mycoplasmal pneumonia and Q fever. The infection may become generalized and is then quite dangerous. Infected cell inclusions (Levinthal-Cole-Lillie bodies) are rather diffuse and ill defined and contain no iodine. These bodies appear in spite of sulfadiazine and cycloserine (compare TRIC agents).

During infection by any of these organisms, *group-specific* CF antibodies are produced. Neutralizing or protective antibodies also appear, though irregularly and in low concentrations, and can be used to differentiate organisms of group A from the organisms of group B. Both groups of organisms are readily recoverable by primary isolation in appropriate cell culture systems (e.g., McCoy cells treated with IUDR and cycloheximide) and are identified by distinctive cytopathologic characteristics and reactions with fluorescent antibody.

ARTHROPODS AS VECTORS OF DISEASE

Many species of insects* transmit disease. Two methods of transmission are observed: (1) mechanical and (2) biologic. The first is illustrated by the transmission of typhoid and dysentery bacilli on the legs of flies, ants and roaches, which crawl first on infectious feces and then on foods, lips of infants, etc. These *coprophagic* insects also can harbor such organisms in their intestines after eating feces, and their fecal deposits can make food infectious.

Biologic transmission is seen in the spread of such diseases as malaria, yellow fever and numerous viral encephalitides by the bites of specific mosquitoes, and the dissemination of European typhus by body lice. Biologic transmission generally involves a period of *extrinsic incubation;* i.e., a period of *development* of the pathogen in the arthropod (e.g., malaria, leishmaniasis) or of *migration* of the pathogen from stomach to biting parts (e.g., yellow fever virus). In either case, during the period of extrinsic incubation the *bite* is not infectious although sometimes, as in yellow fever, the arthropods contain the infective agent at all times.

VIRUSES

A virus may be defined as a particulate infective agent consisting solely of a nucleic acid (NA) genome (or *core*) associated with a protective coating (or *capsid*) made of protein subunits called *capsomers* with or without a more complex outer, host-cell derived covering (or *envelope*). The core with associated pro-

* Used in the ordinary sense to mean any terrestrial arthropod.

tein(s) is called a *nucleocapsid*. The entire particle with any appendages (e.g., the tail of phages or penton fibers of adenoviruses) is called a *virion*.

The first known virus (tobacco mosaic) was discovered in 1892 by Iwanowki, regarded as a living contagious fluid *(contagium vivum fluidum)* by Beijerinck in 1898, and purified as protein in crystalline form by Stanley in 1935. The first known virus of vertebrates (foot-and-mouth disease) was discovered by Löffler and Frosch in 1898; the first known virus of humans (yellow fever), by Walter Reed and his associates in 1899. Studies of animal viruses were laborious, cumbersome and expensive and progressed slowly until the discovery of *bacteriophage* (phage) by Twort in 1915 and d'Herelle in 1917. Because phages could be cultivated easily, quickly, safely and inexpensively in test-tube cultures by allowing them to infect cells of a harmless bacterium (generally *Escherichia coli*), they became a principal experimental subject of virologists. Although bacteria are procaryons, studies of phage have yielded much information directly applicable to virology of animal cells. The development of practical means of cultivating animal tissue eliminated the drudgery and expense of using live animals (and plants) and provided a relatively simple means, now widely used, of studying animal viruses.

All viruses (including the large pox viruses with some experimental manipulation) can pass readily through filters that withhold ordinary bacteria, hence the term "filterable" formerly used to characterize viruses.

Bacteriophage

Studies of phages have provided much of our basic knowledge of mammalian viruses and are therefore discussed in some detail here.

Although phages have been found for many species of bacteria, blue-green algae and some yeasts, the most studied phages are certain types that infect *Escherichia coli, Bacillus subtilis* or *Pseudomonas* BAL-31. There are a score of more of such phages, each identified by number(s) and letter(s), e.g., the "T-even" phages: T2, T4, T6; the "T-odd" phages: T3, T7, etc., γ, ϕ X174, and so on, each with distinctive form, antigenic proteins, capsomers, dimensions, etc. Some have cores of DNA, some of RNA, some single-stranded, some double. Some have 5-hydroxymethylcytosine in place of cytosine; some have uracil of 5-hydroxymethyluracil in place of thymine; some have tails, others do not. Small, tailless phages (24 to 60 nm, e.g., ϕ X174, M12) are icosahedral in form; some (e.g., fl, M13) are filamentous (800 nm. long) with helical symmetry; larger phages (50 to 90 nm.) have tails up to 210 nm. long attached to the "head" or nucleocapsid. The tails of

T-even phages are of very complex structure with terminal spikes and fibers for attachment of the phage to its host cell. Other phage tails are relatively simple. Unlike animal viruses, few phages (e.g., PM2) are enveloped. Small, RNA-containing phages are much like picornaviruses (animal [see Table 5-13]), though they contain RNA only equivalent to about five genes. The RNA of such viruses acts in the host cell as its own mRNA.

In some animal viruses, e.g., herpesviruses, there is also usually an outer *envelope,* often wholly or partly host-cell derived, varying in composition and structure, depending on host-cell membrane structure, but generally containing carbohydrates. These envelopes usually also contain host-derived lipids, making the virus sensitive to lipid solvents such as ether and chloroform and to detergents. These and other properties are useful in the classification of viruses.

Phage Activity.   Phages are very host specific and attach to phage-specific receptors on susceptible cells. Tailed phages absorb to a susceptible bacterium by attaching the tip of the tail, with the aid of *tail fibers,* if present, to a chemicophysically specific receptor on the bacterial surface. By means of enzymic mechanisms localized at the tip of the tail, an opening is made through the bacterial cell wall and cell membrane. Through this, the NA core from the head of the phage enters the cell. The capsid is now an empty shell that may remain attached to the exterior of the cell.

Some phages attach only to F pili and are therefore said to be male specific. Filamentous phages attach endwise; phages lacking tails adsorb at various specific sites. Once inside the bacterium, the phage is no longer demonstrable as such *(eclipse phase).* In some instances the phage NA becomes integrated with the genetic mechanism of the cell as though a part of the bacterial genome, replicating with the bacterial chromosome. There it may remain for many generations, doing no evident harm. It is said to have been reduced to a *latent* state called *prophage.* Phage in this form is said to be *temperate.* The cell containing it is said to be *lysogenic.* The lysogenic cell is sometimes called a *lysogen.* The term lysogeny applies only to phage-infected cells. However, analogous relationships are found between some transforming or oncogenic viruses and their animal host cells.

As a result of various chemical or physical stimuli (e.g., ultraviolet irradiation, certain ions) the prophage in the lysogenic cell may be *induced* or *activated.* It then becomes *virulent.* It multiplies *vegetatively,* injuring the cell. In this state it ceases to be integrated with the bacterial chromosome and takes control immediately of the synthetic mechanisms of the cell.

The phage genome codes for enzymes that cause prompt disintegration of the host DNA to nucleotides, with resulting immediate cessation of cell synthesis, the synthesis of new DNA precursors and "early" replication of phage NA and transcription of the phage genome. Functioning of host-specified mRNA stops, and "late" phage mRNA forms phage materials (NA, enzymes, capsids, etc.) using cell ribosomes. Similar series of events occur in animal cells infected by animal viruses, with modifications depending on the widely varied cell-virus systems.

The new phage NA is *encapsidated;* nucleocapsids and the tails, if present, then combine and the intracellular virions are *mature (end of the eclipse period).* At this point, new phage is *latent* (the *latent period*) i.e., it is demonstrable only by artificial rupture of the cell. The bacterial cell wall is soon disintegrated by the phage *(lysis from within),* liberating new virions (the end of the latent period). (Distinguish between a latent virus and the latent and eclipse phases of intracellular development of phage.) The total duration of the various periods varies from a few minutes with phages to hours or even days with animal viruses.

A cell containing prophage has *prophage immunity,* i.e., it cannot be superinfected by another virion of that phage, although NA of other phages may infect the cell.

When bacterial cells undergo phage lysis, they suddenly liberate many intact virions, producing a "one-step" increase in the number of virions or plaque-forming units (PFU). (Distinguish this type of growth curve from that of bacteria.)

Many phages on entering the susceptible cell proceed immediately to multiplication (vegetative activity) and destruction of the cell as described above. Such phages are said to be *virulent.* Similar or analogous events occur in viral infections in animals. Like phage, the core of mammalian viruses consists of DNA *or* RNA, *never* both.

Regardless of form, animal virions have specific subunits on their surfaces by means of which they attach themselves to receptors on host cells. All exhibit considerable degrees of species, tissue and host cell specificity, which may be modified by passage in other hosts or tissues. The presence or absence of receptors governs to some extent the tissue tropisms of viruses.

Viropexis.   Some mammalian viruses, unlike phages, enter the susceptible cell intact by a process like pinocytosis, with engulfment of the virion in a phagocytic vacuole. Others appear to pass through the cell membrane directly into the cytoplasm without engulfment. Penetration of virion into the cell is called *viropexis.* Other viruses, notably paramyxoviruses and herpesviruses, enter cells by a fusion mechanism whereby viral envelope and cell membrane join to allow passage of the genome into the cytoplasm. Once inside the cell the virion is uncoated, releasing the core. Replicated virus may then either more or less rapidly destroy the cell (e.g., poxvirus and poliovirus) or remain latent until induced (e.g., herpes simplex). The mechanism of such latency remains obscure. Provirus, analogous to prophage, has not been demonstrated. However, integration of viral NA with host genome, in a relationship suggestive of phage lysogeny, is seen in viral malignant transformation.

At maturation some mammalian viruses are formed slowly at or near the cell surface and are given off by "budding" through the cell membrane for considerable periods without destroying the cell (e.g., parainfluenza virus).

Viral Plaque Formation

To demonstrate plaque formation with bacteriophage, a broth culture of bacteria is mixed with a suspension of bacteriophage virions in semisolid agar. The mixture is spread over the surface of nutrient agar in a Petri dish, which is then incubated. Water from the semisolid agar is absorbed leaving a layer of bacteria (including those infected by bacteriophage). After appropriate incubation, small areas of lysis are seen that are called plaques. Each plaque is initiated by an infected bacterial cell in which phage has multiplied and from which progeny virions have been released to infect adjacent cells in the "lawn." Thus the infection spreads from a single cell centrifugally to involve many other adjacent cells. Several cycles of infection are required before a plaque becomes visible. A count of the plaques then gives an idea of the number of particles in the original phage suspension. The term plaque-forming unit (PFU) is used because it is not certain that infection of a single cell is initiated by only a single virion. Similar plaque counts can be made in an analogous manner with poliovirus or other viruses on monolayers of animal cells attached to the surface of a flask. After inoculation of the cell culture with virus, the monolayer is covered with a thin layer of agar containing nutrients and neutral red. The agar immobilizes the virion and, as with bacteriophage, infection spreads centrifugally from initially infected cells. Plaques are revealed as clear areas in which the cells have been lysed and therefore do not take up neutral red, which is a vital dye. Intervening areas of remaining normal cells are therefore stained.

Laboratory Cultivation of Animal Viruses

Avian Embryos. In addition to propagation in their usual natural hosts, many animal viruses may be propagated by serial passage in live, embryonated, avian eggs. The allantoic sac, the amniotic sac or other part of the embryo may be inoculated through small openings in the shell. Bacterial and fungal contaminations are controlled by adding various antibiotics, especially if the inoculum is contaminated (e.g., feces and sputum).

Tissue Cell Cultures. Viruses may also be cultivated in susceptible, living, tissue cells growing in a suitable culture medium. Various normal adult or embryonic cells may be used, or certain neoplastic cells, e.g., the HeLa strain. Culture medium for growth of tissue cells commonly consists of an aqueous solution of essential elements (Na, K, Ca, Mg, S, P) plus glucose, buffered with bicarbonate pH about 7.4 (e.g., Tyrode's, Hanks', Eagle's solutions), with additions of a variety of amino acids, vitamins and other growth essentials. Blood serum is also usually required for *growth* though not for *maintenance*.

Cells for culture are derived from tissue by tryptic digestion treatment with EDTA *(Versene),* and washed in balanced salt solution and suspended in fluid growth medium containing serum and necessary minerals, amino acids, vitamins, glucose and bicarbonate-CO_2 buffer system.

Tissue cell lines attach readily to the surface of glass or plastic and grow in a thin spreading uniform sheet one cell thick (monolayer). Cell lines exhibit density-dependent inhibition, so that when the monolayer has grown out cell division slows down or even stops. Cells in confluent monolayer may be maintained for long periods of time with appropriate maintenance media. Phenol red (phenolsulfonphthalein, PSP) is the indicator most commonly used with a pH change from red to yellow at about 6.8. The presence of virus in inoculated monolayers is signaled by the appearance of cytopathic effects (CPE) manifested as rounding, separation and necrosis of cells, fusion to form syncytia or giant cells, chrosomal damage and/or detachment of cells from the surface. The major groups of viruses may be recognized by characteristic CPE. So-called inclusion bodies are frequently pathognomonic. The site of inclusion bodies, i.e., whether cytoplasmic or nuclear, gives an indication of the general class of infecting agent. DNA viruses with the exception of poxviruses multiply in the nucleus. RNA viruses multiply primarily in the cytoplasm. The nature of inclusions, that is, whether they are clumps of virions, of viral subunits or both, can be determined by cytochemical and immunologic techniques, especially labeled antibody.

Viral Hemagglutination. Many animal viruses, e.g., myxoviruses, paramyxoviruses, adenoviruses, reoviruses, agglutinate different species of erythrocytes. In enveloped viruses, the agglutination is mediated by a glycoprotein in the envelope. The neuraminidase (N) of myxoviruses is a second enveloped glycoprotein that is responsible for elution of myxoviruses from red blood cell surfaces and the liberation of myxoviruses from the surface of infected cells. During elution from the erythrocyte, receptors are destroyed with accompanying release of free N-acetylneuraminic acid. Cells in monolayer cultures infected with myxoviruses and paramyxoviruses adsorb erythrocytes (hemadsorption) due to the presence of viral hemagglutinin in the infected cell membrane. This is a useful diagnostic procedure to detect the presence of these viruses in cell culture. Hemagglutination by poxviruses is mediated by a lipoprotein that is separate from the virion and is liberated into the medium during viral growth. Adenoviral hemagglutination is mediated by specific capsid proteins (penton fibers).

Serologic Tests in Virology. Specific antiviral antibody inhibits hemagglutination or hemadsorption. Hemagglutination inhibition (HI) tests are another form of specific neutralization test used in measuring antibody to viral agents. With myxoviruses, hemagglutination inhibition antibody is type-specific, group-specific antibody being directed against the ribo-nucleoprotein core antigen.

Laboratory Diagnosis of Viral Infection. Diagnosis of viral infection is based on isolation and identification of virus and on serologic responses. Specimens to be examined for the presence of viruses should be delivered to the laboratory as soon after collection as possible. Use of transport medium enhances the probability of survival of any viruses present. Complement fixation (CF) is the type of test most widely used in diagnostic viral serology. In the search for antibody in acute and convalescent sera, viral antigens of known specificity are used. Other forms of neutralization tests are based on the inhibition of cytopathic effects by antibody or inhibition of plaque formation. Neutralization or complement fixation titers are based on serum dilutions with standard quantities of antigen or infective virus.

CLASSIFICATION OF VIRUSES

Older taxonomic systems for viruses were based largely on pathogenic effects on experimental animals and on clinical observations; later systems included supposed tissue tropisms, type of lesion, etc. With advances in all fields of technology, more recent classifications of viruses are based primarily on presence of DNA or RNA; presence or absence of lipid envelopes as reflected by stability to lipid solvents (ether, chloroform or both) or emulsifying surfactants (bile salts, detergents); stability to acid (pH 3.0); thermoresistance

(50 to 60 C.); size, morphology and number of capsomers; thermostabilization by divalent cations (e.g., Mg^{2+}); distinctive CPE; genetic relatedness of nucleic acids; percentage of G + C base composition; production of hemagglutination; pathogenesis; immunologic reactions (Table 5-13).

DNA Viruses

I. Parvoviruses

These viruses require concomitant growth of a helper virus for their complete development. The viral genome is a single strand of DNA, either + or −.

II. Papovaviruses

The group name is derived from *PApilloma, POlyoma* and *VAcuolating* viruses. The group includes rabbit papilloma, human papilloma (warts), polyoma and simian vacuolating virus 40 (SV40). Many viruses induce an early, *transitory,* increased cell proliferation, generally ending in local necrosis, e.g., pox viruses; molluscum contagiosum, myxoma and fibroma of rabbits. The papovaviruses induce cell transformation and malignancy in animals.

III. Adenoviruses

Viruses of this group have been variously called adeno-pharyngeal-conjunctival (APC) or acute-respiratory-disease (ARD) viruses. There are at least 50 serotypes; 31 found in humans, 30 in lower animals. Their morphology is unique in that they possess, in their capsid, 240 *hexons* in an icosahedron, with 12 *pentons,* each supporting a knobbed *fiber* at its apex. The penton fiber mediates attachment to cells. Many of the human adenoviruses can cause malignant transformation in cells of lower animals. However, none has been found in association with any human neoplasm.

IV. The Herpes Group

This group includes the viruses of herpes simplex, varicella-zoster, pseudorabies, cytomegalovirus, equine abortion virus and Epstein-Barr (EB) virus.

Infection with herpes simplex viruses causes local cell proliferation and formation of multinucleate cells or *syncytia* (some strains).

Two forms of herpes simplex virus are recognized: type 1, causing stomatitis, upper respiratory and CNS diseases; type 2, affecting the genitalia. The roles of types 1 and 2, however, can be reversed.

In immunes, herpes simplex virus tends to latency, with recurrent mild herpetic episodes ("fever blister," vesicles on gums, genitalia, etc.) due to *activation of latent virus in ganglionic cells.*

The varicella and the zoster viruses are identical (V-Z virus), the clinical picture depending on the age and the immunity status of the patient, appearing as chickenpox in children and zoster (recrudescent V-Z infection, shingles) in adults. Shingles can be a source of chickenpox in nonimmune children.

V. The Poxviruses

This group includes the human poxviruses (variola, vaccinia, alastrim) and various lower-animal poxviruses (fowl pox, cowpox, etc.). These are the largest of the animal viruses. (200 to 350 nm).

The viruses of vaccinia and *cowpox* are closely related and cross-react sufficiently with variola virus so that vaccination confers solid immunity to smallpox.

RNA Viruses

VI. Picornaviruses

As indicated by the group name, Picorna-(*Pico* = L. for small + *RNA*) viruses are very small, and the specifically active core material is RNA. Several large, immunologically distinct groups having different physicochemical properties (Table 5-13) and embracing nearly 200 more or less distinct viral types, are included. All are associated with the gastrointestinal and respiratory tracts and with a wide variety of clinical conditions. The group includes (A) Enteroviruses (polioviruses, Coxsackie viruses, ECHO viruses) and (B) Rhinoviruses.

During early infection these viruses may be found in oropharyngeal secretions; later in feces. Enteroviruses may invade the blood from the intestinal tract.

A. Enteroviruses. 1. *Propagation of polioviruses* in non-neural tissue cultures by Enders, Weller and Robbins in 1949 led to the development of hypodermically administered, formalin-inactivated, cultured-virus vaccine—highly effective in preventing paralytic polio and very effective in preventing much nonparalytic polio. Later, development independently by A. B. Sabin and by H. R. Cox at the Lederle Laboratories of clones of attenuated polioviruses led to active-("live") virus, orally administered vaccines (3 serotypes).

Active-virus polio vaccines produce enteric inapparent, immunizing infection with only limited dissemination of the attenuated immunizing virus to contacts.

2. *Coxsackie Viruses*. These were named for the town of Coxsackie, New York, where they were first recognized and described by Dalldorf. They produce distinctive lesions in experimentally inoculated immature animals, especially suckling mice. Two groups, A (Enteroviruses 4-46) and B (Enteroviruses 27-32), are dif-

ferentiated by (a) neutralization (N) tests in infant mice or in cell cultures, (b) CF tests, and (c) pathology in suckling mice. In man, they cause pleurodynia, meningitis, common colds, etc.

3. *ECHO Viruses* (Enteric Cytopathic Human Orphan viruses). These are clinically heterogeneous and variable. Only a few are immunologically cross-reactive (1–8, 22–23). Diseases produced in man by various serotypes include aseptic (viral) meningitis and neuronal injury (17 serotypes); encephalitis (2, 9); paresis (2, 4, 6, 11, 16); rash (9, 16); respiratory illnesses (8, 11, 20, 22, 25, 28); infant diarrhea (6, 7, 8, 14, 18).

B. Rhinoviruses. Viruses of this group have been variously called coryzaviruses, ERC viruses. At least 100 serotypes are known. These viruses are generally peculiar in being readily cultivable in human embryo kidney cells at 33 C or human diploid cells. They are most frequently found in nasal washings, *rarely* in feces. They are one of the most, of not the most, frequent cause of common colds in adults.

VII. Reoviruses

These are widely distributed among humans and lower animals and occur in both *Re*spiratory and *En*teric tracts, their role in human disease still being unclear (*O*rphan). (hence REOvirus). In young mice their effect is diagnostically distinctive: jaundice, oily fur, retarded growth, encephalomyelitis, alopecia. Biologically related, though antigenically distinct, rotaviruses cause infantile diarrhea (Table 5-13).

VIII. Togaviruses

A. Rubivirus. This virus causes German measles, (rubella) a mild disease in children and adults but very destructive to various fetal tissues during the first 3 or 4 months of pregnancy.

Infection induces solid, durable immunity, with N antibodies specific for rubella virus, measurable as HI antibody. Live attenuated rubella virus vaccine should be administered to young children (under 12) as part of the standard immunization program (Table 5-21). *No active virus vaccine of any* kind should be administered to pregnant women.

B. Arboviruses. *Arbo* (*arthropod-borne*) viruses typically (a) infect mammals and other vertebrates (notably birds) and (b) are transmitted in nature only by hematophagus arthropods, principally mosquitoes. To become infected the arthropods must bite animals (e.g., birds, horses, pigs, man) during viremia. Viremia may or may not be clinically evident and may last from a few hours to several days.

True arboviruses actually multiply in, or migrate from stomach to mouth parts of, their transmitting arthropod(s). Viruses transmitted mechanically only

TABLE 5-13. Classification of Viruses

DNA Viruses:

Family	Viruses	Diseases
Naked (Unenveloped)		
Parvoviruses ss positive strand; complementary (+ or −) in separate virions, icosahedral symmetry	Parvoviruses (Kilham rat virus, minute virus of mice, H viruses)	(Animals only)
	Adenosatellite viruses (4 serotypes)	Indigenous, no recognized disease
	Densoviruses (insects)	
	?Norwalk-like agents	Gastroenteritis
Papovaviruses ds, circular DNA naked, icosahedral symmetry	Papilloma virus	Verruca vulgaris, condyloma accuminatum
	Simian virus 40 (SV40), SV40-like human viruses (?) (JC)	(Rodent tumors) (?Progressive multifocal leukoencephalopathy)
	Polyoma virus	(Multiple tumors in hamsters)
Adenoviruses ds, icosahedral	Adenoviruses (33 serotypes)	URTI
	Common CF antigen (hexon), type specific antigens (penton), H	? "Pertussis" syndrome, conjunctivitis, lymphadenitis (certain types oncogenic in hamsters)
	(Animal adenoviruses)	
Hepatitis virus ds	Hepatitis B (HB) virus [Surface (s), core (c) and e antigens; Dane particle = virion]	Acute, chronic and inapparent infection ("long incubation," "serum").
Enveloped		
Herpesviruses ds, icosahedral capsid	Herpes simplex, types 1, 2	Herpes labialis, herpes genitalis, encephalitis, keratoconjunctivitis
	Simian herpesvirus (herpes B)	Latent, recurrent infection (oncogenic transformation in animals)
		Type 2: ?cervical carcinoma-associated, sexually transmitted
		Encephalitis
	Epstein-Barr (EB) virus	Infectious mononucleosis, (non-Forssman heterophile antibody) Burkitt lymphoma (lymphoma, malignant neurolymphomatosis), (?nasopharyngeal carcinoma), hepatitis
	Varicella-zoster (VZ) virus	Chickenpox–shingles; VZ pneumonia, postinfectious encephalitis (?Reye's syndrome)
	Cytomegalovirus (CMV)	Congenital, neonatal systemic infections; compromised host, hepatitis, mononucleosis (no heterophile antibody)
	Pseudorabies	(Equines)
Poxviruses ds, complex, lateral bodies, separate HA	Variola virus	Smallpox (variola major, minor; alastrim)
	Vaccinia virus	Eczema vaccinatum, generalized vaccinia, postvaccinal encephalitis (rare complications of vaccination)
		Cowpox
	Parapoxviruses	Milkers' nodes, Orf (sheep)
	Molluscum contagiosum	Multiple skin lesions
	Yaba virus	Localized skin lesions (monkeys)

RNA Viruses:

Family	Viruses	Diseases
Naked (Unenveloped)		
Picornaviruses ss, positive, icosahedral symmetry	Enteroviruses (poliovirus), ECHO & Coxsackie viruses, 70+, H serotypes	Meningitis, meningoencephalitis, poliomyelitis, inapparent infection (lower GI tract), herpangina, URTI, pleurodynia, myocarditis, exanthemata
	Rhinoviruses (100+ serotypes)	URTI, CCS
Reoviruses ds, segmented, linear icosahedral symmetry, double shell capsid inner icosahe-	Reoviruses (3 serotypes), H	Lower gastrointestinal tract, ?disease
	Orbiviruses (all are arboviruses)	Colorado tick fever, (various ungulates)
	Rotavirus	Infantile diarrhea (winter)

Togaviruses	Alphaviruses (group A arboviruses), H	Encephalitis
ss, positive, icosahedral symmetry	Flaviviruses (group B arboviruses), H	Hemorrhagic fever, yellow fever, dengue fever
	Rubivirus (rubella), H	Rubella, with arthritis in adults, congenital rubella syndrome
Orthomyxoviruses	Influenza viruses	Epidemic (group A) and sporadic influenza, CCS, (Reye's syndrome, group B)
ss, segmented, negative, helical symmetry	Serologic groups A, B, C, H–N types	
Paramyxoviruses	Parainfluenza viruses (4 serotypes), HN	URTI, croup, bronchiolitis, pneumonia
ss, negative, helical symmetry	Mumps virus, HN	Parotitis, orchitis, meningitis
	Respiratory syncytial virus	URTI, bronchiolitis, pneumonitis
	Measles (rubeola) virus, H	Measles, subacute sclerosing panencephalitis
Rhabdoviruses	(Vesicular stomatitis virus)	
ss, helical symmetry, bullet shaped	(Kern Canyon [bat] virus)	
	Rabies	Rabies
	?Marburg virus (simian)	Hemorrhagic fever (?nosocomial spread)
	?Ebola virus	
Retraviruses	Oncoviruses, leukoviruses	Host-specific leukemias, sarcomas, mammary tumors
ss, RNA-dependent DNA polymerase in virion, inner icosahedral shell, helical core	(Foamy viruses)	(Persistent infection in different mammalian species)
	(Maedi-Visna group of viruses)	("Slow" viral diseases in sheep: panleukoencephalitis, multiorgan involvement, nononcogenic)
Arenaviruses	Lymphocytic choriomeningitis virus	Choriomeningitis
spherical virion, genome ss, segmented, ribosome-like particles	Lassa virus (?rats)	Lassa fever (nosocomial spread)
	Tacaribe complex (?rodents)	Hemorrhagic fevers
Coronaviruses	Coronavirus (3 serotypes) (different animal species)	Respiratory infections, CCS
ss, enveloped, positive, helical symmetry, cytoplasm, ER		
Bunyaviruses	Bunyamwera virus, H	Mild encephalitis, hemorrhagic fever, sandfly fever, Rift Valley fever
helical symmetry, genome ss, 3 circular segments	California encephalitis viruses	
	Group C arboviruses	

Abbreviations

ss = single stranded; ds = double stranded.
DNA = deoxyribonucleic acid.
RNA = ribonucleic acid.
URTI = upper respiratory tract infection.
LRTI = lower respiratory tract infection.
CCS = common cold syndrome.
H = hemagglutinin.
N = neuraminidase.

Definitions

Virion: The intact (infectious) viral particle.
Genome: Nucleic acid core, embodying genetic information required for viral replication.
Capsid: Protein associated with the genome in cubic or helical symmetry or in complex configuration. Capsids of unenveloped viruses contain protective antigens.
Capsomeres: Structural subunits of the capsid.
Nucleocapsid: Viral nucleic acid combined with capsid protein. Intact nucleocapsid of unenveloped viruses is the infectious unit.
Envelope: Lipoprotein coat that surrounds noninfectious nucleocapsid, contains virus-coded protective antigens, and is essential for infectivity.

by contaminated external parts are not considered true arboviruses.

The *geographic distribution* of arboviral diseases depends on climate, which, in turn, determines distribution of arthropod vectors and of susceptible animal reservoirs. All of these factors are subject to change (e.g., migration of birds, changes in season or climate, etc.) and thus constantly modify eqidemiologic patterns. Arboviruses now subsume several distinct taxonomic groups (togaviruses, Bunyaviruses and orbiviruses, the latter reoviruses with double-stranded RNA) (Table 5-13).

Prevention of arboviral diseases depends on (1) eradication of vector arthropods and their breeding places (often difficult); (2) eradication of animal reservoirs (sometimes impossible); (3) prevention of contact between susceptible humans and vector arthropods; and (4) vaccination (yellow fever only).

IX. Myxoviruses

The term is derived from the affinity of these agents for glycoproteins that are found in secretions and that are similar to if not identical with cell "receptors" for viral hemagglutinin and infection. Characteristically these viruses mature by budding at the cell surface where they are enveloped by a lipid-containing membrane (envelope) into which structural subunits (hemagglutinin, H, neuraminidase, N) are inserted. Viral glycoprotein and lipids are host-specific; the polypeptide portions and the enzymes required for glycosylation are virus-coded.

A. Orthomyxoviruses (influenza virus). These are smaller (80 to 100 nm.) than the paramyxoviruses (100 to 150 nm.) and are divisible into three major serogroups based on the specificity of the ribonucleoprotein (S) antigens with complement-fixing antibody that is not protective (the ribonucleoprotein is internal). Each group, particularly group A, is subdivisible into many serotypes based on the separate antigenic identities of H and N glycoproteins. The latter are subject to antigenic drift and shift resulting from complex genetic reassortments (the viral genome comprises eight segments) in response to immunologic pressures in the individual and herd environments. Group A viruses include swine, equine and avian viruses; the human strains have hitherto been the cause of all epidemic influenza. Group B strains cause continuing sporadic incidence of influenza and are pecularily related to the serious and often fatal complication of Reye's syndrome. Group C viruses are of apparently low intrinsic virulence and account for an unknown, but probably appreciable, proportion of minor respiratory illness, particularly in young children and the elderly.

Antibodies to all the major groups are widespread in the adult population.

For diagnosis, orthomyxoviruses are readily recovered by the inoculation of throat washings into primary monkey kidney or human embryonic kidney cells. Hemadsorption indicates the presence of virus, which is then typed by hemagglutination inhibition with sera of known specificity.

Retrospective serodiagnosis is achieved by complement fixation with group-specific ribonucleoprotein antigens or with hemagglutination inhibition with standard viruses. Nonspecific inhibitors (nonimmunoglobulin sialoprotein receptor analogues) universally present in normal sera must be inactivated with receptor-destroying enzyme (RDE), which leaves specific antibody present to account for any HI activity in the serum. Influenza vaccine grown in the chorioallantoic membrane of the chicken embryo and inactivated (i.e., killed) by formalin is 90% effective in preventing infection if the vaccine matches the strain(s) prevalent in the population. Seasonal immunization is indicated in the elderly, especially those with cardiopulmonary embarrassment or other chronic debilitating diseases, and in the very young. Universal routine immunization is not indicated.

B. Paramyxoviruses. These are large enveloped viruses in which the genome is a single strand of unsegmented RNA. This accounts for their antigenic stability. The lipid envelope contains a major glycoprotein with hemagglutinating activity. In parainfluenza, mumps and Newcastle disease viruses, the same glycoprotein contains neuraminidase activity, which is not found in measles, canine distemper or rinderpest viruses or in respiratory syncytial virus. A second glycoprotein in the viral envelope accounts for cell-fusing activity, which characterizes the cytopathology of some of these viruses (measles and respiratory syncytial). Routine childhood immunization with attenuated measles virus vaccine is now recommended as highly effective in controlling this potentially serious infection.

X. Rhabdoviruses

Viruses of this group are elongated like bullets or rods, hence the name; Gr. *rhabdos* = rod. The Marburg agent (hemorrhagic fever) is probably in this biologic group. The most important member of the group is rabies virus.

Rabies virus gains entrance via bites or other breaks in the skin. Rabies occurs commonly among lower mammals of all species, rarely (in the U.S.) in man. Rabid animals tend to bite. The disease is a typical zoonosis, recently occurring epizoötically in Texas. Without disinfection of the wound, infiltration with hyperimmune human serum and vaccination, survival is extremely rare.

The virus travels along nerve trunks from places of entry and localizes mainly in the CNS and the salivary glands and, sometimes, in visceral tissues. In bats it localizes in the interscapular brown fat. In caves inhabited by bats it seems to have been airborne to other animals by infected guano or by respiratory secretions.

Diagnosis is commonly based on clinical data (history of animal bite, neurologic disturbances, excitation, encephalitis, salivation and drooling, paralysis) and on demonstration of Negri bodies in smears of Ammon's horn of the hippocampus; fluorescent antibody techniques; and inoculation of suspected brain tissues, medulla and thalamus, intracerebrally into mice or guinea pigs. The virus is also cultivable in a variety of cells *in vitro*.

XI. Retraviruses

Retraviruses (RNA genome) are so named because the virion contains RNA-dependent-DNA polymerase (*reverse tra*nscriptase). Retraviruses are oncogenic in one or more animal species other than man and include mammary tumor viruses, leukosis and sarcoma viruses as well as "foamy" viruses and certain "slow" viruses.

XII. Arenaviruses

These are so named for the granular or sandlike internal structure (L. *arena* = sand). One of the group is the cause of lymphocytic choriomeningitis characterized by infiltration of meninges and choroid plexus, the first-recognized viral, aseptic meningitis. The symptomology is varied, and the disease is usually mild, rarely involving the CNS, being mainly referable to the respiratory and enteric tracts. The virus is enzoötic in domestic mice, the source of tangential human infection.

More serious diseases of the hemorrhagic fever type, with neurotropic involvement and hemorrhagic necrosis, and frequently fatal, involve the worldwide Tacaribe group of arenaviruses. Many are arthropod borne. Lassa fever virus is an arenavirus.

XIII. Coronaviruses

These are named for the "crown" of large, club-shaped projections from the envelope, said to resemble the solar corona. They are the cause of respiratory and coldlike diseases. They have no antigenic relationship to the myxoviruses. Isolation is difficult because they grow poorly or not at all in any but ciliated epithelial organ culture (OC) or in particularly sensitive cell lines. There are 3 serotypes.

XIV. Hepatitis Viruses

Hepatitis A (HA) virus purified from human feces appears as a 27-nm. particle that contains RNA. The polypeptides have not been characterized, except to know that they are antigenic. Antibodies to HA are detected by RIA and immunoelectronmicroscopy. The complete hepatitis B (HB) virion is the Dane particle, surrounded by the surface (S) antigen containing at least five antigenic specificities (a group antigen, two pairs of subtypic determinants, d/y,w/r, which are mutually exclusive). A variety of subtypes have been recognized. S antigen may appear free in the blood early after infection. The Dane particle contains a core that is circular, partially double-stranded DNA as well as two additional distinct antigens (c and e). HA viruses are worldwide in distribution. Infection is usually followed by hepatitis of varying severity indistinguishable clinically from infection with B virus or so-called non-A, non-B infection. Spread of HA is by the fecal–oral route and is related to socioeconomic status and crowded living conditions with poor sanitation. Antibody is prevalent in a high percentage of most population groups. Percutaneous transmission of HA virus is infrequent. Diagnosis rests on the identification of A particles in feces and/or serodiagnosis with RIA. Pooled normal immunoglobulin affords effective post- or preexposure prophylaxis against both A and B viruses. HBV infection is acquired percutaneously (transfusions, blood-contaminated injection apparatus), more rarely by contact with body effluvia (e.g., semen, saliva). The disease is most frequently self-limited (virus and HBs antigen disappear, antibody appears) but may evolve into persistent hepatitis (HBs antigen and/or Dane particles and/or HBc antigen persist, little or no antibody appears). Hepatic injury in persistent HB infection may be immunogenic including both cell-mediated immunologic mechanisms and antigen–antibody complex disease. Diagnosis is by detection of HBs antigen and/or antibody and HBc antigen in the serum by radioimmunoassay. Active immunization with HBs purified from the plasma of persistently infected patients is noninfectious and is being tested in man for prophylactic efficacy. Other control measures are obvious from the known modes of transmission from both A and B viruses. Most post-transfusion hepatitis is caused by non-A, non-B hepatitis virus(es).

Chemotherapy of Viral Infection

A few agents are presently available for antiviral chemoprophylaxis and chemotherapy, each with restricted application. Amantadine (Symmetrel) prevents infection with group A influenza viruses and mollifies active disease. Its utility is greatest in situations in which vaccine is either contraindicated or is not available. DNA analogues have been shown to be effective in certain kinds of herpetic disease. Topical IUdR (5-diodo-2-deoxyuridine) is used to treat the early prestromal stages of keratitis caused by herpes simplex virus; it cannot be used systemically. Ara-A (adenine arabinoside) and Acyclovir (acycloguanosine) have been shown to be effective by systemic administration in the therapy of encephalitis proven by brain biopsy to be due to herpes simplex virus. No other DNA or RNA viruses are known to be affected by any of these compounds, with the possible exception of varicella-zoster in the immunocompromised host. Human interferon is receiving renewed attention as a potential chemotherapeutic agent. Large-scale production by bacteria is now possible due to purification of interferon, identification and isolation of human genes coding for its synthesis and dramatic advances in genetic engineering and cloning techniques.

PROTOZOA (PHYLUM PROTOZOA)

Protozoa are unicellular animals. Their cell structure is representative of eucaryotic metazoan cells in general, with the exception of the ameboe. They contain typical eucaryotic endoplasmic reticulum and exhibit meiosis in gametogenesis when present. Multiplication of protozoa is generally by transverse binary fission; flagellates divide longitudinally. Some species of protozoa, notably malaria parasites, have well-differentiated gametes. The protozoan cell exemplifies the extreme of performance, by organelles in the single cell, of all the vital functions seen in organized metazoa.

Classification of major groups of protozoa is based primarily on morphology and on type of motility.

BLOOD AND TISSUE PARASITES

Developmental stages of these protozoa occur in vertebrate hosts and sanguivorous arthropod vectors.

Trypanosomes (Genus Trypanosoma)

Protozoa of this genus may occur in one or more of four forms: trypanosomal (trypomastigote), leptomonad (promastigote), crithidial (epimastigote), or leishmanian (amastigote), depending on species and whether in arthropod or mammalian host. The adult trypanosomes are spindle shaped, with an undulating, keel-like membrane, edged with an anteriorly projecting flagellum, parallel to the long axis. They are about 15 to 30 nm. in length and exhibit active lashing movements. The trypaniform stages of the parasites occur in febrile mammalian blood, furnishing a means of microscopic diagnosis and also of transmission by arthropod vectors, in which they occur in the immature or epimastigote form. The trypanosomes are also found in tissues and spinal fluid and may be cultivated in special blood media.

1. Trypanosoma gambiense. This is transmitted by *bites of tse-tse flies* (*Glossina* sp.) and causes East African trypanosomiasis, characterized by toxemia, wasting and emaciation, and by mental deterioration and stupor ("sleeping sickness") when the CNS is invaded, and is usually fatal. There is an extensive reservoir of infection in both wild and domestic animals. Diagnosis may be made with Giemsa-stained smears of blood, lymphnode aspirates or spinal fluid or animal inoculation.

2. Trypanosoma rhodesiense. Similar to (possibly identical with) the above; Central Africa. It appears to be restricted to man. It causes a more acute and rapidly fatal disease. Suramin sodium is useful in therapy of *early* cases of both infections.

3. Trypanosoma cruzi. This causes Chagas' disease in dry, warm, parts of South and Central America and rarely in the United States. The life cycle includes trypomastigote and amastigote forms in the mammalian host and trypomastigote and epimastigote forms in the arthropod vector. In man it invades myocardium, endocrine glands and CNS.

T. cruzi is transmitted in *feces* of infected reduviid (cone-nosed, kissing or assassin) bugs, e.g., *Panstrongylus megistus, Triatoma infestans* and others, to and from an extensive wild and domestic animal reservoir and human beings. The parasite is primarily intracellular in the reticuloendothelial system and CNS, producing splenomegaly, hepatomegaly, etc.; hence histologic diagnosis is feasible. Distinctive megacolon and megaesophagus are common. Diagnosis in acute stages is made by blood smear, culture or animal inoculation, and in chronic disease by complement-fixation tests. Immediate type allergy can be demonstrated with skin tests. Romaña's sign (edema of face and eyelids) is suggestive but not diagnostic. Drug therapy is of little value. Mortality is high.

Genus Leishmania

These protozoa cause various forms of leishmaniasis. They are ovoid, about 3 by 1 nm. in size, and occur circumterrestrially in warm, moist areas. The amistigote form (no free flagellum) occurs in the mammalian host; the promastigote form, in the arthropod vector. Canines are the major animal reservoir, and *bites* of infected sand flies (*Phlebotomus* sp.) are the principal vectors. Laboratory diagnosis is by microscopic examination of ulcer scrapings, bone marrow or blood smears, depending on species. The parasites may also be isolated in the promastigote stage in pure culture on special blood-agar medium at 20 to 25 C. Although morphologically identical, species may be differentiated by complement-fixation tests. Pentavalent organic antimony compounds like neostibosan or aromatic diamidine are effective in treatment. Secondary bacterial infections may occur in these (or any) ulcerous conditions.

1. Leishmania tropica (cutaneous leishmaniasis, Oriental sore, Delhi boil, etc.).   Infection by *L. tropica* is characterized by a large ulcer at the site of the sandfly bite and is usually self-limited unless secondary bacterial invasion occurs.

Two forms of the disease occur. *L. tropica,* var. *major,* is enzootic among gerbils and is transmitted to man by *Phlebotomus papatassii. L. tropica,* var. *minor,* is enzootic in canines and is widespread in young humans. Solid immunity follows recovery, which is usual.

2. Leishmania donovani (visceral leishmaniasis, kala-azar).   *L. donovani* is morphologically like *L. tropica.* The local ulcer is inconspicuous, but the organism is invasive. It has a predilection for reticuloendothelial cells of the viscera; hence hepatomegaly, splenomegaly and adenopathy are marked. Diagnosis is mainly clinical, by complement-fixation test, or by bone marrow biopsy. Visceral leishmaniasis is often acute and usually is fatal (90 per cent) unless treated.

3. Leishmania brasiliensis (American leishmaniasis, mucocutaneous leishmaniasis, espundia, uta, etc.).   This form of leishmaniasis occurs in tropical South and Central America. The organism is morphologically virtually identical with *L. donovani.*

A local ulcer occurs like that due to *L. donovani,* but the organism tends to invade mucocutaneous junctions, especially in the lips and the nasal septum, blocking lymphatics and causing extensive indurations, ulcerations and large granulomata. Skin tests are much used for diagnosis. The prognosis is good unless metastases have occurred.

Genus Plasmodium

In nature the malarial parasites of man are transmitted only by infected females of certain species of *Anopheles* mosquitoes. They can also be transmitted by blood transfusion or by the use of common injection apparatus, as occurs among drug addicts, who serve as a reservoir for mosquito-borne infections. The life cycle of *Plasmodium* sp. is complex and involves (a) asexual phases in man (*schizogony* and early *gametogony*) and (b) sexual stages in the mosquito.

Asexual development in man begins with the entrance of *sporozoites* from saliva in the proboscis of a mosquito. These first invade liver cells, undergoing replicative schizogony, the *exoerythrocytic stage.* In infections by *P. vivax* and *P. malariae* these may become latent and account for long-delayed relapses. Recrudescences may occur in inadequately treated *P. falciparum* infections. Many *merozoites* are liberated from the liver cells. The merozoites enter erythrocytes and become *trophozoites,* which undergo further schizogony. The erythrocytes rupture, liberating many new merozoites that either attack new erythrocytes or develop into young *gametocytes* awaiting necessary maturation in an *Anopheles* mosquito. Massive destruction of erythrocytes produces anemia, pigmentation of phagocytic cells by *hemozoin* (iron-bearing malarial pigment), anoxia of tissues and consequent difficulties. The cyclical destruction of erythrocytes during schizogony periodically releases pyrogens causing quartan, tertian, etc. (see below), chills, and fever. The cycles are often quite irregular. The time from the mosquito bite to the first febrile attack is called the *intrinsic incubation period.* Hepatomegaly and splenomegaly are typical of malaria.

The sexual cycle occurs only in the mosquito and the period from infection of the mosquito to infectivity comprises the *period of extrinsic incubation* (10 to 14 days). As soon as blood enters the mosquito, male gametes exflagellate and fertilize female gametes, each pair producing a *zygote* that develops into a motile *ookinete.* This invades a cell of the stomach wall and forms an *oocyst* containing many sporozoites. These are liberated on rupture of the oocyst and migrate to the proboscis, ready to infect man.

Laboratory diagnosis of malaria is most often based on Giemsa-stained blood smears (thick or thin or both) and recognition of the parasites.

1. Plasmodium falciparum (malignant tertian or estivoautumnal malaria).   This is mainly tropical. The cycle of schizogony in man is variable, around 36 to 48 hours. Falciform gametocytes are diagnostic; schizonts are rarely seen. Clinically, this is the most severe and dangerous form of malaria, in large part because these parasites invade erythrocytes of all ages, often in multiples, resulting in very heavy parasitemias. There is much capillary obstruction, probably because of adherence of parasites to capillary walls.

2. Plasmodium malariae (quartan malaria).   This is mainly subtropical. The usual cycle of schizogony is 72 hours but is subject to variations in clinical effect. Morphologically *P. malariae* resembles *P. vivax* and *P. ovale* (see below), except that no Schuffner's stippling is present, the erythrocyte is not enlarged and the parasite is more compact. Pigment is darker and more conspicuous than that of *P. vivax.* There is very little ameboid activity. *P. malariae* attacks only mature erythrocytes, with consequent, relatively mild parasitemias. Chronicity is frequent, and glomerulonephritis may occur.

3. Plasmodium vivax (tertian malaria). This is found in temperate zones as well as in the tropics. The cycle of schizogony is 48 hours, but the clinical periodicity of chills and fever is quite variable. Active ameboid motion of the trophozoites and enlargement of the erythrocytes are diagnostic. Schuffner's stippling is conspicuous in the cytoplasm. Gametocytes are large and appear early. *P. vivax* attacks only reticulocytes, with consequently limited parasitemias.

4. Plasmodium ovale. Similar in most respects to *P. vivax,* but there is more Schuffner's stippling; erythrocytes are much enlarged and distorted; *P. ovale* infection is clinically milder than tertian malaria.

Treatment of malaria is made difficult by the occasional emergence of mutants resistant to drugs, especially chloroquine. Sulfonamide combinations (sulfalene-trimethoprim and sulformethoxine-pyrimethamine) have been useful against *P. falciparum* infections in Thailand.

Several species of simian malaria parasites, e.g., *P. cynomolgi, P. brasilianum* and *P. knowlesi,* are also transmissible to man by *Anopheles* mosquitoes under natural conditions.

INTESTINAL PARASITES

The Amebae

The intestinal amebae multiply only by binary fission. The life cycles of many species alternate between very fragile, vegetative *trophozoites,* intermediate precysts and dormant cysts. Some do not form cysts. Many species are minor pathogens or commensals: *Entamoeba coli, Endolimax nana, Iodamoeba butschlii, Dientamoeba fragilis.* These are of importance mainly because of possible confusion with *Entamoeba histolytica,* the only important pathogenic ameba of man, during microscopic examination of stools.

Entamoeba histolytica causes amebiasis, including amebic dysentery. The fragile, pleomorphic, motile trophozoites, around 8 to 60 nm. in size, are seen *only* (except when cultivated in special media) in acute diarrheic (or purged) stools and in invaded tissues. They sometimes contain ingested erythrocytes. The more resistant, *diagnostically distinctive* cysts (5 to 20 nm.) are the forms most commonly seen in normal feces: round, quadrinucleate (when mature), with chromatoids and thick, cyst membrane. Stained with iodine the nuclei are diagnostically distinctive in appearance.

The *trophozoites* secrete histolytic enzymes and penetrate the mucosa of cecum and colon, producing undermining ulcers and sometimes intestinal perforation.

The amebae sometimes enter the portal venules or lymphatics, invading other tissues, notably liver and brain, with expanding abscess formation. Symptomatology then depends on the location of the lesion. Clinically, intestinal amebiasis ranges from subclinical (carriers) to severe dysentery characterized by bloody, mucoid stools, anemia and dehydration. The so-called small-race of *E. histolytica* may or may not be pathogenic.

Transmission of amebiasis is only by cysts: fecal-sewage-food-oral; "hand-to-mouth."

Diagnosis is commonly by microscopic examination of stools for cysts. The *cysts* of the harmless *Entamoeba coli* are recognizable by their larger size and eight distinctive nuclei (when mature). *E. coli* ingests few if any erythrocytes.

Genera Trichomonas and Giardia

1. Trichomonas hominis. The trophozoites of these pear-shaped flagellates are 7 to 15 nm. by 5 to 15 nm. with three to five anterior flagella and a keel-like, laterally attached, undulating membrane with marginal flagellum. A prominent axostyle extends from the anterior (large) end through the center and projects posteriorly as a spike. *T. hominis* occurs in the lumen of the cecum. Transmission is fecal–oral. Pathogenicity is debatable. Diagnosis is by microscopic examination of the stool for the trophozoites. No cysts are formed.

2. Giardia lamblia. This flagellate occurs in people living in warm, moist climates as well as in dry cold regions (e.g. Colorado, Russia). It is sometimes associated with mild intestinal irritation and, rarely, with cholecystitis. Transmission and diagnosis are as for *T. hominis* except that *G. lamblia* forms distinctive cysts that appear in stools.

The trophozoites, which live mainly in mucosal crypts at the duodenal level, are fantastic in appearance, being dorsoventrally flattened, and have two large, eyelike nuclei, eight active flagella and a ventral sucking depression for attachment to intestinal epithelial cells.

Genus Balantidum

Balantidium coli is a pear-shaped ciliate about 75 to 55 nm., with a ciliated mouth *(cytostome),* anal opening, prominent pulsating vacuole and macronuclei and micronuclei. Multiplication is usually by transverse binary fission. There are many saprozoic and commensal ciliates that may be morphologically confused with *B. coli,* the only ciliate protozoan of importance as a human pathogen.

B. coli occurs in the colon, producing dysentery and ulcers that resemble, but are less penetrating than, those due to *Entamoeba histolytica.* Transmission is fecal-oral, chiefly among hogs, occasionally to man. In man, clinically, balantidiasis ranges from (usually) asymptomatic to (rarely) fulminating and fatal.

GENITOURINARY PARASITES

Trichomonas vaginalis, a cause of vulvovaginitis, is slightly larger than *T. hominis* but otherwise closely resembles it. No cysts are known. *T. vaginalis* occurs in the human vagina and prostate, occasionally in urine. Transmitted usually by coitus, trichomoniasis may also be transmitted by moist, freshly contaminated clothing, wash cloths, etc.

Genitourinary trichomoniasis is usually asymptomatic in males and sometimes in females, but in the latter often causes mild to severe vulvovaginitis. Diagnosis is by microscopic examination of exudates for the trophozoites. Cysts have not been seen.

TOXOPLASMOSIS

The worldwide protozoan that causes this disease was observed originally in North African rodents called gondi, hence its name, *Toxoplasma gondii.*

Toxoplasma gondii has a multiphasic life cycle, somewhat like that of the malaria parasites, to which it is distantly related. The sexual stage develops in the intestine of cats; the asexual stage, in the muscles and other tissues of numerous feline and nonfeline mammals, including man. The crescentic, pear-shaped asexual trophozoite is motile by bending and gliding movements.

In the cat, the sexual stage of the parasites results in production of drought- and starvation-resistant infective *oocysts* that are passed in the cat's feces. The oocysts may be ingested by many different warm-blooded vertebrates. If ingested by a cat, new trophozoites develop, the sexual process is repeated, and more infective oocysts are produced. If ingested by man or any animal other than cats, the oocysts develop into trophozoites. These multiply asexually by fission and invade the tissues where they may produce an inflammatory reaction of greater or lesser severity, commonly subclinical. They may eventually form cysts (not sexually produced oocysts as in the cat) and remain encysted in the tissues, causing chronic toxoplasmosis, also usually subclinical, which usually subsides. In any forms, cyst, oocyst or trophozoite, animals eating them may become infected. Man becomes infected most often by ingestion of undercooked meat containing cysts.

A large proportion of persons when tested show serologic evidence of having (had) subclinical toxoplasmosis. Any mammal or bird eating raw or "rare" flesh containing the asexual cysts will contract the infection.

Birds and mammals (except cats) do not pass infective oocysts so far as is known. Their flesh is infective but not their feces. Infected pregnant women can infect the fetus, sometimes with serious results: hydrocephalus, eye and brain damage, etc. The disease appears to be worldwide in distribution and generally unnoticed.

Diagnosis of chronic toxoplasmosis is based on finding the pear-shaped parasites in tissues. Definitive identification may be made by indirect fluorescent antibody tests on material that should be sent to the Center for Disease Control for this purpose. Rising complement fixation titers are suggestive. IgM antibody to *T. gondii* in cord blood establishes the presence of fetal (congenital) infection.

HELMINTHS

The term helminth is commonly used to mean parasitic worms. There are two principal groups: (a) Phylum Platyhelminthes or flatworms, which include class Cestoidea (tapeworms) and Trematoda (flukes); (b) Phylum Nemathelminthes, class Nematoda or roundworms, which includes hookworms, pinworms, etc.

FLUKES (CLASS TREMATODA)

The life cycles of all flukes parasitic in man are complex, details varying with species. In general, fertilized eggs are produced by sexually mature adults in the definitive host, i.e., the host that harbors the sexually mature stage of any parasite. All flukes are hermaphroditic except schistosomes, which are diecious.

Eggs are discharged in feces (in *Schistosoma hematobium,* mainly in urine). Eggs hatch in polluted fresh water, each liberating a free-swimming ciliated larva *(miracidium)* that penetrates an intermediate host, usually a species of snail, in which it becomes a *sporocyst* and (except in schistosomes) produces numerous *rediae* and daughter rediae or sporocysts. These finally become minute, tadpole-like *cercariae* (with forked tails in schistosomes) that penetrate the definitive host (see below), losing their tails and becoming *metacercariae* (incomplete in schistosomes). They enter the definitive host by (a) direct penetration of the skin of swimmers, waders, rice planters, etc. (schistosomes); (b) encysting on aquatic plants, e.g., water cress, water chestnuts, lotus, etc., that are eaten raw (liver flukes: *Fasciolopsis buski; Fasciola hepatica*); (c) penetration of, and encystment in, tissues of aquatic animals (fish, crustacea) that are eaten raw (liver fluke *Clonorchis sinensis* and lung fluke, *Paragonimus westermani*).

After ingestion by the definitive host and excystation

(except schistosomes, which penetrate skin and do not form cysts), migration to specific organs occurs via blood and lymph channels and penetration through intestinal walls and other tissues. Diagnostically distinctive eggs of all species occur in stools, but those of *Schistosoma hematobium* appear mainly in urine and those of *Paragonimus westermani* also in sputum.

Pathogenesis by all flukes is due principally to *obstruction* of various vessels and ducts, to *trauma* due to tissue penetration and burrowing, abscess formation around dead worms, to *intense inflammatory reaction* with *fibrosis* and *stricture,* and to more or less *toxic action* depending on species. Symptoms depend largely on tissue of localization.

Blood Flukes (Genus Schistosoma)

These are distinguished from other human flukes by their slender, cylindrical form, separate sexes and the prominent, longitudinal, copulatory canal of males, which enfolds the female during copulation. Males range in length from 10 to 20 mm. Adults most commonly live in the mesenteric, the portal or the vesical venules, whence eggs enter the intestine or the urinary bladder and appear in feces or urine, depending on species. Intradermal tests for specific allergy with schistosomal antigens are useful in diagnosis. Eggs are not operculate.

1. Schistosoma japonicum (Oriental blood fluke) causes intestinal and hepatic schistosomiasis, chiefly in Japan, North China and adjacent lands and islands. Eosinophilia is marked. This is the most dangerous form of schistomiasis, as the worms are widely disseminated in the body. Distinctive eggs, with rudimentary lateral spikes covered with adherent fecal material appear in the stools.

2. Schistosoma mansoni causes schistosomiasis mansoni or Manson's schistosomiasis in Africa and adjacent lands, the Caribbean Islands and Brazil. The diagnostically distinctive eggs are *laterally spiked* and appear mainly in *stools.*

3. Schistosoma haematobium (vesical blood fluke) causes vesical bilharziasis or urinary schistosomiasis in Africa and adjacent lands. Eggs with one *polar* spike appear mainly in *urine.*

4. Schistosomal dermatitis or swimmers' itch is due to preliminary penetration, into the skin *only,* by cercariae of various species of avian and mammalian flukes other than human. These do not develop further in man. Swimmers' itch is annoying but self-limited.

Control of schistosomes involves elimination of vector snails: *Bulinus* and *Physopsis* for *S. haematobium; Biomphalaria glabrata* for *S. mansoni; Oncomelania* for *S. japonicum.* Treatment involves antimony compounds.

TAPEWORMS (CLASS CESTOIDEA)

Adult tapeworms are typically intestinal parasites of vertebrates. They are attached to the lining of the small intestine of the host by the worm's head or scolex, which is equipped with suckers, and by multiple hooklets in some species. The scolex narrows posteriorly to form a neck from which are produced, by budding, a series of new "segments" or flattened, roughly rectangular proglottids that remain attached to the neck and to each other to form a ribbon-like strobila, which may be millimeters to meters in length, depending on species.

Each proglottid later becomes a sexually mature, hermaphroditic, egg-producing parasite. The older (most distal, and gravid with eggs) proglottids break off and are carried out in feces along with ova (except *Taenia* sp. and *Dipylidium caninum*). Most ova and proglottids have diagnostically distinctive morphology. The scolex remains attached to produce more proglottids. Neither flukes nor tapeworms have alimentary systems. Nutrition is osmotrophic, i.e., by absorption through the surface structures. The life cycles and the intermediate hosts vary with species.

1. Taenia saginata. The beef tapeworm, 4 to 9 m. in length, is found in peoples that eat raw beef, almost never in the United States. Herbivores acquire the embryonated eggs, each containing a six-hooked *onchosphere,* in sewage-polluted pasturage. The freed embryos invade the muscles and remain as encysted larvae *(Cysticercus bovis)* until eaten uncooked by man. The scolex is about 3 mm. in diameter and has four sucking disks but no hooklets (although hooklets are present in the egg). The eggs (*not* species distinctive) are found free by microscopic examination of feces of man and in the proglottids that appear in the stools.

2. Taenia solium. The pork tapeworm occurs in the encysted larval (cysticercus) stage in pork. Infection is rare in the United States. The distinctive scolex has four sucking disks and a *rostellum* with a double row of 26 to 28 hooklets. The species is recognized by counting the number of uterine branches, which in *T. saginata* range from 15 to 20 (average 18) on each side; *T. solium* has 7 to 13 (average 9) on each side. The ova are not distinguishable from those of *T. saginata.* The life history and man-pork relationship are analogous to the man-beef relationship of *T. saginata.* In addition, man may ingest eggs via fecally polluted foods and drink and develop cystercerci in the muscles. Hogs acquire eggs from foods polluted by human feces.

3. Hymenolepis nana, the dwarf tapeworm (about 2 to 4 cm. long and 1 mm. wide) is the smallest and most common tapeworm of man in the United States, occurring most frequently in children. The head has a rostellum with 24 to 30 hooklets and four suckers. There are from 150 to 200 segments.

No intermediate host is necessary. The diagnostically distinctive eggs are passed in feces and are transmitted to the mouth of the same host *(autoinfection)* by soiled hands, underclothing and unclean habits in regard to feces. The *cysticercoid* larvae develop in the intestinal villi and the adults then fasten to the duodenal or the jejunal mucosa and repeat the cycle. Personal cleanliness and sanitary disposal of feces are the best preventives.

Diagnosis depends on the discovery of ova in the feces.

4. Diphyllobothrium latum, the fish tapeworm may reach 12 m. in length, with thousands of proglottids. The head, about 1 by 2 to 3 mm., has no hooklets but has two longitudinal sucking grooves. Each diagnostically distinctive egg has a small hinged lid or operculum at one end, suitable for hatching in water, and demonstrable by pressure on the coverglass on a slide.

Eggs from human feces in cool fresh water produce free-swimming embryos. These are swallowed by copepods ("water fleas" [*Cyclops* or *Diaptomus*]), where a larva forms. The copepod is eaten by a plankton-eating fish and forms a *sparganum* in the muscles. When the fish is eaten undercooked by man, the larval tapeworm matures and attaches in the proximal jejunum. Competition with the host for vitamin B12 may cause profound anemia. Eosinophilia is frequent.

Control involves (1) avoidance of sewage pollution of waters in which the intermediate hosts breed and (2) the cooking of all fish to be eaten.

5. Echinococcus granulosus and *E. multilocularis* (unilocular and multilocular or alveolar echinococcosis respectively; hydatid disease). The definitive hosts of these tapeworms are not man but other carnivorous mammals, especially canines. Cattle, sheep, swine and man are intermediate hosts; i.e., these species harbor the larval cyst stage *(hydatid cyst)* that is analogous to the cysticerci of *Taenia* sp.

Adult *Echinococcus* tapeworms are 2 to 6 mm. long. In dogs, etc., they produce *Taenia*-like eggs that appear in the animal's feces and are swallowed by a wide variety of intermediate hosts with polluted fodder. In the case of man, they are acquired from accidentally soiled hands, food or both, especially among persons closely associated with dogs: Eskimos, sheep herders, etc.

The eggs produce larvae that penetrate via venules to liver, brain, etc., where they usually slowly form either unilocular hydatid cysts *(E. granulosis)*, often amenable to surgery, or alveolar or multilocular cysts *(E. multilocularis)*, rarely amenable to surgery. The cysts may become very large and destructive and usually contain many infective daughter scolices that become adults when the cyst is ingested by a carnivore.

Diagnosis of echinococcosis or hydatid disease in man may be made with hydatid-cyst-fluid antigen by (1) complement-fixation or precipitin tests; (2) cutaneous allergic reaction; (3) the finding of hooklets or scolices in the cyst fluid if surgical procedures are feasible.

PHYLUM NEMATODA

Adult roundworms parasitic in man generally attach to the intestinal mucosa except (1) *Ascaris,* which remains free in the intestinal lumen and (2) filarial worms, which inhabit blood, tissues (especially skin) and lymph spaces. Female nematodes usually are larger than males.

1. Hookworms (*Necator americanus* and *Ancylostoma duodenale*). Male hookworms range around 8 by 0.4 mm. in size. Hookworm infection is widely endemic in circumterrestrial tropics and subtropics, especially in extraurban populations. Adults, attached to duodenal and jejunal mucosa by suckers and cutting plates, digest the mucosa and blood and produce diagnostically distinctive eggs that appear in feces. On warm, moist soil the eggs hatch and undergo 10 to 15 days of development through four larval stages. The last larvae are *filariform* and penetrate exposed skin of bare feet, causing ground itch.

The larvae migrate via blood vessels and lymphatics to the lungs with relatively little pneumonitis; thence, after further development, via trachea, esophagus and stomach to the intestine where, as adults, they attach and renew the cycle.

Pathogenesis involves continuous intestinal irritation and hemorrhage, with resultant anemia, and debilitation, both physical and mental.

Control is based mainly on sanitary disposal of feces and avoidance of direct contact with feces-polluted soil. As in any control program, elimination of sources of infection by treatment of infected persons is essential.

2. Giant roundworms *(Ascaris lumbricoides).* These are worldwide in distribution, and among the most prevalent nematodes of man, except in cold, dry climates.

Male *A. lumbricoides* may attain lengths of over 30 cm. and diameters of 8 mm. Adults live mostly in the small intestine and may migrate *post mortem* into various parts of the gastrointestinal tract (bile and pancreatic ducts, stomach, etc.). They do not attach to the intestinal mucosa. They may perforate the intestinal wall or migrate out of anus, mouth or nares.

They die out after about a year but, in endemic areas, are replaced constantly.

Diagnostically distinctive eggs, passed in stools, mature in warm, moist soil in from 2 to 3 weeks. Ingested, the mature eggs hatch in the small intestine. (Compare with hookworms, eggs of which hatch on the soil, not in the intestine.) The larvae migrate actively to the lungs by way of blood, lymphatics or both, with accompanying pneumonitis, possibly allergic, get into the alveoli and thence to pharynx and esophagus, where they are swallowed. In the small intestine they mature, produce eggs and recommence the cycle. Large numbers can cause serious difficulties by mechanical obstructions. General symptoms of gastrointestinal irritation and malnutrition are common.

3. Whipworms *(Trichuris trichiura).* Males are about 40 by 5 mm. Infection is circumterrestrial, mainly tropical. Adults attach to the cecal mucosa and produce diagnostically distinctive eggs in the feces. The eggs do not hatch, but on warm, moist soil the intraoval embryos become larvae. Under unsanitary conditions they are ingested by man. The eggs hatch in the intestine, and the freed larvae migrate to the cecum, mature and repeat the cycle. A heavy burden of worms causes mucosal inflammation and erosion, diarrhea and hemorrhage, mostly in children. A light worm burden may not cause symptoms.

Diagnosis depends on recognizing the species-distinctive eggs in the stool.

Control is dependent on sanitary disposal of feces and avoidance of feces-polluted soil, food, or objects contaminated with such soil or feces, and is potentiated by adequate treatment of infested patients.

4. Pinworms or seatworms *(Enterobius vermicularis).* Males are about 3 by 0.2 mm. The worms are circumterrestrial in temperate areas. Adults are attached in cecum and colon. Gravid females migrate to the anal and perianal area and deposit diagnostically distinctive eggs that may be picked up for microscopic examination on clear adhesive tape. Sometimes the adult worms may be seen on the skin. Eggs are carried to the mouth on hands or on contaminated dust from clothing, etc., to the same *(autoinfection)* or another host. The eggs hatch in the intestine, and the freed worms attach and repeat the cycle.

Occurring mainly in children under unsanitary conditions, *E. vermicularis* causes perianal pruritus, local irritation, and scratching that invites transmission via hands and secondary bacterial infection. Eosinophilia is marked.

Control involves personal cleanliness and eradication of the worms by chemotherapy.

5. Trichina worm or pork worm *(Trichinella spiralis).* These worms cause trichinosis. Most carnivorous animals are susceptible, and the disease is enzootic in rats and swine. Both eat infected pork as municipal garbage or slaughterhouse offal. Trichinosis occurs in man as a result of eating undercooked pork containing live, encysted larvae.

Once ingested, the larvae excyst and mature in the crypts of duodenum and jejunum as small, slender worms about 1.5 mm. long (males). After copulation the males die, and the females penetrate deeply into the mucous membranes where they produce large numbers of larvae (larviparous) that migrate via veins and lymphatics to the striated muscles. There the larvae grow and, about 3 weeks after ingestion of the infected meat, become encapsulated, coiled in the distinctive arrangement from which the species name is derived. In this condition they can remain viable for 12 years or more, although usually the cysts become entirely calcified in 10 to 12 months.

The early period of invasion by the *newly ingested* larvae is accompanied by local inflammation and gastroenteritis for several days and sometimes also by hemorrhage. The period (1 to 3 months) during which the *newly produced* ("second generation") larvae are migrating through the tissues and muscles is marked by fever, edema (especially of the face; periorbital), myositis or "muscular rheumatism" and general symptoms, including pain. Eosinophilia is marked. Severity depends on the numbers of larvae. Many mild, unrecognized cases occur; others may be fatal.

Diagnosis depends on finding the encapsulated larvae in bits of teased-out muscle after sectioning or digestion with trypsin. Immunologic tests are useful and include precipitin and complement-fixation tests using trichina extracts as antigen and the agglutination of antigen-coated latex particles. Intradermal tests for allergy with similar antigens are also valuable.

Control centers in (a) cooking all garbage fed to swine; (b) eliminating rats from garbage dumps and piggeries; (c) adequate veterinary condemnation of infected swine (difficult); (d) freezing of pork for *at least* 36 hours at -27 C. or *thorough* cooking or both.

6. Filarial Worms. Various species of these worms and their microscopic larvae (*microfilariae,* c. 275 by 7 μm.) cause various forms of filariasis in tropical and some subtropical areas. Geographic distribution of the various species depends on distribution of arthropod vectors (various mosquitoes, gnats, and biting flies) specific for each.

Although distinctive clinical features, epidemiology, etc., depend on the species of filarial worm involved, all forms of filariae and of filariasis have some basic similarities. In general, adult filariae inhabit fibrous subcutaneous or deep lymph nodules or other tissues of man where they produce long, thin microfilariae.

In some species these migrate into peripheral capillaries at hours (*diurnal* or *nocturnal periodicity*) when the arthropod vector specific for that species of worm bites.

After a series of maturation changes in the arthropod, the microfilariae migrate to the proboscis of the arthropod, ready to infect the next person bitten.

Active and extensive migrations of the microfilariae in the human host, their gathering together in large masses, and the allergic reactions consequent to chronic infection, result in pain, blindness (*Onchocerca volvulus*) and various distinctive types and locations of swellings.

Diagnosis before microfilariae appear in the peripheral blood is based on history of exposure, clinical picture and intradermal sensitivity tests with filarial antigens. Later, microfilariae of some species are demonstrable microscopically in the peripheral blood during hours of periodicity or in "skin snips" macerated in saline solution *(O. volvulus). O. volvulus* does not circulate in the bloodstream.

Chemotherapy against *O. volvulus* is not universally employed because of intense reactions that occur in the skin to the sudden release of large quantities of antigen. In Central America, nodules containing the adults are periodically removed as a means of control. Elimination of arthropod vectors is not always practicable, because the larvae grow in fast streams in which pesticides wash away quickly. Diversion of streams is often impossible, because coffee-growing areas are dependent on them.

FUNGI (EUMYCETES)

Fungi pathogenic for man may cause one of three general types of fungal disease (mycosis):

a. Cutaneous mycoses (dermatophytoses). These are superficial and generally not dangerous per se. They involve only the skin, hair and nails, alone or in combination. These mycoses are due to keratin-metabolizing, filamentous *dermatophytes* and sometimes to yeast-like *Candida albicans.*

b. Deep or systemic mycoses. These are usually serious, sometimes fatal.

c. Subcutaneous mycoses. These are usually chronic, localized infections of the skin, underlying dermis and occasionally the deep tissues, such as bones and muscles, principally of the extremities but also occasionally involving any exposed body surface. A variety of fungi, both dimorphic and monomorphic, are responsible.

Pathogenic fungi were previously grouped together under the term Fungi Imperfecti because a sexual or perfect mode of reproduction was not known. The discovery of a sexual reproductive cycle for many of these fungi prompted the adoption of Deuteromycetes (Gr. = *deutero* second) as their Class name. Although identification of the sexual cycle resulted in a reclassification of the fungus according to the type of sexual spores produced, the name of the asexual form was retained and the organism in this form remained in the Class Deuteromycetes. A sexual stage has been identified for several *Microsporum* species, assigned to the genus *Nannizzia,* several *Trichophyton* species, assigned to the genus *Arthroderma, Histoplasma capsulatum,* assigned the name *Emmonsiella capsulata, Blastomyces dermatitidis,* assigned the name *Ajellomyces dermatitidis,* and *Cryptococcus neoformans,* assigned the name *Filobasidiella neoformans.* Excepting *Filobasidiella neoformans,* which is placed in the Class Basidiomycetes, all are grouped in the Class Ascomycetes.

In general, the etiologic agents are recovered from pathologic material by cultivation on various artificial media. Sabouraud's glucose (or maltose) agar, pH 5.6 or 7.0, with and without antibacterial and antifungal drugs (chloramphenicol; cycloheximide) added is the basic medium. Blood agar and other selective and diagnostic media are used when indicated. Incubation is for 1 to 4 weeks at 22 and/or 37 C.

Fungi are studied in much the same manner as bacteria, though low-power or high-dry lenses are generally used to examine undisturbed mycelial formations (spirals, favic chandeliers, raquet hyphae), distinctive asexual spores (conidiospores, aleuriospores, chlamydospores), and color, texture and topography of colonies, all of which are diagnostically distinctive. Filamentous and yeast-like fungal forms may be demonstrated in cutaneous tissues, biopsy material from deeper lesions or pus from abscesses by mounting the material on slides in 10 per cent KOH under a coverslip. Stains used to demonstrate fungi in pus and tissues are Gram's, methylene blue, acid-fast, lactophenol cotton-blue, periodic acid-Schiff, Gridley, Gomori's methenamine silver nitrate, and others.

THE CUTANEOUS MYCOSES

Dermatophytoses are caused principally by species of three closely related genera of keratin-metabolizing filamentous fungi called dermatophytes. Dermatomycoses are caused by a variety of yeasts and filamentous fungi, such as *Candida albicans, Pityrosporum furfur.*

Typically the dermatophytes grow in cutaneous tissues or in cultures in mold-like, branching, mycelial form. Asexual spores of dermatophytes, though little more thermostable than vegetative cells, survive for long periods in soil, shower-bath mats, floors, and hair brushes. Some dermatophytes *(Microsporum canis, Microsporum gypseum, Trichophyton mentagrophytes, Trichophyton verrucosum)* infect domestic animals and are readily transmissible to man. Some species can at times cause any of the conditions listed below subject only to restrictions as to skin, hair or nails as noted. Person-to-person or animal-to-man transmission is common.

Common Dermatophytes

1. Involve skin and hair; nails rarely
   Microsporum audouini, M. canis, M. gypseum cause various forms of tinea (ringworm), especially in preadolescents; *M. canis* causes it in domestic animals also. The first two fluoresce yellow-green in ultraviolet light (Wood's light); *M. gypseum* fluoresces poorly or not at all. These species produce spores and hyphal elements outside the hairshaft, hence are called ectothrix infections.
2. Involve skin and nails; not hair
   Epidermophyton floccosum causes tinea pedis (athlete's foot), tinea cruris (jock itch) and tinea unguium.
3. Involve hair, skin and nails
   Trichophyton mentagrophytes, T. rubrum, T. tonsurans, T. schoenleini cause tinea pedis, favus sycosis, tinea unguium. The last two produce endothrix infections of hair and the first two produce ectothrix infections of hair.

Common Dermatomycoses

1. Candidosis
   Candida albicans and other *Candida* species can cause otomycosis, onychomycosis, thrush, perlèche, vulvovaginitis and skin lesions; *Candida* infections are some of the most frequently encountered mycoses.
2. Tinea versicolor
   Pityrosporum furfur causes a superficial skin infection characterized by the formation of white-, brown-, or fawn-colored lesions; very common infection.

Orally administered griseofulvin is effective against dermatophytoses. Topical agents such as miconazole nitrate, clotrimazole, and the nonprescription tolnaftate are effective against skin lesions, but less effective against nail infections. Nystatin is the drug of choice for dermatomycoses caused by *Candida species.* Keratinolytic ointments and scrupulous personal hygiene are recommended for tinea versicolor.

THE DEEP OR SYSTEMIC MYCOSES

These diseases are caused chiefly by soil-inhabiting, dimorphic or diphasic fungi, that is fungi capable of existing in two phenotypically distinct forms. In general, the free-living or saprobic form is a filamentous mold whereas the pathogenic, tissue-invading form is unicellular and yeast-like. Exceptions are *Candida albicans,* which is indigenous in man and forms mycelia and pseudomycelia when it becomes invasive, *Coccidioides immitis,* which produces sporangiospores in mammalian tissues, and *Cryptococcus neoformans,* which is a monomorphic yeast. The two forms of these fungi may be reproduced on artificial media in the laboratory by manipulating environmental conditions such as pH, temperature, CO_2/O_2 ratios, humidity, and nutrients—amino acids, carbohydrates and vitamins.

As would be expected in the case of soil-inhabiting organisms, infections are acquired by inhaling spores, resulting in primary pulmonary lesions, or by traumatically implanting spores into the skin, resulting in relatively localized infections involving the cutaneous and deeper tissues and occasionally the lymphatics of the affected areas. Systemic mycoses are slowly evolving, chronic diseases characterized by granulomatous reactions, abscess formation, necrosis, and the development of a cell-mediated immune response. Agglutinins, precipitins and complement-fixing antibodies are formed and are useful in diagnostic and prognostic procedures, including latex agglutination, immunodiffusion, complement fixation and immunofluorescent staining techniques.

In contrast to dermatophytoses, person-to-person transmission of systemic mycoses is rare.

Systemic mycotic infections may also be caused by diverse, saprobic, monomorphic, filamentous fungi, e.g., *Aspergillus* species, aspergillosis; *Mucor* and *Rhizopus* species, phycomycoses; and others less frequently encountered. Modern medical practice sometimes requires the use of immunosuppressants, antibiotics, hormones and other drugs in conjunction with certain types of surgical and therapeutic procedures, thus compromising the patient and providing a target for these opportunistic fungal pathogens.

Candidosis

Candida albicans, more frequently the etiologic agent of this mycosis than any other *Candida* species, is a common commensal of the human alimentary tract and vagina. Although *Candida* infections may involve any area of the body, those that involve the deep tissues and organs may be life threatening and are therefore the most serious.

Candida albicans is a nutritionally dependent dimorphic fungus growing as a yeast in its natural habitat or *in vitro* in the presence of glucose and as pseudomycelia and mycelia when it invades tissues and organs or *in vitro* in the presence of dextran, glycogen or starch. Pathologically it is usually a secondary invader of injured, moist, superficial tissues, causing thrush (oral or vaginal), intertrigenous dermatomycoses, perlèche and paryonychia. Rarely, deep invasions may occur producing pneumonias and meningitides. *C. albicans* may produce a serious enteritis as a result of suppression of the normally competitive intestinal bacterial flora by antibiotics following surgery. *C. albicans* is also a significant cause of endocarditis in surgical patients following cardiac valve replacement and in mainline drug addicts.

Coccidioidomycosis

Coccidioides immitis, the etiologic agent of this mycosis, reproduces in tissues as a sporangium, exhibiting endogenous sporulation, that is, a nucleus undergoes many divisions inside a thick-walled diagnostically distinct sporangium or spherule that ruptures in the tissues at maturity, liberating the spores to repeat the process. The soil-inhabiting, saprobic phase is truly mycelial, producing many highly infectious arthrospores on special hyphal branches from the vegetative mycelia. When disturbed, these arthrospores become airborne, and commingled with dust, are inhaled by animal and human hosts. *C. immitis* is common in hot arid areas of the United States and northern Mexico.

As in tuberculosis, most infections are short, asymptomatic and pass unnoticed; however, they are both immunizing and sensitizing. Symptomatic pulmonary coccidioidomycosis with allergic hypersensitivity has been called San Joaquin Valley fever and desert rheumatism. Arrested pulmonary lesions seen in roentgenograms may be confused with those of tuberculosis. A generalized, chronic, progressive, and often fatal form of coccidioidomycosis called coccidioidal granuloma occurs, especially in dark-skinned peoples.

Coccidioidin, an antigen prepared from culture filtrates of *C. immitis,* is used in the coccidioidin skin test, which is analogous in all respects to the tuberculin test. A positive coccidioidin test in patients with significant shadows on chest roentgenograms is extremely suggestive, especially if they have been in the southwest United States or other endemic areas, if there is no clinical evidence of tuberculosis and if the tuberculin test is negative. The skin test is most valuable when conversion from negative to positive reactions occur and when positive to negative reactions occur in conjunction with a rising complement-fixation test titer. Such anergy, as demonstrated by this latter example, is seen in progressive, disseminated cases and is associated with a grave prognosis. The antigen is no longer commercially available because it has been shown to interfere with the diagnostic value of the complement-fixation test.

Primary pulmonary coccidioidomycosis, whether asymptomatic or symptomatic, has a high recovery rate, and therapy usually consists of bed rest or activity restriction and judiciously administered steroids to control the allergic manifestations of erythema multiforme and erythema nodosum. Amphotericin B is the drug of choice when antifungal therapy is indicated. There is no effective method of artificial immunization.

Histoplasmosis

The etiologic agent of this mycosis, *Histoplasma capsualtum,* is commonly found in the Ohio and Mississippi River Valleys in soil of damp, fertile areas polluted by birds, especially chickens, bats, dogs, and skunks. This disease is unique among the systemic mycoses in that it primarily involves the reticuloendothelial system in which the yeast-like, oval parasite is found almost exclusively intracellularly within macrophages and histiocytes. Parasitic phase cells may be grown *in vitro* under CO_2 at 36 C. in artificial media enriched with blood, glucose and cysteine. Diagnostically distinctive infective tuberculate macroconidiospores are produced in soil and *in vitro* on artificial media at 22 C. Inhaled spores give rise to primary pulmonary infections that, like coccidioidomycosis, are often silent, immunizing and sensitizing. In overt or progressive disease, pneumonitis occurs, and lymphadenopathy may be generalized, with splenomegaly and skin lesions. Roentgenograms of arrested pulmonary lesions may be confused with those of tuberculosis and coccidioidomycosis. Progressive disease is severe and often fatal.

Dermal reactivity to histoplasmin is in all respects analogous to the tuberculin and coccidioidin reactions. Although histoplasmin is not in itself immunizing, its intradermal administration has been shown to elevate the complement-fixation titers in marginal reactors to diagnostically significant levels, thus obfuscating the value of the test. For this reason, histoplasmin is no longer commercially available as a skin-test antigen.

Serologic tests with diagnostic and/or prognostic value are latex agglutination, immunodiffusion and complement-fixation and counterimmunoelectrophoresis. The immunodiffusion test is particularly useful because the development and presence of certain precipitin bands, H and M, are indicative of active and chronic or healed histoplasmosis.

Most cases of primary pulmonary histoplasmosis heal uneventfully, with bed rest and supportive therapy prescribed for the moderately severe cases. Chronic, cavitary or progressive systemic disease is treated with amphotericin B.

A clinically distinct form of histoplasmosis, African histoplasmosis, is caused by a large species of the genus *H. duboisii.* This mycosis is characterized by the development of granulomatous and suppurative lesions in the cutaneous, subcutaneous and osseous tissues. The lungs are rarely involved. Untreated cases can progress to a fatal outcome. Amphotericin B is the drug of choice.

A close antigenic relationship between the two *Histoplasma* species has been demonstrated.

Blastomycosis

Blastomyces dermatitidis, the etiologic agent of this mycosis, appears in lesions as large, ovoid to spherical, thick-walled, single budding, multinucleated, yeast-like cells. This organism is thermally dimorphic; therefore, the tissue phase may be obtained *in vitro* by inoculation onto most laboratory media and by incubation of the culture at 36 C. At 22 C. in soil or on artificial media, the organism is filamentous. Infections are probably acquired by inhaling dust-borne spores.

Blastomycosis most often begins as a primary pulmonary infection and, unlike histoplasmosis and coccidioidomycosis, if untreated, progresses to a severe, disseminated, often fatal disease. Cutaneous lesions are common and probably result from the hematogenous metastasis of organisms from a pulmonary or abdominal site. These skin lesions begin as small papules and progress to confluent, granulomatous, verrucous ulcerations and swellings to abscesses. Rare primary cutaneous infections develop from indurated ulcers that necrotize into chancriform lesions accompanied by lymphangitis, lymphadenitis and regional lymphadenopathy. In contrast to paracoccidioidomycosis, the mucocutaneous tissues and viscera are usually spared.

Dermal reactivity to blastomycin is not specific and serologic tests are generally unsatisfactory for the same reason. Diagnosis is dependent upon finding the organism in a pathologic specimen and on clinical and roentgenographic evidence.

Blastomycosis responds quickly to therapy with amphotericin B, which is recommended for all forms of the disease. For those patients who cannot tolerate this drug, 2-hydroxystilbamidine has been used with some success.

Cryptococcosis

Cryptococcus neoformans, the etiologic agent of this mycosis, is a monomorphic, spherical, thin-walled, encapsulated yeast found in debris and accumulated filth of pigeon roosts, such as attics of old buildings, cornices, and cupolas. The yeasts, which are virtually unencapsulated in their saprobic existence, quickly acquire a demonstrable capsule following entry into a mammalian host; therefore, it appears that virulence is more closely associated with the potential for encapsulation than with the degree of encapsulation. Infec-

tions that progress to symptomatic diseases are most often seen in compromised patients.

It is well accepted that the primary lesions are probably pulmonary; however, these are usually silent and asymptomatic. Central nervous system cryptococcosis, particularly cryptococcal meningitis, is by far the most frequently diagnosed form of the disease, and *C. neoformans* exhibits a distinct predilection for this area. The yeasts elicit a feeble immune response in infected patients producing a histologic reaction consisting of numerous histiocytes, in which the organisms multiply profusely, and occassional giant cells, lymphocytes and fibrosing stroma. Encapsulated organisms may be demonstrated by staining tissue preparations with mucicarmine or alcian blue stains.

C. neoformans may be detected in direct slide preparations of clinical specimens, especially spinal fluid, by mixing a drop of specimen with a drop of nigrosin or India ink, placing a cover glass over the preparation and observing microscopically for encapsulated yeasts. The organisms may be readily isolated from clinical specimens by inoculating Sabouraud's glucose agar or any good bacteriologic media. Because of the prevalence of nonpathogenic *Cryptococcus* species, isolates should be subjected to further identification procedures: growth at 37 C., mouse pathogenicity, pigment production, and carbohydrate fermentation and utilization tests. Serologic tests are virtually valueless; immunofluorescent staining using rabbit antiserum to *C. neoformans* has a specificity paralleling that of the mucicarmine stains.

Amphotericin B, given parenterally, is the drug of choice for central nervous system cryptococcosis. Dermal or pulmonary disease may respond to the less toxic 5-fluorocytosine (flucytosine, 5 FC), administered by the oral route. Clinical studies indicate that optimal therapy may be a combination of these two antimycotics. The recommended therapy regimen is 0.3 mg./kg./day of amphotericin B combined with 150 mg./kg./day of 5-fluorocytosine for 6 to 10 weeks. Overt untreated cryptococcosis is often fatal.

Paracoccidioidomycosis

Paracoccidioides brasiliensis, the etiologic agent of this mycosis, is a thermally dimorphic fungus, appearing in tissues and *in vitro* at 37 C. as a spherical, multiple-budding, yeast-like cell and in nature and on agar as a filamentous mold. The organism is endemic in Central and South America. Inhalation of dust-borne spores produces a mild, often asymptomatic pulmonary infection. Dissemination produces secondary lesions of the oronasal mucosa and skin, with lymphangitis of the involved area, and viscera, including liver, spleen, intestines and lymphatics.

Untreated cases are often fatal. Amphotericin B is recommended for all forms of the disease.

THE SUBCUTANEOUS MYCOSES

Sporotrichosis

Lymphocutaneous sporotrichosis is the most common form of this disease, and the cutaneous form without lymphatic involvement is second in frequency for this reason. Sporotrichosis is sometimes grouped with chromomycosis, maduromycosis and rhinosporidiosis as localized infections of the skin and subcutaneous tissues that rarely metastasize to distant sites. Primary pulmonary sporotrichosis, once extremely rare, is being reported with increasing frequency especially from large urban hospitals, probably because of increased awareness and improved diagnostic procedures. The rare disseminated form, which has a grave prognosis, involves multiorgan systems and is usually seen in compromised patients.

Typically, infection is initiated following the traumatic implantation into the skin of spores found on the bark and thorns of trees and shrubs and in garden mulches. An ulcerated, chancriform lesion developes at the inoculation site followed by the development along the lymphatic chain of multiple subcutaneous nodules that in turn become necrotic and ulcerate. The infection usually does not extend beyond the regional lymph nodes.

The etiologic agent, *Sporothrix schenckii*, is dimorphic, reproducing in tissues and *in vitro* at 36 C. on blood agar enriched with glucose and cystine as oval, round or elongated yeast-like cells and in nature and on agar at 22 C. as a mold composed of septate mycelia bearing typical rosettes of small pyriform microconidiospores. There is usually a paucity of demonstrable organisms in biopsy material, even using special histologic stains; however, positive cultures of the same material are readily obtainable. Organisms have been demonstrated in tissues by immunofluorescent staining when none were seen using conventional techniques.

Infections are immunizing and sensitizing and elicit a cell-mediated immune response detectable by the intradermal sporotrichin test. Serologic tests using the yeast-cell antigen were found to be more specific than those in which sporotrichin was used.

Orally administered potassium iodide is used to treat lymphocutaneous and cutaneous forms of the disease. Local heat applications have been shown to promote healing. Amphotericin B is recommended for relapsed lymphocutaneous disease and disseminated sporotrichosis. 5-Fluorocytosine at a dosage of 100 mg./kg./day has been used with some success.

Chromomycosis

This mycosis, caused by a variety of dematiaceous, soil-inhabiting fungi belonging to the genera *Phialophora*, *Fonsecaea*, and *Cladosporium*, is usually seen as an infection of the subcutaneous tissues, that is, verrucous dermatitis, but cases of cerebral chromomycosis, i.e., Cladosporiosis, have been reported.

Verrucous dermatitis is a chronic painless disease characterized by marked pseudoepitheliomatous hyperplasia. Granulomas with neutrophils, lymphocytes, plasma cells and giant cells containing the sclerotic brown bodies of the tissue form of the fungus or strands of pigmented hyphae constitute the histologic picture. Secondary bacterial infection with resulting lymphostasis and elephantiasis is a complication.

Cerebral chromomycosis is characterized by single or multiple brain lesions, usually encapsulated abscesses formed around masses of brown pigmented hyphae. Symptoms are diverse, depending on the location of the lesions.

Surgical excision of lesions in the early stages of verrucous dermatitis is the most reliable treatment. However, most cases are not seen until the disease is well advanced and more refractory to antimycotics. Amphotericin B, used topically or by intralesion injection, thiabenzadole, used orally and topically, and 5-fluorocytosine have been used with varying degrees of success.

Maduromycosis

This disease, clinically identical to mycetoma caused by actinomycetes, is characterized by the development, usually on the extremities, of tumefactions, abscesses, fistulas and sinuses that involve the deep tissues and bones. The lesions contain granules or grains composed of spores and hyphal strands of the offending fungus. A variety of fungi have been isolated as etiologic agents, among them *Madurella* species and *Allescheria boydii*. The disease is extremely refractory to antimycotic therapy; amphotericin B, griseofulvin and nystatin have had limited success even in early cases (mycetoma, on the other hand, responds to sulfa drugs, penicillins and tetracyclines). Excision of early localized lesions or amputation of the affected extremity is recommended for those cases that do not respond to antimycotics.

Rhinosporidiosis

Rhinosporidium seeberii, the etiologic agent of this infection, appears in tissues as large, thick-walled sporangia, producing by successive nuclear divisions, endogenous sporangiospores that, at maturity, exit the sporangia through a "pore" (actually a thinned area of the sporangium wall). The organism has not been cultured *in vitro*. Rhinosporidiosis is a chronic granulomatous disease principally of the mucocutaneous tissues characterized by the formation of friable, sessile and pedunculated polyps. As the name implies, the disease most often involves the nose. Obstruction of passages by large, unsightly polyps may be relieved by careful surgical excision. Superficial lesions may be removed completely; recurrence of surgically removed deep lesions is not uncommon. Local injection of amphotericin B is used as an adjunct to surgery to prevent spread. Other antimycotics are generally ineffective.

VIRULENCE OF MICROORGANISMS

Virulence is the ability of an organism to initiate and maintain an infection in a host, to invade the host from the initial site of infection and to damage the host. Thus, virulence is a combination of infectiousness, invasiveness and pathogenicity. Each factor is a complex of other factors.

Infectiousness enables the parasite to establish and maintain a foothold or beachhead by evading or killing (or both) local defensive mechanisms such as phagocytes, fibroblasts, acid secretions and even specific antibodies. However, infectiousness does not necessarily imply virulence or great pathogenicity. Silent or latent or subclinical infection is common. For example, *infection* with poliovirus can be widespread, but clinical poliomyelitis resulting from *invasion of the CNS, relatively rare*. The same is true of infection by *Neisseria meningitidis*.

Invasiveness enables the parasite to gain access to, and to grow in, blood and tissues *other* than the immediate site of the initial infection as in typhoid fever, brucellosis, bubonic plague or erysipelas. When invasion of the bloodstream by bacteria occurs, *bacteremia* or *septicemia* is said to be present. *Viremia* occurs in many viral diseases, e.g., yellow fever; *parasitemia* occurs in malaria.

Invasion depends (in part, at least) on the ability of the organism to live under the conditions of temperature, pH, etc., of the human body, to escape, repel or kill leukocytes; it depends also on its resistance to antibodies and its ability to grow rapidly in spite of them. Pneumococci furnish examples of invasiveness associated with capsules, and typhoid bacilli examples of other cellular toxic substances (Vi [virulence] antigen). Some organisms, e.g., *Clostridium perfringens, Streptococcus pyogenes* and *Staphylococcus aureus,* may possess enhanced invasiveness because they produce a number of cytotoxic substances, toxins (see specific organisms).

Dosage is another factor of critical importance in determining infection. Large doses of an infective organism of even very low virulence may overcome almost any degree of resistance. Resistance lowered by other factors (alcoholism, chronic diseases, etc.) also increases susceptibility to any infection.

Pathogenicity may depend on any or all of the above mentioned factors or on only one, e.g., toxigenicity. For example, tetanus bacilli remain localized in dead tissues around a wound and do not invade normal tissues. They secrete exotoxin, which is absorbed by the nerves. *Clostridium botulinum* forms potent exotoxin in foods but has no invasive or infective properties.

The Carrier State

A carrier is an animal or person who has recovered from infection (whether subclinical, mild or severe) with certain microorganisms and who continues to harbor the infecting organisms in a fully virulent form although remaining in apparent good health. Apparently healthy carriers can transmit pathogenic organisms to other people.

NONSPECIFIC IMMUNITY

Nonspecific effector mechanisms involved in resistance to infection (not dependent on *specific* immune response) include mechanical barriers, chemical and cellular factors and interferons.

Mechanical barriers. These include (1) contiguous epithelial cells of skin; (2) hairs in nasal and auditory openings; (3) secretion flow (tears, urine, saliva, mucus); and ciliated epithelium in lower air passages.

Chemical factors. These consist of (1) low pH of gastric juice and vaginal secretions; (2) lysozyme in tears and saliva; (3) fatty acids in sweat; (4) detergent action of bile salts in the intestinal tract; and (5) alternate-complement pathway.

Cellular factors. Leukocytes of different types constitute an important defense against a wide variety of infectious agents. Their mode of action may be dependent upon or be enhanced by *specific* factors of the immune response (antibody, complement) even though they are themselves *nonspecific.*

Phagocytic cells can ingest and in many cases destroy infectious agents by the release of lysosomal constituents including proteolytic enzymes, lysozyme, peroxidases and cationic basic proteins. The importance of phagocytic cells can be seen in children who have defects in intracellular killing (Chédiak-Higashi) syndrome and chronic granulomatous disease). Examples of phagocytic cells include the following types:

1. *Macrophages:* fixed macrophages of the reticuloendothelial system and circulating monocytes of the blood.
2. *Polymorphonuclear leukocytes:* neutrophils, which are prominent in acute inflammatory conditions; eosinophils, which are associated with type I allergy, immune complex ingestion and helminthic infections; and basophils, which, along with connective-tissue mast cells, are the source of histamine when cell-bound IgE is triggered by the appropriate antigen.
3. Certain *lymphoid cells* have nonspecific activity in eliminating infectious agents that express new antigens on the cells of the host. Viruses, intermediate forms (chlamydiae), mycoplasmas and bacteria may be involved under certain circumstances.
4. *Natural killer (NK) cells* can nonspecifically (in the absence of antibody and serum complement) cause the lysis of cells bearing new surface antigens in the absence of antibody and complement.
5. *K cells* can bind to the Fc portion of immunoglobulins that are attached to antigens expressed on cells of the host. K cells thus bound then cause lysis of the "sensitized" infection-modified cells without the assistance of complement. This is called antibody-dependent, cell-mediated cytolysis, or ADCC, and is in fact a specific effector mechanism.

Interferons. Interferons are glycoproteins that are produced by cells in vertebrate hosts in response to an inducer. Interferons are not antigenic in the homologous species. Inducers include double-stranded RNA of a virus or a viral replicative intermediate, certain polyanionic or polycarboxylic copolymers, and a variety of obligate intracellular parasites. Lymphocytes stimulated by mitogens or antigens also produce interferon. Interferon may therefore be considered a lymphokine. Differences in the character of interferons produced in response to different inducers depend at least in part on the cell type that has been stimulated. Its synthesis requires *de novo* synthesis of DNA-dependent RNA and of protein, followed by glycosylation and extracellular transport. The mechanism of action is thought to involve binding to a ganglioside and to a second, more specific receptor on the cell membrane that initiates synthesis of a second protein that in turn inhibits translation and/or transcription of viral messenger RNA. In general, the action of interferon is limited to animals of the same species in which it has been produced; it is, however, effective against any virus in the same spcies. Genes coding for interferon in humans appear to be on chromosome 5. Chromo-

some 21 controls the development of the antiviral activity of interferon in humans cells. There are now many preliminary and ongoing trials of its efficacy against viral diseases and malignancies. The two viral diseases showing most promise of yielding to interferon treatment are V-Z infection in patients with cancer and chronic active hepatitis (hepatitis B). The mode of interferon action in malignancies is wholly unknown. The significance of interferon goes well beyond its antiviral action to include immunoregulation. The non-antiviral effects include numerous cell regulatory mechanisms such as interference with attachment of hormones and toxins to ganglioside receptors; feedback inhibition of interferon production; enhancement of phagocytosis, cytolysis and migration of macrophages; increase in the expression of histocompatibility antigens on cell surfaces that depresses delayed-type hypersensitivity thereby prolonging survival of allogeneic skin grafts, modulation of the antibody response, and inhibition of the growth of nonviral intracellular parasites.

SPECIFIC IMMUNITY

Specific immunity is the result of effector mechanisms directly involving antibodies and specific cellular elements of the lymphoid system. The immunologically specific host respones to infections as well as to stimulation by other chemical or biologic molecules involves two basic effector mechanisms: "humoral" (antibody) and "cell-mediated" (lymphocytes and macrophages). Both specific immune responses originate in the lymphoid system, each effector mechanism being primarily associated with a distinct subset of lymphocytes. For example, the production of antibody involves lymphocytes called B cells, whereas the cell-mediated response involves lymphocytes designated T cells.

Antigen

Antigen may be *any* chemical or biologic molecule that under the proper circumstances is capable of inducing a humoral or cell-mediated response. The product of that response (antibody or T lymphocytes) will react specifically with the original antigen. Antigens may vary in their capacity to induce an immune response. This degree of effectiveness is called immunogenicity. The most immunogenic antigens are usually molecules that are completely "foreign" to the host such as microbial products or components. Tissue components from animals of another species (xenoantigens) are in turn much more immunogenic than equivalent components derived from members of the *same* species (alloantigens). An exception to the latter statement is the extremely strong cell-mediated allograft rejection

TABLE 5-14. Sexually Transmitted Diseases

Disease	Causative Agents	Diagnosis	Immune Response	Treatment
Gonorrhea	*Neisseria gonorrheae* (colony types 1,2) (*N. meningitidis*)	Gram stain, culture, F ab	Antibody to pili	Penicillin (PPNG) (spectinomycin)
Syphilis	*Treponema pallidum*	Darkfield (1°,2°)	RPR, FTA-ABS	Penicillin
Vaginitis* (nontrichomonal)	*Hemophilus vaginalis*	Gram stain, "clue cells"		Tetracycline, (sulfonamide)
Chancroid (soft chancre)	*Hemophilus ducreyi*	Gram stain		Sulfonamide
Lymphogranuloma venereum (LGV)	*Chlamydia trachomatis* Immunotypes L_{1,2,3}	Smear and Giemsa stain, inclusions, F ab	CF antibody	Tetracycline (sulfonamide)
Cervicitis	Immunotypes D,E			
Nongonococcal urethritis (NGU)	D,E Ureaplasma urealyticum ("T" mycoplasma)	Culture	Mycoplasmacidal test (metabolic inhibition)	
Pelvic inflammatory disease (PID)	*N. gonorrheae* Polymicrobial: Bacteroides and other anaerobes, Chlamydiae	Culture (endocerv.) & culdocentesis		Depends on cultures; penicillin
Herpes genitalis	Herpes simplex, type 2, (1)	Primary isolation	Neutralizing antibody	
Condyloma accuminatum	Papovavirus (serotype distinct from wart virus)			Podophyllin (fetal toxicity)
Molluscum contagiosum	Poxvirus			
Hepatitis	Type A (B)	B: immunodiffusion, RIA HBs ag, ab		
INTRAUTERINE AND PERINATAL INFECTIONS	**Toxoplasma** (**O**ther-e.g., group B strep. GC lues) **Rubella** **Cytomegalovirus** *Herpes genitalis*	Fa ab, CF test HI (IgM) Inclusion bodies	Primary vs. secondary	

* Also *Trichomonas vaginalis*; candidosis.

observed in immunologically unrelated members of the same species. Under certain conditions, even one's own tissue components can be immunogenic (autoantigens). For example, individuals with collagen diseases may make a variety of antibodies to their own DNA (systemic *l*upus *e*rythematosus, SLE), immunoglobulins (rheumatoid factor), and various other components (smooth muscle).

Very low molecular weight substances (including chemicals) that are not immunogenic by themselves can induce an immune response if combined with immunogenic complex molecules (protein) of higher molecular weight. The low-molecular-weight substance or chemical compound is called a "hapten," whereas the immunogenic complex molecule to which it is bound is called a "carrier." Antibody made in response to a hapten–carrier complex binds specifically to the free hapten in the absence of the carrier. In a similar manner, certain small sequences of amino acids (proteins) or saccharides (carbohydrates) that are an *innate part of complex immunogenic molecules* can elicit an immune respone to those specific areas of the molecule except that the remainder of the complex molecule acts as its own carrier. These integral small groupings of amino acids or saccharides are called *antigenic determinants* and, like haptens, determine the specificity of antibodies reacting with that particular antigen.

Some drugs, cosmetics, antibiotics and industrial chemicals appear to act as haptens and utilize the host's own plasma or tissue proteins as carriers. These combinations can give rise to specific allergic reactions involving IgE antibody in immediate-type hypersensitivity. These must be distinguished from drug idiosyncrasies that have *no* immunologic basis, but in which signs suggestive of hypersensitivity may appear (rash, arthralgias). In addition to the formation of antibody, other haptens (such as heavy metals and certain chemicals) when bound to host tissue elicit *cell-mediated responses* to the *combined antigenic determinant* of hapten and adjacent host amino acids. In this case, free haptens are *not* able to react specifically with T lymphocytes in the absence of host carrier proteins. Examples that can give rise to cell-mediated, delayed-type hypersensitivity reactions include contact dermatitis and poison ivy.

Heterophile antigens contain cross-reactive or similar antigenic determinants occurring in certain tissues, organs, or erythrocytes, and shared by a wide variety of phylogenetically unrelated species of plants and animals: dogs, sheep, turtles, spinach, cell walls of gram-negative bacteria (e.g., *Salmonella*), guinea pigs and hamsters. These Forssman heterophile antigens do not normally occur in pigs, frogs or humans; antibodies to them are found in most human sera as agglutinins for sheep erythrocytes. Forssman heterophile antibodies can be absorbed out with guinea pig kidney tissue (rich in Forssman antigen). The heterophile antibody (sheep cell agglutinin) found in infectious mononucleosis (EB virus) reacts with equine erythrocytes (Monospot test) and cannot be absorbed with guinea pig kidney tissue. The mononucleosis observed in CMV infection is not associated with a heterophile antibody response.

Antibody

In the electrophoretic analysis of serum, the major proteins are segregated into four principal portions: the alpha, beta and gamma globulins, and albumin. Antibodies appear almost exclusively in the gamma portion and are commonly spoken of as gamma globulins or, more exactly, since they are not absolutely restricted to the gamma portion, as immunoglobulins (Ig). The immunoglobulins occur in five major molecular forms, designated as IgG, IgA, IgM, IgD and IgE. There are several subclasses: $IgG_{1,2,3,4}$, $IgA_{1,2}$, $IgM_{1,2}$. The basic structure of IgG exemplifies the unit structure of all immunoglobulins (Fig. 5-1).

Each molecule of IgG is Y shaped, consisting in part of a pair of identical polypeptide chains intertwined and held together by covalent disulfide bonds. Near the midlength, each chain bends away from the

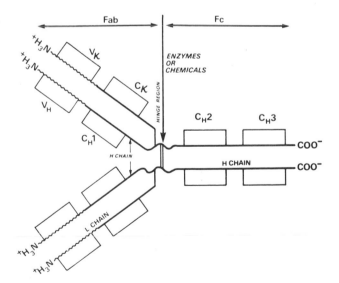

Fig. 5-1. A simplified model for an IgG1(κ) human antibody molecule showing the 4-chain basic structure and domains. V indicates variable region; C, the constant region; and the vertical arrow, the hinge region. Thick line represents H and L chains; thin lines represent disulfide bonds. (Goodman, J. W. and Wang, A.: Immunoglobulins: Structure and diversity. In Fudenberg, H. H., Sites, D. P., Caldwell, J. L. and Wells, J. V.: Basic and Clinical Immunology, 2nd ed., Los Altos, CA, Lange Medical Publications, 1978)

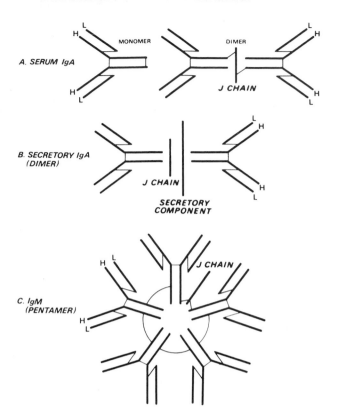

Fig. 5-2. Highly schematic illustration of polymeric human immunoglobulins. Polypeptide chains are represented by thick lines; disulfide bonds linking different polypeptide chains are represented by thin lines. (Goodman, J. W. and Wang, A.: Immunoglobulins: Structure and diversity. In Fudenberg, H. H., Sites, D. P., Caldwell, J. L. and Wells, J. V.: Basic and Clinical Immunology, 2nd ed., Los Altos, CA, Lange Medical Publications, 1978)

other to make the arms of the Y (hinge region). Each of these chains consists of about 440 amino-acid residues, whose sequence (primary structure) is determined genetically. The total molecular weight of each chain is from 53,000 to 75,000, depending on the class. These chains are called the heavy (H) chains. Attached to each of the divergent arms of the Y-shaped molecule is a shorter polypeptide chain of about 220 amino-acid residues, with a molecular weight of about 22,000 per chain. These are called the light (L) chains and are identical in any given molecule and may be of a κ or λ type. The entire structure (including tertiary) of each immunoglobulin molecule or unit is maintained by disulfide bonds.

On both L and H chains, the distal portion (N-terminal ends) is variable in amino acid sequence from one immunoglobulin to another, which enables it to conform to the antigenic determinant for which it is specific. Within the variable regions are primary sequences of amino acids that show even greater variability in

sequence composition and that are called hypervariable regions. The primary structure of the rest of the L and H chains (COO$^-$ terminal end) is constant except for differences between IgG, A, M, D, and E heavy chains or κ and λ light chains as well as some alloantigenic differences (Inv on light chains and Gm on IgG heavy chains). The "arms" of the molecule are flexible through a "hinge" region at the point of divergence of the arms to allow better binding for each antigen binding site. The hinge region is also vulnerable to enzymatic digestion with papain, which yields two Fab (ab for antigen binding) fragments and one Fc (c for crystalizable) portion. The Fc fragment binds to certain cells that have *receptors* for this portion of the immunoglobulin molecule such as mast cells (IgE), K cells (IgG), macrophages (IgG and IgM), and others. Components of serum *complement* are "fixed" or activated by regions in the Fc fragment. (Complement is discussed in more detail later).

IgG as described previously is representative of the various classes of antibody molecules. It is a relatively small, bivalent monomer and is late in appearing in response to initial infection. It is the most plentiful immunoglobulin and is active in agglutination, precipitation and complement activation. It is the only form of antibody that can pass the placenta. IgA occurs as a monomer or dimer of the IgG form, the units being held together at the C ends by covalent bonds of an extra component called J chain. The molecule is equipped with a supplementary secretory piece that facilitates its transportation across membranes. It appears in secretions such as lung exudate in pneumonia or coproantibody (lumen of the gut) in cholera (Fig. 5-2).

IgM is a pentamer of subunits linked together by covalent bonds initiated by interaction with J chain. Because of its polyvalency IgM is especially effective in forming lattices with antigens. It is also active in complement activation and is the first to appear in response to infections. IgE is functional in antibody-mediated (anaphylactic type) of hypersensitivity reactions); little is known of the functions of IgD. However, it is known that IgD is required as an antigen-binding immunoglobulin on B lymphocytes (along with IgM) during early stages of immunologic ontogeny and that most unstimulated B lymphocytes in the body express both IgD and IgM (pre-B lymphocytes).

Antigen/antibody reactions: The reciprocal structural relationship between molecules of antigen and antibody is the basis of immunologic specificity. The antigenic determinant of a molecule and its corresponding specific antibody must "fit" accurately together in order for a specific and effective antigen–antibody reaction to occur. In effect, the better the "fit" is, the stronger are the bonds between antigen and antibody molecules. Antigen–antibody interactions do not involve covalent bonds but depend upon hydrogen bonds, ionic bonds and Van der Waals forces, all influenced by ionic concentrations, pH and temperature.

Since an antigen molecule may contain more than one type of antigenic determinant, an immune response directed against the antigen consists of a group of heterogeneous antibodies, each reacting with its own antigenic determinant on the antigen molecule. As previously discussed, antibody is at least bivalent; and now antigens (especially complex molecules) may also be polyvalent with multiples of the *same* antigenic determinant or an assortment of *different* antigenic determinants. It is these complex interactions that allow visualization of antigen–antibody reactions such as precipitation and agglutination. The detectable or visible result of an antigen–antibody (Ag-Ab) reaction is dependent also on the type of antigen (soluble or particulate) and on the type of immunoglobulin (IgG, IgM, IgA).

1. *Precipitation* involves molecules of soluble antigen in optimal concentration in relation to concentration of antibody molecules (i.e., neither in great excess of the other). A "lattice" is formed consisting of several molecules of polyvalent antibody, such as IgM or IgG, joined to several molecules of polyvalent antigen. Such complexes may form large, visible precipitates whose size and form depend in part on the relative concentrations of antigen and antibody, the ionic content, temperature and other properties of the fluid in which the reaction occurs.

When antibody and antigen are present in ratios of 1:1 or slightly higher, for example, 3:1 or 3:2 ("optimal proportions"), aggregation of antigen and antibody is maximal and lattice formation is most rapid and copious.

2. *Agglutination* involves intact cells or antigen-coated particles (latex agglutination) and optimal electrolyte concentration. Agglutination is best achieved with IgM through multipoint binding of the pentameric antibody, but IgG and IgA can also agglutinate particles. Because of the large size of certain cellular antigens (e.g., erythrocytes), IgM antibodies, being large and pentavalent, are most effective in their agglutination. IgG molecules, being small and only divalent, often fail to "bridge the gap" between large cells, and lattice formation therefore fails. However, they (IgG) may combine with receptors on the cells, preventing the combination of IgG antibodies, thus acting as "blocking" antibodies (see Coombs test).

3. *Neutralization* of soluble toxins (and viruses) basically involves the blocking of reactive sites on the toxin

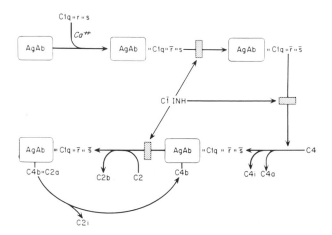

Fig. 5-3. Classic pathway of complement activation. This pathway is initiated by antigen–antibody (Ag-Ab) complexes and is controlled by the C1INH. (Austen, K. F.: The classical and alternative complement sequence. In Benacerraf, B. and Unanue, E. R.: Textbook of Immunology. Baltimore, Williams and Wilkins, 1979)

(or virus) by antibody, thereby preventing expression of its toxic quality (or virus binding to host cells).

4. *Opsonization.* Antibodies directed against microorganisms and other foreign cells make them more readily phagocytosed by macrophages and polymorphonuclear leukocytes. IgG antibodies bound to organisms or cells facilitate their adherence to the membranes of the phagocytic cells that possess specific surface receptors for the Fc portion of the immunoglobulins.

5. *Complement.* Complement (C) is a system of seventeen proteins in the serum. When activated by Ag-Ab reactions, it mediates such diverse biologic functions as cytolysis of mammalian cells and gram-negative bacteria, increased vascular permeability, release of chemotactic factors and increased opsonization for phagocytosis. Binding of antibody to an antigenic determinant, whether on a cell surface or soluble molecule, causes distortion and unveiling of a site on the Fc portion of immunoglobulins (IgG, IgM); this event in turn starts the "classic" cascade effect with the binding of the first component (C1) (Fig. 5-3). The C cascade is in its simplest terms a series of enzyme precursors that are acted on in succession and converted to active enzymes. In addition to classic activation, C may be activated by aggregated IgA, lipopolysaccharides and yeast cell walls (zymosan). This process is called "alternate" activation and includes the components properdin (P), B factor and D factor (Fig. 5-4). Both types of activation lead to the "effector" series of components C3 to C9. The split products of C3 to C7 with biologic activity are shown in Fig. 5-5).

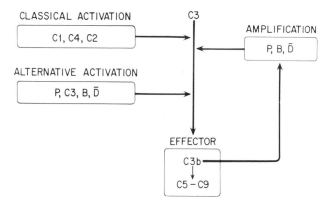

Fig. 5-4. Segregation of the complement proteins into four functional units: two pathways for initial cleavage of C3, the classic and alternative, the C3b-dependent amplification pathway for augmentation of C3 cleavage, and the effector sequence from which are derived most of the biologic activities of the complement system. (Austen, K. F.: The classical and alternative complement sequence. In Benacerraf, B. and Unanue, E. R.: Textbook of Immunology. Baltimore, Williams and Wilkins, 1979)

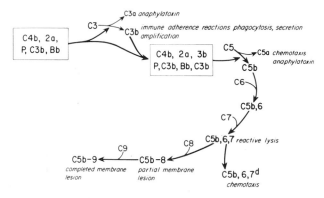

Fig. 5-5. The effector sequence of the complement system. The biologically active fragments and complexes are generated as a result of cleavage of C3 and C5 by the classic and amplification of C3 and C5 convertases, respectively. (Austen, K. F.: The classical and alternative complement sequence. In Benacerraf, B. and Unanue, E. R.: Textbook of Immunology. Baltimore, Williams and Wilkins, 1979)

Cytolysis of cells requires the interaction of C8 and C9, which cause lesions in the membranes. Complement is regulated by extrinsic inhibitors (C1 inhibitors) and by the intrinsic short half-life of the activated components. The absence of C1 esterase inhibitor is the cause of the disease, angioedema.

Cells of the Immune Response

It is apparent that an individual has a diverse number of both T and B lymphocytes that are capable of recognizing a large number of antigenic determinants. In a modification of Burnet's original theory, Jerne has proposed that each cell has a limited number of genes that code for appropriate allotransplantation antigens including (one's own) antigens (germ line theory). Because we cannot tolerate cells that would recognize our own antigens, these cells are suppressed as they appear by the overwhelming amount of our own antigens (immunologic tolerance). Diversification for recognition of all foreign antigens may come from somatic mutation of these cells so that mutant genes code for a variety of new antigenic determinants (somatic mutation theory). The combination of the two theories seems best to fit the evidence of immunologic tolerance, strong graft rejection and the fact that cells are available that recognize synthetic antigens not involved in evolution. (This is considered to be an extreme oversimplification.) The interaction of a cell with its specific antigen leads to blastogenesis and replication (clonal expansion).

As discussed earlier, the specific immune response is mediated by the lymphoid system of cells consisting of two basic types, B and T lymphocytes. Precursor immunologically uncommitted lymphocytes of both types originate from bone marrow stem cells and migrate to either of two primary lymphoid organs. The microenvironment of the primary organ called the bursa of Fabricius (in birds) and diffuse lymphoid structures of the gut or bone marrow itself (in mammals) influences differentiation of lymphocytes into immunologically competent cells (B cells) that recognize a single antigenic determinant. These cells eventually, upon antigenic stimulation, differentiate further into antibody-producing plasma cells. B cells recognize antigen through membrane-bound immunoglobulins on the cell surface. The class of immunoglobulin depends on the state of ontogeny. The specificity of that immunoglobulin (variable region) was determined during exposure of the cell to the bursa of Fabricius (or equivalent) microenvironment. B lymphocytes then migrate to populate the secondary lymphoid tissue such as the germinal center of lymph nodes and the spleen. The thymus is the other primary organ that provides a microenvironment for migrating precursor cells to differentiate into immunologically competent cells called thymus-dependent lymphocytes or T cells. There are numerous subpopulations of T cells that (1) provide "help" for B cells to produce antibody (T helper); (2) react in delayed type hypersensitivity reactions; (3) lyse cells expressing new antigens on their surfaces (T cytotoxic); and (4) regulate or "suppress" the extent of immune response to both antibody production and cell-mediated immune responses (T suppressor). T cells populate the deep cortex of lymph nodes, the periarterial sheaths of the spleen, and comprise the major cell population of lymph and blood. Antigen recognition by T lymphocytes is specific but is *not* mediated by immunoglobulins. There is evidence, however, that the hypervariable regions of immunoglobulins on B cells are the same as those of T-cell antigen receptors on T and B cells that recognize the same antigenic determinants.

The Major Histocompatibility Complex

The genetic control of graft rejection resides on the sixth chromosome in a complex of closely linked genes that is now called the major histocompatibility complex (MHC) (Fig. 5-6). Some of the gene products of this locus are expressed on the surface of most cells of the body and stimulate primarily a cell-mediated allograft rejection; but in later stages of rejection antibodies to these gene products are also produced. More importantly, the MHC is now known to contain genes that control B factor, the fourth component of complement (Bf, C4), certain blood group substances (Chido, Roger) and immune response genes (Ir) (i.e., ragweed atopy).

The alloantigens expressed on the surface of cells are designated human leukocyte antigens (HLA) and are controlled by at least four distinct gene loci (HLA-A, B, C, D). Another locus related to HLA-D (HLA-DR) may be the same as HLA-D or closely linked. The known allelic forms for each locus in this extremely polymorphic system vary from thirty-three (HLA-B) to only six (HLA-C). These genes are autosomal as well as codominant and segregate in progeny with one set of linked (on same chromosome) alleles (haplotype) from each parent. HLA-A, B and C locus antigens are detected by reacting alloantiserum (usually from multiparous women) with peripheral blood lymphocytes in the presence of complement. The HLA-D locus antigens are not as widely distributed as the others and are limited to B lymphocytes, macrophages, sperm and epithelial cells. These antigens are at present being detected by mixing peripheral blood lymphocytes of one individual (containing some B lymphocytes) with those of another. Differences at the HLA-D locus on stimulator B lymphocytes cause blastogenesis of responder T "helper" lymphocytes. If the HLA-A, B and C locus antigens are also different, then responder T "cytotoxic" lymphocytes are induced that will lyse target cells that bear the same HLA-A, B, C antigens as the stimulator cells. The induction of cytotoxic T lymphocytes is *greater* if HLA-D locus disparity occurs and T "helper" lymphocytes are produced. These *in vitro* processes are the basis of primary graft rejection.

Important linkage exists between disease states and specific HLA-B and HLA-D phenotypes. Some of the

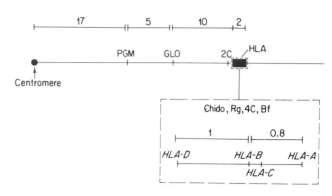

Fig. 5-6. Chromosomal localization of the human major histocompatibility complex. (MHC) (Benacerraf, B. and Unanue, E. R.: Transplantation Immunology. In Textbook of Immunology. Baltimore, Williams and Wilkins, 1979)

strongest linkage occurs between the allele HLA-B27 and ankylosing spondylitis, Reiter's syndrome and acute anterior uveitis. *Salmonella* and *Yersinia* entercolitis, arthritis and *Shigella* arthropathy have strong associations with HLA-B27. Several diseases have significant association with HLA-Dw3 including juvenile-onset diabetes, dermatitis herpetiformis, and idiopathic Addison's disease. These strong associations are mostly limited to HLA-B and D loci (see Fig. 5-6), which may indicate the existence, in this area of the MHC, of numerous Ir genes controlling immune regulatory mechanisms.

Induction and Regulation of the Immune Response

The induction of both humoral and cell-mediated immune responses requires macrophages for "antigen processing" for optimal results. When small amounts of an antigen on the surface of macrophages are presented to T helper cells that have receptors for that antigen, blastogenesis and clonal expansion occur. The release of soluble factors from these cells that are specific for this antigen induces a specific B-cell response to the same antigen (i.e., clonal expansion). Both cells may or may not respond to the *same* antigenic determinant on the antigen molecule; however, if different antigenic determinants are involved, they must be located on the *same molecule*. In the case of a "hapten" conjugated to "carrier" protein, B cells may recognize the hapten, whereas T helper cells may recognize an antigenic determinant on the carrier protein. Antigens that require this process are called T-dependent [Fig. 5-7(1)]. Most complex antigens fall into this category. Antigens that bear identical *repeating* antigenic determinants may stimulate B cells *without* T helper cells [Fig. 5-7(2)]. Examples of these T-*in*dependent antigens include gram-negative bacterial lipopolysaccharide, pneumococcal polysaccharide and viral capsids

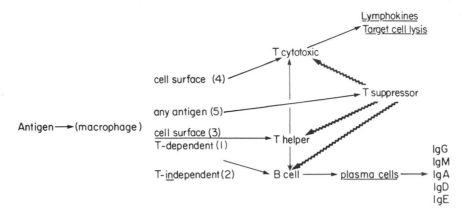

Fig. 5-7. Induction and regulation of the immune response.

(protein coats). Unlike the T-dependent process, only IgM immunoglobulins are formed without T cell help. Cell surface antigens can induce T helper cells (i.e., viral cell surface antigens, tumor antigens, HLA-D alloantigen in previous section) [Fig. 5-7(3)] to provide amplification of the T cytotoxic cell response [Fig. 5-7(4)] to the same (viral,tumor) or other antigens on the cell surface (HLA-A, B, C alloantigen). T-cell helper factors may be both specific and nonspecific in this instance.

Regulation of immune responses is the responsibility of another T cell called T suppressor [Fig. 5-7(5)]. Antigen also induces the T suppressor to replicate and undergo clonal expansion so that it can exert a negative or regulatory influence on B-cell, T-helper, and T-cytotoxic replication. When antigen is no longer available to stimulate the aforementioned cells, it is thought that the remaining cells of the expanded clone revert to small lymphocytes and remain in the individual as long-lived "memory" cells. Memory cells are then available on reexposure to the antigen to provide a rapid immune response, without the need for clonal expansion. An example of this expression is the result of "booster" immunizations that require less antigen and a shorter time for an effective immune response.

Another regulatory mechanism involves "antibody feedback" that governs the amount of antigen available to stimulate the immune respone. In this situation, as antibody is produced, it is available to bind to "free" antigen and form Ag-Ab complexes that are rapidly removed from the circulation by cells of the reticuloendothelial system. An example of this system is the passive administration of Rh immunoglobulin to Rh-negative pregnant women who may be threatened with sensitization to fetal Rh antigen(s). The antibody to Rh "coats" Rh-positive erythrocytes from the fetus, thus promoting their rapid removal from the maternal circulation before they can induce a primary immune response, in the mother, to Rh.

Immunologic Tolerance

The acquired inability of an individual to express an immune response to a molecule that would normally evoke active cell-mediated or humoral responses is called "tolerance" or "immunologic unresponsiveness."

1. Antigens that stimulate an immune response in adults can induce a state of tolerance in newborns with undeveloped immunologic competence. In 1945, Owen observed that during fetal life of dizygotic (heterozygous) twin calves, blood and erythrocytes of each fetus circulated freely in both and, though non-self (foreign), were tolerated throughout adult life as if they were "self" (native); each twin was an erythrocyte chimera. This exemplifies permanent, antigen-specific immunologic tolerance under natural conditions. The studies of Burnet and Medawar extended Owen's work. They injected viable spleen cells of one strain of mice (A) into neonates of another strain of mice (B), thus artifically inducing in adult (B) mice complete, permanent and strain-specific immunologic tolerance to skin grafts from adult (A) mice.

2. T-independent antigens in extremely large doses can induce a state of "paralysis" or tolerance in an individual. Pneumococcal polysaccharide at 10 to 100 times the immunizing dose induces tolerance in animals. Challange with immunizing doses does not induce an immunologic response. Because pneumococcal polysaccharide is a T-independent antigen, the tolerance is probably due to B-cell unresponsiveness.

3. T-dependent foreign protein antigens can be tolerogenic under the following circumstances: (a) if the host is newborn or an immunosuppressed adult; (b) if very low or very high doses of a low-molecular-weight molecule in soluble, monomeric physical form are used; (c) if introduction is by the intravenous route; and (d) if antigen is inherently a weak immunogen in its native form. High doses of antigen probably in-

volve tolerance by *both* B and T cells. Low-dose tolerance apparently involves T-suppressor-cell induction in the absence of a response by T helper or B cells, which effectively prevents the induction of an immune response by excessive negative regulation.

4. Tolerance can be induced to new antigens if they are bound to the surface of the host's own cells. It has been demonstrated that haptens or glycoproteins covalently bound to the surface of autologous cells, when reintroduced into the host, can induce a state of functional tolerance with respect to the induction of the humoral response. T-suppressor-cell induction evidently is the main reason for unresponsiveness in this case, although T-helper tolerance may be involved under certain conditions.

Nonspecific Immunosuppression

This may be produced by various immunosuppressive measures, several of which are used in connection with organ "transplants" because there is as yet no generally acceptable and feasible means of inducing antigen-specific immunologic unresponsiveness to allografts. In general, they suppress proliferation and remove or destroy all clones of antibody-producing lymphocytes nonspecifically and indiscriminantly. Most of these measures have undesirable, often dangerous, side effects and also greatly enhance vulnerability to infection:

1. Whole body x-irradiation may be made specific under certain conditions and depends on injury to macrophages rather than to small lymphocytes.
2. Cannulization of the thoracic duct for mechanical removal of lymphocytes
3. Beta-irradiation of blood; destruction of lymphocytes only
4. Potent, equine, cytolytic, antihyman-lymphocyte globulins (ALG), especially in conjunction with thymectomy to delay regeneration of all antibody-producing lymphoid cells
5. Drugs such as azathioprine, prednisone (and other corticosteroids) and cyclophosphamide.

Immunodeficiencies and Gammopathies

The primary specific immunodeficiency diseases result from an absence or lack of maturation of T and/or B cells. A complete list of lymphocytic defects is shown in Table 5-15.

1. *X-linked agammaglobulinemia* (congenital agammaglobulinemia, Bruton's disease). Affected males have no B lymphocytes, no detectable IgM, IgA, IgD, IgE (only 10 per cent of normal IgG), and no response to immunizations. There is little development of lymph-node germinal centers and tonsils are abnormally small. These individuals do have a normal cell-mediated response with respect to delayed-type hypersensitivity and allograft rejection.

2. *Congenital thymic aplasia* (DiGeorge syndrome). Thymic aplasia results from a congenital defect and is not hereditary. Individuals have no T cells and hence no delayed-type hypersensitivity or allograft rejection capability. Germinal centers are normal with normal numbers of plasma cells in lymphoid tissue. Serum immunoglobulins are normal, the result most likely of T-independent antigen stimulation from infectious agents. The lack of a cell-mediated response makes these individuals susceptible to fatal viral infections.

3. *Severe combined immunodeficiency* (SCID) (Swiss type agammaglobulinemia). This disease is characterized by a lack of both T and B lymphocytes. It is hereditary, being transmitted by x-linked or autosomal recessive genes. Individuals with SCID are agammaglobulinemic and are incapable of rejecting allografts or of mounting delayed-type hypersensitivity.

Complement defects are known for all components of the classic complement cascade except for C1a, C15, and C9. The deficiency of C1 inhibitor is associated with hereditary angioneurotic edema. The lack of C3b inactivator results in patients with recurrent infection with pyogenic bacteria.

Neutrophil phagocytic defects in either the ability to kill intracellular organisms (chronic granulomatous disease, CGD) or degranulation of lysosomes (Chédiak-Higashi syndrome) result in severe recurrent infections. In addition, lowered phagocytic activity may also be observed in recurrent infections due to lack of opsonins (antibody or complement).

Gammopathies are the opposite of deficiencies, being characterized by the abnormal proliferation of cells involved in the humoral response. The result is that excessive amounts of immunoglobulin are produced. Table 5-16 shows the more important monoclonal gammopathies with their associated immunoglobulin classes.

1. *Multiple myeloma* is a malignant proliferation of plasma cells with the following characteristics: (a) cell-mass expansion; (b) immunoglobulin protein elaboration; and (c) the concomitant suppression of normal antibody synthesis. The whole immunoglobulin (M component) may be found in the serum with or without "free" light chains in the urine (Bence Jones proteins). The disease involves osteolytic lesions and pathologic fractures, anemia due to displacement of myeloid elements in the bone marrow by plasma cells, renal failure and nervous system involvement.

2. *Macroglobulinemia* (or Waldenström's macro-

TABLE 5-15. Lymphocyte Defects and Genetic Aspects of Selected Primary Immunodeficiency Syndromes

Disorder	Affected Lymphocyte Populations				Mode of Inheritance
	T Cells		B Cells		
	Stage 1*	*Stage 2**	*Stage 1*	*Stage 2*	
Disorders apparently affecting stem cells					
Reticular dysgenesis	Yes	Yes	Yes	Yes	Unknown
SCID† (thymic alymphoplasia)	Yes	Yes	(Yes)‡	(Yes)	X-linked
SCID (Swiss type)	Yes	Yes	(Yes)	(Yes)	Autosomal recessive
SCID with ADA deficiency	Yes	Yes	(Yes)	(Yes)	Autosomal recessive
SCID with ectodermal dysplasia and dwarfism	Yes	Yes	Yes	Yes	? Autosomal recessive
SCID (sporadic)	Yes	Yes	Yes	Yes	Unknown
Disorders mainly affecting B cells					
Congenital hypogammaglobulinemia (Bruton type)	No	No	Yes	Yes§	X-linked
Congenital hypogammaglobulinemia	No	No	Yes	Yes	Autosomal recessive
Common variable immunodeficiency	No	(No)	No	Yes§	? Autosomal recessive
IgA deficiency	No	(No)	No	No§	Variable
IgM deficiency	No	No	No	?	Unknown
IgG subclass deficiency	No	No	No	?	X-linked
Immunodeficiency with elevated IgM	No	No	No	(Yes)	X-linked
X-linked immunodeficiency with normal globulin count or hyperglobulinemia	No	No	(No)	(Yes)	X-linked
Hypogammaglobulinemia with thymoma	No	No	No	Yes§	Unknown
Disorders mainly affecting T cells					
Thymus hypoplasia (Nezelof's syndrome)	Yes	Yes	(No)	(No)	Variable
DiGeorge's syndrome	Yes	Yes	No	No	Variable
Nucleoside phosphorylase deficiency	Yes	Yes	No	No	? Autosomal recessive
Chronic mucocutaneous candidiasis with endocrinopathy	No	Yes	No	No	? Autosomal recessive
Complex immunodeficiencies					
Wiskott-Aldrich syndrome	Yes	Yes	No	(Yes)	X-linked
Ataxia-telangiectasia	(Yes)	Yes	No	(No)	Autosomal recessive
Hyper-IgE syndrome	No	Yes	No	No	Unknown
Cartilage-hair hypoplasia	?	Yes	No	(No)	Autosomal recessive

* indicates first or second stages of lymphoid cell differentiation.

† SCID = severe combined immunodeficiency.

‡ Statements enclosed in parentheses indicate defects that are variable in severity or expression.

§ Recent evidence indicates the presence of excessive suppressor cell activity.

globulinemia) is characterized by the production of a homogeneous single immunoglobulin (IgM). Clinically, increased viscosity of the blood caused by large amounts of IgM results in thrombosis and bleeding (petechiae) in the skin, nasal mucosa and gastrointestinal tract. Retinal hemorrhages may eventually cause blindness.

3. *"Heavy chain disease"* was first described as being caused by the elaboration of a protein (55,000 daltons) apparently consisting of an incomplete IgG heavy chain and having the antigenic determinants of IgG, but no detectable light chains. Subsequently, IgA and IgM heavy chain diseases have been described. The syndrome is characterized clinically by frequent infections due to impairment of antibody production.

Allergy and Hypersensitivity

Allergy (Gr. *allos* = changed; *ergon* = action) or hypersensitivity is an altered state of reactivity of cells and tissues manifest through specific pathogenic immune reactions occuring *in vivo* (Table 5-17). Most of the manifestations of hypersensitivity are now explicable in terms of molecular and cellular interactions. The principal mechanisms underlying the clinical man-

TABLE 5-16. Monoclonal Gammopathies

Disorder	Class of Protein	Light Chain
Multiple myeloma	IgG, IgA, IgD or IgE	κ or λ
Macroglobulinemia	IgM	κ or λ
Heavy-chain disease	IgG, IgA or IgM	None

ifestations of allergy can be grouped conveniently under four principal headings:

Type I: anaphylactic type allergy, entirely mediated by IgE

Type II: cytotoxic type, dependent on antibody and complement

Type III: immune complex disease (serum sickness)

Type IV: cell-mediated immune reactions

Types I, II and III are all referred to as "immediate hypersensitivity," being mediated by specific antibody. Type IV hypersensitivity is essentially independent of antibody, all reactions being mediated by specifically sensitized T lymphocytes. Types I and IV are independent of complement. It will be evident that more than one of the four types may be operating in a given clinical situation. Moreover, implicit in each type of hypersensitive manifestation is a first experience with a given set of antigens constituting the primary immunization or sensitization. Subsequent exposure to the same or related sets of antigens evokes tissue reaction(s) in the previously "sensitized" host. The manner and route of primary sensitization are not always evident and may be respiratory (e.g., hay fever), contact (poison ivy) or oral (food allergies). Atopic persons are those who inherit (MHC) a tendency to become allergic very easily to many different antigens by synthesizing abnormally high levels of IgE.

Type I Hypersensitivity. "Immediate" type hypersensitivity refers to atopic allergy, manifested by a rapidly developing (minutes) wheal and flare (hives, urticaria) reaction in the skin in response to the intradermal injection of specific antigen(s), exemplified by hay fever (e.g., ragweed allergy). There is no perceptible local cytotoxicity or leukocytic response. The same antigen given systemically (usually inadvertently) causes anaphylactic shock. IgE formed in response to primary (sensitizing) immune responses attaches, by the Fc portion, to specific Fc receptors on mast cells, basophils and platelets, that is, become tissue-fixed and remain *in situ* for months or years. Reactions of homologous antigens with this fixed antibody trigger transmembranally the release of the vasoactive amines responsible for all of the manifestations of "immediate" hypersensitivity, namely, histamine, bradykinin, slow-reacting-substance of allergy (SRS-A), all of which cause smooth-muscle contraction, vasodilatation and increased capillary permeability. Increased coagulation time is due to heparin released from mast cells. Liver damage occurs, and cartilage and collagen tissues are affected. Edema and smooth-muscle contractions in large blood vessels, air passages and elsewhere are frequently the immediate cause of death. Commonly, the active substances are quickly decomposed in the body and the manifestations of immediate allergy are therefore short-lived (2 to 48 hours). Fatal anaphylaxis, which is not unusual, can result from bee stings or from injection of avianized vaccines and antibiotics (especially penicillin), particularly in an atopic individual. Histamine release is under the control of AMP. Falling levels (blockade of adenylcyclase) promote histamine release; promotion of cAMP synthesis by increased adenylcyclase activity (stimulated by epinephrine) reduces histamine release. Xanthines (used in therapy of type I hypersensitivity) block phosphodiesterase, which is responsible for the destruction of cAMP. Eosinophil-chemotactic factor A (ECF-A) is among the products released by basophil–mast cell activation. Eosinophils secrete their granular enzyme (arylsulfatase), which splits SRS-A, providing a feedback control mechanism. These reactions are summarized in Figure 5-8.

Type II Hypersensitivity. This type usually results from the cytotoxic or cytolytic action of complement on cells (tissue cells, erythrocytes) to which specific antibodies to cellular components (e.g., blood group antigens) have attached. These cells are said to be "sensitized" to immune lysis, which is the mechanism underlying hemolytic disease of the newborn (HDN) (q.v.) and incompatible transfusion reactions. Some drugs (e.g., Sedormid, penicillin) bind to tissue proteins and thereby become antigenic, the resulting antibody being specific for the drug (hapten). The same or related drugs adsorbed nonspecifically to cells make them the target for cytotoxic antibody (hemolytic anemia, thrombocytopenic purpura).

Type III Hypersensitivity. The term "serum sickness" refers to the older observation of anaphylactic and immediate allergic manifestations in persons receiving foreign serum therapeutically (e.g., diphtheria antitoxin as horse serum). The term as now used connotes type I or III allergy caused by any foreign antigenic substances, which may include low-molecular-weight compounds (haptens) bound in the circula-

TABLE 5-17. Hypersensitivity: Pathogenic Immune Reactions in Vivo

Designation, Type*	Route of Primary Antigenic Stimulation	Specificity	Skin Test	Clinical Examples	Mechanism	Prevention
I. Anaphylactic, "immediate"	Respiratory GI tract Subcutaneous	IgE (reaginic antibody; distinguish from Wassermann ab)	(Intradermal) "immediate" wheal/flare sec.–min. Transferable with serum	Allergic rhinitis (hay fever); insect venom sensitivity (phospholipase A) *DRUGS* (e.g., penicillin). Hives (urticaria), asthma	Histamine SRS-A, ECF-A from sensitized mast cells, basophils, ?platelets. No tissue damage	"Blocking" IgG
II. Cytotoxic, ADCC	Parenteral, Infection, Drugs as haptens, Altered "self"	IgM, IgG (systemic)	(Systemic reaction, transferable with serum)	Transfusion reactions Hemolytic disease of the newborn (HDN) Hemolytic anemia (DRUGS) Infection Autoimmune diseases Thrombocytopenic purpura	C ("immune") lysis of sensitized cells (rbc, platelets) (tissue damage)	HDN: Rhogam prophylaxis against primary sensitization (not desensitization)
III. Antigen-antibody complex disease, "Serum sickness"	Foreign protein, parenteral, infection	IgG, IgM ("Gatekeeper" IgE)	Arthus type (experimental passive)	Poststreptococcal AGN Rheumatoid arthritis SLE, hepatitis B Drugs, infections	Deposition of Ag/Ab/C in tissues evokes acute inflammatory reaction (pmn, platelets) Tissue damage	None specific
IV. "Delayed," tuberculin type, CMI	Persistent chronic intracellular infection (bacterial, fungal, viral, protozoal) Tumors Tissue grafts	T lymphocytes	(Intradermal) "Delayed" tuberculin type (PPD) 24–48 hours	Tuberculosis, other bacterial infections All mycoses, some viruses Contact dermatitis (e.g. poison ivy, (DRUGS) Tumor and graft rejection	T lymphocytes specifically stimulated to release lymphokines (nonspecific) Transfer factor (specific) Tissue damage	None

*Types I, II and III are all referred to as *Immediate type hypersensitivity*, and all are mediated by specific antibody. Type IV is essentially independent of antibody, and all reactions are mediated by specifically sensitized T lymphocytes.

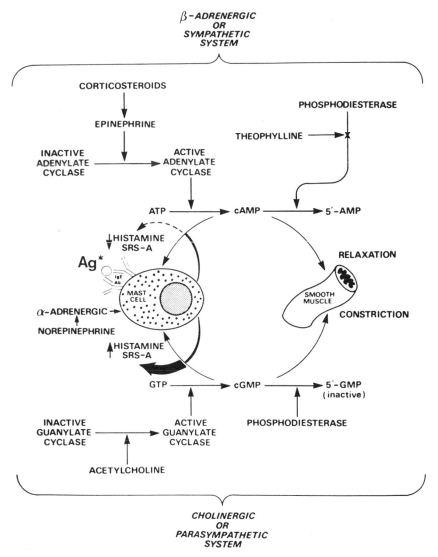

Fig. 5-8. The balance theory of sympathetic and parasympathetic regulation, indicating points of pharmacotherapeutic attack. [* Union of antigen with cell-fixed IgE antibody can be blocked by reaction with homologous IgG (blocking) antibody produced in response to "desensitization."] (Modified from Frick, O. L.: Immediate hypersensitivity. In Fudenberg, H. H., Sites, D. P., Caldwell, J. L. and Wells, J. V.: Basic and Clinical Immunology. Los Altos, CA, Lange Medical Publications, 1978)

tion to serum or to tissue proteins to become complete antigens. Classically, "serum sickness" type hypersensitivity (type III) in a previously unsensitized individual follows 7 to 10 days after systemic injection of foreign antigen, that is, the period necessary to mount a primary antibody response. At a critical level of antigen, enough excess antigen–antibody complexes (IgM, IgG) are found deposited in the tissues, especially in the renal glomerular basement membrane, to cause accretion of complement and initiation of the complement cascade and inflammatory response, accompanied by release of anaphylatoxins (C3b, C5b), which

activate directly (degranulate) basophils and mast cells to release vasoactive amines. Some IgE is inevitably formed in this primary immune response. This IgE sensitizes mast cells and basophils to react with circulating antigen with the same result. At its peak, serum sickness is a constellation of reactions resulting from the relatively protracted systemic release of vasoactive amines. Symptoms and signs subside as antibody appears in excess. Anaphylactic shock occurs in a person already sensitized (e.g., to penicillin) who may or may not have had clinically evident serum sickness but in whom all basophils and mast cells have previously been sensitized (i.e., IgE antibody may remain attached to basophils and mast cells for years following primary sensitization with the offending antigen). The sudden union of massive amounts of antigen with widely scattered sensitized mast cells effectively provides a sudden large systemic charge of histamine, with all of its consequences.

Desensitization. A severe immediate-type allergic reaction may be avoided in foreign serum injections (e.g., equine diphtherial antitoxin) if desensitization is carried out. This consists of a series of very minute (0.001 to 0.01 ml.) subcutaneous doses of the serum given at intervals of half an hour for several hours before the main dose. This in effect gradually saturates all IgE attached to mast cells, thus blocking access by antigen subsequently administered in therapeutic amounts. However, new IgE antibody eventually is formed and perpetuates the state of hypersensitivity so that there can be no permanent amelioration of the atopic state. By the subcutaneous administration of carefully graded doses of antigen (active desensitization), sufficient IgG and IgA antibody can be produced to compete with antigen for fixed IgE antibody and thereby prevent or reduce the triggering of histamine release (e.g., prophylactic treatment of hay fever allergy during the "off" season) (See Fig. 5-8).

Cell-mediated Immune Response (CMIR) and Delayed Hypersensitivity

In the CMIR, "afferent" and "efferent" limbs serve, respectively, to bring the antigen(s) into the immunologic mechanism and to mediate the responses. When exposed to antigen processed by macrophages, a proportion of T lymphocytes in the afferent limb becomes sensitized, that is, has the potential to activate the efferent limb of the CMIR when reexposed to the same antigen. Antigens involved in the CMIR include (1) certain microorganisms (*Mycobacteria, Listeria, Brucella, Chlamydiae* fungi, viruses) and tumor and transplantation cell-surface antigens; and (2) simple chemicals (contact hypersensitivity). In the efferent limb of the CMIR, sensitized T lymphocytes reexposed to the sensitizing antigen may undergo blast transformation and then proliferate. The subsequent progeny of sensitized lymphocytes produce a variety of lymphokines that mediate the associated inflammatory response. The lymphokines themselves are nonspecific with respect to antigen, in contrast to antibody, which is antigen specific. These lymphokines include chemotactic factor, which attracts monocytes and macrophages to the scene of action, migration inhibition factor (MIF) and macrophage-activating factor (MAF), which hold and "activate" macrophages in the area, and lymphablastogenic factor, which stimulates nonspecifically other lymphocytes in the area to undergo blast transformation. The release of lymphokines from stimulated T lymphocytes is extremely important in "activating" macrophages toward enhanced microbicidal activity with those organisms resistant to intracellular killing (i.e., *M. tuberculosis*). Some of these specifically sensitized lymphocytes become long-term "memory" cells that circulate in blood and lymph, retaining reactivity for years. Sensitized T lymphocytes (T cytotoxic) exposed to the appropriate antigen may also produce certain lymphokines (e.g., MIF or interferon) without undergoing transformation or proliferation. Thes nontransforming cells may lyse target cells that have an appropriate antigen on their surface (e.g., viral, transplantation).

The prototypic "delayed" type CMIR is the positive reaction to the injection of tuberculin in patients or animals infected with *M. tuberculosis.* In response to the injection of antigen, there is an accumulation of T cells at the site of injection during the ensuing 24 to 48 hours, resulting in the formation of a palpable area of induration. This is in contrast to the "immediate" wheal and flare reaction caused by histamine release (type I) from IgE-sensitized tissue mast cells or basophils that follows within seconds or minutes the exposure to antigen. The tuberculin (type IV) CMIR accounts for the predominantly round-cell histologic appearance of tuberculous and other chronic infectious lesions (e.g., mycoses). Contact hypersensitivity results from constant exposure of the skin to simple chemicals or heavy metals. These materials form antigenic complexes with host proteins that evoke a delayed hypersensitivity reaction whenever the host is exposed to the chemical or metal.

IMMUNOHEMATOLOGY

Human erythrocytes (rbc) have at their surfaces a variety of genetically determined and usually dominant antigens (alloantigens, isoantigens, Table 5-18). Among the many clinically important rbc antigens are those discovered by Landsteiner in 1900 and called A and B. Numerous others (e.g., A_1) have been discovered since. The A and B antigens are enzymically formed from a precursor antigenic substance that is cross-reactive with type XIV pneumococcal polysaccharide (SXIV). The basic antigenic structure is contained in a branched oligosaccharide. Addition to fucose to both branches confers H (heterogenetic) specificity. Addition of N-acetylgalactosamine (GalNac) to the terminal galactose (Gal) of both branches confers A_1 specificity. Addition of Gal only to the terminal Gal of branch II confers A_2 specificity. Alternatively, an additional Gal at the end of both branches confers

TABLE 5-18. Immunohematology

Blood Group System (Genes)	Genotype	Phenotype		Frequency (%)	Antibody in Serum
			Major blood groups		
ABO	O(H) O(H)	O(H)	*Ags on rbc mem- brane & secretions*	44	Anti-A, anti-B
	A_1A_1	A		42	Anti-B
	A_1A_2				
	A_1O				
	A_2O				
	BB	B		10	Anti-A
	BO				
	A_1B	AB		4	None
	A_2B				
Lewis		Le^a		22	
		Le^{b*}		78	
Se	SeSe	secretors		80	
	Sese				
	sese	nonsecretors		20	
			Ags in rbc only		
MN	MM	M		27	
	NN	N		24	
	MN	MN		50	
S	SS	S		55	
	Ss				
	ss	s		45	
Rh†		DCe,DCE,DcE,Dce		85 ("Rh+")	
		dce,dCe,dcE,dCE		15 ("Rh—")	

Minor Blood Groups
Lutheran (Lu^a, Lu^b), Kell (K^+, K^-), Duffy (Fy^a, Fy^b)
Kidd (JK^a, Jk^b)
P (P_1,P_2,p) Paroxysmal cold hemoglobinuria (Donath-Landsteiner antibody, "cold" IgG)

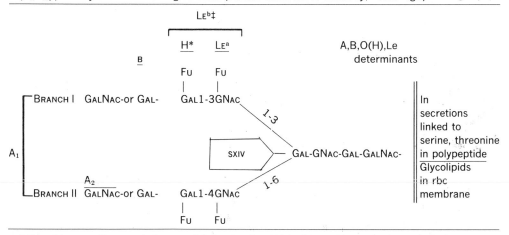

* Found in secretions and plasma of "secretors"; adsorbed to erythrocytes from plasma.
† Based on reactivity with 5 commonly available antisera: anti-D (anti-Rh 1), anti-C (anti-Rh 2), anti-E (anti-Rh 3), anti-c (anti-Rh 4), anti-e (anti-Rh 5)
‡ Se gene function required.

B specificity (see diagram in Table 5-18). Inheritance of glycosyl transferases provides the basis for phenotypic expression of blood-group antigens. In the absence of A or B genes, H remains an unaltered antigen. Persons having both A and A_1 antigens are assigned to blood group A; those with A antigen only, to group A_2; those with B antigen, to group B; those with A, A_1 and B, to group AB; those with A and B antigens but not A_1, to group A_2B; those without A, A_1, or B but with H antigen, to group O (i.e., cells are inagglutinable by anti-A or anti-B).

Rarely, persons originally found in Bombay, India, have none of the above antigens; they are assigned to the Bombay or Oh group. For preliminary and routine clinical purposes only the major groups of the ABO systems are determined, commonly by direct slide agglutination tests.

A or B antibodies (generally IgG) are continuously evoked by contact with specific A- or B-specific oligosaccharides from foods, and microorganisms and may be actively induced by transfusion with blood of the opposite group (A vs. B; B vs. A) or, in some cases, by pregnancy with a fetus of the opposite (incompatible) group.

Subdivisions (A_1, A_2, A_1B, A_2B and others) within each group account for unexpected occurrence of transfusion reactions. With specially prepared, adsorbed, monovalent sera containing *agglutinins* against Group A or against Group B erythrocytes, all 4 major groups may be identified.

In addition to A, B and H antigens there are a score or more of other blood-group antigenic systems, some common, some very rare, all genetically and independently determined: Duffy, Kell, P, Kidd, Lutheran MNSs. Though occasionally involved in transfusion reactions and certain other conditions, most are of more importance in resolving problems of paternity and in genetic studies. The Lewis (a and b) antigens, when present, are found in plasma and in the saliva of secretors (SeSe, Sese) and are adsorbed to erythrocytes without contributing to the structure of the cell membrane.

Antigens of the ABO(H) system occur in soluble form in sputum, colostrum, secretions of the gastrointestinal tract, semen, tears and sweat. They appear there in response to a secretor gene (Se) that is present in about 80 per cent of persons and that is required for expression of the Le^b gene.

Rh Antigens: Erythroblastosis Fetalis

In 1940 Landsteiner and Wiener found agglutinogens on *Rhesus*-monkey rbc that evoked agglutinins against rbc of about 87 per cent of Caucasians and about 95 per cent of Negroes, North American Indians and Chinese. The same antigen was found in many human rbc and is known as Rh agglutinogen. Persons with such rbc antigens are said to be Rh positive (Rh+); those lacking it, Rh negative (Rh−). Unlike the "natural," exogenously stimulated agglutinins of the ABO system, agglutinins against Rh antigen occur only if an Rh− person is actively sensitized by transfusion with Rh+ blood or by pregnancy with an Rh+ fetus.

Fetal erythrocytes from the placental circulation may gain access to the maternal blood during the late stages of pregnancy and parturition and in a first heterospecific pregnancy thus sensitize the mother. On subsequent pregnancies, the mother produces IgG antibody that crosses the placenta to react with the homologous antigen in fetal erythrocytes. Maternal Rh antibodies cause extensive agglutination and hemolysis in the fetus or neonate, resulting in death due to erythroblastosis fetalis or hemolytic disease of the newborn (HDM).

Of all pregnancies erythroblastosis fetalis occurs in an estimated 1 per cent. Of these about 66 per cent are said to be due to ABO incompatibilities and are usually mild. About 30 per cent, due to Rh incompatibility, are usually severe and are often fatal unless promptly treated by exchange transfusion. A small percentage is due to other incompatibilities. Rh erythroblastosis fetalis is entirely preventable by the administration of "rhogam," which is obtained from Rh− males immunized with Rh+ erythrocytes. The globulins are given to Rh− mothers *within 3 days* after the birth of an Rh+ infant or fetus. The antibodies combine with and eliminate Rh+ erythrocytes of fetal origin that have passed into the maternal circulation, thus preventing the primary maternal immune response (sensitization). This must be done after each subsequent Rh+ pregnancy in order to avoid risk of maternal sensitization.

Two systems of nomenclature, each based on a different genetic interpetation, are in use for the Rh antigens. One, the Wiener system, is based on the view that some ten or more genes or gene complexes (multiple allelic genes) occupy a single locus (Rh locus), coding for some 28 or more antigen mosaics or complexes on rbc. Another system (Fisher and Race) assumes the existence of three linked loci with two alleles each, coding for six antigens (C, D, E, c, d, e). Numerous variants and "compound" antigens, e.g., C^wE, C^wDE, ry^w, R^{zw}, also are found (Table 5-19). Rh_o and D are identical.

From a clinical standpoint the RH_o antigen and a variant of D, D^u ("weak D") are most important because, being both the most common and the most potent antigenically, they are most often involved in

TABLE 5-19. Relations of Wiener and Fisher Nomenclatures

Antigens		Genes	
Wiener Blood Factors	Fisher Agglutinogens	Wiener Genes	Fisher Gene Linkages
rh'	C	Rz	CDE ⎫
Rh₀	D	R¹	CDe ⎬ D present =
rh"	E	R²	cDE ⎬ RH +
hr'	c	R⁰	cDe ⎭
hr"	e	r^y	CdE ⎫
		r'	Cde ⎬ D absent =
		r	cde ⎬ Rh −
		r"	cdE ⎭

hemolytic disease of the newborn (HDN). Administration of D^u cells should be restricted to D+ (RH+) recipients because D^u cells can evoke anti-D (Rh₀) antibodies. Conversely, D^u persons should receive only D− (Rh−) cells.

Because the complex Rh antigenic pattern is genetically controlled its determination has great significance in resolving questions concerning parentage and other relationships. For example, two Rh+ persons, one or both heterozygous, may have an Rh− child but two Rh− persons (always homozygous) cannot have an Rh+ child. Transfusions of Rh− females should always be with Rh− blood.

The Direct Coombs Test

Immunoglobulin molecules evoked by rbc antigens are commonly IgG (relatively small, monomeric, bivalent); less commonly they are IgM (relatively large, pentameric, usually pentavalent). Both, especially IgM, can cause agglutination. However, the IgM molecules are often present in low concentration. They are found in the fetal circulation only in reponse to fetal infection, and they do not pass the placental barrier in either direction. The relative ineffectiveness of IgG molecules in hemagglutination is due, in great part, to their small size; they have difficulty in attaching simultaneously to two rbc that are (as is commonly the case) widely separated by negatively charged ions (zetal potential) when suspended in saline. Direct agglutination by IgG antibody can sometimes be made to occur if the effect of the zeta potential is reduced by mechanical force (centrifugation) or by suspending the cells in high concentrations of salt or protein. These measures often bring the rbc sufficiently close together to permit lattice formation by the IgG molecules.

When IgG antibodies attach to erythrocytes without causing lattice formation, they occupy cell receptors (antigens) and block the action of agglutinating IgM or IgG. The attached, nonagglutinating antibodies are called "blocking" antibodies, because they interfere

with agglutination and can be detected only with the Coombs test.

Immunoglobulins are antigenic in heterologous species, in which antibody to human immunoglobulin can be easily produced. Antiglobulin (Coombs serum, named for R. R. A. Coombs, who first described the principle) agglutinates erythrocytes coated with blocking antibody that does not by itself agglutinate the cells. This is the direct Coombs test used to detect sensitization of fetal (cord) erythrocytes by maternal antibody.

The Indirect Coombs Test

Antibody to Rh and other minor blood group antigens can be detected by the "indirect Coombs" test, in which the serum is mixed with erythrocytes of known antigenic specificity and then with antiglobulin. Agglutination indicates the presence, in the first serum, of antibody to the suspected blood group antigen. The test may be reversed by using "known" serum with "unknown" red blood cells.

It should be noted that in the foregoing discussion the term "sensitization" has been used in two distinct contexts. Erythrocytes to which antibodies are specifically adsorbed (e.g., Rh+ cells coated with anti-Rh) are said to be sensitized to the lytic action of complement, that is, immune cytolysis, the basis for HDN, or to agglutination by antiglobulin (Coombs serum). Sensitization is also used as the functional equivalent of the primary IR, as in a first untreated heterospecific pregnancy. In the latter instance, subsequent exposure of the maternal immune system to the same fetal (i.e., paternal) antigens evokes antibody in an anamnestic response, mostly IgG (type II hypersensitivity).

IMMUNOPROPHYLAXIS

The primary locus of infection (whether extracellular, or facultatively or obligately intracellular) has a profound effect on the character of the immune re-

TABLE 5-20. The Immune Response in Relation to Infection and Immunoprophylaxis

	Extracellular	Intracellular	Immune Response: Humoral	Cell-mediated
Parasites (active infection)	*Obligate*—acute Pyogens* Mycoplasma		Protective antibody, opsonins Type III HS	
	Faculative acute–chronic *Brucella Francisella Mycobacteria Listeria* Fungi		Agglutinins CF antibody, not (?) protective	Cellular immune mechanisms, T_c, NK, K (ADCC) Type IV HS
		Obligate acute–persistent *Chlamydia Rickettsia** Viruses**	Neutralizing and CF antibody Type III HS	
Nonreplicating antigens	*Toxins* (toxoids)* Tetanus Diphtheria Botulinum Enterotoxins Anthrax *Killed vaccines** Pertussis Influenza Rabies		Antitoxin Protective antibody	
Abnormal responses associated with infection	*Enzymes* Clostridial Streptococcal *Autoimmune–cross-reactive* (?) Mycoplasma pneumoniae SSPE, ?PRP Infectious mononucleosis Rheumatic fever Lues and other (e.g., i.m., malaria, SLE)		Anti-enzymes Cold agglutinins Antiviral Heterophilic antibody Wassermann, antibody, (BFP)	Cellular immune mechanisms

* See Table 5-21 for immunoprophylactic reagents.
 Abbreviations
 ADCC = antibody-dependent cellular cytotoxicity.
 BFP = biologic false positive.
 CF = complement-fixing.
 HS = hypersensitivity.
 IM = infectious mononucleosis.
 K = killer cells.
 NK = natural killer cells.
 PRP = progressive rubella panencephalitis.
 SSPE = subacute sclerosing panencephalitis.
 T_c = cytotoxic T lymphocytes.

TABLE 5-21. Immunoprophlaxis of Infectious Diseases

Disease	Vaccine	Indications & Age Group
Routine Universal Immunization		
Active	*DTP (APtoxoids, killed B. pertussis phase I)*	Normal infants & children:
Diphtheria, tetanus, pertussis	Trivalent oral (Sabin) live attenuated viruses	DTP, OPV at 2, 4, 6, 15 months
Poliomyelitis (paralytic)	(human diploid cell culture) (Oral polio vaccine, OPV)	4–6 years
German measles (rubella)	Live attenuated virus (RA 27/3, human diploid cell culture)	Over 1 year
Measles (rubeola)	Live attenuated virus (chicken embryo fibroblast culture)	Over 1 year
Mumps	Live attenuated virus (chicken embryo fibroblast culture)	Over 1 year
Restricted Immunization		
Active		
Pneumonia	Multivalent pneumococcal polysaccharide	Individually assessed risk, compromised patients
Meningitis	Meningococcal A,C polysaccharides	
Typhus	Killed *Rickettsia prowazeki*	Special circumstances
Influenza	Influenza virus (groups A,B) of current H–N formulation grown in chicken embryos and formalin-inactivated	Infants and 65 years and over; also compromised patients and special risk groups
Rabies	Rabies virus grown in human diploid cells, inactivated with tri-n-butyl phosphate, subunit	Individually assessed risk; combine with human hyperimmune globulin
Yellow fever	Attenuated 17D strain, grown in chicken embryos	Individually assessed risk of exposure
Smallpox (variola)	Live vaccinia virus (lyophilized)	Not required in United States. Individually assessed risk of exposure
Passive	*Preparation*	
Hepatitis A,B	Pooled normal human immunoglobulin	Individually assessed risk of exposure
Varicella-zoster pneumonia	Zoster immune globulin (ZIG)	Justified by severity of proven infection in high-risk patients
Rabies	Human rabies hyperimmune globulin (RIG)	In conjunction with vaccine

AP = alum precipitated

sponse(s) as well as on the approach to specific immunoprophylaxis. Some of these considerations are summarized in Table 5-20, which includes a list of abnormal antibodies that are elicited in certain infections and that may have antigenic specificities distinct from the microbial agents involved (e.g., Wasserman antibody).

A. Active immunization:
   (1) *Natural:* due to naturally acquired infection
   (2) *Artificial:* due to antigenic stimulation by vaccines made with
      (a) live or active attenuated microorganisms (e.g., oral poliovirus vaccine; vaccinia virus; BCG)
      (b) dead or inactivated microorganisms (e.g., *B. pertussis,* influenza vaccine, Salk-type polio vaccine)
      (c) toxoids (e.g., diphtheria and tetanus toxoids)

B. Passive immunization: due to antibodies passively received from an extraneous source
   (1) *Natural:* transplacental passage of maternal antibodies
   (2) *Artificial:* injection of antibodies preformed in animal sreum, e.g., diphtheria and tetanus antitoxins, gamma globulins of immune humans for prophylaxis of tetanus, epidemic hepatitis, rabies after severe bites, erythroblastosis fetalis (See Table 5-21.)

In producing active immunity against specific infectious diseases several sorts of antigen are used, the type depending on the disease against which immunity is desired. Antigens for this purpose may be classified as follows.

Bacterial vaccines are standardized saline suspensions of selected antigenic strains of bacteria killed by heat or chemicals (or both) such as phenol or formaldehyde. Typhoid and cholera bacterial vaccines are of limited value; pertussis vaccine is very effective. Bacterial polysaccharides (pneumococcal, meningococcal) are highly antigenic.

Toxoids are bacterial exotoxins (diphtheria or tetanus) that have been treated with formaldehyde. This eliminates toxicity without affecting immunogenicity.

Toxoids are produced by cultivating the desired organism in broth, filtering the broth culture to remove bacteria, adding formaldehyde, and holding some days at about 37 C. Such toxoid is referred to as *fluid toxoid.* It may be purified and concentrated by precipitating it from the filtered broth with alum (or $Al(OH)_3$). The sediment (called alum-precipitated toxoid or "toxoid, AP") is resuspended in buffered saline solution.

The advantage of toxoid (AP) lies in the fact that the alum precipitate remains in the tissues unabsorbed, releasing the attached toxoid slowly over a period of days, thus enhancing the antigenic stimulus. AP diphtheria and tetanus toxoids are mixed with killed *Bordetella pertussis* (DTP).

Primary dosage schedules for children 2 months to 6 years of age vary with manufacturers but are commonly three doses intramuscularly at 4- to 6-week intervals and a dose 1 year later. A booster dose is given on entering school. For persons over 6 years of age dosages are of adult-type (Td) toxoid at intervals of 6 weeks and 1 year. Booster doses for persons over 12 are one dose of Td intramuscularly at intervals of 10 years.

Td toxoid and long intervals between booster doses are used to avoid severe allergic reactions, especially with diphtherial toxoid. Td is less concentrated and is used only after preliminary skin tests for allergy. Passive immunization is used therapeutically in established cases of diphtheria. Because equine serum is generally used, all precautions must be taken in regard to (a) detecting sensitivity of the recipient to equine proteins and (b) inevitable primary sensitization (serum sickness) of the initially nonsensitive person.

In dealing with wounds likely to produce tetanus in persons previously immunized with tetanus toxoid, an immediate booster dose of toxoid is sufficient. Concomitant passive prophylaxis with hyperimmune human globulin may be necessary in the absence of known primary immunization with toxoid.

Human immune serum globulin (ISG), standard, concentrated, for prophylactic use, available commercially, contains antibody against measles, hepatitis virus(es), and poliovirus. It is free of infectious hepatitis viruses A and B.

Living or Active, Attenuated Agents

Bacteria. Excepting BCG, in the United States immunizing preparations of living, attenuated bacteria (e.g., *Brucella* vaccine) are used only in veterinary practice.

Viruses. Smallpox immunization (vaccination) is no longer required because of the global elimination of the disease.

Vaccines made from active, attenuated measles virus cultivated in chick tissue (Edmonston strain), are very effective and safe, though many children develop relatively mild febrile reactions.

Rubella can be prevented by use of rubella vaccine in all prepubertal children over 1 year of age. Older females may be immunized if serologically susceptible and if they agree to prevent pregnancy for 2 months after vaccination. Under no circumstances should a pregnant woman be vaccinated with *any* active-virus vaccine.

In the treatment of bites by animals suspected of being rabid, hyperimmune human antirabies serum is injected around the site of the bite and is also given intramuscularly. Rabies virus used in the vaccine is cultivated in human embryonic diploid lung cells and is inactivated with beta-propiolactone.

Other avianized living attenuated vaccines include those for yellow fever and mumps. Influenza viral vaccines are grown in the chorioallantoic membrane of chicken embryos and are inactivated (rendered noninfectious) by treatment with formalin. Persons with allergy to egg protein should not be given any egg-grown vaccine. Current recommendations for immunization are summarized in Table 5-21.

QUESTIONS IN MICROBIOLOGY AND IMMUNOLOGY

The following review questions are designed to correlate specific information with concepts that frequently cross disciplinary lines. In reviewing, the student should attempt to answer the questions as accurately and succinctly as possible. There follow four (4) sets (A to D) of objective (multiple choice) questions, each set in a different format. Instructions for answering the questions precede each section. Answers are given at the end of the chapter.

Define and explain the mechanism of: Koch's phenomenon, serum sickness, erythroblastosis fetalis, acquired or immunologic tolerance, phagocytosis, zone phenomena, complement fixation, immune-adherence phenomenon, anaphylaxis, Coombs test.

Define: cestode, L_f unit, immunity unit, toxoid AP, endotoxin, virus, bacterium, *Rickettsia, Chlamydia,* zoonosis, nematode, enzootic, sulfur granules, parrot fever, microaerophil, virion, procaryon.

What is a plasmid? What is the relation between antibiotic resistance and plasmids?

What is meant by lysogenic conversion, and how does it relate to virulence of certain bacteria?

List the principal anatomic features of bacteria.

How does muramic acid relate to bacteria, rickettsias, chlamydias, protozoa, Eumycetes?

Where is lipopolysaccharide commonly found in certain species of bacteria, and what is its relation to their pathogenicity?

Why are gram-positive bacteria commonly susceptible to penicillin and why are most gram-negative bacteria much less so?

Why are viruses insusceptible to commonly used antibiotics?

Why are protozoa insusceptible to penicillin in ordinary therapeutic doses?

Compare SST and FTA-ABS tests as to technique and significance in infections by *Treponema pallidum*.

Give the basic principle and the mode of application of BCG. What are the prinicipal indications and contraindications for its use in the United States?

What is the relation of homologous serum hepatitis (HB) to therapy with human serum or blood? to drug addiction?

Distinguish between the mechanisms of active and passive immunity. Give an example of each.

Mention four diseases in which serum therapy or prophylaxis is of proved value.

Discuss the function of a primary stimulus and of a secondary stimulus in the development and maintenance of immunity.

What is meant by booster doses? When are they used? What do they accomplish?

Describe methods for cultivating anaerobic bacteria.

List pathways involved in, and products of, glucose energy metabolism by strictly aerobic bacteria; facultative bacteria; strictly anaerobic bacteria. Compare with human muscle in these respects.

Describe the distinctive features and the mechanism of the electron microscope and the scanning electron microscope and compare with visible light microscopy.

Compare fluorescence microscopy and fluorescent antibody staining as to mechanisms and uses.

What are antibiotics? How are they prepared?

Give examples of broad-spectrum antibiotics. What are the tetracycline antibiotics?

What are semisynthetic penicillins? Why are some of them of special value in staphylococcal infections? What is ampicillin? cloxacillin? oxacillin?

Name 2 antibiotics that are: (a) mainly bactericidal in action; (b) mainly bacteriostatic in action.

Discuss the need for, and one method of, antibiotic sensitivity testing.

What is meant by antibiotic resistance, drug fastness, drug dependence? How may these properties originate in microorganisms?

Compare the mode of action of penicillin with that of chloramphenicol; of chlorine.

Give 3 examples of (a) arthropod-borne, (b) feces-borne, (c) saliva and mucus-borne diseases. Name vector and etiologic agent in each.

What is meant by immunologic unresponsiveness? induced immunologic tolerance?

What is the basis of heterograft reactions? What general types of measures are used to minimize them?

What is meant by isograft? allograft? autograft?

On what general types of media are viruses, rickettsias, heterotrophic bacteria, fungi and human tissue cells cultivated?

Mention 3 immunizing agents for human beings consisting of living microorganisms of attenuated virulence.

What are factors determining (a) whether or not an infection shall occur and (b) the virulence of infectious agents?

What is the role of histamine in allergic reactions? In which types of allergy are antihistaminics likely to be of value? Why?

Outline the development of prophage, lysogeny and phage lysis.

What are virus plaques? How are these used in virology?

What is plaque inhibition? hemagglutination inhibiton? Explain the mechanisms and uses.

Define and give specific uses of the CF and N tests in virology.

Explain fully the etymology of Picornavirus; Myxovirus; Arbovirus; ECHO virus; Papovavirus; Respiratory Syncytial virus; Rhinovirus; Reovirus. Rhabdovirus, Coronavirus, Arenavirus, Parvovirus. Give an example of each.

Name 4 species of pathogenic spore-forming bacteria.

Explain the relation of bacterial spores to operating-room procedure.

What is a bacterial capsule? What relation has it to virulence? immunologic specificity?

What is pathogenicity? virulence? On what does each depend?

Discuss the pathogenesis of gas gangrene. What is the value of bacteriologic diagnosis in gas gangrene? of immune serum therapy? hyperbaric oxygen?

Describe 3 pathogenic, strictly anaerobic, non-spore-forming bacteria, and tell how they produce disease and how these diseases may be prevented or treated.

If any saprophytic species of bacteria can cause disease, give examples and explain pathogenesis.

Give the technique of Gram's stain.

Name 10 gram-positive and 15 gram-negative pathogenic bacteria.

Describe the Kinyoun stain. Name 3 pathogenic acid-fast bacteria.

What is meant by the resolving power of an optical or ordinary microscope? On what does it depend?

Give the minimal time and temperature for sterilization by compressed steam; oven.

Explain the mechanisms of microbicidal or microbistatic action of cresols; $HgCl_2$; penicillin; sulfonamide drugs.

Why is bacteriostasis an inexact term?

Name 10 diseases due to viruses. What is a virion? How are viruses cultivated? What is an inclusion body? What is meant by CPE?

In virology, what is meant by syncytium formation?

Mention 5 viral diseases for which effective immunizing agents are available. How and when is each administered? How may immunity in each disease be determined?

What are interferons and what is their probable mode of action? Mention 2 general types of agents that induce production of interferon. Discuss specificity of interferons.

What vaccine against measles is available?

What are the hepatitis viruses? How is infection by each transmitted? prevented?

Is rubella vaccine contraindicated for males? Why?

Name and describe the organisms tha cause lymphogranuloma venereum; psittacosis. How is each transmitted? prevented? treated?

What is meant by TRIC agents?

What is the status of serum and/or serum derivative for the therapy and/or prophylaxis of serum hepatitis? epidemic hepatitis? influenza? syphilis? measles? rabies?

Of viruses, what is a capsomer, core, envelope? What is the origin of the envelope, and why may it vary in composition?

Name the etiologic agent, the vector, and mention a means of prevention of 4 diseases caused by different species of rickettsias.

Mention rickettsial diseases transmitted by lice; ticks; fleas; mites.

What immunizing agents are available for rickettsial diseases?

Name 5 distinct morphologic types of pathogenic bacteria. Give an example of each type and a disease caused by it.

Discuss the role of mutation of procaryons in epidemiology; in antibiotic therapy.

Describe 3 mechanisms whereby genetic information is transferred in bacteria.

What is the significance of coliform bacteria in drinking water? How is their presence proved? Name the important coliform bacteria.

Which pathogenic bacteria may be transmitted by milk? How does each gain entrance to the milk?

How may transmission of communicable disease by milk be prevented?

What bacteriologic tests are used commonly to measure the sanitary quality and the cleanliness of milk? How may mastitis in cattle be detected by examination of pasteurized milk?

How is a microorganism examined for motility?

In what stage of typhoid fever is *Salmonella typhi* recoverable from the bloodstream? the stools? Mention media used.

In the serologic diagnosis of a disease, is a high titer in a single examination of greater or lesser significance than an increase in titer at much lower levels on two successive examinations? Explain.

Differentiate typhoid fever from typhus fever as to etiologic agent, vector, laboratory diagnostic tests used.

How is bacillary dysentery differentiated from amebic dysentery by laboratory methods?

What is the most common cause of food *infection* in the United States?

How is food infection differentiated from bacterial food poisoning? Mention 3 bacterial causes of food poisoning.

What is the purpose of pasteurizing cream-filled baker's goods in relation to food *poisoning?* food *infection?*

What is streptodornase? fibrinolysin? streptokinase? hyaluronidase?

How is septic sore throat related to scarlet fever?

For what pathologic conditions are alpha-type hemolytic streptococci frequently responsible?

What is meant by Lancefield group B streptococci? group A?

How do pneumococci resemble and differ from beta-type hemolytic streptococci?

What is the significance of the staphylococcal coagulase reaction?

What is the role of *Escherichia coli* as pathogen?

What are 4 major groups of streptococci, and how are they differentiated?

What is the role of enzymes in microbial physiology? action of antibiotics or sulfonamides? microbial pathogenesis? Give examples of each.

What is a dimorphic (or diphasic) pathogenic fungus? Give 3 examples.

Mention 2 pathogenic protozoa (1 intestinal and 1 blood); fungi (dermal and systemic); helminths (1 intestinal and 1 blood); cestodes. For each give life history (brief outline), vector, pathogenesis, diagnostic methods, control methods and geographic distribution.

Describe the etiologic agents of filariasis. What is meant by nocturnal and diurnal periodicity? What is the pathologic basis of filarial elephantiasis?

What is toxoplasmosis? What is the best diagnostic test for toxoplasmosis?

For *toxoplasma gondii,* what are intermediate hosts? definitive hosts?

Describe the genus *Neisseria.*

What is the value of cultures in attempting a diagnosis of gonorrhea-like disease in adult women with no admitted history of or exposure to gonorrhea? in pre-adolescent girls? in cases of acute urethritis in adult males?

How are such cultures made and examined?

How is the gonococcus distinguished from the meningococcus? from *N. catarrhalis?* What is the pathologic action of each?

What are causes of and prophylactic measures against ophthalmia neonatorum?

What organisms may cause meningitis?

What spinal fluid findings confirm a diagnosis of epidemic meningitis? How are the necessary data obtained?

What is the value of cultural methods for establishing *therapy* in meningitis? gas gangrene? botulism? tetanus?

Discuss immunoprophylaxis of meningococcal meningitis.

Discuss the relation of undulant fever to Malta fever, relapsing fever, infectious abortion of cattle, brucellosis.

Discuss the pathogenicity of *Hemophilus influenzae.* In what respects do they resemble pneumococci? How do they differ from *Bordetella pertussis?*

What is viropexis? How is it achieved?

How may the type of pneumococci, hemophilus, meningococci, be determined?

Discuss the role of pertussis carriers in the spread of the disease.

How is active immunity to pertussis produced?

What is the use of DDT and/or dieldrin in the control of plague? pertussis? murine typhus? malaria? typhoid fever?

What is sylvatic plague? pneumonic plague? tularemia?

Describe the causative organism of soft chancre and the typical lesion.

How is chancroid distinguished from luetic chancre?

Describe a method of cultivating and identifying virulent diphtheria bacilla.

How does *Corynebacterium diphtheriae* affect the body?

How is diphtheria antitoxin produced and standardized?

Describe active, artificial immunization against diphtheria; against tetanus. How effective is each? How administered?

How is the tubercle bacillus identified in sputum? in urine?

When is the examination of gastric washings of particular value in the diagnosis of tuberculosis?

Which organisms may cause confusion in each of the above materials, and what are their origin and pathologic significance? How may they be differentiated from tubercle bacilli?

What are scotochromogens? atypical acid-fasts?

What are diagnostically distinctive differences in animal pathogenicity between bovine and human tubercle bacilli? Compare the methods of transmission and location of lesions in infection of man by each.

What is the significance of allergy in tuberculosis? How is it related to resistance? to the tuberculin test? to BCG? to leprosy?

Give the morphology, cultural characteristics and staining reactions of the tetanus bacillus.

What are the morphology, cultural characteristics and staining reactions of *C. botulinum?* How is it a source of disease, and why are its symptoms often unrecognized? Discuss prophylaxis and therapy.

Give the morphology, cultural characteristics and staining reactions of *C. perfringens.* What is its pathogenic action? How is its presence in wounds indicated, and what treatment is indicated?

Describe the anthrax bacillus. What is the basis of its pathogenicity? How is it transmitted to man? What are its typical lesions? How is anthrax prevented?

What is the significance of rubella in relation to congenital defects? How may such defects be prevented?

What is homologous serum hepatitis? How is it transmitted and prevented.

Mention 3 diseases due to spirochetes and name the cause of each.

Mention 2 diagnostic tests for syphilis depending on specific antibodies.

Describe the appearance of *Treponema pallidum* in the darkfield. How is the material for this examination obtained?

Compare bejel, syphilis and yaws as to the causative agent, mode of transmission and characteristic lesion.

What is leptospirosis? canicola fever? swineherd's fever? Weil's disease? How is each transmitted? how diagnosed in the laboratory?

What is the characteristic lesion in actinomycosis? Name and describe the organism.

What is coccidioidomycosis? histoplasmosis? Name and describe the causative agent of each disease and discuss the relation of each disease to the diagnosis of tuberculosis. How is each disease diagnosed? transmitted? What are histoplasmin and coccidioidin, and how are they used?

Describe the typical lesion of European blastomycosis. Describe the organism. How is the disease diagnosed?

How is *Entamoeba histolytica* identified in diarrheal stools? in formed stools? How are amebic and bacillary dysentery differentiated by laboratory methods?

Describe the life cycle of a tapeworm common in man. Why is it necessary to recover the head to ensure a cure?

Compare *Taenia saginata, Taenia solium, Echinococcus granulosus* and *Diphyllobothrium latum* morphologically. What is an intermediate and definitive host of each? Describe the dwarf tapeworm.

What laboratory procedures are used in the diagnosis of hydatid disease?

Give the life cycle of *Necator americanus* and its route from the site of infection to its final locus in the body. Give 2 laboratory procedures for its diagnosis.

What is ancylostomiasis, and how is it prevented?

What is the cause of trichinosis in man? How may it be diagnosed? prevented? Describe the encysted organism and give its usual infective location.

Describe briefly the life cycle of *Wuchereria bancrofti*.

How is filariasis diagnosed? Describe its pathogenesis. What is "Calabar swelling"? How is filariasis related to blindness? elephantiasis?

Outline the life history of the malaria parasite. Name the species of malaria parasites. Explain the difference in severity of infection by the different species. How is malaria transmitted? How is it prevented? What are the principal sources of infection? How may these be eliminated?

How is malaria diagnosed? What is the origin of the terms *tertian, quartan, estivoautumnal, vivax* and *falciparum*?

What is an RT (or RTF) plasmid of bacteria, and how is it related to chemotherapy?

What single organic compound is common to all bacteria, and how is it related to antibiotic therapy?

What structural components of bacterial cells are related to their immunologic specificity? their pathogenicity? genetic recombination? Explain.

What is the relationship between antibiotic therapy, L forms of bacteria and latent infection?

What is the presumed basis of immunologic tolerance in neonates? How may it be induced in adults? Explain its relationship to transplantation of tissues or organs.

Give 2 reasons, based on immunologic data, for delaying until the second to fourth month of age the artificial immunization of infants to diphtheria, tetanus, etc.

What is the role of immunoglobulins in infectious disease? How do they relate to erythroblastosis fetalis?

In the structure of antibodies, what is meant by heavy chain? light chain?

MULTIPLE CHOICE QUESTIONS

SECTION A

For each of the following (1 to 40), select the *single best answer* to the question or the *single item* which best *completes* the statement.

1. Cells specifically involved in cutaneous delayed hypersensitivity reactions
   (a) are B lymphocytes from germinal centers of the spleen white pulp.
   (b) probably recirculate from lymph nodes through the thoracic duct to the blood and back to the lymph nodes by the postcapillary venules.
   (c) migrate from germinal centers to the medullary cords of lymph nodes and red pulp cords of the spleen.
   (d) originate in the bone marrow and differentiate in the "bursa equivalent" microenvironment.
   (e) are derived from bone marrow precursors and reside in the germinal center caps.

2. Evidence for T-cell involvement in the induction of an antibody response stems from the requirement for the following mixture of cells to be injected into x-irradiated, syngeneic mice prior to antigen challenge:
   (a) Thymic cells and macrophages
   (b) Adherent and nonadherent cells
   (c) Thymic cells and bone marrow cells
   (d) Thymic cells and peripheral blood lymphocytes (PBL)
   (e) Lymph node cells and spleen cells

3. The *most reliable* surface determinant for detection and enumeration of human B lymphocytes is
   (a) Fc receptors detected by EA rosettes.
   (b) C3 receptors detected by EAC rosettes.
   (c) sheep erythrocyte receptors detected by plain E rosettes.
   (d) surface Ig detected by immunofluorescence.
   (e) "antigen shared with brain" detected by fluorescein-conjugated anti-Thy-1 antibody.

4. The cell-mediated immune response to a specific antigen may be best transferred from one individual to another by
   - (a) serum antibody and complement.
   - (b) T lymphocytes and transfer factor.
   - (c) macrophages with specific macrophage arming factor (SMAF).
   - (d) bone marrow cells and thymus cells.
   - (e) fetal liver cells.

5. Which of the following clinical entities is *most* likely to involve a haptenic reaction in its etiology?
   - (a) Systemic lupus erythematosus
   - (b) Rheumatoid arthritis
   - (c) Autoimmune hemolytic anemia after administration of cephalosporin
   - (d) Multiple myeloma
   - (e) Post-transplantation kidney rejection

6. The immunologic mediator of type I (atopic) hypersensitivity is
   - (a) cytotropic IgG (IgG2) fixed to mast cells by the Fc portion.
   - (b) cytotropic antibody of the autoimmune type (as in SLE) fixed to "self" antigens on leukocytes.
   - (c) IgE attached to mast cells and basophils, which fixes complement and triggers the complement cascade.
   - (d) IgE (reaginic) antibody fixed to tissue mast cells.

7. Type I (atopic) allergy to ragweed antigens is passively transferable from a sensitive to a non-sensitive subject
   - (a) by either serum heated to 56 C for 30 minutes in order to destroy complement or peripheral lymphocytes.
   - (b) by serum and peripheral lymphocytes combined, but by neither alone.
   - (c) by serum alone.
   - (d) by washed peripheral blood lymphocytes in the absence or serum.

8. In the pathogenesis of type III disease, the complexes that are most likely to be trapped in the renal glomerular basement membrane are
   - (a) those formed in moderate antigen excess.
   - (b) those formed in large antibody excess.
   - (c) complexes of antibody (particularly IgM) with complement and no antigen.
   - (d) those composed of antigen with IgE.

9. In attempting to "desensitize" a person suffering from hay fever due to ragweed, graded injections of antigen are given subcutaneously over a period of weeks during the time of year in which the air is free of pollen. The mechanism underlying the amelioration of symptoms during the subsequent ragweed season is thought to be
   - (a) elaboration of broadly specific IgE that "saturates" all potential binding sites, leaving none free to bind inhaled pollen.
   - (b) stimulation of IgG antibody of the same specificity.
   - (c) competitive suppression of the IgE locus of the Ir gene.
   - (d) stimulation of IgM (primary immunization) that would bind to mucosal cells and act as blocking antibody.

10. Mother is group O, Rh negative; father is group B, Rh positive and the infant is group B, Rh positive. In this situation, the ABO incompatibility between the parents
    - (a) enhances the chances of maternal elaboration of anti-D antibody.
    - (b) lessens the chances of maternal iso(allo) immunization with Rh antigen(s).
    - (c) increases the chances of isoimmunization with minor blood-group antigens (e.g., Kell, Duffy).
    - (d) increases the risk of hemolytic disease of the newborn, particularly because there is also maternal-fetal Rh incompatibility.

11. The "convertase" most closely resembling $\overline{C3bBb}$ of the alternate pathway is
    - (a) $\overline{C1}$.
    - (b) $\overline{C42}$.
    - (c) $\overline{C567}$.
    - (d) $\overline{C89}$.
    - (e) $\overline{C56789}$.

12. Enhanced intracellular levels of cAMP, induced by agents such as prostaglandins, will
    - (a) have no effect on phagocytic processes.
    - (b) retard phagocytosis.
    - (c) enhance phagocytosis.

13. The antigenic determinants that define antibody class (isotype) would be best described as occurring
    - (a) in constant regions.
    - (b) in the variable region.
    - (c) in the hinge region.
    - (d) in Fab.
    - (e) in the carbohydrate moiety.

14. Histamine, which is a vasoactive amine initially involved in immune complex disease tissue destruction, is released from
    - (a) polymorphonuclear neutrophils.
    - (b) RBCs.
    - (c) platelets.
    - (d) lymphocytes.
    - (e) macrophages.

15. The presence of cryoglobulins in a patient's serum may indicate that the patient has
    (a) anemia.
    (b) circulating immune complexes.
    (c) Hashimoto's thyroiditis.
    (d) pernicious anemia.

16. A Coombs test is the most important laboratory aid for the diagnosis of
    (a) myasthenia gravis.
    (b) autoimmune hemolytic anemias.
    (c) Waldenström's macroglobulinemia.
    (d) rheumatoid arthritis.
    (e) systemic lupus erythematosus.

17. The most important antibody playing a role in the pathogenesis of systemic lupus erythematosus is
    (a) antibody to thyroglobulin.
    (b) antibody to DNA.
    (c) antibody to mitochrondria.
    (d) rheumatoid factor.
    (e) antibody to smooth muscle.

18. The currently available vaccine against pneumococcal infection contains
    (a) heat-killed pneumococci of the 14 serotypes most frequently encountered.
    (b) cell wall antigen(s), chiefly C substance.
    (c) type-specific polysaccharide of 14 serotypes.
    (d) attenuated pneumococci of the 14 serotypes most frequently encountered.

19. In the syndrome of poststreptococcal glomerulonephritis
    (a) streptococcal nucleases and streptolysin accumulate in the glomerular basement membrane.
    (b) streptococcal capsular antigen (hyaluronic acid) and glucuronic acid subunits precipitate with antibody and are deposited in the glomeruli in "lumpy" patterns.
    (c) immunoglobulin and complement localize in the glomerular basement membrane.
    (d) hematuria is due to the action of streptolysin O.

20. In group A beta hemolytic streptococci, types are determined by the antigenic specificity of
    (a) the capsule.
    (b) the mucopeptide layer.
    (c) the M and/or T proteins.
    (d) the extracellular products, such as streptolysin O, which is produced only by group A streptococci.

21. Prompt and adequate treatment of acute streptococcal pharyngitis constitutes prophylaxis of acute rheumatic fever because
    (a) the immune response is enhanced.
    (b) the immune response to streptococcal antigens is aborted.
    (c) viable streptococci do not persist in the early rheumatic lesions.
    (d) there is an antibody response to streptolysin and other streptococcal exoenzymes.

22. In the test for C reactive protein (CRP) in patients' sera, the reagent used to precipitate the protein is
    (a) group specific cell wall antigen in *Streptococcus pneumoniae*.
    (b) group specific C antigen of beta hemolytic streptococcus.
    (c) factor C3 in the alternate complement pathway.
    (d) rabbit antiserum.

23. Recurrent staphylococcal infection in children with "chronic granulomatous disease" occurs because
    (a) the responsible organism almost always is found to produce penicillinase.
    (b) no antibodies to staphylococcal teichoic acids are formed.
    (c) there is a heritable defect in intraleukocytic killing of bacteria.
    (d) these patients are prone to diabetes mellitus, which predisposes to bacterial infection.

24. The triple vaccine (DTP) routinely used in childhood immunization contains
    (a) killed *Corynebacterium diphtheriae*, *Bordetella pertussis* "toxoid," tetanus toxoid.
    (b) diphtherial toxin exactly neutralized with antitoxin, *Bordetella pertussis*, tetanus toxoid.
    (c) diphtherial toxoid, killed phase 1 *Bordetella pertussis*, tetanus toxoid.
    (d) diphtherial toxoid, avirulent *Bordetella pertussis*, tetanus toxoid.

25. Congenital rubella can be diagnosed in a week-old infant by
    (a) demonstration of maternal IgM antibodies to rubella virus.
    (b) testing for HI antibodies specific for the virus in the infant's serum.
    (c) demonstration in the infant of circulating IgG antibodies to rubella virus.
    (d) demonstration of rubella IgM antibodies in the infant.
    (e) the presence of infant IgA antibodies to rubella virus.

26. Caesarian section has been found to eliminate neonatal complications due to which of the following viruses?
    (a) Varicella-zoster

(b) Cytomegalovirus
(c) Poliovirus
(d) Echovirus
(e) Herpes simplex virus

27. The pasteurization process could be expected to kill all of the following *EXCEPT*
(a) *Brucella abortus.*
(b) *Mycobacterium tuberculosis.*
(c) group B streptococci.
(d) *Bacillus anthracis.*
(e) *Leptospira icterohaemorrhagiae.*

28. To prevent hemolytic disease in a newborn with an A-positive mother and an O-negative father, one would
(a) administer Rhogam to the mother after the birth of her first child.
(b) administer Rhogam to each of her subsequent children.
(c) administer Rhogam to the mother after her first A-positive daughter.
(d) administer Rhogam to her first O-negative child.
(e) do nothing—there is no danger to any of her children.

29. Dermatophytes that infect special keratinized areas of the body, skin and nails only, are likely to belong to which genus?
(a) *Epidermophyton*
(b) *Trichophyton*
(c) *Microsporum*
(d) *Trichosporum*
(e) *Pitysporum*

30. In the currently accepted immunization schedule for children over the age of 6 years, one is advised to give "adult strength toxoid" instead of DTP. This is done
(a) to prevent severe reactions to tetanus and/ or pertussis antigens, to which children of that age already have developed antibody.
(b) only as a booster in children who have already had primary immunization with DTP at an earlier age.
(c) to avoid hypersensitivity reactions to corynebacterial protein(s).
(d) because susceptibility to diphtheria increases with age.

31. The most significant difference between viruses and all other microbiologic agents is
(a) reproduction by multiplication of subunits rather than by binary fission.
(b) obligate intracellular parasitism.
(c) the involvement of the cellular immune response in recovery.

(d) the inability to produce ATP.
(e) the absence of any enzymes in virions.

32. In 1977, a U.S. Navy ship experienced a sudden outbreak of acute respiratory disease three days out of Manila, with 67 per cent of the crew and 100 per cent of those age 18 to 25, showing signs of respiratory disease in a 24-hour period. Armed forces epidemiologists flown to the scene isolated virus from transtracheal aspirates but not from the feces of those severely ill. The most likely agent of this outbreak was
(a) adenovirus, type 7.
(b) measles virus.
(c) respiratory syncytial virus.
(d) influenza of group A.
(e) influenza of group C.

33. The central nervous system is an area of predilection for one of the following organisms that also infects the lower respiratory tract:
(a) *Actinomyces israelii*
(b) *Histoplasma capsulatum*
(c) *Candida albicans*
(d) *Nocardia asteroides*
(e) *Mycobacterium kansasii*

34. Most respiratory and intestinal infections by picornaviruses result in
(a) localized acute disease.
(b) latent infections.
(c) inapparent infections.
(d) recurrent infections.
(e) disseminated disease.

35. Which one of the following is a binding site for amphotericin B?
(a) Cell wall mucopeptide
(b) 50s ribosomal subunit
(c) 30s ribosomal subunit
(d) sterol-containing site in the membrane
(e) DNA

36. Sera may be titrated for neutralizing antibody to virus by
(a) the radial immunodiffusion technique.
(b) determining the equivalence point in the precipitin curve.
(c) determining the highest dilution that specifically inhibits infectivity of the virus.
(d) determining the highest dilution of antibody that will specifically enhance the neuraminidase activity of the virus.
(e) determining the highest dilution of antibody that results in complete hemagglutination.

37. Rickettsia differ from free-living bacteria in that the former
(a) contain DNA but no RNA.
(b) contain RNA but no DNA.

(c) are too small to be seen with the light microscope.

(d) customarily have arthropod vectors.

(e) cannot generate their metabolic energy requirements.

38. Togaviruses
   (a) are DNA viruses.
   (b) cause diseases marked by a viremia during the early stages of infection.
   (c) are spread directly from horses to man.
   (d) are spread by person-to-person contact.
   (e) are carried usually by tick vectors.

39. The lipid envelope characteristic of some animal viruses
   (a) contains proteins specified by the host-cell genome.
   (b) contains lipids specified by the viral genome.
   (c) is resistant to extractions by ether or detergents.
   (d) contains lipids and carbohydrates determined by the host cell.

40. *Only* virulent strains of *Neisseria gonorrhoeae* produce
   (a) endotoxin.
   (b) oxidase.
   (c) capsular carbohydrates.
   (d) pili.
   (e) IgA proteases.

SECTION B

In each of the following test items (1–13) there are multiple choices of which only one is *not* correct. Choose this *EXCEPTION*.

1. All of the following modes of therapy have been shown to be effective in the management of rheumatoid arthritis *EXCEPT*
   (a) vaccination.
   (b) thoracic duct drainage.
   (c) immunostimulation.
   (d) plasmaphoresis.
   (e) lymphophoresis.

2. Evidence is fairly good that a tumor may escape the host defense by all of the following mechanisms *EXCEPT*
   (a) by lacking any immunorecognizable tumor-associated antigens on the tumor cell surfaces.
   (b) by growing at a more rapid rate than the host immune response is capable of handling.
   (c) by immunologic blockade or "enhancement" of the tumor with antibody or antigen–antibody complexes.

(d) by inhibition of a good host immune response with T suppressor cells.

(e) by protection of the tumor due to tumor architecture or secretions that prevent the immune response.

3. *In vitro* assays for delayed hypersensitivity or a cell-mediated immune response may involve all of the following factors *EXCEPT*
   (a) release of migration inhibition factor from sensitized T lymphocytes.
   (b) blastogenesis of peripheral lymphocytes measured by uptake of ^{3}H-thymidine.
   (c) release of histamine from peripheral blood basophilic polymorphonuclear leukocytes.
   (d) release of chemotactic factor from sensitized T lymphocytes.
   (e) cytotoxicity of target cells bearing specific antigen on the surface by direct contact with cytotoxic T lymphocytes.

4. Contact dermatitis may be described by all of the following characteristics *EXCEPT*
   (a) it is a cell-mediated immune response.
   (b) it involves binding of low-molecular-weight "haptens" to host proteins to form an immunogenic complex.
   (c) it involves skin-fixing antibody (IgE) that causes allergic reactions.
   (d) materials such as lead, nickle and phenolic compounds may be involved.
   (e) a "patch test" on the skin may be used to detect hypersensitivity to the suspect compound.

5. Certain HLA alloantigens are strongly linked to diseases such as ankylosing spondylitis. This linkage has all of the following characteristics *EXCEPT* that it
   (a) is primarily related to D and B loci.
   (b) may be the result of closely linked immune response genes.
   (c) is primarily related to A and C loci.
   (d) may be the result of cross-reactivity between the alloantigen and the antigen of an infectious agent.
   (e) indicates an increased risk for a specific disease for those individuals with the linked alloantigen.

6. All of the following are characteristic of the major blood group substances (ABO) *EXCEPT*
   (a) that they are defined by reagent antibody.
   (b) genes for either A or B and H code for a protein molecule.
   (c) secretions of either A or B and H substance are coded for by Le gene.
   (d) absence of an H gene does not necessarily indicate the absence of an A or B gene.

(e) determinants that react with reagent antibody are carbohydrate moieties.

7. Pneumococcal vaccine (Pneumovax) is of clinical usefulness in connection with all of the following conditions *EXCEPT*
(a) sickle cell disease.
(b) following splenectomy.
(c) Chédiak-Higashi anomaly.

8. A young 35-year-old black man has end-stage renal disease (serum creatinine >10 mg.%, creatinine clearance <5 cc./min.) and is being evaluated as to his suitability for a renal transplant. All of the following statements are true *EXCEPT*
(a) if sibling donors are available, you would like him to have a living related transplant since this is better than the cadaver graft.
(b) you would like him to receive a transplant *even* if he is known to be diabetic but is otherwise suitable.
(c) you would not like him to receive a transplant now since he has active pulmonary tuberculosis.
(d) you would not like him to receive a transplant since the quality of life is better on hemodialysis compared to that following a successful transplant.

9. All of the following factors are characteristic of chronic granulomatous disease *EXCEPT*
(a) recurrent infection.
(b) it is caused by organisms of high virulence.
(c) infected eczematoid dermatitis.
(d) chronic lymphadenitis.
(e) death in early infancy.

10. All of the following characteristics of rheumatoid factor are correct *EXCEPT*
(a) an IgM antibody directed to IgG.
(b) an IgG antibody directed to thyroglobulin.
(c) an IgG antibody directed to IgG.
(d) it is occasionally found in normal individuals recovering from influenza.

11. All of the following are true of protein A of *Staphylococcus aureus EXCEPT*
(a) it binds to the Fc portion of immunoglobulins.
(b) it depletes complement in the presence of serum.
(c) it inhibits opsonization.
(d) it interferes with the attachment of staphylococcal bacteriophage.

12. The group-specific antigens of *Streptococcus pneumoniae* include all of the following *EXCEPT*
(a) Forssman antigen.
(b) C polysaccharide.
(c) capsular polysaccharide.
(d) neuraminidase.

13. All of the following are aminoglycoside antibiotics *EXCEPT*
(a) neomycin.
(b) streptomycin.
(c) kanamycin.
(d) amikacin.
(e) erythromycin.

SECTION C

Using the key shown below, answer questions 1 to 29 by selecting the best choice in each case according to the number letters.

(a) a, b, and c are correct.
(b) a and c are correct.
(c) b and d are correct.
(d) d only is correct.
(e) all are correct.

1. Virulence is attributable to the antiphagocytic properties of the capsules of
(a) *Neisseria meningitidis,* groups A and C.
(b) *Yersinia pestis* with V/W and Fl antigens.
(c) *Haemophilus influenzae,* type b.
(d) *Neisseria gonorrhoeae,* Arg⁻.

2. Which of the following is/are true regarding the mode of action of diphtheria toxin?
(a) the combined fragments of the toxin molecule act as an enzyme and bind to translocation factor EF-2.
(b) NAD is required to split the toxin molecule into two fragments.
(c) Fragment A attaches to receptors on the cell membrane.
(d) Antibodies to fragment B block the action of the toxin.

3. Which of the following are characteristic(s) of *Nocardia asteroides?*
(a) The organism is normally found among the oral flora of man.
(b) Benign pulmonary lesions often precede the development of metastatic brain abscess.
(c) Nocardiosis often manifests as a necrotizing infection of the extremities.
(d) Nocardiosis responds best to treatment with sulfadiazine or sulfamerazine.

4. Characteristics of actinomycosis include which of the following?
(a) Infection may follow a tooth extraction.
(b) Abdominal infection may simulate appendicitis.
(c) Sulfur granules with peripheral clubbing may be present in exudates.
(d) Penicillin is the drug of choice.

5. The following are characteristics of the genus *Clostridium:*
   (a) Ability to grow in the presence of oxygen ranges from aerotolerant to obligate anaerobes.
   (b) Ability to utilize a wide variety of carbohydrates for energy
   (c) Production of large amounts of carbon dioxide (CO_2) by most species
   (d) Production of some species of exotoxins that aid in the spread of organisms in tissue

6. Optimal recovery of anaerobic bacteria from clinical specimens may be promoted by
   (a) addition of reducing agents and growth factors to media.
   (b) addition of aminoglycosides to the media.
   (c) prompt transport of specimens to the laboratory.
   (d) use of candle jar to increase the level of CO_2 required for growth of obligate anaerobes.

7. Anaerobic bacteria would *not* be expected to play a major role in which of the following?
   (a) Nongonococcal pelvic infections
   (b) Septic arthritis and osteomyelitis
   (c) Lung abscess and empyema
   (d) Urinary tract infections

8. Anaerobic bacteria should be considered in which of the following conditions?
   (a) Myonecrosis
   (b) Septic thrombophlebitis
   (c) "Sterile pus" (no growth on blood agar in a candle jar)
   (d) Debrided decubitus ulcer

9. Specimens that would be acceptable for culture of anaerobic organisms from infection of the female genital area are
   (a) vaginal.
   (b) cervical.
   (c) urethral.
   (d) culdocentesis aspirate.

10. Which of the following apply to *Staphylococcus aureus?*
    (a) Normal flora of nasal passages of most humans
    (b) A frequent cause of nosocomial infections
    (c) Usually susceptible to specific phage
    (d) 20% or less of strains seen in family practice and outpatient populations are sensitive to penicillin G.

11. Cytomegaloviruses are
    (a) usually acquired before age 15.
    (b) usually acquired as an inapparent infection.
    (c) capable of causing fatal generalized infections in neonates.
    (d) oncogenic in several animal hosts.

12. "Nonspecific" effector mechanisms against infections (in contrast to the specific immune response) include
    (a) interferon.
    (b) lymphokines.
    (c) lysozyme of tears and saliva.
    (d) alternate complement pathway.

13. Which of the following are associated with the immune response to a primary infection by *Mycobacterium tuberculosis?*
    (a) Forty-eight to 72 hours after an intradermal injection of purified tuberculoproteins, an induration of 5 mm or more will appear at the inoculation site.
    (b) a tubercle or granuloma will eventually form at the sites of bacillary proliferation.
    (c) Tubercle bacilli survive and multiply within host macrophages.
    (d) The host develops a relatively high antibody titer to tuberculoproteins.

14. The etiologic agents of brucellosis, bubonic plague and tularemia have which of the following characteristics in common?
    (a) Produce a pneumonia form of the disease that is highly lethal
    (b) Produce a bacteremia during the acute stage of the disease.
    (c) All transmitted by arthropod vectors
    (d) Produce infections in animals that are subsequently transmitted to humans

15. The mode of action of diphtherial toxin on mammalian cells is analogous to the action of fusidic acid on bacterial cells at which of the following stages of macromolecular synthesis?
    (a) Reversible inhibition of DNA synthesis
    (b) Binding to the ribosome resulting in inhibition of mRNA synthesis
    (c) Inhibition of membrane integrity
    (d) Inhibition of mRNA translation mediated by inactivation of an elongation factor

16. A patient is diagnosed by the physician as having a deep abdominal abscess. The laboratory report identifies the causative agent as *Bacteroides fragilis.* Which of the following antibiotics could be used for therapy?
    (a) Chloramphenicol
    (b) Penicillin G
    (c) Clindamycin
    (d) Erythromycin

17. Chemotherapeutic agent(s) that is(are) safe and effective for systemic treatment of herpetic meningoencephalitis is(are)
    (a) adenine arabinoside.
    (b) iododeoxyuridine.

(c) acyclovir.

(d) isatin-β-thiosemicarbazone.

18. Cell-mediated immunity is most important in recovery from primary infections with
    (a) *Herpes simplex virus.*
    (b) *Streptococcus pyogenes.*
    (c) *Mycobacterium tuberculosis.*
    (d) *Corynebacterium diphtheriae.*

19. Which of the following organisms exhibit a yeast-like form in infected tissues and in culture at 35 C. and a mycelial form in the environment and in culture at 22 C?
    (a) *Blastomyces dermatitidis*
    (b) *Coccidioides immitis*
    (c) *Sporothrix schenckii*
    (d) *Cryptococcus neoformans*

20. Chronic infections may be the result of defects in
    (a) B lymphocytes.
    (b) phagocytosis.
    (c) T lymphocytes.
    (d) intracellular killing mechanisms in phagocytes.

21. The source of virus that leads to an eruption of herpes zoster in an elderly person may be
    (a) vesicular fluid from an adult with herpes zoster.
    (b) reactivation of virus in respiratory secretions of another person.
    (c) respiratory secretions from a child with chicken pox.
    (d) reactivation of virus from the patient's own spinal ganglia.

22. The source of infection leading to a case of chicken pox may be
    (a) vesicular fluid from another child with chicken pox.
    (b) respiratory secretions from another child with chicken pox.
    (c) vesicular fluid from a elderly patient with herpes zoster.
    (d) respiratory secretions from an elderly patient with herpes zoster.

23. Outbreaks of the common cold due to a rhinovirus are
    (a) frequently followed by lower respiratory disease.
    (b) most frequent in September and May.
    (c) caused mostly by a few epidemic serotypes.
    (d) caused more or less equally by a large number of serotypes.

24. The disease diphtheria
    (a) may present as a cutaneous, ulcerative lesion.
    (b) is caused primarily by the action of an exotoxin.

(c) may be prevented in the human population by immunization of children with DTP and boosters.

(d) may be treated effectively in the early stages of the disease with penicillin.

25. *Bordetella pertussis*
    (a) is a small, gram-negative, cocco-bacillus and is usually isolated on special agar medium (Bordet-Gengou agar).
    (b) is invasive, resulting in a high recovery rate from the blood after the second week of the disease.
    (c) probably does not induce the carrier state.
    (d) virulence is associated with a potent exotoxin and effective therapy must include treatment with specific antitoxin.

26. Which of the following are characteristic of *Neisseria gonorrhoeae?*
    (a) Some strains isolated in the United States are known to have a reduced sensitivity to penicillin.
    (b) Infection stimulates local immune response with production of IgG and IgA.
    (c) Currently about 1% of cases in the United States are caused by beta-lactamase-producing strains.
    (d) Infection in the female tends to involve the anal region as well as the endocervical area.

27. *Mycoplasma* organisms and L forms differ in that L forms
    (a) have a cell membrane that is chemically and structurally the same as that of the bacterial cell.
    (b) have not been incriminated as virulent forms, though they may be the tissue-persisting forms of pathogenic bacteria.
    (c) may retain some cell wall material other than mucopeptide.
    (d) may revert to bacteria with cell walls.

28. Regarding hemolytic disease of the newborn:
    (a) It is a cytotoxic type II allergic reaction.
    (b) The mother forms Ab against fetal erythrocyte antigens which she lacks.
    (c) Anti-Rh globulin can suppress sensitization of Rh mothers soon after Rh-positive cell introduction into the mother.
    (d) The fetus forms Ab against maternal erythrocytes and destroys its own red blood cells.

29. The period during which infectious mononucleosis may be contagious can be as long as
    (a) 6 hours, only during initial respiratory stage.
    (b) 6 days, during the salivary gland stage.
    (c) 6 weeks, until the patient begins to recover.
    (d) 6 months, since virus is excreted long after recovery.

(e) 6 years, since virus is persistently released indefinitely.

SECTION D

Select one (1) of the lettered items that best relates to each of the subsequent words or statements (1–73).

(a) Mycoplasma
(b) L forms
(c) Spheroplast
(d) Protoplast
(e) All of the above

1. Can be described as insensitive to antibiotics affecting cell wall synthesis
2. Can be produced from gram-positive or gram-negative bacteria by β-lactam antibiotics
3. Cannot revert to a bacterium with a cell wall

(a) *Klebsiella pneumoniae*
(b) *Proteus mirabilis*
(c) *Escherichia coli*
(d) *Pseudomonas aeruginosa*
(e) None of the above

4. The leading cause of urinary tract infections among hospitalized patients
5. Kidney stones possibly induced by alkaline pH of urine associated with urinary tract infections
6. Associated with conjunctivitis acquired by use of contaminated make-up
7. Responsible for respiratory infections in cystic fibrosis patients

(a) *Shigella dysenteriae*
(b) Enterotoxigenic *E. coli*
(c) *Salmonella typhi*
(d) *Salmonella enteritidis*
(e) *Vibrio cholerae*

8. Produces enterotoxin and neurotoxin
9. Pneumonia is a complication of the infection
10. Infectious dose may be less than 500 bacteria
11. Often produces (ST) heat stable type of enterotoxin
12. Variations in O antigen produced by lysogenic conversion

(a) Temperate phage
(b) Virulent phage
(c) Neither
(d) Both

13. Produces enzymes mediating phage DNA insertion into the bacterial chromosome
14. Useful in phage typing of *Salmonella typhi* Vi antigen
15. Employable for gene isolation techniques

(a) Mumps virus
(b) Rabies virus
(c) Measles virus
(d) Rubella virus
(e) Hepatitis B virus

16. Australia antigen
17. Koplik spots
18. Orchitis
19. Congenital cardiopathies

(a) Inhibition of viral DNA synthesis
(b) Inhibition of viral attachment
(c) Inhibition of viral RNA and/or protein synthesis
(d) None of the above

20. Iododeoxyuridine
21. Interferon
22. Acyclovir

(a) *Neisseria meningitidis*
(b) *Neisseria gonorrhoeae*
(c) Both
(d) Neither

23. Associated with pelvic inflammatory disease (PID)
24. Produce(s) IgA₁ protease
25. Receives and maintains R factors
26. Transmitted to susceptible host by asymptomatic human carriers.
27. Children under 5 years of age and young men 15 to 25 years old are especially susceptible to infection
28. Fulminating septicemia with high fever and rash, proceeding to disseminated intravascular coagulation and circulatory collapse

(a) Brucella
(b) Francisella
(c) Yersinia
(d) All of the above
(e) None of the above

29. Cause disease in animals, humans secondarily involved
30. Associated with "rabbit fever"
31. Causes "undulant fever"
32. Acute and convalescent serum antibody titers are useful in diagnosis of disease
33. Etiologic agent of plague
34. Control associated with vaccination of female calves
35. Pathogenicity depends upon ability to survive phagocytosis and multiply intracellularly

(a) *Bacteroides fragilis*
(b) *Clostridium perfringens*
(c) *Bacteroides melaninogenicus*

(d) *Actinomyces israelii*

(e) *Fusobacterium nucleatum*

36. Infection characterized by multiple draining lesions

37. Produces black discoloration of blood-containing exudates, pus may fluoresce red under UV light

38. Most strains produce β-lactamase

39. Primary etiologic agent of myonecrosis

40. Toothpick-shaped, gram-negative rod associated with upper respiratory infections

(a) *Listeria monocytogenes*

(b) *Nocardia brasiliensis*

(c) *Actinomyces israelii*

(d) *Bacillus anthracis*

(e) *Nocardia asteroides*

41. Etiologic agent of neonatal meningitis

42. Etiologic agent of mycetoma

43. Infections may simulate tuberculosis

44. Organism is indigenous to man

45. Industrial infection is a necrotizing pneumonia

(a) Penicillin V

(b) Cephalothin

(c) Oxacillin

(d) Carbenicillin

(e) Any of the above

46. Allergic reactions occur in less than 10% of individuals who are allergic to ampicillin

47. Drug most likely to cure the "scalded-skin syndrome"

48. Drug most likely to cure conjunctivitis involving *Pseudomonas* or *Enterobacter*

(a) Cefoxitin

(b) Bacitracin

(c) Vancomycin

(d) All of the above

(e) None of the above

49. Nonprescription drug limited to topical application

50. Binds cross-linking enzyme

51. Bacteriostatic, not bactericidal, action

(a) Spectinomycin

(b) Gentamicin

(c) Tetracycline

(d) All of the above

52. Binds to the 30S portion of the ribosome inhibiting the binding of tRNA to the ribosome–mRNA complex

53. Effect is more bacteriostatic than bactericidal

54. Employed for control of penicillinase-producing strains of *N. gonorrhoeae*

55. Capable of inducing an allergic state

(a) Sulfone

(b) Amphotericin

(c) Rifampicin

(d) Polymyxin

(e) Lincomycin

56. Drug that has a detergent-like action on bacterial membrane

57. Drug that has a detergent-like action on fungal membrane

58. Drug used for *M. leprae*

59. Drug that is used for treatment of *M. tuberculosis*

60. Inhibitor of protein synthesis used for gram-positive infections

(a) Penicillin V

(b) Ampicillin

(c) Carbenicillin

(d) Oxacillin

(e) Cephalosporin

61. Designed for use against penicillinase-producing staphylococci

62. Designed for use against gram-negative bacteria but sensitive to many β-lactamases

63. Designed for use against gram-negative bacteria that produce β-lactamase, e.g., pseudomonas

64. Individuals allergic to penicillin G are not necessarily allergic to this drug

(a) *Chlamydia trachomatis*

(b) *Rickettsia rickettsii*

(c) *Coxiella burneti*

(d) *Chlamydia psittaci*

(e) None of the above

65. Associated with eye infections

66. Associated with urethritis, thin discharge and genital elephantiasis

67. Can cause high fever and rash with 90% mortality rate in untreated cases

68. Etiologic agent of ornithosis

(a) Reagin of syphilis

(b) Anti-*Treponema pallidum* antibodies

(c) Both

(d) Neither

69. Are present in the serum of patients with secondary syphilitic lesions

70. Decline in titer as the patient responds to treatment

71. Are identified in sera of patients with biologic false-positive reactions in screening tests for syphilis

72. Are measured by the VDRL and RPR screening tests

73. Are measured by the FTA-ABS test

ANSWERS TO MULTIPLE CHOICE QUESTIONS

Section A

1. (b)	11. (b)	21. (b)	31. (a)
2. (c)	12. (b)	22. (d)	32. (d)
3. (d)	13. (a)	23. (c)	33. (d)
4. (b)	14. (c)	24. (c)	34. (c)
5. (c)	15. (b)	25. (d)	35. (d)
6. (d)	16. (b)	26. (e)	36. (c)
7. (c)	17. (b)	27. (d)	37. (d)
8. (a)	18. (c)	28. (e)	38. (b)
9. (b)	19. (c)	29. (a)	39. (d)
10. (b)	20. (c)	30. (c)	40. (d)

Section B

1. (a)	5. (c)	8. (d)	11. (d)
2. (a)	6. (c)	9. (b)	12. (c)
3. (c)	7. (c)	10. (b)	13. (e)
4. (c)			

Section C

1. (a)	9. (c)	16. (b)	23. (c)
2. (d)	10. (e)	17. (b)	24. (a)
3. (c)	11. (a)	18. (b)	25. (b)
4. (e)	12. (e)	19. (b)	26. (e)
5. (e)	13. (e)	20. (e)	27. (e)
6. (b)	14. (c)	21. (d)	28. (a)
7. (c)	15. (d)	22. (a)	29. (d)
8. (b)			

Section D

1. (e)	20. (a)	38. (a)	56. (d)
2. (b)	21. (c)	39. (b)	57. (b)
3. (a)	22. (a)	40. (e)	58. (a)
4. (c)	23. (b)	41. (a)	59. (c)
5. (b)	24. (c)	42. (b)	60. (c)
6. (d)	25. (b)	43. (e)	61. (d)
7. (d)	26. (c)	44. (c)	62. (b)
8. (a)	27. (a)	45. (d)	63. (c)
9. (c)	28. (a)	46. (b)	64. (e)
10. (a)	29. (d)	47. (b)	65. (a)
11. (b)	30. (b)	48. (c)	66. (a)
12. (d)	31. (a)	49. (b)	67. (b)
13. (a)	32. (d)	50. (a)	68. (d)
14. (b)	33. (c)	51. (e)	69. (c)
15. (a)	34. (a)	52. (d)	70. (a)
16. (e)	35. (d)	53. (c)	71. (a)
17. (c)	36. (d)	54. (a)	72. (a)
18. (a)	37. (c)	55. (d)	73. (b)
19. (d)			

6

Pathology

Jack P. Strong, M.D.

Professor and Chairman, Department of Pathology, Louisiana State
University School of Medicine-New Orleans, Louisiana

This chapter is designed to assist the student or candidate in preparing for medical licensing examination in pathology. It was prepared with the assumption that the reader has completed an adequate course in pathology at some time in the past and has access to and is familiar with a good standard textbook of pathology. This review was therefore designed to emphasize those areas that would be most helpful in preparing for qualifying examinations.

Pathology is that branch of biology concerned with disease (Gr. pathos, disease). Disease can be taken to mean any departure from the normal condition of a living plant or animal. Thus, disease is an abnormal condition of a living thing, and pathology is that branch of biology that involves the study of living things in their abnormal forms and conditions.

The broadest definition of pathology is that it is the study of disease. Pathology is the science dealing with diseases: their essential nature, causes and development, and the structural and functional changes produced by them. Pathology is a biological discipline and a branch of the practice of medicine. In pathology as a scientific discipline, the pathologist investigates the causes, mechanisms and effects of disease by observing tissues and organs at postmortem examination and correlating with clinical findings; by examining tissues removed at surgery; by using animal experiments; and by using other methods in the laboratory. In practice, the pathologist acts as a consultant to other physicians in diagnosis of disease during life and after death of the patient by methods of the laboratory—chemistry, microbiology, serology, hematology, examination of surgically removed specimens, and autopsy or postmortem examination.

Disease and Illness

Illness is the reaction between the disease and the individual. In other words, individual plus disease equals illness. This is a useful consideration for the student of pathology: that he is *learning* of *disease,* as such. On the wards and in the clinics he learns about illness as he studies interaction of disease and patient. Obviously, one must know about disease to study and treat illness.

Disease, at least in its initial stages, is no more than a slight departure from the normal condition. While the student usually learns from study of advanced disease, he should always keep in mind that the disease process is a condition that arose from normal or healthy tissue and cells and that even in a severe disease—one with the greatest disruption of structure and deformity—many of the cells of the body or of the affected organ system are still within "normal" limits.

Etiology, Pathogenesis, and Lesions

In pathology, the terms etiology, pathogenesis and lesions are used as key words to the study of disease.

Etiology refers to the cause of disease. There usually is a primary cause of a disease, but often there are many predisposing or contributing factors. For lobar pneumonia in a skid row alcoholic patient who is malnourished, has poor oral hygiene, and who was exposed to the elements while sleeping on a doorstep, the main etiologic agent is the pneumococcus organism, but the other factors have also contributed to the disease.

Pathogenesis refers to the mechanism of development of disease, or the stepwise development of disease.

A *lesion* is the result of disease, or the characteristic change in an organism produced by disease. From the viewpoint of recognition of disease, it is fortunate that constant and characteristic changes in the tissues and cells are frequently produced by disease. Many of them can be recognized grossly with the naked eye or microscopically. The electron microscope has greatly extended the ability to recognize the changes of disease. However, many diseases produce lesions at the level of the constituent metabolic units, the molecules. The classical example is sickle cell disease, which is due to an abnormal hemoglobin molecule with an abnormal pattern of amino acids in the protein. To encompass all of these changes, a lesion can be defined to be a tissue, cellular, or molecular alteration which develops as a result of disease-producing or pathogenic agents.

Some examples: Lobar pneumonia is a lesion. A myocardial infarct is a lesion. A mole is a lesion of the skin. A cataract is a lesion. A tumor of the lung is a lesion. A hemorrhoid is a lesion. A fractured rib is a lesion. An abrasion is a lesion. A boil is a lesion. A tumor of bone is a lesion. The hemoglobin molecule in a sickle cell disease is a lesion. The coating of an infant's red blood cells with antibody in erythroblastosis fetalis is a lesion.

In a specimen of diseased tissue, whether obtained by surgery or at autopsy, one is examining an instant only—a piece in a continuous progression, a frozen section of time, a single frame of a motion picture. The student of disease must study disease processes at many different stages so that he can reconstruct the development of the disease.

GENERAL PATHOLOGY

THE CELL

The human body is a vast, highly organized and complex accumulation of living cells. It is the condition of these cells that determines the state of health of the body or any of its parts. When the cells are normal and healthy, the body is healthy; when cells or specific groups of cells become disturbed or disorganized for any cause, then that part of the body, or under certain circumstances the entire body, is said to be the seat of disease. It seems wise, therefore, to start our discussion of pathology at the level of the cell.

The Normal Cell

Every organ of the body consists of recognizable basic histologic patterns of cells of different types and the associated stroma. The cell is therefore regarded as the basic unit of multicellular organisms, including man. The basic structural and functional components of the cell can be divided into two groups: those that are essential for survival of the cell and those that serve specialized functions characteristic of the differentiated cell type. The former group, which can be regarded as basic components, consists of plasma membrane (maintenance of intracellular environment), the nucleus and nucleolus (site of genetic information and expression), mitochondria (energy production and storage through oxidative phosphorylation of compounds derived from nutrients), endoplasmic reticulum and ribosomes (protein synthesis), and centrioles (cell division). Soluble proteins of the cytoplasm, which contain the enzymes of the glycolytic pathway and other essential systems, also belong to this group. Although the Golgi bodies (transport of the products of protein synthesis) and lysosomes (storage of hydrolytic enzymes) are more specialized organelles, their widespread distribution in cells of different types justifies their inclusion in the group of basic cellular components. The group of specialized cell products includes striated and smooth myofilaments of skeletal and smooth muscle cells, zymogen granules of exocrine cells, neurofilaments of the nerve cell, hemoglobin of the erythroid cells, and others.

Although most cell organelles can be demonstrated by a battery of special methods in cytologic preparations used in light microscopy, detailed structural organization can be observed only with the electron microscope. Basic structural elements, seen at such high resolution, are the systems of membranes of molecular dimensions and well-defined particulate materials. The former, present in the plasma membrane, motochondrial envelope, endoplasmic reticulum, Golgi vesicles, and nuclear membrane, consist of lamellae of lipid and protein molecules in fine distribution such that the macroscopically invisible substances do not segregate into larger droplets of vacuoles. The presence of large aggregations of lipids is therefore a sign of differentiation (cells of adipose reserve and the adrenal cortex) or of a disease process. The particulate elements include chromatin material in the nucleus, nucleolus, and ribosomes, all of which contain nucleic acids.

To perform its specialized functions adequately, the normal cell must have sufficient basic structural and metabolic components to remain alive and to produce its specialized products. The numbers of different organelles and the amounts of soluble enzymes must vary according to the physiologic requirements as well as to the local environment. The normal state consists of a range of successful adaptive changes, rather than a rigid, idealized condition.

In routine histologic reactions used for light microscopy, the tissues are stained with a combination of an acidic and a basic dye. The cytoplasmic organelles are usually not demonstrable. Macromolecules with amphoteric properties stain differently according to the balance of the acidic and basic groups. Structures rich in acid groups of nucleic acids and certain mucopolysaccharides have strong affinity for the basic dye, while proteins are usually stained with the acid dye. The nucleus and ergastoplasms (large accumulations of ribosomes in rough endoplasmic reticulum) are thus basophilic, while the cytoplasm and many differentiated structures are acidophilic.

Cellular Adaptation

Cells adapt to alterations in their environment. The term cellular adaptation is applied to those changes which are intermediate between the normal unstressed cell and the overstressed injured cell. An example is the increase in muscle size in laborers or body builders in which there is an increase in size of individual muscle bundles as a response to increased work load. The most important changes of cellular adaptation include induction of endoplasmic reticulum or hypertrophy of endoplasmic reticulum, hypertrophy, atrophy, hyperplasia, and metaplasia. Three terms that are commonly considered in conjunction with these adaptive changes, even though they are not adaptive in nature, but are related to failure of an organ to develop—hypoplasia, aplasia, and agenesis—will also be considered in this section.

Induction of Endoplasmic Reticulum. The livers of patients who have received repeated administration of barbiturates over a period of time will develop more endoplasmic reticulum in response to the drug adminis-tration. As a result they are able to detoxify a given amount of the barbiturate more rapidly. Once an increased amount of endoplasmic reticulum is present in the liver, the liver cells can also detoxify certain other drugs as well. This adaptive change is protective for the cell.

Atrophy. Atrophy is shrinkage of a cell by loss of cell substance, or decrease in the size of an organ due to decrease in the size of cells. The causes of atrophy include decreased work load, loss of innervation, diminished blood supply, inadequate nutrition, or loss of endocrine stimulation. Examples of atrophy are the muscles of a limb that has been immobilized in a cast, decrease in size of the testes or ovaries with old age, a decrease in the size of the thymus in the normal aging process. In atrophic tissue, in addition to the decrease in size apparent by gross inspection, microscopic changes are also apparent where autophagic vacuoles, or residual bodies, occur as a result of sequestration of cell organelles due to focal injury within the cells. The residual bodies are seen as lipofuscin granules under the light microscope. Lipofuscin is the so-called wear and tear pigment associated with aging and atrophy. It imparts a brown color to atrophic tissue such as the heart and liver.

Hypertrophy. Hypertrophy refers to increase in size of cells with resultant increase in the size of an organ. New cells are not formed in hypertrophy; there is enlargement of preexisting cells. The striated muscle cells hypertrophy in the muscles of a body builder. The myocardial muscle fibers increase in size in response to elevated blood pressure and increased peripheral resistance as well as to valvular disease that produces stenosis or insufficiency.

Hyperplasia. When stressed, cells capable of mitotic activity may respond by increasing in number. Hyperplasia is the increase in the number of cells in an organ or tissue, which usually results in increased size or volume. Hyperplasia and hypertrophy sometimes, but not always, develop concurrently. Hyperplasia may occur physiologically in response to changes in endocrine stimulation. The breast during puberty, pregnancy, and lactation is an example of an organ that undergoes hyperplasia of its component cells. In the gravid uterus there is both hyperplasia and hypertrophy of smooth muscle of the myometrium. Pathologic hyperplasia may follow excessive hormonal stimulation, e.g., endometrial hyperplasia, thyroid hyperplasia, adrenal hyperplasia.

Cell Injury and Response

Because of our greatly increased knowledge of the structure and function of living cells, a consideration of the pathologic changes that result following injury and disease calls for more intensive study of disease processes at a deeper and more fundamental level. Since the cell is the basic functional unit of the organism, all abnormalities in the normal processes of the body that result from injury or disease must originate in the cell.

The causes of injury to cells may be grouped as follows:

1. Physical agents, such as trauma, heat, cold, electrical energy and radiant energy from different sources may affect cells in a variety of ways—simple destruction of cells, burning or freezing of cells or effects on the molecular structure of cell constituents such as water, enzymes and proteins.

2. Chemical agents, such as acids, alkalies and various poisons may destroy cell membranes, alter cell functions and even cause death of the entire organism.

3. Living agents such as bacteria, viruses, rickettsiae and protozoan parasites of various kinds cause cell damage and death in a variety of ways. Viruses, for example, may actually compete for essential substances such as enzymes required for normal cell metabolism and convert them to their own use, thus indirectly destroying the cell.

4. Nutritional disturbances, especially the deprivation of protein or essential vitamins, but also nutritional excesses that may lead to obesity.

5. Genetic defects transmitted as hereditary diseases or resulting from mutations in the developing embryo.

6. Disturbances in arterial circulation leading to loss of blood supply and hypoxia.

7. Derangements in the immune mechanism based on exogenous or endogenous antigenic stimuli.

8. Aging, with widespread regressive changes occurring in the brain, muscle, and gonads, sometimes suggesting a "genetic clock."

General Features of Cell Injury. Changes that occur following injury may affect both the cell cytoplasm and the nucleus, alterations in the latter being the more serious. It must be borne in mind, however, that, in the light of present knowledge, recognizable morphologic changes indicative of injury follow by a considerable time the first damaging effects that occur at the molecular level and are therefore not recognizable by any method yet available. The first recognizable changes are found in the cytoplasm, may be reversible and are manifested by an increase in fluid content and swelling of the mitochondria. If the injury is more severe the endoplasmic reticulum becomes swollen and

vacuolated, and the ribosomes of the granular endoplasmic reticulum dissolve and disintegrate, leading to impaired protein synthesis. The lysosomes in the cells that contain them may rupture and undergo hydrolysis. Lipoprotein production is impaired, and lipid droplets may accumulate from cytoplasm degeneration or from damage to the cell membrane. Injured or damaged cytoplasmic organelles may become isolated in vacuoles or even digested by lysosomal enzymes.

Even if these changes appear severe in the cytoplasm they may still be reversible if the nucleus remains relatively unimpaired and the injurious agent is removed or destroyed before nuclear damage is excessive. Irreparable damage to the nucleus is manifested by changes usually recognizable by light microscopy. These are the shrinkage in size of the nucleus and the accumulation of the chromatin into a dense homogeneous shrunken mass *(pyknosis)*, the disintegration of the chromatin into fine granular fragments that are extruded through the ruptured nuclear membrane *(karyorrhexis)* and the swelling of the nucleus with disappearance of the chromatin *(karyolysis)*. These nuclear changes are characteristic of cell death.

As the degenerative changes progress in the damaged cell the DNA is impaired and the metabolic and synthetic activities of the cell, particularly the replication of DNA and the synthesis of RNA and protein, which are very sensitive to injury, are seriously interfered with and with cell death cease altogether. In spite of the fact that early and reversible, as well as late and irreversible, morphologic degenerative changes can be recognized in some cells by ordinary light microscopy, it is not possible, even with the elaborate methods of study that exist today, to follow stage by stage the biochemical alterations from slight to fatal cell injury. This is due to the fact that these changes take place at the molecular level where they are impossible to detect or observe.

Reversible Cell Injury and Degenerations. The most common reactions of the cell to injury are swelling, with or without the accumulation or appearance of abnormal substances in the cytoplasm and, later, changes of various kinds in the nucleus. Whether or not a change is reversible depends usually upon the severity of the injury to the nucleus.

Cloudy swelling, or *parenchymatous degeneration* or, still better, *cellular swelling,* since the first two designations refer especially to the gross appearance of the affected organ, is a reversible phenomenon observed most commonly in the parenchymal cells of the heart, the kidneys and the liver. It occurs in these and other organs in most cases of acute infection or poisoning and is the most common type of acute degeneration. The affected organ is swollen, the capsule is tense and the cut surface bulges. The tissue is opaque, pale, soft and more friable than normal. The usual vascular markings may be retained. Microscopically the cells appear swollen, and their outlines may, or in some cases may not, be distinct. The swelling is due to the imbibition of water, and the granularity results from changes occurring in the finer cytoplasmic structures such as swelling, vesiculation or rupture of the endoplasmic reticulum, swelling, distortion and disruption of the mitochondria and damage to the plasma membrane.

Hydropic degeneration is a more advanced, but still reversible, form of cellular swelling in which there is a greater degree of imbibition of water by the cell. In the gross, the general appearance resembles that of cellular swelling. Microscopically the parenchymal cells involved show fine and coarse vacuolization of the cytoplasm, due primarily to dilatation of the sacs of the endoplasmic reticulum and disaggregation of the ribosomal clusters. This form of degeneration may be seen as the result of any form of infection or poisoning, especially in the epithelial cells lining the convoluted tubules of the kidneys. The best examples of hydropic degeneration are seen in these cells after intravenous administration of hypertonic sucrose or ingestion of diethylene glycol or in patients with hypokalemia.

Fatty Change. Many terms have been used for abnormal accumulation in the cytoplasm of parenchymal cells, including fatty degeneration, fatty metamorphosis, fatty phanerosis, however fatty change is the most widely accepted term. There is general agreement about the following statements concerning fatty change. The appearance of fat vacuoles within cells represents an absolute increase in intracellular lipids. Fat accumulation in cells is not related to the type of injury but to an imbalance in production, utilization or mobilization of fat. Many varied derangements lead to fatty change; thus, fatty change is a common expression of many types of cell injury or cell overload. Fatty change may be preceded by cellular swelling and imbibition of fluid. While reversible itself fatty change may be followed by cell death and is often seen in cells adjacent to necrotic cells.

Fatty change is seen most often in the liver, heart and kidney. The liver enlarges and becomes yellow and greasy. Microscopically the process begins with development of small membrane-bound inclusions closely applied to the endoplasmic reticulum. As seen by light microscope, small vacuoles occur first in the cytoplasm; they later coalesce to form large clear spaces on hematoxylin and eosin-stained sections. The vacuoles displace the nucleus to the periphery. In advanced cases the liver may almost resemble adipose tissue. Sometimes the cells rupture and fat globules coalesce to from larger fatty cysts.

After moderate but prolonged hypoxia such as may be seen in long-standing severe anemia, the heart may grossly have a "flush breast" or "tabby cat" appearance with alternating bands of yellowish myocardium and darker red-brown myocardium. The yellow areas represent myocardium with fatty change and the darker areas are normal fibers. These changes are related to vascularization of the myocardium with the uninvolved area being closer to blood vessels and less subject to hypoxia. Histologically fat in the myocardial fibers is distributed in minute cytoplasmic vacuoles best seen after fat stains.

The kidneys also may be involved with fatty change. They become enlarged, pale and yellow. The proximal convoluted tubules are most often affected with fat accumulation. Chemical poisonings and profound anemia are among the causes of fatty change of the kidneys.

Hyaline Degeneration. This is an unsatisfactory term usually applied to a variety of changes, some of which cannot be classed as true degenerations. The term *hyaline* is a descriptive term applied to any material that has a structureless, smooth, homogeneous, almost glassy appearance and that stains pink by hematoxylin and eosin stains. The normal colloid of the thyroid gland is hyaline in appearance. Amyloid also appears hyaline, but it is not a true degeneration but rather an abnormal product of cell activity about which more will be said later. But there are changes that can be classed as degenerative or as the result of degeneration to which the term hyaline degeneration can be applied. Scar tissue anywhere, expecially as it gets older, may become the seat of hyaline change, and a similar alteration can be found in the dense fibrous tissue of arteriosclerotic plaques. Hyalinization of the walls of renal arterioles is typical of a severe form of chronic hypertension. Foci of hyaline degeneration can be found in neoplasms and, under certain conditions, e.g., as a result of mercury poisoning, in the epithelial cells of the proximal convoluted tubules of the kidneys where the hyaline material occurs as droplets. Similar hyaline droplets can be seen in liver cells as a result of infection (yellow fever) or in the form of cirrhosis common in alcoholics. *Zenker's hyaline degeneration* is a special form that affects striated muscles and occurs as a complication of typhoid fever, influenza and sometimes pneumonia. It is most common in the rectus muscle of the abdomen and may result in rupture of the fibers of this muscle. Microscopically, there is hyaline transformation of the affected muscle fibers with loss of their characteristic striations.

Amyloid Degeneration; Amyloidosis. Amyloid is one

of the hyalins that has certain more or less definite chemical properties and characteristic staining reactions with iodine, Congo red and methyl violet. The chemical composition is not known; it is probably not a single substance but rather a group of related compounds that consists primarily of a protein polysaccharide complex. Amyloid is insoluble in water but soluble in strong alkalies and slightly soluble in strong acids. It is apparently an abnormal synthetic product of cells and begins as a deposit in the spaces between the cells. As it increases in amount it causes pressure atrophy and sometimes disappearance of the adjacent cells and in some organs, specially the kidneys, may result in severe and even fatal injury.

Although amyloid appears to be a smooth, glassy, hyaline material when viewed through the light microscope, electron microscopic studies show it to be a complex accumulation of fine fibrils and rodlike structures, the fibrils predominating. The most common form appears as a complication of longstanding chronic infections, especially tuberculosis, leprosy, chronic osteomyelitis, and occasionally in other wasting disease. The condition may be focal or diffuse and microscopically appears in the form of an accumulation of a hyaline, structureless material in the region of the basement membrane of epithelial cells and surrounding capillaries or in the form of nodules replacing lymphoid tissue, as in the spleen. Most of the manifestations of amyloidosis are of this *secondary* type, occurring in parenchymatous organs or lymphoid tissue, mainly liver, kidneys, adrenals or spleen. There is a form of *primary* amyloidosis, however, that occurs without any obvious cause. In this form the deposits are found in the mesenchymal tissue of the tongue, larynx, myocardium or adipose tissue. A third form of amyloidosis may also occur in association with multiple myeloma. Finally, rare localized amyloid tumors, which occur without any known predisposing cause, are known.

Mucinous Degeneration. Mucin is also a hyaline-like material, being structureless and clear but viscid or slimy rather than firm. It is composed of both carbohydrate and protein, is slightly acid and therefore stains faintly blue with basic stains. Mucinous degeneration occurs most commonly in association with catarrhal inflammation, and mucus is secreted in excess into the lumina of ducts. It is particularly common in mucinous carcinoma in various sites. An epithelial tumor cell filled with mucin in its cytoplasm, with the nucleus pushed aside, is another good example of a signet-ring cell.

Mucoid Degeneration. This is a hyaline change that occurs in connective tissue. It is found most commonly in subcutaneous regions in the myxedema of thyroid deficiency and in myxomatous neoplasms of bone, breast and other organs. It differs significantly from mucin only in its higher sulfur content.

Irreversible Cell Injury (Necrosis).   Necrosis is the term applied to cell or tissue death in the living body. It is difficult to determine exactly when death of a cell takes place for cells vary in their susceptibility to injury, and, as noted above, the earliest changes, being at the molecular level, are not detectable. Presumably certain powerful toxins or noxious agents can cause immediate cell death. Most probably, however, death comes more gradually, the cell first manifesting the cytoplasmic changes that characterize degenerations of various types and going on, with continuation of the injurious effect, to loss of cell structure, fragmentation of organelles and liquefaction of the cytoplasm and the typical nuclear changes (pyknosis, karyolysis and karyorrhexis) that are indicative of actual cell death. Necrosis of tissue is merely the sum total of the necrosis of masses of cells. The causes of necrosis include injurious agents of many kinds, physical, chemical, bacterial or viral, etc., as well as any cause of anoxia. From a morphologic standpoint necrosis may be of several types:

Coagulation necrosis, seen best in early infarction, is characterized by the general preservation of the architectural features of the organ, but with loss of cellular detail.

Liquefaction necrosis is characterized by the softening and eventual liquefaction of the dead tissue, such as is seen in infarcts of the brain or in the center of a furuncle or boil.

Caseous necrosis is characterized by its soft, cheesy gross appearance and is typical of tuberculous necrosis.

Gummatous necrosis resembles caseous necrosis; however, it is not soft, but rubbery and firm. It is typical of tertiary lesions of syphilis.

Fat necrosis is associated with pancreatic injuries or diseases such as the uncommon but serious condition known as acute hemorrhagic pancreatitis and is due to the liberation of pancreatic enzymes, notably lipases, amylases and proteases, which act on the intraabdominal, mesenteric, omental and even pancreatic fat, forming minute, circumscribed chalky white spots in these tissues. Microscopically these foci of recent necrosis usually are surrounded by extravasated red blood corpuscles and polymorphonuclear leukocytes. Later, they may become the seat of deposition of calcium, with surrounding foreign-body type of inflammatory reaction.

Gangrene is massive death with putrefaction of a part of the body. *Moist gangrene* occurs in parts that are moist and congested. *Dry gangrene,* or mummification, develops in parts that are anemic or dry at the time of tissue death. It is most common in the extremities, in which, if caused by arteriosclerosis, it may develop slowly, but it may occur with great rapidity when a thrombus, forming on the roughened intima of an artery, or a large embolus from the left heart, cuts off the circulation suddenly. *Diabetic gangrene* results from arteriosclerosis. Gangrene in Raynaud's disease and ergot poisoning is caused by a spasm of the small arteries; that of thromboangiitis obliterans is due to endarteritis of toxic or infective origin and may be unilateral. Gangrene may also be caused by trauma, pressure, freezing or infection, particulary infection caused by *Clostridium perfringens* in which it is associated with the formation of gas bubbles (hydrogen) within the tissues, producing the typical crepitus of this infection.

Zonal necrosis refers to conditions in which the injurious agent selectively affects a certain "zone" of a unit structure, e.g., carbon tetrachloride causes necrosis of the efferent part of the lobule (contrilobular necrosis), yellow fever is reported to affect the middle zone of the lobules, and phosphorous poisoning affects the peripheral (efferent) portion of the lobule.

Focal necrosis consists of minute foci of dead tissue and is characteristic of lesions found typically in the liver in typhoid fever.

Sequelae of necrosis. Inflammation occurs as a reaction to the injurious agent and to the components of necrotic tissue. Regeneration may occur particularly if the supportive stroma is not damaged irreversibly and if some parenchymal cells capable of regeneration survive. Repair with granulation tissue and subsequent scarring will fill a defect and replace necrotic tissue in many instances. Dissolution of tissue with cavity or cyst formation may occur as in pulmonary tuberculosis. Deposition of mineral salts (calcium and phosphorus) may occur if the necrotic tissue remains for an extended time leading to dystrophic calcification.

Calcification (Pathologic). In all sites where degenerated or necrotic tissues are found, especially following old infections such as tuberculosis, histoplasmosis or coccidioidomycosis or almost any focus of old, chronic infection, calcification is referred to as dystrophic and is determined in great part by the local relative alkalinity of the tissue. The deposit is mainly calcium phosphate and carbonate. Dystrophic calcification is not caused by hypercalcemia. *Metastatic calcification* is a form in which previous degenerative or necrotizing changes in the tissues do not occur; it is associated with hypercalcemia from any cause, such as the destruction of bone and the solution of its deposit of calcium, hyperparathyroidism, hypervitaminosis D or even excessive intake of calcium. The calcium is deposited wherever acid is being eliminated and there is relative alkalinity of tissues, such as in the kidney (phosphoric acid), the stomach (hydrochloric acid) and the lungs (carbonic acid).

Somatic death is death of the organism. In somatic death, rigor mortis refers to stiffening of skeletal muscles after death; algor mortis refers to gradual cooling of the body; and livor mortis refers to reddish discoloration of the dependent portions of the body due to gravitational sinking of the blood.

Hypoplasia, aplasia and agenesis are usually defined in conjunction with adaptive changes even though they are developmental abnormalities. Hypoplasia is failure of an organ to reach full adult size. Hypoplasia is a less severe developmental arrest than aplasia and agenesis. The organ, usually a lung or kidney, remains small rather than reaching full adult size. Aplasia and agenesis refer to total failure of an organ to develop.

Progressive Tissue Changes. *Hypertrophy* is an increase in size of an organ or a part as well as of certain cells, such as muscle cells, as a result of increased activity. The increased size of an organ may result either from an increase in the size of its component cells or an increase in their number, usually associated with an increase in functional capacity.

Hyperplasia is a controlled increase in the number of cells of an organ or part. The cells may be mature or embryonal, but they are not neoplastic. Hyperplasia may be *physiologic,* as occurs in breast epithelium in puberty and pregnancy; *compensatory,* as occurs in one paired organ when the other is removed or destroyed by disease; of *pathologic,* such as may be seen in the endometrium under excessive estrogen stimulation. The first two types of hyperplasia serve a useful purpose and never become neoplastic; pathologic hyperplasia may sometimes change to true neoplasia.

Metaplasia is a reversible change in which one adult cell type is replaced by another adult cell type usually as a result of chronic irritation. The change from normal pseudostratified ciliated columnar epithelium in the tracheobronchial tree to stratified squamous epithelium in the habitual cigarette smoker is an example of metaplasia. Change to stratified squamous epithelium from mucus-producing columnar epithelium in the endocervix is an example of metaplasia. Dysplastic and anaplastic changes representing a progression from normal adult cell types are covered in the section on neoplasia.

INFLAMMATION, REGENERATION AND REPAIR

Inflammation is the local reaction of the living body to any injury. Whether the tissues are bruised, cut, burned, invaded by pathogenic microorganisms or in any other way hurt or damaged, a complicated and well-coordinated series of vascular and cellular reactions occurs at the site of injury. The object of these reactions is to destroy or remove the injurious agent if possible or to limit its spread, to neutralize toxins, to remove the remnants of destroyed tissues and to prepare the area for the final repair of the damage that was done. The injurious agents may be physical, mechanical, chemical, bacterial, viral, toxic or nutritional.

Repair, on the other hand, is the process whereby an attempt is made to restore to a normal, or approximately normal, state, the part of the body that has been injured. Cells that have been destroyed are either replaced by healthy cells of the same type growing in from adjacent living tissue *(regeneration)* or by the replacement of the dead cells by fibrous tissue and new blood vessels that also come from uninjured neighboring tissues *(granulation tissue* or *scar tissue* formation). There is a gradual merging from inflammation to repair. The repair process is one of the end stages of the inflammatory reaction just as it is for tissue necrosis.

Inflammation

The Fundamental Mechanisms of Inflammation.

Nearly 100 years ago Cohnheim gave such a clear and vivid account of the microscopic changes that occur at the site of acute inflammation that little can be added as a result of modern studies. He noted the dilatation of the local arterioles, venules and, ultimately, capillaries in the region of injury, the initial acceleration and later slowing of the blood flow, the escape of fluid from vessels into the surrounding tissue spaces, the margination of leukocytes along the endothelial linings followed by the emigration of these cells through the vessel walls into the region of injury. We can now attempt to explain these changes in some detail.

The main features of the acute inflammatory reaction can be divided into four broad headings: (1) active hyperemia; (2) increased microvascular permeability; (3) cellular exudation; and (4) reversal of these changes, resolution, regeneration and repair.

The Inflammatory Cells

The inflammatory cells are derived from leukocytes of the blood and certain tissue cells. The normal proportions of leukocytes of the blood are as follows: neutrophils 54 to 73 per cent, eosinophils 2 to 4 per cent, basophils 0 to 1 per cent, monocytes 4 to 8 per cent, and lymphocytes 21 to 35 per cent. The proportion of these cells changes in disease states and with inflammatory conditions. The large variety of changes with disease states is beyond the scope of this review. Only

the basic characteristics of the inflammatory cells will be summarized.

A. Blood Cells
  1. Polymorphonuclear leukocytes (granulocytes)
     a. Neutrophils—short lived, end-stage cells remaining in the blood for 18 to 36 hours. They are mature when released from bone marrow with no further proliferation. Neutrophils are the first cells to accumulate in the acute inflammatory response. They are removed from the inflammatory site by phagocytic activity of macrophages or by dissolution and removal of lymph channels. They are actively motile and have directional mobility in the presence of chemotactic agents. They are actively phagocytic and are aided in phagocytosis by antibodies that coat the infectious organisms (opsonins). They contain receptors for IgG. They are the chief cells in pus and are sometimes called pus cells when found in tissues or urine. Neutrophils contain two types of granules, large azure granules containing acid hydrolases, neutral proteins, myeloperoxidase, cationic proteins and lysozyme (muramidase) and smaller specific granules which contain alkaline phosphates, lactoferrin and lysozyme.
     b. Eosinophils—short-lived cells with many functions in common with neutrophils, including motility and phagocytosis. They respond chemotactically to split products of C3 and C5 and to the trimolecular complex of C567. Eosinophils phagocytize antigens and antibody complexes. They are commonly seen in allergic responses and in the healing phase of inflammation. They also respond to eosinophil chemotactic factor of anaphylaxis, which is secreted by basophils (ECF-A). Ultrastructurally they contain characteristic crystalloid granules.
     c. Basophils—similar to tissue mast cells but less numerous. They have metachromatic granules which contain heparin and histamine in the performed state (and in some species, not man, serotonin).
  2. Monocytes—the blood phase of the monocyte-macrophage system. They have a much longer life span than polymorphonuclear leukocytes and they may progress in maturation after liberation from the bone marrow. In

some instances they may divide and proliferate. Most of the monocytes leave the blood stream to become tissue macrophages. Both monocytes and macrophages are avidly phagocytic, taking up both small and large particles, dead cells, cellular debris, and erythrocytes. They are markedly responsive to chemotactic agents C3a and C5a but are not responsive to C567. They also respond to certain lymphocyte products (lymphokines) and are modified by other lymphocyte products. Monocytes sometimes, but not always kill the organisms they ingest.

3. Lymphocytes—small round cells that are less motile than neutrophils and monocytes and are not responsive to the usual chemotactic agents. They are related to the immune system and there are two basic types. The T cells originate in the thymus and are related to cell-mediated immunity. The B cells are related to plasma cells and are involved with immunoglobulin production and humoral immunity. The small or medium lymphocytes mediate antigen recognition and cellular immunity. The sensitized lymphocytes recognize and react with the antigens that stimulated their appearance.

B. Tissue cells

1. Mast cells—similar to basophils. They contain heparin, histamine, and eosinophil chemotactic factor of anaphylaxis (ECF-A). Mast cells also produce the slow reacting substance of anaphylaxis (SRSOA). They also have a platelet activating factor.

2. Tissue histiocyte or macrophage—the tissue counterpart of the blood monocyte and part of the reticuloendothelial system. These cells have great phagocytic activity especially when particulate matter is to be removed. Many macrophages are derived from monocytes and some are derived from other tissue macrophages. They may become modified by what they have ingested. For example, hemosiderin-laden macrophages are seen in congestive heart failure secondary to mitral stenosis when they have ingested erythrocytes which have entered the alveolar spaces. They may contain carbon particles, parts of necrotic cells, and microorganisms, some of which can live symbiotically within the cells.

3. Giant cells—multinucleated cells found in tissue formed by fusion of histiocytes. They may contain 50 or more nuclei.

4. Plasma cells—not normally found in blood and not phagocytic. They are rich in endoplasmic reticulum and active in protein synthesis. Plasma cells produce large quantities of immunoglobulins. They arise from B-lymphocytes in the germinal center of lymph nodes, spleen, and the gastrointestinal tract.

Sequence of Events in Acute Inflammation

The chronological sequence of events that occurs in acute inflammatory reactions from onset to termination with resolution is as follows:

Transient vasoconstriction
Dilatation of arterioles
Speeding of blood stream
Increase in permeability of venules and capillaries
Exudation of fluid rich in proteins—albumin and globulins, followed by fibrinogen (largest molecular weight)—between the junctions of endothelial cells of venules
Concentration and packing of erythrocytes
Slowing of blood stream, stasis, loss of laminar axial flow
Peripheral orientation of leukocytes (neutrophils) with margination and pavementing
Emigration of neutrophils first, monocytes second, and then other cells
Diapedesis of erythrocytes if injury is severe enough
Accumulation or aggregation of leukocytes and fluid in area of irritant
Phagocytosis of irritants by neutrophils and monocytes
Killing of microorganisms if present
Reversal of vascular changes
Neutrophils and monocytes carry off debris
Fluid reabsorbed by venules and by lymphatic drainage
Repair by ingrowth of capillaries and fibroblasts

This list of changes is essentially what Cohnheim saw and described those many years ago.

Mediators of Inflammation

The two main classes of inflammatory mediators for acute inflammation are vasopermeability factors, and leukotactic (chemotactic) factors. Vasopermeability factors have to do with increasing the permeability of the microvasculature and leukotactic factors have to do with stimulating the unidirectional migration of white blood cells toward an attractant. Chemotaxis is the process in which inflammatory cells move toward a chemical attractant in an unidirectional manner with responsiveness to gradients.

Vasopermeability factors. Vasopermeability is transient and temporary and only occurs when mediators are present. Increased permeability of the microvasculature begins in the venules and venular end of the capillary loops. Most investigators have concluded that it occurs because of changes in the endothelial cell junctions, which become open to the passage of fluid. Permeability factors apparently work by loosening endothelial cell junctions. All the vasopermeability factors that have been described cause smooth muscle cells to contract. They cause periendothelial cells (modified smooth muscle cells) and endothelial cells to contract, thus widening the endothelial cell junctions. Vasopermeability effects are temporary. They go away when the chemical mediators are no longer present. They do not lead to loss of erythrocytes and leukocytes from the vascular lumen.

There is a biphasic response for vasopermeability in the mild acute inflammatory response, an immediate and a delayed response. The first immediate phase of vasopermeability is histamine dependent and can be blocked by the administration of antihistamine drugs. Mast cells contain vasoactive amines (histamine). Several reactions can cause liberation of histamine from mast cells, including cytotoxic reaction and anaphylactic reaction. Certain products of the complement system, anaphylatoxins ($C3_a$, $C5_a$ cleavage products), can cause secretion of vasoactive amines by mast cells and increased vasopermeability.

The second or delayed phase of increased permeability is totally independent of the first. Antihistamines do not block the action. There is no clear single cause; probably multiple factors are involved. Those agents suspected of being involved in the delayed phase of vasopermeability include kinins, protaglandins, and products of the complement system.

The common features of all vasopermeability factors are that they are reversible and temporary, acting only when present. They cause contraction of smooth muscle cells and opening of endothelial cell junctions.

The following is a list of suspected vasopermeability factors:

Vasoactive amines—histamine, serotonin

Kinins—bradykinin, a simple basic peptide generated by activation of the kinin system (involves Hageman factor XII, kallikrein, and kininogen). (Note: review kinin generating system and Hageman factor involvement in the coagulation cascade, kinin generating system, and fibrinolytic system.)

PF/dil—activated form of Hageman factor

Leukokinins—peptides generated by enzymes from leukocytes

Basic (cationic) peptides—performed in lysosomals granules of leukocytes

Slow reacting substance of anaphylaxis (SRA-S)—recently found to be a form of prostaglandin, and named leukotriene

Prostaglandins (prostaglandins, prostacyclins, thromboxanes)—Family of substances having profound effects on smooth muscle cells and multiple effects on tissue.

Anaphylatoxins ($C3_a$, $C5_a$)

Leukotactic (Chemotactic) Mediators. The major substances that have been shown to attract white blood cells and which might play a role in acute inflammation include the following:

Leukotactic factors of host origin

(1) Complement derivatives (review complement cascade). Some chemotactic factors affect only neutrophils, some affect only monocytes, and others affect both. Fragments of C3 and C5 are chemotactic for both neutrophils and monocytes. The trimolecular complex of C567 is chemotactic for neutrophils but not for monocytes.
(2) Activated plasma enzymes. Probably not very important to chemotactic factors.
(3) Lymphocyte products—lymphokines. The most important of these is MIF (migratory inhibitory factor).
(4) Tissue products—collagenase, tissue enzymes which are capable of cleaving C3 and C5

Leukotactic factors of microbial origin

Soluble bacterial products from staphylococcus, streptococcus, and pneumococcus as well as certain other organisms.

Leukotactic factors by inflammatory cell type

A list of factors which are chemotactic for neutrophils and monocytes follows:

Chemotactic factors for neutrophils

(1) Activated trimolecular complex of C567
(2) A plasmin-split fragment of C3
(3) Fragments of C3 which are found after cleavage by tissue proteases
(4) A fragment of C5
(5) Soluble bacterial factors from filtrates

Chemotactic factors for monocytes

(1) A plasmin-split fragment of C3
(2) A fragment of C5
(3) Soluble bacterial factors
(4) A soluble factor derived from sensitized lymphocytes (a lymphokine)
(5) Serum factor from serum treated with immune complexes
(6) Cationic protein—basic peptides

Chemotactic factors for eosinophils are essentially the same as for neutrophils with an additional factor, ECF-A (eosinophilic chemotactic factor of anaphylaxis).

Classification of Inflammation

The process of inflammation may be classified based on duration (acute, subacute, chronic, healed), etiology (bacterial, viral, chemical, physical, etc.), types of reaction produced (exudative, proliferative), and type of exudate produced. Types of inflammation based on types of exudate are:

Serous—extensive outpouring of watery inflammatory edema fluid

Fibrinous—containing large amounts of fibrinogen which precipitates

Catarrhal—containing large amounts of mucus

Purulent or suppurative—exudate characterized by large amounts of pus

Hemorrhagic—containing erythrocytes in addition to other elements of the exudate

Fibrinopurulent—a mixture of large amounts of fibrinogen and pus Mucopurulent—a mixture of mucin and pus

Pertinent Definitions

Pus—thick inflammatory fluid composed of living and dead polymorphonuclear leukocytes and necrotic debris.

Exudate—inflammatory edema fluid characterized by high protein content, high cell counts, specific gravity over 1.018, low glucose content, sometimes clots due to fibrinogen content. This is to be contrasted with:

Transudate—a noninflammatory edema fluid resembling an ultrafiltrate of plasma with certain characteristics: specific gravity about 1.010 (certainly less than 1.018), low protein content, low cell content, normal glucose content, clear, does not clot on standing. Transudates are related to circulatory disorders; exudates are related to inflammatory disorders.

Opsonins—a collective term for humoral factors, including antibacterial and antifungal antibodies, components of complement and other heat-labile substances which promote phagocytosis of bacteria.

Microscopic Features of Acute Inflammation

Microscopically the acute inflammatory lesion shows varing proportions of (1) serous exudate, (2) fibrin, (3) polymorphonuclear leukocytes and (4) large mononuclear cells. According to the character of the exudate, they are classified as follows:

1. *Acute serous or serofibrinous* inflammation occurs on serous membranes such as the pericardium, the pleura or the peritoneum. The exudate is largely serous, with fibrin resulting from coagulation of plasma, and it may be absorbed completely or organized by the ingrowth of young connective tissue, often resulting in fibrous adhesion of visceral and parietal layers. In lobar pneumonia the pleural exudate is mainly serofibrinous. In this condition the exudate undergoes lysis and is either absorbed directly or, in part at least, removed by macrophages.

2. *Acute purulent, seropurulent or fibrinopurulent* inflammation is characterized by the predominance of pus cells (polymorphonuclear leukocytes) and is the most frequent type outside of the serous membranes. It may be either (1) circumscribed or suppurative, to form an abscess, which heals by the walling off of fibrous tissue and scar formation, or (2) diffuse or phlegmonous, acute inflammation, often caused by streptococci, pneumococci, etc., that extends into the surrounding tissues and tends to invade the bloodstream.

3. *Acute hemorrhagic* inflammation is characterized by intense capillary injury, with rupture, permitting large numbers of erythrocytes to escape into the tissues, as in hemorrhagic cystitis and some forms of glomerulonephritis. The red cells must be removed by the leukocytes.

4. *Acute catarrhal* inflammation is relatively mild; it is characterized by a seromucinous exudate on the mucous membrane, which later becomes mucopurulent, as in catarrhal inflammations of the upper respiratory and the alimentary tract.

5. *Pseudomembranous or diphtheritic* inflammation is formed by a fibrinous exudate over a necrotic layer of mucosa. It never organizes but is sloughed off or digested. This type of inflammation is seen in diphtheria and has been observed fairly frequently at autopsy in the alimentary tract of individuals who had been receiving large quantities of some antibiotics. A type of staphylococcus resistant to antibiotics is the usual cause in these cases.

Chronic inflammation differs from acute inflammation in that the cellular reaction consists primarily of lymphocytes, plasma cells, and macrophages together with newly formed collagenous fibers. This chronic process often follows an acute inflammatory one. When pus is associated with a chronic lesion, as in chronic suppurative osteomyelitis, it is termed chronic suppurative inflammation. When the formation of new connective tissue is prominent, the lesion is called chronic productive inflammation. Some inflammatory processes, such as syphilis, never show the features of acute inflammation.

Granulomatous inflammation is a reaction to injury in which a proliferative response rather than an exudative response dominates the reaction. A small but important group of biological agents and physical and chemical agents characteristically induce the aggregation and proliferation of macrophages in addition to the usual changes of simple inflammation. Because macrophages have a strong tendency to arrange themselves in small nodules or granules, this group of conditions have come to be known as granulomas. Some of the disorders that characteristically call forth a granulomatous response include tuberculosis, leprosy, syphilis, sarcoidosis, many mycotic infections including histoplasmosis, blastomycosis, coccidioidomycosis. Foreign bodies also call forth a granulomatous response. The most characteristic inflammatory cell of granulomatous inflammation is the epithelioid cell, which is a macrophage that has been altered in response to the inflammatory agent. Multinucleate giant cells sometimes but not always occur in the granulomatous reaction and they are formed by macrophages becoming fused.

Repair

Repair consists of the replacement of dead or damaged cells by new healthy cells derived either from the parenchymal or connective tissue stromal elements of the injured tissue. Repair and healing are practically synonymous. Repair takes place through parenchymal regeneration and repair by connective tissue. Parenchymal regeneration can be remarkably complete when the preexisting stroma is not seriously damaged and when the residual cells have the capacity for active regeneration. When damage is severe and parenchymal regeneration cannot restore the organ, the repair process takes the form of connective tissue scarring. Scar tissue fills the defects and restores some of the bulk of the organ, but specialized functioning cells are replaced with nonfunctioning connective tissue. An example of this process is healing of a myocardial infarct in which contractile myocardial cells are replaced by nonfunctioning scar tissue.

Repair by regeneration is basically replacement of cells lost through injury or physiological wear and tear by cells of the same type. The ability to regenerate is greater in some cell types than in others. Cells of the body have been divided into three groups based on their capacity for regeneration: labile, stabile, and permanent. Labile cells are cells which continue to multiply under normal conditions and which can respond rapidly by regenerating when damaged.

Labile cells include cells of the epithelial surfaces of the skin, oral cavities, the mucosa of the gastrointestinal tract and genitourinary tract, and cells of the hematopoetic system. When these cells are lost, they are rapidly replaced by regeneration of adjacent cells. Stabile cells do not normally replicate but have the ability to divide when injured. The stabile cells include

the parenchymal cells of most of the glandular organs (liver, tubular cells of the kidney, endocrine glands) and connective tissue cells such as fibroblasts, chondroblasts and osteoblasts. The parenchymal cells can regenerate after damage has occurred and are most effective in replacing preexisting structure when the basic framework of the organ or tissue is unaffected.

Some muscle cells are capable of some degree of regeneration, but certainly not as much as other connective tissues. Regeneration of smooth muscle occurs in the wall of the intestine, urinary bladder and uterus. Skeletal muscle makes some attempt at regeneration, although never complete. Cardiac muscle has no significant regenerative capacity.

Permanent cells are highly specialized cells which do not undergo mitotic division in post natal life even after injury. The nerve cells in the central nervous system are permanent cells and are not replaced when irreversibly damaged. With regard to the peripheral nerves, when the cell body is destroyed, the entire nerve degenerates. If the peripheral axon is injured and the cell body is not damaged, regeneration may proceed from the cell body or from the proximal axonal segment. The distal segment degenerates entirely, and the proximal segment degenerates to the nearest node of Ranvier. The proximal segment then regenerates until it meets the distal channel, in which case the integrity of the nerve may be reestablished. Cardiac muscle fibers, since they do not regenerate, are also considered permanent cells.

Repair by fibrous tissue or scar formation is really the replacement of injured or destroyed tissue by a simpler form of tissue, namely, loose, vascular fibrous tissue, generally known as *granulation tissue* (fibroblasts and proliferating capillaries), which is at first very soft and delicate but which soon becomes more dense and compact, forming a fibrous patch or scar that takes the place of the original tissue destroyed as the result of injury. This form of repair commonly occurs following extensive damage with the loss of much of the original tissue. The healing of wounds illustrates these reparative processes admirably.

Healing by first intention is favored by apposition of the tissues in the absence of infection. There is slight exudate between the apposed surfaces. In 24 hours in the case of a tissue with an epithelial covering, there are mitoses in the epithelial cells and fibroblasts, and some leukocytes are present. In a few days the continuity of the epithielium is restored, and granulation tissue fills in from below the defect in the subepithelial tissue. The strength of the healing area is determined by the amount of collagen fiber that has formed.

Healing by second intention in noninfected wounds, in which tissue apposition cannot occur, begins with a thin surface exudate. In a few days the floor of the wound is covered by granulation tissue, consisting of capillary loops surrounded by fibroblasts and leukocytes, which gradually fills in from the side and the floor of the wound and is finally covered by epithelium. The exuberant granulation tissue in an open wound is called "proud flesh."

In *infected* open wounds there is a purulent exudate on the surface, and complete healing by granulation does not occur until the infection subsides.

ABNORMAL GROWTH AND DEVELOPMENT

Many disease processes are initiated during embryonic life as the consequences of genetic, developmental, and intrauterine abnormalities. Some of these conditions become evident in early pregnancy, resulting in spontaneous abortions, while others do not manifest themselves until later pregnancy and postnatal periods. Of all live-born infants, the highest mortality rate occurs during the neonatal period (the first four weeks). Such mortality is closely correlated with prematurity of the infants at birth. In later infancy (up to one year), the survival rate increases sharply. The major causes of death, roughly in the order of frequency, are infections and their complications, congenital malformations, and malignant neoplasms. Accidental deaths, including those that occur in the home and the automobile, predominate during childhood. In the adult, developmental and genetic factors contribute significantly to a certain proportion of morbidity and mortality, although they may not be easily recognized by the attending physician.

Neonatal Diseases

The development of the fetus can be regarded as a preparation for extrauterine existence. There is a period in early gestation when the fetus is absolutely incapable of survival in the external environment. If pregnancy is spontaneously or artifically terminated during this stage of development, the result is an abortion. Later, the development is chronologically reflected by the growth of organs, which become progressively more adapted for independent life. For practical and statistical purposes, the birth weight of the infant is used as an estimate of the gestational age or the degree of developmental "maturity" with a fair degree of reliability. Because infants weighing 500 to 1000 gm. rarely survive the neonatal period, they are regarded as being "immature" by a number of authorities. "Premature infants" are defined as those whose birth weights are between 1001 and 2500 gm. In this group, the survival rate increases progressively with birth weight. Although histologic evidence of immaturity can be dis-

cerned to some extent in infants weighing less than 1500 gm., these features represent a stage of development, rather than a conclusive evidence of the cause of death. The appearance of terminal air spaces lined by cuboidal cells in the lungs of an immature infant, for example, show only that effective respiration has not taken place. Infants of the same gestational age and birth weight that survive longer show a progressive flattening of the alveolar lining cells in the lungs after respiration has been adequately established. Although branching of the bronchial tree is completed by the eleventh week of gestation, additional terminal air spaces continue to form until at least the eighth year of life, according to quantitative studies made with the use of plastic casts of the air ways. Immaturity is thus a quantitative problem determined by the number of the alveoli and the need of the infant.

In a significant proportion of stillborn infants and in those that die during the first few days of life, autopsy findings consist mainly of petechial and, occasionally, ecchymotic hemorrhages in the visceral pleura, pericardium, and in the thymus. In some cases, petechiae are also demonstrated in the subependymal and subarachnoid spaces. In very severe cases, the immediate causes of death are massive hemorrhages in the pulmonary alveoli, in the subarachnoid and ventricular spaces of the brain. All these changes are ascribed to *intrauterine anoxia* (asphyxia neonatorum), which increases the permeability of the capillary endothelium and other membranes. Known causes of the disease include abruptio placentae, placenta previa, exposure to sedative or hypnotic drugs derived from the maternal blood stream, and umbilical cord compression during labor. It must also be noted that a prolonged uterine contraction, which is clinically associated with a marked drop in the fetal heart rate, is also an important cause of anoxia.

In some stillborn and newborn infants with a similar history, intrauterine aspiration of excessive amounts of amniotic fluid and its contents are demonstrated. In some cases, meconium is present in the fluid and in the lungs. In others, large numbers of squames, derived from vernix caseosa, fill the tracheobronchial tree and the terminal air spaces, preventing an adequate exchange of gases. Certain authors ascribed such *aspiration syndrome* to fetal anoxia, which towards the end of prematurity and at full term, stimulates the respiratory center in the brain and reflexes the anal sphincter.

The most common cause of death during the neonatal period is *hyaline membrane disease*, which is never found in stillborn infants. The disease occurs most frequently in the premature, but it is also significant in full-term infants of diabetic mothers and in those delivered by cesarean section. It is characterized by respiratory difficulty, beginning soon after birth, which becomes progressively worse with time. Clinically, there is progressive rise of pCO_2 and fall of pO_2, which is unresponsive to 100 per cent oxygen. Pulmonary function studies show a marked decrease of the residual volume of the lungs. At autopsy, the lungs are heavy, airless, reddish-purple in color, and sink in the fixing fluid. Histologically, all the alveoli are collapsed, leaving no residual air spaces, while the alveolar ducts and terminal bronchioles are markedly dilated and are lined with eosinophilic, amorphous material, which is regarded as hyaline membrane. This material consists essentially of fibrin, plasma proteins, and some necrotic debris. The mortality rate is high; only a very few infants survive more than a few days.

Evidence is accumulating that the lungs of infants with hyaline membrane disease produce inadequate amounts of an alveolar surfactant, which is required for an effective inflation of the alveoli. This substance has been shown to be lecithin, secreted by pneumocyte II of the alveolar lining. It is also released into the amniotic fluid by the normal intrauterine respiratory movements. The determination of lecithin-sphingomyelin ratio of the amniotic fluid has been used as an indicator of pulmonary maturity of the fetus before a cesarean section or an induced labor.

The most common complications of hyaline membrane disease are subarachnoid and intraventricular hemorrhages, which are occasionally massive in amounts. In some series, these complications are found in about 50 per cent of fatal cases. Intraalveolar and interstitial hemorrhages in the lungs are also not infrequent. These hemorrhages represent the consequences of postnatal anoxia due to an extremely inadequate exchange of gases.

The term *respiratory distress syndrome* has been used clinically to describe progressive dyspnea in newborn infants. Most of these cases correspond to hyaline membrane disease, although some represent cases of the aspiration syndrome, intrauterine pneumonia, and rate congenital anomalies of the lungs.

The most common serious infection in the stillborn and newborn infants that die during the early neonatal period is *intrauterine pneumonia.* The disease is strongly associated with premature rupture of fetal membranes and with prolonged labor, even with intact membranes. Microscopically, the terminal air spaces are filled with neutrophils, macrophages, and necrotic debris. The etiologic agents can be any organisms that reach the maternal genital tract. In the preantibiotic era, group A hemolytic streptococci were the most common cause. Subsequently, *E. coli* became the most frequent agent causing the pneumonia. More recently,

group B hemolytic streptococci are emerging as the most common causative organisms. Intrauterine pneumonia is frequently complicated by septicemia and meningitis.

Rare transpacental infections leading to a generalized disease with necrotic foci in various organs, including the liver, kidneys, adrenals and brain, are cytomegalic inclusion disease, herpes simplex, listeriosis, and toxoplasmosis. In congenital toxoplasmosis, foci of calcification can occasionally be observed in roentgenograms of the head, due to the presence of lesions in the brain.

Hemolytic disease of the newborn (erythroblastosis fetalis) is a group of diseases of considerable interest because of the immulogic mechanism of pathogenesis, which can be prevented by an appropriate measure. The most severe type is due to an Rh incompatibility between the maternal and fetal bloods. When the mother is Rh negative and the fetus is Rh positive, the fetal red blood cells occasionally enter the maternal blood stream, inducing an immunologic response which is initially associated with IgM formation. Because of its large molecular size, the antibody cannot enter the fetal circulation and the first child is therefore usually unaffected by the disease. In subsequent pregnancies, however, IgG is produced in increasing quantities. Since this immunoglobin can readily enter the fetal circulation, the fetus develops a hemolytic anemia, which is variable in severity. In the most severe form, *hydrops fetalis,* the fetus manifests general anasarca due to cardiac and liver failure, with consequent decrease of plasma albumin and osmotic disturbances. *Icterus gravis,* which is a slightly less severe variety, is characterized by a severe hemolytic anemia with a marked bilirubinemia, which must be treated promptly by a complete exchange transfusion. In fetal cases, the basal ganglia, cerebellum and other areas of the brain are yellow, due to the passage of bilirubin through the ineffective blood-brain barrier of the fetus. Such pathologic change, which is not found in the adult brain, is called kernicterus.

Hemolytic disease of the newborn due to ABO incompatibilities is more frequent but the manifestations are much milder than those of the Rh factors.

Traumatic injuries of the newborn are most commonly associated with molding of the head of the infant in its passage through the pelvic canal during delivery. These are usually insignificant, such as caput succedaneum and cephalhematoma, which are eventually resorbed. More severe consequences include subdural hemorrhages, due to tears of the dural sinuses, falx cerebri, and tentorium cerebelli, which can lead to a fatal outcome. Occasionally, subcapsular hematoma and rupture of such hematoma into the peritoneal cavity complicate the breech extraction procedure. Fractures of the clavicle and long bones during delivery are very rare obstetric complications.

Diseases of Pregnancy

This review will be limited to diseases of pregnancy that are of general interest. More specialized topics are covered in the chapter on obstetrics and gynecology.

The most common complication of pregnancy is *spontaneous abortion*, which is defined as an expulsion of the fetus before it has developed sufficiently for extrauterine existence. It usually takes place in the first trimester, although an arbitrary dividing line between abortion and stillbirth has been set at 28 weeks of gestation. Because of the usually poor state of preservation of the products of gestation, pathologic studies are difficult. In the cases in which conclusions can be made, multiple and severe malformations are found in more than 50 per cent of the cases. Karyotype studies also show a similar incidence of severe chromosomal abnormalities, such as tetraploidy, triploidy, and aneuploidy of large chromosomes, which are usually incompatible with life.

Extrauterine implantation of the fertilized ovum, or *ectopic pregnancy*, occurs most frequently in the fallopian tube (tubal pregnancy). It invariably terminates in a rupture of the tube and intraabdominal hemorrhage, usually before the patient realizes that she is pregnant. It is therefore an important consideration in the differential diagnosis of an acute abdominal emergency in the female of a child-bearing age. In rare circumstances, ectopic pregnancy may occur in the abdominal cavity, which is compatible with a long survival of the fetus. The most common predisposing cause of ectopic pregnancy is chronic salpingitis.

Toxemia of pregnancy is a syndrome characterized by hypertension, massive proteinuria, and edema, usually initiated during the third trimester of pregnancy. In some cases, the condition terminates in episodic convulsions and coma, which is called *eclampsia*. The term *preeclampsia* is used when toxemia of pregnancy is of such severity that eventual development into eclampsia can be justifiably suspected. It serves as an indication that an appropriate preventive measure must be taken.

Eclampsia is frequently associated with *disseminated intravascular coagulation* (DIC), which is characterized by multiple fibrin thrombi in small blood vessels with a marked bleeding tendency. In the peripheral blood, fibrinogen, prothrombin, and many coagulation factors are markedly depleted. The appearance of fragmented erythrocytes (schistocytes) is also characteristic of the condition. In addition to hemorrhages in various organs, autopsy findings ocassionally include peripheral necrosis of the liver and cortical necrosis of the kidneys.

In *hydatidiform mole*, the placental villi become large, cystlike structures that are readily recognized on gross inspection. Microscopically, there is a severe edema of the villus with a complete or partial absence of the fetal vascularization. Atypical changes in the trophoblasts of different degrees are the usual findings. In more atypical cases, trophoblasts can be demonstrated in the myometrium. Such condition is called an *invasive mole (chorioadenoma destruens)*. Malignant transformation of trophoblasts corresponds to a malignant neoplasm, *choriocarcinoma*, which is a vascular neoplasm with a strong tendency to spread hematogenously. It is sensitive to a chemotherapeutic regime of methotrexate.

Congenital Malformations (Teratology)

It has been estimated that about two per cent of fetuses and newborn infants are affected with significant malformations; many of these are compatible with life. Musculoskeletal anomalies, which are usually not fatal, are the most common. In those that die during the neonatal period, cardiovascular defects and multiple malformations predominate.

Many congenital anomalies are due to point mutations with typical mendelian distribution. These include multiple polyposis of the colon, polydactyly, albinism, ectodermal dysplasia, xanthoma tuberosum, and many others. Some congenital malformations are associated with chromosomal abnormalities (trisomy 21 of Down's syndrome, Klinefelter's and Turner's syndromes, Trisomy 18 and 13). Most of these are consequences of mitotic errors. Environmentally induced malformations include the well-known rubella syndrome and phocomelia due to thalidomide, both acting during the critical period of morphogenesis (the first trimester). Other drugs and chemical or physical agents acting during this gestational period have also been strongly suspected as possible causes of congenital malformations, but they have not reached the epidemic proportions of the two agents mentioned. It must be noted that maternal rubella during the third trimester is occasionally followed by a generalized infection in the infant, rather than by congenital malformations.

Aging

Man and other animals have limited life spans. In man, many changes that are associated with aging are readily observable on external examination. These include the thinning and wrinkling of the skin, graying of hair, alterations of the general body form due to skeletal changes, and the frequent development of cataracts. Anatomically, atrophy of the heart and brain in older individuals is common. Microscopically, the accumulation of lipofuscin pigment in hepatocytes, myocardial fibers, and certain neurons with age has been observed since the beginning of the science of pathology. The apparent loss of neurons in the aging human brain has been corroborated by actual counting in the brains of aging rats. To this list must be added the increasing incidence of cardiovascular and neoplastic disease with age.

All the changes mentioned above, and the others that remain to be discovered, must depend on one basic mechanism which is responsible for the functional integrity of all the cells and tissues of the body. This mechanism is the regulated expression of gene activities in response to external and internal environments. Most modern theories of aging are based on this mechanism.

In one theory, the limited life span, and therefore the aging process, is programmed in the genetic constitution of the species and is therefore transmitted from one generation to the next. Other theories are based on somatic events in different cells of the body. Thus, one theory postulates somatic mutations, which may be spontaneous or environmentally induced, as the causes of differential alterations, of the activities of some cells or tissues of the body. These alterations which reside in the DNA of differenct cells, account for the different manifestations in aging. Other theories are based on occasional failures of transcription and translation of the genetic information. The pathogenesis of cell aging must therefore reside in the synthesis of mRNA and of the various proteins, including enzymes. It must be noted that these theories are not mutually exclusive. In the final analysis, it is highly probable that all of them may participate in the aging process.

Evidence in favor of these theories has been accumulating in the past few decades. First, extensive studies in a number of laboratories have shown that normal diploid cells of the species that have been investigated have limited life spans in culture. The life span is measured by the number of divisions that the cells can undergo. Thus, human cells have a replicative life span of approximately 50 generations, after which most of them fail to survive. Cells from other animals also have definite replicative capacity. Current data show that the number of divisions that cultured cells can undergo is correlated with the maximal life span of the species. Thus, cells of the turtle, which may live for more than 150 years, can survive 75 to 100 divisions, while those of the mouse, only 10 to 20 generations. In rare circumstances, certain cells in successive cultures become the so-called permanent cell lines, such as the Hela cells, originally derived from a human source. Such permanent cell lines, however, are no longer normal diploid cells. Their chromosome constitution varies greatly even in the same culture; some may be tetraploid and others, octaploid. This phenomenon has been called heteroploidy.

Evidence for somatic mutation is more difficult to obtain because these cells are not readily amenable to conventional genetic analysis. That the phenomenon exists has been shown in certain traits in animals and man. Evidence for altered gene expressions in somatic cells is readily obtained in immunologic data related to the "clonal" responses of lymphoid cells to different antigens.

NEOPLASMS (TUMORS)

Processes of Neoplasia

Neoplasms are aberrations of growth characterized by the abnormal, unregulated, excessive and uncontrolled multiplication of cells with the formation of a mass of new growth of tissue. The mass that develops serves no useful purpose, grows at the expense of normal structures, may even destroy normal tissues and, with rare exceptions, is of unknown cause. The mass that forms as a result of this abnormal cell proliferation may be localized, as in benign tumors, or spreading and invasive, as in malignant tumors, in which case the new growth not only invades and infiltrates the normal tissues in the region in which the neoplasm arose, but may also spread to more distant parts of the body via blood or lymph vessels. While the terms "tumors" and "neoplasm" are sometimes used interchangably, a tumor really refers to a swelling or mass, while a neoplasm is specifically an autonomous new growth. Thus, a neoplasm gives rise to a tumor, but all tumors or masses are not necessarily neoplasms.

Many varieties of neoplasms are known, for virtually all body cells may give rise to their development. In the benign and slowly growing tumors, the nature of the specific cellular origin is usually easy to determine because the cells tend to resemble the normal cells from which they were derived. In the more rapidly growing neoplasms, however, in which the rapidity of cell growth interferes with cellular differentiation, the cell of origin is often difficult, if not impossible, to recognize.

Neoplasms receive their nutrition from the blood, but their growth is autonomous and not controlled by the normal regulatory mechanisms of the host's body. Moreover, because growth is uncontrolled, the tumor cells grow faster than the normal cells around them, and a mass forms that increases in size. In the benign tumors the mass grows slowly and centrifugally, that is, from the center outward, pressing the normal tissues about it and compressing them to form a kind of enveloping membrane or capsule, unless the tumor is on a surface, in which case the new growth projects from the surface in papillary fashion, without a capsule. Malignant tumors, on the contrary, invade and infiltrate the surrounding tissues, the neoplastic cells resembling the roots of a plant in that they insinuate themselves between the adjacent normal tissue cells, often causing their atrophy and destruction.

Metastasis

Metastasis is the formation of new growths from a malignant tumor at locations removed from the original growth. Spread may be via lymphatics or blood vessels, or, in serous cavities, by implantation. Spread may also occur by direct extension within a tissue, or, by traversing fascial planes, by extension into surrounding tissues. In general, neoplasms seldom change in character and the metastases resemble the primary growth. Occasionally, however, a benign tumor may become malignant, and the metastases may differ considerably from the primary growth. Some malignant tumors tend to metastasize to specific organs or structures. Thus, carcinoma of the stomach, the large intestine, the pancreas and the breast frequently metastasize to the liver, while carcinoma of the prostate, the breast, the thyroid, the kidney, and sometimes the lung, are likely to metastasize to the bones. Carcinoma of the lung, one of the most malignant and rapidly growing of all tumors, also frequently metastasizes to the brain, adrenal, liver, and bones. Carcinomas most often metastasize by way of lymphatics, and sarcomas most often metastasize by way of blood stream (hematogenous spread).

Benign and Malignant Neoplasms

There is a succinct contrast between benign tumors and malignant tumors according to the criteria of differentiation, rate of growth, type of growth, and tendency to metastasize. Benign tumors are well differentiated, and the neoplastic cells resemble their normal cell of origin. Malignant tumors have a range of differentiation from well-differentiated tissue resembling the tissue of origin to a poorly differentiated or almost completely undifferentiate appearance. Benign tumors grow slowly and may stop growing or regress. Evidence of cell division, such as mitotic figures, is scarce. In malignant tumors, growth is usually rapid, mitotic figures are frequent, and there may be abnormal mitoses. Benign tumors expand by centripetal expansive growth and sometimes form capsules. Malignant tumors are characterized by infiltrative growth, and encapsulation is rare. Benign tumors do not metatasize. Almost all malignant tumors metastasize; the presence of metastases is definite evidence of a tumor's malignancy. Those malignant tumors that do not usually metastasize, such as gliomas of the central nervous system and basal cell carcinoma of the skin, are invasive and locally destructive even though they do not metastasize.

Growth, Grading, and Staging of Malignant Tumors

A malignant tumor is a progressive growth of poorly differentiated tissue that tends to invade surrounding normal tissues and spreads to other parts of the body by way of lymphatic channels or blood vessels. Eventually death ensues for one reason or another—from loss of appetite, weight and strength (the wasting away of cachexia), intercurrent infection such as bronchopenumonia, loss of function of an important organ, intoxication from tissue destruction, massive hemorrhage, etc.

Malignancy depends on many factors: (1) the type of tumor, (2) the cellular characteristics, such as the degree of anaplasia or differentiation, (3) the location, (4) the extent of the tumor, (5) the rate of growth, and (6) the age and condition of the patient. Ulceration and infection, although they do not influence the malignant process itself, may affect the outcome by hastening death. In general, the more undifferentiated the tissue, the greater the malignancy. These neoplasms are characterized by loss of cellular polarity, loss of natural architecture, variation in the shape and size of the cells, large chromatin-rich nuclei with large nucleoli, large numbers of mitoses that are abnormal in type and lead to irregular and distorted daughter cells, and little or no evidence anywhere of cellular maturity.

The malignancy of a tumor may be judged by the tumor's most anaplastic part rather than by its average structure. Invasion is also an important criterion of malignancy, but metastasis is absolute proof of it. From a clinical standpoint, it is valuable to have methods for estimating the biological behavior and extent of spread of a given neoplasm. Grading and staging of malignant tumors are done for this purpose. Grading of a tumor is done to provide an estimate of its aggressiveness based on differentiation of the tumor cells. Staging of a malignant tumor is based on the size of the primary lesion and the extent of spread by metastasis to regional lymph nodes and to distant sites. Tumors are usually graded on a scale of I to IV based on the degree of undifferentiation or anaplasia of the tumor cells. Staging is accomplished according to standardized staging systems developed by national and international cancer organizations.

Etiology

No single cause for the development of neoplasms is known. Various factors that seem to play a part in the production of new growths are well recognized, some of them inherent in the host, such as age, sex and heredity (intrinsic factors); others are forms of irritants extraneous to the host, such as the chemical agents, physical agents and living agents such as viruses or viruslike substances (extrinsic factors).

Definitions of terms necessary for understanding causative factors in cancer follow:

Carcinogen—any substance that will produce cancer.

Cocarcinogen—any substance that, acting alone, will not produce cancer, but when acting in conjunction with another substance, will produce cancer.

Procarcinogen—any substance that may be metabolized in the body and converted to act as a carcinogen.

Direct-acting carcinogen—any substance that will produce cancer without undergoing metabolic conversion (such a carcinogen is usually potent and has carcinogenic action in many species). Examples are beta propiolactone and nitrosamines.

Ultimate carcinogen—any active substance that is the metabolic conversion product of a chemical carcinogen and is ultimately responsible for initiation of the process of neoplasia.

Two additional definitions are related to Berenblum's two-stage hypothesis of cancer:

Initiator—any substance that initiates the process of neoplasia without necessarily producing a neoplasm.

Promoter—any substance that enhances the process of neoplasia once the process is initiated. An example of these two terms occurs in breast cancer in mice. A virus acts as an initiator in the presence of normal estrogen levels, the promoter. If the ovaries of the mice are removed to decrease estrogen levels, breast cancer will not develop in response to the tumor virus.

The major causative factors thought to be involved in the production of cancer are chemical carcinogens, tumor viruses, and carcinogenic irradiation. Certain hormones may also have some role in carcinogenesis. At least one parasitic organism, the blood fluke *(Schistosomia haematobium)* has been linked to one form of human cancer (cancer of the urinary bladder).

Chemical carcinogens are probably the primary cause of human cancer, especially in industralized nations. The first example of chemical carcinogenesis was observed by Percival Pott in 1775 when he recognized that carcinoma in the scrotal area of chimney sweeps was due to irritation caused by the accumulation of soot in this area of the body.

Polycyclic hydrocarbons act as procarcinogens which are broken down to ultimate carcinogens that bind to DNA. Examples are 3,4-benzpyrene (in cigarette smoke), 9,10-dimethylbenzanthracene, and cholanthrene. Aromatic amines such as butter yellow, (dimethylaminobenzine), 2-naphthalamine, and 2-acetoimmunofluorene cause tumors in some experimental animals. Alkylating agents such as nitrogen mustards, cyclophosphamide, and several other chemotherapeutic drugs are direct-acting carcinogens. Nitrosamines are potent direct-acting carcinogens that affect a variety of animal species. These may be formed when nitrates in the diet combine with proteins. Aflatoxins produced in stored peanuts by aspergillus fungus are potent carcinogens that act in several species. Exposure to metals such as chromium, uranium and and nickel has been associated wtih increased incidence of lung cancer. Asbestos, particularly in combination with habitual cigarette smoking, causes a greatly increased risk of lung cancer. Exposure to asbestos has also been associated with the development of mesothelioma of the pleura, a very rare tumor.

A recently discovered chemical carcinogen is vinyl chloride (or polyvinyl chloride), which produces a very rare malignant lesion in man called angiosarcoma of the liver. Incidence of this tumor is almost entirely due to exposure to vinyl chloride, and is an occupational risk of some workers in the plastics industry.

Radiation carcinogenesis includes the effects of solar or ultraviolet radiation, as well as ionizing radiation from x-rays, nuclear fission, and radionuclides. Radiation injury is a well documented carcinogen. Ultraviolet rays from the sun may lead to squamous cell carcinoma and basal cell carcinoma of the skin. Actinic keratosis (senile keratosis) is a recognized precursor of skin cancer. Light-complexioned individuals are more susceptible to the development of skin cancers than are dark-skinned individuals. These skin cancers obviously tend to occur on the exposed surfaces of the skin.

The carcinogenic effects of ionizing radiation have been known for many years. Radiologists have a higher incidence of leukemia than the general population, and before proper precautions were observed, radiologists developed skin cancers on the hands, when they personally positioned patients while roentgenograms were taken. Radioactive strontium, a product of nuclear fallout from atomic testing, is a source of ionizing radiation to humans and is suspected of causing osteogenic sarcoma. Strontium-irradiated experimental animals have been found to develop osteogenic sarcoma. Radium workers who painted radium onto watch dials were found to have a higher than normal incidence of osteogenic sarcoma. Thorotrast, a radioopaque drug now banned in the United States and previously used in radiocontrast studies of the liver and spleen, is a low emitter of radioactivity and is suspected of causing hepatoma. The practice of treatment of enlarged thymus in children by irradiation during the 1950s has resulted in the development of papillary carcinoma of the thyroid by some of these patients. Individuals exposed to the Hiroshima atomic bomb have a higher rate of leukemia and carcinoma of the thyroid, breast and lung as compared to unexposed individuals. Ionizing radiation produces mutations by damaging DNA.

Tumor Viruses

Viruses are well established as causes of a variety of benign and malignant tumors in many animal species. While certain viruses have been closely associated with several human neoplasms, viruses have not been conclusively established as a definite cause of a single form of human cancer to date. Tumor viruses include DNA viruses and RNA viruses. Both can insert themselves into the host genome as DNA sequences. Oncogenic RNA viruses are known as oncorna viruses—a contraction of oncogenic RNA viruses. The oncorna viruses have been shown to cause leukemia and the Rous sarcoma in chickens, leukemia and sarcoma in mice, mouse mammary tumor (Bittner tumor) in mice, leukemia and sarcoma in cats, and sarcomas, lymphosarcoma and mammary carcinoma in monkeys. No human RNA viruses have been shown to cause human cancer or to transform human cells or other cells.

DNA viruses include the papova viruses (papilloma, polyoma, and vacuolating virus), adenoviruses, and herpes viruses. They all have the capacity to insert themselves into the DNA of host cells and cause neoplastic transformation. Among the papova viruses, papilloma viruses cause papillary tumors in animals, e.g., Shope papilloma in rabbits. They also cause warts and laryngial papillomas (benign tumors) in man. The polyoma virus is widespread in mice. It is so named because it is capable of inducing a large variety of tumors in newborn hamsters. The simian virus 40 (SV40) is derived from rhesus monkey cells. It induces tumors in hamsters in vivo and also transforms human, monkey, mouse, and rat cells in vitro.

Herpes viruses induce a number of tumors in chickens, frogs, and monkeys. One of these herpes viruses, the Epstein-Barr virus (EBV), has strong, but not proven, associations with Burkitt's lymphoma (a highly malignant lymphomatous neoplasm of children, first discovered in Africa) and with nasopharyngeal carcinoma. The EBV is the established cause of infectious mononucleosis, a benign hematological disease. Another herpes virus suspected of being related to the development of human cancer is herpes simplex II (HSV-II), which is implicated in carcinoma of the uterine cervix. There is no proof that the strong associations between Epstein-Barr virus and Burkitt's lymphoma or nasopharyngeal carcinoma and herpes simplex II and cervical carcinoma are definitely causative.

Classification of Neoplasms

Tumors are generally classified on the basis of the type of cell or tissue from which they arise, as well as from their characteristic structure. (see Table 6-1 for this classification.)

Important Tumors, Malignant and Benign, of Different Organs

Lip, Tongue and Mouth. Carcinoma occurs frequently in these areas and is highly malignant. About 75 per cent of these cases are found in males and practically all are of squamous cell type. Fissures, ulcers, papillomas and areas of leukoplakia should receive prompt attention because malignant growths not infrequently develop at the site of such lesions, and, by the time the malignant nature of the process is recognized, the lesion is rarely curable for metastases to the deep cervical lymph nodes have usually occurred. Most of these tumors are related to use of tobacco in one form or another.

Esophagus. Esophageal carcinoma is of frequent occurrence, about 75 per cent being found in males. It usually is of squamous cell type, frequently with cornification, though adenocarcinoma originating in mucous glands also occurs. The tumor may perforate into the trachea, the larynx or the mediastinum or it may metastasize locally. If it is situated at the cardiac orifice, it may metastasize to the liver.

Stomach. Although carcinoma of the stomach is still a very important and lethal form of malignant disease, it has diminished in incidence in the United States in recent years but is common in a number of other countries, e.g., Japan, Chile and Iceland, where the increased incidence may be related to dietary customs. Up to 30 years ago it was the most frequent form of cancer in males in this country but is now a less frequent cause of death than cancer of the lung, colon and breast. The incidence of cancer of the stomach in females is about half that in males. Roughly 90 per cent of these carcinomas occur after the age of 40. About 60 per cent are pyloric, causing stenosis and obstruction. Massive hemorrhage from such tumors is rare. The evidence that gastric carcinoma can originate in a chronic peptic ulcer is only suggestive, and the vast majority of these neoplasms appear to arise independently. The most common type is ulcerat-

TABLE 6-1. Classification of Neoplasms

I. Tumors of Epithelial Tissues

Benign	Malignant Counterpart
Papilloma	Carcinoma
Squamous papilloma	Squamous cell carcinoma
	Basal cell carcinoma
Transitional cell papilloma	Transitional cell carcinoma
	Mucoepidermoid carcinoma
Adenoma	Adenocarcinoma
Cystadenoma	Cystadenocarcinoma
	Adenoacanthoma
Keratoacanthoma	
Hydatidiform mole	Choriocarcinoma

II. Tumors of Nonhematopoietic Mesenchymal Tissues

A. Soft Tissue

Benign	Malignant Counterpart
Lipoma	Liposarcoma
Myxoma	Myxosarcoma
Fibroma	Fibrosarcoma
Fibrous histiocytoma	Malignant fibrous histiocytoma
Fibroxanthoma	Malignant fibroxanthoma
Desmoid fibromatosis	Fibrosarcoma
Leiomyoma	Leiomyosarcoma
Rhabdomyoma	Rhabdomyosarcoma
Hemangioma	Hemangiosarcoma
Lymphangioma	Lymphangiosarcoma
Hemangioendothelioma	Malignant hemangioendothelioma
Hemangiopericytoma	Malignant hemangiopericytoma
Synovioma	Synovial sarcoma
Paraganglioma	Alveolar soft part sarcoma

B. Bone and Cartilage

Benign	Malignant Counterpart
Osteoma (Exostosis)	Osteogenic sarcoma
Chondroma	Chondrosarcoma
Osteochondroma	Chondrosarcoma arising in osteochondroma
Chordoma	Malignant chordoma
Osteoblastoma	Osteogenic sarcoma
Chondroblastoma	Chondrosarcoma
Giant cell tumor	Malignant giant cell tumor
	Ewing's sarcoma

III. Tumors of Hematopoietic Tissues

Benign	Malignant Counterpart
Primary polycythemia	Leukemia
"Pseudolymphoma"	Malignant lymphoma
	a) Malignant lymphoma, histiocytic
	b) Malignant lymphoma, lymphocytic, well differentiated
	c) Malignant lymphoma, lymphocytic, poorly differentiated
	d) Malignant lymphoma, undifferentiated (Burkitt's)
	e) Malignant lymphoma, Hodgkin's type
	f) Multiple myeloma
	g) Mycosis fungoides

IV. Tumors of Neural Tissues

Benign	Malignant Counterpart
Neurilemoma, Neurofibroma	Malignant Schwannoma, Neurofibrosarcoma
Ganglioneuroma	Ganglioneuroblastoma
Meningioma	Meningeal sarcoma
	Neuroblastoma
	Retinoblastoma
	Astrocytoma
	Oligodendroglioma
	Glioblastoma multiforme
	Medulloblastoma
	Ependymoma
Pheochromocytoma	Malignant pheochromocytoma
"Neuroma" (Traumatic)	

V. Germ Cell Tumors

Benign	Malignant Counterpart
	Seminoma (Dysgerminoma)
	Embryonal carcinoma
	Choriocarcinoma
Benign teratoma	Malignant teratoma

VI. Miscellaneous

Benign	Malignant Counterpart
Mixed tumor	Malignant mixed tumor
Melanocytic nevus	Malignant melanoma
	Carcinosarcoma
	Wilm's tumor (nephroblastoma)

ing adenocarcinoma, which invades the stomach wall and may extend into the lumen. It may be medullary or mucinous in part. Nearly as common is the fungating or polypoid type that projects as a large cauliflower-like mass into the gastric lumen. Somewhat less common is the diffusely infiltrating form that may spread superficially in the mucosa but more commonly invades the entire gastric wall, causing great thickening and hardening and leading to the designation *linitis plastica carcinoma*.

Gastric carcinoma spreads through the lymphatics to the peritoneal cavity, with secondary growths in the ovaries or the rectovesical pouch. Extension through the veins to the liver is very common, as well as invasion of the transverse colon, the pancreas and the spleen. The outcome is almost invariably fatal.

Small Intestine. *Carcinomas of the duodenum and the jejunoileum are rare.* They may be adenocarcinoma or scirrhous carcinoma.

Appendix. Carcinoid of the appendix or other portions of the intestinal tract occurs rarely. The cytoplasm of the cells has an affinity for chrome and silver salts (chromaffin, argentaffin). This neoplasm is at least locally malignant and, especially when it occurs in sites other than the appendix, is locally invasive and may metastasize.

Carcinoid Syndrome. When a carcinoid arising in a site outside the appendix metastasizes to the liver or the lungs, or to both, a group of symptoms and pathologic changes that has been termed the carcinoid syndrome may occur: flushing of the skin, a peculiar type of cyanosis, bronchial constriction with asthma-like attacks, and diarrhea. For some time these symptoms were attributed to the release by these tumors of *serotonin* (5-hydroxytryptamine), but this is questionable and the cause of this syndrome must await further study.

Large Intestine. Cancer of the large intestine is now one of the most malignant tumors. The incidence is about equal in males and females. This tumor now ranks with the lung and the breast as one of the most common sites of malignant disease. Although carcinoma of the large intestine occurs most often in older age groups, a number of cases of carcinoma of the rectum or colon have been reported in individuals from 3½ to 20 years of age. The majority of colonic cancers occur in the sigmoid colon and rectum, the cecum being less often involved. These are columnar cell adenocarcinomas, often producing much mucus. In the sigmoid colon the neoplasm may be quite fibrous and contractile, thus causing stenosis and obstruction. Some carcinomas represent malignant change in villous polyps or adenomas. If the lymph nodes are not involved, carcinomas above the rectum are more likely to be operable, with a more favorable outcome than carcinoma of the rectum itself. Bleeding is the most common first symptom. Carcinoma of the anal canal is of the squamous cell type and is highly malignant. A small cell type of carcinoma of the colon and the rectum also occurs, but it is rare, and the prognosis is better than for other types.

Pancreas, Gallbladder and Liver. *Carcinoma of the Pancreas* forms about one per cent; of the gallbladder, from two to four per cent; of the bile ducts and the liver, less than one per cent of all carcinomas. Pancreatic carcinoma is usually in the head. In this site it may invade or compress the pancreatic ducts and the common bile duct, with the consequences of obstruction in the pancreas (digestive disturbance, emaciation) and the liver (icterus). The majority are of the scirrhous type, frequently complicated by suppuration. Metastasis to the lymph nodes occur early, and metastasis to the liver is common. The outcome is fatal.

Respiratory Tract. *Carcinoma of the larynx* is about ten times as common in males as in females and is usually found on the true vocal cords, although about one fourth of the cases are extrinsic, that is,

external to the laryngeal mucosa and potentially more serious. The intrinsic lesion is squamous cell in type and may be cured, if superficial, by conservative surgery and, if invasive, by laryngectomy. Metastases may involve the cervical and submaxillary lymph nodes. Direct invasion of the esophagus may occur. Primary carcinoma of the trachea is rare. The relative risk of developing carcinoma of the larynx is five times greater in cigarette smokers than in nonsmokers.

Carcinoma of the lung is one of the most common and most lethal of malignant diseases, being today the leading cause of death from cancer in men and the rate in women appears to be increasing. The disease occurs chiefly in men in the 40- to 60-year age group and is usually of bronchial origin but may arise in bronchioles as well. Adenocarcinoma of mucous gland origin sometimes occurs but is uncommon.

With the development of bronchoscopy, the cytologic technique of Papanicolaou and early biopsy, in association with roentgenographic visualization, the existence of such growths is being detected earlier, and more cases are being recognized. One of the first clinical symptoms of bronchogenic carcinoma is the insidious development of a persistent hacking cough. Pleuritic pain, dyspnea and sometimes pleural effusion may occur, but in some cases the disease develops so insidiously that the first signs are loss of weight and appetite, and by this time the disease is widespread. Inflammatory processes of the bronchi, by stimulating epithelial proliferation, may be an etiologic factor. Recently, great emphasis has been placed upon cigarette smoking as the most important cause of bronchogenic carcinoma, especially of the squamous and "oat cell" types, because, in both male and female patients, a history of chain smoking (two packs or more a day) and deep inhaling of the smoke has been elicited in a large percentage of the cases. Although a direct causal connection has not yet been established, a merely fortuitous relationship is most unlikely since recent statistical studies have shown that bronchogenic carcinoma is approximately 20 times more frequent in men who are heavy cigarette smokers than in nonsmokers. It may be, too, that carcinogenic compounds that are present in air polluted by automobile exhaust fumes and other hydrocarbon-containing agents play a role, since this form of carcinoma is more common in heavy-smoking city dwellers than in those who live in rural areas. Pipe and cigar smokers do not often develop carcinoma of the bronchi since they rarely inhale the smoke, but even they, as well as cigarette smokers who have given up the habit, run a greater risk than those who never smoked.

The possible part played by chemical carcinogens that have been isolated from the tarry extracts of cigarette smoke is at present still the subject of considerable controversy and much investigation, both statistical and experimental, and all that can be said at the moment is that cigarette smoking is markedly implicated in the clinical causation of cancer of the bronchus in men and women.

Histologically, bronchogenic carcinoma, arising from the bronchial mucosa, is the most common type of lung cancer. The most frequent histologic type is the squamous cell or epidermoid carcinoma, followed by adenocarcinoma and the highly undifferentiated forms such as the small cell undifferentiated carcinoma (including "oat cell type"), the pleomorphic type and the giant cell type.

Mediastinal metastases may compress the thoracic viscera, and pleuritic effusions, pneumonia, lung abscess and bronchiectasis are frequent complications. Metastases usually occur to the bronchial and the mediastinal lymph nodes and to the cervical nodes, the adrenals, the brain and the bones, but they may develop in other sites.

Breast. Carcinoma of the breast is the most common malignant tumor in women, accounting for nearly 25 per cent of all malignant neoplasms. It is rare under the age of 25. Nulliparous women or women whose first full term pregnancy occurs late in their reproductive life are at an increased risk. This suggests that prolonged estrogen activity unbroken by the hormonal changes that take place during pregnancy may play a significant role in the development of the disease. Extension to the axillary lymph nodes occurs early, often before the tumor is discovered or the axillary nodes are palpable. Axillary metastases are found in about two-thirds of the patients at operation.

Trauma plays no part in the etiology of cancer of the breast. Some evidence supports the hypothesis that high fat diet increases the risk, especially for postmenopausal tumors. Premenopausal tumors have a higher frequency of familial aggregation, the susceptibility being genetically transmitted by either of the two parents.

The main morphologic types of breast carcinoma are the following:

1. Infiltrating ductal carcinoma, composed of solid cords of epithelial cells, probably of ductal origin, usually surrounded by dense collagen reactive bands (desmoplasia) which gives the tumor a hard consistency (sclerosing or scirrhous) and often leads to nipple retraction and adhesions to the skin (peau d' orange).
2. Infiltrating lobular carcinoma, made up of smaller epithelial cells resembling those of the mammary lobules which invade the stroma, forming "indian files". Prognostically, it behaves like infiltrating ductal carcinoma.

3. Mucinous (colloid) carcinoma, characterized by abundant mucous secretions.
4. Medullary carcinoma, formed by solid masses of atypical epithelial cells that do not form ducts or glands and have abundant lymphoid stroma.
5. Intraductal carcinoma, corresponds to the in situ variety of ductal carcinoma. It most frequently has a papillary or a "comedo" pattern, characterized by necrosis of the neoplastic cells at the center of each cystic duct.
6. Lobular carcinoma in situ, precursor of the invasive lobular type.
7. Paget's disease is characterized by chronic eczematoid lesion of the nipple, produced by invasion of the epidermis by large, clear, neoplastic epithelial cells presumably originating in the collecting ducts.
8. Less frequent types of breast neoplasms are the cystosarcoma phyllodes, which tends to metastasize via the blood stream; the metaplastic carcinomas, which may have squamous, cartilaginous or osteoid components; tubular carcinoma, which carries a better prognosis; and secretory carcinoma, the predominant variety on the rare occasion that the tumor occurs in children. The so-called inflammatory carcinoma, clinically characterized by redness and pain, is due to massive permeation of lymphatic channels and carries a very poor prognosis.

Metastatic Breast Tumors. In addition to the axillary lymph nodes, carcinoma of the breast may metastasize to the mediastinal and other distant lymph nodes, as well as the lungs, the liver, bones, adrenals, and brain. Widespread invasion of the skin of the thoracic wall also occurs. If biopsy reveals no metastasis in the axillary nodes, 65 per cent are curable. With axillary metastasis, only approximately 20 per cent are curable.

Uterus. Carcinoma of the cervix uteri is less frequent than breast carcinoma and its incidence has been decreasing steadily during the last decade. Carcinoma in situ is more frequent in the 30s; while the invasive carcinoma is more frequent after age 40. It mostly originates around the squamocollumnar junction and is preceded by dysplastic changes whose detection by vaginal cytology helps prevent invasive disease. The great majority of cervical carcinomas are of the squamous cell type. Endometrial carcinoma, a postmenopausal neoplasm, is becoming the most common invasive carcinoma of the uterus.

Ovary. The most common and important tumors of the ovary are cystadenoma, dermoid cyst, fibroma, Brenner tumor and dysgerminoma, which are nonfunctioning, and granulosa cell tumor, theca cell tumor (thecoma) and arrhenoblastoma, which have some functional properties.

The cystadenoma is a nonfunctioning tumor that may be serous, simple and papillary or pseudomucinous. Any one of these types may undergo malignant change.

The dermoid cyst is a benign teratoid tumor, usually cystic, with a grayish-yellow sebaceous material, mixed with a variable amount of hair, in the cavity. Skin and skin appendages and a variety of other tissues, including teeth and bone, may be found in at least a portion of this type of tumor. Unless representatives of all three embryonic layers are present, it is not a true teratoma. Chorionepithelioma of the ovary does occur very rarely and resembles similar tumors of the testis.

The fibroma of the ovary is like fibroma in any other portion of the body. It may be present in both ovaries. The association of ascites, and especially of hydrothorax (Meigs' syndrome), with this type of tumor is an interesting but unexplained phenomenon. Removal of the tumor results in disappearance of the serous effusion.

The Brenner tumor usually is found after the menopause and has no endocrinogenic function. The tumor is mainly fibrous, with islands or strands of epithelial cells throughout the stroma. The origin of this epithelium is not established.

The dysgerminoma is a nonfunctioning tumor and is analogous in origin and similar in appearance to the seminoma of the testis but usually is less malignant. It is found frequently in both ovaries.

The granulosa cell tumor is the most common of the functioning tumors of the ovary. It is characterized by the production of excessive estrogenic hormone. In a child, this results in precocious sexual development, both anatomic and functional, that disappears when the tumor is removed, and it may cause either amenorrhea or excessive menstruation in an adult. If it occurs after the menopause, resumption of menstruation is a characteristic feature. This is associated with endometrial hyperplasia. Some of these tumors may undergo malignant change.

The theca cell tumor resembles in some respects the granulosa cell tumor and in others a fibroma. Irregular uterine bleeding associated with endometrial hyperplasia is characteristic of this condition in the adult. The characteristic feature is the presence of doubly refractive lipoid material in fine droplets in the cells.

The arrhenoblastoma is the masculinizing tumor that is supposed to arise from embryonic cell rests. Amenorrhea, sterility and atrophy of the breasts, associated with hirsutism, deep voice and hypertrophy of the clitoris, are characteristic features. These effects resemble those of some forms of adrenal cortical tumor. Ana-

tomically these tumors vary from the well-differentiated type, characterized by the presence tubules, like those of the testis, to the highly undifferentiated sarcomatous type.

For other tumors of female genital tract, see the chapter on obstetrics and gynecology.

Testis. Tumors of the testis are almost all malignant and comprise less than one per cent of the malignant tumors in males. When this occurs they usually involve men in their 20s, 30s, and 40s.

Benign tumors of the testis are rare. The interstitial (Leydig) cell tumor is masculinizing, and the Sertoli cell tumor is a feminizing neoplasm. In addition to their hormonal qualities, they have in common the presence of lipoid or lipochrome in the cytoplasm of the tumor cells. In both, the cells are uniformly round or polygonal, with relatively clear cytoplasm and no mitoses or abnormal nuclear forms unless they undergo malignant change.

Malignant tumors of the testis may be divided into well-differentiated teratoma, seminoma, embryonal carcinoma and chorionepithelioma.

Teratoma contains different types of tissue, varying from the well-differentiated adult form to highly undifferentiated malignant tissue. Cartilage, bone, muscle, and adenoid, myxomatous and adipose tissue may be found. However, in many of these tumors, foci of seminoma, embryonal carcinoma or even chorionepithelioma also may be discovered if sought for diligently by section of the tumor into thin slices.

Seminoma is composed of fairly uniform polygonal cells with a moderate amount of light-staining cytoplasm. The cytoplasm of these cells may be granular or chromophobic. There may be a considerable number of lymphoid cells between the large polygonal cells (seminoma with lymphoid stroma), and there may be foci of necrosis and hemorrhage throughout the tumor tissue. The corresponding ovarian tumor is called dysgerminoma and is less malignant than the seminoma.

Embryonal carcinoma shows many pseudoacinic structures, slits or irregularly shaped spaces, all lined by one or more layers of high cuboidal epithelial cells and suggesting glandular structures. Between these structures there may be large and small masses of polygonal and round cells, which vary in size and shape, containing mitoses and abnormal nuclear forms. All of these epithelial structures are supported by a dense or a loosely arranged fibrous stroma. Occasionally there are syncytial masses of epithelial cells growing in sheets. *Teratocarcinoma* refers to a mixture of embryonal carcinoma and teratoma.

Choriocarcinoma is composed of tissue similar to that of choricarcinoma in the female, with syncytiotrophoblasts and cytotrophoblasts present as essential components of the tumor. The tumor is unusually vascular and at times shows only focal areas of highly atypical trophoblastic tissue, in association with a teratoid tumor.

The blood and urine of some patients with one of the above malignant teratoid testicular tumors may contain a pituitary-like gonadotropic hormone that, when injected into appropriate animals, will give a positive pregnancy test. Detection of the hormone in such cases can be helpful in diagnosis.

Prostate. Carcinoma of the prostate is one of the four most common malignant tumors in men. It is described more at length in the section on the male genital system.

Thyroid. Tumors of the thyroid gland are mainly the microfollicular (fetal), and macrofollicular (colloid), the papillary and the solid (Hürthle cell) adenomas and carcinoma. These are described at greater length in the section on the Endocrine System (pp. 535 and 536).

Pituitary Gland. Most neoplasms of the pituitary gland arise in the anterior lobe, and are benign. They are traditionally classified according to light microscopic criteria as chromophobic, eosinophilic, or basophilic adenomas. Functional classifications according to endocrine activity as determined by clinical findings, measurement of hormone levels and responses, histochemical studies of the tumor cells, and electron microscopy are under investigation. Most adenomas are inactive hormonally and are chromophobic, i.e., the tumor cells contain no stainable granules. They cause symptoms by overgrowing and destroying normal pituitary tissue and the adjacent optic and hypothalamic structures. Hypopituitarism, blindness, and hypothalamic dysfunction may result. The tumor cells may be arranged in diffuse, sinusoidal, or pseudopapillary patterns. The cells tend to be uniform and polygonal with a richly vascular stroma. These neoplasms may expand the sella turcica, erode its walls, and escape from its confines to encroach on adjacent structures. They are gray-red and encapsulated, sometimes undergoing cystic and hemorrhagic changes. They occur most commonly in middle-aged adults and affect both sexes.

Adenomas, inducing gigantism and acromegaly, are usually composed of cells with acidophilic granules. They are usually smaller than chromophobic adenomas, and the cells are often pleomorphic. Prolactin-secreting adenomas may be acidophilic or chromophobic. Adenomas secreting adrenocorticotropic hormone are usually small and composed, at least partly, of cells with basophilic granules. The granules are PAS positive. These tumors are one of the causes of Cushing's syndrome. Thyrotropin-secreting adenomas may be chromophobic or basophilic.

Craniopharyngiomas are intimately related to the pituitary gland and its stalk. They are thought to be derived from remnants of Rathke's pouch and most commonly occur as suprasellar cystic lesions with calcified walls containing brown fluid rich in cholesterol. They appear in childhood, adolescence, and adult life. Endocrine disturbances may be produced by encroachment of the encapsulated lesion on the hypothalamus and pituitary gland, and the optic system may be damaged by gradually expansive growth of the lesion. Protrusion into the third ventricle may cause hydrocephalus. Microscopically these tumors are usually composed of nests of benign stratified squamous cells surrounded by basal cells in a loose fibrovascular stroma somewhat resembling the adamantinoma or ameloblastoma.

Carotid Body Tumor. This tumor, which develops in the carotid body, is relatively rare and occurs most frequently in the third to the seventh decades. Usually it is unilateral and is associated closely with the region of the bifurcation of the common carotid artery. It grows slowly, is of variable size, frequently appears lobulated, has a definite capsule, is movable from side to side, but not up and down, and may appear to pulsate. Although the tumor usually is benign, it may be locally invasive and may recur if it is not removed completely. Macroscopically the parenchyma is divided by bands of well-vascularized fibrous stroma that merge with the capsule. Microscopically the alveolar masses of parenchyma are composed of large, polygonal cells with a granular eosinophilic, sometimes vacuolated, cytoplasm. The nuclei usually are uniform but may vary in size and shape and may be hyperchromatic.

Malignant Melanoma

This is one of the most malignant of neoplasms, originating in melanoblasts of the ectoderm. The cutaneous form often develops from a flat, hairless mole or nevus that may be light or dark brown in color. Usually these nevi are benign, but if such a lesion begins to darken, to show unusual growth activity or to break down, ulcerate and bleed, malignant transformation should be suspected. Often such a nevus may have become malignant and actually have developed metastases before it attracts the attention of the patient. In general, the hairy, elevated, papillary moles uncommonly become malignant. It should also be noted here that malignant melanomas are uncommon before puberty.

Dissemination occurs through the lymphatics and the bloodstream as well as through the skin. The amount of pigment is no indication of malignancy, which is shown rather by an increase of cytoplasm, hyperchromatic nuclei and mitoses, especially abnormal ones. The regional nodes always are involved before the growth spreads to other parts of the body. Metastasis may occur anywhere but is most frequent in the regional lymph nodes, the skin, the liver and the lungs. It is one malignant tumor that occasionally metastasizes to the myocardium. The eye is a frequent primary site, the growth developing in the choroid, the iris or the ciliary body. Occasionally, melanomas are primary in the meninges or in the anal or the rectal mucosa. The prognosis in all cases is grave.

Malignant Lymphoma

The term malignant lymphoma is applied to lymphomas other than Hodgkin's disease. Malignant lymphomas are usually considered as neoplastic disorders; however, their true nature is not completely understood. They behave as neoplasms in that they progressively spread and cause death unless controlled by treatment. The lymphomas usually begin in lymph nodes, however, they are also found in extranodal lymphoid tissue.

The classification of malignant lymphomas is a controversial subject, and details of various classifications are beyond the scope of this review. The Lukes-Collins classification is based on the origin of lymphomas from T or B lymphocytes and subclassification under these categories. The Rappaport classification of lymphomas is based on the basic pattern of growth, nodular (follicular) lymphomas and diffuse lymphomas with subclassifications according to cell type. The importance of classification is related to prognosis and therapy. In addition to these two classifications, there is a grading of lymphomas by degree of differentiation with grade I (the nodular variants and lesions composed of well differentiated lymphocytes) having a better prognosis, and grade II lymphomas having a poorer prognosis and being made up of poorly differentiated or undifferentiated cells.

Hodgkin's Disease

Hodgkin's disease usually begins in a lymph node or chain of nodes. The mediastinal, cervical and retroperitoneal nodes are frequently the first chains involved. With time, the disease spreads to contiguous chains of nodes and to other parts of the body in a largely predictable pattern.

The gross appearance of the nodes depends upon the histological classification (see Table 6–2 for histological patterns). The nodes are enlarged, soft, with a uniform fish-flesh appearance in the lymphocyte predominance pattern. Enlarged nodes with foci of opaque, yellowish areas of necrosis are characteristics of the mixed cellularity pattern. In the nodular sclerosis

TABLE 6-2 Classification of Hodgkin's Disease

Type	Relative Frequency	Five Year Survival
Lymphocyte predominance	10%	90%
Mixed cellularity	35–60%	70%
Nodular sclerosis	35–60%	50–70%
Lymphocyte depletion	5–10%	20%

and lymphocyte depletion types the involved nodes are usually firm and uniformly gray white.

The histologic features of each of the four types of Hodgkin's disease are capsulized in the nomenclature. The diagnostic feature of all of these is the presence of Reed-Sternberg cells. The Reed-Sternberg giant cell is usually bilobed or binucleate with the nuclear halves appearing as mirror images. There is a large amount of amphophilic cytoplasm and prominent nuclei with large nucleoli usually surrounded by a clear halo (owl-eyed nuclei). Lacunar Reed-Sternberg cells with single-lobed nuclei and pale-staining cytoplasm are characteristic of one of the four patterns, the nodular sclerosing type.

The histologic classification system is important both for prognosis and therapy. In general the more numerous the lymphocytes, the more favorable the prognosis.

Chloroma

This rare tumor occurs primarily in association with myelocytic leukemia, usually the acute type. It is composed of cells of the lymphocytic, monocytic or myelocytic types. In the gross, the striking feature of this tumor is its light green color, which probably is caused by some breakdown product of hemoglobin, perhaps protoporphyrin.

Multiple Myeloma

Multiple myeloma is a multicentric tumor of plasma cells that develops in the red bone marrow of many parts of the skeletal system. Any bone may be involved, but those most commonly affected are the vertebrae, the ribs, the skull, the pelvis, the femur and, to a lesser extent, the ends of the long bones, the sternum, the clavicles and the scapula. The tumors are multiple, small, soft, gelatinous, shiny, pinkish-red and vascular. They largely replace the marrow tissue at the sites of involvement and erode and destroy the adjacent compact or cortical bone, leading in the long bones to spontaneous or pathologic fracture with resulting deformity and in the flat bones to punched-out areas of bone destruction. Extension into adjacent soft tissue is not uncommon, and in the late stages of the disease widespread metastases may develop.

Histologically the tumors are composed of vast numbers of cells that have all the characteristics of plasma cells in that they have small, dark eccentric nuclei in which the chromatin is radially or peripherally arranged and adjacent to which there may be the typical clear zone in the cytoplasm. Mitoses are uncommon, but the neoplastic character of the growths is shown by the presence of abnormal multinucleate or giant plasma cell types. Myeloma cells may infiltrate the kidneys, liver and spleen, sometimes even simulating leukemic infiltration of these organs.

A curious characteristic of these tumors is the elaboration of a variety of gamma globulins, some of which appear to be abnormal, that accumulate in the blood. In addition, in about half of the cases the urine is found to contain a globulin-like substance known for many years as Bence Jones protein but now believed to be a polypeptide, presumably of gamma globulin origin. This substance coagulates at low temperatures (40 to 60 C), dissolves on boiling but reprecipitates on cooling to 60 C. Many cases are also associated with a form of amyloidosis that resembles primary systemic amyloidosis in its incidence, general distribution and variability of staining reactions. There may be severe renal damage as a result of the precipitation of the Bence Jones protein in the tubules. Casts of the precipitated protein fill and obstruct the lumina of the tubules, with consequent atrophy of the nephrons. A feature characteristic of myeloma is a foreign-body type of reaction around the casts in the lumina of the tubules. Multiple myeloma usually terminates fatally. Plasmacytoma is a solitary tumor of plasma cells.

Neoplasms of the Central Nervous System

Various neoplasms affect the central nervous system by arising from the nerve cells or glia of the brain and spinal cord, the meninges, or the nerve roots. Gliomas of astrocytic, ependymal, aligodendroglial and microglial derivation occur in characteristic patterns, locations, and age groups. Neoplasms of nerve cells are rare. Meningiomas and neurilemomas are usually benign surface lesions indenting but not invading the parenchyma. Metastatic neoplasms involve the central nervous system much more commonly than primary neoplasms and may originate anywhere in the body. These will be discussed in greater detail in the section on the nervous system.

IMMUNOPATHOLOGY (HYPERSENSITIVITY, AUTOIMMUNITY, IMMUNOLOGIC DEFICIENCIES, GRAFT REJECTION)

The principles of immunity and the effectiveness of the immune system in man are described in detail in the chapter on microbiology and immunology. However, since disorders of this system are an important part of pathology, some of them will be considered briefly here with the main emphasis on immunologic tissue injury or hypersensitivity reactions, immunologic deficiency and graft rejection.

Hypersensitivity Reactions

Classification of immunologic tissue injury or hypersensitivity reactions includes anaphylactic hypersensitivity, cytotoxic hypersensitivity, immune complex hypersensitivity and cell-mediated hypersensitivity.

Anaphylactic hypersensitivity is a rapidly developing immunologic reaction that occurs almost immediately after the contact of an antigen within an individual previously sensitized to the antigen. The reaction may be systemic or local. Systemic reactions may produce shock that may be fatal. Local reactions may be manifest as hives, allergic rhinitis or bronchial asthma. Anaphylactic hypersensitivity reactions are mediated by IgE antibodies which are found in the serum and also are bound to mast cells and basophils. Mediators released in the anaphylactic reaction include histamine, eosinophilic chemotactic factor of anaphylaxis (ECF-A), slow reacting substance of anaphylaxis (SRA-A) and platelet activating factor. Histamine and ECF-A are preformed and stored in granules of mast cells and basophils, while SRA-A and platelet activating factors are generated during the anaphylactic process.

Cytotoxic hypersensitivity is mediated by complement and occurs when an antibody reacts with antigen on the surface of a cell and activates the complete sequence of the complement cascade which results in direct membrane damage and lysis of the cells. This reaction is the type that occurs in transfusion reaction, erythroblastosis fetalis and autoimmune hemolytic anemia, as well as in some adverse reaction to drugs.

Immune-complex hypersensitivity is a result of antigen-antibody complexes which produce tissue damage by activating mediators in the complement system. The antigen-antibody complex localizes in the glomerulus of the kidney or in blood vessel walls to produce disease. The immune complex diseases include the generalized form, the classic example of which is acute serum sickness, as well as forms that may localize to the kidney, joints or blood vessels. The mechanism of injury is similar once the complexes have been deposited and involves the activation of the complement cascade and the participation of polymorphonuclear leukocytes and monocytes, which release lysosomal enzymes capable of damaging tissue. One of the morphological features of this type of injury on light microscopy of hematoxylin and eosin stained sections is a smudgy eosinophilic change in the blood vessel walls due to the presence of complement, immunoglobulins, and fibrinogen. This change is usually called "fibrinoid" necrosis but is not really truly necrosis, nor is the morphologic appearance specific for an immunologic reaction.

Cell-mediated hypersensitivity is the result of lymphocytes which are sensitized to specific antigens. The sensitized lymphocytes may cause delayed type hypersensitivity such as that occurring in the tuberculin reaction or the sensitized lymphocytes may have cytotoxic effects when they contact a target cell. This cytotoxic effect is the main mechanism responsible for acute allograft rejection. It also is involved in certain viral infections.

Autoimmune Disease

Autoimmune diseases are thought to occur when there is loss of tolerance to self antigens and the body has an immune reaction to these self antigens. The diseases that are usually considered to be due to autoimmune mechanisms include systemic lupus erythematosus, progressive systemic sclerosis (scleroderma), rheumatoid arthritis, dermatomyositis, Sjogren's syndrome, mixed connective tissue disease, and polyarteritis nodosa. These disorders are systemic disorders of multisystem disorders. In addition, there are autoimmune disorders which affect primarily one system or one organ and these include autoimmune hemolytic anemia, idiopathic thrombocytopenic purpura (ITP) and neutropenia, Hashimoto's thyroiditis, pernicious anemia, myasthenia gravis, primary biliary cirrhosis, autoimmune Addison's disease of the adrenal gland, and others.

Basically autoimmunity is simply hypersensitivity against antigens of "self." Both genetic factors and viruses seem to have a role in susceptibility or triggering of autoimmune reactions.

Systemic lupus erythematosus is the classical example of a systemic autoimmune disorder in which there is injury to the kidney, joints, skin, and serosal membranes. This disorder occurs predominantly in young women and involves the development of a number of autoantibodies which are involved in the pathogenesis of the disease and also are laboratory markers for diagnosing the disease. The autoantibodies include antinuclear antibodies against double-stranded and single-stranded DNA, RNA, deoxyribonucleoprotein and antibodies against the Sm antigen. Some of these antibodies can be found in other systemic autoimmune disorders, but antibody to the Sm antigen and antibody to native double-stranded DNA are almost specific for the diagnosis of systemic lupus erythematosus. In fact, anti-Sm antigen, which is found in about 30 per cent of patients with lupus, is considered to be almost pathognomonic of lupus when present. The morphologic

features of SLE include characteristic changes in the skin, particularly in the butterfly area of the face, a variety of patterns of involvement of the kidneys including focal, diffuse and mesangial changes, inflammation of the joints, pericardium and pleura, nonbacterial verrucous endocarditis of the heart valves and endocardium, and involvement of blood vessels in many of the organs throughout the body.

Progressive systemic sclerosis (scleroderma) is characterized by inflammation and fibrosis involving the skin, the gastrointestinal tract, kidneys, heart, muscles, and lungs.

Sjögren's syndrome consists of dry eyes, dry mouth, and arthritis. It may occur by itself or in conjunction with another connective tissue disease such as rheumatoid arthritis.

Polymyositis is an autoimmune disorder characterized by myositis with degeneration of individual groups of muscle fibers and infiltration of chronic inflammatory cells. There is also involvement of the skin and in connective tissue and of the organ systems. This disorder is associated with an increased risk of developing malignant tumors.

Mixed connective tissue disease, as the name implies, has features of several of the connective tissue diseases. The two most distinctive features are high titers of antibody to ribonucleoprotein (RNP) and lack of serious renal involvement. This disease has a better prognosis than systemic lupus erythematosus.

Polyarteritis nodosa, in its broadest definition, includes noninfectious necrotizing vasculitis involving vessels of any types. The broad definition includes the classical polyarteritis nodosa with macroscopic lesions of medium sized and smaller arteries of differing ages and stages, as well as hypersensitivity angitis that is detectable only microscopically. Hypersensitivity angitis is frequently distinguished from polyarteritis nodosa because smaller vessels are affected with all lesions appearing to be of the same age. Drugs such as penicillin and sulfonamides have been associated with the development of vasculitis, usually of the hypersensitivity small vessel type.

Immunologic Deficiency Disorders

A number of primary immunodeficiency diseases that are genetically determined have now been described. Those disorders which best illustrate the different mechanisms of these immunodeficiencies include (1) X-linked agammaglobulinemia (Bruton's disease) in which B lymphocytes are absent or decreased and there is a resultant deficiency in immunoglobulins, T lymphocytes are normal in this disorder; (2) thymic hypoplasia (DiGeorge's syndrome) in which B lymphocytes and immunoglobulins are normal and T lymphocytes are deficient; (3) severe combined immunologic deficiency (Swiss type) in which B lymphocytes and immunoglobulins are absent or decreased, T lymphocytes are absent or decreased, and (4) combined variable immunodeficiencies, a poorly defined but common form of immunodeficiency in which there are abnormalities of B lymphocytes and immunoglobulins and sometimes abnormalities of T lymphocytes.

Secondary immunologic deficiencies may be caused by immunosuppression, irradiation, chemotherapy, malnutrition, and infections.

Graft Rejection

Among the most exciting surgical procedures of recent years have been tissue and organ transplantations, particularly of such organs as kidneys, heart, liver, lungs and certain important, and sometimes life-preserving, tissues like bone marrow. While the technical aspects of organ transplantation have reached a high state of perfection, a more subtle cause for failure of the procedure has been the development of tissue and organ rejection based upon the effectiveness of the immune system in bringing about the destruction of the transplant.

The causes of rejection have been subject to intensive study and cannot be dealt with in any detail here. Suffice it to say, however, that many elements enter into the matter of histoincompatability, especially the genetic makeup of the recipient and donor as far as tissue antigen components are concerned. Tissue grafts from one part of the body to another in the same individual are readily accomplished because no immune reaction is provoked. In similar fashion a tissue or organ can be successfully transplanted from one identical or monocular twin to the other. In those cases tissue compatibility can be taken for granted.

Rejection in humans occurs between individuals whose genetic backgrounds are different, and the process is generally most marked the more different these backgrounds are. Rejection is less marked, for example, between members of the same family, particularly mother and offspring, but tends to be pronounced when the donor and recipient are totally foreign to each other. The rejection process is now known to involve both humoral and cellular mechanisms, and there is good evidence that complement may play a role. It is the effectiveness of these immune processes that one attempts to suppress when organ or tissue grafts are contemplated.

The rejection of transplanted renal grafts is a very complex process in which both circulating antibodies and cell-mediated immunity are involved. The T lymphocytes are the cells causing injury to grafted tissue in the cell mediated immune mechanism. The cytolytic T lymphocytes may be the major cause of tissue damage; specifically activated T lymphocytes may also cause damage by production of lymphokines that cause the attraction and activation of other cytotoxic cells such as macrophages and neutrophils. Humoral antibodies also may have a role in rejection of human kidney transplants. Circulating antibodies have a role in several types of rejection of human kidney transplants. In one instance, circulating antibodies have been preformed in the transplant recipients because they have encountered a particular foreign antigen before transplantation, may occur as a result of previous blood transfusions, previous pregnancies or certain infections. There may also be escape of antigens from the transplanted kidney after transplantation into the recipient's circulation so that the recipient then produces circulating antibodies. Circulating antibodies may lead to injury by several mechanisms, namely, the deposition of antigen-antibody complexes, complement-dependent cytotoxicity and antibody-dependent cell-mediated cytolysis. These antibodies appear to attack the graft vasculature as the initial point of attack.

There are three principal types of rejection reaction, the hyperacute rejection, the acute rejection, and the chronic rejection. The *hyperacute rejection* is the result of preformed circulating antibodies due to previous sensitization to some of the donor-specific antigens. It occurs almost immediately after transplantation. The histologic lesions are similar to those of the Arthus reaction with large numbers of neutrophils infiltrating the vasculature and with immunoglobulin and complement found in the vessel wall.

The *acute* type of rejection may be due to a combination of both cell-mediated immunity and humoral damage by circulating antibodies. This type of reaction may occur within a few days of transplantation if the patient is not given immunosuppressive therapy or may occur after immunosuppressive therapy has been used and then discontinued. At the microscopic level, acute rejection is characterized by mononuclear cell infiltration of the glomeruli and vasculature of the kidney. Acute rejection due to humoral mechanisms involves extensive vasculitis with neutrophilic infiltration, arterial necrosis, and deposition of complement, immunoglobulins, and fibrin. These changes lead to thrombosis of small vessels.

Chronic rejection may occur in patients in whom phenomena of the acute graft rejection are prevented by immunosuppressive treatment. In these patients there is usually progressive renal failure over a period of months. Changes include intimal fibrosis of cortical arteries and ischemic manifestations in the glomeruli and tubules leading to atrophy of the kidney. In some cases there are changes of acute arteritis with presence of immunoglobulins and complement, and in other cases there are interstitial infiltrates of plasma cells and lymphocytes indicating a cell-mediated mechanism of rejection.

The use of bone marrow transplantation in the treatment of leukemia and other hematologic disorders in which immunologically competent cells are transplanted into the marrow of a diseased recipient gives rise to the possibility of two types of immunologic problems for rejection phenomena. The first is the rejection of the grafted bone marrow material by the host; such rejection follows the mechanisms previously described. In the other type of reaction, *graft-versus-host disease* (GVH), T cells in the transplanted normal marrow can react against the recipient's tissue, leading to serious disease usually of an infectious nature.

CIRCULATORY DISORDERS

Edema is the accumulation of abnormal amounts of fluid in intercellular or interstitial spaces or body cavities, especially the natural mesothelium-lined cavities, such as the pleura, the pericardium and the peritoneum. Generalized edema, that is, accumulations of fluid in the subcutaneous tissues and the body cavities so that the body is literally waterlogged, is referred to as *anasarca*. In general, edema is found most commonly in association with cardiac failure, in which blood is dammed back into the venous system, thus increasing the hydrostatic pressure and forcing fluid through the capillary walls into the interstitial spaces, or in certain forms of renal disease in which protein loss through the kidneys lowers the plasma protein to a point that the plasma osmotic pressure drops, permitting the escape of fluid from the blood vessels into the tissues. This fluid is low in protein content and is a *transudate*. It differs from inflammatory edema, which is generally localized, is rich in cells and protein, and is associated usually with infection. Its accumulation is due to the increased permeability of the endothelial lining of the capillaries and small venules brought about by direct injury to the vessel walls. This fluid, often containing inflammatory cells, is an *exudate*.

Nutritional edema results, in part at least, from a loss of plasma proteins following prolonged severe malnutrition or starvation.

Hyperemia means an increased amount of blood in an organ or part, and it may be localized or generalized. It may be caused by active or passive dilatation of blood vessels, especially capillaries and the venules. *Active hyperemia* occurs physiologically in a muscle that is exercised and pathologically in acute inflammation as one of the first local responses to injury. *Passive hyperemia* or *congestion* results from obstruction of venous outflow of blood from a part. This may be brought about by venous thrombosis or any other condition that constricts or obstructs a vein. Passive congestion may be generalized when the venous return to the heart is impaired, as in cardiac failure. The cyanosis, the dyspnea and the edema that occur in this condition are directly referable to the stasis. The "nutmeg" liver, with the congested central and midzonal regions of the lobules, and the enlarged red firm spleen that results from splenic vein obstruction are good examples of chronic stasis in an organ. In the lung, the liver and the spleen, as well as in other organs that may be the seat of chronic venous stasis, there may be a considerable deposit of hemosiderin in the interstitial tissue. In the lung small hemorrhages occur into the alveoli. The red cells are phagocytized, and the hemoglobin is converted into hemosiderin. These hemosiderin-containing macrophages are called *heart-failure cells*. In all organs that are the seat of chronic venous stasis or chronic passive congestion there also may be a considerable increase of fibrous tissue, which, in the liver, accumulates about the central veins of the lobules. This condition is called *cardiac cirrhosis*. In the lung such tissue leads to thickening of the alveolar walls, in which, as well as in the alveoli themselves, hemosiderin-containing macrophages (so-called brown induration) accumulate.

Ischemia is a decrease in the amount of blood flowing into a tissue. It may be the result of functional or organic arterial disease, such as spasm, arteriosclerosis or thromboangiitis obliterans, thrombosis or even pressure on an artery from some external cause. Sudden deprivation of blood may result in infarction, with necrosis of the organ or part; a gradual reduction of the blood supply may result in atrophy of the parenchyma with replacement fibrosis.

A *thrombus* is a semisolid mass, composed of blood platelets, red and white cells and fibrin, formed within the heart or the blood vessels during life. It is caused by: (1) injury to the vascular endothelium; (2) slowing, stasis or eddying of the blood flow; or (3) changes in the composition of the blood. A roughening of the endothelial lining caused by trauma or arteriosclerosis permits the adherence of platelets, to which red and white cells attach themselves. Fibrin is laid down sometimes, but not always. Sclerosis of the veins, malignant tumors penetrating their walls and endocardial scars are common sites. Infection may cause thrombosis by the direct extension of a suppurative process, such as valvular and mural thrombi in the heart, or thrombophlebitis following typhoid or puerperal sepsis. Most common sites are in the veins, particularly in the lower extremities, in which the bloodstream is slow. Substances that agglutinate red cells tend to form capillary thrombi. Some of the factors that have been shown to cause platelet aggregation include adenosine diphosphate (ADP), collagen fibers, and thromboxane A$_2$.

The fate of a thrombus varies. If it is a bland uninfected thrombus it may, after a few days, be lysed by enzyme activity. If this form of resolution does not occur, fibroblasts and new capillaries invade the thrombus from the adjacent intima, not only attaching it firmly to the vessel wall but converting it to a fibrous scar—*organization* of the thrombus. If the thrombus is occlusive in type, that is, it completely obstructs the vessel lumen, newly formed vascular channels may pass through the fibrous tissue to form communications that serve to restore some degree of circulation in the vessel. Occasionally some venous thrombi become calcified and form phleboliths in the vessel lumen. If, on the other hand, bacteria are present, suppuration may occur, giving rise to bacteremia, in which minute, bacteria-laden embolic fragments of the thrombus circulate in the blood.

The other common sequelae of thrombosis include (1) embolism, (2) infarction, (3) edema, and (4) gangrene.

Embolism is the partial or complete obstruction of the lumen of a blood vessel by any mass that is carried to it in the circulating blood. The mass is called an *embolus*. Detached fragments of thrombi are the most common forms of emboli. If they originate in a noninfected thrombus their effects depend upon their size and the degree of vascular obstruction they cause. If they had their origin in an infected thrombus, however, they contain microorganisms and may cause inflammation, and even abscess formation and infarction, at the site of lodgment. In the pulmonary or renal capillaries they may form embolic abscesses without infarction. Emboli from a thrombus on the valves or mural endocardium of the left heart cause infarctions of the brain, kidney, spleen, intestines and other organs. Those in the right heart may produce pulmonary infarcts, but these usually do not occur unless the lung is also the seat of passive congestion.

In *fat embolism* minute globules of fat may be liberated into the bloodstream during an operation on an obese individual or following contusion or laceration of subcutaneous fat tissue. An important cause is trauma to bones, especially fractures of the long bones of the lower extremities. In the latter circumstance, emboli of actual bone marrow, as well as fat, may be found in the vessels of the lungs, brain, and kidneys.

Air embolism may occur as a result of the entrance of air by way of veins and may be of traumatic or surgical origin. Caisson disease, or the bends, occurs in divers and other individuals who work in atmos-pheres where the pressure is much higher than at sea level. If the pressure about them is lowered too quickly, bubbles of gas, chiefly nitrogen, develop in the blood, and they may coalesce to form larger bubbles that may cause vascular occlusion. In fatal cases of air embolism, frothy fluid may be found in the right side of the heart and in the larger veins.

An *infarct* is a localized focus of ischemic necrosis resulting from the occlusion of an artery or, less commonly, a vein. It may be caused by (1) embolism of the artery supplying the part, (2) thrombosis of the artery supplying the part, (3) thrombosis of a major vein, or (4) occlusion of the vessels supplying a part from external pressure. Grossly, infarcts are recognized by their conical or pyramidal shape, the base being at the surface of the organ. At first the region is red, but the center undergoes coagulation necrosis, and the infarct finally becomes pale, owing to depigmentation and to organization by fibrous tissue.

Infarcts of the spleen and the kidneys often are multiple and usually are caused by emboli from the left heart. Infarcts of the brain more commonly result from thrombosis of sclerotic cerebral arteries, causing *encephalomalacia*. Infarction of the lungs results from emboli from the systemic veins or the right heart but may be caused by thrombosis of the pulmonary vessels in a lung that is the seat of passive congestion. Intestinal infarcts are commonly the result of thrombosis of the mesenteric vessels. Infarction of the myocardium is almost always caused by thrombosis of a branch of the coronary arteries superimposed on an atherosclerotic plaque.

Infarcts of the myocardium, kidney, and spleen are "pale" infarcts because the organs are supplied by end arteries. Infarcts of the lungs and intestines are "red" infarcts because of collateral circulation.

Shock

An exact definition of shock has not been established, but shock basically is a decrease in effective blood volume with decreased perfusion of vital organs and tissues. Shock may affect the brain, heart, kidney and lungs, as well as the endocrine system and gastrointestinal tract. Because of decreased perfusion of these organs there is inadequate oxygen delivered to the cells and inadequate removal of metabolic products. One of the most characteristic morphologic findings of shock is tubular necrosis of the kidney.

Disseminated intravascular coagulation (DIC) is a condition that occurs in a variety of disorders in which there is activation of the intrinsic pathway of blood clotting. These disorders include eclampsia, abruptio placenta, amniotic fluid embolism, thrombotic thrombocytic purpura, septicemia and widespread carcinomatosis. As a result of activation of the coagulation cascade, there is consumption of coagulation components and depletion of many of the clotting factors, including platelets, factor I (fibrinogen), factor II (prothrombin), and factors V, VIII and X. The fibrolytic system is also activated producing clot lysis which aggrevates the bleeding tendencies that occur because of the clotting factor deficiencies. The fact that there are small vessel thrombi in addition to bleeding can produce widespread and serious damage to the cardiovascular system, central nervous system, lungs and kidney.

PROCESSES OF INFECTION AND INFECTIOUS DISEASE

Infectious disease is caused by living microorganisms, which may be bacteria, viruses, rickettsiae, fungi, protozoa or metazoa. The incidence of many of these infections has been greatly reduced in recent years as a result of the preventive administration of very effective vaccines or toxoid preparations and, in a few instances, the use of live but attenuated agents (vaccinia inoculations against smallpox and inoculations against poliomyelitis and rubella). Effective treatment is now also provided by the use of broad-spectrum antibiotics.

Pyogenic Infections

The most common pus-producing microorganisms are the staphylococci, pneumococci and gonococci. All may produce local infections, as well as septicemia, and generalized, as well as localized, manifestations of acute suppurative inflammation in other parts of the body. Friedlander's bacilli (Klebsiella pneumoniae) and Klebs-Loffler's bacilli (Corynebacterium diptheriae) also are capable of producing acute suppurative inflammation.

Staphylococcal Infection

This is the most common cause of furuncles or boils, which are localized abscesses of skin around hair follicles, and of carbuncles, which also are circumscribed but deep seated and of more extensive foci or suppurative inflammation in the skin and the subcutaneous tissue. Food poisoning frequently is caused by the toxin produced by the growth of *Staphylococcus aureus* in contaminated food. Osteomyelitis, bronchopneumonia, endocarditis and acute suppurative nephritis are also some of the manifestations of generalized staphylococcal infection. Ninety per cent of *Staphylococcus aureus* are resistant to penicillin G, however most strains remain sensitive to synthetic penicillins and other newer antibiotics.

Streptococcal Infection

The two main forms of pathogenic streptococci are *Streptococcus viridans* (alpha-hemolytic streptococcus), the most common cause of subacute bacterial endocarditis, and *Streptococcus hemolyticus* (beta-hemolytic streptococcus, Lancefield group A), the cause of erysipelas, acute ulcerative endocarditis and scarlet fever, to name only some of the conditions that result from this ubiquitous microorganism.

Erysipelas is a diffuse streptococcal infection of the skin characterized usually by large and small mononuclear cell infiltration, hyperemia and edema of the corium, with suppuration a relatively uncommon complication.

Scarlet fever is also caused by streptococci capable of producing erythrogenic toxin. Sore throat, fever and a widespread erythematous skin rash are the first manifestations of this condition. Acute interstitial glomerulonephritis and otitis media are complications. In this case, too, the inflammatory infiltrate is mainly lymphocytic. Suppuration is relatively uncommon.

Meningococcal Infection

Disease due to *Neisseria meningitidis* probably always begins as a mild upper respiratory infection that is rarely recognized as such. In a small percentage of individuals, usually children or young adults, this leads to a bacteremia with localization of the infection in the CNS, resulting in purulent meningitis. In other individuals, the infection takes the course of rapidly fulminating meningococcemia with circulatory collapse and death.

Meningococcemia is accompanied by a rash, which is petechial, purpura, or ecchymotic hemorrhages, scattered over the entire body surface. These hemorrhages are the result of microthrombi in the small vessels. There is a generalized Swartzman-like reaction and disseminated intravascular coagulation due to endotoxemia. Bilateral adrenal hemorrhage, the Waterhouse-Friderichsen syndrome, occurs in some cases of acute meningococcemia.

Pneumococcal Infection

Streptococcus pneumoniae is the most common cause of bacterial pneumonia. The organism is found as part of the normal flora in the upper respiratory tract. Infection of the lower respiratory tract occurs most often in children under 5 years of age and the elderly. Prior viral infection or alcoholism predispose to serious infection. Meningitis, sinusitis, and otitis media are also frequently caused by this organism. Pneumococcal disease of all kinds is common in persons with sickle-cell anemia and in the asplenic. Of the 83 capsular types of pneumococci, fourteen cause most of the serious pneumococcal disease. A commercial polyvalent vaccine composed of capsular polysaccharide from these fourteen types is now available.

Gonococcal Infection

Gonorrhea, a venereal disease caused by *Neisseria gonorrhoeae,* usually is characterized by acute suppurative urethritis in the male and the female, and by acute cervicitis and bartholinitis in the female. In the male the condition may spread to the posterior urethra and involve the prostate, the seminal vesicles and the epididymis. In the female it may spread to the fallopian tubes and to the peritoneum. The condition may become generalized and lead to local manifestations in other sites, especially acute suppurative arthritis, usually monarticular. Acute, ulcerative and vegetative endocarditis, usually on the right side of the heart, also may complicate the condition. The infection also occurs in newborns, as conjunctivitis, and in infants, as vaginitis. Blindness may result from involvement of the cornea, with resultant opacity.

Nonpyogenic Infections

Diphtheria

The cause of diphtheria is *Corynebacterium diphtheriae,* a microorganism that produces acute membranous inflammation locally and serious generalized symptoms as the result of toxemia. The infection affects primarily the oropharynx, often with extension to the nose and larynx and occasionally the trachea, major bronchi and even the esophagus. The typical local lesion is characterized by the presence on the affected mucous membrane of a dirty whitish or grayish pseudomembrane composed primarily of a fibrin layer in which are enmeshed leukocytes, numerous microorganisms and groups of necrotic epithelial cells. The underlying tissues are hyperemic, edematous and inflamed, with numerous minute ulcerations, at which points the pseudomembrane is attached. If stripped from the mucosa, the fibrinous membrane leaves a focally bleeding, raw mucosal surface. The generalized symptoms of diphtheria are due to the profound toxemia caused by the toxin elaborated by the microorganisms that remain localized in the upper respiratory passage. The most serious effects of the toxin are found in the myocardium where they may be severe enough to lead to cardiac failure and death. Rarely, death may result from mechanical obstruction of the trachea or bronchi by the pseudomembrane. Upon the patient's recovery, the pseudomembrane disappears and the mucosa returns to normal.

Rheumatic Fever

Rheumatic fever is an acute nonsuppurative inflammatory disease involving a variety of tissue structures and organs of the body, particularly the heart and joints, but the tendons, subcutaneous tissues, the larger arteries and even parts of the central nervous system may also be affected. Although the pathogenesis of the disease is not yet fully understood, it is quite clear that it results from hypersensitivity associated with a prior infection due to group A beta-hemolytic streptococci. The first symptoms develop usually from 2 to 4 weeks after the inciting hemolytic streptococcus infection, which occurs nearly always in the throat or pharynx. By this time the local lesions may have cleared completely, though serologic evidence of a recent hemolytic streptococcus infection is demonstrable in a great majority of cases. While the local lesions in the throat or pharynx, while active, actually harbor the streptococci, the systemic lesions of rheumatic fever are bacteria free. The characteristic lesions in the heart are described more at length in the section on the circulatory system.

Typhoid Fever

This is an infectious disease caused by a bacillus, *Salmonella typhi.* The microorganism gains entrance into the body by means of contaminated food or water, although the five Fs most related to the spread of the disease should be borne in mind: food, fingers, flies, fomites and feces. The microorganism may be cultured from the blood, feces, the wall of the intestines, the spleen and lesions in other organs that may complicate the disease. Pure cultures of the inciting agent may even be obtained from rose spots, the skin lesions characteristic of this disease. The important pathologic lesions are the ulcerations in the ileum, the severe mesenteric lymphadenitis, splenomegaly and focal necroses in the liver and bone marrow. The lymphoid tissues in the lower ileum and the cecum are affected earliest and show the most severe changes. In Peyer's patches, the earliest changes are hyperemia and edema, soon replaced by the exudation and the infiltration of large numbers of mononuclear cells, which are characteristic of this condition. These cells exhibit phagocytosis of fragments of lymphocytes, of plasma cells and even a typhoid bacilli. Necrosis then begins, with ulcers forming where the necrotic tissue near the surface sloughs off. These small foci of infection finally coalesce to form round or elliptical ulcers that coincide with a Peyer's patch, the long axis of the ulcer being in the direction of the long axis of the intestine. This is in contrast with the tuberculous ulcer, which tends to run transversely. The important complications of typhoid fever are severe intestinal hemorrhage from an eroded blood vessel in an ulcer, perforation of the intestinal wall as a result of deep extension of an ulcer and rupture of the spleen. Death from severe hemorrhage or from peritonitis may occur. During healing, no stenosis occurs at the site of the ulcer, and in the mucosa the region of the ulcer becomes covered with epithelium, but gland follicles do not reform at that site. Statistically, about two per cent of patients who recover become carriers, that is, individuals who harbor the microorganisms at some site, usually the gallbladder, and who exhibit no signs of clinical disease.

Pertussis (Whooping Cough)

In the pathogenesis of pertussis, the microorganism *Bordetella pertussis* is transmitted from one individual to another by respiratory droplets. The droplets enter the respiratory tract, and there the Bordet-Gengou bacilli proliferate, becoming enmeshed in the delicate cilia of the tracheal mucosa. Laryngitis, tracheitis, bronchitis, bronchiolitis and interstitial pneumonitis may follow. The cough probably results from the irritative effects of the products of disintegration of the specific microorganisms, possibly aggravated by the presence of the bacilli on the mucosal surface.

Viral and Rickettsial Diseases

Details of viral and rickettsial diseases are covered in the Microbiology chapter; a few comments about pathologic findings in selected diseases will be covered here.

Influenza

Influenza is the most common viral disease. It is caused by several antigenically different strains of influenza virus, including types A, B and C, which may be identified by complement fixation and neutralization tests. The disease is characterized by acute inflammation of catarrhal type affecting the air passages, sometimes with necrosis and desquamation of the lining cells. In some cases interstitial pneumonitis may be present, and occasionally bacterial pneumonia may be a complication. In neither human nor experimental influenza have inclusion bodies been demonstrated. In some cases localized alveolar or interstitial emphysema may be present. Resolution of the pulmonary lesions, if severe, may be by organization of the alveolar exudate.

Typhus Fever

The cause of epidemic typhus fever is *Rickettsia prowazekii,* which is transmitted to man by the body louse. There is an endemic type, which is transmitted to man by the bite of the rat flea; it is characterized by immunologic differences from the epidemic, or louse-borne type. In the gross, hyperplasia of the spleen and cloudy swelling of the parenchymatous organs are present; microscopically, endothelial proliferation of the small blood vessels, with or without thrombosis, and perivascular infiltration of large and small mononuclear cells (typhus nodules) are characteristic of the disease. These lesions are most common in skin, brain, and heart muscle. In the heart there may be degeneration of the myocardial fibers, with diffuse interstitial infiltration of large and small mononuclear cells. Interstitial pneumonitis may occur, and in the brain there may be petechiae, perivascular infiltration of lymphactyes and small foci of gliosis.

Other rickettsial diseases include Q fever, caused by *Coxiella burnetii,* probably tickborne; the spotted fever group of which Rocky Mountain spotted fever is an example, caused by tick-borne *R. rickettsii;* tsutsugamushi disease caused by *R. orientalis,* transmitted by a tropical mite; and rickettsial pox caused by *R. akari* transmitted by a rodent mite. The pathologic, and to a less extent the clinical, manifestations of all of these diseases resemble somewhat those of typhus fever.

Infectious Granulomata

Tuberculosis

Tuberculosis is a chronic communicable disease caused by *Mycobacterium tuberculosis.* It involves most commonly the lungs but may occur in other organs. The incidence of the disease in this country has declined markedly in the past 50 years, but it still is a leading cause of death in other countries. Far more individuals may be infected with the microorganism than develop clinical disease, since only about 1 in 20 of those who have actually been infected come down with clinical tuberculosis.

The mode of infection of the lungs by the tubercle bacillus is usually by inhalation of droplets expelled from the mouth (coughing, sneezing or even talking) of a patient with active lesions, or contained in particles of dust. Inhalation is the most important route. Direct infection of the skin or mucous membranes may also occur. In the case of the bovine tubercle bacillus, infections may occur through the alimentary tract from the ingestion of contaminated milk from infected cows. In this case the microorganism enters the body by way of either the cervical or the mesenteric lymph nodes.

The Tubercle. The peculiar character of the tissue reaction to *M. tuberculosis* in the newly infected host results in the formation of a *tubercle*. This is probably due chiefly to the presence of the waxy envelope of the microorganisms, for no toxic substances are either present or produced, and the reaction at first is typical of that excited by insoluble, inert foreign bodies. After a week or two, however, the host's body becomes sensitized, the reaction becomes intensified and along with these changes partial immunity develops and persists.

The first reaction to the tubercle bacilli is the appearance of large mononuclear cells, histiocytes, which become the characteristic large epithelioid cells with vesicular nuclei and abundant cytoplasm, fusing to form multinucleated giant cells that ingest but often fail to destroy the microorganisms. The Langhans' type of multinucleate cell, with central eosinophilic zone and nuclei at the periphery, is most common in tuberculous inflammatory tissue. Surrounding these epithelioid and giant cells is a peripheral zone of lymphocytes. Soon, however, as hypersensitivity develops, the exudate becomes softer, central necrosis occurs, and the macrophages and giant cells become more effective in preventing proliferation of, or in actually destroying, phagocytized bacilli. In most cases of initial infection, healing of the tuberculous focus occurs with the infiltration of reticulin fibers, which become collagenous and finally surround the tubercle with scar tissue. The caseous center remains indefinitely, but after a long time it may become calcified. The bacilli may remain alive indefinitely in the necrotic and calcified center. From a clinical standpoint, however, the individual with these healed lesions does not suffer from clinical tuberculosis.

Because hypersensitivity and some degree of immunity develop as a result of the first infection with *M. tuberculosis,* later infection will provoke a very different response from that following the first. For this reason we speak of *primary infection* and *secondary infection* due to this microorganism.

Extension of tubercles may occur by several processes. In active lesions, the zone of peripheral epithelioid cells is killed by toxic substances, the caseous center enlarges, and a new zone of epithelioid cells is formed. This may be repeated until large masses are caseous. Extension also occurs through the lymphatics to the regional lymph nodes and thence to the bloodstream through the thoracic duct, or by invasion of veins with the formation of infected thrombi, which form disseminating emboli. The coughing up of infected sputum from one bronchus and inhalation of it into another bronchus or the swallowing of tuberculous sputum may disseminate the lesions. Tuberculous sputum may cause lesions through skin abrasions.

Miliary tuberculosis may result from bloodstream invasion, either direct or via the lymphatics. The primary source usually is the lungs or the bronchial lymph nodes. The miliary tubercles are found especially in the lungs, the spleen, the liver and the meninges. Miliary tuberculosis is most common in children, particularly miliary tuberculous meningitis. Tuberculosis of the kidney, the adrenal, the epididymis or the fallopian tube usually arises as a hematogenous infection from the lung.

Pulmonary Tuberculosis. The *primary* type of pulmonary tuberculosis, once called "childhood" tuberculosis because it commonly developed in children, now may occur in young adults because, as a result of the greatly lowered incidence of the disease, the number of individuals in this age group who have never had contact with *M. tuberculosis* outnumbers those who have. Infection results from the aspiration of tubercle bacilli into the lung and the development of a primary focus, the Ghon tubercle. This lesion, measuring about 1 to 3 cm. in diameter, is usually situated in the subpleural region of almost any part of the lung except the apices. Small tubercles develop along the lymphatics to the bronchial lymph nodes draining the region infected. These show active caseation, and the process usually extends to other mediastinal lymph nodes. The lesion in the periphery of the lung, together with the involved tracheobronchial lymph nodes, is called the *primary complex*. In the great majority of cases, the primary focus heals and appears in later life as a calcified lesion in the lung and the regional bronchial nodes. Less commonly, the primary complex, instead of regressing and healing, may progress to tuberculous bronchopneumonia and, by dissemination of the microorganisms via the bloodstream, to generalized miliary tuberculosis.

Secondary or adult type pulmonary tuberculosis may be caused by reactivation of a primary focus, which is rare, or by endogenous or exogenous reinfection. It is much more serious than the primary type and differs from it anatomically and clinically. The primary infection, which occurs in the host who has never previously been infected, no only confers some degree of immunity in most cases but also sensitizes the body to the protein fractions of the microorganism. Thus the host's reaction to *M. tuberculosis* if it invades the body at some later time provokes a more intense reaction because of this hypersensitivity.

Secondary tuberculosis usually begins in the subapical portion of a lobe and extends downward from the apex; extension usually is from the coughing up and the inhalation of caseous material from one bronchus to another. The same lung simultaneously may show tuberculous pneumonia, nodular lesions with caseous necrosis, cavities and scar tissue. The nodular lesions are the prevailing type and vary in size from miliary tubercles to massive lesions formed by the confluence of smaller ones. The larger nodules show much caseous necrosis, surrounded by the typical epithelioid and giant cells with small lymphocytes.

Cavities may arise from the sloughing of a tuberculous bronchus or extension of nodular lesions into a bronchus, with discharge of the caseous material by coughing. There usually is a secondary pyogenic infection that leads to suppuration and increased caseation. Erosion of blood vessels in the wall of a cavity causes hemorrhage, but this is not so common a complication as might be expected, because the local blood vessels, sometimes actually crossing the cavity, frequently are the seat of obliterative endarteritis. Cavities may undergo partial or complete arrest by the formation of fibrous tissue in their walls.

Healing of the pulmonary lesions, especially if cavitation is not present or is minimal, occurs slowly as a result of fibrosis and sometimes focal calcification. The presence of cavities complicates the healing process, and in some cases healing does not occur. If the tuberculous lesions extend to the pleural surface of the lungs, tuberculous pleuritis with or without effusion may occur, and healing results in fibrous adhesions.

Tuberculous Pneumonia.   Whenever large numbers of tubercle bacilli are aspirated from a tuberculous cavity that is in direct communication with a bronchus, tuberculous bronchopneumonia may develop. This may be of the gelatinous, the caseous or the mixed variety. The gelatinous type is characterized by edema of the interalveolar septa, fluid and large mononuclear cells in the alveoli and the bronchioles; the striking feature of the caseous type is the necrosis of the exudate, and even of the pulmonary tissue.

Extrapulmonary Tuberculosis.   The pleura is nearly always involved in pulmonary tuberculosis, with resultant adhesions or effusions. Many cases of fatal secondary pulmonary tuberculosis are limited to the lungs, but involvement of the intestine, the larynx, the adrenals, the meninges and the kidneys is common.

The characteristic tubercle occurs in tuberculosis elsewhere in the body. Tuberculosis may invade practically any organ but is most common in the lungs, the pleura, the pericardium, the peritoneum, the larynx, the lymph nodes, the intestine, the epididymis, the seminal vesicles, the kidneys, the bladder, the skin, the fallopian tubes, the bones and joints and the meninges.

Syphilis

Once one of the most important of diseases affecting man because of its protean and widespread manifestations, syphilis has shown a marked decline in incidence since the introduction of antibiotic therapy. Neverthe-

less, it still remains a major public health problem because of the recent marked upsurge in the number of cases, especially in the 15-to-24-year-age group, in many parts of the United States.

Syphilis is certainly the most serious of the venereal diseases. It is caused by a spirochete, *Treponema pallidum,* which is present in the lesions it causes. Although the infection, once the incitant is in the body, is continuous, it manifests itself clinically in three stages, that of the initial infection, the chancre, a generalized secondary stage with a rash and various tertiary manifestations that may occur years later.

Primary Chancre.   The primary chancre develops, within 2 to 6 weeks after inoculation, from a macule into a papule with eroded or ulcerated surface, and from a few millimeters to several centimeters in diameter. The base of the single, circular ulcer is indurated but painless, and from the surface a nonpurulent serous fluid exudes. It usually is located on or near the genital organs, though extragenital chancres on the lips, the tongue and other parts of the body do occur. The treponemata are widely disseminated throughout the bloodstream within 48 hours after inoculation (hence before the appearance of the chancre). Shortly after the chancre appears, the regional lymph nodes become enlarged and firm, but not tender. Diagnosis is confirmed by darkfield examination of serum from the chancre or a bubo since the treponemata are usually abundant in these situations. Microscopically the chancre is a shallow ulcer with a dense accumulation of mononuclear cells in the corium and subcutaneous tissue, with perivascular infiltration of plasma cells and lymphocytes. The base of the ulcer is composed of well-vascularized dense granulation tissue, also infiltrated with lymphocytes and plasma cells, with small numbers of granulocytes near the ulcerated surface. The histologic appearance is not specific or diagnostic. The necrosis and ulceration usually are superficial, unless the condition is complicated by secondary infection. Healing is complete in 2 months or less, and only a relatively small epithelialized scar remains to mark the site of the lesion.

Secondary Stage.   The secondary stage results from the dissemination and proliferation of the treponemata throughout the body. The typical lesions occur on the average 6 or 7 weeks after the chancre and may be accompanied by the symptoms of acute infection. The characteristic secondary phenomena are (1) the eruption on the skin and (2) on the mucous membranes, (3) sore throat, and (4) adenopathy. The cutaneous eruption is often inconspicuous but may be very marked. The most frequent lesion consists of generally distributed ham-colored macules, caused by perivascular and diffuse infiltration of the skin, which may be raised as papules. Pustules are uncommon, and vesicles are rare. All of these lesions contain numerous treponemata. Papules on hairy surfaces cause loss of hair. Condylomata, or venereal warts, may appear on the genitals and the perineum or in the axilla. Histologically the secondary lesions are characterized by perivascular infiltration of lymphocytes and plasma cells. Unless there is secondary infection, there is no destruction of tissue, and healing occurs without scarring.

Sore throat, often severe and chronic, is common. Mucous patches are commonly found on the mucous membrane of the mouth, the tongue, the palate and the tonsils, as well as between the labia, and correspond to the secondary skin lesions.

Localized periostitis, especially on the anterior surface of the tibia, sometimes occurs. There usually is moderate adenopathy of the inguinal, the posterior cervical, the occipital and epitrochlear lymph nodes, which show diffuse hyperplasia.

In the secondary stage both complement fixation and flocculation tests are positive in almost 100 per cent of cases. The treponemal immobilizing antibody test (TPI) is highly specific, becomes positive early but is difficult to carry out. Increase in the spinal fluid cell count and the globulin occurs in about 25 per cent. Treponemata in the spinal fluid may be demonstrated by animal inoculation before these changes.

Tertiary Stage. Tertiary syphilis may occur from a few months to as long as 50 years after the chancre. The lesions involve the internal organs principally and are of two types: (1) the gumma and (2) diffuse chronic inflammatory lesions in which obliterative endarteritis with perivascular infiltration of inflammatory cells, chiefly plasma cells, predominates.

The gumma is the most characteristic but not the most common lesion of tertiary syphilis. It may occur in any tissue, but its most frequent sites are skin, liver, testes and bones. Gummata vary in size from the miliary gumma to those several centimeters in diameter. They usually are single but may be multiple and consist of a firm, elastic, central, necrotic portion surrounded by a dense fibrous or cellular zone. Microscopically, epithelioid cells are present, mixed with lymphocytes and some plasma cells, around the central focus of necrosis, but they are less conspicuous than in tubercles, and giant cells also are less common. In the necrotic zone, tissue structure still may be recognizable, at least in outline, and, in its center, especially in the later stages, fibroblasts may be present.

Diffuse chronic inflammatory lesions without necrosis and characterized by obliterative endarteritis, perivascular cuffing with plasma cells and even local vascular proliferation are the most common type of tertiary reaction. They are found chiefly in the cardiovascular and the central nervous systems.

Cardiovascular syphilis affects the aorta more than the heart itself, the lesions occurring as endarteritis of the vasa vasorum, involving chiefly the region just above the aortic valve and the ascending portion of the arch. Necrosis of the media with secondary fibrosis follows, the inflammatory reaction frequently extending down to involve the aortic valve itself. The wall of the aorta is thicker than normal at first, because of lymphocytic infiltration and proliferation of fibrous tissue, chiefly in the adventitia but also involving the media. In the larger arteries of the adventitia there is likely to be obliterative fibrous proliferation of the intima. Later, the wall is weakened, thinned and dilated and a typical syphilitic aneurysm may develop although such aneurysms are less common than they were some years ago. Other effects are: (1) narrowing of the coronary orifices, causing angina pectoris, and (2) involvement of the aortic valves, with insufficiency, which may occur as a result of dilatation of the ring, thickening and shortening of the leaflets and fusion of the leaflets with the wall of the aorta at the site of their attachment, so that there is abnormal separation of the cusps at the commissures. Syphilis of the myocardium is rare.

Central nervous system syphilis manifests itself in several different ways, all of which are described in the section on the nervous system. One form, meningovascular syphilis, is characterized by the typical chronic inflammatory and vascular changes that resemble those in the aorta and coronary arteries, together with fibrous thickening of the meninges.

Multiple gummata of the liver were relatively frequent before effective treatment was developed, and the scarred liver (hepar lobatum) is now also a comparative rarity.

Bones. In the bones, syphilis may lead to perforations of the hard palate and destruction of the nasal septum, destruction of the calvaria and, in the long bones, gummata or diffuse destructive osteoperiostitis. In congenitally syphilitic children, osteochondritis used to be common, but this is less frequent since prenatal treatment of the mother has become almost the rule.

Congenital Syphilis. Syphilis may be transmitted from the infected mother to the fetus. Infection of the fetus may occur at any time during intrauterine life.

The *fetal type* includes all stillborn syphilitic infants and all those who die soon after birth. The body is undersized, the skin macerated or covered with bullae, particularly on the palms and the soles. The chief gross findings are enlargement of the spleen and the liver, with disintegration of the hepatic cords, and portal fibrosis and infiltration of lymphocytes, plasma cells and blood-forming cells. At the epiphyseal ends of the long bones, osteochondritis is common. In the liver, the pancreas, the kidneys and the lungs, signs of delayed development are characteristic of congenital syphilis. An unusual amount of undifferentiated mesoblastic tissue is present. In the lungs the condition is known as pneumonia alba. In addition to the increase of interalveolar mesoblastic and fibrous tissue, the alveoli are small and lined by cuboidal epithelium.

The *infantile type* is a less severe manifestation of the infection, which is evidenced about the second month by snuffles, pemphigus, splenomegaly and anemia. Often there are jaundice, rhagades, paronychiae and alopecia.

The *late type* (lues tarda) is characterized by deafness, hutchinsoian teeth (tapered or bulbous incisors, with a notch in the middle of the biting edge), saddle nose, periostitis, keratitis, splenomegaly and neuroretinitis. Occasionally neurosyphilis may develop.

Serologic tests are not invariably positive in infants with congenital syphilis.

Brucellosis (Undulant Fever)

This is an acute or remittent infectious disease caused by any species of Brucella, but most commonly by *Brucella abortus* or *B. suis.* The usual source of infection is occupational exposure to infected animal tissue in meat processing plants. Infection with *B. melitensis* has occurred following consumption of imported, unpasteurized goat-milk cheese. Brucella infection is characterized by invasion of the reticuloendothelial system with resultant hyperplasia and the formation of miliary granulomas resembling those found in tuberculosis, sarcoid, or tularemia.

Tularemia

Tularemia is a subacute infectious disease caused by *Francisella (Pasteurella) tularensis* in man. It is transmitted by the handling of infected rabbits, but the condition also occurs in ground squirrels, mice and rats. The transfer of the infection between animals is effected by the wood tick. The condition may also be transferred to man by the bite of a blood-sucking insect, especially the wood tick and the deer fly. The most common type of the disease is the ulceroglandular, characterized by a primary lesion at the site of the inoculation and enlargement of regional lymph nodes. The results of the oculoglandular type are primary involvement of the conjunctiva and regional or distant lymph node enlargement. The acute type shows no identifiable primary lesion, and there is no obvious enlargement of lymph nodes. In man, the anatomic lesions are granulomatous foci characterized by a necrotic focus surrounded by large mononuclear cells. In the older lesions, fibrosis occurs around such a focus. These lesions are most common in the lymph nodes. They may be present also in the spleen and the lungs, in which there usually is also confluent of nodular bronchopneumonia.

Listeriosis

Human infection with *Listeria monocytogenes* occurs most frequently in neonates or in adults who have some underlying debilitating disease or who are immunosuppressed. In experimental animals and in some early reported cases, a peripheral monocytosis occurred, thus the species name. This is not, however, found consistently. Infection in either group is usually manifest as septicemia and purulent meningoencephalitis. The mortality rate in debilitated adults is usually high, with focal abscesses being found in liver, spleen, lungs and other organs. Infection occurring during the first trimester of pregnancy usually results in abortion, while colonization of the infant from the birth canal may lead to meningitis at seven to ten days of age. The organism is known to affect many animals and to survive in soil for long periods, the epidemiology of the infection in humans is still poorly understood.

Actinomycosis

This is a chronic, granulomatous, inflammatory disease caused by the anaerobe *Actinomyces bovis.* The disease manifests itself mainly in the face and the neck, the intestine or the lungs. The lesion is a granuloma. Microscopically, colonies of the organism (branching filaments) are present in the inflammatory and fibroblastic region surrounding the necrotic focus. In the gross, the granules appear yellow and are referred to as sulfur granules.

Histoplasmosis

The causative agent of histoplasmosis is *Histoplasma capsulatum,* a minute parasitic fungus, occurring in soil and animals. In the human body it is found in the reticuloendothelial cells. Fever, leukopenia, anemia and loss of weight are the main symptoms, and it may be fatal. Granulomatous lesions are present in liver, spleen, lymph nodes and lungs. The nodules become calcified when healing occurs, and can be confused roentgenographically and histologically with calcified tuberculous foci. The concentric lamination of the calcium deposits is characteristic of histoplasmosis.

Coccidioidomycosis

Coccidioidomycosis results from infection with a fungus, *Coccidioides immitis.* Most cases occur in Texas, Arizona and California. In warm dry climates the chlamydospores are carried in dust, and the infection occurs by inhalation. Entrance of the microorganism through the skin has been reported. The clinical manifestations may be slight or like those of influenza or pneumonia. A specific diagnosis may be made by detection of precipitins or by complement fixation test. In the progressive form (coccidioidal granuloma) the condition resembles tuberculosis or blastomycosis. The anatomic manifestations are similar to those of tuberculosis or blastomycosis, with the formation of granulomatous lesions, diffuse fibrosis and even ulceration and cavitation. The differentiation from blastomycosis depends upon the study of the microorganism. *Coccidioides immitis* exhibits endosporulation, whereas Blastomyces reproduces by budding. The microorganisms may be found in giant cells or free.

Other Fungal Diseases

Other fungal diseases beyond the scope of this section for detailed consideration are North American blastomycosis caused by *Blastomyces dermatitidis,* a thick-walled yeast form with a thick refractile wall which reproduces by single budding; South American blastomycosis caused by *Paracoccidioides brasiliensis,* a double-contoured organism that produces multiple buds around the periphery; *Cryptococcus neoformans* in which the causative organ is a small yeast form with a heavy gelatinous capsule; opportunistic fungus infections caused by *Candida albicans, Aspergillus fumigatus,* and the organisms causing mucormycosis (Rhizopus, Mucor, and Absidia).

Leprosy

Leprosy (Hansen's disease) is a chronic, infectious granulomatous disease caused by the acid-fast bacillus *Mycobacterium leprae.* There are approximately 10,000,000 cases worldwide but only 2,000 to 3,000 cases in the United States. The acid-fast organism is very difficult to culture but has been successfully grown in foot pads of mice. The organism has a low degree of infectiousness and usually is thought to require long periods of contact before transmission is possible from one person to another. Exposure to the organism in a normal individual frequently does not lead to progressive disease. In a susceptible host with decreased resistance, the disease may be progressive. It involves principally the skin, mucous membranes, and nerves. The two principal types of reaction in leprosy are the tuberculoid and lepromatous types. In tuberculoid leprosy, there are firm, raised, hypopigmented, sharply demarcated skin lesions. There is involvement of the nerves and sensory loss. A granulomatous inflammation occurs in the dermis, and perineural inflammation of cells, epithelioid cells, and lymphocytes. Acid-fast bacilli may or may not be seen in sections of the nerves. In lepromatous leprosy there are macular, erythematous, nodular skin lesions with indistinct borders. There is massive dermal infiltration by leprae cells, (vacuolated mononuclear cells containing acid-fast bacilli). There is also perineural inflammation. The main complications of leprosy are those caused by nerve damage, mucous membrane changes, and secondary effects of longstanding chronic infection. Amyloidosis is one of the complications of leprosy. In tuberculoid leprosy, T lymphocyte function is normal. Lepromatous leprosy occurs in those patients with low host resistance due to impaired T cell function. While the prognosis of tuberculoid leprosy is good with adequate treatment, the prognosis of lepromatous leprosy is poor.

Noninfectious Granulomata

Boeck's Sarcoidosis

Boeck's sarcoidosis is a systemic disease with granulomatous manifestations in skin, lymph nodes, lungs, bone marrow of phalanges, liver, spleen, parotid, eyes and other sites, but not tendon sheaths, joints, bursae, adrenals or genitalia. The striking difference from tuberculosis is the absence of necrosis in the granulomatous nodules and the absence of a peripheral wall of lymphocytes around the granulomas. Also, the multinucleated giant cells are not usually of the Langhans type and are mostly smaller, with nuclei grouped toward the center. Some contain star-shaped crystal rosettes, asteroid bodies, in their cytoplasm and rod-shaped elastic fibers encrusted with calcium and iron, so-called Schaumann bodies, but they are not specific for this condition.

Other Granulomatous Lesions

Granulomatous lesions similar to Boeck's sarcoid are produced by beryllium if it enters a wound. Magnesium silicate, present in talcum powder, can also produce similar lesions. The most common source of beryllium at one time was beryllium phosphor from fluorescent bulbs, but this source no longer exists. Inhalation of beryllium dust (usually the oxide) from ores may produce acute or chronic pulmonary berylliosis. Even powdered starch (from rubber gloves) may induce the formation of granulomatous inflammation, especially of the peritoneum.

GENETIC ABNORMALITIES

Among the significant advances of the past decade or two have been the disclosures of the importance of the hereditary constituent in determining man's physical and metabolic well-being. The study of genetics has therefore become of major importance, and already our knowledge of disorders based on genetic abnormalities has increased enormously. A detailed account of these genetic derangements and their clinical manifestations is beyond the scope of this chapter, but a brief overview can be given. For more details a standard text on genetics should be consulted.

Genetic disorders may be due to (1) morphologically detectable chromosomal abnormalities that are present and can be recognized in the karyotype or (2) the mutation of a gene or a group of genes either during gametogenesis or after zygote development to affect the initial victim. The resulting disorder, if the original victim survives, can often be transmitted to some, possibly all, offspring either as a trait or as a full-blown disease. However, the genetic defect is not subject to chromosomal analysis and cannot be recognized by any technique presently available.

Disorders of the first group can be recognized by analysis of the chromosomes found in individual cells in the metaphase stage of division. In practice, since cells in mitosis are not found often enough in normal tissues to provide material for study, tissue culture techniques are employed. Leukocytes from the peripheral blood, bone marrow or skin are the cells cultured. After incubation the proliferating cells are fixed so as to arrest cell division in the metaphase stage, and smears or spreads of the cells are prepared and appropriately stained and are ready for study. Usually at least 10, and better 50 or more, counts are made. The orderly and systematic arrangement of the chromosomes found in the metaphase stage of an individual cell is called the karyotype.

The second group is much larger than the first and includes many diseases that manifest their presence in infancy or childhood. The initial defect results from gene mutations that may occur spontaneously during cell division or may originate as a result of some external stimulus such as ionizing radiation, the influence of certain drugs or even in association with virus infection. While the genetic defect is not subject to chromosomal study by any method now available, it is capable in the original patient of causing serious, sometimes even lethal, consequences, including many defects that may be transmitted to offspring, either as dominant or recessive syndromes.

A dominant trait is that which is expressed in both the homozygous and heterozygous conditions, while a recessive trait is expressed only in the homozygous. Dominant and recessive disorders can frequently be recognized in the family pedigree. A dominant disease is transmitted vertically; at least one of the parents of the proband must be afflicted with the same disorder. Horizontal distribution among siblings is the rule in recessive diseases, which are usually the consequences of consanguinity in the parental and more remote generations.

The normal human karyotype consists of 22 paired chromosomes, or autosomes, and two sex chromosomes, X and Y, making a total of 46 chromosomes. The pairs are divided into seven groups, A to G, each group containing from two to six autosomes classified primarily according to their size and the position of the centromere and identified by numbers from 1 to 22. With banding techniques the exact chromosome number can now be determined and the grouping by A to G is no longer needed.

When at least two X chromosomes are present, one becomes inactive and is condensed into a chromatin mass (Barr body), which is cytologically recognizable in the interphase nucleus of the cell. The inactive X chromosome may be paternal or maternal in origin even in adjacent areas of tissues (mosaicism).

Chromosomal abnormalities may be of two kinds: Either the chromosomes are present in abnormal numbers or one or more are defective in morphology; occasionally both types of defects may be present.

Diseases Due to Known Chromosomal Abnormalities

1. *Due to autosomal defects*

   Down's syndrome (Mongolism). Usually in children of older mothers. Due most often to trisomy 21. Important symptoms: mental retardation; mongoloid features; high incidence of certain conditions such as congenital heart disease, acute leukemia, thyroid autoimmune disease.

   Patau's syndrome (trisomy 15). Usually also in children of older mothers. Symptoms: microcephaly; heart abnormalities; hare lip and cleft palate; possibly capillary hemangiomas; mental retardation. Child usually dies in infancy.

   Edward's syndrome (trisomy 18). Mother also usually in older age group. Symptoms: mental retardation; multiple anomalies of heart, kidney, intestine, bones, etc.; organic brain damage often present.

   Cri du chat syndrome. Due to defect in chromosome 5. Rare. Unrelated to age of mother. Symptoms: mental retardation; small larynx (cause of typical cry); sometimes microcephaly. Child rarely survives to adult life.

2. *Due to sex chromosomal defects*

About 50 per cent of chromosomal anomalies found in liveborn infants involve sex chromosomes.

Turner's syndrome (XO). Due to single X chromosome. No relationships to mother's age. Affects females. Symptoms: short stature; infantile ovaries; amenorrhea; negative sex chromatin (no Barr body).

Klinefelter's syndrome. Due to extra X chromosome—XXY. Mothers tend to be older. Affects males. Symptoms: Eunuchoid body habitus; testicular atrophy; female distribution of body hair; possibly gynecomastia. X polysomy may be triple or quadruple. The affected individual has at least one Barr body in the nucleus of the nondividing cell but is phenotypically a male.

X polysomy. Due to extra X chromosome—may be XXX or XXXX. Mothers tend to be in older age group. Symptoms: Body habitus normal female; possibly infertile; possibly mental retardation.

Y polysomy. due to extra Y chromosome—XYY. Maternal age usually normal. Symptoms: Body habitus normal but patient is usually a tall, aggressive male. Some question whether or not there is a higher incidence of this defect in criminals.

Possible Relationship of Chromosomal Abnormalities to Cancer

It is known that nearly all, if not all, cancers show variations from the normal chromosomal patterns, but in only a few cases have specific abnormalities been associated with certain malignant diseases. Only one, the Philadelphia chromosome (usually representing a translocation from chromosome 22 to chromosome 9), has some importance, having been found in association with chronic myelogenous leukemia. In a less definite manner the Melbourne chromosome has been related to Hodgkin's disease and Christ Church chromosome, to chronic lymphatic leukemia.

Diseases Due to Gene Mutation

These disorders, which far outnumber those with demonstrable chromosomal abnormalities, are due to influences that act at the molecular level, often affecting only a single gene and thus leading to changes that are not detectable on chromosomal analysis. Although mutations may be spontaneous, that is, the cause may be some error or defect occurring during cell division, it is known that external influences, such as ionizing radiation, certain drugs and possibly even some viruses may, under appropriate conditions, injure one or more genes. Such mutant genes may be dominant or recessive. If dominant, the effect may be evident in the offspring; if recessive, the effect is usually expressed only in the homozygote, the heterozygote exhibiting no recognizable manifestation of its presence.

Among the genetic disorders due to gene mutations are the following:

1. *Due to autosomal gene defects*

Acute intermittent porphyria—dominant. Abnormal excretion of porphyrobilinogen, neurologic distrubances, abdominal pains

Alkaptonuria–recessive. Impaired synthesis of homogentisic oxidase, ochronosis

Phenylketonuria—recessive. Known as PKU, deficiency of phenylalanine hydroxylase, early mental retardation

Galactosemia–recessive. Deficiency of galactose-1-phosphatase uridyl transferase, inability to convert galactose to glucose, galactose present in urine, early mental deficiency

Glycogen storage diseases–recessive. At least 10 varieties, some due to abnormal accumulation of glycogen, others to defect in synthesis of glycogen

Tay-Sachs disease–recessive. Due to deficiency of hexosamidase, excess storage of gangliosides in ganglion cells of CNS, early onset, red spot in macula, rapidly fatal

Cystic fibrosis A very common metabolic defect in whites; a recessive condition in which the primary biochemical defect remains undertermined.

Niemann-Pick disease–recessive. Deficiency of sphingomyelinase, accumulation of sphingomyelin and cholesterol in reticuloendothelial system and neurons of CNS, hepatosplenomegaly.

Sickle cell anemia–recessive for syndrome. Affects mainly blacks, due to substitution of valine instead of glutamic acid in position 6 of the amino acid sequence.

Other autosomal disorders (dominant) include Marfan's syndrome, certain types of Ehlers-Danlos syndrome, osteogenesis imperfecta, Osler's telangiectasia hemorrhagica, tuberous sclerosis, cystic kidneys of the adult, multiple exostoses, and certain types of hypercholesterolemia.

2. *Due to sex gene defects*

Hemophilia-X–linked recessive. Type A is due to deficiency Factor VIII; Type B (also known as Christmas disease) is due to deficiency Factor

IX. In both cases there is a defect in blood clotting mechanisms.

Granulomatous disease of childhood. Red-green colorblindness.

Common Diseases in which Heredity Plays an Important but not Precisely Definable Role

This group includes diabetes mellitus, essential hypertension, certain allergies, duodenal ulcer, asthma, and hay fever. Diabetes mellitus has been considered for a long time as a model example of metabolic disease, but so far the primary defect has not been discovered. Dominant, recessive, and polygenic hereditary modes have been supported with variable emphasis.

HLA Types as Genetic Markers

The fields of transplantation biology, histocompatibility, and immunogenetics have found genetic markers that in some cases, are associated with increased risk of developing certain disease. Certain HLA types, as determined by lymphocyte toxicity procedures or mixed lymphocyte cultures, have been found to be related to the increased risk of developing certain diseases. Most notable among these are HLA type B27, associated with greatly increased risk of developing ankylosing spondylitis, Reiter's disease and psoriatic arthritis; HLA type B13, associated with increased risk of developing psoriasis vulgaris; B8, associated with dermatitis herpetiformis, insulin-dependent diabetes, thyrotoxicosis, and Addison's disease of the adrenal glands; and B7, associated with multiple sclerosis. Other diseases associated with HLA types include celiac disease, chronic active hepatitis, myasthenia gravis, Sjögren's syndrome, and Hodgkin's disease.

NONGENETIC SYNDROMES (CHEMICAL POISONS, VITAMIN DEFICIENCIES AND RADIATION INJURY)

Chemical Poisons

In fatal *carbon monoxide poisoning* the blood and the tissues have a striking so-called cherry-red color, due to the carbon monoxide hemoglobin. In the brain there may be symmetric foci of petechial hemorrhages and of encephalomalacia, most common in the basal ganglia, especially the lenticular nucleus and the globus pallidus.

Aside from the bright red color of the blood and the mucous membranes, which at first might suggest carbon monoxide poisoning, there is no distinctive morphologic feature of *hydrocyanic acid* or *cyanide poisoning*. The peach kernel or bitter-almond odor of the blood and the tissues is characteristic.

In the later stages of *methyl alcohol poisoning,* atrophy of the optic nerves is the only anatomic feature characteristic of the disease.

In *acute ethyl alcohol poisoning,* cerebral edema and hyperemia, with petechial hemorrhages of the mucosa of the stomach, are the only features. In *chronic alcoholism,* chronic catarrhal gastritis, fat infiltration of liver and Laennec's cirrhosis are the most common findings. Laennec's cirrhosis is considered by some to be due to the direct toxic effect of alcohol on the liver cells, but others attribute the liver damage primarily to nutritional deficiencies in the inadequate diet of the chronic alcoholic. There is much good evidence for both points of view.

In the acute case of *mercury poisoning,* in which the poison is taken by mouth, there is corrosion, mainly mucosal, of the stomach and of the duodenum. The mucosa is white and opaque and shows a variable amount of erosion or ulceration. In the later stages, hemorrhagic membranous ulcerative inflammation of the colon is common, and, necrosis of the proximal convoluted tubules of the kidney is a characteristic and usually fatal feature.

In *chronic lead poisoning,* the so-called blue line of the gums is characteristic, and the basophilic stippling of the red blood corpuscles is another feature. Atrophy and fibrosis of muscles of the extremities and degeneration of the testes and of the anterior horn cells of the spinal cord are common. Lead usually can be demonstrated by chemical tests in the epiphysiodiaphyseal ends of the long bones, the kidneys, the liver and the central nervous system.

In *sulfonamide poisoning* the outstanding effects are acute nephrosis with interstitial edema and infiltration of lymphocytes between the tubules, showing the degenerative change and internal hydronephrisis that result from obstruction of some of the collecting tubules by the precipitation of cyrstals. In this type of nephrosis, the portion of the nephron that begins with the distal part of the loop of Henle shows the greatest degenerative change. This has been referred to as *lower nephron nephrosis,* although it is not limited to the distal portion of the nephron. Interstitial myocarditis with infiltration of leukocytes and eosinophils has been reported commonly. Panvasculitis, especially in the myocardium, and focal necrosis of the parenchymatous organs have been described. The changes in the bone marrow are characteristic of acute anemia and agranulocytosis. A skin rash, presumably on an allergic basis, may occur. Of the various sulfonamides, sulfathiazole is the most likely to injure the kidney.

TABLE 6-3 Vitamin Deficiency in Man

Vitamin	Deficiency State	Characteristic Pathologic Changes
Fat soluble		
A (Retinol)	Night blindness; xerophthalmia; keratomalacia; epithelial keratinizing metaplasia; disturbances in bone growth	Xerophthalmia; hyperkeratosis of skin; deficient regeneration of visual purple; keratinizing squamous metaplasia of epithelium lining ducts and glands
D₂	Rickets (children)	Deficient calcification and endochondral ossification: Excess of osteoid tissue and of metaphyseal cartilage
Calciferol	Osteomalacia (adults)	Counterpart of rickets in the adult, except for absence of endochondral abnormality
K	Hypoprothrombinemia; hemorrhagic diathesis	Increased tendency to bleeding; prolonged coagulation time
Water soluble		
C (Ascorbic acid)	Scurvy	Hemorrhagic manifestation in various parts of the body; deficient osteogenesis and osteoporosis; intercellular cement substance deficient
B Complex B₁ (Thiamine)	Beriberi	Degeneration of peripheral nerves; polyneuritis; edema; cardiac dilatation, especially of right side, with decompensation; Wernicke's encephalopathy; degeneration of mamillary bodies
B₂ (Riboflavin)	Cheilosis; glossitis; dermatitis; occular lesions	Cracks or fissures at corners of mouth; atrophy of tongue; scaly dermatitis; superficial interstitial keratitis
Nicotinic acid (Niacin)	Pellagra	Dermatitis with redness, thickening, hyperkeratosis and scaling; glossitis; colitis with diarrhea; degenerative changes in central nervous system with dementia
B₁₂ (Cobalamin)	Pernicious and other megaloblastic anemias	Pernicious anemia (B₁₂ is extrinsic factor necessary, together with intrinsic factor from gastric mucosa, to prevent pernicious anemia)

Chronic fluoride poisoning occurs most commonly in the southern and the western sections of the United States but is also observed in all areas in which the drinking water contains excessive amounts of fluorides. Mottled tooth enamel, alternating patches of chalk-white and gray enamel, caused by patchy hypoplasia of this tissue, is the earliest and the chief effect of this poison. The fluorine acts directly upon the enameloblasts. Osteosclerosis also occurs. Of interest and importance, however, is the fact that proper fluoridation of drinking water protects against dental caries.

Acute fluoride poisoning is rare and is usually the result of the accidental ingestion of sodium fluoride that has been mistaken for sugar, flour or powdered milk. Less than 1 gr. can be fatal.

Acute mushroom poisoning, most commonly with *Amanita phalloides,* is characterized by acute gastroenteritis, acute nephrosis (with fatty degeneration of the kidney) and fatty degeneration of liver, heart and skeletal muscles. Foci of degeneration may occur in the brain if the condition is not immediately fatal.

Food poisoning, usually caused by the contamination of food with microorganisms of the *Salmonella* group or with toxin-producing staphylococci, commonly causes acute enteritis. A special form of food poisoning is botulism, caused by exotoxin of *Clostridium botulinum,* an anaerobic bacillus that may grow and produce its toxin in certain canned or preserved foods that have been inadequately cooked and sterilized before sealing. The principal effects of the toxin are on the nervous system, and death, which occurs in a high percentage of cases, is usually the result of respiratory failure. There are no specific morphologic changes characteristic of this highly potent toxin.

Vitamin Deficiencies

The diseases or pathologic changes listed in Table 6-3 are known to be caused by vitamin deficiencies. Some of the pathologic conditions that have been attributed to vitamin deficiency in animals have not been observed in man.

Radiation Injury

Radiation injury may result from radiation therapy, exposure of personnel involved in diagnostic radiology and radiotherapy, and accidental exposure due to nuclear accidents. Extensive investigation of victims of the atom bomb explosions in World War II increased knowledge about radiation injury. Forms of radiation include: alpha particles containing two protons and two neutrons, the least penetrating of radiant energy forms; beta particles, electrons which may penetrate through only a few millimeters of the body; gamma rays, emitted naturally from radium, uranium, and man-made radioisotopes, which penetrate deeply into tissue; and x-rays, machine generated gamma rays, which may also have alpha and beta particle effects as they penetrate tissues. Radiation injury is thought to occur either as a result of indirect action in which free radicals and peroxides are formed by ionization of tissue; or by direct action with radiant energy directly damaging vital macromolecules in the cell. The body tissues are sensitive to the effects of radiation approximately in order of their capacity for regeneration, with labile cells being most sensitive, stabile cells being of medium sensitivity, and permanent cells being least sensitive.

Acute radiation injury, such as would occur with atom bomb explosions or accidental overexposure of the whole body to radiation, may produce: the cerebral syndrome, with coma setting in immediately and death following in a few hours; the gastrointestinal syndrome, with necrosis of intestinal epithelium, nausea, vomiting, diarrhea and dehydration; and the hematopoietic syndrome, in which the white blood count begins dropping and different cell types are depleted in a characteristic fashion. Lymphocytes are depleted within 24 to 36 hours, platelets within 2 to 3 days, neutrophils within 5 to 7 days, and anemia becomes evident in a matter of weeks or months if the patient survives. Damage to the hematopoietic tissue in the bone marrow may result in bleeding problems, immunologic deficiencies, and susceptibility to infection.

Chronic radiation injury may lead to radionecrosis of the skin and sloughing. Radium implants used to treat carcinoma of the cervix may lead to rectovaginal fistula because of radionecrosis. Thus, necrosis of normal tissue is a complication of radiotherapy of cancer. Some of the other complications of radiation are sterility, aplastic anemia, cataracts, developmental defects in fetuses exposed in utero, and an increased incidence of leukemia, thyroid cancer and lung cancer.

SYSTEMIC PATHOLOGY

CARDIOVASCULAR SYSTEM

Cardiovascular disease, which includes diseases of the heart as well as vascular lesions of the central nervous system, is the most important cause of morbidity and mortality in the United States and other highly developed countries. The disorders comprising cardiovascular diseases account for over half of all deaths in the U.S. Coronary heart disease is by far the most common cause of death. Vascular lesions of the central nervous system (stroke) are the third leading cause of death following cancer, which is second. Among diseases of the heart, coronary heart disease is the leading cause of death, hypertensive heart disease next, followed by the less frequent causes of rheumatic heart disease, congenital heart disease, syphilitic heart disease and other primary and secondary types of heart disease. There is obvious overlap among coronary heart disease, vascular disease of the central nervous system and hypertensive heart disease because of the interrelationships between atherosclerosis and hypertension.

Congenital Heart Disease

This subject is also covered in the sections on internal medicine and pediatrics; only selected aspects will be presented here. The most important concept about etiology is that the injury producing congenital heart disease always occurs during the first trimester of pregnancy, because that is the period in which the development of the heart is completed. Etiologic agents include maternal disease, such as rubella and possible other viruses, teratogenic agents, such as the antimetabolite drugs and the obsolete drug thalidomide, chromosomal defects, such as those that occur in mongolism and Turner's syndrome, other single gene abnormalities which predispose to atrial septal defect, tetralogy of Fallot, and pregnancy at high altitude.

Congenital abnormalities of the heart are usually the result of abnormal communications and/or obstruction. The defects may result from abnormal septation, abnormal rotation, abnormal endocardial differentiation, and malformation of the aortic arch syndrome.

The major types of congenital heart disease are usually classified according to whether or not cyanosis (implying right-to-left shunt) is present. Those disorders with a left-to-right shunt and no cyanosis include: ventricular septal defect (the most common of *all* congenital heart malformations), atrial septal defect (including ostium primum defect, ostium secundum defect and patent foramen ovale), common atrial ventricular canal or persistent ostium atrioventriculare, and patent ductus arteriosus. Those defects without shunt or cyanosis include: pulmonary stenosis; coarctation of aorta; (adult type with narrowing below the origin of the ductus, 95 per cent of all cases of coarctation; infantile type with obstruction above the origin of the ductus, 5 per cent); aortic stenosis; vascular rings from anomalies of aortic arch, and anomalous origin of the coronary arteries. Congenital heart defects with cyanosis and right-to-left shunt include: tetralogy of Fallot (pulmonary stenosis, interventricular septal defect, overriding of aorta, and right ventricular hypertrophy), the most common form of *cyanotic* congenital heart disease; tricuspid atresia; transposition of great vessels; truncus arteriosus; Taussig-Bing heart; single ventricle; and hypoplastic left ventricle (underdevelopment of left side of heart or mitral aortic atresia).

Congential heart disease may also occur in which cyanosis develops only late in the course of the disease usually as the result of reversal of a left-right shunt. The term Eisenmenger's complex or syndrome, now obsolete, has been used to describe those cases in which left-to-right shunts from ventricular septal defects undergo reversal of after pulmonary hypertension has developed.

Rheumatic Heart Disease

While rheumatic fever may cause arthritis, subcutaneous nodules, chorea, and other manifestations, the most serious sequelae of rheumatic fever result from involvement of the heart. Rheumatic fever causes pancarditis, involving all layers of the heart: pericardium, myocardium, and endocardium, especially the valves. Rheumatic fever and rheumatic carditis are not always fatal, however, patients who die during the first attack of rheumatic carditis usually die as a result of myocarditis with myocardial failure. Patients who die after repeated attacks of rheumatic carditis usually die from the complications of valvular disease. The most widely accepted theory concerning the etiology of rheumatic fever is that it is due to hypersensitivity to group A beta-hemalytic streptococci. (See the section on infectious disease.)

The valves involved most often are the mitral and aortic with the tricuspid and particulary the pulmonary valves being less commonly affected. The mitral valve is involved in the vast majority of cases and the aortic valve is affected with the mitral valve in about 50 per cent of the cases.

Characteristically, multiple minute, firm, wartlike nodules are found on the atrial surface of the mitral valve and on the tricuspid valve when it is involved, situated about 1 to 3 mm. from the free margins, and on the ventricular surface of the aortic valve. In the acute state the vegetations seldom are large enough to interfere with valvular function. The inflammatory process involves practically the entire thickness of the valve structure. In the early stages the valve is swollen and thick, with the verrucous nodules on its surface close to the line of closure. Microscopically the ground substance of the valve is increased and fibrinoid necro-

sis is present near or beneath the verrucous nodules. The inflammatory exudate is not abundant. About the zones of necrosis, palisades of inflammatory cells, often of Anitschkow myocyte type, are present, and sometimes monocytes or polymorphonuclear leukocytes or both may be present.

There are no bacteria in the verrucous nodules on the valve leaflets. In time they become organized and finally covered by a layer of endothelial cells that grow in from the intact endothelium surrounding them. Healing of the valvular inflammation occurs by fibrosis, which causes thickening, stiffening, and retraction of the leaflet. Recurrent inflammation of damaged valves is common. The chordae tendineae also are involved and, as organization proceeds, become thickened and shortened as well as fused. Retraction, deformity and calcification of the scar tissue cause various degrees of valvular stenosis and insufficiency, with hypertrophy of the myocardial walls, the work of which is increased by these lesions. In mitral stenosis, the left atrium and the right ventricle become hypertrophic and dilated, but in aortic stenosis, there is hypertrophy of the left ventricle.

Aschoff bodies are found in the myocardium in about 80 per cent of cases of acute rheumatic fever. These are localized, usually perivascular, foci of a proliferative inflammation that is composed of large mononuclear and multinuclear cells, with so-called owl-eyed vesicular nuclei and some lymphocytes surrounding a focus of collagenous degeneration or necrosis, especially in the early stage of the lesion. The lesion is specific for rheumatic inflammation in the myocardium or other tissues in which it has been observed.

In addition to the rheumatic lesions of the endocardium and myocardium, the pericardium in a majority of cases is also involved, particularly in the active phase. The characteristic lesion is a diffuse fibrinous or serofibrinous inflammation of nonspecific type.

Bacterial Infective Endocarditis

Anatomically, infective endocarditis is characterized by soft, friable vegetations on the affected valve, very different from the firm, granular verrucous nodules of rheumatic valvulitis. The course of the disease may be acute or subacute, but this method of classifying the disease is not as important as classifying by the etiologic agent. The morphologic findings in the heart are quite similar regardless of the etiologic agent or clinical course. About 50 per cent of the cases that develop in a subacute fashion are caused by *Streptococcus viridans* and in many of these cases there has been previous damage to the heart by preexisting rheumatic heart disease or congenital heart disease. Many of the cases that develop rapidly are due to *Staphylococ-*

cus aureus. A large number of infectious agents have been identified as causing infective endocarditis in addition to these two prototype organisms. They include large number of bacteria: other streptococcal species, gonococci, enterococci, coliform organisms, *Hemophilus influenzae,* proteus, salmonellae, as well as mycotic organisms such as candida, aspergillus and mucor. Infective endocarditis is a serious risk of drug addition with intravascular injection of unsterile drugs, and it is also a serious complication of open heart surgery with valve replacement.

The typical lesion is a form of valvulitis, with large, soft, friable platelet and fibrin thrombi on the valve surface with numerous microorganisms both within and on the surface of the vegetations. Portions of this type of friable thrombus break off readily and, if on the mitral valve, may give rise to septic emboli that may be carried by the blood to other parts of the body. This type of endocarditis is extremely serious. Before antibiotics the mortality rate was high, close to 100 per cent. Now a cure is possible in a majority of these cases as a result of intensive treatment with appropriate antibiotics.

Syphilitic Heart Disease

Syphilis of the heart affects primarily the aortic valve, resulting in dilatation of the valve ring with insufficiency and often causing narrowing of the orifices of the coronary arteries. The myocardium is occasionally involved, especially the smaller arteries, which may show low-grade endarteritis and periarteritis. The structure most commonly affected is the aortic arch, the wall of which, along with the distended aortic valve ring, shows inflammation of the vasa vasorum. Aortic stenosis is never found unless there is associated chronic rheumatic valvulitis or arteriosclerotic calcification to account for it. The aortic insufficiency may be brought about by (1) separation of the valve cusps at the commissures, (2) thickening and retraction of the cusps themselves, and (3) stretching of the aortic ring. The cusps show diffuse proliferative inflammation, with thickening of the free margins that roll inward toward the ventricular chamber. Artificial valves made of plastic have been developed and now can be inserted in the aortic ring for correction of the insufficiency.

The inflammatory process may involve the coronary orifices in the aortic sinuses as well as the first portions of the arteries, causing narrowing of the lumina and producing myocardial ischemia, fibrosis and angina pectoris.

In rare instances syphilis may cause gummata or diffuse exudative and proliferative inflammation within the myocardium, with consequent effects on conduction and muscular function.

Coronary (Atherosclerotic, Ischemic) Heart Disease

This is the most common and the most important form of cardiac disease, being responsible for approximately 30 per cent of deaths from all causes in the United States. Coronary atherosclerosis is the underlying cause of 95 to 99 per cent of all cases of coronary heart disease, the rare exceptions being due to narrowing of the coronary ostia by aortic atherosclerotic plaques or syphilitic involvement or emboli to the coronary arteries. The clinical spectrum of coronary heart disease includes sudden death (presumably due to cardiac arrythmias) as a result of coronary occlusion or severe coronary stenosis with ischemia, myocardial infarction as a result of coronary atherosclerosis with occlusion (usually due to thrombosis), and angina pectoris as a result of severe narrowing of the coronary arteries and intermittent ischemia resulting therefrom. Almost all patients with coronary heart disease have extensive involvement of the coronary arteries with advanced stages of the atherosclerotic process—fibrous plaques, calcified plaques, and complicated plaques with necrotic softening, hemorrhage, thrombosis, or ulceration. In the unusual case, coronary heart disease and even sudden death may result from an isolated but significantly placed atherosclerotic plaque with superimposed thrombus. This situation occurs in less than 1 to 20 cases.

The atherosclerotic lesions are scattered throughout the coronary system but occur most frequently in the more proximal portions of the major branches of the coronary arteries. The most common sites of significant atherosclerotic involvement are the first part of the anterior descending branch of the left coronary artery just after its bifurcation and the right coronary artery in the first few centimeters after its origin and another site in the right coronary artery just before it reaches the posterior interventricular septum.

Coronary atherosclerosis may lead to the ischemic complications listed above in the following ways in decreasing order of frequency: (1) slow buildup of atherosclerotic lesions over years and decades with a sudden occlusive event, usually thrombus, superimposed on a ruptured or ulcerated atherosclerotic plaque; (2) progressive narrowing of the coronary lumen by extensive atherosclerotic lesions until ischemia is produced; (3) ulceration of an atherosclerotic plaque producing atherosclerotic embolism in the distal coronary artery.

Risk Factors for Coronary Heart Disease. Epidemiologic studies have shown that there are markers or individual characteristics which are associated with an increased risk of developing coronary heart disease. Three strong and independent risk factors that have been shown to be related to increased risk or coronary heart disease are elevated serum lipids (serum cholesterol, especially cholesterol carried in low density lipoproteins), elevated blood pressure (either systolic, diastolic, or both), and cigarette smoking. Other significant risk factors include diabetes or glucose intolerance, hypothyroidism, obesity, a family history of coronary disease, and sedentary jobs or physical inactivity. Other suspected but somewhat controversial risk factors include "stress," use of oral contraceptives and elevated uric acid levels.

Myocardial Infarction

The site of myocardial infarction is usually determined by which of the coronary arteries are involved and the portion of the vessel that is occluded. Occlusion of the anterior descending branch of the left coronary artery produces infarction in the anterior interventricular septum and anterior left ventricle. Occlusion of the circumflex branch of the left coronary artery produces infarction of the lateral wall of the left ventricle. Occlusion of the right coronary artery typically produces infarction of the posterior interventricular septum, the posterior portion of the left ventricle, and very rarely in a small portion of the right ventricle. The right ventricle is usually spared from myocardial infarction.

Complications of myocardial infarction include cardiac arrhythmias (the most severe being myocardial fibrillation), mural thrombi with distal embolism, myocardial failure, and myocardial rupture with hemopericardium and cardiac tamponade.

Myocardial scars, especially large scars greater than 1 cm. in diameter, are nearly always the result of ischemia from coronary heart disease. They represent healing and replacement of necrotic muscle fibers by fibrous connective tissue. Any disease that produces myocardial necrosis followed by healing will obviously produce a scar, but coronary disease is by far the most common cause of such myocardial necrosis.

Hypertensive Heart Disease

This is a common form of cardiac disease which is the result of prolonged and continued systemic hypertension. Mortality from hypertensive heart disease and other hypertension related diseases has declined in the United States in recent years. Nevertheless, more than 50,000 deaths occur annually as a result of hypertensive heart disease with cardiac failure, and there are many more deaths in which hypertension is an underlying or aggravating cause. Such conditions include two forms of stroke, hypertensive cerebral hemorrhage and cerebral infarction, coronary heart disease (because hypertension is one of the major risk factors), and renal failure from advanced arteriolar nephrosclerosis which occurs in conjunction with hypertension.

The typical findings at autopsy in a person who dies of hypertensive heart disease are a large heart and small kidneys. The heart in hypertension exhibits the major changes of extreme hypertrophy of the left ventricular myocardium (concentric hypertrophy) and an increase in the weight of the heart to 500 or 750 grams and in some cases even higher. The kidneys are small because of the associated arteriolar nephrosclerosis which occurs with prolonged and sustained hypertension.

The only microscopic changes of note in the myocardium are marked hypertrophy of the muscle fibers as well as their nuclei. There may be foci of interstitial fibrosis as a result of sclerosis of small branches of the coronary arteries or there may be some of the previously described changes from coronary atherosclerosis since hypertension aggravates coronary atherosclerosis. Cardiac hypertrophy is the result of increased peripheral resistance resulting in increased work load for the heart over a long period of time. Once the increased demand of the heart cannot be met, there is cardiac dilatation and cardiac failure as a terminal event.

Endocardial fibroelastosis is a form of heart disease usually occurring in children in the first two years of life and characterized by marked thickening of the mural endocardium especially of the left side of the heart. While fibroelastic thickening sometimes occurs in conjunction with other forms of heart disease, particularly congenital anomalies, the condition in its primary form occurs typically in patients presenting with large globular hearts and cardiac failure and without evidence of valvular or other underlying disease. Theories of causation abound; however, the etiology is obscure.

The diagnosis of *primary cardiomyopathy* is made primarily by excluding known causes of myocardial disease. These cardiomyopathies are usually divided into three types: (1) congestive cardiomyopathy, characterized by marked enlargement of the heart, cardiac dilatation and congestive heart failure; (2) hypertrophic cardiomyopathy, characterized by marked myocardial hypertrophy which is frequently asymmetrical, most striking in the interventricular septum, and without significant dilatation; and (3) restrictive or constrictive cardiomyopathy with associated endocardial fibroelastosis or endomyocardial fibrosis. Cardiac abnormalities that mimic some of these primary cardiomyopathies may have been caused by a variety of etiologic agents, including alcohol, metabolic disorders, autoimmune connective tissue disease, amyloidosis, and others.

Myocarditis has been produced by almost all forms of microorganisms, including bacteria (both as a result of direct bacterial involvement and toxins produced by bacteria at distant sites), viruses, rickettsiae, and parasitic organisms. Worthy of special mention is diphtheritic myocarditis, one of the major complications of diphtheria and a result of toxin elaborated by the organisms, whether they be in the respiratory tract, genital tract, or elsewhere. Viral agents cited as frequent causes of myocarditis include the Coxsackie and ECHO viruses.

Congestive Heart Failure

The mechanisms and causes of congestive heart failure are discussed in the chapter on internal medicine. Basically, congestive heart failure occurs either because of a decreased myocardial capacity to contract or because of an increased pressure-volume load imposed on the heart. This section will include only the most significant pathological findings in patients with congestive heart failure. In the heart there is dilatation of the affected chambers. The left ventricle and left atrium are dilated in left heart failure, and the right ventricle and right atrium are dilated in right heart failure. Failure of the left side of the heart also causes pulmonary congestion and pulmonary edema, and the histologic hallmark is the presence of hemosiderin-laden macrophages in the aveoli and hyperemic alveolar capillaries. Failure of the right side of the heart leads to chronic passive congestion of the liver (giving it a nutmeg appearance), congestion of the spleen and other abdominal viscera, and peripheral edema and ascites.

Pericardial Disease

Transudation of fluid into the pericardial sac, which may occur in cardiac failure or the nephrotic syndrome, is called *hydropericardium,* or pericardial effusion. *Hemopericardium,* blood in the pericardial sac, may be due to myocardial infarction with rupture, rupture of a saccular aneurysm of the aortic arch or rupture of a dissecting aneurysm into the pericardium, penetrating wounds, and more rarely tuberculosis or malignant tumor involving the pericardium. Sudden massive hemorrhage into the pericardial sac from any of these causes can interfere with the action of the heart *(cardiac tamponade)* and is usually fatal.

Pericarditis. Acute pericarditis may be caused by both infectious and noninfectious agents. Organisms may involve the pericardium by direct extension from surrounding structures or by the blood stream. Among the bacteria that may cause pericarditis are staphylo-coccus, pneumococcus, streptococcus, and many others. The pericardium may be involved in tuberculosis. A variety of viral agents also may involve the pericardium. Rheumatic fever, characteristically produces fibrinous or sero fibrinous pericarditis. Fibrinous pericarditis may be a result of uremia.

Chronic, or Healed, Pericarditis. Healed pericarditis may be the result of organization of previous involvement of suppurative or granulomatous inflammation. Significant healed pericarditis producing constrictive pericarditis most commonly occurs following infections with staphylococcus and the tubercle bacillus. *Constrictive pericarditis* may prevent adequate filling of the heart during diastole and may cause marked congestion of the liver and spleen, as well as ascites. Another form of chronic pericarditis, *adhesive mediastinopericarditis,* leads to increased workload of the heart and cardiac hypertrophy and dilatation because of adhesions between the pericardium and surrounding mediastinal structures.

Diseases of the Blood Vessels

Aneurysm. A true aneurysm is a localized dilatation of an artery involving all coats of the vessel. Aneurysms are described according to their shape as saccular, fusiform or cylindrical. Three types of aortic aneurysms are *syphilitic aneurysm,* most commonly occurring in the aortic arch; *atherosclerotic aneurysms,* usually occurring in the abdominal aorta; and *dissecting aneurysms,* resulting from *idiopathic cystic medial necrosis.* Dissecting aneurysms usually begin in the arch of the aorta and may dissect throughout its length. The misnomer *mycotic aneurysm* refers to an aneurysm of an artery due to weakening of the wall by bacterial infection, frequently from an infected embolus. A *congenital* or *berry aneurysm* is the type that may form in the circle of Willis when the intravascular pressure causes bulging out from an area of congenital weakness at branching sites, especially at the junction of the internal carotid and middle cerebral artery. A false aneurysm is an extravascular hematoma communicating with the lumen of a blood vessel and is usually traumatic in origin.

Buerger's Disease (Thromboangiitis Obliterans). This is a obscure disease which characteristically involves arteries, veins and nerves of the lower extremity with areas of inflammation and thrombosis. The upper extremities are also sometimes involved. It occurs almost exclusively in men who are heavy cigarette smokers. It causes intensive pain and may lead to gangrene. There is a close similarity of some of the features of Buerger's disease to other conditions such as peripheral atherosclerosis or embolization to the lower extremities; but it seems that the entity of

Buerger's disease actually exists as a distinct condition.

Polyarteritis Nodosa (Periarteritis). Because of the nature of the lesions, polyarteritis nodosa is now classed with the autoimmune diseases, involving primarily the smaller branches of the arterial system, especially in the internal organs, such as the heart, the kidneys, and even the brain, as well as in the skin and in striated muscle. The inflammatory reaction in the affected vessels is a violent one, and marked degeneration and necrosis are followed by intense leukocytic infiltration. Fibrinoid necrosis is usually marked. Polyarteritis nodosa is generally considered to be a response to autoimmune antigen-antibody complexes. In the later stage of the disease, perivascular inflammation is most pronounced, forming characteristic nodules or nodes. Thrombosis may complicate the lesions with obliteration of the vessel lumina, and aneurysmal dilatation may occur, sometimes with resulting hemorrhage.

Phlebitis. Phlebitis often results from an extension of a localized suppurative process, with the formation, in a local vein, of a thrombus that may extend into the larger veins. The vessel wall is infiltrated by leukocytes with thrombus formation at the sites where the intima is involved. Before the thrombus is completely organized, emboli may break off and lodge in the lungs and sometimes even in other organs. If infected, these emboli may set up new foci of inflammation, which may result in the formation of abscesses.

Arteriosclerosis. Arteriosclerosis or "hardening of the arteries," is the term given to those changes that result in thickening, hardening and loss of elasticity of arterial walls. There are three main morphologic types of arteriosclerosis: (1) atherosclerosis; (2) Mönckeberg's medial sclerosis, characterized by ring-like zones of calcification of the media in certain peripheral arteries, especially of the lower extremities; and (3) arteriolar sclerosis, characterized by proliferative fibromuscular or intimal thickening of the small arteries and arterioles.

Atherosclerosis. Atherosclerosis is of great interest because of its clinical significance in causing heart attacks and strokes. It is a specific form of arteriosclerosis. Atherosclerosis primarily involves the intima (innermost coat) of large elastic arteries and the medium-sized muscular arteries with characteristic accumulation of lipid in the lesions. In addition to the accumulation of lipid, there is accumulation of connective tissues and various blood products. A number of complications can result from an atherosclerotic lesion, such as thrombosis, hemorrhage into a plaque, and ulceration. The hallmarks are that atherosclerosis is intimal and that it is characterized by the accumulation of fat. The importance of atherosclerosis is that it is the most prominent form of arteriosclerosis in causing clinically significant disease.

The principle lesions of atherosclerosis recognizable on gross examination of arteries are fatty streaks, fibrous plaques, complicated plaques with ulceration, hemorrhage or mural thrombi, and calcified plaques. Studies of the natural history of atherosclerosis have shown that fatty streaks begin in childhood as fat accumulation in a slightly thickened intima. Fibrous plaques develop early in adult life with connective tissue accumulation around the intimal fat. Complicated lesions leading to arterial occlusion and ischemia occur in later adult life, decades after the initial arterial lesions. Thus, the occlusive consequences of atherosclerosis (myocardial infarction, angina pectoris, cerebral infarction) indicate the end stage of a process usually active for three decades or more.

While the etiology and pathogenesis of atherosclerosis are not completely understood, the role of elevated plasma lipoproteins is well documented. The mesenchymal response with connective tissue accumulation in the arterial intima is also an important element. The two oldest theories of atherosclerosis are the encrustation theory of Rokitansky (incorporation of organized mural thrombi into the intima with development of atherosclerotic plaques) and the lipid infiltration theory of Virchow (imbibition of lipid from the plasma into a damaged intima). Some modern theories encompass aspects of both of these early hypotheses. For example, both plasma lipoproteins and platelet factors are thought to cause connective tissue proliferation in the atherosclerotic process.

Intimal fat in human and experimental atherosclerosis is both intracellular and extracellular. At least two cell types are important in atherosclerosis. Intimal smooth muscle cells accumulate lipid and may also elaborate collagen, elastin, and glycosaminoglycans. Lipid-containing macrophages (foam cells) are prominent features of atherosclerotic lesions and are quite distinct from the lipid-containing smooth muscle cells. While the exact role of endothelial cells (or endothelial damage) and elements of the coagulation system are not completely known, they may also have a role in the pathogenesis of atherosclerosis.

Clinical Significance of Atherosclerosis. Atherosclerosis is the main underlying cause of coronary heart disease, stroke, gangrene of the extremities, and aneurysm (dilatation) of the abdominal aorta. Atherosclerosis produces clinically significant disease by various mechanisms. First, it may narrow the lumen of arteries, thereby producing ischemia (deficiency of blood) to some degree. This change occurs in angina pectoris, for example, in which the coronary arteries are stenotic or partially occluded, and the myocardium becomes ischemic under certain conditions. Second, atherosclerosis sets the stage for sudden complete occlusion with more severe ischemia and resultant death of tissue in an organ such as the heart (in which case, there is sudden death of myocardial infarction) or the brain (in which case, there is stroke) or the leg (in which case, there is infarction and gangrene). Third, atherosclerotic lesions in the aorta can be a source of emboli (thrombi or blood clots which break off from the vascular wall) to the extremities. Fourth, atherosclerosis can produce clinical sequelae by weakening the wall of the aorta. Even though atherosclerosis is primarily a disease of the intima, the media of the aorta may be secondarily weakened, and the result is an aneurysm or ballooning of the vessel wall.

Mönckeberg's Medial Sclerosis. In this form of sclerosis, which affects small- to medium-sized arteries, ringlike bands of calcification accumulate in the medial coats, particularly those of the arteries of the extremities. These changes usually are of relatively little clinical importance.

Arteriolar Sclerosis (Arteriolosclerosis). This change is limited primarily to the arterioles, and sometimes the smaller arteries. It may be of hyaline or hyperplastic type. The former, when it affects the arterioles of the kidneys (and rarely other abdominal organs), may be associated with slowly rising blood pressure of moderate type; the latter, often referred to as the onion-skin type of vascular lesion, may be associated with acute and severe elevation of blood pressure such as occurs in rapidly progressing hypertension. Whether the arteriolar involvement in the kidneys precedes the development of hypertension and even whether the hemodynamic disturbance in the renal circulation bears a primary causative relationship to the production of the elevated blood pressure are still unsettled questions.

Anemia

Anemia is the condition in which there is a reduction in the number of red blood cells per cubic millimeter or of the hemoglobin content of the red cells, or both, with corresponding reduction in the oxygen-carrying capacity of the blood. The main causes are (1) blood loss due to hemorrhage either external or internal; (2) excess red cell destruction, as in hemolytic anemias; and (3) diminished or defective red cell production as in iron deficiency anemias, vitamin C deficiency anemia, pernicious anemia, and bone marrow toxicity anemias.

Anemia from Blood Loss. Hemorrhage with loss of blood from the body removes cell forming elements, especially iron, and blood replacement is necessary. Chronic blood loss is the most common cause of iron deficiency anemia in adults.

Hemolytic Anemias. The hemolytic anemias with excess destruction of red cells include those due to intracorpuscular defects in the erythrocytes (usually inherited) and those due to extracorpuscular factors which cause increased hemolysis or erythrocytes (usually acquired).

Hemolytic anemias due to intracorpuscular defects include the hemoglobinopathies, hereditary spherocytosis, and other genetically determined abnormalities of erythrocytes. The *hemoglobinopathies* include those conditions in which there is (1) a quantitative defect in the synthesis of a specific polypeptide chain such as occurs in β and α thalassemia; (2) a biochemical alteration in the structure of hemoglobin, such as occurs in hemoglobin S, hemoglobin C, hemoglobin D; and (3) combinations of these such as in hemoglobin S/β thalassemia, hemoglobin D/β thalassemia. The prototypes of the hemoglobinopathies are sickle cell anemia and thalassemia.

Sickle cell anemia is determined by the presence of SS hemoglobin and occurs mainly in blacks, but many also occur in persons of Mediterranean ancestry. This inherited disorder leads to the formation of sickle-shaped red blood cells (sicklemia) and is accompanied by severe anemia in those persons who inherit the trait from both parents. The classical laboratory finding of hemolysis is present, and there is hemosiderosis in various organs. Pathological findings in sickle-cell disease occur as a result of both severe anemia as well as a tendency for the abnormal blood cells to cause vascular stasis and thrombosis. In long-standing cases of sickle cell disease, the spleen is usually small and fibrotic because of the multiple episodes of infarction and healing.

The thalassemia syndromes are a group of hereditary disorders characterized by a deficiency in the synthesis of one or other of the normal polypeptide chains. In β thalassemia the synthesis of β chains in decreased, and α thalassemia is a result of inadequate synthesis of α chains of hemoglobin. β thalassemia is the most widespread inherited abnormality of hemoglobin synthesis. Examples have been found in virtually every population studied, although it seems to occur most frequently in the areas that border the Mediterranean Sea.

In *homozygous β thalassemia (thalassemia major),* the clinical picture includes anemia, jaundice and splenomegaly beginning early in life. There is profound erythroid hyperplasia and anemia with hypochromic red cells, leptocytes, and numerous normoblasts in the peripheral blood smear. Excessive iron deposits occur in the marrow, liver, spleen and pancreas. In *heterozygous β thalassemia,* the clinical picture may range from a completely asymptomatic person to a syndrome with moderate anemia, intermittent jaundice, splenomegaly, and changes in hemoglobin concentration. In addition to these thalassemia syndromes, there are combinations of sickle cell disease and β thalassemia.

Hereditary spherocytosis is an autosomal dominant disorder characterized by an intracorpuscular defect that causes the erythrocytes to be spheroydal in shape, more fragile than normal, and vulnerable to splenic sequestration and destruction. Splenomegaly is a characteristic; and splenectomy results in improvement.

Hemolytic anemia due to glucose-6-phosphate dehydrogenase (G-6-PD) deficiency is a condition in which sex-linked inheritance of the mutant enzyme causes the production of red cells which are vulnerable to injury which may be triggered by numerous oxygen drugs such as the antimalarials, sulfonamides, nitrofurans, aspirin and phenacetin, as well as by infection. The hemolytic phases are episodic and do not produce the extensive secondary changes that may occur in other chronic hemolytic anemias. Other enzyme deficiencies may predispose to episodes of hemolysis. Among these is *pyruvate kinase deficiency.*

Acquired hemolytic disorders (principally extracorpuscular defects) include autoimmune hemolytic anemias, usually due to warm autoantibodies to patient's erythrocytes, with positive direct Coombs' test, and occurring secondarily in patients with diseases such as systemic lupus erythematosus; hemolytic anemias mediated by isoantibodies, occurring in transfusion reactions and erythroblastosis fetalis; hemolytic anemias caused by drug-induced antibodies to quinidine, penicillin, alpha methyldopa; hemolysis caused by septicemia, malaria, and various other infections; and hypersplenism in which a greatly enlarged spleen from almost any cause may sequester and destroy erythroctes.

Diminished or Defective Red Cell Production.
Iron deficiency anemia, perhaps the most common form of anemia, is due to inadequate supplies of iron in the blood-forming tissues. Causes may be blood loss from the body, defective absorption of iron, diet deficient in iron-containing foods. Anemia is of the microcytic, hypochromic type and is more common in women than in men.

Pernicious anemia is the classic form of chronic, insidious, megaloblastic (addisonian) anemia, which is caused by a deficiency of vitamin B_{12}. It appears most commonly in individuals over 40 years of age.

In about one fourth of the cases there is a family history of the disease. Most patients have atrophic gastritis or a gastric neoplasm or have had a major portion of the stomach removed surgically. The cause of the disease is the failure of the atrophic gastric mucosa to secrete amounts of an "intrinsic" factor sufficient to bring about absorption of vitamin B_{12}, the "extrinsic" factor or the so-called antipernicious anemia factor. The nervous system is not infrequently involved as well.

The anemia is macrocytic, and normochromic. Usually there is leukopenia with relative lymphocytosis, macrocytosis, poikilocytosis, and anisocytosis. The bone marrow demonstrates megaloblastic red cell maturation. An early distinctive feature of the peripheral blood morphology in this disorder is the presence of large hypersegmented neutrophils. Regeneration is indicated by an increase in reticulated red cells following therapy with vitamin B_{12}.

Iron-containing blood pigment accumulates in the spleen, the liver and the kidneys (hemosiderosis). The spleen usually is enlarged and engorged with red blood corpuscles. Glossitis is common, with atrophy of the mucous membrane of the gastrointestinal tract, resulting in achylia or achlorhydria in 93 per cent of all cases. Subacute combined sclerosis, peripheral neuritis and degeneration in the brain are common.

The blood picture of pernicious anemia is sometimes found with gastric carcinoma, *Diphyllobothrium latum* infestation, sprue and pregnancy. In sprue, this picture is due to folic acid deficiency. A combination of folic acid deficiency and iron deficiency is a common cause of anemia in pregnancy.

Aplastic anemia, or bone marrow failure, is characterized by pancytopenia with a normocytic, normochromic anemia, neutropenia, and thrombocytopenia. About half of the cases are idiopathic. Known causes include whole body radiation, chemical agents and drugs. Aplastic anemia is one of the most feared complications of treatment with chloramphenicol and careful monitoring of the blood is necessary during therapy with this drug. Alkalating agents, antimetabolites and benzene may lead to bone marrow failure. There may occasionally be idiosyncratic reactions with pancytopenia in certain patients being treated with organic arsenicals, penicillin, tetracycline, methylphenylethyl hydantoin, trimethadione, phenylbutazone, and certain other drugs.

Myelophthisic anemia refers to marrow failure caused by space-occupying lesions that cause destruction of large amounts of bone marrow. Metastatic carcinoma, multiple myeloma, and leukemia are the principal causes of myelophthisic anemia.

Hemophilia

Hemophilia is a hereditary disease affecting males only, but transmitted exclusively by females as a sex-linked recessive gene defect. It is characterized by a tendency to hemorrhage that is not easily controlled and may be severe. There are two main types: classical hemophilia (hemophilia A), which is caused by a deficiency in Factor VIII (antihemophilic globulin or AHG), and Christmas disease (hemophilia B), in which Factor IX is deficient. Clinical differentiation is difficult, and both forms exhibit a tendency to hemorrhage that is not easily controlled and may be very severe, even fatal. In these diseases a degree of trauma that is of no significance in a normal individual may result in hematoma formation, and a small puncture or incision in the skin may result in profound loss of blood. The blood platelets are not diminished, and the capillary resistance is normal. The coagulation time is greatly increased. The partial thromboplastin time (PTT) is prolonged. Bleeding time is normal, and the blood vessels retract and contract normally. Another condition, less common than the above, in which defects in one or more of the functional components of Factor VIII are present, is von Willebrand's disease. Prolonged bleeding time and prolonged coagulation time are present. The components of Factor VIII that may be deficient are Factor VIII-related antigen, von Willebrand's cofactor, and the clot-promoting fraction of Factor VIII.

Purpura

Purpura occurs in a group of diseases characterized by spontaneous hemorrhages into the skin and the mucous membranes, a great reduction of platelets in the blood, lengthening of the bleeding time and an increase in the fragility of the capillaries and the smaller vessels.

Symptomatic, or secondary, purpura may occur in (1) leukemia or aplastic anemia, (2) carcinomatosis of the bone marrow, (3) severe sepsis, (4) chemical poisonings, and (5) scurvy.

Schönlein-Henoch purpura is apparently the result of a form of hypersensitivity reaction in which small blood vessels are injured and focal and diffuse hemorrhages occur. The blood itself is normal, but the lability of the vessels leads to petechial hemorrhages in many organs and tissues.

Essential, primary or *idiopathic thrombocytopenic purpura* includes all purpuras of unknown etiology. It is primarily a disease of children and young adults, about 80 per cent of cases being found in the first two decades of life. Epistaxis and uterine bleeding are very frequent; gastrointestinal and urinary tract bleeding is less common. The platelets are greatly reduced during attacks, but may be normal in the intervals. The prothrombin, antithrombin and coagulation times are normal, but the bleeding time is prolonged, especially during attacks, and the capillary resistance usually is diminished. Some victims of this condition are improved greatly by splenectomy. The spleen is moderately enlarged, but the bone marrow is normal.

Leukemia

Leukemia is a form of malignant disease that is characterized by marked hyperplasia of the leukocyte-forming centers, with qualitative and quantitative alterations in peripheral blood leukocytes. This results in a permanent marked increase in white cells, both mature and immature, in the circulating blood. Remissions may occur, but usually the disease leads to anemia, thrombocytopenia and death. Although the cause is unknown, the theories of etiology include the possibility of oncogenic viruses or excessive exposure to ionizing radiation (witness the increased incidence of leukemia in survivors of the atomic bombing of Hiroshima and Nagosaki) and the possibility that genetic (chromosomal) factors may play a role.

Acute leukemia may be myeloblastic, myelomonocytic, monocytic, or lymphoblastic in type, though the specific type often cannot be determined because of the immaturity of the cells. It occurs chiefly in the young. The principal features are bleeding from the gums and the mucous membranes, weakness, anemia and fever. The peripheral leukocyte count may not be markedly elevated, as in the chronic form, and the spleen, the liver and the superficial lymph nodes may not be enlarged.

Acute leukemias have characteristically been classified by the appearance of the cell types in the peripheral blood smear and bone marrow based on Romanowsky-stained preparations. More precise classification can now be obtained by using the results of cytochemical staining with peroxidase, various esterases, Sudan Black B, and Periodic Acid Schiff (PAS) to distinguish among myeloblastic, myelomonocytic, monocytic and lymphoblastic leukemias. Candidates for examination, particularly for specialty examinations, should familiarize themselves with the new French-American-British (FAB) classification of leukemias, which is beyond the scope of this review.

Chronic myelocytic leukemia occurs chiefly in middle life. Weakness, splenomegaly, leukemia and anemia are the prominent features. The leukocytes in the blood may increase to between 100,000 and 500,000 per cu. mm. in typical cases with a wide variety of granulocytes and their precursors, including stem cells, leukoblasts, premyelocytes and myelocytes, and usually an increase in basophils in the circulation. Nucleated red cells may occasionally be seen, and, because the red cell-forming centers may be invaded and destroyed by white cells, severe anemia is usually present. The granulocytes in chronic myelocytic leukemia contain greatly decreased levels or no alkaline phosphatase in contrast to normal granulocytes.

The spleen, the liver, and the lymph nodes are usually enlarged, though the peripheral nodes are not commonly involved. Leukemic infiltration is common in the kidneys and the liver and may even involve the skin, the periosteum, the intestine, and the stomach.

Chronic lymphocytic leukemia involves primarily the lymphatic system, including the peripheral lymph nodes as well as those in the mediastinum and abdomen. The spleen and liver are only slightly to moderately enlarged. The leukocytes in the blood are not as abundant as in chronic myelocytic leukemia, varying between 20,000 and 200,000 per cu. mm. In general they tend to be of one type in any given case, large, medium or small, with varying numbers of immature lymphocytes, though the vast majority of the cells are mature. Anemia is generally uncommon except in the terminal stages when severe anemia may develop.

The spleen shows enlargement of the lymphoid follicles with obliteration of the pulp and the normal architecture of the follicles. The lymph nodes are enlarged and often fused, with hyperplasia obliterating the lymph sinuses. The bone marrow is heavily infiltrated by lymphocytes, with a corresponding decrease of myeloid cells. Nodular leukemic tumors may occur in the skin.

Myeloproliferative Syndrome

The myeloproliferative syndrome provides a unifying concept for several abnormalities of the bone marrow involving one or more of the stem lines. It implies overlap and, in some cases, crossover from one of these conditions to another. For example, the rare case of polycythemia vera (an idiopathic condition characterized by greatly elevated red cell mass) may give rise to myeloid metaplasia, or chronic myelocytic leukemia, or erythroleukemia (Di Guglielmo's syndrome). Conditions that comprise the myeloproliferative syndrome include polycythemia vera, erythroleukemia, chronic granulocytic leukemia, megakaryocytic myelosis, megakaryocytic leukemia, and myelofibrosis (including myeloid metaplasia, and agnogenic myeloid metaplasia). The final common pathway of many of these conditions is the terminal development of an acute "blastic" leukemia.

RESPIRATORY SYSTEM

Pneumoconioses

The pneumoconioses are characterized by the deposition of dust particles (with or without fibrosis) in the lungs. This deposition is related to the concentration of the particle in the air; its size and shape; its chemical nature and solubility; and the duration of exposure.

Anthracosis. Carbon pigmentation of the lungs (anthracosis) is present to some degree in all city dwellers, especially cigarette smokers. In most cases, it is a relatively unimportant form of pneumoconiosis in that it does not stimulate the formation of fibrous tissue and there is not correlation between the existence of anthracosis and any other pathologic process in the lung.

Silicosis. Silicosis is an occupational disease (sandblasting, stone cutting and polishing, glass manufacturing, etc.) that is due to the inhalation of silica particles. The onset is insidious and exposure for 10 to 15 years is usually necessary to produce severe disease. The affected lung contains fibrous nodules which tend to be located in the upper lobes and hilar regions. Eventually, a more diffuse fibrosis may occur and replace large areas of parenchyma. Hilar lymph node involvement is similar to that of the lung. Polariscopic examination of the nodules reveals birefringent particles of silicon dioxide. Serious complications of silicosis include tuberculosis, emphysema, right-sided heart failure (cor pulmonale) and pneumonia.

Asbestosis. Inhalation of asbestos fibers may not only stimulate diffuse interstitial fibrosis, but may also result in a markedly increased incidence of bronchogenic carcinoma and mesothelioma. Significant asbestos exposure is relatively common due to its widespread usuage, brake linings, insulation material, roofing shingles, acoustical products, etc.). In most cases, manifestations of the disease appear 10 to 20 years after exposure. The basal portions of the lower lobes and the pleura are particularly involved. Asbestos bodies, (ferruginous bodies) consisting of asbestos fibers coated with iron, are identified microscopically. Emphysema, bronchiectasis and cor pulmonale are additional complications.

Berylliosis. Berylliosis primarily occurs in workers who extract beryllium metal from ores or who handle it in making alloys. Hypersensitivity probably plays some role in the toxicity of this metal. Acute berylliosis is essentially a chemical pneumonitis with microscopic features of bronchopneumonia. The chronic form is characterized by the formation of large numbers of granulomas in the lung and other organs. These granulomas must be distinguished from tuberculosis and sarcoidosis. Eventually, interstitial fibrosis may result.

Hyaline Membrane Disease

Hyaline membrane disease (respiratory distress syndrome of the newborn) occurs primarily in premature infants, particularly those delivered by cesarean section or those of diabetic mothers. The fundamental defect is now considered to be a deficiency of pulmonary surfactant. The appearance of the lungs has been described in the section on abnormal growth and development.

Hyaline membranes can occur in adults in the adult respiratory distress syndrome (acute alveolar injury). This syndrome occurs as a complication of numerous conditions including pulmonary infections, severe burns, oxygen toxicity, inhalation of irritants, narcotic overdose, uremia, cardiac surgery, etc. The basic lesion is alveolar wall injury resulting in pulmonary edema and hyaline membrane formation. Interstitial fibrosis may result.

Bronchial Asthma

Bronchial asthma is characterized by bronchial obstruction resulting from bronchospasm and tenacious mucous plugs. Most cases are considered to develop on an allergic basis but attacks may be produced by respiratory tract infection, chemicals, etc.

Grossly, the lungs are hyperinflated with occlusion of bronchi and bronchioles by thick, tenacious mucous plugs. Microscopic features include epithelial basement membrane thickening, infiltration of the bronchial walls by eosinophils, enlargement of the submucosal mucous glands, muscle hypertrophy in bronchial walls and mucous plugs containing numerous eosinophils.

Bronchiectasis

Bronchiectasis is a chronic necrotizing infection of bronchi and bronchioles which results in permanent abnormal dilatation of these structures. It usually develops as a result of bronchial obstruction and infection in conditions such as foreign body aspiration, bronchial tumors, scarring, asthma, chronic bronchitis, emphysema and cystic fibrosis. Both lower lobes are usually involved but the involvement may be segmental when resulting from tumors or foreign bodies. The affected bronchi and bronchioles are dilated and filled with purulent exudate. Bronchiectasis may be complicated by lung abscess, pneumonia, empyema and amyloidosis.

Chronic Bronchitis

Chronic bronchitis is a chronic disease characterized by persistent cough with sputum production which is particularly common in habitual smokers and city dwellers. The most characteristic microscopic feature of chronic bronchitis is the increase in thickness of the submucosal mucous gland layer in the trachea and bronchi. Increased numbers of goblet cells, chronic inflammation of the bronchial wall and mucous plugs are additional features. Complications of long-standing disease include cor pulmonale and bacterial infections.

Emphysema

Emphysema is defined as an abnormal permanent enlargement of the air spaces distal to the terminal bronchiole, accompanied by destruction of their walls. Emphysema is more common and more severe in males and the disease is clearly associated with heavy smoking. In the centriacinar type, the proximal portion of the acinus is involved and distal alveoli are spared. Centriacinar emphysema is most common in the upper lobes, especially in the apical segments. In panacinar emphysema, the entire acinus is involved. This type is more severe in the lower portions of the lobes and is the type of emphysema associated with alpha1-1-antitrypsin deficiency. In advanced cases, adjacent alveoli fuse to produce large air-filled spaces and occasionally blebs or bullae. Severe emphysema frequently results in right-sided heart failure, respiratory acidosis and pneumothorax. Peptic ulceration is found in up to 20 per cent of emphysema patients.

Pneumonia

Bronchopneumonia (lobular pneumonia) is characterized by patchy or focal consolidation of the lung and usually represents an extension of bronchitis or bronchiolitis. The disease is especially common in infancy and old age and may be produced by numerous pathogenic bacteria and occasionally fungi. Microscopically, the involved alveoli contain neutrophils, fibrin and necrotic debris. Alveoli located in adjacent areas may be entirely normal. Bronchopneumonia may be complicated by abscesses, empyema and bacteremia with possible abscess formation in other organs.

Lobar pneumonia is characterized by consolidation of a large portion of a lobe or of an entire lobe. This form of pneumonia is seen much less often now because of the effectiveness of antibiotic therapy. It occurs predominantly in chronic alcoholics, the elderly and the debilitated. Most cases are due to pneumococci but klebsiella and other bacteria may also be responsible. Infection occurs via the bronchial tree and spread occurs through the pores of Kohn.

Four stages of the disease are classically described: (1) congestion, in which the alveolar capillaries are distended and the alveoli are filled with a serous exudate containing numerous bacteria and few neutrophils; (2) red hepatization, in which the lung is solid and airless, and the alveoli are filled with neutrophils fibrin and erythrocytes; (3) gray hepatization, in which the alveoli contain fibrin together with disintegrating neutrophils and erythrocytes; (4) resolution, in which the exudate undergoes enzymatic digestion and resorption restoring the parenchyma to its normal state. Complications of lobar pneumonia include abscess formation, empyema, exudate organization (organizing pneumonia) resulting in scar formation and bacteremia with possible abscess formation in other organs.

Atypical (Viral and Mycoplasma) Pneumonias

The clinical and radiological features of atypical pneumonia syndromes are characterized by subacute onset, prominent extrapulmonary features, such as headaches, sore throat and pharyngeal exudate, minimal or disparate chest signs, lung infiltrate that is not lobar or segmental, no clinical response to penicillin, no significant leukocytosis, and a slow clinical course. *Mycoplasma pneumoniae* is probably the most frequent cause of this syndrome, especially in school age children and young adults; however, some of the viral agents that affect the lung may produce this syndrome. While psittacosis is uncommon in the United States, it should be considered in patients with this syndrome because it responds to tetracycline therapy. Influenzal pneumonia is usually observed and associated with recognized outbreaks or epidemics of influenza-like disease.

There are scores of viral agents that may affect the lung, and many of these may cause the atypical pneumonia syndromes. Among the more prominent of these viruses are influenza A and B, adenoviruses, parainfluenza virus, rhinovirus and respiratory syncytial virus.

The principal pathological finding is interstitial inflammation of the lungs with infiltration of mononuclear cells in the alveolar walls and around the bronchioles and bronchi. The alveoli may contain some fluid with a few neutrophils. Hyaline membranes may be present in alveolar ducts and alveoli. In some stages, the lining cells of the alveoli may undergo hyperplasia and metaplasia. Inclusion bodies may be present in some of the viral diseases. The atypical pneumonias are sometimes complicated by secondary bacterial infection and exudative pneumonia.

Tuberculosis and Carcinoma of the Lung

Tuberculosis and carcinoma of the lung were discussed earlier in this chapter.

GASTROINTESTINAL SYSTEM

Esophagus

The most common pathologic changes in the esophagus are atresia, tracheoesophageal fistula, varices, diverticula, both congenital and acquired (pulsion and traction types), and the effects of corrosive poisons and tumors. The early effect of corrosive poisons is necrosis, followed by inflammation of the lining of the esophagus; the late effect, as a result of the healing process, may be stricture.

The most common tumor of the esophagus is squamous cell carcinoma, which usually occurs in males over 50 years. The combination of excessive alcohol intake and heavy cigarette smoking increases the risk of developing esophageal carcinoma. The three most frequent sites of this tumor are (1) at the level of the cricoid cartilage; (2) at the level of the bifurcation of the trachea (about 50 per cent); and (3) at the level of the diaphragm (about 25 per cent). This tumor does not metastasize early but does extend to surrounding structures and kills mainly by causing obstruction of the lumen of the esophagus. Adenocarcinoma is rare but does occur in the lower end of the esophagus, where, in the majority of cases, it originated in the adjacent gastric mucosa.

Stomach

Hypertrophic Pyloric Stenosis. Stenosis occurs in the newborn infant and is the result of idiopathic hypertrophy of the circular layer of smooth muscle of the pylorus. The hypertrophic muscle and spasm together produce the stenosis and the obstruction.

Gastritis. *Acute gastritis* is common, is usually of minor import and is caused by such local irritants as excess alcohol, certain drugs, notably aspirin and other salicylates, and in much more acute and serious form by staphylococcal toxin in contaminated food. In the severe cases the gastric mucosa is hyperemic, edematous and may even show slight to severe superficial mucosal erosions.

Atrophic gastritis is a form of chronic gastritis in which the mucosa becomes atrophic and inactive. The parietal and chief cells diminish in number, and the antipernicious naemia factor is not produced. In many patients there is evidence of a derangement of the immune system with the production of autoantibodies against certain elements of the parietal cells. Histologically there is marked atrophy of the glandular epithelium, low-grade inflammatory cell infiltration of the gastric mucosa and a curious deformity of the surface lining cells.

Peptic Ulcer. Peptic ulcers, especially the acute types, can occur anywhere in the stomach or duodenum; the chronic form is rather sharply limited to specific areas. These ulcers occur in three forms: (1) hemorrhagic erosions, (2) acute ulcers, and (3) the true, classic chronic peptic ulcer.

Hemorrhagic erosions may be found in all parts of the stomach, usually in association with acute gastritis and caused by excessive alcohol, severe vomiting, infection, certain drugs or chemical or unknown factors. The hemorrhage is superficial at first, but the affected tissues may undergo necrosis, after which, chiefly as a result of the digestive action of the acid gastric juice, a superficial ulcer forms. Usually these superficial ulcers heal, but in a few cases they may lead to the development of a true chronic ulcer.

Acute ulcers of the stomach or duodenum penetrate the muscle layer and may later become subacute or chronic. An example is Curling's ulcer, which sometimes develops, usually in the duodenum, as a complication of severe cutaneous burns.

True chronic peptic ulcer, by far the most important of the ulcers that occur in this part of the gastrointestinal tract, develops in the lower stomach or the first part of the duodenum, being much more common in the latter situation. In the stomach it is located in the prepyloric region, on the posterior wall, within about 5 cm. of the pyloric ring and near the lesser curvature. In the duodenum it is situated above the ampulla of Vater, in that portion bathed by acid fluids coming from the stomach, and, in general, acid production is greater in patients with duodenal ulcers than in those with gastric ulcers.

Typically the ulcer is round or oval, punched out, and deeply penetrating. It forms a sharply demarcated cavity or crater with indurated walls. These walls are covered on the surface by a layer of fibrin, beneath which is necrotic tissue resting on granulation tissue, which forms the deepest layer. The ulcer usually measures from 1 to 3 cm. in greatest dimension and extends to the muscularis or—more usually—even deeper. There is seldom any acute inflammatory cellular exudate, but lymphocytes are found in the adjacent tissues in those ulcers that tend to penetrate the wall. Chronic ulcers of this type are almost always single; rarely is more than one found.

The cause of chronic peptic ulcer is not established, but in approximately half of the patients there is associated atrophic gastritis, which is thought to have antedated ulcer formation and perhaps to have contributed to its development. The most important factor that plays a role in chronicity, if not specific etiology, is the highly acid gastric juice, which prevents the healing of ulcers that may have been caused by some other agent. The latter may include mechanical and chemical irritation of foods, the irritating effect of highly spiced foods or of alcohol, infarction of the mucosa by embolism, or thrombosis of arteries of the gastric wall or infection.

Complications of chronic peptic ulcer include (1) hemorrhage from erosion of a large vessel, especially an artery; (2) perforation of the gastric or duodenal wall with consequent discharge of contents into the peritoneal cavity, which may result in peritonitis, or into the retroperitoneal tissues, with possible abscess formation; (3) penetration of and adhesion to the liver or the pancreas; (4) pyloric spasm or stenosis with obstruction; and (5) malignant change in the chronic ulcer, which, on the basis of observed cases, occurs very rarely.

Gastric Polyps. These benign papillary adenomas, may occur in the stomach. They are villous, papillary glandular structures, usually single but occasionally multiple. They are important because polypoid adenocarcinoma may develop from them.

Carcinoma of the Stomach. Once one of the most common tumors, especially in men, carcinoma of the stomach is now decreasing, especially in North America. It is still one of the most common types of cancer in Japan, Iceland, and some of the technicologically underdeveloped countries of Latin America. Stomach cancer may differ in histologic and cytologic characteristics. A useful classification of the most typical forms is the following: (1) polypoid or fungating adenocarcinoma, (2) flat, superficial ulcerative adenocarcinoma and (3) diffuse carcinoma (linitis plastica), which may, in its later stages, convert the stomach into a firm, thick-walled, hard, contracted structure sometimes called the leather-bottle stomach. Spread of gastric cancer is by direct extension to adjacent structures and by metastasis to regional lymph nodes and liver and, rarely, to the left supraclavicular lymph nodes (Virchow's pilot node).

Small Intestine

In *typhoid fever* the entire mucosa of the ileum is hyperemic, but the specific lesions are found only in Peyer's patches and in the solitary follicles, which are largely limited to the lower 50 to 60 cm. of the ileum. The follicles are swollen by an increase of lymphocytes and macrophages filled with phagocytized degenerated cellular debris, followed by the appearance of small necrotic foci that enlarge and coalesce and finally slough off, leaving rough, ragged ulcers. The ulcer extends to the muscle layer or through it, even into the serosa, which may perforate. The long axis of the typical typhoid ulcer lies parallel to the length of the intestine. Healing of these lesions occurs without cicatrization or contraction of the tract.

Regional Enteritis (Crohn's Disease). This involves the distal portion of the ileum, as a rule, often in segmental fashion with so-called skip areas of uninvolved normal mucosa between the involved portions, and the process may extend into the first part of the colon as well. In the gross there is great thickening of the wall, mainly of the submucosa (ropy intestine), with stenosis of the lumen and ulceration of the mucosa. The neighboring lymph nodes are hyperplastic. Microscopically there is a granulomatous type of inflammation characterized by the infiltration of a variety of inflammatory cells, but especially by the presence of foci of epithelioid cells and giant cells in the submucosa. Similar foci occur in the regional hyperplastic lymph nodes. The earliest stage may be characterized mainly by pronounced edema of the submucosa. In the later stages, there may be diffuse infiltration of the entire wall with a variety of inflammatory cells, and there may be an increase of fibrous tissue throughout the wall. The healing stage of regional ischemia of the small intestine from any cause (usually arterial thrombosis) may simulate regional enteritis.

Tuberculous Ulceration. This occurs most frequently in the ileum near the ileocecal valve. Tuberculous ulcers have a characteristic ragged, irregular and undermined border with the long axis usually transverse. In the serosa, at the site of the ulcer, miliary tubercles are commonly found. Perforation and peritonitis may occur. but adhesions to adjacent structures are more common, and scarring may lead to stenosis of the intestine.

Appendicitis

Acute Appendicitis. Probably the most important cause of acute appendicitis is obstruction in some portion, usually the proximal part, of the lumen by a fecalith. Obstruction leads to interference with the circulation and local erosion of the mucosa with entrance of microorganisms that cause infection of the wall. The most common microorganisms are those normally found in the region, *Escherichia coli* or the enterococci, though streptococci may sometimes be found. Which of these processes, obstruction or infection, comes first is often not determinable.

Colon

Ulceration of the colon may be (1) bacillary, (2) amebic, or (3) idiopathic. In the bacillary type the colon is usually involved throughout its entire course. The lesions are at first catarrhal or fibrinous in character, with necrosis beneath the exudate forming a false membrane that rubs off, leaving superficial or deep ulcers, the edges of which are not undermined. The mucosa may be hemorrhagic or gangrenous. Cicatriza-

tion follows severe ulceration, but perforation is rare.

Amebic Dysentery. This condition usually is confined to the upper colon but may involve the sigmoid and the rectum. The parasite *(Entamoeba histolytica)* that causes this disease is present mainly in the tunica propria of the mucosa. Nodules are produced from swelling and cellular infiltration in the mucosa and the submucosa, followed by the formation of ulcers with indurated, undermined edges that may become confluent. Suppuration may extend beneath the mucosa from ulcer to ulcer. Perforation occurs. Healing takes place by the formation of granulation tissue. The mesenteric lymph nodes may be enlarged, and the organisms pass through the lymphatics into the portal vein to form liver abscesses.

Idiopathic Nonspecific Ulcerative Colitis. This is a common and serious inflammatory condition that occurs most frequently in adults in the third to fifth decades. Etiology is not clear, although bacteria, viruses and parasites, as well as allergic states, nutritional deficiencies and even psychogenic factors have been suspected. Recent studies would seem to imply a defect in immune body production since autoantibodies against colonic epithelial cells have been demonstrated in these patients. Whether these play an etiologic role or merely perpetuate the condition is not known. The affected colon, often the entire length, is contracted, and its mucosa is hyperemic, dark red and velvety, with irregular, coalescent ulcerations that are frequently undermined and have ragged margins. The underlying muscle is thickened and rigid. Remissions and exacerbations are common.

Tumors of the Colon and Rectum. These benign and malignant tumors are common, the adenocarcinoma being high on the list of all malignant neoplasms. Among the benign lesions are the *adenomatous polyps* (pedunculated adenomas), the *villous adenomas* and the less common *familial polyposis.* The adenomatous polyp is common, especially after the age of 50, usually small, soft and pedunculated. It consists of hyperplastic glandular structures grouped about a vascular fibrous stalk. It rarely becomes malignant. The villous adenoma, on the other hand, is much less common but is larger than the pedunculated type, has a broad, sessile base and appears as a fungating, plantlike mass rising from the mucosa. Histologically it is composed of villous glandular structures lined by epithelial cells that often appear atypical, even actually malignant. This lesion, therefore, may often develop into adenocarcinoma. The familial type of polyposis is rare, though serious. Multiple small pedunculated adenomatous polyps may occur throughout the colon and sometimes are found as well in the stomach and small intestine. They are to be considered precancerous since more than 70 per cent may become malignant if not resected.

Adenocarcinoma of the colon and rectum is one of the most common of all malignant neoplasms. In the United States, mortality for adenocarcinoma of the large intestine is second only to lung cancer in men and second only to breast cancer in women. It is found most often in the sigmoid colon and rectum—about 28 per cent in the sigmoid and 40 per cent in the rectum. In men only cancers of the skin and the lungs are more common while in women only cancers of the breast and uterus occur more frequently. In the sigmoid colon the neoplasms often encircle the colon in napkin-ring fashion, cause constriction and then obstruction of the lumen and lead to obstipation, constipation and narrow, stringy stools. In the rectum their gross appearance varies from round or oval ulcerated growths with raised edges to flattened, infiltrating lesions, both of which ulcerate easily and tend to bleed. About half of these lesions occur sufficiently close to the anus to be palpable by the examining finger while about 65 per cent of the sigmoidal and rectal lesions can be visualized by the sigmoidoscope. Histologically these lesions are typical adenocarcinomas, often with much mucin production.

Adenocarcinoma may also occur less frequently in other parts of the colon. Of special interest is the right-sided lesion occurring in the cecum and ascending colon. It is a polypoid, fungating lesion that produces symptoms late and is difficult to diagnose and is therefore more frequently fatal. The first suspicion of such tumors may be raised by iron deficiency anemia due to chronic blood loss.

PANCREAS

Congenital Anomalies. These are uncommon or of little significance. *Agenesis,* if it occurs, is associated with other malformations that are usually incompatible with life. *Aberrant* or *ectopic* pancreatic tissue is sometimes found in the stomach, in the duodenum or in a Meckel's diverticulum.

Atrophy of the Pancreas. Atrophy may be caused by impaired circulation that results from arteriosclerosis. It affects both exocrine and endocrine structures, but generally is so slight that function is not significantly affected. More important is atrophy resulting from obstruction of the pancreatic duct. The effect of sudden obstruction of the main pancreatic duct may be acute pancreatitis if infection of the intraductal pancreatic secretion and injury to the lining of the ducts are present. But if the obstruction develops slowly or lasts for a long time, atrophy and destruction of the parenchyma, interstitial fibrosis and cyst formation

may occur. Islet tissue usually remains well preserved. The main functional disturbance of such obstruction is interference with the exocrine secretions of the pancreas, the most important of which is trypsinogen.

Cystic Fibrosis (Fibrocystic Disease). This is a hereditary disease transmitted as a mendelian recessive gene that may have serious consequences. Evidence of its presence may be apparent soon after birth with the development of meconium ileus, or later, when chronic bronchitis and upper respiratory infections, steatorrhea and the secretion of sweat with a high concentration of sodium and chloride are discovered. The abnormality affects all mucous glands of the body, but especially of the pancreas, and the mucus produced is abnormal, being more thick and viscid than usual so that the pancreatic secretions do not reach the duodenum. The term *mucoviscidosis* has been given to the disease process. Histologically both the acini and the ducts of the pancreas are filled with mucus, the stroma is increased and the exocrine glands are atrophied, but the islets of Langerhans are normal. The small intestine may be obstructed by inspissated meconium that results from the lack of pancreatic enzymes, and the intestinal glands are filled with thick mucoid secretion. The respiratory tract shows striking changes. Mucopurulent exudate is present in both trachea and bronchi, and bronchiectasis is often present. The mucus-secreting glands of the trachea and bronchi are dilated with inspissated mucus, and the bronchial and bronchiolar walls are acutely and chronically inflamed. Foci of emphysema, alternating with foci of atelectasis and even consolidation, are present in the lung tissue, apparently because of partial or complete obstruction of the bronchi and bronchioles by thick, viscid mucus complicated by secondary infection.

Pancreatitis. *Acute hemorrhagic pancreatitis,* perhaps better known as *acute pancreatic necrosis,* because of the extensive hemorrhagic necrosis caused by liberated pancreatic enzymes, is so commonly associated with infection of the gallbladder and ducts that it is generally considered to be related to these conditions. It may be caused by regurgitation of infected bile into the pancreas when a gallstone lodges in the common opening of the bile and pancreatic ducts, the infected fluids injuring duct tissues and probably activating pancreatic enzymes. The condition sometimes follows an attack of acute alcoholism. The pancreas is enlarged, softened and permeated with foci of hemorrhagic necrosis, not only of pancreatic parenchyma but also of peripancreatic fat, because of the digestive action of the pancreatic enzymes. The hemorrhage and the chalky white spots of fat necrosis are the most striking findings in this condition. Serofibrinous peritonitis also is present. Large portions of pancreatic tissue may become gangrenous. In the acute stage of the disease (within 48 hours following the onset of the process), the serum amylase usually is elevated greatly, and this is diagnostic.

Chronic suppurative pancreatitis occurs in pyemia but usually is secondary to primary carcinoma of the pancreas. Chronic interstitial pancreatitis is characterized by increase of fibrous tissue between or within the lobules and most commonly is associated with diabetes.

Carcinoma of the Pancreas. The most common site of carcinoma of the pancreas is in the head where approximately 60 to 70 per cent occur. As the neoplasm grows larger, it gradually causes pressure upon the pancreatic ducts, with consequent interference with the entrance of the external pancreatic secretion into the intestine and with resultant digestive disturbances and inanition. It usually also causes obstruction of the common bile duct with resultant jaundice and its consequences. Pain is usually an early symptom, but its presence means invasion of, or pressure upon, adjacent structures.

Carcinoma of the body and tail of the pancreas is less common but is often more difficult to diagnose until weakness, weight loss and cachexia have set in. It tends to be larger than carcinoma of the head because of the paucity of early signs and symptoms.

Practically all pancreatic cancers are adenocarcinomas of duct origin. They are hard, fibrous, gritty masses in which the epithelial cells grow in nests, cords or atypical ducts embedded in dense stroma.

Diabetes Mellitus. This is a disturbance in carbohydrate metabolism characterized clinically by an elevated blood glucose level and associated glycosuria. There are two typical forms: juvenile diabetes and adult diabetes, the first developing usually before the age of 15, the second after the age of 40 or 45. Juvenile diabetes begins acutely, is controlled with difficulty and in many cases leads to blindness and to death in early adult life from cardiovascular complications. The adult type begins more slowly and responds better to treatment but may be associated with obesity and arteriosclerosis and its complications—not infrequently, impaired circulation to the lower extremities and gangrene.

The disease is the result of a deficiency, or lack of normal potency, of the hormone insulin, which is produced by the beta cells of the pancreatic islets of Langerhans, but the underlying cause of the condition is unknown. Because of this insufficiency of insulin, excess glucose accumulates in the blood, and much of the excess is eliminated in the urine. There is also incomplete oxidation of fat, so that ketone bodies are found in the blood, and acidosis results. Usually some

evidence of damage to the beta cells can be demonstrated, but in about 20 per cent of cases no recognizable pathologic changes are demonstrable in the islets.

In juvenile diabetes the number of islets is usually reduced, the beta cells contain few or no granules, and fibrosis of many islets may be present, together with evidence of mild, low-grade inflammation. In the adult diabetic the number of islets is about normal, the degree of granulation of the beta cells usually shows little variation from normal, but the islets exhibit varying degrees of hyalinization with compression atrophy of many islet cells. In some cases hydropic degeneration of the beta cells, shown recently to be caused by accumulation of glycogen within them, is prominent. Often there is no evident relationship between the severity of the clinical manifestations and the extent of the abnormal changes in the islets. Other changes in the pancreas are sometimes found, such as diffuse fibrosis and atrophy of the entire organ and evidence of chronic pancreatitis. Another condition, hemochromatosis, with diffuse fibrosis and hemosiderin and hemofuscin deposits, may sometimes be associated with diabetes.

In other organs pathologic changes may also be found. Recent electron microscopic studies have disclosed rather widespread changes in the smaller blood vessels, especially the capillaries of the skin and skeletal muscles. The basement membranes of the capillary walls are irregularly thickened, sometimes by a homogeneous deposit and sometimes by a doubling of the membrane itself. Glycogen may be demonstrated in many tissues, particularly the kidneys, in which the epithelial cells of Henle's loops and some of the convoluted tubules may be distended with glycogen. Other manifestations of diabetes in the kidneys are nodular thickenings of the basement membranes of the glomerular capillaries (the glomerulosclerosis of Kimmelstiel and Wilson) and hyaline thickening of the walls of the afferent and efferent arterioles. In the liver the storage of glycogen is decreased within the cytoplasm of the liver cells, but the nuclei may have an increased amount and may appear vacuolated. Arteriosclerosis is more marked in diabetics than in nondiabetics of the same age group and, in the heart and lower extremities especially, may lead, respectively, to coronary heart disease and diabetic gangrene of the toes and feet.

LIVER

Congenital Lesions

Congenital anomalies are rare, but some may be of great consequence. Congenital hepatic fibrosis, characterized by a great increase of bile ducts in a fibrous stoma with linkage of portal areas, frequently eventuates in portal hypertension and its sequelae. Polycystic disease of the liver occurs with or without concomitant polycystic renal disease. The prognosis usually depends primarily on the severity of the renal disease. Choledochal cysts involving the extrahepatic biliary tree and segmental intrahepatic dilatation of bile ducts (Caroli's disease) may lead to cholestasis, choledocholithiasis, and cholangitis. Biliary atresia of both the intrahepatic and extrahepatic varieties have been thought to be congenital or developmental anomalies due to failure of formation or canalization of bile ducts. Recent evidence suggests that many cases represent acquired destruction of ducts associated with infectious, metabolic or chromosomal abnormalities. The extrahepatic type is usually severe, leading to marked cholestasis, portal fibrosis and ductular proliferation, and eventual biliary cirrhosis. The liver in the intrahepatic variety shows cholestasis and an absence of bile ducts. Patients may survive many years before developing cirrhosis.

Storage and Pigmentation

Storage of lipid in hepatocytes, designated fatty metamorphosis, appears in conventional histologic sections as large cytoplasmic vacuoles which displace the nucleus to the periphery. Associated conditions include malnutrition, obesity, diabetes mellitus, alcoholism, malabsorption, some metabolic disorders, postjejunoileal bypass surgery, and exposure to some drugs (most commonly corticosteroids). Glycogen is normally stored in hepatocytes, but is stored in excess in the glycogen storage diseases. A marked increase in copper content (frequently visible by special stains), characterizes Wilson's disease (hepatolenticular degeneration). Alpha-l-antitrypsin globules accumulate in periportal hepatocytes in alpha-l-antitrypsin deficiency. Severe cases are associated with the progressive development of periportal fibrosis and sometimes cirrhosis.

Lipofuscin pigment progressively accumulates with aging. An excess of pigment may follow chronic ingestion of some drugs. Hemosiderosis is the accumulation of hemosiderin (iron) in an organ. The term hemochromatosis usually refers to hemosiderosis plus tissue damage and fibrosis. Hemosiderin deposition results from blood transfusions, various hematologic disturbances, excessive dietary iron intake, and an inheritable condition, idiopathic (primary) hemochromatosis. The latter is most likely to be associated with hepatic fibrosis and even cirrhosis and tissue damage in other organs.

Vascular Disorders

Chronic passive congestion is a result of chronic congestive heart failure. The liver develops a "nutmeg" appearance, owing to the intense red-brown color of the congested central zones which contrasts with the tan peripheral lobular regions. Microscopically, the central zones show dilatation and congestion of sinusoids, atrophy of hepatocytes, and sometimes fatty metamorphosis. Cases of long duration may show fibrous linkage of central veins, a pattern sometimes labeled "cardiac cirrhosis". Acute severe congestive heart failure or shock may produce centrilobular coagulative necrosis.

The Budd-Chiari syndrome results from obstruction of the major hepatic venous outflow (hepatic veins and/or inferior vena cava). Thrombi, tumors, congenital venous webs are responsible. Most cases are fatal. A related disorder, venoocclusive disease, follows restricted outflow from the central veins of the liver. The most common causes are ingestion of pyrollizidine alkaloids in various "bush teas" and radiation damage. The liver in venous outflow obstruction is enlarged, tense, and red purple. Rapidly accumulating ascites is common. Microscopic changes resemble those of severe congestive heart failure, except that changes in outflow veins (e.g. thrombi, intimal proliferation, fibrosis) are more likely found.

Hepatic infarcts are rare, since the organ possesses a dual blood supply. Occlusion of the hepatic artery or one of its branches by thrombi, inadvertent ligature, or polyarteritis nodosa is the most common cause.

Hepatocellular Injury and Necrosis

Patterns of Necrosis. Central necrosis (i.e., necrosis chiefly localized about the central vein) is characteristic of injury associated with certain drugs and toxins. Carbon tetrachloride, acetaminophen in large doses, and the toxin associated with mushroom poisoning are the most notable examples. Midzonal necrosis, a rare phenomenon, is associated with yellow fever. Peripheral or periportal necrosis is found in eclampsia, disseminated intravascular coagulation, and toxic injury associated with phosphorus or ferrous sulfate. Focal necrosis is seen in various infectious processes, such as typhoid fever. In diffuse necrosis or massive hepatic necrosis, virtually the entire parenchyma is lost and the outcome is usually fatal. The collapsed, flabby parenchyma is red and is enclosed by a wrinkled capsule. Occasional islands of yellow to green regenerating parenchyma may be found. Less extensive involvement is termed submassive hepatic necrosis. The most common cause is viral hepatitis, although a variety of other drugs and toxins may be at fault. The more usual form of viral hepatitis produces "panlobular injury" in which all zones of the lobule are affected but not all cells are necrotic. Some cells show degenerative changes such as ballooning degeneration, others regenerative changes, and others necrosis in the form of acidophilic bodies.

Viral Hepatitis. Three types of viral hepatitis are currently recognized. A,B, and non-A, non-B. The last is the least well understood. It is termed "type C" by some investigators, but may represent disease caused by more than one virus.

Hepatitis A (infectious hepatitis) is transmitted by the fecal-oral route. Infection usually results from close contact with infected individuals, ingestion of contaminated food or water, or swimming in contaminated waters. Following an incubation period of about 2 to 6 weeks, there is an abrupt onset of symptoms. Viral particles, 27 nm. in diameter, have been identified in the stools of infected individuals by immunoelectron-microscopy, a technique too cumbersome for routine use. Antibodies to hepatitis A virus of the IgM class are indicative of acute viral hepatitis, type A; tests for such antibodies have been recently developed and are becoming more refined and more available. Microscopically, the usual case shows panlobular injury as described above. Cholestasis is sometimes present and may be marked. Fatty metamorphosis is usually absent. An inflammatory infiltrate of predominantly lymphocytes is present in the lobules and in the portal tracts. Viral particles have been identified in the cytoplasm of hepatocytes by electron microscopy. The usual case resolves without sequelae. Rarely, submassive or massive hepatic necrosis, sometimes fatal, occurs. Chronic hepatitis or a chronic carrier state associated with hepatitis A is not recognized.

Hepatitis B (serum hepatitis) is classically transmitted by direct innoculation of blood or blood products (as by transfusion or by inadvertent injury with contaminated needles or instruments). More recent evidence indicates that transmission also occurs by the fecal, oral, and venereal routes. The incubation period is about 6 weeks to 6 months. A 42 nm. spherical particle appears to represent the virus of hepatitis B. It is composed of 27 nm. core (hepatitis B core antigen), which is produced in the nuclei of hepatocytes, and a 20 to 25 nm. coat (hepatitis B surface antigen), which is synthesized in the cytoplasm and added to the core. An excess of the surface antigen is released into the circulation during acute hepatitis and frequently in chronic hepatitis. Serologic tests for the surface antigen (formerly Australia antigen) have received widespread clinical application in diagnosis and in detection of potentially infectious blood donors. Tests for antibodies to the surface antigen and the core antigen are providing more insight into the disease and are of clinical value. The histologic findings in acute hepatitis are identical to those of hepatitis A. A small percentage of patients develop chronic hepatitis of variable severity. A benign form, chronic persistent hepatitis, is char-

acterized by chronic inflammation in portal tracts and focal necrosis. Chronic active (aggressive) hepatitis has a worse prognosis and shows, in addition, periportal degeneration and necrosis of hepatocytes and periportal fibrosis. In some cases, the fibrosis is progressive and may eventuate in cirrhosis. Cirrhosis may also follow acute submassive necrosis in some instances. Patients with cirrhosis or with chronic hepatitis may have "ground-glass hepatocytes", a morphologic indicator of hepatitis B infection. The ground-glass appearance is accounted for by the presence of hyperplastic endoplasmic reticulum, which contains an excess of surface antigen. Special stains are available to confirm the presence of the antigen.

Non-A, non-B hepatitis was recognized by the development of transfusion-associated hepatitis in patients without serologic evidence of hepatitis A or B. This type of hepatitis apparently accounts for approximately 90 per cent of cases of posttransfusion hepatitis in the United States. The incubation period is approximately two to fifteen weeks. Specific serologic tests have not been developed; the diagnosis remains one of exclusion. Lots of Factor VIII, which were implicated in human disease, have been used to produce hepatitis in chimpanzees. Viral particles, 27 nm. in diameter, were recovered from a homogenate of liver obtained from an infected animal. Further study is necessary to determine if such particles are the responsible agent. A morphologic spectrum of hepatic disease similar to that of type B hepatitis is observed in non-A, non-B hepatitis.

Alcoholic Liver Disease. Fatty metamorphosis may be caused by a short-term increase in alcohol consumption, but severe hepatocellular injury and cirrhosis follow many years of heavy intake. The precise role of nutritional deficiency in the production of injury is not established, but most investigators believe that alcohol itself is toxic to the liver. Some individuals are less susceptible to hepatic damage than others, but the protective factors are not known. Hepatocellular injury first develops in the central zones. Some hepatocytes show ballooning degeneration, and a neutrophilic infiltrate around degenerating cells and foci of necrosis are characteristic. Mallory's hyaline (alcoholic hyaline, Mallory bodies) is commonly found in degenerating hepatocytes; it consists of irregular cytoplasmic clumps of hyaline material. With continued damage, fibrosis appears around the central vein and extends radially into the lobule. Ductular proliferation and periportal fibrosis also develop, and fibrous linkage of the portal tracts and central veins eventually dissects the lobules into microunits resulting in a pattern of micronodular cirrhosis. Considerable parenchymal regenerative activity may be noted. Fatty metamorphosis is commonly present during all active stages of this disease process.

Cirrhosis. Many classifications of cirrhosis have been devised, but none has received universal acceptance. This discussion will adhere to the recently adopted classification of the World Health Organization. Cirrhosis is the extensive alteration of the hepatic architecture resulting from extensive fibrosis in areas of parenchymal degeneration and necrosis with the formation of "pseudolobules" of parenchyma bounded by fibrous septa. The pseudolobules frequently show evidence of hepatocellular regeneration. Three basic morphologic patterns have been defined: micronodular, macronodular, and mixed. In the micronodular variety, most of the pseudolobules are less than 3 mm. in diameter. The macronodular type is characterized by a predominance of pseudolobules greater than 3 mm. in diameter. The mixed type contains approximately equal numbers of micronodules and macronodules. A cirrhotic liver may be classified into one of the three basic categories and then subclassified according to etiology. Altered vascular relationships, impediment of blood flow through the microcirculation, and arteriovenous shunting are probably responsible for portal hypertension that accompanies many cases of cirrhosis. Portal hypertension may be followed by splenomegaly and collateral circulation between the portal and systemic circulation, the most important manifestation of which is esophageal varices. Such varices may rupture, producing serious hemorrhage.

The cirrhosis associated with alcoholic liver damage (formerly called Laennec's cirrhosis, portal cirrhosis, or nutritional cirrhosis) is the most common form of micronodular cirrhosis.

Biliary cirrhosis is also micronodular and follows prolonged obstruction of and/or infection of the biliary tree. In adults, tumors or calculi are the most common causes. Biliary atresia and choledochal cysts are the most likely etiologies in infants and children. Prominent cholestasis and/or cholangitis are the dominant morphologic manifestations of the obstruction in the liver. In time, there are prominent ductular proliferation and periportal fibrosis with linkage of adjacent portal tracts and formation of irregular micronodules. An idiopathic type of biliary cirrhosis (primary biliary cirrhosis) affects some middle-aged persons, usually women, and has some features of an autoimmune process. The disease is characterized morphologically by the gradual destruction of the intrahepatic bile ducts with eventual formation of micronodular cirrhosis.

The cirrhotic stage of hemochromatosis (pigment cirrhosis) is usually micronodular.

Cardiac cirrhosis is a very rare sequel of chronic congestive heart failure. Fibrous linkage of central veins results in a micronodular pattern.

The cirrhosis associated with viral hepatitis is typically macronodular. Usually the fibrous septa are thick and contain remnants of several collapsed adjacent lobules. The pattern has also been called "postnecrotic cirrhosis." In type B, ground-glass hepatocytes may be found in some pseudolobules.

Macronodular patterns are typically found in cirrhosis associated with Wilson's disease and alpha-l-antitrypsin deficiency. Mixed cirrhosis may sometimes be observed in those conditions that ordinarily produce a macronodular pattern and also in alcoholic liver disease.

Other infectious diseases, such as syphilis and schistosomiasis, may produce extensive hepatic fibrosis. Although formerly classified as cirrhosis, such disorders lack the diffuse architectural reorganization and pseudolobule formation characteristic of cirrhosis.

Tumors. The *hepatocellular adenoma,* although benign and rare, is receiving increasing attention because it may rupture and cause fatal hemorrhage and because of its apparent association with prolonged use of oral contraceptives in many cases. Hepatoblastoma is a malignant tumor of children. In addition to proliferation of immature hepatocytes, mesenchymal elements (e.g. bone, cartilage) may be found. Hepatocellular carcinoma most commonly develops in livers with cirrhosis due to hemochromatosis, viral hepatitis, or alcoholism.

Bile duct adenomas are rare and are usually of no clinical consequence. Cholangiocarcinoma (bile duct carcinoma) usually develops in noncirrhotic livers. The tumors resemble adenocarcinomas of other organs. Some cases in the Far East appear to be associated with Chlonorchiasis.

The cavernous *hemangioma* is the most common benign tumor of the liver. Infantile hemangioendotheliomas commonly produce congestive heart failure because of arteriovenous shunting. *Angiosarcoma* (malignant hemangioendothelioma) is a highly malignant neoplasm that may be produced by exposure to vinyl chloride, arsenic, or thorotrast in some cases. Other cases are idiopathic. Most hepatic tumors are metastatic. Tumors of the gastrointestinal tract, biliary tract, and pancreas are common sources, but almost any organ may be a primary site.

GALLBLADDER

Cholecystitis, inflammation of the gallbladder, is usually associated with *Escherichia coli* infection pyogenic cocci or *Salmonella typhi,* but the route of infection is not definitely established. It may be hematogenous or ascending. Biliary calculi usually predispose to infection but may sometimes be secondary to it. Typhoid bacilli, if present, are usually residual from an old infection, and the host is considered to be a chronic carrier.

Acute cholecystitis may be catarrhal, phlegmonous

or gangrenous, with edema and leukocytic infiltration of the wall. Perforation may occur. In subacute and chronic cholecystitis, the wall is thickened, indurated and opaque, with chronic exudative and proliferative inflammation, resticted usually to the outer layers.

Cholesterolosis (strawberry gallbladder) results from the deposition of cholesterol in the hyperemic mucosa.

Empyema of the gallbladder is a form of acute or chronic suppurative cholecystitis in which the cavity is filled with pus and the duct is occluded.

Cholelithiasis is found in at least 75 per cent of all forms of definitely diseased gallbladders. Obesity probably plays a predisposing role, as does pregnancy. Infection, stagnation and supersaturation of the bile combine to determine the precipitation of cholesterol, bile salts, bile pigment and calcium carbonate that accumulate around desquamated epithelial cells, bacteria and organic detritus to form calculi. Some calculi may be primarily of pigment type, others of cholesterol, but the majority are of mixed type. The pigment type is composed of calcium bilirubinate and is usually associated with a hemolytic process. Biliary calculi may be present without producing symptoms, but occasionally, if caught in a duct through which they cannot pass, they may cause especially extreme pain (biliary colic). Biliary calculi that escape from the gallbladder and reach the common duct before being stopped may also cause severe icterus. The presence of calculi in the gallbladder may determine the presence of hydrops, empyema, fistula formation, cholecystitis (if not already present) and cholangitis. In some cases calculi have apparently played a role in inducing carcinoma of this organ.

ENDOCRINE SYSTEM

Some aspects of endocrinology are covered in the sections on biochemistry, physiology, internal medicine, pediatrics, and obstetrics and gynecology. Emphasis in this section will be on the pathologic changes in the endocrine system which are most frequent and most significant. Endocrine disorders are usually the result of increase or decrease of the hormone secretions of the endocrine glands, which may be the result of disease processes affecting the endocrine organs or from alteration of feedback and other mechanisms controlling hormone secretion. The endocrine organs may be affected by destructive lesions, neoplasms with varying degrees of autonomy, and changes reflecting altered control mechanisms. The decrease of hormone secretion can result from genetically determined enzyme defects, such as those that occur in cretinism and the adrenogenital syndromes, destructive lesions, such as those involving the adrenal, pituitary and thyroid, and destructive lesions of the adenohyphysis and hypothalamus which produce releasing and trophic factors. Increase in hormone secretion can result from autonomous tumors and hyperplasia of the endocrine organs, increased production of hypothalamic and adenohypophysial trophic factors, secretion of trophic hormones from ectopic sites, such as tumors, and substances that compete for endocrine receptors. A description of selected endocrine disorders follows.

Thyroid Gland

This endocrine organ actively traps iodine from the blood, binds it to tyrosine residues to form mono and diiodotyrosine (MIT and DIT) which are later coupled to form the thyroid hormones triiodotyronine (T3) and thyroxine (T4). These are incorporated to the thyroglobulin molecule and stored in the follicle. These hormones are released when needed by phagocytosis and proteolysis of thyroglobulin. When this process is interrupted, hypothyroidism results. In the adult, it is manifested by *myxedema,* a syndrome characterized by slowing of intellectual and motor performances, cold intolerance, peripheral edema, macroglossia, low basal metabolic rate, and low levels of T3 and T4 in the blood. *Primary myxedema* may occur after total thyroidectomy, radiotherapy, severe chronic thyroiditis, or maybe idiopathic. In such cases TSH levels are elevated. *Secondary myxedema* is usually associated with pituitary deficiency (Sheehan's syndrome or destructive tumors) and is accompanied by low blood levels of TSH and TRH (thyroid-releasing hormone). Severe iodine deficiency during pregnancy is believed to lead to *cretinism* in the offspring, characterized by mental and physical retardation, as well as deafness. Iodine deficiency in a community is associated with endemic goiter and sometimes, but not always, with *endemic cretinism.* Other nutritional deficiencies are believed to be contributing causes of endemic cretinism. *Sporadic cretinism* may be due to agenesis of the thyroid gland or to enzymatic defects which block one or several of the steps required for thyroid hormone synthesis and release. In the latter cases multinodular goiter is observed, presumably due to continuous stimulus to cellular replication unchecked because of failure of the feedback mechanism which depends on the blood level of thyroid hormones.

Insufficient supply of iodine in a community results in *endemic goiter,* which used to be very prevalent in some areas of the United States, especially around the Great Lakes, but has practically disappeared since adequate iodine supply had been available. Several forms of goiter are observed in endemic areas. The most common is characterized by multiple solid nodules composed of proliferating follicular cells which compress the surrounding parenchyma and form a pseudocapsule. They may form follicular structures of different size or solid cellular cords. These nodules may attain a maximal size of 5 to 6 cm. and usually involute because of central atrophy and fibrosis, intranodular hemorrhage or cystic degeneration. This type is called *nodular parenchymatous goiter, or NBG.* The second type is characterized by excessive colloid accumulation diffusely distributed throughout the gland, so-called *diffuse colloid goiter, or DCG.* The third type, called *nodular colloid goiter, or NCG,* is characterized by excessive colloid accumulation present in all follicles but leading to pseudonodules which compress each other but are not surrounded by a capsule. Mixed forms (parenchymatous and colloid nodules) are also frequent in endemic areas. After iodine supplementation, within the same generation, colloid goiter decreases in prevalence in children and diminishes in size in adults; the colloid component of mixed goiters is considerably reduced but the NPG of adults does not decrease in frequency. The second generation with adequate iodine supply is free from endemic goiter and does not differ in this respect to people living in areas where iodine supply has always been plentiful. Goiter is still to be found in such populations at lower frequency (sporadic goiter) and the same basic histologic types are represented. The cause is unknown but borderline enzymatic defects and goitrogenic substances in the environment are suspected. Nodules histologically identical with those of parenchymatous nodular goiter when found in populations free of endemic goiter are usually called adenomas. There is no proof that they are more or less premalignant than endemic goiter nodules. The majority of multinodular goiters cause no physiologic disturbances though occasionally one nodule may become hyperfunctional and lead to mild hyperthyroidism, usually not accompanied by exophthalmos.

Exophthalmic goiter (diffuse hyperplastic goiter; Grave's disease or Basedow's disease) makes up about 75 per cent of all cases of hyperthyroidism. It is four to five times as common in females as in males, occurs chiefly in young adults or in middle age, and is characterized by exophthalmos (the cause of which is not understood), tachycardia, increased metabolic rate, systolic hypertension, fine tremor and moderate enlargement, usually symmetric, of the thyroid gland. The cause of Grave's disease has long been uncertain. An unusual finding in a large number of cases has been the presence of a long-acting stimulating substance which may be responsible for the hyperactivity of the gland.

Microscopically there is hyperplasia, usually marked, of the parenchymatous tissues. The epithelial cells lining the acini are columnar, with deeply stained cytoplasm, and there are many papillary projections into the acinar spaces. The colloid is decreased in amount and shows peripheral vacuolation. Foci of lymphocytes are frequently present. If preoperative treatment with iodine is given, the excised gland may show only slight hyperplasia or even moderate degree of colloid involution.

Acute thyroiditis may develop in the course of infectious diseases. The gland is large and tender. There may be fever and rapid enlargement of the gland, if it occurs, may cause dyspnea, dysphagia and hoarseness. Mild hyperthyroidism may occasionally result.

Chronic thyroiditis is characterized by excessive lymphocytic infiltration and fibrosis. The gland may be larger or smaller and is usually firmer than normal. A common form of chronic thyroiditis is *struma lymphomatosa (Hashimoto's disease),* in which the gland is moderately but symmetrically enlarged, is markedly infiltrated by lymphocytes even to the point of actual lymph follicle formation and is usually moderately underactive, though in some cases function is normal. Fibrosis, while present, is not marked in the typical case. There may be varying degrees of atrophy of the acini, many of which are often embedded in broad fields of lymphoid cells and show deeply acidophilic cytoplasm. A sclerosing form of chronic thyroiditis with marked stony-hard fibrosis, sometimes mistaken for scirrhous carcinoma, has long been known as Riedel's struma.

Struma lymphomatosa is one of the early diseases to be attributed to the effect of autoantibodies, and antibodies against colloid antigens, as well as epithelial cell elements, have been demonstrated in the blood of many patients.

Granulomatous thyroiditis (subacute or giant cell thyroiditis) is characterized by the presence of a foreign body type of multinucleated giant cells and macrophages in addition to lymphocytes and plasma cells. The etiology is unknown and most of the times the disease resolves by itself without sequelae.

Tumors. The most common malignant thyroid tumor in the United States is the papillary carcinoma. It is more frequent in women and tends to occur at younger ages than other malignant neoplasms. Its clinical course is slower than most carcinomas and can be controlled by surgery in a large proportion of cases. It is composed of epithelial cells which characteristically have clear (ground glass) nuclei and tend to organize themselves in well-defined papilla but may also form well-structured follicles. The cells invade by direct extension the thyroid gland and its neighboring structures, penetrating lymphatic channels and producing local lymph node metastasis. Most of the time the tumor elicits marked desmoplastic reaction but is not detained by this fibrosis. Follicular carcinomas are second in frequency and are usually found in glands previously affected by goiter or adenomas. The tumor cells form follicles or solid cords, grow by centrifugal expansion and are surrounded by a capsule which usually contains numerous telangiectatic blood vessels which are frequently invaded by tumor emboli. Spread is predominantly via blood-borne metastasis but lymph node metastasis may also occur. Anaplastic carcinomas are characterized by rapid growth and aggressive local and distant spread. They are frequently found in older individuals of both sexes who usually have a long-standing goiter.

In addition to the thyroid hormone-producing cells, the thyroid gland harbors the parafollicular cells that secrete thyrocalcitonin, which lowers the level of calcium in the blood. These cells may give rise to a special type of tumor called medullary carcinomas with amyloid stroma, which belong to the family of the APUD tumors. There is a tendency for familial aggregation and the patients frequently have pheochromocytomas and small cutaneous and mucosal neuromas.

Exposure of the neck organs to irradiation, such as occurred in the past when irradiation of "enlarged" thymus in children was in vogue, is implicated in the development of cancer of the tyroid.

Parathyroid Gland

The chief pathologic changes exhibited by this organ are hyperplasia and adenoma or carcinoma, all of which frequently are accompanied by the clinical signs and symptoms of hyperparathyroidism. Hypercalcemia, osteitis fibrosa cystica, metastatic calcification, increased alkaline phosphatase in the blood, excessive excretion of calcium in the urine and formation of urinary calculi are the most important changes that characterize this condition. The adenomas are composed most frequently of chief cells. The hyperplasia may be primary, cause unknown, or secondary to renal excretory insufficiency, rickets or osteomalacia. Destruction of the parathyroids from any cause including surgery results in symptoms of hypoparathyroidism.

Thymus Gland

At various times functional activities of various kinds have been attributed, without adequate evidence, to the thymus gland. However, a lymphopoietic function is generally recognized, and evidence of erythropoietic and myelopoietic activities has been noted during fetal life. As a result of studies recently carried out in thymectomized animals there is good reason to believe that the thymus plays an important role in some immune reactions. The immunologic incompe-

tence that follows extirpation of the thymus, especially in young animals, is accompanied by depletion of the small lymphocytes from the blood, spleen and lymph nodes. Indeed, thymectomy is being performed to aid in preventing the rejection of homotransplants. *Hyperplasia of the thymus* is known to be associated with myasthenia gravis in nearly three fourths of the cases and, in association with actual lymph follicle formation, with such autoimmune (collagen) diseases as systemic lupus erythematosus and rheumatoid arthritis as well as hypogammaglobulinemia, thrombocytopenia, etc. *Tumors of the thymus (thymoma)* are rare but may be of epithelial, spindle cell and lymphoid types, though an occasional teratomatous variety has been reported. Thymomas may also be found in association with myasthenia gravis, and the latter condition appears to have an autoimmune origin, for autoantibodies against muscle tissue have been found in about one third of these patients. The indications, therefore, are that the thymus plays an important role in the body, and is not surprising to find abnormalities of this gland associated with many of the diseases considered to be of autoimmune origin.

Pituitary Gland

This organ may exhibit a variety of pathologic changes, such as parenchymatous degeneration, atrophy, necrosis, infarction from embolism or thrombosis, inflammation, hyperplasia and neoplasia, some of which are associated with hypofunction and others with hyperfunction of the organ.

Hypopituitarism (Fröhlich's syndrome; Dystrophia Adiposogenitalis).   In the young, this is characterized by obesity, genital hypoplasia and faulty skeletal growth. Because of deficiency of the anterior lobe hormone, which normally stimulates the growth of connective tissue, especially bone, there is bony underdevelopment; the head is small, the pelvis is broad, the teeth are flattened, the knees are knocked, the hair is scanty and of the female type, and there is general obesity of female distribution. The condition may be produced by invasive adenoma of the hypophysis or by other hypophyseal tumors or by diseases injuring the base of the skull. *Pituitary dwarfism* of Lorain type, in which the stature is small but normal bodily proportions are maintained, may also result from the destruction of the anterior lobe in a child. Body form is thin and delicate, and secondary sex characteristics are usually defective. In some cases the cause of dwarfism is not destruction of the anterior lobe but rather a congenital deficiency of acidophil cells of the lobe. These latter patients are sexually and otherwise quite normal.

In the adult the result of severe hypopituitarism is called *Simmonds' disease.* This occurs mostly in females and usually is caused by postpartum necrosis of the pituitary. It is characterized by profound cachexia (the result of fibrosis and atrophy in many other endocrine organs), loss of sexual function, weakness, low basal metabolic rate, loss of hair and of skin turgor, pigmentation of the skin, premature senility, low blood pressure and hypoglycemia.

Hyperpituitarism. Overactivity of the pituitary gland before adolescence causes a symmetric overgrowth of the skeleton resulting in *giantism.* Hyperpituitarism after adolescence, when the epiphyseal junctions have fused, results in *acromegaly,* characterized by overgrowth of the orbital ridges, the lower jaw, the hands and the feet, with thickening of the nose and the lips, the affected individual having some of the features of an ape. The sella turcica usually is enlarged. In mild cases there is only hyperplasia of the acidophil cells, but in severe progressive cases there is practically always an acidophil adenoma of the anterior lobe. Pressure on the optic chiasm may cause bitemporal hemianopsia and, later, complete blindness.

Tumors of the Pituitary Gland. These were described earlier in this chapter in the section on tumors.

Adrenal Glands

Lesions of the adrenal glands may be divided into two categories, namely, those due to abnormal function of the cortical tissues, which are much more important, and those involving the medullae.

Adrenal Cortex—Hyperactivity (Hypercorticism). *Congenital adrenal hyperplasia* involves a number of distinctive clinical syndromes caused by complete or partial deficiency of a specific enzyme involved in the biosynthesis of adrenal steroids. The two most common forms are virilizing congenital adrenal hyperplasia, caused by partial deficiency of 21-hydroxylase, and salt-losing congenital adrenal hyperplasia, caused by complete deficiency of 21-hydroxylase. Other less common types are: deficiency of 17-hydroxylase; a hypertensive type, due to deficiency of 11-hydroxylase; and several lethal forms of congenital adrenal hyperplasia from other enzyme deficiencies. The hyperplasia in the congenital adrenal hyperplasia syndromes is bilaterally symmetrical and may either be diffuse or nodular. It is impossible to differentiate congenital adrenal hyperplasia from some of the other forms of primary hyperplasia, such is seen in the other primary hyperplasias.

Cushing's syndrome, induced by excess elaboration of cortisol, is characterized by typical form of central buffalo-type obesity, affecting especially the face and trunk with prominent dorsal and supracavicular back pads, thin legs, hypertension, osteoporosis, impotence or amenorrhea muscular weakness, facial hirsutism and virilism in women. There are four principal causes of the excessive elaboration of cortisol: (1) prolonged treatment with glucocorticoid drugs, (2) excess stimulation by pituitary ACTH only sometimes associated with a pituitary tumor, (3) a cortisol-producing tumor of the adrenal cortex (either malignant or benign), and (4) ectopic production of ACTH by a nonpituitary tumor, such as carcinoma of the lung, bronchial adenoma, thymoma, pancreatic carcinoma and others.

Hyperaldosteronism, most common in adults, especially women, in the fourth and fifth decades, may be primary or secondary. The symptoms include moderate hypertension, polyuria, some muscular weakness, hypokalemia with alkalosis and sometimes parasthesias or even tetany. The primary form is usually produced by an aldosterone-producing adrenocortical adenoma (Conn's syndrome) or by hyperplasia of the zona glomerulosa of the adrenal. The secondary form is in reality an appropriate response of increased aldosterone as a result of renal ischemia, renin-producing neoplasms, or generalized edema.

Adrenal Cortex—Hypoactivity (Hypocorticism). *Addison's disease,* due to adrenal cortical deficiency, is characterized by asthenia, pigmentation of the skin and mucous membranes, anorexia, gastrointestinal disturbances, hypotension and nervous symptoms. It is due to the destruction of all, or almost all, of the cortical tissue of both adrenals. Up to 30 or 40 years ago most cases were due to bilateral massive tuberculosis of the glands or, more rarely, replacement of the cortical tissues by amyloid deposits. Today most cases of Addison's disease are included with the autoimmune disorders, and the affected glands are extremely small, difficult to recognize grossly and so contracted that the capsules seem to surround only the medullary portions which may still be recognized. Cortical tissue is usually not detectable. In significant numbers of these cases circulating autoantibodies against adrenal tissue have been demonstrated. In children *acute adrenal insufficiency* may be observed in the course of overwhelming septicemias, especially with meningococcal septicemia. The gland shows massive hemorrhagic necrosis (Waterhouse-Friderichsen syndrome).

Adrenal Medulla. The adrenal medulla is less important from a pathologic point of view than the cortex, and the only lesions of major significance are tumors. Of these the neuroblastoma and the pheochromocytoma are noteworthy.

Neuroblastoma. This is a highly malignant tumor occurring in infants and children. It is composed of vast numbers of small, dark, lymphocyte-like cells that sometimes exhibit a rosette-like arrangement about a network of fine neurofibrils. Widespread metastases usually occur early. Rarely *spontaneous regression* has been noted, or the neoplasm slows in growth and matures to form the more differentiated ganglioneuroma.

Pheochromocytoma. Composed of the cells that normally are found in the adrenal medulla, the pheochromocytoma is a (usually) benign functioning tumor that may occur in childhood or middle age. Usually unilateral, the tumor may reach a fairly large size—up to 10 cm. or more in diameter. Symptoms are produced by the secretion of catecholamines, chiefly norepinephrine, and include paroxysmal hypertension, nervousness, tachycardia, sweating, trembling and variations in pulse pressure. Catecholamines and their breakdown products are found in the urine.

KIDNEY AND URINARY SYSTEM

Congenital Malformations of the Kidney

Agenesis of the kidneys is rare. If bilateral, it is incompatable with life. *Hypoplasia* is also rare and usually unilateral. The hypoplastic kidney is smaller than normal, and the opposite kidney shows compensatory hypertrophy. *Horseshoe kidney* results from the fusion of the two organs across the midline, usually at the lower pole. This malformed organ generally functions normally.

Polycystic kidneys are a much more serious congenital defect. This may result in death at birth, or soon thereafter *(infantile polycystic disease),* if little or no functioning renal tissue is present. If functioning renal parenchyma is sufficient, the patient may live for some years *(adult polycystic disease).* However, sooner or later, usually before the fifth and sixth decade, death results from renal failure, either because of changes in the vascular system or because of an increase in the size or the cysts, with resulting compression atrophy of functioning renal tissue. The adult form of polycystic disease is more common, and is inherited as an autosomal dominant.

Pyelonephritis

Pyelonephritis is characterized by inflammation of the renal pelvis, as well as the interstitial tissue of the kidney, caused by infection by one of several types of microorganisms. Infection may reach the kidneys by one of two ways. By the ascending route, in which case the bladder, ureter, and renal pelvis are infected first, and the process spreads in a retrograde fashion to involve the renal tubules and the stroma; or by the hematogenous route, in which the microorganisms reach the kidneys via the bloodstream. The former route is more common. It is often associated with a vesicoureteral reflux of infected urine during micturition, and/or with obstruction, as in benign prostatic hypertrophy in males or cystitis and pregnancy in fe-

males. In both cases urinary obstruction may play an important role. Probably every case of pyelitis is accompanied by a certain amount of pyelonephritis.

In *acute pyelonephritis* the kidney is greatly enlarged, the surface smooth, and the capsule nonadherent. In both cortex and medulla there may be obvious foci of suppuration even with abscess formation. Microscopically, the subepithelial portion of the mucosa of the pelvis is infiltrated by polymorphonuclear leukocytes, and there may be leukocytes between the epithelial cells lining the pelvis. Similar interstitial exudation may be present in the adjacent medullary pyramids, and frank necrosis of renal papillae (necrotizing papillitis) may occur. There is exudate in the lumina of the tubules and obstruction of these tubules by the exudate may lead to dilation of the proximal portion of the tubules, some of which are filled with masses of homogeneous pink-staining material or exudate.

In *chronic pyelonephritis,* the characteristic changes are seen on gross rather than microscopic examination. The kidney is usually smaller than normal, though rarely it may be normal or slightly enlarged in size. The capsular surface is scarred with a variable number of rather flat, shallow depressions, some of which may be quite large. The organ is firm, cuts with resistance, and the incised surface usually shows distortion of the normal architecture particularly the calyces. Small foci of suppuration may be seen in the cortex or medulla. The pelvis is thicker and rougher than normal, and its surface may be hyperemic or covered with exudate. Microscopically the most striking features are atrophic, dilated tubules filled with hyaline deposits, so-called colloid casts, especially in the proximal convoluted tubules of the cortex. In the collecting tubules, there may be some exudate consisting of polymorphonuclear leukocytes, Similar cells are also present between the tubules. Subepithelial lymphoid aggregates with germinal centers may be seen under the mucosa of the pelvis. A variable number of glomeruli show sclerotic changes. A common accompaniment of the condition is proliferative endarteritis, characterized by layers of fibroblasts and elastic fibers, the so-called onion-skin type of intima, in the larger intrarenal arteries. In "healed" pyelonephritis, the signs of active inflammation subside. When chronic pyelonephritis precedes the development of arteriolosclerosis or complicates existent nephrosclerosis, it may induce renal excretory functional impairment and the development of the malignant phase of hypertension. It is an insidious disease, often mistaken clinically for chronic glomerulonephritis.

Chronic Interstitial Nephritis

This is an interstitial inflammatory disease which may be morphologically indistinguishable from chronic pyelonephritis, but which is definitely not caused by bacterial infection. It has been related to the excessive intake of drugs particularly analgesics (e.g., phenacetin) which results in chronic interstitial inflammation, fibrosis, tubular atrophy, and medullary papillary necrosis. The papillae are affected bilaterally but irregularly.

Glomerular Diseases

Glomerulonephritis. Glomerulonephritis may be a primary or secondary renal disease and may be either focal or diffuse. The characteristic lesion is an inflammatory reaction in the glomeruli with accompanying tubular injury. The glomerular changes vary with the etiology of the condition, but in all cases there will be varying degrees of swelling and proliferation of capillary endothelium, mesangial proliferation, leukocytic invasion, thickening of the glomerular capillary basement membrane (GBM) and proliferation of the capsular glomerular epithelium. The result of these reactions is a narrowing or closing of the glomerular capillaries that determines the resultant structural and functional changes.

The major clinical syndromes that result may either be *nephrotic* (proteinuria, hypoalbuminemia, hyperlipidemia, and generalized edema), or *nephritic* (hematuria, red blood cell casts, azotemia, hypertension, and oliguria).

Recent techniques have elucidated that immune mechanisms are implicated in the majority of glomerulopathies. Both circulating immune complexes, which may be trapped in glomerular capillaries, and antibodies directed against GBM antigens are responsible for activating secondary immune responses leading to glomerular injury. Further details of these immune mechanisms are beyond the scope of this review.

Nephrotic Syndromes. The hallmark features of these glomerulopathies is marked proteinuria, and this finding usually reflects changes in the glomerular basement membrane (GBM). *Membranous glomerulonephritis* is the major cause of nephrotic syndrome in adults and is characterized by the presence of numerous electron-dense immunoglobulin deposits in the GBM, causing marked thickening and distortion of the GBM. The GBMs have a "spike and dome" appearance due to the visualization of the separate deposits, and the distorted GBM. The etiology of membranous glomerulonephritis may be idiopathic or related to autoimmune disease, infection, or drugs. The precise pathogenesis remains obscure.

Lipoid nephrosis or *minimal change disease* is the major cause of nephrotic syndrome in children. The only morphologic alteration noted is fusion or loss of the foot processes of the glomerular epithelial cells seen only by electron microscopy. The glomeruli other-wise appear normal. The etiology remains unknown, but a prominent clinical feature is the dramatic response of the disease to corticosteroid therapy. Prognosis is usually good with long term remissions.

Focal and segmental glomerulosclerosis use to be considered a variant of minimal change disease but is now considered a distinct entity because of its markedly worse prognosis and failure to respond to steroid therapy. The morphologic lesions predominantly affect juxtamedullary glomeruli and are focal-segmental in distribution. Their distribution is spotty and sometimes only affects a portion of a tuft rather than the whole glomerulus. Progression to renal failure occurs at variable rates. This disease has been noted to recur in patients who receive renal allografts.

Membranoproliferative glomerulonephritis or *mesangiocapillary glomerulonephritis* describes a group of disorders that are characterized by alterations in the basement membrane and the proliferation of cells in the mesangium. The clinical manifestations are variable with two-thirds of the patients being nephrotic and the remainder having elements of the nephrotic and/or nephritic syndrome. Serum complement levels are characteristically persistently decreased. The morphologic alterations include mesangial interposition into the capillary loops, giving the GBM a "double contour" or "train track" appearance, and by the presence of occasional immune deposits in the GBM, or by a uniform, ribbonlike deposition of immune deposits in the GBM (dense deposit disease) without a doubling of the GBM. Immune mechanisms including both circulating immune complexes as well as activation of the alternate complement pathway have been postulated to explain the mechanism of the glomerular injury. This disease has also been noted to recur in patients who receive renal allografts.

Nephritic Syndrome. The hallmark feature of these glomerulopathies is hematuria, and this usually reflects a proliferative type lesion. The classic example of a primary nephritic glomerulopathy is *acute poststreptococcal glomerulonephritis*. The association of hemolytic streptococci of group A, particularly types 4, 12, 25 and Red Lake, as well as, though less commonly, pneumococci, staphlococci, and even certain viruses with acute glomerulonephritis, make it practically certain that these microorganisms, especially streptococci, must play some role, be it direct or indirect, in causing some cases of diffuse glomerulonephritis. The disease is most common in children and young adults. In the majority of cases of acute glomerulonephritis, especially in the young, recovery is complete; a few die of uremia; and a smaller number, about two per cent, progress to chronic glomerulonephritis.

It has been shown that soluble immune complexes of antibody and streptococcal-related antigen (exogenous antigen) circulating in the blood stream become trapped in glomerular capillary basement membranes and evoke an exudative inflammatory response. Immunofluourescent studies and electron microscopy visualize these "humps" of immune deposits and demonstrate GBM injury.

Goodpasture's syndrome (pulmonary hemorrhage with hemoptysis and associated renal failure) is an example of a condition in which autoantibodies to basement membrane are present, and these antibodies react uniformly not only along the basement membranes of the glomeruli and also to the basement membranes of the pulmonary alveoli.

Another form of nephritic syndrome is *rapidly progressive glomerulonephritis* (RPGN) which is characterized by proliferation of glomerular epithelial cells that form crescents around glomeruli within Bowman's capsule, and rapid deterioration of renal function leading to renal failure and possible death in uremia. This morphologic pattern does not describe a singular entity but can be a common pathway for several distinct etiologies, which may involve either deposition of circulating immune complexes, anti-GBM disease, or be idiopathic. Thus, RPGN can occur as a form of poststreptococcal glomerulonephritis, Goodpasture's syndrome, or in secondary glomerulopathies such as lupus nephritis, Henoch-Schonlein syndrome, and others which are described below as secondary glomerulopathies.

Secondary Glomerular Diseases

Many systemic diseases are associated with renal lesions. The clinical manifestations and the morphologic lesions are varied, and on pure morphologic grounds may be indistinguishable from primary glomerulopathies. Lupus nephritis (systemic lupus erythematosus) may cause glomerular changes which are focal or diffuse, membranous or mesangial. Diabetes mellitus may cause nodular or diffuse glomerulosclerosis. Likewise, amyloidosis, subacute bacterial endocarditis, polyarteritis nodosa, Henoch-Schönlein purpura and various microangiopathic disorders all may cause renal disease, and their etiologies and manifestations are too varied to be considered here. They are distinguished from primary nephropathies by ancillary clinical and laboratory findings. Many secondary glomerulopathies may have a focal, (rather than diffuse, spotty) glomerulonephritis as their initial morphologic pattern. The reason for the random distribution remains unclear, although immune mechanisms are thought to be involved.

Chronic Glomerulonephritis

This is the end stage of glomerular disease and may have as an etiology any of the diseases listed above.

Only occasionally is there a history of preceding definite acute glomerulonephritis. The urine in these cases contains albumin and casts in varying amounts. In the subacute stage, before the condition becomes truly chronic, oliguria may be present, but in chronic cases large amounts of urine with low specific gravity are passed. Edema may be present, and sometimes fluid collects in the serous cavities. Hypertension is common. Moderate left ventricular hypertrophy occurs, but rarely is there pronounced cardiac insufficiency. Diminished renal function is indicated by decreased clearance of the blood urea nitrogen and elevated creatinine. Later, there is the development of albuminuric retinitis, uremia, and an ultimately fatal outcome. Secondary anemia may be pronounced. The kidneys are small, symmetrically contracted, firm, diffusely granular, and the glomeruli may show the residua of a primary disease progressing to global hyalin obliteration of glomeruli. Except for patients maintained on dialysis or who receive renal transplants, the outcome is invariably death.

Vascular Disturbance

In addition to the diseases described above, hematuria and/or proteinuria may occur in association with other conditions which do not have the same consequences or sequelae. Orthostatic albuminuria may be caused by a marked fall in the pulse pressure in the upright position, by compression of the left renal vein in visceroptosis, or by kyphosis. It is of no clinical significance. Chronic passive congestion of the kidneys from heart failure may cause albuminuria and casts and sometimes diminished urea nitrogen excretion or clearance. These changes disappear when the heart becomes compensated. Furthermore, it is well known that transitory hematuria may result after vigorous exercise. None of these conditions are indicators of progressive renal disease.

Vascular Disease of the Kidneys

Acute Arteritis.   This can be idiopathic or part of generalized polyarteritis nodosa. It also may be the result of lodgement of infected emboli or be secondary to acute suppurative inflammation in the kidney.

Renal Arterial Disease.   In recent years, mainly as a result of arteriography, a stenotic lesion of the main renal artery, either due to fibromuscular dysplasia or atheromatous plaque of one or both kidneys, has been recognized with increasing frequency in patients with hypertension. In such patients, it is now generally admitted that hypertension is due to renal ischemia with secondary activation of the renin-angiotensin system, and corrective surgery has been performed. Favorable results are to be expected only in those individuals who have a stenotic lesion of one or both main renal arteries and who lack an intrarenal cause of ischemia in either kidney as determined by biopsy.

Arterial Nephrosclerosis. Arterial nephrosclerosis is caused by obliterative arteriosclerosis of the extrarenal or the larger intrarenal arteries. The kidney usually is roughly nodular, with irregularly shaped deep depressions of various sizes in the cortex that correspond to foci of atrophy of the parenchyma and replacement fibrosis. The visible arteries show obvious thickening of wall and reduction in the size of the lumen. The functional changes are usually minimal but may be significant if the degree of parenchymal atrophy is great.

Arteriolar (Benign) Nephrosclerosis. The kidney may be of normal size, but more commonly it is reduced in size and may be very small, especially if the larger intrarenal arteries are also involved. As a rule the capsule is not adherent. The outer surface is usually finely and uniformly granular with the small nodules of parenchyma projecting slightly above the reddish gray or gray network of connective tissue which is usually depressed. The organ is firm and cuts with increased resistance, and the cut surface usually shows a narrow cortex. If the larger vessels are also affected, and they usually are, the walls of these visible arteries may be thick and the lumens smaller than normal. Microscopically, there are the changes of ischemic atrophy. The walls of arterioles, particularly the preglomerular ones, and smaller arteries are thickened, fibrous, and hyalinized. In the arterioles the entire wall may be hyalinized. In the small arteries, the intima alone is involved. Special stains may reveal lipoid material in the hyalinized intima. The glomeruli vary from many that are normal to some that are transformed into completely fibrotic, hyalinized structures. Even in many of the glomeruli that appear normal, the basement membranes may be thickened and wrinkled. Focal glomerulitis or chronic pylonephritis may complicate the picture and play an important part in the development of so-called malignant nephrosclerosis. Parenchymatous and fatty degeneration of the lining epithelium of the tubules is common in the foci of atrophy. The tubular units are either atrophic or entirely absent. Some of the tubules may be moderately or greatly dilated. Persistent hypertension is a frequent accompaniment of this condition, usually without associated significant disturbance of renal excretory function. In this type, called benign hypertension, the cause of death is usually either heart failure or apoplexy.

Malignant Nephrosclerosis. This condition may develop from the benign form of arteriolar nephrosclerosis, sometimes from chronic glomerulonephritis, chronic pyelonephritis, or it may arise, sometimes quite rapidly, without apparent previous clinical renal disease. It is extremely serious, being characterized by markedly elevated arterial pressure, renal insufficiency, failure with uremia, and characteristic vascular changes in the eyegrounds. Grossly the kidneys may show little, except for minute hemorrhages in the cortices, to account for the severity of the clinical symptoms. Histologically however, the changes are characteristic and marked. Most striking is the severe necrotizing arteriolitis affecting the interlobular and afferent arterioles. The walls are thickened and sometimes hyalinized. There is reduplication of the intima with concentric ring formation (onion skin). There are fibrinoid deposits and sometimes actual thrombi in the lumens, and occasionally extension of the degenerative process into some glomerular tufts. Otherwise the glomeruli show little and inflammatory cells are few.

Urinary Calculi (Urolithiasis)

Calculi in the urinary system are relatively common, especially in the renal pelvis and calyces. The majority are calcium containing. They are composed of varying mixtures of calcium oxalate, calcium phosphate, ammonium phosphate, uric acid, and cystine that are precipitated from the urine under varying conditions, especially high concentrations of these substances. The most common calculi are mixtures of phosphates and oxalates, though pure phospate and oxalate stones, as well as lesser numbers of calculi in which mixtures of these substances with uric acid and cystine are present, may also be found occasionally. Infection may play a role, and bacteria may even serve as the nidus on which the above elements are precipitated, particularly ammonium phosphate. Calculi may also cause hemorrhage, secondary infection, obstruction with hydronephrosis, or ureteral colic. In the renal pelvis, calculi tend to be irregular in shape and may form a cast of the pelvis called a *stag-horn calculus.* These are usually composed of ammonium phosphates.

Hypervitaminosis D also may be complicated by the formation of urinary calculi, and in both man and animals, hyperparathyroidism frequently is associated with the occurrence of urinary calculi. In both hypervitaminosis D and hyperparathyroidism, hypercalcemia occurs and is probably the determining factor.

Bladder

Cystitis usually is secondary to diseases that cause obstruction and stagnation of urine, such as enlarged prostate, urethral stricture, tumors, calculi, or paralysis of the bladder. Bacteria that produce ammonia are particularly irritating to the mucosa. Less commonly cystitis results from a descending infection. In acute cases, the mucosa swells and reddens with a small amount of exudate that may become hemorrhagic or purulent. The inflammation may be ulcerative, gangrenous, or pseudomembranous. In chronic cystitis the lesion is less severe, but the walls are thickened by fibrosis and there is lymphocytic infiltration. In some cases of chronic cystitis not caused by infection with a virus or a fungus, histiocytic phagocytosis or fatty acids, polysaccharides, or both, with subsequent calcification, results in the development of granulomatous submucosal plaques referred to as *malacoplakia.*

Hypertrophy of the musculature of the bladder is caused by any obstruction of the urethra with the bulging of the hypertrophic musculature causing trabeculation of the mucosa.

Paralytic bladder may be caused by (1) tabes or (2) lesions of the lumbar cord (multiple sclerosis, tumors, myelitis, or trauma) that interrupt the reflex arc.

Urethra

Gonorrheal urethritis is very common in the male. It begins in the fossa navicularis and extends rapidly over the mucosa towards the bladder. The prostate usually is involved. The mucosa of the urethra is reddened and swollen with a rather profuse purulent exudate. Frequent complications include suppuration of the prostate, epididymis, the seminal vesicles, and the bladder. Rarely, gonorrheal arthritis of endocarditis results. Urethral stricture, usually in the membrane portion, is a late sequel that may occur as long as 20 years after infection.

Gonorrheal urethritis in the female usually is relatively mild. Infection with *Escherichia coli* is more frequent.

Tumors of the Urinary Tract

Benign adenomas of the renal cortex are relatively common. The most important malignant tumors are renal cell (clear cell) carcinoma, carcinoma of the bladder and renal pelvis, and the relatively uncommon Wilms' tumor of children. Renal cell carcinoma is the most common, occurs chiefly in males of middle to late age, and usually is quite large when discovered because it can remain symptomless for a long time. Major symptoms are painless hematuria, sometimes dull pain, or a mass in the flank, or both, and even occasional low grade fever that is difficult to explain. Histologically most of these neoplasms are composed of "clear" or vacuolated epithelial cells that resemble cells of the adrenal cortex, a characteristic that has led to the inaccurate diagnosis of hyperneophroma. The tumor has a tendency to invade the renal vein, and blood-borne metastases to the lungs and other sites, such as bone, are common. Transitional cell papillomas may develop in the pelvis and other portions of the urinary tract, especially the bladder where they are most common and most dangerous, since some of these are actually early carcinomas when first discov-

ered, or may become so. Indeed, the differentiation between benign and malignant bladder tumors is difficult and often depends on the degree of invasion of the wall. Wilms' tumor, a massive malignant neoplasm reproducing primitive renal tissue embedded in fibromyxomatous stroma, is most common in children under 10 years of age. It is sometimes present in the newborn. Wilms' tumors currently respond well to combined surgical, radiotherapeutic, and chemotherapeutic treatment.

GENITAL SYSTEM

Male

Congenital anomalies of the urethra, such as *hypospadias,* in which the urethral opening is on the ventral surface of the penis, or *epispadias,* in which it is on the dorsal surface, are important since infertility and bladder infections are common complications. *Phimosis* is the condition in which the prepuce, because of a small and contracted orifice, will not retract normally to uncover the glans, so that an accumulation of smegma, secretions, desquamated epithelial cells, etc., collect beneath, sometimes leading to infection that may at times be confused with gonorrhea. The most important infections of the penis are gonorrhea, syphillis, chancroid, and sometimes, pyogenic infections of the glans and the prepuce that lead to ulcerative or gangrenous *balanoposthitis.*

Condyloma accuminata is a benign squamous papilloma of the penis caused by a virus. The most important malignant tumor is *squamous cell carcinoma* of the glands; a tumor that occurs in association with the accumulation of smegma or foci of infection or inflammation that have been present for a long time beneath the prepuce of men in older age groups (from 50 to 70 or more years). This form of cancer is extremely rare in Jewish men who practice circumcision, which effectively prevents accumulations of the secretion since the prepuce has been removed.

Testis and Epididymis. The most important anomaly of the testis is *cryptorchidism,* or undescended testis. Although opinions differ somewhat, the undescended testis is considered by some to be more susceptible to the development of malignant disease.

Various forms of *orchitis* may occur. The most common are caused by gonorrhea, syphilis, and sometimes in adults who suffer from mumps, a form of mumps orchitis that may be serious enough to lead to sterility.

Although testicular tumors are not very common, they are usually serious, and in young adult males between 25 and 35 they are almost the most common form of malignant disease. Among the more important of malignant neoplasms are the *seminoma,* a fairly well-differentiated, relatively slowly growing malignant tumor; the *embryonal carcinoma* of high malignancy, with a varying but always poorly differentiated histologic pattern and poor prognosis; and the *teratoma* of immature of adult type. *Choriocarcinoma,* usually of high malignancy, rarely occurs. These tumors are described more at length in the section on neoplasms.

Epididymitis usually is caused by infection spread from the urethra. Abscesses may form, and the ducts may be occluded in the healing process. Bilateral epididymitis may result in sterility. Tuberculosis often involves the epididymis, but seldom the testis. Syphilis, on the other hand, rarely affects the epididymis, but *gumma* of the testis may occur. The passage of spermatozoa into the interstitial tissue of the epididmyis, most likely on a traumatic basis, results in the formation of a granulomatous lesion in which degenerated spermatozoa, usually only the heads, are recognized.

Prostate Gland. Benign enlargement (hyperplasia) is by far the most common disease of the prostate gland, causing obstructive symptoms in about eight per cent of men over 60. The enlargement involves mainly the central and lateral areas of the gland. A nodule of the median lobe may project into the trigone of the bladder and cause obstruction of the internal urethral orifice, the chief cause of obstruction being narrowing and angulation of the urethra. The nodules are composed chiefly of hyperplastic, hypertrophic, and cystic glands that may form adenomalike foci alternating with many small nodules composed mainly of smooth muscle and fibrous tissue.

Prostatitis in young men usually is caused by gonorrhea; in old men it frequently is caused by infection and injury from catheterization. The glands are filled with pus cells and desquamated epithelium, and abscesses may form that rupture into the urethra, the bladder, the rectum, or the pelvic connective tissues.

Carcinoma of the prostate is one of the most common malignant tumors occurring in men. Like benign hyperplasia, the incidence of cancer increases with age, though the two conditions appear to be independent and unrelated lesions. Carcinoma usually originates in the posterior lobe, is most often subcapsular in location, and may be present for a long time without being suspected. Histologically, carcinoma of the prostate can vary greatly. The simplest form is the latent type that grows slowly, causes no symptoms, and is usually found by chance at autopsy. A common form is also slowly growing but exhibits definite hyperplasia, sometimes atypical, and evidence of malignancy by invasion along nerve sheaths. Finally, there is the very cellular, rapidly growing medullary anaplastic growth that replaces most of the gland. Metastases develop in the regional lymph nodes, the pelvic bones, and the spine. When metastases are present in the skeleton, the *acid phosphatase* level in the blood is greatly increased.

Female

Diseases of the female genital system are very common and will be considered in more detail in the chapter on obstetrics and gynecology. Some of the more important will be mentioned here.

The *vulva* may be the site of inflammations of which the luetic chancre is the most important, but more important still are tumors, both benign and malignant, of which there are a considerable variety. Papillomas, inflammatory condylomas, leukoplakia, which must be considered at least a precancerous lesion, carcinoma-in-situ, and invasive squamous cell carcinomas are the most important examples.

The *vagina* in general is not commonly affected by primary disease, though moderate infections such as trichomonal or *Candida albicans* vaginitis not infrequently occurs. Primary carcinoma is rare.

The *cervix* is perhaps the most important part of the female genital tract because of the fact that it is a very common site of malignant disease. Next to carcinoma of the breast, carcinoma of the cervix is the most common malignant disease in women. The disease may occur at almost any age, but is most frequently between the ages of 30 and 50, and married women are more frequently affected than are single women. The neoplasm is a form of squamous cell or epidermoid carcinoma, and from a pathologic point of view, it can be divided into five categories based upon the extent of the growth. It may vary from simple preinvasive or intraepithelial carcinoma (carcinoma-in-situ), to carcinoma confined to the cervix itself, and then to stages of invasion extending beyond the cervix to involve the vagina, the pelvic wall, the bladder or rectum, or both, and perhaps the ureters and even more distant organs.

In the *uterus* proper, endometrial inflammation is uncommon, but *endometriosis,* the presence of endometrial glands and stroma in abnormal locations, is a more important abnormality. Endometriosis may involve the myometrium (adenomyosis), but more important is external endometriosis in which foci of endometrial tissue are found in the pelvic peritoneum, in or on the surface of the fallopian tubes, and on the ovary.

Tumors of the uterus include the common leiomyoma, almost always benign, but often multiple and varying in size from a few millimeters to 15 to 20 centimeters, and the more serious endometrial adenocarcinoma. These tumors, too, are described in greater detail elsewhere.

The *ovaries* are the site of various types of tumors, the most important of which were described in the section on neoplasms. Of the diseases that occur in association with pregnancy, the most important are eclampsia, ectopic pregnancy, hydatidiform mole, and choriocarcinoma, all of which are described in more detail elsewhere.

Although the *breast* is not a part of the female genital tract, it is a closely related organ and a brief summary of the more important lesions may be given here. Congenital abnormalities occur but are not of clinical significance. Supernumerary nipples and foci of breast tissue that develop in the mammary line are not infrequently seen. Of all breast lesions, *fibrocystic disease* or *mammary dysplasia* is perhaps the most common. It results from some abnormality of the cyclic changes that occur in association with the menstrual cycle. The breast tissues are more fibrous than normal and with varying numbers of cysts, small or large or a mixture, filled with yellowish, turbid, blood-tinged, or partly coagulated and gelatinous material. It is said that women who suffer from this condition are somewhat more susceptible to the development of breast carcinoma.

Benign tumors of the breast include—as the most common type in younger women—the *fibroadenoma,* a slowly growing, probably estrogen-induced fibroepithelial encapsulated nodule that is usually solitary but may be multiple and even bilateral. It rarely exceeds four centimeters in diameter. One typical manifestation of this tumor is the intracanalicular capillary fibroadenoma in which the stroma is more actively growing than the epithelial element. A most unusual form is the giant intracanalicular fibromyxoma, more generally known as cystosarcoma phyllodes, which, in spite of its name, can be either malignant or benign. Intraductal papillomas may also occur in older women, and their relationship to the development of carcinoma has been suggested although not proved.

Malignant breast tumors are described in the section on neoplasms.

NERVOUS SYSTEM

Congenital Malformations

Various harmful influences, genetic or environmental, acting at crucial times during embryonic development, can result in failure of normal formation of nervous system structures. Similar malformations can result from different causes, and a variety of malformations can be produced by a single cause. Anencephaly (absence of the brain) and amyelia (absence of the spinal cord) represent extreme degrees of arrested development. Failure of fusion of the neural tube can result in craniorachischisis (unfused central nervous system, including meninges, skull, and spine) or porencephaly (complete defect through brain tissue). Protrusion of nervous tissue and leptomeninges through a defect in bone and dura mater can involve the cranium (encephalocele) or spine (myelocele). Such defects may involve bone and meninges only (meningocele) or bone only (spina bifida occulta). Excessive fusion can result in such anomalies as cyclopia, arhinencephaly and other examples of failure of cleavage of nervous tissue into symmetrical paired structures. Aqueduct atresia is a common form of this process. The Chiari malformation includes a mixture of fusions and cleavages, displacements, and distortions, including dysplasia of the cerebral cortex, hydrocephalus, aqueduct atresia, malformation and caudal displacement of brain stem structures, cerebellar tonsillar displacement, and meningomyelocele. Errors of migration lead to abnormal location of nerve cells (heterotopias), disarranged cerebral cortex (polymicrogyria, macrogyria, lissencephaly or agyria, and pachygyria). Nervous system anomalies are frequently accompanied by anomalies of other body structures.

A peculiar group of diseases having genetic and neoplastic features are included in the phakomatoses (tuberous sclerosis, von Hippel-Lindau disease, von Recklinghausen's disease, and Sturge-Weber disease). In addition to anatomic malformations, congenital abnormalities of nervous tissue metabolism leading to structural and functional changes may occur (phenylketonuria, lipid storage diseases, and leucodystrophies).

Hydrocephalus

Most cases of hydrocephalus producing clinical manifestations are the result of obstruction of flow of the cerebrospinal fluid. When this obstruction is congenital it most frequently involves the aqueduct (stenosis or atresia), less commonly other areas such as the outlets of the fourth ventricle (Dandy-Walker syndrome), and results in enlargement of the head by separation of the cranial sutures. Brain damage is slowly progressive due to pressure and distortion. When the obstruction is acquired, it most frequently involves the subarachnoid space around the brain stem, where postmeningitic obliterative adhesions are most likely. Less commonly, the ventricular system may be obstructed by neoplasm. Rapidly progressive increased intracranial pressure and brain damage occur if the cranial sutures have closed.

Communicating hydrocephalus exists when the obstruction is between the outlets of the ventricular system and the arachnoid villi, allowing flow of cerebrospinal fluid from the ventricles into the lumbar subarachnoid space but preventing reabsorption.

Noncommunicating hydrocephalus results from obstruction of the ventricular system.

Cerebral Palsy

Cerebral palsy is a broad term that refers to a heterogeneous group of nervous system disorders apparent from birth or early infancy characterized by diffuse, usually bilateral brain damage of variable severity associated clinically with various combinations of abnormal movements, spastic paralysis, and intellectual deficit. More than two per 1000 births are affected to some degree. Pathologic changes vary with the multitude of etiologic factors, including genetic abnormalities, intrauterine damage (hypoxia, infection, toxicity, deficiency, x-ray exposure), birth injury (hypoxia, trauma), kernicterus, and early infantile diseases (infection, seizures).

Inflammatory Diseases

Except for direct implantation through open skull fractures and during surgical procedures, microorganisms reach the central nervous system by spreading from a focus of infection elsewhere. Routes of infection are by continuity, blood stream, or along nerve roots. Infections may involve the meninges, the parenchyma, or the nerve roots. Almost any organism can be involved. Leptomeningitis is the most common type of central nervous system infection. It may be acute, subacute, or chronic. Most commonly it is due to bacterial infection. Coliform organisms are most frequently involved in newborn infants and in old and debilitated patients; Hemophilus influenzae, in infants; Neisseria meningitidis, in children and young adults (epidemic meningitis). Other organisms are less influenced by age than by predisposing conditions such as lowered resistance, debilitating diseases, or loci of infection elsewhere in the body (pneumococcal, streptococcal, staphylococcal, tuberculous, mycotic, and parasitic). Gross pathologic changes consist of hyperemia of the piaarachnoid membrane followed by purulent subarachnoid exudate. Microscopically the leptomeninges show acute inflammatory changes, and microorganisms can be detected by special techniques. Complications of bacterial meningitis may occur during active infection (cerebritis with herniation, arteritis with infarction, thrombophlebitis with venous infarction) or as postmeningitic sequelae (obstructive hydrocephalus, cranial nerve palsies, parenchymal destruction, and gliosis) leading to motor, sensory, and intellectual deficits and epilepsy. Tuberculous leptomeningitis is usually subacute, associated with pulmonary or miliary tuberculosis, and tends to concentrate around the base of the brain as a fibrinous mononuclear exudate causing severe vasculitis. Tuberculomas in the parenchyma are rare. Neurotuberculosis is more common in children than in adults. Fungus infections of the leptomeninges tend to be chronic, occurring most often as opportunistic infections in debilitated patients. Cryptococcus neoformans is the most common organism. This causes mucinous exudate due to its thick capsule, and inflammatory reaction is feeble. As in other, rarer, fungus infections (mucormycosis, histoplasmosis) the nervous system involvement is secondary to infection in other systems.

Brain abscess results from hematogenous dissemination of organisms usually from pulmonary suppuration or bacterial endocarditis or from contiguous spread from middle ear, mastoid, or paranasal sinus infections. The most common locations are frontal, temporal, or cerebellar.

Parasitic infections of the nervous system of greatest importance are malaria (capillary occlusions by parasitized erythrocytes), cysticercosis (parasitic cysts in the parenchyma, meninges, or ventricles), amebiasis (cerebritis, abscess), echinococcosis (cyst), and toxoplasmosis (granulomatous meningoencephalitis).

Viral infections of the central nervous system may be acute, subacute, or chronic and may affect the meninges or parenchyma. Various viruses tend to focus their destructive effect at particular levels in the central nervous system: nerve roots and ganglia, herpes zoster; spinal cord, poliomyelitis; brain stem, rabies; basal ganglia, encephalitis lethargica, Japanese B, St. Louis, equine encephalitis; cerebral cortex, herpes simplex; leptomeninges, lymphocytic choriomeningitis, mumps, and infectious mononucleosis. The involved tissue is congested and swollen but usually intact. Intense inflammatory changes are evident. Distinctions between different types of infection may be possible on the basis of the location of major involvement, destructiveness, and inclusion bodies and by correlating pathologic changes with clinical manifestations. Subacute viral infections, such as those due to rubella, cytomegalovirus infection, progressive multifocal leucoencephalopathy, measles, and subacute sclerosing panencephalitis, may persist for months to years and produce extensive destruction of gray and white matter. Slow virus infection, in which a long latency period precedes the onset of clinical manifestations, is thought to be involved in kuru and Creutzfeldt-Jakob disease. Neurosyphilis may occur in meningitic or meningovascular forms or during tertiary stages as general paresis affecting the cerebral cortex or tabes dorsalis involving the spinal cord.

Traumatic Lesions

Concussion is a form of injury to nervous tissue due to physical force that causes temporary impairment of function without structural alteration. Contusion produces traumatic disruption of small blood vessels within the tissue of the brain or spinal cord at the site of injury. Brain contusions may be of the coup or contrecoup type. Lacerations of brain or spinal cord are often associated with fracture of overlying bones and are followed by scarring and permanent defects. Regeneration of nerve cell processes is possible in the peripheral nervous system. Traumatic neuroma may result from improper healing. Focal subarachnoid hemorrhage is a frequent result of physical injury to the head or spine. Subdural hematoma results when head injury produces disruption of surface blood vessels, particularly veins. The hematoma may accumulate rapidly, causing acute displacement of brain tissue, or slowly, resulting in gradual encapsulation. Most subdural hematomas are traumatic, but occasional bleeding in this area results from ruptured arterial aneurysm or neoplastic infiltration of the dura.

Epidural hematoma, usually intracranial, is caused by laceration of a meningeal artery when the overlying bone is fractured. This most commonly occurs in the temporal region. The hemorrhage accumulates rapidly and must be evacuated promptly.

Posttraumatic syndromes result from combinations of these structural lesions with functional impairment frequently associated with subtle emotional factors.

Peripheral Neuropathies

Although peripheral nerve lesions may have different causes, the reactions are very limited and often nonspecific. Myelin sheaths and/or axis cylinders may be affected. Sensory, motor, or combined effects may result. Metabolic disorders (porphyria, carcinoma, amyloidosis), nutritional deficiencies (beriberi, pellagra, pernicious anemia), vascular diseases (polyarteritis nodosa, diabetes mellitus, systemic lupus erythematosus), intoxications (heavy metals, diphtheria, drugs, and industrial poisons), infection (herpes zoster, leprosy), heredity (peroneal muscular atrophy, hypertrophic interstitial polyneuropathy, hereditary sensory radicular polyneuropathy), neoplasia (neurilemoma, neurofibroma), postinfectious, postvaccinal, and immune states (acute infective polyneuropathy), and trauma (contusion, compression, avulsion) may be involved. Regeneration of peripheral nerve fibers is possible under optimal circumstances.

Toxic and Nutritional Disorders

The number of exogenous poisons capable of damaging the nervous system increases yearly and includes environmental, occupational, and medicinal substances. Carbon monoxide poisoning causes nervous system lesions by combining with hemoglobin and impairing oxygen transport. Widespread hypoxic nerve cell damage results. Symmetrical necrosis of the globus pallidus nuclei is characteristic. Lead intoxication results in encephalopathy (infants) or peripheral neuropathy (adults). Lead encephalopathy causes massive swelling and widespread damage in brain tissue. Peripheral neuropathy mainly involves motor nerves. In arsenic poisoning, acute encephalopathy with multiple petechiae in the white matter is mainly due to the toxic effect on small blood vessels. Peripheral neuropathy, associated with chronic intoxication, damages myelin sheaths and axis cylinders and affects predominantly sensory nerves. Manganese intoxication causes widespread neuronal damage concentrating in the basal ganglia and is associated with extrapyramidal signs. Mercury poisoning causes nerve cell loss characteristically severe in the granular layer of the cerebellum. Dementia, ataxia, and tremor are prominent clinical signs. Acute alcoholic intoxication causes reversible physiologic (depressant) effects on nerve cells often associated with congestion and edema. Chronic alcoholism may result in encephalopathy which is the effect of alcohol and nutritional deficiency. The cerebral cortex, periventricular gray matter, and particularly the mammillary bodies are characteristically involved by acute followed by chronic nerve cell changes. Korsakoff psychosis is the typical clinical manifestation of Wernicke's encephalopathy. Cerebellar cortical atrophy, central pontine myelinolysis, central necrosis of the corpus callosum, and peripheral neuropathy may be seen under these circumstances.

Vascular Diseases

Vascular diseases of the central nervous system mainly concern atherosclerosis, which causes narrowing and occlusion of major arteries; hypertensive arteriolar sclerosis leading to hyperplasia, stenosis, occlusion with small infarcts, and necrosis with spontaneous hemorrhage; aneurysms; vascular malformations; venous occlusions; and rare inflammatory lesions of arteries and veins producing occlusions, ruptures, or focal dilatations, "mycotic aneurysms," due to inflammatory necrosis. Ischemic infarction is the most common parenchymal lesion of vascular type and is much more common in the brain than in the spinal cord. Following a sudden episode of total ischemia, there is a delay of several hours before characteristic nerve cell changes become apparent microscopically and the brain begins to swell. Maximal swelling is reached in 24 to 36 hours. As swelling subsides, liquefaction of the necrotic tissue occurs and is followed by phagocytic activity, shrinkage of the lesion, and gliosis leaving a permanent cavitated indurated scar associated with atrophy of interrupted tracts. Thrombotic occlusion of arteries characteristically produces ischemic infarcts. Embolic occlusions, much less common, cause hemorrhagic infarcts. The emboli usually originates in the heart or major arteries supplying the brain. Saccular or berry aneurysms are outpouchings of the walls of intracranial arteries usually at bifurcations or branching sites near the circle of Willis. These usually measure less than 1 cm. in diameter and occur in two to three per cent of normal adults. They cause symptoms when they rupture or impinge on adjacent nerve roots or brain tissue. Multiple aneurysms are found in 10 to 12 per cent of patients. Venous occlusions characteristically cause hemorrhagic infarction of brain and spinal cord tissue and are most likely to occur during dehydration, hemoconcentration, and hypercoagulability in infants with diarrhea, postpartal women, and patients with advanced debilitating disease. Vascular malformations are collections of abnormal arteries, veins, or capillaries in brain or spinal cord parenchyma that may produce clinical signs by rupturing or distorting nervous tissue. Most are asymptomatic, but some may cause recurrent bleeding and focal seizures.

Demyelinating Disorders

Demyelinating diseases are those in which myelin failure is the primary lesion, as opposed to the more common myelin destruction secondary to vascular, inflammatory, toxic, traumatic, or degenerative diseases. In demyelinating disorders there is selective deterioration of normally formed myelin or basically abnormal myelin. Oligodendroglia and myelin are the focus of the abnormality. Neurons and their processes are relatively spared. In multiple sclerosis, foci of myelin dissolution are scattered rapidly through the brain, spinal cord, and optic nerves during recurrent clinical episodes. Evolving lesions usually contain lymphocytes. Old lesions are overgrown by astrocytes. All lesions are permanent because of their destructive effect on oligodendroglia, although clinical deficits may improve during remissions as inflammatory changes subside, some myelin is spared, and compensatory mechanisms are utilized. Lesions vary in size, shape, age, and completeness of demyelination, but tend to concentrate in periventricular white matter. The cause is unknown but viral infection and immune mechanisms are suspected. Demyelination may occur after systemic viral infections or immunizations and may affect central and peripheral myelin, resulting in postinfectious, parainfectious, or postvaccinal encephalopathy, myelopathy, radiculopathy, or neuropathy. Sudden damage to myelin causes clinical manifestations that vary with the location of the lesions. The most common form of this process is polyradiculopathy resulting in ascending paralysis associated with increased cerebrospinal fluid

protein and few inflammatory cells, Landry-Guillain-Barré syndrome with albuminocytologic dissociation. Rare forms of demyelination, mainly affecting children, also of unknown cause, involve large confluent areas of cerebral white matter and progress over months to years to involve the entire nervous system. Based on the age of onset, manner of progression, histologic and chemical features, and detectable enzymatic deficiencies, they may be divided into those that result from deterioration of formed myelin (diffuse sclerosis) and those due to abnormal myelin formation (leucodystrophy).

Neoplasms

Neoplasms involving the nervous system may be primary or metastatic. Primary neoplasms may arise in any of the cell types of the parenchyma or coverings. Metastatic neoplasms may arise in any tissue. Intracranial neoplasms most frequently involve the parenchyma, less often the meninges or nerve roots. Intraspinal neoplasms are most often extramedullary and usually involve the meninges or nerve roots. Neoplasms involving the central nervous system are more often malignant; those in the peripheral nervous system are usually benign. Of the primary neoplasms of the brain, astrocytomas are most common. They are usually malignant in adults (glioblastoma multiforme) and more benign in children. The malignant forms in adults usually involve the cerebral hemispheres; the benign forms in children usually involve the brain stem or cerebellum. Ependymomas involve the ventricular lining and are most frequent in the fourth ventricle. Oligodendrogliomas are most common in middle life in the white matter of the cerebral hemispheres, frequently extending to the surface. Characteristic calcification may be visible on x-ray examination. Medulloblastoma is a neoplasm of the midline cerebellum in childhood and is composed of primitive, undifferentiated, rapidly growing cells which are sensitive to irradiation. Meningiomas are extrinsic lesions arising in the arachnoid membrane, usually benign and slow growing, amenable to surgical cure. They become attached to the dura and indent the underlying parenchyma from which they are distinctly demarcated. They are typically composed of whorled and interlacing patterns of arachnoid cells. Malignant forms are rare. Nerve sheath tumors are common lesions of nerve roots and peripheral nerves and are usually benign. Intracranial forms usually arise in the acoustic nerve and produce hearing impairment. Intraspinal forms usually involve the posterior nerve roots. They are composed of spindle cells often arranged in palisades. Neurofibromatosis (von Recklinghausen's disease) is a familial disorder in which multiple neurofibromas are associated with pigmentation of the skin and sometimes with meningiomas and gliomas.

Epilepsy

Epilepsy is a clinical syndrome characterized by recurrent episodes of convulsive seizures and/or alterations of consciousness due to abnormal discharge of nerve cells within the gray matter of the brain. The pathologic substrate of epilepsy is twofold and consists of predisposing factors, about which little is known, and a brain lesion that may be of any type, generalized or focal, structural or functional. In symptomatic epilepsy a structural lesion may be demonstrated. In idiopathic epilepsy there is no such demonstrable lesion. Focal epilepsy with jacksonian seizures is usually associated with focal structural abnormality in an appropriate location. Temporal lobe epilepsy causing psychomotor seizures is usually produced by a lesion in or near the medial temporal cortex. Petit mal epilepsy is not associated with any known pathologic change in brain tissue.

Degenerative Diseases

During adult life there is gradual attrition of nerve cells even in healthy individuals. Advancing age is accompanied by atrophy of nervous tissue. This is most apparent in the brain where a slowly progressive loss of nerve cells and their processes results in shrinkage of gray and white matter and enlargement of the ventricular system. The frontal and parietal lobes are most affected. Microscopically the most characteristic change of aging is atrophy of nerve cells with the accumulation of lipochrome granules in their cytoplasm. Neurofibrillary degeneration and deposits of neurofibrillary debris, senile plaques, are expected after the sixth decade. Excessive degenerative changes of this type result in senile dementia. In Alzheimer's presenile dementia these changes begin early and progress at an excessive rate. Presenile dementia in Pick's disease is due to lobar sclerosis in the cerebrum with argyrophilic neuronal inclusions. Huntington's chorea is a heredofamilial disease which becomes manifest in middle life as dementia and chorea and is characterized by widespread degeneration of gray matter, particularly affecting the caudate nuclei, putamens, and cerebral cortex, accompanied by intense gliosis. The clinical syndrome of tremor, rigidity, and hypokinesis referred to as paralysis agitans or parkinsonism may be due to several causes. Usually idiopathic, this syndrome may be due to encephalitis, vascular disease, trauma, and poisoning. Pathologic changes are widespread but most constant in the substantia nigra and locus ceruleus, where pigmented neurons undergo degeneration and develop cytoplasmic inclusion bodies

(Lewy bodies). Degenerative disease of motor neurons is of unknown cause and occurs in three main forms, amyotrophic lateral sclerosis, progressive bulbar palsy, and progressive spinal muscular atrophy. Motor neurons and their processes deteriorate selectively and result in atrophy of nerve cell processes and denervation of muscle.

Various combinations of degeneration of the cerebellum and spinal cord occur, most having a hereditary tendency. The most common form is the spinal type, Friedreich's ataxia, in which the predominant changes are atrophy of the posterior columns, corticospinal and dorsal spinocerebellar tracts. Cystic cavitation of the spinal cord (syringomyelia) or of the brain stem (syringobulbia) is of unknown cause, most probably due to malformation or degeneration of the central parenchyma. In some cases there are neoplastic features. Dissociated anesthesia due to stretching of crossing nerve fibers is a characteristic clinical manifestation.

OSSEOUS SYSTEM

Generalized Osteitis Fibrosa Cystica (von Recklinghausen's Disease)

This is a disease of bone (long bones, vertebrae, pelvis, skull) characterized by distortion of the architecture, due to osteoclastic resorption of the bony trabeculae and replacement of bone and bone marrow by connective tissue. Poorly developed and poorly calcified foci of new bone form in the connective tissue. Hemorrhage into the fibrous tissue results in the deposition of hemosiderin in phagocytes, which imparts a brown color to the tissue. Nodular foci of this tissue are referred to as brown tumors. Cysts lined by connective tissue may result from hemorrhage and degeneration. The condition is due to excessive secretion of parathyroid hormone, the result of parathyroid hyperplasia or, more commonly, adenoma. Hypercalcemia, hypophosphatemia, increased phosphatase in the blood and nephrocalcinosis, as well as other manifestations of metastatic calcification, occur as complications of this condition.

Osteitis Deformans (Paget's Disease of Bone)

As in the case of osteitis fibrosa, there is osteoclastic resorption of bone, but there is simultaneous formation of abundant, poorly calcified bone in both the spongiosa and the cortex. Therefore, the bones may be thick but soft and deformed. The calcium and the phosphorus in the blood are unchanged, but the blood phosphatase is high. There is no abnormality of the parathyroid glands. Microscopically the diagnostic feature of this condition is the so-called mosaic appearance of the bone due to the wide irregular lines of ground substance between the trabeculae of poorly calcified new and old bone. Approximately one out of four patients with this disease develops sarcoma of bone.

Eosinophilic Granuloma

This condition occurs in children and in young adults. The lesion frequently is monostotic but may occur in several bones. The lesion consists of soft brown tissue, with foci of hemorrhage, degeneration and even cyst formation. Microscopically it consists mainly of collections of large mononuclear cells that exhibit phagocytosis and may have a foamy cytoplasm, with an abundance of eosinophilic leukocytes and some multinucleated giant cells, plasma cells and lymphocytes. In the late stages eosinophils may not be abundant. It is considered that eosinophilic granuloma is a form of histiocytosis.

Osteoporosis

This is a relatively common metabolic bone disease that affects older men and women, the latter more seriously. It is characterized by generalized thinning of cortical bone due to a loss of bone tissue that may be accompanied by pain and sometimes pathologic fractures.

Tumors of Bone

Osteoma. Composed of dense, normal-appearing bone, this is a benign tumor found most frequently in the frontal region of the skull. The neoplastic character of some of these bony lesions that appear to be tumors is questioned by some who, because of the very slow growth, or apparent lack of it, consider the lesion to be the reaction to previous injury.

Osteogenic Sarcoma. This is a highly malignant, usually rapidly growing, primary neoplasm of bone that is found most commonly in young patients between the ages of 10 and 20 years. The most common sites are about the knee—lower end of the femur or upper end of the tibia, and the shoulder—upper end of the humerus. The average survival time after diagnosis is from 1 to 2 or 3 years, 5-year survivals being about 10 per cent or less. Rarely, osteogenic sarcoma may develop in older individuals who suffer from osteitis deformans (Paget's disease.).

Histologically these neoplasms vary greatly, from rapidly growing, anaplastic, poorly differentiated forms in which recognizable bone formation is slight or missing to sclerosing types in which calcified osteoid tissue is fairly abundant. The former are often difficult to recognize as of bone origin. Metastases occur early via the bloodstream, and pulmonary metastases are not infrequently present when the original diagnosis is made.

Chondromas and Chondrosarcomas. These benign and malignant tumors, respectively, of cartilage, may be found occasionally in bone. The former may appear in the small bones of the hands or feet, occasionally elsewhere, like the multiple enchondromas of childhood (Ollier's disease). Chondrosarcomas, on the other hand, while malignant, are more common in men over 25, may arise from enchondromas and, if adequately excised, offer a better prognosis than malignant bone tumors. Growth is slower than that of osteogenic sarcoma, and metastases, if they occur, appear late. Occasionally, if foci of calcification are found, differentiation from osteogenic sarcoma may be difficult.

Giant Cell Tumor. This is usually a benign tumor of long bones characterized histologically by the presence of multinucleate giant cells resembling osteoclasts or foreign body giant cells and occurring generally in young to middle-aged adults. About one third of the tumors recur locally after excision, while approximately 10 per cent may actually metastasize, occasionally very widely.

Ewing's Sarcoma. This tumor is a rare, highly malignant bone tumor occurring in patients in young adulthood. It arises in the marrow cavity, usually in the metaphysis or diaphysis, but never in the epiphysis. It usually involves the long tubular bones, but may also involve bones of the pelvis, thoracic cage, and skull. The tumor consists of undifferentiated sheaths of small round or oval cells. The histogenesis of the tumor is unsettled.

Arthritis

The most important forms of arthritis are infectious, rheumatic, gouty, rheumatoid and osteoarthritic. Of these, by far the most important, are the rheumatoid and the osteoarthritic types.

Rheumatoid Arthritis. This is a common systemic disease, often with a familial predisposition, commonly affecting young adults, especially women, and involving primarily the joints, though muscles, blood vessels, skin, and even the heart may be affected. While the cause is unknown, there is much evidence that an autoimmune mechanism plays a role. There are similarities, for example, to known hypersensitive states, like rheumatic fever and serum sickness. The disease may sometimes occur in association with systemic lupus erythematosus. Hyperglobulinemia is a fairly constant finding. Finally, a complex substance recognized as rheumatoid factor, shown to be an antibody against gamma globulin, can be found in the blood serum of nearly 90 per cent of patients. The disease usually has an insidious onset, but it may be acute. It most commonly attacks the joints of the hands and feet. The larger joints are swollen and painful, and eventually there is deformity and limitation of motion. In the region of the joints there are often subcutaneous nodules that microscopically may contain structures resembling Aschoff nodules. It is characterized by a thick synovial membrane, the seat of diffuse inflammation that may be complicated by necrosis, hemorrhage and formation of synovial villi. Ankylosis due to fibrous adhesions, which may later become calcified and ossified, is a common complication. Cartilage is involved only secondarily. Periarticular inflammation also occurs.

Osteoarthritis. This form of arthritis, also called hypertrophic, degenerative or senile arthritis, primarily is a degenerative process involving joint cartilage associated with hypertrophic overgrowth of underlying bone. It is not primarily infectious or inflammatory. It occurs more commonly after the age of 40 and affects large joints. Deformity and limitation of motion may occur, but anklyosis does not, although the degenerated cartilage may become ossified and eburnated. Overgrowth of subchondral bone results in the characteristic condition called lipping at the edges of the joints. When it affects the spine (spondylitis deformans), kyphosis may result, and the back usually is stiff, although true ankylosis of vertebrae does not occur.

Gouty Arthritis. Arthritis is the salient clinical feature of gout. Hyperuricemia, which is key to the pathogenesis of gout, leads to precipitation of urates into the synovial membranes of joints with characteristic tophus formation—a mass of urates surrounded by an inflammatory reaction with characteristic large foreign body giant cells. The joints most frequently involved are the great toe, bones of the feet and ankle, and knee. Primary gout is a familial disease due to a disorder of purine metabolism. Secondary gout occurs when uric acid levels are increased for prolonged periods whether by increased cell breakdown, decreased excretion, or other causes.

Pyogenic Arthritis. Any of the pyogenic organisms may occasionally cause suppurative arthritis; however, the gonococcus is the organism which most frequently causes pyogenic arthritis in young adults.

QUESTIONS IN PATHOLOGY

Choose the one best answer or completion in the following multiple choice questions. The answers are at the end of this chapter.

1. The edema of acute inflammation involves the exudation of protein-rich fluid:
   (a) primarily through venules and capillaries
   (b) primarily through arterioles
   (c) only through capillaries
   (d) through lymphatic vessels
   (e) through all microvessels more or less equally

2. In inflammatory reactions, the presence of hemorrhage implies:
   (a) the action of chemotactic mediators
   (b) the action of vasopermeability mediators
   (c) the action of lymphocyte mediators (lymphokines)
   (d) structural damage to blood vessels
   (e) none of the above

3. The principal chemical mediator of enhanced vessel permeability from neutrophils is:
   (a) a basic peptide
   (b) an acid phosphatase
   (c) beta glucuronidase
   (d) cholesteryl oleate
   (e) a mucopolysaccharide

4. All of the following are characterized by granulomatous inflammation EXCEPT:
   (a) sarcoidosis
   (b) tuberculosis
   (c) histoplasmosis
   (d) diptheria
   (e) leprosy

5. The most characteristic feature of granulation tissue is the:
   (a) resemblance to a granuloma
   (b) growth of fibroblasts and new capillaries
   (c) character of the exudate
   (d) granular scar that results
   (e) presence of monocytes and fibroblasts

6. Petechiae on pleural and pericardial surfaces and squames in alveoli of an autopsied neonatal infant suggest:
   (a) a transplacentally acquired viral infection
   (b) intrauterine anoxia
   (c) a metaplastic epithelial response to oxygen therapy
   (d) a marked decrease in pulmonary surfactant
   (e) an inherent clotting defect

7. Spontaneous maturation of tumor cells and a more benign clinical course potential is occasionally observed in which of the following neoplasms of childhood?
   (a) Medulloblastoma
   (b) Osteogenic sarcoma
   (c) Nephroblastoma
   (d) Neuroblastoma
   (e) Retinoblastoma

8. The most common malignant neoplasm in women between the ages of 30 and 55 years occurs in the:

(a) breast
(b) colon
(c) lung
(d) cervix
(e) ovary

9. Which of the following combinations cause the greatest mortality from cancer in Americans?
(a) Carcinoma of lung and stomach
(b) Carcinoma of lung and large intestine
(c) Carcinoma of stomach and large intestine
(d) Carcinoma of breast and stomach
(e) Carcinoma of breast and kidney

10. The immunoglobulin class responsible for sensitization of man for local and systemic anaphylactic reactions is:
(a) IgA
(b) IgD
(c) IgE
(d) IgG
(e) IgM

11. Of the following, the earliest step in the formation of a thrombus is:
(a) formation of fibrin
(b) adherence of platelets to vascular intima
(c) activation of Hageman's factor
(d) trapping of erythrocytes
(e) none of the above

12. Which of the following statements about alcoholic liver disease is correct?
(a) It is rarely associated with fatty metamorphosis.
(b) It invariably develops in individuals who consume large amounts of alcohol for more than three months.
(c) It produces extensive hepatic fibrosis rather than true cirrhosis.
(d) Mallory bodies and neutrophilic infiltrates are morphologic features of the early stages of the disease.
(e) It is not directly related to toxic effects of alcohol but rather to nutritional disturbances.

13. Autopsy of a 42-year-old white male found dead and suspected of suicide demonstrated numerous ulcerations of the mucosa of the stomach and ascending colon, along with marked coagulation necrosis of renal tubules. The most likely diagnosis is poisoning with:
(a) bismuth
(b) mercury
(c) arsenic
(d) phosphorus
(e) inorganic acid or alkali

14. Chronic salpingitis is considered to be a significant condition predisposing to:

(a) ectopic pregnancy
(b) carcinoma of the cervix
(c) leiomyomata
(d) cystic hyperplasia of the endometrium
(e) choriocarcinoma

15. All of the following statements regarding viral hepatitis are true EXCEPT:
(a) Most cases resolve without clinical or morphologic sequelae.
(b) All three recognized types (A, B, and non-A, non-B) may progress to chronic active hepatitis.
(c) "Ground glass" hepatocytes are found in association with type B but not with types A and non-A, non-B.
(d) Chronic active hepatitis is more likely to progress to cirrhosis than is chronic persistent hepatitis.
(e) In the United States, posttransfusion viral hepatitis is caused by type non-A, non-B more frequently than by type B.

16. In the majority of cases of infectious hepatitis, one year after recovery the liver most often would appear:
(a) coarsely nodular
(b) finely nodular
(c) with residular fibrosis in the portal areas
(d) with only minimal pseudolobule formations and increased fibrous tissue in portal areas
(e) histologically normal

17. Rickettsial diseases primarily affect:
(a) endothelial cells
(b) nerve cells
(c) renal tubular cells
(d) hepatocytes
(e) fibroblasts

18. Most of the tissue damage evoked by fungi is due to:
(a) exotoxins
(b) their ability to modify the metabolic and reproductive activity of the cells of the host
(c) progressive development of sensitization to the fungal antigens
(d) endotoxins
(e) obstruction of ducts, blood vessels or lymphatics

19. The organ system that is most severely affected in *fatal* histoplasmosis is the:
(a) central nervous system
(b) genitourinary system
(c) alimentary tract
(d) respiratory system
(e) reticuloendothelial system

20. Occlusion of the right coronary artery near its

origin by a thrombus would most likely result in:

(a) infarction of lateral wall of right ventricle and the right atrium
(b) infarction of the anterior left ventricle
(c) infarction of lateral left ventricle
(d) infarction of posterior left ventricular wall and the posterior septum
(e) infarction of the anterior septum

21. A decrease in the number of granular leukocytes in the blood occurs most commonly following exposure to:

(a) chlorine
(b) salicylic acid
(c) benzene
(d) cobalt
(e) mercury

22. The type of Hodgkin's disease with the best prognosis is:

(a) nodular sclerosis
(b) mixed
(c) reticular
(d) lymphocyte depletion
(e) lymphocyte predominant

23. Silicosis is most often complicated by:

(a) asthma
(b) carcinoma of lung
(c) mesothelioma
(d) tuberculosis
(e) bronchial-alveolar cell tumor

24. The most common site of carcinoma of the colon is:

(a) cecum
(b) ascending colon
(c) transverse colon
(d) splenic flexure
(e) rectosigmoid

25. The fate of acute poststreptococcal glomerulo-nephritis is usually:

(a) development of chronic glomerulonephritis
(b) development of membranous glomerulone-phritis
(c) development of lobular glomerulonephritis
(d) development of subacute glomerulonephri-tis
(e) complete recovery

26. Nodular hyperplasia (benign hypertrophy) of the prostate involves principally the:

(a) anterior lobe
(b) lateral lobes
(c) posterior lobe
(d) verumontanum
(e) prostatic utricle

27. Bleeding from the nipple in a 45-year-old woman without a palpable breast mass should suggest:

(a) fibroadenoma
(b) sclerosing adenosis
(c) intraductal papilloma
(d) fat necrosis
(e) medullary carcinoma

28. Spontaneous intracranial hemorrhage in hypertension is most closely related to:

(a) rupture of venous structures in the subdural space
(b) laceration of arterial vessels in the epidural space
(c) fibrinoid necrosis of small penetrating arteries
(d) inflammatory necrosis of small veins
(e) atherosclerosis of medium-sized arteries

29. Cerebral infarcts most frequently occur in the:

(a) amygdala
(b) hypothalamus
(c) corpus striatum and internal capsule
(d) corpus callosum
(e) nucleus subthalamicus

For each numbered item, select the one heading most closely associated with it. Each lettered heading may be selected once, more than once, or not at all.

(a) Neutrophils   (d) Monocytes
(b) Eosinophils   (e) Lymphocytes
(c) Basophils

30. Streptococcal cellulitis
31. Typhoid fever
32. Bronchial asthma
33. Pneumococcal pneumonia
34. Trichinosis

(a) Retinoblastoma
(b) Squamous cell carcinoma of skin
(c) Basal cell carcinoma of skin
(d) Carcinoma of esophagus
(e) Renal cell carcinoma

35. Rarely metastasizes
36. Frequently occurs in siblings
37. Associated with alcoholism and smoking
38. Contains abundant lipid
39. Frequently spreads by invading veins

(a) Rapidly progressive glomerulonephritis
(b) Minimal change disease
(c) Chronic glomerulonephritis
(d) Acute poststreptococcal glomerulonephritis
(e) Membranous glomerulonephritis

40. Increased mesangial and endothelial cells with neutrophilic infiltrate
41. Fusion of foot processes by electron microscopy
42. Epithelial crescents in Bowman's space
43. Thickened glomerular basement membranes with spike and dome immunofluorescence pattern

    (a) Chancroid
    (b) Chancre
    (c) Granuloma inguinale
    (d) Lymphopathia venereum
    (e) Condyloma acuminatum

44. Donovan bodies
45. Spirochetes
46. *Hemophilus ducreyi*

    (a) Amyotrophic lateral sclerosis
    (b) Syringomyelia
    (c) Multiple sclerosis
    (d) Cervical spondylosis
    (e) Diffuse sclerosis

47. Scattered foci of myelin damage with relative preservation of axons
48. Tubular cavitation of the spinal cord
49. Motor neuron degeneration

For each numbered item, indicate whether it is associated with:

    (a) A only   (c) Both A and B
    (b) B only   (d) Neither A nor B

    (A) Rheumatoid arthritis
    (B) Osteoarthritis
    (C) Both
    (D) Neither

50. Proliferative synovitis
51. Immune complex deposition
52. Primarily an articular cartilage degeneration
53. Blood-borne infection of joint

    (A) Healing by first intention (primary union)
    (B) Healing by second intention (secondary union)
    (C) Both
    (D) Neither

54. Granulation tissue
55. Reepithelialization by eight days
56. Proud flesh

    (A) Squamous cell carcinoma of skin
    (B) Basal cell carcinoma of skin
    (C) Both
    (D) Neither

57. Predisposed to by chronic exposure to sunlight
58. Rarely, if ever, metastasizes

    (A) Scurvy   (C) Both
    (B) Rickets   (D) Neither

59. Subperiosteal hematomas
60. Failure of osteoid mineralization

The gallbladder from a 26-year-old white female was found to contain multiple irregularly shaped black stones (nonfaceted) approximately 5 mm. in diameter which cut easily with a knife and were uniformly black throughout.

61. The stones most likely are composed principally of:
    (a) cholesterol
    (b) calcium bilirubinate
    (c) calcium carbonate
    (d) mixed cholesterol and calcium bilirubinate
    (e) mixed cholesterol and calcium carbonate

62. A likely cause of these stones is:
    (a) chronic hemolytic processes
    (b) hypercholesterolemia
    (c) stasis of bile
    (d) infection of the gallbladder
    (e) typhoid fever

A 28-year-old man was admitted to the hospital because of severe shortness of breath and cyanosis. The patient died before treatment could be instituted. An autopsy was performed and the final pathological diagnosis was as follows:

1. High interventricular septal defect in the heart (1.0 cm. in diameter)
2. Bicuspid aortic valve
3. Bacterial (vegetative) endocarditis of the aortic valve (*E. coli* was cultured from vegetations)
4. Hypertrophy and dilatation of right heart (severe)
5. Hypertrophy and dilatation of left heart (moderate)
6. Mural thrombi in right atrium of heart
7. Chronic passive congestion of liver (severe)
8. Chronic passive congestion of lungs (moderate)
9. Recent and old pulmonary infarcts
10. Septic infarcts in spleen and both kidneys
11. Arteriosclerosis of coronary arteries and aorta

63. The most likely underlying cause of the bacterial endocarditis was:
    (a) old rheumatic heart disease
    (b) congenital cardiac anomalies
    (c) transient *E. coli* bacteremia
    (d) probable dental manipulations prior to admission
    (e) septic infarcts in the kidneys

64. Hypertrophy and dilatation of the right heart was most likely due to:
    (a) chronic pulmonary congestion

(b) bicuspid aortic valve

(c) bacterial endocarditis of the aortic valve

(d) interventricular septal defect

(e) left ventricular hypertrophy and dilatation

65. Chronic passive congestion of the liver was most likely due to:
    (a) failure of the right heart
    (b) failure of the left heart
    (c) septicemia
    (d) chronic pulmonary congestion
    (e) none of the above

66. Which of the following is the most likely cause-effect relationship?
    (a) $8 \rightarrow 4$
    (b) $1 \rightarrow 4$
    (c) $2 \rightarrow 4$
    (d) $6 \rightarrow 10$
    (e) $2 \rightarrow 8$

A 45-year old white male was a known alcoholic admitted with hematemesis (vomiting blood) and a shocklike state. He had a history of melena (black, tarry stools) for one week prior to admission. He expired soon after admission. An autopsy was performed.

67. The liver was small, nodular and yellowish-brown in color, divided into small, uniform nodules on cut surfaces. The most likely diagnosis is:
    (a) portal cirrhosis
    (b) postnecrotic cirrhosis
    (c) cardiac cirrhosis
    (d) biliary cirrhosis
    (e) all of the above

68. Which of the following microscopic changes would you *not* expect to see in his liver?
    (a) Fatty change of parenchymal cells
    (b) Acute cholangitis
    (c) Alcoholic hyaline in parenchymal cells
    (d) Pseudolobule formation
    (e) Fine fibrous bands connecting the portal triads

69. Esophageal varices in this case are most likely the result of:
    (a) increased blood flow to the liver
    (b) right-sided heart failure
    (c) decreased albumin in blood
    (d) thrombosis of portal vein
    (e) portal hypertension

Please answer questions 70 to 91 using (a) to (e) as follows:
    (a) only *1, 2, and 3* are correct
    (b) only *1 and 3* are correct
    (c) only *2 and 4* are correct
    (d) only *4* is correct
    (e) *all* are correct

70. Tissues highly sensitive to ionizing radiation include:
    (1) brain
    (2) intestinal mucosa
    (3) liver
    (4) lymphoid tissue

71. Vasopermeability factors that are generated by cleavage of plasma substrates include:
    (1) histamine
    (2) anaphylatoxins
    (3) slow reacting substance of anaphylaxis (SRS-A)
    (4) kinins

72. Significant chemotactic agents for neutrophils include:
    (1) soluble bacterial products
    (2) histamine
    (3) components of the complement system
    (4) bradykinin

73. Organisms that sometimes cause disseminated infections in the fetus include:
    (1) cytomegalovirus
    (2) Herpes simplex virus
    (3) *Toxoplasma gondii*
    (4) *Treponema pallidum*

74. Viruses capable of inducing neoplasms in experimental animals include:
    (1) polyoma virus
    (2) measles virus
    (3) SV 40
    (4) influenza B virus

75. Tumors that may produce substances with hormone activity include:
    (1) oat cell carcinoma of the bronchus
    (2) medullary thyroid carcinoma
    (3) granulosa-theca cell tumor of the ovary
    (4) renal cell carcinoma

76. In general, rickettsial infections are characterized by:
    (1) obligate intracellular parasitism
    (2) localization of organisms in endothelial cells
    (3) transmission of arthropods
    (4) phlegmonous inflammation

77. *Intranuclear* inclusion bodies occur in:
    (1) smallpox
    (2) chicken pox
    (3) herpes simplex
    (4) rabies

78. The Chédiak-Higashi syndrome is characterized by:
    (1) hypopigmentation of skin, eyes and hair
    (2) large abnormal lysosomes in polymorphonuclear leukocytes
    (3) predisposition to chronic infections

(4) abnormal response to delayed type of hyper-sensitivity

79. In patients with alpha-1-antitrypsin deficiency:
    (1) symptoms appear at birth
    (2) enzyme activity is decreased but not totally absent in persons with homozygous state
    (3) there is increased risk of developing bronchogenic carcinoma
    (4) emphysema usually develops

80. Ostium primum defects:
    (1) are commonly associated with a cleft mitral valve
    (2) arise from abnormalities of rotation
    (3) occur commonly in Down's syndrome
    (4) occur at various locations in the intra-atrial septum with approximately equal frequency

81. Cyanotic congenital heart diseases include:
    (1) tetralogy of Fallot
    (2) transposition of the great vessels
    (3) total anomalous pulmonary venous return
    (4) Taussig-Bing anomaly

82. Hereditary spherocytosis is characterized by:
    (1) decreased osmotic fragility
    (2) autosomal recessive inheritance pattern
    (3) a small contracted spleen
    (4) a cell membrane defect

83. Features of ulcerative colitis include:
    (1) superficial mucosal ulcers
    (2) crypt abscesses
    (3) pseudopolyps
    (4) marked thickening of the gut wall

84. Hypertension may result from:
    (1) an adrenal medullary tumor
    (2) Addison's disease
    (3) an adrenal cortical tumor
    (4) amyloidosis of adrenal gland

85. Papillary necrosis of the kidney may be associated with:
    (1) acute pyelonephritis in combination with partial obstruction
    (2) diabetes mellitus
    (3) phenacetin abuse
    (4) benign nephrosclerosis

86. Leiomyomata of the uterus:
    (1) frequently undergo sarcomatous change
    (2) are sharply circumscribed
    (3) are encapsulated
    (4) rarely arise after the menopause

87. Serous cystadenocarcinoma of the ovary:
    (1) is bilateral in approximately 66 per cent of cases
    (2) frequently results in widespread abdominal implantation
    (3) is commonly papillary with psammoma bodies

(4) is derived from the coelomic epithelium covering the ovary

88. Massive intracerebral hemorrhage characteristically:
    (1) is preceded by long-standing hypertension
    (2) occurs in the lenticulostriate region
    (3) is due to rupture of small vessels
    (4) is fatal more frequently than cerebral infarction

89. In a patient who dies with severe presenile dementia (Alzheimer's disease) the diagnostic histologic findings in the brain include:
    (1) severe arteriolar sclerosis
    (2) abundant senile plaques
    (3) multiple cortical microinfarcts
    (4) neurofibrillary tangles in neurons

90. Organisms frequently responsible for meningitis in the newborn period include:
    (1) group B streptococcus
    (2) *Neisseria meningitidis*
    (3) *Escherichia coli*
    (4) pneumococcus

91. Characteristics of degenerative joint disease (osteoarthritis) include:
    (1) pannus formation
    (2) degeneration of articular cartilage
    (3) ankylosis
    (4) involvement of weight-bearing joints

ANSWERS TO MULTIPLE CHOICE QUESTIONS

1. (a)	24. (e)	47. (c)	70. (c)
2. (d)	25. (e)	48. (b)	71. (c)
3. (a)	26. (b)	49. (a)	72. (b)
4. (d)	27. (c)	50. (a)	73. (e)
5. (b)	28. (c)	51. (a)	74. (b)
6. (b)	29. (c)	52. (b)	75. (e)
7. (d)	30. (a)	53. (d)	76. (a)
8. (a)	31. (d)	54. (c)	77. (a)
9. (b)	32. (b)	55. (a)	78. (a)
10. (c)	33. (a)	56. (b)	79. (c)
11. (b)	34. (b)	57. (c)	80. (b)
12. (d)	35. (c)	58. (b)	81. (e)
13. (b)	36. (a)	59. (a)	82. (d)
14. (a)	37. (d)	60. (b)	83. (a)
15. (b)	38. (e)	61. (b)	84. (b)
16. (e)	39. (e)	62. (a)	85. (a)
17. (a)	40. (d)	63. (b)	86. (c)
18. (c)	41. (b)	64. (d)	87. (e)
19. (e)	42. (a)	65. (a)	88. (e)
20. (d)	43. (e)	66. (b)	89. (c)
21. (c)	44. (c)	67. (a)	90. (b)
22. (e)	45. (b)	68. (b)	91. (c)
23. (d)	46. (a)	69. (e)	

7

Pharmacology

JAMES A. RICHARDSON, PH.D.*

Professor of Pharmacology, Medical University of South Carolina

SCOPE OF PHARMACOLOGY

The word pharmacology is derived from two Greek words, *pharmakon,* which is equivalent in modern parlance to "drug," and *logia,* meaning "study." In the broadest sense, this discipline is concerned with the history, source, physical and chemical properties, biochemical and physiologic effects, mechanisms of absorption, distribution, action, biotransformation and excretion, compounding, and therapeutic and other uses of drugs. Since a drug is a substance used in the diagnosis, prevention, treatment or cure of disease the subject of pharmacology is obviously quite extensive. In addition to its many diverse ramifications, this discipline forges a strong link between the basic and clinical medical sciences.

GENERAL TYPES OF DRUG NAMES

Drug therapy, as currently practiced, depends on selection from a prodigious number of cataloged drug

* I wish to express my thanks to those members of the Pharmacology staff who assisted me in the preparation of this section, with special thanks to Dr. Glen R. Gale.

names. This massive list of drug names is a product of the remarkably accelerated pace of investigative medicine and the combined influence of intensified commercial activity. The actual number of basically valuable drugs is relatively small, but this number undergoes progressive multiplication by several processes. Simple chemical variations of the basic drugs are produced by numerous commercial firms, and, although these sometimes prove to be independently valuable in a new area of effects, most often they do not alter significantly the pattern of the original basic drug, except in minor features of dosage, absorption, excretion, etc. However, these new drug variants have been claimed to be a necessity of competitive survival, and the extent of their continued production is one of the chief issues now being faced by the Food and Drug Administration. At least, their existence must be recognized as a reality, and the multiplicity of names follows naturally, since each has a chemical name, a generic name and one or, possibly, several proprietary or trademarked names. Additionally, some may have had a code name during the investigational stage. A trademark may be owned indefinitely (subject only to renewal), although control of any given chemical for commercial sale may be monopolized only for 17 years through protective patents. A generic, nonproprietary or public name is selected after discussion by committees or representatives of the American Medical Association, the United States Pharmacopeia, the World Health Organization, the National Formulary and the commercial sponsor of the drug. Since 1961 the names finally selected have been known as United States Adopted Names (USAN), and they are intended to provide the features of brevity, easy recall and some syllable or stem that indicates the group to which the drug belongs. International recognition of the USAN reduces the occasion for worldwide multiplicity of names.

The older nomenclature bodies that now participate in selection of the USAN continue to operate in their special areas. Since 1820, the US Pharmacopeia has engaged in the selection of drugs based on therapeutic merit and has specified their standards of purity. The designation USP after a drug name is legal testimony on the part of the manufacturer that the product meets the published purity standards and that the drug has been considered to have therapeutic merit by revision committees acting every 5 years. The National Formulary designation NF is associated usually with older drugs and combinations of declining importance that are used sufficiently to satisfy an arbitrary standard. In 1975, the United States Pharmacopoeial Convention acquired all rights to the National Formulary. As a result, the present USPXX and NFXV appear together in a single binding. Standards for essentially every chemical entity marketed as a drug in the United States, as well as many combination products, are found in this volume.

A publication, AMA Drug Evaluations, prepared by committees and consultants of the AMA is a valuable source of information on most drugs that are available in the United States. It is particularly useful in checking on available preparations and currently accepted therapeutic practices.

REGULATORY CONTROL OF DRUGS

The Food and Drug Administration is charged with protection of the public interest insofar as it is affected by the sale and the distribution of drug products. This agency, founded in 1906 through the missionary-type efforts of Dr. Harvey Wiley, was, for many years limited to the control of the sanitary state of manufacturing premises, the detection of adulteration and the correction of minor features of labeling. The greater part of the staff was engaged in the inspection of meat.

Food and drug promotions with obvious fraudulent intent were liable to restraint or prosecution, but there was no authority to halt sales of disastrously dangerous drugs, and there were no governmental standards for proof of efficacy. Congress empowered the FDA in 1938, to require demonstrations of reasonable safety and, in 1962, to require proof of efficacy. In both instances, legislation followed spectacular incidents—in one case, the "elixir of sulfanilamide" tragedy, which cost over 100 lives because of unexpected toxicity of diethylene glycol, the solvent; in the other, the thalidomide experience, in which teratogenic effects of an apparently harmless sedative occurred in several thousand cases, almost all of them outside the United States.

Practical difficulties in the enforcement of such legislation are obvious when it is recognized that a "dangerous" drug must be defined in terms compatible with the use of drugs such as insulin and digitalis, which, recognizably, must be used as calculated risks. Again, for new drugs, the proof of efficacy, to be meaningful, may be expected to require statistically significant indices of improvement over older drugs, based on procedures such as double-blind controlled studies, and these call for academically directed projects much more elaborate than those that were practiced previously.

In 1971, the FDA in collaboration with the National Academy of Sciences and National Research Council, began rating the efficacy of drug products in an effort to provide the prescriber with the best possible clinical judgment in choosing drugs for patients. The efficacy ratings are commonly referred to as DESI (Drug Efficacy Study Implementation) ratings.

In 1951, an amendment to the US Federal Food, Drug and Cosmetic Act established specific regulations in regard to prescription practices. A number of situations were clarified, such as the procedure of placing prescriptions by telephone, which is now acceptable under some conditions. Clear distinctions are made between drugs that may be dispensed on prescription only ("legend" drugs) and those that may be sold over the counter by any merchant. The first category bear the prescription legend "Caution: Federal law prohibits dispensing without prescription." Among the prescription-legend drugs, certain ones can be refilled for the time specified by the prescriber, as indicated by his "refill" instructions; however, it should be noted that such instructions as "refill prn" or "refill ad lib", or other notations that place no limit on the length of time in which the prescription may be refilled, have no recognition by the FDA as valid refill authorizations.

The Comprehensive Drug Abuse Prevention and

Control Act (Contolled Substances Act) of 1970, which supersedes the Harrison Narcotic Act, places further limitations on the prescribing and refilling of certain depressant, stimulant and hallucinogenic drugs. The Controlled Substances Act places such drugs in five different "schedules." Those drugs that have no legal use (such as heroin and LSD) are all placed in schedule I. Those drugs in the remaining schedules (II through V) are rated according to their decreasing potential for addiction or habituation. Prescriptions for drugs in schedule II (morphine, cocaine, and methamphetamine, for example) cannot be refilled. Prescriptions for drugs in schedules III and IV may be refilled, if the prescriber authorizes, not more than five times nor for longer than 6 months after the prescription is issued. Drugs in schedule V (formerly referred to as "exempt narcotics") may be refilled according to the prescriber's instructions; if no refill instructions are supplied, the prescription may not be refilled.

When prescribing controlled substances, the prescriber must include the full name and address of the patient, must sign the prescription in ink or indelible pen and must show his own address and BNDD (Bureau of Narcotics and Dangerous Drugs) registration number. It is illegal for a pharmacist to fill a prescription for a controlled substance unless all these requirements are met.

The Food and Drug Administration, first operated under the Department of Agriculture, is now part of the Department of Health and Human Services (formerly Health, Education and Welfare), as a part of the Consumer Protection and Environmental Health Service. Other regulatory agencies include: the National Microbiological Institute of the National Institutes of Health, which regulates vaccines, sera, antitoxins, etc., under the broad class of "biologicals."

The Federal Bureau of Narcotics and Dangerous Drugs, which has operated successively under the aegis of the Treasury Department, and then the Justice Department, has been merged with the Food and Drug Administration's abuse control program.

The Federal Trade Commission exercises control over direct public advertising of drug products that move in interstate commerce. Validity of advertising claims is judged in terms of possible direct injury and, also, of indirect hazard brought about by encouraging the use of ineffective remedies.

The Drug Regulation Reform Act of 1979 was the culmination of several years of effort on the part of members of Congress, the Administration, industry, academic researchers, and consumer activists. It is a major revision of the way in which new drugs are brought onto the market and includes provisions for their surveillance after marketing.

GENERAL PRINCIPLES

Drugs attach to receptor sites, which in some cases are enzyme molecules, and there is a high degree of spatial specificity in this process of apposition. The kinetics of attachment and release depend on forces such as covalent electron sharing, electrostatic charges, hydrogen bonding and van der Waals forces, these being listed in order from highest to lowest energy equivalents. The bond energy of a covalent bond may be 100 kcal. per mole; that of electrostatic forces, 5; hydrogen bonds, 2 to 5; and van der Waals forces, about 0.5 kcal. per mole. Ester formation is a chemically weak covalent reaction, but it is potent in terms of drug and protoplasm reactions; examples occur in the attachment of conversion products of dibenamine to alpha-adrenergic receptors and diisopropyl fluorophosphate to acetylcholinesterase, both of these being pharmacologic reactions with exceptionally slow recovery requiring several days. In acetylcholine, the quaternary ammonium group acts as a cationic site that binds electrostatically with anionic sites in its relevant receptors. Attachment of morphine and of histamine to receptor sites illustrates the operation of weaker hydrogen bonding and van der Waals forces. The spatial separation of these binding sites can usually be expressed in terms of distances that may amount to a few Angstrom units, and these interatomic distances represent guides in synthesis of drugs with a high degree of specificity. An example is the 7 Å distance between the nitrogen and carbonyl groups of acetylcholine; this amounts to a spatial entity that is repeated in the analogs and blocking agents of acetylcholine.

Although many drug effects are due to interaction with enzyme receptors and follow the Michaelis-Menten formulation of enzyme kinetics, there are other more general effects that relate primarily to membrane permeability. Here dominant influences are relative lipoid-water solubilities and pH changes. A high lipoid-water solubility coefficient favors passage of drugs through lipoid-protein cell membranes and, in case of ionizable compounds, those pH changes that reduce ionization favor penetration by shifting the equilibrium toward the less polarized, less water-soluble form. Alkalinity favors the passage from aqueous media into the cells in the case of alkaloids and other basic substances; acidity increases the ionized, water-soluble state of basic drugs and, accordingly, retards their passage into cells or accelerates their excretion in aqueous urine. The reverse is true of organic acids such as salicylic acid, penicillin and barbiturates; these are notably increased in their excretion rate when urine is alkalinized. Relative ionization characteristics determine relative influences of these pH effects, and this is simply compared in terms of pK_a values. Highly ionized salicylic acid, with a low pK_a of 3.0, is more responsive than barbital, with a higher pK_a of 7.8. With basic substances in which high pK_a values indicate high degrees of ionization, it can be shown that acetanilid, with a pK_a of 0.3, is less affected than mecamylamine, with a pK_a of 11.2.

Graphs of the relationship between stepwise increases in drug doses and the percentage of subjects exhibiting an all-or-none response delineate characteristically S-shaped or sigmoid curves. Similar dose-response curves are observed when graded reponses are plotted against doses. When the doses of the drug, which are plotted on the X axis, are expressed as logarithms, the curve becomes more linear and easier to interpret. These graphs can be used to show the interaction between two or more drugs. For example, competitive antagonism or inhibition between drugs results in a parallel shift of the curve to the right, with no diminution in the height or efficacy. This shift of the curve to the right illustrates the necessity for a larger dose of the agonist in the presence of an antagonist to achieve the same effect. The distinction between competitive and noncompetitive antagonists can be brought out by plotting reciprocals of drug concentration on one axis and reciprocals of responses on the other. Known as Lineweaver-Burk charts, such graphs can be used to distinguish between competitive and noncompetitive types of inhibition.

Because the position of the dose-response curve on the X axis indicates the relative potency of a drug, shifts of the curve to the left indicate an increase in potency. If a second drug is added and the efficacy of the combination is greater than that of either drug for a given dose, the drug effects are said to be additive. This effect is reflected in an elevation in the curve for a given dose.

Potentiation and synergism are terms used to denote that the efficacy of the combination is greater than the sum of the individual effects, although the term synergism is often used to indicate a simple additive effect. Potentiation is usually associated with drugs acting by different mechanisms to produce the same final effect. Examples are the potentiative effects of thiosulfate and methemoglobin-formers in detoxifying cyanide poisoning; the effect of physostigmine in potentiating the action of acetylcholine on isolated muscle strips; the antispirochetal action of oxophenarsine and penicillin; the antimalarial action of sulfonamides and folic acid antimetabolites.

Variability in drug responses is conspicuously greater than in the precisely consistent results that can be obtained in experiments in the physical sciences. The most rigorously conducted drug experiment can be expected to exhibit quantitative variabilities greater than $\pm$ 10 per cent of the mean value. For example, in a group of 10 animals, determinations of the lethal dose of digitalis in individual animals will usually give values ranging from 0.5 to 1.5 the mean value. Because of practical limitations, it is usually necessary in therapeutic trials to accept as significant P values that are higher than would be considered in most scientific observations. As occurs at times with drugs used in psychiatry, responses do not follow the usual dose-response relations, in which case a high degree of "placebo" or psychologic effect can be presumed. Also, there is little benefit in development of a drug with relatively high potency unless there is an increase in its efficacy or maximal effect. As long as a dose is low enough to be conveniently administered, there is no practical advantage in making a similar drug with still lower dosage. Most significant is an improvement in "therapeutic index," which relates the dose producing a therapeutic effect to the dose producing toxic or fatal effects. Commonly the latter is expressed as the LD_{50}/ED_{50}, designating the dose that is lethal to 50 per cent of a group, compared to the dose that is effective (or therapeutic) in 50 per cent of a similar group. Significance can be attached to other ratios such as LD_1/ED_{99}, which can be less reliable mathematically but more meaningful in terms of safety.

Many obvious factors, such as age, sex, nutritional status, genetic traits and intercurrent pathologic states, contribute to drug variability. A special example is the manner in which one drug may affect the potency of a subsequent drug through action on metabolic enzymes. For instance, disulfiram (Antabuse) inhibits hepatic microsomal enzymes needed for the metabolism of the coumarin anticoagulants and thus potentiates the action of anticoagulants. Conversely, phenobarbital and 3,4-benzypyrene increase the activity of drug-metabolizing enzymes, and bishydroxycoumarin has been shown to be much less potent following previous administration of phenobarbital.

AUTONOMIC DRUGS

A number of drugs are particularly characterized by actions that mimic the effects of stimulation of parts of the autonomic nervous system, while others typically block these same effects. They are reasonably consistent in that their actions resemble either augmentation or inhibition of the parasympathetic (cholinergic) or the sympathetic (adrenergic) system. Consequently, when the basic action of one of these drugs is known, a considerable number of its specific effects can be recognized or anticipated. The nerve impulses are transmitted largely by chemicals liberated at the nerve endings, and the drugs of this group closely resemble, or may be identical with, these chemicals.

Norpinephrine is liberated at sympathetic nerve endings. Similarly, acetylcholine is the chemical liberated at the nerve endings of the parasympathetic system. Acetylcholine also is a chemical mediator of nerve impulses to skeletal muscle, to the adrenal medulla and at the ganglionic synapses of both the sympathetic and the parasympathetic systems.

Parasympathomimetic Drugs

Acetylcholine is essentially an experimental drug. Its administration produces effects typical of stimulation of the parasympathetic system: miosis; ciliary muscle spasm; salivation; lacrimation; sweating; heart slowing; peripheral vasodilation; bronchial, gastric and intestinal secretion; and stimulation of the smooth muscle of the bronchi, the stomach, the gut, the ureters and the urinary bladder. These effects are typical but vary according to the mode of administration. The ocular effects, for instance, are obtained only by local application. Also, the primary effects just listed may be counterbalanced by other effects, depending on dose and conditions. This is particularly evident in the case of heart rate changes. The primary effect of acetylcholine is rate slowing equivalent to vagal stimulation. At the same time, this chemical mediator is acting on chromaffin tissue in the heart, which liberates significant quantities of norepinephrine. If the dose is sufficient, there may be action at the adrenal medulla, liberating epinephrine, and there also may be action on autonomic ganglia. In isolated heart preparations treated previously with atropine, acetylcholine causes marked stimulation of rate and force along with demonstrable release of norepinephrine. Acetylcholine is unstable and is inactivated by body cholinesterase with extreme rapidity. It is not effective orally.

Synthetic variations with clinical usefulness include: carbachol (carbamylcholine); bethanechol (carbamylmethylcholine, Urecholine); and methacholine (Mecholyl). These are characterized by greater stability, longer period of action and satisfactory effectiveness by oral administration. They also may be given subcutaneously, but intravenous administration may be disastrous because of marked bronchospasm and heart slowing, along with copious salivary and bronchial secretions. Atropine usually is an effective antidote after such accidents. Methacholine has about the same pattern of action as acetylcholine and is used chiefly for its vasodilating effect in peripheral vascular disease and for its heart-slowing effect in paroxysmal tachycardia. Carbachol and bethanechol have relatively less cardiovascular action and more predominant effects on the gastrointestinal tract and the urinary bladder. They are used mostly in atonic conditions of these viscera.

Pilocarpine, a naturally occurring alkaloid, has effects that mimic those of parasympathetic postganglionic stimulation. It is used as a miotic (one to four per cent locally) in the management of glaucoma.

Muscarine is similar in action and is of interest as one of the toxic agents in one type of mushroom poisoning *(Amanita muscaria).* It is treated effectively by atropine. The actions of this drug so faithfully mimic the effects of stimulation of effector cells supplied by postganglionic nerve endings that the term *muscarinic* has general application. It signifies this particular action of acetylcholine with exclusion of its actions at autonomic ganglia and at the motor end-plate of skeletal muscles. The latter actions of acetylcholine usually are termed *nicotinic,* referring to the minimal actions of nicotine at low doses and being distinct from the paralytic actions of nicotine at higher concentrations.

Physostigmine (eserine) is a naturally occurring alkaloid that is parasympathomimetic in action. It is an inhibitor of acetylcholinesterase, the enzyme that normally destroys acetylcholine, and its presence at nerve endings thus serves to intensify and prolong the effects of the acetylcholine formed at this point. Overdoses produce fibrillary tremors of skeletal muscle and convulsions. Physostigmine is useful as a miotic (0.25 to 0.5 per cent locally) after refractions and occasionally in the medical management of glaucoma. Presumably, spasm of the sphincter iridis and the ciliary body serves to open the spaces of Fontana and the canal of Schlemm and, by improved drainage, to relieve intraocular pressure.

Neostigmine (Prostigmin) is a synthetic variation of physostigmine that has a more suitable pattern of parasympathomimetic action for clinical use (less heart slowing and salivation for a given degree of gut stimulation). It is used for combating atonic conditions of the gut and the urinary bladder (1 to 2 ml. of 1:2,000 solution parenterally). It is also useful in the treatment of myasthenia gravis (orally in 15 mg. tablets; subcutaneously or intramuscularly, 0.5 to 2.0 mg.). Its demonstrated usefulness in myasthenia supports the concept of a similarity in the chemical mediation of nerve impulses at the skeletal muscle end plate and at autonomic ganglionic synapses. Some of the actions of neostigmine are caused by cholinesterase inhibition, whereas others are the result of a combination of enzyme inhibition plus a direct acetylcholine-like effect. Atropine will antagonize the muscarinic effects but not the neuromuscular nicotinic actions of this agent.

Benzpyrinium is closely similar to neostigmine in

action and has been used in abdominal distention and in bladder atony. Other related compounds used in the management of myasthenia are pyridostigmine (Mestinon) and ambenomium (Mytelase). Overdosage with these agents may produce a cholinergic crisis if a patient in a refractory phase of the disease is given increasing doses in an attempt to control symptoms.

Edrophonium (Tensilon) also is closely related in actions to neostigmine and is significant because of its predominant action at the skeletal neuromuscular junction. It inhibits cholinesterase at this site, acts directly on the motor end plate and also accomplishes competitive displacement of curare. These effects can be obtained at doses producing relatively minimal muscarinic actions. Accordingly it has proved to be a very satisfactory antagonist to curare, and the prompt but brief improvement in myasthenia gravis is of diagnostic value. It is useful in emergency treatment of myasthenic crises. Brevity of action and lack of cumulative effects are characteristic. Administration of atropine to abolish muscarinic effects is usually not necessary during diagnostic tests, but atropine should be readily available.

DFP (diisopropyl flourophosphate), a product of chemical warfare experimentation in World War II, has the effect of irreversibly inactivating cholinesterase. Accordingly, it produces long-sustained parasympathomimetic effects. Its uses in myasthenia gravis has not been successful because of toxic effects, but results in the management of primary openangle glaucoma and in accommodative esotropia have been more promising. Echothiophate iodide (Phospholine) is a related compound that has produced critical systemic effects when used locally in glaucoma. With prolonged administration of either drug, iridic cysts may develop. Demecarium (Humorsol) has similar uses and toxic properties. Other alkyl phosphate anticholinesterase agents that have been tested in the treatment of myasthenia gravis are hexaethyl tetraphosphate, tetraethyl pyrophosphate and octamethyl pyrophosphoramide.

DFP is available under the trade name of Floropryl. Its USP designation is isoflurophate. Tetraethyl pyrophosphate is available as an insecticide under a variety of trade names, such as Bladex, Fosvex, Hexamite, Nifos, Tetron and Vapotone. TEPP, along with parathion and other similar phosphoric acid esters, has numerous chemical variants in use as insecticides. They are highly lipid soluble compounds, rapidly absorbed by all routes including the skin.

Cholinesterase Reactivators. Even though under ordinary circumstances cholinesterase inactivation by organophosphates such as DFP is irreversible, compounds have been developed that are capable of reactivating the enzyme. One such agent is pralidoxime (Protopam; PAM). To be useful, it must be administered soon after poisoning occurs. It is most effective at skeletal neuromuscular sites, whereas atropine, the time-honored antidote, abolishes symptoms arising from muscarinic sites and to a moderate extent those associated with the central nervous system.

Drugs Blocking Parasympathomimetic Effects

Atropine, from the belladonna root or leaf, is the racemic form of *hyoscyamine*. It blocks the action of acetylcholine on the cells innervated by the postganglionic cholinergic system, and its typical effects then include mydriasis; cycloplegia; mouth and skin dryness; acceleration of heart rate; diminution in secretory activity of bronchi, stomach and gut; and relaxation of smooth muscle of bronchi, stomach, gut, biliary tract, ureters and urinary bladder. However, most of these effects are not striking until toxic overdoses are given. Overdoses are characterized additionally by cerebral excitation and hyperpyrexia. Flushing of the face is an anomalous effect obtained with atropine poisoning.

Atropine competes with acetylcholine for attachment to the receptor cells. Quantitatively, these cells supplied by the postganglionic cholinergic nerves are blocked much more readily than are the cells of the skeletal muscles or ganglionic synapses, and although atropine can accomplish blocking action at these latter locations, the doses required are much beyond those occurring in ordinary use. Apparently, with some of the synthetic atropine variants, there is not such a wise spread between the concentrations producing blocking effects at these three locations.

Atropine is used to neutralize excessive overactivity of the cholinergic system, and this may be obtained with doses below the toxic level. It is used to diminish secretions preoperatively and to overcome spasm of the gut, the bronchi (as in bronchial asthma), the biliary tract, the ureter (as in colic) and the urinary bladder (as with irritability due to cystitis or to mental disturbances). Atropine and related alkaloids have special value in overcoming the excessive rigidity and salivation of parkinsonism. They also are used locally as mydriatics and as cycloplegics. Mydriasis may block drainage, and in glaucoma the increased intraocular pressure may permanently damage the retina. The USP dose of atropine (0.5 mg.) is approximately equivalent to 1.5 ml. of the tincture of belladonna. Mouth dryness usually is obtained with 1 to 2 mg. of atropine given orally; impaired accommodation, with somewhat larger doses.

As contrasted with the usual atropine salts, atropine

methylbromide, apparently because of its electrostatic charge, does not penetrate as readily through the blood-brain or placental barriers.

Hyoscine (scopolamine) is a natural alkaloid with similar actions on the parasympathetic nervous system. Cerebral effects from small doses are largely depressant. Combination of morphine with hyoscine, as has been used in obstetrics, produces a special type of narcosis with amnesia.

Tincture of stramonium and tincture of hyoscyamus contain atropine and atropine-like alkaloids. Numerous synthetic variations of atropine are available. When these compounds are selected as mydriatics, usually it is on the basis of a shorter period of action; when selected for spasmolytic effects, usually it is on the basis of a relatively lesser degree of mouth dryness and heart acceleration. Spasmolytic action on the gastrointestinal tract may be claimed to be associated with less paralysis of the bladder, and, on the other hand, urinary tract relaxation may be claimed to be associated with less mydriatic and mouth dryness (xerostomia) effects. In the case of some, such as methantheline (Banthine), the additional blocking effects at ganglionic synapses and at skeletal myoneural junctions are recognized. Relatively little cholinergic blocking action but a more direct action on the muscle cells is described in the case of others.

Synthetics that have been used most in ophthalmology are: eucatropine (Euphthalmine), homatropine (novatropine), cyclopentolate (Cyclogyl) and dibutoline (Dibuline). A considerable number of synthetics are being offered for relief of gastrointestinal hypermotility and hypersecretion; some of these are recommended at the same time for the reduction of hyperhidrosis.

Compounds in this category are easily synthesized, and at least 30 variants of atropine are available under trade names. The quaternary ammonium compounds have less central nervous system effects than the tertiary drugs, and some act to block transmission at the ganglionic synapse. Some relax smooth muscle primarily by exerting a nonspecific direct action on the muscle fiber. A common claim is that of selective reduction of gastric hypermotility without corresponding urinary retention, increased intraocular tension, disturbed accommodation, tachycardia or mouth dryness. Unfortunately, animal studies do not make a reliable guide for predicting the relative response of the different systems in the human; reliable demonstration of preferential effects in the patient is controlled with great difficulty. For the most part, documentation is generally inadequate for claims that any of these anticholinergics are preferable to atropine in its clinical uses.

The multiplicity of these products is related to the fact that they can be synthesized much more easily than they can be evaluated clinically. Laboratory and clinical measurements of their critical properties are less decisive than with most drug groups. Their absolute doses vary widely. When promoted on the basis of lesser side effects, the sponsor might be expected to recommend relatively weaker biologic doses; when promoted on the basis of greater effectiveness, relatively higher biologic doses may be recommended.

The muscular rigidity and tremors of parkinsonism are relieved by the administration of large doses of belladonna or of stramonium alkaloids. Benefits of this long-established therapy also extend to other manifestations such as the oculogyric crises and excessive sweating and salivation. The large treatment doses, sometimes reaching phenomenal levels, necessarily produce distressing side effects. The belladonna alkaloids, therefore, have been largely supplanted by synthetic anticholinergic drugs that are equally effective but produce fewer peripheral side effects. Drugs of this type include trihexyphenidyl (Artane), cycrimine (Pagitane), benztropine (Cogentin), caramiphen (Panparnit), procyclidine (Kemadrin) and biperidin (Akineton). Some antihistamines have mild antiparkinson activity that has been attributed to their central cholinergic blocking action. A similar action has been postulated for a phenothiazine derivative, ethopropazine (Parsidol). The antiviral agent amantidine is moderately effective, presumably by the release and inhibition of reuptake of dopamine and other catecholamines from neuronal storage sites. Its action is characterized by a rapid onset with optimal benefit occurring within 2 weeks. Levodopa, an intermediate in the synthesis of norepinephrine and epinephrine, is an effective agent in treating parkinsonism. The nigrostriatal dopaminergic system plays an important pathogenetic role in parkinsonism. In this disease, the level of dopamine is decreased in the substantia nigra and in the striatum. Conversion of L-dopa to dopamine corrects the deficiency. Dopa decarboxylase inhibitors, such as carbidopa, are used to eliminate the need for large doses of L-dopa and thus to decrease the incidence and severity of peripheral side effects. Since these inhibitors do not readily cross the blood-brain barrier, they block the conversion of L-dopa to dopamine in peripheral tissues but do not interfere with this reaction in the central nervous system. Consequently, smaller doses of L-dopa are required. The most common adverse reactions to L-dopa are gastrointestinal disturbances, involuntary movements, psychiatric disturbances and cardiovascular symptoms. A hypertensive crisis may occur if the drug is given with a monoamine oxidase inhibitor. The therapeutic effect of L-dopa is reduced or abolished by administration of pyridoxine in amounts commonly found in daily multiple vitamin preparations.

Bromocriptine (Parlodel) is an ergot derivative approved for treatment of the amenorrhea-galactorrhea syndrome. It can also relieve akinesia, rigidity and tremor in patients with Parkinson's disease. It crosses the blood-brain barrier and stimulates dopaminergic receptors. Its main disadvantage is a high incidence of mental symptoms, including nightmares, hallucinations, and paranoid delusions.

Experimental drugs such as Tremorine mimic the tremors of parkinsonism and, additionally, have cholinergic side-effects.

Sympathomimetic Drugs

An understanding of the actions of sympathomimetic drugs requires knowledge of present concepts of the effects of adrenergic receptor stimulation. Such receptors are categorized as $alpha_1$, $alpha_2$, $beta_1$ and $beta_2$. $Alpha_1$ adrenergic receptors are the classic postsynaptic alpha receptors, such as those that mediate the effects of alpha-adrenergic agonists in constricting smooth muscle. $Alpha_2$ receptors are found on presynaptic nerve terminals where they mediate feedback inhibition of norepinephrine release. $Alpha_1$, and $alpha_2$ receptors can be distinguished because of differences in affinities for various selective adrenergic agonists and antagonists. For example, prazosin appears to be relatively $alpha_1$ selective, whereas yohimbine, a plant alkaloid, is an $alpha_2$ selective blocker. Drugs which stimulate $alpha_1$ receptors produce vasoconstriction, bronchoconstriction, increased hepatic glycogenolysis, sphincter constriction in the gastrointestinal tract and bladder, and contraction of pilomotor muscles. Stimulation of $beta_1$ receptors results in cardiac stimulation (inotropic and chronotropic) and increased lipolysis while $beta_2$ stimulation produces bronchodilation, vasodilation, skeletal muscle tremor and increased muscle glycogenolysis. Although some drugs such as epinephrine stimulate all receptor types, other compounds are highly selective in their action.

Epinephrine (3,4-dihydroxy-alpha-methyl-aminomethyl benzyl alcohol), *norepinephrine* (arterenol), its precursor before methylation, and isopropyl arterenol, in which an isopropyl group is substituted for the methyl group, have basically similar types of adrenergic action. They are of considerable clinical value and might be used interchangeably, but, because of secondary pharmacodynamic distinctions, each has its particular area of usefulness. Epinephrine normally represents the major catecholamine output of the adrenal gland and is secreted in large amounts as a response to hypotension, hypoxia or other sources of sympathetic stimulation. Norepinephrine also occurs in the adrenals to the extent of about 10 to 20 per cent of the total catecholamines, although the norepinephrine usually predominates in tumors of the pheochromocytoma type. Isopropyl arterenol has been reported to occur in the adrenal in small amounts. Norepinephrine is the chemical mediator liberated at the peripheral sympathetic nerve endings and is also an important mediator within the central nervous system. The sympathetic nerve ending structures at peripheral sites in the myocardium and the vascular bed have the capacity for rapidly removing norepinephrine from the circulation, an occurrence that has been demonstrated by infusions of tritiated norepinephrine with subsequent radioautography. This storage mechanism is part of the rapid inactivation mechanisms; in these and other locations, norepinephrine is stored in discrete granules that also contain ATP in a fairly constant ratio of four to one. Storage of the norepinephrine in the nerve ending structure is affected by reserpine (chronic depletion) and tyramine (acute discharge).

Epinephrine and norepinephrine are stored and metabolized rapidly in the body, and their plasma levels, whether from endogenous or exogenous sources, are reduced about as rapidly as the disappearance of their pressor effects. Their metabolic conversion is accomplished largely by two enzymes: (1) catechol-o-methyltransferase, which converts one of the hydroxyl groups of the benzene ring to a methoxyl group, the products being termed, respectively, metanephrine and normetanephrine; and (2) monoamine oxidase, which converts the terminal amino groups to carboxyl groups. The usual final product with either of the catecholamines is 3-methoxy-4 hydroxy-mandelic acid (vanillylmandelic acid, VMA). The urinary excretion of the latter is an index of catecholamine production and is significantly increased in conditions such as pheochromocytoma. These metabolites show little or no pharmacodynamic activity.

Epinephrine (adrenalin) was isolated in 1901 from the adrenal gland, in which it occurs as the levo form. The synthetic racemic mixture, prepared a few years later, exhibits about half the activity, since the dextro form is only about 1/15 as active. Both natural and synthetic forms are distributed commercially. Aqueous solutions of the hydrochloride are specified in the USP as a 1:1,000 solution for injection and a 1:100 solution for inhalation by spray. Dosage is in terms of the free base. The bitartrate salt presumably is less irritant and is used in ointments. The free base is used in a 1:500 oil suspension. Epinephrine is not effective by oral administration, although infants may show some absorption by this route.

The more conspicuous effects of epinephrine, after

the usual clinical doses, include mydriasis, peripheral constriction of the arterial and the venous beds, cardiac acceleration, increased force of myocardial contraction, tendencies to increased arrhythmia, splenic contraction, increased blood levels of free fatty acids by mobilization from fat depots, discharge of glucose from the liver, and relaxation of the smooth muscle of the bronchi and alimentary canal (sphincter muscles of the alimentary canal may be stimulated). Effects of the alimentary canal are not of clinical significance, and this is also true of some limited increase in salivary secretion and sweating, as well as some pilomotor stimulation. Effects on the uterus are not distinctive, although there may be some relaxation of bands of contraction. Rate of oxygen consumption is increased, as are blood lactic acid and potassium levels; eosinophil counts are decreased. Blood flow is usually increased in the coronary arteries and the skeletal muscles, without much change in cerebral vessels; these vasodilator effects, when they occur, may be largely a result of passive dilation due to the increased pressure head in the large central arteries and, also, can be secondary to increased oxidative metabolism. With minimal doses of epinephrine, vasodilation may occur that is not secondary to these effects. Repeated administration of epinephrine to animals can cause them to develop a high grade of tolerance to large intravenous doses.

The hypertensive response following usual doses of epinephrine may be expected to initiate baroreceptor reflexes that can overcome direct cardiac accelerating effects, with resulting bradycardia. Palpitation and tremulousness occur commonly. The usual subcutaneous dose of 0.5 ml. of 1:1,000 epinephrine as the hydrochloride may be thought of as a type of depot administration, since intense vasoconstriction localizes the drug to a marked extent. Intravenous administration should involve a grossly extended time interval to deliver the same amount of drug and is ordinarily accomplished as a carefully monitored infusion of a diluted solution. In cases of cardiac standstill, in extremis, direct intraventricular injection of epinephrine, with several aspirations, may restore contractions, since there is a direct action on the effector cells at the endocardial surface.

Levarterenol bitartrate (norepinephrine, Levophed) has been manufactured synthetically and has been used extensively in various hypotensive states, particularly in those states with myocardial depression. The pronounced cardiac stimulation is in contrast with the effect of other pressor amines used for the same purpose, such as phenylephrine and methoxamine, which have little or no cardiac effect at pressor dose levels. In contrast with epinephrine, levarterenol produces fewer metabolic effects and has no component of vaso-

dilation, as occurs with small doses of epinephrine; there is less apprehansion, and tremors are less marked. In its extensive use by venoclysis, levarterenol occasionally has caused sloughs, and this is to be taken as evidence of relativley intense local vasoconstriction. The sloughing is most frequently due to faulty technique with perivascular infiltration; it can be antagonized by adrenergic blocking agents such as phentolamine and may be prevented by incorporation of such agents in small amounts in the infusion. As with epinephrine, prolonged infusion can lead to acidosis, with steadily increasing refractoriness or lack of pharmacodynamic responses; some return of responsiveness can be obtained by administration of sodium bicarbonate or THAM. Levarterenol, as well as other vasoconstrictors, is much used in combination with local anesthetics in dental work.

Dopamine hydrochloride (Intropin) is the immediate biochemical catecholamine precursor of norepinephrine. Acting on β_1 receptors, it exerts a positive inotropic effect on the myocardium, resulting in increased cardiac output. It increases glomerular filtration rate, renal blood flow and sodium excretion presumptively by activation of a dopaminergic receptor responsible for dilatation of the renal vasculature. Dopamine is indicated for management of the shock syndrome due to myocardial infarction, openheart surgery, trauma and endotoxic septicemia. Correction of hypovolemia should be instituted or completed prior to its use.

Dopamine should be infused into a large vein whenever possible to prevent the possibility of extravasation into tissue adjacent to the infusion site. Untoward effects include nausea, vomiting, headache, dyspnea, precordial pain and vasoconstriction as indicated by a disproportionate rise in diastolic pressure. Ventricular arrhythmia is the most serious adverse effect. Prior use of monamine oxidase inhibitors substantially reduces dosage requirements. The drug is inactivated in alkaline solutions.

Isoproterenol (isopropylnorepinephrine, Isuprel) differs from epinephrine and levarterenol chiefly in its relatively marked degree of vasodilation and its ability to be absorbed systemically by the sublingual mucosa. The latter feature is due probably to increased fat solubility, contributed by the isopropyl group, and to the relatively smaller degree of local vasoconstriction. Also, isoproterenol is considered to be relatively more potent in its bronchodilator action and undoubtedly causes fewer hypertensive responses than epinephrine when used in bronchial asthma. However, its use in patients with preexisting cardiac arrhythmias associated with tachycardia is generally considered contraindicated because its cardiac stimulant effect may aggravate such disorders. This beta-sympathomimetic stimulant is administered as an aerosol mist by inhalation.

The major differences between epinephrine or isoproterenol and the new selective beta$_2$ sympathomimetic drugs, metaproterenol, solbutamol, terbutaline, rimilerol, salmefamol, fenoterol, and carbuterol are that the more selective beta$_2$ agonists (a) are active when swallowed, (b) have a slower onset of action, (c) some have a much longer duration of action, (d) and generally do not directly stimulate the myocardium unless adminstered in large doses or intravenously. The selectivity of the newer drugs may be most important during an exacerbation of asthma when tachycardia is common.

Dobutamine (Dobutrex), a new synthetic catecholamine, is indicated for short-term intravenous treatment of cardiac decompensation due to cardiac surgery or refractory heart failure. It increases myocardial contractility by a direct action on cardiac beta$_1$ adrenergic receptors. Unlike norepinephrine, it produces little vasoconstriction at usual therapeutic doses, and unlike isoproterenol, it only occasionally causes tachycardia. Dobutamine does not selectively dilate mesenteric and renal vascular beds as dopamine does, but mesenteric and renal blood flow may increase as a consequence of improved cardiac output. Except for occasional reports of nausea, vomiting, and headache, adverse reactions to this drug have been confined to the cardiovascular system. Premature ventricular contractions have been reported in about five per cent of patients. An excessive increase in heart rate and blood pressure has occurred in some instances. Dobutamine can precipitate angina in patients with coronary artery disease. It is contraindicated in patients with idiopathic hypertrophic subaortic stenosis because it can increase the obstruction of cardiac outflow. As with other catecholamines, cyclopropane and, to a lesser extent, halothane may aggravate the arrhythmic effects of the drug.

Comparison of Epinephrine-Type Adrenergic Agents. The three adrenergic agents levarterenol and its methyl and isopropyl derivatives (norepinephrine, epinephrine and isopropylnorepinephrine, respectively) have in common an exceptionally intense myocardial stimulation at low dose levels. They differ chiefly in the relation of vasodilator to vasoconstrictor effects, with isoproterenol having a marked vasodilator component, epinephrine a slight vasodilator component and levarterenol having no action of this sort. The respective differences in their effects on cardiac output and heart rate can be interpreted on the basis of these features. The differences in composite results are most marked at low dose levels.

Many of the physiologic responses elicited by catecholamines have been linked with activation of the adenyl cyclase system. These drugs, or their endogenous equivalents, have been termed a first messenger, which activates adenyl cyclase to catalyze the conversion of ATP into cyclic 3',5'-AMP (second messenger). This second messenger in turn activates other enzyme systems to increase circulating levels of glucose and free fatty acids. There is also some evidence to implicate cyclic AMP in the initiation of the inotropic response to catecholamines. Glucagon, a known hyperglycemic hormone, has also been shown to possess inotropic activity, which is slower in onset and longer in duration than that of the catecholamines. Glucagon is an activator of adenyl cyclase but apparently acts at a different site from the catecholamines, inasmuch as its action on this system is not blocked by betaadrenergic blocking agents.

Therapeutic Uses. Epinephrine has been of longstanding service in bronchial asthma and other histamine-release type of disorders, including pruritus, urticaria, angioneurotic edema and anaphylactic shock. In acute anaphylactic shock, vasodilation and bronchoconstriction are almost precisely antagonized. In bronchial asthma, epinephrine possibly is helpful in counteracting edema, as well as through its bronchodilating action. Selective beta$_2$ agonists are presently favored in asthma. As compared with epinephrine, the lower grade of hypertension produced is a clear advantage in the use of isoproterenol to improve automaticity in heart block conditions. In shock, particularly with a cardiac depression component, levarterenol has been most used, and here, as compared with epinephrine, the lower grade of apprehension is an advantage. The same may be true when these compounds are used as vasoconstrictors with local anesthetics, as is done extensively in dental work.

Other Adrenergic Drugs

Since ephedrine was introduced in 1923 as a product of plant origin, a considerable number of synthetic adrenergic agents have been developed, and, in some cases, their patterns of action have provided some useful advantage. This is particularly true of compounds that can be given orally and are used for their effect as central nervous system stimulants. In contrast with the three epinephrine-type agents described in the previous section, some of this group do not act directly on effector cells but depend, to greater or less degree, on release of norepinephrine from sympathetic nerve endings. Tyramine acts totally in this manner; it is not used clinically. Drugs acting by this indirect mechanism are usually tachyphylactic, and, presumably, this is due to exhaustion of norepinephrine stores.

Ephedrine is a naturally occurring alkaloid, known to ancient Chinese medicine, that mimics many of the important effects of epinephrine but differs chiefly in that it has a more prolonged period of action, is more stable and is effective by oral administration. In addition, ephedrine has marked stimulating effects on the central nervous system. On administration of a series of large doses, both pressor and positive inotropic responses decrease and even may be reversed.

Ephedrine, in doses of 20 to 50 mg., is useful in the prevention and treatment of asthmatic attacks and may give symptomatic relief in hay fever. For such purposes it is combined advantageously with a barbiturate to antagonize the cerebral effects, which, in this case, are undesirable. Because of its prolonged local vasoconstrictor action, ephedrine is used widely for application to the nasal mucosa. Shrinkage of the congested mucosae temporarily opens the nasal passage and permits drainage through the ostia of the paranasal sinuses. However, undesirable effects may be local irritation, depression of ciliary activity and effects from systemic absorption (cerebral excitation). Ephedrine is a satisfactory shortacting mydriatic. It also is used in the management of narcolepsy and of myasthenia gravis.

Ephedrine has two optically active carbon atoms; accordingly, six different d-, l- and racemic forms are obtainable. The USP form is levorotatory. There are no great differences in the activity of any of these forms.

Amphetamine (Benzedrine) is characterized by marked central nervous system stimulation, which, in favorable doses, is mildly euphoric. It is used in the treatment of narcolepsy and minimal brain dysfunction in children, as adjunctive therapy to other remedial measures (psychological, social, educational). As a short-term adjunct in a regimen of weight reduction based on caloric restriction, its limited usefulness should be weighed against possible risks inherent in its use. Dextro amphetamine (Dexedrine) has similar uses. Its potential for drug abuse seriously limits its usefulness. Methamphetamine (desoxyephedrine) has the same uses and actions as amphetamine with less circulatory action for the same degree of central nervous system stimulant effects.

The use of these compounds as nasal vasoconstrictors has led to the introduction of an unusually large number of chemical variants for this purpose. These include phenylephrine (Neo-synephrine), methoxamine (Vasoxyl), cyclopentamine (Clopane), mephentermine (Wyamine), metaraminol (Aramine), phenylpropanolamine (Propadrine), tuaminoheptane (Tuamine) and propylhexedrine (Benzedrex). Usually they are administered in isotonic salt solution or, since some are volatile, by inhalation. Chemically different compounds used for the same purpose contain an imidazoline ring (Privine, Tyzine, Otrivin). With all of these compounds, aftercongestion and side-effects on

the nervous and the cardiovascular systems are common complications.

The circulatory stimulant actions of these synthetic adrenergic agents has led to their use in somewhat the same conditions for which levarterenol is used. For instance, ephedrine, and metaraminol and mephentermine have distinct pressor and cardiac stimulant effects but are more prolonged in action than levarterenol or epinephrine. Disadvantages are central nervous system stimulation, in the instance of ephedrine, and tachyphylaxis, in the instance of mephentermine. These pressor-inotropic agents are most useful when there is a component of myocardial depression. They are critically distinct from those agents that have little or no myocardial stimulant action at ordinary doses, as is true of phenylephrine and methoxamine. The latter, by their hypertensive effects, can add a dangerously increased work load to an already incompetent myocardium. On the other hand, phenylephrine and methoxamine may be favored in conditions such as hypotension of spinal anesthesia, in which the myocardium is not depressed; in such cases, there is an advantage because of the lesser tendency to arrhythmia, a feature that is associated with increased myocardial contractility.

Several variants of this group have had clinical interest. Methoxyphenamine (Orthoxine) has been used chiefly for its bronchodilator action. Isoxsuprine (Vasodilan) is adrenergic in type, but vasodilator action is present to the extent that peripheral blood flow is increased under some conditions; it has been used in peripheral vascular disease and, somewhat unexpectedly, as a uterine relaxant. Nylidrin (Arlidin) also is used in occlusive conditions of the extremities. Phenmetrazine (Preludin) is related chemically to amphetamine, the difference being that the former has an oxazine ring instead of the usual side chain. Like amphetamine, it has anorexic effects and is used in weight reduction schedules.

Drugs Blocking Sympathetic Effects

Ergotamine and ergotoxine, which have practically identical actions, block some of the effects typical of epinephrine. The phenomenon is chiefly of academic interest, and the important clinical effects of ergotamine and ergotoxine (relief of migraine headache and stimulation of uterine muscle) are considered to be due to a direct stimulation of smooth muscle and not to autonomic systemic effects. Ergotamine, in doses of 0.25 to 0.50 mg. subcutaneously, will relieve migraine headache in some patients. The best explanation of the effect is based on the assumption that the drug acts on smooth muscle of the blood vessels to overcome excessive pulsations and dilation of the cerebral arteries.

Both of these drugs are derivatives of lysergic acid. A more recently introduced derivative of this acid, methysergide (Sansert), also is used for prophylaxis of migraine. Its action as a serotonin antagonist is emphasized. Retroperitoneal fibrosis is a surprising late complication, sometimes occurring after prolonged use; incidence has been quoted at about one per cent. Presumably the initial mechanism is the same as in another observed complication, acute limb ischemia due to protracted vascular spasm.

Ergotamine and ergotoxine, along with yohimbine, may be thought of as naturally occurring compounds that were the predecessors of the later synthetic adrenergic blocking agents. Both natural and synthetic types act on effector cells to block the action of injected epinephrine and its variants; with more difficulty, they block the action of chemical mediators liberated at sympathetic nerve endings.

Phenoxybenzamine (Dibenzyline), a synthetic drug related to the nitrogen mustard war gases, is an exceptionally effective agent in blocking the pressor effects of epinephrine. This is due to a direct action on both alpha$_1$ and alpha$_2$ adrenergic receptors. It does not block the inhibitory effects of epinephrine on the gut, nor does it block the hyperglycemic response to epinephrine. The type of block produced is nonequilibrium in nature and is due to the formation of a reactive carbonium ion following an in vivo cyclization of the tertiary amine. This accounts for the slow development and the persistence of the block. In man, effects may persist for 1 to 4 days. Miosis, disorientation and orthostatic hypotension may be elicited by clinical doses.

Phentolamine (Regitine) is an imidazoline derivative with weak competitive alpha-adrenergic blocking effects and, also, some histamine-like vasodilator effects. As with tolazoline, it may be administered orally.

Phentolamine appears to have most usefulness in conditions that require direct antagonism of adrenergic action; examples are accidental leakage of norepinephrine during intravenous infusions and extreme hypertension during operative removal of pheochromocytoma.

Tolazoline (Priscoline) has some adrenergic blocking actions similar to those of phenoxybenzamine. In addition, it produces distinct and direct vasodilating effects, some stimulation of gastrointestinal activity, apparent myocardinal stimulant effects, pilomotor effects and gastric secretory stimulation, the last resembling the effect of histamine. Tolazoline has been used extensively in various peripheral vascular diseases, in spite of the variety of undesired but characteristic effects, which, however, may be minimized by the use of common parasympatholytic drugs as antagonists.

For the much more common problem of managing decreased circulatory function as occurs particularly in the extremities, several drugs are considered, in addition to tolazoline. These include: Azapetine (Ilidar), which has generally similar structure and activity but produces fewer side effects; nylidrin (Arlidin) and isoxsuprine (Vasodilan), both of which dilate vessels in the muscles more than in the skin and have distinct positive inotropic action; nicotinic acid (niacin), which has marked vasodilating properties evidently due to a type of histamine release; its conspicuous skin-flushing effect decreases with repeated doses; and Roniacol, which is the carbinol equivalent of nicotinic acid and has similar actions. These agents may be generally helpful when a vasospastic element is involved; they may be harmful when fixed mechanical obstruction exists.

Another application for compounds of this type, particularly phenoxybenzamine, is in experimental efforts to treat shock. Similarly, this adrenergic blocking agent has been tried as pretreatment for cardiac bypass and other conditions in which a condition of shock may be expected to develop. Presumably the antagonism of overactivity of endogenous catecholamines provides an improved grade of tissue perfusion.

Beta-Adrenergic Blocking Agents

Phentolamine, phenoxybenzamine and the ergot alkaloids are more or less specific in blocking the vasoconstrictor effects of the epinephrine group and have little effect on the marked increase in contractile force and heart rate that is produced by the epinephrine group; further, they have little effect on the vasodilator or depressor effects that are noted particularly with isoproterenol and to some extent with small doses of epinephrine. A working classification has been developed that designates the vasoconstrictor effects as a response of alpha receptors and the cardiac and vasodilator effects as a response of beta receptors. This classification has been completed by the recognition of compounds that block the latter responses. The first compound recognized as having beta receptor-blocking properties was dichloroisoproterenol (DCI). This compound has intrinsic cardiostimulant effects that preclude its clinical use. However, its discovery led to subsequent development of propranolol (Inderal). Propranolol, through its beta-blocking effect, has been found to be efficacious in angina pectoris, hypertrophic subaortic stenosis and in reducing arrhythmias due to excess catecholamine liberation such as occurs in pheochromocytoma. In addition, propranolol exhibits a membrane-stabilizing or local anesthetic effect on cardiac cells that endows the compound with antiarrhythmic properties in addition to those attributable to receptor blockade. It is effective in the management of hypertension. When vasodilator drugs such as hydralazine, minoxidil, diazoxide, or nitroprusside are given, the lowering of pressure brings about increased cardiac output and tachycardia through reflex mechanisms. Propranolol prevents these undesirable reflex effects. Its precise antihypertensive effect is unresolved. One metabolite of the drug, 4-hydroxypropranolol, found only after oral or intraportal administration, has blocking activity similar to that of the parent compound. Propranolol is now being promoted for prevention of migraine headache. The majority of short-term trials have been favorable. Whether the drug is effective over a long period of time remains to be determined. It is not recommended for the treatment of migraine attacks, nor for the prevention or treatment of cluster headaches. Upon withdrawal of the drug a rebound in migraine attacks can occur. Bronchial asthma and congestive heart failure are special contraindications to the use of propranolol.

It is now possible to separate the cardiac and peripheral beta receptors into two components. These are now commonly referred to as β_1 and β_2 respectively. Metoprolol (Lopressor), a newer agent, has been shown to have greater affinity for the β_1 receptor, and the term cardioselective has been attached to it. The advantage of metoprolol is that, by having predilection for the heart, the therapeutic results can be attained without incurring the serious side-effects associated with blocking of peripheral β_2 receptors such as precipitation of bronchial asthma in susceptible individuals. The beta-receptor blocking agents may be used alone or in combination with other antihypertensive agents, especially thiazide-type diuretics.

Timolol (Timoptic) is unique in that it is used solely for the management of chronic open-angle glaucoma. When instilled into the conjunctival sac it causes a fall in intraocular pressure, presumably by a reduction in aqueous humor production. Unlike pilocarpine, it does not produce miosis nor interfere with vision even in patients with central lens opacities. Concomitant administration of timolol with epinephrine seems to enhance its ocular hypotensive effect in many patients.

Corgard (Nadolol) is a synthetic beta$_1$-beta$_2$ adrenergic blocking agent recently approved for marketing as a one tablet-per-day medication for the management of angina pectoris and hypertension.

CENTRAL ADRENERGIC CONTROL MECHANISMS

Although it has been known for many years that there are vasomotor centers and autonomic centers of control in the brain which could modify the cardiovascular system, the role of the central nervous system in the pathogenesis of hypertension and its role in the mechanism of action of antihypertensive drugs have been largely ignored until recent times. Today it is recognized that central catecholaminergic neurons have an integral place in central connections of the peripheral nervous system. Furthermore, alpha adrenergic receptors are present in the CNS that, when activated, can modify arterial pressure. A number of antihypertensive drugs including methyldopa and clonidine produce their hypotensive effects through an interaction with these central catecholaminergic neurons or their receptors.

Drugs Blocking Nerve Impulses at Autonomic Ganglia and at Skeletal Muscle

Nicotine has special theoretic interest, because it first stimulates and then paralyzes ganglion cells of the autonomic system and because it blocks responses of skeletal muscles to nerve impulses. The latter effect is of interest in connection with acute poisoning in which the mechanism of death is peripheral paralysis of the respiratory muscles. Less severe poisoning may involve autonomic effects.

Tetraethyl ammonium (Etamon) was introduced in 1946 as an agent capable of blocking autonomic efferent pathways by a relatively specific effect at ganglionic synapses. From this has been developed a class of compounds that have usefulness largely because of their effects on the adrenergic system; usually their action on ganglionic synapses of the cholinergic system are undesirable side-effects. (Drugs have not been developed that selectively block ganglionic synapses of one and not the other autonomic system.) Their chief uses have been as antihypertensive agents (although, for such use, they have been superseded by other types of agents), as antagonists to acute hypertensive crises and as agents for producing controlled hypotension during surgery, with resultant decrease in bleeding.

Subsequently developed agents include hexamethonium (Methium), of British origin; mecamylamine (Inversine), and trimethaphan (Arfonad), which, for controlled hypotension, has the advantages of rapid onset and brief period of action. Other ganglionic blocking agents include pentolinium (Ansolysen), chlorisondamine (Ecolid), trimethidinium (Ostensin) and pempidine (Perolysen). In most of these, the chemical structures have, apparently, spatial similarity to acetylcholine sufficient to suggest that they can reasonably be expected to act competitively at receptors of ganglionic synapses. However, mecamylamine and pempidine do not share this resemblance; they are secondary rather than quaternary amines, and they are thought to penetrate into the cell of the postganglionic neuron. The undesirable side effects of this group are largely manifestations of ganglionic blocking actions.

They include postural hypotension, mouth dryness, ciliary muscle paralysis, difficulty in micturition and bowel movements, gastric anacidity and paralytic ileus. Mecamylamine has been observed to produce mental excitation, with delusions or hallucinations.

Curare, an arrow poison of the South American Indians, was studied by Magendie and by Claude Bernard and has been a common laboratory tool since that time. However, the clinical use of curare was not developed until the early 1940s, about a century later. Clinical use depended on a purified and a standardized supply of the active principles. The first active crystalline product was isolated in 1935 and shown to be an alkaloid with two quaternary ammonium groups. This product, d-tubocurarine, subsequently has been modified to form its dimethyl ether (Metubine, Mecostrin), which is active in about one third the dose of the original compound. The quaternary ammonium groups in these compounds are about 14 Å apart, and this, apparently, is optimal, since it has been deliberately reproduced in some of the subsequently developed synthetic variants. The distance has some critical significance with respect to acetylcholine, in which the loaded groupings are separated by exactly half this distance.

The effect of these compounds is to interfere with transmission of impulses at the myoneural junction of nerves supplying skeletal muscles. Evidently there is competitive attachment to the receptor site in the muscle cell (muscle sole plate), since excess acetylcholine will overcome the blocking effect. Cholinesterase inhibitors (physostigmine, neostigmine or edrophonium) antagonize the blocking effect of curare by retarding destruction of acetylcholine and by their own action, directly on the receptor site, in the same way as acetylcholine. Pancuronium bromide (Pavulon) is a nondepolarizing neuromuscular blocking agent that differs from d-tubocurarine in its greater potency and lack of histamine-releasing or ganglionic blocking actions.

Gallamine (Flaxedil), a synthetic, acts similarly to d-tubocurarine. It has a shorter duration of action, may produce tachycardia and is contraindicated in patients with poor renal function. Pancuronium (Pavulon) resembles d-tubocurarine in pharmacologic activity, but has the advantage of a more rapid onset of action and is less likely to cause bronchial constriction or hypotension.

Decamethonium (Syncurine) and **succinylcholine** (Anectine) generally produce paralysis of the same type at the skeletal neuromuscular junction. However, the mechanism of action differs from curare in that these agents act to prolong the depolarization phase at the junctional tissue, and this constitutes an unresponsive

stage in the usual sequence of stimulation and contraction. The significance of this distinction is that neostigmine and its variants will intensify the paralysis in the case of the depolarizing agents.

Neuromuscular blocking drugs are used commonly as supplements to anesthetics and less frequently to modify convulsions due to electroconvulsive therapy. D-tubocurarine is synergistic with ether, quinidine and certain antibiotics such a neomycin, streptomycin and kanamycin. It may manifest histamine-release phenomena (bronchoconstriction and hypotension). Prolonged administration, as may be employed in antagonizing the spasms of tetanus, can lead to shock, apparently due to a net loss of intracellular potassium.

Decamethonium is not potentiated by ethyl ether, and successive doses do not produce cumulative effects but, rather, produce decreased responses. When comparable limb-paralysis doses are tested in patients, respiratory muscles are most depressed by decamethonium and least depressed by tubocurarine. Succinylcholine is shorter acting than tubocurarine because of its rapid hydrolysis by plasma cholinesterases. Prolonged muscular relaxation and apnea are seen in the occasional patient having a genetic makeup such that the plasma cholinesterases are atypical. It elevates intraocular pressure and can be dangerous in acute glaucoma.

Miscellaneous agents producing neuromuscular blockade through diverse mechanisms include the magnesium ion, botulinus toxin, nicotine, quinine and hemicholinium (HC-3).

Centrally Acting Muscle Relaxants

Pain and disability due to muscle spasm are very common and can be alleviated in varying degree by physiotherapy, placebos, sedatives, analgesics and drugs of the type termed tranquilizers. Theoretically, more precise drug therapy is possible with drugs that interfere at some point of the polysynaptic motor nerve system. A dihydroxypropane derivative (mephenesin) depresses internuncial neuronal synapses in the spinal cord and brain stem, apparently with less cerebral depression than barbiturates and less peripheral paralysis than curare compounds. Mephenesin has a number of variants with related chemical structure, such as mephenesin carbamate (Tolseram), with more effective oral absorption; methocarbamol (Robaxin), reported as long acting; carisoprodol (Soma); phenaglycodol (Ultran); and meprobamate. Central synaptic depression also is described for some of the ring structure tranquilizers, such as chlormezanone (Trancopal), mephenoxalone (Trepidone) and chlordiazepoxide (Librium). Diazepam (Valium) is chemically related to the last named and is used in the same way. The diazepoxides, chlorodiazepoxide and diazepam, are generally viewed as antianxiety agents and are discussed in the section on tranquilizers. No objective data are available to make reliable comparisons of relative effectiveness and safety among these agents. Psychic or physical dependence may develop after long-term use of large doses of some.

Attempts to use these centrally acting relaxants in tetanus have had nominal success and various complications. Mephenesin and meprobamate in concentrated solutions intravenously cause hemolysis; meprobamate also causes thrombosis when given intravenously but has been given intramuscularly in propylene glycol solutions.

DRUGS ACTING ON THE CIRCULATORY SYSTEM

Digitaloids

Several hundred compounds that can be derived from numerous plant sources and limited animal sources are capable of producing actions identified as those of "digitalis" in the classic descriptions of Withering in 1785 of the use of the crude digitalis leaf to produce diuresis and relief of the symptoms of "cardiac dropsy." The compounds currently recognized as producing the same effects under experimental and clinical conditions are glycosides of a cyclopentenophenanthrene structure with a lactone ring at C-17 and sugar attachments at C-3. Removal of the lactone ring abolishes activity, whereas reduction or removal of the sugar attachments reduces but does not abolish activity. When all sugar attachments are removed the resulting aglycone or genin is considered to be more rapid in action than the parent glycoside. Spatial attachment to the receptor site has assumed a structure resembling that of lithocholic acid, and the receptor site has been presumed to be Na^+—K^+ activated adenosine triphosphatase at the cell membrane. A basic pattern of action is postulated in that all of these compounds have essentially the same therapeutic index or relation of therapeutic contractility increase to toxic arrhythmias. They differ considerably in potency on a dose-weight basis, in rapidity of onset and disappearance of action and in percentage of absorption from the gastrointestinal tract.

At the cellular level, the action of digitaloids can be partly interpreted in terms of their relatively specific and potent inhibition of Na^+—K^+ activated ATPase. This enzyme normally acts to hydrolyze high-energy phosphates at the cell membrane, and the resulting energy is utilized by the "sodium-potassium" pump to extrude sodium that enters the cell at the time of depolarization; potassium lost by the cell during repolarization is actively transported back into the cell. Inhibition of this system is associated with arrhythmias of the polymorphous type, which occur at later toxic stages of digitalis and can be interpreted, in some cases, as expressions of increased automaticity in the His-Purkinje system brought on by the abnormal balance of cations; these arrhythmias are identified with a decrease in intracellular potassium and an increase in intracellular sodium. At the therapeutic stages of digitalis action, contractility increases, and the heart often returns toward nearly normal size when failure has been of such degree as to bring on dilation. This is interpreted at the cellular level as being the result of increased calcium availability to the sarcomere upon membrane depolarization. The action of the digitaloids in increasing calcium availability may result from alterations in a cell membrane (sarcolemma) system that catalyzes sodium-calcium exchange. The alteration of such exchange would (by hypothesis) be due to increases in intracellular sodium secondary to inhibition of the sodium-potassium pump by the drug. Such a mechanism assumes that the sodium-potassium pump is the receptor system through which the inotropic response to the digitaloids is mediated. While considerable evidence supports this assumption, some studies appear to suggest that a receptor other than the sodium-potassium pump might mediate the inotropic effect.

The hemodynamic effects of increased contractility in conditions of congestive failure include: increased ventricular activity with increased stroke volume; increased ejection fraction; decreased end-diastolic volume and end-systolic volume; decreased central venous pressure; and generally unchanged arterial pressure. Increased contractility is also manifested as a more rapid rate of contraction, recognized clinically by the use of catheters to record the rate of pressure rise during the period of isometric contraction (dp/dt); by roentgen kymography; and by monitoring the "ejection time index" by external sensing devices.

With normal sinus rhythm in failure, rate is decreased by digitalis, both as an effect of increased vagal activity and as a result of decreased sympathetic activity, which had occurred as a response to failure. The conduction system becomes more refractory, and conduction is slowed as a result of increased vagal activity, decreased adrenergic activity and, in later stages, as a direct action of digitalis on these fibers. In the atrium, the direct effect of digitalis is to lengthen the refractory interval, but an opposing action of increased vagal activity may predominate.

Digitalis increases stroke-work of the ventricle without a correspondingly great increase in oxygen consumption, the latter being an excellent index of energy utilization. This well-documented disparity is probably not due to biochemical phenomena but can be interpreted as a manifestation of the physical advantage of the heart operating at a less dilated state. The mechanical advantage of a contracting sphere is substantially increased by a reduction in radius, and, with unchanged internal pressure, increased pumping performance can be accomplished without a corresponding increase in energy utilization. These hemodynamic principles are applicable to the effects of digitalis in congestive failure when an increase in contractility is accompanied by a decrease in heart size.

An increase in urinary excretion and a reduction of general edema usually accompanies the successful use of digitalis in congestive failure. The effect is considered to be due to circulatory improvement with increased renal blood flow and glomerular filtration rate. Experimental indications that digitalis acts directly on the kidney to decrease, for instance, the tubular reabsorption of filtered salt and water are probably not applicable at therapeutic dose levels.

Increasing doses of digitalis lead to increased conduction block and automaticity with extracardiac effects, which can include nausea and vomiting, diarrhea, disturbed color vision, and bizarre neurologic and psychiatric symptoms. The common predisposing condition is potassium deficiency due to diuretics or corticosteroids. Also, in uremia delayed excretion increases sensitivity. Cardiac effects represent the chief limiting hazard, and, with the various preparations, exhibit a fixed ratio of toxic to therapeutic action, although this feature is commonly obscured by the high variability of clinical conditions. As observed with the ECG, progressive effects variably develop through S-T segment changes, PR interval lengthening, A-V dissociation, paroxysmal tachycardia with block, premature ventricular complexes, nodal rhythms, bigeminy, multifocal ventricular ectopic tachycardia, with polymorphous complexes, and, finally, ventricular fibrillation. Ventricular automaticity is effectively reduced by potassium salts without comparable decrease in contractility. Diphenylhydantoin is somewhat similar in action. Other agents, such as local anesthetics, procainamide, chelating agents and beta-adrenergic blocking agents, are effective in reducing automaticity but are significantly depressant to contractility. All such agents, including potassium salts, carry the hazard of increased block in the conduction system.

Because toxicity to digitalis begins to appear at about double the therapeutic equilibrium serum concentration, intoxication is common and hazardous. The development of methods for determining serum concentrations of digoxin and digitoxin by radioimmu-noassay may be important in the prevention of some cases of digitalis intoxication. However, such determinations should not replace good clinical judgment because numerous factors, such as underlying heart disease and degree of protein binding influence the significance of a given serum concentration.

Approximately equivalent daily, oral maintenance doses are: digitalis powdered leaf, 100 mg.; digoxin 0.25 mg.; digitoxin 0.1 mg. Several multiples of these doses are used initially, depending on the urgency of the condition. Usually absorption from the gastrointestinal tract is about 20 per cent with powdered digitalis, 60 per cent with digoxin and 100 per cent with digitoxin. Intravenous doses given stepwise in occasional emergency treatment are: digoxin, 1.5 mg.; ouabain, 0.50 mg.; deslanoside, 1.2 mg.; digitoxin, 1.5 mg. Clinical dose selections have often deviated widely in actual biologic strengths of these products while the "cat unit" potencies are reliably established as: ouabain 0.1 mg.; digoxin 0.23 mg.; deslanoside 0.23 mg.; and digitoxin 0.33 mg. This unit represents the amount per kilogram that acts fatally in a lightly anesthetized cat infused to termination in about 1 hour. Although this was a long-used official test of biologic potency, the test is now conducted on pigeons because they are more easily available or by spectrophotometric assay using appropriate reference standards. Digitoxin is slowest in onset and the longest in duration of action. Digoxin is chiefly excreted by the kidneys, while digitoxin is subject to a higher degree of destruction in the liver. Since bioavailability of the glycosides varies considerably between products, patients should be maintained on the same brand preparation. Numerous factors affect dosage requirements, among them renal function, electrolyte balance, age, and the thyroid state.

Congestive failure treated with digitalis is most often due to hypertension or to the myocardial ischemia of arteriosclerosis with normal sinus rhythm. In failure with atrial fibrillation, improvement is greatly favored by the slowing and regularization of ventricular rate, which occurs through increased refractoriness and decreased conduction in the A-V node and His bundle; fibrillating rate of the atria is increased, and in atrial flutter the condition may progress to fibrillation. Intravenous administration of digitalis is usually effective in terminating paroxysmal atrial tachycardia, and the effect is evidently through vagal action. Benefit is equivocal or does not occur in mitral stenosis with normal sinus rhythm, or cor pulmonale, with septal defects, in myocarditis, in subaortic hypertrophic stenosis and in constrictive pericarditis. Hyperthyroidism requires the use of higher doses, and hypothyroidism is associated with increased sensitivity; this may be due to the altered rate of destruction and excretion and to other factors. Cardioversion can precipitate arrhythmias during full digitalization, but ordinarily it is safe after maintenance doses have been discontinued about 2 or 3 days. Electric pacemakers used in block, such as following infarction, are compatible with digitalization.

Antifibrillatory Drugs

Several drugs have the effect of diminishing the excitability of the heart muscle. Some have been found to be of practical use; others appear to have potential value in counteracting atrial fibrillation and ventricular arrhythmias that may progress to ventricular fibrillation. The latter occur particularly after coronary occlusion, during cyclopropane anesthesia and during digitalis intoxication. Quinidine is the outstanding drug of this type. Other drugs are procaine, procainamide (Pronestyl), lidocaine, beta-adrenergic blocking agents phenytoin, bretylium, and disopyramide.

Quinidine is an antiarrhythmic agent whose basic effect is depressant at higher dose levels, as may be shown by isolated muscle strips and isolated heart preparations. In some cases of atrial fibrillation, the administration of quinidine may abolish the irregular movements completely. Presumably, the refractory state that follows the impulse is prolonged sufficiently by quinidine so that the advancing impulse falls on unresponsive tissue and is extinguished. It is a common experience that these effects are associated with a brief period of tachycardia; apparently, the atrium, in passing from fibrillation to normal mechanism, goes through a stage of flutter, and the ventricle, responding with possibly a 2-to-1 rhythm, is temporarily accelerated over its previous rate. This tachycardia may be dangerous in a failing heart, and the direct depressant effect of quinidine on the ventricle also may be dangerous. Some deaths have been attributed to delay of the sinoatrial node in resuming normal function after atrial fibrillation has ceased. Another possible development is "quinidine syncope" (ventricular flutter and fibrillation). The daily dose of quinidine is usually not over 3 g., in several installments. Since the advent of DC shock for conversion of arrhythmias, quinidine is used primarily as a prophylactic drug for the prevention of recurrences after shock. Since quinidine is the dextroisomer of quinine, its antimalarial effects are similar, and it has been used successfully in quinine-sensitive patients.

There has been serious challenge of the theory that quinidine abolishes atrial fibrillation by the process of increasing the refractory period of a circus movement. Observations with the oscillograph and high-speed motionpicture cameras indicate that in atrial fibrillation most of the atrial mass is in a state of continuous, asynchronous activity of varying strength and irregular rates. According to the interpretation that has followed, quinidine slows the rate of discharge from such ectopic foci; when this rate is less than normal sinus rhythm, the sinus node takes over as pacemaker. Digitalis increases the rate of discharge from such ectopic foci and thus converts atrial flutter to fibrillation or converts coarse fibrillation to fine fibrillation.

Quinidine, basically, has been considered to increase refractory period and to slow conduction. In the older circus theory of atrial fibrillation, the quinidine effect was attributed to a predominance of the change in refractory period sufficient that the circus movement was extinguished. In the more current concept of atrial fibrillation as an occurrence of multiple ectopic foci, decreased conduction is considered predominant and any actual increase in refractory period under clinical conditions is now questioned. There is good evidence that quinidine decreases the rate of diastolic depolarization in isolated conduction or pacemaker tissue, and (probably not as relevant) quinidine decreases the rate of rise in the rapid depolarization phase.

The antiarrhythmic drugs listed above have at least two common traits: local anesthetic activity and depression of automaticity. In general, these drugs produce a quinidine-like effect. Additionally, the beta-adrenergic blocking agents prevent the increase in automaticity elicited by catecholamines.

Procainamide is used as an alternative to lidocaine in the management of ventricular premature contractions (VPC). It can be given intravenously, intramuscularly, or orally. Its major advantage over quinidine is a relative lack of adverse cardiovascular effects. However, if infused too rapidly hypotension, heart block, and ventricular arrhythmias may occur. Individuals allergic to procaine may have anaphylactic reactions when treated with procainamide.

Lidocaine is considered the drug of choice in the treatment of ventricular premature contractions. Since it is metabolized mainly by the liver, patients with reduced hepatic function or diminished hepatic blood flow should receive half the usual loading dose and lower maintenance doses. Adverse effects include central nervous system depression, stimulation, or seizures followed less commonly by untoward cardiovascular effects.

Phenytoin shares with lidocaine the treatment of choice in digitalis-induced tachyarrhythmias. Since it can precipitate in aqueous infusion solutions, for intravenous administration it must be given undiluted. When given orally, slow accumulations may cause a delay of several days before therapeutic levels are reached in the blood. Ataxia, nystagmus, stupor, and coma can occur with rising blood levels. With long-term use, blood dyscrasias have been noted and gingival hyperplasia occurs in about 20 per cent of patients.

Bretylium (Bretylol), originally used as an antihypertensive agent, has recently been approved for parenteral treatment of life-threatening ventricular tachycardia or fibrillation refractory to other therapy. It is a quartenary ammonium compound with complex pharmacologic actions. It increases the fibrillation threshold of both normal and ischemic tissue in animals and prevents many experimentally induced arrhythmias. Accumulating in postganglionic adrenergic neurons it initially stimulates release of norepinephrine; subsequently, however, it prevents further release of the neurotransmitter and thus acts as a sympathetic blocking agent.

Disopyramide (Norpace) is similar to quinidine and procainamide in its spectrum of antiarrhythmic efficacy. It decreases the rate of diastolic depolarization (phase 4) in cells with augmented automaticity and decreases the upstroke velocity (phase 0) and increases the action potential duration of normal cardiac cells. The major advantage claimed for disopyramide is a lower incidence of adverse effects compared with quinidine. It can, however, cause hypotension, aggravate existing heart failure, and produce heart block and tachyarrhythmias. Because of its anticholinergic properties, urinary retention frequently requires discontinuation of therapy; it should not be used in patients with glaucoma. As with other antiarrhythmic agents, any potassium deficit should be corrected before instituting therapy in order to insure effectiveness.

Propranolol (Inderal), a beta-adrenergic blocking drug with quinidine-like properties, controls the ventricular rate in atrial tachyarrhythmias by increasing the degree of block at the atrioventricular node and depressing the rate at the sinoatrial node. Beta-adrenergic blockade is of unique importance in the management of arrhythmias due to increased circulating levels of catecholamines or enhanced sensitivity of the heart to these biogenic amines (arrhythmias associated with thyrotoxicosis, exercise, pheochromocytoma). Hypotension, acute heart failure with pulmonary edema, and cardiovascular collapse can occur with relatively small intravenous doses, or after several days of oral treatment. It is capable of precipitating severe bronchospasm in patients with bronchitis or asthma. Sudden withdrawal of the drug in patients with angina pectoris can precipitate increasing angina, cardiac arrhythmias or myocardial infarction.

Drugs Affecting Coronary Flow

Since glyceryl trinitrate has long-standing recognition as an agent capable of relieving attacks of angina pectoris, this agent and a number of its variants have been thought of as coronary vasodilators. To some extent this is also the case with the xanthines, particularly theophylline, and with the benzodiazepines. However, coronary vasodilation and coronary flow rates respond secondarily to increased myocardial oxygen consumption and to the head of pressure in the aorta, and these influences overshadow presumed direct and isolated dilation of the coronary arteries. Further, under conditions in which such drugs are most needed, structural changes that greatly reduce the elastic dilating capabilities of the coronary vessels usually have developed. Symptomatic relief of coronary insufficiency can occur through reduction of myocardial oxygen demands without commensurate reduction in coronary flow, and the associated pain can be affected by analgesics, tranquilizers and placebos. Analyses of this circulatory-metabolic complex of events within the myocardium can be assessed in animals, with determinations of PO_2 levels in the coronary sinus outflow and in myocardial tissue, of coronary flow rates with flowmeters and indicators such as dissolved krypton-85; in patients, arteriograms and telemetering of ECG recordings during exercise add information.

Nitrites and nitrates generally relax smooth muscle in all parts of the body, and their action in the circulatory bed results in marked dilation of postarteriolar capillaries and venules, with a lesser effect on veins and arteries. In angina pectoris, the reduction of peripheral resistance, with corresponding reduction of the work load of the myocardium, is an important element in the relief of ischemic pain. Drugs of this class have little or no direct action on the myocardium, although the acute hypotension they sometimes produce may be sufficient to involve sympathetic stimulation, with increased myocardial force.

Glyceryl trinitrate (nitroglycerin) is administered sublingually in tablets containing up to 0.6 mg. Absorption is dependable, since this triester resembles fat and is soluble in it; absorption also can be obtained directly through the skin. Effects are cerebral vasodilation and throbbing of the head and, at times, some fall in arterial pressure; gut and bronchiolar muscles are relaxed. Acute effects subside in 20 to 30 minutes, but headache and relief from ischemic pain may continue for some time. It is the preferred drug for treatment of acute angina.

Amyl nitrite is administered only by inhalation, immediately after a glass pearl containing 0.2 ml. of the drug has been broken. Its effects are rapid and intense. Less intense but more prolonged effects of the same general type are obtained with nitrites and nitrates of sugars and other simple organic compounds. Erythrityl tetranitrate and mannitol hexanitrate are examples.

Xanthines, particularly theophylline, increase coronary blood flow under some conditions, but they have a direct effect also of increasing heart force. The latter is useful in paroxysmal nocturnal dyspnea due to left heart failure. Xanthines are diuretics and have some effect in relaxing visceral smooth muscle—the latter demonstrated by the usefulness of theophylline in relieving bronchial asthma. Intravenous injections are used at times but have caused a number of instances of severe circulatory depression and death; slow, controlled injection is a requisite precaution. Its effectiveness in the treatment of angina pectoris has not been proved.

Papaverine, a non-narcotic opium alkaloid, is capable of producing increased coronary flow in animals when given by intravenous injection, but it also directly increases heart force. Papaverine and several variants have been tried by oral administration but have not proved to be useful in angina pectoris. Dilation of other vascular beds can be obtained with papaverine, and it has been tried in various obstructive and vasospastic peripheral vascular disease with little success.

Dipyridamole (Persantine) has been demonstrated in laboratory animals to produce increased coronary flow through what appears to be a direct metabolic effect in the myocardium. Its alleged beneficial effect in anginal patients is unproved. Because it reduces the adhesiveness of platelets, it is used in open-heart surgery and following myocardial infarction, frequently in combination with aspirin.

Another approach in the management of angina is indicated in the clinical use of beta-adrenergic blocking agents such as propranolol (Inderal). These agents definitely reduce myocardial oxygen demand, as might be expected of agents that are negatively inotropic and hypotensive, although other mechanisms might be involved. It is not useful in abolishing acute attacks, but it may act additively with nitroglycerin given for this purpose. It is contraindicated in patients with asthma or congestive heart failure.

Antianxiety agents are recognized to be useful as adjuncts in certain patients with angina pectoris. Benzodiazepines (e.g., diazepam) through their additional coronary dilating action are particularly effective.

Pressor and Depressor Agents

A number of peptides from both natural and synthetic sources produce profound arterial hypotension when injected intravenously in very low doses. Their cardiac effects are minimal and largely secondary to hypotension. These include bradykinin, with a hypotensive dose (per kg.) in animals of about $1\mu g$. (10^{-6} g.), and eledoisin, with doses about one tenth this value. With physalaemin, the dose is still lower and is expressed in nanograms (10^{-9} g.).

Plasma kinins are generated by a family of enzymes, the kallikreins, acting upon alpha-globulin substrates. Besides being potent vasodilators, plasma kinins such as bradykinin cause constriction of bronchial smooth muscle, increased capillary permeability, and pain when applied to a denuded surface. Other effects of bradykinin include constriction of uterine and most gastrointestinal smooth muscle, release of catecholamines from the adrenal medulla, histamine from mast cells, and prostaglandin from the kidney. Some of the conditions in which the kinins are believed to play a pathogenetic role are acute pancreatitis, arthritis, endotoxin shock, carcinoid syndrome and hereditary angioneurotic edema. Since hypertensive patients excrete less kallikrein than normotensive individuals, the kallikrein-kinin system may be involved in the pathogenesis of essential hypertension.

Prostaglandins derived from tissues comprise a series of fatty acids related to linolenic and arachidonic acids. In animals, some are vasodilator, and some, vasoconstrictor, in doses comparable to those of eledoisin. They have few direct inotropic effects.

Angiotensin amide (Hypertensin) is a potent pressor agent available as a synthetic peptide. Because it does not have important direct inotropic effects at pressor dose levels it has had trials in hypotensive states without myocardial involvement. As a test of function of the left ventricle, it has been used as an "afterloading" agent.

The renin-angiotensin system is thought to maintain elevated systemic vascular resistance in heart failure. Renin released by the kidneys catalyzes the formation of angiotensin I, which is converted to angiotensin II, the active vasoconstrictor, by an angiotensin-converting enzyme found widely in the vascular bed. In severe heart failure, administration of an inhibitor of the converting enzyme causes a reduction in systemic vascular resistance and a rise in cardiac output. Concomitantly, the left ventricular filling pressure falls. Although the mechanism of action of inhibitors of the angiotensin-converting enzyme has not been completely elucidated, some such as captopril, show promise of being useful in the treatment of chronic congestive heart failure poorly controlled by digitalis and diuretics.

Antihypertensive Agents

Essential hypertension suggests overactivity of the sympathetic system, and, in attempted management of this condition, most of the agents are used either to reduce or to antagonize autonomically mediated vasoconstriction. It may be postulated that cerebral inhibition of sympathetic outflow is reduced by phenobarbital, acting as a nonspecific sedative; by reserpine, acting to deplete neuroeffectors in the hypothalamus;

or by veratrum alkaloids, acting reflexly at the vasomotor center. The ganglionic blocking agents effectively interrupt the pathways of the sympathetic system to about the same degree as does surgical sympathectomy but with introduction of side-effects due to parasympathetic blocking. Reserpine, guanethidine, bretylium and alpha-methyldopa, by various ways, reduce the output of the neuroeffector norepinephrine at the sympathetic endings, and the dihydroergot compounds and other adrenergic blocking agents prevent action of the sympathetic receptors. The MAO inhibitors have a hypotensive action possibly by production of a false transmitter. The arteriolar smooth muscle is made less responsive to sympathetic stimulation by the chlorothiazide compounds, through what appears to be some type of electrolyte shift that is independent of the diuretic effect and, in some manner, is possibly related to that of the salt-free diet regimens. A nondiuretic thiazide derivative, diazoxide (Hyperstat), is useful in treatment of hypertensive crises. In such cases the potent diuretics furosemide and ethacrynic acid are useful adjuncts. Sodium nitroprusside is preferred by some for treatment of hypertensive crises. The alpha-adrenergic blocking drugs, phentolamine and phenoxybenzamine, are used only in hypertension caused by an excess of circulating catecholamines. The beta-adrenergic drug, propranolol (Inderal), produces a sustained antihypertensive effect. These various agents are used to some extent in hypertension of pyelonephritis, nephritis, nephrosclerosis, toxemias of pregnancy, pheochromocytomas and the angiotensin-producing effects of renal artery obstruction.

In essential hypertension, the use of drug combinations has lengthened the life span and reduced the incidence or the onset of cerebrovascular accidents, damaged kidney function, myocardial infarction, retinopathy and congestive heart failure. Drug therapy is considered to have reduced sharply the incidence of congestive failure as the cause of death with an increase in deaths from coronary artery disease. The choice of an appropriate drug depends upon the severity of the disease and the patient's response to a therapeutic trial. Thiazides constitute initial therapy, and drug combinations are adjusted according to individual conditions.

Hydralazine (Apresoline) lowers blood pressure principally by acting directly on arteriolar smooth muscle. Two structurally unrelated agents, minoxidil (PDP) and guancydine, have similar peripheral vasodilator action. The combined use of minoxidil and beta blockers appears promising in the treatment of severe hypertension that fails to respond to other forms of treatment. Long-term therapy with high dosage of hydralazine may produce a type of systemic lupus erythematosus or a rheumatoid arthritis-like syndrome

that is a milder, reversible form of the same reaction. Headache, palpitations, tachycardia, and postural hypotension also are encountered. Side effects are dose dependent and, with cautious doses, can be reduced to an acceptably low incidence. Renal blood flow is increased, rather than reduced as it is with most other antihypertensive agents. It is usually prescribed in combination with other antihypertensive agents and is seldom used alone.

Veratrum alkaloids cause reflex hypotension and bradycardia by stimulating pressor receptors in the heart, lungs and possibly other thoracic locations. They are rarely used today because more effective agents are available and because of the narrow margin between the therapeutic and the toxic dose.

Reserpine (Serpasil) is a bradycardiac-hypotensive agent with sedative and tranquilizing effects. It conspicuously depletes from the brain and peripheral sites several biogenic amines, including norepinephrine, epinephrine, dopamine and serotonin. The bradycardia and some other cholinergic side effects can be antagonized by atropine. Equivalent doses are: crude drug (Raudixin), 100 mg.; a partially purified product termed the alseroxylon fraction (Rauwiloid), 1.0 mg; a purified alkaloid reserpine with several trademark names, 0.1 mg. Similar alkaloids from the same source are rescinnamine (Moderil), deserpidine (Harmonyl) and syrosingopine (Singoserp). The onset of action of these products is slow; they have a flat dose-response curve and are recommended only for the milder forms of hypertension. Their numerous side effects are described in the section on tranquilizers. There has been concern in regard to the ability of a reserpinized patient to withstand surgical stress, and it is customary to withhold this agent for 1 week or longer before elective surgery. However, the reserpinized state should not contraindicate needed surgery, since the hazard of hypotension has probably been overemphasized. Claims of carcinogenicity for reserpine are highly controversial.

Thiazides have proved to be highly valuable agents when used in combination with other antihypertensive drugs. Their effect was first thought to be due to their diuretic action, with resultant reduction of plasma volume and total body sodium. However, since the nondiuretic thiazide, diazoxide, has similar antihypertensive effects, a direct effect on vascular smooth muscle has been postulated. Irrespective of the ultimate mechanism, it appears that the diuretic thiazides relax peripheral arteriolar smooth muscle. The diabetogenic action of the thiazides has become a recognized complication as well as their tendency to produce hyperuricemia. Their potassium-depleting effects may intensify digitalis arrhythmias. This can be countered by the administration of supplemental potassium chloride or a potassium-sparing diuretic (e.g., spironolactone, triamterene). Enteric-coated preparations containing a thiazide and potassium chloride may cause small-bowel ulceration.

Diazoxide (Hyperstat) is a safe and effective drug for the emergency reduction of blood pressure. When given by rapid intravenous injection, it produces an immediate fall in blood pressure. The hypotensive effect is attributed to direct relaxation of vascular smooth muscle. Although it is a thiazide derivative, it is not a diuretic and actually causes a retention of sodium and water. Concurrent intravenous administration of ethacrynate sodium or furosemide counteracts this effect and also enhances the hypotensive action. Because of its potent antihypertensive action, close and frequent monitoring of the patient's blood pressure is required during the administration of diazoxide. Infrequent but serious adverse reactions include hypotension to shock levels, myocardial ischemia, arrhythmias and cerebral ischemia.

Monamine oxidase inhibitors were introduced as mood elevators, but the occurrence of orthostatic hypotension led to trial as antihypertensive agents. Pargyline (Eutonyl), a nonhydrazide member of the group, has been found to be effective in moderate to severe hypertension. Orthostatic hypotension and various autonomic side effects greatly limit is usefulness. Its hypotensive action is related to: 1) sympathetic ganglionic blockade, 2) production of a false transmitter, and 3) decreased rate of production and turnover of norepinephrine. Because of the high incidence of untoward effects and availability of superior agents, the monamine oxidase inhibitors are seldom used in treating hypertension.

Pargyline and other MAO inhibitors have been implicated in the "cheese syndrome"—i.e., patients under therapy with these drugs have been known to suffer marked cardiovascular crises on ingestion of some cheeses and wines that contain high levels of tyramine and other active amines. For this reason, this agent is used infrequently.

Methyldopa (Aldomet), introduced in 1963, is a decarboxylase inhibitor. Since the enzyme decarboxylase, which converts dopa to dopamine, is essential for synthesis of norepinephrine and serotonin, it was thought that inhibition would reduce the level of active vasoconstrictor amines. The drug is taken up by adrenergic neurons and metabolized to alpha-methylnorepinephrine. At one time it was postulated that this compound acted as a peripheral false neurotransmitter to reduce blood pressure. Subsequently it was found that decreased peripheral stores of norepinephrine did not correlate with the hypotensive response. It is now generally accepted that the hypotensive action of methyldopa is a consequence of its influence on central adrenergic mechanisms through the stimulation of central alpha receptors by alpha-methylnorepinephrine. Additionally, it lowers plasma renin activity. Drowsiness is a common side effect, and nasal stuffiness and dry mouth also occur. Postural hypotension is one of the side effects but is not as severe as it is with the use of guanethidine. With prolonged treatment, some patients develop a positive Coombs' test, and a few cases of hemolytic anemia have been reported. Thiazides potentiate actions of methyldopa. When given intravenously, it is useful in hypertensive crises.

Guanethidine (Ismelin) produces a long-sustained hypotensive effect, which is relatively slow in onset. It produces adrenergic neuronal blockade. It has no ganglionic blocking action but depletes norepinephrine at the sympathetic nerve ending. It does not block the effect of injected catecholamines. Side-effects include diarrhea, bradycardia, drooping eyelids, retrograde ejaculation and orthostatic hypotension. Since the drug causes sodium and water retention a diuretic should always be administered concurrently. It should not be used in patients suspected of having a pheochromocytoma, as severe hypertension may occur as a result of massive release of endogenous catecholamines.

Bretylium (Bretylol) acts as a sympathetic blocking agent by preventing release of norepinephrine from neuronal sites. Formerly used as an antihypertensive drug, it is currently administered parenterally in the treatment of life-threatening ventricular tachycardia or fibrillation refractory to other therapy.

Prostaglandin (PGA$_2$), a potent vasodilator, is under investigation for the treatment of essential hypertension. Its use is based on the concept that some cases of essential hypertension may not be due to increased activity of blood pressure-raising mechanisms but rather to a deficiency of circulating vasodilators.

Clonidine (Catapres), initially developed as a nasal decongestant, is an antihypertensive agent that acts by direct stimulation of central nervous system alpha-adrenergic receptors located in medullary centers and possibly the hypothalamus. The result is a decrease in sympathetic outflow and a concomitant decrease in blood pressure. Hemodynamic effects include a decrease in cardiac output, heart rate, stroke volume and total peripheral resistance in the erect position only. The most commonly encountered side effects are drowsiness and dry mouth. A rebound increase in blood pressure may follow its rapid withdrawal.

Nitroprusside (Nipride) is an immediate acting, potent intravenous hypotensive agent. This action is probably due to the nitroso (NO) group. Its effect is almost immediate and ends when the intravenous infusion is stopped. The brief duration of action is due to rapid conversion to thiocyanate. The hypotensive effect is caused by peripheral vasodilation as a result of a direct action on vascular smooth muscle. The drug is indicated for the immediate reduction of blood pressure in hypertensive crises and also for producing controlled hypotension in order to reduce bleeding in certain surgical procedures. For short-term management of congestive heart failure, the peripheral vascular effects of nitroprusside are considered beneficial. The drug should be used only when the necessary facilities and equipment for continuous monitoring of blood pressure are available. Since the drug is very sensitive to light, the infusion system should be protected against light. Excessive dosage can produce cyanide intoxication.

Propranolol (Inderal) is generally well tolerated when used in the management of mild, moderate or severe hypertension usually in combination with other drugs. The mechanism of its hypotensive effect has not been clearly established. Among the factors that may be involved are diminution of tonic sympathetic nerve outflow from vasomotor centers in the brain, decreased cardiac output, and inhibition of renin release from the kidneys. Although total peripheral vascular resistance may increase initially, it readjusts to the pretreatment level, or lower, with chronic use. Dosage must be individualized. Among the contraindications to its use are bronchial asthma and congestive heart failure.

Metoprolol (Lopressor) represents a new generation of beta blockers whose actions are relatively selective because of preferential blockade of beta$_1$ receptors in cardiac tissue rather than the beta$_2$ receptors in bronchial and vascular tissues. Because of this selective action, metoprolol has certain advantages over earlier beta blockers such as propranolol. These include: 1) relatively less danger of provoking undesirable bronchoconstriction in patients with asthma and other forms of chronic obstructive pulmonary disease, 2) less likelihood of temporary rise in peripheral resistance at the start of therapy, 3) less likelihood of sudden and pronounced rises in blood pressure after physical exertion and emotional stress, 4) less likelihood of side effects caused primarily by blockade of beta receptors. Metoprolol is generally well tolerated. The most common adverse reactions are tiredness or dizziness, depression, diarrhea, and shortness of breath with bradycardia. As with other beta blockers, there have been reports of exacerbations of angina pectoris and, in some cases, myocardial infarction following abrupt cessation of therapy. The drug is contraindicated in sinus bradycardia, heart block greater than first degree, cardiogenic shock, and overt cardiac failure.

Prazosin (Minipress) is a peripheral alpha-receptor blocking antihypertensive compound derived from quinazoline. Its hypotensive effect results from relaxation of peripheral arterioles as a consequence of blockade of post-synaptic alpha adrenergic receptors rather than by direct relaxation of arteriolar vascular muscle. The most important hemodynamic effect is a reduction in total peripheral resistance, but in contrast to hydralazine, tachycardia is seldom produced. It differs from phentolamine, which acts at both pre- and postsynaptic alpha adrenergic receptors, and from diazoxide and hydralazine which directly affect vascular smooth muscle. Prazosin appears to have no central action on blood pressure and does not affect neuronal adrenergic function. The plasma half life is reported to be about 1 to 2 hours; it is extensively metabolized with only a small fraction being excreted unchanged. Prazosin is effective in lowering blood pressure in all grades of hypertension: in mild and some cases of moderate hypertension when used alone and in moderate and severe hypertension when used in combination with other agents. The most important side effect is marked postural hypotension after the initial dose and sometimes after a rapid dose increment. This effect can be minimized by beginning treatment with a low dose and increasing dosage gradually.

Promising early results have been obtained with the use of prazosin in the treatment of heart failure refractory to digitalis and diuretic therapy.

Ticrynafen (Selacryn) is a new oral antihypertensive and diuretic compound chemically related to ethacrynic acid. Initially, ticrynafen causes a reduction in blood pressure through reduction of plasma volume. The long-term antihypertensive effect may involve both renal and extrarenal mechanisms. Ticrynafen resembles the thiazides in its diuretic potency and antihypertensive effects, but, in contrast, lowers serum uric acid levels instead of raising them through its uricosuric effect. Unfortunately, the compound was removed from the market because of severe hepatic complications.

DRUGS THAT RETARD DEVELOPMENT OF ATHEROSCLEROSIS

There is much documentation and some guarded acceptance of the association between elevated serum lipid levels and the development of atherosclerosis. Similarly, it is generally agreed that there are some advantages in prophylactic therapy that reduces serum lipids. Since hyperlipidemia usually is a combination of increased triglycerides and cholesterol, therapies differ accordingly. Heparin given parenterally in daily doses of 100 or 200 mg. activates a clearing factor (lipoprotein lipase) and transiently reduces triglyceride levels. It is not indicated for therapy of either acute or chronic manifestations of hyperlipoproteinemia. Cholesterol levels are reduced by a high proportion of unsaturated dietary fats and by aluminum nicotinate. Nicotinic acid has caused disappearance of cholesterol deposits in the skin. Its usefulness is greatly limited by its side effects which include flushing, pruritus, gastrointestinal complaints and disturbances in liver function. Thyroxin analogs, which to a degree are hypocholesteremic and less calorigenic than *l*-thyroxine, should not be used in patients with coronary artery disease and ectopic premature beats. Estrogens are thought to have some protective effect against atherosclerosis, as judged by the lower incidence of the condition in premenopausal women, but are not useful because of feminizing effects and increased incidence of thromboembolism. Triparanol and some other synthetics (structural analogs of cholesterol) have the effect of blocking endogenous cholesterol synthesis at the desmosterol level, but their toxic actions and the atherogenic influence of desmosterol itself make this a matter of purely theoretic interest. Experimentally, neomycin lowers serum cholesterol levels primarily by an increase in fecal excretion of sterols and bile acids. Sitosterols (plant sterols) also lower serum levels of cholesterol, probably by interfering with its alimentary canal absorption. Some synthetic esters have been shown to interfere with cholesterol synthesis, and it has been hypothesized that they act at a step before the sterol nucleus is formed.

Clofibrate (Atromid S) is thought to reduce net triglyceride output from the liver and to decrease the rate of cholesterol synthesis in the liver. When compared with other therapies in clinical trial series, clofibrate reduces serum cholesterol and is conspicuous in its hypotriglyceridemic effect. Side effects of clofibrate administration include increased sensitivity to coumarin anticoagulants and gastrointestinal upset. Cholestyramine (Questran) is a quaternary ammonium anion exchange resin that absorbs bile acids in the intestinal tract. The net effect is a lowering of serum cholesterol. Cholestyramine is used primarily for the relief of pruritus associated with biliary tract obstruction. The drug may interfere with the absorption of numerous drugs and fat-soluble vitamins. A combination of diet and drug therapy may be useful in retarding atherosclerosis. However, long-term efficacy has not been demonstrated.

Probucol (Lorelco) is indicated as an adjunctive therapy to diet for the reduction of elevated serum cholesterol in patients with primary hypercholesterolemia. Its mechanism of action is unknown.

DIURETICS

Developmental History

Renal effects of purine bases, caffeine, theobromine and theophylline were intensively studied during the first part of this century and, along with salts such as ammonium chloride, these diuretics were about the only means of removing edema fluid by direct mechanisms. Chance observation during antiluetic therapy led to the use of organic mercurials in 1920. A similarly unexpected observation during antibacterial sulfonamide therapy led to the introduction of carbonic anhydrase inhibitors that have in common the—SO_2NH_2 grouping, which is also represented in the later thiazide class of diuretics. This latter class, introduced in 1957, is not primarily dependent on carbonic anhydrase inhibition; it now constitutes a considerable group, ranging in effective oral dose from the original chlorothiazide (0.5 to 1.0 g.), down to those thiazides with doses of 1 to 2 mg. Still more potent agents, such as furosemide and ethacrynic acid, promote the excretion of 20 to 30 per cent of sodium chloride in the glomerular filtrate during their peak effect, as contrasted with 10 per cent in the case of the thiazides. In the case of furosemide, the sulfamyl group is present, but ethacrynic acid contains neither sulfur nor nitrogen; it was developed in a search for compounds that would inhibit sulfhydryl-catalyzed renal sodium transport systems.

General Mechanisms

Current analysis and localization of drug action within the nephron involves micropuncture techniques, radioautography and stop-flow experiments. Special methods have attempted perfusion of isolated segments of single nephrons.

Generally it is thought that the net sodium excretion produced by the more effective diuretics is chiefly by inhibition of the active sodium transport system located at the basal surface of the tubular epithelial cells. This occurs after the sodium of the glomerular filtrate diffuses passively from the tubular lumen into the epithelial cells and is then pumped outward into the interstitial space by this active transport mechanism. Water in the filtrate is reabsorbed passively, depending on permeability of the tubular epithelium, which varies considerably in different segments of the nephron. Diuretic action in the proximal tubular segment can be obscured by local adjustments and, later, by adjustments in more distal segments, depending on tubular volume and flow velocity. The most critical net effects probably occur in the ascending loop of Henle, and the important diuretics, furosemide, the mercurials, ethacrynic acid and, to a lesser degree, the thiazides, act at this site, although the thiazides also act more distally. Higher doses of the more potent agents have more generally distributed effects on other parts of the nephron. Because the Na^+—K^+ and Na^+—H^+ exchange mechanisms occur mostly in the distal segment with less opportunity for further adjustment, the net effects are critical, and significant potassium losses occur with most diuretics.

Osmotic Diuretics

Crystalloids that increase urinary volume by osmotic effects have only limited effect on excretion of electrolytes. The extent to which they increase excretion of toxic agents such as barbiturates is a matter of question. Sucrose, which was used previously as an osmotic diuretic, was discontinued after it was found to produce a foamy vacuolization of the renal tubules. Urea has been used widely but does have the disadvantage of crossing cell membranes with relative ease.

Mannitol is a hexahydric alcohol that remains confined to the extracellular spaces, is not metabolized, is filtered freely by the glomerulus and is not subject to significant tubular absorption or secretion. Since it produces only a minimal effect on the excretion of electrolytes, it is not used as a diuretic agent in the classic sense, i.e. mobilization of edema fluid. Perhaps one of the most important indications for its use is in the prophylaxis of acute renal failure. A closely related use is in the evaluation of acute oliguria. It is also used for the reduction of pressure and volume of the cerebrospinal and intraocular fluids.

Xanthines

The xanthines were first recognized as diuretics through the observation of the action of caffeine-containing beverages. *Theophylline,* which produces less stimulation of the central nervous system, is the agent most used. Solubility is much enhanced in the combination theophylline-ethylenediamine (aminophylline).

Although the segment of the nephron is uncertain, aminophylline is considered to depress the renal tubular reabsorption of sodium, and the effect is additive with thiazides and with mercurials. The response is independent of metabolic acidosis and possibly is augmented in metabolic alkalosis. Xanthines are myocardial stimulants and vasodilators, and these effects may sufficiently increase the glomerular filtration rate to explain most of the diuretic effect.

Mercurials

The effective mercurial diuretics produce a sustained excretion of sodium and chloride ions and the osmotically equivalent amount of water. The mechanism of action involves interaction of the mercury ion with a sulfhydryl-containing protein necessary for the active reabsorption of sodium and chloride. The known sites of action include the proximal and distal tubules, with an additional proposed site in the ascending limb of the loop of Henle. Excretion of chloride ion can preponderate, since there can be some distal tubular reab-

sorption of sodium ion in exchange for potassium and hydrogen ions. Excessive action is characterized by hypochloremic alkalosis. Cellular mechanisms probably involve degradation of the organic structures in the presence of adequate hydrogen ion concentrations, with release of small quantities of mercury ions and their subsequent reaction with —SH groups in the enzyme systems. The enzyme systems most involved are those that accomplish the active reabsorption of sodium. Unquestionably the presence of various compounds with available —SH groups can be shown to reduce or abolish the diuretic action. Dimercaprol (BAL) has been used as treatment for toxic kidney effects. Monothiols such as cysteine antagonize cardiac arrhythmias that are produced when these diuretics have been given inadvisedly by the intravenous route. Diuretic effects of mercurials are intensified by acidity and reduced by alkalinity.

Common examples are mercaptomerin (Thiomerin) and meralluride (Mercuhydrin). They are most effective when given intramuscularly and have some limited usefulness when administered orally or in suppositories. Generally they are reserved for refractory instances of cardiac edema, nephrotic edema and ascites. They are being displaced by the later orally effective and highly potent agents.

Mercurials are contraindicated in most forms of renal disease; damage to proximal convuluted tubules has been observed.

Carbonic Anhydrase Inhibitors

Acetazolamide (Diamox) was developed subsequent to the observation that the acidosis caused by sulfanilamide and its variants was due to inhibition of carbonic anhydrase. This enzyme greatly accelerates the reaction of CO_2 and H_2O, leading to H^+ and HCO_3^-. Since this inhibition could be correlated with diuretic activity in a series of compounds, a number of effective analogs were subsequently developed. These include dichlorphenamide (Daranide), ethoxzolamide (Cardrase) and methazolamide (Neptazane). The characteristic effect is distal tubular depression of H^+ ion synthesis and also depression of reabsorption of bicarbonate ion, with resulting alkalinization of the urine and metabolic acidosis. The development of acidosis reduces or eliminates the diuretic action, presumably by presenting the kidney with sufficient H^+ for Na exchange, even without the carbonic anhydrase synthesis. With H^+—Na$^+$ exchange reduced by the drug, the distal tubule excretes increased amounts of K to exchange for Na. Both acidosis and hypokalemia are characteristic effects of the action of these drugs.

Acetazolamide is absorbed promptly on oral administration and is excreted in the urine, to the extent of about 80 per cent in 8 to 12 hours. Before the advent of the thiazides, it was a useful diuretic in ambulatory patients with mild to moderate cardiac decompensation. It is valuable in the management of acute glaucoma, probably by inhibiting carbonic anhydrase in the ciliary body in which the aqueous humor is formed. It has been demonstrated that acetazolamide decreases intraocular inflow and also the production of cerebrospinal fluid. The drug is used to a limited extent in managing reduction of epileptic seizures.

Thiazides

These compounds, developed as an extension of the carbonic anhydrase inhibitors, have several unique characteristics and currently represent a very widely used class of drugs. All contain the sulfamyl group, to which is attached a thiadiazine ring. Chlorine in position 6 is replaced by a CF_3 grouping in some of the variants. Other more varied forms of these compounds include chlorthalidone, which has a typical but longer period of action; quinethazone, which is typical; and diazoxide, which has no diuretic action, but is antihypertensive and has remarkable relaxant action on the uterus.

Chlorothiazide (Diuril) and its several common variants are potent diuretics, with the capability of inhibiting 5 to 10 per cent of the sodium and chloride normally reabsorbed from the glomerular filtrate. These ions are excreted in approximately equal proportions, and acid-base balance is not usually affected. The action is relatively independent of acidotic or alkalotic conditions and can be demonstrated as an additive effect with the action of mercurials. Paradoxically these drugs decrease urine volume in diabetes insipidus. They exhibit hyperglycemic effects capable of aggravating diabetes mellitus, probably through inhibiting release of insulin from the pancreas. Similarly, they can intensify the symptoms of gout, and it is thought that they compete for the same transport mechanisms in the tubules that excrete uric acid, the penicillins and PAH.

These thiazides cause significant potassium loss, and the action is in part due to carbonic anhydrase inhibition, with resultant decrease in the amount of H^+ available at the distal tubule sites for exchange of Na^+. Potassium loss has been a particularly disturbing complication during digitalization. It proved difficult to prevent hypokalemia by administration of oral potassium in coated solid form because the resulting release in the small gut led to local irritation and scarring. The potassium deficit can be met by administering spironolactone, which interferes with aldosterone action, or by administering triamterine, which acts directly to retain potassium. Both are weak diuretics that act suitably in combination with thiazides.

The thiazides have wide use in the management of hypertension because their addition to other drugs has had the general effect of lowering blood pressure more than when these agents are used alone. Even when used alone, however, the thiazides have been of benefit, and the variant, diazoxide, which is not diuretic, has been of benefit. This latter agent has been shown to sharply decrease motility in the nongravid uterus, and some type of magnesium-like antagonism of calcium has been suggested. The question of antihypertensive action remains unsettled, but included among mechanisms are a possible direct decrease in vascular reactivity of hypertensive patients, some renal mechanism producing an effect similar to that of the low-salt diet, the hypovolemic effect, and a possible direct effect of sodium depletion.

Ethacrynic Acid and Furosemide

Ethacrynic acid (Edecrin), an unsaturated ketone derivative of phenoxyacetic acid, has had considerable trial since its experimental recognition in 1962. Both ethacrynic acid and furosemide (Lasix) are highly effective in conditions relatively refractory to other diuretics. In both cases, the action is an inhibition of sodium transport in the ascending limb of Henle's loop, to a degree that is considered unique. This inhibition results in decreased medullary hypertonicity and eliminates the osmotic gradient responsible for the reabsorption of free water. The marked natriuresis produced by these agents also indicates that, at time, reabsorption in the proximal tubule is somewhat inhibited. These so-called "high ceiling" diuretics are satisfactorily absorbed orally, are rapid in onset of action, are independent of changes in acid-base balance and produce distinct K^+ loss. In the presence of liver disease, ethacrynic acid has produced hepatic coma; also, excessive, rapid dehydration has led to severe hypotension, hypovolemia and hypokalemia. With ethacrynic acid too, hearing losses have been reported, some of which occurred very suddenly and others led to permanent deafness in patients with renal failure.

Ticrynafen (Selacryn), a new oral diuretic chemically related to ethacrynic acid, also possesses antihypertensive and hypouricemic effects. As a diuretic, it acts in the cortical diluting segment of the distal tubule. Like the thiazides, it blocks the reabsorption of sodium and thereby enhances the excretion of sodium and water. It lowers serum uric acid levels by inhibiting the reabsorption of uric acid at both pre- and postsecretory sites in the proximal tubule. The drug is rapidly absorbed. (This agent was recently withdrawn from the market, however, because of hepatic complications.)

Metolazone (Diulo) and chlorthalidone (Hygroton)

are diuretic/saluretic/antihypertensive drugs. They act primarily to inhibit sodium reabsorption at the cortical diluting site and in the proximal convoluted tubule, and are approximately equal to thiazides in diuretic potency. Their longer duration of action is attributed to protein binding and enterohepatic recycling. They are indicated for the treatment of sodium and water retention and in the management of hypertension either as the sole therapeutic agent or to enhance the effectiveness of other antihypertensive drugs.

PLASMA VOLUME REPLACEMENT

There are occasions in which survival depends upon a prompt increase in circulating plasma volume. This occurs particularly after severe hemorrhage, burn shock, crush injuries or sepsis. Since the acute, critical need is for replacement of circulating fluid, it follows that saline or dextrose solutions or plasma would be used under emergency conditions when blood transfusions are not available or when the need for red cells and other blood components is not of prime importance. Saline and dextrose are readily diffusible crystalloids of low molecular weight, and experience has shown that their capacity to maintain blood volume is distinctly less than that of solutions containing nondiffusible colloids of high molecular weight. Comparative experiments in animals following massive blood losses show about 60 per cent of the original blood volume 3 hours after replacement with saline or glucose and approximately 100 per cent of the original blood volume when dextran or similar colloid solutions were used as replacement fluids. Colloids of the dextran type have been developed to meet the need for a cheap, stable, compatible, noninfectious substitute for blood colloids. Other products that have been tried include, particularly, acacia, which was introduced by the physiologist Bayliss in World War I, and polyvinylpyrrolidone (PVP), which was used widely in Germany in World War II and is still used in some foreign countries. Both of these products are chemically dissimilar to body colloids; they give a high incidence of histamine-release phenomena, they are incompletely metabolized and their prolonged storage in the body is considered undersirable but has not been found to be a practical hazard. Other products with some degree of trial include pectin, isinglass, gelatin, and oxidized gelatin and a Japanese seaweed product, Alginon.

The plasma substitute that has been studied and used most extensively is the Swedish product, *dextran,* obtained by the action of *Leuconostoc mesenteroides* on sucrose solutions. This enzyme-produced polymer of dextrose units with predominantly 1,6 linkages is in the form of flexible coils, with branching at 1,3:1,4

and 1,6 positions, and reaches molecular weights up to 10 million. The molecular weight is reduced by acid hydrolysis to an average of 75,000 for clinical use in this country and a somewhat higher figure for use in Europe. A lower viscosity product, roughly of 40,000 mol. wt., is used in peripheral vascular disease for its presumed effects in preventing aggregation of red cells. It is also used as a priming fluid (alone or as an additive) for pump-oxygenators during extracorporeal circulation. Large volumes of this product have had the effect of producing anuria, probably by viscous obstruction to flow in kidney tubules. Dextran is distributed as a 6 per cent solution in isotonic saline. The colloid, in this case, produces less than 1 per cent of the total osmotic pressure, but this is critical because it represents a differential between intravascular and interstitial osmotic pressures. The dextrans of medium molecular weight (75,000) contain about 10 per cent dextrans with less than 20,000 mol. wt. and 10 per cent with more than 200,000 mol. wt. The smaller molecules are eliminated rapidly, and the larger produce a higher incidence of side-reactions. Typical side reactions include histamine-release phenomena, bleeding tendencies (when more than 1 liter is administered), elevation of erythrocyte sedimentation rate and erythrocyte aggregation, which, to a moderate degree, interferes with blood grouping and crossmatching. Dextran has a low but recognizable degree of antigen-antibody type of reactions. The half-life of dextran in the circulation is 12 to 24 hours, and storage in the reticuloendothelial system is no longer present after 1 or 2 weeks. Dextran solutions when shelf-stored for years have shown flaking, probably due to hydrogen bonding of the linear chain portions; the flakes can be redissolved on heating, and the phenomenon is probably of minor toxicologic significance.

Hetastarch (Volex) is a glucose polymer of related type. This hydroxyethyl starch is prepared by ethylene oxide treatment of waxy sorghum starch and is largely amylopectin; in its characteristic branching, it is more closely related to glycogen. Because of its resemblance to a naturally occurring polymer, it is virtually nontoxic and free of sensitivity reactions. Plasma expansion is persistent. The 6 per cent solution does not develop flaking on storage. The adjunctive use of hetastarch in leukophoresis has been shown to improve harvesting and increase the yield of granulocytes by centrifugal means.

Plasma protein fraction, a 5 per cent solution of stablized human plasma proteins in sodium chloride solution, is used for the treatment of hypovolemic shock and as a source of protein in patients with hypoproteinemia. The incidence of adverse reactions is low. Normal human serum albumin is used for the same purposes in either a 5 or 25 per cent solution that has been free from hepatitis virus by heating for 10 hours at 60°C.

It was proposed that adequate volume replacement could be obtained if lactated Ringer's solution were to be used in amounts substantially larger than the calculated blood loss. The result in many cases was either inadequate replacement or pulmonary edema.

Blood Products

In addition to the blood products that have been used for plasma replacement, there are others with different uses.

Fibrinogen (Parenogen) is used for restoring fibrinogen levels that may be reduced after a number of conditions such as premature separation of the placenta and extensive surgical procedures. This product carries the hazard of hepatitis virus. It can cause thrombosis when it is administered rapidly or in high concentration.

Immune serum globulin is a sterile solution of globulins (chiefly gamma globulin) prepared from pooled normal human plasma. It contains many antibodies normally present in blood. It is administered intramuscularly to prevent infectious hepatitis, poliomyelitis, chickenpox and rubella. Measles may be modified or temporarily prevented by administration of immune globulin of known measles antibody titer.

Hepatitis B immune globulin (Human; H-Big) is a sterile solution of immunoglobulin containing a high titer of antibody to hepatitis B surface antigen. The U.S. Public Health Service Advisory Committee on Immunization Practices unequivocally recommends this blood product for only one circumstance, namely, a one-time exposure to blood containing hepatitis B virus, either by accidental needle-stick or by contact with mucous membranes, such as might occur in a pipetting accident.

Rhô (D) immune globulin is used to prevent formation of active antibodies in RH-negative mothers after delivery of an RH-positive infant or abortion of an RH-positive fetus. To be effective, it must be given within 72 hours after delivery or abortion. *Tetanus immune globulin* is an effective prophylactic agent in patients with woulds potentially contaminated with *Clostridium tetani.*

DRUGS AFFECTING BLOOD COAGULATION

Drugs Decreasing Coagulability

There has been considerable controversy in regard to the use of anticoagulants in coronary artery disease. However, they may be of value in the majority of patients with acute infarction, especially "poor-risk" patients; in long-term therapy of 1 to 5 years after acute myocardial infarction, with possible reduction of reinfarction and mortality, particularly in younger patients; in angina pectoris, with younger patients and in cases in which there has been recent increase in intensity and frequency. Further, anticoagulants are indicated in patients with pulmonary or peripheral emboli and in severe congestive failure with peripheral edema. They are used also in advancing thrombophlebitis, occlusive perhipheral vascular disease and in cardiac and vascular surgery. Conditions with high hemorrhage potential are contraindications. Heparin, by parenteral administration, is the agent of choice when rapid anticoagulant action is needed, while the coumarin derivatives are used by oral administration in long-term therapy.

Heparin sodium USP (Liquaemin) is present in mast cells; it is obtained from the lungs and intestines of cattle, although originally it was obtained from the liver. Heparin is a polymer of about 20,000 mol. wt. made up of paired units of acetylated glucosamine and glucuronic acid sulfated at two to three points of attachment. This highly acidic, negatively charged product has not been separated as a wholly pure entity; it is assayed to contain 120 USP units per mg. or more. The solutions for injection contain 1,000 to 40,000 units per ml. Primarily, heparin inhibits thromboplastin generation and thus interferes with the conversion of prothrombin to thrombin. A globulin in plasma is necessary as a cofactor. Heparin also acts as an antithrombin. Platelet agglutination is decreased, and fibrinolysis possibly is potentiated. Its clinical action is monitored by coagulation time determinations as by the Lee-White method or by assessment of activated partial thromboplastin time. Desirably, clotting time is increased to two to three times normal, i.e., about 20 to 35 minutes. Because of considerable variation in potency in commercial preparations, dosage should always be indicated in units rather than milligrams. Transient action of the drug necessitates frequent administration. Management typically consists of intravenous injection of 5,000 to 10,000 units every 4 hours. Continuous intravenous infusion is the most reliable means to keep clotting time constantly elevated when rigorous control is advisable. Adjustment of dosage and neutralization of effect are more difficult when subcutaneous or intramuscular routes are used. The repository mixtures of gelatin and dextrose give irregular absorption and may produce hematomas. Heparin administered sublingually or orally is not absorbed.

Intravenous administration of heparin causes prompt clearing of the turbidity of alimentary lipemic serum, and clearing of the same type also occurs if the lipemia has been produced by fat emulsions injected intravenously. Factors are contributed by both the tissues and the plasma to develop this lipemia-clearing factor, which appears to act as a lipolytic enzyme and to be capable of demonstration in vitro. The visible clearing of lipemic serum is accompanied by the disappearance of the large aggregates of low-density lipoproteins and the appearance of smaller lipoproteins of higher density. The requisite doses of heparin are lower than those necessary for prolonging clotting time. Another effect of heparin and its variants is increased sodium excretion, due to suppression of formation of aldosterone; this has occurred in patients with and without edema. Osteoporosis and damage to the adrenal zona glomerulosa have been associated with prolonged heparin administration.

Toxic effects of heparin are largely hemorrhage; subintimal hemorrhage, massive hematuria or activation of any bleeding lesion. Sulfates of various carbohydrates have been tried as heparin substitutes; some caused alopecia, and none is routinely used. Heparin action can be neutralized by basic substances such as protamine. Paradoxically, it has anticoagulant action of its own, and in the absence of heparin it prolongs clotting time. Although usually well tolerated, toxic manifestations include dyspnea, hypotension and bradycardia.

Bishydroxycoumarin (Dicumarol), available as a synthetic chemical, was first identified about 1940 by a study of the hemorrhagic disease caused in cattle by the eating of spoiled sweet clover hay. Other coumarins and phenylindandiones have been introduced as improvements in terms of dependability of oral absorption and rapidity of action. They result in decreased synthesis of prothrombin, and, in therapeutic use, prothrombin levels are reduced to about 20 per cent of normal according to the one-stage method of Quick (this corresponds to a clotting time of about 27 seconds, as contrasted with a normal of about 12 seconds). These compounds appear to act as antagonists of vitamin K, which is part of the enzyme system producing prothrombin; the action is reversible, and the prothrombin-reducing effect can be overcome by excess of vitamin K. The chemical structure of these anticoagulants suggests that they may act as competitive analogs of vitamin K. The prothrombin reduction is a delayed effect and is not demonstrable in vitro. There is also decreased synthesis of proconvertin (Factor VII), plasma thromboplastin component (Factor IX), and Stuart-Prower Factor (Factor X). Maintenance dose of coumarin and indandione derivatives should be reevaluated periodically in patients with impaired liver or kidney function, when the patient receives new drugs (e.g., phenobarbital) or when a drug is being

withdrawn. Coumarin compounds are relatively free of untoward effects and have been given for long periods without signs of toxicity. Occasional adverse effects include dermatitis, urticaria, diarrhea, alopecia and leukopenia. Indandione derivatives carry a greater risk for severe reactions. Clinically useful variants of the coumarin structure are warfarin sodium (Coumadin) and acenocoumarin (Sintrom). Variants of the indandione structure are phenindione and diphenadione. These may produce an orange color in alkaline urine that may be mistaken for hematuria. Overdose of these compounds, with bleeding, is treated with vitamin K preparations, with transfusions of fresh whole blood or with Factor IX complex (Konȳne) consisting of purified Factors II, VII, IX and X. To avoid serious hypersensitivity reactions, a test dose should be administered before the full dose is given. Water-soluble vitamin K preparations are slow in action, and some consider them inadequate. When anticoagulant therapy is resumed after the administration of vitamin K, larger than usual doses may be required initially.

Fibrinolysin, Human (Plasmin) promotes the dissolution of intravascular thrombi. It is prepared by activating a human blood plasma fraction with streptokinase; it exhibits profibrinolysin-activator and fibrinolytic properties. Evidence of clot lysis has been shown by radiographic techniques. It is used in phlebothrombosis, pulmonary embolism, thrombophlebitis, and thrombosis of arteries except those involving the coronary and cerebral vessels. The drug is contraindicated in the presence of hypofibrinogenemia or a hemorrhagic diathesis.

There is currently marked interest in drugs that inhibit platelet adhesiveness and aggregation and thus might prevent thrombus formation. The vasodilator drug dipyridamole (Persantine) inhibits platelet aggregation in vitro. There are several other compounds, including prostaglandin E_1, aspirin, and pyrazole drugs, that affect platelet function in vitro and may prevent platelet aggregation induced by collagen. The in vivo effectiveness of these drugs in the prevention of thrombosis is under intense investigation; much further work is needed before the in vivo effectiveness of antiplatelet drugs is clearly established.

Hemostatics

Capillary bleeding may be retarded by the local application of various substances. Arterial bleeding is not affected, and the value of these products generally is limited. Epinephrine, alum, tannic acid and tincture of ferric chloride have been used most in the past as local styptics.

Local application of materials with extensive surface areas also has the effect of checking hemorrhage. Absorbable, nonirritant substances now being used are special forms of gelatin sponge (Gelfoam), oxidized cellulose (Oxycel), thrombin as powder or in solution, thromboplastin and fibrin foam. Except for the immediate control of hemorrhage, oxidized cellulose is not recommended as a surface dressing, as it is considered that such application inhibits epithelization.

Antihemophilic factor preparations (Factor VIII) are used in the treatment of classical hemophilia as well as in patients who are not true hemophiliacs but who have acquired circulating Factor VIII inhibitors. Fibrinogen (Parenogen) may be indicated in extensive surgical procedures and in certain obstetric complications. Plasma concentrates in general carry a relatively high risk of acute viral hepatitis. Calcium salts, used preoperatively and under conditions of internal hemorrhage, have not been shown to be valuable.

Vitamin K. The administration of vitamin K represents a special circumstance in which decreased coagulability may be returned to normal. Decreased coagulability in this case is due to a prothrombin deficiency. This arises most commonly in the condition of obstructive jaundice or biliary fistula draining to the outside. Lacking bile in the alimentary canal, vitamin K, a fat-soluble material, is not absorbed adequately. A normal supply of vitamin K is needed by the liver for the production of prothrombin and other factors. A lowering of these factors in the blood has marked effects on coagulation time, particularly after the prothrombin level is decreased below 20 per cent of normal. This decreased coagulability occurs when the normal supply of bile to the gut is interrupted, when the liver is damaged to a degree that prevents the formation of prothrombin, and when absorption from the gut is deficient. A lowered prothrombin level also exists in certain hemorrhagic diseases of the newborn. Vitamin K products are strikingly effective in correcting the hemorrhagic tendency of these conditions, except in instances of severe liver damage. High doses of vitamin K cause hyperbilirubinemia in the newborn.

Synthetic Variations. Naturally occurring vitamin K is a naphthoquinone derivative obtained from plant and animal sources and is a product of bacterial fermentation in the gut. Numerous synthetic variations are available, some oil soluble for intramuscular injection and some water soluble for intravenous injection. They may be given orally, usually along with 1 to 2 g. of bile salts to facilitate absorption. Menadione and menadione sodium bisulfite are oil soluble and water soluble, respectively; they are given in doses of 0.5 to 2 mg. daily. A highly water-soluble product is menadiol sodium diphosphate (Synkayvite). It can be given orally, subcutaneously, intramuscularly or intrave-

nously and usually is given in doses about three times those of menadione. Like menadione, it will hemolyze red blood cells in individuals deficient in glucose-6-phosphate dehydrogenase (G6PD) as well as in newborn, especially premature infants. Vitamin K_5 (Synkamin) is water soluble and has actions and uses similar to those of phytonadione and menadione.

The naturally occurring product termed vitamin K is composed of two substances, both with a naphthoquinone nucleus and similar physiologic properties. They are referred to as vitamin K_1 and vitamin K_2, of which the former is available as phytonadione (Mephyton). It is dispensed in 1-ml. ampuls containing 50 mg. of vitamin K_1 as a highly dispersed emulsion. The emergency use of these emulsions by intravenous injection has led to severe reactions in some cases. They do not antagonize heparin-produced incoagulability.

Aminocaproic acid (Amicar) inhibits fibrinolysis and is used in bleeding states with excessive fibrinolytic activity such as occur in open-heart surgery, bleeding of the urinary tract, neoplastic diseases, liver cirrhosis and abruptio placentae. This amino acid, which is related to lysine, inhibits the conversion of plasminogen to plasmin and also, to a less degree, directly inhibits the action of plasmin, which is the active fibrinolytic enzyme. In abruptio placentae, its administration may be followed by fibrinogen and whole blood. If hemorrhage is caused by diffuse intravascular coagulation (DIC), its use can be dangerous. Generalized peripheral thrombosis and thrombophlebitis have occurred following its administration. It should not be administered without a definite diagnosis, and/or laboratory findings indicative of hyperfibrinolysis. Safe use has not been established with respect to adverse effects upon fetal development. Aminocaproic acid may be given intravenously or orally and is excreted rapidly in the urine.

DRUGS USED FOR THEIR EFFECT ON BLOOD CELLS

Iron-Deficiency Anemias

The daily intake of available iron in the usual diet is from 10 to 20 mg., and only about 10 per cent of this is absorbed. In anemia, a daily one per cent rise in hemoglobin values can be accomplished if about 25 mg. of absorbed and completely utilized iron is provided. It is evident that food iron cannot supply the necessary utilizable iron following any serious loss. The amount of a medicinal salt, administered orally, needed to result in systemic absorption of 25 mg. of iron varies according to the percentage of ionized ferrous iron made available in the intestinal environment. A widely favored form is ferrous sulfate in tablets of 0.2 or 0.3 g. each, given in daily doses of about 1.0 g. Other widely used ferrous compounds include the gluconate, fumarate and lactate. These are well absorbed, but therapeutically equivalent doses produce gastrointestinal side-effects with about the same frequency as does the less expensive sulfate. More complex iron forms, such as the chelated ferric choline citrate, have shown no therapeutic advantage.

It is reasonably clear that iron is absorbed chiefly in the ferrous form, and ferric salts must be converted to the ferrous form to be absorbed and utilized. Absorption occurs chiefly from the duodenum, and the process involves a combination of the ferrous iron with the protein apoferritin. The combined product ferritin acts to regulate the intake of iron; in iron-deficiency anemias a relatively high proportion of medicinal iron is absorbed, whereas a mucosal block is interposed when there is no iron deficiency.

Iron preparations often cause abdominal cramps, loose stools or constipation. The formation of iron sulfide may make the stools black. Large accidental doses in children have caused intense gastrointestinal irritation with black, bloody stools. Serum Fe concentrations may rise to more than ten times normal values, with hypotension, hypoprothrombinemia and circulatory depression. Treatment consists of forming iron chelates, which are readily excreted in the urine. The most specific available iron-chelating agent is a bacterial product, deferoxamine (Desferal). Although not absorbed from the gastrointestinal tract, it is given orally to inhibit further iron absorption. Given parenterally, it will strikingly enhance renal iron excretion. The older chelating agent, calcium disodium edathamil, has also been used effectively.

Complex iron salts may be given intravenously or intramuscularly, but there is considerable local irritation, and excessive doses can lead to a condition resembling hemochromatosis. The rate of utilization of parenteral iron generally is not significantly greater than that following oral administration. Therefore, parenteral iron is indicated only when gastrointestinal complications exist. The body does not have an effective mechanism for removing rapidly the excess iron that can accumulate from parenteral administration.

An iron-dextran complex (Imferon) containing 50 mg. per ml. of elemental iron is available for intramuscular and intravenous administration and has had particular use in pediatric practice. Tattooing may occur unless it is given by deep intramuscular injection. The possibility that this agent might be carcinogenic has been discounted.

The addition of small amounts of other metals to antianemia preparations has been proposed from time to time. Generally, this is not considered to be necessary, although small amounts of copper may be of value in the case of infants receiving only cow's milk that is deficient in this element. Further, a zinc-deficiency syndrome along with iron anemia has been described in young males in localities of the Near East.

The response to iron medication depends chiefly on the level of hemoglobin values and the red cell count. A maximum response corresponds approximately to a one per cent rise in hemoglobin values daily and 250,000 red cells weekly. Reticulocyte counts may show as much as a 5 to 10 per cent increase during the first days of treatment.

Megaloblastic Anemias

The maturation defect in pernicious anemia and certain other megaloblastic anemias is considered to be the result of a deficiency of either folic acid or vitamin B_{12}. Vitamin B_{12} is essential to the functional integrity of parts of the central nervous system. Although folic acid can produce satisfactory hematologic responses, it does not prevent, and may even accelerate, the neurologic degeneration associated commonly with pernicious anemia.

Folic acid (pteroylglutamic acid) functions in the methylation of deoxyaridylate to thymidylate catalyzed by thymidylate synthetase. Thus, folate deficiency results in reduced deoxyribonucleic acid synthesis, which is quantitatively proportional to the rate of cellular turnover. This includes particularly the gut mucosa as well as the hemopoietic apparatus of the bone marrow. Its action depends on its enzymic conversion to the citrovorum factor (folinic acid), which is an N^5-formyl, tetrahydro derivative of folic acid. The 4-amino-N^{10} analog of folic acid (methotrexate) blocks this conversion as well as acting directly to antagonize the reduction of folic acid to the active form. Folic acid in 5 mg. tablets is administered orally for the management of nutritional macrocytic anemias and the anemias associated with tropical sprue and idiopathic steatorrhea. Folic acid is the preferred treatment in the macrocytic anemia of pregnancy and is useful in the megaloblastic anemia of infancy that occurs in conditions of ascorbic acid deficiency. Calcium leucovorin injection is an approved preparation of N-5 formyl FH_4 (folinic acid, citrovorum factor) of value in reversing the effects of folate antagonists (methotrexate).

Cyanocobalamin (vitamin B_{12}) is one of several compounds termed cobalamins that differ in that the cyano group may be replaced by a hydroxo group, a nitrito group or other groupings. These forms are convenient for administration but apparently must be converted in vivo to the active form, deoxyadenosylcobalamin.

Deoxyribonucleic acid production is reduced in human cells as a consequence of cobamide deficiency, but the exact mechanisms can only be inferred at present from pathways demonstrated in bacterial systems. One such reaction involves a reduction of ribonucleotides to the corresponding deoxyribonucleotides. A second important reaction involves the conversion of N_5-methyltetrahydrofolate to FH_4, with the transferred methyl being used in methionine synthesis. A requirement for B_{12} in proportionate catabolism in animals infers that this may be the cause of the neurologic defects observed in pernicious anemia. In support of this, humans with this disease have elevated urinary levels of methylmalonate and acetate.

Vitamin B_{12} is not synthesized in mammalian metabolism, and microorganisms represent the original natural source. *Streptomyces griseus*, the mold that produces streptomycin, is capable of high levels of production, and the residues from streptomycin furnish the present commercial source of cyanocobalamin.

In pernicious anemia patients, initial treatment may consist of intramuscular doses of 100 to 200 μg. of vitamin B_{12} daily with progressively decreasing doses, which may stabilize at 100 to 200 μg. per month. These doses, which are multiples of minimally effective doses, are considered justified by virtue of the nontoxicity of the agent and the seriousness of the condition being treated. Reticulocyte responses peak at 5 to 7 days. Iron preparations are sometimes used in the several weeks before erythrocyte counts reach normal levels. Maintenance of hematologic remission and protection against neurologic degeneration are accomplished by continued parenteral administration at intervals of about 2 to 4 weeks continued for the remainder of the life span. Orally administered, very large doses of cyanocobalamin with or without added intrinsic factor are not dependably absorbed, but such therapy is tried when parenteral administration is not available.

In the Schilling test for intrinsic factor, 2.0 μg. of cyanocobalamin-^{60}Co administered orally is followed in the next 24 hours by about 10 per cent excretion in the urine of normals and 2.5 per cent or less in patients with pernicious anemia. A flushing dose of 1 mg. of nonradioactive cyanocobalamin subcutaneously is necessary, because this agent has considerable binding affinity after absorption but can be displaced by a type of mass action.

Megaloblastic anemia following gastrectomy is slow in developing because of the high retention of stores of vitamin B_{12}. Fish tapeworm infestation apparently removes vitamin B_{12} and produces a megaloblastic anemia. Both of these conditions are treated effectively with cyanocobalamin. Other megaloblastic anemias that respond more suitably to folic acid, with possibly vitamin B_{12} in addition, include megaloblastic anemias of sprue, celiac disease, pregnancy, infancy, intestinal surgery and liver disease.

GENERAL ANESTHETICS

Principles

The basic mechanisms by which drugs produce a reversible depression of nervous activity are not clear. It has been proposed that anesthetics affect electrical charges, membrane permeability, colloidal aggregation or oxidative processes of nerve cells. The Meyer-Overton theory is simply a correlation between potency and the fat-water distribution coefficient of an anesthetic. According to this, the potency of anesthetics within a given series parallels their fat-water distribution coefficient. This has been shown to hold with fair consistency, for instance, with the volatile anesthetics, the barbiturates, the local anesthetics of the cocaine group and the experimental hypnotics of the substituted urea group. It may be considered as a correlation that explains the ability of a drug to leave aqueous body fluids and concentrate in the fat-rich nervous system. Again, the correlation may be related to the lipid of cell membranes in general. The correlation has been applied only to the potency of chemicals known to have anesthetic action and not to lipid-soluble agents with little or no anesthetic action. Some more mechanistic interpretation is needed to explain a common anesthetic effect among those agents known to produce anesthesia.

Pauling has proposed a concept that is based on formation of crystal hydrates (clathrates). These microcrystalline structures contain the anesthetic molecule in the center, as in a cage held together with physical bonding of a type that is much weaker than the usual covalent or ionic bonds. The formation of these structures is considered to reduce energy of electrical oscillations of a stimulant nature, or, again, catalytic activity of enzymes may be decreased by formation of the crystals in the neighborhood of their sites. Factors involved in crystal formation may include hydrogen bonding of water molecules; van der Waals interactions between the anesthetic and water molecules; size and shape of the anesthetic molecules and stabilization of the crystals by protein sidechains. Crystal formation is favored by lower temperatures and increased concentrations of the anesthetic agents. These interpretations have the merit of providing an acceptable concept for the reversibility of anesthetic effects.

The most intensive studies attempting to relate metabolism and anesthesia have demonstrated that some oxidative reactions are not affected by anesthetics, whereas others appear to be sensitive to anesthetics; possible blockade just preceding the cytochrome system has been suggested as being characteristic of anesthetics. Both the generation of high-energy phosphate compounds and the synthesis of acetylcholine have been shown to be depressed during anesthesia, and these reactions are related, respectively, to the energy of functional activity and to the permeability of cell membranes. Any explanation offered as a possible mechanism of anesthetic action is complicated by the difficulties in reconciling in vitro and in vivo observations, in proving that inhibitions are the cause and not the result of anesthetic depression and in extending the explanation to the widely diverse group of chemicals that can produce anesthesia. This group is impressive in its heterogeneity and includes aliphatic ethers (diethyl and divinyl); halogenated hydrocarbons (chloroform, ethyl chloride, trichloroethylene, halothane); halogenated ethers (methoxyflurane and fluoroxene); halogenated alcohols (tribromoethanol, chloral hydrate); paraldehyde; unsaturated hydrocarbons (ethylene, cyclopropane—the three-member cyclic structure of cyclopropane giving it these characteristics); noncombustible, relatively inert gases, nitrous oxide and xenon; barbiturates; magnesium salts; a steroid (hydroxydione); and a substituted thiazane. Some of the latter agents are not fully qualified as practical general anesthetics but appear to be capable of permitting surgical operations under some conditions. The same is true generally of intravenously administered morphine, meperidine and ethyl alcohol.

Stages of Anesthesia

Ordinarily the general anesthetics produce a descending depression of the central nervous system; however, the descending order is not strictly regular, since the cord is depressed before the medullary centers. The chief site of drug activity has been thought to be the reticular activating system of the brain stem. This multisynaptic pathway has been shown to be primarily responsible for the control of awake and sleep patterns as well as the integration of prolonged behavioral response to sensory perception. Anesthetic action at this level serves the dual purpose of producing sleep and decreasing sensory perception by reducing neural transmission to the cortex. Apparently this system is inactivated at lower anesthetic concentrations than are the classical spinothalamic and medial lemniscus pathways to the cortex, which are responsible for the immediate reflex response to sensory stimulation.

During administration of an inhalation anesthetic agent, the attainment and maintenance of a steady state of anesthesia depend primarily upon the equilibration of the partial pressure of the anesthetic in the tissues, blood and aveoli. Factors governing the rate at which a given partial pressure can be attained include the inspired concentration of the agent delivered to the alveoli and the solubility of the agent in the blood and tissues. The Ostwald solubility coefficient is often used to express the concentration of an agent in blood (liquid phase) relative to its concentration in the alveoli (gaseous phase). Agents exhibiting high Ostwald values such as diethyl ether (15) are highly soluble in blood, and the attainment of a high partial pressure and equilibrium is delayed. On the other hand, cyclopropane is relatively insoluble in blood (Ostwald coefficient 0.415), and equilibration of partial pressures and anesthesia are rapidly attained.

Anesthesia depth is judged by observing the patient's responses to stimuli; these responses include changes in rate and depth of respiration, heart rate, arterial pressure, skeletal muscle tone, and color and bleeding of incision. For purposes of identification, an arbitrary series of stages and planes has been defined according to the following progressive order:

Stage I (Analgesia and Altered Consciousness). Minor surgical operations and the second stage of parturition are possible.

Stage II (Delirium). Begins with loss of consciousness. Pupil often is dilated but reacts to light. Coughing and vomiting may occur, with danger of aspiration. Muscular tone may be increased. The patient should not be stimulated in any way during this stage.

Stage III (Surgical Anesthesia). Begins with onset of regular automatic breathing and muscular relaxation. Is further divided into the following planes:

Plane 1. Conjunctival, swallowing and pharyngeal (gag) reflexes abolished. Eyeballs eccentric, often roving.

Plane 2. Eyeballs fixed centrally. Excellent relaxation of skeletal muscles. Laryngeal reflex (cough) abolished. Most surgery is conducted in planes 1 and 2.

Plane 3. Intercostal activity begins to decrease or is delayed. Depth of respiration reduced. Reflex to light decreases. Pupillary dilation may occur with ether.

Plane 4. Intercostal activity paralyzed. Only diaphragmatic jerk (or gasp) present. Pupils dilated wide with most anesthetics. Lacrimation absent.

Stage IV (Respiratory Arrest, Medullary Paralysis). Diaphragmatic movements cease. The pulse is slow and feeble, and blood pressure is at shock level. These signs become progressively less discernible, and the stage is terminated by cardiac failure and death.

During recovery the patient goes through the same planes and stages in the reverse order.

This descriptive definition of the various levels of anesthesia is essentially that presented by Guedel in

1937. Similar descriptions have been presented by numerous other observers at intervals since the period of Morton's anesthesia demonstration in 1846. The conditions are primarily those of ether anesthesia without premedication, and with cyclopropane, for instance, anesthesia may proceed so rapidly that some of these signs will be missed. With thiopental, respiration may be depressed relatively more than the reflex responses. Similarly, although stage I usually is not considered to be a basis for major surgery, highly specialized conditions have permitted, for instance, cardiac surgery at this level of depression.

Volatile Liquid Anesthetics

Ether boils at slightly more than ordinary room temperature (35° C.) and is flammable. Although its use has declined in recent years, it is probably safest in the hands of the less experienced. It produces good muscular relaxation with relatively slight cardiac effects. As contrasted with chloroform, it has longer periods of induction and recovery. In common with chloroform, it increases respiratory minute volume in the early planes of stage III. This is an effect of medullary stimulation or pulmonary reflexes followed by depression as anesthesia deepens. Also in common with chloroform, it causes nausea and vomiting and significant metabolic disturbances (acidosis, hyperglycemia). The hyperglycemia and other metabolic changes during ether anesthesia have been shown to be due to increased plasma levels of epinephrine and norepinephrine brought about by sympathoadrenal discharge. This occurs with some other inhalation anesthetics but does not occur with barbiturates. Cardiac depression by volatile anesthetics would be manifested more conspicuously if this counterbalancing sympathoadrenal effect were not present. Ether and most other general anesthetics cause temporary oliguria due largely to increased secretion of the pituitary antidiuretic hormone.

Vinyl ether (Vinethene) was used at one time rather extensively for induction of general anesthesia and for short operations. It is now obsolete.

Chloroform is characterized by special cardiac and hepatic toxicity. It is seldom used today as a general anesthetic.

Halothane (2-bromo-2-chloro-1,1,1-trifluoroethane, Fluothane) chemically and pharmacologically is closely similar to chloroform. It is nonflammable, boils at 50.2° C., does not react with the usual carbon dioxide adsorbents and is rapid in onset and recovery. Hypotension is pronounced, especially at deeper levels of anesthesia. Apparently the hypotension is due, in part, to myocardial depression, which is of about the same degree as occurs with chloroform. Liver damage is less severe than with chloroform and is more nearly of the same order as with ether; however, this agent is not recommended for use in biliary surgery or in patients with a history of liver disease. There have been reports that halothane sensitized the heart to epinephrine and other inotropic sympathomimetic amines, and caution should be used when these drugs are used during halothane anesthesia.

Fluroxene (2,2,2-trifluoroethyl vinyl ether) has anesthetic potency similar to that of ether. Its boiling point is 43.2° C., and it is flammable in concentrations above four per cent. The flammability limit is raised somewhat when it is used in a closed system, because of the accumulation of water vapor. Tachypnea is a common occurrence during light surgical levels of anesthesia.

Methoxyflurane (2,2-dichloro-1,1-difluoroethyl methyl ether) (Penthrane) is characterized by a slow induction and a prolonged recovery period. The recovery time can be shortened markedly by discontinuing the use of the agent about 30 minutes before the completion of the procedure. Because of the high boiling point (104.8° C.), vaporization of methoxyflurane is somewhat difficult. The effects on the cardiovascular and the respiratory systems are similar to those of halothane. Postoperative analgesia is reported to be good, and the need for postoperative narcotics is reduced. An ashen skin color postoperatively is somewhat characteristic, even in those patients who have normal blood pressure. A nephrotoxic effect has been associated with methoxyflurane that is apparently due to the liberation of free fluoride ions. This syndrome is a high output renal failure consisting of hypernatremia, increased serum osmolarity and BUN, and a delayed return to a normal renal concentrating ability.

Enflurane (2-chloro-1,1,2-trifluoroethyl difluoromethyl ether) (Ethrane) is a relatively new halogenated hydrocarbon anesthetic with a boiling point of 56.5° C. It is characterized by fast induction and a rapid recovery time. Its effects on the cardiovascular and respiratory systems are similar to those observed with halothane. Metabolic degradation of enflurane with the liberation of free flurorine is less than that observed with other halogenated agents, and no serious liver or renal toxicity has been attributed to its use. Increased motor activity has been reported at deep levels of anesthesia and appears to be exacerbated by low arterial levels of carbon dioxide.

Anesthetic Gases

The ordinary anesthetic gases are very rapid in their action and do not produce metabolic disturbances as profound as those of ether or chloroform. They must be mixed with oxygen or air in definite proportions, by means of special machines. Closed-system arrangements, using a tightly fitting mask or tracheal catheter and a canister of soda lime for absorption of carbon dioxide, enormously reduce the amount of gas needed for anesthesia.

Nitrous oxide is nonflammable but will support the combustion of flammable anesthetics in the same way as oxygen. Explosions have occurred with the mixtures obtained after the addition of ether to reinforce the effect of nitrous oxide. Induction and recovery are exceptionally rapid with nitrous oxide, which is frequently used for short operations requiring only slight relaxation. Muscular relaxation with nitrous oxide is obtained only after heavy preanesthetic medication or in the extremely debilitated. Nitrous oxide is relatively free from any direct toxic effects; hence, its dangers are chiefly those attributable to anoxia (cerebral degeneration and cardiovascular accidents).

Ethylene is flammable and, in mixtures with oxygen, has been the cause of disastrous explosions. It is generally similar to nitrous oxide in action but is more potent, and, in the usual anesthetic mixtures with oxygen (80:20 to 90:10), it does not present such serious disadvantages of anoxia.

Cyclopropane is chemically related to ethylene, and its pharmacologic actions generally approximate those of ethylene, with a significantly increased anesthetic potency. Anesthetic mixtures with oxygen (10:90 to 40:60) carry no disadvantage of anoxia and even may introduce some minor complications due to the excess oxygen present. The mixtures are flammable and explosive. Unlike chloroform and ether, cyclopropane does not stimulate respiratory movements, and respiration proceeds smoothly until depressed in deep anesthesia. Cyclopropane causes cardiac arrhythmias recognizable by pulse irregularities, and this happens more frequently with deep anesthesia than with light anesthesia. These arrhythmias may be related to the increased sympathoadrenal activity that occurs in deep cyclopropane anesthesia. Epinephrine or a sudden sharp stimulus may produce ventricular fibrillation in a heart sensitized by cyclopropane. At the same level of anesthesia as with ether, even ten times the dose of epinephrine will not produce arrhythmias. The arrhythmias induced by epinephrine under cyclopropane anesthesia can be induced by other sympathomimetic amines also. Pressor amines not exhibiting this sensitizing effect are characterized also by the absence of positive inotropic actions.

Ethyl chloride is a gas at ordinary room temperature but may be stored as a liquid under moderate pressure (boiling point 12.5° C.). Induction and recovery are especially rapid, although it does not give smooth relaxation. It is not suitable for long operations but has been used in the past for induction and for short proce-

dures. Cardiac irregularities have been observed during ethyl chloride anesthesia, and, apparently, ethyl chloride sensitizes the myocardium to epinephrine in the same way that cyclopropane does. An incidental use is based on its local anesthetic action when it is used as a refrigerating spray. However, a drawback of this practice is that occasionally it produces tissue necrosis.

Ethyl chloride burns with a green flame, giving off HCl.

Trichloroethylene (Trilene) has been used as a general anesthetic since about 1944, but ordinarily its use is limited to stages no deeper than plane 1. Disadvantages are tachypnea, hepatic damage and cardiac arrhythmias with occasional arrest. Although the commercial product is well purified and stabilized, it decomposes under some abnormal conditions of storage, yielding dichloracetylene and other toxic products that injure cranial nerves and, in extreme cases, cause a type of encephalitis. High boiling point (87° C.) and reactivity with soda lime prevent its being used by the usual routine methods. Soda lime accidentally exposed to trichloroethylene should be discarded. Trichloroethylene is most favored as an analgesic in about 0.5 per cent concentration in air, and self-inhalers are in common use. Since about 1915, it has been used for trigeminal neuralgia and in some cases is highly effective at early stage I levels. It is not flammable, except at high concentrations of oxygen.

Nonvolatile General Anesthetics

In contrast with the volatile inhalation anesthetics, drugs that are administered by vein or by rectum always carry the special danger of a drug whose action cannot be recalled. The danger is obviated to some degree by cautious administration in installments, depending on the symptomatic condition of the patient.

Barbiturates were introduced first as sedatives or hypnotics and were not considered seriously as anesthetic agents until the later development of shorter-acting variations with a better margin of safety. Historically the first representatives, barbital (Veronal) and phenobarbital (Luminal) were introduced in the early 1900s and were used only as sedatives during the considerable period before the development of various shorter-acting types in the late 1920s.

In barbital and phenobarbital, the ethyl and the phenyl groupings substituted in the malonic acid of barbituric acid (malonyl urea) are relatively stable in both the test tube and the metabolic processes of the body. Accordingly these compounds are metabolized relatively little by the body and are excreted largely by the kidney. Barbital can be recovered unchanged from the urine to the extent of about 75 per cent of dose; phenobarbital, to about 20 per cent. The slower rate of elimination is manifested in a prolonged period of action, and if these compounds should be given in anesthetic doses, recovery will not take place for several days.

If the ethyl and the phenyl groupings of these compounds are substituted by less stable groupings, containing, for instance, double bonds, side-chains and saturated cyclic structures, the resulting products are metabolized more rapidly by the body, the greatest destruction taking place in the liver. The period of action of such compounds is briefer, and in the more favorable examples, the margin of safety is greater than in the older, more stable class. The ultrashort-acting barbiturates pass with special rapidity into the fat depots, from which location they later may be released slowly. These shorter-acting compounds have proved to be useful as intravenous anesthetics. The danger inherent in such fixed anesthetics as against inhalation anesthetics is minimized by cautious administration of the barbiturate in installments as the symptomatic condition of the patient changes.

In general, it is considered to be most suitable to obtain basal narcosis with these agents and to complement the anesthetic effect with nitrous oxide or curare preparations. When these compounds are administered to the point of surgical anesthesia, recovery to near normal occurs ordinarily in 12 to 18 hours with amobarbital (Amytal); in 4 to 6 hours with pentobarbital (Nembutal); and in 1 to 2 hours with thiopental (Pentothal). These products with progressively shorter periods of action were developed in that order.

There is a special use for amobarbital in conditions requiring relatively prolonged depression, as in tetanus, status epilepticus, status asthmaticus or violent psychoses. Thiopental is the anesthetic used most routinely. In this group of ultrashort-acting anesthetics, an older drug of European origin is hexobarbital (Evipal), and later drugs are thiamylal (Surital) and methohexital (Brevital). Thiamylal is claimed to exhibit less of the side-effects of thiopental, which are laryngospasm, occasional bouts of sneezing and wheezing and particularly the intense respiratory depression. With thiopental the usual signs of anesthetic depth are not reliable; occasionally, first-plane reflexes may occur with fourth-plane respiratory depression. Porphyria contraindicates the use of barbiturates.

Secobarbital (Seconal) is essentially similar to pentobarbital, with a slightly larger dose and a slightly shorter period of action.

Any of these barbiturates can be used as sedatives or hypnotics if they are administered orally in small fractions of the anesthetic dose. Besides those already mentioned, a considerable number are in common use.

The characteristic action of these compounds is a relatively uniform depression of central nervous system activity. In sedative doses they are not analgesic, and, in the presence of severe pain, a patient may exhibit greater restlessness because of the mild paralysis of inhibitory cortical centers. Sedative doses are combined commonly with analgesic drugs.

In contrast with the use of small oral doses, moderate doses given intravenously can provide relief from pain. Pentobarbital sodium, in doses of 60 mg. given intravenously, relieves postoperative pain in about half the instances, whereas morphine, in doses of 8 mg. given intravenously under the same conditions gives relief to about 80 per cent of patients.

There are few individual distinctions among barbiturates other than the speed of action, the dose and the margin of safety. Thiopental tends to sensitize the vagus; amobarbital and pentobarbital tend to paralyze the vagus. Phenobarbital specially raises the threshold of cortical excitability, which is a late-experimental justification of its long-standing use in epilepsy. Mephobarbital has effects of the same type.

The free barbituric acid or the sodium salt of these compounds may be prepared in oral dosage forms. The free acid is water insoluble, and usually the liquid dosage form is prepared in an elixir vehicle. The sodium salts of barbiturates are relatively unstable in aqueous solution, and such solutions must be prepared fresh when they are to be used with anesthetics. The rectal route of administration has been used to a considerable degree with hexobarbital and to a lesser degree with thiopental.

Intramuscular or subcutaneous injection of the soluble sodium salts is complicated by the considerable degree of local irritation, with possible resulting abscess formation. Sodium phenobarbital is an exception, and the suitability of injecting sodium phenobarbital by these routes probably has been the basis for its widespread popularity as a sedative, a preoperative medicant and an anticonvulsant, all despite its being notably the longest acting of the barbiturates, often not taking effect as quickly as desired and maintaining an effect much longer than desired. For such use, stable solutions of sodium phenobarbital in 60 per cent propylene glycol in water are available commercially. The need for a short-acting barbiturate suitable for intramuscular administration is very obvious. To some extent the need has been met by an ampul preparation of pentobarbital sodium in propylene glycol, alcohol and water. This preparation can be tolerated satisfactorily, but occasionally it produced abscesses.

The use of these compounds as sedatives, which is widespread, carries the same possibility of habit formation as does that of any group of depressant drugs with minimal side-effects. Such use represents an escape mechanism in the same way as does the use of alcohol. A true physical dependence now is recognized among the chronic users of barbiturates. This has been observed chiefly in the U.S. Public Health Service hospitals at Lexington and Fort Worth, where there has been a special concentration of patients addicted to drugs. Withdrawal symptoms include convulsions and psychotic states; no characteristic anatomic damage remains.

Overdose of barbiturates is common, due both to accident and to suicidal intent. Treatment is essentially the maintenance of oxygenation, as the respiratory center is depressed at considerably lower concentrations of the drug than is the heart. A patent airway (endotracheal catheter, if tolerated) and artificial continuance of external respiratory movements are the basic treatment. Besides the conventional respirators acting on the thoracic cage, there are several mechanical devices that act directly on the atmosphere leading into the airway, thereby providing interrupted positive pressure or alternating positive and negative pressures. Oxygen administration can be helpful, as long as mechanical respiration is continued; it can be harmful in the absence of mechanically assisted respiration, since it may remove the stimulus arising from the chemoreceptors of the carotid and the aortic bodies. The artificial kidney has been used effectively to reduce blood levels of barbiturate by hemodialysis. Mannitol diuresis and alkalinization of the urine may hasten elimination. Such measures may be especially helpful in the case of overdoses of phenobarbital, which notoriously is prolonged in its action. Spectrophotometric determinations of blood levels can be decisive in establishing the diagnosis of barbiturate poisoning. Present methods of determining intensity of absorption in the ultraviolet are capable of estimating blood levels as low as one tenth the fatal level. Identification and measurement of barbiturates in the blood by gas chromatography may be done.

SELECTIVE PAIN CONTROL

By contrast with agents capable of total depression of the central nervous system, there have been numerous attempts to selectively diminish central pain perception and conduction, particularly in relation to surgical conditions that do not require a high degree of muscular relaxation. Earliest trials included intravenous administration of alcohol or opiates or, again, traditional general anesthetics at stage I levels. Considerable experience has developed with the morphine-scopolamine twilight sleep method; the promethazine combinations termed lytic cocktail; and tranquilizers

such as haloperidol, a butyrophenone. A recent combination of a potent butyrophenone tranquilizer (droperidol) with a narcotic analgesic (fentanyl) has resulted in a compound (Innovar) that produces a state termed neuroleptanesthesia. This state is characterized by reduced motor activity and profound analgesia without a complete loss of consciousness. A phencyclidine compound (Ketamine) acts as a dissociative type of drug, with apparent predominant activity in the cortical frontal areas. These agents are especially subject to psychic alterations in the emergence period, producing vivid dreams, delirium and hallucinations.

OTHER CENTRAL NERVOUS SYSTEM DEPRESSANTS

Alcohols

Ethyl alcohol is a central nervous system depressant, acting generally as a weak anesthetic, most of which is eliminated by slow metabolic destruction. Oxidation to acetaldehyde is the first metabolic stage and is due to action of alcohol dehydrogenase, with nicotinamide adenine dinucleotide as the hydrogen acceptor; acetaldehyde in turn is converted to acetate by adlehyde oxidase, and the acetate is metabolized, through the tricarboxylic cycle, to carbon dioxide. The average oxidation rate (about 10 ml. per hour) allows about 1,300 calories per day as a theoretic maximum—an appreciable energy value but only a fraction of the total caloric requirements. Alcohol cannot be utilized in tissue formation, and most alcoholic drinks contain only slight amounts of accessory food values, hence malnutrition and vitamin deficiencies may be the most prominent features of chronic alcoholism. Gastritis, kidney damage and liver cirrhosis may occur in the chronic alcoholic, but the incidence is not spectacularly greater than among nonalcoholics. Mental disorders occur with significant frequency and may include Korsakoff's syndrome and delirium tremens.

Institutional management of the chronic alcoholic has involved the use of various nauseants intended to create conditioned reflexes that favor abstinence. The drug tetraethythiuram disulfide (Antabuse), if ingested in adequate dosage, will produce a highly disagreeable and, at times, dangerous reaction when there is subsequent ingestion of alcohol. Alcohol ingestion 12 hours after intake of Antabuse results commonly in intense erythema of the upper body, pulsating headache, tachypnea and tachycardia. The effect is thought to be due to the formation of considerable amounts of acetaldehyde, possibly by antagonism of aldehyde oxidase.

In ordinary individuals, blood levels of alcohol approximately parallel the state of acute intoxication and are accepted as medicolegal evidence. A subjective sensation of stimulation (release from control by higher centers) and euphoria occur with concentrations up to 80 mg. per 100 ml.; emotional instability and motor incoordination occur with 80 to 100 mg. per 100 ml.; "legal" drunkenness, with 150 mg. per 100 ml.; approach of paralysis, with 200 to 400 mg. per 100 ml.; and death with 700 mg. per 100 ml.

Because of the characteristic vasomotor paralysis and dilation of peripheral vessels, some recommend moderate amounts of alcohol in peripheral vascular disease and coronary disease. Gastric secretion is stimulated by moderate doses, and for this reason, alcohol sometimes is recommended before meals. However, in this case, the psychologic effects of relaxation probably are more important. Diuresis observed in drinkers of alcoholic beverages is due to ingestion of fluid and also to inhibition of release of antidiuretic hormone from the posterior lobe of the pituitary.

Methyl alcohol resembles ethyl alcohol in its depressant action. However, it is detoxified more slowly and has a special propensity for the optic nerve and the retinal cells, occasionally causing blindness. Its wide use as an industrial solvent is largely responsible for its frequent implication in cases of occupational or accidental poisoning. Methanol is converted into formic acid and produces acidosis. Therapy consists of alkalinization; correction of the acidotic state with sodium bicarbonate given intravenously or orally is the most important antidotal procedure. Since ethanol retards conversion to formic acid, its use has been proposed in the treatment of methanol poisoning—a suggestion more interesting than practical.

Isopropyl alcohol is a byproduct of the petroleum industry and is used extensively as a substitute for ethyl alcohol in external medicinal preparations principally for disinfection of the skin. Its physiologic actions resemble those of ethyl alcohol, although it is distinctly more potent. The fatal dose is about 120 to 240 cc. In severe, nonfatal cases marked renal impairment occurs.

Sedatives and Hypnotics

A considerable number of drugs, varying widely in their chemical types, are used for promoting or producing sleep. When their doses are increased beyond the sedative or hypnotic range, in some cases they may produce surgical anesthesia. Ordinarily, however, they are not used for this purpose because of an unsuitable range of safety, too prolonged period of action, incomplete muscular relaxation or other reasons. Selection of these compounds as sedatives or hypnotics usually is based on opinions as to their period of action, their

smoothness of action, their freedom from after effects (such as confusion and headache) and their relative incidence of toxic reactions (such as dermatitis, blood dyscrasias and asthmatic seizures). All drugs producing such narcosis of the higher centers result in the tendency to develop habit formation, particularly among neurotic individuals given to self medication. Occasionally, large doses are taken by accident or with suicidal intent and may cause death by respiratory depression or prolonged coma and late bronchopneumonia. Such cases are treated by gastric lavage, if oral ingestion was recent, and by artificial respiration, oxygen, general supportive measures (heat, intravenous saline and mannitol) and the very cautious use of analeptics.

Commonly used short-acting hypnotics are chloral hydrate (usual dose 1 g.) and pentobarbital sodium (usual dose 0.1 g.). Intermediate in duration of action is paraldehyde (usual dose 10 ml.). Longest in duration of action are such drugs as phenobarbital (usual dose range 30 to 100 mg.). Numerous proprietary barbiturates are available. These differ from one another chiefly in their period of action. Phenobarbital is used to lessen the incidence and the severity of epileptic seizures. Glutethimide (Doriden), with a glutaramide structure, resembles phenobarbital, and, although it has been used only as a sedative, its overdose effects are typical of barbiturates.

All of these sedatives produce anesthesia at high dose levels. A few compounds have been used that produce sedating or quieting effects without being truly anesthetic in higher doses. In this category may be listed bromides, ethchlorvynol (Placidyl), methyprylon (Noludar), ethinamate (Valmid), carbromal, methaqualone (Quaalude) and flurazepam (Dalmane).

Monoamine oxidase inhibitors may potentiate the depressant effects of barbiturates. In general, doses of the sedative-hypnotics must be reduced when given with other central nervous system depressants (e.g. antihistamines, alcohol, antianxiety agents).

Tranquilizers

The antipsychotic agents (neuroleptics), formerly termed major tranquilizers, modify the symptoms of acute and chronic psychoses. They include the substituted phenothiazines, the substituted thioxanthenes, the substituted butyrophenones and the alkaloids of Rauwolfia. The term minor tranquilizers, or antianxiety agent, is used for those drugs that are useful in the treatment of anxieties and neuroses but are not effective antipsychotic agents. The principal drugs in the latter group are the benzodiazepines and meprobamate. The phenothiazine group is credited generally with a substantial reduction in the institutional care needed for psychotic patients. Double-blind studies of institutionalized schizophrenic patients have shown significant superiority of these drugs over placebo treatment. For the noninstitutionalized neurotic patient, there is not much documentation of results that differ significantly from those obtained with traditional sedatives.

The antipsychotic agents produce a wide variety of adverse reactions. Some are allergic or idiosyncratic in nature, and others result from their secondary action on the central and autonomic nervous systems.

Chlorpromazine (Thorazine) was the first of the phenothiazine derivatives to receive clinical trials. Its introduction about 1951 followed the observation that the antihistaminic, promethazine (Phenergan), with a phenothiazine nucleus, exhibited sedative and calming effects. Chlorpromazine reduces emotional activity and in animals has a taming effect similar to that of reserpine. It causes some drowsiness, increases the sleeping time of general anesthetics and increases the subjective relief associated with typical analgesics. Certain types of vomiting, as with apomorphine, are antagonized by chlorpromazine through blockage of the chemoreceptor trigger zone, although it is not effective against motion sickness or digitalis-induced vomiting. Chlorpromazine is a weak-to-moderate sympatholytic, parasympatholytic, local anesthetic and antihistaminic. On the circulatory system it is hypotensive, accelerates heart rate, antagonizes pressor-receptor reflexes and suppresses cardiac arrhythmias. Although it can be given intravenously or intramuscularly, chlorpromazine usually is given orally. The timed-release preparation has no significant advantage over ordinary oral dosage forms since the drug has a prolonged half-life. Most of the drug is metabolized by several routes: sulfoxidation, demethylation, ring hydroxylation and glucuronide conjugation, or oxidation at the terminal nitrogen of the side-chain. The liver is the chief site of destruction and can metabolize substantial amounts of the drug in the anuric state. Side effects include parkinsonism-like states, drowsiness, orthostatic hypotension (especially after parenteral administration), jaundice, skin eruptions and bone marrow depression; although the last named is recognized, there is a relatively low incidence of agranulocytosis. Loss of ejaculation develops occasionally. Miosis with pinpoint pupils has occurred with large doses. Endocrine types of effects, such as polyuria, polydipsia and weight gain, have been reported. Like reserpine, it causes nasal stuffiness and dry mouth. The jaundice appears to be obstructive in type, usually is not associated with important changes in liver function tests and may disappear during continued administration of the drug. Jaundice in the newborn has been thought possibly to be due to phenothiazines administered to mothers during labor; evidence indicates this is likely only in the instance of premature infants. In addition to its use in anxious, agitated states, chlorpromazine is used in preanesthetic medication, in combination with analgesics and as an antiemetic.

One of the chemical variants, trimeprazine (Temaril), exhibits relatively greater antihistaminic activity than promethazine and finds special indication in pruritus. Another, methotrimeprazine (Levoprome) is a strong analgesic, having an analgesic potency about half that of morphine on a milligram basis. Other phenothiazines are promoted chiefly as antiemetics.

Attached to the nitrogen atom of the phenothiazine nucleus in chlorpromazine is a straight three-carbon chain with terminal substituted amino grouping; this is also true of promazine (Sparine) and triflupromazine (Vesprin). In treatment of neuroses, the oral daily dose of these derivatives is in the range of 150 to 400 mg.; in psychoses, the dose is about doubled. Mepazine (Pacatal) and thioridazine (Mellaril), each with a piperidine side-chain, are somewhat similar both in dose range and in general characteristics. Promazine and mezapine have produced an unusually high incidence of seizures.

The introduction of additional halogens increases the potency of phenothiazine derivatives. Generally, lower doses are used with the group containing a piperazine side-chain; doses range downward through prochlorperazine (Compazine), thiopropazate (Dartal), perphenazine (Trilafon), trifluoperazine (Stelazine) and fluphenazine (Permitil). This group with a piperazine side-chain produces less sedation but a higher incidence of extrapyramidal symptoms (parkinsonism, motor restlessness, etc.); however, these side-actions are not requisite for or parallel to therapeutic results. The side actions occur about twice as often in women as in men. Extrapyramidal effects frequently respond well to antiparkinsonism agents of the anticholinergic type. Tolerance or addiction is not characteristic of this group of drugs. It is current belief that the antipsychotic mechanism of action is through a central adrenergic blocking action that prevents the release of the amines from storage sites.

Reserpine is one of about 20 alkaloids that have been obtained from *Rauwolfia serpentina,* a long-time medicinal plant of Indian folklore. The alkaloid, synthesized in 1956, has a chemical nucleus resembling yohimbine and, like sertonin and lysergic acid derivatives, contains an idole moiety. The whole dried root (Raudixin), the extracts (Rauwiloid) and the alkaloid have had prominence both as tranquilizing and as bradycardiac-hypotensive agents.

It was recognized in 1955 that reserpine reduces

the concentration of serotonin (5-hydroxytryptamine) in the brain and, later, that it reduces the concentration of norepinephrine in the brain, the adrenals, the heart and the blood vessels. In human atrial appendages, assays have confirmed the observations in animals, with a clear demonstration of norepinephrine depletion in reserpinized patients. In blood platelets, reserpine reduces the serotonin either in vitro or in vivo. Reserpine acts as an analog, combining with the serotonin receptors and, thus, displacing this agent. Effects of depletion continue for some time after reserpine is no longer present. (By contrast, *chlorpromazine* does not deplete serotonin or norepinephrine but does interfere with the action of serotonin. Similarly, it interferes to some degree with the action of histamine, epinephrine or norepinephrine. Some interpretations of the action of chlorpromazine are based on its being a strong electron donor.) Although the antipsychotic effectiveness of both the substituted phenothiazines and reserpine depend upon an adrenergic blocking effect, these agents are antagonistic because the antiadrenergic effects of reserpine are accomplished by transmitter depletion, while those of the phenothiazines are accomplished by preventing the release of the transmitter.

In animals, a taming effect, with markedly reduced hostility responses, can be demonstrated. Relaxation of the nictitating membrane, ptosis and miosis are characteristic, and the last named has been used as a type of bioassay; these effects can be overcome readily by sympathomimetic drugs. In patients side effects include nasal stuffiness (relieved by nose drops of atropine solutions), postural hypotension, parkinsonism-like effects with rigidity and tremors, gastrointestinal hypermotility and increased secretory activity. Peptic ulcers are activated by the increased secretory activity. More extreme nervous reactions include marked fatigue, paradoxical agitation and paranoid and suicidal tendencies. There is an enormous range between the usual dose and the amounts that have been taken by individuals who survived after taking excessive amounts.

Reserpine preparations are not much favored now as psychiatric agents, although they are of considerable mechanistic interest. Some of these preparations are listed in the section on antihypertensive agents.

Thioxanthenes.   The substituted thioxanthenes are structural analogs of the phenothiazines, and the overall range of activity and side effects is similar. Two drugs in their class are marketed currently. They are chlorprothixene (Taractan) and thiothixene (Navane).

Butyrophenones.   The substituted butyrophenones have certain structural similarities to GABA, but interactions with this agent are not thought to be involved in the mechanisms of action. Haloperidol (Haldol) is equivalent in effectiveness to that of some of the phe-

nothiazines, to which it is pharmacologically but not chemically related. It is recommended for use in the manic phase of manic-depressive psychosis, in schizophrenia and involutional, senile, organic, and toxic psychoses. It is a potent antiemetic. Adverse effects suggest the same pattern of actions as seen with phenothiazines. They may appear with low doses but in general seem to be dose related.

Lithium carbonate is effective in the treatment of the manic phase of manic-depressive psychosis. Flurothyl (Indoklon), a convulsive agent, is used occasionally in treating severe depressive psychosis. Given by inhalation, it has the same indications and attendant risks as electroconvulsive therapy.

Benzodiazepines.   Currently, a growing number of drugs in this class are used in the US: chlordiazepoxide (Librium), diazepam (Valium), oxazepam (Serax), clorazepate (Tranxene), prazepam (Nerstran), and lorazepam (Ativan). These constitute the most important class of antianxiety agents. In addition to their effects on anxieties, benzodiazepines have pronounced skeletal muscle-relaxing and anticonvulsant properties. These agents have a high therapeutic index and produce less cortical depression than barbiturates. Their site of action is believed to be in the limbic system. Present evidence suggests an interaction between the benzodiazepines and the allosteric protein modulator of GABA recognition sites. They increase the affinity of GABA receptors for GABA, an inhibitory transmitter in the CNS.

Although benzodiazepines are considered most useful in the unagressive, anxiety-ridden individual, they have been observed to induce anxiety in individuals not initially anxious and have induced hostility reactions in anxious individuals with inadequate control of impulses. Long-term use of larger than usual therapeutic doses may cause psychic and physical dependence. In recent years they have become associated with widespread drug abuse. With chlordiazepoxide, extreme care must be used in giving it to patients with impaired hepatic or renal function.

Meprobamate (Miltown, Equanil), a substituted propanediol dicarbamate, exhibits a blocking action on the interneurons of the spinal cord and a relatively pronounced effect on the thalamus. Electrical recordings from the thalamus show that low doses produce a slowing of frequency and an increase in voltage. The cortex, the hypothalamus and the autonomic systems are not affected much. The drug has been used extensively in the anxiety and tension states and in conditions requiring muscle-relaxant effects. However, meprobamate is little different from other sedatives, and the described tranquilizing and muscle-relaxing effects are not unique. Adverse reactions are usually of a minor nature. Like the barbiturates, meprobamate has been observed to cause true addiction after prolonged administration of high doses. Numerous other antianxiety drugs are marketed. They include phenaglycodol (Ultran), tybamate (Solacen), hydroxyzine (Atarax), azacyclonol (Frenquel), and benactyzine (Suavitil).

Anticonvulsants; Antiepileptics

Drug management of epilepsy began with the observation in 1857 that bromides would reduce the incidence and the severity of seizures. The use of bromides for this purpose became very general, and about 1900 the annual consumption by one English hospital was estimated at 2 tons. Phenobarbital was introduced for the same purpose in 1912, and these two drugs constituted the sole treatment until the observation in 1938 that diphenylhydantoin (Phenytoin) raised the threshold of electrical excitability in animals without producing the same degree of somnolence and ataxia as phenobarbital; clinical trials demonstrated that this chemical was highly effective in grand mal epilepsy. This successful experimental approach to the problem of epilepsy quickly resulted in the introduction of trimethadione (Tridione) as the drug of choice in management of petit mal, and, in turn, has been followed by the development of a considerable number of synthetics with varying patterns of usefulness. Experimental screening procedures include the use of electric shock techniques in animals and determinations of threshold convulsive doses of drugs such as pentylenetetrazol and strychnine. Low sodium levels, thyroid or cortisone lowers the threshold for convulsions, while high sodium levels, thyroidectomy and DOCA raise the threshold; these features may be regulated or varied deliberately in conjunction with the various tests of cortical excitability. EEG patterns are helpful indicators in the experimental procedures.

Bromides no longer are considered important in the management of epilepsy, and their current interest is related chiefly to frequent instances of bromide intoxication, which develops most commonly after self-medication with proprietary sedative mixtures. The cumulative characteristics of bromides are responsible for this type of chronic intoxication. Their body distribution is largely extracellular, although the bromide ion readily enters red blood cells. The ratio of bromides to chlorides is relatively uniform in the extracellular fluids and is about the same in the urine, which is the predominant route of excretion. The lack of preferential secretion of bromide over chloride by the kidney is the basis for its relatively slow elimination and its ready cumulation on continued ingestion. The toxic level of serum bromide is about 150 to 200 mg. per 100 ml. (20 to 25 mEq. per liter), while twice that level usually is fatal. Neurologic disturbances and acneiform dermatitis are common toxic effects. Sodium chloride excess will hasten elimination of bromides. Hemodialysis by the artificial kidney has been used to reduce extreme levels of serum bromides.

Phenobarbital, more than most barbituates, raises the theshold for electroshock seizures. This was not recognized until after it had been found empirically to be useful in grand mal epilepsy. Two other barbiturates have had some similar use but with more suitability for the petit mal type of epilepsy; these are mephobarbital (Mebaral) and metharbital (Gemonil). Primidone (Mysoline) is related chemically to phenobarbital, the only difference being the presence of two hydrogen atoms in place of oxygen in the urea grouping. It has been favored in grand mal and in psychomotor seizures.

Diphenylhydantoin (Phenytoin) probably acts to prevent the spread of excessive discharges in the motor cortex and of those originating in the thalamus. In experimental animals, it does not effectively antagonize convulsive drugs such as pentylenetetrazol but modifies greatly the character of electroshock convulsions. The interseizure EEG in patients with grand mal or with psychomotor seizures may be improved in terms of diffuse abnormalities, while an abnormal focus may be defined more sharply. The maximum daily oral dose usually is considered to be 0.6 g. Characteristic toxic effects include hirsutism and gum hyperplasia, the latter resembling a vitamin C deficiency; excessive overdoses produce excitation; mephenytoin is a close chemical variant of Phenytoin; bone marrow depression is a serious hazard in its use.

Trimethadione (Tridione), an oxazolidine derivative, is conspicuous for the degree to which it raises the threshold dose of pentylenetetrazol-induced convulsions. Commonly, in petit mal it abolishes both seizures and the characteristic spike-and-wave EEG abnormality. Oral doses range from 1 to 2 g. daily. Photosensitivity, blood dyscrasias, nephrosis, hepatitis and dermatitis may occur during its administration. Paramethadione (Paradione) is closely related and sometimes may be used as a replacement when the response to trimethadione is not satisfactory.

The succinimides, phensuximide (Milontin) and methsuximide (Celontin) have a structural chemical resemblance to trimethadione, and their spectrum of anticonvulsant action is similar. Another member of this group, ethosuximide (Zarontin) has successfully controlled the attacks in patients who have been resistant to trimethadione and other forms of therapy.

Phenacemide (phenylacetylurea, Phenurone) has a relatively broad spectrum of effectiveness both in experimental testing procedures and in the various forms of epilepsy. Toxic potentialities are high and include personality changes.

Magnesium compounds have the effect of depressing nervous and muscular activity. However, orally administered compounds, such as magnesium salts for catharsis, have no important systemic effects, since they are very poorly absorbed from the gut, and such amounts as are absorbed are excreted readily by the kidney. Traditionally, magnesium sulfate by intravenous and intramuscular injection has been used to antagonize the convulsions of eclampsia. However, animal experiments indicate a very low margin of safety, with death by respiratory depression. Calcium salts (chloride or gluconate) by intravenous injection act as a prompt and spectacular antidote for magnesium depression.

Carbamazepine (Tegretol), a tricyclic compound related to imiprimine, was originally introduced for the treatment of trigeminal neuralgia. It is recommended for the treatment of grand mal and psychomotor epilepsy. It appears to be as effective as phenytoin, and may prove to be better tolerated. Carbamazepine is usually well tolerated but can cause nystagmus and drowsiness. Other adverse effects include anorexia, ataxia, dizziness, and diplopia. More serious adverse effects are rare but aplastic anemia, hepatitis, heart block, and a lupus erythematosus syndrome have been reported. The drug should first be given in low dosage with gradual increments.

Valproic acid (depakene) is a new antiepileptic approved by the US Food and Drug Administration for treatment of petit mal seizures. Experience with this drug abroad and recent studies in this country indicate that valproic acid is also effective for treating generalized tonic-clonic and photosensitive seizures, and particularly for myoclonic seizures, which are often refractory to other anticonvulsants. Its mechanism of action has not been established, although increased brain levels of GABA have been implicated as an explanation. The drug is rapidly absorbed when orally administered, has a serum half life of 8 to 12 hours, and is strongly bound (90 per cent) to plasma proteins. Valproic acid can increase phenobarbital levels when the two drugs are taken concurrently. The most common adverse effects are nausea, vomiting, and diarrhea. Temporary hair loss and weight gain can occur and weight loss, rash, hypersalivation, headache and insomnia have been reported. Valproic acid can interfere with platelet function; spontaneous bleeding or bruising are indications for stopping the drug. Severe hepatic toxicity has occurred rarely.

Diazepam (Valium) is now the drug of choice in the treatment of status epilepticus. Since it is short acting, dosage can be readily titrated. It is administered by slow intravenous injection or intramuscularly if necessary. Phenytoin and phenobarbital are effective alternatives for treatment of status epilepticus. Any of the drugs used can be lethal if they are given too rapidly or in overdosage. If these drugs do not suppress the continuous seizure activity, general anesthesia may be necessary.

Acetazolamide (Diamox), a carbonic anhydrase inhibitor, is used occasionally. Its effectiveness is thought to be related to inhibition of carbonic anhydrase in the central nervous system. Although effective in all types of epilepsy, its usefulness is limited by the rapid development of tolerance.

Clonazepam (Clonopin), a benzodiazepine, is particularly useful for myoclonic and akinetic seizures, which may be resistant to treatment with other anticonvulsants. It is also effective for treatment of absence attacks, but generally less so than ethosuximide or valproic acid. Like diazepam, tolerance may develop to its anticonvulsant effects; frequent adverse effects such as behavioral changes, drowsiness, and ataxia may outweigh the benefits in some severely retarded or disabled patients.

Analgesics and Antipyretics

A number of drugs have the common property of a depressant action that is generally limited to the area of the thalamus and the hypothalamus. Their effect is to block pain sensations and to lower body temperature without causing other important effects in the nervous system. The analgesic action, presumably due to thalamic depression, is moderate compared with the more powerful action of the opiates. There is now increasing evidence that the analgesic action may also be due, at least in part, to interactions with chemical substances at peripheral sites. Blockade of the pain elicited by bradykinin injection has been demonstrated, and reduced activation of prostaglandins is seen in some preparations. For example, the analgesic effect of aspirin is due, in part, to a direct peripheral action as a result of inhibition of prostaglandin synthetase. The antipyretic action, presumably due to effects on the hypothalamus, is obtained chiefly by increased heat dissipation through peripheral vasodilation. Although sweating is an additional important factor in heat dissipation, the antipyretic effect is not significantly altered when sweating is prevented by atropine administration. The proposed mechanism for reversal of fever by aspirin is through inhibition of prostaglandin synthetase in thermoregulatory centers of the anterior hypothalamus. Ingestion of even small doses of aspirin, but not sodium salicylate, prolongs the bleeding time, presumably by inhibiting platelet function. The mode of action of aspirin in blocking platelet aggregation and its significance in the prevention of thrombosis are being investigated. Aspirin has been used in several clinical trials for the secondary prevention of myocardial infarction, but results of these studies have been inconsistent and subject to varying interpretation. Recent findings concerning thromboxane (TXA_2) and prostacyclin (PGI_2) systems may explain why aspirin's effect in preventing thrombosis has not been dramatic. Because platelet aggregation is stimulated by thromboxane, inhibiting its formation is potentially beneficial. However, this benefit may be lost if synthesis of prostacyclin, which is carried out by the vascular endothelium, is also diminished, with the resultant loss of its inhibitory effect on platelet aggregation. The postulated beneficial effect of aspirin appears to be based on the assumption that it has less effect on the vessel wall than on the endothelium.

Antipyretics are chiefly effective against abnormally elevated or febrile temperatures and do not significantly lower normal temperatures. Aspirin, sodium salicylate and acetophenetidin are commonly used in the usual dose of 0.3 g. (5 grains). A metabolite of acetophenetidin (Phenacetin) is acetaminophen (Tylenol), which is more soluble in water. Acetophenetidin may cause mild methemoglobinemia and when chronically abused has been associated with serious nephrotoxicity. Acetaminophen has not shown these effects and so has largely replaced acetophenetidin. Due to its increased availability, there has been an increase in the number of acute overdoses with acetaminophen, most commonly in adults with suicidal intent. An investigational drug, N-acetylcysteine (Mucomyst) is a safe and highly effective antidote.

In ordinary antipyretic-analgesic doses the chief toxic effect of aspirin is allergic, and this occurs with particular frequency in asthmatics; doses of salicylate commonly used in rheumatic fever and arthritis may produce reversible auditory, visual and gastrointestinal disturbances. Acetanilid produces methemoglobinemia, and aminopyrine has been charged with a number of instances of agranulocytosis so that the use of these agents has been largely abandoned.

Phenylbutazone (Butazolidin), dispensed in tablets of 100 to 200 mg., is an effective analgesic in the treatment of rheumatoid arthritis but has a high incidence of toxic effects, including blood dyscrasias. Oxyphenbutazone (Tandearil) and sulfinpyrazone (Anturane) are chemically and pharmacologically similar to phenylbutazone. Indomethacin (Indocin) is chemically different but used for the same purposes; it has about the same effectiveness as aspirin in rheumatoid arthritis but has more serious toxic effects.

Although the mechanism has not been delineated,

sulfinpyrazone (Anturane) significantly reduces the incidence of sudden cardiac death during the high-risk period shortly after an acute myocardial infarction; there is no further apparent effect beyond the seventh month after infarction.

Colchicine is administered in 0.5 mg. tablets for relief of the pain of gout and has special interest because of its unique ability to arrest mitosis in the metaphase.

The analgesic action of salicylates is not demonstrable by laboratory tests with the same consistency as with morphine derivatives. This supports the view that its practical analgesic action is due partly to an anti-edema effect at the site of the pain. Ordinarily the analgesic action of salicylates is considered to be more effective in instances of pain from integumental structures, while the analgesic action of morphine is relatively more effective in painful conditions of the viscera.

The large doses of salicylates (about 10 g. daily) used in rheumatic fever evidently act through additional mechanisms. Pain, swelling and tenderness in the joints are reduced; joint, pericardial and pleural effusions are absorbed more quickly; sedimentation rate, leukocytosis and content of C-reactive protein decrease; however, the incidence of damage to cardiac structures does not appear to be influenced by salicylates. Analgesic doses of salicylate reduce renal excretion of uric acid by reducing tubular secretion. Higher doses have an opposite uricosuric effect, largely by blocking tubular reabsorption. This effect is of little practical significance in treating gout at present because of the availability of more potent uricosuric agents. Salicylates increase the oxygen consumption of isolated tissues in much the same way as dinitrophenol. Doses of salicylate at maximum therapeutic or higher levels increase oxygen consumption and depth and rate of external respiratory movements; cardiac output is increased, and there is moderate positive inotropic action at some stages. Hyperventilation of central origin (salicyl dyspnea) produces alkalosis and compensatory buffer-base depletion. Later, associated with a markedly increased metabolic rate and uncoupled oxidative phosphorylation, acidosis may supervene with accumulated salicylate, carbon dioxide and metabolic acids. Hyperpyrexia and circulatory collapse are commonly exhibited in fatal overdoses. Methyl salicylate is extremely irritating to the gastric mucosa and so is used only topically in liniments. Salicylates do not produce methemoglobinemia, although the highly reduced hemoglobin may produce cyanosis. Reduction of prothrombin as a basis for occasional bleeding tendency probably has been overemphasized.

Altering urinary pH from 5.0 to 7.5 tends to convert free salicylic acid to the water-soluble sodium salicylate and, in actual demonstration, increases renal clearance about eight-fold. The response is considerably greater than would be predicted from the shift in urinary pH alone and may reflect an intracellular pH effect.

A number of potent nonsteroidal antiinflammatory drugs have been developed recently. They include ibuprofen (Motrin), naproxen (Naprosyn), fenprofen (Nalfon), and tolmetin (Tolectin). All inhibit prostaglandin synthesis and are indicated for the treatment of rheumatoid arthritis. Ibuprofen is also approved for treating osteoarthritis. As compared with aspirin, a lower incidence of gastrointestinal toxicity is claimed. A recently marketed nonsteroidal antiinflammatory drug is sulindac (Clinoril). Like other members of this group it inhibits prostaglandin synthesis and this is probably the mechanism of its antiinflammatory activity. It appears to be effective for short-term treatment of arthritic disorders; its safety for long-term use remains to be determined.

Opium and Related Drugs

Opium, the dried exudate of the incised unripe poppy capsule, contains morphine ordinarily in a concentration averaging about 10 per cent. The other alkaloids present (codeine, thebaine, papaverine, etc.) are not in sufficient amounts to have clinical significance. There are several simple chemical variations of morphine whose actions resemble those of the parent compound but with some moderate distinctions. For instance, codeine is a methylated derivative of morphine; heroin is a diacetylated derivative; hydromorphone (Dilaudid) has had one double bond hydrogenated and one hydroxyl reduced to the ketone form; hydrocodone (Dicodid, Hycodan) is obtained by comparable changes in the codeine molecule; metopon is a methylated form of hydromorphone; levorphanol (Levo-Dromoran) differs in structure from morphine by the absence of the oxygen bridge, the alcoholic hydroxyl and one double bond; oxymorphone (Numorphan) is used in a dose about one-tenth that of morphine. Pentazocine (Talwin), a benzomorphan derivative, appears to be a potent analgesic with lessened tendency to produce opiate dependence. Hallucinatory side effects have been disturbing

Morphine blocks pain impulses, probably by a depressant action in the thalamus in addition to the characteristic cortical effect. Its pain-blocking action is exceptionally powerful but is more effective against dull chronic pain than against sudden sharp stimuli. Other actions of morphine are moderate cortical depression (euphoria, sleep), moderate to marked medullary depression (dulling of cough and emetic reflexes and slowed respiration) and a group of peripheral manifestations that suggest a parasympathetic or cholinergic mechanism (miosis, heart slowing, diaphoresis and moderate spasm of the smooth muscles of the bronchioles, the gastrointestinal tract, the biliary tract, the ureters and the urinary bladder). There is some evidence that a release of intestinal 5-HT may follow morphine administration and contribute to the intestinal response obtained. The effect of checking diarrhea and causing constipation is due to the nonpropulsive spasm of smooth muscle, which possibly may be followed by a period of inactivity. Hyperglycemia and antidiuretic effects can be demonstrated. Morphine does not elevate the threshold for electroshock convulsions. Multineuronal reflexes are generally depressed, while monosynaptic cord reflexes may be enhanced or not affected. Other effects of ordinary doses of some morphine compounds are nausea and occasional vomiting (principally in ambulatory patients), dilation of skin vessels, pruritus, sneezing, allergic reactions and occasional cerebral excitation (the last most frequently in women). Codeine differs from morphine in that large doses usually cause excitement, especially in children. These alkaloids are active in releasing histamine when injected intravenously, a property not shared by methadone.

Morphine, for the most part, is conjugated in the liver to the glucuronide and excreted in the urine. Methylation also occurs, and there is some elimination in the feces.

Morphine is used chiefly to diminish pain, promote rest, obtund the cough reflex, check diarrhea and, in dyspnea such as "cardiac dyspnea," to bring about slower and more efficient respiratory movements. Comparable analgesic doses are morphine, 10 mg.; codeine, 64 mg.; dihydromorphinone, 1 mg.; and pentazocine, 30 mg.

Common doses of the older opium preparations are intended to be comparable with 6 mg. morphine. Such doses are: powdered opium 60 mg., used chiefly for diarrheas; and opium tincture (laudanum) 0.6 ml.; camphorated tincture of opium (paregoric) contains 1.6 mg. morphine in its usual dose of 4 ml.; Pantopon (Omnopon) is an injectable mixture of opium alkaloids, about half of which is morphine.

Toxic overdose effects of morphine compounds are characterized by pinpoint pupils, slowed respiration and coma, from which the subject usually may be aroused temporarily.

Continued use of morphine may lead to greatly increased tolerance and physical dependence or addiction. Tolerance may be explained partly by an increased ability of the body to destroy or conjugate morphine. However, this does not explain the manner in which tolerance to large intravenous doses can be developed or the type of tolerance and dependence that can be developed in tissue cultures using epithelial cells. Withdrawal symptoms may be minimized by controlled gradual decrease in the dose or by substituting other narcotic drugs, none of which has any specific value. Addiction liability is greatest with heroin, least with codeine.

Papaverine has no analgesic or sedative action. It has had some clinical trial because of its general depression of smooth muscle, with suggestively favorable results in asthma, the anginal syndrome, peripheral vascular disease and pulmonary embolism

Meperidine (Demerol, pethidine) is chemically related to atropine (piperidine nucleus) but exhibits no consistent spasmolytic actions similar to those of atropine. Meperidine exhibits analgesic and sedative actions similar to those of morphine, although the actions are not as intense or as long lasting. Excessive doses of meperidine may result in cerebral excitability. As an analgesic, 100 mg. of meperidine approximates 10 mg. of morphine. In spite of earlier claims, comparison of respiratory and smooth muscle side effects following equianalgesic doses of meperidine and morphine indicate that no significant differences can be clearly defined. There is less likelihood of the development of physiologic dependence on it than on morphine because addiction usually develops more slowly. Alphaprodine (Nisentil) and anileridine (Leritine) are congeners producing analgesia equal to meperidine at lower dosage levels. No advantage has been demonstrated for these agents. Another variant of the meperidine structure, diphenoxylate, is combined with atropine in a tablet or liquid preparation (Lomotil) which has been much used in the control of diarrhea.

Methadone (amidone, Dolophine), a German synthetic studied particularly in the United States, is simpler chemically than morphine but resembles it in several ways. It raises the pain threshold and, under conditions of large dosage, is highly euphoric and depressant to respiration. In therapeutic doses (from 2.5 to 10 mg.) it has effects of sedation, respiratory depression and constipation similar to morphine. It acts for a longer period than morphine. Methadone is effective rapidly when given orally, and, when given intramuscularly and subcutaneously, frequently it proves to be irritant. Nausea often follows oral administration. Withdrawal symptoms are less marked than with morphine, largely because methadone is more highly protein bound, and tissue concentrations dissipate slowly. For this reason, it has been used as a substitute for morphine in institutionalized addicts and in large-scale substitution programs for control of opiate abusers. At present, it is not available for analgesic use and is limited to use in abuse programs.

Levorphanol is more closely related to morphine than the other commonly used synthetic narcotic analgesics. Its subcutaneous or oral dose of 2 to 3 mg. is considered to be equal in analgesia to the usual therapeutic dose of morphine, but typical opiate side-effects and addiction liability are proportionately increased.

Levorphanol is the *l*-isomer of the racemic racemorphan (methorphinan, Dromoran). The *d*-isomer dextrorphan exhibits less analgesic and more antitussive effects. Its methyl ether, dextromethorphan (Romilar), is used exclusively for this purpose, and appears to be a satisfactory substitute for codeine.

Propoxyphene (Darvon) is a synthetic analgesic chemically very similar to methadone that is widely used as a substitute for codeine. It does not require a narcotic prescription, although addiction to Darvon has been reported. Like codeine, it is commonly used in combination with aspirin. Although the potential for physical dependence on propoxyphene is relatively low, the actual abuse potential appears to be fairly high.

Nalbuphine (Nubain) is a narcotic agonist-antagonist analgesic, available only for parenteral use. It is related structurally and pharmacologically to the narcotic oxymorphone (Numorphan). After intravenous injection, analgesic effects begin within two to three minutes, and within fifteen minutes after subcutaneous or intramuscular administration. The duration of analgesia is comparable to morphine, lasting from three to six hours. Tolerance probably develops more slowly to nalbuphine than to morphine.

Butorphanol (Stadol) is a potent, narcotic analgesic belonging, like morphine, to the phenanthrene series. Its site of action is thought to be subcortical, possibly in the limbic system. The duration of analgesia is generally 3 to 4 hours and is approximately equivalent to that of morphine. Additionally, it possesses narcotic antagonist activity similar to that of nalorphine. Caution should be exercised in its use in patients with head injuries, since it, like other morphine-like analgesics, tends to elevate cerebrospinal fluid pressure.

Nalorphine (N-allylnormorphine, Nalline) is uniquely effective in antagonizing morphine, methadone, meperidine and their simple variants with narcotic activity. Nalorphine does not antagonize the action of barbiturates and the volatile anesthetics. This specialized ability to interrupt and abolish effects of the narcotic analgesics strongly suggests both a structural blockade at the receptor cells and a spatial chemical similarity in the several narcotic analgesics, despite their diverse structural formulas as represented in the conventional manner. A phenyl methylpiperidine grouping has been proposed as the common moiety in this group, although this requires special interpretation in the instance of methadone; the receptor site can then be visualized as possessing three points of attachment: an anionic site, a cavity and a flat-surface cationic site.

When given to man or to animal without previous medication, nalorphine produces weak morphine-like effects with some moderate differences such as dysphoria, diuresis and decrease of gut tone. It is used to overcome respiratory center depression in newborn infants following administration of narcotics to the mother during delivery. Intravenous doses of 10 mg. of nalorphine counteract narcotic overdoses in the adult and can precipitate the withdrawal syndrome in narcotic addicts. Under these conditions the syndrome may be more severe than that following withdrawal. Similarly, withdrawal symptoms can be produced in individuals who have had only a few doses of narcotics and have not yet exhibited tolerance to the narcotic.

A synthetic congener, N-allyl levodromoran (Levallorphan, Lorfan), generally has similar actions to nalorphine.

Naloxone (Narcan) is a newer agent with prominent opiate-antagonist properties and virtually no agonistic activity. It is presently favored in abuse treatment programs where an attempt is made to induce refractoriness to opiates. Single daily doses can effectively block the euphoric responses to large doses of the opiates. At present, naloxone is considered the drug of choice for the treatment of opioid-induced respiratory depression.

Synthetic narcotic drugs in the United States are subject to the same legal restrictions as are opium and compounds derived from opium alkaloids. About 20 such synthetics have been defined as "opiates," meaning in this case that they have addiction characteristics similar to those of morphine or cocaine.

In recent years, in an effort to elucidate the basic mechanism of action of narcotic analgesics, the study of morphine receptors in the brain and endogenous morphine-like compounds has been intense. The brain contains a variety of opioid peptides (endorphins) which bind to morphine receptors. These opioids seem to act as neurotransmitters of specific nerve pathways that process information relating to pain, emotional behavior, and other bodily processes known to be affected by opiates. Their spectrum of activity is similar to that of morphine and other narcotic agonist drugs. When a placebo is administered, they are released from storage sites and produce analgesia.

CENTRAL NERVOUS SYSTEM STIMULANTS

The various drugs used for stimulation of the central nervous system differ considerably in their pattern of action. Some, for instance, act most intensely on the cortex, others on the medullary centers, and still others on the spinal cord. With large doses they produce convulsions that are characteristic of the chief site of action. These drugs also differ considerably in their degree of direct action on the cardiovascular system and in their range of safety. They tend to oppose the action of sedatives and hypnotics, and, when used for their awakening or arousal effect, they are termed *analeptics*. Drug-produced stimulation or overactivity necessarily is followed by the physiologic sequel of depression, and this may intensify the existing state of depression. Some analeptics have, in addition, a direct paralytic effect in high doses.

Although these drugs antagonize general depressants such as barbiturates, the effect is not dependable except at light stages of anesthesia. At deep levels of anesthesia, their effects are equivocal. For instance, the respiratory paralyzing dose of barbiturates is only moderately increased by optimally selected doses of picrotoxin, pentylenetetrazol or bemegride. By contrast, mechanical respiration permits the injection of about three respiratory-paralysis doses before circulatory depression supervenes. Accordingly the essential feature in treatment of overdose of such depressants is mechanical maintenance of respiration, since there is a wide margin between respiratory failure and circulatory failure produced by these depressants.

Strychnine, from the nux vomica seed, has its chief effect on the spinal cord, where its action may be interpreted as a general lowering of synaptic resistance. Both strychnine and tetanus toxin act to block the inhibitory effects of the Renshaw cells. A dose of 2 mg. taken orally may increase cord reflexes and visual and auditory acuity. Larger doses produce reflex, bilateral, symmetric, tonic convulsions. Stimulation of the respiratory center and direct effects on the cardiovascular system are slight at the ordinary therapeutic dosage level. It has no demonstrated therapeutic value.

Caffeine acts chiefly on the cortex and, to a lesser but appreciable degree, on the medullary centers. It is a suitable antagonist to depression by morphine and by alcohol (dose of caffeine sodium benzoate, 0.5 gm.). There is moderate direct stimulation of the myocardium. Stimulation of the vasoconstrictor center is approximately counterbalanced by direct dilation of peripheral vessels. Theophylline (aminophylline), a related xanthine, may afford some relief of Cheyne-Stokes respiration apparently because of its stimulating action on the medulla.

Ephedrine is a cortical stimulant, characterized by a relatively long period of action; its effects include dilation of the bronchioles and marked peripheral vasoconstriction. The effect that it has of raising the blood pressure on occasion may be an objection to its use as a stimulant drug.

Pentylenetetrazol (Metrazol) acts with fair uniformity on the central nervous system, although probably with greatest intensity on the cortical areas. Occasionally it may have a slight direct stimulant action on experimental isolated heart preparations, but the observed instances of clinical improvement in circulatory functions are due in most cases to central nervous system stimulation. It is recommended by some as a cerebral stimulant for treatment of mental depression or senility; however, there is not adequate evidence to support its effectiveness for these purposes.

Nikethamide (Coramine) stimulates the central nervous system, its chief action being on the medullary centers. In addition, it may have a direct stimulative action on the chemoreceptors of the carotid and aortic bodies. Circulatory effects probably are secondary to those of medullary and respiratory stimulation. Its use in drug-induced coma is of no value.

Picrotoxin is chiefly a meduallary stimulant that was formerly used in treating overdoses of central nervous system depressants, particularly barbiturates. Because of its ineffectiveness in hastening arousal and the possibility of severe convulsions, it has become obsolete.

Bemegride (Megimide) has analeptic actions similar to those of pentylenetetrazol.

Ethamivan (Emivan) is used also as a respiratory stimulant; its circulatory actions are due in part to a direct stimulation of the adrenal medulla, with release of epinephrine. Doxapram (Dopram) is proposed for use in hastening arousal during the postoperative recovery period and in management of drug-induced respiratory depression. As with other analeptics, its use appears inadvisable for such purposes.

Psychomotor Stimulants

These drugs increase behavior manifestations, and, when this is not accompanied by an anxiety component, they are spoken of as mood elevators. The term psychic energizers also has been used. Although these compounds antagonize barbiturates to a certain degree, this feature is not as pronounced as with the analeptic group just described, and this psychomotor stimulant group is less convulsant in character. Older examples such as cocaine and amphetamine (Dexedrine) have been followed by drugs such as pipradol (Meratran) and methylphenidate (Ritalin). The later drug is useful in the treatment of narcolepsy and of the hyperkinetic syndrome in children. A still later group is that which followed the accidental observation that, when derivatives of isonicotinic acid hydrazide were used in tuberculosis management, the patients also exhibited conspicuous mood elevation. Most of these compounds have also proved to be inhibitors of the enzyme monoamine oxidase, and this presumably has bearing on the accumulation or the destruction of brain metabolites. Examples are a benzylcarboxamide derivative of INH (nialamide, Niamid); isocarboxazid (Marplan); and phenelzine (Nardil). These are being recommended for essential depressions including manic-depressive psychoses and involutional and reactive depressions; with schizophrenics some consider that they should be combined with a phenothiazine tranquilizer. These compounds also are used in angina pectoris and in primary hypertension. Orthostatic hypotension occurs with some and is attributed to ganglionic blocking actions. A bizarre complication has been a reversible impairment of red-green color discrimination.

Hepatic toxicity with high serum transaminase values has occurred often enough to bring about withdrawal of some of these drugs from general distribution. This has occurred with iproniazid and others less commonly used. Since the symptoms resemble those of infectious hepatitis, the true incidence is difficult to evaluate. Tranylcypromine (Parnate) has been implicated in hypertensive crises and deaths from the "cheese syndrome." Because the monoamine oxidase inhibitors are more toxic than the tricyclic compounds, they should be reserved for only those patients not responding to tricyclic agents or electroconvulsive therapy.

Antidepressant agents that have chemical structure closely resembling the phenothiazines and that are without MAO-inhibiting effects are imipramine (Tofranil) and amitryptyline (Elavil). The latter is described as having atropine-like activity and as being incompatible with MAO inhibitors. Others of this type are desipramine, protriptyline, and doxepin. Caution is advised in prescribing these tricyclic antidepressants to patients with hypertension taking guanethidine or similar compounds whose mechanism of action involves gaining entrance into the postganglionic nerve ending. The tricyclic compounds will inhibit that action and result in higher pressures.

PSYCHOTOMIMETIC DRUGS

Cannabis (hashish, marihuana) is an ancient drug that is now used in the United States as a drug of indulgence. It produces a peculiar type of cerebral disturbance, involving distortion of the sense of time and space with waves of emotional instability that may be euphoric or of an agonizing type. Motor function is affected and moderate dose-dependent increases in blood pressure and heart rate are seen at usual doses, e.g., one-cigarette tolerance to this agent has been clearly demonstrated. Decisive findings concerning the neurochemical basis for its behavioral effects are lacking. Although habit formation may occur occasionally, it ordinarily does not lead to a condition of physical dependence. Active constituents of the crude drug have been isolated (Δ^9 and Δ^8 tetrahydrocannabinol), and synthetic compounds (dibenzopyrane derivatives) with typical activity have been prepared.

Some potential medical applications for marihuana exist. For example, cannabinoids lower intraocular pressure in patients with wide angle glaucoma. Since effective glaucoma medications already exist, what the cannabinoids might offer is either potentiation of the established medications or effectiveness in those patients who are unresponsive to conventional treatment. In cancer patients, receiving chemotherapy, marihuana has proved to be effective in controlling the nausea, vomiting, and loss of appetite associated with treatment. A number of synthetic cannabinoids have been developed and are now being studied for anticonvulsant, tranquilizing, analgesic, and intraocular pressure-lowering properties.

Mescaline, the best-known alkaloid from peyote (mescal) has hallucinatory effects that have been used as an experimental form of schizophrenia. After oral doses of from 200 to 500 mg., the subject experiences disturbed auditory and visual sensations, the latter suggesting multicolored lights and varied geometric patterns; consciousness and insight are not grossly disturbed; anxiety, tremors and nausea may be pronounced.

Lysergic acid diethylamide (LSD 25) has effects somewhat similar to those of mescaline and is remarkable for the small doses that produce a pseudohallucinatory state. These range from 50 μg. upward. Tolerance is rapidly developed and rapidly lost. Chlorpromazine, diazepam and phenobarbital have been used to counter the effects. However, street preparations of LSD are often contaminated with unknown substances (e.g. strychnine), and drug therapy is not recommended for overdose. The wide extent of its use has precipitated psychoses among a considerable number of individuals, many of whom were probably predisposed to mental disturbances.

Morning glory seeds, readily purchasable, contain compounds similar to LSD. Following ingestion, symptoms include drowsiness, confusion, perceptual distortion, and hallucinations. Giddiness and euphoria may alternate with intense anxiety.

Phencyclidine (PCP; angel dust) is licitly manufactured as a veterinary tranquilizer. It is becoming one of the most frequently used adulterants and hallucinogens available on the illicit drug market and is often misrepresented as Δ^9 tetrahydrocannabinol (THC). Despite the fact that PCP produces severe toxic psychosis and violent behavior, its use has increased steadily because of its availability both alone and in combination with LSD, amphetamines, and local anesthetics. Depending on dosage, route of administration, and time lapsed since ingestion, PCP can produce symptoms ranging from a comatose state to agitated, violent behavior. In addition, the mental state may fluctuate over a period of several days, because of the rather long half life of approximately 11 hours.

Nutmeg, a spice used throughout the world, contains a hallucinogen thought to be myristicin. Ingestion of large amounts produces euphoria, hallucinations, and an acute psychotic reaction. Side effects, similar to atropine poisoning, include tachycardia, decreased salivary secretion, and flushing of the skin. Unlike atropine, nutmeg may produce early miosis.

Psilocybin and psilocin are extracted from mushrooms that occur principally in Mexico where native cults use them in religious rites. The effects produced are similar to those seen with mescaline.

Anticholinergic agents which are commonly abused include preparations or plants containing scopolamine, atropine, and synthetic atropine substitutes. In high doses these agents induce disorientation, confusion, hallucinations, and eventually coma. Anticholinergic agents abused for their psychotomimetic effects are sometimes falsely marketed as LSD.

Numerous gases and highly volatile organic compounds are inhaled for their effects. Among the most popular inhalants are lighter fluid, gasoline, model airplane glue, paint thinners, cleaning fluid, and nail polish remover. These agents contain a variety of volatile aliphatic and aromatic hydrocarbons, including acetone, amyl acetate, naphtha, benzene, toluene, carbon tetrachloride, and chloroform. Many have serious toxic effects. For example, carbon tetrachloride and chloroform are toxic to the liver, kidney and myocardium. Exposure to high concentrations of toluene may result in bone marrow suppression, renal tubular acidosis, acute hepatic failure and permanent encephalopathy. Fatal aplastic anemia can result from glue sniffing.

LOCAL ANESTHETICS

Cocaine is the oldest of a considerable number of compounds that reversibly depress or paralyze function in peripheral nerve structures. Sensory nerves usually are paralyzed more quickly or at lower concentrations than motor nerves, probably because sensory nerves, with a smaller fiber size, present relatively more surface to the anesthetic. Cocaine and others of this group appear to act at the lipoprotein membrane to interfere with depolarization and passage of the impulse. Temporary stabilization of the membrane is accomplished in some way to prevent the normal influx of sodium as it occurs during depolarization. It now appears likely that the local anesthetic molecules compete with calcium ions for receptors on the nerve membrane. Sodium ions, the physiologic competitor for these calcium sites cannot displace the more strongly bound local anesthetic molecules. Local anesthetics must be sufficiently lipid soluble at tissue hydrogen ion concentration to facilitate uptake by the nerve membrane. However, the intracellularly active form appears likely to be the ionized cationic form.

Based on knowledge of the chemical structure of cocaine, many local anesthetics have been synthesized that differ from cocaine both chemically and pharmacologically.

Cocaine is a benzoic acid ester of the base ecgonine and, in that respect, resembles atropine. Most of the synthetic variants are benzoic acid esters and are hydrolyzed by cholinesterases; all contain a secondary or tertiary nitrogen. By virtue of this basic nitrogen, they all form salts with acids and, accordingly, are more ionized in an acid than in an alkaline medium.

Selection or choice of anesthetics is based on differences in onset and duration of action, penetration through mucous membranes, incidence of systemic toxicity and local irritation.

Procaine (Novocain) was synthetized in 1905 and is of simpler chemical constitution than cocaine. It has been the longest time in general use and is regarded as the safest of the local anesthetic group. The incidence of severe central nervous and cardiovascular toxicities after its use is conspicuously lower than after other local anesthetics that have had substantial periods of clinical trial. However, the limitation of procaine is its relatively slight penetrability through mucosae and, correspondingly, its ineffectiveness as a topical anesthetic. In recent years its popularity has declined and it has been replaced by lidocaine as a standard local anesthetic. Another product in this category is butethamine (Monocaine). Most of the synthetic variants of procaine are the results of trials that have developed compounds with reasonably adequate penetration of mucosa and, in some cases, with reasonable safety on injection. Products in this category are piperocaine (Metycaine), tetracaine (Pontocaine), butacaine (Butyn) and phenacaine (Holocaine).

Lidocaine (Xylocaine) has an amide linkage instead of the more common ester and has gained particular prominence because of its safety record, which rivals that of procaine. Also, lidocaine has more favorable lipid solubility resulting in rapid onset of action and excellent tissue penetrance. It is probably the most widely used of the local anesthetics at present in routine dental and medical infiltration techniques. Other amides that are both topical and injection anesthetics are mepivacaine (Carbocaine) and prilocaine (Citanest).

Because of relatively low water solubility, some local anesthetics have been used for surface anesthesia over prolonged periods with little or no incidence of systemic effects; they are not intended as operative anesthetics but rather for painful ulcers, burns, etc. Examples are ethylaminobenzoate (benzocaine, Anesthesin) and butyl aminobenzoate (Butesin), used commonly as the picrate. These agents are responsible for an appreciable incidence of skin-sensitivity reactions.

More recent variants include: chloroprocaine (Nesacaine), with a shorter period of action than procaine; amolanone (Amethone), a topical anesthetic used for intraurethral installation before instrumentation; benoxinate (Dorsacaine) and proparacaine (Ophthaine), surface anesthetics used in opthalmology; cyclomethycaine (Surfacaine), dimethisoquin (Quotane), dyclonine (Dyclone) and paramoxine (Tronothane), general surface anesthetics.

There are numerous other suitable local anesthetics available. However, the needs of most physicians can be met by the use of only two or three different agents chosen for different purposes.

Toxic Effects

Systemic toxicity may follow the use of topical or injection anesthetics and may be of the excitatory or the depressant type, or, as frequently happens, the toxic reaction may show phases of both types. Excitation is similar to that seen in the criminal abuse of cocaine and in laboratory demonstrations of overdose in dogs. This cerebral excitation is characterized by restlessness, hypermotility, hyperpyrexia and, finally, clonic convulsions. This pattern of toxicity has been most frequent in association with applications to large mucous surfaces, as in bronchoscopic procedures. A wide variety of agents have been implicated, with tetracaine probably having the highest incidence of involvement.

The depressant type of toxicity is more common and dangerous and may be a hypersensitivity reaction to relatively small doses. Characteristically the patient experiences shortness of breath, palpitation and faintness and becomes pale or cyanotic. Recovery is promoted most effectively by artificial respiration and circulatory support.

The incidence of such reactions is reduced by the addition of epinephrine (2 to 10 μg. per ml.) or other local vasoconstrictors to the anesthetic solutions. This procedure helps to retain the local anesthetic at the point of injection ("chemical tourniquet") and thus produces anesthesia of longer duration with less systemic effects.

Types of Local Anesthesia

Injection anesthesia is accomplished by (1) the *infiltration technique,* in which a large volume of a weak solution (procaine about 0.5 per cent) is injected into the operative area, or (2) *conduction block* or *regional block,* in which small volumes of a relatively concentrated solution (procaine 1 to 2 per cent) are injected around nerve trunks supplying the operative area.

Spinal anesthesia may be regarded as a special form of block anesthesia in which the local anesthetic is deposited in the subdural space. Puncture usually is made just below the level of the conus medullaris (L2 to L3), and the anesthetic is made to reach the desired level by varying the volume introduced, by barbotage or by the position of the patient. Sensory and sympathetic nerve structures are paralyzed for a longer time and at lower concentrations than are motor nerve roots. An orthodox conservative dose is 1 mg. of procaine per pound body weight. Piperocaine, tetracaine and dibucaine also have been used. Tetracaine is by far the most commonly used agent for spinal procedures today. Dibucaine has the longest period of action and the lowest absolute dose; it is seldom used because of a significant incidence of persistent paresthesias.

Spinal anesthesia provides good muscular relaxation with a minimum of metabolic disturbances and no pulmonary irritation. Post operative distention is less than with general anesthetics, partly because the sympathetic inhibitory innervation of the gut is paralyzed, while vagal tone is unaffected. Disadvantages include postpuncture headache (presumably due to meningeal leakage) and some paralysis of bladder function (due chiefly to paralysis of sacral autonomics supplying the detrusor muscle of the bladder).

Deaths from spinal anesthesia are rare and usually attributed to rise of anesthetic in the spinal canal, and corresponding paralysis of various nerve structures affecting respiration and circulation. Artificial respiration is the most effective treatment of impending cardiorespiratory collapse.

Epidural or Peridural Anesthesia. The disadvantages of meningeal puncture are avoided by epidural or peridural anesthesia, in which the anesthetic is deposited in the peridural space and passes out with the nerve trunks through the intervertebral foramina. Large amounts of anesthetic are needed (20 to 50 ml. of 2 per cent procaine); hence, there is a special danger of systemic drug affects.

Continuous caudal anesthesia is a special form of extradural block used chiefly in obstetrics. The anesthesia is delivered in installments through a needle or a catheter inserted into the caudal canal through the sacral hiatus.

Local anesthetics also have special usefulness in producing *sympathetic block* for release of vasoconstrictor impulses in the head or the extremities and for relieving pain in localized areas *(therapeutic nerve block).*

HISTAMINE AND HISTAMINE-ANTAGONIZING AGENTS

Histamine has interesting theoretic significance in that it has been shown to be liberated in appreciable amount during anaphylactic shock. Its experimental injection stimulates the picture of anaphylactic shock, i.e., bronchial spasm and dilatation of arterioles and capillaries. Gastric secretion, particularly of HC1, is powerfully stimulated by histamine, which is routinely used for diagnostic purposes in doses of about 0.5 mg. subcutaneously. Betazole (Histalog) is an analog that is used in a dose about 100 times as great; it has the same effect in stimulating gastric secretion but has a much lesser degree of side effects.

Histamine in the body is located chiefly in the mast cells; it is stored in subcellular granules in combination with heparin. Various drug agents can bring about a release of histamine by disruption of these cells, while IgE-antigen release is through an energy-requiring system. Associated heparin release is recognized in the dog and, in some species, serotonin release also is recognized. When given intravenously, effective histamine-release agents include high polymer colloids such as dextran, acacia and polyvinyl pyrrolidone, as well as morphine and curare types of alkaloids and the condensed organic base, compound 48/80.

5-Hydroxytryptamine (5-HT, serotonin) was originally studied as the vasoconstrictor substance of serum. Whereas, most usually its intravenous injection produces pressor effects, this may be phasic, tachyphylactic or variable, according to species; its positive inotropic and chronotopic effects are more consistent. On visceral smooth muscle its effects commonly resemble histamine, and similarly its occurrence and release from various tissues have been postulated to have functional significance.

Antihistamine Compounds. The recognized role of histamine in various allergies has attached special significance to the laboratory development of drugs that antagonize most of the common pharmacologic effects of histamine. These compounds, developed first in French laboratories, have been improved and employed extensively in general clinical practice. The first representatives of this group to be used widely were diphenhydramine (Benadryl) and tripelennamine (Pyribenzamine). Other USP products of this type are chlorpheniramine (Chlor-Trimeton), doxylamine (Decapryn), pyrilamine (Neo-antergan), and promethazine (Phenergan). Chlorcyclizine (Perazil) is chemically distinct, containing a piperazine ring instead of the common ethylenediamine or aminoethyl ether grouping. Its period of action is claimed to be greater.

The antihistamines have recently been classified as H_1 receptor antagonists and H_2 receptor antagonists. By far the largest number of antihistamines, including those above, are H_1 receptor antagonists. In 1977, an H_2 receptor antagonist, cimetidine, was introduced in this country for the treatment of duodenal ulcer. It antagonizes those responses to histamine, such as gastric secretory effect, that are uninfluenced by H_1 receptor antagonists.

Experimental work has demonstrated that the action of these compounds is to combine with cellular receptor substances on which histamine acts ordinarily. The usual action of subsequently injected or released histamine thereby is nullified through inability of histamine to combine with its usual receptor substance in the effector cell. The blocking action is accomplished without any necessary stimulant or depressant action by the antihistaminic drug. Some side actions are obtained by these compounds, but they are independent of the primary blocking action. In the laboratory, previous injections of H_1 receptor antagonists will block the usual action of histamine in producing bronchospasm in the guinea pig, histamine whealing in the skin, hypotension in the cat or the dog and contraction of isolated gut strip from the guinea pig. Several of these compounds have in common some degree of local anesthetic action, some weak atropine-like action, and some smooth muscle spasmolytic action. H_1 receptor antagonists do not block histamine-induced gastric secretion. The duration of action of these compounds is short; generally they do not have cumulative effects. Doses must be repeated every 3 to 6 hours in order to maintain the therapeutic effects. Clinically the H_1 receptor antagonists are most effective in diminishing the symptoms of seasonal hay fever, urticaria, angioneurotic edema, serum sickness, drug reactions, atopic and contact dermatitis, pruritus, insect bites and the allergic cough of asthma. The most common side-actions of these compounds are sedation and weakness, although they may produce tremors and excitation also. Mouth dryness is common; gastrointestinal disturbances occur occasionally. Agranulocytosis and hemolytic anemia have been reported in a few cases, due largely to the widespread indiscriminate use of these compounds as a fancied preventive of the common cold. Methapyri-

lene, an ingredient in several over-the-counter sleep aids and other formulations, causes liver cancer in rats and mice and is presumed to do so in humans.

One of the antihistaminics, phenindamine (Thephorin), has little sedative action and may act as a central nervous system stimulant. Promethazine (Phenergan) is the antihistaminic from which the phenothiazine tranquilizers evolved; it is relatively long acting and has unusual capacity to block serotonin effects on smooth muscle. Cyproheptadine (Periactin) is a newer antihistamine with potent antiserotonin activity.

Dimenhydrinate (Dramamine), a salt of diphenhydramine and chlorotheophylline, had proved to be of value in reducing the incidence or the intensity of motion sickness. Usually it is administered in oral tablets of 50 mg. Other antihistamines have this characteristic, but it is absent in some, and, accordingly, the anti-motion-sickness effect is not considered to be related to the antihistaminic action; most probably the sedative and the atropine-like actions are involved in this effect. Other antihistaminics used in this way and as antiemetics are cyclizine (Marezine), meclizine (Bonine), pipamazine (Mornidine) and trimethobenzamide (Tigan).

Cimetidine (Tagamet) competitively inhibits the action of histamine at the H_2 receptors of the parietal cells. Despite the extensive list of actions of histamine on H_2 receptors in many tissues, there is only one practical clinical application of the H_2 antagonists—the suppression of gastric acid secretion. Historically, burimamide, introduced in 1972, was the first effective H_2 receptor blocker, followed by metiamide, abandoned because it produces granulocytopenia. Cimetidine inhibits both daytime and nocturnal basal gastric acid secretion. It also inhibits secretion stimulated by food, histamine, pentagastrin, caffeine and insulin. It is indicated in short-term treatment of duodenal ulcer, and in the treatment of pathological hypersecretory conditions (i.e., Zollinger-Ellison Syndrome, systemic mastocytosis, multiple endocrine adenomas). A rather large number of seemingly unrelated adverse effects have been reported. These include pancytopenia, impotence, mental confusion, gynecomastia, and fever. Hypoprothrombinemia has been noted in patients receiving cimetidine and warfarin concurrently. Perforation of duodenal, esophageal, and gastric ulcers has been reported following abrupt discontinuance of the drug.

HORMONES

Adrenal Cortex

Extracts of adrenal cortex can maintain life in adrenalectomized animals and have been useful in Addison's disease and other forms of adrenal insufficiency. Their effects essentially reverse the derangements of adrenal insufficiency since they bring about increase in strength and weight, sodium retention, potassium excretion. Aqueous extracts have been given intravenously in crises, and more concentrated oily solutions have been given intramuscularly for prolonged effects. Standardization in the USP was defined in terms of hydrocortisone acetate. These extracts are now used very infrequently, since the more important hormones of the adrenal cortex are available synthetically. Extraction of these hormones had been considered a relatively poor yield procedure, since little was actually stored in the gland, synthesis in the gland being followed by rapid release into the bloodstream. Desoxycorticosterone and aldosterone are the chief salt-retaining hormones of the adrenal cortex and hydrocortisone the chief glycogenic and anti-inflammatory agent. Whereas the salt-retaining hormones possess little activity of the other type, hydrocortisone has activity of both types. The adrenal cortex also secretes androgens and, to a very limited degree, progesterone and estradiol.

Salt-Retaining Cortical Hormones (Mineralocorticoids)

Desoxycorticosterone acetate (DOCA), which occurs in the adrenal cortex in small amounts, was synthesized in 1937 and is now available under a number of registered names (Cortate, Percorten, etc.). Its usefulness is limited to conditions of adrenal insufficiency in which it is used commonly to supplement administration of hydrocortisone and substantial doses of sodium chloride. Its activity is limited singularly to water and electrolyte effects, sodium ion and water being retained and potassium being excreted through direct effect on the kidney tubules. There is a decrease in nitrogen retention; an increase in absorption of fat and glucose from the intestine. Toxic manifestations are largely those of water retention and increased blood volume. Hypertension develops after prolonged administration. Potassium depletion may require adjustment. Microcrystalline suspensions in oil are given intramuscularly, and pellets implanted under the skin provide an effective dose for months.

Aldosterone increases sodium and chloride reabsorption by the renal tubules, and its sodium-retaining activity is 25 to 100 times that of DOCA. The resulting increased salt levels and osmolarity of intracellular fluids may be presumed to increase secretion of the antidiuretic hormone, with correspondingly increased reabsorption of water from the glomerular filtrate. While retaining sodium, aldosterone increases excretion of potassium, magnesium and hydrogen ions. Aldosterone is secreted by the outer zone of the adrenal cortex, one of the most important stimuli being angiotensin originated by the juxtaglomerular apparatus. Unlike the glucocorticoids, its secretion is not much influenced by stimulation from the anterior pituitary (ACTH). Hypoaldosteronism occurs in adrenal insufficiency, and hyperaldosteronism is associated with generalized edema and hypertension, including toxemia of pregnancy, congestive heart failure, hepatic cirrhosis and the nephrotic syndrome. These conditions are considered secondary causes leading to the increased secretion of aldosterone; primary aldosteronism is due to an adrenal cortical adenoma or hyperplasia of the gland. Aldosterone secretion is decreased by heparin and by metyrapone, the latter interfering with biosynthesis. The sodium-retaining effect on the renal tubules is directly blocked by some structurally related drugs; spironolactone (Aldactone) is a clinically useful blocking agent that is most effective in removing edema fluid when it is combined with a mercurial or thiazide diuretic. Aldosterone itself is not used clinically.

The susceptibility of aldosterone to blocking action by spironolactone and some similar relations that have been demonstrated experimentally with DOCA lead to speculations in regard to the possible type of attachment of these compounds to a receptor site. A close association with the alpha surface of rings A, C and D and with the side chain seems to be essential.

Glucocorticoids

Hydrocortisone, cortisone and some of their highly active, clinically useful analogs have generally similar actions, and this can also be true of corticotropin (ACTH), which acts on the adrenals to stimulate secretion of hydrocortisone. Actions are: provision of resistance to stress in conditions of adrenal insufficiency; provision of antiinflammatory and antiallergic effects, both systemically and locally; promotion of glycogen deposition, gluconeogenesis, hyperglycemia and glycosuria; promotion of breakdown of protein, possibly inhibiting synthesis of proteins; inhibition of activity by the lymphatic system, with leukopenia and reduction in size of lymph nodes; the reduction of counts of circulating eosinophils; inhibition of fibroblast proliferation and increase in collagen breakdown; stimulation of erythropoiesis and production of platelets; maintenance of muscle strength in physiologic amounts and induction of muscle wasting in excessive amounts; stimulation of gastric acid production; inhibition of bone growth, matrix formation and calcification; suppression of ACTH release by the anterior pituitary; suppression of production of endogenous steroids by the adrenal cortex.

The first therapeutic application of these compounds

was in the active rheumatoid arthritis. Although they accomplish temporary suppression of most manifestations of this condition, they are used ordinarily only after an adequate trial of salicylates, phenylbutazone or even gold therapy. This reservation is based on the side effects associated with the necessarily prolonged therapy of this condition. Other indications for these compounds are rheumatic fever with carditis; idiopathic thrombocytopenic purpura; temporary benefit in acute leukemia; serum sickness and angioneurotic edema; generalized eczema; exfoliative dermatitis; pemphigus; topically, in numerous inflammatory skin and ocular conditions; pulmonary fibrosis, sarcoidosis and emphysema; ulcerative colitis; nephrotic syndrome; systemic lupus erythematosus; cerebral edema. Prolonged administration in these conditions initiates side-effects, which, in variable degree, may be manifested as Cushing's syndrome symptoms (moon face, central obesity, lipemia, diabetes, protein depletion, osteoporsis, hypertension, cutaneous striae, fragility of blood vessels, mental aberrations). Infectious processes may be intensified. Activation of peptic ulcers has been relatively frequent. There is lowered threshold to epileptic seizures. Aseptic necrosis of the femoral head has developed, probably through suppression of osteoblastic activity.

Cataracts, with minimal loss of vision, have been reported, with substantial incidence in patients receiving cortocosteroids for periods longer than 2 years. Intraocular pressure is increased, and thinness of the cornea, with perforation, has occurred. Increased intracranial pressure, with mild papilledema, has been found, particularly in children. Corticosteroids suppress secretion of ACTH, with resulting adrenal insufficiency to the point of atrophy; this effect may persist for months following administration for stressful conditions, particularly surgery. Mothers taking corticosteroids should be advised not to nurse since these drugs appear in breast milk and could suppress growth, interfere with endogenous corticosteroid production or cause other untoward effects in the infant.

Contraindications to systemically administered glucocorticoids are considered to be active tuberculosis, malignant hypertension, uremia, psychoses and active peptic ulcers. Contraindications to ophthalmic preparations include viral, tuberculous and fungal infections of the eye.

Glucocorticoids as well as mineralocorticoids are metabolized largely in the liver by a variety of degradations, the products of which are excreted in the urine; oxidation and conjugation as sulfates and glucuronides take place. Radioisotope tagging of orally administered hydrocortisone discloses that its breakdown products can be recovered in the urine to the extent of about 90 percent in 48 hours. Before its degradation, transport in the blood involves some protective combination with albumin and globulins.

Cortisone acetate was synthesized in 1948 and was the first of this group to be used extensively. It is administered parenterally, orally or topically.

Hydrocortisone is administered usually in moderately smaller dose. Its acetate is less water soluble and its cypionate ester still less water soluble, while the sodium succinate salt (Solu-Cortef) is highly water soluble. Prednisone, prednisolone and their fluoro and methyl derivatives (triamcinolone, dexamethasone, betamethasone, etc.) are effective in smaller doses and have much higher ratios of anti-inflammatory action to salt-retaining properties. Some of these are esterified to reduce water solubility and others are modified as phosphates or succinates to increase water solubility. Of those used exclusively by local application for inflammatory and allergic dermatoses, fluorometholone and hydrocortamate do not cause systemic effects; these effects do occur with fludrocortisone acetate, which is used chiefly but not exclusively by topical application. This last-named compound, which is the 9-fluoro derivative of hydrocortisone acetate, is essentially a more potent form of hydrocortisone, with high sodium-retaining action. The other fluorinated derivatives in common use are generally without these electrolyte effects.

Inhibition of Adrenal Cortex

The adrenals are peculiarly damaged by the insecticide, tetrachlorodiphenylethane (DDD), and are inhibited by an aniline type of derivative, amphenone. Synthesis of adrenal hormones is inhibited by metyrapone (Metopirone), and this is used as a test of anterior pituitary function; in the presence of functioning adrenals, urinary excretion of hormone precursors will be increased. In deficient anterior pituitary function, metyrapone will not increase urinary metabolites of the precursors of hydrocortisone, corticosterone, and aldosterone. Aminoglutethimide (Elipten) blocks steroidogenesis by interfering with the conversion of cholesterol to pregnenolone.

Anterior Pituitary

The anterior pituitary gland has been shown to secrete agents that promote growth (GH); thyroid function (TSH); adrenal cortex function (ACTH); diabetic tendencies; and gonadotropic effects, which include primarily maturation of ovarian follicles (FSH), luteinization of ovarian follicles (LH or ICSH); progesterone secretion by the corpus luteum, and lactation (LTH) and, in the male, spermatogenesis and stimulation of interstitial cells. The secretion of these hormones is stimulated by hypothalamic-releasing factors also known as hypophysiotropic hormones. The anterior pituitary preparation commonly used therapeutically is corticortropin (ACTH).

When *corticotropin* (ACTH) is administered to animals or human subjects with responsive adrenal glands, several cortical hormones are secreted. Effects are generally similar to those produced by cortisone, with additionally more pronounced changes in electrolyte metabolism and androgenic function. A decrease in eosinophils in the peripheral blood (Thorn test) is an index of ACTH action. Concomitantly, there is also a decrease in lymphocytes and an increase in neutrophils. With a functioning adrenal cortex, the administration of ACTH measurably increases plasma and urine 17-hydroxycorticosteroids and 17-ketosteroids. In contrast with cortisone, ACTH causes adrenal hypertrophy. Also, ACTH is considered to be more likely to produce hypertension and virilism. Allergic sensitivity to ACTH has developed in a small percentage of patients, the reactions varying from anaphylactoid shock to giant urticaria.

Although it is ineffective in Addison's disease, ACTH is used for treatment of generally the same conditions as cortisone. However, therapy with ACTH is less convenient and less predictable and appears to possess no advantages over glucocorticoid therapy in most diseases. It does have an accepted role in the management of severe myasthenia gravis.

Numerous influences release ACTH from the anterior pituitary; one of these is a decapeptide termed corticotropin-releasing factor.

ACTH is an open-chain polypeptide consisting of 39 amino acids and has been synthesized as an experimental demonstration of its structure. It is obtained commercially from the pituitaries of domestic animals and is bioassayed by measurement of the marked diminution it produces in the ascorbic acid content of the adrenals in hypophysectomized mice. (The cholesterol content of adrenals is decreased also.) Activity is expressed in terms of a standard powder, 1 international unit corresponding to 1 mg. of standard powder. It is available as a stable dry powder but is dispensed most usually in solutions with 10 to 40 units per ml. Repository forms for intramuscular injection are made up with gelatin or a zinc hydroxide suspension.

Synthetic ACTH analogs containing subunits of the 39 amino acid polypeptides have been prepared. Cosyntropin (Cortrosyn) contains the first 24 amino acids in the natural sequence. It is used as a diagnostic agent in patients believed to have adrenal insufficiency. Response is determined by plasma cortisol levels or urinary excretion of steroids. The incidence of sensitivity reactions to cosyntropin is less than with ACTH since synthetic polypeptides containing 1 to 24 amino acids have little immunologic activity.

Human growth hormone is not commercially available, and the limited supply has been used for clinical investigation in replacement therapy of hypopituitary dwarfism. Pituitary growth hormone (GH) secretion is controlled by two separate hypothalamic regulatory hormones with direct actions on the pituitary cells, one that stimulates and the other that inhibits its release. Growth hormone-release and inhibitory hormone (GR-IH, "somatostatin") has been purified from extracts of ovine hypothalami. An unexpected effect of this decapeptide is its action in inhibiting glucagon and insulin from pancreatic alpha and beta cells. Its effects on glucagon may have special significance, since its injection causes moderate hypoglycemia. The therapeutic usefulness of somatostatin in diabetes, acromegaly, and other diseases is being explored. Recent reports indicate that it is effective in the treatment of bleeding esophageal varices, presumably through its ability to reduce splanchnic blood flow, and therefore portal pressure, in patients with cirrhosis of the liver.

Thyrotropin (TSH, Thytropar) acts upon the functioning thyroid to increase iodine uptake and the formation and secretion of thyroid hormones. Used primarily as a diagnostic agent, it can be employed to determine mild forms of hypothyroidism. It also is possible to differentiate thyroidal (primary) hypothyroidism from pituitary (secondary hypothyroidism) by giving TSH, which will cause a response in thyroid function when the defect is in the pituitary. A more sensitive method of distinguishing primary from secondary hypothyroidism is to measure serum levels of TSH by radioimmunoassay technique, which is high in primary and low in secondary hypothyroidism. The thyroid-releasing hormone (TRH) has been synthesized and is undergoing various clinical applications. In normal persons, it causes release of thyrotropin and prolactin. It may be useful as a diagnostic agent in evaluation of pituitary reserve and differentiation of hypothalmic hypothyroidism from that resulting from pituitary destruction. Hypothyroid patients respond to TRH with a marked elevation of serum thyrotropin. Patients with hyperthyroidism do not respond to TRH. Follicle-stimulating hormone (FSH) has been isolated from the anterior pituitary of swine, sheep and humans. The use of porcine or bovine FSH in humans results in an antihormone response.

Luteinizing hormone (LH) is available in limited quantities for clinical investigation. It has been used in conjunction with human chorionic gonadotropin to stimulate ovulation. Luteotropic hormone (LTH), also known as prolactin or lactogenic hormone, exists in quantities available only for research in humans.

Bromocriptine (Parlodel), a peptide ergot alkaloid derivative, is a potent dopamine receptor agonist that inhibits prolactin secretion. The tuberoinfundibular dopaminergic neurons modulate the secretion of prolactin from the anterior pituitary by stimulating the release of prolactin inhibitory factor. Since it activates post-synaptic dopamine receptors bromocriptine significantly reduces plasma levels of prolactin in patients with hyperprolactinemia. It is indicated for the short-term treatment of amenorrhea and galactorrhea associated with hyperprolactinemia.

Posterior Pituitary

The posterior lobe of the pituitary body contains hormones having oxytocic, antidiuretic and vasoactive properties. Two fractions are identified. One contains most of the antidiuretic and vasoactive activity while the other is predominantly oxytocic. Both fractions, vasopressin and oxytocin, have been synthesized. Both are peptides containing eight amino acids; six of these amino acids are common to both peptides. Oxytocin preparations are assayed for oxytocic activity by measuring the blood pressure fall that they produce in domestic chickens. Vasopressin (Pitressin) is assayed by measuring the blood pressure rise that it produces in rats. It also has antidiuretic and gut-stimulating effects. Vasopressin, notwithstanding its suggestive name, is not used as a pressor agent. It is used in the management of diabetes insipidus. Its mode of action as an antidiuretic is attributed to an increase in the size of pores or channels for the flow of water along osmotic gradients. This is mediated by increases in the concentration of adenosine-3′, 5′-monophosphate, which then alters permeability.

Posterior pituitary antidiuretic hormones and their synthetic analogs are effective only for diabetes insipidus caused by deficient secretion or release of antidiuretic hormone (ADH) resulting from tumors, trauma, or infections. "Nephrogenic" diabetes insipidus, characterized by unresponsiveness of the kidney to antidiuretic hormone, does not respond to ADH replacement. Lypressin (Diapid), a synthetic lysine vasopressin nasal spray is used two to four times a day; its duration of action may be too short for patients with severe disease. Repository intramuscular vasopressin is effective for 24 to 48 hours, but can cause pain and sterile abscesses at the site of injection. Desmopressin (DDAVP), a new synthetic analog of arginine vasopressin, has a longer duration of action than previously available synthetic preparations, and appears to have a low incidence of adverse effects. It

probably is the drug of choice for treatment of severe central diabetes insipidus.

Pancreas

Insulin is a crystalline protein obtained from pancreatic extracts. It is composed of two chains of amino acids, linked by two disulfide bridges, with additionally one cyclic S-S bridge attached to one of these peptide chains. Even limited hydrolysis destroys its biologic activity. A widely held view is that insulin promotes the entry of glucose into skeletal and heart muscle cells, fat and leukocytes. Some basic aspects of its action may involve induction of enzyme synthesis. Its action is exerted on specific receptors in cell membranes. In addition to the older in vivo bioassays, which depend on the production of convulsions in mice or the lowering of blood glucose in rabbits, several more sensitive, in vitro methods have been developed. One such method is based on the capacity of insulin to increase the glycogen content or the glucose uptake of the rat diaphragm; another is by radioimmunoassay.

Crystalline zinc insulin (regular, CZI) is absorbed rapidly from subcutaneous tissues leading to peak activity in 2 to 4 hours.

Protamine zinc insulin (PZI) is a buffered suspension of water, the maximum hypoglycemic action of which usually is obtained in about 18 to 20 hours following its subcutaneous injection. The corresponding period is about 12 hours with globin zinc insulin. *NPH* (neutral protamine Hagedorn) *insulin* is a modification of protamine zinc insulin but differs in that it contains relatively less protamine and still less zinc; also the insulin is crystalline rather than amorphous. The USP designation for NPH insulin is *isophane insulin.* This preparation has both a rapid and a sustained action. Since it does not contain an excess of protamine, regular insulin can be added to it without losing its rapid, intense action. This is in contrast with protamine zinc insulin, which has sufficient excess of protamine to combine with and retard some of the regular insulin with which it may be mixed.

Lente insulin is a mixture of insulin (of specially regulated particle size) with sufficient zinc chloride to make it relatively insoluble. Three varieties have been made available, and various periods of sustained action can be obtained by mixing these varieties. These preparations have the advantage of freedom from any modifying foreign protein. In order to avoid confusion concerning volume, concentration or correct syringe to be used, the American Diabetes Association has recommended that all insulin preparations should be marketed in a concentration of 100 units per cc. Current predictions are that, by 1980, about 90 per cent of the units used in this country will be U-100.

In addition to the generally available insulins, some highly purified, single component preparations are obtainable for special cases. These preparations are useful in insulin "allergy" and atrophy of fatty tissue at the site of injection.

Sulfonylurea compounds have hypoglycemic actions in both normal and diabetic subjects and, under some conditions, make it possible to manage diabetics without insulin injections. Their mode of action is probably that of increasing insulin secretion from the beta cells; they are not active in the total absence of endogenous insulin. Analogs of this group are tolbutamide (Orinase), chlorpropamide (Diabinese), acetohexamide (Dymelor) and tolazamide (Tolinase). Duration of action is the principal difference in members of this group. Profound, uncontrolled hypoglycemias have developed in some cases, and this has occurred particularly in the aged. An intolerance to alcohol similar to the disulfiram (Antabuse) reaction may occur following ingestion of tolbutamide. The sulfonylureas should be used only in patients with adult-onset diabetes that cannot be controlled by diet or weight loss and in whom the use of insulin is impractical. Phenformin (DBI), a biguanide, lowers blood sugar by potentiating the action of endogenous and exogenous insulin, particularly on adipose tissue. DBI has numerous contraindications, including severe hepatic and renal disease.

Diabetic or hyperglycemic coma, commonly occurring in association with some infection, is treated with intravenous and subcutaneous insulin, saline infusions, dextrose and, possibly, pressor agents. Gross deposition of glycogen carries with it potassium removal, and hypokalemia is a common secondary complication of treatment.

Ovary

Estrogens of the steroid type are obtained from the urine of stallions, pregnant women, and pregnant mares. *Estrone* (theelin) was the first estrogen to be isolated in pure form, and this accomplishment in 1929 was shortly followed by isolation of estriol, the trihydroxy analog of the ketone, estrone. Both are thought to be formed naturally from estradiol, the dihydroxy analog. *Estradiol* is used in ester form as the benzoate and the dipropionate and as the ethinyl derivative. Other esterified derivatives of estradiol are the cypionate and the valerate.

Conjugated estrogens (Premarin) are a combination of the sodium salts of the sulfate esters of estrogenic substances, principally estrone and equilin. They are effective parenterally, orally and topically.

In addition to these natural modified steroids, it has been possible to produce, at lower cost, synthetic compounds that have typical estrogenic activity and are effective on oral administration. The earliest of this group and one of the most potent, *diethylstilbestrol,* is based on modification of a stilbene nucleus, and of the several others available, such as *Dienestrol,* most have an obvious spatial relationship.

Estrogenic activity is usually typical regardless of the selection from this group, and the chief difference is in dosage and in rates of absorption and excretion. With diethylstilbestrol, incidence of anorexia and nausea has been thought to be higher. The primary effects of estrogens involve growth stimulation of the endometrium, the vaginal epithelium and the mammary duct glands, through inhibition of secretion of the anterior pituitary gonadotropin, FSH. Estrogens are used for control of symptoms of the menopause and in amenorrhea, senile vaginitis, kraurosis vulvae and pruritus vulvae. They have some restraining influence on metastases of prostatic and mammary carcinoma. On the other hand, they have been reported to increase the risk of endometrial carcinoma in postmenopausal women. They are metabolized largely in the liver, and a relatively small fraction of these compounds can be recovered from the urine in conjugated form.

Progesterone, produced by the corpus luteum, can be obtained by extraction of the ovaries and has been prepared synthetically. It has the effect of converting the proliferating endometrium to the secretory phase and prepares the uterus for nidation of the ovum; contractile activity of the myometrium is decreased. It is not effective orally, and, when injected intramuscularly, its action in preventing threatened abortion and reducing uterine bleeding and dysmenorrhea is not very clearly documented. Orally effective synthetic variants, known as progestogens, are used more frequently, and these have variable degrees of associated androgenic and estrogenic actions. These synthetic compounds include several variants with the C19 carbon (ethisterone, hydroxyprogesterone, medroxyprogesterone) and several nor-compounds without this carbon (norethindrone, norethynodrel). The latter are effective in antagonizing production of FSH and thereby preventing ovulation. Virilizing effects on the fetus can occur with the use of some of these compounds during pregnancy.

Several contraceptives are available in which orally effective synthetic progestational agents are combined with an estrogen. Examples are: norethynodrel with mestranol (Enovid), norethindrone with mestranol (Ortho-Novum, Norinyl), norethindrone acetate with ethinyl estradiol (Norlestrin) and medroxyprogesterone acetate with ethinyl estradiol (Provest). These combinations are taken on the 5th through the 24th days of the cycle, and is thought that they suppress ovulation by inhibiting pituitary gonadotropin release (FSH). However, there is evidence that they are effective in doses lower than those necessary to suppress gonadotropins, and there may also be a direct effect on the ovary or interference with transport of ova or with nidation: cervical mucus is made less penetrable to sperm.

Such combination of estrogen-progestogen first was tried in 1956; it has been generally available since and has been used satisfactorily in millions of women, but there has been increasing recognition of numerous side effects. One of the more serious of the possible side effects is thrombophlebitis; however, its presence has been considered by some to be coincidental. Effects that are more clearly related are nausea, breakthrough bleeding, retention of salt and water with weight gain, hypertension in susceptible individuals, skin effects, and breast tenderness. In less frequent instances there have been reports of loss of hair, increase in size of fibroids, masculinization of female newborn infants and estrogen aggravation of hepatitis. Cigarette smoking increases the risk of serious cardiovascular side effects from oral contraceptive use. When used during early pregnancy, birth defects/and or malignancy in off-spring may occur. Another regimen is: an estrogen for 16 days, followed by a progestational agent for 5 days; this is considered to simulate the usual cycle more closely. However, such sequential oral contraceptives are less effective than combination products. The "minipill," which contains only a progestogen, is even less effective than the sequential formulations. In large doses, estrogens or progesterones may be used as contraceptives.

Clomiphene (Clomid) is a nonsteroidal agent that may stimulate ovulation in anovulatory women who have potentially functional hypothalamic-pituitary-ovarian systems and adequate endogenous estrogen. It is used in women with amenorrhea who desire pregnancy. With its use, the incidence of multiple pregnancies is eight times the normal. Blurring or other visual symptoms may occasionally occur and may render such activities as driving a car or operating machinery more hazardous than usual, particularly in variable lighting.

Placenta

Chorionic gonadotropin, obtained from the urine of pregnant women, is used in cryptorchidism; descent of the testis usually results if there is no anatomic obstruction. In infertile women in whom anovulation is caused by absence of or a low level of gonadotropins, it may produce ovulation.

Menotropins (Pergonal) are pituitary hormones (FSH and LH) prepared from the urine of postmenopausal women. They are used to treat anovulatory women whose ovaries are capable of responding to pituitary gonadotropins but whose gonadotropins are decreased or absent. Results of clinical experience are varied because of considerable difference in individual response and different dosage regimens employed.

Testes

Methyltestosterone and testosterone propionate, as well as enanthate, cypionate and phenylacetate, are synthetic androgens that provide effective replacement therapy when there is deficiency or lack of internal secretion of the testes, as in eunuchoidism, hypogonadism and surgical castration. Their use temporarily suppresses spermatogenesis. In the female it is used in control of menorrhagia and metrorrhagia and in post-partum inhibition of lactation or breast engorgement. Large doses (from 150 to 300 mg. testosterone propionate weekly) have been used for palliation of breast cancer. Fluoxymesterone is used for the same purpose. These androgens accelerate growth of prostatic carcinoma. Side effects include hirsutism, voice deepening, increase in libido, enlargement of the clitoris and flushing or acne. Unusually prolonged administration of androgens may lead to hypercalcemia or, because of electrolyte retention, to edema and cardiac failure. Methyltestosterone, even in moderate doses, has produced jaundice in a number of instances. Some of the androgens can be given by sublingual administration.

Characteristically, androgens increase protein synthesis, along with a measureable degree of nitrogen retention and weight gain. Creatinuria is produced by methyltestosterone but is decreased by testosterone. This protein anabolic effect can be considered to be a desirable type of supportive therapy, and efforts have been made to develop steroids in which the anabolic effect is obtained with a relative absence of the effects on secondary sex characteristics. One such product is norethandrolone; others are nandrolone, oxymethalone, stanolone and stanozolol. Fluoxymesterone is used not only as an anabolic steroid but also for androgen deficiency.

The anabolic steroids have numerous adverse effects. They may cause sodium retention, aggravation of carcinoma of the prostate, and masculinization of the fetus if used in pregnant women. When used in children to stimulate growth, they may lead to premature epiphyseal closure.

Thyroid

The activity of dried thyroid usually is related to its iodine content, and the USP specifications require this content to be about 0.2 per cent. Additionally, it is common commercial practice to bioassay the preparations by determining the increase in oxygen consumption in guinea pigs. Another less common test is based on the increased sensitivity to hypoxia produced in small animals. One milligram of crystalline thryroxine given intravenously corresponds in activity to approximately 60 mg. dried thyroid given orally. Only the latter preparation is used routinely in treatment of myxedema, cretinism and other conditions, such as nephrosis and menstrual irregularities. Since metabolic stimulation develops slowly, continued administration has cumulative effects.

Sodium levothyroxine (Synthroid) represents the levo isomer of thyroxine and is administered orally in doses of 0.1 or 0.2 mg.

Thyroxine, which is tetraiodothyronine, apparently is converted in the tissues to triiodothyronine, which is four or five times as active as thyroxine and is more rapid in its action. Triiodothyronine is available as the levo form, sodium liothyronine, usually in tablets containing 5 or 25 μg.

Calcitonin (thyrocalcitonin) is a single-chain polypeptide isolated from thyroid glands of several mammalian species. Low doses experimentally have reduced serum calcium levels. LATS, a long-acting thyroid stimulator unrelated to the thyrotropin, has been recognized in the serum of patients with hyperthyroidism. It is considered to be a gamma globulin antibody developed as an autoimmune reaction against thyroid protein. Propylthiouracil is also highly effective in reducing the manifestations of hyperthyroidism and is considered to act through blocking thyroxine synthesis. Under the influence of propylthiouracil, the gland undergoes an extreme hyperplasia because of the increased action of the pituitary thyrotropic hormone, an activity that follows the low levels of thyroglobulin or blood thyroxine. If iodides are administered along with propylthiouracil, the vascularity and the sponginess of the gland are reduced greatly. Another compound used in the same way is methimazole, (Tapazole). Iothiouracil (Itrumil) has been inferred to combine the actions of iodides and the thiouracil compounds.

Although the reduction of hyperthyroid symptoms by iodides is one of the most reliable and valuable therapeutic maneuvers, the mechanism has been obscure. It has been proposed that iodides directly inhibit the thyrotropic hormone or, again, that they interfere with the enzymic conversion of thyroglobulin to thyroxine just before thyroxine leaves the gland to appear in the serum as protein-bound iodine. Drugs of the thiouracil type are thought to interfere with the enzymic conversion of iodides to elemental iodine; in the presence of elemental iodine, tyrosine is converted to diiodotyrosine, which is a direct precursor of thyroxine.

Parathyroid

Parathyroid increases blood levels of calcium chiefly by mobilization of calcium from the bone; it has been proposed that osteoclasts are stimulated to produce organic acids, which have a solubilizing effect on bone calcium. This hormone also appears to have some actions in the intestine, to promote absorption of calcium, and in the kidney tubules, to increase calcium reabsorption and to decrease phosphorus reabsorption. The hormone is thought to be a protein, although an active peptide has been reported. When obtained in extracts of the parathyroid glands, it is assayed in terms of USP units, 100 of which raise blood calcium levels in dogs by 1 mg. per 100 ml. The only therapeutic value of this preparation is in the management of parathyroid deficiency, which, at the state of tetany, calls for intravenous therapy. Refractoriness develops rapidly, and sustained treatment is carried out most effectively with dihydrotachysterol USP, which has actions somewhat between those of the hormone and vitamin D. As a diagnostic test, parathyroid extract is useful in establishing the diagnosis of idiopathic and postoperative hypoparathyroidism.

Calcitonin, a hormone secreted by the parafollicular cells of the thyroid, is also involved with calcium homeostasis. It produces hypocalcemia by inhibiting bone resorption and promotes urinary excretion of calcium and phosphate. It has been used clinically in osteoporosis, osteitis deformans (Paget's disease) and a variety of hypercalcemic states. Its short duration of action limits its usefulness. Etidronate (Didronel), a synthetic compound, with a longer duration of action, slows the rate of bone resorption and new bone accretion and is used in treating Paget's disease.

PROSTAGLANDINS

Prostaglandins are a group of cyclic, unsaturated fatty acids originally found in seminal fluid but occurring in many tissues. All are derived in the body from "essential" fatty acids (e.g., linoleic, linolenic) of the diet. They are derivatives of prostanoic acid, a C-20 acid that contains a five-membered ring. They do not exist free in tissues in appreciable amounts but rather are biosynthesized and released in response to many varied stimuli. Once formed, they are rapidly metabolized, especially by the lungs. Therefore, they may serve as "local hormones," acting either in the tissue where formed or on nearby tissue. Their trivial names are by letter and subscript number. The prostaglandins (PG)PGE_1, PGE_2, PGA_1, and PGF_2 alpha have been most widely studied. They are among the most active natural substances known. Although similar in structure, their actions differ both quantitatively and qualitatively. Their major pharmacologic activity is exerted on the uterus, gonads, bronchi, kidneys, cardiovascular system, platelets, gastrointestinal system, nervous system and inflammatory and immune mechanisms. Such widespread activity suggests an action on some basic control mechanism. Those actions of prostaglandins that have been investigated clinically include induction of labor and abortion (PGE_2 and PGF_2 alpha), bronchodilation (PGE_1 and PGE_2), inhibition of gastric secretion (PGA_1), vasodilation and diuresis (PGA_1), and inhibition of platelet aggregation for harvesting and preservation of platelets for transfusion (PGE_1). The principal prostaglandins (the "2" series) are formed from arachidonic acid via a cyclic peroxide intermediate. This intermediate can also be converted to thromboxane A_2 (TXA_2). Formed primarily by platelets, this latter compound is a potent vasoconstrictor and platelet aggregating agent. Prostacyclin (PGI_2), synthesized by the vessel and endothelium, is a potent vasodilator and antiaggregating agent. The balance between these two members of the prostaglandin family has tremendous significance for the state of health or disease within the cardiovascular system. Drugs modifying their action are currently under investigation.

Some of the prostaglandins are now synthesized industrially. Dinoprost (prostaglandin F_2 alpha, Prostin F_2 alpha) is used for preparation of instrumental abortion during the first trimester of pregnancy, and also for induction of abortion beyond the 12th week of gestation. Following its use, cardiopulmonary failure and eventual death have been reported.

ANTISEPTICS

External and Irrigation Antiseptics

Many chemicals damage the cytoplasm of pathogenic organisms by general mechanisms that restrain their growth (antisepsis) or cause their death (disinfection). Relatively nonspecific chemicals of this sort are used routinely for external disinfection and for irrigation of the urethra, the bladder, the draining sinuses, etc. Common examples are phenols, cresols, oxidizing agents, chlorine compounds, mercury compounds, silver compounds, furan derivatives, dyes and surface-active agents. These last compounds lower surface tension substantially at the interface of their water solution and air. This property is based on the fact that they are made up of a water-attracting ion and a water-repelling ion. The water-repelling (hydrophobic) component projects partially from the water into the air phase and thereby concentrates the chemical at the interface. Since hydrophobic components usually are fat soluble, they tend also to concentrate at the surface of organisms because of the fat in their membranes. Their surface activity may be considered to be associated usually with ability to concentrate at surfaces of organisms and thereby improve any inherent antiseptic action of a given compound.

Some surface-active agents are ineffective as antiseptics. In a surface-active compound with effective antiseptic action an added advantage comes from the detergent action and the ability to enter small crevices when applied topically. Soap is an example of a surface-active antiseptic whose hydrophobic component carries a negative charge and is anionic; numerous synthetic detergents contain a hydrophobic anionic component. One of these latter, which is used as a surgical antiseptic, is sodium octylphenoxyethoxyethyl ether sulfonate (pHisoderm). This is incorporated with the biphenol derivative, hexachlorophene USP, in the product pHisohex. Practical antiseptics that contain a hydrophobic cationic component have been obtained from quaternary ammonium derivatives. Examples are benzalkonium chloride (Zephiran chloride), benzethonium chloride (Phemerol chloride) and cetyl pyridinium chloride (Ceepryn chloride). Anionic and cationic antiseptics undergo considerable loss of activity if intermixed because of neutralization of opposite charges.

Formaldehyde and sulfur dioxide were used in the past as gaseous disinfectants. Current gaseous sterilization of hospital equipment is accomplished more satisfactorily with ethylene oxide. At workable concentrations, it is effectively bactericidal and virucidal after 4 or more hours exposure at room temperatures. The chemical mechanism is by alkylation.

Urinary Tract Antiseptics

Numerous compounds with antibacterial action are sufficiently concentrated in the urine to exert powerful antiseptic or even disinfectant action. Most of them are taken orally for this purpose, although on occasion they may be given intravenously to obtain maximum urinary concentration. The antibiotics and the sulfonamides are the most effective antiseptics used in urinary tract infections. The sulfonamides are given ordinarily in daily doses that are about half those used for critically dangerous systemic infections. Some of the more prominent of the urinary antiseptics in the period before the sulfonamides and the antibiotics are used occasionally at the present time. One of these, mandelic acid, is given in daily doses of about 10 g., usually as the ammonium, sodium or calcium salt. Commonly it causes gastric irritation; occasionally it causes hematuria; and it may cause acidosis if kidney function is deficient. Methenamine (Urotropin) in an acid urine liberates sufficient quantities of formaldehyde to have an antiseptic effect, which is irritant and frequently causes hematuria. Acidification of the urine is obtained with acid sodium phosphate or ammonium chloride. Methenamine mandelate (Mandelamine) is a combination of mandelic acid and methenamine. The azo dye phenazopyridine (Pyridium) has little antiseptic action, but it has unique qualities of prompt and high concentration in the urine, where it has some local anesthetic action. Nitrofurantoin (Furadantin) has a wide spectrum of antibacterial activity and has been recommended particularly for resistent Proteus and Pseudomonas strains. Following oral administration, about half of this product is excreted unchanged in the urine; it is largely secreted by the tubules. Effective concentrations can be obtained in an acid urine.

Quinoline derivatives, nalidixic acid and oxalinic acid, have been particularly effective in inhibiting growth of gram-negative bacteria in the urinary tract. They appear to act by interference with DNA synthesis. Daily oral doses up to 4.0 g., continued for several days, have been given with occasional side effects related to the gastrointestinal, visual and central nervous systems. Rapid emergence of restraint bacterial strains occur.

SULFONAMIDES

Historical

In 1932, the azo dye prontosil was found to be effective in protecting mice against several lethal doses of hemolytic streptococcal infections. This observation, along with favorable clinical reports and the description of a soluble form, neoprontosil, was reported in 1935 by Domagk of the I.G. Farbenindustrie in Germany. Shortly after that, French workers at the Institut Pasteur demonstrated that these compounds were effective in these types of infections largely through the presence of the relatively simple compound paraamino-benzene-sulfonamide. This compound, later called sulfanilamide, was shown to be effective when administered alone. Both sulfanilamide and the soluble red dye neoprontosil subsequently were demonstrated by clinicians in Britain and the United States to be effective in several types of coccal infections. Chemical substitution in the sulfanilamide molecule has resulted since in the development and the study of several thousand related compounds. Sulfapyridine and sulfathiazole were among the first useful representatives of this group. For various reasons most of these compounds

have been superseded by similar derivatives such as sulfadiazine and sulfamerazine. Other derivatives that have been claimed to have particular advantages over the earlier compounds are *sulfamethazine* and *sulfisoxazole* (Gantrisin). An additional group of sulfonamides has been developed for use as intestinal antiseptics, used largely as preoperative preparation for bowel surgery. They are absorbed poorly from the gut, and large oral doses produce relatively low concentrations in the blood. Examples of this type are: *phthalylsul-fathiazole* USP (Sulfathalidine) and *succinyl sulfathiazole* USP (Sulfasuxidine). These are used also in the bacillary dysenteries and in instances of ulcerative colitis. Sulfapyridine, although no longer used as a general bacteriostatic, has special use in dermatitis herpetiformis.

Another more recent type of sulfonamide variant has longer sustained blood levels after oral administration; their antibacterial range is essentially the same as the other common sulfonamides. Examples are sulfamethoxypyridazine (Kynex, Midicel); sulfadimethoxine (Madribon), and sulfamethizole (Thiosulfil). This group has been particularly identified with occurrence of the Stevens-Johnson syndrome.

Mechanism of Action, Absorption, Distribution, Acetylation, Excretion

The sulfonamides restrain the multiplication of bacteria and, in higher concentrations, may kill bacteria. Ordinarily the restraint of multiplication is assisted by leukocytes and other body-defense mechanisms, and the final result is elimination of the infection. The sulfonamides do not stimulate defense mechanisms or confer immunity to subsequent infections. Growth restraint has been attributed to several possible mechanisms, but most attention has been given to the process by which paraaminobenzoic acid (PABA) is synthesized to pteroylglutamic acid, the latter being a necessary growth factor for several organisms. Sulfonamides presumably interfere with bacterial utilization of PABA by processes of competitive inhibition. This conception is supported by the observation that small amounts of PABA oppose the antibacterial action of sulfonamides. (The same effect is obtained with procaine, which chemically is related closely to PABA). The organisms that are sensitive to sulfonamides are probably incapable of taking up folic acid from their medium and must depend on synthesis of this agent after penetration of PABA and other components. Organisms that can take up folic acid from the media and mammalian systems that take up folic acid as a vitamin are not affected by sulfonamides.

In 1942 an examination of some 50 sulfanilamide types of compounds in terms of acid constants and in vitro bacteriostatic activity showed that bacteriostatic activity was correlated with the negativity of the SO_2 group. Sulfadiazine represented a near optimum, and it was predicted that its range of effectiveness would not be exceeded by other derivatives. This generally has proved to be true, and subsequent variants have differed chiefly in more or less secondary characteristics.

Sulfonamides are most effective in diffuse, nonsuppurative inflammations with maximal tissue invasion and minimal tissue destruction. In the presence of pus or necrotic tissue, the value of sulfonamides is limited chiefly to protection of uninvolved tissues.

Sulfadiazine and related sulfonamides other than the gut antiseptic group are all absorbed well after oral administration. Sulfanilamide is absorbed the most completely, and only during conditions of severe diarrhea does any important quantity of orally administered sulfonamide appear in the feces. The administration of 8 g. sulfadiazine on the first day and 4 g. on subsequent days ordinarily produces a blood level of about 15 mg. per 100 ml., which is considered to be the therapeutic optimum. Higher levels do not achieve important therapeutic advantage and may favor development of toxic effects. Commonly, somewhat lower doses are used. Sulfanilamide is distributed through all body fluids with exceptional uniformity. Sulfadiazine and sulfamerazine appear in the spinal fluid and the ocular fluid in substantial but reduced fractions of the level in the bloodstream. Under conditions of meningeal inflammation, high levels appear in the spinal fluid, and there is no clear indication for intrathecal administration.

Although sulfanilamide is soluble to the extent of one per cent in water at body temperature, the other sulfonamides are relatively insoluble. The influence of the various substituted groups in salfadiazine, sulfamerazine, etc., is to confer a degree of acidity on the unsubstituted hydrogen atom of the sulfonamide group. When such acidity is neutralized by alkali, the resulting salts are soluble readily in water. Sodium salts of sulfadiazine, etc., may be administered intravenously in five per cent solutions. Such solutions are strongly alkaline (pH 9 to 11) and correspondingly are irritant if injected into tissues, although 0.5 per cent solutions can be safely injected subcutaneously. Neoprontosil is relatively nonirritant and is available in 2.5 percent solutions.

Shortly after the introduction of sulfanilamide, Marshall and co-workers developed a practical method for determination of sulfonamide concentrations in body fluids. Protein-free filtrates were treated with diazotization reagents to form red dyes similar to the earlier neoprontosil. The intensity of red coloration was found to be proportional to the concentration of sulfonamide.

As sulfadiazine and sulfamerazine represent higher molecular weight compounds than sulfanilamide, and yet for each molecule have the same quantity of free amino grouping to give the red diazo coloration, equivalent color readings represent higher absolute concentrations. For instance, a color reading indicating a level of 10 mg. per 100 ml. sulfanilamide would represent 15 mg. per 100 ml. sulfadiazine. The other sulfonamides commonly used have about the same relation.

After absorption, circulating sulfonamides are subjected to a process of acetylation in the liver that may continue until a high proportion of circulating sulfonamide is acetylated. The proportion varies with each compound, and if a completely acetylated sulfonamide is introduced directly, it may be deacetylated to some degree. The acetylated form is not active therapeutically but may give the usual or even more intense toxic effects, and usually it is considered to be a therapeutic liability. Acetylation takes place at the free amino group, the same grouping involved in the diazo color reaction, hence the ordinary determination of blood levels does not recognize the presence of acetylated or conjugated sulfonamide. This can be recognized by an additional determination of free sulfonamides after a process of hydrolysis with acid. The total sulfonamide thus determined, minus the free sulfonamide determined before hydrolysis, represents the amount of acetylated or conjugated sulfonamide. In cases of anuria due to toxic effects of sulfonamides, there may be relatively complete conjugation and corresponding absence of free sulfonamide in the bloodstream.

Both free and acetylated sulfonamides are excreted by the kidney, although there are considerable differences in the rate of elimination of various sulfonamides and their acetylated forms. Urinary concentration may reach levels greater than the solubility of the compounds, and crystalluria develops frequently. With sulfadiazine and sulfamerazine, the acetyl derivatives are more soluble than the free sulfonamide. The reverse is true of sulfapyridine, and particularly true of sulfathiazole. Alkalinization of the urine increases greatly the solubility of sulfadiazine and sulfamerazine and their acetyl derivatives. Sulfisoxazole, sulfadimetine and sulfacetamide exhibit relatively high solubility in acid urines, which has favored their use as urinary antiseptics. The rapidity of excretion of sulfisoxazole is attributed principally to its extracellular distribution. The use of sulfonamide mixtures lowers the individual dose of each and, correspondingly, the incidence of crystalluria, although it may increase also the possibilities of sensitivity reactions. However, it is claimed that sensitivity is more related to dose than to the number of sulfonamides. Oral trisulfapyrimidines suspension

USP contains about equal amounts of sulfadiazine, sulfamerazine and sulfamethazine.

Sulfacetamide (N¹-acetylsulfanilamide) has been used particularly as a urinary antiseptic because of ready absorbability and relatively high urinary solubility even under acid conditions. This compound is not to be confused with the metabolic product, acetyl sulfanilamide, in which the free amino group has been acetylated; with sulfacetamide, an acetyl substituent has been introduced into the amide or sulfonamide grouping. This compound, in the form of its sodium salt, is used in 30 per cent solution for topical application in the eye.

Therapeutic Applications

Sulfonamides are indicated chiefly in meningococcal infections, in urinary tract infections, in bacillary dysentery and in instances of antibiotic toxicity. Their relatively low cost, high stability on storage and reliable oral absorption are favorable practical considerations. Their effectiveness extends in varying degree to the beta-hemolytic streptococci, gonococci, pneumococci, staphylococci, Shigella, *Klebsiella pneumoniae, Vibrio cholerae, Pasteurella pestis, Haemophilus ducreyi, Bacillus anthracis,* Brucella, *Haemophilus* influenzae, Actinomyces, *Donovania granulomatis;* urinary and meningeal infections with *Escherichia coli, Aerobacter aerogenes,* Proteus and *Pseudomonas aeruginosa;* the viruses of trachoma, psittacosis, ornithosis and lymphogranuloma venereum. In serious infections with these organisms, combined therapy with antibiotics is often employed. Development of sulfonamide resistance was most conspicuous in the instance of gonococci; however, it has been observed with pnemococci, streptococci and shigellae, and more recently with meningococci. Resistance to sulfonamides once acquired has been permanent. However, the organisms remain sensitive to penicillin. There has been some correlation between this development of resistance and the ability to synthesize abnormally large amounts of para-aminobenzoic acid.

Toxic Effects

Sulfanilamide produces toxic effects that are relatively distinctive and characteristic. These include cyanosis, acidosis and acute hemolytic anemia. Sulfapyridine administration was characterized particularly by nausea and vomiting. Sulfathiazole produced a relatively high incidence of conjunctivitis, skin sensitivity reactions and crystalluria. Sulfadiazine and sulfamerazine are not characterized by distinctive toxic effects and show a relatively low incidence of those side effects common to all sulfonamides. These include skin rash, fever, disorientation, nausea, vomiting, weakness, hepatitis, leukopenia, and agranulocytosis. Renal damage may vary through milder effects, such as microscopic hematuria and crystalluria, to severe tubular necrosis with complete anuria. The severe effects are not due necessarily to physical action of crystals on the tubules but may be a specific direct cellular action somewhat similar to that produced by mercuric chloride. It is recognized also that sulfonamides produce a characteristic type of necrotizing arteritis in the viscera that resembles periarteritis nodosa; this is usually believed to have an allergic basis. An increase in the number of diagnosed cases of periarteritis nodosa has been attributed to the widespread use of sulfonamides.

A fixed dosage preparation contains sulfamethoxazole and trimethoprim. This latter drug is an inhibitor of bacterial, but not mammalian, dihydrofolate reductase. Currently used only for urinary tract infections, this combination appears to have a distinct advantage over either drug used alone.

ANTIBIOTICS

Inasmuch as antibiotics are the products of microorganisms, reference is made at this point to Chapter 5, *Microbiology and Immunology,* in which there is description of the source organisms, the history of antibiotics and the various biologic aspects of their behavior.

Penicillin. *Penicillin G* USP (benzylpenicillin) effectively restrains bacterial growth in much more dilute concentrations than are required with sulfonamides. The basic action is that of blocking synthesis of the cell wall. Thus, the protoplast is exposed to great osmotic forces that destroy the cell. This general concept is in agreement with the observations that radioactive penicillin is rapidly bound by a component of the cell membrane; that penicillin action is evident only in dividing cells; that the rate of bactericidal action is not increased beyond a certain maximal rate regardless of the amount of penicillin present; that the giant, bizarre forms of the organisms can be obtained with certain penicillin concentrations, and that penicillin has been shown to cause accumulation of nucleotides that otherwise would have been used in manufacture of the cell wall. Penicillins inhibit the final cross-linking reaction in bacterial cell-wall synthesis by inhibiting the action of a transpeptidase reaction. Consequently, the monomeric units are not incorporated into the cell wall polymer responsible for structural integrity of the cell. Another group of closely related antibiotics, the cephalosporins, have a similar mechanism of action.

Penicillin G is usually the agent of choice in infections caused by streptococci, nonresistant staphylococci, pneumococci, meningococci, gonococci and *Treponema pallidum*. (Staphylococcal infections, particularly those occurring in hospital environments, have developed a high incidence of resistance to penicillin, and commonly this has been associated with a high level of the enzyme penicillinase, which converts penicillin to an inactive form. Some limited resistance, with necessity of increasing doses, has been reported in gonorrheal infections). Other organisms that are effectively inhibited are the etiologic agents of tetanus, gas gangrene, diphtheria and anthrax.

The natural penicillins have been identified as types G, X, F and K, which contain, respectively, the groups benzyl, hydroxybenzyl, pentenyl and heptyl attached to a thiazolidine-lactam nucleus. Although the synthetic demonstration of the structure of penicillin was accomplished in 1946, and variants could be obtained by adding compounds to the culture broths, the synthetic approach to new variations was not widely available until 1959, when the intermediate, 6-amino-penicillanic acid, was obtained in quantity by modification of the usual fermentative production process. This structural unit made possible a wide variety of semisynthetic derivatives and has provided typically active penicillins that are resistant to gastric acidity (penicillin V and phenethicillin), that are resistant to the enzyme penicillinase (methicillin, cloxacillin, oxacillin and nafcillin), or that exhibit a broader spectrum of activity (ampicillin and carbenicillin). Although resistance to degradation by gastric acidity can provide more uniform absorption after oral administration, about the same effect can be obtained if the less resistant penicillin G is given in multiple doses and given on an empty stomach.

Penicillin G is highly acid and forms water-soluble sodium and potassium salt. Intramuscular injections or intravenous infusions are followed by exceptionally rapid excretion in the urine, since penicillin is actively secreted by the kidney tubules. After intramuscular injection, some can be detected in the urine in 10 minutes, and most is excreted unchanged in 4 hours. In circumstances in which exceptionally high levels must be maintained, probenecid is used to block tubular excretion. For the prolonged maintenance of lower levels, repository forms are used, the most usual being procaine penicillin G and benzathine penicillin G (Bicillin). The last named, on intramuscular injection of 1 million units, can give detectable concentrations for periods up to 4 weeks. (A unit corresponds to 0.6 µg.) The sodium or potassium content can be significant, since relatively heavy doses may be given at times, amounting to 60 g. daily dose in some instances. Distribution in the body is irregular, and low concentrations appear in the spinal fluid; in the presence of meningitis,

however, this is substantially increased. There is seldom any indication for intrathecal administration of penicillin. The average therapeutic blood level is about 0.3 to 1.0 unit per ml. Generally it is considered that intermittent blood level peaks are effective since the organisms are sensitive only when multiplying, and a recuperative period of several hours is postulated. Further, penicillin concentrations are sustained more uniformly in the lymph and the tissues than in the blood. The relatively low blood levels obtained over long periods with repository forms such as benzathine penicillin are suitable in prophylaxis against hemolytic infections in rheumatic fever patients; this is also true in the treatment of syphilis.

Penicillin toxicity is largely that of sensitivity, and this has a high incidence. Approximately five per cent of all patients have reactions of some sort ranging from mild transitory allergic phenomena to angioneurotic edema, periarteritis nodosa and anaphylactic shock. Skin rash is frequently noted following administration of ampicillin but not with other penicillins. Hypoxia associated with anaphylactic shock can lead to irreversible brain damage, and estimates of the incidence of such are serious. Probably most hypersensitivity reactions, including fatalities, are now due to this agency rather than foreign sera, which was once the most common cause. There is little basis for considering one of the penicillins much different from the others in this respect. The most promising method of predicting sensitivity is based on a reaction between a drop of the patient's serum, a penicillin solution and a suspension of leukocytes. Basophilic degranulation occurs in positive reactors. Another predictive test employs intradermal administration of a penicillin-polylysine conjugate. Skin testing of suspected penicillin reactors by intradermal injection of penicillin alone is never indicated, since even the small amount injected may induce an anaphylactic reaction. Penicillinase (Neutrapen) is available as a specially purified enzyme from *Bacillus cereus*. Since it has the effect of promptly reducing blood penicillin levels to near zero and maintains this effect for several days, it is used in severe but delayed penicillin reactions. The enzyme itself is rather strongly antigenic and is ineffective against the penicillinase-resistant forms of penicillin. It is most applicable to the long-acting injectable forms such as benzathine penicillin.

Cephalothin (Keflin) and **cephaloridine** (Loridine) are structurally closely related to penicillin and exert a bactericidal action through the same mechanism. They are considerably more active against various gram-negative bacteria than is benzylpenicillin but must be given parenterally. They are not destroyed by penicillinase and are consequently active against most penicillin-resistant staphylococci. Patients who are sensitive to penicillin may display a corresponding sensitivity to these two antibiotics. Cephalexin (Keflex) and cephaloglycin dihydrate (Kafocin) are available for oral administration. The former is indicated for certain systemic infections, while the latter is indicated primarily for urinary tract infections. Nephrotoxicity is produced by high doses.

Cefaclor (Ceclor) is a new cephalosporin antibiotic that is readily absorbed from the gastrointestinal tract. It has been found effective in the treatment of otitis media, upper respiratory tract infections caused by *S. pyogenes,* urinary tract infections, and skin infections. Unlike caphalexin, it is indicated in infections of the lower respiratory tract due to susceptible strains of *H. influenzae.*Cefamandole (Mandol) is a semisynthetic cephalosporin antibiotic for parenteral administration. In vitro studies and clinical experience indicate that it has a broader antibacterial spectrum than earlier compounds in this family.

Streptomycin is an organic base containing three cyclic structures (streptidin, streptose and glucosamine) connected by glucosidic linkages. It forms water-soluble and relatively stable salts with the common inorganic acids and also forms a water-soluble double-salt complex with calcium chloride. Unitage is expressed in terms of the pure, crystalline base. Various chemical methods are used in assaying streptomycin, and the USP specifies two microbiologic assays using respectively *Bacillus subtilis* and *Klebsiella pneumoniae.*

Oral administration of streptomycin provides only limited and irregular absorption, and substantial fractions of the drug appear in the feces. Since this provides significant antibacterial action in the gut, oral administration is sometimes used in preoperative disinfection of the gut for elective surgery. The intramuscular route is most usual, although streptomycin may be given intravenously and subcutaneously. An intramuscular injection of 0.5 g. may be expected to maintain therapeutic serum levels for as long as 12 hours. From one half to three fourths of the injected drug is excreted in the urine in 24 hours. Excretion is slower than with penicillin and involves only glomerular filtration. Streptomycin distribution in the body is confined to extracellular fluids. Distribution is irregular, being high, for instance, in intraperitoneal fluids and low in spinal and ocular fluids. In acute infections, total daily doses of 2 to 4 g. are given by intramuscular injection at 6- to 12-hour intervals. Repository forms are not used.

Streptomycin acts by preventing protein-chain initiation at the bacterial ribosomal level. Relative impermeability prevents the drug from having the same effect on the host cell.

Mycobacterium tuberculosis and other gram-negative organisms *rapidly develop resistance* when streptomycin is administered continuously; this has been explained on the basis of constantly occurring chance mutations. In some instances organisms may develop dependence on the presence of the drug. It has been thought in these cases that streptomycin is essential for messenger attachment to ribosomes in the dependent cells.

Streptomycin is effective against a number of gram-negative organisms that are not readily susceptible to penicillin. Tularemia, brucellosis and plague are special indications for the use of streptomycin. Lymphogranuloma inguinale responds to streptomycin, but this condition can also be treated with the less toxic tetracyclines. Gram-negative bacillary infections of the urinary tract are treated effectively with streptomycin so long as there is adequate renal function and the organisms have not developed resistance. Alkalinity of the urine favors the action of streptomycin. Some bacillary meningitides respond similarly to streptomycin if resistance has not developed.

Streptomycin was the first clinically effective drug in the treatment of tuberculosis. Along with isoniazid (isonicotinic acid hydrazide) it is considered to be one of the primary drugs in the management of the variety of infections produced by *M. tuberculosis.* A secondary drug is PAS (para-aminosalicylic acid), the action of which is synergistic with either of the two primary drugs. This potentiation of action is probably an effect of delaying emergence of resistant forms. Ordinarily these primary drugs are not combined advantageously, although the combination is used sometimes in acutely critical infections. Thiosemicarbazones occupied a place in this regimen, but because of a high incidence of toxicity, they are not used now. Ethambutol (Myambutol) is a dibutanol derivative used with primary drugs to retard development of resistance to these drugs. Kidney damage and disturbed visual function occur with higher doses.

The large doses of isoniazid used in these treatments has produced neuropathies, which possibly may be prevented by concurrent use of pyridoxine. Hepatic dysfunction is likely to occur in approximately one per cent of all patients who receive isoniazid.

Streptomycin produces typical allergic reactions in sensitive patients and has caused an abnormally high incidence of skin reactions in personnel handling the drug. Eighth nerve and labyrinthine toxicity are most characteristic; vertigo, tinnitus and deafness appear in about that order, and some such symptoms develop in nearly all patients receiving prolonged administration of the drug.

Dihydrostreptomycin prepared by catalytic hydrogenation of streptomycin, does not differ greatly in activity from the parent compound. It is less injurious to the vestibular apparatus but more readily causes tinnitus and deafness. It is not generally used now.

Neomycin is an unusually stable antibiotic that is effective against a variety of both gram-positive and gram-negative organisms. *M. tuberculosis* that has become resistant to streptomycin retains sensitivity to neomycin. Neomycin can be given by intramuscular administration; if given orally, very little is absorbed, and on this basis it has been used as an intestinal antiseptic.

Neomycin has been observed in a number of instances to produce paralysis of external respiratory movements. The effect appears to be synergistic, with ether and with curare types of agents.

Kanamycin (Kantrex) is another antibiotic of the aminoglycoside group. Its sprectrum of activity is similar to that of neomycin, but its toxicity is somewhat less. It must be given by parenteral administration. It is used chiefly against gram-negative bacteria and drug-resistant staphylococci and in the treatment of tuberculosis.

Gentamycin (Garamycin) is another member of the aminoglycoside group of antibiotics. It differs from the other aminoglycosides in that cross resistance is unidirectional. Most bacteria resistant to gentamycin are resistant to other aminoglycosides, but organisms resistant to streptomycin and kanamycin, for example, may be sensitive to gentamycin. In addition, it is useful in combination with carbenicillin in the treatment of Pseudomonas septicemia (the two drugs should not be mixed in the same intravenous solution, however), and it has a higher degree of activity against strains of Serratia than any other antibiotic.

Spectinomycin (Trobicin) is an inhibitor of protein synthesis in the bacterial cell; it interacts with the 30S ribosomal subunit *reversibly*. It is used clinically for only one infection, acute, uncomplicated gonococcal infection of the genitalia or rectum. Administered intramuscularly, side effects include urticaria, dizziness, nausea, chills, and fever.

Tobramycin (Nebcin) is a bactericidal aminoglycoside antibiotic for parenteral administration. It is similar to other aminoglycoside antibiotics in physiologic distribution and in pharmacologic and in vitro *activity;* however, it is more active in vitro against Pseudomonas. **Amikacin** (Amikin) is another member of the aminoglycoside group. It is indicated in the short-term treatment of serious infections due to susceptible strains of gram-negative bacteria. Despite ototoxicity, nephrotoxicity, and neuromuscular blockade, properties shared by other aminoglycoside antibiotics, tobramycin and amikacin are among the most valuable antibiotics in severe infections. The concurrent use of potent diuretics such as furosemide and ethacrynic acid should be avoided as they may cause cumulative adverse effects on the auditory nerve and kidney.

Tetracyclines. The tetracyclines and chloramphenicol have been termed broad-spectrum antibiotics because they are effective against a much wider variety of organisms than penicillin or streptomycin. They act by preventing attachment of the tRNA-amino acid to the mRNA-ribosome complex, thus conferring inhibition of protein synthesis. Closely similar chemical structures occur in chlortetracycline (Aureomycin), oxytetracycline (Terramycin), tetracycline (polycycline, Achromycin, Tetracyn, Steclin), methacycline (Rondomycin) and doxycycline (Vibramycin). Demethylchlortetracycline (Declomycin), produced by a mutant of the strain of *Streptomyces aureofaciens,* Duggar, is more potent on a weight basis than tetracycline, the average adult daily dose being 600 mg.; it is claimed to give longer sustained levels of antibacterial activity in the serum, but its use is occasionally accompanied by a reversible syndrome virtually identical with diabetes insipidus. The broad-spectrum antibiotics have in common a four-ring nucleus containing amide, amine and hydroxyl groups; they form soluble salts and hydrochlorides, the latter being the form in which they are most stable and the most commonly dispensed. Tetracycline has been obtained directly from microorganisms and also can be obtained semisynthetically from chlortetracycline by removal of the chlorine atom through catalytic hydrogenation. The tetracyclines have closely similar antibacterial and related biologic actions. Tetracycline and demethylchlortetracycline are the newest of the group and have a number of apparent advantages. These include greater water solubility; greater stability in acid and alkaline solutions; higher and more sustained blood levels from a given dose; less nausea, vomiting and diarrhea.

Ordinarily, the tetracyclines are given by oral administration in doses repeated every 6 hours and totaling about 4 g. daily in severe infections. Peak blood concentrations are obtained in 2 to 4 hours from single doses. Absorption is not complete, and appreciable amounts appear in the bile and the feces. Urinary excretion accounts for 5 to 30 per cent, the most stable (tetracycline) being the most completely recovered. The tetracyclines can be given intravenously and also can be applied topically. Local irritation has been observed when they are given intramuscularly, intrathecally, by nebulization and by rectal administration.

The tetracyclines are effective against a number of gram-positive and gram-negative bacteria, the rickettsiae, the Eaton agent of primary atypical pneumonia and the psittacosis-lymphogranuloma venereum group of viruses. Bacterial resistance develops but is more gradual and stepwise, as with penicillin. Disturbing side actions have been gastrointestinal symptoms and development of monilialike infections. Photosensitization has occurred after administration of demethylchlortetracycline, while this is rarely observed with the other tetracyclines. Tetracycline localized in proliferating osseous tissue and bone tumors has been identified by its fluorescence in ultraviolet light. It also localizes in epiphyses and deciduous teeth in children, and it has stained teeth in children and has been charged with defects in enamel. Tetracycline given during the last trimester of pregnancy traverses the placenta and deposits in the fetal skeleton; it has been shown to retard skeletal growth in premature infants. Large doses of tetracycline given in pyelonephritis have led to serious liver damage. On storage of the drug, degraded forms of tetracycline have developed; their use led to a syndrome (Fanconi-like), which, at the outset, resembles lupus erythematosus and, later, may include nausea, vomiting, proteinuria, acidosis, glycosuria and aminoaciduria. Various observations indicate that tetracycline is antianabolic, and the decreased utilization of amino acids in protein synthesis is considered to present an excessive load for kidney excretion.

Minocycline (Minocin) is effective against some staphylococci and Nocardia that are resistant to other tetracyclines. An expensive drug, with a high incidence of vertigo associated with its use, its therapeutic blood levels are sustained for prolonged periods of time.

Chloramphenicol (Chloromycetin) is a relatively simple chemical consisting of a nitrobenzene nucleus with a propane derivative attached para to the nitro group. Like chlortetracycline it contains nonionic chlorine in the molecule. It has been prepared by large-scale synthetic methods, the product being identical with that obtained from microorganisms. It acts by inhibiting protein synthesis. The highly insoluble palmitate ester has been used as a means of obviating its highly bitter taste. A water-soluble sodium succinate is available for parenteral administration. Chloramphenicol prevents peptide bond formation at the bacterial ribosomal level.

Chloramphenicol is absorbed somewhat better and distributed more uniformly in the body than the tetracyclines. The greater penetration into the cerebrospinal fluid has proved to be a particular advantage. It is largely metabolized in the body, only a small percentage appearing unchanged in the urine. The general antimicrobial spectrum is similar to that of the tetracyclines. However, with typhoid fever its effectiveness is outstanding, and frequently it is preferred in the treatment of typhus and other rickettsial infections. In typhoid fever daily oral doses totaling about 3.0 g. are given in four to six installments; the drug is continued for a few days beyond the period of fever. It has been used effectively in cystic fibrosis not responsive to other antibiotics.

Considerable attention has been given to the incidence of aplastic anemia and agranulocytosis that may be caused by chloramphenicol. The incidence of such is statistically low when it is recognized that chloramphenicol has been given in millions of courses of treatment. The bone marrow depression is generally related to dosage and duration of treatment and is usually reversible on discontinuance of the drug. Besides the usual monitoring of blood counts, it has been shown that the effect can be predicted by recognizing a delay in turnover of radioactive iron. This toxicity appears to be more frequent in the presence of renal and liver disease. The aplastic state following use of this drug is probably idiosyncratic and not a direct extension of its predictable leukopenia.

Erythromycin (Ilotycin, Erythrocin) is similar to penicillin in its bacterial spectrum. It is effective on oral administration and is considered to produce less alteration of the normal intestinal flora than the usual broad-spectrum antibiotics. Oleandomycin and carbomycin have about the same spectrum and cross resistance as erythromycin. These agents differ from penicillin in that they have some action against the rickettsiae and the ptissacosis-lymphogranuloma venereum group of viruses. The estolate salt is occasionally implicated as inducing an allergic cholestatic hepatitis.

Tyrothricin, polymyxin, colistin, methane-sulfonate and **bacitracin** are relatively insoluble peptides with sufficient systemic toxicity so that their therapeutic use has been predominantly by topical application. However, because of developing resistance to other antibiotics, there have been increasing instances of the systemic use of each of these except tyrothricin.

Tyrothricin contains two substances: gramicidin and tyrocidine. It is highly active against most gram-positive pathogenic cocci and is inhibitory to some fungi. Its hemolytic and neurotoxic action precludes systemic use.

Polymyxin B (Aerosporin) is a potent antibiotic in the control of infections with gram-negative bacteria. It has special value in Pseudomonas and Proteus infections, which often are insensitive to other antibiotics. Injury to the kidney and to the central nervous system has been observed during its therapeutic use.

Bacitracin is thought to be less nephrotoxic than formerly because of improved purification of the commercial product. Its antimicrobial specrum resembles that of penicillin.

Lincomycin (Lincocin) and **Clindamycin** (Cleocin) are two closely related antibiotics with broad antibacterial spectra. Both are available as oral and parenteral preparations. The potentially life-threatening pseudomembranous enterocolitis associated with these two drugs (as well as occasionally with ampicillin, tetracyclines, and chloramphenicol) is probably due to a toxin elaborated by a strain of lincosamide-resistant *Clostridium difficile* which proliferates inordinately when susceptible gastrointestinal flora is suppressed. Recent evidence shows that administration of the nonabsorbable antimicrobial vancomycin can prevent or ameliorate the colitis. Both drugs appear to be highly useful in the treatment of anaerobic (Bacteroides) infections.

Viomycin is an adjunctive antibiotic used in the treatment of tuberculosis. Both viomycin and neomycin are nephrotoxic and neurotoxic. Cycloserine is another adjunct in tuberculosis treatment.

Several antibiotics have been introduced on the basis of greater effectiveness against strains resistant to more common antibiotics. These include: novobiocin (Albamycin, Cathomycin), which was introduced in 1955 for use against resistant strains of *Staphylococcus aureus* and *Proteus vulgaris;* it may produce a yellow pigment in plasma and thus increase the icteric index; vancomycin, which is used in the same way; kanamycin (Kantrex), which resembles neomycin in antibacterial spectrum, side effects and negligible grade of absorption from the gut; oleandomycin (Matromycin), derived from *Streptomyces antibioticus;* and its triacetyl derivative (TAO, Cyclamycin).

Rifampin is a semisynthetic derivative of rifamycin B produced by *Streptomyces mediterranei.* In far-advanced tuberculosis, a combination of rifampin and isoniazid is as effective (or more so) than isoniazid, ethambutol, and streptomycin combined. Rifampin is very active against mycobacteria, gram-positive organisms, and Neisseria species. It inhibits RNA synthesis by interacting directly (1:1 molar ratio) with DNA-dependent RNA polymerase. In the US, it is used to treat mycobacterial infections and meningococcal carriers. When used alone in treating tuberculosis, emergence of resistance is rapid. In the treatment of lepromatous leprosy, it is more effective than dapson. It is well absorbed from the gastrointestinal tract; therapeutic levels are achieved in cerebrospinal and pleural fluids. Its most common side effects are nausea, vomiting, and diarrhea; headache, ataxia, and dizziness may occur, as well as skin rashes, eosinophilia, leukopenia, and liver damage.

Selection of Antibiotic or Sulfonamide

The multiplicity of drugs effective in combatting infections has emphasized the limitation of lists that may attempt to indicate the agent of choice for each given infecting organism. It is considered to be more pertinent to have a direct test of the sensitivity of the infecting organism against a selected series of the most likely antibacterial agents. A practical procedure of current value is the use of filter-paper disks soaked in representative antibiotics and sulfonamides and laid directly on the streaked culture of the infecting organism. Drug sensitivity is indicated by a halo around the corresponding disk. Since this measure is considerably conditioned by the diffusibility of the antibiotic, it is desirable to conduct at the same time other tests, such as determination of sensitivity in liquid media. Following determination of the initial effectiveness of an antibiotic or a sulfonamide, other considerations arise, such as the development of acquired resistance, observed particularly with penicillin and streptomycin; the development of virulence, observed particularly with sulfonamides; and the development of overgrowing Monilia and other yeastlike organisms, observed particularly with tetracyclines.

Antagonism between the antibiotics has been suggested but is not a frequent practical consideration. On the other hand, additive and synergistic effects may occur. On occasion, members of the following group have been thought to be synergistic with each other: penicillin, streptomycin, bacitracin, neomycin, polymyxin B. There is a second group in which there is no synergism, but any member of the group may show synergism or, again, antagonism, when combined with a member of the first group. This second group includes tetracycline, chloramphenicol, erythromycin and sulfonamides.

ANTIMYCOTIC AGENTS

For fungus infections of skin, several drugs of low irritant value are used in addition to the time-honored and still valuable keratolytic, salicylic acid. The later drugs are related to the natural acids of perspiration. These include undecylenic acid, propionic acid and caprylic acid. Various combinations of these acids, their zinc salts and salicylic acid derivatives are known by names such as Desenex, Sopronol, Propion Gel and Naprylate. Their fungistatic action is more pronounced in acid than in alkaline media. As much as 20 to 30 g. of these acids can be taken orally without harm, as was shown in an older, bizarre treatment for psoriasis. Since they exhibit fungistatic action at concentrations as low as 0.01 per cent, their therapeutic index is exceptionally high.

Griseofulvin (Fulvicin, Grifulvin) is an orally effective antibiotic used in management of superficial fungus infections (tinea corporis, pedis and capitis and onychomycosis). It can produce leukopenia, headaches and skin rashes.

Amphotericin B (Fungizone) has been used for systemic fungus infections. Other antifungal agents are hexetidine and hydroxystilbamadine isethionate. Amphotericin B combines with sterols in the fungus membrane, leading to loss of selective permeability. This affinity for sterols is largely responsible for its toxicity (hemolysis, azotemia).

Nystatin (Mycostatin) is chemically similar to amphotericin B, but is used only for topical treatment of Candida infections of the skin and the oral and vaginal mucosa.

5-Fluorocytosine, a fluorinated pyrimidine, has limited usefulness in the treatment of systemic infections due to *Candida albicans* and *Cryptococcus neoformans*.

Miconazole and clotrimazole, both substituted imidazoles, have been used extensively for treatment of cutaneous candidiasis. More recently, a parenteral form of miconazole (Monistat IV) has been introduced for treatment of systemic fungal infections. It appears to be more effective than amphotericin B, and is considerably less toxic. It has been shown to be effective in treatment of coccidioidomycosis, cryptococcis, and systemic candidiosis, and paracoccidioidomycosis. Its major mode of action is by an alteration of fungal membrane permeability; it also inhibits fungal peroxidases and catalases.

CHEMOTHERAPY OF RICKETTSIAL AND VIRAL INFECTIONS

Chloramphenicol was the first antibiotic to be used in treatment of rickettsial diseases; its value in epidemic and murine typhus was demonstrated in Mexico and South America in about 1948. Chlortetracycline and oxytetracycline were soon shown to have parallel effects. These broad-spectrum antibiotics have since proved to be effective in Brill's disease, scrub typhus, Rocky Mountain spotted fever, rickettsial pox, African tick-borne typhus and Q fever. Ordinarily, oral doses of 2 to 4 g. are followed by daily doses of about half that amount until fever subsides, which may require from 2 to 5 days. With scrub typhus, the average duration of fever has been reported to be about 30 hours after treatment with antibiotics, about 90 hours after PABA and about 2 weeks with no treatment. Early institution of therapy is followed by a greater incidence of relapses. Since the rickettsial agent develops no resistance to the antibiotic, relapses can be controlled by a brief second treatment. Late treatment is followed by a lower incidence of relapses, since the antigenic stimulus of infection has more opportunity to provide immunity. On the other hand, early treatment significantly reduces mortality, which is notably high in epidemic typhus. In murine typhus with early treatment, discontinuance of treatment at the time fever subsides has been followed by prompt, severe relapses; this has led to the recommendation that in murine typhus therapy should be continued for about 2 weeks.

As mentioned above, the broad-spectrum antibiotics have common usefulness in infections with the biologically related rickettsiae and the large viruses of the LGV-P group. Tetracycline is the agent of choice in psittacosis (ornithosis) and is useful in lymphogranuloma venereum, although, in the latter instance, there is equal or greater value in the use of sulfisoxazole in daily oral doses of 4 g. for 2 to 3 weeks.

In the treatment of trachoma virus infections, administration of tetracycline along with oral sulfamethoxypyridazine is currently favored.

The rickettsiae and the LGV-P group of large viruses may be responsible for a primary pneumonia, as may also the pleuropneumonia-like organisms (PPLO, Eaton agent), and "atypical" or "viral" pneumonia of the latter type responds to tetracycline. Clincially, similar pneumonia due to other known and unknown true viruses is not specifically affected by broad-spectrum antibiotics.

The numerous small viruses pathogenic to man have been generally insensitive to chemicals in concentrations that can be tolerated by the host. Nevertheless, a number of relatively specific inhibitors in experimental systems have been developed, and there is practical value in the use of iododeoxyuridine (Idoxuridine, IDU) in human herpes simplex keratitis. Experimental screening of an enormous number of chemicals is being conducted, particularly with tissue culture systems, chick chorioallantoic and amniotic membrane cultures and small animals inoculated with multiple infective doses of the viruses. Biologic products that have shown ability to interfere with intracellular stages of viral replication are various protein-like bacterial constituents and a product termed interferon, which has been shown to exhibit a dose-response relationship in the inhibition of polio virus. Effective inhibitory chemicals have fallen largely into four groups: benzimidazoles, guanidine derivatives, thiosemicarbazones and acridine compounds. Both hydroxybenzyl-benzimidazole and guanidine inhibit members of picornavirus group; these are RNA viruses and include poliovirus, Coxsackie B and the majority of Echoviruses. Possibly they inhibit synthesis of viral RNA and protein by retarding production of virus-induced RNA polymerase. Sulfhydryl reagents such as chlormercuribenzoate reduce the infectivity of several enteroviruses, and it is postulated that SH groups facilitate adsorption of virus to host cells. It has been suggested that acridines interact with DNA through electronic binding to the bases of the nucleotides. Both benzimidazoles and thiosemicarbazones have strong intramolecular hydrogen bonds, with possibilities of specific protein binding.

In instances of smallpox exposure, methisazone (a thiosemicarbazone), administered promptly before the maturation stage in replication of the pox virus, has had the effect of markedly reducing the incidence and the severity of resulting cases of smallpox. Vaccination alone under these conditions is often ineffective.

Idoxuridine (IDU), an analog of thymidine, has been shown to inhibit DNA synthesis in vaccinia and herpes simplex in cell culture experiments. Both the fluoro- and the bromo-derivatives are also inhibitory at low concentrations. Topical application of idoxuridine is not beneficial in cutaneous herpes simplex, but its aqueous solution is effective in most instances of acute corneal inflammations due to this virus. It appears to be most useful in dendritic keratitis and in geographic ulcers and apparently is of doubtful value in disciform keratitis and herpetic iritis. A related antimetabolite product, cytosine arabinoside, also blocking the synthesis of viral DNA but at a different metabolic site, has been reported to act favorably in experimental herpetic keratitis.

Amantadine (Symmetrel) has found limited use in the prophylaxis of viral infection, principally against the Asian A_2 strain of influenza. Such prophylaxis may be desirable in certain populations (schools for retarded children and nursing homes), but such a practice cannot be considered to be universally practical. Since amantadine blocks viral penetration into host cells, it may prove to be a prototype of a class of drugs with extensive practical applications.

Adenine arabinoside (Vidarabine) was introduced recently for systemic use. It differs in structure from naturally occurring adenosine only by the relative positions of a hydrogen and an hydroxyl group on the five-membered sugar constituent. In vivo, it is metabolized to the triphosphate, and the resulting anabolite is a potent inhibitor of viral DNA polymerase. Part of the administered dose is metabolized to hypoxanthine arabinoside, which also has antiviral activity following conversion to the triphosphate. Its major indication is in the treatment of herpes incephalitis, but its utility in management of herpes zoster is being investigated. It is also available as a three per cent topical preparation for treatment of herpes keratoconjunctivitis.

CHEMOTHERAPY OF MALIGNANT DISEASE

In some instances, chemicals provide a useful degree of growth restraint and alleviation of symptoms in neoplastic processes. Growth restraint is based on the greater sensitivity associated with more rapid cell division and on antagonistic hormonal effects. The sensitivity of neoplastic processes to x-rays and radioisotopes has parallels in the sensitivity to radiomimetic agents such as alkylating agents and to metabolic inhibitors such as folic acid and purine metabolic antagonists. Normal tissue processes suffer necessarily in varying degree and, commonly, in direct relation to rapidity of cell division. Drug effects frequently appear to depend on inhibition of nucleic acid systems. Hematopoietic elements, intestinal mucosae and germinal epithelium are affected most prominently, with corresponding manifestations of decrease in formed blood elements; hemorrhagic and ulcerative gastrointestinal lesions; amenorrhea and decreased spermatogenesis. Chemotherapy has been most useful in choriocarcinoma, Hodgkin's disease, lymphomas and lymphosarcoma. Hormonal antagonisms have been most significant in the instances of cortisone and ACTH, which bring about significant remissions in some of the leukemias and malignant lymphomas, and in the instance of estrogens in prostatic carcinoma and both estrogens and androgens in mammary carcinoma.

Laboratory screening tests for antineoplastics include protozoal culture systems; tissue cultures of human epidermoid carcinoma cells; inoculated tumor growths in embryonated eggs; transplanted rodent tumors and leukemias either of spontaneous origin or induced by viruses, radiation or carcinogens. Ascites tumors and the lymphocytic lymphoma L1210 are among the most frequently used in the current massive search for effective agents.

Laboratory screening tests for sensitivity of human tumors to antineoplastics include such maneuvers as incubation of tumor slices and determination by autoradiography of the rate of uptake of tritiated thymidine or deoxyuridine into DNA; inhibition of uptake by antineoplastics is, in some cases, correlated with tumor sensitivity to the same drug.

Alkylating Agents

The alkylating agents are not localized preferentially in tumor tissues and do not show unusual specificity for tumor enzyme systems. In the preferential action on tumors, the primary site of alkylation appears to be DNA, with attachment of the 7-position of adjacent guanine moieties resulting in interference with strand separation of chains of DNA. When tested at minimal concentrations, this appears to be the most sensitive and critical system. Since the synthesis of DNA is considered generally to be a requisite for cell division, this may be the basis for the high sensitivity of mitotic processes to alkylating agents. On the other hand, general cytotoxic effects are much less specific and probably are the result of alkylation of a wide variety of tissue constituents.

Nitrogen mustard (methyl bis (beta-chloroethyl)

amine) (mechlorethamine USP; Mustargen) reacts rapidly with water and most organic compounds under physiologic conditions. On intravenous injection its primary reaction with tissues is completed in 2 to 3 minutes. Involution of lymph nodes, thymus and spleen is prompt and conspicuous and occurs more rapidly than it does from the same tissue-injury doses of total body radiation. There is less edema response in tissues than with equivalent x-ray treatment. Because of its vesicant action it is usually injected into a freely flowing intravenous infusion system. Venous thromboses can occur even after careful injection. Nausea and vomiting occur commonly, and the side-effects have cholinergic characteristics. Treatment consists of courses of about 25 mg., repeated after several weeks.

Nitrogen mustard effects are increased by high temperatures and high oxygen tensions and, correspondingly, decreased with lowered temperatures and oxygen tensions. Systemic and local effects are antagonized by sodium thiosulfate. These features are sometimes invoked when regional arterial perfusion procedures are tried; thiosulfate should be promptly instilled into the affected area if an intravenous injection inadvertently is extravasated into the subcutaneous tissues.

Other *mustard analogs* include uracil mustard, phenylalanine mustard, chlorambucil (Leukeran). Phosphamide esters of nitrogen mustard are inactive alkylating agents until converted by an enzyme present in increased amounts in liver; a compound of interest in this connection is cyclophosphamide (Cytoxan). Other compounds with basically similar alkylating actions are the ethylenimines (triethylenemelamine [TEM] and triethylenethiophosphoramide [thio-tepa], sulfonic esters (busulfan [Myleran]), and 1,3-*bis* (2-chloroethyl)-1-nitrosourea (BCNU). A European product of this type is dibromomannitol. Because of less intense immediate reactions, some of these can be given by oral and intramuscular routes.

Antimetabolites

Folic Acid Antagonists. These compounds are of considerable value in acute leukemias, more particularly in children. The 4-amino analog of folic acid (aminopterin) and its methyl derivative (amethopterin, methotrexate USP) have been used most. These antagonists interfere with nucleic acid synthesis, possibly by inhibition of the enzyme that reduces dihydrofolic acid to tetrahydrofolic acid (folic acid reductase). This, along with other reactions, is vital to the synthesis of nucleic acid. Amethopterin is not itself reduced by folic acid reductase and is largely excreted unchanged in the urine. These antagonists are given orally or intravenously. Folinic acid (citrovorum factor, leu-

covorin) reduces the toxicity of these compounds if given shortly after their administration.

Frequently the folic acid antagonists are administered to the point of toxicity, which includes: ulceration in the mouth and the digestive tract, bone marrow depression, alopecia and hyperpigmentation. During pregnancy they may cause fetal abnormalities and fetal death, a feature that has led to their trial as abortifacients.

Purine and Pyrimidine Antagonists. Analogs of naturally occurring purines also produce remissions in acute leukemia and are useful in adults. Additionally, they have been of value in chronic myelogenous leukemia. 6-mercaptopurine (6MP, Purinethol) is the best example in common clinical use. They interfere with the formation of nucleic acids and other purine-containing substances, the mechanism being essentially different from that with the folic acid antagonists. Purine antagonists may be effective when folic acid antagonists have developed a refractory state; the reverse is also true. They exhibit a characteristic liver toxicity.

Other antimetabolites of similar interest include analogs of guanine (6-thioguanine) and pyrimidine (5-fluorouracil [FU], 5-fluoro-2-deoxyuridine [FUDR], cytosine arabinoside, 5-fluoro-orotic acid and glutamine antagonists (azaserine and diazo-oxo-norleucine [DON]). FU and FUDR have had extensive clinical use. FU is metabolized in the same way as uracil, and the resulting 5-FUDR phosphate is a potent inhibitor of thymidylate synthetase, the enzyme that converts UdR phosphate to thymidylic acid.

Antibiotics

Actinomycin D (Dactinomycin) is being used in various carcinomas, and **Daunomycin** (Rubidomycin) in leukemias. The latter, originating in Italy and France, has exhibited myocardial depression during infusions.

Doxorubicin (Adriamycin), a complex structure of microbial origin, is used extensively in many combination chemotherapy regimens. It intercolates by hydrogen bonds into the DNA double helix structure and effectively prevents synthesis of DNA and RNA. Its dose-limiting toxicity is a cumulative effect on the myocardium. At total doses of about 550 mg. per sq. meter, it induces congestive failure which does not respond readily to cardiac glycosides.

Bleomycin (Bleocin) is a widely used antitumor antibiotic with a rather broad antineoplastic spectrum. It induces strand breaks in DNA and retards repair of these molecular lesions. In addition to the customary side effects usually associated with cytotoxic chemotherapeutic agents, it induces a fairly high incidence of pulmonary fibrosis.

Other Antimitotic Drugs

These agents are relatively specific in affecting dividing cells while leaving unaffected the resting cells. Their evident action is that of blocking mitosis in the metaphase. Effects may be on DNA synthesis during the preparative phase, on some of the energy factors required for mitosis or on cytoplasmic viscosity. Agents that have been of experimental interest because of metaphase arrest are, particularly, colchicine, vinblastine, podophyllotoxin, griseofulvin and some of their derivatives. Vinblastine (Velban) has been used in leukemias and reticuloendothelioses. Another alkaloid, *vincristine,* from the same source, the periwinkle, has had favorable clinical results in leukemias, lymphomas and Hodgkin's disease.

Hydroxyurea (Hydrea) is recommended for the management of melanoma and resistant chronic myelocytic leukemia. It has also shown some usefulness in management of carcinomas of the head and neck when used in combination with radiation. It is described as inhibiting DNA synthesis without interfering with the synthesis of RNA or protein. Action is only on those cells that actively synthesize DNA, and there is no direct effect on the mitotic process. Adverse effects are altered hemopoiesis and hyperuricemia, and teratogenic effects have been seen in laboratory trials.

Procarbazine (Natulan), a hydrazine derivative, is particularly effective in treatment of Hodgkin's disease.

L-asparaginase, an enzyme that deaminates asparagine, exploits the asparagine-dependent characteristic of certain tumor cells. Its use is associated with a significant number of hypersensitivity reactions as well as induction of diabetes mellitus.

Immunosuppressive Drugs

Organ transplantation is limited by the immune response of the host, and grafts are actively rejected after an interval unless identical twins are involved or the immune response is reduced by drugs. These usually are the conspicuous members of the antimalignancy drug group or simple variants of these. Among the latter may be mentioned azathioprine (Imuran), an imidazole derivative of 6-mercaptopurine. Corticosteroids are given in large doses. Under these conditions, infections commonly require intensive use of antibiotics.

Experimental Carcinogens

Compounds most used for production of experimental tumors include particularly: polycyclic hydrocarbons (methylcholanthrene, dimethylbenzanthracene, benzpyrene); aromatic amides and amines (acetylaminofluorene, naphthylamine dimethylaminobenzene, benzidine, aminostilbene); azo dyes and their intermediates (dimethylaminoazobenzene, aminoazotoluene), and a variety of miscellaneous agents such as urethane, podophyllin, dimethylnitrosamine, croton oil, thioacetamide, nickel and chromium powder. With some of these, one oral dose will dependably produce tumors in rats in a few weeks; others require prolonged feeding and special rodent strains. Either synergism or inhibitions can occur when these agents are combined.

Potency among the polynuclear aromatic hydrocarbons is correlated with steric resemblance to active steroids and to behavior as electron donors. With members of each group there is a correlation of potency and avidity of binding with characteristic proteins of the cytoplasm; these bound proteins tend to disappear during subsequent development of the tumor. Dimethylbenzanthracene produces selective necrosis of the adrenal cortex and corpora lutea, and, since these are sites of steroid synthesis, this effect provides further inferences in regard to the interrelationships of steroids and hydrocarbon carcinogenicity.

Hormones

In some manner, cortisone, prednisolone and prednisone reduce proliferative activity in acute leukemia, and they are the agents of choice if acute symptoms are severe. They represent a third type of useful compound along with the folic acid antagonists and mercaptopurine; these agents are alternated in sequence as refractoriness is developed.

Estrogens can bring about some degree of regression in prostatic carcinoma. This may be a direct action but more probably is due to suppression of androgenic secretion with consequent regression of androgen-dependent cells. At times, subjective responses are very favorable, and objective effects on biopsy specimens and plasma phosphatase levels are demonstrable. Diethylstilbestrol is given in oral doses of 5 mg. daily.

Mammary carcinoma has been treated with large doses of androgens or estrogens. Estrogens usually are reserved for postmenopausal patients. Androgens have been indicated most in bony metastases; estrogens, in soft tissue metastases. The responses are mostly subjective and are difficult to demonstrate morphologically. General metabolic effects may be the most important element in the treatment. Doses are sufficiently large to develop characteristic side effects. Hypercalcemia from androgens may be treated with intravenous EDTA. The progestational hormone, methylhydroxyprogesterone is used in endometrial carcinoma. Tamoxifen (Nolfadex), a nonsteroidal agent, is used empirically in breast carcinoma with response rate of

20 to 40 per cent. In postmenopausal patients whose estrogen receptor assay is positive, the response rate is about 60 per cent. Acute adverse effects are nausea and vomiting; delayed untoward reactions include hot flushes, thrombocytopenia, leukopenia, vaginal bleeding, hypercalcemia, and corneal opacities. Adrenal cancer shows specific response to o,p'DDD, a derivative of the insecticide DDT.

Heavy Metal Compounds

Cisplatin (Platinol) is the first totally inorganic compound to have a rational role in cancer chemotherapy. Chlorides in the compound dissociate (as in bis-chloro-ethyl nitrogen mustards) and the resulting, double, positively charged species binds tenaciously with negative sites on DNA, RNA, and protein. The binding to DNA is probably its principal mode of action. It is quite effective in the treatment of testicular and ovarian carcinoma. It has also been used for the treatment of other tumors with some preliminary success in cancer of the head and neck, bladder, and cervix, and in osteogenic sarcoma. For testicular tumors, cisplatin is used in combination with vinblastine and bleomycin; in ovarian tumors, it is recommended for combination therapy, particularly with doxorubicin. Renal damage is dose-related and cumulative, and can be severe. Nephrotoxicity can be ameliorated by brisk prehydration, mannitol diuresis, and posthydration. Cisplatin is also ototoxic, causing tinnitus and high-frequency hearing loss that may be irreversible. Combined with furosemide, the ototoxicity of the two drugs may be superadditive. Marked nausea and vomiting occur in almost all patients. Presently, other platinum compounds for the treatment of cancer are undergoing extensive trials.

Combination Therapies

The use of as many as four to five antimalignancy drugs simultaneously has shown impressively favorable results and opens a promising area for experimental studies. A preferred combination in diffusely metastatic solid tumors and in Hodgkin's disease is made up of cyclophosphamide, vincristine, amethopterin, 5-fluorouracil and prednisone.

ANTHELMINTICS

Modern chemotherapy principles have not been applied as extensively in this field as may be justified in terms of the wide distribution of worm infestations. The numbers of individuals subject to low-grade infestation runs into the hundreds of millions and, although only a low percentage of these represent life-threatening situations, such infestation is a grave threat to world health. Because of the type of populations involved, government-supported professionals have been most active in evaluating efficacy and judging toxicity potentials. Effective anthelmintics, beginning with the ancient oleoresin aspidium, were first developed largely as the result of chance empiric observations. Current new drugs are based more on recognition of differing metabolic sensitivities of the helminths and the mammalian hosts. For instance, it is recognized that helminths in the gastrointestinal tract and tissues are usually anaerobic in terms of survival even though they can consume oxygen in a somewhat incidental manner. A number of nematodes, cestodes and protozoa produce succinic acid and other low molecular weight aliphatic acids in contrast to the lactic acid end product of mammaliam anaerobic metabolism. Enzymes such as the phosphofructokinases of helminths are more sensitive to certain anthelmintic drugs than are the corresponding mammaliam enzymes. In some instances, anthelmintics inhibit the uptake of glucose by the worm, and in others there is a neuromuscular type of blockade resembling that of curare.

The choices of treatment commonly accepted are:

Hookworm

Necator americanus (New World Hookworm)
    Pyrantel pamoate (Antiminth)
    Tetrachlorethylene
    Bephenium (Alcopara)
    Thiabendazole (Mintezol)
Ancyclostoma duodenale (Old World Hookworm)
    Bephenium (Alcopara)
    Pyrantel pamoate (Antiminth)
    Thiabendazol (Mintezol)
    Tetrachlorethylene
Larva migrans
    Local sprayed ethyl chloride
    Systemic thiabendazole

Pinworm

Enterobius; Oxyuris
    Pyrantel pamoate (Antiminth)
    Piperazine
    Pyrvinium (Povan)
    Thiabendazole (Mintezol)

Roundworm

Ascaris
    Piperazine
    Pyrantel pamoate (Antiminth)
    Thiabendazole (Mintezol)
    Hexylresorcinol

Threadworm

Strongyloides
    Thiabendazole (Mintezol)
    Pyrvinium (Povan)

Whipworm

Trichuris
    Mebendazole (Vermox)
    Hexylresorcinol
    Thiabendazole (Mintezol)

Large Tapeworm

Taenia saginata, T. solium
Diphyllobothrium latum
    Niclosamide (Yomesan)
    Paromomycin (Humatin)
    Quinacrine (Atabrine)
    Oleoresin aspidium

Dwarf Tapeworm

Hymenolepis nana
    Niclosamide (Yomesan)
    Paromomycin (Humatin)
    Hexylresorcinol

Trinchinosis

Trichinella
    Thiabendazole (Mintezol)
    Corticosteroids for severe symptoms

Piperazine (diethylenediamine), particularly as the citrate, has been favored for both roundworms and pinworms. It produces a reversible, flaccid paralysis of the muscle of the worm and the myoneural blocking effect can be competitively antagonized by acetylcholine. Metabolic production of succinic and volatile fatty acids is sharply reduced as a result of decreased muscular activity rather than by specific metabolic inhibition. The drug is given in the form of tablets or syrup. Occasionally, urticaria and dizziness are associated with its use.

Tetrachlorethylene was first used in veterinary medicine for the elimination of hookworm, and it is currently of significant value in both human and animal infestations with this worm. This effect is that of direct anesthesia, and the worms may or may not be recovered alive. Side effects have been those of early central nervous system depression and have not been serious. When given in the presence of roundworm, the latter may be caused to migrate and, because of their large bulk, may produce intestinal obstruction. Occasionally they have entered the bile ducts. Com-

monly, with such a mixed infection, one of the roundworm treatments is given first.

Pyrvinium pamoate (Povan) is administered in suspension as a single-dose treatment for pinworm and is also used for strongyloides. It colors stools bright red and resembles another cyanine dye, dithiazinine, which produces a deep blue coloration. The alternating double bonds in pyrvinium identify a type of chemical resonance that appears to be associated with interference with the active transport of glucose into the worm. Gentian violet, once used for pinworm and strongyloides, is thought to have chemical similarities that are relevant.

Thiabendazole (Mintezol) was developed first in veterinary medicine, but in the form of mint-flavored tablets has proved useful in a number of human nematode infections. Most favorable results have been reported in roundworm and pinworm infestations, and it has been considered the agent of choice in strongyloides infestations and cutaneous larva migrans. Results with hookworm and whipworm have not been so favorable. Dizziness lassitude, headache and gastrointestinal symptoms frequently occur. It is the only agent used for systemic treatment of trichinosis, although corticosteroids are used as palliative treatment in the management of severe symptoms.

Bephenium hydroxynaphthoate (Alcopara) is effective against both species of hookworm. It is also useful for treating mixed roundworm and hookworm infections. Due to its bitter taste, it may cause nausea and vomiting. No serious toxic effects have been reported.

Hexylresorcinol was used as an antiseptic because of its surfactant properties and, as one of the early urinary tract antiseptics, it demonstrated a low incidence of systemic toxicity. Lamson demonstrated its effectiveness against roundworm in the 1930s, and its wide use since that time has proved it to be an essentially safe drug. When the solid was chocolate coated it produced mouth burns, which healed promptly, but the product was withdrawn and then was reintroduced in its present form, with a gelatin coating. Although less effective than other drugs, it may be useful in some mixed infections because of its wide anthelmintic spectrum.

Quinacrine is an effective drug in the treatment of large tapeworm infestations. It is given in relatively large doses as compared to the dosage in malaria treatment and is preceded by and followed by a purge. It has more or less replaced the dangerous oleoresin aspidium, which was used for some 20 centuries despite its recognized toxicity.

Pyrantel pamoate (Antiminth) in a single oral dose is highly effective in the treatment of pinworm and roundworm infections. In hookworm infections, three consecutive daily doses are generally required. Fasting before treatment is not necessary. Adverse reactions include anorexia, vomiting, abdominal pain, dizziness and rashes.

Mebendazole (Vermox) is considered effective and safe for treatment of whipworm infection; no equally effective oral treatment is available. It is also effective for infections caused by Enterobius, Ancylostoma, Ascaris and Strongyloides, but suitable alternative drugs exist for these indications, and these are recommended until there is more clinical experience with mebandazole.

Niclosamide (Yomesan) is under clinical investigation in the United States. It is highly effective against large and dwarf tapeworms. It causes the worm to be disintegrated in the gastrointestinal tract, an action possibly mediated through intestinal proteolytic enzymes. In the process, viable eggs are released. Therefore, if it is used in a patient with pork tapeworm (Taenia solium) infection, a purge should be given within 1 or 2 hours after treatment to avoid the possibility of cysticercosis.

Paromomycin (Humatin), a broad-spectrum antibiotic used principally as an amebicide, is an investigational drug in the treatment of large and dwarf tapeworm infections. In such cases, it acts similarly to niclosamide. Nephrotoxicity may result from the absorption of the drug.

Diethylcarbamazine (Hetrazan) is a derivative of piperazine that has proved useful in some types of filariasis. Suramin (Bayer 205) and various arsenicals and antimonials have also been used.

AMEBICIDES

Drug therapy for amebiasis can be divided broadly into the following categories: (1) treatment of acute symptoms of amebic dysentery (fever, myalgia, arthralgia, diarrhea); (2) treatment of tissue invasion of trophozoites (intestinal ulceration, hepatitis, liver abscess and, less frequently, metastases in lung and brain); (3) prevention of relapse by removing all cysts from the gut; (4) elimination of cysts in symptomless carriers, thereby preventing development of active amebiasis in the individual and removing the source of infectious transmission to others. Because of differing body locations and differing chemical susceptibilities of the active, motile trophozoites as contrasted with the encysted forms, no single drug has proved to be curative.

Ipecac. The root of this tropical plant has been used for centuries as a medicinal by South American Indians. Its specificity in amebiasis followed the demonstration by Vedder in 1911 that its infusions were directly lethal to *Entamoeba histolytica* in low concentrations and that one of its alkaloids, emetine, was effective in still lower concentrations. An associated alkaloid, cephaeline, has similar actions but is less suitable for therapy. Before the advent of synthetic amebicides, the crude ipecac was used extensively for treatment of symptoms as well as removal of cysts. Large doses were administered as pills with enteric coatings (the coatings are necessary because of the intense local irritant action of ipecac). Use of the crude drug now is limited largely to its status as a nauseant and an expectorant. Ipecac syrup USP, by virtue of the vagal reflexes that it induces, has a place in current treatment of paroxysmal tachycardia.

Emetine was shown by Rogers in 1912 to have conspicuous value in relieving the symptoms of acute amebiasis and in treating amebic hepatitis. It is characterized by unusual stability in the body with preferential concentration in the liver; most of the alkaloid is excreted in the urine but at a slow rate that continues for several weeks. Toxicity is common, particularly if certain dose levels are exceeded, the effects being due in considerable part to direct cellular injury in the myocardium and the skeletal muscles. Manifestations are ECG irregularities, precordial pain, tachycardia, weakness and muscular pain, nausea, vomiting and diarrhea. The cardiac toxicity dictates against its administration by the intravenous route. Because it is an intense local irritant, usually it is given by deep subcutaneous injection. The recommended dose is 1 mg. per kg. of body weight daily for 10 days. Commonly, a total dose of 600 mg. is fixed as an upper limit. Because of its cumulative characteristics, a second course is not given for several weeks.

Usually the administration of emetine produces prompt alleviation of symptoms such as fever, arthralgia and myalgia; enlargement and tenderness of the liver are reduced; liver abscesses are resolved or reduced in size with much greater safety in subsequent drainage procedures. Motile forms and cysts disappear from the gut, but the cysts reappear in most cases, and emetine alone is not considered to be curative.

Emetine bismuth iodide is insoluble, and its oral administration has been used particularly by the British.

Chloroquine is highly effective in amebic hepatitis and, because of lesser toxicity, usually is favored over emetine for this type of extraintestinal amebiasis. It does not have the effectiveness of emetine in treating the acute, severe symptoms of amebic dysentery, and it has little value in freeing the gut from cysts. Chloroquine is concentrated in the liver to levels that are several hundred times greater than in the plasma. Dosage is considerably higher than in malaria treatment and amounts to about 10 g. over a 2 week period.

Quinacrine also has had some trial in the same way.

For removal of cysts, a series of halogenated oxyquinolines has been used since the introduction of *chiniofon* in 1921. This product, an iodohydroxyquinoline compound, also is known as anayodin and yatren. The other two products introduced subsequently, *Vioform* and *Diodoquin,* contain additional halogens, Diodoquin being diiodohydroxyquinoline. Their effectiveness is limited to intestinal amebiasis. They are favored particularly in the treatment of chronic, symptom-free cyst carriers. Oral doses of 10 to 50 g. are given over periods of 1½ to 3 weeks, the larger doses being used only with Diodoquin. Toxic effects are limited mainly to diarrhea; less frequently, to anal pruritus; occasionally, to sensitivity reactions.

A series of arsenical compounds has been available for the same purpose and over about the same period as the halogenated oxyquinolines. The first of these arsenicals was the French antiluetic acetarsone. Subsequently, *carbarsone* and *thiocarbarsone* were introduced with claims of lower toxicity; glycobiarsol (Milibis), a related arsenical that also contains bismuth, was introduced in 1949. Their order of doses is lower than with the quinoline derivatives, from 3 to 8 g. being used over a week or 10 days. They are subject to the same toxic potentialities as the arsenicals that have been used in syphilis treatment, exfoliative dermatitis being the most serious hazard.

Antibiotics have significance in the treatment of amebiasis because of their value in checking secondary bacterial invaders and because *Entamoeba histolytica* may be influenced unfavorably by inhibition of the associated bacterial flora of the gut. Chlortetracycline, oxytetracycline, chloramphenicol, erythromycin, carbomycin and bacitracin have been used in amebiasis and probably act through one or both of these secondary mechanisms. Paramomycin (Humatin) resembles neomycin, restrains various pathogenic bacteria in the gut and has proven useful as an intestinal amebicide.

Metronidazole (Flagyl) is amebicidal at both intestinal and extraintestinal sites; it appears to be the drug of choice for all of the commonly encountered amebic infections with the possible exception of asymptomatic intestinal amebiasis. Unlike other amebicides it is used alone. Since it is a nitroimidazole, it is contraindicated in patients with a history of blood dyscrasias.

CHEMOTHERAPY OF OTHER PROTOZOAL INFECTIONS

Schistosomiasis (bilharziasis) has been recognized for some time as being peculiarly susceptible to antimony compounds. The simple tartar emetic (potassium antimonyl tartrate), given intravenously, is considered to be one of the most effective treatments, but it carries a high incidence of side effects such as coughing, arthralgia, ECG changes and liver damage. The organic forms of antimony such as stibophen (Fuadin), a pyrocatechol compound, and the mercaptosuccinate can be given intramuscularly and are generally considered less toxic but less effective. They produce selective inhibition of schistosome phosphofructokinase essential to the anaerobic production of lactic acid from glucose. This inhibition of carbohydrate metabolism by trivalent antimony compounds is reversible in intact worms or their extracts. In experimental animals, these compounds have the effect of shifting the worms from the portal system into the liver, from which they return later, following drug effects. Despite the kinship of arsenic and antimony, it appears that the action of arsenicals is on a different enzyme system, and specifically on sulfhydryl groups of enzymes such as hexokinase.

Nonmetallic synthetic compounds are being tried extensively in the management of schistosomiasis. These include lucanthone (miracil D), a substituted thioxanthone, and one of its metabolic products considered to be more active. Another such product is Niridazole (Ambilhar), a nitrothiazole derivative. This latter produces mild central nervous disturbances, which have been reduced by concomitant administration of phenobarbital.

Transmission is reduced by the organized use of molluscicides such as copper salts. This reduction of prevalence of the intermediate snail hosts is increasingly important in view of the increasing construction of inland dams and irrigation canals.

Trichomonas, particularly *T. vaginalis,* is a pathogen of routine significance because of its common occurrence in the vagina, urethra and prostate. A systemic trichomonicide is metronidazole (Flagyl), and other antiprotozoan agents are variably successful. Topical amebicides are used, in addition to the older treatment with lactose tablets, that are intended to change acidity conditions.

ANTIMALARIALS

Drugs used in malaria therapy can be broadly categorized into those groups that act on: (1) the schizonts or merozoites in the erythrocytic phase (suppressive agents for all forms of malaria); (2) the gametocytes in the plasma phase and (3) the secondary tissue schizonts and trophozoites (antirelapse agents for vivax, ovale and malariae infections). Drugs acting on the asexual erythrocytic phase are alleviative when given during the acute attack, and they suppress development of clinical symptoms. Before the development of chloroquine-resistant strains these drugs generally produced a radical cure for *Plasmodium falciparum* infections. Quinine, quinacrine, chloroquine and amodiaquine have this action, and they have in common a quinoline nucleus with a significantly weighted grouping attached to the 4-position. They are without important action on the tissue phase, and relapses are common in infections due to *P. vivax* and *P. malariae* when these drugs are used alone. They are thought to form molecular complexes with DNA and to block DNA replication. The chlorguanides and diaminopyrimidines have generally similar actions, and their mechanism is that of folic acid antimetabolites; sulfonamides have a similar effect by blocking the formation of folic acid in the parasite. Drugs that act on both the gametocytes and the tissue phases are particularly pamaquine, pentaquine and primaquine, which were developed in that order. They render a patient noninfectious, act to prevent relapses, and each one is an 8-amino quinoline.

Quinine, first prepared synthetically in 1944, is naturally obtained from cinchona bark, where it occurs with other alkaloids such as its optical isomer quinidine. The other alkaloids have similar actions, and an extract containing the crude mixture of alkaloids, termed totaquine, has proved to be effective and economical. Its action on the malaria plasmodia is considered to be some direct type of growth restraint such as that shown by the sulfonamides on bacteria. It has moderate action as a general antipyretic and analgesic. After oral administration, rapidity of absorption is chiefly governed by the solubility of the particular salt being used. It does not concentrate in the liver and erythrocytes in the same degree as do the later synthetic antimalarials. Excretion in the urine takes place rapidly, and cumulative effects do not ordinarily develop. About two thirds of the quinine is metabolized (chiefly by the liver), and one third is excreted in the urine. Toxic effects (cinchonism) include auditory and visual disturbances that may progress to permanent deafness or blindness. Tremors and palpitation also occur. When used in falciparum malaria it has been implicated in the development of blackwater fever. Quinine has no gametocidal activity against falciparum malaria but has effect against gametocytes of vivax and quartan malaria.

Quinacrine (mepacrine, Atabrine) was introduced in 1930 and is a synthetic acridine derivative. It is absorbed rapidly after oral administration, is excreted very slowly in the urine and the feces and, being a yellow dye, imparts a yellow color to the skin. It may be given by intramuscular injection, but it is considered to be dangerous by intravenous administration. Quinacrine acts on the asexual forms of all types of malaria and terminates the acute attacks. The ordinary dose is 2.5 to 3.0 g., administered orally in 0.1 g tablets during the course of a week. It was used extensively in World War II with usually only minor toxic effects. The extent of use can be recognized when it is recalled that there were about 500,000 cases of malaria in US troops in the South Pacific. Psychoses and atypical lichen planus leading to exfoliative dermatitis occurred in a small number of instances. The drug is no longer important as an antimalarial agent but is still employed to some extent as an anthelmintic.

Chloroquine (Aralen) is a product of government-supported research in the United States during the latter period of World War II. Its effectiveness is considered to be greater and its toxicity less than with quinacrine. It terminates the acute attack of vivax and falciparum malaria and eradicates the infection in the latter case. It alleviates rapidly the symptoms of quartan malaria. Chloroquine can be given intramuscularly. Toxic symptoms ordinarily are mild, and there is no skin coloration. Absorption and excretion generally are the same as with quinacrine. For treatment of acute attacks of vivax and falciparum malaria, 2.5 g. usually is administered orally during the course of 3 days. The drug is given in 0.25 g. tablets of the diphosphate.

Chloroquine is one of the agents used in the treatment of chronic discoid lupus erythematosus.

Amodiaquin (Camoquin) is a later variant of chloroquine and is used for the same purpose, i.e., treatment of the acute attack. It is active only against the erythrocytic, asexual forms, and relapses occur after medication is discontinued. However, the interval before relapse is much greater than with quinacrine or quinine. Like chloroquine, it does not produce discoloration of the skin.

Pamaquine (Plasmochin) was the first of the important synthetic substitutes for quinine. It was introduced in 1926, and was recognized to have special value in destroying the sexual forms of the plasmodia. Because of serious toxic effects and relative ineffectiveness, its use was discontinued during World War II.

Pentaquine and **Primaquine** are chemical variants of the earlier pamaquine. Pentaquine and primaquine were reinvestigated with the expectation of finding a "radical cure," i.e., an agent that would prevent relapses. Primaquine usually is considered to be relatively more effective and less toxic. Primaquine is combined suitably with quinine or chloroquine, but there have been warnings against combination with quinacrine.

Primaquine and the other 8-aminoquinolines, pentaquine and the older pamaquine have in common the propensity for producing methemoglobinemia. Characteristically this is associated with hemolytic anemia and hemoglobinuria. This occurred in suppressive therapy used in Vietnam; the episode is not life threatening, and the red cell counts can return toward normal in a few weeks even while primaquine therapy, 30 mg. daily, is being continued. This propensity to methemoglobinemia is a genetically linked trait that occurs with particularly high incidence in dark-skinned ethnic groups in various geographic areas. It is associated with a deficiency of enzymes involved in maintaining reduction of methemoglobin to hemoglobin; these enzymes include particularly glucose-6-phosphate dehydrogenase, although deficiencies in glutathione reductase, diaphorase and the coenzyme, nicotinamide adenine dinucleotide are also involved.

Pyrimethamine (Daraprim) and chloroguanide (Paludrine) inhibit folic acid reductase, resulting in cessation of DNA synthesis and ultimate death of the parasite. Their use as antimalarials followed extensive experimentation in British laboratories about 1945, and the findings of this work added the concept of a potentiative action with sulfonamides. Chloroguanide, which is inactive in vitro, is converted in the body to its active form, cycloguanide, which closely resembles the structure of pyrimethamine. These agents are active against the erythrocytic asexual froms of the plasmodia and have been reasonably effective as alleviative and suppressive agents. Rapid development of resistance has limited their effectiveness when used alone, and the requisite doses have approached those producing folic acid deficiencies. A variant, trimethoprim, developed in studies of antibacterial agents, has been reported to be more suitable, both in terms of lesser development of plasmodial resistance and reduced host toxicity. In monkeys and man it has been shown that folinic acid can reverse the toxicity of folic acid antimetabolites without affecting the efficacy against plasmodia.

Drug Development Methods

The use of canaries as test systems for malarial infections began as early as 1926 in German laboratories and has since been extended to other avian species.

Of the model test systems now in use, infections with *Plasmodium berghei* in mice comes closer to predicting reactions of human malaria than the earlier experimental avian infections. *P. cynomolgi* and *P. knowlesii* in rhesus monkeys have proved to be suitable for advanced testing. In the late 1950s *P. falciparum* was successfully transmitted to the chimpanzee, and since then *P. vivax* has also been transmitted to simians, thus providing test systems for human strains of malaria in nonhuman hosts.

Therapeutic Selections

Before the advent of the German synthetic antimalarials, malaria therapy commonly consisted of administration of quinine sulfate in 10 grain capsules, three the first day and one each day for a variable number of weeks. This frequently alleviated symptoms and acted as a suppressant, while providing some nominal assistance to natural processes acting against the tissue phase. More intensive initial therapy with quinine, including intravenous administration, was recognizably necessary with the cerebral manifestations of *P. falciparum,* and, because this does not involve a persistent tissue phase, the treatment could be curative. Pamaquine, introduced in 1926, variably reduced the incidence of relapses; and quinacrine, massively used in World War II, was more effective as an alleviative and suppressant. The latter, in turn, was replaced by chloroquine after intensive research in the US, which involved the screening of some 15,000 potential antimalarial compounds; this program also introduced primaquine as an improved variant of pamaquine. During the Korean conflict and at the beginning of operations in Vietnam, the standard oral regimen was 1.5 g. chloroquine base in 3 days, with primaquine base 15 mg. daily for 14 days. This was effective as a radical cure for most instances of vivax malaria. An adopted regimen for exposed personnel was 300 mg. base chloroquine and 45 mg. primaquine base weekly, which was effective as suppressant of vivax malaria.

About 1966 it was recognized in Vietnam, as it had been recognized a few years earlier in South America, that these regimens were occasionally inadequate, largely because of the incidence of falciparum malaria with refractoriness to chloroquine. Quinine was reintroduced, and its intravenous use was necessary in acute, cerebral involvement, with oral administration later. Refractoriness to quinine developed in some cases, and therefore, pyrimethamine was often added to the regimen. Since that time, there has been clinical application of earlier experimental observations in bird malaria, indicating the potentiating value of sulfonamide variants and folic acid antimetabolites. Diaminodiphenylsulfone (DDS), when used in leper colonies, had been observed to act as a malaria suppressant; because of this and earlier experimental observations it was added to the suppressive regimen of service personnel in Vietnam in an effort to prevent recrudescences due to drug-resistant *P. falciparum.*

When long-acting sulfonamides such as the methoxypyridazyl derivative (sulfalene) were combined with pyrimethamine or trimethoprim, the combination acted as a radical cure for normal falciparum malaria as well as for that which had proved resistant to chloroquine. Both the sulfonamides and the folic acid antimetabolites have their special dose-related toxic manifestations: the Stevens-Johnson syndrome in the case of the sulfonamides and megaloblastic and other anemias in the case of the folic acid antimetabolities. By virtue of sequential metabolic blockade in the parasite, however, synergistic action occurs with these combinations such that sufficiently low doses can be employed to minimize toxicity.

During the Vietnam war it was found that troop personnel returning to this country exhibited a significant number of recrudescences, usually of vivax malaria. These occurrences in individuals who had had the standard therapy for a "radical cure" indicate that the tissue phase of *P. vivax* is often difficult to eradicate.

Antimalarials for Rheumatoid Arthritis and Dermatologic Conditions

Antimalarials are used in relatively high doses and for prolonged periods in rheumatoid arthritis and some chronic dermatologic conditions. Chloroquine, quinacrine and amodiaquine have been most used. Side actions have been numerous, the most serious being retinopathy, corneal opacities, neuromyopathy and psychoses. Psoriasis is intensified or initiated by these agents. Ophthalmologists have attempted to discover early indications of visual disturbances through the use of electroretinography. Retinal lesions are said to be irreversible, although the corneal lesions are reversible. Chloroquine is excreted very slowly in the urine, some being detected for years; acidification hastens urinary excretion of these organic bases.

ANTILUETICS

Penicillin G now is the dominant agent in the treatment of syphilis in most of its stages. However, older therapy with arsenicals, bismuth, mercury and iodides constitutes a background for comparison of results and represents probably the most massively extended application of chemotherapy in medical history. The best recommended regimen for treatment of early syphilis before the advent of penicillin consisted of about 12 months of continuous therapy with weekly injections of alternating courses of arsenical and a heavy metal. Attempts to shorten the period to a few weeks of intensive treatment were effective in rendering patients noninfectious but were associated with a high incidence of toxic reactions. With penicillin, the schedule consisted first of intramuscular injections of aqueous solutions every 3 hours for several days. Repository forms of penicillin have permitted schedules with fewer injections and have placed the therapy on an ambulatory basis.

Other common antibiotics have antiluetic value but have not been shown to be superior to penicillin.

Arsenicals

The various arsphenamines, which were the first clearly effective agents used in the treatment of syphilis, are colloidal and are rapidly flocculated on injection, with deposition chiefly in the reticuloendothelial system. Arsenoxide, a conversion product, was considered to be the active form; it presumably acts to inactivate the glutathione respiratory mechanism. Tryparsamide, a pentavalent arsenical, penetrates the central nervous system and has some usefulness in the treatment of trypanosomiasis. Its conspicuous toxic effect is optic atrophy.

Mercury

Mercury compounds have been used in the treatment of syphilis since the first orthodox descriptions of the disease about AD 1500. In early transfer experiments calomel ointment was seen to have special value in preventing transmission, and it has been used extensively in local prophylaxis. Oral administration was accomplished by a solution or tablet containing mercury bichloride in an excess of potassium iodide—the once widely used "mixed treatment."

Iodides

Potassium iodide has been used routinely in the treatment of syphilis since its introduction in 1836. It is not directly spirocheticidal, and its only clearly established value is in accelerating resolution of gummata and in acute meningeal involvement. Iodides are excreted rapidly in the urine.

Penicillin

Penicillin has proved to be a highly effective antiluetic according to short-term criteria—disappearance of spirochetes, healing of early surface lesions and serologic reversal. A relapse rate less satisfactory than with heavy metals was obtained in the first extended trials with penicillin. In considerable part this has been attributed to inadequate dose or inadequate proportions of penicillin G in the products used. The Jarisch-Herxheimer reaction is obtained with relatively high incidence after penicillin administration. This reaction is a flare-up of symptoms thought to be due to sudden release of products from killed spirochetes; its intensity is reduced by cortisone.

Apparently, adequate therapy can be provided by one single intramuscular injection of 2,400,000 units as benzathine penicillin G (Bicillin). Late neurovascular, cardiovascular and gummatous syphilis is treated with schedules totaling about 10,000,000 units; fever may be combined with penicillin in treatment of late neurosyphilis. Treatment of the mother during pregnancy is especially successful in preventing luetic involvement of the infant. However, treatment of congenital syphilis calls for more intensive treatment, and results are less satisfactory.

A number of generalities have evolved from experience with these treatments. For instance, a relatively minute concentration of penicillin has been found to be effective if maintained for periods of 4 days or longer. Much greater than ordinary doses, as much as 25,000,000 units, are ineffective if penicillin concentrations are not maintained for at least 4 days. The period for remultiplication of the treponema is estimated at about 30 hours, in contrast with 20 to 30 minutes in the instance of ordinary bacteria. Penicillin is effective only when the organisms are multiplying. There is little advantage in combining penicillin with other antiluetic agents. Defense mechanisms of the host provide the treponemicidal action of penicillin with very limited assistance. The organism does not develop resistance to penicillin. Doses of penicillin or related antibiotics that are used for treating other types of infections may be less than with the usual treatment schedule for syphilis but nevertheless may be adequate for preventing the infection in exposed cases or for rendering a case noninfectious; these features have reduced considerably the reservoir of infectious syphilis among the population.

RADIOACTIVE COMPOUNDS

A radioactive element is one that gives off ionizing energy because of spontaneous internal rearrangement of the nucleus. Naturally occurring radioactive isotopes are limited to those elements with atomic number greater than 83, or with mass number greater than 209; better-known examples of such are polonium ($^{210}_{84}Po$), radium ($^{226}_{88}Ra$), thorium ($^{232}_{90}Th$) and uranium ($^{238}_{92}U$). Subscripts designate the atomic number (denoting number of nuclear protons or orbital electrons), and the superscript designates the mass number or the total number of nuclear mass particles (protons plus neutrons). By a practice officially recognized in 1964, such subscripts and superscripts are placed to the left of the atomic symbol; a subscript to the right is used to designate atoms per molecule.

In 1934, radioactivity was induced in light elements by bombardment with alpha particles and by the cyclotron accelerator. In 1938, ^{32}P as sodium radiophosphate was introduced for the therapy of polycythemia, and in 1942, ^{131}I, for the control of hyperthyroidism. Fission reactions, as generated in the atomic pile, led to availability of a profusion of isotopes with a wide variety of medical uses.

Selection of isotopes for specific purposes is based on the half life of their radioactivity, type and energy of radiation and on absorption and excretion characteristics of the molecular compounds in which they can be incorporated. The last-mentioned feature can be expressed as biologic half life and, with the known physical half life of the isotope, which identifies the rate of radioactive disintegration or decay, provides a basis for estimating the effective half life, which is a measure of the time a tissue is exposed to the radioactive material. Biologic effects of such exposures are similar to those produced by x-rays and are presumed to result from the action of ionizing radiation on water, with production of active radicals and compounds such as hydrogen peroxide; effects resemble the reaction of nitrogen mustards with cells. There may be direct cell death, depression of functional activity or depression of mitotic activity, and, in the case of germ cells, there may be mutations. Late effects of ionizing radiation may be carcinogenic, as has been demonstrated in the past subsequent to ingestion of radium and the use of thorium dioxide as a contrast medium. In man, the most radiosensitive tissues are, in decreasing order, the lymphoid tissues, the bone marrow, the epithelium of the small intestine, the gonads and the basal cells of the epidermis.

Dosage exposures are expressed in terms of *rads* when the energy is due to emission of alpha or beta particles, this unit corresponding to 100 ergs absorbed per gram of absorbing material. The exposure dose unit is the roentgen (r) when the energy is due to emission of γ radiation of x-rays, and these electromagnetic radiations are defined in terms of ionization produced in air. The energy absorption in tissue is approximately the same for 1 rad and for 1 roentgen. For calculations of total accumulated dose over lifetime periods the unit *rem* is used, which, again, is about the same as the r or the rad but allows for possible differences in biologic effectiveness of the radiations. Radioactive compounds are administered in dosage units of curies, millicuries, microcuries or, occasionally, nanocuries, each unit being progressively $\frac{1}{1000}$ of the preceding unit. The curie corresponds to the emission activity of 1 g. of radium per second or 3.7×10^{10} disintegrations per second.

A striking feature of radioactive elements is the constancy of type and energy of the radiation emitted. Similarly there is constancy in regard to the rate of disintegration, with a fixed percentage of all atoms disintegrating per unit of time. Alpha particle emission occurs only among the heavy, naturally radioactive nuclides and a few others of relatively obscure nature. These heavy elements are bone seekers and, although alpha particles, which are equivalent to helium nuclei, do not penetrate more than 70 microns in tissue, they act with considerable energy on immediately adjacent tissue. The biologic effectiveness of these heavy particles is, under some conditions, about four times as great as that of beta emissions so that the dose in rems is about four times that in rads. Beta emissions, which more commonly are electrons (i.e., negatively charged), penetrate tissues only a few millimeters. Their energies for any given element vary over a wide spectrum and must be calculated as a maximum or an average; the radiation energies vary widely from element to element, and different counting equipment is required for "hard" and for "soft" beta emissions. Usually, both beta radiation and gamma radiation are produced, although there are a number of important pure beta emitters, such as ^{14}C, ^{3}H, ^{32}P, ^{90}Sr and ^{35}S.

Isotopes in Radiation Therapy

Sodium iodide (^{131}I), with radioactive half-life of 8 days, is given in average doses of 4 to 8 millicuries for the treatment of *hyperthyroidism*. Recurrence of symptoms is infrequent. Myxedema occurs in a significant number of instances (variably reported at 40 per cent or more at 20 years) and must be treated with thyroid extract. Possibilities of a late incidence of leukemia, carcinoma or genetic mutations have tended to restrict use to those over age 40; in the absence of convincing evidence that these actually have resulted from the treatment, there is increasing selection of the treatment in younger age groups. Euthyroid patients with intractable angina pectoris or congestive heart failure have been given large doses of the radioiodide as a desperate measure. In thyroid cancer, doses of 30 to 100 millicuries have been given and repeated as long as uptake is appreciable. Since many such malignant conditions have a low uptake, thyroid-stimulating hormone also is used. Bone marrow depression limits this therapy, which is only nominally successful.

Sodium phosphate (^{32}P), with a radioactive half life of 14.3 days, is given in intravenous doses of about 4 millicuries in *polycythemia*. Because of some limited selective localization in hematopoietic tissues as well as high sensitivity of these cells in radiation, there is suppression of hematopoietic activity without serious body radiation effects. There is controversy whether or not the subsequent incidence of leukemia is increased by this treatment. The same agent is used in the attempted management of leukemias. Colloidal chromic phosphate with ^{32}P was used in neoplastic pleural effusions and, in contrast with previously used ^{198}Au, did not expose attendants to gamma radiation. Another pure beta emitter, ^{90}Yt is now more used in the same way. The same considerations apply to the management of ascites. Other forms of interstital implantations and intracavity applications of radioisotopes have been used in malignant disease, as was done previously with radium and radon. Cobalt (^{60}Co), with a half-life of 5.2 years, is used in the form of wire or

needles. Bladder tumors have been irradiated with radioactive tantalum wire, and brain tumors have been treated similarly with iridium. Boron compounds show some degree of localization in brain tumors, and ^{10}B emits alpha particles when subjected to neutron bombardment; this procedure is more indicative of possibilities than an accepted practice. Since antibodies to tumor tissue can be prepared, their tagging with radioactive isotopes is being tried as another means of localizing radiation, particularly in the instance of brain tumors.

Diagnostic Radioisotopes

Since compounds tagged with radioactive isotopes can be measured easily and with high accuracy, there are numerous ways in which these procedures can be applied to clinical diagnosis. A conspicuous example is the thyroid, in which the high concentrating capacity for iodine and the easy recognition of ^{131}I, with its substantial gamma radiation, make it possible to measure function in a number of ways. In hyperthyroidism, as contrasted with normal or reduced thyroid activity, intravenous or oral administration of about 5 microcuries of sodium iodide (^{131}I) is followed by measurably reduced excretion of radioactivity in the 24 hour urine, by increased uptake of radioactivity as monitored over the thyroid gland and an increased level of serum protein-bound iodine (^{131}I); red blood cells in vitro take up an increased amount of triiodothyronine labeled with ^{131}I. Serum competes more actively for this compound when it is absorbed on a resin–sponge combination. Urinary excretions of less than 30 per cent of the tracer dose in 24 hours are consistent with the diagnosis of hyperthyroidism. More usually, diagnoses are based on gamma counts taken over the region of the gland at 2 to 24 hours after administration. Normally, 5 to 12 per cent of activity is picked up at 2 hours and 15 to 45 per cent at 24 hours. Each of these various tests is subject to error, one of the most important sources being previous administration of iodine-containing compounds. Functional studies with radioisotopes are in common use for evaluation of the cardiovascular system, the liver, the gut and the kidney. Examples are: determinations of red cell mass, by tagging cells with sodium chromate (^{52}Cr); of plasma volume, with serum albumin labeled with ^{131}I or ^{125}I (RISA); of circulation times, with ^{24}Na and ^{42}K; of cerebral blood flow, with dissolved ^{133}Xe; of blood flow of muscles in the leg and coronary arteries, with dissolved ^{133}Xe; of body water compartmentalization, with tritium (^{3}H)-labeled water; of kidney function, with ^{131}I-labeled urographic agents; of liver function, with similarly labeled rose bengal dye; of intestinal absorption, with ^{57}Co- or ^{58}Co-labeled cyanocobalamin, in pernicious anemia (urinary collection or Schilling test is one procedure); of utilization and storage of iron, with ^{55}Fe and ^{59}Fe.

Most of the above methods use fixed monitoring probes over one point of the area in question. As an extension of this, automatic scanning devices provide a sketch of radioactivity over a considerable area. This is useful in that it indicates "hot spots" or "cold spots" when a tumor, an abscess or a hematoma is either more active or less active than the organ in concentrating the tagged compound. These maneuvers include the use of ^{131}I for recognition of malignant nodules in the thyroid: ^{75}Se, as selenomethionine similarly, in the pancreas; liver abscesses can be distinguished from hepatitis with sulfur colloids of ^{99m}Tc; pulmonary emboli can be localized with an aggregated albumin preparation tagged with ^{99m}Tc; bone metastases can be recognized with ^{18}F; kidney localization can be aided and clearance values obtained without catheterization by use of ^{131}I-tagged iodohippurate or imaged with ^{99m}Tc-labeled chelates. Tumor imaging and abscess localization are aided by the use of ^{67}Ga citrate. Ischemic heart disease may be studied with ^{201}Tl as thallium chloride. An elaborated technique for brain tumor localization uses either of the positron emitters ^{11}C or ^{14}N, which have the characteristic of setting up radiation that moves equally in opposite directions in a straight line; two counters recording only simultaneous impingements (coincidence counting) indicate the precise line in which the disintegration occurred; two such lines establish a fix on the radiation source that is highly accurate. The same principle has been used with ^{84}Rb in scanning studies of coronary blood flow.

Selection of progressively more suitable isotopes is illustrated in the instance of iodine with about two dozen radionuclides, some half of which are considered to be of biomedical usefulness. With a half life of 60 days, ^{125}I gives better shelf storage convenience; with no beta emissions the subject is spared this useless radiation; its gamma-ray "merit rate" is high, that is, its ratio of target to nontarget radioactivity. Also, ^{123}I, with a 13.3 hour half life, absence of beta emission and high specific activity (1900 curies per mg.), is peculiarly suitable for some studies. Similarly, ^{121}I, with a half life of 2.1 hours, low photon energy and a high degree of directionality, is specially adapted for use with the positron scintillation camera.

Whether the moving detector devices (scanners) or the stationary type of cameras are used, image intensity depends upon the number of emerging photons, and this leads to search and selection among the short-lived radionuclides. They have become more available now through the generator systems or "mother-daughter" systems, from which the short-lived radionuclides can be removed from time to time. A particular example is technetium-99m from the parent nuclide ^{99}Mo. It has a 6 hour half life, satisfactory gamma radiation, absence of beta radiation and is stable in aqueous solutions as the pertechnatate ion. It is particularly suitable for brain scanning and thyroid scanning. Combined with sulfur colloid, it is rapidly removed by the reticuloendothelial system and has been used to visualize the liver, spleen and bone marrow. Combined with albumin, it has been used for blood pool, and lung scanning. Combined with pyrophosphates or phosphonates, it is used for imaging the skeletal system. A still shorter-lived radionuclide is indium-113m, obtained from the parent nuclide ^{113}Sn in a similar generator system. This ^{113m}In can be used in much the same way as ^{99m}Tc and may have advantages over it. (The m designation used here refers to metastability, which rapidly decays to a stable form.)

Drug Metabolism

Drug absorption and excretion as well as drug metabolic pathways can be followed precisely by tagging with a radioactive isotope. The availability of isotope-tagged organic compounds has been extended greatly by the Wilzbach procedure of exposure to tritium (^{3}H); ^{3}H carries significant soft beta activity and has a half life of 12 years. With or without a catalyst, tritium is incorporated directly into organic compounds in amounts producing up to 56 curies per g. The tritium is usually localized in the more labile portions of the molecule.

Intracellular localization of isotope-tagged compounds can be accomplished by radioautography, in which thin sections of frozen tissue are placed on specially prepared photographic film for comparatively long periods and the isotope (usually a beta emitter) produces the radiograph directly.

Stable isotopes can be measured by the mass spectograph, as has been done with ^{15}N incorporated in the pentobarbital molecule.

Ordinarily it has been considered that there are no available radioactive isotopes of carbon, oxygen or nitrogen that are relevant to diagnostic and therapeutic applications. However, it has more recently been possible, under highly specialized conditions, to set up small accelerators that produce ^{15}O, ^{13}N and ^{11}C. These are short-lived isotopes with half lives of ½ to 20 minutes; they decay with positron emission and thus can be monitored by coincidence counting. When used to measure regional distribution and blood flow in the lungs, for instance, they reveal diagnostically significant differences in blood flow rates and ventilation in upper and lower lung zones.

THERAPEUTIC GASES

Oxygen administration is most valuable in conditions that limit the amount of oxygen passing from the pulmonary atmosphere to the blood (anoxic anoxia); it is of some value in conditions of impaired circulation that fail to expose enough blood to the pulmonary atmosphere (stagnant anoxia); it is of less value in conditions of deficient oxygen-transporting blood pigment (anemic anoxia); and it is almost valueless in tissue poisonings that render the cells incapable of utilizing oxygen (histotoxic anoxia). Conditions of anoxic anoxia include pneumonia, pulmonary edema, emphysema, atelectasis and pulmonary obstruction. Any condition lowering the oxygen content in the alveoli produces anoxic anoxia; this occurs most frequently now in high-altitude flying. Anoxic anoxia is also a matter of frequent concern in the administration of anesthetics. Congestive heart failure, coronary occlusion and shock may cause stagnant anoxia and may be benefited by oxygen administration.

Oxygen may be dangerous when the medullary respiratory center is grossly depressed by anesthetics, narcotics or prolonged anoxia. Under these conditions the more primitive and resistent chemoreceptors, the carotid and the aortic bodies, furnish the drive for the respiratory mechanism, and this drive is dependent on the existing anoxia. Accordingly, administration of oxygen removes the final remaining stimulus for the respiratory mechanism. This "chemical denervation" of the carotid and the aortic bodies necessitates the immediate institution of mechanical respiration. Its occurrence is recognized readily by any significant depression of respiratory movements that follows the administration of oxygen.

Oxygen, when helpful in the anemic anoxias such as monoxide poisoning and methemoglobinemia, acts chiefly through its physical solution in plasma. The maximum solubility with 100 per cent oxygen as the inspired gas is 2.0 volumes per cent, which is thus an appreciable fraction of the oxygen carried by normal amounts of hemoglobin (20 volumes per cent). Oxygen is frequently given along with inhalation or intravenous anesthetics, since, in addition to its respiratory and circulatory benefits, it has been shown to protect against liver damage.

With the usual methods of administration, approximate figures for oxygen concentrations in inspired air are: tents, 25 to 50 per cent; nasopharyngeal catheters, 40 to 60 per cent; hoods, 50 to 80 per cent; oronasal masks, 80 to 100 per cent. The higher figures in each case are obtained by increased flow rates; with catheters, a flow rate greater than 8 liters per minute usually produces an unacceptable degree of irritation of the oropharynx. Oronasal masks equipped with a demand valve supply 100 per cent oxygen at a rate equal to the respiratory minute volume. Regardless of the concentration provided by the oxygenating system, monitoring of the arterial blood for oxygen saturation is the only means of assuring that therapy is effective.

In premature infants the occurrence of retrolental fibroplasia has been attributed to excessive administration of high oxygen concentrations followed by sudden withdrawal of administered oxygen. The minimum use of oxygen in premature infants usually is recommended.

Hyperbaric oxygen chambers have been constructed in which patients may be placed and fully manned surgical operations may be performed. This provides the advantages of high-oxygen therapy at levels of 2 to 3 atmospheres pressure. At the higher pressure, 6.6 ml. of oxygen is present in free solution in 100 ml. of blood. Hyperbaric oxygen is currently used in the treatment of obstructive lung disease, gas gangrene, acute myocardial infarction, burns, shock, carbon-monoxide poisoning and peripheral vascular diseases. It is utilized as an adjunct to radiation therapy of cancer and during corrective surgery for cyanotic congenital heart diseases.

Prolonged exposure leads to lung damage as well as to symptoms of cardiac and central nervous system toxicity.

Carbon dioxide, being the physiologic respiratory stimulant, is very effective in increasing the depth of the external respiratory movements. Its effect is chiefly on the respiratory center, although there may be some slight effect on the carotid body. As ordinarily administered it is mixed with oxygen in concentrations of 5 to 10 per cent. Carbon dioxide is of value in only a few situations. It is added to pump oxygenators to avoid reduction of the CO_2 tension of the blood. It is introduced around the heart, kidney and other organs to delineate these for x-ray examinations. Because of its rapid absorption, it is the safest of gases to use for these purposes. However, respiratory acidosis can occur if large quantities are insufflated into the body. The solid form is used by dermatologists to cauterize certain skin lesions. Because carbon dioxide is the most potent cerebrovascular dilator known, it should not be used in patients with increased intracranial pressure or head injury.

Helium is a completely inert gas under body conditions and has relatively low water and fat solubility. It is, next to hydrogen, the lightest gas available and exhibits an exceptionally rapid rate of effusion through narrow orifices. A mixture of 20 per cent oxygen and 80 per cent helium has one-third the specific gravity of air; the work of breathing may be reduced as much as 60 per cent. This is especially desirable in patients with obstructive pulmonary disease. Since helium is much less soluble than nitrogen in the body fluids and tissues, it can be used in decompression chambers to shorten the period of decompression. On emergence to normal atmosphere there is much less likelihood of caisson disease, as less of the inert gas has been dissolved in the body, and it is eliminated much more rapidly. At high atmospheric pressures, helium-oxygen mixtures are much better tolerated than are nitrogen-oxygen mixtures, which exhibit narcotic effects.

CATHARTICS

Drugs that increase frequency of stools or promote their softening or fluidity are termed variously laxatives, cathartics or purgatives. Their intensity of action increases in about the order named.

Some act by irritating the gut to produce increased propulsive movements and restricted absorption of fluids. The most popular of the irritant group have common features of action, i.e., they are relatively nonirritant until acted on by the contents of the gut and then are automatically removed and thereby prevented from excessive overactivity. Castor oil, for instance, is ordinarily a bland emollient, but in the gut is converted to ricinoleic acid, which is an active irritant. Changes with other popular cathartics are not as well understood as the simple lipolytic splitting of a fat; nevertheless, they have about the same rate of conversion and the same irritant intensity of the final products. Examples are bisacodyl (Dulcolax), calomel, aloes, cascara, senna, phenolphthalein, rhubarb and sulfur.

Some cathartics maintain an abnormal volume of intestinal contents, and the resulting distention serves as a stimulus for propulsive activity. An example is carboxymethylcellulose, which is an indigestible, synthetic, hydrophilic colloid. Solutions of certain salts retain abnormal bulk and fluidity because of the fact that they are poorly absorbed and tend by osmotic force to hold or attract water into the intestinal lumen. Liquid petrolatum is an indigestible hydrocarbon that is dispersed along the walls of the gut and through gut contents as oily globules that are not absorbed and, by their insoluble coating effect, tend to prevent the normal absorption of water. The oil itself also adds extra fluid bulk. The increased bulk and fluidity hasten the passage of gut contents.

A generally different type of action is involved in the use of surface-active or wetting agents that counteract the formation of hard, dry fecal masses. Dioctyl sodium sulfosuccinate and poloxalkol have been used in this way in patients with cardiovascular disease or hernia to lessen the strain of defecation.

In general, cathartics rarely are indicated. Forced evacuation of the lower gut is obtained more satisfactorily by enemas or suppositories. The common practice of taking carthartics for undiagnosed abdominal complaints has frequently caused perforated appendices and spreading peritonitis.

ANTACIDS AND ADSORBENTS

Mildly alkaline salts are used to relieve the discomfort of hyperacidity and peptic ulcer. They are also used to alkalinize the urine, since this sometimes is of value in combating urinary infections and in preventing precipitation of substances such as the sulfonamides, hemoglobin and uric acid. Healing of peptic ulcer may be accelerated by the use of alkaline powders, although their value is probably less than some of the other components of the usual treatment such as rest, frequent feedings of a bland diet, aspiration of stomach contents and administration of anticholinergic drugs.

Continued administration of alkalies may lead to alkalosis, may produce either diarrhea or constipation and may predispose to the formation of kidney stones. Antacids containing magnesium can produce severe toxic effects in patients with impaired renal function. A soluble alkali such as sodium bicarbonate is more likely to produce alkalosis than the water-insoluble alkalies such as magnesium oxide and calcium carbonate—although all of these may produce alkalosis on occasion. Alkalosis produced in this way is treated by withdrawal of the alkali, parenteral administration of sodium chloride and possibly oral administration of an acid-forming salt such as ammonium chloride.

Magnesium oxide or carbonate may cause diarrhea; calcium carbonate may cause constipation. Magnesium trisilicate, aluminum hydroxide and aluminum phosphate both adsorb and combine with acid. The latter two are used commonly as a four per cent gel or suspension in water.

EMETICS AND ANTIEMETICS

Drugs that cause vomiting may act through nonspecific irritation of the digestive tract or, more specifically, may stimulate the emetic center in the medulla or some other area in the nervous system that acts secondarily through the emetic center. A chemoreceptor "trigger zone" for emesis has been described in the *area postrema* of the medulla. Apomorphine is conspicuous in its specific action at this point, and its 5 mg. subcutaneous dose usually produces vomiting very promptly. Several drugs produce vomiting as an undesired side effect and independent of any action on the digestive tract. This is particularly true of morphine, digitalis, salicylates and veratrum. Drugs that produce vomiting by direct action on the gastrointestinal tract are copper sulfate, zinc sulfate, mustard and strong sodium chloride solution, the latter two being considered effective household emetics. Antimony potassium tartrate (tartar emetic) and ipecac apparently act both by local irritation in the digestive tract and by central action. All emetics, whether local or systemic, can be profoundly depressant and now are used rarely as a means of emptying the stomach, although this was a common practice in the past. They are contraindicated after ingestion of caustic substances or petroleum distillates.

The suppression of vomiting frequently is desired. Such antiemetic action may be obtained to some degree by the use of insoluble powders or relatively insoluble local anesthetics that act to reduce impulses arising from the stomach. Systemic agents include barbiturates, scopolamine, butyrophenones, antihistaminics and the phenothiazine derivatives. The latter are the most potent and effective; they should be prescribed only when vomiting cannot be controlled by less hazardous drugs. Benzquinamide (Emete-con) is a nonaminedepleting antiemetic chemically unrelated to the phenothiazines and to other antiemetics. The mechanism of action in humans is unknown. It is indicated for the prevention and treatment of nausea and vomiting associated with anesthesia and surgery. Morphine has a potent antiemetic effect as an intermediate phase of its action, i.e., there may be an early and also a late emetic effect with an intermediate interval of emetic center depression. Caution should be exercised in the use of antiemetics because they may mask the toxic effects of other drugs or an underlying organic disease.

ANTITUSSIVES

The cough reflex is a protective mechanism that rids the respiratory tract of a mechanical or pathologic irritation. At times, however, cough suppressive therapy is indicated to permit rest, facilitate sleep and reduce the irritation to the respiratory tract that tends to make cough self-perpetuating. The objective is to decrease both the intensity and frequency of the cough while still permitting adequate elimination of respiratory tract secretions and exudates. Antitussives act centrally, peripherally or both. The centrally active suppressants include narcotic agents (e.g., codeine and hydrocodone), non-narcotic agents (e.g., dextro-

methorphan (Romilar) and levo-propoxyphene (Novrad). Those acting peripherally include the demulcents (e.g., acacia, glycerin, licorice, honey) and the expectorants and mucolytics.

Expectorants are used orally to increase flow of respiratory tract secretions. Their use is based primarily on tradition and the widespread subjective clinical impression that they are effective. The group encompasses terpin hydrate, ammonium chloride, potassium iodide, and glyceryl guaiacolate. Some emetics, such as syrup of ipecac, in small doses act as expectorants. Mucolytic agents are used by inhalation to reduce the viscosity of respiratory tract fluid as an adjunct to systemic therapy in the management of acute respiratory diseases. Humidification can be accomplished by the nebulization of water or sodium chloride solution. Detergents such as tyloxapol (Alevaire) increase wetting and thereby supposedly increase liquefaction of mucus. Acetylcysteine (Mucomyst) reduces the viscosity of mucus by depolymerizing mucopolysaccharides; pancreatic dornase (Dornavac) acts by hydrolyzing deoxribonucleoprotein in purulent mucus.

OXYTOCICS

Ergot, from a rye fungus, has been used since 1807, usually in the form of its fluid extract. The USP dose of 2 ml. or larger amounts was given orally with fairly prompt effects. Subsequently, ergotamine (Gynergen) and ergotoxin, which are virtually identical in action, were separated and administered intramuscularly in doses of 0.25 mg. These active principles are obtained from the alcohol-soluble fractions of the crude drug. At a later date the water-soluble fraction was found to contain a principle that acted more rapidly and was effective by oral administration. This principle, officially termed ergonovine, also is known by the proprietary name Ergotrate. It produces less vasospasm than ergotamine and has been credited with less toxic side effects on prolonged administration. The lesser degree of vasospasm probably is related to its lesser degree of effectiveness in treating migraine headaches. Its obstetric dose as ergonovine maleate is 0.5 mg. intramuscularly. Frequently, smaller doses are used intravenously. The administration of ergonovine by sublingual administration sometimes is recommended. However, it is not absorbed through the buccal mucosa, and the impression of effective absorption by this route has been developed because of very rapid absorption after swallowing.

Methylergonovine (Methergine) is a synthetic variant of ergonovine with essentially similar properties. Ergotism is characterized by dry gangrene of the extremities and is considered to be due to prolonged excessive vasospasm. Lesions of the intima develop, and there is stasis thrombosis in the smaller arteries and arterioles. Cyanosis of roosters' combs has been used as a bioassay of ergot products. Ergotism has occurred most widely following ingestion of fungus-contaminated rye bread. Prolonged administration during the puerperium has also produced gangrene in a few cases not attributable to the usual causes. Prolonged administration of ergot alkaloids for migraine and other conditions in which peripheral vascular disturbances were absent has indicated a relatively slight incidence of gangrene and an acceptable degree of safety.

Acute symptoms of ergot poisoning include anginal pains, tingling in extremities, cerebral excitation and nausea and vomiting.

Posterior pituitary preparations have as principal actions smooth muscle spasm and antidiuretic action. The smooth muscle spasm is manifested most prominently on the pregnant uterus at term. The contractions may be so powerful as to rupture the uterus, injure the fetus or lacerate the cervix and the perineum. Effects are obtained quickly after subcutaneous or intramuscular injection, and they pass off rapidly. The intestinal muscle also responds, and posterior pituitary preparations have been used to combat abdominal distention. The effect here is chiefly the expulsion of flatus from the large gut, with relatively little effect on the small gut. Coronary spasm as a dangerous side effect has occurred often enough to lead to discontinuance of this practice. Another prominent effect is spasm of arterioles and capillaries, which is shown in anesthetized animals as a marked blood pressure rise on intravenous injection. Ordinarily, in the human subject, no blood pressure rise is obtained, as a result of compensatory reflexes and possibly coronary constriction.

The antidiuretic action is due to some special effect of posterior pituitary in increasing water reabsorption by the renal tubules. This effect is useful in the management of diabetes insipidus. It may be an objection to the use of pituitary in toxemic patients.

Both oxytocin and vasopressin are composed of eight amino acids, six of which are common to each. These peptides both contain disulfide linkages, and reduction to the sulfhydryl forms destroys biologic activity. The extremely high potency of these peptides is illustrated by the fact that antidiuretic effects can be obtained in man with doses of about $\frac{1}{1000}$ of a microgram.

The USP preparation of *oxytocin* and *vasopressin* represent, respectively, nearly complete separation of the oxytocic effects and the vasopressor, gut-stimulating and antidiuretic effects. The lack of complete separation of these effects is not a matter of residual

contaminants but an inherent characteristic of these two closely related peptides. Both oxytocin injection and *posterior pituitary solution* are given in doses of about 1 ml. intramuscularly. Only synthetic oxytocin is now available. Paradoxically, the nonpregnant uterus is much more sensitive to vasopressin than to oxytocin.

Oxytocics are used principally for controlling postpartum hemorrhage. The drug-induced spasm of the emptied uterus produces a tamponading effect that significantly reduces the average amount of blood loss.

Another interpretation is that uterine muscle bands are entwined around arterial vessels in a type of figure-of-eight loop; drug-induced muscle spasm then has the effect of occluding the arterial blood supply of the uterus. Oxytocics may be given after the delivery of the shoulder in normal deliveries, at the end of the second stage or, more safely, after expulsion of the placenta. For this purpose, pituitary acts most quickly and has the briefest period of action, while ergotamine is relatively slow in developing its effects and has the most prolonged period of action. Ergonovine is intermediate in both respects.

The use of oxytocics during the first or the second stages of labor carries extreme hazards to both mother and fetus and is generally condemned. During the puerperium, daily administration of ergot preparations is thought to hasten involution of the uterus and diminish the lochial discharge. During the medical induction of labor, pituitary solution may be used but only with special caution. Oxytocin solutions in great dilution have been used by intravenous infusions. Besides uterine tetany, coronary constriction appears to be one of the hazards of this type of administration.

Prostaglandins, (PGE$_2$ and PGF$_2$ alpha) are used for the purpose of inducing or accelerating labor. Dinoprost tromethamine (Prostin F$_2$alpha) is the first prostaglandin product to become available for use by physicians in this country. It is used for preparation of instrumental abortion during the first trimester of pregnancy, and also for induction of abortion beyond the 12th week of gestation. When administered intra-amniotically it stimulates the myometrium of the gravid uterus to contract in a manner that is similar to the contractions seen in the term uterus during labor. A high incidence of vomiting, abdominal cramps and uterine pain occurs. Less frequently, posterior cervical perforations, grand mal convulsions and uterine rupture have been noted. Dinoprostone (Prostin E2), administered intravaginally, is indicated for the termination of pregnancy from the 12th gestational week through the second trimester as calculated from the first day of the last regular menstrual period. The most frequent adverse reactions observed are related to its contractile effect on smooth muscle.

Angiotensin amide (Hypertensin) is a nonadrenergic, synthetic octapeptide pressor agent that has had trial in counteracting hypotensive states of varied etiology. It is mainly of value in controlling acute hypotension during administration of general anesthetics that sensitize the heart to catecholamines. Pressor action is obtained with lower dose ranges than are possible with levarterenol and, with infusions, can be maintained for long intervals. Further, angiotensin acts directly on the arteriolar smooth muscle; it has little direct cardiac effect at ordinary pressor doses; it causes constriction mainly at arteriolar sites, with little venoconstriction; it is not affected by autonomic blocking agents; it has little metabolic effect; it stimulates the adrenal cortex to increase aldosterone secretion and ordinarily decreases urinary secretion but, under conditions of anesthesia, causes an increase in urine secretion. The last-mentioned renal effect is due possibly to hemodynamic effects, or it may be related to a blocking action of the antidiuretic hormone, also an octapeptide. Angiotensin is not tachyphylactic. Excessive doses may produce a marked increase in myocardial oxygen demand, and, hence, myocardial hypoxia.

The synthetic manufacture of this agent followed the recognition of its production in the body as a result of decreased renal blood flow or lowered pressure in the renal artery; under these conditions, the juxtaglomerular apparatus secretes renin, a proteolytic enzyme, which reacts with a serum globulin to yield the decapeptide angiotensin I, which, after cleavage to two amino acids, is recognized as angiotensin II, representing then the active peptide.

TERATOGENIC DRUGS

From late 1959 through 1961, several thousand instances of phocomelia occurred that were attributed to the administration of the sedative thalidomide (phthalimido-glutaramide) during the first trimester of pregnancy. Phocomelia, or "seal extremities," was recognized previously as a rare malformation affecting particularly the limb buds of the upper extremities. In these instances it was considered to be a nongenetic pathologic modification of the mesenchymal structures of embryos without recognizable chromosomal aberrations, occurring most critically between the third and the sixth weeks of pregnancy. The malformations bore resemblances to riboflavin deficiency in rodents, and it has been suggested that thalidomide forms an inactivating combination with some of the vitamin B mechanisms. The intensified animal experimentation following this incident has provided a "teratogenicity" index for most of the commonly used drugs. The cancer chemotherapy drugs, certain pesticides, salicylates, antihistaminics and serotonin have proved to be highly active. Treatment of leukemias and lymphomas during pregnancy has been reviewed, with the conclusion that malformations are associated largely with the use of aminopterin or combinations of other antineoplastic drugs administered during the first trimester of pregnancy. The latter drugs, used alone, appear to be relatively safe.

VITAMINS

Vitamin deficiency syndromes are described in other sections of this volume. Therapy with vitamin replacements is highly effective. The infrequency with which these primary syndromes are found in the United States at the present time may be regarded as part of the picture of progress—from deficient diets to overconsumption. As current medical problems, obesity and atherosclerosis appear to outweigh, in seriousness, scurvy, pellagra, beriberi, night blindness and rickets, combined. However, manifestations of vitamin-deficiency states are produced by bizarre diets of food faddists and by malabsorption syndromes, extensive surgery, and the metabolic antagonisms of certain drugs. Further, the use of vitamins as a type of blanket prophylaxis and as therapy for subclinical deficiency states, actual or presumed, has led to widespread distribution of highly potent preparations. Ingestion of gross amounts and excessive selfadministration may induce specific toxic actions.

Vitamin A. This fat-soluble vitamin is available as fish liver oil with high content of the vitamin, as concentrates from such sources and as manufactured synthetic products. Vitamin A and water-miscible vitamin A are standardized by a spectrophotometric procedure in terms of the USP unit. The recommended daily dietary allowance for adults of about 5,000 units is greatly exceeded in some of the therapeutic applications, as in hyperkeratotic conditions. Toxicity from excessive doses causes vague symptoms of irritability, headache, arthralgias, gingivitis, etc; there may be clear demonstrations of enlargement of the liver, since the vitamin is stored tenaciously in this organ; also, there may be significant degrees of periosteal new bone formation. Premature closures of epiphyses have occurred, with serious alterations of skeletal development. Dermatologic changes resemble those of vitamin A deficiency. The toxic syndromes have been observed in the Arctic in persons who have eaten polar bear liver, which has been reported to contain as much as 8,000,000 units of vitamin A per pound. Hypervitaminosis A has occurred also in numerous instances of excessive self-medication with high-dosage preparations.

Vitamin D. The term vitamin D originally referred to the antirachitic component in cod liver oil, and the bioassayed unit corresponded to about $\frac{1}{100}$ the amount in 1 ml. of average medicinal cod liver oil. The latter amount is approximately equivalent to 0.025 μg. of calciferol (vitamin D_2, viosterol), which is formed commercially by irradiation of ergosterol. The bioassay is based on changes in the skeletal calcification in rachitic rats. Irradiation of 7-dehydrocholesterol yields vitamin D_3, the naturally occurring antirachitic factor present in fish liver oils and formed in the skin by the ultraviolet of sunlight. Microgram for microgram, the D_2 and the D_3 forms are considered equivalent. The designation vitamin D_1 is no longer in use. One of the potent irradiated sterols is dihydrotachysterol (Hytakerol), which has, typically, the effect of raising calcium levels in the blood but has only weak antirachitic effects; its use is primarily in hypoparathyroidism, although it may also have value in rickets resistant to other activated sterols. Dihydrotachysterol acts chiefly by phosphate diuresis and has only moderate influence in increasing intestinal absorption of calcium.

Vitamin D preparations correct the defective bone formation of rickets by increasing intestinal absorption of calcium and also by exerting regulatory effects on blood phosphatase and on calcium and phosphate ratios occurring in mobilization of mineral from the bone and excretion of these ions by the renal tubules.

Synthetic oleovitamin D contains 10,000 units of vitamin D per gram. The childhood and adult daily requirement is about 400 units. Supplemental calcium administration is particularly important in the diet of premature infants and, in the treatment of rickets, may be necessary to control or prevent hypocalcemic tetany. Prophylactic doses in the ordinary ranges have been reported to produce hypercalcemia of infancy in special cases, and the total intake of vitamin D from all sources is considered to be a feature requiring attention. Instances of marked variability in sensitivity are not uncommon.

Calcitriol (Rocaltrol) occurs naturally in humans and is synthetically manufactured for oral administration. The two known sites of action of this active form of vitamin D_3 are intestine and bone. Additional evidence suggests that it also acts on the kidney and the parathyroid gland. It is indicated in the management of hypocalcemia in patients undergoing chronic renal dialysis.

Vitamin E (the tocopheroles). This vitamin exhibits an antioxidant action and is an essential nutrient apparently having a role in heme synthesis. Clinical vitamin E-responsive states include macrocytic megaloblastic anemia in some children with severe protein-calorie deficiency, hemolytic anemia in premature infants and autohemolysis of red blood cells in vitro from patients with genetic low-density lipoprotein deficiency.

Vitamin B Complex. As a matter of historic development, this term was applied to the water-soluble vitamins, excluding ascorbic acid. Individual members of the group now are identified more with specific therapies rather than by their similarity in regard to this minor feature. The roles of cyanocobalamin (B_{12}) and the folic acid group in anemias; of nicotinic acid compounds as blood cholesterol-lowering agents, and of the now superseded use of para-aminobenzoic acid in typhus and Rocky Mountain spotted fever are examples. Several of the water-soluble vitamins, such as folic acid, nicotinic acid, pyridoxine, riboflavin and thiamine, are readily available as synthetic manufactured products, and these can be administered now in precise dosages in dietary deficiencies.

Thiamine (vitamin B_1) was synthesized in 1936. Shortly thereafter, at a time when there were thousands of cases of beriberi in the Orient and South America, it was manufactured on a large scale. Food-enrichment programs have all but eliminated beriberi in many parts of the world where it was once a serious problem; nevertheless, there is frequent reappearance of this condition, and this sometimes is associated with overrefinement of foods. Usual daily requirements are 1 or 2 mg., based on age, relative carbohydrate consumption and factors such as febrile states, muscular activity and pregnancy that exhaust thiamine stores.

Thiamine is converted to its diphosphate in the body, and this acts as the coenzyme of pyruvate decarboxylase, transketolase and, presumably, other enzymes of general metabolism. Monophosphate and triphosphate esters also occur in the body. Antimetabolites that block the actions of thiamine are oxythiamine, neopyrithiamine and thiochrome. Thiamine is virtually without pharmacodynamic effects in doses that are usual in therapy. Daily doses of 500 mg. have been administered for weeks without distinctive toxic effects, although sensitivity reactions have occurred. In some manner, thiamine is necessary to the functional integrity of peripheral nerves and has had therapeutic trial in a great variety of neuropathies other than beriberi. Evidence now available indicates that thiamine deficiency is the cause of Wernicke-Korsakoff syndrome. Usually the conditions in which the best results are obtained are those that involve thiamine deficiency, as in the case of chronic alcoholism. There have been many studies of this nature, particularly in the period about 1955, and equally numerous studies have centered on various metabolic disorders, again with little clear definition of specific benefits.

Riboflavin (vitamin B_2) is an essential component of coenzymes involved in the removal of hydrogen from metabolites. It was first isolated from milk; it was synthesized in 1936 and is manufactured commercially in large quantities. A synthetic analog containing two chlorine atoms in place of two methyl groups is antagonistic. Usual daily maintenance doses are the same as with thiamine (1 to 2 mg.), while doses of 5 to 15 mg. are given in riboflavin deficiency.

Pyridoxine (pyridoxine HCl, vitamin B₆) occurs as pyridoxal, pyridoxine and pyridoxamine, which have the common structure of a substituted pyridine ring with, respectively, aldehyde, alcohol and amine attachments. Deficiencies result in convulsive seizures; this has occurred particularly in infants and in patients receiving isoniazid. A rare syndrome has been described, namely, a pyridoxine-responsive anemia that handles tryptophan abnormally in the same manner as develops during pregnancy. The vitamin is indicated for the prevention or treatment of peripheral neuritis caused by administration of certain drugs (e.g. isoniazid, penicillamine, hydralazine). It interferes with the beneficial effects of levodopa.

Nicotinic acid (niacin) and nicotinamide are specifics in the treatment of pellagra but are without effect on the polyneuritis of this condition, which usually is treated with thiamine. In 1956 it was reported that large doses of nicotinic acid (but not nicotinamide) effectively reduced elevated serum cholesterol levels, particularly in the beta-lipoprotein fraction. In view of the evidence of a relationship between elevated cholesterol levels and coronary artery disease, this has been used in therapy. Nicotinic acid in doses of 3 to 6 g. has been administered orally daily over prolonged periods, with apparent inhibition of synthesis of cholesterol and fatty acids at the acetate level and with an enhancement of oxidation of cholesterol. Changes in hepatic function and uric acid metabolism occur, limiting its usefulness. An acute effect that occurs frequently is similar to the effect of histamine release and includes flushing, pruritus and nervousness. Since histamine blood levels are not increased, this explanation is based on the assumption of a localized site of release. The effect is reduced substantially by the use of a preparation of aluminum nicotinate (Nicalex).

Other compounds that usually are considered to be components of the water-soluble vitamin B complex are pantothenic acid, biotin, inositol, choline and para-aminobenzoic acid.

Ascorbic Acid (vitamin C). This is a lactone of hexuronic acid; it is essential for many physiologic functions, among them collagen formation, a function that ceases in severe scurvy. It is heat stable but susceptible to oxidation. Normal adult daily requirement is about 30 mg., and doses up to 1,000 mg. are used in treatment of scurvy. Evidence to support claims that massive doses are effective in preventing and aborting colds is unconvincing. Because ascorbic acid is not stored regularly in the body, replacement is indicated after diarrheal and febrile disorders and following severe burns. Because of its role in wound healing, severely traumatized patients may benefit from its administration.

SPECIAL POISONINGS

Carbon monoxide is an agent to which exposure is exceptionally common, since it is a product of most forms of combustion as well as a constituent of artificial fuel gases. It combines with the hemoglobin of the blood, forming carboxyhemoglobin, which is incapable of carrying on the usual oxygen transport. When approximately 20 per cent of the blood pigment is thus combined, the subject experiences headache and "dizziness"; with 40 per cent combined, there is collapse; with 60 per cent, coma; higher proportions of combined pigment are likely to be fatal. The dissociation pressures of the remaining oxyhemoglobin are less than normal under these conditions. Carboxyhemoglobin is a red pigment, and cherry-red flushing of the skin may be a helpful diagnostic point. Large skin blisters may occur. This combination of monoxide and hemoglobin is subject to dissociation, but at a slow rate, since the affinity of monoxide for hemoglobin is 200 to 300 times greater than the affinity of oxygen for hemoglobin. Exposure to a monoxide concentration of 0.1 per cent can be fatal in about 2 hours. Treatment consists of artificial respiration and oxygen administration with or without carbon dioxide. Transfusions might be helpful but usually cannot be carried out during the critical period. The same might be said for the use of hyperbaric oxygen.

Cyanides and **hydrocyanic acid** represent a special danger because of their use in industries and fumigation procedures. They are also encountered as suicidal poisons. Cyanides directly inhibit the respiratory mechanism of the tissue cells by a highly sensitive inactivation of the cytochrome oxidase system. Hyperpnea is pronounced, apparently owing to histotoxic anoxia in the thoracic chemoreceptors. The convulsions, probably anoxic in character, are followed by respiratory failure. Experimental poisoning, even up to 20 lethal doses, can be antagonized effectively by intravenous injection of sodium nitrite and sodium thiosulfate. This combination has been used effectively in human cases. Methylene blue is less effective but may be more readily available in an emergency. Thiosulfate supplies excess sulfur for the conversion of —CN to the relatively nontoxic —CNS. Methemoglobin, by virtue of exceptional affinity for —CN, diverts the —CN from its intracellular complex with cytochrome oxidase.

Methemoglobin is formed by the action of certain

inorganic substances (chlorates, nitrites), aniline dyes and some of the common drugs that are aniline derivatives, such as acetanilid and sulfanilamide. It is a converted form of hemoglobin that is incapable of transferring oxygen. Ferrous hemoglobin iron is converted to the ferric state. A characteristic chocolate-brown color is readily recognizable in drawn samples of blood that contain substantial quantities of the pigment; it is responsible for the characteristic cyanosis noted, particularly in the lips and the oral mucosa and under the nail beds. The severity of the symptoms increases with the proportion of methemoglobin in the total blood pigment and, as with carboxyhemoglobin, may have a fatal result when greater than 60 per cent. Since blood P_{O_2} is not substantially decreased, respiration is not stimulated.

Susceptibility to methemoglobin formation is increased in newborn and premature infants. In adults, susceptibility follows genetic trends and is associated with deficiency of enzymes such as glucose-6-phosphate dehydrogenase. Normally, reduction by methemoglobin diaphorase maintains the physiologic relations of hemoglobin and methemoglobin.

Methemoglobin is partially eliminated in the urine and partially reconverted to normal hemoglobin over the course of several hours. Red cells are hemolyzed. Chronic methemoglobinemia is associated with anemia. Treatment of the acute poisoning consists of oxygen administration and methylene blue (1 to 2 mg. per g. intravenously or 10 times this amount orally).

Kerosene poisoning is chiefly a problem of pneumonitis due to aspiration. Therefore, vomiting should not be induced, and gastric lavage must be carried out with extreme caution. There is evidence also that kerosene produces pulmonary inflammation by virtue of transport through the bloodstream from the alimentary canal. Turpentine has about the same effects, with a more conspicuous degree of kidney inflammation and urinary suppression.

Boron hydrides such as pentaborane and decaborane have been responsible for acute and chronic toxicities. Mild symptoms resemble those of the common respiratory infections and allergies. In more severe cases, muscle spasms convulsions disorientation and coma develop, frequently after a latent period of several hours. Liver tenderness and abnormal liver function tests may continue for some time.

Lead is widely distributed and offers numerous possibilities of chronic exposure. Toxic effects may be obtained after ingestion of a few milligrams daily over several weeks. The most rapidly dangerous route of entry is through the respiratory tract (inhalation of dusts and of the volatile tetraethyl lead), although poisoning also results from oral ingestion and through absorption of organic compounds through the skin.

Lead resembles calcium in the manner of its circulation in the bloodstream and ultimate deposition in the long bones. A greater amount is excreted in the stools than in the urine. Signs and symptoms include: stippling of red cells, reticulocytosis, anemia, pallor, lead line on the margin of teeth and gums, neuritis, colic and encephalopathy. X-ray density at the epiphyseal line is diagnostic in infants. Infants more commonly exhibit cerebral and meningeal symptoms.

In the treatment of chronic lead poisoning the most effective efforts are those directed at finding and eliminating sources of lead intake.

The elimination of stored lead can be significantly hastened by use of the chelating agent calcium disodium salt of ethylenediamine tetraacetic acid (EDTA, Versene, Sequestrene). This product forms a soluble nonionized compound with the circulating lead, and this, in turn, is excreted in the urine in relatively high concentrations. Though not considered routine, dimercaprol (BAL) (British Antilewisite) may be added to the regimen in order to further facilitate excretion.

Another effective chelating agent is penicillamine (dimethyl cysteine), which is capable of removing copper as well as lead. This feature has led to its use in hepatolenticular degeneration for which it is approved by the FDA. It is effective orally. Individuals sensitive to penicillin respond similarly to penicillamine.

Mercury in soluble ionized form is intensely corrosive, and after absorption it has conspicuous toxic effects in the kidney tubules. Mercuric chloride (corrosive sublimate) is the most common form that results in acute poisoning. Usually it is ingested orally, but it may also act through vaginal absorption. The episode is characterized by two stages: the first of chemical trauma due to corrosive action in the alimentary canal, and the second (a later effect) due to damage of the kidney tubules and to colitis. Anuria, acidosis and shock may be seen in fatal cases.

Treatment consists of stomach lavage, proteins as local protection, and parenteral fluids. Surgical efforts have included cecostomy with colon lavage and kidney decapsulation. Sodium formaldehyde sulfoxylate has specific detoxifying action, but the usual poisoning case is seen too late for it to be of much value. The same is true for BAL (British antilewisite, dimercaptopropanol). BAL, being a dithiol, competes with cellular SH (sulfhydryl groups) for those heavy metals that combine with and block the function of these essential cellular agents. Gold and antimony poisonings, for instance, also are influenced favorably by the use of BAL. D-Penicillamine counteracts the lethal effects of mercuric chloride.

Arsenic in simple inorganic form has been a frequent cause of accidental and suicidal poisonings. Acute poisoning may result from ingestion of as little as 100 mg. of arsenic trioxide (white arsenic). It is characterized by gastrointestinal disturbances, usually with severe vomiting and diarrhea. The chief systemic action is capillary dilation, most marked in the splanchnic area. Symptomatic treatment is directed toward replacement of fluids and salt. BAL may prevent further systemic action of the arsenic. The encephalitis and the dermatitis of organic arsenicals have responded favorably to administration of BAL. They symptoms of acute and chronic antimony poisoning are similar to those of arsenical poisoning.

Beryllium. Chronic beryllium poisoning was once of special interest, largely because of its incidence in the early days of the fluorescent-lamp industry. Presently it is used in alloys, atomic energy technology and in ceramics. Skin granulomas may develop following direct contact. Small amounts of inhaled beryllium produce nodular and diffuse granulomas, replacing lung parenchyma. Symptoms of weakness, dyspnea, cough and weight loss may develop at considerable intervals following exposure. Polycythemia has been reported. Administration of prednisone, in some instances, has resulted in measurable improvement.

Cigarette Smoking. The toxic exposures of the cigarette smoker include particularly nicotine, carbon monoxide, tars containing known carcinogenic hydrocarbons, pesticides and polonium 210 (^{210}Po); the last-mentioned emits alpha particles and is volatile at temperatures below that of a burning cigarette. Concern over these health hazards has been emphasized by the report of the advisory committee to the Surgeon General of the Public Health Service. Conclusions were that cigarette smoking is causally related to lung cancer in men, is a significant factor in the incidence of cancer of the larynx and may be related to cancer of the mouth, the esophagus and the urinary bladder. It is considered to be the most important cause of chronic bronchitis in the United States and to have a causative relation to pulmonary emphysema. Mortality figures from these nonneoplastic conditions are significantly greater among cigarette smokers than among nonsmokers. Graded epithelial changes have been observed in the tracheobronchial tree in approximate dose-response relationships to cigarette smoking. These changes include loss of cilia, basal cell hyperplasia and atypical cells with hyperchromatic nuclei; bronchial glands also exhibit hyperplastic changes. Women who smoked during pregnancy have been reported to have babies with smaller birth weights. Smoking is also associated with an increased incidence of peptic ulcer and myocardial infarction.

Radiation Exposures. Doses of the order of 50,000 rads at high dose rates are followed by immediate injury and death, presumably as the result of damage to the central nervous system; exposure to about 1,000 rads leads to death in several days, owing to loss of the gut epithelium; total body irradiation with several hundred rads is followed by profound effects on the hematopoietic system, with death in 2 to 4 weeks; smaller doses of 100 rads or less may produce only equivocal acute symptomatology and may have long-term effects such as cataracts, decreased life span or increased incidence of degenerative disease, and tumors, long after the initial radiation insult. It has been estimated that the dosage requirement for equivalent shortening of life is about five times as great for chronic as for acute irradiation.

The testing of nuclear weapons has fastened interest on radiation exposures of population groups, with intensive monitoring in various parts of the world. The predominant longlived nuclide from fusion reactions is tritium; from fission reactions, ^{90}Sr. ^{90}Sr and ^{137}Cs appear in plants through uptake from soil, usually at depths greater than several inches below the surface. The fallout behavior of ^{131}I differs because of the short half life and usually is related to rain and the surface area of plants; transfer of ^{131}I to man occurs principally through milk.

Protection against radiation injury is difficult to achieve, although some limited degree of success has been obtained with —SH-containing compounds (e.g., mercapto-ethylamine and cysteine). They must be given in nearly toxic amounts to be effective. Since the free radicals formed on irradiation of water are mainly oxidants, it follows that reducing substances administered prior to exposure may be expected to confer some protection. Hypoxia by diverse means is a mechanism for achieving protection against radiation injury, and chemical agents, generally, show a correlation of these two features; presumably intracellular oxygen tensions are the critical factor.

RODENTICIDES AND INSECTICIDES

Chemicals of this group have been made increasingly effective, and the consequent greater use has increased the hazards of public exposure to these agents.

Rat Poisons. *Red Squill* is one of the oldest and most common rodenticides. It contains cardiac glycosides (scillaren) and other glycosides. It produces alternating convulsions and paralysis in rats. Household pets and man usually vomit the poison before a lethal dose is absorbed.

Sodium fluoroacetate (1080) is volatile and stable and can be absorbed through the skin in toxic amounts. It is used only by specially trained commercial exterminators. The mechanism of death is by ventricular fibrillation.

Alpha-naphthol-thiourea (ANTU) stimulates powerfully the flow of lymph and kills by massive pulmonary edema and pleural effusion.

Warfarin, a coumarin derivative resembling Dicumarol in its chemical and anticoagulant properties, is effective as a rodenticide because of its extreme potency. Concentrations of 0.025 per cent in cornmeal bait produce fatal cumulative effects in Norway rats after small amounts are ingested over 3 to 4 days. Vitamin K is considered to be an effective antidote.

Insecticides. *Pyrethrum* is a mixture of esters from a plant source. It is effective as a "knockdown" agent but not as a killer. It is a central nervous system stimulant. Oral ingestion by man results in hydrolysis of the esters to inactive compounds, which gives it a wide margin of safety. However, its allergenic properties are marked in comparison with other insecticides.

Rotenone is a crystalline neutral principle from the derris root. It causes death in mammals through convulsions and respiratory depression.

Some *chlorinated hydrocarbons* are unusually effective against a considerable variety of infestations. Usually they are applied in kerosene solution and, when ingested accidentally, the symptoms of poisoning may be those of kerosene. Chlorophenothane (DDT) is a central nervous stimulant and sensitizes the heart to fibrillation. Chronic poisoning is characterized by nervous system symptoms and severe liver damage. DDD, TDE and Methoxychlor are similar. Isomers of benzene hexachloride are extremely potent; the gamma form (gammexane, lindane) is the most potent. Its toxic effects are stimulant in character, whereas the beta and the delta isomers are depressant to the central nervous system. Chlorinated camphene (Toxaphene) produces reflex excitability and convulsions; barbiturates are effective with antidote. Chlordane, a chlorinated indane derivative, has action similar to DDT with greater skin absorbability and greater incidence of chronic toxicity. Dieldrin and aldrin also are chlorinated hydrocarbons related in action and uses to chlordane and toxaphene.

The chlorinated hydrocarbons cumulate tenaciously in body fat, but their excretion rate increases as the level of body concentration increases, and mass surveys indicate a relatively stabilized uniform concentration. Gas-liquid chromatography methods have provided means of recognizing the considerable degree of body conversion of DDT to DDE (dichlorodiphenyl dichloroethylene), as well as the identification of stored traces of related compounds.

The organic phosphate insecticides were developed first in Germany and are used principally as contact poisons for insects infesting crops. The common representatives are hexaethyl tetraphosphate (HETP), tetraethyl pyrophosphate (TEPP), and diethyl nitrophenyl thiophosphate (Parathion), all of which are incorporated into various trade-name insecticides. HETP and TEPP hydrolyze rapidly to form nontoxic compounds in the presence of water and accordingly do not usually leave dangerous residues. Ordinarily they do not produce cumulative toxic effects in man. Parathion, on the other hand, is more stable and also is more liable to develop cumulative poisoning in those chronically exposed. TEPP is acutely two or three times more toxic than HETP and is several times more toxic than nicotine.

Less toxic variants are Malathione, Dipterex and Diazinon. All of this group inhibit cholinesterase, and symptoms are parasympathomimetic. Atropine, accordingly, is the specific antidote and is frequently given to the point of typical atropine excitation; this latter can be controlled by the cautious use of barbiturates. Since atropine is only moderately effective against the central respiratory depressant action of these organic phosphates, artificial respiration can be a critical necessity. Reactivation of cholinesterase can be accomplished by pralidoxime (PAM), which unites with the organic phosphorus compound to break the enzyme-phosphorus bond. There have been numerous deaths among farming personnel, due to inhalation or skin absorption of these compounds. Presently expanding use of these pesticides because of the ban on DDT makes this a matter of increasing concern.

These organic phosphorus insecticides are related to the "GB nerve gas" or Sarin, which is a phosphonofluoridate. Minute quantities of this compound cause marked and prolonged inhibition of cholinesterase.

QUESTIONS IN PHARMACOLOGY

REVIEW QUESTIONS

Give some points of distinction between generic and proprietary drug names.

What governmental agencies are concerned with drug regulations and what is their degree of authority?

What information must be included in all prescriptions for controlled substances?

What types of information can be derived from dose-response curves?

What forces commonly determine the attachment of drugs to their receptors?

What mechanism is commonly involved in potentiation between drugs?

Give one practical therapeutic example of potentiative drug action.

List typical effects of acetylcholine and indicate the

manner in which the action of pilocarpine, physostigmine, and neostigmine differs from that of acetylcholine.

Explain the marked stimulation of the isolated perfused heart that occurs after successive administration of atropine and acetylcholine.

List acceptable therapeutic uses for drugs of the parasympathomimetic group.

Discuss the use of anticholinesterases in the management of glaucoma.

Discuss the role of cholinesterase reactivators in the treatment of poisoning by organophosphate insecticides.

Define the basic action of atropine and list individual effects.

List four common disturbing side effects associated with the use of cholinergic blocking agents in the treatment of peptic ulcer.

Discuss the mechanism of action of the various drugs used in the management of parkinsonism.

Which two enzymes have been considered primarily as hastening the metabolic inactivation of epinephrine?

List various effects produced by epinephrine when used in the treatment of bronchial asthma.

Contrast the effects of epinephrine and ephedrine.

List some of the therapeutic uses of ephedrine and name three other drugs of the same general type.

Contrast the actions of epinephrine, norepinephrine and isopropyl arterenol.

Name two of the sympathomimetic pressor drugs that have a marked positive inotropic effect. Name two in which this characteristic is not pronounced.

Discuss the use of ergotamine in the treatment of migraine.

Indicate the practial applications of ganglionic blocking agents and name two in common use.

Discuss the clinical applications of beta-adrenergic blocking agents.

Which adrenergic amines act directly on receptors and which act secondarily through release of norepinephrine?

Which adrenergic amines are predominantly pressor and which are pressor-inotropic? Indicate where this may be critically important.

Outline a scheme illustrating the circulatory effects of alpha and beta-adrenergic blocking agents.

Discuss the relationship between certain antihypertensive drugs and central adrenergic control mechanisms.

Discuss the actions and uses of dopamine.

Give some of the acute effects and mechanism of action of nicotine and of curare.

Outline briefly the development of the curare compounds now being used.

Discuss the difference in tubocurarine and decamethonium with respect to blocking actions produced by agents such as neostigmine or edrophonium.

What drugs act synergistically with d-tubocurarine?

What are the important differences between pancuronium and d-tubocurarine?

Outline the sequential steps of digitaloids at the cellular level, including inhibition to membrane ATPase and calcium effects on myofibrils.

Explain the hemodynamic mechanism of digitalis action when given in the condition of congestive heart failure with normal rhythm. Include both cardiac and systemic effects.

Outline the progressive development of digitalis intoxication, including the associated ECG changes.

Discuss the relative value of digitalis in different heart conditions.

Discuss dosage schemes with digitalis, meaning of the USP "digitalis unit," and various available preparations with a similar action.

Contrast the cardiac effects of digitalis and of quinidine in the treatment of atrial fibrillation.

Interpret digitalis-produced ventricular automaticity in terms of depolarization of Purkinje cells.

Discuss the use of potassium salts in antagonizing digitalis arrhythmias.

What are the hazards of parenteral quinidine or diphenylhydantoin when used to antagonize digitalis arrhythmias?

Discuss the role of bretylium, disopyramide, and propranolol as antiarrhythmic agents.

Discuss the uses of nitroglycerin, its mechanism of action and its toxic effects.

Discuss the role of captopril in the treatment of congestive heart failure.

Give mechanisms by which Veratrum alkaloids produce bradycardia and hypotension.

Discuss hydralazine with respect to mechanism of action and adverse effects.

Discuss the thiazides with respect to mechanisms of action and adverse effects.

What are the indications for the use of diazoxide?

Discuss clonidine with respect to mechanism of action and adverse effects.

Discuss methyldopa with respect to mechanism of action and adverse effects.

Discuss guanethidine with respect to mechanism of action and adverse effects.

Discuss the mechanism of action and indications for the use of nitroprusside.

What are the advantages of metoprolol over earlier beta-adrenergic blocking drugs?

Discuss prazosin with respect to mechanism of action and untoward effects.

Discuss the indications and the method of use of heparin and of bishydroxycoumarin.

Discuss the effect of heparin in clearing lipemia and indicate the possible value of this action.

Indicate the conditions of prothrombin deficiency in which vitamin K is most valuable. Give some details of its administration.

Discuss the basic mechanisms of action of heparin and bishydroxycoumarin.

What are some of the adverse reactions associated with the use of heparin?

Discuss aminocaproic acid with respect to actions, indications and possible untoward effects.

Name some of the postulated mechanisms explaining the basic action of general anesthetics.

Describe the microcrystalline hydrate theory of anesthesia.

Give several examples of the diverse chemical nature of substances that can produce anesthesia.

Outline the stages and the planes of anesthesia according to a generally accepted scheme.

Contrast advantages and disadvantages of ether, halothane and vinyl ether when used as general anesthetics.

Give some distinctive characteristics of anesthesia with nitrous oxide, with ethylene and with cyclopropane.

Compare the actions of halothane with some other highly halogenated anesthetic.

Give a list of the common inhalation anesthetics and designate which are flammable and which non-flammable.

What manifestations of sympathoadrenal activity occur during ether anesthesia?

What is the relation of ether anesthesia to the antidiuretic hormone of the pituitary?

Discuss the use of barbiturates as general anesthetics.

List some features of barbiturate addiction.

What is the effect of anesthetics on the reticular ascending system?

Discuss the factors determining the size and frequency of doses of iron salts in the treament of anemia.

Discuss the use of parenteral iron preparations.

Discuss the biochemical effects of vitamin B_{12} in pernicious anemia.

Contrast the action of folic acid and vitamin B_{12} in the treatment of pernicious anemia.

List the characteristics of acute intoxication with ethyl alcohol. Mention briefly the status of methyl alcohol and isopropyl alcohol in the same connection.

Describe the conditions of chronic alcoholism.

Name two typical tranquilizing drugs and contrast their actions with that of barbiturates.

Name four major toxic effects of phenothiazine tranquilizers.

Name three general types of drug action that are represented to some extent in the actions of phenothiazine tranquilizers.

Name two drugs that can be considered psychomotor stimulants and give a special characteristic of each.

What types of epilepsy respond to carbamazepine? What are its adverse effects?

Contrast the clinical and the laboratory spectrum of activity of two drugs used commonly in the management of epileptic conditions.

A patient receiving antiepileptic drugs may show one of the following toxic effects. Indicate in each case which drug is the most probably causative agent: gingival hyperplasia, photosensivity, hirsutism, acneform eruptions, drowsiness.

What is the proposed mechanism of action of valproic acid?

What influence does it have on serum levels of phenobarbital?

Give characteristic toxic effects of salicylates, acetophenetidin and phenylbutazone.

List possible mechanisms by which salicylates can act in rheumatic fever.

What is the effect of combining orally administered sodium bicarbonate with sodium salicylate?

List typical actions of morphine in therapeutic doses. When possible, suggest a mechanism of action.

What are the special characteristics and the uses of methadone?

Give comparable therapeutic doses and some points of distinction among morphine, codeine, dihydromorphinone and meperidine.

Give some of the features of morphine addiction.

Describe the mechanism by which N-allylnormorphine antagonizes the action of morphine.

Distinguish between the types of depressants that are antagonized by N-allyl-normorphine and those that it does not antagonize.

Cite the advantages of naloxone over the older narcotic antagonists.

Discuss the uses of central nervous system stimulants.

Name two drugs that can be considered psychomotor stimulants and give a special characteristic of each.

Define the action of strychnine on the Renshaw cells.

Discuss the role of sodium and calcium in the present theory of the mechanism of local anesthetics.

Give the advantages of lidocaine as a substiute for procaine.

Discuss toxic effects of local anesthetics, their prophylaxis and treatment.

List advantages and disadvantages of spinal anesthesia.

Characterize briefly epidural anesthesia, continuous caudal anesthesia and sympathetic block.

What is the theory of action of antihistamine compounds?

Name two typical antihistaminic drugs and state the typical toxic effects characteristic of this group.

Discuss the role of cimetidine in the treatment of duodenal ulcer.

Differentiate renal mechanisms of action of mercurial diuretics, carbonic anhydrase inhibitors and thiazides.

Characterize the mechanism of the diuretic action of ethacrynic acid and indicate its special type of hazard.

Name two diuretics likely to produce a potassium deficit and indicate by what two different means it can be prevented.

Characterize briefly and give examples of three different types of hallucinogens.

What are some potential medical applications for marijuana and synthetic cannabinoids?

Briefly give characteristics and plan of treatment for acute poisoning with: (1) carbon monoxide, (2) cyanides, (3) sodium nitrite, (4) mercuric chloride, (5) arsenic trioxide.

Discuss the chemical variants of cortisone that are useful clinically.

Discuss the use of cortisone and ACTH in treatment of the leukemias and malignant lymphomas.

When a patient has been receiving cortisone regulary and is to undergo surgery, what is a recommended procedure for continued cortisone dosage?

Discuss undesirable side effects associated with prolonged administration of glucocorticoids.

List contraindications to the use of glucocorticoids.

Discuss cosyntropin as a diagnostic drug in suspected adrenal insufficiency.

Discuss vasopressin with respect to usage and mechanism of action.

Which hormones with potent circulatory effects are present normally in the adrenal medulla?

Explain why small amounts of regular insulin will not act with usual rapidity when mixed with protamine zinc insulin.

What is the mechanism by which the sulfonamide type of oral hypoglycemic compounds reduces blood sugar?

What fundamental action is involved in the reduction of blood sugar by insulin?

Identify insulins of short, intermediate, and long duration of action.

Discuss the mechanism of action of oral contraceptives.

What are the uses of dinoprost?

Discuss the uses of estrogens.

Discuss adverse effects of androgens.

Name two orally administered thyroid preparations given in much smaller dose than thyroid USP.

Indicate the mechanism by which the following agents reduce the manifestations of hyperthyroidism: potassium iodide, propylthiouracil, radioactive iodine.

List some of the types of preparations used in the treatment of pernicious anemia.

Contrast the action of folic acid and vitamin B_{12} in the treatment of pernicious anemia.

List a number of types of chemicals used as external antiseptics; give a specific example of each type.

Differentiate and give examples of anionic and cationic surface-active antiseptics.

What conditions are effectively treated with griseofulvin?

Mention some of the common urinary antiseptics, omitting the sulfonamides and the antibiotics; give a distinguishing characteristic of each.

Discuss the mechanisms and the general principles of the antibacterial action of sulfonamides.

Outline important points regarding the absorption, distribution, conjugation and excretion of sulfonamides.

Indicate some of the conditions in which sulfonamides have proved to be most valuable, mentioning both systemic and local infections.

Differentiate the mechanism of antibacterial action of penicillin and streptomycin.

Give briefly methods of administration and standardization and fields of usefulness of penicillin.

Compare the spectrum of activity of penicillin with that of streptomycin.

Discuss the development of bacterial resistance to antibiotics.

Discuss additive and potentiating actions by antibiotics.

Discuss the use of broad-spectrum antibiotics in treatment of the rickettsioses.

Which types of viral infections can be expected to respond favorably to chemotherapy?

List and discuss briefly drugs that have tuberculostatic effects.

Discuss the uses and side effects of rifampin.

Outline a scheme of treatment for acute amebiasis. Indicate the toxic potentialities of each drug used.

Which hormone has been useful in reducing the intensity of Herxheimer reactions occurring during penicillin treatment of syphilis?

In what instances have effective antiviral agents been used?

Which laboratory procedures are used most in screening compounds for potential value as viricidal agents?

Contrast the actions of nitrogen mustards with x-ray effects.

Name the four organ systems that are conspicuously sensitive to folic acid antagonists. Indicate the relative order of sensitivity.

Which agent can be used to protect against the toxic action of folic acid antimetabolites?

Which laboratory procedures are used in screening compounds for potential value in the restraint of malignant disease?

Discuss the role of cisplatin in cancer chemotherapy.

Which drugs are special tetatogenic hazards and at what stage of pregnancy are they most critical?

Indicate the relative doses of radioacitve iodine (^{131}I) used in diagnosis of thyroid conditions, treatment of hyperthyroidism and treatment of malignant disease of the thyroid.

Give examples of effective use of radioisotopes in diagnostic scanning procedures.

Briefly discuss radiation exposures from the fallout of nuclear explosion tests.

Indicate some of the uses of radioactive phosphorus (^{32}P).

Indicate some diagnostic and therapeutic uses of radioactive cobalt (^{57}Co).

Name two conditions in which radioisotope therapy may be sufficiently intense to represent a hazard to personnel attending the patient.

Give an acceptable scheme of treatment for hookworm infestation. Indicate possible toxic effects from the drug used. Give similar information for roundworm, tapeworm, pinworm.

Give an acceptable scheme of treatment of acute symptoms of vivax malaria and also a schedule for suppressive (prophylactic) treatment.

Do the same for chloroquine-resistant falciparum malaria.

Name a currently favored antimalarial drug that is effective against *Plasmodium vivax* (1) when in the asexual, erythrocytic form, (2) when persisting in the tissues and (3) when in the sexual (gametocyte) form.

Indicate the reasons for special value of a combination of sulfonamides and folic acid antimetabolities in malaria treatment.

Outline the conditions for which oxygen is administered, indicating the relative value of oxygen in each case.

Discuss the mechanism by which oxygen may cause apnea in severe barbiturate depression.

Discuss various techniques of oxygen administration.

Give the basis for the use of carbon dioxide and some estimates of its indications and value.

What are the special characteristics of helium and in what conditions is it useful?

Define the following, giving a common use and example of each: demulcents, emollients, ointments, dusting powders, counterirritants, astringents, corrosives.

Discuss the treatment following contact with strong acids and alkalies.

Briefly give dose and indicate mechanism for the cathartic action of phenolphthalein, magnesium sulfate, mineral oil, dioctyl sodium sulfosuccinate.

List some undesirable features attending the use of cathartics in general and list some particular toxic effects associated with two commonly used cathartics.

Name and give dose of two drugs used as emetics that act through stomach irritation and one that acts by direct stimulation of the emetic center. List some measures used to counteract vomiting.

Name two synthetic drugs that are clinically useful in stimulating uterine contractions.

Give some characteristic side effects of ergot and of posterior pituitary. Name some of the preparations of each that are used in obstetrics.

Indicate possible explanation for the occurrence of retroperitoneal fibrosis following the continued use of ergot products.

Discuss the indications for the use of oxytocics in obstetrics.

Give some of the hazards involved in the use of oxytocin by intravenous infusion in the first and the second stages of labor.

Discuss the use and hazards of prostaglandins in obstetric practice.

Discuss the actions and uses of angiotensin.

What toxic effects are associated with excessive doses of vitamin A?

How does vitamin D correct the defective bone formation of rickets?

What are some conditions responsive to therapy with vitamin E?

What are some indications for the use of large doses of vitamin C?

Briefly give characteristics and plan of treatment for chronic poisoning with lead compounds.

Discuss the action of chelating agents in lead poisioning.

What are some of the more common types of insecticides and rodenticides?

Give the basic steps in treating poisoning with insecticides of the organic phosphate, anticholinesterase type.

MULTIPLE CHOICE QUESTIONS

Select *one* best answer. Answers are listed at the end of this chapter.

1. Which compound would be most ionized in pH 5 urine?
   (a) acid drug, pKa 5.0
   (b) basic drug, pKa 5.0
   (c) acid drug, pKa 3.0
   (d) basic drug, pKa 8.0

2. A patient is established on a dosage regimen of drug X which is highly bound to plasma proteins. Beginning concurrent therapy with drug Y which is also highly bound might be expected to result in:
   (a) a need for increased dosage of X
   (b) an excessive effect from the regular dose of X
   (c) a need for a higher than normal dose of Y
   (d) no interaction expected

3. Coadministration of a drug metabolizing enzyme inducing drug would require what change in dosage of a chronically used medication?
   (a) a possible increase in dose
   (b) a possible decrease in dose
   (c) no change unless both drugs were acids or both were bases
   (d) no change unless the drugs were congeners

4. A weakly basic drug of pKa 6.4 is present in plasma:
   (a) more than half ionized
   (b) less than half ionized
   (c) half ionized
   (d) more than 99 per cent ionized
   (e) more than 99 per cent nonionized

5. Urinary excretion of probenecid (a carboxylic acid drug) could be enhanced by administration of:
   (a) penicillin
   (b) sodium bicarbonate
   (c) ammonium chloride
   (d) a cathartic
   (e) charcoal

6. Atropine, an organic base of pKa 9.6, would be *most* ionized in:
   (a) pH 8 urine
   (b) pH 8 intestinal contents
   (c) pH 5 urine
   (d) pH 1 stomach contents

7. Which tissue would be the slowest to *equilibrate* with a drug in the blood?
   (a) brain
   (b) liver
   (c) muscle
   (d) fat

8. Drug-receptor interactions typically initiate a sequence of events which culminates in a biological response to the drug. The first event in the sequence is probably:
   (a) dissociation of the drug from the receptor
   (b) denaturation of the receptor by the drug
   (c) alteration in the shape of the receptor by the drug
   (d) transfer of the drug to a second receptor
   (e) inhibition of protein synthesis by the drug

9. The major mechanism for inactivation of neurotransmitter released at postganglionic parasympathetic neuroeffector junctions:
   (a) enzymatic degradation by monoamine oxidase
   (b) reuptake into nerve ending
   (c) enzymatic degradation by catechol-o-methyl transferase
   (d) enzymatic degradation by acetylcholinesterase

10. Released during nerve stimulation from nerve endings by the process of exocytosis:
    (a) norepinephrine
    (b) acetylcholine
    (c) both
    (d) neither

11. The long duration of action of diisopropyl fluorophosphate and echothiophate is due to their ability to:
    (a) combine irreversibly with acetylcholine receptors
    (b) inhibit the synthesis of acetylcholinesterase enzyme
    (c) inhibit acetylcholine synthesis
    (d) form extremely stable covalent bonds with the active site of acetylcholinesterase enzyme

12. The single most important agent in the drug management of organophosphate poisoning is:
    (a) pralidoxime
    (b) pilocarpine
    (c) atropine
    (d) succinylcholine

13. Which of the following agents acts by promoting reactivation of phosphorylated acetylcholinesterase?
    (a) pralidoxime
    (b) atropine

(c) pilocarpine

(d) neostigmine

14. The clinical use of neostigmine to antagonize d-tubocurarine is generally preceded by atropine in order to:

    (a) minimize fasciculations of skeletal muscle

    (b) block the muscarinic effects of d-tubocurarine

    (c) minimize the central nervous system effects of neostigmine

    (d) minimize muscarinic effects of neostigmine

15. Atropine poisoning would be best antagonized by:

    (a) pralidoxime

    (b) neostigmine

    (c) cyclopentolate HCl

    (d) physostigmine

16. A patient undergoing surgery for a pheochromocytoma suddenly spikes a dangerously high blood pressure. Which one of the following drugs should be administered to lower the pressure?

    (a) phenoxybenzamine

    (b) propranolol

    (c) atropine

    (d) phentolamine

17. Which one of the following drugs maintains renal blood flow best during the therapy of shock?

    (a) dopamine

    (b) norepinephrine

    (c) isoproterenol

    (d) epinephrine

18. Epinephrine reversal is due to the fact that phentolamine blocks:

    (a) both the alpha and beta effects of epinephrine

    (b) the alpha effects of eprinephrine but not the beta

    (c) the beta effects of epinephrine but not the alpha

19. The drug of choice in acute anaphylactic shock is:

    (a) diphenhydramine

    (b) cortisone

    (c) epinephrine

    (d) isoproterenol

20. Stimulation of alpha-adrenergic receptors in the medullary area of the brain:

    (a) will produce vasoconstriction and bradycardia

    (b) will produce an elevation of blood pressure and a tachycardia

    (c) will produce a decrease in blood pressure and a bradycardia

    (d) will produce a vasodilatation and a tachycardia

    (e) none of the above

21. Which one of the following drugs would be most useful in the management of hypertension due to pheochromocytoma?

    (a) alpha methyldopa

    (b) propranolol

    (c) phenoxybenzamine

    (d) isoproterenol

22. Epinephrine is efficacious in:

    (a) prolonging the duration of local anesthetics

    (b) reducing localized bleeding

    (c) bronchial asthma

    (d) (a) and (c) only

    (e) all of the above

23. The drug of choice in treating severe anaphylactic shock due both to its vasoconstriction in restoring circulation and its relaxation of bronchial smooth muscle, is:

    (a) epinephrine

    (b) norepinephrine

    (c) isoproterenol

    (d) phenylephrine

24. Which one of the following drugs is contraindicated in bronchial asthma?

    (a) ephedrine

    (b) aminophylline

    (c) propranolol

    (d) isoproterenol

25. Bromocriptine is:

    (a) an alpha-adrenergic receptor agonist

    (b) a dopaminergic receptor agonist

    (c) a beta$_1$ adrenergic receptor agonist

    (d) a beta$_2$ adrenergic receptor agonist

26. A dopadecarboxylase inhibitor used as an adjunct in the management of Parkinson's disease is:

    (a) carbidopa

    (b) gallamine

    (c) carbachol

    (d) deprenyl

27. A mydriatic that is sometimes used to treat open angle glaucoma is:

    (a) epinephrine

    (b) atropine

    (c) pilocarpine

    (d) propranolol

28. Dopamine administration to a patient in shock can cause:

    (a) renal vasodilation via dopaminergic receptors

    (b) generalized peripheral vasoconstriction via alpha-adrenergic receptors

    (c) greater increments in cardiac output than norepinephrine

    (d) the less likely appearance of cardiac arrhythmias than isoproterenol

    (e) all of the above

29. A hypertensive crisis after ingestion of certain cheeses by a patient under treatment with a monoamine oxidase inhibitor would be most logically treated with:
    (a) phentolamine
    (b) amphetamine
    (c) propranolol
    (d) intravenous monoamine oxidase

30. Which of the following inhibits the uptake and storage of norepinephrine by the storage vesicles?
    (a) desipramine (tricyclic antidepressant)
    (b) alpha-methyl-p-tyrosine
    (c) reserpine
    (d) none of the above

31. A drug which is contraindicated in bronchial asthma is:
    (a) phentolamine
    (b) salbutamol
    (c) propranolol
    (d) epinephrine

32. The advantages of metoprolol over propranolol include all of the following *except:*
    (a) less likely to provoke bronchoconstriction
    (b) more likely to be effective in sinus bradycardia
    (c) less likely to produce temporary rise in peripheral resistance at the start of therapy
    (d) less likely to produce sudden rises in blood pressure after physical exertion

33. Dobutamine:
    (a) is a potent vasoconstrictor
    (b) is indicated in idiopathic hypertropic subaortic stenosis
    (c) increases myocardial contractility by a direct action on beta$_1$ receptors
    (d) is frequently used during cyclopropane anesthesia

34. The selective beta$_2$ sympathomimetic drugs differ from epinephrine in all of the following *except:*
    (a) they are active when administered orally
    (b) they have a slower onset of action
    (c) they have a shorter duration of action
    (d) generally do not stimulate the myocardium directly

35. Timolol:
    (a) reduces intraocular pressure by a reduction in aqueous humor production
    (b) produces marked miosis
    (c) is contraindicated in combination with epinephrine
    (d) is similar in action to pilocarpine

36. Neuromuscular blocking effect may be enhanced by diethyl ether:
    (a) d-tubocurarine
    (b) succinylcholine
    (c) both
    (d) neither

37. Neuromuscular blocking effect can be antagonized by neostigmine:
    (a) d-tubocurarine
    (b) succinylcholine
    (c) both
    (d) neither

38. All of the following are true of pancuronium *except:*
    (a) is similar to succinylcholine in mechanism of action
    (b) is more potent than d-tubocurarine
    (c) is devoid of ganglionic blocking action
    (d) is devoid of histamine-releasing action

39. The diuresis produced by digitalis is primarily due to:
    (a) a direct action on the proximal renal tubule to decrease sodium reabsorption
    (b) production of hyperchloremic acidosis
    (c) improvement in cardiac function
    (d) increase in renal kallikrein production
    (e) none of the above

40. Digitalis glycosides are effective in treating patients with atrial flutter because they:
    (a) produce a positive inotropic effect
    (b) prolong refractory period of A-V node
    (c) increase conduction velocity in atrial muscle
    (d) prolong the atrial refractory period

41. The increase in ventricular automaticity produced by the cardiac glycosides:
    (a) is responsible for the positive inotropic effect
    (b) is considered a toxic action of the drug
    (c) is responsible for the slowing of sinus rate
    (d) is considered a therapeutic action of the drug
    (e) none of the above

42. In terms of therapeutic usefulness, the most important pharmacological action of digoxin in congestive heart failure is:
    (a) the reduction in cardiac size
    (b) the increase in ventricular contractile force
    (c) the slowing of heart rate
    (d) the diuretic effect
    (e) the increase in arterial pressure

43. Potassium antagonizes the toxic effects of cardiac glycosides by:
    (a) inhibition of active sodium-potassium transport
    (b) stimulation of active sodium-potassium transport
    (c) increasing the binding of sodium to the sarcolemma

(d) stimulation of the synthesis of ATP via oxidative phosphorylation

44. Which of the following is (are) useful in the treatment of ventricular tachycardia:
    (a) lidocaine
    (b) digitalis
    (c) both
    (d) neither

45. Of drugs useful in treatment of congestive heart failure, which is most specifically directed at the underlying pathology?
    (a) chlorothiazide
    (b) spironolactone
    (c) digoxin
    (d) nitroglycerin
    (e) furosemide

46. The appearance of ventricular tachycardia with the use of quinidine in the treatment of atrial fibrillation is usually prevented by prior administration of:
    (a) phenoxybenzamine
    (b) epinephrine
    (c) digitalis
    (d) atropine

47. Bretylium:
    (a) inhibits release of acetylcholine from post-ganglionic cholinergic neurons
    (b) is indicated in the treatment of ventricular tachycardia
    (c) is indicated in the treatment of congestive heart failure
    (d) is a potent dopaminergic receptor agonist

48. Disopyramide:
    (a) increases the rate of diastolic depolarization (phase 4) in cells with augmented automaticity
    (b) frequently causes hypertension
    (c) effectiveness is increased when moderate hypokalemia exists
    (d) urinary retention is an undesirable side effect

49. Of the drugs listed below, the most effective drug to provide chronic prophylaxis in the treatment of angina is:
    (a) propranolol
    (b) oral pentaerythritol tetranitrate
    (c) oral sustained releasing nitroglycerin preparations
    (d) dipyridamole

50. Relaxation of vascular smooth muscle by the nitrites is:
    (a) blocked by phenoxybenzamine
    (b) antagonized by atropine
    (c) antagonized by propranolol
    (d) none of the above

51. Of the vasodilators listed below, the drug of choice for treatment of acute anginal attacks is:
    (a) nitroglycerin
    (b) acetylcholine
    (c) papaverine
    (d) propranolol
    (e) sodium nitrite

52. A significant problem in the chronic administration of nitrates is the development of:
    (a) supersensitivity
    (b) cycloplegia
    (c) tolerance
    (d) cardiac arrhythmias

53. The principal mechanism by which nitroglycerin exerts a beneficial effect in the treatment of angina is because:
    (a) nitroglycerin causes a redistribution of coronary blood flow
    (b) nitroglycerin is a coronary vasodilator
    (c) nitroglycerin dilates systemic and pulmonary veins which results in a decreased venous return
    (d) nitroglycerin causes a shift in the oxyhemoglobin dissociation curve

54. Which of the following can relieve angina pectoris by decreasing myocardial work, but may precipitate congestive heart failure:
    (a) phentolamine
    (b) phenoxybenzamine
    (c) propranolol
    (d) atropine
    (e) none of the above

55. Clonidine and methyldopa appear to:
    (a) stimulate central alpha-adrenergic receptors in the area of the nucleus of the solitary tract
    (b) produce a peripherally-mediated decrease in arterial pressure
    (c) lower arterial pressure by blocking alpha-adrenergic receptors
    (d) lower arterial pressure by stimulating cholinergic receptors in the brain

56. All of the following are true of prazosin *except:*
    (a) it relaxes periperal arterioles by blocking post-synaptic alpha-adrenergic receptors
    (b) marked postural hypotension after the initial dose can be minimized by beginning treatment with a low dose
    (c) It is useful alone or in combination therapy in lowering blood pressure in all grades of hypertension
    (d) marked tachycardia is a frequently encountered undesirable side effect

57. All of the following are true of nitroprusside *except:*

(a) its hypotensive action is the result of a direct action on vascular smooth muscle

(b) cyanide intoxication may occur with excessive dosage

(c) its hypotensive action is the result of an action on central adrenergic control mechanisms

(d) it should be protected against light

58. Cholestyramine:
    (a) is the drug of choice for elevated triglycerides
    (b) increases the absorption of fat soluble vitamins
    (c) increases the fecal excretion of bile acids
    (d) is responsible for the reduction in ischemic heart disease in the United States.

59. The metabolic alkalosis associated with prolonged use of mercurial diuretics is due to excess excretion of:
    (a) Na^+
    (b) Cl^-
    (c) K^+
    (d) HCO_3^-

60. Acetazolamide:
    (a) is a long acting diuretic
    (b) inhibits distal Na^+ uptake
    (c) causes metabolic alkalosis
    (d) has a persistent effect on aqueous humor production during chronic use
    (e) causes the production of urine with high chloride content

61. Therapy with the thiazide diuretics may result in:
    (a) hyperuricemia
    (b) hyperglycemia
    (c) hypokalemia
    (d) all of the above

62. Permanent hearing loss is most usually associated with the administration of:
    (a) furosemide
    (b) furosemide and streptomycin
    (c) ethacrynic acid
    (d) mannitol

63. Acute hypovolemia and possible shock would most likely be associated with the administration of:
    (a) mannitol
    (b) mercurial diuretics
    (c) thiazide diuretics
    (d) furosemide

64. The characteristic of chlorothiazide that is *most important* to consider in concommitant therapy with digitalis is its tendency to produce:
    (a) hypokalemia
    (b) hyponatremia

(c) hyperuricemia

(d) hyperglycemia

65. All of the following are true of ticrynafen *except:*
    (a) resembles the thiazides in diuretic potency
    (b) lowers serum uric acid levels
    (c) potentiates the action of coumarin anticoagulants
    (d) efficacy is enhanced when administered in combination with triamterene

66. Which of the following is true of heparin?
    (a) strongly basic compound
    (b) a synthetic polysaccharide of low molecular weight
    (c) half life of 24 to 48 hours
    (d) placental transfer may damage fetus
    (e) not antagonized by vitamin K

67. The value of anticoagulation with warfarin has been *established* for:
    (a) immediate therapy of pulmonary emboli
    (b) chronic therapy of venous thrombosis
    (c) prevention of thrombosis on prosthetic valves
    (d) prevention of recurrent heart attacks
    (e) both (b) and (c)

68. The absorption of iron from the gastrointestinal tract is limited because:
    (a) it is bound to food in the gastrointestinal tract
    (b) it is destroyed by the acidity of the gastrointestinal tract
    (c) of the lack of intrinsic factor
    (d) of the mucosal block
    (e) none of the above

69. Both folic acid and vitamin B_{12}:
    (a) are effective in the treatment of megaloblastic anemia of pregnancy
    (b) can be used in treating the anemia caused by the fish tapeworm
    (c) may correct the neurological manifestations of pernicious anemia
    (d) will produce hematologic remission in pernicious anemia
    (e) are poorly absorbed after oral administration

70. It is generally agreed that the most effective oral iron therapy is obtained with iron in the form of:
    (a) ferrous salts
    (b) ferric salts
    (c) iron chelates
    (d) colloidal iron

71. Pernicious anemia may be distinguished from folic acid deficiency by:
    (a) the greater degree of hemopoietic suppression
    (b) neurological damage
    (c) atrophy of the gastrointestinal tract

(d) megaloblasts present in the bone marrow

(e) none of the above

72. According to Guedel's signs and stages of anesthesia, Stage II is the stage of:

(a) excitement or delirium

(b) surgical anesthesia

(c) analgesia

(d) medullary depression

73. Ketamine produces the type of anesthesia known as:

(a) regional

(b) narcotic

(c) dissociative

(d) none of the above

74. Which of the following produces the greatest degree of muscle relaxation?

(a) diethyl ether

(b) halothane

(c) nitrous oxide

(d) ethrane

75. Which one of the following anesthetics potentiates the effects of curare?

(a) halothane

(b) methoxyflurane

(c) ether

(d) ethrane

76. Diffusion hypoxia is most often associated with:

(a) halothane

(b) nitrous oxide

(c) ether

(d) thiopental

77. Which agent should *not* be used with adrenalin or adrenalin-like drugs?

(a) nitrous oxide

(b) cyclopropane

(c) diethyl ether

(d) thiopental

78. The short duration of action of thiopental is thought to be due primarily to:

(a) metabolism of the drug

(b) redistribution of the drug

(c) excretion of the drug

(d) tachyphylaxis or tolerance

79. The major factor in terminating the action of ethanol is:

(a) biotransformation

(b) excretion through lungs

(c) excretion unchanged in urine

(d) excretion in feces

(e) none of the above

80. Secobarbital and ethanol when given together show:

(a) additive sedative action

(b) reduced sedative action

(c) competitive antagonism

(d) chemical antagonism

(e) none of the above

81. Ethanol may be useful in the treatment of methanol intoxication because it:

(a) reverses acidosis

(b) retards oxidation of methanol

(c) enhances excretion of formaldehyde

(d) stimulates gastric secretion

82. When listing barbiturates in order from shortest acting to longest acting, which of the following is correct?

(a) thiopental, phenobarbital, pentobarbital

(b) phenobarbital, pentobarbital, thiopental

(c) pentobarbital, phenobarbital, thiopental

(d) thiopental, pentobarbital, phenobarbital

83. Which of the following hypnotics may be given to a patient with marked respiratory insufficiency?

(a) diazepam

(b) glutethimide

(c) flurazepam

(d) methaqualone

(e) none of the above

84. Chlorpromazine is effective as an antiemetic by:

(a) quieting nervous stomach

(b) blocking the chemoreceptor trigger zone

(c) depressing the vomiting center

(d) decreasing nervous input from the vestibular apparatus to the vomiting center

85. Hyperplasia of the gums is a common side effect of long-term therapy with:

(a) diphenylhydantoin

(b) diazepam

(c) trimethadione

(d) phenobarbital

86. Each of the following agents is used therapeutically to suppress epileptic seizures except:

(a) diazepam

(b) reserpine

(c) phenytoin

(d) phenobarbital

(e) ethosuximide

87. Which drug is preferred in the treatment of status epilepticus?

(a) diazepam

(b) ethosuximide

(c) trimethedione

(d) chlorpromazine

(e) primidone

88. All of the following are true of carbamazepine *except:*

(a) is useful in the treatment of grand mal and psychomotor epilepsy

(b) was introduced originally for the treatment of trigeminal neuralgia

(c) can cause nystagmus and drowsiness

(d) initial dosage should be high

89. All of the following are true of valproic acid *except:*
    (a) its mechanism of action may be related to increased brain levels of GABA
    (b) is indicated in the treatment of petit mal seizures
    (c) decreases phenobarbital levels when the two drugs are administered concurrently
    (d) can cause spontaneous bleeding

90. Which of the following drugs is *least* effective as an antiinflammatory agent?
    (a) indomethacin
    (b) aspirin
    (c) acetaminophen
    (d) phenylbutazone

91. Therapeutic uses of acetylsalicylic acid include:
    (a) analgesia, antipyresis and the lowering of arterial pressure.
    (b) anticonvulsant activity and the healing of peptic ulcers
    (c) acute rheumatic fever and stimulation of platelet aggregation
    (d) rheumatoid arthritis
    (e) hepatic damage induced by an overdose of acetaminophen

92. The mechanism of action of acetylsalicylic acid may involve:
    (a) stimulation of prostaglandin synthetase
    (b) stimulation of adenylate cyclase
    (c) inhibition of prostaglandin synthetase
    (d) stimulation of the sodium-potassium pump
    (e) inhibition of NADH cytochrome c reductase

93. A patient complains of dizziness, confusion and ringing in his ears. This is consistent with toxicity due to:
    (a) digitalis glycosides
    (b) imipramine
    (c) propranolol
    (d) acetylsalicylate
    (e) procainamide

94. Therapeutic uses of the narcotic analgesics include:
    (a) relief of pain, cough and diarrhea
    (b) reversal of the depressant effects of the phenothiazines, monoamine oxidase inhibitors and the tricyclic antidepressants
    (c) increasing respiratory reserve in patients with emphysema and cor pulmonale
    (d) production of euphoria in mentally depressed patients
    (e) relief of anxiety in disturbed patients

95. Placebos can cause analgesia because:
    (a) the active ingredient can bind to the opiate receptor
    (b) they decrease pain thresholds
    (c) they release endorphins
    (d) they are nocioceptive

96. Potential therapeutic uses for marijuana include all the following *except:*
    (a) antinauseant
    (b) analgesia
    (c) antibacterial agent
    (d) treatment of glaucoma

97. Local anesthetic drugs:
    (a) are more effective under acidic conditions
    (b) specifically affect sensory nerves
    (c) significantly increase potassium conductance across the nerve membrane
    (d) all of the above
    (e) none of the above

98. The mechanism of action of antihistaminic agents is:
    (a) inhibition of histidine decarboxylase
    (b) inhibition of histamine release from mast cells
    (c) competition with histamine for the receptor site
    (d) depletion of histamine from storage granules

99. Pretreatment with diphenhydramine would attenuate which of the following responses to injected histamine?
    (a) fall in blood pressure
    (b) increased gastric HCl production
    (c) both of the above

100. Sedation is a property of
    (a) H_1 blocking agents
    (b) H_2 blocking agents
    (c) both of the above

101. H_2 blocking drugs such as cimetidine have therapeutic value for patients with:
    (a) gastric hypersecretion
    (b) seasonal rhinitis
    (c) allergic dermatosis
    (d) urticaria

102. The primary mechanism of action of ACTH is:
    (a) stimulation of CRF release
    (b) stimulation of steroidogenesis
    (c) release of stored cortisol
    (d) antagonism of aldosterone activity
    (e) blockade of the renin-angiotensin system

103. Which of the following is not an adverse effect of cortisone therapy?
    (a) osteoporosis
    (b) psychoses
    (c) peptic ulcer
    (d) hypoglycemia
    (e) hypertension

104. Which drugs are effective in the absence of a functioning adrenal gland?
    (a) cortisone
    (b) dexamethasone
    (c) both
    (d) neither.

105. A patient with truncal obesity, muscle weakness, and hypertension is admitted to the hospital. Which of the following medications could have caused these problems?
    (a) aldosterone
    (b) prednisone
    (c) desoxycorticosterone
    (d) insulin

106. Which of the following best describes the action of desoxycorticosterone (DOC)?
    (a) is a potent antiinflammatory agent
    (b) promotes K^+ reabsorption in distal renal tubule
    (c) has no effect on water or electrolyte excretion
    (d) promotes Na^+ reabsorption in the distal renal tubule

107. The mechanism of action of sulfonylureas as hypoglycemic agents is:
    (a) decrease gluconeogenesis
    (b) increase conversion of protein to amino acids
    (c) stimulate peripheral utilization of glucose
    (d) increase secretion of insulin from pancreas

108. All of the following are true of calcitriol *except:*
    (a) occurs naturally in humans
    (b) is administered intravenously
    (c) is an active form of vitamin D_3
    (d) is indicated in the management of hypocalcemia

109. Used for possible destruction of the thyroid gland as a primary treatment of hyperthyroidism:
    (a) multiple dose of iodine in microgram amounts per day
    (b) multiple dose of iodine in milligram amounts per day
    (c) single dose of radioactive iodine
    (d) multiple dose of propylthiouracil
    (e) none of the above

110. Used to decrease the vascularity of the thyroid gland prior to surgical treatment of toxic goiter:
    (a) multiple doses of iodine in microgram amounts per day
    (b) multiple doses of iodine in milligram amounts per day
    (c) single doses of iodine-131
    (d) multiple doses of propylthiouracil
    (e) none of the above

111. The drug which acts by the release of formaldehyde in the urinary tract is:
    (a) nitrofurantoin

(b) ammonium chloride
(c) methenamine mandelate
(d) nalidixic acid
(e) ascorbic acid

112. A surface active germicide:
    (a) castor oil
    (b) benzalkonium chloride
    (c) undecylenic acid
    (d) methylene blue
    (e) DDT

113. All of the following are true of sulfonamides *except:*
    (a) are generally effective in urinary tract infection
    (b) are rendered less effective by paraaminobenzoic acid
    (c) are less effective in the presence of necrotic tissue
    (d) are more effective in the acetylated form

114. The most serious side effect of penicillin therapy is:
    (a) CNS stimulation
    (b) anaphylactic shock
    (b) renal tubular necrosis
    (d) eighth cranial nerve damage
    (e) fatty liver

115. A drug which is used in a fixed dose combination with sulfamethoxazole for treatment of urinary tract infections is:
    (a) triacetyloleandomycin
    (b) trihydantoin
    (c) trimethoprim
    (d) triamcinolone
    (e) tyrothricin

116. Pulmonary blastomycosis would most logically be treated with:
    (a) amphotericin B
    (b) chloramphenicol
    (c) amikacin
    (d) griseofulvin
    (e) nystatin

117. A drug useful for treatment of corneal herpes virus infections is:
    (a) amantadine
    (b) griseofulvin
    (c) nystatin
    (d) iododeoxyuridine
    (e) hydroxyurea

118. Nalidixic acid is most commonly used in treatment of:
    (a) dermatophytosis
    (b) pseudomonas infections
    (c) shigellosis
    (d) urinary tract infections
    (e) moniliasis

119. A drug frequently used with carbenicillin in treatment of pseudomonas septicemia is:
    (a) ampicillin
    (b) gentamycin
    (c) polymixin B
    (d) erythromycin
    (e) chloramphenicol

120. Sustained blood levels of benzyl penicillin can be achieved by the concurrent administration of:
    (a) procarbazine
    (b) probanthine
    (c) proteomycin
    (d) prolactin
    (e) probenecid

121. The most serious side effect of tetracycline therapy is:
    (a) photosensitization
    (b) fatty liver
    (c) staphylococcal suprainfection
    (d) osteoporosis
    (e) ulcerative colitis

122. If a patient with enterococcal endocarditis were treated with penicillin plus streptomycin:
    (a) antibiotic antagonism would be expected
    (b) the antibiotics should be mixed prior to use
    (c) antibiotic synergism may be observed
    (d) toxicity would be intolerable
    (e) none of the above

123. Gastric irritation is most commonly encountered following oral administration of:
    (a) griseofulvin
    (b) phenethycillin
    (c) sulfonamides
    (d) tetracycline
    (e) methenamine mandelate

124. Which of the following is *not* an inhibitor of cell wall synthesis in microorganisms?
    (a) methoxycillin
    (b) isoniazid
    (c) cycloserine
    (d) cephalosporin
    (e) nalidixic acid

125. A bactericidal drug would be preferred over a bacteriostatic drug in a patient with:
    (a) renal insufficiency
    (b) reduced immunocompetence
    (c) liver damage
    (d) uncontrolled nausea
    (e) a history of hypersensitivy reactions

126. Colonic ulceration would be most likely to occur following administration of:
    (a) chloramphenicol
    (b) carbenicillin
    (c) clindamycin
    (d) chlortetracycline
    (e) colistin B

127. The inhibitory action of nystatin on susceptible microorganisms depends upon:
    (a) blood levels achieved
    (b) the presence of sterols in the plasma membrane of the microorganism
    (c) the presence of mycolic acid in the cell wall of the microorganism
    (d) the replicative state of the microorganism
    (e) all of the above

128. The most serious side effect of isoniazid administration is:
    (a) hepatotoxicity
    (b) nephrotoxicity
    (c) monoamine oxidase inhibition
    (d) convulsions
    (e) anaphylaxis

129. A useful drug for treatment of uncomplicated streptococcal infections in patients who are hypersensitive to penicillin is:
    (a) nitrofurantoin
    (b) chloramphenicol
    (c) erythromycin
    (d) amikacin
    (e) amantadine

130. Host response to antimicrobial therapy is influenced by:
    (a) renal function
    (b) age
    (c) hepatic function
    (d) genetic background
    (e) all of the above

131. An extensive infection with *Trichophyton rubrum* would usually be treated with:
    (a) tolnaftate
    (b) griseofulvin
    (c) nystatin
    (d) amphotericin B
    (e) micronazole

132. The antimicrobial action of paraaminosalicyclic acid (PAS) on susceptible mycobacteria can be antagonized by:
    (a) isoniazid
    (b) sulfanilamide
    (c) paraaminobenzoic acid
    (d) metaaminosalicylic acid
    (e) streptomycin

133. Reversible leukopenia is most often detected following the administration of:
    (a) chloramphenicol
    (b) tobramycin
    (c) trimethoprim

(d) griseofulvin

(e) nitrofurantoin

134. A *direct* inhibitor of bacterial nucleic acid synthesis is:

(a) sulfamethosazole

(b) kanamycin

(c) cycloserine

(d) rifampin

(e) griseofulvin

135. Which of the following exerts a bactericidal action by interacting with the bacterial 50s ribosomal subunit?

(a) erythromycin

(b) kanamycin

(c) chloramphenicol

(d) streptomycin

(e) none of the above

136. Allopurinol is sometimes given to patients receiving cancer chemotherapy:

(a) to synergize the antitumor activity of purine antimetabolites

(b) to reduce the level of uric acid in the glomerular filtrates

(c) to counteract the marrow suppression caused by the chemotherapy

(d) to increase serum creatinine levels

(e) to enhance uric acid excretion

137. An antineoplastic agent which undergoes biotransformation to form a potent inhibitor of thymidylate synthetase is:

(a) 5-fluorouracil

(b) 6-mercaptopurine

(c) methotrexate

(d) hydroxyurea

(e) cyclophosphamide

138. Selective inhibition of mammalian riboside phosphate reductase occurs following administration of:

(a) 5-fluorouracil

(b) 6-mercaptopurine

(c) methotrexate

(d) hydroxyurea

(e) cyclophosphamide

139. The cumulative dose-limiting toxicity of adriamycin (doxorubicin) is:

(a) alopecia

(b) renal proximal tubular necrosis

(c) cardiomyopathy

(d) hepatic necrosis

(e) convulsions

140. The typical nitrogen mustard antineoplastic agents:

(a) are highly cell cycle specific

(b) are active only during cell mitosis

(c) form cross links between adjacent strands of DNA

(d) are never effective if given orally

(e) rapidly cross the blood-brain barrier

141. Peripheral neuropathies are most frequently observed following administration of:

(a) cyclophosphamide

(b) chlorambucil

(c) L-phenylalanine mustard (melphalan)

(d) L-asparaginase

(e) vincristine

142. An antimetabolite which undergoes biotransformation to form an inhibitor of DNA polymerase is:

(a) cytosine arabinoside

(b) chlorambucil

(c) methotrexate

(d) 5-fluorouracil

(e) vinblastine

143. Cisplatin:

(a) is devoid of renal toxicity

(b) should be administered in combination with furosemides

(c) is effective in the treatment of testicular carcinoma

(d) interacts with DNA-dependent RNA polymerase

(e) none of the above

144. The agent of choice in treatment of ascariasis, also effective against *Enterobis vermicularis,* is:

(a) tetrachloroethylene

(b) thiabendazole

(c) piperazine

(d) metronidazole

145. Piperazine or pyrvinium pamoate are useful drugs in the treatment of:

(a) pinworm infections

(b) amebiasis

(c) protozoal infections

(d) all of the above

(e) none of the above

146. Least toxic and most effective treatment for the symptoms of acute amebic dysentery:

(a) metronidazole

(b) emetine hydrochloride

(c) chiniofon

(d) carbarsone

(e) paromomycin

147. Which one of the following laxatives is a surface-active agent that eases defecation principally by softening the stool?

(a) dioctyl sodium sulfosuccinate

(b) phenolphthalein

(c) magnesium hydroxide

(d) senna

(e) bisacodyl

148. Possesses cathartic action which limits its use as an antacid:
    (a) sodium bicarbonate
    (b) magnesium hydroxide
    (c) aluminum hydroxide
    (d) all of the above
    (e) none of the above

149. Which of the following antacids would be most likely to produce depression of mental function in a patient with poor renal function?
    (a) sodium bicarbonate
    (b) magnesium trisilicate
    (c) calcium carbonate
    (d) aluminum hydroxide

150. Which of the following is a laxative antacid?
    (a) aluminum hydroxide
    (b) magnesium carbonate
    (c) calcium carbonate
    (d) phenolphthalein
    (e) sodium sulfate

151. Inhibits absorption of phosphate from the gut:
    (a) diphenoxylate
    (b) dioctyl sodium sulfosuccinate
    (c) castor oil
    (d) aluminum hydroxide gel
    (e) none of the above

152. Which of the following is a constipating antacid?
    (a) sodium bicarbonate
    (b) bran
    (c) cascara
    (d) magnesium hydroxide
    (e) calcium carbonate

153. Which of the following adverse reactions is associated with sodium bicarbonate?
    (a) severe skin eruptions
    (b) fluid retention in patients with renal, hepatic or cardiac disease
    (c) aspiration pneumonia
    (d) somnolence in patients with renal disease
    (e) hypophosphatemia in chronic use

154. In the third trimester of pregnancy uterine smooth muscle becomes more sensitive to stimulation by:
    (a) oxytocin
    (b) ergonovine
    (c) both
    (d) neither

155. Ergonovine is most commonly used for:
    (a) induction of labor during the first trimester
    (b) induction of labor during the second trimester
    (c) induction of labor during the third trimester

(d) inhibition of postpartum bleeding

(e) control of high blood pressure

156. Used to induce labor:
    (a) perchlorate
    (b) oxytocin
    (c) probenecid
    (d) colchicine
    (e) none of the above

157. Moderate-to-severe toxic effects occur most frequently as a result of overdosage with:
    (a) vitamin E
    (b) vitamin D
    (c) ascorbic acid
    (d) riboflavin
    (e) thiamine

158. Cures wet beriberi:
    (a) ascorbic acid
    (b) pantothenic acid
    (c) pyridoxine
    (d) riboflavin
    (e) thiamine chloride

Answers to Multiple Choice Questions

1. (d)	30. (c)	59. (b)	88. (d)
2. (b)	31. (c)	60. (d)	89. (c)
3. (a)	32. (b)	61. (d)	90. (c)
4. (b)	33. (c)	62. (b)	91. (d)
5. (b)	34. (c)	63. (d)	92. (c)
6. (d)	35. (a)	64. (a)	93. (d)
7. (d)	36. (a)	65. (d)	94. (a)
8. (c)	37. (a)	66. (e)	95. (c)
9. (d)	38. (a)	67. (e)	96. (c)
10. (c)	39. (c)	68. (d)	97. (e)
11. (d)	40. (b)	69. (d)	98. (c)
12. (c)	41. (b)	70. (a)	99. (a)
13. (a)	42. (b)	71. (b)	100. (a)
14. (d)	43. (b)	72. (a)	101. (a)
15. (d)	44. (a)	73. (c)	102. (c)
16. (d)	45. (c)	74. (a)	103. (d)
17. (a)	46. (c)	75. (c)	104. (c)
18. (b)	47. (b)	76. (b)	105. (b)
19. (c)	48. (d)	77. (b)	106. (d)
20. (c)	49. (a)	78. (b)	107. (d)
21. (c)	50. (d)	79. (a)	108. (b)
22. (e)	51. (a)	80. (a)	109. (c)
23. (a)	52. (c)	81. (b)	110. (b)
24. (c)	53. (c)	82. (d)	111. (c)
25. (b)	54. (c)	83. (e)	112. (b)
26. (a)	55. (a)	84. (b)	113. (d)
27. (a)	56. (d)	85. (a)	114. (b)
28. (e)	57. (c)	86. (b)	115. (c)
29. (a)	58. (c)	87. (a)	116. (a)

117. (d)	123. (d)	129. (c)	134. (d)	139. (c)	144. (c)	149. (b)	154. (c)
118. (d)	124. (e)	130. (e)	135. (c)	140. (c)	145. (a)	150. (b)	155. (d)
119. (b)	125. (b)	131. (b)	136. (b)	141. (e)	146. (a)	151. (d)	156. (b)
120. (e)	126. (c)	132. (c)	137. (a)	142. (a)	147. (a)	152. (e)	157. (b)
121. (c)	127. (b)	133. (a)	138. (d)	143. (c)	148. (b)	153. (b)	158. (e)
122. (c)	128. (a)						

Part 2

Clinical Sciences

8

Surgery

CHARLES ECKERT, M.D.

Distinguished Professor of Surgery,
Albany Medical College of Union University

In this chapter, first, those subjects common to all branches of surgery and, second, the surgical lesions encountered in various organs and anatomic sites will be discussed.

WOUNDS

The ability of the organism to recover from wounds by means of the process of fibroplasia and epithelial proliferation is of fundamental importance. Considerable progress has been made in our understanding of the basic biological and molecular changes involved in the process of fibroplasia.

Hydroxyproline and *hydroxylysine* are amino acids identified in the collagen molecule, but in no other biologic protein that has been studied except for minute amounts in complement. The enzyme protocollagen *proline hydroxylase* is responsible for the hydroxylation of proline. Ascorbate has been identified as a necessary cosubstrate in this system. The rate of hydroxyproline formation from ^{14}C-labeled proline in healing wounds has been used as an index of the rate of collagen synthesis.

The collagen molecule is stabilized by polymeriza-tion, and there is good evidence that cross linkage between the three helices in the molecule is important in fibrogenesis.

In addition to collagen, the healing wound contains considerable quantities of proteoglycans (mucopoly-saccharides). These substances are largely polysaccha-rides composed of chains of repeating disaccharide units that are in turn composed of glucuronic acid or iduronic acid and a hexosomine. The units are called glycosaminoglycans, they rarely exist free in the body, but instead couple to proteins to form proteoglycans. The hexosamine fraction gives a metachromatic stain-ing reaction to healing wounds. This reaction reaches a peak on the fifth or sixth day after wounding and thereafter gradually subsides. The role of proteoglycans in the process of wound healing is not understood, but it appears that they play an important role in colla-gen fiber formation by binding polymer chains of colla-gen by electrostatic interactions. Fiber orientation and size may be influenced by the characteristics of specific proteoglycans.

The relation between deficiencies in various nutrients and wound healing has been studied extensively. Blood flow adequate to provide a sufficient quantity of oxygen and removal of metabolic end-products is certainly necessary. Hypoproteinemia is probably a significant factor only where local edema occurs and interferes with blood flow.

Collagen synthesis and wound healing are suppressed by corticosteroids, but collagen synthesis and tensile strength can be returned to normal by the administration of Vitamin A.

Tensile strength in the healing sutured skin wound decreases slightly from the time of suturing until the fourth day, when it begins to increase. The increase in tensile strength continues progressively up to 150 days. In fullthickness wounds of the abdominal wall, the rate of increase in tensile strength is greatest from the fourth to the twenty-first day; thereafter, although it still increases, the rate is slower.

The type of suture material used influences wound healing, inasmuch as all sutures are foreign bodies. Absorbable sutures elicit a greater inflammatory response than nonabsorable sutures. Both cellular and humoral factors are responsible for the absorption. No suture material produced for clinical use is devoid of tissue reaction, although inert metals and plastics stimulate a minimal reaction. The eventual fate of nonabsorbable sutures is encapsulation. In the presence of infection, nonabsorbable sutures act as foreign bodies and perpetuate the infection until they are extruded or removed. However, monofilament sutures are less conducive to infection than are multifilament sutures of the same material.

Efforts to regulate the process of fibroplasia or accelerate the process of healing have not been rewarding to date. Cleanly incised wounds that are properly sutured will heal unless infection supervenes. Bleeding points must be ligated carefully, because the development of a hematoma predisposes to infection. Careful obliteration of dead space is necessary to minimize the collection of serum in the wound.

Traumatic wounds that are associated with a large amount of contamination and destruction of soft tissue should be debrided. If the wounds are seen early and cleaned properly, primary closure may be feasible. The use of antibiotic therapy in conjunction with debridement has reduced markedly the massive infection rates previously seen in contaminated wounds and has permitted early secondary closure and plastic procedures heretofore impossible.

In wounds that are unsutured, or in wounds with loss of substance, there is initial retraction of the wound margins owing to the elasticity of the normal skin. As the process of healing progresses, contraction of the wound occurs which narrows the size of the defect. This appears to result from the migration of normal skin at the margins. Primitive mononuclear cells in the healing tissues may differentiate into fibroblasts or myofibroblasts. Both can form collagen fibers, but the myofibroblast also has contractile properties. These properties are thought to play a part in the process of wound contraction.

Infection

Inflammation is a response of the body tissues to a noxious agent, such as a microorganism. It manifests itself by the presence of heat, redness, swelling and tenderness. Spontaneous pain also may be present. If the response progresses to destruction of tissue and development of pus, fluctuation also is demonstrable.

The early stage of the inflammatory response in soft tissue is known as cellulitis. This may subside spontaneously or may progress to formation of an abscess. Extension of the infection along the course of the lymphatics is manifested by the development of red streaks with local tenderness. The regional lymph nodes become enlarged and tender. These conditions are known as lymphangitis and lymphadenitis. The *Streptococcus pyogenes* is the organism most frequently causative of cellulitis, lymphangitis and lymphadenitis. It does this by virtue of its production of hyaluronidase and streptokinase. Contrarily, the *Staphylococcus* is more likely to produce localized abscesses.

Erisepelas is a special type of cellulitis also usually caused by the *Streptococcus pyogenes* and characterized by a red, raised advancing margin. ·

Treatment of cellulitis consists of the application of heat locally to the part, adequate immobilization and elevation. In addition, antimicrobial agents, such as penicillin and the broad-spectrum antibiotics, often are of value in arresting the spread of the infection and in shortening the course of the disease. In the modern treatment of infection the antimicrobials hold a very prominent place. The surgeon chooses the antimicrobial on the basis of the organisms that he believes will most likely be present in a given situation, which choice is based on clinical judgment aided by Gram stains of smears. Cultures should always be obtained and antimicrobial therapy adjusted according to the proven sensitivity of the predominant organisms.

Tetanus. This is an infection caused by a strict anaerobe, *Clostridium tetani.* It is found in puncture wounds and in wounds in which there is dead tissue or poor blood supply. The organisms are found in the excreta of animals, especially cows and horses; hence, wounds contaminated by street dirt and fertilized soil are more susceptible to infection by the tetanus organism.

The organism produces an exotoxin that is absorbed by the peripheral nerves and carried to the spinal cord. The sensory nerves react to the slightest stimuli, and the hypersensitive motor nerves carry impulses that produce spasms of the muscles they supply. The extensor muscles in spasm produce a convulsive contraction, with the head pulled back, called opisthotonos. Death occurs from asphyxia, due to diaphragmatic spasm or exhaustion.

Meticulous wound care is the greatest prerequisite for tetanus prophylaxis. This includes irrigation, thorough debridement of dead and devitalized tissues and the removal of foreign bodies.

Table 8–1 is a guide to the use of active and passive tetanus immunization prophylaxis following the recommendations of the United States Public Health Service Committee on Immunization Practices. In all patients who have not previously had a complete course of immunizations (three or more injections of tetanus toxoid) tetanus toxoid is given. In patients with clean minor wounds, the interval since the last dose should not exceed 10 years. In all other wounds this period must not exceed five years. An accurate history is essential, and if there is any doubt, the patient needs an immunizing course. Basic immunization with adsorbed toxoid requires three injections; the second injection is given 4 to 6 weeks after the first and the third is given 6 to 12 months later.

In major wounds, antimicrobial prophylaxis should also be considered in the previously nonimmunized patient. In those not sensitive to penicillin, 1,200,000 units of benzathine penicillin G (Bicillin) is administered by deep intramuscular injection. Penicillin-sensitive patients should be given tetracycline 0.5 g. four times a day by mouth for 3 weeks.

Gas Gangrene. This infection results following injuries in which there are destruction and death of soft tissue. These tissues serve as a culture medium for the growth of the anaerobic gas-forming organisms. Gas gangrene spreads rapidly along fascial planes, destroying large segments of soft tissue, especially muscle. It is a serious infection requiring prompt and radical treatment. This consists of wide excision of the involved part, with amputation if necessary. It also includes the use of massive doses of antitoxin and penicillin. Good results have been reported with the use of oxygen under pressure. The patient is placed in a sealed tank, and oxygen is supplied under 3 atm. of pressure.

Necrotizing Fascitis. This is a serious infection characterized by extensive necrosis of the superficial fascia with widespread undermining of surrounding tissue and severe toxicity. Although it may be seen following surgical wounds in most instances the infection follows comparatively mild injury outside the hospital. A variety of microorganisms including anaerobes, have been cultured, the diagnosis depends on the presence of widespread necrosis of the superficial

TABLE 8–1. Guide to Tetanus Prophylaxis in Wound Management

History of Tetanus Immunization (Doses)	Clean Minor Wounds		All Other Wounds	
	Tetanus Toxoid	Tetanus Immune Globulin	Tetanus Toxoid	Tetanus Immune Globulin
Uncertain	Yes	No	Yes	Yes
0–1	Yes	No	Yes	Yes
2	Yes	No	Yes	No*
3 or more	No†	No	No‡	No

* Unless wound is more than 24 hours old.
† Unless more than 10 years have elapsed since the last dose.
‡ Unless more than 5 years have elapsed since the last dose.

fascia rather than on the causative organism. Treatment consists of adequate drainage, thorough debridement, and antimicrobials effective against both streptococci and penicillinase producing staphylococci.

Carbuncle. This is a soft tissue infection, usually staphylococcal in origin, in which there is diffuse destruction of the subcutaneous tissues with the development of multiple sinuses presenting on the skin surface. Antistaphylococcal antibiotics, administered parenterally in adequate doses, may abort the infection and allow it to subside spontaneously. However, with the formation of extensive slough and pus, operative excision of the area or incision and drainage is necessary. In these cases, the resulting defects may be so massive as to require subsequent skin grafting.

Rabies. In all patients who have sustained animal bites or have been in contact with bat feces, rabies prophylaxis must be considered. The decision for or against rabies prophylaxis is based on the severity of the wound and the availability of the animal for observation and autopsy purposes to substantiate the diagnosis of rabies. Prophylaxis consists in a course of duck embryo vaccine and the administration of rabies antiserum. The latter is of equine origin; therefore the danger of anaphylaxis exists when it is used, and the usual precautions must be taken.

Insect Bites. Bees, wasps and hornets inject a venom that may cause sensitization, and in sensitized people, anaphylaxis that may be fatal. The black widow spider venom is a neurotoxin that causes severe muscle spasm; death may occur. The brown spider bite produces ischemic necrosis and a slough that may necessitate skin grafting.

Snake Bites. The poisonous snakes in the United States are, with the exception of the coral snake, pit vipers. The venom is both neurotoxic and hemolytic. The bite is painful, and fang marks are the first external evidence. Swelling, pain and ecchymosis rapidly follow. The use of a tourniquet as an emergency measure to prevent lymphatic spread is important. Definitive treatment is early excision of the bite wound; this can remove most of the venom and eliminates the need for antiserum. The defect is repaired by either a local flap or graft.

THE CONTROL OF BLEEDING

Nothing is more important in surgery than the ability of the surgeon to control hemorrhage, either in wounds or at operation. In addition to the skill of the surgeon, the control of bleeding depends upon the complex process of coagulation of blood, local vascular factors and a balance between coagulation and fibrinolysis.

Defects in the clotting mechanism most often encountered by the surgeon are thrombocytopenia, vitamin K deficiency, hemophilia (Factor VIII deficiency) and those of iatrogenic cause such as the administration of heparin or the coumarin drugs.

The local vascular factors that influence the control of bleeding include such things as the ability of a cut blood vessel to contract, the state of the vascular bed with regard to the existing degree of vasodilatation or vasoconstriction and the hydrostatic pressure within the vascular bed. Capillary oozing under normal circumstances is controlled by the agglutination of platelets. Defects in platelet function can result in excessive bleeding from capillaries. An artery that is completely transected will contract, its lumen will be narrowed, and clot will form at the end, with control of bleeding. If the same artery is partially transected, it cannot contract; hemorrhage will continue to the point of near-exsanguination. Surrounding scar tissue or sclerosis of the vascular wall will also limit contraction of the blood vessel and increase the amount of hemorrhage. This is frequently the case in arterial bleeding from chronic duodenal ulcer. Anesthetic agents such as cyclopropane may cause vasodilatation and increased blood loss. Bleeding is also more profuse in patients with arterial or portal hypertension.

Disseminated intravascular coagulation is a syndrome that may complicate shock, massive hemorrhage, septic abortion, prolonged use of the pump oxygenator and large cavernous hemangiomas. As the name implies, there is diffuse intravascular coagulation that results in a depletion of the factors essential for clot formation. Fibrinogenopenia, thrombocytopenia, prothrombinemia and a deficiency in Factors V and VIII are all noted. Split fibrin products are likely to be found in the blood, and activation of the fibrinolytic system is likely to be present. Bleeding is the clinical manifestation. The process usually follows release of

thromboplastic material into the circulation. Treatment is directed toward relief of the underlying disease state and the maintenance of capillar blood flow. Intravenous fluids are indicated to maintain plasma volume and if myocardial function is impaired digitalis or isoprotercuol may be indicated. Heparin has been used to prevent intravascular coagulation, but it must be given cautiously while monitoring the levels of platelets and fibrinogen. Use of fibrinogen or epsilon aminocaproic acid is contraindicated for uncontrolled progression of the disseminated intravascular coagulation may result.

SHOCK

Shock is characterized by decreased tissue perfusion secondary to either heart failure or reduction in circulating blood volume. In either case, decreased tissue oxygenation and the retention of metabolites will follow. Depending on the effectiveness of compensatory mechanisms and treatment, failure in function of major organ systems will lead to death. The reduction in circulating blood volume may be absolute in terms of hemorrhage or may be relative owing to an increased capacity of the vascular bed. At times a combination of factors will intensify the physiologic abnormality. Clinically, shock is most frequently seen in patients with massive hemorrhage, burns, acute myocardial infarction with heart failure or bacterial sepsis.

Elucidation of the physiologic abnormalities is best accomplished by direct measurements of the central venous pressure, left atrial pressure, blood volume and cardiac output. The history and physical findings will be of help, but accurate and effective treatment must be assisted by physiologic monitoring. Monitoring the central venous pressure by inserting a suitable catheter into the superior vena cava is not difficult, and it is of considerable help in managing fluid and blood replacement. A low central venous pressure indicates an unfilled vascular bed, but a high central venous pressure indicates a venous volume greater than the heart can pump. In older people with a tenuously compensated myocardium, sudden increases in blood volume may precipitate heart failure even though the increase is slight. In most hospitals today intensive care units are equipped with monitors that make it possible to use the information available by passage of the Swan-Ganz flow directed catheter. This information includes right atrial and ventricular pressure, pulmonary artery and wedged pulmonary artery pressure. The latter is the equivalent of left atrial pressure. A thermistor tip also permits determination of cardiac output by the thermal dilution technique. The information available by use of the Swan-Ganz catheter is considerably more useful than is the simpler measurement of central venous pressure. Its use is particularly indicated in the unstable patient.

In septic shock the most important aspect of therapy is the control of infection; however, attention to the maintenance of adequate tissue perfusion is also essential.

NUTRITION

Inasmuch as many surgical patients are unable to eat or drink for varying periods, they must be protected against serious alterations in body composition by parenteral therapy. Over short periods, changes in water and electrolyte balance are of little importance, however all too frequently a short-term problem turns into one requiring protracted parenteral support. Under these circumstances caloric intake, along with sufficient fat, protein and vitamins, becomes significant. The routine use of flow sheets, upon which intake and output are charted on a cumulative as well as a daily basis, will he helpful in management. The source, composition and volume of all known losses and increments should be individually noted.

Daily basal requirements of an average-sized adult man in the temperate zone are: water, less than 2,000 ml.; sodium chloride, 2 to 3 g.; calories, 1,600. Insensible water loss through skin and lungs increases with fever, increased environmental temperature, etc. With vomiting, diarrhea, fistulas, etc., losses of water, sodium chloride, potassium and bicarbonate increase. The latter losses are measurable and should be replaced in equal volume of water and concentration of salts. Most abnormalities in electrolyte concentration are iatrogenic, resulting either from improper ingestion of fluid by the patient, or most often, incorrect replacement by the surgeon.

In the prolonged vomiting of pyloric obstruction, hypochloremic-hypokalemic alkalosis usually develops. Treatment with sodium and potassium chloride will restore the potassium and chloride deficits as well as the acidbase imbalance. Sodium will be excreted by the kidneys.

The symptoms and signs of specific electrolyte deficits are at times characteristic:

Hyponatremia is manifested by restlessness, mental confusion with delusions or hallucinations.

Hypokalemia results in decreased tone and contractility of smooth, striated and cardiac muscle. Adynamic ileus may be present. The electrocardiogram shows a depressed S-T segment, a prolonged QT interval, small T waves fused with V waves.

Hypochloremia, most frequently secondary to vomiting, paradoxically causes nausea and vomiting.

Hypocalemia increases muscle tone and irritability leading to tetany. Early symptoms include perioral numbness and tingling of the digits.

Intravenous Hyperalimentation

In patients who are unable to use their alimentary tract for the maintenance of their nutritional state, intravenous hyperalimentation has been shown to be a suitable substitute. The technique is also applicable to patients in whom for one reason or another it is desirable to rest the alimentary tract. The feeding mixture consists of a hypertonic solution of glucose and amino acids, vitamins and minerals infused into the superior vena cava through a catheter placed usually percutaneously into the subclavian vein. Each 1,000 ml. contains approximately 1,000 kcal. Twice a week solutions of fat (Intralipid) are given in order to prevent essential fatty acid deficiency. The infusate, 2,500 to 3,000 ml. in volume, is delivered slowly over a 24 hour period. Nitrogen equilibrium, positive nitrogen balance, weight gain and growth are possible when this route is used as the sole source of food. The complications include sepsis caused by both bacteria and fungi, of which *Candida albicans* is most frequent. Prophylaxis is most important, consisting of care in the insertion of the catheter and strict asepsis in the dressing of the skin at the point of puncture as well as in the preparation and changing of solutions. Complications resulting from catheter placement include: pneumothorax, hemothorax or hydrothorax; injury of the subclavian artery; air embolism and catheter breaks. Arrythmias may occur if the catheter enters the heart and perforation of the myocardium has been reported. Metabolic complications include hypophosphatemia, hyperosmolarity, nonketotic hyperglycemia, convulsions, and coma. In diabetics, ketoacidosis may develop. When the intravenous hyperalimentation is stopped, rebound hypoglycemia may occur. Deficiencies of trace elements has also been reported. Prevention, of course, consists of the addition of these elements to the solution.

Peripheral veins can also be used for intravenous feeding by using less concentrated solutions of amino acids and glucose with added fat. Eventually, however, thrombosis occurs.

Another approach to the management of patients with small intestinal fistulas, Crohn's disease or the short bowel syndrome is the use of elemental diets for feeding. A number of commercially prepared mixtures of medium-chain triglycerides, protein hydrolysates, glucose, minerals and vitamins, in variable proportions, are available. Some of the preparations contain no fat. Most of the preparations are unpalatable and may require a small polyvinyl feeding tube if they are to be given for prolonged periods.

TRANSPLANTATION

Burgeoning interest in tissue and organ transplantation has given rise to the development of a series of new specialties in biology, including transplantation immunology, transplantation genetics, transplantation pathology and transplantation surgery. A new vocabulary has evolved, and the field becomes increasingly complex. Certain tissues such as aorta, bone, cartilage, and fascia are transplanted as dead tissues. They are replaced by the process of creeping substitution and are called *homostructural* grafts. The transplantation of complex organs, however, involves the maintenance of viability by connecting the blood vessels of the transplant to those of the host. This is a *homovital* graft. With the exception of grafts between identical twins, such grafts will undergo necrosis through a recognizable sequence of steps, and this process is called rejection.

A second graft from the same donor is rejected faster—a second set response. This can be likened to the anamnestic response familiar in classical immunology.

The phenomenon of rejection is caused by antigenic differences between host and graft. The strength and number of antigens in a given case will alter the speed of rejection. Cellular aspects of rejection are prominent in terms of the infiltration of lymphocytes. Humoral factors, not at first apparent, are now proving also to play a significant role in the process of rejection. Allografts of skin have been used for many years in the management of burns in infants; usually they were obtained from the mother and were permitted to take as lifesaving measures to control evaporative water loss and infection. Today xenografts as well as allografts are used as biologic dressings.

Immunosuppressive agents are used to ablate or retard rejection. They include (1) azathioprine—an antimetabolite originally used in cancer chemotherapy; (2) corticosteroids; (3) actinomycin C—an antibiotic-like agent produced by actinomyces, used mainly when rejection appears to be taking place in an attempt to abort the episode: (4) ionizing radiation to graft, host blood, host spleen, etc.: (5) antilymphocyte serum. Of these, azathioprine, steroids and antilymphocyte serum are the mainstays of immunosuppressive therapy in clinical organ transplantation.

Transplantation of all organs and tissues has been investigated, but among these only renal transplantation has achieved widespread clinical use. However, both liver and cardiac transplantation are done with improving success rates.

GENERAL CONDITIONS OF THE EXTREMITIES

LOWER EXTREMITIES

Ulcers

The most common ulcer of the lower extremities results from venous statis secondary to deep thrombophlebitis with reversal of flow between the deep and superficial venous systems. The valves in the communicating veins are incompetent. The skin of the lower medial leg develops a brawny induration that is brownish in color, the result of accumulation of hemosiderin pigment. Usually varicosities of the greater saphenous system are also present. Extreme or neglected cases may show circumferential ulcers. The diagnosis is made on the basis of the history and physical findings. It is confirmed by venography, which shows recanalized channels with destroyed valves and flow from deep to superficial veins. Treatment consists of stripping of the superficial varicosities, along with ligation of all incompetent communicating veins. Ulcers are treated by the application of split-thickness skin grafts after excision of devitalized skin and the scarred base of the ulcer.

Ulcers on the legs and feet may also occur as a result of syphilis or arteriosclerosis obliterans. Luetic ulcers are mainly of historical interest. Ulcers resulting from decreased arterial flow will be considered subsequently.

Varicose Veins

Abnormally dilated veins, seen most frequently in the lower extremities, are spoken of as varicose veins. Varicosities appear more frequently in women than in men, occurring most often following pregnancy and in those engaged in occupations demanding that the patient be on her feet for long periods. In some patients there is a familial tendency toward varicosities; in others the varicose veins are the result of deep thrombophlebitis. The valves in the involved veins become incompetent. The Trendelenburg test is used to demonstrate such incompetency of the valves. This is carried out by applying a tourniquet to the upper thigh, with the patient lying supine with the leg elevated and the veins empty. Upon the patient's standing and removal of the tourniquet, the entire vein fills immediately from above. With the tourniquet in place and the patient erect, filling from below indicates incompetence of valves in the communicating veins. Application of the tourniquet at different levels will help to localize these channels.

The treatment of varicose veins involves either high ligation—with multiple excision of segments in which incompetent communicating veins are present—or stripping of the entire varicose vein. Injection therapy with sclerosing solution is seldom used at present. In patients with a history of thrombophlebitis or with stasis changes in the skin, a period of compression with elastic bandages or well-fitting elastic stockings is a useful test to indicate whether the stripping of varicose veins will be tolerated or will give satisfactory symptomatic results. Perthes' test also may be used to determine the competency of the deep veins. It is carried out by placing a rubber tube tourniquet snugly around the lower thigh. Then the patient is asked to walk or exercise the leg. If the deep veins are competent, contraction of the calf muscles will suck the blood in the superficial varices through the communicating veins into the deep veins, and the varicose veins will become less prominent. On removal of the tourniquet the veins will refill from above.

Venous Thrombosis (Phlebitis)

In this condition the veins are involved by intravascular clotting. Phlebitis has been divided into two types.

Thrombophlebitis. By this is meant an acute inflammatory reaction in the wall of the vein associated with production of a thrombus within the vein. This type of phlebitis is seen in the puerperal period, postoperatively and after trauma and debilitating disease such as myocardial infarction or cancer; in its most common form it is called milk leg. There is marked swelling of the leg because of the block of the deep venous circulation, and the edematous white leg is called phlegmasia alba dolens. The entire lower extremity is swollen, pale and cold. This is the result of reflex arterial spasm and can in great measure be improved by lumbar sympathetic block. More extensive involvement of the venous system leads to a dusky purple discoloration of the skin associated with painful swelling. This condition, called phlegmasia cerulea dolens, is a much more serous manifestation, with gangrene as a potential sequela. Treatment, in addition to sympathetic block, is mainly with anticoagulant therapy, usu-

ally introduced by the use of heparin intravenously, either by continuous drip or intermittent injection. The clotting time is monitored with the objective of maintaining it at approximately twice normal. The activated partial thromboplastin time has generally supplanted the clotting time as a measure of heparin dosage.

Heparin is usually continued for 7 to 14 days following which one of the coumarin drugs is continued. Since at least 48 hours is necessary before a significant effect on the clotting mechanism is observed, whichever drug is selected is begun several days before heparin is to be discontinued. Stopping heparin abruptly may be followed by a rebound increase in clotting potential. For this reason the dose is gradually reduced over a 48 to 72 hour interval. The coumarin drugs are continued for a variable time, usually 3 months. The prothrombin time is used to adjust dosage and optimally is kept at twice normal. Dicumarol and coumarin are also used. They are given orally and require 24 to 48 hours for full therapeutic effect. The dosage of these drugs is adjusted by trying to keep the prothrombin time between 20 and 30 per cent of normal.

Phlebothrombosis. This is another type of intravascular clotting, seen most often following abdominal operations. It probably results from a slowing of the blood flow in the veins. It occurs without symptoms in the veins of the calf and the thigh. Often the first indication is pulmonary embolism. Careful examination may show calf tenderness, slight increase in calf diameter and calf pain on dorsiflexion of the foot (Homans' sign). Frequently all signs are absent. In this type of intravascular clotting there is a minimal reaction in the walls of the veins, and the clot is soft and loosely attached to the intima. It is complicated by pulmonary embolism, which is frequently the first manifestation of the process. The diagnosis of phlebothrombosis should be confirmed by venography.

In patients with suspected pulmonary embolism, further confirmation of the diagnosis should be obtained by isotopic injection and pulmonary scanning. The most certain means of diagnosis, however, is pulmonary angiography. Recurrent pulmonary embolism in a patient receiving adequate anticoagulant therapy is an indication for interruption of the inferior vena cava either by ligature or one of the techniques for narrowing the vena cava for the trapping of emboli. In the postpartum female both ovarian veins must also be ligated. Septic thrombophlebitis with embolization is an indication for complete interruption of the vena cava. Anticoagulant therapy also is given to prevent further intravascular clotting. It may be necessary for these patients to wear supporting stockings or bandages to prevent swelling when they are back on their feet.

A number of prophylactic measures have been shown to be effective in the prevention of clot formation in the veins following operation. They are elevation of the legs during and after operation, low-dose heparin therapy given subcutaneously and prophylactic use of the coumadin drugs. Early ambulation, relied upon by some, is not as effective for prophylaxis of thrombophlebitis as it is in improving respiratory mechanics. The exercise is also of nutritional help in attaining positive nitrogen balance.

Peripheral Arterial Disease

Arterosclerosis Obliterans. This is a degenerative disease occurring in older people, and in diabetics at a younger age. Its clinical manifestations are those of impaired arterial flow. In the muscles, intermittent claudication—pain on activity relieved by rest—constitutes the clinical picture. Impending gangrene, manifested by rest pain, rubor on dependency and extreme pallor on elevation, is another means of presentation. Atrophy of the distal fat pads on the plantar surface of the toes, loss of growth of hair, thin shiny skin and actual necrosis of the distal toes may all be seen. The onset may be gradual or abrupt. Arteriography is the most important method of study. Noninvasive methods are also useful. These include evaluation of the flow signal and determination of ankle blood pressure by means of doppler flowmetry and pulse volume recordings. Frequently segmental occlusion is seen. This may be correctable by direct surgical means. Bypass grafting, preferably using autologous veins, or short thromboendarterectomy yields good results. Anastamoses to increasingly small vessels are surprisingly effective in salvage of limbs. Lumbar sympathectomy is used in patients with signs of sympathetic overactivity—particularly excessive sweating—or in an effort to prevent gangrene of the skin. Arterial flow in muscle is not improved by sympathectomy.

Thromboangitis Obliterans (Buerger's Disease). There is considerable question as to whether this exists as a clinical and pathologic entity. As originally described, it is a syndrome in which there is hypersensitivity to tobacco, with venous and arterial spasm, followed by thrombosis. Its onset is in the third decade of life, and migratory venous thrombosis may be the first clinical manifestation. Involvement of middle-sized vessels and associated nerves by an inflammatory process is supposedly characteristic. Involvement of vessels in the upper extremities and viscera are end states. Complete avoidance of tobacco is the most important therapeutic measure. These patients should be studied by arteriography if gangrene threatens.

Raynaud's Disease. This is a vasospastic disease primarily of women, which usually involves the fingers, and is precipitated by cold and relieved by warmth. Frequently it is associated with scleroderma. Preganglionic sympathectomy may be used in treatment when loss of tissue threatens. Good results are frequently only temporary, and eventual recurrence is common, particularly when scleroderma is also present. In *Raynaud's phenomenon* both sexes are afflicted; frequently there is a predisposing factor such as the use of the typewriter or high-frequency vibratory tools. Vasospasm triggered by cold is also present in this condition. The results of sympathectomy are generally more favorable than in Raynaud's disease.

Peripheral Embolization. The breaking off of a thrombus on the myocardial wall or a valve may lead to its passing through the arterial circulation until it lodges in a vessel, depending on its size. Sudden obliteration of arterial flow to a part results in pain, pallor, anesthesia and, depending upon the extent of collateral circulation, gangrene. The level depends upon the point of occlusion of the arterial circulation, as well as upon the condition of the arterial bed with regard to primary degenerative changes. Immediate embolectomy is the treatment of choice, followed by anticoagulant therapy. Removal under local anesthesia is usually possible and Fogarty catheters (long plastic catheters with inflatable balloons of varying dimension) passed proximally and distally are valuable adjuncts in the complete removal of clots. Major arterial occlusion may occur without gangrene, but the end results are best when normal flow is restored. The temptation to treat such patients with sympathetic block and anticoagulation should be avoided.

Arteriovenous Fistula. This is a communication—usually traumatic in origin—between artery and vein, shunting arterial blood into the venous system, in which there is a lower pressure. It is evidenced clinically by swelling of the extremity, associated with the increased collateral circulation and a continuous bruit heard over the fistula. The cardiovascular effects often are severe. Increased blood volume, diminished pulse pressure, cardiac hypertrophy and locally increased venous pressure occur. Digital pressure over the fistula causes an increase in peripheral resistance, resulting in a temporary rise of blood pressure with a decrease in pulse rate. This is called Branham's sign. Modern treatment consists of the restoration of arterial flow by excision and grafting. Quadruple ligation after suitable collaterals have developed is of historic interest only.

Arterial Aneurysm. The most frequent type of aneurysm in civilians is the result of arteriosclerotic weakening of the wall. The vessels most frequently involved are the abdominal aorta below the renal arteries, the common iliacs, the femorals, and the popliteals. Aneurysms of the thoracic aorta are most frequently traumatic from deceleration tears in high-speed automobile accidents. Syphilitic aneurysms are still seen but are less common than prior to penicillin therapy for syphillis. Spontaneous rupture and occlusion are serious complications, and in most instances repair by resection and grafting is indicated. Traumatic aortic aneurysm is treated by excision and direct suture and when necessary by insertion of a prosthesis.

Frostbite

This injury results from prolonged exposure to cold. Depending on the degree of cold and the length of exposure, the damage may range from the most minimal superficial changes all the way to frank gangrene. Fingers, toes, hands, feet and ears are the common sites of involvement. Rapid warming of the frostbitten tissue using warm water (40 to 44° C) for a period sufficient to return the tissue temperature to normal is important. In minor degrees of frostbite, complete recovery will occur. However, in extensive injury gangrene may set in and require local amputation after demarcation has been established. Paresthesias may follow this injury. Sympathectomy early after severe frostbite will reduce the amount of tissue loss. When paresthesias are present, sympathetic block may give relief.

HAND

Paronychia

This is an infection between the nail and the eponychium usually caused by *Staphylococcus aureus.* It usually arises from a hangnail or from too vigorous manicuring. Elevation of the eponychium by incising it at the nail edge will drain a small abscess in the early stages. Infection can progress around the base of the nail between the eponychium and the nail, later extending underneath the nail to form a subungual abscess. The eponychium should be incised and turned back, and the base of the nail should be excised in order to provide adequate drainage.

Distal Closed Space Infection or Felon

An infection of the pulp of the palmar surface of the distal phalanx of the finger is very common. It usually arises from injury. Because of the anatomic characteristic of this space, a small infection rapidly may shut off the blood supply and lead to necrosis of the pulp and extension of the infection to the bone. To drain the abscess adequately, all of the septa between the dermis and the periosteum of the distal phalanx must be cut. Bilateral incisions may be necessary,

but through-and-through drains should be avoided. Bone involvement is treated conservatively and bone removed only if it is free in the abscess cavity.

Tenosynovitis of the Flexor Tendon Sheaths

Flexor tendon sheaths of the index, the middle, and the ring fingers end at the distal palmar crease, but those of the fifth finger and the thumb extend upward to the bursae at the wrist. Infection of these sheaths usually occurs as the result of injury and is characterized by pain, swelling and immobility of the finger. Early incision and drainage on the lateral sides of the finger are indicated if necrosis of the tendon is to be avoided. Infections of the fifth finger and the thumb spread to involve the radial and ulnar bursae. In postoperative care, splinting from the forearm to the fingertips, hot wet dressings and a synthetic penicillin not destroyed by penicillinase such as methicillin, oxacillin, or dicloxacillin are indicated.

Infections of the Palmar Spaces

The palmar spaces are hypothetical areas in the palm lying between the metacarpal bones and the overlying tendons and palmar fascia. They are infected by direct implantation or extension of infection from tenosynovitis or from infections along the lumbrical muscles arising under calluses at the distal part of the hand. The thenar space lies to the thumb side of the middle metacarpal, and the middle palmar space lies to the ulnar side. Infection of these spaces lies to the ulnar side. Infection of these spaces is characterized by swelling of the palm and marked swelling of the loose tissue of the dorsum of the hand. Drainage of the middle palmar space is obtained through the web between the middle and the fourth fingers. Drainage of the thenar space is through the web between the thumb and the index finger.

Mouth Wounds of the Hand

Frequently these wounds are sustained by a blow of the fist in which the teeth lacerate the skin, usually over the fingers or the knuckles. Anaerobic organisms are implanted in the contused lacerated wound. These give rise to an extensive, suppurative, destructive infection unless it is checked adequately. Treatment of these wounds, if seen early, should consist of thorough cleansing and debridement. The wound should not be closed; the part should be splinted, and prophylactic antibodies are advisable. If the infection is well established, vigorous antibiotic therapy is indicated, using drugs effective against both gram-positive and gram-negative organisms. However, in spite of this, gangrene may set in and necessitate amputation of a portion of the hand.

Treatment of Infections of the Fingers and Hand

In all the infections of the finger, the tendon sheaths and the palmar spaces, intensive antibiotic therapy may abort the infection if given early. Incision and drainage may be necessary only if the infection does not subside before suppuration takes place. Incision and drainage for infection of the major spaces should be done under general anesthesia using a tourniquet to ensure a bloodless field.

SHOULDER

Acute Subdeltoid Bursitis

This is a fairly common and very painful condition of the shoulder. It often follows moderate trauma, such as prolonged use of the arm in unaccustomed activities, but may occur without any history of such injury. A deposit of amorphous calcium soaps is found within the bursa when it is exposed at operation. Injuries to adjacent tendons—particularly the supraspinatus and long head of the biceps, followed by chronic tendonitis—are frequent associated lesions.

On roentgenographic examination, one may find evidence of calcium deposition in the region of the bursa. The acute pain may be relieved by infiltration of the area with a local anesthetic agent such as procaine. Injection of a corticosteroid is helpful in certain patients. Local heat and adequate sedation also are of value. Complete immobilization of the shoulder is undesirable, because fixation may result. This is especially likely to occur following repeated acute attacks in which the patient refuses to move the shoulder because of pain. In such cases it is necessary to carry out manipulation under anesthesia in order to break up the adhesions and permit return of function to the shoulder. At times excision of the calcified mass is necessary, but such areas may disappear spontaneously under treatment. X-ray therapy has been used in certain cases with satisfactory results. Indomethacin, aspirin or butazolidin for short periods in adequate dose may also be helpful.

In addition to the bursae about the shoulder, other sites may be involved, such as those over the olecranon process and the ischial tuberosity and beneath the Achilles tendon. Effusion into the prepatellar bursa is known as housemaid's knee.

AMPUTATIONS

Among the indications for amputation are extensive infection, gangrene and malignant tumor. It is indicated also in cases of extensive trauma with so much destruction of bone or soft tissues that preservation or conservation of the part is impracticable. On rare occasions, amputation is carried out as an elective procedure in order to improve the function of a part for cosmetic reasons, or to facilitate nursing care. Primary amputation is carried out early after injury when there is irreparable tissue damage or loss of viability. In selecting the site of amputation, in general one attempts to preserve as much of the extremity as possible. Considerations that alter this are the suitability of the level for fitting a functional prosthesis, resistance of the tissues at the stump to long-term trauma and cosmetic ones. In the upper extremity length is particularly important. At least 7.5 cm. of radius and ulna are necessary for a functioning prosthesis if the elbow joint is to be preserved, and a similar length of humerus is needed at the shoulder. Amputation through the flare of the humeral condyles should be avoided. Above all, however, if there is the possibility of salvage of anything resembling a functioning hand everything possible should be done to preserve it. In amputation of digits or portions of digits articular cartilage should be removed. Amputation through the carpus or tarsus is generally unsatisfactory.

In the lower extremity transmetatarsal amputation leaves a very satisfactory functioning foot. Weight-bearing stumps such as that left by the Syme's amputation at the ankle or the Gritti-Stokes at the knee are satisfactory. Amputations through the leg are best done at the junction of the upper and middle third. Amputation through the femur may be carried out at any site. Supracondylar amputation, which is largely tendinous, is particularly satisfactory, and a minimum of 5 cm. below the greater trochanter is necessary for satisfactory fitting of a lower limb. If a patient has had an amputation through the femur on one side every effort should be made to preserve the knee joint should amputation become necessary on the other side.

In diabetics conservative amputation is frequently possible. Either amputation of a toe or transmetatarsal amputation yields good functional results. When wet gangrene with systemic manifestations of sepsis is present, either in diabetics or patients with arteriosclerosis, refrigeration along with use of a tourniquet and antimicrobial therapy will permit control of sepsis. Thereafter, guillotine amputation with skin traction and secondary closure is the treatment of choice.

BURNS

Burns are classified according to their severity. First-degree burns involve only the superficial layers of the skin and are marked by erythema. Second-degree burns are somewhat deeper, and blisters or bullae develop.

In third-degree burns there is destruction of all layers of the skin, and a granulating surface results.

Mortality rate depends upon the age of the patient and the surface area involved, particularly in deep second- and third-degree burns. Large amounts of serum are lost to the body in the burn wound by exudation from the surface. Early mortality in burns is the result of burn shock. This is controlled by the replacement of lost extracellular fluid and electrolyte. At present we use a continuous infusion of lactated Ringer's solution and five per cent dextrose in water, adjusting the rate according to urinary output, hematocrit, pulse rate, blood pressure and state of consciousness. A minimal output of urine of 25 ml. per hour must be maintained.

The local treatment of the burn wound consists of gentle cleansing and debridement followed by the application of 0.5 per cent silver nitrate, Sulfamylon silver sulfadiazine (Silvadene) ointment. These agents have reduced the mortality rate from burn sepsis, particularly in patients with 30 to 50 per cent body surface burns.

First- and second-degree burns should be healed in a period of 10 to 14 days. Third-degree burns require skin grafting as soon as the surface is sufficiently free of necrotic tissue and infection. Burns of the face may involve the upper respiratory tract; tracheostomy and assisted respiration may be necessary in these cases.

FRACTURES AND DISLOCATIONS

Delayed Union or Nonunion of Fractures

Delayed union of a fracture is prolongation of healing beyond the time that normally would be required for union to occur at that particular site. Nonunion is indefinite delay in healing. Certain fracture sites are particularly likely to develop delay in union. Among these are fractures at the junction of the lower and the middle thirds of the tibia, the neck of the femur and the carpal scaphoid. Factors that contribute to delay in union include: inadequate reduction, for example, undue separation of the fragments or interposition of soft tissue; improper immobilization, which permits excessive movement; and poor blood supply. The position of the fracture relative to the point or points of entry of the nutrient artery and the extent of periosteal injury are both important in the development of delayed union or nonunion of fractures. Rarely, constitutional disease may contribute to delay in union.

Delayed union should be prevented insofar as possible by adequate reduction and fixation of the fragments at the time of the original injury. However, once it has been developed, delayed union may be managed by: (1) prolonged immobilization, such as in a carpal

scaphoid fracture; (2) application of splints that permit active use of the parts to improve the blood supply—for example, a walking caliper splint; (3) physiotherapy; (4) drilling of the fracture site; and (5) the use of bone grafts to bridge the fracture site.

UPPER EXTREMITIES

Clavicle

Fracture of this bone usually occurs at the junction of the middle and the outer thirds. The proximal fragment is drawn upward by the sternocleidomastoid muscle. The outer fragment is carried downward, inward and forward by the weight of the shoulder. The fracture is reduced by lifting the shoulder upward, outward and backward. It usually can be held in a satisfactory position by the use of a posterior figure-of-eight dressing of plaster or a posterior clavicular T splint. Delayed union or nonunion is almost unknown in this region. Immobolization for 4 weeks usually suffices.

Greenstick fractures are partial fractures without significant displacement and may be managed by the use of a Velpeau dressing or an axillary pad, a sling and a swathe dressing.

Humerus

Fractures of the Greater Tuberosity

This is a not infrequent complication following dislocation of the shoulder. Under any circumstances the displacement usually is not great, and satisfactory position may be obtained by the use of an axillary pad, a sling and swathe dressing or by use of an abduction splint.

Fracture of the Anatomic Neck

Fracture of the anatomic neck or of the lesser tuberosity of the humerus is uncommon. Prolonged immobilization of fractures of the upper end of the humerus is undesirable. Active and passive motion should be started after 10 days.

Fracture of the Surgical Neck

The upper fragment is abducted, and the lower fragment is drawn upward and inward into the axilla. At times, the fragments may be impacted with very little displacement. In contrast with dislocation of the shoulder, the contour of the shoulder is maintained because the humeral head is still in place. With adequate anesthesia, reduction usually can be accomplished by abduction of the arm, bringing the lower fragment outward to meet and engage the upper fragment. Following impaction of this sort, the arm may be brought partially down to the side. In some instances an axillary pad and a sling and swathe dressing may suffice for fixation, but the most frequently used method of treating stable fractures of the surgical neck of the humerus and humeral shaft is the so-called hanging cast. This consists of a plaster cast from the upper portion of the arm to the metacarpal heads. The elbow is at 90 degrees of flexion, and the forearm is in midposition with regard to pronation and supination. A supporting sling goes around the neck and is passed through a ring incorporated at the wrist. The long tendon of the biceps must be intact if this method of management is to be successful. The patient is instructed to keep the arm hanging freely as much of the time as possible. While he is in bed, about 2.25 kg. of traction is maintained through a second ring formed at the elbow. This method permits abduction and circumduction exercises relatively early, thereby preventing disabling shoulder stiffness.

Separation of the Upper Humeral Epiphysis

This injury results in a deformity similar to that of a fracture of the surgical neck of the humerus. Accurate reduction is necessary in order to minimize interference with growth of the bone. Following reduction of the separation, a dressing similar to that used for fracture of the surgical neck of the humerus is satisfactory.

Dislocation of the Shoulder

This injury usually follows acute abduction of the arm, with resultant tearing of the head of the humerus through the weak inferior portion of the capsule of the joint. The displaced head then comes to lie in the subglenoid position but rarely remains there. Instead, it is carried forward to lie in the subcoracoid position, which is the most common location for the head following dislocation in this region. More rarely the humerus may be displaced even further medially, and the head then occupies the subclavicular position. Posterior dislocation of the humerus is extremely rare and upward displacement almost unknown. Under adequate anesthesia this dislocation is reduced readily by either the Cooper or the Kocher method. In the Cooper method the foot is placed in the axilla, while gentle traction is maintained on the outstretched hand and forearm. Moderate adduction and internal and external rotation in association with traction usually result in prompt replacement of the dislocation. In the Kocher maneuver, the elbow is flexed to a right angle, and the humerus is rotated outward as far as possible. With external rotation maintained, the elbow is carried medially, and then the hand is brought to the point of the opposite shoulder. A Velpeau or axillary pad, a

sling and a swathe dressing provide adequate immobilization following reduction. After a week or 10 days a simple sling should suffice; however, abduction of the arm should be avoided for a period of 6 to 8 weeks.

Following initial dislocation of the shoulder, subsequent dislocations are much more likely to occur, and eventually dislocation may take place as the result of extremely minor trauma. Under such circumstances, an operative procedure to prevent such recurrence is desirable.

Fracture of the Shaft of the Humerus

This fracture may be complicated by radial nerve injury, inasmuch as the nerve follows a winding course about the shaft of the humerus. This injury is manifested by the presence of wristdrop. Following reduction of the fracture, a hanging plaster cast may be applied. Union usually is obtained in 6 to 8 weeks, though delayed union or nonunion of the shaft of the humerus occasionally results. An abduction cast or an intramedullary pin also may be used in the management of fractures of the shaft of the humerus.

Fractures of the Lower End of the Humerus

The most common fracture in this region is supracondylar. This occurs usually in children and results in posterior displacement of the distal fragment. Satisfactory reduction usually can be accomplished by flexing the elbow acutely and at the same time bringing the distal fragment forward into line with the upper. For older children, a lateral hyperflexion plaster dressing holding the arm in this position may be applied, provided that the radial pulse is not obliterated as the result of swelling. Volkmann's ischemic contracture is a dreaded complication of supracondylar fractures treated by acute flexion. If the radial pulse is weak or disappears the arm should be extended beyond 45 degrees, and as the swelling subsides it may be returned to acute flexion of 45 degrees or greater. It may be preferable to resort to traction. In young children, flexion of the elbow may be maintained by the use of Jones's position, in which the wrist is suspended by a short sling about the neck. In general, this dressing will be satisfactory for most fractures in the region of the lower end of the humerus, though occasionally displacement is such that open reduction will be necessary. Fractures in this region occasionally are associated with ossifying hematoma. This is the development of a calcified mass in the soft tissues as a result of calcium deposit in the hematoma. Bone formation may take place. As a rule, these ossifying hematomas tend to disappear gradually over a time.

Dislocations of the Elbow

Though anterior and lateral dislocations of the elbow may occur, the common deformity in this injury is that of posterior displacement. This is manifested by prominence of the olecranon posteriorly, loss of the lower humeral posterior concavity and fullness in the antecubital fossa. Reduction is accomplished under anesthesia by hyperextension and traction. Immobilization by means of an internal right-angle splint for 1 week, followed by use of a sling for another week or 10 days, should suffice.

Forearm

Fractures Through the Olecranon Fossa

These often are associated with sufficient displacement that results from pull of the triceps tendon, to necessitate open reduction. Otherwise, immobilization in moderate extension for a period of several weeks is required.

Fracture of the Head of the Radius

This is often associated with comminution and tearing of the orbicular ligament, so that the fragments lie either free in the joint or outside the orbicular ligament. Fractures of this type are treated best by excision of the head of the radius, though linear or compression fractures may be managed by simple immobilization for a few days, followed by guarded function. Other fractures of the radial head requiring operation are marginal fractures with displacement toward the elbow joint, fracture involving more than one-third of the articular surface of the radial head and fractures of the neck with angulation.

Fractures of the Shafts of the Radius and Ulna

Fracture of only one bone of the forearm usually may be reduced without undue difficulty, inasmuch as the other serves as a splint. However, fracture of both bones of the forearm with displacement sometimes presents a problem in reduction. Occasionally, open reduction must be restored to. Intraosseous pins frequently are employed to maintain reduction. Unless satisfactory reduction is obtained, the interosseous space may be narrowed, thus interfering with supination and pronation. Synostosis between the radius and ulna may also occur, similarly limiting function. The interosseous space can be preserved by applying padded board splints and incorporating them in the cast. Following reduction it is necessary to immobilize the hand, the wrist and the elbow in order to avoid loss of position.

Colles' Fracture

This is a fracture of the radius at the suprastyloid level that often is associated with a fracture of the styloid process of the ulna. This is an extremely common site of bone injury. It results from a fall on the outstretched hand. In the typical displacement there is a silver-fork deformity, the distal fragment of the radius being displaced upward and backward. The articular surface of the radius is displaced upward, and the interstyloid line lies at right angles to the forearm. Reduction usually is accomplished readily, and immobilization is maintained for 4 weeks with plaster splints or a cast. In dressing these cases, the wrist frequently is held in a position of moderate flexion and ulnar deviation. Reduction is deemed adequate when length is normal and the distal articular surface of the radius has regained palmar deflection.

Hand and Wrist

Fractures of the Carpal Bones

These injuries are not common. The only one of particular interest is that of the scaphoid. Frequently it is missed, inasmuch as there is no significant displacement, and roentgenographic examination often is not undertaken at the time of the initial injury. Instead, a diagnosis of sprain of the wrist is made, and the patient is treated for such an injury. Careful roentgenographic examination, including oblique views at the time of the accident, should reveal the nature of the injury. This is a common site for nonunion. Therefore, prolonged immobilization in a plaster cast for 12 weeks or more should be carried out, including immobilization of the proximal phalanx of the thumb and utilization of a small amount of radial deviation in order to impact the fragments.

Fractures of the Metacarpals

These usually result from a blow with a closed fist. Healing takes place readily, and satisfactory position can be obtained by pressure over the flexed proximal phalanx. Diagnosis in this injury usually can be made by the local tenderness at the fracture site and the presence of a dropped knuckle when the patient tries to make a fist.

Fractures of the Phalanges

Often these injuries are associated with insignificant displacement and are treated readily for both conditions by simple immobilization with a tongue depressor, a hairpin or a plaster splint. However, the displacement occasionally is such that a satisfactory position is obtained only by elastic or spring traction utilizing a banjo splint.

Dislocation at the metacarpophalangeal or the interphalangeal joints is quite evident on physical examination. Usually, reduction is accomplished readily, and immobilization by means of a hairpin or tongue depressor splint for a period of a week to 10 days should suffice.

VERTEBRAL COLUMN

The usual injury to the vertebral column results from forcible flexion of the spine, such as may result from a fall from a height, jolting of the patient while riding in a car, and so on. The region most commonly involved is the lumbar or lower thoracic spine. As a rule, there is no cord damage, and the patient's only complaint is of pain. On examination there are tenderness and localized muscle spasm. However, the diagnosis must be made by roentgenographic studies, and lateral views of the spine especially demonstrate the compression deformity of the vertebral body. The treatment consists of rest in bed for 2 to 3 weeks followed by ambulation, with the patient wearing a back brace for support until the fracture is stable. Hyperextension, previously used, requires a long period of disability and does not give better results than the simpler method of management. Occasionally the articular facets also are damaged, and fracture-dislocation results. This is a much more serious injury and frequently is associated with damage to the cord which is likely to be permanent. Cord damage is evidenced by findings on neurologic examination and the presence of bloody spinal fluid, associated at times with evidence of block. Prompt reduction of the fracture-dislocation is necessary in order to minimize the damage to the nervous system. Operative treatment may be necessary in order to accomplish this. In the lower spine, extension may be obtained by the application of traction to the lower extremities. In the cervical region, extension may be obtained by the use of traction through the skull. In either circumstance it must be prolonged, and, even after the patient is allowed out of bed, partial immobilization is necessary for several months, either by means of a neck or a back brace, as the case may be.

In patients who have sustained head injuries from automobile accidents or falls from a height, fracture of the cervical spine should be suspected until excluded by satisfactory roentgenograms. The head and neck should be immediately immobilized with sandbags until roentgenograms have been reviewed.

Fracture of the Coccyx

This is a rare injury, and only gross deformity requires correction. Often healing—whether by bony or by fibrous union—will be satisfactory, but occasionally pain persists. In these circumstances, excision of the coccyx is justified, inasmuch as this bone serves no useful purpose.

Herniated Nucleus Pulposus

This injury may follow a fall or attempts at lifting heavy objects. There is pain in the back with radiation down the leg, usually along the course of the sciatic nerve. The reflexes are altered, and sensory impairment can be elicited. The pain is produced by pressure of the herniated cartilaginous disk on the spinal nerves. Roentgenographic examination, including myelography, will demonstrate the herniated disk.

Treatment has consisted of conservative management by bed rest and traction on the lower extremities, or of operative removal of the herniated disk.

PELVIS

Fractures of the pelvis result from a fall from a height, a direct blow or a crushing injury. Common sites for fracture of the pelvis include the symphysis and the rami of the pubis and the ischium. These may be bilateral, and, in addition, there may be fractures of the sacrum and the ilium. In general, no marked displacement is evident, though pressure over the greatest trochanters or the crests of the ilia is likely to give rise to pain at the fracture site. The diagnosis must be made by roentgenographic examination. The amount of displacement usually is not great, and satisfactory union results. Not infrequently there are soft-tissue injuries of serious degree. The most common of these is a tear of the bladder or the urethra. This is manifested by inability to void or by the passage of bloody urine. A tear of the bladder may be demonstrated by instillation of sterile salt solution through a catheter and subsequent inability to recover all this fluid, or by instillation of a radiopaque solution such as sodium iodide and x-ray demonstration of the extravasation. A tear of the bladder must be repaired promptly by operative means. A tear of the urethra may be managed by the use of an indwelling catheter—either alone or associated with a suprapubic cystostomy. Tears of the vagina and the rectum are less common. Fractures of the pelvis should be managed by bed rest for 6 to 8 weeks. Approximation of the fragments may be maintained by the use of a tight binder or sling.

LOWER EXTREMITIES

Femur

Fracture of the Neck of the Femur

This usually occurs in elderly persons. It is a common site for nonunion, and even after apparently satisfactory union has occurred, aseptic necrosis of the head of the femur may develop. The diagnosis is suspected on the basis of the history and physical examination and confirmed by roentgenograms. The history usually is that of a fall in an elderly person who subsequently is unable to rise. The lower extremity is externally rotated, abducted and the heel cannot be lifted from the bed. Shortening may be obvious on inspection, or it may be slight and only demonstrated by measurement. In impacted fractures the patient may be able to walk, the posture may be normal, and the heel may be lifted from the bed. The degree of displacement is important with respect to the frequency of avascular necrosis and consequently, to treatment.

In the usual case the greater trochanter will lie above Nelaton's line (a line drawn from the anterior superior spine of the ilium to the ischial tuberosity). There is also shortening of the horizontal line of Bryant's triangle. (This triangle is formed by one line projecting downward from the anterior-superior spine of the ilium perpendicular to the table. The second side is formed by a line passing from the anterior-superior iliac spine to the greater trochanter. The third side is a line joining the first two at the level of the table.) Since this fracture occurs in the elderly, death frequently results from intercurrent infection, such as brochopneumonia. For this reason, older methods of treatment, such as the application of an abduction plaster cast or the use of balanced traction, have been displaced by internal fixation after adequate reduction. In some older patients immediate resection of the femoral head and neck with insertion of a prosthesis may be indicated.

Intertrochanteric Fracture of the Femur

This occurs frequently in the elderly from a direct fall on the hip. The blood supply is excellent and delayed or nonunion is almost unknown. The fracture is unstable with considerable shortening and external rotation. The fracture should be reduced under anesthesia with fixation by means of a nail and plate such as the Jewett blade plate.

Dislocations of the Hip

These are uncommon. The displacement of the head of the femur may be either anterior or posterior to the acetabulum. The latter is the more common deformity. In this injury the patient lies with the knee and the hip flexed and the leg rotated internally, so that the affected extremity overlies the normal side. There is apparent shortening, and the foot on the involved side rests on the opposite instep. Occasionally there is sciatic nerve injury.

In anterior dislocations the extremity is abducted and rotated externally. The head of the femur is palpable in the groin. As a rule, the deformity in either condition is reduced readily under adequate anesthesia. The knee is flexed, as is also the hip. With traction in this position, and with internal and external rotation, abduction and adduction, the head of the femur usually returns readily to the acetabulum (methods of Bigelow and Allis). In posterior dislocations of the hip, the deformity at times may be reduced without anesthesia by placing the patient prone on a table with the thighs extending over the edge at right angles. The knee on the affected side is flexed. The weight is applied to the calf. As the muscles gradually tire, spontaneous reduction may occur.

Following reduction of a dislocation of the hip, the patient should be kept in bed for a period of 2 to 3 weeks. The ankles may be strapped loosely together during this time, or simple Buck's extension may be applied to the involved extremity. Weightbearing may be begun after this time if extreme range of motion is not undertaken. Prolonged followup is indicated because of the possible occurrence of avascular necrosis of the head of the femur and of arthritis.

Congenital Dislocation of the Hip

This deformity occurs much more frequently in the female than in the male. It may not be recognized until the age of about 1 year, because the first symptom is a limp when the child starts to walk. It may be a bilateral deformity. There is shortening of the extremity as shown by the displacement of the greater trochanter above Nelaton's line. On roentgenographic examination the head of the femur may be deficient, and the acetabulum may be malformed. Treatment should be begun as early as possible. Initially, reduction may be obtained under anesthesia. Then the child is dressed in a wide abduction plaster cast for a period of many months. If closed reduction is unsatisfactory, operative therapy is indicated. If conservative treatment is unsatisfactory, some form of reconstruction ultimately must be undertaken.

Fracture of the Shaft of the Femur

This fracture may occur anywhere in the shaft and may be transverse, spiral, or comminuted. The principal deformity is one of shortening and angulation. In most cases, satisfactory reduction can be obtained and the definitive treatment carried out by the use of balanced traction (Russell). Either skin or skeletal traction may be used. In the latter, a Thomas or a Hodgen splint with a Pierson attachment may be used. Alternate forms of treatment consist of closed reduction and immobilization by means of a plaster spica, or open reduction and internal fixation by means of a bone plate or by intramedullary nail.

In supracondylar fractures of the femur the distal

fragment is displaced posteriorly and may damage the vessels and the nerves in this region to such an extent that vascular occlusion and gangrene set in. In order to accomplish reduction of the fracture in this area, the hip and knee must be well flexed. Though the actual progress of healing must be followed by repeated roentgenologic examinations, one should anticipate a period of immobilization of 8 to 12 weeks.

Patella

Fracture of the patella may be either transverse or comminuted. In either event, the bony injury is associated with a tear of the quadriceps tendon. For this reason, open reduction with repair of the laceration and approximation of the fragments is necessary, unless the roentgen films show no significant displacement of the fragments and the power of extension of the extremity is maintained. In badly comminuted fractures, excision of the patella fragments and tendon suture give good results. Following operation, the knee should be immobilized for about 6 weeks in plaster in almost complete extension, though weight bearing may be begun after 4 weeks.

Knee

Injuries to the knee joint are of particular interest to surgeons responsible for the care of athletic teams. Football players are especially liable to incur serious injuries to the knee joint. Injuries to the collateral ligaments of the knee, particularly the medial collateral ligament, are the most frequently seen major injury. They may occur alone or in combination with injuries of the semilunar cartilages or the cruciate ligaments. Early repair of major injuries of the knee is an important new concept, which has reduced the disability incident to these injuries. Early exercise of the muscles around the knee joint also contributes to the lessened disability.

Injuries of the menisci can be evaluated by arthrography, in which air and an absorbable contrast media are injected into the joint. Arthroscopy is also useful for evaluating tears of the menisci as well as of the cruciate ligaments.

Tibia

A common site for fracture of the tibia is at the junction of the lower and the middle thrids. Frequently, there is an associated fracture of the fibula, though this may occur at a different level. Because of the subcutaneous position of the tiba in this region, compounding is seen frequently. Under fluoroscopic guidance and with adequate anesthesia, satisfactory reduction usually can be obtained and the position maintained by means of plaster splints or a plaster cast extending from the toes to the upper thigh. Occasionally it may be necessary to resort to open reduction and internal fixation by means of a bone plate or an intramedullary pin.

This is a common site for delayed union, but ultimate union is to be anticipated. If adequate healing has not taken place after 8 to 12 weeks, a walking caliper splint should be used.

Fractures of the upper portion of the tibia may extend into the joint (plateau fracture) with downward displacement of a portion of the weight-bearing surface. This may be associated with a fracture of the head or the neck of the fibula. If there is no displacement in a plateau fracture of the tibia, the injury may be treated by immobilization in plaster. If there is displacement of the joint surface, open reduction and internal fixation may be necessary in order to obtain a satisfactory weight-bearing-surface. Fractures of the upper portion of the fibula occasionally are associated with foot drop as a result of damage to the peroneal nerve as it curves about the neck of the fibula.

Ankle

Pott's Fracture

This is a common fracture in the region of the ankle, with the foot in eversion and abduction. As a result the internal malleolus is torn off, and the fibula is fractured, usually at a level somewhat above the external malleolus. Lateral displacement of the foot results. This is known as bimalleolar fracture. Occasionally the posterior lip of the tibia is also torn away, resulting in a trimalleolar fracture with posterior displacement of the foot. Swelling is marked in this injury, and the deformity is evident. The bone injury may be confirmed by roentgenologic examination. Prompt reduction is desirable. Satisfactory position ordinarily can be obtained by closed reduction after anesthesia. It is desirable to achieve anatomic reduction in oder to completely correct the displacement. Immobilization in plaster for 6 to 8 weeks is required. It may be necessary to resort to internal fixation of the fracture in order to obtain satisfactory reduction, including replacement of the separation of the distal tibia and fibula.

A *sprain* is a more common injury in the region of the ankle. However, this normally results from inversion of the foot. There is no bony deformity, and the tenderness lies in the region of the ligaments that are injured, usually below, and anterior to, the external malleolus.

If fractures of the lower portion of the lower extremity are well reduced and adequately immobilized by plaster, a walking iron may be incorporated in the cast to permit weight bearing during the period of healing. This minimizes the disability and promotes healing.

Os Calcis

Fracture of the os calcis results from a fall from a height, the individual landing on his feet and suffering a crushing injury of the os calcis. Comminution is frequent, and there is flattening of the bone with decrease in Böhler's angle. Böhlers angle is the angle formed by the axis of the subtalar joint and the superior surface of the tuberosity. Accurate reduction of these fractures is extremely difficult and often impossible. With minimal displacement, simple immobilization for several weeks should suffice. However, if there is marked flattening of the os calcis, skeletal traction through the posterior and inferior fragment may be necessary in order to improve the position.

JOINT REPLACEMENT

Prosthetic joints have been developed to replace interphalangeal joints, metacarpophalangeal joints, the hip joint, knee joint and scapulohumeral joint. The usual indications are avascular necrosis and rhematoid arthritis. Considerable rehabilation has been accomplished with these measures in patients otherwise incapacitated by their joint disease.

SOFT TISSUE SARCOMAS

These tumors present challenging problems in diagnosis and treatment. Most of them arise in areas in which early diagnosis and treatment should be simple. Despite this they are frequently large and have been present for months before the patient seeks medical advice. In some instances, that advice is poor, in that simple reassurances is offered on the fallacious assumption that a given lump is a lipoma or some other innocent lesion. Obviously at some point in their clinical evolution all soft tissue sarcomas should be curable by wide local excision. Nevertheless, the curability rate in many histologic types is low, and amputational surgery is necessary for local control of the growth. The end results of treatment depend on (1) the "biologic potential" of the tumor in terms of its speed of growth and capacity to invade blood vessels and thereby to metastasize to distant sites; (2) resistance of the host; (3) the anatomic site of occurrence; (4) the type and

adequacy of treatment. The only clue to the biologic potential of a given soft tissue sarcoma is in its histology. It is therefore most important to assess this by preliminary biopsy, before the method of treatment is decided upon.

Because soft tissue sarcomas grow expansively they are surrounded by an adventitious capsule, which is never complete. The temptation to remove these growths by "shelling them out" is great. This never constitutes adequate removal, which minimally consists of the removal of surrounding normal structures in such a way that the growth is not seen during the course of its removal. The influence of the anatomic site of origin on curability is great, particularly for lesions of the extremities. If a highly malignant tumor encroaches on the blood and nerve supply of an extremity, the need for amputation is quite evident. A similar tumor that arises in the lateral thigh might well be locally excised with surrounding normal muscle, leaving a functional extremity. Lesions on the trunk obviously must be locally excised, with as adequate a margin as possible. The decision as to proper therapy in a given soft tissue sarcoma, then, is a synthesis of knowledge of pathology and of anatomy.

These tumors arise from the mesenchymal supporting tissues. Exact classification may be difficult, but an expert tumor pathologist can usually provide the surgeon with a reasonable assessment of the biologic aggressiveness of a given sarcoma: (1) Fibrosarcoma—extreme variability in the degree of malignancy, metastasizes infrequently to lymph nodes, radioresistant. (2) Malignant fibrous histiocytoma—many of the previously unclassified soft tissue sarcomas and anaplastic fibrosarcomas fall into this group. The growth pattern is variable as is the degree of malignancy. Metastasis to lymph nodes is infrequent. (3) Liposarcoma—also variable in behavior; is frequently moderately radiosensitive. (4) Synovial sarcoma—arises in the region of joints, but direct connection to synovial membrane is infrequent. In children its behavior is more benign than in adults. This type metastasizes to regional lymph nodes with greater frequency than other sarcomas. (5) Rhabdomyosarcoma—embryonal form in children may respond to combined surgical removal and chemotherapy (Vincristine). In adults it is highly malignant. (6) Malignant schwannoma—tumor of nerve sheath origin, seen alone or in patients with von Recklinghausen's disease. Local persistence following removal is frequent; metastases to lungs is usually late. (7) Kaposi's sarcoma—of vascular origin, it is frequently multicentric. Individual lesions can be controlled with radiotherapy or surgical excision.

The cure rate of embryonal rhabdomyosarcoma of childhood has been greatly increased by the combined use of surgery, radiation therapy and chemotherapy. As a result other soft tissue sarcomas are being treated by multimodal therapy in an effort to increase the cure rate and to avoid amputation in some lesions of the extremities. High dose radiation therapy alone is also in use.

EAR

Meniere's Syndrome

This is characterized by attacks of vertigo, nausea and vomiting, along with progressive loss of hearing and tinnitus in one ear. Occasionally the opposite ear becomes involved. The underlying pathology consists of hydrops of the vestibular and cochlear labyrinth. It should be differentiated from other causes of vertigo, particularly those cases that arise from decreased blood flow in the basilar artery.

Facial Nerve Paralysis

Facial nerve paralysis is the result of (1) exposure to cold; (2) direct extension from acute or chronic otitis media; (3) operative trauma (more common in radical mastoidectomy); and (4) a lesion of the central nervous system. When it is caused by the last-mentioned condition, the patient ordinarily can close the eye and wrinkle the brow on the affected side, and there is no change in the sense of taste, because the chorda tympani nerve is not involved.

Peripheral facial nerve lesions (Bell's palsy) produce marked facial muscle paralysis on the side of the lesion, loss of sense of taste and lesions of the eye because of inability to close the lids on the involved side.

SALIVARY GLANDS

The major salivary glands include the parotid, submaxillary and sublingual glands. Minor salivary glands are distributed throughout the submucosa of the buccal mucous membrane and tongue.

Suppurative infection involves primarily the parotid; it is caused by staphylococci and occurs in dehydrated, debilitated patients. Treatment consists primarily of the synthetic penicillin drugs, to which nearly all staphylococci are sensitive. If suppuration occurs, incision and drainage are necessary.

In Sjögren's syndrome, enlargement of the parotid gland results from lymphocytic infiltration. This must be differentiated from the congenital anomaly (frequently misclassified as a neoplasm) papillary cystadenoma lymphomatosum. Primary lymphosarcoma occurs but is unusual.

Primary tumors are seen in both major and minor salivary glands. Pleomorphic adenoma (mixed tumor) is the most frequent variety. It is essentially a benign lesion that persists locally after inadequate removal. In five per cent of cases mixed tumors are malignant. The mucoepidermoid tumors are malignant but may be very low grade and therefore quite curable by surgical removal. The cylindromatous variant of adenocarcinoma is a distinctive tumor with a long clinical course. It characteristically invades nerve sheaths, and for this reason local recurrence after surgical removal is the rule. Poorly differentiated adenocarcinoma, epidermoid carcinoma and undifferentiated carcinoma all occur; they are generally of high malignancy and infrequently cured.

THROAT

Vincent's Angina (Trench Mouth)

This is caused by two organisms—a spirochete and a fusiform bacillus. It is characterized by one or more painful ulcers, usually found on the tonsils, the gums, the faucial pillars, the buccal membrane of the cheeks and the pharyngeal wall. These ulcers are undermined, have sharp irregular edges and bleed easily. If they are present on the gums, pyorrhea results. The diagnosis depends on the foregoing clinical picture and on the finding of the two organisms on a smear obtained from the ulcer. Treatment consists of perborate gargles, penicillin or five per cent neoarsphenamine in glycerin applied directly to the ulcer. Penicillin lozenges are of value.

Peritonsillar Abscess (Quinsy)

An infection of the peritonsillar tissues with abscess formation, peritonsillar abscess is more common in adults than in children. Symptoms are (1) pain, usually radiating to the ear of the affected side; (2) fever; (3) malaise; and (4) great difficulty in swallowing. Examination reveals swelling or bulging of the tonsil and the soft palate and cervical adenitis. Treatment consists of incision and drainage of the abscess when it is pointing. Hot saline throat irrigations are helpful before and after incision. The incision should be made at the junction of an imaginary line along the free border of the anterior pillar at its most bulging point and at another line along the free edge of the soft palate.

Ludwig's Angina

This is an acute inflammatory process involving the cellular tissues of the floor of the mouth and the submaxillary region of one or both sides of the neck. Symptoms include pain in the floor of the mouth, difficulty in swallowing and talking, and excessive salivation. The tongue is elevated, and there is brawny induration beneath the jaw. Dyspnea and edema of the glottis may necessitate tracheotomy. Treatment consists of bed rest, intravenous fluids, chemotherapy—preferably penicillin in large doses—and incision and drainage when indicated.

Retropharyngeal Abscess

An accumulation of pus between the posterior wall of the pharynx and the vertebral column, retropharyngeal abscess is most common in young children. The staphylococcus is the microorganism usually found in cultures of the abscess. Signs of general sepsis are present, with local symptoms of dysphagia, dyspnea, aphonia, cough and regurgitation. The head is in an extended position, and the mouth is open. Palpation reveals a soft fluctuant swelling of the posterior pharynx that occasionally is palpable at the sides of the neck. Unless prompt diagnosis is made and treatment instituted, the prognosis is grave.

NECK

Branchiogenic Cysts

These arise from embryonic remnants of the branchial clefts. Although they may appear in childhood, they are more frequently seen after puberty and may first be evident in the fifth and sixth decades of life. They arise anterior to the sternocleidomastoid muscle, although the highest ones arise anterior to the tragus of the ear. Treatment of these cysts consists of complete excision. If they become secondarily infected, or are incompletely drained or removed, a fistula will develop.

Thyroglossal Cysts

Congenital cysts that arise in the midline of the neck as a cystic remnant of the thyroglossal duct, these cysts may be seen in the region extending from the suprasternal area to the suprahyoid area. Remnants of thyroid tissue are frequently present. The cysts are lined by stratified squamous, pseudostratified columnar or ciliated columnar epithelium. Lymphoid tissue is also usually prominent. The thyroglossal duct originates in the foramen cecum at the base of the tongue and frequently passes through the hyoid bone. For this reason a portion of the midline of the hyoid bone should be excised.

Lymph Node Enlargements in the Neck

In former years tuberculosis lymphadenitis was the most frequent cause of enlarged cervical lymph nodes. Since the compulsory pasteurization of milk and the destruction of tuberculous herds, this is no longer so. In childhood, lymphadenitis related to regional infection in tonsils, gums or middle ear is most frequent. In girls in the late teens to twenties, metastatic carcinoma from the thyroid is the most likely explanation for persistent cervical lymph node enlargement. In middle-aged and older males metastatic carcinoma from the upper digestive or respiratory tract is common.

Malignant lymphoma including *Hodgkin's disease* is an additional cause of lymph node enlargement. The staging of Hodgkin's disease is important in deciding upon the correct course of therapy. Lymphography and abdominal exploration are the methods whereby staging is accomplished. Splenectomy, liver biopsy and lymph node biopsy of the most suspicious periaortic nodes on lymphography are the basis for histologic grading. In women the ovaries and tubes should be mobilized and transposed behind the uterus. Radiation therapy in adequate dosage is now known to be curative in early stages, whereas combination chemotherapy is of considerable value in systemic disease.

ORAL CAVITY

Carcinoma of the Tongue

Found predominantly in the male, carcinoma of the tongue usually is of the squamous cell type and occurs along the edges. These lesions present as ulcerating infiltrating areas, often with palpable metastatic involvement of the regional cervical lymph nodes at the time that patient is first seen. Predisposing factors in the development of carcinoma of the tongue include chronic irritation from poor dental care, poorly fitted dental plates, chronic inflammation, pipe smoking, leukoplakia and syphilis.

Surgical excision is recommended for small lesions that occupy the anterior third of the tongue. If cervical lymph nodes are suspiciously enlarged, combined jaw-neck resection should be done. For larger cancers and lesions that involve the posterior third of the tongue, radiation therapy is usually indicated.

Carcinoma of Buccal Mucosa

Squamous cell carcinoma arising from the buccal mucosa is treated by wide local removal. If lymph nodes are clinically involved, combined resection of the primary lesion and radical neck dissection is indicated. A variant known as verrucous carcinoma, seen in tobacco chewers, seldom metastasizes, but it may extend entirely through the cheek to the skin surface.

Carcinoma of Floor of the Mouth

Carcinoma in this area frequently requires resection of both mandibular rami if surgical treatment is elected. Primary reconstruction should be performed to avoid the crippling deformity that may otherwise result. Lymph nodes metastases are frequent in this anatomic site of origin, and when clinical evidence of lymph node involvement is present, primary surgical treatment is indicated.

Gingival Carcinoma

Either primary surgical resection or radiation therapy with a supervoltage source is indicated for gingival carcinoma, again depending to a great extent on the status of the regional lymph nodes.

Cancer of the Lips

On the lower lip any sore that does not promptly heal should be considered squamous cell cancer until proven otherwise by biopsy. On the upper lip the usual malignant lesion is basal cell carcinoma. Metastases from squamous cell carcinoma of the lower lip to regional lymph nodes occur in approximately 10 per cent of cases. For this reason elective node dissection is not indicated. The curability of squamous cell carcinoma is high, even when lymph node metastases exist. For lesions that require sacrifice of most of the lower lip along with extensive reconstruction, primary radiation therapy should be elected instead of surgery.

Larynx

Overuse of the voice may result in development of fibrotic nodules, which cause hoarseness, on the vocal cords. Epidemiologically the use of tobacco and alcohol is associated with the development of squamous cell carcinoma of the larynx. These tumors are classified according to the exact site and extent of involvement along with the status of the regional nodes. Cancer limited to the vocal cord with continued mobility of the cord is curable in over 90 per cent of cases by radiation therapy. More extensive lesions are treated by partial or total larynegectomy. Whether or not neck dissection is done depends on the exact anatomic area of involvement as well as the clinical status of the lymph nodes.

NOSE

Sinusitis

The paranasal sinuses may be involved in an acute or chronic infectious or allergic process or by neoplasia. Acute or chronic infectious processes are the most common forms, and the symptoms vary according to the sinus or group of sinuses involved. Headache or periodic pain and nasal discharge are the usual complaints. Suppurative sinusitis may arise (1) as a complication of the common cold; (2) from infected water that enters a sinus of a swimmer; (3) from obstruction to the sinus ostia by intranasal foreign bodies, polyps, neoplasms or a deviated septum; (4) from an infected tooth; and (5) from rapid changes in barometric pressure, as in an aerosinusitis. One or all the sinuses may be involved.

The diagnosis is made by (1) inspection and palpation, which may reveal swelling and tenderness over the involved sinus; (2) intranasal examination, which may reveal pus in the middle meatus if the anterior sinuses (frontal, maxillary and anterior ethmoid) are involved or in the sphenoethmoid recess if the posterior sinuses (posterior ethmoids and sphenoids) are involved; (3) transillumination; (4) roentgenologic examination; and (5) diagnostic puncture of a maxillary sinus.

Treatment of acute suppurative sinusitis should be conservative and should consist of (1) vasoconstrictors, which improve ventilation and promote drainage; (2) heat applied to the involved sinus; (3) analgesics; (4) forcing of fluids; and (5) chemotherapy if the attack is severe. Maxillary sinus irrigation is reserved for those cases that are in the subacute or the chronic stage. Operative procedures should not be done until conservative therapy has been given a trial.

THYROID

Goiters may be nodular or diffuse and toxic or nontoxic. The most common is the diffuse nontoxic gland caused by iodine deficiency that occurs in endemic goiter belts. With the public acceptance of iodized table salt, the incidence of iodine deficiency in these areas has been decreased greatly. Such glands are removed only when pressure symptoms appear or for cosmetic reasons.

Nodular goiters usually are removed because of the significant incidence of carcinoma in such glands. Carcinoma occurs in from 10 to 20 per cent of solitary nodules.

Nontoxic goiters produce pressure symptoms because of their size, causing dyspnea, hoarseness, dysphagia and disfigurement. Toxic goiters are characterized by overproduction of thyroxine, and the symptoms are nervousness, sweating, tremor, loss of weight, exophthalmos and an increase of body metabolism.

The functional status of the thyroid gland is elevated

by determination of the plasma level of thyroxine (T_4), the triiodothyronine (T_3), uptake of red blood cells, or the ^{131}I uptake.

Patients with diffuse toxic goiter (Graves' disease) are treated by subtotal thyroidectomy, prolonged use of antithyroid drugs or with ^{131}I. The decision is based on the age of the patient and the preference of the physician. Generally in patients under 35 years of age ^{131}I should be avoided. Patients to be operated upon should be restored to a euthyroid state by the use of antithyroid drugs such as propylthiouracil in adequate dosage. Iodine, as potassium iodide or Lugol's solution, is given for 10 to 14 days before operation. The procedure used today is subtotal thyroidectomy. Some patients are treated with propylthiouracil for 1 to 2 years in the hope that a permanent remission will result. The recurrence rate is 30 to 40 per cent. Therapeutic use of radioactive iodine is reserved for patients over 35 years of age. Fear of the development of thyroid cancer is the reason for avoiding radioactive iodine therapy in the young, however, there are no published reports of the development of thyroid cancer in the patients treated for hyperthyroidism with ^{131}I.

Carcinoma of the thyroid is treated by total thyroidectomy and radical neck dissection if the nodes are clinically involved. Radioactive iodine has proved to be of benefit after total thyroidectomy.

Thyroiditis

This rather obscure group of nonspecific inflammations of the thyroid is encountered occasionally by the surgeon. Hashimoto's disease, or struma lymphomatosa, signifies a firm gland infiltrated with lymphocytes. The process is usually seen in middle-aged women; it is bilateral and associated with reduced thyroid function. The titer of autoantibodies to thyroglobulin is usually high in Hashimoto's disease. Riedel's struma is an unusual process that consists of a woody, hard fibrosis involving the surrounding muscles as well as the thyroid. Subacute granulomatous thyroiditis is frequently made manifest by acute pain in the lower neck, dysphagia, etc. Frequently it can be dramatically improved by corticosteroid therapy. Thyroidectomy sometimes is necessary to relieve pressure symptoms or to exclude malignancy.

PARATHYROIDS

Parathormone has a dual function; first, it mobilizes calcium from bone; second, it increases renal tubular excretion of phosphate. Excessive parathormone secretion is seen in hyperplasia of the parathyroid glands and in functioning tumors. Benign adenoma greatly exceeds carcinoma in frequency. Clinically, two clinical pictures are produced by parathormone excess. Most frequent is renal calculus formation or nephrocalcinosis. The second is osteitis fibrosa cystica (von Recklinghausen's disease of bone). Frequently seen today are examples of parathormone excess without clinical manifestations, diagnosed by the increased serum calcium concentrations found on routine screening study. Duodenal ulcer and pancreatitis are also seen with parathormone excess. Primary hyperparathyroidism is usually caused by an adenoma, but hyperplasia may also be causative. Differentiation between the two may be difficult. Secondary hyperparathyroidism is caused by renal failure.

Hypoparathyroidism is seen either as a congenital process or, more commonly, as a complication of operations on the thyroid gland. It is manifested early by paresthesias of the lips and digits. There may be signs of increased neuromuscular excitability (positive Chvostek's or Trousseau's sign) and frank tetany. Tetany is due to hypocalcemia, resulting from hypophosphaturia and hyperphosphatemia. Treatment consists of vitamin D and a high calcium diet. Dihydrotachysterol (A.T. 10), which possesses the properties of both vitamin D and parathormone, is reserved for prolonged cases. Parathormone may be used for brief periods.

THE BREAST

Examination

Examination of the breasts should be conducted in a well-lighted room with the assistance of a chaperone. Inspection in the sitting position may demonstrate subtle changes that may be significant, such as irregularities in contour, changes in the configuration or axis of the nipple or dimpling of the skin. These may be further accentuated by having the patient raise her arms over her head, bend forward with the hands supported or contract the pectoral muscles. Palpation should be conducted with the side to be examined elevated by a pillow, feeling the breast tissue against the chest wall. The patient should be instructed in self examination, which should be done once a month preferably at the end of the menstrual period.

Mammography and xeroradiography are screening techniques of value in demonstrating some early cancers of the breast. Based on the increased frequency of breast cancer in woman survivors of the atomic bombing of Hiroshima, and the increased frequency of breast cancer in women with pulmonary tuberculosis who had repeated fluoroscopic examinations of the chest, as well as in theoretical models, mammography and xeroradiography have been used in more restricted manner than formerly. Routine screening is now advised only in women age 50 or older. Younger women should have mammography only when they have one or more factors increasing their risk of breast cancer. These "risk factors" include, in decreasing order of importance, cancer of one breast; a family history of breast cancer in siblings or on the maternal side of the family, the presence of fibrocystic disease or nodular breasts, nulliparity, first pregnancy after age 30, and early menarche.

Fibroadenoma of the Breast

This is a benign tumor, usually occurring in a girl in her late teens or twenties. It manifests itself by the appearance of a solitary lump in the breast, usually associated with little or no discomfort. The tumor appears to be well encapsulated, freely movable and not attached to the skin and the subcutaneous tissue. Treatment consists of simple excision of the tumor. Complete removal is not followed by recurrence.

Chronic Cystic Mastitis

This is an extremely common condition, appearing usually in the late 20s, 30s, or 40s. The symptoms tend to subside after the onset of menopause. Women with cystic disease are likely to complain of discomfort in the breast bilaterally, especially around the time of their menstrual period (mastodynia). In addition, masses (known as blue-dome cysts of Bloodgood) often develop; they usually are cystic in nature. These cysts can be treated safely by aspiration. However, aside from the solitary mass, the breast presents an irregular, diffuse, shotty induration as a result of multiple cysts, many of which are microscopic in size. In case of doubt, any breast mass should be excised and examined microscopically to obtain a definite diagnosis. The formation of other cysts in the same or opposite breast is not uncommon.

Duct Papilloma

In general these lesions are quite small and often cannot be felt on examination of the breast. They usually manifest themselves by the appearance of intermittent bleeding from the nipple. Their relation to cancer is not clear cut, but when they can be localized by compression of the duct their removal is indicated. Although Paget's disease of the nipple, which is intraductal carcinoma with invasion, may present without a palpable mass, seldom indeed will a patient with *only* a bloody discharge from the nipple have cancer.

Carcinoma of the Breast

This is now the most frequent lethal cancer in women. Although occurring usually in middle and older age groups, it is not unknown in the 20s. It is almost always unilateral. Except on rare occasions the presenting symptom is a painless lump that has developed insidiously. In contrast with fibroadenoma, these tumors are not readily movable and early show evidence of infiltration and fixation to the surrounding structures. This is manifested by dimpling of the skin, retraction or deviation of the nipple and elevation of the breast. As the disease progresses, the overlying skin becomes involved to such an extent that there is frank infiltration with development of edema and an orange-peel type of skin. Extension inward leads to fixation of the breast to the pectoral muscles and eventually to the chest wall. Along with the local extension, there is a lymphatic spread of the disease. The axillery nodes are involved early. They become enlarged, hard, and eventually, matted together. The lymphatic drainage of the breast also may lead to enlargement of the supraclavicular nodes and those in the thorax along the course of the internal mammary vessels. Eventually, widespread metastasis takes place with involvement of bone, the liver, lungs, and the brain. Unfortunately, local pain is a very late symptom in the disease. In untreated cases, ulceration often takes place with secondary infection, purulent and foul drainage and repeated episodes of hemorrahge.

Treatment of the disease consists of radical mastectomy in operable cases. This involves removal of the entire breast, along with a generous ellipse of skin, the pectoralis major and minor muscles, and the axillary lymph nodes. If these nodes show no evidence of metastatic spread at the time of operation, about 80 to 90 per cent of the patients will survive 5 years. On the other hand, if these nodes are involved at the time of operation only about 35 to 45 per cent will survive that long.

In this country modified radical mastectomy has largely supplanted the radical operation, the modification consists of sparing the pectoralis major muscle or the pectoralis major and minor muscles. Partial mastectomy is practiced by some and partial mastectomy combined with radiation therapy is advocated by others.

When the initial biopsy is done tissue should be assayed for the presence of estrogen receptor protein. When significant levels are present alteration of hormonal balance is likely to be beneficial in treatment of patients with disseminated disease.

X-ray therapy has been used both preoperatively and postoperatively, but controlled studies have not shown prolonged survival in the treated group. Generally, radiation therapy is reserved for the treatment of recurrent or metastatic disease. The role of surgical or roentgen castration in premenopausal women who have this disease is debatable, but is contraindicated when the cancer is estrogen receptor negative.

Unfortunately, when a patient presents herself for care, frequently the disease has progressed so far that radical surgery cannot hope to extirpate it. In these circumstances such patients often are treated by x-ray therapy alone. This also is true for the aged. However, for these older people and also for those who present with ulcerated, bleeding masses or masses threatening to break down, simple mastectomy occasionally is carried out as a palliative procedure. Attempts to treat women with locally inoperable or disseminated breast cancer by the administration of estrogens or androgens, or by the removal of the ovaries, adrenals and anterior pituitary depend, as above mentioned, on the presence or absence of estrogen receptor protein in the cancer cells. Progesterone receptors are also being sought and this test gives promise of even greater reliability than does the test for estrogen receptors. Combination chemotherapy and a newer drug, adriamycin, are now producing remissions of greater or lesser extent and duration in up to 50 per cent of women with disseminated breast cancer.

In this disease cure can be expected only with early recognition and prompt treatment. Therefore, all women should undergo frequent careful physical examinations. However, during the intervals they should examine their own breasts each month and report immediately for attention if any lump develops.

Paget's disease of the breast should be considered a special form of carcinoma in which there is an eczematoid lesion of the nipple and the areola with an associated carcinoma beneath. The management of this condition is the same as that of any carcinoma of the breast.

Sarcoma of the Breast

This is an uncommon type of malignant neoplasm in the breast. It occurs usually in middle-aged women and appears as a mass in the breast, normally undergoing rather diffuse enlargement. The consistency may be quite soft, and the overlying vessels often are prominent. In contrast with carcinoma, this disease does not spread to the lymphatics. If it is treated early by wide excision, the results are excellent.

THE THORAX

Trauma

Alterations in Basic Physiologic Mechanisms.
An understanding of the alterations in basic physiologic mechanisms is vital to the treatment of patients with chest trauma.

Frequently, penetrating wounds of the thorax cause *pneumothorax* or *hemothorax,* or a combination of both. The effect is similar. If one pleural space is filled with air or blood, respiratory exchange may be embarrassed seriously. This burden can be tolerated by the patient unless the air or the blood causes displacement of the mediastinum toward the normal side, thereby further hindering respiration and impairing venous return to the heart.

Treatment consists of insertion of a thoracostomy tube attached to either a water seal drainage bottle or to a suction apparatus. When air in the pleura is under tension (tension pneumothorax), immediate aspiration is life-saving.

Defects in the chest wall give rise to "sucking" wounds, so named because of the inrush of air through the wound with each inspiratory effect. Aeration of the lung on the involved side is impossible in these circumstances. The heart and the mediastinal structures are pushed from side to side with each respiratory movement (mediastinal flutter). Emergency measures require that the defect be plugged immediately.

Crushing injuries of the thoracic cage in which there are multiple rib fractures ("flail chest") create paradoxic respiration, that is, collapse of the chest wall with inspiration and expansion with expiration. Flail chest producing respiratory embarrassment, as judged by inspection and the finding of a low oxygen tension and a high carbon dioxide tension in arterial blood, is splinted today by use of a cuffed endotracheal tube and use of a volume-cycled mechanical ventilator.

Of great importance in all chest injuries is maintenance of an open airway and the clearing of bronchial secretions.

With severe thoracic injuries pulmonary contusion is very likely to occur. If suspected, arterial blood gases should be monitored. A falling PaO_2 and/or a rising $PaCO_2$ are indications for ventilatory support with a volume-cycled ventilator. The O_2 in inspired air (FiO_2) is raised in increments to a maximum of 60 per cent depending on response of the PaO_2. If elevated inspiratory pressure and FiO_2 fail to correct abnormalities in blood gases, positive end expiratory pressure (PEEP) should be instituted also, in increments from 5 to 15 cm. of H_2O, depending upon response. Antibiotic therapy is also indicated.

Cardiac Tamponade. Penetrating wounds of the heart that are not immediately fatal may result in death by cardiac tamponade. A relatively small amount of bleeding into the pericardial sac may embarrass the diastolic filling of the heart, giving rise to a classic triad of symptoms—increased venous pressure, distant heart sounds and increased diastolic blood pressure with narrowed pulse pressure.

Treatment consists of immediate pericardial aspiration, followed by operation if bleeding continues. The pericardium is exposed by a median sternotomy incision.

Cardiac Arrest

The cessation of the heart beat can be caused by many factors, but essentially two mechanisms are involved: (1) Simple arrest occurs with potassium intoxication and sometimes in hypoxia; (2) ventricular fibrillation most frequently attends acute myocardial infarction, but may be seen with hypothermia and hypoxia. Treatment must be rapidly and skillfully executed in order to be effective. An adequate airway must be provided by removal of vomitus or other foreign material and keeping the tongue forward. Next, artificial respiration is instituted, preferably by an anesthesia machine using oxygen, but if this is not available, by mouth-to-mouth technique. Cardiac output is maintained by closed-chest cardiac massage at a rate of 80 to 100 per minute. Intravenous infusion of Ringer's lactate solution should be started, if necessary, by cutdown. The mechanism of arrest is determined by obtaining an electrocardiogram. If the heart is beating weakly and ineffectively, norepinephrine is added to the intravenous infusion. If an effective heart beat does not return, calcium chloride should be injected into the heart. If the heart is in standstill, epinephrine should be injected into the right ventricular cavity. If ventricular fibrillation is present, the defibrillator must be used. Metabolic acidosis develops rapidly and should be combated by adding sodium bicarbonate to the intravenous infusion. If blood loss was responsible for the cardiac arrest, blood is rapidly transfused.

Open cardiac massage is seldom used today except when cardiac arrests develops during thoracotomy. If heart action does not return with closed-chest massage in patients who are in the operating room, open massage may be effective.

THE HEART AND THE GREAT VESSELS

Great strides have been made in the surgical correction of congenital and acquired lesions of the heart and the great vessels. The development and refinement of pump oxygenators that permit total cardiopulmonary bypass without an unacceptable physiologic insult permit more leisurely and extensive intracardiac manipulations. This was essential to the expansion of this field and constitutes one of the fascinating chapters in the history of modern surgery. Common lesions that are amenable to surgical techniques will be listed and described briefly.

Patent Ductus Arteriosus

The persistence of the embryologic shunt from aorta to pulmonary artery is associated with symptoms caused by left heart strain and pulmonary hypertension. There is a classic machinery murmur heard to the left of the sternum. The treatment of choice is ligation and division of the ductus.

Coarctation of the Aorta

This is a narrowing of the arch of the aorta just past the origin of the left subclavian artery. It may range from severe stricturing incompatible with life to minor degrees of narrowing. The clinical picture may range from symptoms of heart failure to the incidental finding of hypertension in the upper extremities. In most cases there is hypotension in the trunk and the legs. Death results from heart failure or cerebrovascular accidents.

Surgical treatment entails resection of the narrowed segment and end-to-end anastomosis or grafting. This is usually accomplished with partial bypass.

Tetralogy of Fallot

This complex anomaly includes pulmonary valve stenosis, overriding of the aorta, interventricular septal defect and hypertrophy of the right ventricle. Its presence is obvious in infancy or early childhood because of the cyanosis (blue baby).

Treatment is directed toward increasing pulmonary arterial flow. To this end, two procedures were developed: anastomosis of aorta and pulmonary artery (Potts) or anastomosis of the subclavian and the pulmonary arteries (Blalock). The long-term prognosis following these procedures is poor. More recent methods involve direct repair although the shunt operations are still done as temporizing procedures.

Atrial Septal Defects

These defects must be differentiated from a patent foramen ovale that is a normal defect in up to 25 per cent of adult hearts. Because of its slitlike opening, the patent foramen ovale permits shunting only from right to left. Left-to-right shunting of blood is characteristic of atrial septal defects, but is also seen with anomalous pulmonary veins and atrioventricular canal malformations. The atrial septal defects are divided into ostium secundum and ostium primum types. The former is the more frequent and more readily repaired. Mitral and tricuspid insufficiency accompany ostium primum defects and atrioventricular canals. The diagnosis of ostium secundum defect is seldom made early in life because the symptoms and physical signs are not sufficiently distinct. With the passage of time a soft systolic murmur is heard in the second or third left intercostal space along with fixed splitting of the second pulmonic sound. Pulmonary blood flow is increased and eventually pulmonary hypertension develops. Repair is indicated when the shunt is large and the volume of flow in the pulmonary circuit is one and one-half to two times greater than the systemic circuit.

Ventricular Septal Defects

These are frequent congenital anomalies of the heart comprising 20 to 30 per cent of all cases of congenital heart disease. Because of the great difference in pressure between the left and right ventricles, the left-to-right shunt is likely to be very large, depending on the size of the defect and the pulmonary vascular resistance. The volume of blood flow in the pulmonary and systemic circuits is determined by cardiac catheterization. As in atrial septal defects, when pulmonary blood flow is one and one-half to two times systemic flow, operation is indicated. Severe pulmonary hypertension, seldom seen in children, is a contraindication.

Transposition of the Great Arteries

This is one of the more common serious anomalies. In the lethal form there is no communication between the pulmonary and systemic cercuits. Palliative procedures are directed toward increasing the communication in order to increase the flow of oxygenated blood in the systemic circuit. Nonoperative opening of the foramen ovale by balloon fracture is one method; the Blalock-Hanlon operation, another. The most successful method of definitive correction is the technique developed by Mustard.

Acquired Valvular Lesions

These are the result of either rheumatic valvulitis or arteriosclerosis. In some instances direct repair (such as mitral commissurotomy) of damaged valves is possible; in others the damage to valves is so extensive that repair is not feasible. In the latter situation, resection and replacement by prosthetic valves gives good functional results, provided that the myocardium remains in good condition. Multiple replacements are frequently necessary.

Myocardial Revascularization

The main indication is intractable angina not responsive to medical therapy or so-called crescendo angina (preinfarction angina). Coronary and cardiac angiography permit an exact assessment of the state of the coronary arteries and the myocardium. Satisfactory examination is essential for the selection of patients for myocardial revascularization procedures. Most fre-

quently used today are direct anastomoses between the internal mammary artery to a coronary artery and bypass vein grafts to the aorta and one or two coronaries, as indicated. Some surgeons use only bypass vein grafts. Although this procedure remains controversial, there is agreement that patients with occlusion of the left anterior descending coronary artery do better with surgical shunting than with medical therapy.

Pulmonary Embolism

This catastrophe often occurs during a postoperative or postpartum period. It results from a breaking off of a segment of thrombus in the venous circulation, the separated portion then being swept into the heart and carried into one of the pulmonary arteries, where it lodges. The symptoms of pulmonary embolism consist of a sudden onset of chest pain and cough, bloody sputum, dyspnea and extreme anxiety. If the embolism is large, shock sets in, and death occurs promptly. In cases of small emboli, spontaneous recovery usually takes place, although repeated pulmonary embolism is common, and eventually death may result. Although the symptoms and signs may be typical, great difficulty in differential diagnosis between pulmonary embolization and acute myocardial infarction exists. Inasmuch as the therapy for the one condition differs so from that for the other, a need exists for rapid and accurate methods of establishing the correct diagnosis. Selective pulmonary angiography is the most accurate method of making the diagnosis of pulmonary embolism. In patients who are not in shock and have had no previous episodes, anticoagulant treatment with intravenous heparin is used. In patients who have previously had emboli, ligation of the inferior vena cava below the renal arteries is indicated. This can be complete or, as previously mentioned, one of the methods of narrowing or segmentation of the vena cava may be used. Patients who develop a pulmonary embolism while receiving adequate heparin therapy should also have inferior vena caval interruption. In poor risk patients transjugular placement of an umbrella type device (Mobin-Udin or Greenfield) is well tolerated and has given good results. Patients in shock should be treated by embolectomy during cardiopulmonary bypass. This is followed by partial or complete occlusion of the inferior vena cava.

THE LUNG

Respiratory Failure

Respiratory failure is a major cause of death in surgical patients, but owing to improved methods of ventilatory support, improved diagnosis, and better understanding of pulmonary physiology many who heretofore would have died are being saved. The causes include hypoventilation, diffusion defects, ventilation-perfusion imbalance, abnormalities in oxygen carriage or release, and right-to-left shunting. Clinically pulmonary insufficiency is seen in post operative patients, patients with multiple organ injury, in the presence of long bone fractures, with fluid overload, fat embolization, and so forth. Preexisting pulmonary disease will compound the problem and sepsis appears to be a frequent common denominator.

The diagnosis is made by monitoring arterial blood gases. A falling PaO_2, a rising $PaCO_2$ in the absence of metabolic alkalosis are the findings. The patient may have tachypnea, a low-tidal volume, expiratory effort and in extreme instances, cyanosis. Physiologically, in addition to changes in blood gases studies show a low function residual capacity, low vital capacity and inspiratory force.

Treatment consists of endotracheal intubation with ventilatory support. The oxygen content of inspired air (FiO_2) is increased and positive end expiratory pressure (PEEP) should be given, in increments from 5 to 15 cm. of water, depending upon improved PaO_2 and $PaCO_2$.

Tumors of the Lung

Bronchial Adenoma. There are two histologic types of bronchial adenoma. The cylindromatous variety, which resembles the similar tumors of salivary gland origin, and the carcinoid type. The latter may secrete serotonin and cause the carcinoid syndrome. Both lesions are really low-grade carcinomas and may metastasize. When metastasis occurs it is most frequently to regional lymph nodes and liver.

Bronchogenic carcinoma is one of the most frequent cancers in men and it is increasing in women. The correlation between smoking and lung cancer appears to be irrefutable evidence of a causative relationship. The most frequent symptoms are cough, hemoptysis, weight loss and weakness. All of these are late manifestations, and by the time they appear the tumor is usually incurable. The diagnosis is at times made on incidental chest roentgenogram. In addition to chest roentgenography, sputum cytology and bronchoscopy with biopsy are usually done for diagnosis. The fiberoptic, flexible bronchoscope extends the range of visibility of the examination. When combined with brush biopsy the diagnostic accuracy is considerably enhanced. Treatment consists of pulmonary resection, the extent depending on the location and size of the primary lesion.

At times bronchogenic tumors have an endocrine function, producing a parathormone-like substance, an antidiuretic hormone, and even an inappropriate ACTH secretion that causes the clinical manifestations of Cushing's syndrome.

Tuberculosis

The antituberculous drugs have made possible a direct attack on the disease process. Surgical emphasis has shifted from thoracoplasty to resection in instances in which the lung involvement is confined and the disease is not controlled by chemotherapy alone.

Empyema

Empyema may be a complication of pneumonia, particularly in children. It is common during epidemic influenza and may occur from contiguous infection (tuberculosis, gangrene, abscess of the lung) or from chest wounds.

The most common organism is the pneumococcus. The streptococcus causes a virulent form. Staphylococcus, *Haemophilus influenzae,* Friedlander's bacillus and the colon bacillus are rarely the primary invaders. If there is communication with an abscessed, gangrenous or bronchiectatic lung, the pus is foul. Empyema is rarely bilateral. It may be encapsulated. Physical examination, roentgenograms and aspiration give the diagnosis.

Treatment. With the use of effective antimicrobial agents, empyema is less common. When needle aspiration yields watery material, the antimicrobial to which the organism is sensitive should be administered by direct intrapleural instillation. This will usually need to be repeated. If the pus is thicker, loculation may occur. At times the enzymes streptokinase and streptodornase will be useful in direct antimicrobial treatment. More frequently, underwater seal drainage—using an intercostal tube and systemic antibiotics—will be used. When an abscess develops, open thoracotomy and adequate drainage will usually lead to expansion of the lung and obliteration of the cavity. At times, decortication or thoracoplasty may be necessary for cure.

Massive Collapse of the Lung

This is the term applied to the condition that results from a plugging of one of the bronchi with mucus. Air cannot reach the lung parenchyma, the residual air in the pulmonary alveoli is absorbed, and the portion of lung aerated by the plugged bronchus collapses. The collapse may involve an entire lobe or an entire lung, depending on the air passage that is blocked. Massive collapse is not uncommon immediately following abdominal operations, when respiration and coughing are depressed because of anesthesia, pain and medication. Increased respiratory rate, absence of breath sounds and fever are signs that point to this complication. The tenacious mucous plug may be removed by aspiration through a bronchoscope or through a catheter inserted into the trachea through the nose.

THE ESOPHAGUS AND DIAPHRAGM

Carcinoma of the Esophagus

The manifestations of carcinoma of the esophagus are difficulty in swallowing and weight loss. Roentgenograms obtained during the ingestion of barium and direct esophagoscopic examination will usually establish the diagnosis. In some instances, patients with preexisting esophagitis develop cancer and the diagnosis is more difficult. It arises anywhere in the esophagus, but involvement of the lower third is most frequent. Early lymph node metastasis, not uncommonly at some distance from the primary tumor, limits curability. In the middle third, invasion of the carina of the trachea may accentuate pulmonary symptoms. Bronchoscopy is essential for the evaluation of lesions in this area. In the lower third, surgical removal is generally the treatment of choice. Elsewhere surgical resection and supervoltage radiation therapy. The results in terms of cure are poor with either modality.

Diverticulum of the Esophagus

Traction diverticula usually are not symptomatic. The most important pulsion diverticula are those arising at the pharyngoesophageal juncture. Regurgitation of undigested food, gurgling in the neck and dysphagia are the usual symptoms. When visualized radiographically, they present in the left lower neck. Excision with closure of the mucosal and muscular defect is the recommended treatment. Cricopharyngeal myotomy should also be done.

Diaphragmatic Hernia

Hernias about the esophageal hiatus are of two types—the "sliding" and the paraesophageal. The former is an acquired separation of the diaphragmatic crura associated with weakening of the esophageal attachments to the diaphragm, permitting the esophagocardiac junction to slide up and down with changes in posture and intraabdominal pressure. Pressure studies show the presence of a functional lower esophageal sphincter that may become incompetent in the presence of a sliding type of hiatus hernia. In some instances it is incompetent in the absence of a hiatus hernia. When incompetence develops, reflux of gastric juice leads to esophagitis. Muscle spasm, ulceration and scarring with stricture formation eventually result. Once a fixed stricture develops treatment is much more

difficult; therefore, patients who do not respond promptly to medical therapy should be advised that operative treatment is indicated. The operations in greatest favor today are the Nissen fundoplication or the Belsey repair. Both appear to be satisfactory, providing the technical details are carefully observed. When duodenal ulceration and gastric hypersecretion are present along with reflux esophagitis, control of hypersecretion is an essential part of the operative treatment.

Subdiaphragmatic Abscess

An abscess in this location is secondary to infection elsewhere in the peritoneal cavity, such as acute appendicitis. Fever and leukocytosis persist. There may be discomfort in the region of the abscess, and tenderness usually can be elicited by pressure or jarring over the abscess. Pain may be referred to the shoulder. Fluoroscopic examination reveals limitation of movement and elevation of the diaphragm and a sterile pleural effusion.

The treatment for this disease is adequate surgical drainage.

THE ABDOMEN

Abdominal Injury

Two types of abdominal injury are seen; the first, the result of blunt forces; the second, penetrating injuries from stab wounds or gunshot wounds.

Blunt Injury.   The usual cause today is automobile accidents. Properly worn seat belts minimize such injuries, but if the force is sufficient, may actually cause them. Industrial accidents, falls, sports injuries, etc., are less common causes. Frequently blunt injuries of the abdomen are seen in association with multiple organ injury, especially of the brain, as well as injuries of the thorax and osseous fractures. Lacerations of the spleen and liver are frequently associated with fractures of overlying ribs. Both results in hemorrhage; shock is frequent. The pancreas, despite its protected location, may also be injured. Contusion or laceration may cause extravasation of pancreatic juice with resulting pancreatitis and pseudocyst formation. Elevation of serum amylase is a usual accompaniment of such injuries. Tears in the mesentery and blowout injuries of the small intestine occur. The most frequent site of intestinal injury is at the duodenojejunal juncture. Renal injuries are seen with all types of abdominal trauma, but for some reason are particularly common in football players. A distended bladder may be ruptured by a seat belt or kick, so also may a gravid uterus. Fractures of the pelvis may cause secondary lacerations of the bladder or urethra. Displaced fractures of the pelvis are prone to tear large pelvic veins with resultant potentially exsanguinating hemorrhage.

When intraabdominal injury is suspected, but the indications for abdominal exploration are not clear, aspiration is useful. We prefer a small midline incision below the umbilicus with insertion of a small peritoneal dialysis catheter. Aspiration of blood that does not clot is a significant finding. If no aspirate is returned, isotonic saline is injected, aspirated and examined microscopically for leukocytes.

Stab Wounds. If signs of bleeding or peritonitis are not present the insertion of a small catheter, held in place by a purse-string suture in the skin, followed by injection of a water-soluble radiopaque medium for evidence of peritoneal penetration, has been useful in deciding which patients can be safely observed.

Gunshot Wounds. All gunshot wounds of the abdomen should be operated upon. The extent of injury is related to the velocity of the missile; high-velocity missiles produce great tissue damage, while injury from low-velocity missiles is much less. Fortunately in civilian life the latter are most frequently seen. Holes in the small intestine are usually debrided and closed. Small puncture wound of the colon with minimal contamination may also be closed. More extensive injuries, however, as well as a greater degree of contamination or questionable viability of tissues are all indications for exteriorization.

THE STOMACH AND DUODENUM

Gastric Ulcer

The etiology of benign gastric ulcer is not completely understood. Pyloric obstruction is a factor contributing to increased antral stimulation of gastrin, which in turn plays a part in the pathogenesis of benign gastric ulcer. Prepyloric ulcers have the same secretory pattern as duodenal ulcers. The resting level of acid production in most benign gastric ulcers in low, but in prepyloric as in duodenal ulcer the fasting level is increased. Acute gastric ulcers occur as complications of sepsis, burns, extensive fractures, etc. A relation to acid secretion is doubtful.

The surgical treatment of gastric ulcer usually consists of partial gastrectomy with gastroduodenostomy or gastrojejunostomy. When pyloric obstruction is present, pyloroplasty or gastrojejunostomy may suffice. If the ulcer is not removed, four-quadrant biopsy is mandatory to exclude cancer. Prepyloric ulcers should be treated similarly to duodenal ulcer, as should other gastric ulcers in which fasting hyperacidity exists or in which a scar of active or healed duodenal ulcer

is present. Acute gastric ulcer is usually manifested by massive hemorrhage. Treatment is directed toward control of hemorrhage and removal or healing of the ulcerative process. Many benign gastric ulcers will heal with conservative therapy, which is empirical inasmuch as the etiology is usually not clear cut. The recurrence rate is high; this, along with the difficulty in differentiating benign gastric ulcer from ulcerating cancer, is a strong indication for surgical management.

Gastric Carcinoma

Carcinoma of the stomach has decreased in frequency in the United States for reasons that are unclear. It occurs twice as often in men as it does in women. It usually appears at the age of 45 or beyond and is characterized by rather indefinite digestive symptoms—indigestion, malaise, lack of appetite and so forth. As the disease progresses, it produces more marked symptoms—obstruction when the tumor becomes large enough to obstruct the pyloric end of the stomach, bleeding, anemia and the presence of a mass in the epigastrium. Many patients with gastric carcinoma have pain that may be almost exactly like that of peptic ulceration. Carcinomatous ulcers may not be distinguishable from benign ulcers. The combined use of roentgenograms, gastric analysis, gastric cytology and gastroscopy with biopsy or a complete survey with the gastrocamera increases diagnostic accuracy. In a good laboratory the frequency of false-positive reports on gastric cytology is practically zero. Neither the location of the ulcer nor roentgenographic criteria are as useful in diagnosis as formerly believed.

Surgery is the only known method of cure for carcinoma of the stomach. The prognosis usually is poor because the patients are referred for operation when complete removal of the tumor is no longer possible. The extent of the stomach to be removed depends upon the operative findings, but as a rule a very radical gastrectomy is performed, including also the areas of lymphatic extension, that is, the gastrohepatic and greater omentum and the lymphatic areas of drainage around the pylorus and around the left gastric vessels. Some authors believe that a total gastrectomy should be performed in all cases in which carcinoma is present or suspected. The principle behind this theory is the radical excision of the tumor, but there is no convincing evidence that such radical operation produces better results, and the morbidity associated with total gastrectomy is much greater than with subtotal resection of the stomach.

Duodenal Ulcer

Duodenal ulcer is generally associated with acid pepsin hypersecretion, particularly in the interdigestive phase. With recurring exacerbations of the ulcer and healing, changes that produce organic complications may take place. Indications for surgical therapy are these symptoms: (1) bleeding; (2) obstruction of the pylorus; (3) intractability, i.e., unsatisfactory response to medical treatment; and (4) perforation.

In the treatment of rupture of a duodenal ulceration, early operation with closure of the perforation or plugging of the perforation with an omental graft is indicated. It has been found that the results depend upon the lapse of time between perforation and the performance of surgery. Thus, those who are operated upon soon after perforation have an excellent prognosis, whereas those who have had a continuing leak over a period of 12 hours or more have generalized peritonitis and a less favorable prognosis. Patients with a prolonged history of ulcer disease prior to perforation may be treated by a definitive operation to control the ulcer diathesis, providing severe peritonitis is not present. In patients with few or no preceding symptoms, closure of the ulcer with an omental flap is the operation of choice. Conservative treatment of perforated ulcers is associated with a higher mortality risk than is operative treatment.

Because duodenal ulcers are believed to be the result of the action of the acid and pepsin of gastric juice upon the mucosa of the duodenum, operations have been proposed that would reduce the secretion of this juice in order to cure ulcer. Some operations are designed to remove the factors that stimulate the production of gastric juice. One of these entails division of the vagus nerve (vagotomy), thereby blocking the impulses that produce the nervous phase of the stimulation of gastric juice. Another consists of removal of the gastric antrum, which is the area of the stomach in which the acid-stimulating hormone gastrin is produced. Other operations may remove not only the antrum but also a fairly generous portion of the body of the stomach. In such a case, not only is the hormonal stimulating area (antrum) removed but also a large part of the stomach—that part in which the cells that produce gastric acid juice are located. These various factors that are concerned with the production of acid gastric juice may be combined in a single operation. Thus, the vagus nerve may be divided and partial gastrectomy performed.

In those operations in which the vagus nerve is divided, some form of drainage of the stomach must be provided, because the vagus nerve not only influences the secretion of gastric juice in the stomach but also serves as the motor nerve to the stomach.

Heineke-Mikulicz pyloroplasty, Finney pyloroplasty and Jaboulay pyloroplasty are all used in drainage procedures, as is gastrojejunostomy. If gastrojejunostomy is undertaken it should be placed close to the pylorus in order to provide good drainage of the antrum.

Highly selective (or parietal cell) vagotomy is under investigation at present. Since it spares the innervation of the pylorus (nerves of Latarjet) a drainage procedure is unnecessary. It is hoped that this operation will result in minimal disturbance of gastric physiology while controlling the ulcer diathesis. At present, the early excellent results of this procedure appear to be sustained. If this proves to be correct on further followup, highly selective vagotomy will supplant other operations that are all associated with physiologic deficits that are undesirable.

The operation that has been most effective, in that the rate of recurrence of ulcers is lowest after it, is truncal vagotomy with antrectomy. Subtotal gastrectomy is no longer justifiable.

Operations that ablate the pyloric mechanism may lead to the dumping syndrome. This syndrome is characterized by a feeling of faintness, sweating, palpitations and nausea coming on during or shortly after the ingestion of food. The cause appears to be related to the rapid passage of hyperosmolar liquids into the duodenum or jejunum. Fluid passes from the vascular compartment into the intestinal lumen. The symptoms result from distention of the intestine and reduction in plasma volume. Hypoglycemia is seen in some patients but not until some time later. Treatment is directed at reducing the hyperosmolarity of the material leaving the stomach; fat is increased, carbohydrate decreased, and liquids are given between meals. This syndrome was seen in severe form much more frequently when radical subtotal gastrectomy was the operation of choice. It leads to crippling nutritional depletion so every effort should be made to avoid it by the selection of operations that are less likely to produce it.

Stress Ulcers

This term refers to acute gastroduodenal ulceration that occurs after shock, sepsis, complicated operations, burns, serious fractures and head injuries. The etiology is uncertain, but gastric hypersecretion is not present. Ischemia appears to play a part and back diffusion of hydrochloric acid has also been incriminated. In spite of the apparent decrease in hydrochloric acid secretion, prophylaxis with antacids, and the H_2 inhibitor, cimetidine, have been effective in reducing the frequency of this complication.

GALLBLADDER AND BILE DUCTS

Cholelithiasis

Calculus cholecystitis is a chronic disease, frequently subject to acute exacerbations, known as biliary colic.

This disease usually occurs during middle life and is more common in the female than in the male. It often follows pregnancy. Stasis and infection probably predispose to gallstone formation, but probably of greater importance are abnormalities in the composition of bile. Most important is maintenance of a normal ratio between bile salts and phospholipid (lecithin) and cholesterol. An increase in cholesterol or a reduction in the bile salt pool is a potential cause of a derangement in this association. The bile salt pool can be reduced by resection or bypass operations on the ileum. The type of bile salt is also of importance since lithocholate is insoluble and deoxycholate is soluble. In experimental studies in which chenodeoxycholate has been fed to patients with asymptomatic stones there has been evidence of decrease in size and disappearance of stones after prolonged feeding.

Cholecystitis

Acute Cholecystitis.   If a stone obstructs the cystic duct, an attack of acute biliary colic results. In general, these attacks occur at night and are more likely to follow some dietary indiscretion, such as overeating. The pain is severe and is present in the epigastrium or the right upper quadrant. However, in addition, it frequently radiates to the back, the scapular region or the right shoulder. Nausea and vomiting are common. During the attack, in most cases, tenderness occurs in the region of the gallbladder, and there is some muscleguarding. As a rule these attacks subside in a few hours with the aid of opiates and atropine or similar drugs. Residual soreness in the region of the gallbladder often persists for 1 or 2 days after the attack has subsided.

Although these acute attacks may subside, not infrequently the stone becomes so impacted in the cystic duct that it cannot be released spontaneously. In addition to the factor of obstruction, bacterial infection sets in, with marked fever and leukocytosis. Frank pus forms in the gallbladder, and eventually gangrene of the gallbladder wall occurs. However, this process is much slower than such a development in acute appendicitis. Unless operative intervention is resorted to, perforation of the gallbladder may take place, with the development of peritonitis, either spreading or localized. Occasionally the perforation takes place into an adjacent viscus, such as the stomach, the duodenum, or the colon, with a resulting internal biliary fistula.

The following conditions must be considered in differential diagnosis: (1) acute appendicitis, (2) perforated peptic ulcer, (3) acute pancreatitis or pancreatic lithiasis, (4) renal colic or pyelitis, (5) pneumonia, and (6) coronary artery occlusion.

Chronic Cholecysitis.   During the intervals between the acute exacerbations there may be no symptoms at all, or a sense of fullness and distention in the upper abdomen may be present, with a tendency toward belching. There may actually be some epigastric distress. These symptoms usually occur after large meals or ones containing fatty foods.

During the interval phases, stones may be demonstrated in the gallbladder by means of a cholecystogram. Examination of the bile obtained by duodenal drainage may reveal crystals of cholesterol or bile salts.

The ideal treatment consists of cholecystectomy as an elective procedure between attacks of acute biliary colic. Should an attack of colic fail to subside promptly with administration of opiates and atropine, continuous gastric suction drainage and intravenous fluids, operation is indicated. Occasionally, because of obliteration of normal anatomic planes, the best procedure will be cholecystostomy, though usually it is possible to remove the gallbladder even during an acute attack.

Common Duct Obstruction

If a stone reaches the common duct but is unable to pass the ampulla of Vater, obstructive jaundice results. There may be upper abdominal distress, nausea and vomiting, or the patient may present little in the way of symptoms aside from icterus. However, there frequently is associated infection, with chills and fever. The stools become claycolored as the result of the absence of bile pigments, and the urine is very dark. The direct van den Bergh reaction is immediate. The degree of jaundice may be measured either by the indirect van den Bergh determination or by the icterus index. Bilirubin and bile salts appear in the urine.

In prolonged jaundice the prothrombin level falls and hemorrhagic tendencies develop. This results from failure of absorption of vitamin K from the intestinal tract, because this vitamin requires the presence of bile salts for absorption. In preparing these patients for operation, it is necessary to make repeated determinations of the prothrombin level and to supply vitamin K parenterally or to administer it by mouth in conjunction with bile salts, so as to provide for its absorption. In addition, the hepatic damage associated with jaundice should be combated by providing these patients with a high-calorie, high-protein, high-carbohydrate and high-vitamin diet that is low in fat content. Treatment consists of choledochostomy and removal of the stones. Ordinarily the gallbladder also is removed at this time. Prior to removal of the drainage tube, patency of the ductal system should be demonstrated by means of a cholangiogram.

Frequently a common duct stone has a ball-valve-like action, producing bouts of fever, chills and jaundice. (Charcot's intermittent hepatic fever). A progressive relentless jaundice should suggest the possibility of carcinoma, primary in the ductal system or in the head of the pancreas.

Operative cholangiography is being increasingly used today as a supplement to the clinical history and palpation of the common bile duct when the surgeon is deciding if operative exploration of the choledochus is necessary. Usually the procedure is done through the cystic duct, but it may be done through the gallbladder or the choledochus itself; 15 to 20 ml. of dilute contrast material is injected. The indications for exploration of the common bile duct at operation include: a history of jaundice, associated pancreatitis, dilatation of the common duct, sludge in an aspirate of the common bile duct, palpation of a stone and a stone seen on the cholangiogram.

When stones in intrahepatic ducts cannot be removed or when recurrent stones or sludge is present either side-to-side choledochoduodenostomy or sphincteroplasty should be considered. Choledochoduodenostomy may also be indicated when stones impacted at the ampulla of Vater cannot be removed.

Retained stones require removal either by secondary operation or by extraction through the tract of a T tube.

PANCREAS

Acute Pancreatitis

Though the etiology of this condition is not understood clearly, it often has been surmised that it results from reflux of bile into the pancreatic ducts, with resultant activation of the pancreatic enzymes and subsequent autodigestion of this organ. Others believe that the significant factors in the etiology of acute pancreatitis are obstruction of the pancreatic duct and the presence of an actively secreting gland. The obstruction may occur at the ampulla because of edema or a common duct calculus when there is a "common channel" shared by the common and the pancreatic ducts.

This disease manifests itself by the sudden onset of severe upper abdominal pain, commonly associated with nausea and vomiting. The pain may be referred also to the back. On examination one finds tenderness and muscle guarding over the region of the pancreas; if the disease progresses, these findings become more diffuse, and generalized distention sets in. There is a moderate febrile response, frequently with tachycardia that is quite out of proportion to the temperature elevation. Polymorphonuclear leukocytosis is present. However, the distinctive laboratory finding in this disease is the prompt elevation of the serum amylase and lipase levels. These values usually show a definite increase within a few hours of the onset of the disease, and though the former may return to normal after 24 hours, the latter usually is elevated for several days.

There are two distinct types of acute pancreatitis that are of great importance, because the prognosis is so different in the two. The first is known as the acute edematous or interstitial type. This is marked by an intense edema of the retroperitoneal tissues in the region of the pancreas. There is an outpouring of free peritoneal fluid, which is bile tinged and at times somewhat hemorrhagic in character. There are yellowish-white areas of fat necrosis, most marked in the region of the pancreas. This condition is usually a mild self-limited disease and carries with it a low mortality. However, in contrast, acute hemorrhagic or necrotizing pancreatitis is marked by areas of frank hemorrhage and necrosis that frequently destroy almost the entire pancreas. This type is extremely serious and carries with it a high mortality.

In the milder cases, if one can rule out a catastrophe such as perforated peptic ulcer, conservative treatment is justified. This includes the use of a gastric tube with continuous suction drainage, intravenous fluids and supportive measures, such as transfusions. On the other hand, in the more severe cases, or in those in which the diagnosis cannot be made with certainty, surgical exploration is justified. The purpose of operation is first to confirm or refute the diagnosis, secondarily, if bile-tinged hemorrhagic peritoneal fluid is present, cholecystostomy should be done and the lesser peritoneal sac should be drained.

The operative measures used in patients with chronic pancreatitis are directed toward correction of the specific etiologic factors involved. Since there is a high incidence of related gallbladder or common duct stones, or both, cholecystectomy and common duct exploration may be sufficient. Transduodenal sphincterotomy is done if the sphincter of Oddi is spastic or fibrotic. If the pancreatic duct is obstructed close to the sphincter and is otherwise normal, caudal pancreaticojejunostomy should be considered. When multiple points of obstruction of the duct of Wirsung produce the "chain-of-lakes" appearance, lateral pancreaticojejunostomy may give relief. It may be easier, as well as more effective, to carry out 95 per cent pancreatectomy.

Cysts

Three types of pancreatic cysts are seen: (1) congenital, (2) pseudocysts, and (3) neoplastic. Of these the pseudocyst is most common. Congenital cysts are of little clinical importance except when they are multiple and part of the systemic disease, cystic fibrosis. Pseudocysts follow leakage from a torn major pancreatic duct in which the secretory products become walled off. This is caused by blunt or penetrating injuries or acute necrotizing pancreatitis. Cysts without a persistent communication with the pancreatic ductal system can be cured by simple drainage. These are infrequent, however, and a more reliable method of management is drainage to the stomach or jejunum by cystogastrostomy or Roux-en-Y cystojejunostomy.

Carcinoma of the Pancreas

Usually the head is involved in pancreatic carcinoma. Unfortunately, there are few symptoms early in this disease. However, as it progresses to involve the region of the common duct, obstructive jaundice sets in, is usually relentless, and gradually increases in intensity. The stools become acholic, and the urine is dark. Frequently, the icterus is associated with extreme itching that is almost intolerable and may be the most distressing feature of the disease. Other symptoms include vague indigestion, nausea, vomiting, weight loss and, eventually, cachexia.

Epigastric disease often is present, but severe pain is not ordinarily a feature early in this disease. The differential diagnoses include carcinoma of the ampulla of Vater, ductal carcinoma, calculous common duct obstruction and hepatitis. The usual roentgenograms are seldom diagnostic, although widening of the duodenal loop, straightening of the descending duodenum and the "reversed-three" signs are suggestive. Newer procedures include hypotonic duodenography and selective angiography. A distended gallbladder in the presence of obstructive jaundice suggests carcinoma of the head of the pancreas, whereas a contracted gallbladder suggests calculous common duct obstruction (Courvoisier's law).

Carcinoma arising in the body or tail of the pancreas is usually asymptomatic until invasion of somatic nerve fibers leads to pain. The pain is nonspecific in character and the usual roentgenograms and laboratory studies are negative leading to prolonged delays in diagnosis. Selective angiography will frequently show encasement of vessels in the region of the tumor and the body section computerized scans may outline the mass. With newer techniques the diagnosis may be suspected earlier, leading to exploratory operation, but it is unlikely that many such tumors will be found to be surgically resectable.

Islet Cell Adenoma

These tumors manifest themselves by the symptoms of hyperinsulinism. These symptoms following fasting, not the ingestion of food. To make the diagnosis, Whipple's triad should be present. This includes: (1) central nervous system symptoms such as weakness, nervousness and, at times, convulsions, coming on usually several hours after eating; (2) blood sugar 50 mg. or less per 100 ml.; and (3) prompt relief of symptoms following ingestion of glucose or its administration by vein. These tumors are too small to be felt on physical examination and cannot be demonstrated by roentgenography. The diagnosis is confirmed by determination of the plasma insulin levels, using the radioimmunoassay technique. The tolbutamide tolerance test is also of value. Treatment consists of excision of the adenoma. Complete relief of symptoms should result. At times more than one lesion has been found. Most lie in the body and the tail of the pancreas and, in general, are readily felt on palpation of the pancreas at operation. However, in some cases no tumor has been palpable, and subtotal pancreatectomy has been carried out. The results in such cases are often unsuccessful.

Not infrequently, these islet cell tumors are malignant.

Ulcerogenic Tumors (Non-Beta Cell Tumors, Zollinger-Ellison Syndrome)

Some tumors of the pancreatic islets are associated with the secretion of a gastrin-like substance that induces maximal and continued secretion of hydrochloric acid by the stomach. This results in ulcers of the stomach and duodenum that are atypical in location and refractory to the usual medical and surgical methods of treatment. Diarrhea is a frequent associated symptom, and, in some non-beta cell tumors of islet origin, diarrhea without hyperacidity or ulceration has been reported. The most important laboratory procedure for substantiation of the diagnosis is the finding of elevated levels of gastrin in the serum as determined by the radioimmunoassay technique. Gastric analysis shows increased volume and acidity without further increase when histamine is given. The tumors may be benign or malignant, but the most important feature of surgical treatment is total gastrectomy. Solitary and resectable tumors should be removed, but this is not a substitute for total gastrectomy. Surprisingly regression of metastases has followed total gastrectomy and the subsequent nutritional state remains very good. In some children growth and development have been perfectly normal after total gastrectomy for the Zollinger-Ellison syndrome, even though metastases to liver were present.

Another syndrome caused by secretion of a humoral agent by a pancreatic tumor consists of watery diarrhea, hypokalemia, and gastric hypochlorhydria or achlorhydria (WDHA syndrome or pancreatic cholera). The active agent appears to be vasoactive intestinal peptide. Removal of the pancreatic tumor is curative.

THE SPLEEN

Indications for Splenectomy

Rupture of the Spleen. This injury results either from a fall from a height, the individual landing on his feet or buttocks, or from direct trauma to the region of the spleen, as in an automobile accident. The patient complains of severe left upper quadrant pain, frequently with reference to the left shoulder. There are tenderness and muscle guarding in the left upper quadrant, and shifting dullness may be demonstrable. Leukocytosis is promptly evoked. If the bleeding is severe, a shocklike picture results. Abdominal paracentesis should demonstrate blood in the peritoneal cavity. Scanning the spleen using 99m technesium sulfur colloid is a useful diagnostic procedure; it is of particular help in instances of subcapsular bleeding that may give rise to delayed rupture. Angiography is also of value.

Treatment consists of surgical exploration as promptly as possible. Splenectomy, formerly routine surgical treatment is now avoided whenever possible, particularly in children. This change is the result of the incidence of pneumococcal sepsis following splenectomy. Should splenectomy be necessary in childhood, pneumococcal vaccine should be used as prophylaxis against infection. Large amounts of blood should be available for transfusion during operation in order to maintain the patient in satisfactory condition.

The most common indication for splenectomy today is iatrogenic injury produced by the surgeon in the course of operation around the spleen.

Congenital Hemolytic Icterus. This disease is due to a congenital tendency to form abnormally shaped red blood cells (spherocytes) that are more fragile than normal. The spleen filters out and destroys these abnormal cells, producing a hemolytic type of jaundice. Occasionally, the hemolyzed pigments are excreted in the bile in sufficient quantity to form pigment stones in the common bile duct; splenectomy is curative.

Idiopathic Thrombocytopenic Purpura. This is a bleeding tendency characterized by a low platelet count and prolonged bleeding time. Bleeding may occur into the skin, the kidneys, the gastrointestinal tract or the brain. In children, idiopathic thrombocytopenic purpura usually is an acute self-limited process that responds promptly to adrenal steroids. In adults it follows a chronic course, with frequent remissions and exacerbations. In the absence of a response to corticosteroids splenectomy is indicated. It is also indicated when, after a satisfactory response, it is impossible to withdraw corticosteroids without an exacerbation. This is true regardless of age, although the need arises more frequently in adults than in children.

Hypersplenism. Enlarged spleens occasionally are hyperactive, causing a decrease in one or all of the cellular blood elements. When there is associated active bone marrow, splenectomy may be of benefit.

Other Indications. Tumors or cysts of the spleen are uncommon but may cause pressure symptoms and should be removed.

THE LIVER

Portal Hypertension

Increased pressure in the portal bed may result from an intrahepatic (cirrhosis) or an extrahepatic (thrombosis of the portal or splenic vein) block. Naturally occurring collateral venous channels between the portal circulation and the cava proximal to the liver are utilized in an effort to bypass the block. Peptic erosion, or rupture of such collateral veins in the esophagus, gives rise to serious gastrointestinal hemorrhage, with death following rapidly if the hemorrhage is not controlled. Emergency treatment consists of control of hemorrhage by esophageal tamponade. During this time studies of hepatic function are carried out. The tendency today is to carry out portacaval shunt early in the course of bleeding from varices resulting from hepatic outflow block of cirrhosis. Extrahepatic portal bed block frequently occurs in childhood; if conservative measures fail, transesophageal ligation is a useful temporizing measure. Splenorenal shunt is not possible until growth has progressed to the point at which a splenic vein has developed of sufficient size to effectively decompress the portal bed when anastomosed to the renal vein. If splenectomy has already been done, a shunt should be created between the vena cava and superior mesenteric veins either by end-to-side anastomosis between the inferior vena cava and the superior mesenteric vein or by use of a so-called H graft using a Dacron prosthesis between the same vessels.

An alternate shunting procedure is the Warren operation of central splenorenal shunt in which the spleen is left in place, and the central end of the divided splenic vein is anastomosed to the renal vein. The operation is technically difficult, but Warren reports satisfactory reduction in portal pressure without the usual deleterious effect of portal-systemic shunting.

Another complication of increased portal pressure is splenomegaly and hypersplenism. When there is appreciable depression of the cellular elements of the blood despite active bone marrow, splenectomy and splenorenal shunt are indicated.

INTESTINES

Intestinal Obstruction

Intestinal obstruction may be either mechanical (dynamic) or paralytic (adynamic). Mechanical obstruction results from any factor, extrinsic or intrinsic, that encroaches on the lumen of the bowel. These factors include tumors, adhesions, hernias, volvulus and intussusception, and the obstruction may be either partial or complete. The patient suffers intermittent crampy abdominal pain. Peristalsis is visible and audible, and the crampy pain may be correlated with bouts of borborygmus. On auscultation, peristalsis is heard in rushes, and the note frequently is high pitched, metallic and tinkling. Distention is evident. Vomiting is frequent, and the vomitus actually may be intestinal in character. As a result of repeated vomiting, dehydration, electrolyte deficits and alterations in acid-base balance may be present. A survey film of the abdomen reveals distention. If the film is taken with the patient in the erect or lateral recumbent position, it reveals air and fluid levels in the gut (stepladder pattern). Constant severe pain in contrast to simple intermittent crampy pains should suggest strangulation of the bowel.

Paralytic ileus results from reflex paralysis of the musculature of the intestinal tract without actual mechanical obstruction of the lumen. It may follow any intraabdominal procedure, especially if there is trauma to the intestines, peritonitis, retroperitoneal hemorrhage or operative procedures, renal calculi or pneumonia. Hypokalemia may also result in paralytic ileus. In contrast to mechanical obstruction, no peristaltic sounds are heard on auscultation. The abdomen may show marked distention, and yet the patient has no pain aside from that associated with the extreme tension. Repeated vomiting occurs.

After the diagnosis has been established and the patient is suitably prepared the treatment of mechanical intestinal obstruction is by operation. The stomach should be emptied by passage of a Levin tube with continued suction drainage. Intravenous fluids are given to correct dehydration and electrolyte losses. At least 100 g. of glucose are provided in order to correct ketosis. The urine output is monitored, along with the specific gravity. An hourly urine output of over 25 ml. is desirable, and the specific gravity should be decreasing. During operation the distended intestine is decompressed, either by passage of a Leonard tube (a long tube passed through the mouth—a coiled spring aids passage; the surgeon guides it manually) or by passage of a Baker tube through a jejunotomy opening.

During the course of colonic obstruction the intraluminal pressure rises gradually. When complete obstruction of the colon develops with the ileocecal valve being competent for retrograde flow, it is a closed-loop obstruction. Therefore, immediate operative decompression is required to prevent rupture of the cecum. The operation of choice is transverse loop colostomy or cecostomy.

In contrast to mechanical obstruction, paralytic ileus often may be managed by intubation of the gut with the Miller-Abbott tube alone. During this period of decompression, administration of parenteral fluids, vitamins and transfusions must receive the same attention that is given to operative cases. Hypokalemia, if present, must be corrected.

A postoperative complication closely resembling paralytic ileus is known as acute dilation of the stomach. This usually follows some major abdominal procedure. Marked upper abdominal distention develops, associated with discomfort in this region. The patient experiences recurrent vomiting of dark gastric contents. This condition is handled readily by placing an indwelling Levin tube in the stomach and applying continuous suction drainage while maintaining the patient's fluid and electrolyte balance by parenteral means.

Appendicitis

Acute appendicitis is an extremely common disease that occurs most frequently during the second and third decades of life. It is somewhat more common in males than in females. Though there may be a primary diffuse inflammatory change in the appendix, obstruction of the lumen frequently occurs as a result of kinking or a fecal concretion. This seems to be a precipitating or aggravating factor. Secondary bacterial invastion, generally by a mixed infection including streptococci, staphylococci and *Escherichia*, takes place. If progress of the infection is not arrested, gangrene and perforation result.

The first symptom of this disease is abdominal pain. This usually is periumbilical or diffuse in character at the onset, but over a period of hours tends to localize in the region of the appendix. The pain is mild and cramplike, in marked contrast to the severe colic associated with biliary or urinary tract obstruction. Nausea and frequently vomiting follow the onset of pain. Either constipation or diarrhea may be present. The former is somewhat more common; the latter may signify that the appendix lies in the pelvis along the rectum. There is a mild febrile reaction. The temperature is rarely over 100° F., except in children or complicated cases. Moderate leukocytosis also develops, with a definite increase in the polymorphonuclear leukocyte percentage. On examination, the tenderness to palpation is over the area where the diseased appendix happens to lie. If the appendix lies in the pelvis, it may be difficult to elicit abdominal tenderness, but then it can be demonstrated on rectal or vaginal examination. Rigidity or muscle guarding usually is present over the area involved. However, if the appendix lies in a retrocecal position and is protected from the anterior parietal peritoneum, this may be minimal or absent. The disappearance of pain after several hours is not necessarily a good sign, inasmuch as it may indicate perforation of the appendix.

If the disease progresses and remains untreated, perforation eventually takes place. If the disease has been sufficiently slow in its progress, the appendix is likely to have been walled off by surrounding structures at this time, and a localized abscess develops. However, if this walling-off process has not been complete, spreading peritonitis sets in. Other complications of acute appendicitis are secondary abscess of the pelvic, the hepatic or the subhepatic regions, intestinal obstruction and pyelophlebitis. The last should be considered if the symptoms of chills and high fever are added to the picture. If multiple liver abscesses develop, the mortality is high.

The differential diagnosis should include acute mesenteric adenitis, bleeding graafian follicle, acute gastroenteritis, acute diverticulitis involving the sigmoid or Meckel's diverticulum, renal colic, pyelitis, biliary colic, perforated peptic ulcer, salpingitis and pneumonia.

Treatment. Though many cases of acute appendicitis no doubt subside spontaneously, the mortality in delayed treatment is extremely high, and that of prompt operation is minimal. Operation should be undertaken within the first few hours of the onset of the disease. If perforation has already taken place, and an abscess is present, nothing more than simple drainage may be feasible at the time of operation. Following such a procedure, a regimen for postoperative peritonitis should be followed, including continuous gastric suction drainage and intravenous fluids. Antibiotic therapy has greatly reduced the mortality in such cases.

Recurrent or chronic appendicitis is a term that should be reserved for cases of intermittent appendiceal colic, resulting in most cases from a fecalith that intermittently obstructs the appendiceal lumen. Not infrequently, one such attack fails to subside spontaneously and goes on to the typical changes described above with secondary bacterial invasion. When the diagnosis of recurrent appendicitis can be made with reasonable certainty, interval appendectomy is warranted.

Polyposis of the Intestinal Tract

Familial Polyposis. This disease characterized by innumerable polyps of the colon and rectum and is inherited as a Mendelian dominant. The polyps usually appear at puberty and cause bleeding from the rectum, diarrhea, tenesmus, or, less commonly, intestinal obstruction. The most serious complication is malignant change in the polyps. Most untreated patients die before the age of 50 from carcinoma of the colon. Treatment consists of colectomy and ileoproctostomy, or total colectomy and ileostomy.

Gardners Syndrome. This is a variant of familial polyposus, also inherited as a Mendelian dominant, that is associated with osteomas of the skull, multiple sebaceous cysts of the scalp, and desmoid tumors. It involves both large and small intestines, and lesions of the second portion of the duodenum close to the ampulla of Vater have been reported with some frequency. The age at which it is expressed is earlier than polyposis coli, but it also has an inexorable tendency toward malignant change.

Peutz-Jegher's Syndrome. This is a familial disease in which there is an association between hamartomatous polyps of the gastrointestinal tract and pigmented spots on the lips, buccal mucosa and hands. These polyps do not undergo malignant change. The small intestine contains more polyps than other portions of the gastrointestinal tract, but the entire tract may be involved. Symptoms arise from intussusception, which may spontaneously reduce or progress to intestinal obstruction.

Non-Familial Polyps of the Colon

Non-familial adenomatous polyps of the colon may be single or multiple, pedunculated or sessile. Whether benign polyps undergo malignant change remains conjectural, but both benign and malignant polyps occur. There is a correlation between size and malignancy, for example, pedunculated polyps less than 1 cm. in diameter have nearly a zero frequency, whereas the likelihood of a polyp 4 centimeters or more in diameter being malignant is nearly 30 per cent.

The villous adenoma (papillary adenoma) is a polyp of glandular origin with a great tendency to undergo malignant change. Larger lesions may be associated with significant losses of water, sodium and potassium.

Juvenile polyps, as the name implies, are lesions seen predominantly in the first decade of life. They are not neoplasms and are not associated with cancer. The presenting symptoms are bleeding and less frequently, abdominal pain.

Malignant Tumors of the Small Intestine

Cancer of the small intestine is rare. It is manifested by bleeding or obstruction, or both. Adenocarcinoma tends to encircle and obstruct the bowel. Smooth muscle tumors are bulky and polypoid with central ulceration, which gives rise to bleeding. Carcinoid tumors in the small intestine metastasize with greater frequency than carcinoids elsewhere in the alimentary tract; they also give rise to obstruction.

Carcinoid Syndrome

This is a symptom complex consisting of episodic flushing of the skin, abdominal cramps, diarrhea and asthma and is caused by a serotonin-secreting argentaffin tumor that has metastasized to the liver. The primary growth is located most commonly in the gastrointestinal tract, particularly in the distal ileum. The benign, nonfunctioning carcinoid tumor occurs preponderantly in the appendix. The diagnosis of a functioning carcinoid tumor is made by the detection of abnormal amounts of breakdown products of serotonin (5-hydroxy-3-(B-aminoethyl) indole in the urine. Surgical excision of the primary lesion is indicated. Carcinoid tumors of the tracheobronchial tree can also cause the carcinoid syndrome.

Carcinoma of the Colon and Rectum

The large intestine is a frequent site of carcinoma. The type of lesion and the symptoms differ greatly on the two sides of the colon. In the left side of the colon a constricting napkinring-like lesion is found. Associated with it are symptoms of mechanical obstruction, including alternating constipation and diarrhea, crampy abdominal pain and distention of the bowel. Blood may be noticed in the stools, and sometimes there is alteration in their caliber as the result of the constriction. On the other hand, in the right side of the colon the lesions are bulky and cauliflower-like in nature and are less likely to encircle the bowel. In addition, the liquid character of the fecal material on this side also diminishes the likelihood of obstructive symptoms. In this region blood loss is marked, and a profound anemia develops. This and the associated weakness may be the earliest symptoms of the disease in this area. There may be some discomfort in the region, and a mass may be palpable.

Carcinoma of the rectum presents symptoms that resemble more closely those of carcinoma of the left side of the colon. The change in caliber of the stools, alternating diarrhea and constipation, loss of blood and mucus and tenesmus all should suggest this lesion. Carcinoma of the rectum and the sigmoid comprises the largest percentage of neoplasms in the large bowel. Therefore, digital examination of the rectum and sigmoidoscopic examination should establish the diagnosis in a high percentage of cases of neoplasm of the large gut. Biopsy of the tumors in this area confirms the diagnosis. Though lesions above the reach of the rigid sigmoidoscope may sometimes be felt on abdominal palpation, the diagnosis is made by demonstration of the lesions by means of a barium enema. In cases in which carcinoma of the large intestine is suspected, a barium meal should not be given by mouth, inasmuch as complete obstruction may be precipitated by this procedure, and the barium may become inspissated proximal to the point of obstruction.

The flexible fiberoptic colonoscope has revolutionized the diagnosis of colonic carcinoma and polyps. In expert hands it is safe and permits accurate inspection of the entire colon. Biopsy can be obtained and pedunculated polyps can be removed. The examination should be carried out when roentgenograms are equivocal or polyps are present beyond reach of the rigid sigmoidoscope. It should be noted that a flexible, fiberoptic sigmoidoscope is in use that has also improved diagnostic accuracy, as well as permitting endoscopic removal of polyps up to 5 cm. in diameter.

Carcinoma of the colon is not usually a radiosensitive lesion. Operation offers the patient the only hope of cure. The type of resection necessary depends on the location of the lesion and on the factors peculiar to each case.

Below the pectinate line the epithelium becomes squamous in character. Therefore, carcinoma occurring in the anal canal or the anus is a squamous cell lesion, in contrast to adenocarcinoma of the bowel. Carcinoma in this area manifests itself as a persistent ulcer. Diagnosis is established readily by biopsy. Both wide surgical excision and radiation therapy have been used in the treatment of this lesion, but surgical removal is preferable. Metastases involve the inguinal lymph nodes as well as inferior mesenteric and hypogastric lymph nodes.

Diverticular Disease of the Colon

In older persons diverticula of the large intestine are very common. They occur most often in the region of the sigmoid and the descending colon but may appear anywhere in the colon. Though frequently asymptomatic, they may undergo acute inflammatory changes, giving rise to pain, fever, leukocytosis, tenderness and a mass. The inflammatory change in the bowel wall may be sufficient to encroach on its lumen and result in partial obstruction. In some ways the clinical picture resembles that presented by malignant disease in this area. A barium enema demonstrates the irregular constricted lesion. The roentgenologist may or may not be able to establish the nature of the constricting lesion, and, indeed, carcinoma and diverticulitis may coexist.

Mild cases of acute diverticulitis may respond to conservative treatment consisting of rest of the intestinal tract, parenteral fluids and antispasmodic drugs such as atropine and phenobarbitol. Antimicrobial agents are also of value in limiting the infection. If the process subsides completely, nothing more need be done. However, recurrent bouts of diverticulitis should lead to resection of the involved area. Frequently, diverticulitis progresses to the point of perforation with the development of a localized abscess. If the abscess forms in the mesentery, resection and anastomosis are feasible and preferable to drainage. Abscesses other than these will require adequate drainage and proximal colostomy. Resection will subsequently be necessary. Perforation into adjacent viscera, including bladder, small intestine and vagina, leads to fistula formation. This is also an indication for surgical resection.

Hemorrhage from diverticulosis occasionally occurs. This appears most often in the hypertensive older patient. Bleeding from the rectum in profuse amounts is the outstanding symptom.

Selective angiography of the superior and inferior mesenteric arteries is most useful in delineating the site of bleeding. Although diverticula are more frequent in the sigmoid, massive bleeding is frequent from lesions on the right side. For this reasons total colectomy and ileorectostomy may be necessary.

Angiodysplasia is probably a more frequent cause of bleeding from the colon than is diverticular disease. It has been defined by selective angiography of the cecum and ascending colon. Treatment is by resection of the right colon to the splenic flexure. If lesser resections are done, recurrent bleeding is likely.

Ulcerative Colitis

This is a chronic disease subject to acute exacerbations. The etiology is unknown, though the disease appears to be more common in nervous, high-strung individuals. Relapses may be related to periods of emotional upset or nervous tension.

The disease is marked by diarrhea containing blood, pus and mucus. There are marked weight loss and anemia. During exacerbations the patient may be critically ill with high temperature, leukocytosis and tachycardia. Death from peritonitis may result during such a period.

The process begins in the rectum and spreads proximally to successively involve the colonic mucosa. Skip areas do not occur. Involvement, mainly of the mucosa, consists of crypt abscesses, ulcerations, pseudopolyp formation and healing.

On direct inspection of the rectal mucosa, a velvety appearance is seen. There are multiple tiny ulcers that bleed readily from trauma. A barium enema may demonstrate a fuzzy appearance of the mucous membrane, and in late stages the bowel is contracted and rigid.

Differential diagnosis includes consideration of specific diseases, such as amebic and bacillary dysentery. Crohn's disease of the colon is the most frequently seen inflammatory lesion of the large intestine to be confused with idiopathic ulcerative colitis. The cobblestone appearance of the mucosa, presence of granulomas and transmural involvement are distinguishing features of Crohn's disease. It may be segmental, and skip areas may also be present as well as involvement of the small intestine.

Treatment. Every effort should be made to control the disease by medical management, including adequate rest and bland diet from which all foods irritating to the patient's bowel have been excluded. Corticosteroid therapy has been shown to increase the frequency of remissions and to shorten the periods of activity of disease. Mild cases may be controlled in this way. However, many will continue to have so much trouble that surgery becomes necessary. The procedure of choice combines ileostomy and colectomy. Rarely the disease process quiets down sufficiently after ileostomy to permit restoration of bowel continuity. Complications of ulcerative colitis include profuse hemorrhage, perforation, obstruction, arthralgia, uveitis, necrotizing pyoderma and cancer. Toxic megacolon is a complication that frequently necessitates emergency colectomy. Cancer of the colon occurs with greater frequency and at an earlier age in patients with ulcerative colitis. The longer a patient suffers from ulcerative colitis, the greater is the risk of cancer.

Regional Enteritis (Crohn's Disease)

This is an inflammatory disease of the intestinal tract, which usually, but not always, involves the terminal ileum. Skip areas occur, with involvement of jejunum, colon, duodenum, stomach and even the esophagus. As noted above many cases involving the colon have been erroneously called idiopathic ulcerative colitis. The process is characterized by involvement of all layers of the wall of the intestine, granuloma formation with predominantly a giant cell response, and skip areas. The regional lymph nodes are strikingly involved. The etiology is unknown, but the condition may be the result of lymphatic obstruction. Symptoms consist of diarrhea, weight loss, fever and crampy abdominal pain. Blood, pus and mucus may be found in the stool. The acute form may be mistaken for appendicitis.

Treatment is conservative unless one of the complications appears—perforation, fistula formation, obstruction or intractability. If operation becomes necessary, resection of the diseased intestine is done, if possible. Other options include bypass procedures such as ileostomy or ileocolostomy in exclusion. Recurrences are common.

Ischiorectal Abscess

The causative agent in this infection usually is the colon bacillus. It reaches the ischiorectal fossa as the result of extension of an infection in an anal crypt outward into the perirectal space. The disease is manifested by pain, tenderness, induration and redness on one side or the other of the anus. Eventually, fluctuation is demonstrable. The temperature is elevated, and there is leukocytosis. Treatment consists of adequate incision and drainage. Frequently the patient is left with a fistula-in-ano following this procedure, which requires correction by secondary operation. Supralevator abscess is most frequently caused by diverticular disease of the colon.

Fistula-in-Ano

Fistula-in-ano results from extension of infection in an anal crypt outward into the subcutaneous tissues. Having reached this area the infection eventually appears beneath the skin in the perianal region and usually drains spontaneously. Then the patient is left with either a fistula that persistently drains a small amount of pus, and perhaps fecal material, or he is subject to recurrent bouts of superficial healing of the external opening, with subsequent formation of an abscess that opens spontaneously at the site of the previous opening. Treatment of the condition consists of complete excision of the tract, with division of the external sphincter or a portion of it, if necessary, to obtain complete removal. The wound is packed open and allowed to heal secondarily by granulation tissue.

Hemorrhoids

Hemorrhoids are protruding masses of tissue in the region of the anal canal, usually associated with dilation of the venous plexus beneath. Contributing factors in the development of hemorrhoids include back pressure such as results from pregnancy, constipation and straining at stool. The term *external hemorrhoids* is reserved for those hemorrhoids that rise below the pectinate line and the term *internal hemorrhoids* for those rising above this level. Frequently the two types are combined and are known as mixed hemorrhoids. Hemorrhoids may be asymptomatic or give rise to various complaints. Internal hemorrhoids may excite a mucoid discharge. They may prolapse at the time of stool and have to be replaced. They are eroded readily and give rise to rectal bleeding, which is bright red in color. Hemorrhoids may be associated with itching. External hemorrhoids occasionally undergo thrombosis with the development of a painful, tender, bluish swelling at the anal margin. Finally, internal hemorrhoids may prolapse and become strangulated, ulcerated and gangrenous.

The treatment for hemorrhoids in general is surgical excision, which usually calls for sharp dissection and suture, though occasionally the clamp and cautery method is used. Thrombosis of an external hemorrhoid is relieved readily by incision of the thrombosed hemorrhoid with the clot being shelled out under local anesthesia. Surgical excision is the preferred treatment. Though bleeding in hemorrhoids usually is small in amount, its continuance over a long time may give rise to definite secondary anemia. *Sigmoidoscopic examination should always be carried out before hemorrhoidectomy is done.*

Fissure-in-Ano

This is a longitudinal ulceration at the opening of the anal canal. Almost always these ulcerations are located in the midline. Fissure-in-ano is associated with pain and bleeding at the time of defecation, and the pain persists for some time thereafter. There is usually spasm of the sphincter muscle that is responsible for the pain. The usual treatment is excision with packing of the wound. Division of the external sphincter is usually necessary.

Rectal Prolapse

Rectal prolapse is a herniation of the rectum through the anus. It usually occurs in older individuals. The primary etiologic factors are: (1) weakening of the muscular and ligamentous support of the pelvic floor; (2) dilation of the anal sphincters and (3) redundancy of the rectum and the sigmoid. Very often, surgical correction is followed by recurrence. The most successful operation has been the combined abdominoperineal approach in which the redundant sigmoid is resected and fixed to the sacrum, and the perineal supports are plicated.

HERNIA

A hernia is a protrusion of a viscus through the wall of the cavity that ordinarily confines it. Several terms are used to describe various types of hernias. A *reducible* hernia is one in which the contents may be returned entirely to the cavity that ordinarily contains them. This is not possible in an *irreducible* or *incarcerated* hernia, usually because of the development of adhesions between the contents and the hernial sac or between the visceral surfaces of the contents themselves. Incarcerated hernias can be either acute or chronic. A painful acutely incarcerated hernia should be suspected of being *strangulated* until proven otherwise by early operation. A strangulated hernia is one in which the blood supply of the viscus is interfered with so that gangrene ultimately results. A *congenital* hernia is one present at birth and is almost always inguinal or umbilical in type. An *acquired* hernia develops somewhat later in life.

Hernias are described also according to their location. The most common type of hernia is one in the *inguinal* region. It is more common in the male. There are two types, *direct* and *indirect*. An indirect hernia is one in which the sac opens at the internal inguinal ring and passes down the course of the inguinal canal anterior to the structures of the spermatic cord. The neck of the sac lies lateral to the inferior (deep) epigastric artery and vein. If sufficiently large, it then emerges through the external inguinal ring and may actually continue down along the cord into the scrotum. In the female the sac passes along the course of the round ligament of the uterus into the labium majus. The sac is the unobliterated processus vaginalis and follows the course of descent of the testicle and the round ligament.

A direct inguinal hernia is a protrusion directly through the posterior wall of the inguinal canal medial to the deep epigastric vessels. It may also present through the external inguinal ring and usually manifests itself as a rounded swelling of limited size, in contrast with the elongated tubular course of the indirect type. This type represents a bulging of all the structures of the abdominal wall, and, although it may present at the external ring, it does not descend into the scrotum. The direct inguinal hernia usually is seen in older men and is the result of a weakening of the fascial structures. Direct inguinal hernias do not occur in women because of the excellent support of the posterior wall of the inguinal canal.

A *femoral* hernia passes through the femoral canal. Therefore, the sac lies below Poupart's ligament, slightly lateral to the pubic tubercle and medial to the femoral vein, upon the pectineus muscle. The sac may present at the fossa ovalis and be directed upward over Poupart's ligament. In such cases it may be confused with an inguinal hernia. Also, it may be difficult at times to distinguish it from enlarged inguinal lymph nodes in that region.

An *umbilical* hernia is a defect in the region of the umbilicus. A small defect in this area is not uncommon, but usually it fills with scar tissue as the child develops, especially if the hernia is kept reduced by means of adhesive strapping or a truss. Umbilical hernias also are not uncommon in older women. In children especially, umbilical hernia often is associated with separation of the rectus muscles, known as diastasis of the recti. An *incisional* hernia occurs at the site of a previous operative wound and frequently is the result of postoperative infection. This is a type of ventral hernia.

There are various types of internal hernias in which the viscera protrude through openings within the abdominal cavity and therefore, are not manifested externally. A protrusion through the obturator foramen, an *obturator* hernia, is an example of this type.

An *epigastric* hernia is a small nodular mass in the midline of the upper abdomen that results from protrusion of the preperitoneal fat along the course of a vessel penetrating the linea alba. These hernias contain no peritoneal sac.

A *diaphragmatic* hernia is a protrusion of abdominal contents upward through the diaphragm into the thorax. Almost always, these are left-sided, since the right side of the diaphragm is protected by the liver. They may be congenital or acquired. Trauma is the most frequent cause of the latter.

As a rule, the diagnosis of hernia is made readily by the demonstration of a mass in one of the locations described. This mass often transmits an impulse on coughing or on straining. If reducible, the defect in the abdominal wall is demonstrable. Diaphragmatic hernia can be demonstrated by the finding of peristalsis in the thorax on auscultation, the roentgenographic demonstration of intestinal gas patterns or the presence of barium following the administration of a barium meal.

Incarceration and strangulation of hernias constitute surgical emergencies. A strangulated hernia, implying an interference with the blood supply of the contents of the sac, in addition presents a picture of constant severe pain and a tense, tender hernial sac. An attempt may be made to reduce such a hernia by placing the patient in a reclining position with the hips elevated and the knees and hips flexed. With the patient relaxed it may be possible to reduce the hernia by gentle manipulation. This procedure is known as taxis. In attempts to reduce an incarcerated or strangulated hernia, at times the mass is returned to the abdominal cavity en bloc or en masse; therefore, the trouble is not relieved, because the constricting ring of the neck of the hernial sac still imprisons the viscera.

In infants, indirect inguinal hernias are usually not associated with significant abnormalities in the musculoaponeurotic supporting structures. Removal of the patent processus vaginalis is sufficient to cure the hernia and simple closure of the wound in layers is all that is necessary. If the conjoined tendon is sutured to Poupart's ligament anterior to the spermatic cord, a *Ferguson herniorrhaphy* will have been done. When the internal inguinal ring is significantly stretched, a defect in the transversalis fascia of varying size will be present and reconstruction of the posterior wall of the inguinal canal will be necessary. The spermatic cord may be mobilized and the conjoined tendon sutured to Poupart's ligament posterior to the cord, constituting a *Bassini* repair. In large indirect inguinal hernias and in direct inguinal hernias the posterior wall of the inguinal canal is deficient. The *Halsted* herniorrhaphy corrects this by suturing both the conjoined tendon and external oblique aponeurosis posterior to the spermatic cord leaving the cord in a subcutaneous position. The preferred operation by many for large indirect inguinal hernias and direct inguinal hernias is the *McVay* repair. In this operation the transversus aponeurosis is sutured posterior to the cord to Cooper's ligament medially, and the transversalis fascia laterally. A relaxing incision in the rectus sheath is necessary to relieve tension on the suture line.

ADRENAL GLANDS

The indications for surgery of the adrenals are: (1) tumors or hyperplasia of the adrenal medulla or cortex and (2) palliation in metastatic carcinoma of the breast.

Tumors of the Adrenal Medulla

Neuroblastomas arise from nerve cells. They have no endocrine function and are more common in infants and children than in adults. Treatment is surgical excision.

Pheochromocytoma is an endocrine tumor that arises from chromaffin cells and produces norepinephrine and epinephrine. The chief symptom is persistent or paroxysmal hypertension. If untreated, the patient dies from a complication of hypertension or from congestive heart failure. Ten per cent of these tumors arise in an extraadrenal location, primarily along the paravertebral sympathetic chain. A small percentage are malignant. When bilateral pheochromocytomas are present, they are likely to be familial. The thyroid gland may harbor a medullary carcinoma with amyloid stroma in this situation. (Sipple's syndrome)

The diagnosis today is based on the quantitative assay of catecholamines and their metabolic products in the urine. Treatment consists of surgical removal. Preparation with dibenzyline and adequate hydration is helpful.

Tumors of the Adrenal Cortex

Tumors of the cortex may be functioning or nonfunctioning. A functioning adenoma may cause an adrenogenital syndrome that has different manifestations, depending on the age when the hormonal stimulation appeared. Prenatal virilism may cause pseudohermaphroditism at birth. Postnatal virilism causes precocious puberty in the male and heterosexual characteristics in the female.

Cortical tumors and, more commonly cortical hyperplasia may cause Cushing's syndrome. There is a moon face and buffalo obesity. The skin is striated; pigmentation and hirsutism develop. Amenorrhea occurs in females and impotence in males. Removal of the adenoma or total adrenalectomy for hyperplasia results in improvement. Hyperplasia is usually treated today by proton-beam radiation of the pituitary gland.

Hyperaldosteronism

A primary increase in secretion of aldosterone is seen in some functioning cortical adenomas or with cortical hyperplasia. The manifestations are hypertension, muscular weakness, metabolic alkalosis, potassium deficiency, suppressed plasma renin activity, and increased potassium and aldosterone excretion. These findings must be documented in the absence of diuretic therapy, chronic vomiting (or laxative abuse), or renal arterial disease.

Palliation for Advanced Cancer

Total adrenalectomy will provide temporary benefit to many patients with hormone-dependent metastatic carcinoma. This therapy is reserved until castration, radiation and hormone therapy are no longer helpful. Its greatest use has been in cancer of the breast.

PEDIATRIC SURGERY INVOLVING THE DIGESTIVE TRACT

Esophageal Atresia

The most common form consists of discontinuity between proximal and distal esophagus; the proximal esophagus ends blindly, and a fistula is present between the distal esophagus and the trachea. The infant appears to salivate excessively. A tube cannot be passed into the stomach if intubation is attempted. Barium swallow is contraindicated, for it will be regurgitated into the tracheobronchial tree. The preferred treatment is early repair through an extrapleural approach.

Intestinal Atresia

The absence of swallowed vernix cells in the meconium (Farber's test) indicates intestinal atresia. Such atresias occur most frequently in the ileum and the duodenum. Abdominal roentgenograms confirm the diagnosis. There is a characteristic "double bubble" on the roentgenogram in duodenal atresia. The type of operation depends upon the site of the atresia: in the duodenum, either duodenojejunostomy or gastroenterostomy with accompanying pyloroplasty; elsewhere, end-to-end anastomosis using interrupted fine non-absorbable sutures is the procedure of choice. The extremely dilated proximal segment is resected and the distal segment distended by injecting saline solution.

Imperforate Anus

Imperforate anus usually is diagnosed at birth when the absence of an anal opening is apparent. If this defect is not recognized for 36 to 48 hours, the infant presents a picture of colon obstruction.

The common anorectal abnormalities may be grouped as follows: (1) anal stenosis due to incomplete rupture of the anal membrane; (2) imperforate anal membrane; (3) imperforate anus with the rectum ending in a blind pouch some distance from the anal dimple—with associated rectovesical, rectourethral or rectoperineal fistulas in males, and rectovaginal or rectoperineal fistulas in females in a large percentage of cases; and (4) normal anus and lower rectum, with the rectal pouch ending blindly. The treatment varies with the type of abnormality. The third type is much more common than the others. Treatment depends partly upon the distance separating the rectum from the anus. This can be determined by means of a roentgenogram with the infant inverted and a marker on the anal dimple. If the pouch is low or an anal membrane is present primary anal repair is feasible. When the pouch is high a transverse colostomy is performed with elective repair after the baby is 1 year of age. With larger structures more satisfactory positioning of the rectum in relation to the puborectalis sling is possible.

Meconium Ileus

Meconium ileus, caused by impacted meconium as a part of a picture of cystic fibrosis and pancreatic insufficiency, is a form of intestinal obstruction in the newborn with a high mortality rate. Vomiting frequently begins on the first day and is associated with abdominal distention, caused partly by palpable masses of meconium within the dilated loops. Roentgenograms characteristically reveal distended loops of intestine that vary in size. There is a mottled appearance due to inspissated meconium. Volvulus of the involved segment is also frequent. Treatment consists of operation with resection of the distal ileum containing the inspissated meconium. Primary anastomosis is preferable to colostomy, which is reserved for infants who are in extremis.

Pyloric Stenosis

Hypertrophic pyloric stenosis represents a form of pyloric obstruction resulting from hypertrophy of the pyloric muscle. It occurs most commonly in first-born male infants, 2 to 4 weeks of age. The etiology is uncertain. Diagnosis is confirmed by palpation of an olive-sized, firm tumor in the right upper quadrant and by roentgenograms of the stomach. Vomiting may be propulsive and is usually free of bile. Operation consists of dividing the thickened pyloric muscle (Ramstedt operation).

Malrotation

Incomplete rotation of the midgut, due to peritoneal bands across the duodenum, causes duodenal obstruction in infants. The mesentery of the small intestine is elongated and its fixation to the posterior parietes is shortened, because of this, midgut volvulus is frequent. Operation consists of freeing the bands lateral to the duodenum and untwisting the midgut in a counterclockwise direction.

Intussusception

Intussusception is the telescoping of a portion of intestine into another segment. It is the most common cause of obstruction in childhood. The etiology is unknown in most cases. The most common type is ileocolic. The clinical picture consists of a triad of signs: (1) abdominal cramps; (2) a mass in the right lower quadrant; and (3) blood in the stool.

Reduction of the intussusception may be achieved by operation or by barium enema. If reduction is not accomplished, the blood supply to the gut is compromised, and gangrene develops.

Congenital Megacolon

Hirschsprung's disease consists of colon obstruction appearing in infancy or childhood and due to abnormal distal colonic function. Peristaltic waves are ineffective in the involved segment because of the absence of ganglion cells in Auerbach's plexus. The rectum and the rectosigmoid are involved most commonly.

The diagnosis will be suspect if barium studies of the colon and rectum show constriction of the distal aganglionic segment and dilatation of the proximal colon. The diagnosis is established by deep biopsy of the rectal wall that shows absence of ganglion cells in the myenteric plexus.

Considerable abdominal distention may occur, particularly in older children. In these cases, large fecal masses within the colon may be felt through the abdominal wall.

Treatment consists of resection of the aganglionic segment. It may be necessary to perform a preliminary colostomy in infants when obturation obstruction is present.

The Genitourinary System

Hematuria

Hematuria may be:

1. Urethral from: (a) calculus; (b) instrumentation or trauma; (c) acute urethritis; or (d) new growths. Gross blood may be visible at the meatus; though the voided specimen contains blood, the catheterized specimen does not.
2. Prostatic from: (a) calculus; (b) trauma; (c) instrumentation; (d) hypertrophy; or (e) tumor. The urine usually contains blood clots at the end of micturition.

3. Vesical from: (a) papilloma; (b) carcinoma or other tumors; (c) stones or foreign bodies; (d) ulceration; or (e) inflammation. The urine contains clots, mostly at the end of micturition.
4. Ureteral from: (a) calculus; (b) neoplasm; (c) inflammation; or (d) trauma. The bleeding often is slight, and the clots formed in the ureter may appear in the urine as worm-like casts.
5. Renal from: (a) calculus; (b) tuberculosis or other bacterial infections; (c) papilloma; (d) neoplasms; (e) trauma; (f) chemical poisoning; (g) blood disease, or (h) essential hematuria.

In hematuria from systemic disease, such as nephritis secondary to fever, albumin and casts also are found in the urine. Moderate microscopic hematuria following renal colic is almost pathognomonic of a calculus.

THE KIDNEYS

Calculus

Symptoms. A large staghorn calculus anchored in the substance of the kidney does not give rise to obstruction and therefore rarely produces colic. There is rather a dragging ache in the loin. However, pyuria, gross or microscopic hematuria and crystalluria are present. A smaller stone in the pelvis or the ureter is likely to give rise to obstruction. This is characterized by acute agonizing pain in the back and loin, often referred along the course of the ureter to the bladder and the external genitalia. Nausea, vomiting, chills and fever may be present. Unless the ureter is obstructed completely, red blood cells and leukocytes usually can be seen in the urine. Urgency and dysuria often are present. If the calculus is of long duration, chronic or recurrent infection is frequent, and the chief complaints may be those of pyelitis or pyelonephritis.

Diagnosis. The history, physical examination, urinalysis and survey film of the abdomen usually establish the diagnosis. On cystoscopic examinations and catheterization of the ureters, the obstruction may be demonstrated, and scratch marks appear on a wax-tipped ureteral bougie. Differential diagnosis includes acute appendicitis, acute biliary colic and penetrating or perforating peptic ulcers. The milder pain in acute appendicitis and the characteristic initial and subsequent locations of the pain, plus the absence of roentgenographic and urinary tract findings, help to establish the diagnosis of the disease. In biliary tract disease the history of preceding attacks, fatty indigestion and radiation of the pain to the right scapula and shoulder, associated with local tenderness over the gallbladder area, aid in distinguishing this disease from renal calcu-

lus. Usually in peptic ulcer there is a typical history of gastric pain exacerbated by hunger and eased by the ingestion of food prior to the onset of penetration or perforation.

Treatment. Small stones may pass through the ureter, with morphine being given for pain and drugs of the atropine group being given in an attempt to relax the ureter. Frequently, also, hot baths give the patient great comfort during the passage of the calculus. Should the stone become impacted in the ureter, it may be dislodged at times by ureteral manipulation through the cystoscope. Larger calculi require surgical removal by incising the renal pelvis or the ureter. Extremely large stones at times require surgical removal through the renal cortex. If the calculus has been associated with distention of long standing, the kidney is damaged beyond repair.

Hydronephrosis

Hydronephrosis is distention of the renal pelvis and calices secondary to obstruction somewhere in the course of the urinary tract, giving rise to back pressure. If the distention is of sufficiently long standing, there is secondary atrophy of the renal parenchyma. The obstruction may be due to: (1) angulation or kinking of the ureter; (2) stricture; (3) aberrant vessels; (4) calculus; (5) neoplasm; (6) trauma; (7) pressure from external growths; (8) prostatic enlargement; or (9) retroperitoneal fibrosis. It is seen more frequently in women than in men. In the mild form there is discomfort in the region of the kidney. In ureteral catheterization a large amount of urine is obtained on entering the renal pelvis. Hydronephrosis may be demonstrated both by intravenous urography and retrograde pyelography. Hydronephrosis often is associated with secondary bacterial infection, and the primary symptoms then are those of pyelonephritis.

Treatment depends entirely on the cause of the obstruction. Removal of the causative factor usually will result in relief of the hydronephrosis. If the obstruction has been of long standing, and the renal parenchyma is largely destroyed, nephrectomy at times will be necessary. Retroperitoneal fibrosis usually results in bilateral ureteral obstruction. To relieve the obstruction both ureters must be mobilized and transposed to an intraperitoneal position.

Infections of the Kidney

Perinephric Abscess. This condition may result from a primary infection, probably blood borne, or from secondary infection of the urinary tract or extension from an adjacent focus of infection in the kidney. The infection usually lies behind the kidney, though it may involve an extensive area in the retroperitoneal region above and below the kidney. The colon bacillus is a frequent offending organism. If allowed to go untreated, the abscess may dissect well downward toward the pelvis in the retroperitoneal space or upward into the thorax and rupture into the pleural cavity.

The symptoms consist of deep-seated pain in the flank, often radiating downward and increased by pressure, together with local tenderness over the kidney and muscular rigidity. As the result of muscular spasm, the spine may be quite rigid. High temperature and leukocytosis are present, and there may be visible fullness on the involved side overlying the kidney. Redness and edema are seen occasionally. The abscess is likely to be so deep that fluctuation cannot be demonstrated. Unless there is associated pyelonephritis, the urine is likely to be normal. Perinephric abscess often is recognized only late in the course of the disease. Any patient who has a persistent fever and leukocytosis should be examined carefully for evidence of this condition. The obliteration of the psoas shadow on a supine film of the abdomen is a strongly suggestive finding.

As soon as the diagnosis can be established, adequate drainage should be carried out through a posterior approach.

Tuberculosis. Tubercle bacilli may reach the kidney from the bloodstream, the lymphatics or the lower urinary tract. Renal tuberculosis may be one manifestation of the miliary form of the disease. This occurs commonly in children. Primary involvement of the renal parencyhma is unilateral as a rule and is more common in young women than in men. If the parenchyma alone is involved, there are no specific findings in the urinary sediment. However, as soon as the lesion drains into the renal pelvis, the urine contains blood, pus and tubercle bacilli. Renal tuberculosis may result also from extension of the disease upward from the lower urinary tract. This type is more common in men and is often bilateral.

There is bladder irritability with urgency, frequency and polyuria. Hematuria may be profuse without apparent cause. Pyuria is present, and the urine usually contains no bacteria other than tubercle bacilli. There is discomfort in the lumbar region and local tenderness. General symptoms of tuberculosis, such as an evening rise in temperature, loss of weight, night sweats and weakness, may be present. On cystoscopic examination there are redness, swelling and retraction of the ureteral orifice. Occasionally, tuberculosis ulcers of the bladder may be seen. Diminished renal function eventually results. X-ray examination may show calcified deposits in the parenchyma. Both the intravenous urogram and the retrograde pyelogram show distortion of the pelvis, the calices and the ureter. Complications include extension of the infection to involve the perine-

phric area or downward extension to involve the ureter and the bladder. This often results in secondary involvement of the opposite kidney. Mixed infections may ensue eventually. Stricture formation may lead to pyelonephritis.

Irritability of the bladder without adequate explanation and sterile pyuria suggest the possibility of renal tuberculosis. Evidence of the disease may be found elsewhere, as in the bladder, the epididymis and the seminal vesicles. Demonstration of the tubercle bacilli in the urine smear, culture or guinea pig inoculation establishes the diagnosis.

Treatment with antituberculous drugs for a minimum of 2 years is indicated. Surgery is reserved for complications such as abscess formation, a destroyed kidney, etc.

Tumors of the Kidney

Hypernephroma (Clear Cell Carcinoma). This is the most common renal tumor. Usually it occurs in the male in midlife. Embryoma (Wilms' tumor), in contrast with hypernephroma, occurs in children, frequently manifesting itself during the first year of life. Other malignant tumors include papillary carcinoma and epithelioma of the renal pelvis, carcinoma and sarcoma. Occasionally the kidney also is the site of metastatic carcinoma. Benign tumors of the kidney include cortical adenoma papilloma, papillary cystadenoma, angioma and simple or solitary cysts of the kidney. Polycystic disease of the kidney is benign in the true sense of the term. However, the prognosis is poor, because eventually there is so much destruction of renal parenchyma that renal insufficiency develops. The cardinal symptoms of renal tumor are hematuria, a mass and pain. Nonspecific symptoms such as cachexia, anemia and weight loss usually are late manifestations of the disease. Hematuria may be intermittent and therefore demands early and complete investigation. An intravenous urogram and retrograde pyelogram demonstrate deformity of the renal pelvis and the calices. Angiography is extremely helpful, particularly in smaller tumors that do not encroach on the renal collecting system.

If there is no roentgenographic evidence of widespread metastases, exploration should be carried out and nephrectomy performed, if this is feasible. Though some of the malignant lesions, such as embryoma, are radiosensitive, the best results in the treatment of malignant tumors of the kidney have followed early nephrectomy. Benign lesions often can be corrected by local removal or partial nephrectomy. Though repeated aspiration of the cysts in polycystic disease of the kidney has been tried, up to the present time no satisfactory treatment has been discovered.

Wilms' Tumor. Embryoma of the kidney is the most common abdominal tumor in childhood. These tumors are highly malignant and may reach a large size. Metastases are first noted in the lungs. The mass is painless. There is usually associated low-grade fever.

Treatment consists of excision in association with radiation and chemotherapy. Addition of the latter two modalities has greatly improved suvival rates.

Rupture of the Kidney

This injury results from direct trauma. There are local pain and tenderness with splinting of the overlying muscles. The adjacent ribs may be fractured. Blood is found in the urine. On ureteral catheterization, origin of the bleeding from the damaged kidney can be confirmed. In most cases conservative treatment will suffice. If there is evidence of extensive and continued hemorrhage, nephrectomy may be necessary to control the bleeding. Intravenous urography is useful in evaluating the extent of injury and in deciding if an operation is necessary. In patients with multiple organ injury, tears in the kidney may be present. At operation a retroperitoneal hematoma will be present. There is a tendency for bleeding from minor tears, as well as some major ones, to be tamponaded by the peritoneum and fascia with clot formation and cessation of bleeding. If the hematoma is not expanding the peritoneum should be left intact and the kidney not explored. Severe trauma may result in complete disruption of the renal artery and vein. Bleeding is usually massive, but frequently will cease. Pyelography will show absence of function and renal scanning with ^{131}I hippurate will show lack of perfusion. A delayed complication of a perinephric hematoma may be hypertension. This elevated pressure can be normalized by nephrectomy or removal of the encapsulating hematoma.

PROSTATE

Benign Hypertrophy

This is extremely common in men over 50. In many cases of hypertrophy obstructive symptoms of some degree develop, and some ultimately develop carcinoma. The etiology is unknown. The hypertrophy is composed of both glandular and fibrous tissue elements. The prostatic urethra becomes elongated and distorted. As a result of obstruction at the internal meatus, the bladder wall undergoes hypertrophy, trabeculation and dilatation. There is increasing residual urine. Secondary infection ultimately results, involving primarily the bladder. However, as the obstruction gradually involves the upper urinary tract, hydroureter and hydronephrosis set in. Secondary infection also occurs here and, finally, renal insufficiency. The symptoms include diminution in force and size of the urinary stream, delay in starting, frequency, nocturia, bouts of acute retention requiring catheterization and incontinence due to overflow. When chronic cystitis and pyelonephritis develop, the picture of infection is evident. Rectal examination reveals an enlarged firm prostate. Catheterization may be difficult because of elongation and distortion of the prostatic urethra. However, hypertrophy of the prostate gland is best demonstrated by cystoscopic examination. In chronic retention with back pressure of long standing, one should guard against sudden decompression of the bladder by catheterization. Unless decompression is gradual, edema and congestion of the bladder and kidney result, with gross hematuria, suppression of urine and uremia that may be fatal.

Treatment. Obstruction to the outlet of the bladder may be relieved by four methods: (1) suprapubic prostatectomy; (2) perineal prostatectomy; (3) retropubic prostatectomy; and (4) transuretheral resection. Transuretheral resection especially has attained widespread popularity. It consists of removal of the obstructing prostate through a cystoscope by electrosurgery. In advanced disease with uremia, a preliminary period of preparation is frequently desirable, including catheter drainage or suprapubic cystotomy, chemotherapy and increased fluid intake.

Carcinoma

The symptoms of carcinoma of the prostate may be minimal or absent at first or may resemble those of simple hypertrophy if the malignant mass leads to obstruction of the outlet of the bladder. However, on rectal examination, the prostate is firm, hard, nodular and asymmetrical. If the disease is advanced, there may be evidence of fixation to the surrounding structures. If seen early, prostatectomy may be carried out. The acid phosphatase should be measured, elevation is usual with extension and metastasis. Metastasis occurs to the regional lymph nodes, the spine and the pelvic bones. Pain from bony metastasis may be the first symptom of the disease. Radiation therapy has no permanent value. In inoperable cases or in patients with pain from bone metastasis, excellent palliative results may be obtained by bilateral orchiectomy and the use of estrogenic agents. If prostatic obstruction is sufficiently severe suprapubic cystostomy or transurethral resection may be required.

SCROTUM AND GENITALIA

Common enlargements include hydrocele, hernia, acute orchitis, epididymitis, tuberculosis, syphilis, malignant neoplasms and varicocele.

Hydrocele

This is a cystic enlargement of the tunica vaginalis. It may occur at any age. Frequently it is entirely asymptomatic except for the presence of the mass. It may be quite tense or cystic in nature. Transillumination usually confirms the diagnosis. The cystic swelling may obliterate the outlines of the testicle and the epididymis. Aspiration yields a clear fluid. Occasionally, hydrocele may involve a portion of the spermatic cord instead of surrounding the testis.

Repeated aspirations are of palliative value only. The procedure of choice is surgery, consisting of opening the sac and everting it about the testicle.

Scrotal Hernia

Usually this can be demonstrated proceeding downward from the inguinal canal into the scrotum above the testis. Often it is reducible, transmits an impulse when the patient coughs, increases when he stands and may be tympanitic and demonstrate peristalsis on auscultation if it contains bowel. It does not transmit light on transillumination.

Varicocele

An undue enlargement or varicosity of the pampiniform plexus, varicocele is more common on the left side than on the right. Occasionally it is associated with a dragging, aching sensation in the testis on that side. The discomfort may be diminished by the use of adequate support. On examination, the varicosity is evident along the structures of the cord above the testicle. This is most marked in the erect posture. Frequently, it has been described as feeling like a bag of worms. Treatment consists of excision of the varicose portion of the plexus.

Stricture of the Urethra

This is usually the end-result of a gonorrheal infection. On the other hand, it may follow trauma to the urethra, as in fracture of the pelvis. Repeated dilatation of the stricture by a sound usually will maintain an adequate passage, but it may be necessary to resort to transurethral division of the stricture.

Acute Orchitis

This disease may follow mumps or other infectious disease or, occasionally, trauma. The onset is usually rather sudden. The pain is extremely severe and may radiate to the groin and the back. The disease may be sufficiently severe to show associated systemic symptoms. The testis is swollen, hard and tender. An associated history of trauma or parotitis may establish the nature of the orchitis.

Acute Epididymitis

This is a common complication of gonorrheal urethritis. There is a sudden onset of pain and tenderness, frequently with associated systemic symptoms. The epididymis is swollen and tender; the testis also may be involved. A history of gonorrhea and the finding of gonococci in the urethral discharge establish the diagnosis in the usual type.

Tuberculosis occurs in young adults. There is likely to be evidence of tuberculosis elsewhere, especially in the prostate and the seminal vesicles. The epididymis is hard and nodular with coalescent swelling. Sinuses may develop, and tubercle bacilli may be isolated from the pus in these sinuses.

Acute epididymitis may also complicate prostatectomy or instrumentation of the urethra (including catheterization).

Syphilis

A gumma manifests itself as a unilateral, hard, freely movable painless mass in the testis. The history of the primary and the secondary lesions, a positive serologic test and the prompt response to antiluetic therapy establish the diagnosis.

Carcinoma of the Testis

Carcinoma of the testis is a disease of young adult life. The treatment and prognosis vary with the histologic type; therefore, accurate classification is important. The clinical manifestation is, in all forms, the presence of an enlarging tumor that is usually not tender. When such a lesion is found, operation should be performed through an inguinal incision with high ligation of the cord structures and removal when the presence of a tumor is confirmed on gross inspection. Seminoma is then treated by irradiation therapy to the preaortic area and the hilum of both kidneys. Embryonal carcinoma is treated by surgical removal of the lymph nodes. Teratomas are treated by removal of the testis alone. The trophoblastic tumors may be associated with gynecomastia and increased urinary excretion of chorionic gonadotropins. The tumors are highly malignant and infrequently cured.

Cryptorchidism

On examination the scrotum if found to be empty on the involved side. The testis may lie anywhere along the course of the inguinal canal or in the retroperitoneal tissues. It is likely to be small and underdeveloped if the individual is an adult. If the disease is bilateral, sterility is almost always present. Inguinal hernia is often associated. If the condition is not corrected early—before the onset of puberty—atrophy of the testis results, and a high incidence of malignant transformation takes place in these retained testes. For these reasons, the condition should be corrected early in life. Although replacing the testis in the scrotum does not alter the tendency toward cancer it does permit palpation and earlier diagnosis. Some good results have been recorded following the use of pituitary gonadotropins; however, in general, it is necessary to resort to operation with movement of the testis down into the scrotum, anchoring it in this position while healing takes place.

Phimosis

A condition in which the prepuce is elongated and the opening is so constricted that retraction cannot take place, phimosis results in retention of secretions with irritation and secondary infection. Occasionally the opening is so small that the urinary flow is obstructed, with subsequent dilatation of the urinary tract above it. Rarely, cystitis and vesical calculus result. In adults an epithelioma may be found. The treatment for phimosis is circumcision; however, if extensive acute infection is present, the more conservative procedure of making a dorsal slit in the prepuce until the infection is under control is indicated.

Paraphimosis

In this condition the tight retracted prepuce is constricted behind the glans. There are swelling, edema, pain and, at times, ulceration and gangrene. Early reduction fo the paraphimosis may be carried out by manipulation. However, it frequently is necessary to make a dorsal slit in the prepuce in order to accomplish this. Circumscision should be carried out unless infection is so extensive that the procedure must be deferred.

QUESTIONS IN SURGERY

REVIEW QUESTIONS

By what process does the healing of wounds take place?

Name two amino acids found only in collagen.

What functions have been attributed to mucopolysaccharides in wound healing?

Name five local factors that interfere with wound healing. Which one is the most important?

Why is catgut used as ligature and suture material in contaminated wounds?

Discuss the prophylactic and active treatment of tetanus.

What are the indications for rabies prophylaxis?

What is the difference in the clinical manifestations of bites by the black-widow spider and the brown spider?

Describe the modern definitive treatment of poisonous snake bites.

Discuss the systemic and local factors of importance in the coagulation of blood.

Discuss the predisposing factors to disseminated intravascular coagulation.

Define and discuss surgical shock, cardiac shock and septic shock.

What are the daily water and salt requirements of normal man?

Discuss the diagnosis and treatment of water intoxication.

What are the complications of intravenous hyperalimentation?

What alternatives to intravenous hyperalimentation exist for nutritional maintenance in patients with small intestinal fistulas?

What is the pathogenesis of stasis ulceration of the leg?

Discuss the diagnosis and treatment of acute thrombophlebitis and phlebothrombosis. What is phlegmasia cerulea dolens?

How can you determine whether peripheral arterial insufficiency is surgically correctable?

Discuss the management of an embolism to the common femoral artery.

What is Branham's sign?

Discuss the pathogenesis and prevention of Volkmann's ischemic contracture.

Give the indications for amputation of an extremity.

What are the areas of election for amputation of the forearm? the leg? the thigh?

Discuss the treatment of burns.

Describe paronychia and give its treatment.

What is a felon? How is it treated?

What are the anatomic boundaries of the midpalmar space?

Discuss the rejection of allografts.

What agents have been used to prevent the rejection of an allograft (homograft)?

Discuss the management of a liposarcoma 10 cm. in diameter arising in the lateral portion of the thigh.

Discuss delayed union and nonunion of fractures. What are the frequent sites of nonunion?

Describe the most common fracture of the clavicle and its treatment.

Describe fracture of the surgical neck of the humerus; give its complications and treatment. How is it differentiated from dislocation of the shoulder joint?

Describe the primary and secondary positions of dislocations of the shoulder joint. Give Kocher's method of reduction.

What are the common complications of fracture of the shaft of the humerus? Give the treatment of the fracture and the complications.

What symptoms suggest a herniation of an intervertebral disk? What is the treatment for a patient with a herniated disk?

Differentiate fracture of the lower extremity of the humerus from dislocation of the elbow and its treatment.

Describe the appearance of posterior dislocation of the elbow and its treatment.

What is a Colles' fracture?

Describe intracapsular fracture of the femur and its treatment.

How is congenital dislocation of the hip diagnosed?

Describe fracture of the shaft of the femur. What must treatment effect? Describe the treatment.

Give the treatment of fracture of the patella.

Give the diagnosis and the treatment of fracture of the tibia.

Describe Pott's fracture and its treatment.

How is dislocation of the semilunar cartilage diagnosed and treated?

Describe the common fractures of the true pelvis. What are the common complications, and how are they treated?

What are the indications for insertion of a prosthetic joint?

How would you treat surgical parotitis?

What is the most frequent tumor seen in the parotid gland?

How would you treat a peritonsillar abscess?

What is the most likely cause of a persistently enlarged lymph node in the deep cervical chain in a 25-year-old woman?

Discuss the staging of Hodgkin's disease.

Is elective lymph node dissection indicated in cancer of the lower lip?

Describe the preparation for surgery of the patient with thyrotoxicosis.

State the possible results of accidental but serious injury to the parathyroids occurring during thyroidectomy.

Describe the syndrome associated with hyperparathyroidism.

What are the physical signs of breast cancer?

Discuss the pathology, the diagnosis, the routes of metastasis and the treatment of carcinoma of the breast. Describe the palliative measures available in advanced mammary carcinoma.

What is paradoxic respiration? Explain its significance.

What is the treatment of a patient with a flail chest resulting in respiratory embarrassment?

Discuss the signs, the symptoms and the treatment of cardiac tamponade.

Describe the management of acute cardiac arrest.

What are the components of the tetralogy of Fallot?

What is the most accurate method of establishing the diagnosis of pulmonary embolism?

Where do bronchial adenomas most frequently metastasize?

What are the advantages of fiberoptic bronchoscopy?

Give the causes, diagnosis and treatment of thoracic empyema.

What is the preferred treatment of carcinoma of the lower third of the esophagus? The middle third?

Describe the treatment of pharyngoesophageal pulsion diverticulum.

What are the two types of hiatal hernia? Describe their differences.

Discuss blunt and penetrating wounds of the abdomen.

What are the indications for surgery for duodenal ulcer?

Under what conditions should a definitive operation for control of ulcer disease be used in patients with a perforated duodenal ulcer?

Describe the physiologic basis for the common operations for duodenal ulcer.

How should a patient with the Zollinger-Ellison syndrome be treated?

Discuss the etiology, the symptomatology, the differential diagnosis and the treatment of chronic cholecystitis. Give the clinical picture and the treatment of acute gallstone colic; of empyema of the gallbladder.

What substance has been used for the dissolution of gallstones in vivo?

Why is vitamin K given in the treatment of patients with icterus?

Give the etiology, the clinical picture and the treatment of acute pancreatitis.

What is Whipple's triad? Of what is it a diagnostic finding?

What laboratory tests are used for the confirmation of the diagnosis of islet cell adenoma?

Give the differential diagnosis of carcinoma of the head of the pancreas.

Give the signs and symptoms of rupture of the spleen. What is the treatment? What are commonly accepted indications for splenectomy?

What is the rationale of the portacaval shunt operation? What are the indications and contraindications for its use?

What are the causes of subdiaphragmatic abscess?

Describe the management of a patient with mechanical obstruction of the ileum arising from an adhesive band.

How would you treat a patient with complete obstruction of the sigmoid colon resulting from cancer?

What is the cause of acute appendicitis? Give the symptoms and signs in the order of their usual appearance. Give the differential diagnosis and the surgical treatment.

What are the indications for operation in terminal ileitis? What is the operation of choice?

Contrast Peutz-Jegher's syndrome with familial polyposis of the colon.

What are the indications for colonoscopy?

Why is barium by mouth contraindicated in a patient with carcinoma of the colon.

Describe the treatment of carcinoma of the rectum.

Give the clinical picture and treatment of acute diverticulitis of the colon.

Give the causes, the diagnosis and the treatment of ischiorectal abscess; fistula-in-ano; hemorrhoids.

Give the pathology, the symptomatology, the complications, the diagnosis and the treatment of carcinoma of the rectum.

Differentiate indirect inguinal hernia and describe its anatomic features; direct inguinal hernia; femoral hernia.

What is a sliding hernia? Discuss its treatment.

Discuss management of a patient with pheochromocytoma.

What are the clinical manifestations of an aldosteronoma?

What is the Farber test?

Discuss the management of imperforate anus.

What is the pathogenesis of congenital megacolon?

Of what is hernaturia a symptom?

Give the symptoms of ureteral calculus and the conditions to be considered in the differential diagnosis.

What are the symptoms that would suggest benign hypertrophy of the prostate?

What is a transurethal resection of the prostate, and for what is it performed?

What is cryptorchidism? Discuss its treatment.

Classify the causes of hematuria.

Give the clinical picture, the differential diagnosis and the treatment of renal calculus.

Discuss the pathogenesis, the pathology, the diagnosis and the treatment of hydronephrosis.

What is the treatment of Wilms' tumor (embryoma of the kidney)?

Give the causes, the diagnosis and the treatment of perinephric abscess.

What are the common causes of intestinal obstruction in the newborn?

Describe the diagnostic features of duodenal atresia.

Contrast the clinical pictures of hypertrophic pyloric stenosis and duodenal atresia.

What is the triad of signs that make up the clinical picture of intussusception in children?

What is the basic defect in congenital megacolon?

Discuss common tumors of the kidney and give their diagnosis, routes of metastasis and treatment.

Differentiate prostatic hypertrophy and carcinoma of the prostate. What are the early symptoms, the complications and the treatment?

List the common causes of enlargement of the scrotum.

Give the diagnosis and the treatment of hydrocele.

Differentiate the common causes of enlargement of the epididymis and of the testis.

Give the diagnosis and treatment of undescended testis.

Describe phimosis and paraphimosis and their treatment.

MULTIPLE CHOICE QUESTIONS

Select the *best* answer for each question. Answers are at the end of this chapter.

1. Hyperkalemia is most likely to occur:
   (a) with prolonged vomiting
   (b) in renal failure
   (c) with functioning adrenal cortical tumors
   (d) in Boeck's sarcoidosis
   (e) in the Zollinger-Ellison syndrome
2. All of the following are well-recognized inciting factors in thrombophlebitis except:
   (a) prolonged bed rest
   (b) driving an automobile for long distances
   (c) pelvic tumors
   (d) brain tumors
   (e) pelvic operations
3. Raynaud's disease:
   (a) is most frequent in males
   (b) is associated with hypertrophy of the volar carpal ligament
   (c) causes prolonged conduction time in the median nerve
   (d) is caused by spasm of small arteries
   (e) is frequent in the tropics
4. The most frequent complication of delayed treatment of a felon is:
   (a) spread to flexor tendon sheaths
   (b) necrosis of the skin overlying the distal phalanx
   (c) osteomyelitis of the distal phalanx
   (d) septicemia
   (e) none of the above
5. In Colles' fracture of the wrist
   (a) the usual mechanism is a fall on the outstretched hand

(b) A "silver-fork" deformity is characteristic

(c) reduction implies restoration of length and palmar deflection of the distal articular surface of the radius

(d) initial fixation in a long arm cast is essential

(e) all are correct

6. Neoplasms occur most frequently in which of the following salivary glands?.

(a) Submaxillary

(b) Parotid

(c) Sublingual

(d) Buccal

(e) Lingual

7. A 13-year-old girl develops exophthalmos, nervousness, diarrhea and weight loss following the death of her mother. Her blood pressure is 170/90. The most likely diagnosis is:

(a) multiple endocrine adenoma (MEA), Type II

(b) a pheochromocytoma

(c) Graves' disease

(d) retroorbital pseudotumor

(e) none of the above

8. If the diagnosis is MEA Type II, which of the following confirmatory findings would be least likely?

(a) Elevated serum thyrocalcitonin

(b) Elevated urinary metanephrins

(c) Elevated serum calcium

(d) Low serum phosphorus

(e) Elevated T_4

9. Of the following pathological findings in the breast, which is *least* likely to be precancerous?

(a) Fibroadenoma

(b) Intraductal papilloma

(c) Sclerosing adenosis

(d) Lobular hyperplasia

(e) Cancer of one breast

10. A 6-year-old underdeveloped boy is seen because of signs of heart failure. He also has hypertension in the arms, but not in the legs and prominent notching of the lower rib margins. The most likely diagnosis is:

(a) patent ductus arteriosus

(b) tetralogy of Fallot

(c) pulmonary stenosis

(d) patent interventricular septal defect

(e) coarctation of the aorta

11. Open drainage of empyema is indicated only:

(a) in streptococcal infections

(b) when the pus is thick

(c) when the mediastinum is fixed

(d) in bilateral disease

(e) when thoracostomy tube drainage is ineffective

12. Cricopharyngeal myotomy is used in the surgical correction of pharyngoesophageal pulsion diverticulum in order to:

(a) better expose the neck of the diverticulum

(b) restore normal pressure relationships and thereby prevent recurrence

(c) prevent narrowing of the esophagus at this point

(d) eliminate the risk of infection

(e) all are correct

13. Positive findings in suspected subphrenic abscess include:

(a) fixation of the diaphragm

(b) sterile pleural effusion above the abscess

(c) absent Litton's signs

(d) elevation of the diaphragm

(e) all of the above

14. A previous healthy 17-year-old male has had an appendiceal abscess drained. The appendix was not removed. Future management should consist of:

(a) long-term antibiotic therapy

(b) roentgenograms of the small intestine and colon

(c) regular physical examination

(d) weekly complete blood counts

(e) interval appendectomy at three months

15. A 45-year-old man is brought to the emergency room when he fainted after vomiting an undetermined amount of bright red blood. The history and physical examination were uninformative. Laboratory studies: WBC 9,600, RBC 3,200,000, hemoglobin 9 gm. per 100 ml., hematocrit 32 percent. The *next* diagnostic procedure should be:

(a) selective angiography

(b) upper gastrointestinal roentgenograms

(c) barium enema

(d) endoscopic examination of esophagus, stomach and duodenum

(e) none of the above

16. Which of the following is most supportive of the diagnosis of the Zollinger-Ellison syndrome?

(a) 12 hour gastric secretion of 800 ml.

(b) Serum gastrin level of 1,000 nanograms percent

(c) Basal acid output of 12 ml. per hour

(d) A history of recurrent ulcer following three presumably satisfactory ulcer operations

(e) Multiple ulcers of duodenum and jejunem

17. Whipples triad, useful in the diagnosis of insulinoma of the pancreas, consists of:

(a) central nervous system symptoms, fasting blood sugar of 50 mg. per 100 ml., relief following ingestion of glucose

(b) central nervous system symptoms, fasting

blood sugar of 50 mg. per 100 ml., relief following intravenous glucagon

(c) abdominal pain, fasting blood sugar of 50 mg. per 100 ml., relief following ingestion of glucose

(d) abdominal pain, high serum insulin, relief following the ingestion of glucose

(e) fasting nausea and vomiting, positive tolbutamide test, relief following intravenous glucagon

18. A 49-year-old woman has been treated with steroids for ideopathic thrombocytopenic purpura, with return of the platelet count to normal. Following discontinuance of steroids, thrombocytopenia recurs. Treatment at this time should consist of:

(a) splenectomy

(b) repeat steroid administration, if good response continue indefinitely

(c) give azathioprine for one week then recommend splenectomy

(d) repeat steroids, and if no response initially, increase the dosage

(e) none of the above

19. The most frequent adverse effect following otherwise successful portocaval shunting for bleeding esophageal varices in the cirrhotic patient is:

(a) progressive hepatic failure

(b) intolerance to fats

(c) meat intoxication

(d) recurrent bleeding

(e) lactic acidosis

20. Treatment of intestinal obstruction caused by cancer of the rectosigmoid is best accomplished by:

(a) decompressive colostomy

(b) decompression by passage of a long intestinal tube, subsequent resection

(c) immediate resection

21. A 13-year-old boy experiences sudden severe pain in the right testis. On palpation there is exquisite tenderness. The most likely diagnosis is:

(a) spontaneous hemorrhage

(b) torsion

(c) strangulated hernia

(d) epididymitis

(e) seminoma of the testis

For the following, answer:

A if 1, 2 and 3 are correct
B if 1 and 3 are correct
C if 2 and 4 are correct
D if only 4 is correct
E if all are correct

22. Which of the following play an important role in wound healing?

(1) Zinc

(2) Vitamin C

(3) Copper

(4) Cobalt

23. A properly positioned Swan-Ganz catheter will permit determination of:

(1) left artrial pressure

(2) right atrial pressure

(3) pulmonary artery pressure

(4) right ventricular pressure

24. Complications of intravenous feeding include:

(1) non-ketotic hyperglycemic coma

(2) hyperphosphatemia

(3) hyperosmolarity

(4) hypercalcemia

25. Characteristic of renal allograft rejection is:

(1) lymphocytopenia

(2) bradycardia

(3) polyuria

(4) rising serum creatinine

26. Patients with intermittent claudication:

(1) most frequently have a block in the superficial femoral artery

(2) will most likely require an amputation within five years of onset

(3) should be encouraged to exercise

(4) should have an immediate arteriogram

27. Causative in embolization of major arteries is:

(1) mural thrombus following myocardial infarction

(2) ventricular aneurysm

(3) cardiac myxoma

(4) patent ventricular septal defects

28. In a 50-year-old woman with a 35 per cent body surface burn of the trunk:

(1) mortality is mainly secondary to burn shock

(2) the severity of infection can be lessened by topical use of sulfamylon

(3) systemic antimicrobials are of greater efficacy than are topical agents

(4) either lactated Ringers solution or isotonic sodium chloride solution will be effective in combatting burn shock

29. Nonunion is frequent in fractures of:

(1) the carpal scaphoid

(2) the lower third of the tibia

(3) the neck of the femur

(4) intertrochanteric fractures

30. Joint replacement is useful in crippling arthritis involving which of the following joints?

(1) Metacarpophalangeal

(2) Hip

(3) Scapulohumeral

(4) Knee

31. Thyroglossal duct cysts are characterized by:
(1) location beneath the anterior margin of the sternocleidomastoid muscle
(2) absence of thyroid tissue in the wall
(3) disturbances in thyroid function
(4) a tract extending through the hyoid bone to the foramen cecum

32. Pleomorphic adenoma (mixed tumor) of the parotid gland:
(1) is best treated by superficial lobectomy
(2) frequently requires removal of the facial nerve for adequate treatment
(3) has a tendency to locally recur following removal
(4) frequently metastasizes to cervical lymph nodes

33. Which of the following are indicative of inoperability in patients with breast cancer?
(1) Inflammatory cancer
(2) Satellite skin nodules
(3) Parasternal nodules
(4) Involved axillary lymph nodes

34. Signs of cardiac tamponade include:
(1) small pulse pressure
(2) hypertension
(3) distended neck veins
(4) bradycardia

35. Useful methods of study in suspected traumatic splenic rupture include:
(1) scanning with 99m technesium sulfur colloid
(2) AP and lateral roentgenograms
(3) arteriography
(4) ultrasound scanning

36. A 21-year-old man is operated upon for acute appendicitis, the appendix and cecum are normal but the terminal ileum is acutely inflamed. Which of the following statements is correct?
(1) The appendix should be removed
(2) A right hemicolectomy is acceptable treatment
(3) The likelihood of developing chronic regional enteritis is small (less than 25 per cent)
(4) A course of Asulfadine should be given postoperatively

37. Continuous neutralization of gastric acidity with antacids is indicated in which of the following clinical situations?
(1) Perforative appendicitis with localized peritonitis treated by appendectomy
(2) A patient with a 40 per cent body surface burn
(3) Following acute myocardial infarction
(4) A patient comatose, but responsive to painful stimuli following severe head injury

38. A 68-year-old man is suspected to have a carcinoma of the body of the pancreas. Which of the following studies will be helpful in substantiating the diagnosis?
(1) Serum amylase concentration
(2) Selective angiography
(3) 99m Technesium sulfur colloid scans
(4) Computerized tomography

39. Which of the following is precancerous?
(1) The polyps of Peutz-Jeghers syndrome
(2) Juvenile polyps of the colon
(3) A solitary pedunculated adenomatous polyp 5 mm. in diameter of the midsigmoid
(4) Villous adenomas of the rectum

40. Useful studies in the diagnosis of renal cell carcinoma include:
(1) angiography
(2) intravenous pyelography
(3) nephrography
(4) urine cytology

Each set of lettered headings below is followed by a list of numbered words, phrases, or statements. For each numbered word, phrase, or statement the correct response will be:

(a) if the item is associated with (a) only
(b) if the item is associated with (b) only
(c) if the item is associated with *both* (a) and (b)
(d) if the item is associated with neither (a) nor (b)

(a) Carcinoma of the lip
(b) Carcinoma of the tongue
(c) Both
(d) Neither

41. Is (are) radiosensitive

42. Causally related to exposure to sunlight

43. Elective lymph node dissection frequently employed in treatment

44. Highly curable even if cervical lymph nodes are involved

45. Metastases present in 60 per cent or more of patients.

(a) Papillary cancer of the thyroid
(b) Follicular cancer of the thyroid
(c) Both
(d) Neither

46. Frequent multicentric foci in both lobes

47. Cervical lymph node metastases in over 50 per cent of patients

48. Vein invasion and blood born metastases a significant factor

49. Radiosensitive

50. Highly lethal

(a) Sliding hiatus hernia
(b) Paresophageal hiatus hernia
(c) Both
(d) Neither

51. Only indication for repair is esophagitis
52. Require truncal vagotomy for adequate repair
53. Necrosis of the gastric wall may occur

(a) Familial polyposis of the colon
(b) Gardner's syndrome
(c) Both
(d) Neither

54. Polyps also occur in the small intestine with some frequency
55. Age of expression usually latter part of the second or the third decade of life
56. Osteomas of the cranial bones
57. Death from cancer inevitable if untreated
58. Usual treatment total colectomy and proctectomy

(a) Angiodysplasia of the colon
(b) Diverticular disease of the colon
(c) Both
(d) Neither

59. Occult anemia
60. Precancerous
61. Treated by surgical resection when the diagnosis is made
62. Massive bleeding
63. Fistula formation

(a) Meconium ileus
(b) Duodenal atresia
(c) Both
(d) Neither

64. Farber test positive

65. Double-bubble sign
66. Complicated by volvulus
67. Early operation desirable

(a) Benign prostatic hypertrophy
(b) Carcinoma of the prostate
(c) Both
(d) Neither

68. Elevated acid phosphatase
69. May require transurethral resection
70. Most frequently starts in posterior lobe
71. Elevated alkaline phosphatase

ANSWERS TO MULTIPLE CHOICE QUESTIONS

1. (b)	19. (c)	37. (c)	55. (a)
2. (d)	20. (a)	38. (c)	56. (b)
3. (d)	21. (b)	39. (d)	57. (c)
4. (c)	22. (a)	40. (a)	58. (c)
5. (e)	23. (e)	41. (c)	59. (a)
6. (b)	24. (b)	42. (a)	60. (d)
7. (c)	25. (d)	43. (b)	61. (a)
8. (e)	26. (b)	44. (a)	62. (c)
9. (a)	27. (a)	45. (b)	63. (b)
10. (e)	28. (c)	46. (a)	64. (b)
11. (c)	29. (a)	47. (a)	65. (b)
12. (b)	30. (e)	48. (b)	66. (a)
13. (e)	31. (d)	49. (d)	67. (c)
14. (e)	32. (b)	50. (d)	68. (b)
15. (d)	33. (a)	51. (a)	69. (c)
16. (b)	34. (b)	52. (d)	70. (b)
17. (a)	35. (b)	53. (b)	71. (d)
18. (d)	36. (b)	54. (b)	

Internal Medicine

SOLOMON PAPPER, M.D.

Distinguished Professor and Head, Department of Medicine,
University of Oklahoma at Oklahoma City—Health Sciences Center

Note: In order to avoid excessive length and repetition, the following topics, which have been taken up fully in other chapters, are omitted when possible: (1) Vitamins (see Chap. 4, Biochemistry, and Chap. 6, Pathology); (2) Endocrine (see Chap. 3, Physiology); (3) Infections (see Chap. 5, General Microbiology and Immunology, Chap. 6, Pathology, and Chap. 12, Public Health and Community Medicine); and (4) Poisoning (see Chap. 4, Biochemistry, Chap. 7, Pharmacology, Chap. 6, Pathology, and Chap. 12, Public Health and Community Medicine).

DISEASES OF THE CIRCULATION

THE HEART

The heart is a muscular pump that has the function of distributing blood through the systemic and pulmonary circulations. Its efficiency may be impaired by damage to (1) the valves; (2) the myocardium, endocardium or pericardium; (3) the coronary arteries; (4) the conduction system; and (5) the peripheral vessels. Initial symptoms of patients with heart disease result primarily from myocardial ischemia, from distur-bances in myocardial contractility, or from abnormal cardiac rate or rhythm.

A correct and complete diagnosis is essential for the proper management of the patient. As outlined by the New York Heart Association, the diagnosis should consider:

1. Etiology: congenital, rheumatic, hypertensive, atherosclerotic, or unknown.
2. Structural abnormalities: chamber enlargement, valvular involvement, myocardial infarction.
3. Physiologic function: arrhythmia, myocardial perfusion or congestive heart failure.
4. Functional reserve impairment: degree of activity to elicit symptoms.

The most common variety of heart disease in the infant relates to a congenital defect in development; in the adolescent and young adult, valvular heart disease, often due to rheumatic fever; and in the older adult, atherosclerosis and hypertension.

For the sake of simplicity, most pathologic or functional disturbances will be discussed only with the etiologic class in which they are most characteristic, even though they may occur also in other types of heart disease.

Congenital Heart Disease

In approximately 9 births in 1,000 significant cardiovascular abnormalities occur. With appropriate medical and surgical management most of these children may be cured or dramatically improved. The most frequent occurrences are ventricular septal defect, followed by tetralogy of Fallot, transposition of the great arteries, patent ductus arteriosus, atrial septal defect and coarctation of the aorta. Other entities such as single ventricle, valvular atresias, pulmonary stenosis, persistent truncus arteriosus and common atrioventricular canal have less than five per cent incidence in the patients diagnosed with congential heart disease.

The pathogenesis of congenital defects in the development of the heart is unknown, except that many cases apparently are the consequence of maternal rubella during the first trimester of pregnancy. Evidence is accumulating that other illnesses of the mother, especially viral diseases, may have a similar result during the critical first 3 months of pregnancy. Other potential causes include ionizing irradiation, hypoxia, intake of several categories of drugs (including, perhaps, alcohol) and deficiency or excess of several vitamins.

Many patients with congenital heart disease have two features in common: (1) History of early onset of cardiac symptoms such as: birth as a "blue baby," a loud murmur with a thrill along the left sternal border, and the occurrence of cyanosis with intense dyspnea upon exertion early in childhood. Polycythemia and clubbing of fingers are likely to occur in patients with longstanding cyanosis. (2) Failure of normal growth and development.

A clinical classification of congenital heart disease based on the presence or the absence of cyanosis is commonly employed:

I. Without Cyanosis

A. No shunt (normal pulmonary perfusion)

With right ventricular predominance: valvular pulmonic stenosis, pulmonary artery stenosis or primary pulmonary hypertension

With left ventricular predominance: idiopathic hypertrophic aortic stenosis, valvular subaortic stenosis or coarctation of the aorta

B. Left-to-right shunt (increased pulmonary perfusion)

With right ventricular predominance: atrial septal defect with or without mitral stenosis

With left ventricular predominance: ventricular septal defect, patent ductus arteriosus

II. With Cyanosis

A. Right-to-left shunt (normal or decreased pulmonary perfusion)

With right ventricular predominance: tetralogy of Fallot

With left ventricular predominance: tricuspid atresia or Ebstein's anomaly of the tricuspid valve

B. Right-to-left and left-to-right shunts (increased pulmonary perfusion). Complete transposition of great vessels

Another lesion not included in the above classification is congenital heart block, which may occur in the absence of any other abnormality.

The most common congenital heart disease lesions are:

1. Ventricular Septal Defect. The ordinary interventricular septal defect is small in size. The harsh systolic murmur and thrill at the left margin of the sternum are in striking contrast to the usual absence of cyanosis or other evidence of impaired cardiac efficiency. In other instances there may be an overactive heart with biventricular enlargement, an accentuated pulmonic component of the second sound, ECG evidence of left ventricular hypertrophy, and increased pressure within the pulmonary circuit. All gradations of severity may exist, and the septal defect may be complicated by other defects such as patent ductus, atrial septal defects, pulmonic stenosis and coarctation of the aorta. The treatment is surgical if a moderate or large amount of the left ventricular output is shunted to the right side.

2. Tetralogy of Fallot. This is a combination of four defects: (a) pulmonic stenosis, (b) dextroposition of the aorta, (c) ventricular septal defect, and (d) hypertrophy of the right ventricle. The most characteristic diagnostic feature is continuous cyanosis, which nevertheless is compatible with life to adult years. There may be a harsh systolic murmur at the left sternal border, but the location and the intensity of the murmur are variable. Usually the ECG shows right-axis deviation. Secondary polycythemia is usually present. Upon fluoroscopy, the pulsation of the pulmonary artery is much reduced. Complete surgical reconstruction is possible with mortality rates of less than 10 per cent in children. When such correction is not possible, operation to produce an anastomosis between the pulmonary artery and the systemic aorta or one of the great systemic arteries will greatly improve the efficiency of the patient's cardiorespiratory system by increasing the blood flow through the pulmonary circuit.

3. Patent Ductus Arteriosus. The presence of a

continuous loud machinery-like murmur in the pulmonic area is practically diagnostic of this condition. Usually there is a thrill and moderately elevated systolic and depressed diastolic blood pressure. Because of the higher pressure in the systemic aorta, the direction of the blood shunt is from the aorta into the pulmonary artery. The increased volume of blood in the pulmonary circuit increases the work of the right ventricle, and the increased volume of blood returning from the lungs increases the load on the left ventricle so that both sides of the heart are involved. Cyanosis is absent in uncomplicated instances. Elimination of the shunt by surgical ligation of the patent ductus is a highly successful procedure, particularly when done in childhood. In recent years pharmecological therapy, with indomethacin, has met with some success in certain instances in infants with patent ductus arteriosus.

4. Atrial Septal Defect.   This is also a common congenital heart defect and may vary from an open foramen ovale to complete absence of the interatrial septum. A patent foramen ovale persists in a significant percentage of adults, but shunting of the blood does not occur with normal atrial pressures, and no symptoms result. Persistent ostium secundum, midseptal or cephalad in location, allows a left-to-right shunt because left atrial pressure is higher than the right. A systolic murmur results, with splitting of the second sound that does not vary with respiration. Increased pressure within the pulmonary arterial system may be evident from fluoroscopic examination and becomes apparent on the ECG later in the disease. Surgical repair is successful. Persistent ostium primum, one margin of the opening being made up of tissue between the atrioventricular valves, is technically much more difficult to repair. Symptoms usually appear in childhood, with a systolic murmur and evidences of left as well as right ventricular hypertrophy. Mitral or tricuspid regurgitation may be present and favors the diagnosis of ostium primum defect. Pulmonic stenosis may be present and result in a right-to-left shunt.

5. Coarctation of the Aorta.   In the usual type of coarctation, the narrowing of the aorta occurs at the point where the ligamentum arteriosum is attached near the origin of the left subclavian artery. It is generally discovered during examination of an adolescent or a young adult with hypertension. When there is very weak or unobtainable pulse and blood pressure below the diaphragm, the diagnosis is practically established. The murmur (produced at the point of narrowing of the aorta) ordinarily is neglected until the basic diagnostic findings have been discovered. Sometimes coarctation is discovered by the radiologist who notices "scalloping" or "notching" of the lower borders of the ribs. This is produced by the enlarged intercostal arteries, which serve to "detour" circulation around the coarctation. A plastic operation on the aorta produces a dramatic cure. It should not be delayed since the aorta loses its elasticity steadily as the patient becomes older.

6. Pulmonary stenosis varies in severity and degree and may be associated with an atrial septal defect, resulting in a right-to-left shunt. It may lead to heart failure in infancy or cause difficulty only in later life. A systolic murmur in the pulmonic area, splitting of the second sound and right ventricular hypertrophy are found, and the stenosis is verified on cardiac catheterization. The treatment is surgical in the severe form.

7. Eisenmenger Complex.   This consists of a ventricular septal defect, dextroposition and overriding of the aorta and a normal pulmonary artery. This is differentiated from the tetralogy of Fallot by the prominence of the shadow and pulsation. Cyanosis is not so extreme. The use of the term Eisenmenger complex is losing favor because of lack of specific criteria.

In practically all instances of congenital heart disease, confirmation of the clinical diagnosis by such technical procedures as cardiac catheterization and angiocardiography will be desired before any operation is attempted.

Valvular Heart Disease

This group now represents a decreasing portion of all instances of heart disease because of the recognition of rheumatic fever and the prevention of its recurrence. Although not all chronic valvular heart disease is due to rheumatic fever, a significant proportion is a characteristic sequela of rheumatic carditis. About half of all patients with valvular disease present a definite history of acute rheumatic fever. The common factor is regarded as a sensitivity reaction to the hemolytic streptococcus, which produces its damage without actually being present in the heart. There is evidence to suggest that a hereditary factor may determine the susceptibility to rheumatic heart disease. During the acute phase there is pancarditis, with pericarditis, myocarditis (Aschoff bodies) and endocarditis. The first two ordinarily resolve, leaving chronic endocarditis with scarring of the valves.

The mitral valve is the valve most commonly affected (over two thirds of patients), and aortic stenosis is present in one fourth of patients with valvular disease.

In *mitral insufficiency (mitral regurgitation)* there is regurgitation of blood through the incompetent mitral valve when the left ventricle contracts. Consequently the typical murmur is systolic in time. It is heard best at the apex and transmitted to the axilla.

It is "blowing" in character. The left ventricle usually is enlarged as demonstrated by palpation, percussion, and by x-ray examination. Unless acute in onset, or complicated by stenosis, the condition is often well compensated, and the prognosis is fairly good.

The etiology of *mitral valve prolapse (Barlow's syndrome, Click-murmur syndrome)* is poorly understood. It most often occurs in otherwise healthy young women. However, it is also noted in atrial septal defect, Marfan's syndrome, after myocardial infarction and sometimes appears to be familial. Patients may be asymptomatic or have atypical chest pain or arrhythmias. On physical examination there is normal size heart, and a midsystolic click that may be followed by a late systolic murmur. The ECG may show nonspecific ST-T changes and the QT interval may be long. Chest roentgenogram may be normal. Echocardiography may be diagnostic. Mitral valve prolapse generally has a benign course; on occasion severe regurgitation occurs.

Pure *mitral stenosis* occurs in 40 per cent of patients with rheumatic heart disease. The stenosis interferes with the filling of the left ventricle because of the narrowed valve. Therefore the typical murmur is middiastolic, low pitched, diminuendo and best heard at the apex. Often it is associated with a rough, crescendo, presystolic murmur, terminating in a sharp first sound and accompanied by a fine apical thrill. If atrial fibrillation intervenes, the presystolic murmur disappears. The pulmonic component of the second sound usually is accentuated and split, and the first sound at the apex is loud and sharp. There may also be an opening snap at the lower left sternal border. The x-ray picture shows transverse enlargement with prominence of the left atrium and the pulmonary artery segment. The ECG shows right ventricular preponderance. Atrial fibrillation and decompensation are common as late manifestations. The narrowed mitral valve interferes with the flow of blood from the left atrium into the left ventricle. Left atrial pressure increases, the chamber enlarges, and the pressure is transmitted back to the pulmonary circulation. Pulmonary congestion and exertional dyspnea may result. Orthopnea, paroxysmal nocturnal dyspnea, cough and hemoptysis may follow. In a more advanced stage, increased pulmonary pressure occurs with arteriolar changes, increased resistance to blood flow and relative pulmonary valvular insufficiency. Dilatation and failure of the right ventricle may cause tricuspid insufficiency. Evidence of right ventricular failure may appear with increased venous pressure, distended neck veins, engorged liver, and peripheral edema.

The ultimate prognosis is guarded. In patients with pure mitral stenosis, mitral comissurotomy has proved to be a highly satisfactory procedure if the valve leaflets are pliable. Replacement of the valve by a prosthesis has proved to be a satisfactory procedure but is associated with greater operative mortality.

Aortic stenosis is found more frequently in older patients, and calcification of the valve is a common occurrence. Isolated aortic stenosis is rarely due to rheumatic heart disease. Multiple valve disease including aortic stenosis suggests a rheumatic etiology. In patients under age 65 congenital bicuspid aortic valve is the most common cause of aortic stenosis. In patients over 65, the cusps may be sclerotic and calcified secondary to arteriosclerosis. The left ventricle hypertrophies without much dilatation in the early stages. Deficient cerebral blood flow, with fainting, syncope and dizziness, is frequent. Anginal pain may occur. Cardiac failure or sudden death may follow with frequent incidence of ventricular arrhythmias. A harsh or a musical systolic ejection murmur at the aortic area, transmitted to the vessels of the neck, is the classical sign. There is an accompanying thrill and a reduced aortic second sound. The narrow pulse pressure and pulsus tardus are characteristic. The treatment of severe aortic stenosis is valve replacement.

Idiopathic hypertrophic subaortic stenosis (IHSS) is the most common form of subvalvular left ventricular outflow obstruction. The etiology is unknown, although it is believed to be genetic. Anatomically, IHSS is a cardiomyopathy characterized by an asymmetric and thickened ventricular septum. The septal cells are hypertrophied, abnormal in shape and arrangement. If outflow obstruction occurs it is apparently due to anterior motion of the mitral valve into the outflow tract. Although many patients are asymptomatic and referred because of murmur or ECG findings, patients may have dyspnea, angina, syncope, and palpitations. On physical examination there is a left ventricular impulse, and an ejection or regurgitant murmur at the lower left sternal border or apex. The murmur radiates poorly if at all to the carotids, as distinguished from prominent radiation in aortic stenosis. ECG often shows left ventricular enlargement. Chest roentgenogram is commonly normal. Echocardiography is often virtually diagnostic. The course is quite variable. Endocarditis prophylaxis is indicated. Propranolol is often useful in decreasing outflow obstruction. Digitalis may enhance obstruction. Ventral septal myotomy and/or a myectomy may be indicated if symptoms are severe and propranolol is not uniformly effective.

Aortic regurgitation may occur as a result of rheumatic heart disease, but it also may be of syphilitic origin as well as associated with rheumatoid spondylitis, Marfan's syndrome, trauma and bacterial endocarditis. The findings are (1) a soft, high-pitched diastolic murmur in the aortic area transmitted to the left border of the sternum; (2) left ventricular dilatation and hypertrophy; (3) lowered diastolic pressure with a wide pulse pressure; (4) to-and-fro arterial bruits (Duroziez's sign); (5) pistol-shot femoral artery sound; (6) water hammer pulse; and (7) capillary pulsation. There is usually a systolic murmur at the aortic area which, combined with the diastolic murmur, gives a to-and-fro murmur. The left ventricle hypertrophies and may compensate for this defect for many years, but when decompensation occurs it is likely to progress rapidly. Valve replacement is effective therapy.

Pulmonic stenosis has been discussed in the section on congenital heart disease.

Tricuspid insufficiency occurs most frequently as a result of cardiac dilatation and failure—relative tricuspid insufficiency. Organic insufficiency is the result of rheumatic fever or endocarditis often related to drug abuse. Rheumatic tricuspid insufficiency is usually associated with disease of other valves as well. It produces a systolic murmur at the lower end of the sternum accentuated with respiratory inspiration, marked cardiac enlargement to the right, palpable systolic venous pulse in the neck veins and a palpable expansile pulsation of the liver. Tricuspid stenosis is relatively infrequent and seldom recognized by clinical means.

Infective (Bacterial) Endocarditis

Traditionally, distinction has been made between "acute" and "subacute" endocarditis. Although recent years have revealed less sharpness in this separation, there is probably still some clinical value in its consideration.

Acute bacterial ("ulcerative") endocarditis is a rapidly progressive invasion of the endocardium associated with destruction of the affected valves and with signs and symptoms of a fulminating infection. Its differentiation from subacute bacterial endocarditis is primarily on the basis of the virulence of the invading pyogenic organism. The hemolytic streptococcus, the *Haemophilus influenzae,* staphylococci, pneumococci, gonococcus or fungus may be the infecting agent. Prompt and vigorous treatment with antibiotics has made recovery possible in a large number of cases.

Subacute bacterial endocarditis is much more common than the acute type. The alphahemolytic streptococcus and the nonhemolytic streptococci are the most common infecting agents. The infection usually is superimposed upon valves previously damaged by rheumatic fever; the aortic and the mitral valves are most commonly involved. Bacterial endocarditis also occurs in hearts with congenital defects. The symptoms include (1) prolonged fever of a septic type; (2) chills; (3) malaise; and (4) fatigue. Anemia is common. Emboli originating from the valvular vegetations may produce splanchnic, renal or cerebral infarcts; other embolic phenomena include petechial hemorrhages in the skin and mucous membranes and splinter hemorrhages beneath the nails. Tender Osler's nodes of the fingertips also occur. The diagnosis is suggested by a protracted fever in a patient with a valvular defect, particularly if petechial hemorrhages or gross embolic phenomena, marked anemia, microscopic hematuria and a palpable spleen are present. Repeated blood cultures are positive for the alpha-hemolytic streptococcus in about 90 per cent of cases. Vigorous treatment with antibiotics, especially penicillin, will result in a bacteriologic cure in the majority of cases; in the case of infection with penicillin-resistant organisms, combinations of bactericidal antibiotics may be necessary.

Endocarditis in narcotic addicts is increasing. In general, addicts are young, and take drugs intravenously. Staphylococcus is the predominant organism, and although the left side of the heart is more frequently involved, tricuspid insufficiency and pulmonic lesions may be present.

Bacterial endocarditis may result from dental and other surgical procedures in patients with rheumatic or congenital heart disease. When such procedures are undertaken these patients should be protected by antibiotics in therapeutic doses.

Cardiovascular Syphilis

Luetic Heart. In this country, syphilis and, with it, syphilitic heart disease are declining steadily in frequency. Typically, syphilitic heart disease is a complication of syphilitic aortitis, which (1) causes *aneurysm* of the aortic arch; (2) extends backward to involve the aortic valve, with resulting *regurgitation;* and (3) finally causes stenosis of the branches of the aorta, particularly the *coronary arteries.* Men between 45 and 55 years of age are most commonly afflicted.

Luetic aortitis is due to an obliterative endarteritis of the vasa vasorum, with resultant destruction of the media and wrinkling of the intima. The aortic wall is weakened, loses its elasticity and stretches. The lesion is most common in the ascending aorta and is found less often in the arch. *Aneurysm* is caused by the stretching of the thinned walls. A saccular aneurysm is less common than a diffuse dilatation of the ascending aorta with resulting aortic regurgitation. The aortic ring is stretched, and the commissures between the cusps are widened. Since the aortic valves do not completely close at the end of systole, the elastic recoil of the peripheral vessels forces a portion of the ejected blood back into the left ventricle. The findings are the same as in aortic regurgitation of the rheumatic variety. At present, the preferred treatment of syphilitic aortitis is penicillin.

Coronary Artery Disease

Atherosclerosis with narrowing of the lumen is the most common form of coronary artery disease; it is most prevalent in the fifth and sixth decades of life and is found more often in men than in women. Rarely such disorders as polyarteritis nodosa may involve the coronary vessels as well as the systemic arteries. Recently, the phenomenon of spasm of the coronary arteries (without atheroscherotic narrowing) has been recognized and found to be of clinical significance. In the case of coronary artery narrowing but without complete occlusion, the presence or the absence of symptoms has a direct bearing on the relationship between the requirements of the myocardium for oxygen and the ability of the coronary circulation to transport that oxygen. Patients may be asymptomatic at rest, and manifestations of myocardial ischemia may develop only when the demand for an increased work load is placed upon the heart. Not only may myocardial ischemia result from the narrowing of the coronary vessels but it may follow complete occlusion of such a vessel by thrombosis, which may follow ulceration of an atheromatous plaque or subintimal hemorrhage.

Data continue to accumulate about factors that increase risk of coronary artery disease. Hypertension, with both systolic and diastolic pressures of equal risk, obesity, smoking and elevated cholesterol levels contribute to increased risks.

Because the resting ECG may be normal, exercise testing may be useful; however false negatives and false positives do occur.

Angina Pectoris. This is a manifestation of coronary insufficiency characterized by paroxysmal substernal pain usually produced by exertion and relieved by rest. The pain consists of a sense of oppression in the substernal region; it is variously described as a pressure, a squeezing pain or a boring pain. The pain frequently radiates into the neck and along the medial aspect of the left arm and forearm. These episodes usually are of short duration and, as a rule, are relieved promptly by rest. Unstable angina is defined as anginal pain that is increasing in severity, duration and frequency. This is a high risk group of patients. Angina pectoris often precedes coronary thrombosis. The pain in the two conditions is similar but differs in its duration. Physical examination in a patient with angina pectoris often reveals no abnormalities. Exercise testing will usually evoke conspicuous ECG changes suggestive of myocardial ischemia. The frequency of attacks of angina pectoris often can be controlled by reduction in physical activity; attacks often may be aborted or their severity decreased through the use of preparations such as amyl nitrite or nitroglycerin. Those patients with hypercholestrolemia and angina pectoris may benefit from low fat diets. Frequently, angina pectoris associated with severe hypertension will be ameliorated by reduction in the blood pressure toward normal. Propranolol is widely given to patients with angina and reduces frequency of attacks by reducing cardiac work through slowing of heart rate and lowering blood pressure response to exercise. Although the precise indications for coronary bypass surgery are debated, some patients have marked symptomatic improvement following surgery. Patients with left main coronary disease and those who do not respond to medical therapy should especially be considered. Certain patients may spontaneously develop a collateral circulation with relief or at times almost complete recovery from their angina. Angina pectoris has a death rate of 3 to 5 per cent per year.

Myocardial Infarction. Coronary insufficiency may result in myocardial infarction that occurs either with or without occlusion of a branch of a coronary artery. Not all sudden deaths in patients with coronary arteriosclerosis are the result of myocardial infarction; some of these are the results of fatal ventricular arrhythmias precipitated by an episode of myocardial ischemia. The classic symptoms are (1) pain; (2) shock; and (3) dyspnea. The pain is similar to that of angina pectoris in location and in quality; usually it is intense and may persist for hours. It is not caused specifically by exercise, not is it relieved by rest. The hypotension may be of any degree and usually is associated with signs of peripheral vascular collapse; cyanosis and the signs of acute heart failure may be present in massive infarcts. On auscultation, the heart sounds are usually diminished in intensity and the most common extra sound is the S_4 or atrial gallop. A friction rub is heard in a majority of patients at some time in the course. The presence of myocardial infarction also is associated with elevation of temperature, leukocytosis and elevation of the sedimentation rate, as well as by characteristic ECG changes. Certain enzymes are present in high concentration in heart muscles and are released into the blood with infarction. The level of creatinine phosphokinase (CPK) rises and falls most rapidly. Serum glutamic oxaloacetic transaminase (SGOT) is increased in the blood within 6 to 12 hours and reaches a peak in 2 to 3 days, then reverts to normal. Lactic dehydrogenase (LDH) activity in the serum is an index of myocardial necrosis and is of greater specificity than SGOT and is elevated for a longer period.

The classical electrocardiographic findings in leads overlying the infarcted muscle are (1) the presence of significant Q waves in leads that ordinarily would be expected to be dominated by R waves; (2) abnormal elevations of the S-T segments; and (3) abnormal inverted T waves. During the very early phases of myocardial infarction the characteristic electrocardiographic findings may not have evolved fully, and in such instances serial tracings are necessary.

Treatment of acute myocardial infarction consists of:

1. Relief of pain. *Morphine* still is one of the drugs most widely used for this purpose, but other narcotics, such as *meperidine,* may be substituted if the patient has an idiosyncrasy to morphine. Because of potential for producing hypotension, the minimal effective dose should be used. Barbiturates alone are not effective in relieving the pain but should be used for adequate sedation.
2. Oxygen therapy. When the pain does not respond readily to the administration of narcotics, or when cyanosis is present, oxygen therapy should be prescribed either by nasal catheter or mask.
3. The treatment of hypotension may be difficult. First, if possible, the cause should be determined. If there is a volume deficit, careful volume expansion should be used. If the patient is in cardiogenic shock, the choice of vasopressor drugs is controversial, as is balloon assistance and emergency bypass surgery.
4. Digitalis is of uncertain value in acute myocardial infarction with congestive heart failure. Evidence suggests that patients in this category are unusually sensitive to digitalis. During the acute phase diuretics are recommended to control congestive failure.
5. Adequate treatment of arrhythmias. Ventricular premature systoles may be the forerunner of more serious ventricular tachy arrhythmias. Intravenous administration of lidocaine is often effective and may be followed by oral use of procainamide or quinidine sulfate when appropriate.

    Supraventricular arrhythmias are common and are treated with a short-acting glycoside such as digoxin. Electroshock is used if arrhythmia persists and is refractory.
6. Anticoagulants have been used in some centers for the past 25 years, but current evidence of their efficacy remains in doubt.

Shoulder-hand syndrome occurs in 5 to 10 per cent of patients after myocardial infarction any time within a year after the occlusion. It is characterized by pain and tenderness of the shoulder, followed by pain, redness, swelling and stiffness of the hand and fingers, and is occasionally accompanied by atrophy of the muscles of the hand. Aspirin, physiotherapy and an exercise program are helpful.

Postmyocardial infarction (Dressler's) syndrome may occur from 2 weeks to 2 months after the acute infarction. It is characterized by fever, leukocytosis, pleuritis, pericarditis and pneumonitis. Pleural and pericardial exudates, which may be hemorrhagic, occur. The cause is unknown but may be due to sensitization to antigens resulting from myocardial necrosis. It is a benign disorder, which may be mistaken for recurrence of myocardial infarction.

Ventricular aneurysm occurs in about 20 per cent of the cases within weeks or months after the acute infarct. On x-ray examination an abnormal bulge of the ventricular contour is seen, which may be evident on palpation as an abnormal area of pulsations on the chest wall. Ventricular asynergy may also be a complication.

Atherosclerosis

Atherosclerosis is a disease in which atheroma, deposits of lipid-containing material, appear beneath the intima of arteries. Hypertension, diabetes mellitus, hyperlipidemia, obesity, and smoking are major risk factors. It is primarily a disease of the aorta and its branches, rather than of the pulmonary circuit, and is the basic etiologic factor in a high percentage of cases of coronary occlusion, cerebral thrombosis, mesenteric thrombosis and occlusive peripheral vascular disease. The rapidity and the extent of atheromatous changes are modified to some extent by race, hereditary factors, age, sex and previous damage to the vessel walls. The effects of diet and the cholesterol or lipid content of the blood are not fully determined. There appears to be a relationship of the amount and the quality of fat consumed in the diet and the cholesterol and the lipoprotein content of the blood to the death rate from coronary artery disease. The solid saturated fats tend to elevate the blood level of lipoproteins, whereas linoleic acid and some other unsaturated fatty acids from marine and vegetable oils tend to lower it. It seems firmly established that certain dietary fats induce increased blood coagulability and decreased fibrinolysis, but the effect of these factors in coronary heart disease is not established.

Plasma Lipoprotein Abnormalities

The association of atherosclerosis and its accompanying vascular changes with alterations in the plasma cholesterol and lipoproteins has increased interest in lipoprotein abnormalities.

Hyperlipoproteinemia not explained by other primary disease represents metabolic problems that are difficult to classify. Lipoprotein-excess states have been classified in five categories on the basis of plasma appearance, electrophoretic pattern, blood cholesterol and triglyceride concentrations.

Type I hyperlipoproteinemia:
Milky serum (increased chylomicrons in blood) is present with intense chylomicron band on electrophoresis and decreased alpha, beta and prebeta bands. Occurs in infancy, presents with abdominal pain and has no predisposition to coronary artery disease.

Type II hyperlipoproteinemia:
Serum cholesterol and phospholipids are increased but triglycerides are normal. Electrophoresis shows increased beta and prebeta bands. There is strong evidence of accelerated vascular disease in this category. Type II is familial and is autosomal dominant. Xanthomata are frequent. Dietary restriction of saturated fats and use of polyunsaturated fats are desirable as well as drug therapy (cholestyramine) to bind cholesterol in the gut.

Type III hyperlipoproteinemia:
Serum cholesterol and triglycerides are increased with a broad beta band on electrophoresis. Palmar xanthomata are characteristic. Vascular disease is frequent and weight reduction with the use of polyunsaturated fats is recommended. Clofibrate has been used.

Type IV hyperlipoproteinemia:
Serum cholesterol and triglyceride levels are elevated; diabetes mellitus is usually noted, and there is a dense prebeta band on electrophoresis. Premature coronary artery disease is frequent. Weight reduction and decrease in carbohydrate intake and of saturated fatty food is prescribed. Clofibrate will lower triglyceride levels.

Type IV profiles are seen also with hypothyroidism, nephrotic syndrome, obstructive jaundice, dysproteinemias (multiple myeloma) and uncontrolled diabetes mellitus.

Type V hyperlipoproteinemia:
Serum cholesterol and triglycerides levels are elevated. Obesity and eruptive xanthomata, especially on knees, are common. This occurs in late teens and is associated with abdominal pain. Weight reduction is essential.

Hyperlipidemia needs attention when cholesterol exceeds 220 mg. per 100 ml. and triglycerides 140 mg. per 100 ml.

The Cardiomyopathies

The cardiomyopathies are classified clinically as follows:

Congestive: manifested by poor systolic ejection function, cardiac dilatation, heart failure, arrhythmias, emboli and murmurs of mitral and triscuspid regurgitation

Ischemic: diffuse degenerative myocardial changes

Hypertropic: with or without obstruction to ventricular outflow

Cardiomyopathies are considered primary when the heart is the chief target organ and secondary when it accompanies known systemic conditions. Primary and secondary myopathies may fall into the above clinical classification. Amyloid, hemochromatosis, sarcoidosis, scleroderma, lupus erythematosus, neuromuscular disease, and coronary artery disease may be in both the congestive and ischemic categories and are considered secondary cardiomyopathies.

Examples of primary disease are familial, alcoholic, postpartum and endocardial fibrosis and fibroelastosis. These are usually manifested by congestive changes.

Idiopathic hypertropic subaortic stenosis (IHSS) is an example of heart disease due to obstruction to ventricular outflow. IHSS was discussed under Valvular Disorders.

Cor Pulmonale

Cor pulmonale is a right-sided heart enlargement due to disease in the pulmonary circuit, to valvular defects that increase the pulmonary pressure or to congenital defects. Acute cor pulmonale is caused by sudden obstruction of the pulmonary artery or one of its branches, usually by a clot. Chronic cor pulmonale is gradual in its development and may result from left ventricular failure, from mitral stenosis or from a wide variety of pulmonary or vascular lesions resulting in increased pressure and resistance to flow through the pulmonary vascular bed.

The manifestations are cyanosis, polycythemia, clubbing of the fingers, venous engorgement, increased venous pressure, engorgement of the liver and edema. Right ventricular dilatation and tricuspid insufficiency occur. X-ray films show enlargement of the pulmonary artery with increased pulsation. The right atrium and the right ventricle are enlarged. The ECG shows right-axis deviation and evidence of right ventricular hypertrophy. Treatment is that of cardiac failure plus treatment, when possible, of the underlying pulmonary lesion.

Congestive Heart Failure

Heart failure is defined as an abnormality of cardiac function in which the ventricles do not deliver an adequate amount of blood to the tissues at rest or during normal activity. The mechanism of myocardial failure is complex, and even an approximate understanding of it demands knowledge of cardiac function, hemodynamic states, water and electrolyte metabolism and renal and endocrine function. In most patients, heart failure results from anatomic lesions of the myocardial cell, heart valves or pericardium. In addition there are frequently precipitating causes that lead to manifestations of heart failure in the presence of underlying heart disease. These are:

1. Pulmonary embolism
2. Infection
3. Anemia
4. Thyrotoxicosis
5. Pregnancy
6. Arrhythmias
7. Myocarditis
8. Bacterial endocarditis
9. Physical exertion
10. Sodium excess
11. Severe hypertension

When fully developed, the syndrome is characterized by dyspnea, edema, venous hypertension, hepatomegaly and often by pleural effusion. On further inquiry and examination, some or all of the following may be found: orthopnea, paroxysmal cardiac dyspnea, pulmonary rales, enlargement of the heart, murmurs, disturbances in the cardiac mechanism, gallop (ventricular) rhythm, pulsus alternans, a positive hepatojugular reflux and abnormal arterial blood pressure. There will be variation in the details, depending to some extent on the underlying type of heart disease, but the general pattern is consistent.

Often it is difficult or impossible to change the course of many types of heart disease, but cardiac failure sometimes can be delayed for long periods by certain prophylactic measures. As examples: the activity and the habits of some patients must be changed, and the treatment of anemia, thyrotoxicosis, obesity and moderate hypertension, when they exist, will be especially helpful. Furthermore, recurrences of rheumatic fever now are largely preventable, and patients with chronic rheumatic valvular disease should be evaluated for surgery before, not after, cardiac failure appears. Lastly in this regard, prompt recognition and successful treatment of certain cardiac mechanism disturbances often will forestall cardiac failure.

The goal, once cardiac failure is manifest, is to restore adequate cardiac output and to maintain it. Rest is paramount, and individual circumstances dictate the strictness of the program. Sedation may be helpful. Oxygen is indicated for the cyanotic or the severely dyspneic patient. Digitalis continues to be the single most useful drug in cardiac failure, and any of the active, well-standardized preparations are acceptable. Optimum digitalization and maintenance, irrespective

of the preparation used, is the main point. It is seldom necessary to digitalize a patient fully by the single-dose method. Sodium restriction has become almost routine, but seldom does it need to be extremely rigid. A diet containing 800 mg. (35 mEq) sodium (2.0 g. salt) per day will serve for most patients. Injectable "loop" diuretics such as furosemide may be used, but oral diuretics such as the thiazide group, and furosemide are satisfactory in most cases. Spironolactone may be used in persistent therapy, primarily to avoid potassium loss. Care must be taken to guard against serum electrolyte depletion when combined sodium restriction and diuretics are used. These are selected instances when the application of tourniquets to the extremities or venesection will be beneficial, and the utility of occasionally removing large collections of pleural fluid should be remembered. Specific therapy should be directed toward the particular type of underlying heart disease whenever possible. In recent years therapy with peripheral vasodilating agents has been used with some success. Agents that dilate arterioles reduce total peripheral resistance and, hence, left ventricular afterload and aortic impedance. Venodilators reduce cardiac preload and, as a result, of these two effects a new and more effective cardiac function curve may be achieved.

Hypertension and Hypertensive Heart Disease

The upper limits of normal blood pressure are usually defined as 140 mm. systolic and 90 mm. diastolic. Recent life insurance statistics show that any persistent increase in blood pressure above these figures, regardless of age, is associated with a shortened life expectancy. In the United States the average weight and the average blood pressure increase steadily with advancing years. However, extensive studies have proved that at any year of adult life a patient is the best "insurance risk" if both weight and blood pressure are approximately what would be *average for sex and height at the age of 25 years.* Hypertension is an important risk factor in myocardial infarction and stroke. Systolic and diastolic levels are equally considered as risk factors.

Etiology. Over 90 per cent of all hypertension is of unknown cause and is referred to as "Essential hypertension." Secondary hypertension, i.e., when an etiology can be determined most commonly is due to renal artery stenosis, bilateral renal parenchymal disease, or oral contraceptive agents. Less common causes of secondary hypertension include primary hyperaldosteronism, pheochromocytoma, coarctation of the aorta, Cushing's syndrome, renin-producing tumors, and excessive licorice ingestion.

Essential hypertension is an extremely common and important disturbance after the age of 40. Plasma renin activity levels may be high, low, or normal. The relation of renin to vascular complications is debated.

High blood pressure may exist for many years without symptoms, or there may be headaches, vertigo, palpitation, moderate dyspnea or nervous tension states for which no other cause can be found. The effects of hypertension on certain organs should be determined when high blood pressure is first detected and regularly thereafter. This "end-organ" evaluation includes retinal blood vessels, the heart, the kidney and the cerebral vessels. The earliest retinal vascular changes are tortuosity and narrowing of the arteriolar lumen (the normal arteriolar-venous ratio of 3:4 decreases perhaps to 1:2). If therapy is inadequate the lesion will progress to severe arteriolar narrowing, A-V nicking, and copper or silver wire appearance of the vessel. Hypertensive heart disease is first manifest as left ventricular hypertrophy revealed in the ECG, and then enlargement detectable by x-ray and physical examination. Left ventricular heart failure may ensue. Hypertension also is a risk factor in the development of coronary atherosclerosis. The renal vessels develop arteriolar nephrosclerosis. Mild (1+) proteinuria is common and renal functional impairment may develop. Cerebral vascular disease may be manifest as transient ischemic attacks or strokes.

The vast majority of patients with essential hypertension die of cardiac failure and cerebral vascular accidents. Since treatment with potent antihypertensive drugs has become available, the incidence of these complications can be greatly reduced. Early and effective treatment is critical in patients with hypertension. Approximately 5 per cent of patients with hypertension of all causes may develop the malignant phase.

Accelerated or malignant hypertension is characterized by marked blood pressure elevation in association with retinal hemorrhages, exudates, papilledema, and malignant nephrosclerosis. It may also include manifestations of hypertensive encephalopathy such as headache, vomiting, visual disturbances, stupor and coma. As mentioned previously, essential hypertension often involves the kidney with arteriolar ("benign") nephrosclerosis, mild proteinuria, and the possibility of modest and slowly progressive impairment of renal function. This seldom results in renal failure. In accelerated or malignant hypertension, the renal lesion ("malignant" nephrosclerosis) consisting of proliferative endarteritis and necrotizing arteriolitis is devastating if untreated and rapidly results in renal failure. Prior to availability of effective therapy, life expectancy was less than 2 years with death due to uremia, cerebral hemorrhage, and cardiac failure. With therapy prognosis is markedly improved.

Treatment of Hypertension.   There is debate concerning how extensive the search should be for causes of secondary hypertension. Several generalizations may be made: (1) Clinical clues should be pursued; e.g., the results of discontinuing oral contraceptives should be determined; blood pressure differences between upper and lower extremities should be followed by assessment for coarctation of the aorta; "attacks" of hypertension suggest pheochromocytoma; hypokalemia (without diuretics) suggests hyperaldosteronism; subcostal bruits establish the possibility of renal arterial disease as might hypertension under age 20. (2) Only patients who would otherwise be operated on should have a workup for surgically correctable lesions. (3) Where there are no clues to cause or patients are not surgical candidates, it may be well to institute treatment directly. If response to therapy is difficult or changing, a search for cause may be indicated.

Systolic or diastolic hypertension readings, i.e., above 140/90 mm. Hg are indications for therapy. Three categories of antihypertensive drugs are available; diuretics, adrenolytic agents and vasodilators. The diuretics (most commonly hydrochlorothiazide) are most commonly used to begin therapy in mild and moderate hypertension. If this is inadequate, adrenolytic agents (e.g., centrally acting agents such as methyldopa or clonidine; reserpine; prazosin or beta-adrenergic receptor blocking drugs such as propranolol, nadolol, or metoprolol) or vasodilator drugs (e.g., hydralazine, minoxidil) may be added. Guanethidine may also be added.

In hypertensive crisis or malignant hypertension, the direct vasodilator drugs such as hydralazine, diazoxide, or minoxidil may be best. If these are not effective, sodium nitroprusside or trimethaphan may be used.

Hypertensive Cardiovascular Disease.   Cardiac disease secondary to chronic hypertension is a common cause of cardiac failure in the middle-aged. It is equally distributed in males and females. The pathology of the hypertensive heart is primarily a work hypertrophy that first affects the left ventricle, leading to left ventricular dilatation, relative mitral regurgitation and dilatation of the left atrium and, ultimately, of the right ventricle also.

The most common symptom is progressive dyspnea. Paroxysmal nocturnal dyspnea is also common. Pain is unusual unless there is accompanying coronary arterial insufficiency (with or without occlusive arterial disease). The characteristic sign is left ventricular hypertrophy, associated with high blood pressure.

Hypertension with systolic pressure of over 200 mm. Hg may persist for many years. But when the heart no longer can sustain the burden of work, the pressure usually falls, and symptoms of cardiac failure, such as edema, engorgement of the liver and pulmonary edema, develop, with the commonly associated coronary artery disease arrhythmias, especially atrial fibrillation. The most common associated conditions are (1) congestive heart failure; (2) stroke; (3) angina pectoris; (4) coronary thrombosis; and (5) nephrosclerosis.

Cardiac Arrhythmias

Normal Mechanism. The orderly contractions of the atria and the ventricles are controlled (1) by impulses that arise in the sinoatrial node, transmitted through (2) the atria to the (3) atrioventricular node and thence through (4) the bundle of His to the ventricular musculature. As the stimulus passes from the sinoatrial node down the atria, it stimulates atrial contraction; as it passes from the atrioventricular node down the bundle of His, it stimulates ventricular contraction. Abnormal cardiac rhythms are caused by interferences with this mechanism.

Arrhythmias. The clinically important arrhythmias may be divided into three major categories: (1) the atrial arrhythmias, (2) atrioventricular conduction defects, and (3) ventricular arrhythmias. In some instances these arrhythmias may be diagnosed by physical examination, but in most instances electrocardiographic study is essential.

Sinus pauses and sinoatrial block are the result of failure of impulse formation at the sinoatrial node. This form of heart block may be the result of vagal or of carotid sinus stimulation, or it may follow intoxication with substances such a digitalis, potassium salts or quinidine. Progressive disease is due to a destructive process in the sinus node and neighboring tissue. Specifically, coronary artery disease and rheumatic myocarditis may play a role. If the sinoatrial node is quiescent for a prolonged period, and unless another pacemaker initiates impulse formation and ventricular contraction, Adams-Stokes attacks will occur. This condition is known as the "sick sinus syndrome" and may also show periods of tachycardia and bradycardia as well as sinus arrest. Pacemaker installation may be required.

Premature beats may be atrial or ventricular in origin; extrasystoles are uncommon and should be referred to as interpolated beats, since they occur midway between two normal beats and are not followed by a compensatory pause. Atrial and ventricular premature beats cannot be differentiated by physical examination. Premature beats frequently are found in patients with normal hearts and may be precipitated by nervousness or the excessive use of coffee or tobacco. In other instances they are associated with myocardial disease; they may be a manifestation of digitalis toxicity. Treatment usually is not necessary; removal of the offending agent may be indicated; in some instances administra-

tion of quinidine or procainamide will suppress the ectopic focus.

Paroxysmal atrial tachycardia is manifested by the sudden onset of a very rapid regular rhythm with ventricular rates of 140 to 220 beats per minute; this arrhythmia always is abrupt in onset and termination. The attack may be interrupted by vagal stimulation, such as carotid sinus pressure. The Valsalva maneuver or cholinergic drugs may be useful. Both digitalis and quinidine are effective in controlling this arrhythmia if other measures fail.

Atrial flutter is characterized by rapid contractions of the atria at rates of 250 to 350 per minute; however, the ventricular rate is slower. Varying degrees of atrioventricular block exist. If the block is regular, such as 2:1, the ventricular contractions are regular at 150 beats per minute, but an irregularity in the block results in an irregular ventricular response. This arrhythmia is more likely to develop as a complication of some organic cardiac disease. Correct diagnosis requires electrocardiographic confirmation. Treatment consists of digitalization to show the ventricular rate. Electric countershock is often necessary.

Atrial fibrillation (AF) is characterized by a completely irregular ventricular rhythm; the ventricles in this disorder respond irregularly and with varying force to a small portion of rapid, totally irregular, atrial impulses. Atrial fibrillation generally is a manifestation of organic heart disease. Treatment consists of slowing the ventricular rate with digitalis; this is accomplished by increasing the atrioventricular block. After the ventricular rate is controlled, cardioversion to a sinus rhythm with quinidine or electric countershock may be attempted. This is more likely to be effective in AF of recent onset than in chronic AF.

Atrioventricular conduction defects or block may be localized to (1) the A-V node and (2) the infranodal tissue, which consists of the bundle of His, the proximal bundle, and the distal Purkinje fibers. A-V node block is due to digitalis intoxication, inferior myocardial infarction, myocarditis, cardiac surgery and congenital heart block; it is often reversible. Clinically it can be recognized by a narrow QRS complex, occasional Wenckebach periods and an escape rate of 50 or more beats per minute with a form identical with normal beats. Permanent pacemaking is often not needed.

Infranodal block is more serious and is due to destructive process of the bundle and its branches. Clinically the patient shows dropped beats, bundle-branch block, slow idioventricular escape beats with wide QRS. Anterior myocardial infarction may be present, and the treatment of choice is usually permanent implantation of a pacemaker.

Ventricular premature beats are the most common

ventricular arrhythmia and are essentially of the same significance as the atrial premature beats mentioned above.

Ventricular tachycardia is an ominous arrhythmia that may terminate in ventricular fibrillation and death. The ventricular rate is regular or may be very slightly irregular; the rate usually is 150 to 250 beats per minute. Consecutive beats do not sound precisely the same but tend to vary somewhat in intensity. This arrhythmia never is slowed by carotid sinus stimulation. Prompt treatment is necessary and consists of intravenous injection of lidocaine. Precordial electrical countershock may be required to terminate the arrhythmia.

Pericardial Disease

Acute benign pericarditis is probably due to a viral cause and at times to an autoimmune reaction. Viral infection is poorly documented although Coxsackie infection seems frequently implicated in pericarditis. Recurrences are frequent; effusion may occur with tamponade, and eventually constrictive disease may ensue. Steroid therapy is used to relieve symptoms but does not significantly alter the course.

Collagen vascular disease may involve the pericardium and is seen in rheumatoid arthritis, progressive systemic sclerosis and lupus erythematosus, including the syndrome caused by procainamide.

Tuberculosis is difficult to diagnose in pericardial disease since cultures are usually negative; biopsy is needed to confirm the diagnosis. Pericardial constriction is a sequela even after appropriate and prolonged therapy.

Uremic pericarditis is now controlled through chronic dialysis; it occurs in younger patients and does not directly relate to the level of urea nitrogen or creatinine.

Cardiac antigens appear to be involved in the immune mechanism with postpericardectomy syndrome (60 per cent) and postmyocardial infarction syndrome (three per cent).

Miscellaneous Vascular Diseases

Leriche Syndrome. This thrombotic obliteration of the bifurcation of the aorta may result from progressive thrombosis at the bifurcation, which ultimately leads to complete obliteration of the aorta. A similar clinical picture may occur with a saddle embolus lodging at this area. Intermittent claudication with pain in the low back and absence of both femoral pulses with symmetrical atrophy of the legs are the prominent symptoms. Aortograms make the diagnosis definite.

Aortic Arch Syndrome (Pulseless Disease, Takayasu Syndrome). Progressive atherosclerosis or inflammatory changes in the intima may lead to partial or complete obliteration of the major branches of the aortic arch. It may follow severe trauma to the upper chest that damages the media and leads to the intimal atherosclerosis. There is absence of pulses in the upper part of the body, with normal femoral pulses. The clinical features are easy fatigability of the arms and atrophy of muscles and soft tissues. Syncopal attacks may occur.

Dissecting Aneurysm of the Aorta. This occurs more frequently in men and usually starts from an intimal rent in the aorta. The dissection extends proximally to the aortic ring and distally, for a variable distance, into one or several of the branches of the aorta. The symptoms include pain, aortic regurgitation, interference with the blood supply through branches of the aorta, and x-ray evidence of widening of the aorta. Antihypertensive therapy or surgery may be indicated.

(Peripheral vascular diseases are discussed in Chap. 8, Surgery.)

DISEASES OF THE HEMATOPOIETIC SYSTEM

Anemia

Anemia is a reduction in the number of red cells, the amount of hemoglobin, or both. It may be acute or chronic and may arise from: (1) loss of blood, (2) increased destruction of blood, or (3) defective formation of blood.

A classification based on the size of the red cells (macrocytic and microcytic anemias) or upon the hemoglobin content of the cells (hyperchromic and hypochromic) is very useful for descriptive purposes.

Iron Deficiency Anemias

Iron deficiency is the most common cause of anemia; in the United States in the adult this deficiency occurs through physiologic or pathologic loss of blood. Red cell mass is maintained at the expense of iron stores as blood loss occurs. The usual sequence in the development of iron deficiency is (1) decrease in iron stores with increase in iron-binding capacity; (2) decrease in plasma iron; (3) fall in hemoglobin and red cell mass; and (4) lastly, reduction in size of red cell and hemoglobin concentration.

Loss of blood in women regularly occurs in pregnancy and from menses. In men, iron deficiency is almost always due to gastrointestinal blood loss, acute or chronic. Hypochromia and microcytosis are the morphologic findings in advanced iron deficiency but may also be found in chronic inflammation and malignant disease, hemoglobin C disease and in cases of lead poisoning.

Treatment is directed at the cause of blood loss. Oral iron therapy should be maintained for 1 year to replete stores. Parenteral administration of iron is rarely indicated and may cause sensitivity reactions.

Sideroblastic or Iron-overload Anemia. This consists of a heterogeneous, ill-defined group of anemias that are drug-related (alcohol, isoniazide, pyrazinamide), idiopathic or pyridoxine-responsive. These anemias are microcytic and hypochromic in type and refractory to iron and other types of therapy. The plasma iron level is high, tissue hemosiderosis is usually marked, and the iron-binding protein of the blood is almost completely saturated. Erythrocyte precursors in the bone marrow show an increased number of iron granules, and siderocytes in the peripheral bloodstream are common. The nature of the block in hemoglobin synthesis is not known. The treatment consists of elimination of offending drugs and transfusions. Certain patients will respond to pyridoxine.

Hemolytic Anemias

The normal life span of an erythrocyte in the peripheral blood is about 120 days, and any abnormality that shortens this period interferes with the erythroid steady state. The bone marrow is capable of producing erythrocytes at a rate that is six to eight times more rapid than is normal. Therefore, moderate grades of increased hemolysis can be compensated for by increased production, so that anemia does not develop in spite of excessive hemolysis of moderate degree. When the life span of the erythrocyte is shortened to 15 to 20 days, the compensatory mechanism of the marrow is exceeded and anemia develops. The evidence of hemolytic anemia includes (1) increased reticulocytosis; (2) erythroid hyperplasia of the bone marrow; (3) increased excretion of fecal urobilinogen; (4) jaundice; (5) increased polychromasia, (6) the red blood cells may show fragmentation, helmet shapes, may show the specific abnormalities of spherocytes, elliptocytes and target cells, and (7) frequently moderate leukocytosis and thrombocytosis. Rarely, a hypoplastic crisis of the marrow occurs. The life span of the erythrocytes may be measured by tagging a sample of the patient's cells with radioactive chromium and measuring the rapidity with which they are removed from the circulation.

Excessive destruction of platelets and red and white blood cells often is attributed to overactivity of the spleen. However, the spleen serves as the "graveyard" of blood cells. "Hypersplenism" is therefore a diagnosis that is tempting to make simply out of convenience when the cause of a hemolytic anemia is obscure, but such a reaction is not infrequent in lymphomas and lymphocytic leukemia and other conditions associated with splenomegaly. (See the section on the spleen.)

Anemia from excessive destruction of erythrocytes may be of extrinsic or intrinsic origin. Extrinsic factors are those chemicals, drugs and animal or bacterial toxins that act on the normal red cell to cause hemolysis. Malarial anemia is a classic example.

Intrinsic forms of hemolytic anemia are those in which there is a defect in the erythrocytes themselves or in the patient's plasma, which leads to an increased rate of destruction. Hemolytic anemias may be classified as follows:

1. Hereditary or intrinsic causes
   Hereditary spherocytosis (familial hemolytic icterus)
   Hemoglobinopathies, as sickle cell anemia
   Enzyme deficiencies
       Glucose-6-phosphate dehydrogenase
       Pyruvate kinase
2. Acquired or extrinsic causes
   Isoimmune—erythroblastosis fetalis
   Autoimmune
       Primary—idiopathic
       Secondary—lymphoma, leukemia, collagen diseases
       Chemical and physical agents
       Infections
       Hypersplenism
       Paroxysmal nocturnal hemoglobinuria

Hereditary Spherocytosis. This condition, also called familial hemolytic icterus is characterized by the presence of spherocytes in the peripheral blood—erythrocytes that are thicker but of smaller diameter than normal. They appear as small deeply staining cells and are more fragile than normal and hemolyze more readily in hypotonic saline solution. The spleen is enlarged, the patients are jaundiced, pale, and pass dark urine during the episodes of hemolysis, which may be triggered by infection. Cholelithiasis is common in older patients. The more severe forms of the disease appear in childhood, but many cases are so mild as to produce no symptoms. Spherocytosis, reticulocytosis, splenomegaly, jaundice, erythroid hyperplasia of the marrow and increased fragility of the erythrocytes accompanied by varying degrees of anemia characterize the disease. Splenectomy produces a clinical cure, but the increased fragility remains.

Hereditary Hemoglobinopathies. Many abnormal hemoglobins have been demonstrated and are caused by genetically determined abnormalities in the formation of hemoglobin. Only a few of these are of clinical significance. Hemoglobin is composed of globin and four heme radicals. Globin contains two α and two β chains containing 141 amino acids in each α chain and 146 in each β chain. *Hemoglobin S*, which causes sickle cell trait and sickle cell anemia, differs from normal Hb A in that in Hb S one amino acid, glutamic acid, is replaced by valine in the β peptide. Reduced Hb S is less soluble than deoxygenated Hb A and forms tactoids, which distort the erythrocyte; the deformed cells are more fragile than normal and break up more rapidly, and anemia develops. Vascular occlusion and infarction form a common complication, and repeated splenic infarction results in a small fibrotic atrophic spleen. The usual findings of hemolytic anemia are present, plus the severe sickling and bizarre forms of erythrocytes. The disease occurs most frequently in blacks and the sickle cell trait (heterozygous) is more common than sickle cell anemia (homozygous). Hb S apparently gives some protection against malaria.

Hemoglobin SC disease has a combination of Hb S and Hb C. The features are similar to Hb S disease. Hemoglobin C disease is similar to Hb S disease, but target cells are common, splenomegaly is usually present, and there is no sickling of the cells.

Thalassemia syndrome represents deficient hemoglobin production and decreased cell vitality. It produces a chronic microcytic hypochromic anemia, with excess hemolysis, leptocytosis, target cells and splenomegaly. The hemoglobin is normal, and iron stores are adequate. It is a hereditary disease most common on the shores of the Mediterranean Sea. It occurs as thalassemia minor and thalassemia major. In the severe forms all manifestations of hemolytic anemia are present, with increased amounts of Hb F and Hb A_2.

Paroxysmal nocturnal hemoglobinuria is a hemolytic disorder of unknown cause, characterized by excessive nonimmune hemolysis that occurs during sleep, and extensive enough to cause hemoglobinuria and a chronic anemia. The erythrocytes are unusually sensitive to acidified normal serum, and the disease is frequently accompanied by leukopenia and thrombocytopenia.

Erythrocyte Antibodies. Hemolytic disorders may be caused by erythrocyte antibodies and associated with serologic manifestations of the immune process. With the exception of hemolytic transfusion reactions caused by the ABO blood group incompatibility, these serum factors are, for the most part, immunoglobulins. The majority are warm agglutinins, that is, they are most active at 37 C. and produce agglutination rather than hemolysis. Anti-A and Anti-B erythrocyte antibodies are most active in the cold and are complete, attaching to more than one erythrocyte at a time, and as a result clumping or agglutination occurs in saline. In contrast, immune erythrocyte antibodies are incomplete and attach to only one cell at a time and therefore act as blocking antibodies, and red cells to which these substances are absorbed will not agglutinate in saline. The most useful means to detect incomplete erythrocyte antibodies is the Coombs, or antiglobulin, test. Incomplete erythrocyte antibodies are immunoglobulins, and cells coated with these substances will be agglutinated by anti-human globulin antibodies contained in Coombs' serum, which are obtained from rabbits that have been injected with human immunoglobulins. A positive direct Coombs test consists of the agglutination of washed erythrocytes suspended in Coombs' reagent and indicates the presence of an abnormal antigen-antibody complex protein adsorbed to the surface of the cell. A positive indirect Coombs test indicates free antibody in serum. The specificity of Coombs' serum can be increased by injecting the donor rabbits with pure human immunoglobulins.

Acquired Autoimmune Hemolytic Anemias. The acquired autoimmune hemolytic disorders are divisible into two groups—primary or idiopathic, and secondary. A vast majority of the cases are of the secondary type, so that an acquired autoimmune hemolytic anemia practically always means some other primary disease even though that disease remains hidden. The causes of the secondary autoimmune hemolytic anemia are diverse and include (1) hematologic neoplasms such as lymphoma, chronic lymphocytic leukemia, plasmacytic myeloma and macroglobulinemia; (2) collagen diseases such as systemic lupus erythematosus, polyarteritis and scleroderma; (3) nonhematologic neoplasms such as ovarian cysts, dermoid cysts and renal carcinoma; and (4) infections such as infectious mononucleosis, primary atypical pneumonia and infectious hepatitis. The clinical manifestations of the primary and secondary autoimmune hemolytic anemias differ only insofar as the underlying basic disease contributes to the clinical picture. The hemolytic mechanisms are the same regardless of the source of the abnormal protein or antibody or the nature of the stimuli evoking the formation. There are many reasons to implicate normal lymphocytes and plasmacytes as the cells that synthesize immunoglobulins in response to specific antigenic stimuli. There is good evidence that these cells elaborate the abnormal globulins that cause the autoimmune hemolytic anemia.

Hemolytic anemias that are due to genetically determined enzyme deficiencies in the erythrocytes are recognized. A deficiency in pyruvate kinase, a glycolytic enzyme, has been found in some hemolytic anemias, and a deficiency in glucose-6-phosphate dehydrogenase in the erythrocytes is encountered in patients who develop hemolysis on exposure to certain drugs such as primaquine and sulfonamides.

Erythrocyte Production Defects

Aplastic Anemia, Hypoplastic Anemia or Bone Marrow Failure. In the peripheral bloodstream this is represented by a reduction of the platelets, leukocytes and erythrocytes, and in the bone marrow by hypocellularity of the specimen. This may result from external agents (secondary aplastic anemia) such as x-rays, radioactive materials, benzene and related chemical compounds, as well as many commonly used drugs. Bone marrow sensitivity is one of the most important toxic effects to be watched for whenever a new drug is introduced. Idiopathic aplastic anemia represents the same features but occurs without contact with any recognized causative agent. The changes in the peripheral blood, as well as in the bone marrow, are the same in the secondary and idiopathic types. Few therapeutic measures for this condition are available, except to remove the patient from contact with the causative agent when it is recognized and to give blood transfusions. Androgenic steroidal agents are said to be of some value by certain authors. Bone marrow transplantation may be effective in idiopathic aplastic anemia.

The bone marrow may also be depressed by systemic disease such as sepsis, renal failure and hypothyroidism. Anemia from replacement of the normal bone marrow by malignant cells occurs and is designated as myelophthisic anemia.

Megaloblastic Anemias

Pernicious Anemia. This is a progressive disease involving the blood and the blood-forming organs, the gastrointestinal tract and the nervous system. It is characterized by spontaneous remission. The disease is the most common cause of vitamin B_{12} deficiency and is due to absence of an "intrinsic" factor of the gastric secretion (not identical with the known gastric enzymes or acids) necessary to combine with an "extrinsic" substance in the food. This extrinsic factor has been shown to be vitamin B_{12}, and the intrinsic, or gastric, factor is necessary for its proper absorption and utilization. Pernicious anemia is more common in males than in females and occurs chiefly in middle life. Patients appear to be well nourished, with lemon-yellow skin tint. The gastrointestinal symptoms include a painful glossitis, achylia and often diarrhea and anorexia. Most important diagnostically, is the invariable failure of the stomach to secrete hydrochloric acid. The nervous symptoms are those of subacute combined sclerosis of the cord and peripheral neuritis. This is manifested by numbness, tingling and paresthesias. Loss of vibration sense occurs early, but the nervous symptoms may not be present in the early stages of the disease.

The blood picture is characterized by signs of red cell destruction and regeneration. The red cells are markedly reduced—often below 1 million, in untreated cases—with relatively less diminution in the hemoglobin percentage. Smears show marked variation in the size, shape and staining reaction of the erythrocytes, but the predominant cell is the large oval macrocyte. There are a moderate degree of leukopenia but hypersegmentation of polymorphonuclear leukocytes is common and a lowered platelet count. The mean corpuscular volume (MCV) and the mean corpuscular hemoglobin (MCH) are both increased above the normal. Aspiration of bone marrow shows a preponderance of megaloblasts. This is a macrocytic hyperchromic type of anemia.

Pernicious anemia should be suspected in any severe anemia. There are other causes of vitamin B_{12} deficiency. Failure of the stomach to secrete acid is essential to the diagnosis. The dramatic reticulocyte response to vitamin B_{12} confirms the diagnosis. A test for the absorption of vitamin B_{12}, using radioactive cobalt (Schilling test), is helpful in the diagnosis of obscure or partially treated cases.

Proper response to therapy is manifested by a rapid increase in reticulocytes within 3 to 5 days, followed by a slower increase in the red cell count. The hemoglobin increases more slowly, and the morphology of the blood and the appearance of the bone marrow return gradually to normal. The continued use of vitamin B_{12} is necessary to prevent recurrence. The achylia does not disappear, and the cord changes are arrested but not cured. The most convenient treatment consists of intramuscular injection of vitamin B_{12}.

Folic acid, in contradistinction to B_{12}, is not stored and needs replenishment. Therefore, folic acid deficiency is a more common dietary cause than B_{12} deficiency for megaloblastic anemia. It is a complication of hemolytic anemia, pregnancy and alcoholism. It should be considered when drugs such as isoniazid, Dilantin and antifertility agents are given because of metabolic competition. The metabolic inhibitors used in oncology and immunosuppression also cause megaloblastic changes.

Erythropoietin

Erythropoietin is a humoral factor that regulates the quantity of hemoglobin synthesized in the body. This substance is detectable in plasma and in urine and is a glycoprotein that is inactivated by proteolytic enzymes.

Erythropoietin is produced for the most part by the kidney, and its effect is to bring about stem cell–erythrocytic differentiation. Hypoxia, irrespective of the type and method of its production, appears to be the chief determinant of erythropoitin activity. An inappropriate and unexplained increase is erythropoietin is seen in patients with hydronephrosis, renal cysts, renal neoplasm, hepatomas and cerebellar tumors.

Polycythemia

Erythrocytosis or polycythemia (increased red blood cell mass) may be divided into primary and secondary forms. The hematocrit is elevated. However, the hematocrit may also be increased due to a reduction in plasma volume (relative polycythemia, as with diuretics, catecholamine excess, some patients with hypertension, and in "stress" polycythemia).

Secondary polycythemia results from anoxia, which stimulates erythropoiesis. It may accompany certain types of congenital heart disease, some forms of acquired heart disease, chronic pulmonary disease or exposure to certain toxins that produce methemoglobin and certain hemoglobinopathies. Tissue hypoxia is the underlying etiologic factor. Relative polycythemia is not a disorder of red cell production but rather is due to a contracted plasma volume.

Polycythemia vera (primary polycythemia) is a myeloproliferative disease with increases in erythrocyte count, blood volume, hemoglobin concentration and hematocrit, which causes increased viscosity of the blood and sluggish peripheral circulation. The leukocyte count and the platelet count are also often increased. The bone marrow is hypercellular. Total blood volume is substantially increased (150 to 300 per cent of normal). Patients have a dusky-red complexion, dizziness, ringing of the ears, anorexia and dyspnea; itching is common, particularly after bathing. Hemorrhagic tendencies are common as is spontaneous venous thrombosis. Oxygen saturation of the blood is normal. Peptic ulcer and gout are frequent complications. Because of the diffuse venous engorgement in all organs and tissues, the subjective symptoms are widespread. *Treatment* consists of venesection and removal of blood to alleviate the symptoms and administration of radioactive phosphorus to decrease erythrocyte production. Debate about the value and safety of the latter continues.

Leukemia

Leukemia is a systemic disease of unknown cause characterized by rapid and abnormal proliferation of leukocytes in the hematopoietic organs and by the presence of immature leukocytes in the peripheral blood. The total leukocyte count is elevated in most patients, but it may be normal or low. The presence of immature cells in the bloodstream is of more significance than elevation of the leukocyte count. Leukemia is classified according to rapidity of development and to the type of leukocyte that is affected predominantly; therefore, myelogenous, lymphocytic and monocytic leukemia

are the common types. Plasma cell, megakaryocytic and eosinophilic leukemias are encountered rarely. All types of leukemia occur in acute and chronic forms and may have leukemic (elevated white count) or aleukemic (normal or low white count) phases. Invariably, leukemia is fatal. Acute forms are more common in children. Evidence is gradually accumulating to support the probability of viral infection being at least one of the causes of leukemia.

Chronic granulocytic leukemia is most common in young adults; the cause is unknown. The onset is insidious, and the first symptoms may be due to the greatly enlarged spleen or to anemia. Slight fever and moderate hemorrhages are not uncommon. There is no marked enlargement of the lymph nodes. The severity of the disease is reflected by the height of the leukocyte count.

The blood shows mild anemia, and the platelets are reduced only in the late stages of the illness. There is (1) a relative and absolute increase in the white blood cells of the myelocytic series in most cases, (2) immaturity of cells found ordinarily only in the bone marrow—neutrophilic, eosinophilic and basophilic myelocytes, myeloblasts, and (3) the Philadelphia chromosome. Although the percentage of lymphocytes is reduced, their absolute number is not decreased. The number of leukocytes may reach 1 million per cu. mm. The median survival rate is from 2 to 4 years. The chronic course may be interrupted by an acute "blast crisis."

Chronic lymphatic leukemia is characterized by slow, painless enlargements of the cervical, axillary and inguinal lymph nodes, which are discrete and not tender. The spleen and the liver are also enlarged. The onset is insidious. The disease is uncommon under the age of 40. A vague feeling of malaise and fatigue is the most common presenting complaint.

The blood shows moderate secondary anemia, with 100,000 to 200,000 leukocytes per cu. mm., but in some cases the leukocyte count is low. Small lymphocytes form 80 to 99 per cent of the smear. Mild anemia and mild thrombocytopenia are seen. Since this is a disease of older age, death is often due to an unrelated cause. Bacterial infection is a common complication.

In both types of chronic leukemia the most important treatment is directed toward relieving the patient's discomfort, reducing the mass of leukemic cells and using supportive therapy to control complications. In myelocytic leukemia, busulfan is the treatment of choice as well as x-rays to the spleen and radioactive phosphorus. In chronic lymphocytic leukemia, chemotherapeutic agents, corticosteroids and x-ray therapy are used. It is unclear whether therapy prolongs life.

Acute leukemia is a fulminating, fatal disease, occurring most often in individuals under 30. The onset often resembles an acute infection. There are fever, prostration, marked tendency to hemorrhage from gums, nose, stomach, rectum or uterus, purpuric hemorrhages of the skin and swelling and ulceration of gums, cheek, jaw and tonsils. The cervical lymph nodes may enlarge very rapidly. The spleen and the liver may be moderately enlarged. Lymphoblastic leukemia presents more commonly with bone and joint pain. The blood shows numerous very immature cells. It is sometimes impossible to identify acute leukemia as myelogenous or lymphatic in type and such cases have been called stem cell leukemias. Anemia is extreme, and thrombocytopenia is severe. Acute lymphoblastic leukemia is currently treated with combinations of chemotherapeutic agents and prolonged remissions may occur especially in children. Similar therapy with acute myelogenous leukemia has a lower remission rate.

Monocytic leukemia is less common than either the myelogenous or the lymphocytic type and may occur as either an acute or a chronic form, but the acute is more common.

Myelomonocytic leukemia presents immature cells of both the myeloid and the monocytic series in the peripheral blood and occurs usually as an acute leukemia.

Myelofibrosis (Agnogenic myeloid metaplasia; osteosclerotic anemia)

Myelofibrosis generally is considered a myeloproliferative disease and frequently is mistaken for chronic myelocytic leukemia. It is characterized by marked splenomegaly without lymphadenopathy. There is severe and progressive anemia, although early in the disease polycythemia may be present. Marked variations in the size and the shape of the erythrocytes are noted with a prominence of cells shaped like teardrops. The leukocyte count varies and may be low, although usually leukocytosis is present with a shift to the left of the myeloid elements, giving a picture suggestive of chronic myelocytic leukemia. The platelet count is low. Bone marrow aspiration is difficult, and evidence of hypocellularity is found. On biopsy the marrow is fibrotic. The extramedullary hematopoiesis found in the spleen accounts for the splenomegaly. The marrow fibrosis probably is a part of the proliferative process as is the extramedullary hematopoiesis. Treatment is not satisfactory, and repeated transfusions are given. Splenectomy may reduce the hemolytic process in this disease in some very carefully selected patients.

Infectious Mononucleosis

Infectious mononucleosis is a virus disease characterized by fever, sore throat, lymphadenopathy, deterioration in liver function tests and an increase in lymphocytes and monocytes with morphologically atypical forms. Children and young adults chiefly are affected. A temperature of 100 to 103 F. may last for several weeks with headache, sweating, fever, malaise and sore throat. The tonsils and the cervical nodes are enlarged and tender. The blood shows from 10,000 to 30,000 white cells, largely mononuclear, although in the early stage leukopenia may be present. A positive heterophil antibody agglutination test helps to establish the diagnosis. In most instances the patient will recover spontaneously in the course of a few weeks. The etiologic relationship to the Epstein-Barr virus (EBV) has been established.

Lymphoma

The lymphomas comprise a group of pathologic and clinical entities characterized by progressive, painless enlargement of lymphatic tissues. Lymphadenopathy and a large spleen are characteristic. Their etiology is unknown, and their classification is subject to dispute. A leukemic blood picture may develop in many patients, resulting in the picture of lymphocytic leukemia. The clinical features of the lymphomas are similar, and differentiation must be made by histologic examination of tissue. It is common to divide lymphomas into Hodgkin's or non-Hodgkin's lymphomas.

Hodgkin's Disease

Hodgkin's disease is characterized by slow, painless, progressive enlargement of the lymph nodes, often accompanied by fever, cachexia and anemia. Frequently the spleen is enlarged. It is most common in the second and third decades, occurring most often in males. The cause is unknown.

Most frequently the cervical nodes are enlarged, though the tumor masses may be found in mediastinal, axillary, retroperitoneal, mesenteric and inguinal regions. The nodes are discrete and vary in consistency. Pruritus is common. Enlargement of the nodes may cause obstructive symptoms in the mediastinum or obstructive jaundice. Anemia often is found. Occasionally, moderate eosinophilia may be present. Reed-Sternberg cells are found in biopsy material.

There are four major histological patterns in order of worsening prognosis: lymphocyte-predominance; nodular cellularity; mixed cell type; and lymphocyte depletion. Lymphocyte-predominant Hodgkin's disease has the best prognosis (90 per cent 5-year survival).

Diagnosis must be established by biopsy of a lymph node and, in addition to chest roentgenograms, a lymphangiogram and peritonoscopy are commonly obtained to detect involvement of abdominal lymph nodes, which are otherwise undetectable. This is necessary for accurate staging of the disease before treatment.

Stage I Disease limited to one lymph node group of two contiguous groups on one side of the diaphragm.

Stage II Disease limited to two noncontiguous lymph node groups on same side of diaphragm

Stage III Disease on both sides of diaphragm, but limited to involvement of lymph nodes and spleen

Stage IV Involvement of bone marrow, lung parenchyma, pleura, liver, bone, skin or any organ or tissue other than lymph nodes or spleen

All stages are subclassified as A or B to indicate absence or presence of systemic symptoms, respectively.

Treatment. Although there are some variations, in general patients classified as IA, IIA and IIIA receive radiation while chemotherapy is employed in IIIB, IVA and IVB. Patients staged as IB and IIB are often given both radiation and chemotherapy. Such therapy has revolutionized the care of patients with significant remission and cure rates—as high as 90 per cent in favorable situations.

Non-Hodgkin's lymphomas are classified in various ways according to cell type: well-differentiated small lymphocytes; lymphoblastic; histocytic (reticulum cell). The latter has the worst prognosis. Patients are staged as in Hodgkins. In general, non-Hodgkins lymphoma is less responsive to therapy.

DISORDERS OF COAGULATION

Hemophilia

Hemophilia, a hereditary disease transmitted by the female to the male only, is characterized by a tendency to intractable hemorrhage following trauma. The blood picture is entirely normal, except for a markedly delayed clotting time, due to a biologically inactive antihemophilic factor of the plasma (Factor VIII). Bleeding may occur from tooth extractions, bruises or scratches and often occurs into joints and muscles. In contrast with purpura, the bleeding time and the platelet count are normal. The partial thromboplastin time is prolonged, but the prothrombin time is normal. This classic type of hemophilia is also called *hemophilia A.* Treatment consists of administration of concentrates of Factor VIII.

A condition that is very similar from a clinical standpoint is *hemophilia B,* or *Christmas disease,* which is a defect of thromboplastin component (Factor IX) and is benefited by concentrates containing Factor IX.

Von Willebrand's Disease

Von Willebrand's disease is characterized by a prolonged bleeding time, decreased Factor VII level and abnormal platelet adhesiveness; it is distinct from hemophilia A. Fresh frozen plasma will correct the abnormal bleeding time.

DISORDERS OF PLATELETS

Purpura

Purpura is a hemorrhagic disease characterized by extravasation of blood into the skin, subcutaneous tissues and mucous membranes. The most characteristic lesions are the size of a small pinhead, but large extravasations of blood may occur. These manifestations are caused by platelet dysfunction, qualitatively or quantitatively.

Thrombocytopenic Purpura. *Idiopathic thrombocytopenic purpura* is an acute or chronic disease of unknown etiology characterized by reduction in the number of platelets, prolonged bleeding time, a nonretractile clot, a positive tourniquet test and normal coagulation time. Spontaneous hemorrhages occur into the skin and the mucous membranes, and trauma may result in severe hemorrhage. Unfortunately, cerebral hemorrhage is common. The spleen may be enlarged. It is more common in children and young adults and is more frequent in females than males. The bone marrow shows an adequate number of megakaryocytes, but platelet formation is decreased. Antibodies are directed against platelet antigens and cause destruction of platelets. Thrombocytopenic purpura may be an early, or even the first, clinical manifestation of lupus erythematosus, and this possibility must always be considered.

Treatment consists of (1) prednisone, (2) platelet transfusion, and (3) splenectomy if prednisone fails.

Secondary thrombocytopenic purpura has the same clinical and laboratory features, but is secondary to some recognizable disease such as leukemia, aplastic anemia, liver disease or lymphoma or to conditions caused by toxins or drugs. Transfusions and steroid therapy sometimes are of benefit. Splenectomy is not indicated.

Nonthrombocytopenic Purpura. This is a group of vascular defects of diverse nature in which extravasation of blood occurs into the skin and other tissues. In one type of vasculitis (Schonlein-Henoch), hemorrhage may occur into the joints and the gastrointestinal tract. It may occur also in scurvy. The blood findings are normal. Purpura simplex is a condition with purpuric skin lesions only and without obvious cause. Symptomatic purpura is a form occurring in cachetic or senile patients or as a result of hydrostatic pressure (getting out of bed after prolonged rest from coronary occlusion or postoperatively). It is a manifestation of capillary weakness.

Hypercoagulable State

The hypercoagulable state is less well defined, but disseminated intravascular coagulation (DIC) is important clinically. DIC is associated with malignancy, hypoxic states, sepsis, oral contraceptives and pregnancy. In its severe form DIC is manifest by increased clotting and bleeding. Hypofibrinogenemia and thrombocytopenia may be seen in association with increased fibrin split products.

PLASMA CELL DYSCRASIAS

Plasma cell dyscrasias may be benign or malignant. The benign form occurs in two to six per cent of the population and is associated with an asymptomatic monoclonal gammopathy. The most common malignant form is multiple myeloma.

Multiple Myeloma

This is a neoplastic disease with proliferation of abnormal plasma cells characterized by anemia, bone involvement, hypercalcemia and renal disease. In the bones it produces destructive lesions with pain, pathologic fractures, compression fractures of the vertebrae, hematopoietic depression and hypercalcemia. The typical x-ray picture is that of multiple punched-out osteolytic areas, but there may be a diffuse osteoporotic process rather than the sharply demarcated lesions. Marrow aspiration of the sternum, ilium or vertebral spine shows a predominance of myeloma cells. Bence Jones proteinuria occurs in many patients. In the serum the gamma globulin fraction is increased, and a characteristic peak in the electrophoretic pattern is diagnostic. The proteins produced in multiple myeloma are immunoglobulins, identical with normal immunoglobulins but abnormal in amount and in most cases with one specific monoclonal protein in increased density, i.e. IgG, IgA or Bence Jones, (light chain). The sedimentation rate is elevated. Bone or joint pain in an elderly patient with an unexplained anemia should suggest the possibility of this disease. When the abnormal plasma cells (myeloma cells) appear in the peripheral bloodstream in large numbers or hypercalcemia appears, the prognosis is poor. Renal disease with uremia is frequently associated. Solitary myeloma may occur. This usually becomes multiple if it originates in bone, but plasmacytomas of soft tissue may not become generalized. Extramedullary plasmacytomas occur in the upper respiratory tract. X-ray therapy relieves the pain in some patients, and improvement has been noted with melphalan and cyclophosphamide.

Macroglobulinemia (Waldenström) has many similarities to multiple myeloma but is without bone lesions. Waldenstrom's disease has lymphoproliferation, elevated IgM and sometimes Bence Jones protein. The condition is characterized by bleeding tendencies, anemia, thrombocytopenia, leukopenia and hepatosplenomegaly.

DISEASES OF THE LUNG

Acute Respiratory Failure

Acute respiratory failure may occur due to a variety of causes such as chronic obstructive pulmonary disease (COPD), sedative drugs, severe pneumonia, status asthmaticus, brain damage, and adult respiratory distress syndrome (ARDS). The major consequences of acute respiratory failure (ARF) are inadequate oxygenation of organs and respiratory acidosis due to CO_2 retention. ARF may result in death or permanent brain damage.

The goals of therapy are to correct the hypoxemia and acidosis. Properly administered oxygen is required. Intubation, tracheostomy and mechanical ventilation may be needed.

Repeated measurement of pO_2, pCO_2 and pH to monitor hypoxemia, hypoventilation and acidosis are necessary.

Pulmonary Function Tests

In addition to the measurements of blood gases—pO_2, pCO_2 and pH—specific functions of the lung can be measured. Spirometry measures the flow of air per unit time. Useful measurements include: The forced vital capacity (FVC); the forced expiratory volume in 1 second (FEV_1); maximal midexpiratory flow (MMEF); and maximum voluntary ventilation (MVV). Spirometry allows one to distinguish between an obstructive ventilatory defect (chronic obstructive pulmonary disease, asthma) and a restrictive ventilatory defect (interstitial disease, obesity and neuromuscular disorders). In obstructuve disease there is reduced FEV_1, MMEF and usually some reduction of FVC with lowering of the FEV_1/FVC ratio. In restrictive disease the MMEF is normal and the FEV_1 is reduced, but because of significant reduction in FVC and FEV_1/FVC ratio is maintained. Additional tests include the determination of lung volume and lung diffusing capacity.

Chronic Obstructive Pulmonary Disease (COPD)

COPD is usually a combination of chronic bronchitis and pulmonary emphysema, although one or the other may predominate. COPD is usually related to smoking cigarettes, although there may be other causes, such as hereditary alpha$_1$-antitrypsin deficiency. The disease becomes apparent after age 40 with chronic cough and sputum production accompanied by dyspnea and wheezing. These symptoms progress as the disease advances. Physical examination reveals rhonchi, wheezes, and if the disease is advanced, the use of accessory muscles of respiration, cyanosis and right ventricular enlargement. There may be secondary polycythemia, a low PO$_2$, elevated pCO$_2$ and a partially compensated respiratory acidosis. Pulmonary function tests are those of an obstructive defect. Episodes of bronchopulmonary infection are common.

Treatment includes stopping smoking, bronchodilator therapy and the early use of antibiotics for infection. Continuous low flow oxygen is useful in selected patients with severe hypoxemia.

Bronchial Asthma

Asthma is a condition of recurrent dyspnea due to spasmodic reversible obstruction of the bronchi and characterized by wheezing and prolonged expiration. The lungs are filled with squeaking and musical rales, and the large rales of associated bronchitis are often present. Asthma is ordinarily an allergic condition, in which an extrinsic or intrinsic precipitating excitant is superimposed upon a fundamental hypersensitivity. The nature of this sensitivity is generally unknown, but there is a definite familial and hereditary tendency. Hypersensitivity is manifested (1) by the association of the attacks with exposure to the allergen and (2) by specific skin reactions.

In children, asthma is commonly due to food sensitivities; in adults, to pollen, dusts and to other, unidentified factors. Some cases may be initiated by emotional factors.

Treatment. Usually the acute attacks can be controlled by intravenous administration of aminophylline, subcutaneous isoproterenol injections and inhalation of bronchodilator substances. Attention should be directed to hydration of the patient, antibiotic therapy for any associated infection in the lung, bronchial tree or sinuses. These measures failing, steroids may be used as a supplement. Caution is advised in the overuse of propellant-driven nebulizers, which may cause paradoxical bronchospasm and arrhythmias.

Children sensitive to food may be cured by elimination of the offending substances. When offending extrinsic factors cannot be eliminated, desensitization by increasing inoculations with the specific proteins is of value in some cases. In cases in which the causal allergen cannot be discovered or removed, bronchodilator drugs or steroid maintenance therapy or both often provide complete control of the symptoms. The antihistamine drugs usually are disappointing.

Pulmonary Emboli

The most common sources of pulmonary infarction are emboli from the veins of the lower extremities, pelvis, or from the right atrium, that cause obstruction in a branch of the pulmonary artery and a wedge-shaped infarct with its base toward the pleura. These infarcts vary in size from a few millimeters to many centimeters and are often multiple. They most frequently involve the lower lobe. The incidence of pulmonary infarct is 25 to 30 per cent in autopsied patients. Most of these were not detected before death.

The symptoms of pulmonary infarction are (1) sudden onset of dyspnea, often with signs of cardiovascular collapse; (2) sudden development of localized fibrinous pleurisy with pain, friction rub and, if the infarct is large, physical signs of consolidation; and (3) bloody sputum with mucus. The acute onset is characteristic and may cause death immediately, but in some cases the symptoms are much less evident. An electrocardiogram may give evidence of right-axis deviation and is an aid in the diagnosis and particularly in distinguishing pulmonary embolus from myocardial infarction. Chest x-ray, radioisotopic lung scan, and pulmonary angiogram may be used in selected instances in establishing the diagnosis.

Treatment is designed to sustain life and prevent recurrence. Immediate anticoagulation with intravenous administration of heparin is advised. Surgical venous ligation and the placement of vena caval filters is reserved for anticoagulant failures; pulmonary embolectomy may also be considered.

Pleural Effusions

History, physical examination and examination of the pleural fluid usually allow for a diagnosis of the cause of pleural effusion. Although large effusions may cause dyspnea, many effusions do not directly cause symptoms. Physical examination varies, depending on amount of fluid and the condition of the underlying lung. Characteristic findings include decreased expansion, decreased fremitus, flat percussion note, reduced breath sounds and sometimes tracheal deviation to the contralateral side. Examination of the fluid should include gross appearance, cells, stains, cytology, cultures and analysis of transudate vs. exudate. The latter is often critical and an exudate is usually present if (1) the pleural fluid to serum total protein ratio exceeds 0.5; (2) pleural fluid LDH exceeds 200 international units per liter; and (3) the pleural fluid to serum LDH ratio exceed 0.6. Pleural biopsy may be helpful to determine the cause of an unexplained exudate. Treatment depends on the cause.

Interstitial Lung Disease

A variety of diseases afflict primarily the interstitial tissues of the lung. These include environmental inhalants, drugs (nitrofurantoin), infections, granulomatous disorders (sarcoid), collagen vascular diseases, and tumors. Whatever the initial cause of injury, interstitial fibrosis may be the outcome. The most common manifestation is dyspnea which is progressive. Physical examination may be normal except for small basilar rales; later there may be tachypnea, clubbing and cor pulmonale. The laboratory may show secondary polycythemia and evidence of an autoimmune process (i.e., antinuclear antibodies, rheumatoid factor). Chest x-ray is either normal or shows a nodular infiltrate at the basis. Pulmonary function tests reveal a restrictive ventilatory defect, decreased diffusing capacity and reduced lung compliance. The treatment depends on cause. In patients in whom no etiology is identified, i.e., idiopathic interstitial fibrosis, steroids may be tried, although the results are questionable. The prognosis varies with cause and the effectiveness of therapy.

Carcinoma of the Lung

Cigarette smoking plays a major etiological role in the most common varieties of lung cancer, the squamous and undifferentiated cell types, and is less related to adenocarcinoma. Patients may have no symptoms or may have cough, hemoptysis, pneumonia or wheeze. Metastases to local nodes cause superior vena caval obstruction, hoarseness and pleural effusion. Distant metastases involve virtually all organs. Remote manifestations include neuromuscular syndromes, clubbing, ectopic endocrine disorders (ADH, hyperparathyroidism, Cushing's syndrome), and thrombophlebitis. In addition to the clinical picture and the x-ray findings, bronchoscopy, mediastinoscopy and thoracotomy may be required for diagnosis. The overall results of surgery are poor, but the outlook is considerably better for the patient with a solitary, peripheral lesion ("coin" lesion) without metastases. Chemotherapy is not effective except in the poorly differentiated small cell ("oat cell") type.

Lobar Pneumonia

(See discussion in Chap. 5, General Microbiology, and Chap. 6, Pathology.)

Lobar pneumonia occurs most commonly in winter and early spring, and most often in young children and the aged, although it may affect the healthy adult. Over 95 per cent of lobar pneumonia is due to pneumococcus, the remainder being caused by streptococci,

Haemophilus influenzae, klebsiella and staphylococci.

Symptoms. The typical case of pneumonia begins abruptly with sudden onset of: (1) shaking chill, (2) pleural pain, (3) cough with rusty or bloody sputum, (4) fever with temperature above 38 C., or a combination of these. Physical findings in the chest may not be apparent for the first 24 to 48 hours. Therefore, it is important that the diagnosis be made from the symptoms and the type of organism then be determined. The first chest signs of early pneumonia are: (1) slight local dullness; (2) "bronchial" breath sounds; and (3) fine, inspiratory, crepitant rales. Later, typical signs of consolidation occur. Other valuable signs are cyanosis, rapid, shallow breathing, dilation of the alae nasi, herpes of the lips and limitation of motion on the affected side. Leukocytosis is usual, except in very toxic cases, in which leukopenia is found. X-ray examination affords the most conclusive confirmation of the diagnosis.

Complications: These include (1) empyema, (2) pleural effusion, (3) endocarditis, (4) meningitis, (5) pericarditis and (6) arthritis.

Treatment. The preferred treatment is to start large doses of penicillin as soon as a sputum specimen has been obtained. Unless one is dealing with multiple-lobe involvement, the patient's temperature usually will be almost normal in 48 hours to 72 hours. Pulmonary infiltrate may persist for 7 to 10 days.

Bronchopneumonia

The terms *lobar pneumonia* and *bronchopneumonia* disignate anatomic types of pneumonia and should·not be used to imply etiologic diagnosis. From a practical point of view, the classic distinction between bronchopneumonia and lobar pneumonia is much less important than determination of the etiologic agent. Five per cent of pneumonias that are lobar in anatomic type are not caused by the pneumococcus. Of the bronchopneumonias over 50 per cent are caused by the pneumococcus. Furthermore, careful x-ray and pathologic studies have shown that anatomic differentiation often is impossible, since frequently the two patterns coexist.

The majority of cases of bronchopneumonia are secondary to some precipitating factor, such as (1) contagious disease (measles in childhood); (2) debility (terminal pneumonia in cancer); (3) inhalation of irritative gases (phosgene or nitrous oxide); (4) aspiration of mucus or vomitus (postoperative pneumonia); (5) hypostatic congestion and retention of secretions in the bronchi (pneumonia following stroke); and (6) immunologic impairment.

The invading microorganism may be the pneumococcus, the streptococcus, the staphylococcus, gram-negative organisms, viruses or many others that occur less frequently. Sputum cultures should be taken and the sensitivity of the organism to various antimicrobial agents determined as a guide to therapy.

The *symptoms* vary from those of ordinary bronchitis to the severe symptoms found in a severe lobar pneumonia. The physical findings differ from those of lobar pneumonia in that there are scattered patches of roles and impaired resonance instead of a massive area of consolidation.

Types. Some of the types of bronchopneumonia deserve separate mention:

1. *Staphylococcus aureus* bronchopneumonia is associated with a high mortality rate. Formerly it often caused multiple abscesses along the bronchi, but now it usually is controlled by antibiotics, including high-dosage penicillin and others as indicated by drug-susceptibility testing, including penicillinase-resistant penicillin. About 2 per cent of the bronchopneumonias are of this type.

2. Primary atypical pneumonia ("virus pneumonia") has been recognized as a clinical entity. The physical findings may be absent or very slight, and most cases might be considered severe bronchitis, except for the x-ray finding of a cloudy infiltration radiating from the hilus of one lung toward the periphery. The mortality rate is about 2 per cent.

3. Another group of pneumonias comprises the psittacoses. The diagnosis is established by a history of exposure to parakeets, parrots, other exotic birds or fowl, as well as by complement-fixation tests and mouse inoculations with sputum or blood from the patient. The tetracyclines are highly effective in treatment.

4. Nosocomial pneumonitis. Hospital-acquired gram-negative bacillary pneumonias are now frequent and depend on underlying disease, use of antibiotics and duration of hospitalization. Organisms found are *Pseudomonas aeruginosa,* proteus and klebsiella. Contaminated inhalation therapy equipment has also been implicated in spreading infection. Specific therapy is dependent on organism sensitivity in vitro and includes such drugs as cephalin and aminoglycosides.

Bronchopneumonia is particularly dangerous in young infants and very old individuals. For them, supportive treatment is of the utmost importance.

Tuberculosis

(Review discussions in Chap. 5, General Microbiology, and Chap. 6, Pathology.)

The present concept of the common pattern of pulmonary tuberculosis of the adult type is that is has the following pathogenesis:

1. Childhood infection, usually brief, benign and undiagnosed, leaving a calcified Ghon tubercle or hilar node;

2. A long-lasting sensitivity to the tubercle bacillus, manifested by a positive tuberculin test;

3. A reinfection in youth or adult life, with entirely different features, that is the result of the sensitization to the organism and progresses to a chronic phase.

Chronic pulmonary tuberculosis may follow the primary infection after a short or long period of dormancy. Features are (1) absence of recent exposure; (2) tendency to chronicity and cavitation and (3) production of fibrous tissue of repair. The most common site is the apical portion of the lung with spread downward and medially; this is due to the finding of abundant bacilli in the liquid caseum of the tuberculous cavity.

Onset may be insidious; the patient may be asymptomatic and the disease diagnosed only by chest roentgenogram. Early constitutional symptoms are due to absorption of tuberculoprotein in the hypersensitive host. Fever is often present in late evening, leading to night sweats. General malaise, weight loss and cough productive of morning sputum may be noted.

Diagnosis. Pulmonary tuberculosis must be suspected in the presence of one of the following criteria:

1. The history or the presence of pleurisy with effusion
2. History of hemoptysis
3. Moderately coarse rales about the third rib and the third vertebral spine
4. Definite x-ray findings in the same area
5. Tubercle bacilli in the sputum.

Activity is indicated by (1) fever, (2) night sweats, (3) rapid pulse, (4) loss of weight and strength, (5) increased sedimentation rate, (6) hemoptysis, (7) less significantly, cough, and (8) expectoration. Increase of physical signs or x-ray findings at intervals of about 2 months may be the only evidence of progression but indicates what has taken place, as contrasted with symptoms, which indicate present activity. A positive tuberculin reaction does not indicate present activity, but a negative reaction is highly significant in excluding the diagnosis of tuberculosis except in an anergic patient.

Complications include cavitation, making the patient highly infectious; hemoptysis; pleurisy with effusion; tuberculous pneumonia and bronchopleural fistula with empyema. Patients may continue with these symptoms for many years before presenting for treatment.

Extrapulmonary complications of pulmonary tuberculosis include involvement of the larynx, the intestines, the lymph nodes, the bones, the peritoneum, the meninges, the kidneys and the genital area.

Treatment of chronic pulmonary tuberculosis may be summarized under (1) specific drug treatment, (2) surgical treatment and (3) nonspecific measures.

1. All cases of active disease should be treated with a combination of two of the three principal antituberculosis drugs, e.g., isoniazid and ethambutol or isoniazid and rifampin. All three drugs may be used in severely ill patients with large cavities.
2. If rigorous drug therapy fails to arrest the disease or if there is appreciable doubt regarding the permanency of the arrested state, excisional surgery may be employed.
3. Included under nonspecific measures are rest, diet, occupational therapy and rehabilitation. Prolonged hospitalization is not required.

Acute miliary tuberculosis is a blood-borne infection in which the organisms are seeded throughout the body from a primary focus. The lungs are affected principally when the bacilli come through the thoracic duct or systemic veins, while a pulmonary focus that breaks into the veins of the lungs results in a generalized distribution.

Miliary tuberculosis without treatment is uniformly fatal. Lesions are found not only in lung but liver, spleen, bone marrow and meninges. Diagnosis is best made by biopsy of liver, node or marrow, searching for caseating granulomas. The clinical picture is similar to chronic infection due to other causes such as histoplasmosis, coccidioidomycosis, cryptococcosis, or to the picture of diffuse carcinomatosis. Prompt treatment with the three major drugs (isoniazid, ethambutol and streptomycin) has a 95 per cent survival rate. The tuberculin test may be negative.

Tuberculous meningitis usually occurs as part of acute miliary tuberculosis. It is found most often in young children. The diagnosis is suggested by the history and the physical condition and is established by a positive spinal fluid test or by the finding of tubercles in the choroid. The spinal fluid reveals from 25 to 1,000 or more white cells per cu. mm., predominantly lymphocytes. Spinal fluid protein is elevated. Usually tubercle bacilli are found in the cobweb-like clot of fibrin. In young children a positive tuberculin skin test is significant. With the several drugs now available, surivival rates are high, with some incidence of permanent brain injury but relatively little recurrence of the meningitis.

Other Pulmonary Infections

Bronchiectasis. This is seen far less often than in years past, is characterized by cylindrical, fusiform or sacculated dilatation of the bronchi. There are a rare congenital type and a common acquired type. The condition is the result of three factors: (1) softening of the bronchial walls, as in chronic bronchitis secondary to nasal sinus infection; (2) increase in the distending forces, as from a long-continued cough; and (3) traction on the wall, as from pulmonary fibrosis.

The lesion may be unilateral as bilateral. The bases are involved more frequently than the apices, except that tuberculous bronchiectases are usually in the upper lobes.

The *symptoms* are (1) paroxysmal cough; (2) large amounts of fetid sputum, which on standing separates into three layers; (3) dyspnea on exertion; and (4) sometimes hemoptysis. Constitutional symptoms are absent as long as drainage is maintained. Clubbing of fingers is common.

Physical signs are absent in mild cases but there may be rales. Signs of co-existing bronchitis, emphysema and fibrosis may be present. There is often some enlargement of the right heart.

Diagnosis depends upon the history, the physical signs, the characteristic foul sputum and bronchograms. In most cases a roentgenogram following the injection of radiopaque material into the bronchus or direct examination by bronchoscopy is necessary to confirm the diagnosis.

Treatment is directed toward improving the patient's general condition and diminishing the amount of sputum by postural or bronchoscopic drainage. The medical treatment is that of chronic bronchitis and in some cases includes frequent intermittent use of antibiotics on a long-term basis. Some patients with localized bronchiectasis are cured or improved by resection of segments or lobes or combinations of segments and lobes. The prompt diagnosis and treatment of bacterial infections of the lower respiratory tract is the best way of avoiding a chronic complication such as bronchiectasis.

Lung Abscess. Suppuration in the lung may result (1) following pneumonia, particularly aspiration forms of bronchopneumonia; (2) from wounds or operations of the throat, particularly tonsillectomy or dental manipulation in patients with periodintal disease; (3) from infective embolism; (4) from perforating carcinoma; or (5) from perforation of the lung. If abscess occurs during the course of another disease, the symptoms are greatly aggravated at once. If it occurs in a patient previously well, the onset may be insidious, and the first characteristic sign may be the appearance of a large amount of foul sputum when the abscess ruptures into a bronchus. The odor is offensive but at first is not fetid. The sputum contains fragments of elastic tissue from the lung.

Fever, cyanosis, dyspnea and clubbing of the fingers are frequent manifestations.

Diagnosis is based on the history, physical examination and the presence on x-ray of one or more areas of infiltration with air-fluid levels.

Treatment. Intensive antibiotic therapy is the most important factor in treatment. With the exception of bacteroides and staphyloccocus, most of pathogens found are sensitive to penicillin, erythromycin and tetracycline. Bacteroides is sensitive to clindamycin and chloramphenicol. If the abscess is well defined and does not progress steadily to complete healing, segmental or lobe resection should be undertaken, provided that the patient's general condition is reasonably good. Having the patient lie with the affected side uppermost favors endobronchial drainage, and bronchoscopic aspiration may be helpful.

Idiopathic pulmonary hemosiderosis is characterized by widespread pulmonary capillary hemorrhages resulting in repeated hemoptysis and hypochromic anemia. After a variable period pulmonary hemosiderosis and fibrosis develop. Early, there are ill-defined scattered opacities on x-ray films; they vary from day to day and may clear completely. After repeated episodes a diffuse reticular pattern appears. Goodpasture's syndrome presents a picture of pulmonary hemorrhage associated with hematuria.

Alveolar proteinosis is a condition in which large groups of alveoli are filled with proteinaceous material with minimal or no change in the alveolar walls. There is gradually increasing dyspnea with a productive cough, although physical signs are lacking. X-ray examination reveals a diffuse soft density that is similar in appearance to pulmonary edema. The vital capacity is reduced, the oxygen saturation of the hemoglobin is reduced, and complicating infections may be present. The cause is unknown, and treatment is unsatisfactory, although pulmonary lavage may be helpful.

Farmer's lung is a condition, caused by inhalation of spoiled or moldy hay, that is characterized by the sudden onset of dyspnea some hours after exposure to this or other vegetable material. There may be fever, chills and cyanosis, and a roentgenogram of chest suggests diffuse interstitial pneumonia. Histologically there are numerous granulomas involving the pulmonary intestitum, and there may be obliterative bronchitis. The cause of the condition is apparently a hypersensitivity reaction to moldy hay. The disease usually lasts for several days and is followed by complete recovery.

Silo-filler's disease results from inhalation of oxides of nitrogen that are formed within a silo soon after it is filled. The disease is limited to individuals who enter silos within a day or two after filling, and the clinical picture consists of cough and dyspnea immediately after exposure, relative remission of symptoms during the next 2 or 3 weeks, followed by a second phase of the illness with fever, chills and progressive dyspnea and cyanosis. Numerous bubbling rales are heard over the lungs, and there is wheezing respiration during the third phase of the illness. An x-ray examination reveals generalized infiltration of the lungs with innumerable discrete densities. Adrenal steroids are valuable in the treatment of the acute phase of the disease.

Cystic fibrosis or mucoviscidosis is a familial systemic disease characterized by abnormal secretory products of a number of exocrine glands. Involvement of the bronchial glands leads to production of thick viscid pulmonary secretion; consequently, radicals of the tracheal bronchial tree become plugged, and recurrent pulmonary infections and destruction of lung tissue result. Pulmonary infection is most commonly caused by staphylococci. A history of repeated attacks of pneumonia throughout life is characteristic of this disease. The pancreatic secretions are similarly affected, producing pancreatic insufficiency with malnutrition and steatorrhea. The mucous glands of the entire gastrointestinal tract may be involved. The sweat and saliva contain unusually high concentrations of sodium and chloride, and detection of the increase in sweat electrolytes is the simplest means of diagnosis.

Pneumoconiosis refers to the chronic changes in the lung induced by the prolonged inhalation of dust. Mineral dust such as silica and asbestos lead to fibrosis of the lungs, whereas organic materials are more liable to excite an inflammatory or an allergic reaction. The most common form of pneumoconiosis in the United States is silicosis resulting from the inhalation of dust with a high concentration of silica. It is characterized by widespread fibrosis and, clinically, by shortness of breath and greatly increased susceptibility to pulmonary infections. It is a very real hazard in a wide variety of industries in which either quartz or sand is used. The diagnosis is based on the history of exposure to silica, together with the x-ray evidence of the disease. The principal clinical manifestation is dyspnea.

Spontaneous pneumothorax is collapse of the lung in the absence of trauma. This may result from a superficial bulla that ruptures through the pleura with the escape of air directly into the pleural space. Spontaneous pneumothorax is sometimes thought to be associated with chronic pulmonary tuberculosis. Bleeding may occur with development of the pneumothorax, resulting in hemopneumothorax.

DISEASES OF THE KIDNEYS

The kidneys perform two vital functions. The normal *excretory* control of water, electrolytes and metabolic products maintains the volume and composition of body fluids. The *regulatory* (nonexcretory) functions of the kidney play roles in determining red cell formation (erythropoietin), bone metabolism (via generation of 1,25 dihydroxycholecalciferol), and regulation of arterial pressure (renin, prostaglandins). When renal function fails, there are abnormalities secondary to failure of both the excretory and nonexcretory functions.

The methods of evaluation of a patient include those that diagnose disease and those that measure function. In addition to history and physical examination, the urinalysis is critical. Other major tests include: 24 hour urine for protein and determination of creatinine clearance as a measure of glomerular filtration rate (GFR); urine culture, blood urea nitrogen (BUN), serum creatinine, serum electroylytes, x-rays, ultrasound, and radiorenograms.

Renal Failure

Renal failure is defined as that stage of renal function when the kidney cannot maintain the integrity of the internal environment. It may be divided into chronic (CRF) and acute (ARF) forms. The *uremic syndrome* may occur in either CRF and ARF and is a clinical constellation including (1) CNS manifestations (lassitude, memory loss, anxiety, stupor, coma); (2) cardiopulmonary abnormalities including pericarditis and adult respiratory distress; and (3) gastrointestinal symptoms of nausea and vomiting. Uremia is due to retained metabolic waste products and reverses with dialysis.

Chronic renal failure. CRF is the result of a host of chronic renal diseases of diverse cause which have in common the progressive destruction of the kidney. The manifestations may be divided into the following categories:

1. Fluid and electrolyte abnormalities. This includes extracellular fluid excess or deficit, hyponatremia, hypocalcemia, hyperphosphatemia, and hypermagnesemia. Hyperkalemia is uncommon in CRF unless excess potassium is administered or oliguria occurs.
2. Abnormalities of nonexcretory function. Anemia due to marrow failure (erythropoietin deficiency), osteomalacia due to Vitamin D deficiency, and occasionally hypertension due to increased renin production.
3. Metabolic abnormalities such as glucose intolerance and hyperlipidemia may occur.
4. The uremic syndrome.
5. Social and emotional problems of chronic illness.

Treatment consists of (1) searching for treatable disease, e.g., obstruction; (2) searching for reversible factors that might make renal function worse, e.g., volume depletion, heart failure, infection, superimposed obstruction, nephrotoxic drugs; (3) use of appropriate diet and salt and water intake; (4) maintaining normal serum phosphorus by use of aluminum antacids to minimize hyperparathyroidism; (5) being careful about dosage of medications excreted by the kidney. (6) Finally, chronic intermittent dialysis and transplantation may be needed. Clinical guides are primary indicators for dialysis but generally when serum creatinine reaches 12 mg. per 100 ml. and GFR is less than 5 ml. per minute, dialysis should be given serious consideration.

Acute renal failure. Acute renal failure may be divided into three categories: (1) prerenal failure (heart failure, hypovolemia); (2) intrarenal failure; and (3) postrenal failure (obstruction). The most common cause of intrarenal failure is acute tubular necrosis (ATN). ATN is caused by ischemia or nephrotoxic agents, and may or may not be associated with oliguria. Other causes of acute intrarenal failure are acute glomerular diseases; acute interstitial nephritis; and acute vascular disease (vasculitis, malignant hypertension, bilateral arterial occlusion). These various causes can usually be distinguished by clinical examination urinalysis, and the determination in a random urine sample of sodium concentration and osmolality. In prerenal azotemia, urine sodium is less than 20 mEq. per liter and urine osmolality over 500 mOsm. per Kg. while in ATN urine sodium is greater than 40 mEq. per liter while urine osmolality is less than 400 mOsm. per Kg.

Treatment depends on cause. In ATN the goal is to maintain life and nutrition while hoping for spontaneous recovery. In particular, this means careful monitoring of fluid balance to avoid volume overload and hyperkalemia, and dialysis to prevent uremic symptoms and to permit adequate nutrition. Mortality in "surgical" ATN is 60 per cent, in "medical" ATN 30 per cent, and in "obstetrical ATN" 15 per cent.

Glomerular Diseases

Glomerular diseases may be divided according to pathogenesis as follows: (1) immunologic, (2) vascular (polyarteritis, malignant nephrosclerosis), (3) coagulation (DIC, hemolytic-uremic), (4) metabolic defects (diabetes, amyloid), (5) hereditary (Alport's syndrome), and (6) unknown (lipoid nephrosis). The immunologic mechanism is further divided into the more common immune complex variety where a circulating antigen-antibody complex damages the glomerulus and an antiglomerular basement membrane antibody disease (anti-GBM) in which an antibody reacts with antigen fixed to basement membrane.

Glomerular diseases of diverse cause produce certain *glomerular syndromes:* acute glomerulonephritis; rapidly progressive glomerulonephritis, chronic progressive glomerular disease; asymptomatic proteinuria/hematuria; and the nephrotic syndrome. All glomerular syndromes are characterized by proteinuria and many have RBC and RBC casts as well. The particular diseases causing the glomerular syndromes may be *primary* renal diseases or *secondary* to some systemic illness.

Acute glomerulonephritis is characterized by oliguria, edema, hypertension, hematuria, proteinuria and RBC casts. The clinical prototype is acute poststreptococcal glomerulonephritis (immune complex). Multisystem diseases may cause the same syndrome, e.g., SLE, vasculitis, and infective endocarditis.

Rapidly progressive glomerulonephritis (RPGN) has a similar clinical picture as actue glomerulonephritis, but it develops more insidiously and generally results in end-stage renal failure within 1 to 3 months. Pathologically there is epithelial proliferation in the form of crescents. Goodpasture's syndrome (i.e. antiglomerular basement membrane disease with associated lung hemorrhage) is the prototype. There is also an idiopathic form as well as multisystem disease production of RPGN (e.g., SLE, Henoch-Schonlein purpura, vasculitis).

Chronic progressive glomerular disease is the result of many glomerular illnesses of varied causes. It is generally characterized by hypertension, proteinuria, microscopic hematuria and progressive reduction in GFR.

Asymptomic proteinuria and/or hematuria without reduced GFR may occur as an early manifestation of diffuse disease or may represent focal illnesses such as IgA (Berger's) nephropathy. The overall outlook is good.

Nephrotic Syndrome is defined as the renal excretion of 3.5 g. or more of protein in 24 hours. There are usually edema and hypoalbuminemia, and often hyperlipidemia. About 75 per cent of patients have idiopathic nephrotic syndrome, i.e., the disease is of unknown origin and is restricted to the kidney. In children the most common variety of idiopathic nephrotic syndrome is lipoid nephrosis ("minimal" or "nil" lesion). It has a good prognosis. In adults the most common lesion is membranous nephropathy (immune complex) with a 20 per cent spontaneous remission rate. Other types of lesions are membranoproliferative, and focal sclerosis. Only the lipoid lesion is responsive to steroid. For the other lesions, debate persists. Causes of secondary nephrotic syndrome include diabetes, SLE, tumors, amyloid, malaria, drugs, and pregnancy.

Selected Glomerulopathies

Diabetes Mellitus produces a nodular as well as a diffuse lesion. The nodular lesion of Kimmelstiel and Wilson is diagnostic of diabetes. The nephrotic syndrome and chronic progressive syndromes are common clinical expressions. When azotemia develops the prognosis is poor. IVP contrast material may produce acute renal failure especially if azotemia is present. There is no specific therapy. Dialysis is one-half as effective as in non-diabetics. Transplantation of a live donor kidney is also effective.

Systemic lupus erythematosus (immune complex) produces all the glomerular syndromes described. There is a focal lesion which is more benign but may progress into the more destructive diffuse membranoproliferative disease. Treatment with steroids may be followed by arrest of the disease or improvement.

Hepatitis B antigenemia may result in immune-complex glomerular disease producing all the glomerular syndromes.

Interstitial Disease

Diseases that involve primarily the interstitium of the kidney are characterized by only mild proteinuria, pyuria, and variable reduction of GFR. Acute interstitial nephritis includes bacterial pyelonephritis and drug-induced nephritis. The prototype is methicillin-induced nephritis, and in addition to acute renal failure patients may have skin rash and eosinophilia. Discontinuing the drug is usually sufficient therapy. Chronic interstitial nephritis can be due to chronic pyelonephritis, analgesic abuse nephropathy, papillary necrosis, gout, or heavy metals. In all cases of pyelonephritis in children, vesicoureteral reflux should be considered.

Analgesic abuse nephropathy is not rare. It is most often caused by combination analgesics that include phenacetin. Most patients have pain, indigestion, anemia, pyuria, and azotemia. They may have renal calculi and papillary necrosis. Discontinuing the drugs often results in arrest or improvement.

Vascular Diseases

Vascular diseases include (1) "benign" nephrosclerosis, (2) "malignant" nephrosclerosis (see hypertension), (3) renal artery occlusion due to embolism or clot that results in renal infarction or renovascular hypertension, and (4) bilateral renal vein thrombosis associated with the nephrotic syndrome.

Congenital Diseases

Polycystic Kidneys. This is a congenital and familial disease, in which the normal renal tissue is gradually replaced and encroached upon by multiple cysts of the renal parenchyma. The kidneys are enlarged and filled with grapelike clusters of cysts containing clear or hemorrhagic fluid. Ultrasound and intravenous pyelograms reveal the enlarged kidneys with deformed pelvis and flattening of the calyces. Hypertension and renal insufficiency develop later. Puncture of the cysts does not prolong life.

Obstructive Nephropathy

Urinary tract obstruction results in dilatation of the system proximal to the obstruction and ultimately leads to renal atrophy, infection and renal failure. Obstruction may occur at any point in the urinary system and common causes include benign prostatic hypertrophy, cancer of the prostate, bladder, or ureters, neurogenic bladder, pelvic tumors, retroperitoneal fibrosis, stones, and ureteropelvic narrowing. Early diagnosis and surgical treatment are needed. After relief of obstruction there may be a period of postobstructive diuresis; in some instances this is massive enough to cause volume depletion.

Renal Cell Carcinoma (Hypernephroma)

Although this condition is discussed more fully in the urology section, the triad of hematuria, flank pain and a mass occurs in only a small number of patients. However renal cell carcinoma is especially known for its many systemic manifestations, including fever or hormonal abnormalities such as hypercalcemia, hypertension, polycythemia, and Cushing's syndrome. IVP, and arteriography are the basic diagnostic tools.

Renal Stones

Calcium stones are most common and occur most often in hypercalcemic states (hyperparathyroidism, sarcoidosis) and hypercalciuric conditions (idiopathic hypercalciuria, renal tubular acidosis). Uric acid stones are next most common and are radiolucent; they occur in gout and chronic diarrhea. Other types of stones are cystine, and triple phosphate stones. To prevent calculi, hydration and therapy of the underlying cause should be done wherever possible. Idiopathic hypercalciuria can be treated with thiazide diuretics, and gout with allopurinol or benemid.

Selected Electrolyte Abnormalities

Hyponatremia is divided into three categories: (1) extracellular volume (ECFV) deficit due to renal or extrarenal losses of sodium, (2) excess ECFV (edema); and (3) syndrome of inappropriate ADH. In the first category, isotonic saline may be used; for categories two and three, water restriction. Serious CNS symptoms including coma generally develop with serum levels below 120 mEq. per liter.

Hypokalemia is a result of urinary loss as in diuretic therapy or of gastrointestinal loss of potassium. Treatment of the underlying cause and potassium replacement are the basis of therapy.

Hyperkalemia usually results from acute oliguric renal failure. Treatment consists of reduced intake, gastrointestinal resins and dialysis.

Hypercalcemia is seen in primary or ectopic hyperparathyroidism, neoplasm, vitamin D excess, sarcoid, vitamin A excess, thiazide therapy. Malignancy is the most common cause. Treatment in selected patients consists of saline, loop diuretics, and dialysis.

Hypophosphatemia is noted in alcoholics, diabetics receiving insulin and in patients receiving parenteral alimentation. Levels less than 1 mg. per 100 ml. cause rhabdomyolosis, infection, hemolysis, bone pain and encephalopathy. Oral or intravenous replacement is indicated.

Metabolic Acidosis is characterized by a reduction in pH, pCO_2 and serum HCO_3^-. There are two types according to whether the anion gap is increased or normal. In the former acid is added (e.g. diabetic ketoacidosis, lactic acidosis), toxic substances are ingested that generate acids (e.g., salicylates, methyl alcohol, ethylene glycol) or there is a failure to excrete acids (renal failure). In normal anion gap (hyperchloremic) acidosis, there is a loss of HCO_3^- as in diarrhea, ostomies, renal tubular acidosis, or dilutional acidosis. Acidosis can produce Kussmaul's breathing, cardiac malfunction and shock. The treatment is the underlying condition and the administration of alkali.

Metabolic alkalosis is characterized by increased pH, pCO_2 and serum NCO_3^-. It is due either to ECF volume depletion (responds to saline) or to excess mineralocorticoid activity (resistant to saline).

Respiratory acidosis is characterized by reduced pH, increased pCO_2 and increased HCO_3^-. It is due to impaired ventilation. The treatment must be directed at improving air exchange.

Respiratory alkalosis is characterized by increased pH, decreased pCO_2 and decreased NCO_3^-. It is due to overventilation and treatment is directed at its cause.

DISEASES OF THE ESOPHAGUS, THE STOMACH AND THE INTESTINES

The esophagus rarely gives rise to any symptoms unless there is a serious organic lesion. The usual symptoms from esophageal lesions are pain or difficulty in swallowing (dysphagia). The most common ailments are:

1. Stricture of the esophagus from scarring, usually after swallowing lye or other corrosive agents.
2. Cancer of the esophagus. The dysphagia may be intermittent at first but progresses as the growth encroaches upon the lumen.
3. Cardiospasm (achalasia) is not a true spasm but a failure of relaxation of the terminal end of the esophagus. The pressure of the peristalsis in the

upper portion leads to dilatation of the lower part. Treatment, after esophagoscopy, is forceful dilatation.

4. Bleeding esophageal varices.
5. Diaphragmatic hernia—herniation of a portion of the stomach through the esophageal hiatus. Symptoms are aggravated by eating and by lying down.
6. Peptic esophagitis—inflammation or erosion of the esophageal mucosa due to reflux of acid gastric juice. This may occur with diaphragmatic hernia.
7. Diverticula. These are frequently small and asymptomatic but may become ulcerated or so enlarged as to cause dysphagia.
8. Esophageal moniliasis is usually seen in patients with malignant disease who are taking immunosuppressive drugs.

Peptic Ulcer

Peptic ulcer may occur at any age. It is more common in men than women. Duodenal ulcers are more common than those of the stomach.

Peptic ulcers may be acute or chronic and are sometimes multiple. Gastric ulcers are usually situated near the pylorus, most often at the lesser curvature. Duodenal ulcers almost always are within 1 to 10 cm. of the pylorus. Ulcers may be concentric, round, oval or irregular and vary in size from a pinpoint to about 4 cm. They may be superficial or may penetrate through all the layers of the wall, and usually they have a punched-out appearance. Their cause is not definitely established, but gastric acid and pepsin are required.

Symptoms and Diagnosis.   The outstanding features are (1) epigastric pain, usually 2 to 3 hours after eating; (2) hypersecretion of hydrochloric acid by the stomach; and (3) x-ray findings. The pain is characterized by: (1) its circumscribed epigastric location; (2) its tendency to cyclic periods of remission and recurrence; (3) its relation to mealtimes; (4) its increase with alcohol, acids and condiments; (5) its relief by milk, alkali, bland food and vomiting and (6) its gnawing, aching or burning character.

The patient usually localizes the pain with one or two fingers, and there may be muscular resistance, tenderness or hypersethesia over the same area. Hyperacidity after a test meal is usual but not constant. The significant x-ray findings are (1) delayed emptying; (2) pyloric or duodenal spasm; (3) hyperperistalsis; (4) the presence of a crater; (5) a permanent irregularity; and (6) a penetrating cavity. Hourglass stomach may be due to spasm or cicatrization.

Complications.   The most serious complication is perforation, which may lead to generalized peritonitis, perigastric adhesions, abscess and localized peritonitis. Hemorrhage may be the first symptom of ulcer and may be massive. Scarring with resultant pyloric obstruction may occur and require surgical relief. Intractability, despite medical therapy occurs in a few patients.

Treatment.   Perforation requires surgery. Hemorrhage requires rest and sedation. Transfusion may be imperative. The patient is fed either by nasogastric suction or given small hourly feedings of milk and antacid.

Medical treatment of ulcer includes (1) mental and physical rest, (2) correction of hyperacidity, and (3) regulation of diet. Antacids should be given frequently in small doses. Liquid antacid such as aluminum or magnesium hydroxides is the treatment of choice for relief of symptoms. Cimetidine, the H_2 receptor antagonist, lowers gastric acidity. Its long range role in therapy remains to be determined. Anticholinergics may be used to combat excessive secretion of acid as well as muscle spasm. The diet should meet three requirements: (1) It should not contain foods that are chemically or mechanically irritant; (2) it should contain food that combines readily with acid; and (3) it should be nourishing.

The patient with severe symptoms may initially be placed on 2-hourly feedings of milk and cream, sometimes with cereal, to which rice, custard, soft egg, milk toast, purees and gelatins may be added gradually. Proper habits of eating are as important as the food eaten.

Surgical treatment is indicated (1) when there is repeated recurrence or lack of success following medical treatment ("intractability"); (2) after repeated hemorrhage; (3) in progressive pyloric obstruction; (4) when there is evidence or suspicion of carcinoma in a gastric ulcer; or (5) when there is perforation. Vagotomy and pyloroplasty are commonly employed.

With use of endoscopy with fiberoptic cytology and direct biopsy, diagnostic accuracy in gastric ulcer (benign vs. malignant) is excellent.

Cancer of the Gastrointestinal Tract

Neoplasia of the large bowel is the second most common malignancy in American adults and accounts for 20 per cent of all deaths in the U.S. due to malignancy and are twice as frequent as deaths due to cancer of the stomach. They occur equally between males and females and in all age groups, particularly over age 45.

The causes of colonic malignant disease are not established although there is a relationship between adenomatous polyps and carcinoma. Chronic inflammatory bowel disease also predisposes to malignancy. Symptoms of colon carcinoma are usually vague and nonspecific at the onset. Weight loss and malaise are common. Changes in bowel habits and size and frequency of the stool are important. Gross bleeding occurs in over 70 per cent of left-sided colon lesions and is less noticed in right-sided tumors. Pain is an infrequent symptom although it may be accentuated by exercise and leaning forward. Anemia is common. Ten per cent of all colorectal cancers are palpable by rectal examination and up to 50 per cent may be detected by proctosigmoidoscopy. Diagnosis is dependent on x-ray findings of characteristic lesions and is enhanced by fiberoptic-assisted endoscopy. The only readily available therapy is surgery, which has an overall 5-year survival rate of 40 to 50 per cent.

Gastric carcinoma has shown a decline in incidence and still is very often not diagnosed until far advanced when signs of obstruction occur. These include (1) vomiting of stagnant stomach contents containing undigested food and frequently blood, (2) absence of free HC1, (3) cachexia, (4) loss of weight and (5) anemia. In addition (6) a mass may be felt. Occasionally, metastatic glands may be palpable, especially in the left supraclavicular region. Occult blood in the stools is common.

Most cancers of the stomach originate on the lesser curvature and cause only vague distress until extension and obstruction occur. Such early growths should be suspected in any elderly man complaining of digestive disturbances. The x-ray pattern of a gastric ulcer in the absence of free HC1 is helpful, and endoscopy will insure diagnosis. The 5 year survival is less than 10 per cent.

Pancreatic carcinoma appears to be increasing in incidence. Although the tumor may appear in any portion of the pancreas, two-thirds occur in the head. The classic triad occurs late: pain, weight loss and jaundice. The gall bladder or a mass may be palpable. The early diagnosis is difficult despite G-I series, hypotonic duodenography, endoscopic retrograde cholangiopancreatography (ERCP), ultrasound and computerized tomography (CT scan). The 5 year cure rate is well under 1 per cent.

Carcinoid Syndrome

Malignant carcinoid usually develops from a primary lesion in the ileum. It metastasizes to the liver, and to the ovary in the female. Large amounts of serotonin are present in the cells of the primary and the metastatic tumors. A bizarre syndrome develops slowly and consists of paroxysmal flushing of the face and the neck, associated with edema of the eyes, tachycardia, hypotension and respiratory distress. Diarrhea and abdominal pain may be present with nausea and vomiting. Disease of the pulmonary and the tricuspid valves may develop and, ultimately, cardiac failure. The symptoms develop because of the effect of serotonin on smooth muscle, causing vasomotor reactions, hyperperistalsis and bronchoconstriction. Surgical removal is the only satisfactory treatment.

Malabsorption Syndrome

Malabsorption occurs in a variety of pancreatic, biliary and bowel diseases. Sprue refers to an inherent defect of the small intestine and takes the form of celiac disease in children and tropical or nontropical sprue (idiopathic steatorrhea) in adults. Malabsorption also occurs following surgery, particularly gastrectomy and resection or exclusion of a segment of small intestine. Gastrocolic or enterocolic fistulas and involvement of the intestinal wall by regional enteritis, Hodgkin's disease or Whipple's disease may be responsible for secondary impairment of absorption. Malabsorption secondary to deficient digestive enzymes occurs as a result of chronic pancreatitis and complete obstruction of the common bile duct. Lactose intolerance may account for the condition. Steatorrhea or the presence of excess fat in the feces is the characteristic feature of the malabsorption syndrome. Diarrhea is usually, but not always, present, and the stools are typically bulky, soft or liquid, pale in color, frothy and have a pungent and offensive odor. There is usually a history of progressive weakness and weight loss in spite of a good or excellent appetite. The body becomes emaciated, but the abdomen is protuberant and tympanitic. Malabsorption of one or more dietary constituents other than fat is usually evident, and the resulting deficiencies may dominate the clinical picture. Failure to absorb iron or vitamin B_{12} may cause glossitis and a microcytic or macrocytic anemia, and the bone marrow may be megaloblastic. Low serum albumin and edema may result from defective protein absorption, and there may be tetany and osteoporosis due to calcium deficiency. Defective absorption of potassium and sodium also may occur, and even water absorption is sometimes inadequate. The clinical syndromes associated with vitamin B complex deficiency also are found occasionally.

The single best test is a 72 hour stool fat determination while eating 75 to 100 g. of fat daily. Less than 7 g. of stool fat per day are normally excreted. Other tests include a low D-xylose excretion after xylose load, an abnormal Schilling test not corrected by vitamin B_{12}. Low serum calcium, low serum albumin and low serum carotene levels also may be found. The glucose tolerance test shows a low curve, except in pancreatic malabsorption, in which there may be a diabetic curve.

In celiac disease and in many cases of adult sprue, administration of a wheat-free diet brings about rapid improvement. It has been demonstrated that the important factor is gluten, the protein fraction of wheat, and that wheat starch is not harmful. The treatment of secondary causes of malabsorption is that of the primary disease. The diet should be high in protein and low in carbohydrate, and deficiencies of vitamins, iron and calcium should be corrected by parenteral therapy.

Chronic Inflammatory Bowel Disease

This disease is divided into two categories: chronic nonspecific ulcerative colitis and Crohn's disease (granulomatous colitis). Both disorders share clinical features but there are sufficient differences to allow distinction. In ulcerative colitis, rectal bleeding, rectal involvement with friability of the mucosa, continuous mucosal abnormalities and absence of small bowel disease are prevalent; the mucosa and submucosa are chiefly affected. In Crohn's disease, fistula formation, perirectal abscess, skip areas, small bowel disease and transmural findings microscopically with frequent granulomas are the rule; malignant degeneration is rare. The etiology of both diseases is unknown. Fever, abdominal pain and diarrhea, often bloody, may be the presenting complaints, although over 25 per cent of patients have no other symptomatology but weight loss, fatigue and malaise. The disease must be distinguished from tuberculosis, lymphoma, ischemic colitis, diverticulitis and cancer. The diagnosis is confirmed by x-ray findings, sigmoidoscopy and colonoscopy.

The treatment is chiefly through the use of antimicrobials (sulfasalazine), antiinflammatory agents (steroids), sedation and psychotherapy in helping patients adjust to this illness. Colectomy in ulcerative colitis is considered for (1) persistent disease in a fulminant phase despite medical treatment, (2) hemorrhage, (3) perforation, (4) suspected malignancy and (5) prophylaxis for carcinoma in colitis of more than 10 years' duration. Colectomy has a higher recurrence rate in Crohn's disease.

Diverticulosis

Diverticulosis refers to the presence of multiple small diverticula, predominantly in the colon and particularly in the sigmoid and the descending colon. This is usually a silent benign condition producing no symptoms and requiring no treatment. Diverticulitis occurs in a small percentage of these patients. Inflammation may produce pain, fever and evidence of peritoneal inflammation. Perforation and abscess formation may result. Diverticular hemorrhage is the most common cause of massive hemorrhage from the lower gastrointestinal tract.

Mesenteric Vascular Insufficiency

The most familiar form of this illness is acute mesenteric thrombosis or embolism, which is characterized by a sudden onset of severe generalized abdominal pain associated with vomiting, and usually with a short period of bloody diarrhea followed by constipation. Dehydration and shock soon appear, and surgical intervention is indicated. Chronic mesenteric arterial insufficiency, sometimes termed abdominal angina, is more common in elderly men and those who have evidence of obliterative arteriosclerotic changes elsewhere in the body. The symptoms are pain, which is usually in the neighborhood of the umbilicus, and is worse after meals. The patient reduces his food intake and loses weight. Nausea and vomiting may occur. The pain may be controlled by vasodilating drugs, and in some cases thromboendarterectomy is advisable.

Zollinger-Ellison Syndrome

Zollinger-Ellison syndrome is an islet cell tumor (gastrinoma) of the pancreas associated with gastric hypersecretion and intractable peptic ulcer disease. The excessive gastric secretion is caused by gastrin, a hormone that can be extracted from these tumors. Adenomatous involvement of other endocrine glands, parathyroids and pituitary (Multiple endocrine adenoma-I), is seen in many of these patients, in whom there is usually a familial tendency to the disease. Multiple ulcerations in the esophagus, stomach and duodenum are frequently present; the secretion of hydrochloric acid in the stomach is sometimes 10 to 20 times the normal volume. Medical management is often not entirely satisfactory although cimetidine is sometimes effective. Surgical removal of the tumor is often not feasible, but total gastrectomy may result in improvement.

Dumping Syndrome

The dumping syndrome is caused by excessively rapid gastric emptying and usually occurs following gastric surgery. Food and fluid are evacuated rapidly into the small intestine. Extracellular fluid from the plasma moves rapidly into the lumen to achieve isotonicity, thereby decreasing the circulating blood volume and causing compensatory vasoconstriction. The phenomenon results in warmth, sweating, weakness, pallor, nausea and explosive diarrhea. There is frequently a hypoglycemic reaction 2 or 3 hours after a meal. Medical treatment includes multiple feedings of a diet high in protein and fat and low in carbohydrate, with limitation or exclusion of liquids during and immediately after meals.

Peutz-Jeghers Syndrome

Peutz-Jeghers syndrome consists of familial gastrointestinal polyposis with distinctive mucocutaneous pigmentation, which is most noticeable on the lips and buccal mucosa, but also appears in the skin of the fingers, palms and forearms. The polyps accentuate the peristaltic activity and thus lead to intussusception. Abdominal pain, borborygmi and midabdominal colic occur. The polyps are not malignant.

DISEASE OF THE SPLEEN AND THE LIVER

Splenomegaly

Enlargement of the spleen may be understood best in terms of its physiology and pathologic physiology.

The spleen is a part of the reticuloendothelial system and removes abnormal elements from the bloodstream whether they are infectious organisms or otherwise. In this process it enlarges. The infections that most often cause splenic enlargement are typhoid fever, malaria, infectious mononucleosis, subacute bacterial endocarditis, brucellosis and septicemia.

The spleen vein drains into the portal system; hence it enlarges for mechanical reasons when there is back pressure in the portal system, as in cirrhosis of the liver. This syndrome of chronic congestive splenomegaly is characterized by portal hypertension, hemorrhage from the gastrointestinal tract, leukopenia, anemia and thrombocytopenia. Banti's syndrome is a term frequently applied to this condition.

The spleen is a repository for all cellular elements in the blood and removes abnormal cells. The convenient but not universally accepted concept of hypersplenism refers to the theory that the spleen may become overactive and remove cellular elements that are much needed and even apparently normal. In this condition there are: (1) an enlarged spleen, (2) a deficiency of one or all of the formed elements in the cirulating blood, (3) normal or hyperplastic bone marrow is demonstrated by biopsy or aspiration and (4) the possibility of cure by splenectomy. A secondary form of hypersplenism may occur in lymphocytic leukemia, lymphomas and other diseases associated with splenomegaly and results in a hemolytic type of anemia complicating the primary disease.

Splenectomy

Removal may be required as an emergency operation in case of rupture of the spleen—a condition that can result from even mild trauma to an enlarged spleen. Splenectomy may be required only on rare occasions for purely mechanical reasons in splenomegaly of extreme degree. Splenectomy should be of specific value in hypersplenism, and it has established value in two conditions that might fall into this classification: (1) congenital hemolytic jaundice or congenital spherocy-

tosis and (2) idiopathic thrombocytopenic purpura. In idiopathic splenic neutropenia and splenic pancytopenia, splenectomy may also be of value. In one other condition, thrombosis of the splenic vein, splenectomy may be required because of bleeding from distended collateral veins in the stomach.

Jaundice

Jaundice, a yellowish discoloration of skin, mucous membranes and body fluids, is due to an excess of bile pigments. Bilirubinemia—bilirubin content 1.5 per cent or higher—is present before the tissues become discolored, and bilirubinuria often precedes the appearance of jaundice. Bilirubin is a derivative of the iron-free prophyrin of hemoglobin and is formed in the reticuloendothelial system where the erythrocytes are destroyed. When liberated to the bloodstream, it gives an indirect van den Bergh reaction because of its insolubility in water and its nonpolar structure. Ordinarily it is not excreted by the kidney but is taken up by liver cells. In the liver, bilirubin is conjugated with glucuronic acid to water-soluble bilirubin glucuronide, which gives a direct van den Bergh reaction. Elevation of this direct reacting fraction indicates disease of the liver parenchyma or of the bilary tract.

Jaundice is of three types: (1) obstructive, in which excretion of bile pigments is prevented by blocking of the bile ducts; (2) hemolytic, in which excretion of bile pigments is incomplete because of their too rapid formation by hemolysis of red blood cells; and (3) hepatic, in which excretion of bile pigments is impaired by damage or destruction of the hepatic cells.

Obstructive jaundice comprises about 85 per cent of all cases and may be caused by (1) internal obstruction of the bile ducts by gallstones (the most common cause); (2) obstruction due to changes in the walls of the ducts by inflammation, neoplasm or stricture; and (3) obstruction by pressure on the ducts from tumors, cysts, enlarged nodes or adhesions.

Hemolytic jaundice may be due to congenital and acquired hemolytic jaundice, pernicious anemia, malaria, chemicals that produce hemolysis, erythroblastosis fetalis, transfusion with incompatible blood, etc. It is caused by excessive destruction of erythrocytes and liberation of their pigments. Unless there is associated liver damage, it is characterized by absence of bile in the urine, by increased urobilinogen in the urine and the stools and by an indirect or delayed van den Bergh reaction in the serum.

Hepatic jaundice is due primarily to liver parenchymal disease. This may be seen in cirrhosis of any etiology; inflammatory disease of the liver, which includes infectious hepatitis, chronic active hepatitis and toxic and drug-induced hepatitis; and carcinoma or abscess of the liver. Adverse drug reactions of the liver include such agents as: halothane, isoniazid, PAS, chlorpromazine and oral contraceptives.

No single test can be relied upon to distinguish these three types of jaundice. Many tests have been proposed to distinguish the three mechanisms of jaundice. Bile pigments are never absent from the stools in pure hemolytic jaundice, whereas clay-colored stools are characteristic of complete obstructive jaundice and even may be found in the acute phase of hepatic jaundice. The sensitive tests for liver function, SGOT and SGPT, and serum proteins, including albumin, globulin, prothrombin and fibrinogen, are abnormal from the onset of hepatic jaundice. They are not abnormal in hemolytic jaundice and are not abnormal in obstructive jaundice until longstanding biliary obstruction has produced secondary liver damage. Alkaline phosphatase is a good indicator of obstructive hepatobiliary disease. Ultrasound may be useful in detecting dilated ducts in extrahepatic obstruction. In some patients percutaneous cholangiography and ERCP are needed to localize the cause of obstruction.

Acute Viral Hepatitis

Acute viral hepatitis is a systemic infection involving primarily the liver; it occurs in two immunologically different but clinically similar forms, hepatitis A (infectious hepatitis) and hepatitis B (serum hepatitis or Australia antigen-positive hepatitis). Both are characterized by hepatic cell necrosis; the usual picture is that of an anicteric period followed by jaundice and recovery. Many cases are mild and recognized only by abnormal liver function tests. A third category of virus, referred to as "non A, non B" also exists.

The incubation period for hepatitis A is 15 to 50 days and for hepatitis B 50 to 180 days. Transfusion hepatitis may be due to either virus.

The first symptom is usually painless jaundice, associated with a variable fever, malaise and often a mild gastrointestinal upset. The liver and spleen may be slightly enlarged and tender. In hepatitis B disease there may also be urticaria, arthritis, and arthralgia. The disease ordinarily resolves in about 4 weeks. The diagnosis may not be established conclusively until the patient recovers. Some tests of liver function may not return to normal for several months after symptomatic recovery. Patients should rest in bed until acute symptoms have subsided. A high carbohydrate and high protein diet may be advisable. Patients with acute viral hepatitis usually recover completely although infrequently relapse may occur. Chronic liver disease may occur in 10 per cent of hepatitis B and the non A-non B form. It probably does not occur after type A. Two forms of chronic hepatitis are identified by

liver biopsy. Chronic persistent hepatitis is benign and self limited but may cause mild symptoms. Chronic active hepatitis on the other hand often progresses to cirrhosis. Chronic active hepatitis may require steroids.

Cirrhosis of the Liver

Hepatic cirrhosis (fibrosis) is divided as follows: (1) portal cirrhosis, which includes the common alcoholic cirrhosis of Laennec and the rare cases of cirrhosis found with hemochromatosis or with Wilson's hepatolenticular degeneration and (2) postnecrotic cirrhosis.

Portal Cirrhosis.   Portal cirrhosis is a disease of middle life occurring twice as frequently in men as in women. It is found commonly in chronic alcoholism and is believed to be the direct result of alcohol toxicity (alcoholic hepatitis) accentuated by poor protein diet. It is characterized by a tremendous increase in the fibrous tissue of the liver capsule and between the portal lobules, giving the surface the hobnail appearance.

Diagnosis. The early symptoms are (1) indigestion; (2) nausea; (3) anorexia; (4) flatulence; and (5) occasional vomiting, particularly in a chronic alcoholic. As the condition advances, "obstructive" symptoms appear. These include (1) bleeding from esophageal varices with hematemesis and melena; (2) ascites; (3) enlargement of the spleen; and (4) enlargement of the liver. In addition to the esophageal varices, attempts at collateral circulation may result in hemorrhoids, caput medusae and dilatation of the epigastric veins. Usually there is also intermittent mild jaundice. The appearance of spider angiomas are helpful diagnostically. The most significant laboratory findings are a reduction of the serum albumin and abnormal liver function tests.

Treatment requires prohibition of alcohol. The diet should be high in carbohydrates and protein unless hepatic encephalopathy exists. The intake of sodium chloride should be restricted if fluid retention is present. Ascites should be combated by restoring the blood proteins (diet) and by diuretics.

Hepatic Coma. The later effects of hepatocellular failure are widespread. There are endocrine disturbances with testicular atrophy, impotence in males and amenorrhea in women, loss of axillary and pubic hair and gynecomastia. Vascular spiders may appear on the face, the neck and the upper trunk, with erythema of the palms. Dupuytren's contracture and parotid enlargement may also occur. Extensive liver damage may ultimately result in hepatic coma. A flapping tremor (asterixis) may be present with incoordination of the extremities with neurologic and psychiatric disorders. The cause of hepatic coma is not known, but it is associated with elevation of the blood ammonia level.

Wilson's disease (hepatolenticular degeneration) is an

inherited disease with degenerative changes in the brain (basal ganglia) and cirrhosis of the liver. A Kayser-Fleischer ring, a brownish pigmented ring at the corneal margin, results from a deposit of copper and is pathognomonic of the disease, which is manifested by tremor, incoordination, rigidity and dysarthria. Jaundice may be an early symptom, and evidence of cirrhosis of the liver appears. The disease is caused by an increase in absorption of copper and accumulation of this metal in brain, liver and other tissues.

Postnecrotic cirrhosis. This is the most common form worldwide. It should be suspected in nonalcoholic patients with chronic liver disease, especially in the younger age group. It is probably the sequla of viral hepatitis as well as injury from hepatotoxins. The liver is small and markedly distorted and microscopically shows islands of parenchymal cells with mononuclear infiltrations. The clinical course is similar to portal cirrhosis.

METABOLIC AND ENDOCRINE DISEASES

Simple Colloid Goiter

Simple, diffuse, colloid goiter was endemic in inland regions, particularly around the Great Lakes. Usually it starts at the age of puberty. It is characterized by slow, painless, diffuse enlargement of the thyroid without the production of any symptoms except occasionally those of pressure. There is a normal metabolic state, and hypothyroidism or hyperthyroidism rarely develops. The condition is due to a low iodine content in the drinking water and the soil of the endemic area. The condition has become much less frequent since the introduction of iodized salt.

In the presence of an enlarged gland, thyroid hormone often will reduce the goiter by suppressing TSH secretion. Surgery is necessary for pressure symptoms only.

Thyroid Nodules

Nodules may be single or multiple, active (takes up radioiodine) or inactive. The multinodular goiter can often be treated with thyroid hormone suppression. Sometimes pressure symptoms or cosmetic reasons require surgery. The treatment of single nodule is controversial because of the question of cancer. The single active ("live") nodule may be treated initially with thyroid hormone and followed. The single "cold" nodule is often operated on unless there is some other compelling reason not to. In some centers, percutaneous biopsy is employed.

Thyroiditis

Subacute thyroiditis is an inflammatory condition of the thyroid of unknown etiology and associated with swelling and tenderness of the gland with accompanying chills and fever. The iodine uptake is usually depressed to a very low level, but there is transient elevation in T3 and T4 levels. The disease tends to have remissions and relapses for weeks to a few months. Analgesics and thyroid hormone are used; in severe instances, prednisone may be employed.

Hashimoto's thyroiditis, struma lymphomatosa, is a chronic disease manifested by progressive enlargement of the thyroid associated with atrophy of the parenchyma and lymphocytic infiltration. It may now be the most common cause of goiter in the adult. This is considered to be a type of tissue hypersensitivity to a protein or proteins of the thyroid. In advanced disease, hypothyroidism supervenes. Antithyroglobulin antibodies are increased in this disease.

Thyroid Cancer

Thyroid cancers are more often differentiated than anaplastic. The most common of all is the differentiated papillary form. It has a relatively low order malignancy and patients may live for 20 to 30 years even with metastases. Surgery and thyroid hormone replacement are used.

Tests of Thyroid Function

The most important tests are the measurement in the blood of the two active hormones, T_4 (thyroxin), and T_3 (triiodothyronine). Other tests include: radioiodine uptake (RAI); pituitary TSH (thyroid-stimulating hormone) levels; thyroid suppression tests; tests for thyroid antibodies; hypothalamic TRH (thyrotrophin-releasing hormone); and thyroid binding globulin (TBG).

Measurement of T_3 and T_4 are affected by the serum level of TBG. Estrogens in oral contraceptives, pregnancy and as prescribed for postmenopausal women, cause an increase in TBG, and an increase in T_4, which has greater avidity for TBG than T_3. If both T_4 and T_3 are elevated, hyperthyroidism is likely. If T_4 and T_3 are decreased hypothyroidism is probable. If T_4 and T_3 deviate from normal in opposite direction, a decrease or increase in TBG in a euthyroid patient is generally the situation.

Hyperthyroidism

Exophthalmic Goiter. Graves' disease is a constitutional disease of unknown cause that is characterized by expressive thyroid hormone secretion by an enlarged thyroid gland. (Probably there is no fundamental difference between "toxic adenoma" and "toxic diffuse hyperthyroidism" so far as fundamental pathologic physiology is concerned.) It is more common among women than among men and occurs most frequently in young adults, often becoming manifest following emotional trauma. All of the symptoms except exophthalmos and certain nervous manifestations have been produced in both animals and humans by administration of thyroid extract. There is associated hyperactivity of the sympathetic nervous system.

The classic *symptoms* are (1) goiter, (2) exophthalmos, (3) tachycardia, (4) fine tremor, (5) nervousness, (6) loss of weight, (7) excessive sweating and sensitivity to heat, (8) muscular weakness, and (9) frequently, vomiting and diarrhea.

Most of the symptoms are referable to an increased thyroid secretion that causes an increased metabolic rate with excessive oxidation in the tissue cells, resulting in the loss of weight despite increased appetite. The uptake of radioactive iodine by the thyroid gland is increased. Cardiovascular findings include a wide pulse pressure, atrial arrhythmias, systolic murmurs and at times heart failure. Long-acting thyroid stimulation (LATS) is an immunoglobulin (IgG) found in these patients; its relation to disease is unclear. There is other evidence as well for altered immune and genetic mechanisms.

Treatment. Radioactive iodine (^{131}I) will successfully control the manifestations of most patients with exophthalmic goiter. It is less satisfactory in toxic adenoma. It is especially valuable in those with complicating heart disease, which makes operation hazardous, and also in those in whom there is recurrence of the disease after surgery. There is a high and cumulative incidence of permanent myxedema. The long-continued use of antithyroid drugs requires careful and close supervision, but it may control the disease successfully. Antithyroid drugs are also useful in hyperthyroidism in pregnancy. Surgical treatment may be useful in patients with toxic adenoma. To reduce the sympathomimetic activity of Graves' disease and in thyrotoxic crisis, adrenergic blocking agents such as propranolol are used.

Hypothyroidism

Hypothyroidism occurs as (1) endemic cretinism originating from thyroid deficiency during fetal life and infancy and characterized by stunted mental and physical development; and (2) myxedema, which occurs sporadically in adults as the result of thyroidectomy, thyroiditis or atrophy. Both conditions are due to thyroid deficiency.

Cretinism. The symptoms of cretinism are usually noticed after the first year of life because of slow development in stature, intelligence and activity. In addition to the retarded development, there are dry skin, imperfect dentition, flaring nostrils and sunken nasal bridge, potbelly, fatty pads on the shoulders and buttocks and thickening of the tongue.

Prophylactic treatment is all important. In goiter areas iodine should be given to pregnant women. Thyroid extract will produce an amazing physical improvement in a cretin. Unfortunately, however, the condition is often not diagnosed early enough to save the child from permanent mental impairment.

Myxedema. This develops slowly between the ages of 30 and 60. Its symptoms are the antithesis of those found in hyperthyroidism: (1) slowing of bodily and mental activities; (2) increased weight; (3) decreased appetite; (4) dryness and coarseness of the skin and the hair; (5) expressionless facies; (6) edema, most marked in the hands, the feet and the supraclavicular fossae; (7) decreased cardiac output; and (8) commonly, painful joints. The uptake of radioactive iodine by the thyroid is diminished as are the T_3 and T_4 levels.

Treatment. The condition responds well to thyroid replacement by mouth. Patients may be treated with T_3, T_4 or desiccated thyroid which has both T_3 and T_4. Subsequently, for the rest of his life the patient must take a sufficient daily dose of thyroid to maintain a euthyroid state.

Addison's Disease

Chronic primary adrenal cortical insufficiency may result from tuberculous fibrocaseous destruction of the adrenal or from idiopathic bilateral adrenal cortical atrophy. The symptoms consist of weakness, fatigability, weight loss, pigmentation of the skin and mucous membranes and gastrointestinal manifestations. The pigmentation is a diffuse tanning with accentuation in scars, over pressure areas and dark freckles. The blood pressure is low and the heart small. The serum sodium and chloride levels are low, and the potassium high. Serum cortisol levels are low while ACTH levels are increased. Administration of ACTH does not stimulate the adrenal to increase the secretion of plasma cortisol; however, in secondary adrenal insufficiency there is a subnormal increase. Treatment consists of administration of cortisone. The addition of NaCl to the diet may be helpful, or the administration of 9-alpha-fluorocortisol may be necessary at the beginning of treatment.

Acute adrenal cortical insufficiency may occur at the beginning or during the course of the chronic form as a result of infection, operation or other stress. It is manifest by anorexia, nausea, vomiting, diarrhea, abdominal pain and collapse. It requires immediate intravenous infusion of isotonic saline and hydrocortisone.

Cushing's Syndrome

This condition is caused by excessive secretion of glucocorticoids by the adrenal cortex. An identical syndrome is produced by excessive amounts of corticosteroids administered to patients for therapeutic purposes. There is decrease of protein in the bone, causing osteoporosis; muscle weakness; alterations in the skin, causing stria; decreased carbohydrate tolerance, causing mild diabetes; retention of sodium; hypertension and excessive loss of potassium. There is a gain of weight, alteration or cessation of the menses in women, muscle weakness and rounding of the face. Fat pads appear over the upper dorsal vertebra causing a buffalo hump and in the superclavicular fossae. Depressed purple striae appear over the abdomen and hips.

The most common form is bilateral adrenocortical hyperfunction due to excessive and unremitting secretion of pituitary ACTH. The best screening tests are elevated plasma cortisol levels which are not diminished by dexamethasone. Treatment of severe disease is with transsphenoidal resection of a pituitary tumor, pituitary irradiation or bilateral total adrenalectomy with long-term replacement as given in Addison's disease. Adrenal adenoma is much more common in women, onset is more rapid than in the pituitary-dependent form, and virilism is at a minimum. Treatment is removal of the adenoma with recovery occurring through normal function of the remaining gland on the other side. Adrenal carcinoma causes severe Cushing's syndrome, steroid values are high and are not suppressed by dexamethasone. The treatment is similar to that for adenoma. In addition, hypercortisolism can be caused by cancers of nonendocrine organs such as the lungs (oat cell carcinoma), thymus and pancreas.

Primary Aldosteronism

This results from an increase in the secretion of aldosterone by an adrenal tumor, leading to hypertension and increased sodium retention without edema and with some degree of potassium wasting; there is reduced plasma renin activity. The elevated aldosterone and reduced renin levels are very suggestive. In later stages potassium depletion and alkalosis may lead to characteristic attacks of muscle weakness or tetany.

Pheochromocytoma

This is a catecholamine-producing tumor arising from chromaffin cells of the sympathoadrenal system; it is a rare condition but must be considered in differential diagnosis in patients with hypertension. About 80 per cent of pheochromocytomas originate in the adrenal glands; more than 95 per cent of the tumors are located in the abdominal cavity; and the remainder, in the paravertebral areas of the thorax and neck. The manifestations result from increased secretion of norepinephrine and epinephrine. Hypertension is the principal sign and may be either persistent or paroxysmal in nature. Attacks are characterized by severe headache, sweating, palpitation, tremor, pallor, nausea, vomiting, pain in the chest and hypertension. Pheochromocytoma may be associated with medullary carcinoma of the thyroid and hyperparathyroidism (MEA-II).

Hypopituitarism

Resulting from destruction of the anterior lobe of the pituitary, hypopitiutarism is accompanied by secondary atrophy of the gonads, thyroid and adrenal cortex together or individually. Sheehan's disease is hypopituitarism caused by postpartum necrosis of the gland. If tumor (e.g., chromaphobe adenoma) is the cause, transsphenoidal resection or pituitary radiation may be indicated. Hormonal replacement therapy is indicated.

Acromegaly

This is a chronic disease characterized by overgrowth of bone connective tissue in response to excessive secretion of growth hormone by a pituitary tumor, usually a eosinophilic adenoma. It is a disease of adult life, characterized by enlargement of the hands, feet, face and head. *Gigantism* is a childhood counterpart of acromegaly resulting from oversecretion of growth hormone in a child before closure of the epiphyses. Prolonged active acromegaly leads to increased incidence of cardiovascular disease and hypertension and should be treated if possible. Surgery or high-voltage radiation to the anterior pituitary is used.

Hyperprolactinemia

Galactorrhea and amenorrhea may be due to a pituitary prolactin-secreting tumor. Surgery may be indicated. Secondary hyperprolactinemia is associated with certain drug therapy (e.g., reserpine, methyldopa).

Diabetes Insipidus

This disorder results from a deficiency of antidiuretic hormone from the posterior pituitary and causes persistent excretion of large volumes of urine of low specific gravity, which produces extreme thirst and secondary polydipsia. There is no renal disease, and replacement therapy relieves the symptoms promptly. Radioimmunoassay of arginine vasopressin will confirm the diagnosis.

Primary Hyperparathyroidism

This results from overproduction of the parathyroid hormone caused by an adenoma or hyperplastic glands. Osteitis fibrosa cystica may result, as well as hypertension. Elevated serum calcium and urinary calcium and a lowered serum phosphorus levels are present. There are anorexia, weakness, fatigability, difficulty in swallowing, nausea, vomiting, and hypotonicity of muscles. *Hypoparathyroidism* usually results from inadvertent removal of the parathyroid glands during an operation of thyroid disease. There is decreased serum calcium with low urinary calcium excretion and increased serum phosphorus. The lowered serum calcium results in increased excitability of the peripheral nerves, and tetany results.

Diabetes Mellitus

Diabetes mellitus is classically a relative deficiency of insulin secretion by the pancreas, resulting in diminished ability of the organism to metabolize carbohydrates, frequently with associated disturbances in the metabolism of proteins and fats. The cause is unknown, but obesity, racial susceptibility and heredity are possible etiologic factors. Juvenile onset diabetes may be related to viral infection. It may occur at any age. The primary pathologic lesion is described as hyalinization, fibrosis or hydropic degeneration of the beta cells of the pancreatic islands of Langerhans. However, in more numerous cases no lesion can be found in the pancreas. In general, diabetes may be classified as follows: (1) overt diabetes either of ketosis-prone (juvenile) or ketosis-resistant (adult) type. Fasting blood sugar tests are abnormal, and symptoms are easily elicited; (2) chemical diabetes in which there are no symptoms, but the 2 hour postprandial sugar or glucose tolerance test is abnormal. Vascular disease may occur in this phase; (3) latent diabetes brought out only in stress (e.g., pregnancy and infection); and (4) prediabetes, which is anticipated because of hereditary factors.

Symptoms develop slowly as a rule and include: (1) polyuria, (2) polydipsia, (3) polyphagia, (4) loss of weight, (5) weakness, and (6) often pruritus, particularly of the genitalia.

The *diagnosis* rests on the finding of glycosuria and hyperglycemia at the same time. A 2 hour postprandial glucose test (after a meal containing 50 g. of glucose) should yield the same value to be normal. In borderline cases a formal 3 hour glucose tolerance test is needed to establish the diagnosis.

Complications include: (1) ketoacidosis and coma as well as hyperglycemic nonketotic coma, (2) neuritis, (3) furunculosis, (4) carbunculosis, (5) cataract, (6) arteriosclerosis with ulcer or gangrene, (7) retinopathy, (8) coronary artery disease, and (9) diabetic nephropathy.

The *juvenile-onset* type of diabetes is unstable, sensitive to insulin and easily influenced by stress factors. Ketoacidosis is easily produced, and the patient must have an adequate diet and take insulin. Primary complications in a well-controlled patient are cardiovascular and renal. The *maturity-onset* type has minimal symptoms at the onset. Chief complaint may be weight loss or weight gain. Visual disturbances may be the first sign heralding diabetic retinopathy. Uremia and anemia may be the sign of significant nephropathy. Paresthesias, loss of sensation, impotence, nocturnal diarrhea, postural hypotension and neurogenic bladder indicate diabetic neuropathic involvement; peripheral vascular disease may be seen presenting as ulcer or gangrene as an initial complaint.

The goal of *treatment* of diabetes mellitus is to (1) correct underlying metabolic abnormalities to reduce diabetic symptoms, (2) maintain ideal body weight, and (3) prevent, if possible, or minimize complications such as disease of the eye, kidney, nerves and cardiovascular system. Dietary treatment is the main factor in management in most cases; the diabetic patient has the same nutritional requirements as the nondiabetic patient; it should be designed, therefore, to prevent excessive hyperglycemia or hypoglycemia (if the patient is taking insulin); to keep the weight, as well as cholesterol and triglycerides stable; and to prevent or delay early atherosclerosis. Various regimens of partition of calories into fats, carbohydrates and proteins are available for individualized patient programs.

The use of oral hypoglycemic agents, such as the sulfonylureas is controversial because there is some question as to their safety in the presence of cardiovascular disease. They are, however, recommended if insulin is unacceptable to the patient and dietary measures have failed. The use of insulin is clearly recommended in growth-onset diabetes and in the maturity-onset type as noted above. Insulin is required in diabetic ketoacidosis; few patients develop insulin resistance.

Hypoglycemic reaction from an overdose of insulin is manifested by weakness, sweating, mental confusion, incoordination, trembling and sometimes loss of consciousness and convulsions. Sugar or orange juice or any form of carbohydrate usually allays the symptoms, or 10 to 50 ml. of 50 per cent glucose may be given intravenously; recovery is dramatic. The symptoms begin when the blood sugar falls below 70 mg. and become severe when the level falls to 40 mg. per 100 ml.

Diabetic Ketoacidosis. Acute ketoacidosis occurs when the CO_2-combining power of the plasma falls below 15 mEq. per liter and the pH below 7.35. The symptoms are (1) nausea, (2) vomiting, (3) epigastric pain and distress, (4) hyperpnea (Kussmaul breathing), (5) dry skin and oral mucosa, and (6) drowsiness or coma. The mucous membranes are bright red. The breath has a fruity odor of acetone bodies, and the breathing is very labored. Omission of insulin, infection, vascular accidents and alcoholic pancreatitis are prime precipitating causes of ketoacidosis. Beta-hydroxybutyrate and acetoacetate are the ketone bodies responsible for the acidosis. Hypokalemia may result from too vigorous therapy of ketoacidosis.

Hemochromatosis

Hemochromatosis is an iron-storage disease characterized by deposition of iron in the tissues and organs with resultant fibrosis and interference with the function of the organs involved. Hemosiderin is deposited in the tissues, giving a bronze pigmentation at autopsy and giving the skin either a bronze or a blue-gray discoloration. The deposition is greatest in the liver but involves other organs and tissues. Fibrosis is thought to result from the accumulation of iron. Clinically the disease is characterized by skin pigmentation, diabetes, hepatomegaly with evidence of liver insufficiency, cardiac irregularities and cardiac failure. Hemochromatosis may result from an idiopathic metabolic error, from repeated blood transfusions or from excessive iron administration.

(The vitamin deficiency diseases are outlined in Chap. 4, Biochemistry and Chap. 6, Pathology.)

INFECTIOUS DISEASES

Numerous infectious diseases are not described here because all essentials of these diseases are included in other chapters (see Index).

Measles

Measles is a communicable disease of viral etiology, usually epidemic during the winter and the spring. Most cases occur before the 15th year, and about half occur during the first 5 years of life.

The disease has an incubation period of about 12 days and a prodromal period of 2 days. Infectivity is present for only a few days after the rash appears.

The prodrome consists of catarrhal symptoms, including inflammation of the eyes, the nose and the respiratory tract, fever and Koplik's spots. Koplik's spots are seen on the buccal mucosa as bluish-white spots of pinpoint size surrounded by a bright red areola. They are present in practically all cases and are diagnostic before the rash appears. Leukopenia with relative lymphopenia usually is present in the preeruptive stage. Later there is leukopenia with relative lymphocytosis.

The *eruption* appears about 2 days after the temperature has risen. It is noticed first behind the ears or on the forehead and spreads rapidly over the face and the neck and downward, covering the entire body in 2 or 3 days and lasting for 4 or 5 days. The lesions first appear as dusky-red maculopapules, which form blotches and may become confluent. The fever and the respiratory symptoms increase with the rash, which after running its course leaves a fine, branlike desquamation.

Complications result from secondary infection. Laryngitis, bronchitis, bronchopneumonia, otitis media, vomiting and diarrhea are common. Measles may activate latent tuberculosis. The complications are most hazardous in children less than 5 years of age. Rarely, encephalitis is a complication.

Prevention. Active immunization is effective with attenuated live virus vaccine. Gamma globulin in doses of 0.1 to 0.2 ml. per lb. of body weight protects against measles if given within the first 5 days of exposure, but attenuation is more likely if it is given later.

Treatment is largely symptomatic. Careful watch should be made for pulmonary and ear complications. Human convalescent serum usually will modify measles if given during the incubation period. The antibiotics should be reserved for the complications.

Rubella

Rubella (German measles) is an acute contagious disease, usually affecting children and young adults, that is characterized by a skin rash and lymphadenitis. It is of viral etiology and occurs in epidemics. The usual course is mild and of short duration. Immunity is lasting, so that second attacks are rare. The importance of rubella lies not in the course of the disease itself but the frequency with which fetal abnormalities appear when the mother is infected in the early months of pregnancy. Infection of the mother may lead to intrauterine death (stillbirth) or to delivery of a viable fetus with mental retardation or varying degrees of congenital abnormalities.

Women exposed to rubella in early pregnancy should receive gamma globulin or convalescent serum prophylactically. Active immunization with live attenuated rubella vaccine is commonly used in children. It should not be used in women who are pregnant or who might become pregnant within 2 months of immunization.

Rheumatic Fever

Rheumatic fever is a late complication of group A streptococcal infection and therefore a preventable disease. It is most common between the ages of 5 and 30 and is characterized by (1) focal proliferative and (2) diffuse exudative lesions. The focal lesions are typified by Aschoff bodies in the myocardium and periarticular nodules and foci in the endocardium and the central nervous system. The exudative lesions involve (1) the joints, (2) the pericardium and (3) the pleura.

Symptoms. The onset often is preceded by tonsillitis or upper respiratory infection and is followed in about 2 weeks by sudden onset of fever, prostration and polyarthritis. Often the larger joints are affected symmetrically, and there is a definite tendency for the infection to skip from joint to joint. The usual cycle lasts from 10 to 14 days, with localization in each set of joints for 4 to 5 days, but such single cycles may recur, or the manifestations may continue uninterruptedly.

While the joint symptoms are the most striking, the cardiac manifestations are the most dangerous, and the patient should be examined daily for tachycardia, arrhythmia, gallop rhythm, developing murmurs, pericardial friction rub or signs of pericardial effusion. Pleural effusion sometimes occurs. Chorea may occur without any joint involvement. Polymorphonuclear leukocytosis usually is found during acute joint involvement, and an accelerated sedimentation rate is present throughout the active stages of the disease. An abnormal protein that reacts with the C polysaccharide of the pneumococcus also is present during periods of activity (C-reactive protein). Although it occurs in other diseases, it is a useful measure of activity. In the electrocardiogram there may be prolonged PR or QT intervals.

Treatment. Rest in bed, nourishing diet and liberal fluids are indicated. Practically all the acute symptoms *except those of the heart* are relieved by salicylates. From 0.9 to 1.2 g. sodium salicylate may be given every hour for 8 to 10 doses, but the patient should be watched for toxic symptoms (ringing in the ears, deafness, nausea, vomiting and acidosis with deep forced breathing). The following day the dosage should be reduced by half and continued till all signs of activity have been absent for a week. Eradication of the streptococcus from the throat should be attempted with penicillin. Up to 10 days of treatment is required. Followup throat cultures should be taken to make sure that the organism has been eliminated. In certain cases steroid therapy is beneficial.

After congenital heart disease, rheumatic fever is the most common cause of cardiac disease in the young. Prophylaxis with daily administration of oral penicillin (200,000 units) or with monthly injections of benzathine penicillin (1,200,000 units) should be carried out in people who have had rheumatic fever. Prevention of the disease should be attempted by prompt diagnosis of all group A streptococcal infections.

Diphtheria

Diphtheria is caused by *Corynebacterium diphtheriae* and is still common in parts of the world. The lesions of diphtheria are (1) local, due to the action of toxin at the site of infection; and (2) systemic, due to the action of the exotoxin absorbed through the blood and the lymph stream. The typical pseudomembrane may be found in the larynx, the tonsils, the trachea, the epiglottis, the nose, the bronchi and rarely in the esophagus, the vagina or the conjunctiva. Systemic lesions involve (1) the myocardium; (2) the peripheral and the cranial nerves; and (3) the kidneys.

Clinical Diagnosis. Diphtheria occurs chiefly in children and young adults. If scarlet fever, thrush, Vincent's angina or infectious mononucleosis can be excluded and there is a visible membrane in the nose or throat, particularly if more marked on one side, the condition should be treated as diphtheria. A serosanguineous nasal discharge always should be investigated with care.

Fever is relatively slight, and there is usually little pain on swallowing. The throat, if reddened, is of a darker, beefier red than in scarlet fever.

Croup in a young child should be treated as laryngeal diphtheria unless there is a negative Schick test or absence of membrane upon direct laryngoscopy. Throat and nose swabs should be taken on Löffler's medium and examined after 18 to 24 hours for the organism. A single negative culture does not rule out the diagnosis.

Treatment. In any suspected case of diphtheria, antitoxin should be administered without waiting for culture reports since the earlier it is administered the more certain and rapid the effect. The dosage of antitoxin may vary from 8,000 units in mild cases to more than 80,000 units in malignant cases.

It is recommended that mild and moderate cases be treated subcutaneously or intramuscularly; severe cases, intravenously or intramuscularly; and malignant cases, intravenously. Laryngeal diphtheria, moderate cases seen late and cases complicating the exanthemata should be treated as severe.

In neglected cases of laryngeal diphtheria, intubation or tracheotomy may be necessary. Local treatment of the membrane is generally useless and actually may be harmful. Penicillin is helpful but does not replace antitoxin. Fortunately, immunization with toxoid is rapidly making the disease a curiosity.

Complications. Tachycardia, arrhythmia, heart

block, gallop rhythm and cardiac decompensation develop most commonly from 1 to 3 weeks after the onset. The symptoms are due to myocardial degeneration and to degeneration of the vagus. For this reason, rest in bed is essential until the heart action is normal. Digitalis is of singularly little value to the damaged myocardium.

The most common paralyses are those of the palate, constrictors of the pharynx and of the extraocular muscles. The adductors of the larynx and the motor nerves of the upper and the lower extremities and of the intercostals and the phrenics sometimes are involved. Fortunately most of these paralyses are transient. However, tube feeding may be required in grave cases.

Bronchopneumonia is a frequent complication of laryngeal diphtheria. Albuminuria is common, but nephritis rarely is marked. (For *Schick testing* and immunization, Chapt. 5, General Microbiology, should be consulted.)

Acute Streptococcal Tonsillitis, Pharyngitis and Scarlet Fever

These diseases are caused by group A streptococci. Susceptibility and mortality diminish from the first to the tenth year. Epidemics are more common in the fall and the winter and are associated with the school year.

The incubation period is usually 3 to 5 days, but the infection probably is not communicable before the onset. The period of infectivity lasts while there are streptococci in the throat.

Diagnosis. The clinical picture is generally clear. It includes (1) abrupt onset, sometimes with headache and vomiting; (2) rapidly rising temperature; (3) sore throat, often with follicular tonsillitis and marked reddening of the fauces; (4) typical punctate rash on the hard palate; and (5) for scarlet fever, followed in 12 to 24 hours by a finely punctate rash on the neck and the chest, which, in about 48 hours, spreads gradually over the entire body and remains 4 to 5 days; (6) strawberry tongue; and (7) subsequent desquamation, beginning on the chest, 3 to 10 days after disappearance of the rash. The rash may be limited to the groins, the axillae and the elbows. The cervical nodes are usually enlarged.

The common sequelae are (1) otitis media, (2) sinusitis, (3) nephritis, (4) adenitis, and (5) arthritis. Endocarditis, acute articular rheumatism and chorea also are complications of this disease.

The disease should be treated with strict isolation technique until streptococci are absent from the throat. Penicillin is the only drug of established value; 600,000 units intramuscularly of procaine penicillin should be used daily for 7 to 10 days. Follow-up cultures are

necessary. Benzathine penicillin may be used intramuscularly as a single dose of 1,200,000 units. Oral therapy should be continued for 2 weeks.

Erysipelas

Erysipelas is an acute inflammation of the skin, or occasionally the mucous membranes, caused by group A hemolytic streptococcus. Infection with the specific streptococcus begins at the site of a wound, a fissure or an abrasion; it is most common on the face, and less common on the umbilicus of the newborn and on the vulva during the puerperium or around surgical wounds and injuries.

It begins as a small area of red, swollen and tender skin with margins that are sharply marked, elevated and indurated. It extends by contiguity, with involution of the central portion. The onset is abrupt, with chill, high fever, malaise, headache and anorexia. On the face there is often the symmetrical butterfly pattern. The process usually stops at the hairline and very rarely passes anteriorly down the neck. The disease may persist for several days to several weeks, usually terminating by crisis. Relapses and recurrences are not uncommon.

Complications include: (1) subcutaneous abscesses, (2) gangrene of the skin, (3) orbital abscess, (4) pneumonia and, in fatal cases, (5) septicemia.

Treatment. Patients should be isolated. Usually penicillin is dramatically effective. It should be given as described under Acute Streptococcal Tonsillitis, Pharyngitis and Scarlet Fever.

Infections Due to Compromised Host

Fungal infections, particularly Candida, affect the debilitated patient. Predisposing factors include intravascular catheters, prosthetic heart valves and antibiotic therapy. Amphotericin B and 5-fluorocytosine are effective therapeutic agents. Specific therapy is usually not required if a foreign body such as a catheter can be removed. Cryptococcal infection is seen in patients with impaired cellular immunity, as in Hodgkin's disease and sarcoidosis. Aspergillus is also found in this group of patients.

Pneumocystic infection and toxoplasmosis are opportunistic infections in a susceptible host and may be treated effectively, after appropriate diagnostic tests, with pentamidine and sulfonamides respectively.

Following cardiopulmonary bypass or the immunosuppression of a transplantation procedure, cytomegalic inclusion virus and herpes zoster may cause disease representing activation of latent infection. Therapy is not available, but diagnosis is important in the overall management of the patient.

Leprosy (Hansen's Disease)

Leprosy (Hansen's disease) is caused by *Mycobacterium leprae,* which is an acid-fast bacillus. Attempts to grow the organism on culture media have failed, as have attempts to inoculate human volunteers. Adults seem to be practically immune to any type of exposure. Hansen's disease has three forms:

1. The neural, or maculoanesthetic form, manifested by pigmented anesthetic areas on the skin
2. The nodular form, manifested by indolent deep-seated nodules that may become confluent
3. The mixed form, in which both manifestations are present.

The sulfone drugs (Promin and Diasone) have been shown to be a reliable form of treatment.

Typhoid Fever

Typhoid fever is an acute infection with *Salmonella typhosa,* characterized by involvement of the lymphoid tissues, usually with marked hyperplasia and ulceration of Peyer's patches and enlargement of the spleen. Clinically it is characterized by (1) continued fever, (2) leukopenia, (3) relatively slow pulse, (4) crops of rose spots, (5) mental confusion or torpor, and (6) a variety of intestinal symptoms. It is most common in epidemics, which result from fecal contamination of the water or the food (especially milk) supply.

Symptoms. The incubation period averages 10 days, usually followed by 5 to 7 days of prodromal malaise, anorexia and drowsiness. The onset is frequently marked by epistaxis or bronchitis. The pulse rate is disproportionately low for the elevated temperature. In the United States typhoid fever was very common half a century ago but is rare at present.

Rose spots appear in crops over the abdomen toward the end of the first week. They are slightly elevated and fade on pressure. The spleen is usually palpable at the end of the first week. There may be slight leukocytosis during the prodromal period, but there is usually leukopenia with relative lymphocytosis.

Diagnosis depends upon (1) the clinical picture as a whole and (2) laboratory confirmation.

(See Chap. 5, General Microbiology, for the specific laboratory tests.)

The differential diagnosis must exclude (1) miliary tuberculosis, (2) subacute bacterial endocarditis, (3) typhus, (4) trichinosis, and (5) brucellosis.

Complications of typhoid cause three quarters of the deaths. Hemorrhage is most frequent during the third week. It is manifested by (1) tarry stool, (2) chills, (3) marked fall in temperature, (4) pallor, and (5) rapid rise in pulse and leukocytosis. Abdominal pain is rare and suggests perforation. Perforation is most common in the second or third week; its most frequent site is the lower 18 inches of the ileum. As a rule, there is sudden and severe pain involving the entire abdomen, followed by the signs of general peritonitis.

Treatment includes: (1) isolation, (2) proper nursing and disposal of excreta, (3) care of teeth, mouth and skin, and (4) observation for signs of hemorrhage, perforation or other complications. At present it is possible to prevent typhoid and paratyphoid infections by immunizing the patient with vaccines. It is also possible to treat the disease effectively with chloramphenicol, 1 or 2 g. daily for up to 3 weeks. Ampicillin may also be used. After treatment the patient must be observed carefully to see if a carrier state has developed. Most often this is fecal in nature but rarely is urinary in type. Retreatment with chloramphenicol and treatment with large doses of ampicillin or cholecystectomy may result in cure.

(Smallpox and malaria are discussed in Chap. 12, Public Health and Community Medicine. Syphilis is discussed in both Chap. 5, General Microbiology and in Chap. 6, Pathology.)

DISEASES OF THE SKIN

Contact Dermatitis (Dermatitis Venenata)

An acute inflammation of the skin caused by the external application of animal, vegetable or chemical irritants, contact dermatitis is characterized by redness and swelling, frequently by vesicles and bullae, and is accompanied by itching and burning. The lesions are limited at first to the areas of contact but may spread. There is often marked swelling in areas about the eyes and the genitalia.

Common causes are: (1) poison ivy, (2) poison oak, (3) poison sumac, (4) nettles, (5) primrose, (6) lacquer and varnish, (7) dyes and numerous other chemicals met with, especially in industry, as well as (8) phenol, iodine, mercury, sulfur and many other drugs.

Rarely are there systemic symptoms. No internal treatment is required, but the systemic use of steroids may permit continued activity and wage earning during the course of the disease. Avoidance of a known excitant is more important than any medical treatment. Local treatment consists of calamine lotion in mild cases. Analgesics and antipruritics should be applied only with great caution since this form of dermatitis greatly increases the hazard of a local or systemic toxic reaction. The topical use of hydrocortisone or prednisoline is a valuable adjunct for its antiinflammatory and antipruritic effect.

Desensitization for poison ivy may be of value in

protecting against this important offender but *not* during an acute attack.

Dermatitis Medicamentosa

This includes eruptions induced by the internal action of drugs ingested, absorbed through the skin or the mucosa or administered hypodermically. The lesions are not specific but include all lesions from erythema to gangrene. They are usually symmetric. They may appear from hours to weeks after the medicine is taken. The lesions appear suddenly, as a rule, and usually vanish quickly upon withdrawal of the cause. There probably is an underlying hypersensitivity in most cases.

A few drugs produce characteristic lesions. Among them are:

1. Iodides and bromides; acneform pustules
2. Arsenic; "raindrop" pigmentation and palmar and plantar keratoses
3. Arsphenamine: exfoliative dermatitis
4. Silver salts; slate-blue discoloration of the skin
5. Phenolphthalein: lilac-colored blotches (usually "fixed")
6. Serums: urticaria
7. Atropine: scarlatiniform erythema
8. Atabrine: diffuse yellowing of the skin without yellow sclerae
9. Ergot: gangrene of the fingers and toes after prolonged excessive ingestion

Many other drugs may cause dermatitis medicamentosa. The skin lesions most commonly resemble measles, erythema multiforme or urticaria.

Diagnosis is based upon the sudden appearance, symmetric and more or less generalized distribution, history and, as a rule, absence of constitutional disturbances. Treatment depends on identifying and withdrawing the offending substance.

Pediculosis (Louse Infestation)

Pediculosis capitis is commonly limited to the scalp, but occasionally it is seen in the beard and the pubic region. The lesions are those induced by itching and scratching and may result in pustules and crusts. If the lice are not seen, diagnosis depends upon finding the ova (which completely encase the hair, being deposited in a series, away from the scalp).

Pediculosis Corporis. The body louse lodges in the clothing and is seldom found on the body, though occasional ova appear on hairs. The skin lesions consist of a primary puncture wound and secondary excoriations from itching. The clothing should be boiled or baked in an oven at 160 to 175 F.

Pediculosis Pubis. This infestation is ordinarily limited to the pubic regions, though occasionally it is found in the axillae, the eyebrows and the lashes. The louse is firmly attached to the pubic hairs, on which ova may also be found. The lesions result from bites and secondary excoriations and infection from scratching.

Treatment. Lice are destroyed easily with numerous agents, such as sulfur ointment, bichloride or mercury, xylol in petrolatum, and coal oil. However, it must be remembered constantly that each of these agents may produce a serious irritation, especially when applied to areas where the epithelium is thin and the skin is covered with hair and clothing.

Scabies

Scabies is a contagious disorder of the skin produced by *Acarus scabiei,* characterized by intense itching, which occurs chiefly at night, and by multiform lesions.

The characteristic lesion is the burrow produced by the itch mite. The areas involved are the hands, especially between the fingers, the wrists, the axillae, the buttocks and the genital regions. The face is rarely involved.

The burrow resembles a beaded, dotted, yellowish or blackish thread. There is usually a vesicle or pustule at one end. As a result of the itching there are usually papules, pustules, crusts, excoriations and secondary dermatitis.

Treatment with gamma benzene hexachloride is generally effective.

Pityriasis Rosea

Pityriasis rosea is an acute, eruptive disease of unknown cause, characterized by superficial scaling patches of varying size, usually oval, with a pale-red hue and a fawn-colored center, situated chiefly on the trunk. A "herald spot" may antedate the rest of the picture by days to weeks.

The lesions are level with the skin or slightly elevated, and the long axis of each disk corresponds to the lines of cleavage of the skin. The hands and the face generally escape. There may be mild itching. The disease is usually self-limited to a few weeks and requires little or no treatment.

Ringworm (Tinea)

Fungal infections of the skin may be caused by a large number of species of simple fungi. The common forms of tinea may be classified according to their clinical manifestations:

Athlete's foot is the most familiar. There are itching, maceration and crackling and scaling of the skin, especially between the toes. The organism may be spread farther than the toes and involve the instep, where vesicles are not rare. Often the organism produces an allergic response on the hands in the form of multiple vesicles between the fingers or on the palms.

Tinea versicolor gives the picture of multiple slightly scaling, tan macules on the trunk. It is the object of attention only for cosmetic reasons or because it may be mistaken for some more serious ailment.

Tinea of the inguinal and the axillary regions produces a confluent and usually symmetric brownish discoloration of these areas. Usually it is discovered merely by accident.

Deeper tinea infections involve usually the bearded area (tinea barbae) or, in childhood, the scalp (tinea capitis and favosa). There may be plaques or nodules and pustules, which prove difficult to treat even after x-ray epilation.

Treatment. The first three types of tinea are superficial and may respond to topical antifungal agents such as tolnaftate, miconazole, and clotrimazole.

Griseofulvin is an oral antibiotic that is effective in the treatment of fungal infections of the skin. It is highly effective in ringworm of the nails, scalp and skin.

Lichen Planus

Primary lesions of lichen planus are from pinpoint to pinhead in size, polygonal, flat, lilac-colored papules. These are sharply defined and are covered not with a scale but with a thin transparent horny film, giving a waxy appearance. The pinhead-sized papules may become umbilicated but retain their sharply defined polygonal outlines. Larger purplish or reddish areas are formed by the coalescence of these papules, with a characteristic glistening surface. Severe itching is characteristic of the disease (when widespread on the body or hypertrophic on the shins).

The distribution is usually symmetric, with a predilection for the flexor surfaces of the wrists and the forearms and the legs above the ankles. The eruption may appear on only one side of the body and may cover large areas. The face, hands, palms and soles seldom are affected. The cause of the disease is unknown. Frequently, oral mucosa shows reticulate fine white lines, and genital lesions are common. Treatment is difficult.

Psoriasis

Psoriasis is a chronic, benign, inflammatory disease of unknown cause, characterized by reddish-brown flat papules or circumscribed plaques or areas of varying size covered with imbricated silver-white scales. The typical lesions are slightly elevated, sharply defined and covered more or less completely with silvery white or mother-of-pearl-colored scales arranged in thin layers. On removal of the scales, there is a bright red surface with several minute bleeding points. The distribution is usually symmetric and most commonly involves the extensor surfaces of the extremities, the scalp, sacrum, upper chest and abdomen. The hairline of the scalp and the elbows and knees are favorite locations.

There are no systemic symptoms. Itching is usually slight. The general health is not affected.

Psoriatic arthritis, a joint disease practically indistinguishable from rheumatoid arthritis, may accompany the skin manifestation. The terminal interphalangeal joint is commonly involved. The rheumatoid factor is not present in the serum.

Treatment. In mild cases, glucocorticosteroid creams or ointments may help. In more severe involvement, topical coal tar ointments and ultraviolet light may be useful.

Impetigo Contagiosa

This disease is most common in children. It is contagious and is characterized by vesicles, pustules and superficial crusts, usually occurring on the face, ears, neck and hands. There are no subjective symptoms, and the lesions terminate without sequelae.

The early lesion is a flat or erythematous macule or vesicle that rapidly changes into a pustule, drying quickly to leave a superficial crust. The disease is caused by Streptococcus pyogenes distributed by the fingernails.

Treatment with penicillin is indicated.

Discoid Lupus Erythematosus

This is a chronic, sometimes acute, skin disease, characterized by erythematous scaling patches of various sizes and configurations, induce superficial atrophy. The early lesion consists of one or more bean-sized, slightly elevated reddish papules. These do not fade under pressure. They are covered by a grayish, adherent scale. The primary lesion enlarges peripherally to the size of a coin or a saucer. The color is pink to purple, with a red border that is firm to the touch and definitely elevated. The disease is seen most frequently on the face, ears and scalp but may occur anywhere. Often it will spread symmetrically over the nose and the cheeks to produce a butterfly pattern. As the borders advance the centers undergo involution and leave atrophic scars.

The cause of the disease is unknown. Many forms of treatment have been proposed, but none has proved to be consistently reliable. Quinacrine hydrochloride, chloroquine phosphate and hydrochloroquine sulfate have been employed internally with favorable results.

Systemic lupus erythematosus will be discussed later.

Pemphigus

Pemphigus is characterized by the appearance of bullae in successive crops or continuously. The lesions are located in any part of the body, including mucous membranes, and may be localized or widely distributed. The bullae vary in size from that of a split pea to that of a hand and are filled with a serous, seropurulent or hemorrhagic exudate. They often rupture and form crusts, sometimes followed by pigmentation. Sometimes the lesions fail to heal. Constitutional symptoms may be present. The etiology is still unknown, but an autoimmune disease is suspected.

Treatment. Pemphigus is frequently fatal, and the present treatment is only symptomatic and supportive. Steroids, usually in high doses, will control many cases of chronic pemphigus.

Urticaria

Urticaria is characterized by wheals that are rapidly changeable in form, distribution and color. Each crop lasts only a few hours, usually to be replaced by new wheals. The acute type is usually due to ingested food or injection of foreign protein (antitoxin). Among drug causations, penicillin is common. The rare chronic type is of unknown origin. The lesions usually remain small but may coalesce. Itching is severe.

Dermatographism is a common phenomenon. The rapid appearance and disappearance of the lesions, at sites of trauma, are a distinctive feature. Urticaria results from sensitivity to animal or vegetable proteins, certain drugs and insect bites. Treatment includes elimination of the allergen and the use of antihistamine drugs. In severe instances, steroids may be used.

Erythema Multiforme

Erythema multiforme is an acute inflammatory disease characterized by crimson or purplish-red macules, papules or nodules or occasionally by vesicles and bullae. The lesions are isolated or variously grouped and tend to recur. The disease may occur as: (1) an idiopathic eruption of 2 to 4 weeks; (2) a symptom of infection; (3) a skin manifestation of visceral disease; or (4) a reaction to drugs or serums. Like urticaria it is fundamentally due to a specific sensitivity. There is great variation in the shape, size and color of the lesions. Systemic symptoms are mild or absent.

Diagnosis is indicated by the bilateral symmetry, the recurrence of lesions in successive crops, the absence of an external irritant and the brightly colored many-shaped lesions. The iris pattern of the eruption that is present in many cases is very helpful diagnostically. The condition usually clears up spontaneously.

Treatment is the underlying disease or elimination of the causative agent.

Erythema Nodosum and Erythema Induratum

Erythema nodosum and erythema induratum are frequently confused. Erythema nodosum is characterized by the occurrence of painful nodules chiefly on the anterior surfaces of the legs. It is more common in young women. It is associated with Group A streptococcal infections, sarcoidosis, tuberculosis, coccidioidomycosis, histoplasmosis, and oral contraceptive agents. The underlying disease should be treated, and steroids are sometimes useful.

(The skin manifestations of syphilis are reviewed in Chap. 6, Pathology, and the skin manifestations of the common communicable diseases in Chap. 12, Public Health and Community Medicine).

RHEUMATOLOGY AND RELATED DISORDERS

Systemic Lupus Erythematosus

Systemic lupus erythematosus (SLE) is a disease of unknown etiology in which most clinical manifestations are caused by the trapping of antigen-antibody complexes in various small blood vessel systems. The serum of these patients contains many antibodies, collectively termed antinuclear antibodies (ANA); these consist of antibodies to deoxyribonucleic acid (DNA), nucleoprotein and other nuclear components. The immune complexes are deposited in capillaries or the basement membranes of the kidney glomeruli, leading to specific disorders.

SLE is primarily a disease of women and presents most commonly with manifestations of arthritis or arthralgias. In addition, patients may have a variety of abnormalities including skin rash, nephritis, fever, neurologic and psychiatric disorders, Raynaud's phenomenon, pericarditis, pleurisy, hemolytic anemia, leukopenia and thrombocytopenia. The most frequent causes of death are uremia, and lupus cerebritis.

Laboratory confirmation includes positive ANA test, positive LE prep, in 30 to 50 per cent the quite specific antinuclear antibody to double stranded DNA, and immunofluorescent deposits at the junction of dermis and epidermis of normal skin.

The most common form of drug-induced SLE is due to procainamide. Hydralazine, isoniazid and several anticonvulsants (phenytoin and mephenytoin) also cause this disorder. Most symptoms and findings present are similar to those of non-drug-induced SLE with the exception of involvement of the kidneys and brain.

The management of SLE is guided by the degree of activity of the disease as measured by the clinical course, complement levels and amount of DNA antibody present. Aspirin, antimalarials, steroids and cytotoxic agents have been used for therapy with variable results.

Progressive Systemic Sclerosis (Scleroderma)

Progressive systemic sclerosis (PSS) may take a mild form with only sclerodactyly and Raynaud's phenomenon for many years. The disease may be slowly progressive with masklike facies and waxy, smooth fingers. In some cases there is rapid progression with esophageal disease, cardiopulmonary involvement, arthralgias and renal disease. Many patients demonstrate ANA, and some have positive rheumatoid factor. No drug therapy has proven valuable although steroids have improved symptomatology.

Polyarteritis Nodosa

Almost any artery of the body may be involved in classical polyarteritis nodosa, seemingly at random, with the result that the most bizarre series of symptoms may occur on an organic basis. Of all possible manifestations, the combination of renal disease, hypertension and mononeuritis most likely suggests polyarteritis. Occasionally, this disease follows sulfonamide treatment. *Hypersensitivity angiitis* involves smaller vessels especially in the skin and kidney. Steroids may be useful in both conditions. *Wegener's granulomatosis* is a necrotizing arteritis involving the respiratory tract and the kidneys, leading to uremia and death. Cytoxic agents, especially cyclophosphamide have been shown to be beneficial.

Dermatomyositis-Polymyositis

This disease involves the skin and the underlying muscles and is rare. Early in the disease there are pain in the muscles, active inflammation of areas of the skin, discoloration of the affected skin and edema around the eyes. Later in the disease, the skin, especially of the hands and the face, may resemble somewhat that of mild scleroderma. There are also irregularly distributed patches of freckled pigmentation, of depigmentation and of telangiectasia. The muscles are weak and atrophied.

Malignant neoplasm may be associated with a significant number of cases; skin and muscle inflammation improves on removal of the tumor. Steroids and cytotoxic agents may be useful in treatment.

Sjogren's Syndrome

This syndrome consists of dryness of the eyes and mouth and chronic arthritis. It is seen commonly in middle-aged women. The dryness around the eyes and mouth results from lymphocytic infiltration of the lacrimal and salivary glands. This disease should be differentiated from malignant lymphocytic infiltration of the same areas (Mikulicz's syndrome); the treatment is symptomatic.

Mixed Connective Tissue Disease

Some patients, mostly women, have an overlapping of features of SLE, scleroderma, and polymyositis with antinuclear antibody to ribuonuclear protein (RNP). Patients have joint pain, Raynaud's phenomenon. Myositis, impaired esophagel motility, pulmonary disease, splenomegaly. Renal disease is less common than in SLE. Many patients respond to steroids.

ARTHRITIS

The classification of arthritis is difficult. The word arthritis is used to include not only ailments that involve the joint space, its synovial membrane and articular cartilages, but also ailments that affect primarily the adjoining bone, the ligaments and the soft tissues.

The following classification is based so far as possible on etiology:

1. Metabolic arthritis (gout)
2. Traumatic arthritis (acute or chronic)
3. Neurotrophic arthritis (the Charcot joint of tabes dorsalis or syringomyelia)
4. Allergic arthritis (serum sickness)
5. Suppurative arthritis (in which the joint contains pus and the causal organisms—usually various cocci)
6. Arthritis from a hemorrhagic disease (hemophilia or purpura)
7. Chronic rheumatoid arthritis
8. Chronic osteoarthritis

Rheumatoid Arthritis

Rheumatoid arthritis (chronic infectious arthritis; atrophic arthritis; arthritis deformans) includes about two thirds of all chronic arthritides. It occurs twice as often in women as men and at any age; no one is too old to get rheumatoid arthritis. Significant physical impairment occurs in 15 per cent of patients. While an infectious etiology still is disputed, many competent authorities believe that it is an autoimmune disease.

The essential pathology is an inflammation of the synovial membrane, capsule and surrounding soft tissue, leading to destruction of the cartilage, invasion of the capsule and periarticular structure by granulation tissue and ultimately to fibrous or bony ankylosis. The periarthritis is the primary change, and the arthritis is secondary.

In the early stages the condition migrates from joint to joint; most frequently, the knees and the fingers are first involved, although elbows, shoulders, wrists and ankles often suffer early in the disease. The temperature is seldom very high, and the pain is moderate in proportion to the swelling. Still's disease is probably rheumatoid arthritis in children, and Marie-Strumpell disease is a form of rheumatoid arthritis localized in the spine.

In the early stages, x-ray findings may be negative. Later, they may show diminished intraarticular space or even bony contact, with atrophy and rarefaction of the ends of the involved bones.

Secondary anemia, moderate leukocytosis and increased sedimentation rate are common. Cardiac and renal disturbances are unusual.

Present in the serum of these patients is the rheumatoid factor, noted in 70 per cent of cases. Inert particles, such as latex and bentonite or tanned sheep erythrocytes, when coated with human gamma globulin, are agglutinated by rheumatoid serums as a result of this rheumatoid factor.

Treatment includes the following:

1. Rest, especially in early acute stages. However, excessive quiet and immobility lead to ankylosis and muscle atrophy so that a combination of rest and exercise should be adapted to the individual patient.
2. Analgesics. Salicylates are most satisfactory in the dosage necessary to make the patient comfortable. Phenylbutazone is of value, but usually it is no more effective than salicylates, and toxic reactions are frequent.
3. Physiotherapy. Heat, exercise and massage are important in certain stages of the disease.
4. Orthopedic measures to correct deformities in advanced stages.
5. General health. A nutritious diet, especially for those who are underweight, and correction of anemia when present are important.
6. Psychotherapy to counteract the emotional factors inherent in this crippling disease.
7. Gold salts are used for resistant cases and may produce satisfactory remissions in some patients. Toxic reactions are common.
8. Corticosteroids. The synthetic compounds with increased antiinflammatory properties and less effect on electrolyte metabolism are useful. They may be used as the initial treatment (after aspirin).
9. Some patients do better in a warm dry climate.

Degenerative Joint Disease (Osteoarthritis)

The differential diagnosis of the two principal types of chronic arthritis is well illustrated in Table 9-1.

Osteoarthritis is most common in elderly people and appears not to be infectious nor immunological in origin. It is characterized by degenerative changes in the bone and the cartilege, with thickening of the synovial membrane. There are simultaneous bone absorption and production. Most frequently affected are the hip, knee, spine and finger joints. Old age, trauma, overweight, faulty posture and exposure are contributory factors.

An x-ray examination shows characteristic bony lipping and spur formation along the articular margins with erosion in the late stages.

TABLE 9-1. Differential Diagnosis: Rheumatoid Arthritis and Osteoarthritis

	Rheumatoid Arthritis	Osteoarthritis
Average age at onset	Any age	Fifth and sixth decades
Weight	Normal	Usually overweight
Condition of bones	Rarefaction near joints	Condensation of articular margins, with spurs and osteophyte formation
Joints involved	Any joint in body	Chiefly knees, spine and fingers
Appearance of joints	Periarticular swelling	Little swelling
Type	Primarily an inflammation of its soft tissue around the joint with later rarefaction of bone adjoining the joint	Primarily an irregular overgrowth of bone at the joint margin
Special signs	Fusiform finger joints	Heberden's nodes
Streptococcic agglutinins	Often present	Seldom present
Blood count	Secondary anemia and slight leukocytosis	Normal blood count
Sedimentation rate	Considerably accelerated	Normal
Course	Usually progressive	Stationary or slowly progressive
Termination	Ankylosis and deformity (15%)	No ankylosis; usually no deformity

In contrast with rheumatoid arthritis the sedimentation rate is normal.

Treatment includes (1) rest for the affected joint; (2) physiotherapy; (3) orthopedic surgery (when necessary); and (4) weight reduction in the obese patient. Injection of hydrocortisone into the joint sometimes will give temporary relief.

Neither the pain nor the disability is extreme. The patient usually learns to accept his condition as one of the annoyances of advancing years.

Tietze's Syndrome

A costal chondritis of unknown cause, with pain, tenderness and sometimes swelling of one or more costal cartilages. X-ray findings are negative. The pain is accentuated by breathing and coughing and may last for weeks or months.

Gout

Gout is a disease caused by a disturbance of purine metabolism and characterized by severe joint pain, accumulation of sodium biurate with production of hyperuricemia and tophi, and secondary lesions in the kidney. The disease is chronic with acute exacerbations during which the level of uric acid in the blood is elevated, the urates in the urine are increased, and the joint manifestations increase in severity. It is more common in men. The first stage of the disease consists of recurrent attacks of acute gouty arthritis. The joints, frequently of the great toe, become swollen, red and extremely painful. One or several joints may be involved, and the attack may last a few days to a few weeks. Following this, the joints may be painless for several months. The second stage is chronic gouty arthritis, with the acute attacks becoming less severe but more frequent, and with tophi and residual joint changes developing. Early attacks are usually monarticular, but later attacks are polyarticular. In the later stages the joints do not recover completely. The acute episodes develop rapidly. The pain may be extreme; the joint is swollen, tender and red. Edema may develop in the area.

Osseous tophi may be visible on roentgenograms but probably do not depend on the intensity of urate accumulation or on the number of attacks. Areas of erosion may appear in the joints of the hands and the feet.

Acute gouty arthritis is an inflammation of the articular and the periarticular tissues, and relief is obtained from antiinflammatory agents that have no direct effect on urate metabolism. The acute attack of gout occurs when urate crystals within the joint are phagocytosed by leukocytes. Inflammation occurs through the activation of complement or *release* of enzymes from the leukocyte. Colchicine is effective therapeutically by interfering with this mechanism.

Treatment is as follows: Colchicine is used for the acute attacks, with 2 tablets, each containing 0.65 mg., given at the onset and 1 tablet given every 2 hours until gastrointestinal symptoms appear. This is effective if initiated a few hours after the attack. Intravenous administration of colchicine (2 to 3 mg.) may also be extremely useful. Phenylbutazone and indomethacin are valuable in acute gout, particularly in established attacks of 1 to 2 days' duration. Cortisone or prednisone are effective by oral administration if given in large enough dosage. In chronic cases a diet low in purine content is advisable, and probenecid (0.5 to 2 g. daily) may aid in preventing acute attacks by promoting uric acid excretion.

Allopurinol, which inhibits the enzyme xanthine oxidase, thereby blocking uric acid production and reducing both serum and urine urate levels, is an extremely valuable drug for long-term hyperuricemia. The usual dose is 300 mg. daily.

DISEASES OF THE NERVOUS SYSTEM

The Stroke Syndrome

Stroke is a sudden and dramatic onset of focal neurologic impairment due to cerebral vascular disease. It may take a severe form with rapid onset and progress to coma, or it may appear with only minimal neurologic deficits. Stroke may be categorized by course:

1. Transient ischemia attacks (TIA), which last from a few seconds to hours.
2. Stroke in evolution, in which symptoms evolve slowly and intermittently over a period of days.
3. Completed stroke, in which the patient shows partial or complete hemiplegia and alteration of sensorium.

Stroke may result from the following:

1. Ischemic brain disease, usually related to atherosclerosis; (arterial thrombosis; inflammatory arterial disease); hemorrhagic abnormalities (sickle cell disease); cerebral embolism and cerebral venous thrombosis.
2. Hemorrhagic brain disease, due to subarachnoid hemorrhage (from aneurysms, trauma or vascular malformations), hypertensive intracranial bleeding and subdural or epidural hemorrhage.

Sometimes TIAs herald a completed stroke but in many patients are the manifestation of ischemic brain disease. They are related to decreased blood flow and to microemboli from atherosclerotic plaques. Because of their transitory nature they must be differentiated from other focal neurologic signs found in migraine, tumors, arrhythmias and vertigo. Anatomically the lesions may affect the carotid and middle cerebral arteries or the vertebral and basilar artery systems; the former is more favorable for extracranial surgical intervention. Completed stroke is caused by infarction and destruction of brain substance; the extent of symptoms will depend on location and magnitude of the lesion. Increasingly severe vascular headaches or a change in pattern of migraine may precede the occurrence of a stroke. Oral contraceptives have been related to ischemic brain disease in young women.

Specifically, cerebral embolism may occur from heart disease (myocardial infarction, valvular disease, endocarditis, arrhythmias, myxomas), or from ulcerated arterial plaques, as well as air, fat or foreign bodies from instrumentation. Cerebral embolism is probably the cause of over 15 per cent of cerebral infarction; rheumatic heart disease and myocardial infarction are the most common causes of embolism.

Differentiation between embolism and thrombosis is important in regard to therapy and requires angiography. Long-term anticoagulant therapy for embolic TIAs or other causes of cerebral embolism is indicated, particularly before infarction (which may be hemorrhagic) may occur. Endarterectomy may be useful for extracranial disease; aspirin and other platelet aggregation inhibitors, for complete carotid occlusion and vertebrobasilar disease, which are inoperable. Anticoagulation and surgery are useless in completed stroke with infarction; supportive therapy is required.

In hemorrhagic brain disease the prognosis is poorer, the presenting symptoms are severe and the neurologic deficit is large. Primary subarachnoid hemorrhage is usually due to rupture of an aneurysm in the anterior cerebral, anterior communicating, internal carotid, posterior communicating, or middle cerebral areas. Intracerebral hemorrhage is due to hypertensive disease and has a grave prognosis. Treatment consists of reduction of blood pressure and steroid administration. Occasionally, intracerebral hematomas may be evacuated surgically with success.

Hemorrhage, embolism and thrombosis may cause the same picture. Abrupt onset, deep coma and hypertension usually are found with cerebral hemorrhage. Embolism is most often found in younger individuals with bacterial endocarditis and with other evidence of embolic phenomena. Thrombosis should be suspected when hemiplegia comes on gradually without loss of consciousness.

Cerebral angiography is of great value in the differential diagnosis of cerebral vascular lesions and will demonstrate intracranial aneurysms, intracranial clots and occlusion of major vessels distal to the point of injection. It is also of value in distinguishing aneurysms, intracranial tumors and subdural hematomas.

During the acute attack the patient must be treated symptomatically. Later the paralyzed extremities should be treated with massage and passive exercise. Most of these patients must be reeducated to lead a sedentary life.

Epilepsy

Although epilepsy often is diagnosed as a disease, primarily it is a syndrome arising from one of a variety of causes. When a definite cause for seizures is known (as brain injury or tumor), it is termed *symptomatic epilepsy;* when the cause is unknown, it is called *idiopathic epilepsy.* Usually in idiopathic epilepsy the first attack occurs before 20 years of age and practically always before 30.

In about half the cases, grand mal seizures are preceded by a warning, or aura, consisting of sensations often bizarre and usually localized. In other cases there is no warning. The patient falls suddenly, with complete unconsciousness, in a stage of tonic muscular rigidity followed by a stage of clonic muscular jerking. During the attack the patient often injures himself in falling or bites his tongue. Respiration is very stertorous, and loss of sphincter control is common. There is complete amnesia for the seizure, which is followed by deep sleep or sometimes by mental confusion. Status epilepticus consists of a series of rapidly occurring seizures and may end in coma or death.

The clinical evaluation of a patient with epilepsy is based on a careful analysis of the seizure itself and of the immediate postictal state. Epilepsy may be distinguished from hysteria by the signs of previous injuries, complete loss of consciousness and absence of ecstatic attitudes or sounds characteristic of the hysterical seizure. Furthermore, the electroencephalogram usually revels characteristic changes in epilepsy.

Treatment. During the seizure the patient should be protected from injury, and an object should be placed between the teeth to prevent his biting the tongue. No attempt should be made to arouse the patient from the sleep that follows the attack. The activity of the epileptic should be regulated, especially with a view to protecting him from the danger of being involved in industrial or automobile accidents during a seizure. (See Table 9-2 for the typical findings and treatment in the four common forms of epilepsy.)

Brain Tumor

Brain tumor is invariably fatal unless it is removed surgically. Hence, early diagnosis is of the utmost importance. The generic features are (1) headache, (2)

TABLE 9-2. The Four Major Typical* Patterns of Epilepsy

Name	Clinical Pattern	Electroencephalogram	Treatment
1. Grand mal (Generalized: major motor convulsions)	Generalized convulsion	Discharges of rapid spikes	Phenytoin or phenobarbital
2. Petit mal (Generalized: absence attacks)	Momentary simple unconsciousness with amnesia	Slow alternate "spikes and domes"	Ethosuximide
3. Psychomotor (Complex partial seizure)	Sudden series of automatic coordinate activities with amnesia	Slow discharge of "flat-topped waves"	Same as 1. or primidone
4. Jacksonian (Simple partial seizure)	Series of chronic jerks advancing from one point to involve the entire body in regular order	Local point of atypical spike discharges usually found	Same as 1.

* The newer classification is in parentheses.

vomiting and (3) choked discs on ophthalmoscopy. These symptoms suggest merely a space-occupying mass. The localizing features depend on the site of the tumor and may be any of a legion of manifestations. The more frequent are (1) sudden onset of convulsions, (2) visual field defects, (3) unilateral paresis, and (4) behavior disorders, often of a very bizarre pattern. Radioisotopic brain scanning or cerebral angiography is required for diagnosis.

Headache

Migraine refers to periodic, hemicranial, throbbing headaches that begin in early adulthood and occur with increasing frequency as the patient becomes older. They are often preceded by aura, which may be severe neurologic abnormalities (hemianopsia, hemiparesis, aphasia, and hemiparesthetic deficiencies) as well as nausea and vomiting. Symptoms may last for hours or days. In addition, aura may occur even without the headache, and severe headache may occur without preceding aura. Mild cases may be treated with analgesics, but more severe cases should be treated in the neurologic phase with ergot preparations. Cyproheptadine (Periactin) has prophylactic effects as does propranolol.

Muscle-contraction headache is common and is due to tightening of scalp or neck muscles or those involved with chewing; it can be severe or mild, and therapy is directed toward muscle relaxants and toward patient awareness of the situation. *Cluster headaches* occur in men and are nocturnal, retroorbital in nature and accompanied by nasal stuffiness and tearing. Ergot preparations may be useful. Tic douloureux is seen in involvement of the fifth cranial nerve and more rarely in the seventh, ninth and eleventh. Neurosurgery may be needed to control symptoms, but Dilantin and carbamazepine may be successful.

Cranial arteritis is seen in patients who are elderly and manifests itself with severe headache, blindness or field defect, fever and possibly gangrene of the tongue. Elevation of the erythrocyte sedimentation rate and gamma globulin level are seen. Diagnosis is made from temporal artery biopsy, and steroid treatment is effective.

THE DEMYELINATING AND DEGENERATIVE DISEASES

Multiple Sclerosis

Multiple sclerosis is a disseminated disease of the central nervous system characterized by recurrent, patchy demyelination in multiple areas, resulting in widely diversified symptoms, often transient, involving both the sensory and the motor systems. Although the incidence of new cases is low, this disease accounts for much disability; ordinarily the patients live with the disease for many years and die of another cause or from debilitation.

Three features virtually are mandatory for this diagnosis: (1) onset of first symptom between 20 and 40 years of age, (2) multiple sites of involvement of the nervous system and (3) remission and exacerbation of symptoms.

Symptoms may include virtually any dysfunctions of the nervous system *other than persistent pain;* multiple sclerosis is a painless condition. Among the early symptoms noted most frequently are (1) diplopia, (2) disturbed urinary bladder control, (3) numbness in the extremities and (4) disturbed equilibrium. Later in the course of the disease one or more of the following usually develop: (1) spasticity, (2) nystagmus, (3) loss of abdominal reflexes, (4) cerebellar ataxia, and (5) mental or emotional disturbances.

There is no specific increased laboratory test. During exacerbations there may be pleocytosis, increased spinal fluid gamma globulin and first or second zone elevation of the colloidal gold curve. The question of an autoimmune mechanism as the etiologic factor in multiple sclerosis has been raised but not proved. In addition, a "slow" viral etiology has been postulated.

The diagnosis of multiple sclerosis should be made with the greatest caution. Spinal cord tumors, platybasia, cerebellar tumors, porphyria, Guillain-Barré syndrome and many others usually masquerade under the mistaken diagnosis of multiple sclerosis. Only after the systematic elimination of all other possibilities, frequently including utilization of myelography, should the diagnosis be established.

There is no specific therapy, yet much can be done with symptomatic treatment. This is a chronic disease, usually marked by prolonged remissions of months or years. The patients need encouragement and appropriate physical therapy to insure maximum use of preserved functions. A short course of steroid or ACTH therapy may be helpful.

Amyotrophic Lateral Sclerosis

This is the most common form of a group of diseases, including progressive muscular atrophy, progressive bulbar palsy and primary lateral sclerosis, in which there is degeneration of the anterior horn cells, the bulbar motor nuclei and the corticospinal pathways. The cause of the disease is entirely unknown; the principal complaints are weakness and wasting of muscles. The involved muscles show fasciculations, which are spontaneous contractions of groups of muscle fibers that can be felt by the patient and observed as sudden ripples under the skin. The anterior horn cells in the cervical region are usually first affected and lead to wasting and fasciculations in the upper extremities, particularly in the small muscles in the hand. There is preservation of the reflexes in the atrophied muscles, and later spasticity and increased reflexes appear. The characteristic picture of the disease is a combination of diffuse muscle atrophy, fasciculation and retained reflexes in the muscles, with spastic paraparesis of the lower extremities. Sensory changes are absent. the course is progressive, and death usually occurs within 5 years of the onset.

Parkinsonism

Paralysis agitans is a syndrome most often affecting elderly persons. Although the etiology is not well understood, frequently it seems to be a residual of diffuse inflammation within the central nervous system, either infectious or toxic in origin. It is characterized by: (1) muscular hypertonia—"cogwheel rigidity"—without hyperreflexia or other evidence of corticospinal tract involvement and (2) alternating tremor of extremities or head. Though one of these features may be present in much greater degree than the other, almost always both are discernible in some degree. Associated signs and symptoms include (1) stooped posture (generalized flexion), (2) expressionless facies, (3) monoto-

nous speech, (4) short, shuffling steps, and (5) stiffness and slowness of movement (e.g., no arm swing when walking).

Recent findings reveal that there is a high concentration of dopamine in the basal ganglia of the brain and patients dying with parkinsonism have very small amounts of dopamine in the basal ganglia. Present management therefore utilizes levodihydroxyphenylalanine (L-dopa) as a means of relieving signs and symptoms. Further treatment may be given with antihistamine and anticholinergic drugs. For those who do not respond to medication, there may be help in one of the recently developed surgical procedures aimed at destruction of the ansa lenticularis or adjacent basal ganglia.

INFECTIOUS DISORDERS OF THE NERVOUS SYSTEM

Meningitis

Infection of the leptomeninges may be caused by *bacteria*, particularly the meningococcus, the pneumococcus, *Haemophilus influenzae* and *Mycobacterium tuberculosis;* by *viruses* e.g., Echo, Coxsackie, poliomyelitis and mumps; by *fungi,* such as *Actinomyces, Cryptococcus* and *Candida;* and by *spirochetes.* Clinically and pathologically two major groups may be recognized—purulent and nonpurulent meningitis—differentiated primarily on the basis of the number and type of leukocytes found in the spinal fluid. Most of the bacterial meningitides are characterized by a profuse polymorphonuclear response, whereas the tuberculous, viral and mycotic infections are not, mononuclear cells being more typical.

Certain clinical features are generally present; these include (1) stiff neck, (2) headache, (3) fever, and (4) malaise, often with alterations of consciousness varying from irritability to stupor.

Frequently, convulsions are present, especially in infants and small children.

Bacterial meningitis caused by one of the common organisms, such as meningococcus or pneumococcus, produces cloudy spinal fluid with several thousand cells, mostly polymorphonuclear leukocytes, increased protein and low sugar values. Bacteria can be recovered from the spinal fluid or the blood.

Prompt identification of the incitant in bacterial meningitis is indicated so that specific therapy can be carried out. Usually this will be in the form of an antibiotic or a sulfonamide preparation, or combinations. Therapy should be continued until clinical signs have disappeared and the spinal fluid has returned to a normal or a relatively normal level.

Complications include (1) pericarditis, (2) endocarditis, (3) arthritis, (4) pneumonia, (5) pleurisy, (6) empyema, (7) panophthalmitis, (8) epididymitis, (9) peritonitis, (10) adrenal hemorrhage, and (11) otitis media. Hydrocephalus may be a late result of subarachnoid block, particularly in infants.

Tuberculous meningitis deserves special mention because of the difficulties in making an early diagnosis. Usually the cells will be predominantly lymphocytes, the sugar will be low, and organisms may be recovered from the spinal fluid with difficulty. It is important that the treatment be instituted early with isoniazid, ethambutol and streptomycin.

Brain Abscess

Brain abscess is seen in patients with congenital heart disease, lung infections and those taking immunosuppressive drugs who develop lateralizing neurologic signs or focal seizures. Brain scan and EEG are diagnostic. Surgery is the treatment of choice, as well as antibiotics. Subdural empyema occurs most frequently as a complication of frontal sinusitis and resulting osteomyelitis. Evaluation and treatment are similar to those for brain abscess.

Encephalitis

Encephalitis occurs both epidemically and sporadically. The condition has been called sleeping sickness. The etiologic agent may be one of a number of strains of filterable viruses. Specific viruses responsible for encephalitis are as follows: (1) St. Louis type, (2) eastern and western equine types, (3) Japanese B, (4) herpes simplex, (5) Venezuelan type, and (6) others. The brain and the spinal cord show congestion and minute hemorrhages. It is most common in early adult life. Mycoplasma infections can also produce encephalitis with cerebellar ataxia as a prominent symptom.

The symptoms vary greatly, the three most common being headache, lethargy and blurring of vision. The most common abnormal physical signs are: (1) slight bilateral ptosis and (2) ophthalmoplegia, with, sometimes, (3) fine nystagmus; (4) slight facial weakness; (5) signs of meningeal irritation; and (6) mental confusion. The tendon and the abdominal reflexes are diminished, but usually there are no sensory or sphincter disturbances. The lethargy may be constant, or, in some cases, diurnal with nocturnal insomnia or delirium.

The cerebrospinal fluid may be normal, though there are usually 10 to 100 mononuclear cells. The protein often is not increased. Glucose is normal or increased. Gamma globulin may be increased.

Late manifestations were very common and important following the epidemic of 1919–1920 but have been much less conspicuous in recent years. They include (1) derangements of ocular movements, (2) parkinsonism, (3) mental changes, (4) involuntary movements, (5) respiratory disturbances, and (6) lethargy.

Treatment of the acute stage is symptomatic but antiviral agents are becoming available.

Guillain-Barré Syndrome

The Guillain-Barré syndrome may occur as part of an infectious process (infectious mononucleosis) but usually follows a nonspecific respiratory or gastrointestinal infection. It is a form of acute polyneuritis with diffuse weakness of limbs and trunk and associated paresthesias, hypotonia and areflexia. Spinal fluid is acellular and the protein is increased. Treatment is with steroids. A long course of months is common.

Slow Virus Infections

Slow and chronic virus infections are rare but are associated with syndromes of dementia, myoclonus and death in adults (Jakob-Creutzfeldt disease), and a similar picture is seen in children (subacute sclerosing panencephalitis), with high titers of measles antibody and myxovirus found in the brain. No treatment is known for these disorders.

Neurosyphilis

Invasion of the central nervous system by the *Treponema pallidum* is manifested by three types of disorders, depending upon the location of the lesion: (1) meningovascular syphilis, (2) tabes dorsalis, and (3) general paresis. These types overlap and may be combined, as in taboparesis.

Meningovascular syphilis develops within 5 or 6 years of the infection and is characterized by exudative inflammation of the meninges, especially the piaarachnoid, and perivascular infiltration of the cerebral blood vessels.

The symptoms vary with the extent and location of the meningeal and the vascular lesions. Accordingly, meningovascular syphilis may imitate almost any nervous or mental disease. During the first 6 months there may be headache, vertigo and blurred vision, as well as spinal nerve root pains. Occasionally, signs of severe meningitis are also present. The onset may be abrupt, with an epileptiform convulsion. The most serious complication is thrombosis of a large meningeal or cerebral vessel, especially the sylvian and the lenticulostriate arteries, resulting in hemiplegia.

Tabes dorsalis is characterized by degeneration of the posterior column of the cord, the posterior roots and the posterior ganglia.

Either the signs or the symptoms may appear first.

The symptoms are (1) gastric, rectal and other crises, (2) disorders of the sphincters, (3) visual and auditory disturbances, (4) trophic joint degeneration (Charcot), (5) ataxia, and (6) "shooting pains," especially in the lower extremities.

The most important signs are (1) absence of knee and ankle jerks, (2) Romberg's sign, (3) ataxia, (4) Argyll Robertson pupil, (5) loss of sphincter control, (6) Charcot joints, and (7) loss of sense of motion and position of joints.

The tendon reflexes are usually lost before the appearance of symptoms but rarely may persist throughout. The spinal fluid is usually serologically positive before the appearance of marked signs and symptoms.

General paresis is a chronic syphilitic meningoencephalitis characterized by progressive dementia and diffuse, generalized paralysis appearing late in the disease.

Treatment of neurosyphilis depends primarily on appropriate dosages of penicillin. Early detection and treatment of syphilis have decreased the incidence of neurosyphilis.

QUESTIONS IN INTERNAL MEDICINE

CARDIOLOGY

Give a simple method of classifying heart disease.

Describe the most common forms of congenital heart disease and their treatment.

Describe the etiology, the age incidence and the pathology of rheumatic endocarditis.

Name the common extracardiac lesions of rheumatic heart disease.

Give the principal signs and symptoms of congestive heart failure.

Name the frequent precipitating causes of congestive heart failure.

Outline the treatment of congestive heart failure.

Describe the murmur of mitral insufficiency and the mechanism of its production; describe the same for mitral stenosis.

What happens to the presystolic murmur of mitral stenosis if atrial fibrillation intervenes?

Give the etiology signs, symptoms, prognosis and treatment of subacute bacterial endocarditis.

Describe the pathology, symptomatology and diagnosis of cardiovascular syphilis.

Describe the symptoms, diagnosis and treatment of angina and contrast them with those of acute myocardial infarction.

Review the diagnosis and treatment of IHSS and contrast with other cardiomyopathies.

Describe clinical manifestations of cor pulmonale.

What causes are known for hypertension?

What pathologic changes are found in the heart and the arterioles in hypertension?

Describe accelerated hypertension.

Name the principal antihypertensive drugs.

Classify the cardiac arrhythmias and describe the treatment of each.

Name the causes of pericarditis.

HEMATOLOGY

Name the common causes of anemia.

Name and describe an example of each major class of anemia.

Contrast the hereditary hemolytic anemias with acquired hemolytic anemias.

Name the causes of secondary aplastic anemia.

Differentiate primary and secondary polycythemia.

Give the clinical picture and the outstanding pathology of pernicious anemia; describe the gastric contents and the blood picture; outline the treatment of pernicious anemia; explain how the blood picture indicates the response?

Give the clinical picture and the blood findings of chronic myelocytic leukemia; chronic lymphatic leukemia. How are the two differentiated by blood examination; what are their therapy and results?

Describe acute leukemia.

Differentiate infectious mononucleosis from leukemia.

Give the clinical picture, pathology, diagnosis and treatment of Hodgkin's disease.

How is hemophilia transmitted? Give the blood findings and treatment for each syndrome.

Classify the purpuras and their blood pictures. What is the value of splenectomy?

Describe the causation, clinical picture and treatment of agranulocytosis.

Describe the clinical picture of multiple myeloma.

PULMONARY CONDITIONS

Describe the clinical picture of chronic tuberculosis of the lungs.

What are the signs of activity and common complications of tuberculosis?

Discuss the therapy of tuberculosis.

Describe the clinical picture of acute miliary tuberculosis and its treatment.

Discuss the etiology of lobar pneumonia.

Describe the onset and typical symptoms of pneumococcal pneumonia.

What are the common complications of pneumococcal pneumonia?

Describe viral pneumonia.

Discuss the etiology, symptomatology and diagnosis of pulmonary infarct.

Describe of chronic obstructive pulmonary disease.

What is the characteristic respiration of bronchial asthma? Discuss the etiology and treatment.

Name the most common form of pneumoconiosis.

NEPHROLOGY

How do you measure GFR clinically?

List the glomerular syndromes.

What is the nephrotic syndrome?

Describe idiopathic membranous nephropathy.

Discuss lupus nephritis.

What is the natural history of diabetic nephropathy.

Contrast the etiology and course of acute renal failure with chronic renal failure.

Describe the uremic syndrome and outline available treatment.

GASTROENTEROLOGY

Describe the four major diseases of the esophagus.

Discuss the etiology, location, pathology, symptomatology, diagnosis and complications of peptic ulcer.

How is peptic ulcer treated medically?

What are the indications for surgery of peptic ulcer?

Name the causes of the malabsorption syndrome.

Differentiate the two types of chronic inflammatory bowel disease.

Describe the two types of viral hepatitis and discuss the clinical picture of each.

Differentiate three types of jaundice.

Discuss the etiology, pathology and differential diagnosis of cirrhosis.

ENDOCRINOLOGY

Describe thyroid nodules and give reasons for their surgical removal.

Describe the classic symptoms, pathologic physiology, differential diagnosis, laboratory findings and treatment of exophthalmic goiter.

What are the early symptoms of diabetes mellitus?

Discuss the etiologic factors and the pathology of diabetes mellitus and give the common complications.

Discuss the treatment of diabetes mellitus.

Describe the clinical picture, laboratory findings and treatment of diabetic acidosis.

Describe hypothyroidism and its treatment.

Classify hyperadrenalism and the diagnosis and treatment of each category.

What is a prolactinoma?

INFECTIOUS DISEASES

Discuss the incubation period and the infectivity of measles.

Describe Koplik's spots and discuss their diagnostic value; describe the development of the rash.

List the common complications of measles.

Describe the pathology and clinical manifestations of rheumatic fever.

Discuss the diagnosis of diphtheria. What are the principal complications? How is antitoxin used? Discuss prophylactic immunization.

Discuss the etiology, incubation period, infectivity and clinical picture of group A streptococcus infections. What are the common sequelae?

Discuss the treatment of hemolytic streptococcal infection.

Describe the onset, clinical picture, laboratory diagnosis and treatment of typhoid fever.

Discuss the etiology, clinical picture, complications and treatment of erysipelas and wound infections.

Give three examples of opportunistic infections, that is, infections that may develop in a compromised host.

DERMATOLOGY

Differentiate contact dermatitis and dermatitis medicamentosa; give several causes for each condition and describe the treatment.

Describe the typical lesion of scabies and give the treatment.

What are the appearance and distribution of pityriasis rosea?

Describe the appearance and distribution of lichen planus. What is its treatment?

Describe the typical lesion of psoriasis and its distribution.

How is impetigo contagiosa diagnosed and treated?

Describe and differentiate erythema multiforme; erythema nodosum; erythema induratum.

RHEUMATOLOGY

Distinguish rheumatoid arthritis from osteoarthritis pathologically and clinically.

Which laboratory procedures assist in differentiation of rheumatoid and osteoarthritis? How is each condition treated, and what is the prognosis for each?

Describe the immunologic process of systemic lupus erythematosus (SLE).

Name the clinical manifestations of SLE.

What drugs induce SLE?

What is the treatment of SLE?

Describe the clinical picture of progressive systemic sclerosis and differentiate it from dermatomyositis.

What signs and symptoms characterize polyarteritis?
What is Sjogren's syndrome; Mikulicz's syndrome?
What is current therapy for gout?

NEUROLOGY

Describe three types of neurosyphilis.

Discuss the pathology and clinical picture of multiple sclerosis.

Describe the clinical picture of amyotrophic lateral sclerosis.

Describe parkinsonism and discuss its pathology.

Describe epilepsy.

Describe a grand mal epileptic seizure and differentiate it from a hysterical attack.

Differentiate cerebral hemorrhage from cerebral thrombosis and describe the clinical picture of each; give the prognosis and treatment.

What are the etiology and course of transient ischemic attacks?

Contrast the treatment of evolving stroke with completed stroke.

Describe a migraine syndrome.

Describe the clinical picture and diagnosis of cranial arteritis.

Name the causes of bacterial meningitis and review treatment of each.

List the causes of viral encephalitis.

Discuss the clinical picture, laboratory findings and prognosis of tuberculous meningitis.

MULTIPLE CHOICE QUESTIONS

Choose the correct answer. Answers are at the end of this chapter.

1. Mitral valve prolapse:
   (a) occurs equally in men and women
   (b) occurs mostly in women
   (c) is a disease of the aged
   (d) is the end result of rheumatic mitral insufficiency
   (e) is one manifestation of Libman-Sacks disease

2. High blood pressure:
   (a) always needs a thorough search for all possible causes
   (b) never needs a thorough search for all possible causes
   (c) must be treated unless the patient is asymptomatic and is over 40 years of age
   (d) must be treated
   (e) should not be lowered to normal because it may result in renal failure

3. Anemia in women:
   (a) is treated with iron

   (b) is treated with iron and if unresponsive vitamin B_{12} and folic acid are added
   (c) is the autoimmune hemolytic anemia of lupus until proved otherwise
   (d) requires a search for cause
   (e) should not be treated unless the hemoglobin is below 11.5 gm per 100 ml.

4. A 50-year-old man complains of fatigue. History is otherwise negative as is the physical examination. CBC is entirely normal. Urinalysis is normal. The only abnormal finding is a monoclonal IgG gammopathy in the serum. Which statement is correct?
   (a) Bone x-rays and a bone marrow biopsy are indicated.
   (b) The patient has multiple myeloma.
   (c) The patient has a benign monoclonal gammopathy.
   (d) Cytoxan or Alkeran should be started.
   (e) He probably has leukemia and should be followed.

5. A 50-year-old patient previously in good health had sudden onset of right anterior chest pain without chills, fever or cough. On physical examination he was tachypneic and had a temperature of 99.4 F. Over the right lower rib cage there was an inspiratory rub. Chest x-ray was negative. Which statement is correct?
   (a) Viral pneumonia is the most likely diagnosis.
   (b) Pneumococcal pneumonia is most likely and penicillin should be given.
   (c) Pulmonary embolus must be considered promptly.
   (d) Bronchoscopy needs to be done promptly.
   (e) Bronchogenic carcinoma is most likely.

6. Bronchogenic carcinoma:
   (a) may be a largely preventable disease
   (b) has a 50 per cent cure rate
   (c) responds to cytoxan
   (d) is synonymous with "coin" lesion
   (e) responds well to x-rays

7. A 28-year-old woman has the acute onset of oliguria, gross hematuria and nausea and vomiting. On physical examination she has 1+ edema, blood pressure of 180/110. Urinalysis was 3+ protein, red blood cells and red cell casts. BUN is 40 mg. per 100 ml. Which statement is correct?
   (a) She has the nephrotic syndrome.
   (b) She has lupus nephritis.
   (c) She has pyelonephritis.
   (d) She has acute tubular necrosis.
   (e) She has the acute glomerular syndrome.

8. A 50-year-old woman begins to experience fatigue and weakness. Her only past history is severe head-

ache for 20 years. Physical examination reveals a sallow, chronically ill-appearing woman; the remainder of the physical is negative. She is found to have a hemoglobin of 9 gm. per 100 ml. Urine reveals a trace of protein, 10 to 12 white cells and a rare white cell cast. Urine culture is sterile. BUN is 40 mg. per 100 ml. Which statement is correct?

(a) She has chronic glomerulonephritis.

(b) She has lupus.

(c) She has interstitial nephritis, e.g., analgesic abuse, tuberculosis, obstruction.

(d) She has inactive pyelonephritis.

(e) She has multiple myeloma.

9. Which statement is correct?

(a) With cimetadine's availability, antacids have no place in managing peptic ulcer (except in the patient who is allergic to cimetadine).

(b) The indications for peptic ulcer surgery are obstruction, perforation, uncontrolled or recurrent hemorrhage, and intractability.

(c) Everyone with peptic ulcer should have a serum gastrin determination.

(d) Everyone with peptic ulcer should have a parathyroid hormone assay done.

(e) With cimetadine, smoking and alcohol in moderation are less harmful in patients with a peptic ulcer.

10. Which statement is correct?

(a) Crohn's disease never involves the colon.

(b) Ulcerative colitis never involves the small bowel.

(c) Colectomy is good treatment for Crohn's disease.

(d) Cancer of the colon is rare.

(e) Many cancers of the colon can be diagnosed by proctoscopy.

11. Which statement is correct?

(a) An elevated T_4 means hyperthyroidism.

(b) Antithyroid drugs have no place in treatment of hyperthyroidism.

(c) Inorganic iodine should be given to all patients with hyperthyroidism.

(d) Elevation of both T_3 and T_4 generally indicates hyperthyroidism.

(e) Abortion is indicated if hyperthyroidism develops during early pregnancy.

12. Which statement is correct?

(a) Primary hypothyroidism may reverse spontaneously.

(b) Propranolol controls the symptoms in 40 per cent of patients with myxedema.

(c) Myxedema coma is an emergency.

(d) Myxedema is uncommon in an affluent society.

(e) Myxedema is never associated with goiter.

13. Which statement is correct?

(a) SLE is very rare.

(b) Antinuclear antibodies are an almost consistent feature of SLE.

(c) There is no satisfactory treatment of SLE.

(d) Renal involvement with SLE does not respond to treatment.

(e) Arthritis is against true lupus.

14. Which statement is correct?

(a) Gout is rare without hyperuricemia.

(b) Gouty arthritis does not result in crippling.

(c) Gout never occurs in women.

(d) Allopurinol is indicated only after the first uric acid stone is passed.

(e) Hyperuricemia in malignancy does not require treatment.

Answers to Multiple-Choice Questions

1. (b)	**5.** (c)	**9.** (b)	**12.** (c)
2. (d)	**6.** (a)	**10.** (e)	**13.** (b)
3. (d)	**7.** (e)	**11.** (d)	**14.** (a)
4. (a)	**8.** (c)		

10

Obstetrics and Gynecology

ROBERT E. L. NESBITT, JR., M.D.

Chairman and Professor, Department of Obstetrics and Gynecology,
State University of New York, Upstate Medical Center at Syracuse

OBSTETRICS

The word obstetrics is derived from the Latin term *obstetrix,* meaning midwife; it designates that branch of medicine that deals with parturition, its antecedents and its sequelae. The objectives of maternity care set forth by the World Health Organization (WHO) are: to ensure that every expectant and nursing mother maintains good health, learns the art of child care, has a normal delivery, and bears healthy children. In the narrower sense maternity care consists of care of the pregnant woman, her safe delivery, her postnatal examination, the care of her newlyborn infant, and the maintenance of lactation. In the wider sense it begins much earlier in measures aimed to promote the health and well-being of the young people who are potential parents, and to help them to develop the right approach to family life and to the place of the family in the community.

The reduction in maternal mortality over the past half century has been one of the most dramatic and gratifying trends in medicine. Except for two brief periods, the rate has fallen steadily in that time span; maternal mortality has declined from rates of 668.6 per 100,000 live births during the period 1925 to 29, from rates of 245.2 down to 116.6 in the mid 1940s, to the current rate of approximately 15 per 100,000. The maternal mortality rate reflects the quality of obstetric care since studies have shown that up to two-thirds of maternal and between one-third and one-half of perinatal (sum of fetal and neonatal) death rates might have been prevented with modern-day management practices. These same considerations bear upon the likelihood of permanent damage among surviving infants born under adverse circumstances. In addition, these several parameters provide an index of the overall socioeconomic status of the population under study. Despite great overall reduction in maternal mortality in the United States in recent decades, nonwhite populations are still disadvantaged when compared with whites with respect to salvage rates. Currently, maternal mortality rate in the nonwhite population is approximately 34 per 100,000 live births, or about three times that of the white (10.0). The former rate recorded for nonwhite women was achieved in the white population during the mid 1950s. Certain cultural factors and social customs including economic, geographic, and general health considerations create barriers for achieving optimal success in childbearing for all groups. The risk factors tend to be concentrated in a minority segment of the obstetrical population where the socioeconomic standards are lowest.

The many variables relating to higher risks of maternal mortality include such cultural variables as age of marriage, age of first pregnancy, number of children, state of nutrition, degree of health abuse involving adverse drinking, drug and smoking habits, as well as knowledge and cooperation in participating in health care delivery. Despite the considerable progress referred to in reduction in maternal mortality rates, the specific causes of death have remained the same: toxemia, sepsis, and hemorrhage, followed by ectopic pregnancy and abortion. All other causes of maternal death make up little more than one quarter of the cases. In individual health care institutions, notably tertiary care centers, certain causes of death such as heart disease and anesthesia-related deaths may loom relatively larger. The factor of maternal age in relation to the risk of childbearing is particularly noteworthy because aged women tend to be more vulnerable to toxemia (which may be superimposed upon preexisting chronic hypertension), heart disease or chronic cardiovascular disease, as well as for placenta previa and ruptured uterus and postpartal hemorrhage, particularly among those of advanced years who are also highly parous. Past obstetrical history, reflecting on the quality of the reproductive performance in prior pregnancies, is a particularly important prognostic variable for both mother and infant. Traditionally, maternal mortality is lowest at ages 20 to 24, slightly higher under 20 years, and rises dramatically after age 30. Maternal mortality rates triple in women aged 35 to 39 and rise 5 to 10 times higher in the decade of the 40s (10 times after age 45).

Traditionally, it has been customary to attribute the dramatic decreases in maternal mortality to delivery in the hospital and avoidance of traumatic operative procedures, availability of blood, antibiotics, more qualified obstetricians, and effective reviews of maternal deaths at local and state levels. Since 1957, more than 95 per cent of all deliveries in the United States have occurred in hospitals, in contrast with only 37 per cent in 1935. Currently, over 98 per cent of births occur in hospitals, although quite recently interest in alternative birthing options that permit labor and delivery in less formal, homelike, family settings may change that trend. At the same time, the concept of high-risk pregnancy calls for identification of women at risk and provision of increased care, usually by transporting vulnerable mothers to tertiary care centers where there are highly trained personnel and sophisticated resources to handle complex medical problems.

Throughout the 1970s there were rapid developments and changing concepts in medicine generally and in the field of obstetrics and perinatal medicine in particular. Since 1974 the American Board of Obstetrics and Gynecology has awarded a certification signifying special competence in the subspeciality of maternal and fetal medicine. These individuals, with advanced training amounting to two years of postresidency experience, become closely associated with neonatologists and other health professionals who together form the perinatal health care team at regional centers. These combined efforts by professionals with special knowledge of perinatal medicine are beginning to bring about recent reductions in fetal and neonatal death rates that had tended to level off in the 1960s. One of the striking consequences of great capability to sustain the life of immature infants in the nursery, coupled with close liaison between the obstetrician and pediatrician in decision making on timing of delivery, has been the great increase in abdominal delivery during the 1970s. Avoidance of trauma, intervention on a timely planned basis, and extirpation of the fetus from its hostile environment based on objective data gained through continuous fetal monitoring and stress tests, constitute the foundations for these changing attitudes about methods of delivery. Improvement of perinatal and maternal health as a major medical priority has created a sense of direction and a focus for greater effort and prospect for progress. Moreover, recognition that the solution of these health problems necessitates a joint effort of multiple health and health-related agencies, as well as representation by multiple disciplines, has broadened the base of programs directed toward vulnerable groups on a regional basis.

The availability and liberal use of blood probably transcends all other advances in management of hemorrhage and reduction of the risk of maternal death. By the same token, the routine use of ergot preparations and oxytocic agents to improve uterine tone and to minimize postpartal hemorrhage during the past five decades or more has been a significant advance. The availability of an increasing variety of chemotherapeutic agents for specific as well as prophylactic use has made it possible to prevent or control intrapartal or postpartal infections to a large extent. This advance, coupled with strict rules and regulations to establish and maintain appropriate infection-control measures for maternity and newborn services, has caused major reductions in maternal death from infection. A reduction in traumatic obstetrics has resulted in a reduction of maternal and prenatal death from injuries, hemorrhages and sepsis. Increasing safety of cesarean section, so that this operation now can be performed at the optimal time in a variety of medical and obstetric conditions in the best interests of the fetus as well as the mother, has made it possible to spare most women long complicated labors and difficult vaginal deliveries. The status of obstetric anesthesia has improved with respect to choices, techniques and qualified personnel. Moreover, the increasing emphasis on the education of the patient, her emotional support, the use of minimal analgesia and on "physiologic" or "natural" childbirth has minimized the necessity for deep narcosis and general anesthesia and acceptance of the potential risks of such management. The advance of conduction anesthesia, including saddle block and caudal and local pudendal blocks, has added a significant dimension of safety in the conduct of labor and delivery.

The WHO has encouraged uniform reporting practices and the use of standard definitions that can be universally applied. Maternal death is defined as "a woman dying of any cause whatsoever while pregnant or within 90 days of termination of the pregnancy, irrespective of duration of the pregnancy at the time of termination or the method by which it was terminated." When the death results from complications of pregnancy itself, from intervention that is elected or required, or from the chain of events initiated by the complication or the intervention, it is classified as a direct obstetric cause. A death resulting from disease present before or developing during pregnancy that is not a direct effect of the pregnancy, although it may be aggravated by its physiologic effects, is classified as an indirect obstetric cause. There may be a nonrelated cause classification applied to any maternal death in which the fatal condition is totally unrelated to pregnancy, its complications or management. Proper classification is dependent upon accurate and complete record keeping. Traditionally almost one third of all maternal deaths are reported as deaths due to nonobstetric causes. It is customary to group maternal deaths into six major categories as follows: (1) sepsis of pregnancy, childbirth and the puerperium; (2) toxemias of pregnancy and the puerperium; (3) hemorrhage of pregnancy, childbirth and puerperium; (4) abortion without mention of sepsis or toxemia; (5) abortion with sepsis; and (6) other complications of pregnancy, childbirth and the puerperium. Of course, additional subgroup classifications based on specific nature of the disorder, underlying conditions, and stage of pregnancy when death occurred, are applied to provide more clarification.

Unfortunately, vital statistics of the United States are somewhat misleading because maternal deaths associated with maternal heart disease and other coincidental conditions are not included. Moreover, deaths listed by cause based on data derived from certificates are unclassifiable since no specific complication is mentioned in over 40 per cent of the cases. Nevertheless, hemorrhage, toxemias of pregnancy and infection still account for almost 60 per cent of reported maternal deaths in the United States. A direct cause of death such as infection may have a significant predisposing factor such as hemorrhage. Nearly one half of the deaths associated with infection are related to abortion, and most of these are provoked by self-induction or criminal intervention. Recently, liberalized abortion laws in most states, resulting in safer terminations under proper hospital conditions and by qualified personnel, have succeeded in reducing deaths from this cause.

As the mortality rates from toxemia, hemorrhage and infection have decreased, other conditions resulting in maternal deaths have attracted increased clinical attention. Cardiac disease seems destined to become one of the foremost causes of maternal mortality. In some hospitals heart disease already accounts for as much as one quarter of all maternal deaths. Currently, between 10 and 20 per cent of all maternal deaths are considered secondary to vascular catastrophes that may take the form of embolism, hemorrhage or thrombosis. Maternal deaths directly or indirectly related to complications of anesthesia, notably aspiration of vomitus or overdosage of spinal anesthetics, make up a small but important proportion of all deaths related to pregnancy. Acute infectious hepatitis, nonobstetric hypertension, renal diseases, and a variety of other medical disorders loom relatively larger as causes of maternal death as the more traditional obstetric causes are curtailed.

The unfavorable position of the nonwhite group is more marked in maternal mortality than in all but a few nonmaternal causes of death. Moreover, within each geographic division of the United States maternal mortality among nonwhite women is three or four times the rate of loss among white mothers. With respect to cause, the differential between nonwhite and white maternal deaths is fivefold for toxemia, four- to five-fold for abortion (sixfold with sepsis), and eight- to ninefold for ectopic pregnancies.

It is appropriate to consider reproductive losses rather broadly and to recognize that in addition to deaths there will be remote sequelae reflecting damage among surviving infants. The consequences to the mother may be either immediate or remote depending upon the nature and severity of the obstetrical problem. In the United States there are approximately 3 million live births a year, representing an annual "fertility rate" of 66.7 live births per 1000 women of reproductive age and a "birth rate" of 14.8 per 1000 population. Effective family planning practices and methods in the 1970s resulted in a decline in the U.S. birth rate, but the trend has favored white women whose fertility rate is 63.0 compared with 89.2 for nonwhites.

Worldwide, it is estimated that perhaps only about one-third of all conceptions will terminate in a live birth at term by a normal delivery. A pregnancy terminated before 20 weeks of gestational age or passage of a fetus weighing less than 500 gm. is designated an abortion. These may be either spontaneous or induced, either legally (therapeutically) or criminally. Roughly, 10 to 15 per cent of all identified pregnancies are known to terminate by spontaneous abortion. Estimates of the true incidence may be placed much higher, perhaps up to 40 per cent, since many conceptions go unrecognized. The general incidence of chromosomal defects in spontaneous abortion is about 25 to 50 per cent, but the earlier the abortion, the higher will be the incidence of cytogenetic anomalies. The distribution of errors shows that up to one-half take the form of autosomal trisomy whereas about one-quarter exhibit a chromosomal polyploidy, and about one-eighth demonstrate a monosomy for the X chromosome.

A death in utero of a fetus of 20 weeks gestational age or older and/or 500 grams or over in weight is a "fetal" death and the rate is expressed per 1,000 births. The death of a live born infant of any weight within the first 28 days of life is a "neonatal" death and the rate is expressed per 1,000 live births. Some will qualify the definition to exclude any infants of less than 20 weeks gestational age or weighing less than 500 grams (abortions), regardless of any evidence of life at birth. The "perinatal" mortality rate is the sum of the "neonatal" and "fetal" death rates. A special designation is the "immature" birth which represents a pregnancy terminated between 20 weeks and the end of the 27th week and/or the delivery of an infant weighing between 500 grams and 999 grams. Infants of 28 weeks gestational age (up to 36 weeks) or weighing between 1,000 grams and 2500 grams are referred to as "prematures" by the traditional definition. However, these distinctions have less importance at the 28th gestational week since perinatal survival during the immature period is now a realistic potential justifying planned delivery under certain circumstances. Approximately 70 per cent of the neonatal deaths occur in low birth weight infants, which constitutes a rate 20 times higher than in newborns of normal weight. More infant deaths occur in the first 3 days of life than in the remainder of the entire first year. The special vulnerability lies in the risk, first, of respiratory distress, which is the largest cause of concern, but also of importance are intracranial hemorrhage, hypoxia, sepsis, and malformation. Multiple gestation results in a 50 per cent premature birth rate. In addition, to perinatal deaths, there are aftermaths of the birth process and remote sequelae that take the form of anomalies, neurologic deficits, mental retardation, functional disorders, epilepsy, behavioral problems, etc. For example, roughly four or five newborns per 1,000 will exhibit cerebral palsy.

Perinatal results reflect more sensitively upon quality of obstetric care than maternal mortality now that the latter rates have been so dramatically reduced. Some studies show that up to about one-quarter of all pregnancies that come to medical attention end either in fetal death or in the death of an infant during the neonatal period, has a significant anomaly that requires medical care or will interfere with normal functioning, or has a low birth weight that imposes its own special hazards and influences the pattern of growth and development. Women whose last prior pregnancy had a poor outcome are subject to relatively high reproductive loss or damage in subsequent pregnancies, and there is a tendency for the same untoward event to occur.

In recent years the neonatal mortality rate, fetal death rate, and the perinatal mortality rate have fallen substantially. Currently, perinatal mortality rates of about 25 per 1,000 live births are being achieved, and the neonatal segment (roughly 13.0) is not greatly different from the fetal (12.0). There has been about a 20 per cent reduction in these rates in the last decade, which reflects favorably upon perinatal care.

The proportion of fetal deaths among perinatal deaths has remained consistently higher in the black population than among white infants, i.e., 53.6 per cent versus 48.4 per cent. Interestingly, advanced maternal age seems to favor fetal mortality, while young mothers tend to have greater risk of neonatal mortality. In addition to the maternal age factor, many other variables influence outcome; among them, birth order, legitimacy, prior reproductive experience, gestational age, socioeconomic level, birth weight, medical-obstetrical conditions, health care, and nutrition.

Unfortunately, even the most recent studies show that the cause of perinatal death cannot be determined by examination of the mother or infant in about one-quarter of the cases. In another 15 per cent there will be no pathologic findings in the infant but the mother's pregnancy will have been complicated by toxemia, diabetes mellitus, or other diseases. The overall incidence of respiratory distress syndrome now tends to exceed that of placental disease in most studies and so does fetal malformation. Placental disease, complications of labor, and infection are each responsible for 6 to 8 per cent of perinatal deaths. Birth injuries due to trauma are responsible for less than one per cent of the deaths. The incidence of erythroblastosis fetalis, as a cause of death, is similarly low. Meconium aspiration, cord compression, and other conditions give rise to only about 5 per cent of the perinatal deaths as a group.

The infants of young primigravidas are at a greater risk of toxemia; however, in supervised cases, the traditional concern over dystocia should be eliminated by updated monitoring technics. The modern trend of liberalizing abdominal delivery in cases of breech and other malpresentations has likewise reduced the significance of trauma as a cause of perinatal death.

The current practice of evaluating risk factors at the initial prenatal visit and of utilizing a broadly based method of laboratory screening and monitoring, should suffice to identify the patient who is vulnerable for pregnancy and labor.

It is important for the physician to check for and correct significant medical, endocrinologic, metabolic and emotional disorders in women prior to and during their reproductive years, because perinatal problems arise disproportionately and recurrently among vulnerable groups. By so doing, the physician is practicing preventive medicine and at the same time is providing a basis for a continuum of care and supervision throughout the adolescent period and the years of reproduction.

ANATOMY AND PHYSIOLOGY OF FEMALE SEX ORGANS

Pelvis

The upper, or false, pelvis that lies above the linea terminalis has no obstetric significance; it serves merely to support the intestines in the nonpregnant woman and the enlarged uterus in the pregnant state. The linea terminalis forms the boundary between the false pelvis above and the true pelvis below. The true, lower or small, pelvis is intimately concerned in childbirth and defines the shape of the parturient canal. It is tubular and curves slightly anteriorly. The walls of the true pelvis are partly ligamentous and partly bony. The four bones making up the pelvis are: the sacrum, the coccyx and two innominate bones. The innominate bones articulate strongly with the sacrum (sacroiliac synchondroses) and with each other at the symphysis pubis. Anteriorly the pelvis is bounded by the symphysis pubis and posteriorly by the length of the sacrum.

Dimensions.   The entrance (superior strait) and the outlet (inferior strait) of the true pelvis are smaller than the midportion. The roomiest portion of the pelvic cavity (plane of greatest pelvic dimensions) extends from the middle of the posterior surface of the symphysis pubis to the junction of the second and the third sacral vertebrae and laterally passes through the ischial bones over the middle of the acetabulum. Its anteroposterior and transverse diameters measure 12.75 and 12.5 cm. respectively in the normal pelvis. It is customary to delineate also the plane of least pelvic dimensions that extends through the lower margin of the symphysis pubis and the ischial spines. The anteroposterior dimension measures 11.5 cm., while the transverse diameter between the spines (the shortest diameter of the normal pelvic cavity) measures 10.5 cm. The diameters of the plane of the inlet in the normal pelvis are:

1. true conjugate (CV). . . . .   11.0 cm.
2. diagonal conjugate (CD) . . . . . .   12.5 cm.
3. transverse . . . .   13.5 cm.
4. right oblique . . . .   12.75 cm.
5. left oblique . . . .   12.75 cm.

The plane of the outlet passes through the arch and the rami of the pubes, the tuberosities and the tip of the coccyx. Its transverse diameter is 8 to 11 cm., and the anteroposterior diameter, or the distance between the lower border of the symphysis and the tip of the sacrum, is 11.5 cm.

Pelvimetry

External Pelvimetry.   External measurements of the pelvis, as methods of measuring the true pelvis, are of no real value, and these procedures have been eliminated in most obstetric clinics.

Internal Pelvimetry.   The diagonal conjugate, which is measured on the examining hand from the lower border of the symphysis to the promontory of the sacrum, is the most important clinical measurement of the pelvis. The true obstetric conjugate is estimated by subtracting 1.5 cm. from the diagonal conjugate. A diagonal conjugate of 11.5 cm. or more is considered to be normal. The pelvic outlet measurement also is very important (diameter between the ischial tuberosities), and a measurement in excess of 8.0 cm. is normal. The posterior sagittal diameter of the pelvis extends from the midpoint of a line between the ischial tuberosities to the tip of the sacrum. Thoms' rule states that when the sum of the tuber ischii and the posterior sagittal diameters of the outlet exceeds 15 cm., the outlet is considered to be adequate. Clinical estimation of midpelvic capacity is not satisfactory, but these measurements frequently are similar to those of the outlet.

X-ray Pelvimetry.   This possesses certain advantages over manual measurement, as follows: (1) It affords greater precision. (2) It makes possible measurement of certain diameters that cannot be obtained by manual methods. (3) By stereoscopic technique, x-ray pelvimetry permits three-dimensional visualization of the pelvic architecture. (4) Standing films taken in the course of labor yield precise information concerning the presentation, the position, the station and the relative size of the presenting part.

The dose of radiation to the maternal gonads utilizing the usual technics for x-ray pelvimetry is about one to two rads. Even that level of radiation represents potential genetic and oncogenic hazards that restrict the use of x-ray pelvimetry for specific indications. Nevertheless, the more important needs are to measure the anteroposterior and transverse diameters of the inlet, and the anteroposterior, posterior sagittal, and interspinous diameters of the mid-pelvis. Contraction of the transverse diameter of the mid-pelvis is a common problem underlying arrest of progress at the level of the ischial spines. When there are reduced pelvic dimensions or an unusual bony configuration of the pelvis following previous injury or disease, x-ray pelvimetry may be useful. Likewise, malpresentation, notably breech presentation, and unengaged vertex presentation, particularly in a primigravida in labor at term, an excessively sized fetus, or failure to make progress in labor despite normal uterine contractions, represent commonly used indications. However, in many cases, clinical assessments together with a test of labor under careful observation and fetal monitoring will dictate the management of labor and mode of delivery regardless of measurements found on x-ray pelvimetry. In other circumstances, the radiographs merely confirm the presence of an obvious clinical problem that calls for abdominal intervention.

Pelvic Architecture.   There are several types of pelves. Even pelves whose measurements are normal differ greatly in the shape of the inlet, in the proximity of the greatest transverse diameter of the inlet to the sacral promontory, in the size of the sacrosciatic notch, and in their general architecture. These several characteristics have been utilized in the Caldwell-Moloy classification of pelves, as follows:

Gynecoid Pelvis (40 to 45 per cent). This is regarded as the normal female type. Inlet is well rounded in hind pelvis and fore pelvis. Sacrosciatic notch is curved, moderate in width and depth. The bispinous and the bituberous diameters are wide, and the side walls are straight.

Anthropoid Pelvis (20 to 30 per cent). Inlet is deep in hind pelvis and fore pelvis, increased in anteroposterior diameter. Sacrosciatic notch is broad and shallow. The subpubic arch is narrowed.

Platypelloid Pelvis (2 to 5 per cent). Inlet is decreased in anteroposterior diameter. Sacrosciatic notch is curved and small. This is a flat pelvis with wide subpubic angle.

Android Pelvis (25 to 33 per cent). Inlet is wedge shaped with shallow hind pelvis and pointed fore pelvis. Sacrosciatic notch is narrow, deep and pointed. The side walls converge to form the funnel pelvis.

In addition to these pure types, many pelves are of mixed type. The posterior segment determines the type, while the anterior segment may show variations. For example, a gynecoid pelvis may have an android tendency, meaning that the hind pelvis is gynecoid in type and the fore pelvis has characteristics of the android type.

Vagina

The vagina is a musculomembranous tube interposed between the bladder and the rectum and lying in the pelvic floor between the vulva and the uterus. The urethral portion is firmly united to the urethra and the vesicovaginal septum; the vesical portion is loosely attached to the bladder. It is separated above and behind from the rectum by the culde-sac of Douglas. The upper end of the vagina forms a blind vault into which the cervix projects, with its opening looking backward. The vaginal wall consists of three layers: the mucous, the muscular and the connective tissue layers. The mucosa is composed of stratified epithelium, of which the lowest layer is columnar. The submocosa is rich in blood vessels. The sphincter vaginae is a thin layer of voluntary muscle, but for practical purposes the levator ani muscle acts as the sphincter. In the adult the vagina measures 8 to 10 cm. in length. It forms a part of the birth canal at labor, represents the excretory duct of the uterus and is the female organ of copulation.

Uterus

The uterus is a flattened, pear-shaped, hollow, muscular organ, partially covered by peritoneum and lined with mucous membrane. It consists of an upper triangular corpus and a lower cylindrical cervix. The fallopian tubes come off the cornua on either side of the corpus. The adult virgin organ measures 5.5 to 8, 3.5 to 4 and 2 to 2.5 cm. in its greatest vertical, transverse and anteroposterior diameters respectively, as compared with 9 to 9.5, 5.5 to 6 and 3 to 3.5 cm. in multiparous women.

The Cervix.   The *cervix* is the portion that lies below the isthmus and the internal os. Its upper boundary is marked anteriorly by the lowest reflection of the peritoneum. Its intravaginal portion projects into the vaginal fornix and at its tip presents the external os. The cervix is composed of connective tissue containing muscle fibers, some elastic tissue and many vessels. Its mucosa is composed of a single layer of high, narrow, columnar epithelium resting on a thin basement membrane. This epithelium is continued in the lining of the cervical glands, which are branching and racemose. The mucosa covering the vaginal portion of the cervix is directly continuous with that of the vagina and also consists of stratified epithelium.

Pelvic Floor. The pelvic floor creates a resistance that must be overcome in the process of labor before birth can occur. It consists primarily of a strong pelvic diaphragm formed by the levator ani and coccygeus muscles with their fascia, along with a urogenital diaphragm that adds additional strength. The latter is comprised of perineal fasciae, the superficial muscles and the transverse perinei muscles, both superficial and deep, which, together with the fasciae, provide significant support. The endopelvic fascia, which is a continuation of the transversalis fascia of the anterior abdominal wall, is reflected off the pelvic viscera where these organs pierce the pelvic floor. Envelopments of fibrous investments blend with the outer muscular coats of the organs along with other connective tissues to form the ligaments of support. These tubular connective tissue condensations encorporating muscular components give rise to definitive structures. The condensations of tissue on the lateral aspects of the isthmus of the uterus extending to the lateral pelvic wall provide the major support for the uterus and are called the cardinal ligaments. The condensations extending from the posterior aspect of the uterine isthmus to the sacrum are the "uterosacral" ligaments (lateral boundaries of the pouch of Douglas). Attenuation and lateral displacement of these ligaments predispose to the occurrence of a cul de sac herniation in the form of an enterocele. The condensations of fascia between the pubis and urethra give rise to a pubourethral ligament which helps maintain urinary continence through its support to the sphincteric segment. The location of the endopelvic fascia, which forms tightly fitting collars about the several organs, determines its specific designation at the various sites. The fascia between the pubis and cervix is known as the pubocervical fascia; between the bladder and vagina as the vesicovaginal fascia; and between the rectum and the vagina as the rectovaginal fascia. The vesical, uterine and rectal layers become continuous not only with the transversalis fascia from above but also the fascia of the pelvic diaphragm, the iliac fascia, and the obturator fascia.

The *broad ligaments* are two winglike folds of peritoneum that extend from the lateral margins of the uterus to the pelvic walls. The inner two-thirds of the superior margins contain the fallopian tubes, while the lateral third forms the suspensory ligaments of the ovaries and transmits the ovarian vessels. Beneath the fallopian tube the broad ligament contains the parovarium. The parovarium is the remnant of the wolffian duct (Gartner's duct). The caudal portion, called paroophoron, is a vestigial group of mesonephric tubules, which may occasionally give rise to cysts of variable size. Laterally the broad ligament is reflected upon the side of the pelvis. The inferior margin is continuous with the connective tissue of the pelvic floor and transmits the uterine vessels. The uterine end of the broad ligament is triangular, containing uterine vessels in the broad base, with a wide connective tissue attachment adjacent to the cervix called the parametrium. These tissues together with the paravaginal connective tissue provide major uterine support.

The *round ligaments* lie within the broad ligaments on either side and extend from just below the insertion of the tubes in the uterus to the inguinal canal, terminating in the labia majora after coursing through the inguinal canal.

The Body of the Uterus. This is made up of three layers—serous, muscular and mucous. The serous layer is formed by the adherent peritoneum. The peritoneum is nonadherent just above the bladder and laterally where it is deflected to the broad ligaments. Owing to the changes of menstruation, the endometrium varies greatly in thickness, measuring from 0.5 to 3 or 5 mm. It has no submucosa but is attached directly to the musculature. The surface epithelium is composed of a single layer of high, columnar, ciliated cells with a basement membrane and projects below the surface to form large numbers of small, tubular uterine glands. The cilia persist throughout the reproductive era and for some years thereafter, and the current is in the same direction as that of the tubes, namely, from the fimbriated end of the oviducts downward to the external os. The secretory activity of the endometrium is limited to nonciliated cells. The cells in the tubules have the same structure as the surface epithelium and extend down to the muscular layer. Between the glands is a loose stroma of stellate cells with many blood vessels and lymphatics and occasional lymphoid nodules.

The musculature of the uterus is made up of bundles of nonstriated muscle, united by connective tissue containing elastic fibers and richly perforated with blood vessels.

The *blood supply* of the uterus is derived from (1) the uterine artery, which arises from the hypogastric, enters the broad ligament, crosses the ureter and divides into a cervical and a uterine branch; the last divides into fundal, tubal and ovarian branches; (2) the ovarian or internal spermatic artery (a branch of the aorta), which supplies the ovary and, after traversing the broad ligament, anastomoses with the ovarian branch of the uterine artery.

The veins correspond to the arteries and are very abundant. The blood from the ovary and the upper part of the broad ligament collects in the pampiniform plexus; the vessels from this plexus terminate in the ovarian vein. The right ovarian vein empties into the vena cava, while the left empties into the renal vein.

The *lymphatics* of the body of the uterus are distributed to the hypogastric and the lumbar glands; those from the cervix to the hypogastric glands.

Innervation of the uterus is derived principally from the sympathetic nervous system, but partly also from the cerebrospinal and parasympathetic systems. Both systems enter the plexus of Frankenhauser, which consists of ganglia of varying size on either side of the cervix just above the posterior fornix and in front of the rectum. The abundant nerve supply of the uterus appears to be regulatory rather than primary. The sympathetics cause muscular contraction and vasoconstriction, whereas the parasympathetics inhibit contraction and cause vasodilation. Pain from the uterus is carried by sensory fibers in 11th and 12th thoracic nerve roots, and that of the cervix and upper vagina is transmitted through the pelvic nerves to the 2nd, 3rd and 4th sacral nerves. Pain from the lower tract passes through the ilioinguinal and pudendal nerves.

Fallopian Tubes

Each fallopian tube consists of (1) a uterine portion (interstitial), (2) isthmus, (3) ampulla, and (4) infundibulum. It varies in thickness from 2 to 3 mm. at the isthmus to 5 to 8 mm. at the ampulla. Except for the uterine portion, it is entirely enclosed in the peritoneum of the broad ligament. The funnel-shaped fimbriated extermity (infundibulum) opens freely into the abdominal cavity, the fimbria ovarica extending almost to the ovary. It is composed of an inner circular and an outer longitudinal layer and is lined with a single layer of high columnar epithelium resting upon a basement membrane. Cilia occur in patches. The mucosa is arranged in elaborate longitudinal folds resembling a Maltese cross or in complicated treelike folds. Tubal mucosa undergo cyclic histologic changes similar to but less marked than those noted in the endometrium. Spontaneous contractions under the influence of hormones occur, and their greatest frequency and intensity are noted during ova transport at mid cycle. The tubes are richly supplied with elastic tissue, blood vessels and lymphatics.

Ovaries

Each ovary is attached to the broad ligament by the mesovarium and to the uterus by the ovarian ligament. The suspensory ligament of the ovary extends from its upper or tubal pole to the pelvic wall and is really a continuation of the broad ligament, through which the ovarian vessels and the nerves pass. Except for its hilus, the ovary lies freely in the abdominal cavity and is not covered by peritoneum. The size is variable, but usually during the childbearing period the ovary measures about 2.5 to 5.0 cm. in length, 1.5 to 3.0 cm. in breadth and 0.5 to 1.5 cm. in thickness. In later postmenopausal years the ovaries may not exceed 0.5 cm. in diameter.

On cross section the ovary presents an external cortex and an internal medulla, the former containing the ova and the graafian follicles. The outermost portion of the cortex is dull and whitish and is designated tunica albuginea. The surface germinal cuboidal epithelium of Waldeyer forms the outermost layer. The medulla is composed of loose connective tissue continuous with that of the mesovarium. Both sympathetic and parasympathetic nerves supply the ovaries.

Graafian Follicles. Before puberty the graafian follicles are found only in the deeper portions of the cortex. However, later they make their way to the surface, becoming thinner walled and obtaining a larger blood supply. Necrobiosis of the overlying tissues rather than pressure within the follicle gives rise to rupture gradually in an almost bloodless area called the stigma. The whole process of discharge of the ovum along with its zona pellucida and attached follicular cells probably takes only a few minutes. Normally, during each cycle, only one mature follicle makes its way to the surface and discharges its ovum, although this limiting mechanism is unknown.

From the outside inward, the mature graafian follicles consist of (1) a connective tissue covering (theca folliculi); (2) an epithelial lining (membrana granulosa); (3) the ovum; and (4) the liquor folliculi. Just before rupture the ovum separates from the follicular wall as fluid accumulates in the cumulus, and it floats freely in the liquor.

The *theca* is divided into a tunica estrna of ordinary ovarian stroma and a tunica interna of yellow, granular theca lutein cells that play a part in the formation of the corpus luteum.

The *membrana granulosa* consists of a number of layers of small polygonal or cuboidal cells that at one point are massed to form the discus proligerus, in which the ovum is included.

The *follicular fluid* is partly the product of degenerated follicular epithelium and partly a transudate. The fluid is normally clear, albuminous liquor folliculi, which contains the specific internal secetion of the ovary—estrogen.

Ovum. As the ovum approaches maturity, it becomes the largest cell in the body (0.133 to 0.140 mm. in diameter). Primary oocytes, resting in the prophase of their first meiotic division, undergo individual maturation; the process is completed shortly after the release of the egg at ovulation. Usually only one of a group of follicles continues to grow to produce a mature egg, which is extruded at ovulation. Others undergo atresia and develop into irregular hyaline bodies. There is a gradual decline from a mean of 439,000 oocytes in girls under 15 years of age to a mean of 34,000 in women over the age of 36. It is *not* generally accepted that ova are continuously arising from the germinal epithelium throughout maturity.

It is important to recognize some of the essential structures within the mature ovum and in its surroundings. It has an outer enveloping corona radiata; a zona pellucida; a peri vitelline space, which contains the first polar body shortly before ovulation; a small clear zone of protoplasm; a broad, finely granular zone of protoplasm; a central deutoplasmic zone; the nucleus with its germinal spot; and many spheroidal mitochondria. Shortly before ovulation the nucleus achieves a peripheral position and formation of polar bodies begins.

Corpus Luteum. The corpus luteum is formed at the site of a ruptured graafian follicle. When the mature follicle ruptures, the ovum, the liquor folliculi and part of the degenerated membrana granulosa escape, and the walls of the empty follicle collapse. However, in a short time the cavity becomes filled with blood, is rapidly penetrated by proliferating granulosa cells and forms a yellow corpus luteum. In the proliferative stages, strands of so-called K cells of Hertig migrate from the theca to penetrate the membrana granulosa as far as the central coagulum. The peripheral yellow ring enlarges until it almost entirely fills the follicle; this ultimately undergoes hyalinization forming the corpus fibrosum. The mature corpus luteum measures 1 to 3 cm. in diameter (prior to 23rd day of the cycle) and is characteristically bright yellow. The life cycle of the corpus luteum is characterized by stages of proliferation, vascularization, maturity and retrogression; finally, if pregnancy has not occurred, it becomes a fibrosed structure known as a corpus albicans. The active life span of the corpus luteum of menstruation is about 8 days, and thus its secretory function begins to decline some 6 days prior to the next menstruation. In the event of pregnancy, the corpus luteum does not retrogress but becomes even larger, forming the corpus luteum of pregnancy. This structure and its steroid elaborations are necessary for implantation, but there seems to be no critical need for their existence beyond the earliest stages of pregnancy. The early trophoblast appears to secrete sufficient progesterone to sustain the conceptus. Degenerative changes and a diminution in secretion occur in the corpus luteum after the 9th day. Regressive changes take place up to menstruation when the central coagulum has been obliterated by connective tissue and blood pigment has been removed by leukocytes. Thus spaces in the ovary left by the ruptured follicles are obliterated without the formation of scar tissue and progressive gonadal devitalization.

Menstrual Cycle

Menstruation. Menstruation is that part of the menstrual cycle of endometrial changes in which the endometrial lining of the uterus is sloughed off and expelled, together with a discharge of blood. Except during pregnancy and lactation, it normally occurs every 28 days from puberty to the menopause, lasting from 3 to 5 days, though the duration varies considerably. The term cannot be properly applied to anovulatory or dysfunctional bleeding, to the discharge of blood during pregnancy or to that caused by the presence of a neoplasm or some other abnormality.

The menstrual cycle is ordinarily divided into three phases: (1) proliferative, from the 6th to the 14th days; (2) secretory (or progestational or luteal) from the 15th to the 28th days; and (3) menstrual, from the 1st to the 5th days. Although the postovulatory phase of the cycle is usually very close to 14 days, the follicular phase may show normal variations from 7 to 21 days. Changes in the activity of the endocrine glands and response in the uterus are continuous throughout the cycle, and considerable variations in pattern are normally observed. The postovulatory phases can be subdivided according to their histologic features since identifiable characteristics occur on an almost day-to-day basis. These changes have significance clinically since they permit "dating" the endometrium and assessment of sufficiency or insufficiency of progestational development.

Immediately following the menstruation the endometrium is very thin, and during the subsequent week or so, it proliferates markedly. The cells on the surface become taller, while the glands that dip into the endometrium become longer and wider. As the result of these changes the thickness of the endometrium increases sixfold or eightfold. It is during this phase of menstrual cycle (from the 6th to the 14th days) that a graafian follicle each month is approaching its greatest development and is manufacturing increasing amounts of follicular fluid. The estrogenic hormone (estradiol) contained in this fluid causes reorganization, proliferation and growth of the endometrium. It also causes growth of the uterine musculature and sensitizes the myometrium to oxytocic activity. Estrogen stimulates the growth of the spiral arterioles of the endometrium (thus improving blood flow) and induces rhythmic contractions of the fallopian tubes. The estrogenic hormone—in the form of estradiol—is secreted by the maturing follicle and, later, by the corpus luteum. During the preovulatory phase of the cycle, estradiol is produced in increasing quantity.

Following rupture of the graafian follicle (ovulation), between the 13th and the 16th days of the cycle, the cells that form the corpus luteum begin to secrete, in addition to estrogen, another important hormone, progesterone. This supplements the action of estrogen on the endometrium in such a way that the glands become very tortuous or spiral in appearance and greatly dilated. This change is due to the fact that they are swollen with a secretion containing large amounts of glycogen and mucin. Abundant glandular secretion results from the combined action of progesterone and estrogen. Meanwhile, the blood supply of the endometrium is increased, with the result that it becomes very vascular and succulent. Apparently, vascular patterns and physiologic mechanisms observed during the menstrual cycle constitute patterns of behavior and function observable in the myometrium and decidua during pregnancy and are responsible for many vascular and muscular actions and phenomena observed in the gravid state. Similarly, a steroid hormonal milieu underlies these manifestations. Under the influence of progesterone the cervical mucus becomes scanty, viscid, full of leukocytes, unable to form a fern pattern and impermeable to spermatozoa.

Changes in the endometrium are directed at furnishing a bed for a fertilized ovum. Unless the ovum is fertilized, the corpus luteum is short lived, and its activity regresses rapidly after about 8 days (or around the 23rd day of the cycle). This means withdrawal of estrogen and progesterone, the hormones responsible for building up and preparing the endometrium, and the endometrium undergoes a phase of premenstrual ischemia and involution associated finally with vasoconstriction of the coiled arterioles some 4 to 24 hours before the onset of menstrual bleeding. Collapse and desquamation of the superficial layers of the endometrium and both arterial and venous bleeding then occur as constricted vessels relax. There seems to be a well-established sequence of vasoconstriction, relaxation and hemorrhage resulting in a succession of blood extravasations from individual arterioles or capillaries confirming over a variable time. Hemorrhage stops later when the coiled arterioles return to a state of vasoconstriction.

Just prior to puberty the cerebral centers and endocrine tissues reach a critical level of maturity. The central nervous system has a profound effect on the endocrine system and messages are relayed to a specialized part, the hypothalamus, from visual, olfactory and psychological areas. Decoded messages affect the neurohumoral process in the hypothalamus, which is an essential part of the secretion of releasing hormones or factors. For each of the trophic hormones elaborated by the pituitary gland, there is a hypothalamic-releasing hormone; inhibitory factors may also be secreted. Relative to gonadotropins, the hypothalamus secretes a decapeptide-releasing hormone known as leuteinizing hormone-releasing hormone (LHRH) or gonadotropic-releasing hormone (GRH). This hormone has the ability to stimulate the synthesis, as well as the release, of both follicle-stimulating hormone (FSH) and leutinizing hormone (LH) from the pituitary gland. The portal vessels are particularly important in the transmission of the releasing hormones from the hypothalamus to the anterior pituitary. The region of the median eminence and preoptic area of the hypothalamus are the main centers for secretion of LHRH. The preoptic area is the center leading to the cyclic release of LH and FSH necessary for ovulation, whereas the tonic release of both gonadotropins is controlled by the center in the median eminence. The mechanism of neurosecretion in the hypothalamus involves two basic actions. The dominant mechanism under normal conditions involves certain catecholamines that stimulate the secretion of LHRH and prolactin inhibiting factors (PIF). A second mechanism, controlled by a serotoninergic action, will inhibit the gonadotropin secretion and stimulate prolactin secretion. The nature of the latter control mechanism is not as well understood, but at least in animals, there may be gonadotropin-inhibiting activities in the melatonin and serotonin secretions from the pineal gland.

The menstrual cycle is a function of a coordinated, intact hypothalamic-pituitary-ovarian axis. The estradiol signal in the recycling system operates at key moments and plays a critical role in both negative feedback and positive feedback relationships. Thus, the interplay between the ovarian follicle and the hypothalamus represents messages that lead to successful follicular development and triggering of ovulation. First, the negative feedback results in a critical initial rise in FSH during menses. A rapid rise in estradiol at midcycle triggers a surge of LH and ovulation through the positive feedback mechanism. Presumably, the nature of this LH response determines the life span of the corpus luteum; there will be inevitable degeneration unless conception occurs and human chorionic gonadotropin elaborated by the trophoblast emerges as a new luteotrophic stimulus. The latter hormone should become operative at the 8th day after ovulation, which prevents regression. The fourth factor in the scenario is the endometrium, which should have been properly prepared to permit implantation and proper placentation.

If the ovum is fertilized, the first part of the cycle is like that of the normal menstrual cycle, but the collapse of the corpus luteum and the endometrium does not take place. The corpus luteum grows larger and continues its hormonic influence on the endometrium, which becomes the decidua of pregnancy. The integrity and the growth pattern of trophoblast are dependent upon a well-prepared uterus. Extensive ultracytochemical studies have been made of the human endometrial cycle that show that biochemical determinants of intracellular metabolic activity are required to support implantation and early nutrition of the conceptus. Among these are the well-timed appearances of glucose-6-phosphatase around the time of ovulation and early secretory phase and acid phosphatase in the lysosomes of glandular epithelium after the 21st day.

Fertilization of the Ovum. The spermatozoa are carried into the uterine cavity—both by their own motility and by uterine contractions against the ciliary action of the uterus and the tubes. Fertilization usually occurs in the outer third of the tubes, the fertilized ovum normally being carried down the tubes to the uterus, not only by the ciliary current but also by peristalsis of the tubes. The timing of the relaxation that normally occurs at the ampullary-isthmic junction that releases the ovum may be an important factor in transport. Proper synchronization between transport and endometrial preparation is important. Normally the ovum requires 3 to 3½ days to traverse the tube and reach the uterine cavity. The ovum and the sperm undergo a series of changes in the direction of maturation before fertilization occurs. The nuclear events in both oogenesis and spermatogenesis are essentially the same except that, in the former, cytoplasmic division is unequal.

During early embryonic life, the sex cords first break up into distinct clumps of cells, usually by age 6 weeks, and then develop into an organized pattern resulting in primary follicles (16th week), which incorporate germ cells soon to become recognizable as oogonia (7 million by the 20th week). Although most of these undergo atresia, a first meiotic division occurs in many by the time of birth, and at that point these cells, called primary oocytes, number about 1 million. They remain dormant in the prophase until puberty, although by that stage their number has been reduced to about a half million. Ultimately, ovulation consumes less than 500, and fertilization involves only a few.

The first maturation division (meiotic division) results in the formation of a large secondary oocyte and the minute first polar body. The polar body, which has scant cytoplasm, lies between the zona pellucida and the vitelline membrane of the secondary oocyte and is cast off while still in the ovary. Following this process and before the nucleus of the secondary oocyte returns to a resting stage, the second meiotic division begins, which results in the formation of a large mature oocyte and a second polar body. Ovulation occurs as the spindle begins to form in the secondary oocyte. In the second maturation division, the paired chromosomes separate so that half go into the polar body and half remain in the egg or ootid. In every species each individual cell normally has a characteristic number of chromosomes. The set number for the normal human being is 46, consisting of two each of 22 different autosomes in addition to the sex chromosomes X or Y. The constancy of this chromosome number is assured by the process of meiosis. Upon penetration of the vitelline membrane, male and female pronuclei, each with 23 chromosomes, unite to form the segmentation nucleus and restore the original 46 chromosomes. The primary sex ratio is established. Normally, fertilization of an ovum bearing the X chromosome by an X-bearing sperm results in a zygote with the XX constitution. A Y-bearing sperm fertilizing the same ovum would result in a male zygote with the XY constitution. The sex ratio of infants at birth favors the male (106 males to 100 females), and this numerical difference may be even greater at conception. The process of fertilization initiates the sequence of mitotic divisions resulting in cell cleavage and development of the zygote.

Only one of many millions of spermatozoa deposited actually penetrates the ovum, presumably by enzymatic action. Failing to meet a spermatozoon within 24 hours of ovulation, the ovum begins to degenerate. When fertilization does occur, the ovum continues to develop up to the stage of implantation and shedding of the zona pellucida.

Implantation of the Ovum. This usually occurs on the upper part of the anterior or posterior wall of the uterus on about the 6th or 7th day after fertilization. The full decidual response of the endometrium is not elicited until the trophoblast has eroded the superficial uterine epithelium, presumably the result of histamine or histamine-like substances at the site of the blastocyst attachment. The early ovum is covered on all sides by shaggy chorionic villi, but very shortly those villi, which invade the decidua basalias, enlarge and multiply rapidly. This portion of the trophoblast is known as the chorion frondosum (leafy chorion). On the other hand, the chorionic villi covering the remainder of the fetal envelope degenerate and almost disappear, leaving only a slightly roughened membrane. This is called the chorion laeve (bald chorion).

The majority of the villi are aborescent structures whose free endings do not reach the decidua. A certain proportion extend from the chorionic membrane to the underlying decidua, attaching the ovum to it; hence, they are designated as fastening villi. Where the invading trophoblast meets the decidua, there is a zone of fibrinoid degeneration called Nitabuch's layer. An inconstant deposition of fibrin, Rohr's stria, is found at the bottom of the intervillous space surrounding the fastening villi. After day 21 there is progressive proliferation of cellular trophoblast at the tips of the villi, and these columns anchor to the decidual plate to form the floor of the intervillous space. These anchoring villi give rise to proliferating "free" villi within the intervillous spaces; while capillary blood vessels multiply within them. The sprouting, free-floating, tertiary villi become the major surfaces for fetomaternal exchange.

Embedding of the ovum is the work of the trophoblast, which possesses the peculiar enzymatic property of being able to digest or liquefy the tissues with which it comes in contact. In this manner these cells not only burrow into the decidua and eat out a nest for the ovum but also digest the walls of the many small blood vessels that they encounter beneath the surface. Villi penetrate even relatively large maternal vessels, setting free maternal blood to form large placental blood spaces. Trophoblast invades some 40 to 60 spiral arterioles by the 6th week after conception. While the trophoblastic cells invade maternal endometrium and tap maternal blood vessels, the cytoplasmic vacuoles coalesce to form lacunae that rapidly become filled with maternal blood. The ovum finds itself deeply embedded in the decidua with lacunae of blood in its immediate environment. Progesterone, which stimulates blastocystic expansion, may serve as a mechanism for removing CO_2 by augmenting carbonic anhydrase activity. The fetal and the maternal blood systems, the former being developed by the 17th day, are separated only by the trophoblastic epithelium and a delicate layer of mesenchyme. Mitotic figures are noted in the cytotrophoblast, but they are absent in the syncytium. The rapid accumulation of nuclei in the syncytium is probably due to cellular proliferation in the cytotrophoblast followed by coalescence of daughter cells in the syncytium. The nourishment of the fetus is accomplished by the passage of foodstuffs from the maternal blood in the intervillous spaces through the walls of the chorionic villi to the fetal blood, and through the destruction and absorption of parts of the uterine decidua by the trophoblast, which is the parenchyma of the placenta.

Upward pressure from the pulsatile arteriolar spurts at the placental base exerts its force upon free-floating villi, creating a relatively hollow center within tentlike walls made up of closely packed secondary and teritary villi (intervillous space). In effect, each fetal cotyledon is a terminal arterial glomus from which blood spurts and then filters slowly through the surrounding fetal villi into the intervillous space proper. By the 225th day the basal plate is pulled up between major cotyledons by anchoring villi to form septa, and there is continued growth and development of the definitive placenta. The chorionic frondosa contain some 200 primary and anchoring stem villi, although about 150 become functionless. Placental transfer occurs across the placental membrane by simple diffusion, active transport mechanisms and by the passage of whole particles via fluid-filled vacuoles through a phagocytic syncytial process known as pinocytosis. A virtually continuous line of vesicles and vacuoles is present between the suncytial surface and the fetal capillaries.

Placenta

The placenta is the organ through which the embryonic mass is attached to the uterine mucosa and through which the embryo receives its nourishment. Collectively the ancillary organs of the developing conceptus consist of the placenta itself, the chorion, the amnion and vestigial structures representing the allantois and yolk sac. In addition, there is the umbilical cord uniting the placenta with the fetal body. A number of anatomic arrangements or types of placenta are found in mammals to serve as the union between fetal and maternal tissues for purposes of physiologic exchange. When the chorion is vascularized by the allantois or its derivatives, as it is in man, the placentation is referred to as the chorioallantoic type. More specifically, according to the Grosser classification, man's placenta is termed hemochorial, since the trophoblast is directly exposed to maternal blood. Other classifications of the human placenta refer to it as villous because of its villi; deciduate because of maternal decidua, which is shed along with the fetal placenta at birth; and discordal because of its circular shape.

The Chorion.   The chorion arises from a single layer of ectodermal cells forming the wall of the blastodermic vesicle. The wall of the blastocyst, at first entirely smooth, develops polypoid projections known as trophoblastic buds. Initially these are quite solid, but later they are penetrated by a core of mesenchyme to form the early villi. Villi in primitive form are distinguishable as early as the 12th day of development, but it is not until the 14th day that maternal blood enters the intervillous space and the 17th day before both fetal and maternal blood vessels are functioning. Villous structures after in situ angiogenesis are termed tertiary. The embryo is connected with the connective tissue layer of the chorion by the abdominal pedicle, the forerunner of the umbilical cord, and in it the fetal blood vessels develop.

The Amnion. This begins as a small sac covering the dorsal surface of the embryo but eventually enlarges and completely surrounds it, thus lining the interior of the chorion. The two membranes are slightly adherent but are separated readily at the end of pregnancy. The amniotic cavity is filled with amniotic fluid in which the embryo is suspended.

The Decidua. The mucous membrane of the uterus that has undergone certain changes under the influence of the ovulation cycle to fit it for the implantation and the nutrition of the ovum, the decidua is usually divided into (1) the decidua vera that lines the main cavity of the uterus; (2) the decidua basalis beneath the ovum; and (3) the decidua capsularis that surrounds the ovum. However, at the 12th week of pregnancy the growing ovum entirely fills the uterine cavity, so that the capsularis and the vera are brought into intimate contact.

The decidua vera is composed of three layers: (1) a compact surface layer made up of large oval or polygonal cells with large lightly staining vesicular nuclei, (2) a spongy layer of dilated hyperplastic uterine glands, and (3) a zona basalis.

Sexual Differentiation. Genetic or chromosomal sex is determined at the moment of fertilization, but the gonads remain in an indifferent stage until about the 7th embryonic week. At that time, one set of differentiation is stimulated preferentially in response to gonadal development while the other set undergoes atrophy. The Y chromosome carries the testicular inductor in the human fetus. In the absence of the testicular inductor, the indifferent gonad develops as an ovary. Under androgenic influence (testosterone), there will be medullary dominance and midline fusion forming the scrotum and penile shaft; development within the wolffian system gives rise to the seminal vesicles, vas deferens, epididymus, and collecting system in the testicle itself. Without this androgenic influence, there will be a crotical dominance that results in preservation of the müllerian system. Apparently, there are also unidentified organizing substances, but the X chromosome does not appear to possess a counterpart gene opposite to the testis-inducing one in the Y chromosome. There must be two X chromosomes for the ovary to differentiate, since gonadal dysgenesis occurs if the second X is either missing or deformed. The germ cells of XO individuals (45 XO karyotype) reach the gonads in the normal manner, but are apparently lost through some unknown mechanism.

The consensus view about the derivation of the vagina is that the organ develops from the müllerian ducts in its upper four-fifths, and from the epithelium of the urogenital sinus in its lower fifth. The sinus epithelium forms a cord growing upwards to displace, at least in part, the müllerian epithelium craniad and establishes the anlage of the future hollow tube. In the absence of a vaginal mass, the hymen is not formed. Incomplete fusion of the distal portions of the müllerian ducts results in various forms of partial or total duplication of the uterus as well as septation of the vagina. The vagina is the last genital organ to be completed embryologically; masculinizing effects beginning relatively late may result in aberrations in its formation. Development of the external genital system and structures of the hind end are so closely related that isolated anomalies are rare.

PREGNANCY

Physiologic Changes

Water retention is one of the most characteristic biochemical changes in late pregnancy, and this factor, plus retention of sodium caused by steroidal sex hormones, is responsible in part for weight gain. There is a net gain in nitrogen, hyperlipemia, increased plasma insulin, increased maternal requirements for insulin, more rapid destruction of insulin, diminished maternal hypoglycemic effect of insulin and a tendency for oral dextrose tolerance tests to show hyperglycemia for a longer period than in the nonpregnant woman. Consequently, this taxing of the body economy may evoke a diabetic state in pregnancy. Normally the pregnant woman hyperventilates and develops mild respiratory alkalosis (lowered pCO_2). The maternal blood volume may be increased at term by nearly 50 per cent over nonpregnant levels. There is an increase in both the plasma and erythrocytes. (450 ml.). Although the volume of circulating erythrocytes may be increased by 33 per cent or more, there may be a slight decrease in the concentrations of hemoglobin and erythrocytes as well as the hematocrit during the course of pregnancy. There is accelerated production of erythrocytes but not an increase in their life span. A failure to mobilize sufficient iron from body stores during pregnancy will cause the hemoglobin concentration and the hematocrit to decrease as gestation advances. Blood leukocytes range from 5,000 to 12,000 per cu. mm. but in labor the count may rise substantially. Several blood coagulation factors are increased, notably fibrinogen (by 50 per cent) and Factors VII, VIII, IX and X. Arterial blood pressure shows little change. There is reduced blood flow and increased venous pressure in the legs. Glomerular filtration rate and renal plasma flow increase early in pregnancy, the former remaining elevated to term; the latter decreases toward the nonpregnant range during the third trimester. There is an increase in the release of antidiuretic hormone. The supine position and, to a greater extent, the standing position cause reduction in urinary flow, sodium excretion, GFR and RPF. The elevated GFR causes an increase in the clearance of urea, and the blood concentration is somewhat lower during pregnancy. Some dilatation of the ureters and renal pelvis associated with stasis of urine is a natural result of pregnancy. Glycosuria may develop because of the increased GFR without a corresponding increase in tubular reabsorption capacity. The vital capacity and maximum breathing capacity are not significantly altered in pregnancy, but elevation of the diaphragm causes a decrease in the functional residual capacity. The pulmonary compliance is also slightly reduced. There is usually decreased motility of the gastrointestinal tract and prolongation of gastric emptying time in pregnancy. There is a decrease in the A/G ratio, decrease in TSP, increase in serum alkaline phosphatase activity and slight decrease in the capacity of the liver to secrete Bromsulphalein into bile. The basal metabolic rate progressively increases during normal pregnancy to as high as +25 per cent. Protein-bound iodine and BEI rise (2nd month), thyroxine-binding proteins increase, T_3-resin uptake falls, but unbound thyroxine is not increased. There is also an increase in plasma cortisol, transcortin and aldosterone. Virtually all systems are affected and require maternal adjustments, adaptations and compensations to establish normal physiologic functions and proper efficiency within the organism.

Prenatal Care

This term has a wider application than the words imply and may be defined as such supervision and care of the pregnant and parturient woman that will enable her to pass through the dangers of pregnancy and labor with the least possible risk, to give birth to a living child and to be discharged in such a condition that she will be able to nurse it. Women who have demonstrated disproportionate obstetric problems should have the benefit of preconceptional workup and care and interpregnancy supervision, which includes responsible family planning. Every effort should be exerted to identify all risk factors and to program patient management on an individualized basis, as determined by the various adverse factors uncovered and estimates of the level of prenatal vulnerability.

Proper antepartal care requires a preliminary medical and obstetric history and a complete physical examination, including blood pressure, weight, measurement of the pelvis, urinalysis, blood type, Rh deter-

mination, complete blood count and serologic test for syphilis. It is advisable to screen patients for a metabolic disorder by obtaining a 2 hour postprandial blood sugar. Detection of anti-Rh antibodies should be attempted in all Rh-negative patients; the zygosity of the husband should be evaluated. Patients with blood group O should have the husband's blood group determined for possible ABO incompatibility in the fetus. A screen for bacteriuria is helpful, and is mandatory if there is a history of urinary infection or abnormal urine sediment. A check for the presence of glucose in the urine should be made repeatedly during pregnancy and, if present, or if the 2 hour postprandial blood sugar level is borderline or elevated, a glucose tolerance test is indicated. A routine chest roentgenogram (with proper pelvic shielding) is sometimes rewarding as a screening procedure, and such evaluations are mandatory when chest symptoms are present.

The patient should be instructed regarding diet, rest, exercise, bowel habits, bathing, clothing, smoking, alcohol, douches, breast care, coitus, recreation and dental care. She should also be cautioned tactfully about certain danger signals that include vaginal bleeding, however slight; edema; persistent headaches; visual disturbances; pain; persistent vomiting; chills and fever; urinary discomfort; sudden escape of fluid from the vagina; and persistent constipation. Vaginal and cervical smears should be obtained for cancer and hormonal screening. A careful colpocytogram is a screening method that is helpful in giving some indication of the degree of progestational domination and of the likelihood of abortion. A high proportion of cornified karyopyknotic, eosinophilic cells appearing in the smear portends poorly for the pregnancy if this pattern persists. Determination of urinary steroid may also provide valuable information in selected cases.

The normal patient should be seen at least once a month for the first 7 months, then semi-monthly until the last month, when weekly visits are essential to her safety. Patients with particular problems are seen more often during the earlier stages of pregnancy. Any of the standard immunization procedures can be safely administered in pregnancy, including those for poliomyelitis and influenza, and these should be instituted in susceptible women at the time of epidemics.

Patients recognized as being at risk of toxemia should be supervised at intervals beyond the routine. At each visit the blood pressure should be taken and the urine examined carefully, especially for albumin. The patient should be weighed at each visit, since sudden weight gain may be regarded as a sign of oncoming toxemia. Sudden and excessive weight gain may occur as the first warning sign before hypertension, edema and albuminuria develop. Total weight gain in pregnancy for most women in the United States is about

24 pounds, although there is considerable variability. Curtailment of weight gain must not impair the quality of the diet. Moreover, the underweight or malnourished patient must be supported nutritionally to assure an optimal weight gain. The demands of metabolism, fetal growth, uterine growth, breasts, increased blood volume, lactation, etc., require that protein consumption be emphasized, along with adequate intakes of vitamins and minerals. It now seems clear that past emphasis on strict weight control and actual weight loss in pregnancy seems to be at least potentially hazardous and gives rise to low birth weight infants in the extreme. The fact that, at least in animals, the presence of undernutrition causes a reduction in the brain cell number calls for intensified effort to test the effects of nutritional states upon the human fetus. Some available epidemiologic evidence suggests that these same organic brain changes may occur in the human. Nutritional deficits may be either intrinsic or extrinsic in type. Each category may result in fetal growth retardation. Extrinsic causes such as placental vascular insufficiency give rise to asymmetric growth patterns in which the fetal brain is spared while other organs are undergrown. Intrinsic defects caused by maternal malnutrition may give rise to symmetrically retarded growth, including the brain. Both types of conditions obviously present problems in management, but the prognosis is different.

A carefully controlled diet, usually high protein, low fat, low carbohydrate, rest regimens, or even periodic hospitalization for study, rest and control measures, may be required to combat excessive or sudden weight gain and water retention (see section on Toxemia). It should be emphasized that fluid retention manifested as sudden weight gain (particularly in the last trimester) may be a manifestation of toxemia of pregnancy; however, there is no evidence that excessive weight gain predisposes to that complication. The growth pattern of the uterus should be noted at the time of each clinic visit, and any abnormality of shape, size or tone should be noted. The fetal heart beat should be checked regularly after it appears. Supplemental iron therapy is indicated, since most women have marginal iron stores available that are insufficient to meet the increased demands of pregnancy. Calcium and vitamin supplements may be given as indicated. Fluoride administration may be desirable for women not drinking fluoridated water to help reduce dental caries in the offspring. Since the high phosphorus content of milk may depress diffusible serum calcium and lead to muscular tetany, milk ingestion may be restricted and phosphorus-free calcium and vitamin D administered.

Attention is directed to any of the common complaints experienced during pregnancy. These include backache, varicosities, hemorrhoids, heartburn, pica, ptyalism, fatigue, somnolence, headache, leukorrhea, nausea and vomiting, etc. If mild in degree, of temporary duration and unattended by worrisome associated complaints, they are easily treated symptomatically, and the patient is reassured about their nature. Psychosomatic complaints during pregnancy and in the puerperium must be given careful attention, especially when there is a history of emotional problems.

About 2 weeks before term, accurate pelvimetric measurements should be obtained, and the presentation and the size of the fetus should be determined by external and internal palpation; this may also reveal any abnormality of the generative tract. A recheck of hemoglobin is indicated in the last month of pregnancy. A more detailed evaluation is performed, if indicated.

Diagnosis of Pregnancy

The diagnostic criteria of pregnancy may be classified into (1) positive signs; (2) probable signs; and (3) presumptive signs, which naturally vary according to the state of pregnancy. The positive signs of pregnancy are (1) hearing and counting the fetal heart beat; (2) perception of active fetal movements by the examiner; and (3) recognition of the fetal skeleton by x-ray examination. Probable signs of pregnancy include (1) positive pregnancy test; (2) outlining the fetus; (3) ballottement; (4) changes in shape, size and contour of the uterus; (5) enlargement of the abdomen; (6) changes in the cervix; and (7) the detection of intermittent contractions of the uterus. Obviously, numbers 4 to 7 can be encountered occasionally with uterine pathology, such as myomata, which can mimic the changes of pregnancy closely. A variety of presumptive signs may also be noted: (1) cessation of menses, (2) changes in the breasts, (3) nausea and vomiting, (4) quickening, (5) Chadwick's sign, (6) pigmentation of skin and abdominal striae, (7) urinary frequency, and (8) fatigue. Obviously, these latter signs merely require that pregnancy be included in the differential diagnosis.

Laboratory Tests.   Chorionic gonadotropin is produced shortly after implantation and is excreted in the urine. It is readily detectable because of its action on the rodent ovary and on the gonads of various amphibia. A large number of pregnancy tests are based on this fact, namely (1) the Aschheim-Zondek; (2) the Friedman; (3) the Xenopus, or Hogben; and (4) the American male frog, or *Rana pipiens*. Simple, rapid immunologic tests have rendered these cumbersome, expensive, time-consuming tests largely obsolete. An immunodiagnostic pregnancy test has been developed that can be interpreted after 2 hours. The test is based on an antigen-antibody reaction that utilizes human chorionic gonadotropin (hCG) as the antigen and an antiserum obtained from rabbits immunized against hCG. When this antiserum is mixed with erythrocytes sensitized to hCG, the erythrocytes agglutinate. If pregnancy (hCG-positive) urine is mixed with the antiserum, agglutination of the erythrocytes fails to occur, and they settle to the bottom as a brown ring. If the urine is not from a pregnant woman, a diffuse yellow-brown sediment is seen, indicating a negative test. The immunologic test is very sensitive and detects not only chorionic gonadotropin but also pituitary gonadotropin and biologically inactivated gonadotropins. In normal pregnancy the diagnostic accuracy is 95 per cent; in absence of pregnancy, it is about 98.5 per cent accurate. The test is reliable in detecting pregnancy as early as 4 days after the date of the missed period (expected date of menstruation).

A commercially available test, based on inhibition of agglutination, employs polystyrene latex particles coated with a purified preparation of hCG as the antigen and antiserum to hCG. When mixed with test urine on a slide and gently agitated, results are obtained in 2 minutes. Several commercial test kits containing latex particles or red cells that are agglutinated by hCG antibodies are available. Failure of agglutination after adding a woman's urine that contains hCG represents a positive test; it may be sensitive to small amounts, amounting to hCG levels of only 1,000 to 4,000 IU/liter. The tests become positive at 10 to 14 days after the first missed menstrual period.

More recently, it has been possible to separate the alpha and beta subunits of hCG. The availability of antisera to the beta subunit makes it possible to detect hCG in the pregnant woman within a week of conception. A highly sensitive test of this type can be useful in cases of suspected ectopic pregnancy. It has its greatest role in following women with evacuated trophoblastic tumors. The specific assay permits the measurement of minute amounts of hCG in the presence of LH. It should be emphasized that hCG titers below 5 mIU./ml. may overlap with physiological levels of LH with less sensitive tests. It is important to distinguish between the two hormones since the earliest rises denoting malignant disease will not be missed.

Ultimately, the definitive diagnosis will be based on detection of the fetus. It is possible to detect a gestational sac within the uterus from about the sixth week after the last menstrual period up to about 10 to 12 weeks. After about the 13th week, the fetal head should be demonstrable within the uterus by this method of study. Utilizing Doppler techniques, it may be possible to detect a fetal heart beat between the 8th and 10th week after the last menstrual period.

Currently a number of screening tests are available for evaluation of fetal environment and in utero welfare. Adjuvants that help to evaluate fetal jeopardy include serial measurements of levels of certain bio-chemical, enzymatic and endocrine determinants such as diamine oxidase (plasma) and estriol or total estrogen (urinary); human placental lactogen; estrogen/creatinine ratios (urinary and plasma); urinary urea nitrogen total nitrogen ratios (estimate of protein intake sufficiency); and urinary formiminoglutamic acid assay. Amniotic fluid analyses have been very helpful in determining degrees of fetal hemolysis in isoimmunization problems (spectral OD at 450 mμ), in estimating fetal maturity (creatinine, per cent of Nile blue sulfate stain and disappearance of peak in spectral OD at 450 mμ), in determining fetal lung maturity be assessing phospholipids (lecithin/sphingomyelin ratio) and in cytogenetic diagnosis by karyotyping fetal cells grown in culture media. Enzymatic studies capable of discovering in utero many inborn errors of metabolism can be made of amniotic fluid. Assessments of certain endocrine analyses, such as 17-ketosteroids, hold promise of detecting adrenogenital syndromes in utero. Scanning techniques utilizing minimal amounts of radioisotope to locate the placenta focus upon placental locations in disease states and upon in utero therapeutics requiring transuterine injections.

Calculation of Term

On the assumption that labor occurs 280 days from the beginning of the last menstrual period, the date of confinement (EDC) is estimated by adding 7 days to the date of the first day of the last menstrual period and subtracting 3 months (Naegele's rule). This is not accurate, but, other things being equal, usually it proves to be correct within a few days, despite the fact that patients with long cycles ovulate relatively later and pregnancy will terminate at a later date. In approximately 40 per cent of cases, a deviation of 1 to 5 days before or after that date may be expected. In over 3 per cent, labor is delayed 3 or more weeks after the calculated date. Ultrasound techniques can be used for fetal cephalometry, to determine fetal growth, distinguish pathology within and outside the uterus, and diagnose many clinical problems requiring prompt attention. Amnioscopy utilized serially in postdate pregnancy or in situations in which chronic fetal distress is suspected may demonstrate meconium-stained liquor amnii. Amniocentesis may be used in a similar fashion to document the presence of meconium in the fluid.

Test of Fetal Maturity and Intrauterine Status

The various tests available are capable of providing important information about several indices of fetal maturity and intrauterine status. Serial cephalometry and measurements of the anteroposterior diameter of the chest, utilizing the ultrasonic method with measurements extrapolated to term, are techniques capable of achieving accuray in predicting the EDC as well as the additional dividends of detecting retardation of fetal growth and hydrocephalus. Generally, it can be assumed that 90 per cent of fetuses with a biparietal diameter greater than 8.5 cm. weigh more than 2500 grams. Fetal lung maturity may be assessed by determination of the ratio of lecithin to sphingomyelin (L/S ratio). These phospholipids are secreted into the amniotic fluid by type II pulmonary alveolar epithelial cells, and up until about the 35th gestational week these substances appear in approximately equal quantities. After that time, the secretion of lecithin rises abruptly while the sphingomyelin remains the same or gradually declines. Respiratory distress syndrome develops in less than two per cent of newborns when the L/S ratio is greater than 2.0. In the range of 1.5 to 2.0, approximately 40 per cent of infants will suffer this respiratory problem. It should be recognized that a rise in the L/S ratio is accelerated over that noted in normal pregnancy in association with a variety of clinical situations that cause fetal distress. The more important examples include placental insufficiency, hypertensive toxemia, and premature rupture of the membranes.

Ultrasonic diagnosis of intrauterine growth retardation has a clinical accuracy of about 75 per cent. Additional reflections on the status can be determined by obtaining frequent serial determinations of estriol levels. A reduction in values either slowly or abruptly may forecast impending fetal death, although a number of pitfalls need to be understood in interpreting data. One of the most remarkable is the finding of essentially zero levels in association with placental sulfatase deficiency that results in inability to hydrolyze steroid sulfates. Thus, there is no substrate for placental aromatization to produce estriol. The pregnancy and fetal growth and development are normal (usually male infant) although the onset of labor may not occur. Recent findings made possible by real-time sonography are the decline in the frequency of respiratory movements in the presence of fetal distress and the appearance of gasps or apnea just before death. Evaluation of the frequency of fetal movements is important, as is the reactive pattern of fetal heart rate (FHR) to these movements in assessing uteroplacental perfusion and fetal reserve. Between the 32nd and the 40th gestational week, almost all normal fetuses (97 per cent) move more than 10 times in 12 hours. In the presence of infrequent fetal movements and a nonreactive pattern of FHR (no acceleration greater than six beats per minute (or lack of beat-to-beat variables), the fetus may be in jeopardy and the perinatal mortality rate among such infants can be expected to be high.

Diagnosis of Presentation

Presentation is determined by the four maneuvers suggested by Leopold:

1. Palpation of head or breech at fundus
2. Palpation of back and nodular extremities through abdominal wall.
3. Palpation of head or breech between thumb and fingers to determine engagement and degree of flexion
4. Deep pressure toward the superior strait, showing the cephalic prominence on the same side as the small parts in vertex presentations; on the same side as the back in face presentations

The examiner can appreciate the presentation from the data thus obtained.

Ascertainment of position from the fetal heart sounds is of disputed value. In excessively fat patients a roentgenogram of the fetus is of value, or, in other circumstances, a combined vaginal and abdominal examination will be helpful in identifying the presenting part.

PHYSIOLOGY AND CONDUCT OF LABOR

Uterine Contractility

From the first trimester onward the uterus undergoes sporadic, nonrhythmic, painless contractions, the intensity of which is not great until near term, when they account for most cases of false labor. These are so-called Braxton Hicks contractions. The uterus also exhibits low-intensity contractions of great frequency and rhythmic pattern that result from an increasing concentration of actomyosin, the contracile muscle protein, and from changes in steroids and in electrolytes. Theories concerning the cause of the onset of labor include (1) progesterone deprivation, with release of the myometrial block and loss of potassium effect at the placental site, which causes hyperpolarization of the cellular membrane; (2) oxytocin theory—increasing sensitivity of the myometrium to oxytocin; (3) uterine stretch theory—any hollow viscus tends to contract and empty itself when distended to a certain point; (4) the fetal adrenal theory—by providing the placenta with C-19 precursors for estrogen metabolism may give rise to an endocrine milieu that favors the onset of labor. Uterine action in labor, like that of the heart, is under intrinsic nervous control originating either in the muscle itself or in ganglia in the uterine wall; however, pacemaker activity is not nearly so defined in the uterus as in the heart, and there is no known bundle of His. Nevertheless, the dependence of normal labor on rhythmic, coordinated contractions suggests that the bioelectrical physiology is an important feature; Also, (5) the prostaglandin theory—in which these hydroxylated 20-carbon fatty acids widely distributed in mammalian tissues are markedly elevated in both the amniotic fluid and the peripheral blood of spontaneously laboring women (eight-fold increase over nonlaboring women). Smooth muscle contraction requires an elevated level of intracytoplasmic free calcium. An ATP-dependent system binds or releases calcium from the sarcoplasmic reticulum that surrounds the myofibril. Prostaglandins E_2 and F_2 alpha inhibit the calcium binding in pregnancy and in nonpregnant women. The resultant rise in intracytoplasmic levels of calcium would promote myometrial contractility.

The character of labor involves intermittent contraction and relaxation phases, and as labor advances the interval betweeen contractions decreases. At the acme of contractions intrauterine pressures may normally reach 50 mm. Hg or more. Proper uterine contraction requires the interaction of a contractile substance (actomyosin), a supply of energy (adenosine triphosphate), a stimulus to initiate contraction and a means of conducting the stimulus to contractile elements (distribution of ions in the membranes). There must be a so-called fundal dominance and downward gradient of force for progress to be made and cervical dilation to proceed normally.

In normal labor there is a latent phase of several hours' duration, during which the cervix effaces but dilates only slightly. An active phase ensues, with great acceleration in progress when the cervix dilates rapidly and progressively. A deceleration or slowing occurs just prior to full dilatation. Prolongation of any one of these three phases, resulting in protraction of labor, may connote a problem.

Normal Labor

In labor, the irregular painless uterine contractions are replaced by regular uncomfortable ones that bring about cervical effacement and dilatation. Pacemaker activity tends to center in the area of the uterotubal junction but excitation points and propagation of electrical impulses may wander or arise in any group of myometrial cells. Differentiation of pattern normally establishes an upper segment that is actively contractile, and a physiologic retraction ring separates this thick powerful area from the thin, more distensible less active lower segment. Normally, before the onset of labor, the fetal head in most primigravidas has settled into the pelvic brim (often 2 or more weeks earlier), this process of fetal descent of the presenting part is referred to as "lightening." There may be associated ineffectual uterine contractions (false labor pains), but

the process of shortening of the cervical canal is usually begun (effacement of the cervix). With the beginning effacement there may be discharge of the cervical plug along with the passage of a small amount of blood known as "bloody show."

Stages. Labor is divided arbitrarily into three stages:

First stage: from the onset of labor to complete dilatation of the cervix.

Second stage: from complete dilatation of the cervix to the birth of the infant.

Third stage: from the birth of the infant to the delivery of the placenta.

The Mechanism of Labor. This is conditioned by the fact that the greatest diameter of the superior strait is oblique, that the midpelvis is larger and permits turning and that in the inferior strait the greatest diameter is the anteroposterior. It is apparent that some process of accommodation of suitable portions of the fetal head to the various planes is requisite to the satisfactory completion of childbirth. The positional changes of the presenting part constitute the mechanism of labor, and the cardinal movements are listed below:

1. Engagement
2. Descent
3. Flexion
4. Internal rotation
5. Extension
6. External rotation
7. Expulsion

(These seven steps occur in sequence)

Anterior rotation of the occiput is caused by the twisting of the head upon the shoulders as the occiput is directed from an oblique diameter to the long diameter of the pelvic outlet, i.e., the anteroposterior. The occiput turns forward 45 degrees in anterior positions, 90 degrees in transverse and 135 degrees in posterior.

Restitution occurs following the birth of the head, which returns to its original position in relation to the shoulders.

External rotation is due to the anterior rotation of the shoulder girdle to bring the shoulders into the anteroposterior diameter of the outlet. The occiput rotates 45 degrees to the transverse position.

In about 20 per cent of patients, the membranes rupture prior to the onset of labor. Delivery should be accomplished 24 to 48 hours thereafter if the fetus is mature in order to avoid chorioamnionitis. Usually there is no fear of prolapsed cord if the presentation is normal and the fetus is not hypoxic. An effort should be made to establish whether or not the membranes are ruptured by demonstrating fetal epithelial cells in the vaginal fluid, vaginal fluid alkalinity, a treelike crystallization of dried fluid, fat globules, or presence of lanugo hair on a smear. Occasionally, only the chorion will rupture while the amnion remains intact. However, collected fluid between the two layers may be lost in a manner similar to rupture of both membranes. This situation does not predispose to intraamniotic infection.

While solid food is not allowed, oral fluids may be offered in early labor. The patient may walk around until an analgesic is required. Later, a lateral recumbent position may relieve uterine pressure on the vena cava. Vaginal examinations may be made at variable intervals in context with supervision of the frequency, duration and intensity of uterine contractions. Fetal heart rate should be recorded every 15 minutes during the time of contraction; and for a short period afterwards there should be no decelerations below 120 beats per minute or accelerations above 160 beats per minute. Currently, there is enthusiasm for monitoring the fetal heart externally by phonocardiographic or Doppler ausculation through the abdominal wall or internally by electrodes attached to the presenting fetal part. Tokodynametric external monitoring of the uterine contractions or monitoring by an internal intraamniotic transcervical catheter attached to an external transducer are also valuable methods of monitoring the labor. Certainly, all patients with high risk pregnancy, suspected fetal distress, passage of meconium, premature labor, in utero growth retardation, or whose fetal heart is abnormal by evaluation with the stethoscope, should have the benefit of these more objective assessments. Fetal hypoxia resulting in fetal acidosis can be detected by demonstrating an abnormally low pH in capillary blood obtained from the fetal scalp. Values below 7.20 are quite worrisome, particularly if the mother's blood gases are normal and there is an abnormal FHR pattern. Passage of thick meconium and risk of meconium aspiration pneumonia are of further concern.

Bladder care is necessary to avoid distension, hypotonia, and infection. When labor is long, intravenous glucose and possibly electrolyte infusion may be required. If the membranes are intact, amniotomy may expedite a desultory labor and may be used selectively if the presenting part is well engaged. Obviously, appropriate analgesia properly timed and given in proper dosage, may help support the labor in addition to the critical emotional considerations. In the second stage of labor, the patient may be instructed to use her abdominal muscles to assist the uterine expulsive effort. Leg cramps from pressure of the fetal head on the pelvic nerves may be diminished by massage or changing the leg position. The patient should be managed in a controlled manner to prevent injury to the fetal head from sudden decompression with rapid expulsion and to avoid significant laceration of the maternal tissues. There is a gaping of the introitus with each contraction and the perineum may be put under great tension. At this time, there is considerable risk of a perineal laceration. A proper episiotomy may prevent this trauma in many instances. A modified Ritgen maneuver is the proper and simplest procedure to follow.

The fetal neck should be checked for a loop of umbilical cord, since this may be observed in about a quarter of deliveries. The cord should be slipped over the fetal head, if possible, or cut between clamps if it is tight. An unrecognized shoulder dystocia is another potential problem in some cases, if aid is not given to the shoulders by depressing the fetal head gently downward and forward until the anterior shoulder appears beneath the pubis. Gentle assistance may be given to the posterior arm after the head is lifted gradually to bring the posterior shoulder over the perineum. This is another point when perineal lacerations are likely to occur.

After delivery, lowering the infant below the introitus of the mother before cord pulsations cease results in a significant transfer of placental blood into the fetus (equivalent to about 50 mg. of iron). The infant's head should be dependent to allow mucus to drain into the nasopharynx where it can be aspirated. The cord is clamped and cut and the infant is warmed, labelled appropriately, and given a one per cent solution of silver nitrate in each eye in an effort to prevent gonorrheal ophthalmia neonatorum.

Delivery of Placenta. The third stage of labor is made up of two phases, namely, the phase of placental separation and the phase of placental expulsion. The sudden diminution in uterine size after delivery of the fetus is accompanied by a decrease in the area of the placental site. The placenta becomes thickened, buckles on itself and becomes separated in the spongiosa layer of the decidua. In the majority of cases this takes place within a few minutes after the birth of the infant. Expulsion of the placenta, aided by downward pressure on the uterus by the operator's hand, may occur sideways into the vagina with the maternal surface appearing first at the vulva (Duncan mechanism) or, much more commonly, by inversion of the sac with the fetal surface of the placenta presenting at the vulva (Schultze's mechanism). These mechanisms apply only to the behavior of the placenta in the vagina, because the placenta is expelled from the uterus through the flabby lower segment in only one manner. Thus, separation of the placenta is due primarily to a disproportion between the static size of the placenta and the reduced size of the placental site, this disproportion being the natural result of the uterine contraction associated with the birth of the baby. The periphery of the placenta is the most adherent portion and, as a result, separation usually begins elsewhere, commonly with the formation of a hematoma in the decidual cleavage plane. No traction should be put on the umbilical cord because of the risk of inverting the uterus. To aid separation, it is customary to administer 10 units of oxytocin intramuscularly immediately after delivery of the anterior shoulder of the fetus. After delivery of the placenta, an ergot preparation is given to promote uterine tone. The placenta should be examined carefully to see that no remnants are in the uterus.

There is current enthusiasm for manual removal of the palcenta and exploration of the uterine cavity to assure that it is clean and intact, even in the absence of specific indications such as long retention, hemorrhage and retained placental fragments or membranes. However, this practice should be avoided if possible in Rh-negative mothers, to minimize the risk of transfusing the maternal blood sinuses with antigenic Rh-positive fetal red blood cells.

A special comment about "inversion" of the uterus is warranted on the basis of its preventability as well as the seriousness of this complication if it is provoked. Strong traction on the umbilical cord, together with vigorous downward pressure on the uterine fundus in instances when the placenta is firmly attached may result in an inverted uterus, partial placental detachment, hemorrhage, hypovolemia with shock, or, occasionally, acute circulatory collapse. Pushing on the central area of the inverted uterus should be avoided. A smooth muscle-relaxing anesthesia (e.g., halothane) should be employed. The uterus can usually be gradually replaced by digitally pressing upward against the junction of the inverted and uninverted position of the uterus. If the placenta is still attached, it should be manually separated but only after replacement and supportive measures consisting of oxytocin administration, blood replacement as needed, fundal massage, and observations for uterine atony. Only rarely is replacement by the abdominal approach necessary, or is incision of the constriction ring in the neck of the inversion in the posterior midline required.

An interesting phenomenon of the immediate puerperium during its first hour is the occurrence of "postpartal chills" which occur in up to a fourth of patients, particularly those who have had an operative delivery under regional anesthesia. One hypothesis is that the chills represent a fetomaternal transfusion reaction, although the cause has not been established.

Episiotomy

Episiotomy is incision of the perineum prior to delivery of the baby. It serves several purposes. (1) It substi-tutes a straight, clean-cut surgical incision for the ragged, contused laceration that is otherwise likely to ensue; such an incision is easier to repair and heals better than a tear. (2) The direction of the episiotomy can be controlled, whereas a tear may extend in any direction, sometimes involving the anal sphincter and the rectum or the vascular periurethral tissues. (3) It spares the baby's head the necessity of serving as a battering ram against the perineal obstruction. (4) The operation shortens the duration of the second stage and spares the maternal soft parts and the pelvic visceral supports.

Episiotomy may be made in the midline of the perineum (median episiotomy), or it may be begun in the midline and directed obliquely away from the rectum (mediolateral episiotomy). The median episiotomy is more easily repaired, is attended by less bleeding and causes the patient less discomfort; however, median episiotomies are attended more frequently by extensions into the rectal sphincter and mucosa than the mediolateral episiotomies. The choice of the type of incision should be suited to the individual circumstances, although, routinely, the median type is preferred.

Care of the Lacerated Perineum

Perineal tears of the first degree implicate the mucous membranes of the fourchette and the skin and the subcutaneous tissue of the perineum; those of the second degree, the skin of the perineum, the constrictor vaginae and the transversus perinei muscles, and sometimes the levator ani; those of the third degree the sphincter ani muscle and, in addition, the anterior surface of the rectum. Involvement of the rectal mucosa is sometimes referred to as a fourth degree perineal laceration.

In all cases, the immediate closure of perineal lacerations and episiotomies by suture is urgently indicated. If the vagina is lacerated, its edges should be brought together by deeply laid chromic catgut sutures. In complete tears the rectum and its mucosa should be united by buried catgut sutures and the sphincter ani firmly sutured by catgut. The operator must make certain that the lateral halves of the sphincter muscle, which usually are retracted laterally, are approximated in the midline.

Care should be taken to inspect the periurethral region since longitudinal tears in this area can bleed profusely. Blood may pour over the perineum, and the precise location of the laceration may not be immediately apparent. Moreover, unattended tears in this area may be a cause of subsequent descensus of the vesical neck and loss of the posterior urethrovesical angle.

Finally, it has become customary to think in terms

of a fourth stage of labor because bleeding and other problems may be of paramount importance after delivery of the placenta. Sometimes there is atony requiring oxytocins, manual massage, compression or evacuation of the uterus, blood transfusion and attention to the prevention of sepsis. In other circumstances, careful attention to bladder atony and other considerations are paramount. It is important to institute perineal exercises in the postpartal period to help reestablish proper pubococcygeal muscle tone and urinary control.

ANESTHESIA AND ANALGESIA IN LABOR

Pain relief in labor may be of two main types: (1) *obstetric anesthesia* and (2) *obstetric analgesia*. Obstetric anesthesia is the administration of certain drugs at the time of delivery for the purpose of rendering the birth of the baby painless; it is employed chiefly in operative deliveries and is the same as surgical anesthesia. Obstetric analgesia is the administration of certain drugs during the first and second stages for the purpose of lessening the suffering caused by the labor pains prior to the actual birth of the baby. Certain drugs may be used both as anesthetic and analgesic agents, but in that event the dosage and the method of administration are quite different in the two types of pain relief.

The techniques used in obstetric analgesia and anesthesia may be grouped as follows: (1) systemic sedation for labor combined with general inhalation anesthesia for delivery (nitrous oxide, Ethrane, ether, halothane, cyclopropane, ethylene and trichloroethylene); (2) systemic sedation for labor supplemented with intravenous barbiturate anesthesia for delivery (Pentothal sodium, Surital sodium, Seconal sodium and Nembutal); (3) systemic sedation for labor with terminal conduction block of spinal, caudal or local for delivery (Nupercaine, Xylocaine, etc.); (4) continuous conduction analgesia-anesthesia for labor and delivery (usually caudal or lumbar peridural block); and (5) psychoanalgesia for labor and delivery, sometimes supplemented with mild systemic sedation for labor and local pudendal anesthesia for repair of the episiotomy. Of course, inhalation and intravenous anesthesia produce unconsciousness; in spinal, caudal and local infiltration the patient is awake, but sensation has been abolished in the areas concerned. By and large, conduction anesthesia is the most popular, since the effects of fetal narcosis are avoided and the patient is spared the several complications of unconsciousness.

The potential hazards of providing pain relief during labor and delivery for both the mother and fetus call for skilled personnel, adequate safety standards and equipment in the delivery room, and resuscitation capabilities. In the mother the emergency complications may take the form of respiratory obstruction, aspiration of gastric contents, or laryngospasm, hypotension, cardiac arrest, drug overdose or sensitivity reactions. The potential of acute problems calls for a secure indwelling plastic catheter for intravenous fluids and drug administrations, and availability of blood. The possibility of hypoxia, depression and subsequent neurologic disturbances in the newborn requires that analgesics and anesthestics be chosen and administered properly and that the minimum effective dose of drugs be offered on a timely basis with respect to the anticipated delivery.

Appropriate childbirth education should be available to all patients and knowledge about pain relief, various methods, and value in good obstetrical practice should be emphasized. During labor, appropriate analgesia can be provided systemically or by regional sensory blockade. The patient is insensitive to pain in a variable degree but she is awake and responsive and the effect upon the fetus should be minimal. The use of a narcotic (meperidine or alpha prodins) often administered in small intravenous doses with or without a tranquilizer is a popular approach. Since all drugs cross the placenta readily, it is important to minimize fetal depression by choosing the proper drug, dosage, route of administration, and time of use based on peak concentrations. In the major regional blocks such as caudals and epidurals, care must be taken to avoid hypotension by maintaining left uterine displacement and preloading the vascular system with appropriate fluids.

For most spontaneous and low forceps vaginal deliveries, a pudendal block is a very safe, effective anesthetic if intravascular injections are avoided and maximum recommended doses are not exceeded. Subanesthetic inhalant or intravenous analgesia may be added to the local block as the need arises. Nitrous oxide, methoxyflurane and intravenous ketamine are popular agents for this purpose. When a general anesthesia is required for specific indications, care must be taken to evaluate the patient for the possibility of a full stomach and to treat her accordingly. Atropine or scopolamine are used to inhibit secretions. An endotracheal tube is inserted to maintain the airway against laryngospasm and aspiration of vomitus. A balanced form of general anesthesia utilizing thiopental for rapid induction, succinylcholine for muscle relaxation, and nitrous oxide for analgesia represents a suitable choice when administered properly because the fetus is not usually greatly affected. Spinal anesthesia is likewise both popular and safe when proper technics and safeguards are followed to avoid hypotension and excessively high levels. Generally, anesthesia limited to the saddle area will suffice for vaginal deliveries. The drug should not be administered intrathecally during a uterine contraction as a safeguard against high levels of anesthesia and systemic ill effects. Spinal anesthesia would not be the proper method if uterine relaxation were to be required. For that purpose, halothane produces rapid uterine relaxation. By the same token, postpartal hemorrhage from uterine atony becomes a risk with its administration. Unless general medical or obstetrical conditions dictate more special handling, anesthesia for cesarean section can be achieved quite satisfactorily by either the balanced general technique described or by regional anesthesia in the form of a spinal or epidural block. Trained personnel in both anesthesia and the specialized care required in managing patients during the period of recovery should be constantly available.

The effects of hypoxia, narcosis, and trauma may be additive or synergistic insults for the newborn; in selecting proper methods of obstetric management, these several factors must be given consideration if the infant is to be spared severe birth damage. The program of pain relief for the mother must be determined in concert with the maturity and status of the fetus as well as the proposed method of delivery and its prospects for provoking hypoxia and/or trauma.

Systemic Analgesia

The purpose of systemic analgesia is to reduce the discomfort to a tolerable level and to relax the patient enough to permit her to rest or sleep during the pain-free intervals. She should also be cooperative and sufficiently responsive to assist the progress of labor in the second stage. Analgesia should usually not be instituted until labor is well established, and the dosage should be timed properly so that the infant is not born during the period of maximal effect. The patient should be observed constantly during the period of analgesia to prevent injury and to note any irregularities of the fetal heart. Systemic drugs should be given in moderation to patients with term-sized infants and avoided altogether, if possible, when the fetus is immature. Moderate analgesia is feasible in patients who are properly prepared for labor and understand the fundamentals of the physiologic process. Some women are suitable candidates for "natural" childbirth, which usually means that a patient can proceed through labor and delivery with little or no pain relief, but most women seek and deserve assistance in accordance with their particular obstetric and psychologic situation. However, emotional support of the patient is a prerequisite for satisfactory analgesia in all cases. Nevertheless, it should be emphasized that a safe, properly chosen program of analgesia suited to the patient's individual needs allows the obstetrician to conduct a safe, orderly labor and delivery without deleterious effects upon the mother or the fetus. No single method can be used in all women during labor.

The most important complication accompanying the use of systemic analgesics is depression of the infant's respiratory center, and this fact must be kept in mind when selecting a program of management. Demerol has been one of the principal drugs employed for obstetric analgesia. In general, this drug has been used in conjunction with an ataractic or tranquilizing drug, thereby permitting the use of smaller amounts of the narcotic. Barbituric acid derivatives have no analgesic properties and are employed principally to arrest the discomfort associated with false labor. The analgesic potency of Nisentil is less than that of Demerol, but it has the advantage of rapid onset and short duration of action.

Continuous Caudal Anesthesia. At the lower end of the sacrum and on its posterior surface, there is an opening resulting from the nonclosure of the laminae of the last sacral vertebra. It is screened by a thin layer of fibrous tissue. This opening is called the sacral hiatus and leads to a space within the sacrum known as the caudal canal, or caudal space. This space is really the lowermost extent of the bony spinal canal. Through it a rich network of sacral nerves pass downward after they have emerged from the dural sac a few inches above. The dural sac separates the caudal canal, below, from the spinal cord and its surrounding spinal fluid.

By filling the caudal canal with a suitable anesthetic solution, pain sense in the sacral nerves is abolished, and anesthesia of the pelvic region is produced. This is called caudal anesthesia. In continuous caudal analgesia a pliable needle with polyethylene tube attached is inserted through the sacral hiatus and into the caudal space and is left there throughout labor. Then the space is kept continuously filled with anesthetic solution. If the procedure is successful, the patient experiences no pain in labor whatsoever and is conscious neither of uterine contractions nor perineal distention.

Caudal analgesia-anesthesia has certain disadvantages that should be recognized. Hypotension, infection and inadvertent spinal injections are dangers. Uterine tone makes intrauterine manipulations difficult, and since the bearing-down efforts during the second stage of labor are largely eliminated, the forceps delivery rate is increased. Moreover, the procedure requires experienced personnel and adequate hospital facilities.

Maternal Hazards of Anesthesia

Maternal deaths directly or indirectly related to anesthesia make up about 5 to 10 per cent of the total. Complications of obstetric anesthesia are generally regarded as the fifth most common cause, although in certain areas or in isolated studies they may rank higher. There is rather general agreement that aspiration of vomitus with inhalation anesthetics and unusually high anesthetic levels with spinals are the prime offenders. The problem of aspiration can be minimized if food is withheld at the initiation of uterine contractions. The dosage employed in spinal and saddle block anesthesia should be less than that utilized for the nonpregnant patient of comparable size and weight. A test dose designed to rule out intrathecal effects is indicated before injecting a full anesthetic dose into the caudal canal. Other avoidable problems are administration of incompatible drugs, failure to administer proper fluid, electrolyte and blood replacements, failure to maintain a proper airway and failure to recognize serious medical diseases. Certain anesthetics such as halothane (Fluothane) produce marked uterine relaxation with the potential of subsequent postpartal hemorrhage and possibly maternal liver damage. In addition, fetal depression is a significant problem. Probably, such agents should be resticted to clinical situations requiring rapid uterine relaxation.

POSTPARTAL CARE OF THE MOTHER

The uterus should be watched for at least an hour after delivery. If it is not firmly contracted, it should be grasped through the abdominal wall and massaged gently and continuously; Ergotrate or Methergine should be administered intramuscularly immediately after delivery of the placenta to promote uterine tone.

The vulva should be washed with sterile water and soap and covered with a sterile pad held in place by a T bandage. If the abdomen is very fat or flabby, a tight abdominal binder will make the patient more comfortable. Severe after-pains may be treated by .5 grain codeine by mouth. An ice bag applied to the perineum will be comforting and reduce the risk of hematoma. The temperature and the pulse should be taken four times a day, as fever is the first symptom of infection. The patient should be encouraged to urinate within 6 hours, but catheterization should be avoided unless absolutely necessary. Early ambulation is helpful in establishing normal urinary and bowel function. A mild cathartic or enema on the third day may be required. The patient should be instructed about proper toilet of the vulva. The diet should be well balanced, containing 2,500 to 3,000 calories. Under normal conditions salt and fluids need not be restricted.

Before and after each nursing the nipples should be washed with sterile water and soap. Full milk production will be achieved in 10 to 14 days, but the quantity of available milk per feeding will vary with the mother's diet, emotional status, fluid intake, drug intake, and other factors. Encrusted nipples are most likely to become irritated or inflamed. If the nipples

become cracked or painful, they should be treated with compound tincture of benzoin, lanolin or penicillin ointment. The use of a sterile nipple shield is of some assistance. If mastitis develops, nursing must be discontinued, and the breasts should be bound tightly and chemotherapy instituted promptly. If fluctuation is felt, the abscess should be incised surgically, the incisions running from the areolar edge to the periphery to avoid cutting the ducts. If appropriate chemotherapy is administered at the first sign of mastitis, abscess formation almost always can be prevented.

The patient should have blood studies on the third postpartum day, and if her hematocrit was low or borderline before delivery or is subnormal after delivery, appropriate studies are performed to determine the type of anemia, usually iron deficiency, and appropriate therapy is employed. Determinations of serum iron and iron-binding capacity are often required and, occasionally, study of the bone marrow to establish the diagnosis.

Puerperal pain in the perineum, area of the episiotomy, vagina, or perirectal area, or problem voiding with or without visible bleeding sometimes accompanied by shock or subsequent anemia should raise the suspicion of puerperal hematoma. A mass is usually visible or easily palpated if the hematoma is below the pelvic fascia. Unrecognized or traumatic rupture of a vessel above the pelvic fascia may create a proximal paravaginal tumor and spread into the broad ligament and retroperitoneally in any direction. There may be a presentation above the inguinal ligament or the hematoma may rupture into the peritoneal cavity. Painful and expanding hematomas of a moderate to large size must be incised, drained, and vessels sought out and ligated. Packing may be required and blood replacement, as well as antibiotic coverage, are essential aspects of management. Recently, circumferential pneumatic compression provided by means of an anti-gravity-type suit has been employed with success in the control of markedly expanding intrapelvic hematomas. Pain, fever, and unexplained shock or anemia or considerable bladder or rectal pressure occurring in the puerperal period calls for an immediate search for this possible underlying cause.

If the patient does not nurse her infant, the breasts should be bound, and ice bags and sedation employed as necessary. A natural or synthetic estrogenic or androgenic hormone can be used to suppress lactation. Most normal women can be safely discharged from the hospital by the fourth postpartal day.

The puerperium is the period of six weeks between the termination of labor and the return of the generative tract to its normal condition, which includes involution of the uterus and placental site, as well as general adaptations involving the breasts, urinary tract, lower generative tract, abdominal wall and peritoneum. In the absence of nursing, menses may resume within 6 to 8 weeks, and, by 3 months, roughly 90 per cent will have had the return of menstruation. It is not unusual for women to have a brownish discharge with even occasional spurts of blood in minimal quantities for several weeks, but usually there is lochia alba after 2 weeks. Complete involution and normal recovery should be assured by a 6-week postpartal checkup. In addition to the history and careful examination, the urine should be checked and a smear should be taken for cytologic study. Follow-up of any abnormal findings noted during pregnancy should be undertaken; e.g., glucose tolerance test, CBC, cardiovascular renal studies. Evidence of cervicitis should be corrected.

Family planning advice and implementation should be offered as desired. These include the rhythm method, spermicidal creams and foams, vaginal diaphragms, but, for the most part, choices today lie between oral contraceptives and application of an intrauterine device (IUD). The choice of method must be suited to the individual case after appropriate evaluation and discussion with the patient and her husband. In general, orally ingested steroids surpass all other methods in efficacy and generally may be slightly superior to the IUD. Other methods and techniques are now under extensive study and hold promise for the future. Ethinyl estradiol and stilbestrol have been used as a "morning-after" pill, but this is a misnomer since either drug is given in high dosage for 5 days. Apparently, their effectiveness is based on the disruption of the synchrony of endometrial maturation. Implanted steroid deposits hold forth some promise as a contraceptive control technique, and, ultimately, the use of antireleasing factor substances may be a method of choice if current trials prove successful. It must be kept in mind that regardless of method, responsible family planning and "wanted" pregnancies are indispensable prerequisites for achieving optimal prerinatal results.

PATHOLOGY OF PREGNANCY

Abortion

Abortion is the termination of pregnancy before the fetus is viable (20 weeks), that is, before it is capable of extrauterine existence. When pregnancy terminates after 20 weeks but before full term (fetus weighing 2,500 g. or more), it should be classified as "premature labor" rather than as "abortion." Abortion may be subdivided into its two main forms: spontaneous and induced. *Spontaneous abortion* is the termination of a previable conception through natural causes and without the aid of mechanical or medicinal agents. *Induced abortion* is the artificial termination of a previable conception, either therapeutically or criminally.

As a consequence of certain variations in the clinical course of abortion, the following conditions may be distinguished:

Threatened Abortion. An abortion is regarded as threatened if a patient in early pregnancy has vaginal bleeding or spotting; this may or may not be associated with mild cramps. The cervix is closed. Presumably, the process has started but may abate spontaneously or respond to suitable treatment, or it may proceed to a more advanced clinical stage. Although about one patient in five will have bleeding of some degree in pregnancy, only about one-half of these will eventually abort.

Inevitable abortion is so called because the process has gone so far that termination of the pregnancy cannot be prevented. Bleeding is marked, and the pains more severe. The membranes may or may not have ruptured, and the cervical canal is dilating. A part of the product of conception is usually palpable within the cervical os. At this stage the institution of hormone or other therapy is worthless as evidenced by a low chorionic gonadotropin titer and abnormal smear indicative of irreversible placental deterioration.

Incomplete Abortion. In incomplete abortion the fetus is passed, but the membranes and placenta, either entire or in part, are retained in the uterus. Bleeding usually persists until the uterus is empty, and infection is common in neglected cases. With the infection confined to the uterus or to the immediate parametrial tissues, an energetic medical program, including appropriate chemotherapy, is carried out until the infection is under good control, and then uterine curettage is performed when the patient has been afebrile for about 36 to 48 hours. Ill-advised and premature intervention will almost certainly cause a spread and exacerbation of the infectious process. An exception to this approach would be the superimposition of evidence of developing endotoxic shock, usually a complication of criminal abortion, when immediate uterine curettage is mandatory. The same intervention is required in *Clostridium perfringens* infection. Abdominal intervention is necessary if a pelvic roentgenogram indicates the presence of a foreign body or if there is evidence or suspicion of uterine perforation or bowel, bladder or other injury.

Immediate blood replacement to combat shock is essential, since, in addition to the immediate problems of circulatory collapse, brain, heart and renal injury, there may be the remote problems of postpartal amenorrhea, polyuria (diabetes insipidus), hypothyroidism and other changes indicative of anterior pituitary insult.

Complete Abortion. Complete abortion is the expulsion of the entire product of conception.

Missed Abortion. In a missed abortion, the fetus dies in the uterus, but instead of being expelled, it is retained indefinitely. Following fetal death three quarters of the women will expel the fetus and placenta within 2 to 4 weeks. When 2 months or more elapse the condition is referred to as a missed abortion. During this period the fetus undergoes marked degenerative changes. Of these, maceration, or general softening, is the most common. Symptoms, except for amenorrhea, are usually lacking, but occasionally such patients complain of malaise, headache, anorexia and a peculiar taste in the mouth. Hypofibrinogenemia tendency may also occur in certain of these cases. In these, the vaginal smear shows a high proportion of cornified cells or, sometimes, of parabasal cells, similar to a postpartal smear, and the chorionic gonadotropin titer is quite low or negative. If the missed abortion terminates spontaneously, as most do, the process of expulsion is quite the same as in any ordinary abortion. The uterus can sometimes be emptied by infusion of gradually increasing concentrations of oxytocin. When the uterus is easily palpable abdominally, abortion may be induced by injecting hypertonic dextrose or saline into the uterine cavity. Although these techniques are generally safe, deaths from infection, especially Welch bacillus with dextrose injections, or from serious cardiorenal reactions from inadvertent injection of hypertonic saline intravascularly, have been reported. Nevertheless, the risks of hypofibrinogenemia and hemorrhage in patients treated conservatively for too long a period are likewise troublesome. Management will be based on weekly fibrinogen determination after the 6th week of fetal death. A falling trend in the level, particularly below 100 mg. per 100 ml., calls for reevaluation and probably timely intervention.

Noncoagulability of the blood, resulting from disseminated intravascular cooagulation (DIC), occurs in about 40 per cent of patients with retention of a dead fetus beyond 2 months. Activation of this consumption coagulopathy is not unlike that encountered with infected abortion, amniotic fluid embolism, and placental abruption; and spontaneous remission can be expected once the underlying problem is eradicated. Intervention and effective uterine evacuation can be achieved by the infusion of oxytocin or prostaglandin $F_2\alpha$. Recently, a vaginal suppository containing prostaglandin E_2 or an intraamniotic infusion of a combination of urea and prostaglandin $F_2\alpha$ has proved to be effective. Overall, current methods should be successful in evacuating the uterus in at least 97 per cent of patients within a 12 hour period.

Habitual Abortion. By this term is meant a condition in which abortion occurs in successive pregnancies (three or more). With proper selective hormonal and other therapy, more than three quarters of these patients who have had three successive spontaneous abortions will go through pregnancy satisfactorily. Specific and supportive therapy in chronic illness, attention to diet, hygiene, emotional needs and habits of the patient and the correction of systemic endocrinologic and anatomic defects constitute an important concept of "preventive medicine" in obstetrics, whereby the faulty maternal environment is corrected prior to conception in anticipation of greater fetal salvage. However, without proper therapy, these patients have a much poorer chance of success in a subsequent pregnancy. It should be noted that the formerly held view that salvage rates deteriorate rapidly with each succeeding abortion is not correct. The abortion rate, even after three prior previable losses, is only about 20 to 30 per cent.

Criminal Abortion. This refers to the instrumental induction of abortion without medical and legal justification. Since these operations are always performed secretly, it is difficult to secure accurate figures concerning their frequency, but the very minimum estimate was 100,000 annually in the United States. Some authorities put the figure at over half a million a year. Quite apart from this destruction of fetal life, criminal abortion carries a substantial risk of maternal death. These clandestine operations usually are performed by hands that are not only unskilled but also unclean. As a result, fatal infections, usually coliform with endotoxic shock or *Clostridium perfringens* in type, are common; of those who survive, many are left invalids, others become permanently sterile. Hemorrhage and uterine perforation are common complications of such procedures. Fortunately, liberalized abortion laws in most states have succeeded in causing a reduction in the incidence of abortions of this type and in the disastrous consequences of such interventions.

In some areas septic abortions represent 20 to 30 per cent of observed abortions, and the death rate among these patients is 2.0 to 2.5 per cent. In most of the fatal cases, endotoxins form and flood the circulation to give rise to endotoxic shock. The etiologic agents are usually either *Escherichia coli* or *Pseudomonas aeruginosa* derived from endogenous sources. Approximately one half of these patients succumb to their illness.

The clinical course may be gradual in onset, but during a period of 8 to 36 hours there is a gradual development of cyanosis, oliguria, hypotension, pulmonary edema and heart failure.

Therapy includes massive chemotherapy, vasopressor drugs, steroids, polyvalent antitoxin, positive-pressure oxygen, rapid digitalization, and anticoagulation should there be embolization. A thorough uterine debridement should be done at the earliest sign of falling blood pressure, rising pulse, diminishing urinary output or mental confusion. An immediate laparotomy is performed if there is a foreign body present in the pelvis or when air is observed within the abdominal cavity secondary to perforation of the uterus. Any delay or laxity in managing these seriously ill patients will be costly. Vital signs and urinary output must be monitored constantly to detect the earliest suspicion of deterioration, because a delay in debridement beyond this optimal period will be attended by a high death rate.

Therapeutic Abortion. This has traditionally meant the instrumental induction of abortion by a physician because of some grave maternal disease that would make continuation of the pregnancy extremely hazardous. As a rule, two or more physicians are called into consultation to make certain that the procedure is absolutely necessary. Modern methods of prenatal care are making the necessity for therapeutic abortion for these causes relatively rare. Advanced chronic hypertensive disease and severe rheumatic heart disease are the more common indications, although modern care of such patients has greatly reduced the need for interruption of pregnancy in these cases. In the recent past, however, many states have sanctioned liberalized abortion laws so that now proper indications have been broadened to include psychiatric illness, attempted suicide, fetal anomaly or genetic defects, or pregnancy occurring in very young adolescents, or by rape or incest. The intent here is to recognize as legitimate indications those situations that jeopardize the health and well-being of the mother and family, not merely those that threaten the life of the mother. Even more recently, certain states have enacted laws permitting abortion upon demand.

Procedures employed to implement the "voluntary" abortions have included suction uterine curettage in the first trimester, and, for the most part, saline inductions, in the second trimester. By and large, these procedures are safe although each has its complications. Generally, such procedures offered to women with unwanted pregnancies have succeeded in reducing maternal mortality attributable to criminal abortion, shock and sepsis. Administration of prostaglandin to produce abortion in the second trimester seems to offer some advantages over intraamniotic hypertonic saline, and this technique is currently being given an extensive trial.

Clinical Picture. About 75 per cent of all spontaneous abortions occur during the 2nd and the 3rd months of pregnancy, that is, before the 12th week. The acci-

dent is very common, it being estimated that about 10 to 12 per cent of identified pregnancies terminates in spontaneous clinical abortion. Almost invariably, the first symptom is bleeding due to the separation of the ovum from its uterine attachment. The bleeding is often slight at the beginning and may persist for days before uterine cramps occur, or it may be followed at once by cramps. Occasionally the bleeding is torrential in character, leaving the patient in shock. The uterine contractions bring about softening and dilatation of the cervix and expel the products of conception, whether completely or incompletely. In most cases, the embryo had been dead for a period of weeks before the abortion is completed. About 10 per cent of abortions will terminate as late as the fourth gestational month.

Causes. Careful microscopic study of the material passed in these cases shows that the most common cause of spontaneous abortion is a pathologic defect in the product of conception. This defect may express itself in an abnormal embryo, an abnormal trophoblast or in both abnormalities. In early abortions, 60 per cent are associated with some defect of the embryo or trophoblast that is either incompatible with life or would result in a grossly deformed child. These are attended by chromosomal anomalies consisting usually of polyploidy, autosomal trisomy and aberrations of sex chromosomes. The incidence of defects in fetuses passed after the 2nd month is somewhat lower, but not less than 40 to 50 per cent. The recognition of the effect of abnormal germ plasm is simpler than explaining its exact mechanism. However, it is clear that the causes can be divided into two main groups: those arising from defective chromosomes and genes and those arising from faults in intrauterine environment. Undoubtedly, a host of factors, such as radiation, viruses and chemicals, can affect both intrauterine environment and the embryo.

Although many spontaneous abortions are due to causes other than defects in the product of conception, little is known about these factors. The conventional major categories depicting the causes of abortion are defective or genetic factors, hormonal imbalance, circulatory impairment (hypertension, diabetes, etc.), mechanical factors (pelvic disease, anatomic defects, congenital anomalies, etc.), psychologic factors, and, in rare cases, trauma.

Treatment. Threatened abortion is usually treated by absolute rest in bed, analgesic or narcotic drugs and sometimes by a progesterone preparation. It is not clearly proved that an energetic program of therapy favorably influences outcome, probably because so many abortions are attended by chromosomal defects. The use of chorionic gonadotropin determinations, the growth pattern of the uterus, a fern test on the cervical mucus and vaginal smears may be guides to fetal prognosis in individual cases. The clinical factors that are known to influence the outcome in patients who are threatening to abort are: maternal age, previous reproductive difficulties, socioeconomic and nutritional status, the date of efforts at conception, endocrine imbalance, types of previous abortion, general maternal health, local pelvic status and the employment of preconceptional therapy and psychologic support. If the abortion is incomplete, efforts ordinarily are made to aid the uterus in emptying its contents either by the administration of oxytocin or by the instrumental removal of the retained products of conception, particularly if no evidence of infection exists. Active bleeding may make this urgently necessary. If evidence of infection is present (fever, foul discharge or suspicious history of criminal abortion), it is best to withhold any invasion of the uterine cavity until the infection is controlled lest it disseminate bacteria into the venous sinuses of the uterus and thence into the general circulation. On the other hand, bleeding and certain other circumstances may make removal of the uterine contents desirable despite the presence of infection. Complete abortion requires exactly the same care as that given during the postpartal period. As already indicated, habitual abortion may be helped by endocrine therapy, as well as by meticulous attention to general hygiene, rest, vitamin requirements, etc., with emphasis on the preconceptional approach.

Hyperemesis Gravidarum

Hyperemesis gravidarum represents a pernicious exaggeration of the nausea and vomiting that many pregnant women experience. Refractory vomiting leads to starvation, weight loss, marked dehydration, low grade fever, hypokalemic alkalosis, extreme electrolyte imbalance, and finally acidosis. In the past, the gravity of this clinical situation would severely jeopardize the fetus and in some instances the life of the mother would be sufficiently threatened to call for a therapeutic interruption of pregnancy. The most ominous signs included fever, tachycardia, jaundice, delirium, and retinal hemorrhages. These grave cases are not encountered today, undoubtedly because of better emotional preparation and support of patients and because of appropriate family planning practices. Among those with troublesome symptoms, the self-limiting nature of the problem together with simple measures including reassurance, eliminating stressful commitments, adopting multiple small dry feedings, drinking only hot or very cold fluids between meals but often avoiding these altogether in the early morning, and use of an antiemetic drug, usually will be successful. Hospitalization is rarely necessary, and it is unusual to resort to parenteral fluids and electrolyte adjustments. Psychiatric care is seldom necessary. It appears that the height of nausea and vomiting coincides with the maximum peak of hCG production in the first trimester and, perhaps on this same basis, one can associate troublesome symptoms with the relatively higher levels found in molar and multiple pregnancy.

A special note of concern pertains to the clinical problem of late nausea and vomiting appearing after the first trimester. An organic basis for these symptoms should be considered. The same is true of severe and refractory vomiting even in the first trimester. Occasionally, the cause is not related to pregnancy, and possible underlying etiologic factors may include intestinal obstruction, gastrointestinal tumor or other disorders, hyperthyroidism, heavy metal poisoning or other toxic states.

Toxemias of Pregnancy

The toxemias of pregnancy are a group of diseases peculiar to pregnant and puerperal women, characterized in the nonconvulsive stage (preeclampsia) by hypertension, edema and proteinuria, separately or together, and in the convulsive stage (eclampsia) by the same signs with convulsions, coma, or both superimposed. The two stages represent simply degree of severity and the common denominator is the presence of an underlying generalized arteriolar vasoconstriction with an increase in vascular resistance. So-called recurrent toxemia may represent episodes of preeclampsia but, also, may indicate vascular damage. Patients who represent the greatest risk of toxemia include women who are very early or very late in their reproductive life, especially with their first pregnancy, as well as those with chronic hypertensive vascular disease, obesity, diabetes mellitus, multiple gestation and polyhydramnios. Chronic arterial hypertension may be idiopathic or the result of specific disease; but, in either circumstance, there may be superimposed preeclampsia. Patients with preexisting hypertension develop preeclampsia four or five times more frequently than normotensive individuals. Women in low socioeconomic groups with poor nutrition, neglected health and minimal prenatal care are particularly susceptible to development of toxemia. Except for special circumstances such as hydatidiform mole, the disease process occurs typically in the third trimester, often quite early in that period if there is severe underlying vascular damage. Although acute nephritis, chronic glomerulonephritis and nephrosis, nephrosclerosis or nephritis with lupus erythematosus and other conditions are not classified as toxemias, since there is no general vasoconstriction underlying these conditions, they may nevertheless present a similar clinical picture and require intensive supervision and special management.

The "diagnosis" is arbitrarily made when one or more of the following signs appear after the 20th week of pregnancy:

1. A systolic pressure of 140 mm. Hg or more, or a rise of 30 mm. or more above the usual level; a diastolic pressure of 90 mm. or more, or a rise of 15 mm. or more above the usual level. These findings are to be noted on at least two occasions, 6 hours apart.
2. Significant proteinuria (1+ or more) confirmed on catheter specimen and in the absence of pyuria. More specifically, proteinuria in excess of 300 mg. per liter per 24 hours is pathologic. In severe forms, there may be up to 6 to 8 g. per liter of protein excreted in a day. Proteinuria is the last important sign to make its appearance.
3. Edema in the upper half of the body, especially of the hands and the face. This finding is to be suspected when recent weight gain has exceeded 1 pound in a week or as much as 6 pounds in one month.

The differential diagnosis between mild and severe preeclampsia should be deemphasized except retrospectively, since these designations lead to a sense of complacency in the symptomatic woman and fail to emphasize the rapid evolution of the disease process in certain cases. However, in the presence of blood pressure higher than 160 systolic and 110 diastolic, over a 6-hour period at bed rest, proteinuria of 5 gm. or more in 24 hours, oliguria (400 ml. or less per 24 hours), cerebral or visual disturbances and pulmonary edema or cyanosis, the condition is obviously severe.

The physiopathological alterations are these of arteriolar constriction, tissue anoxia, increased capillary permeability, edema, and tissue necrosis. This chain of events in vital organs, such as the kidney, brain, liver and heart, is responsible for the clinical manifestations. A renal glomerular lesion, with capillary constriction, edema of the endothelium, homogeneous fibrinoid deposits between basement membrane and endothelium, and ischemia, appears to be one sensitive lesion when toxemia occurs and persists until the uterus is evacuated. This complication of gestation is seen in 5 to 10 per cent of all gravidas. About two-thirds of the patients have preeclampsia-eclampsia and one-third have hypertension with or without superimposed preeclampsia-eclampsia. Eclampsia (convulsive disorder) occurs in only about one in 1000 to 1500 deliveries.

Although several relatively complicated classifications of the toxemias of pregnancy have been devised, the simplest and perhaps most useful one has been proposed by the American College of Obstetricians and Gynecologists. Since there is no clear "toxicity" or toxin operative, it is more appropriate to classify these conditions as "hypertensive" disorders in pregnancy and the following subsets have been offered by that organization:

1. Preeclampsia and eclampsia
2. Chronic hypertension (of whatever cause)
   a. Essential
   b. Secondary
3. Chronic hypertension with superimposed pre-eclampsia-eclampsia
4. Late or transient hypertension

Special attention should be given to a type of hypertension that makes its appearance for the first time during pregnancy but without the usual signs and symptoms associated with preeclampsia-eclampsia are not present. There appear to be no maternal or perinatal risks, or known sequelae, and the hypertension disappears in the first week or 10 days following delivery. Although the cause is unknown, it seems likely that the condition is a latent manifestation of underlying essential hypertension or perhaps a subclinical stage of preeclampsia.

Recent years have not served to clarify the etiology of preeclampsia-eclampsia precisely, although the uterine ischemia theory is still widely held as a very plausible explanation. Much evidence points to changes in uterine muscular vasculature in preeclampsia or even among women destined to develop a pregnancy-related hypertensive disorder that will affect placentation and alter placental blood flow. The common occurrence of hypoxic and/or in utero growth retardation of fetuses in association with these hypertensive disorders is a supporting argument for the existence of chronic uterine ischemia. However, other factors must be considered. The suppressed pressor effect of angiotensin II, noted in normal pregnancy, is lost totally, or in part in patients with preeclampsia or even in those at midpregnancy who later are destined to become hypertensive. By the same token, altered uteroplacental blood flow may disturb metabolic functions including the conversion rates of steroids. Conversion rates of dehydroepiandrosterone sulfate to estrogens may be sustained at abnormally low rates in some women for several weeks prior to the development of preeclampsia. Recently, it has been demonstrated that the tendency for susceptible women to have vascular hyperactivity can be demonstrated between the 28th and 32nd week, prior to the appearance of clinical evidence of preeclampsia, by utilizing a very simple "roll-over test." The test demonstrates that women who are candidates for preeclampsia will develop a pressor effect in response to a simple roll over from the lateral recumbent to the supine position.

There is histopathologic evidence of fibrin deposition in many organs and at least a low-grade disseminated intravascular coagulation especially in severe preeclampsia-eclampsia. Evidence for this is provided by the increased fibrin monomers and fibrin split products together with a decreased fibrinogen and platelets. The fibrinoid deposits found in the glomerular capillary endothelium stain with immunofluorescent antifibrinogen antibodies.

Generalized segmental narrowing of arterioles becomes sustained resulting in marked increases in peripheral resistance, decreased blood flow and damage involving the uteroplacental bed, kidneys, retina, and central nervous system. There may be lowered endogenous estrogen and progesterone production by the placenta, decrease in creatinine clearance and urinary output with a drop in the glomerular filtration rate, rise in serum uric acid in association with altered tubular function and albuminuria associated with a disturbed glomerular membrane function. Dynamic physiologic alterations noted with the progression of preeclampsia include major shifts of intravascular fluid to the extravascular space (hemoconcentration), increase in total body water with an accompanying but less marked rise in total exchangeable body sodium, and decreased plasma renin activity and aldosterone levels, and hypertension. Patients with preeclampsia excrete less sodium in response to an intravenous load than one observes in the normal pregnant woman. When there is clinical evidence of a reduced blood volume (elevated hematocrit), accentuation of the SGOT level, depressed platelet count, or clinical evidence of vascular hyperreactivity to one of the several prognostic tests, careful supervision is mandatory especially among women with predisposing factors. Diuresis can be promoted by periodic bed rest in the lateral recumbent position along with restricted activity. Stringent dietary controls, inadequate maternal weight gain, salt restriction and the use of diuretics are not preventative measures and may be quite harmful.

Important preventatives consist of control of concomitant disease and an optimal balanced diet. (To assure a 15 pound weight gain in the last half of pregnancy, roughly 1 pound per week), providing adequate daily protein (76 g.), carbohydrate (150 to 200 g.) and fat along with proper intake of foods containing recommended amounts of calcium, phosphorus, iron, iodine,

and vitamins. There need be no unusual restriction of salt. Signs suggestive of incipient preeclampsia call for twice weekly visits for examination and favorable circumstances with respect to fetal maturity, engagement of the fetal head and overall obstetrical situation might justify induction of labor as a preventative in the vulnerable patients, such as prediabetics, postdate pregnancies, suspicion of in utero growth retardation, or an equivocal stress test.

Among chronic hypertensive patients, close supervision for any early signs of a superimposed preeclampsia is imperative. Fetoplacental monitoring is advisable after 28 to 30 weeks of gestation, and non-stress tests to monitor the status of the fetus may be performed after the 34th week. Any warning clinical signs of preeclampsia despite a rest regime calls for hospitalization. The same would be true of signs of fetoplacental jeopardy. Usually, cases of chronic hypertension are managed aggressively when complications arise because further in utero existence in a hostile environment can cost the fetus its life. Even infants weighing less than 1,000 g. at birth may fare better in the nursery under intensive care depending upon the circumstances.

Under all circumstances, the patient is hospitalized once the diagnosis of preeclampsia is made.

Treatment.   There is no ambulatory treatment of toxemia. The general status is evaluated in the hospital, and the patient is observed for retinal spasm, urinary output, proteinuria and weight trends. In mild cases, the blood pressure and the fetal heart tones are checked several times daily. Any patient with the early signs of toxemia who does not respond to the preventive measures may present a problem of faulty uterine environment, even in the absence of further deterioration of maternal status. An active toxemia process is brought to a halt only by delivery, and it is not advisable to sponsor expectant management for any considerable period if any signs or symptoms of preeclampsia persist. After appropriate stabilization, induction of labor is advisable when the obstetric circumstances become favorable, usually about the 38th week. Assurance of fetal maturity can be determined by ultrasound measurements of the biparietal diameter and amniocentesis to determine the amniotic fluid L/S ratio. In severer forms of the disease, delivery by the most expeditious means after a period of stabilization is mandatory even at much earlier stages of pregnancy. The findings on the stress test may dictate the probable safest method of delivery.

Certain tests may be needed to screen patients who may be suspected of having an underlying vascular or renal disorder. These may include blood chemistries, especially BUN, uric acid, total protein, A/G ratio, sodium and potassium; concentration and dilution renal function tests; teleoroentgenogram for heart size; urea clearance test; and Addis count. In special circumstances, the cold pressor test, analysis for catecholamines, determination of total body water, sodium space and plasma volume as well as, occasionally, a renal biopsy, may be valuable in evaluating hypertensive patients. A rising chorionic gonadotropin titer or a falling pregnanediol or estriol urinary excretion may indicate progressive placental deterioration. Measurements of the height and the breadth of the fundus are made regularly to evaluate the growth pattern of the fetus.

In "severe" preeclampsia signs of impending eclampsia may develop rapidly. These include epigastric pain, cerebral or visual disturbances and extreme hyperreflexia. In these serious circumstances the basic objectives of therapy are: to promote diuresis, correct hemoconcentration, promote vasodilatation, provide sedation to allay convulsions, prevent residual vascular damage, establish a stable phase of the disease process and effect delivery at the optimal time in the best interests of mother and fetus.

Acceptable methods of achieving these ends include: complete bed rest, solitude and quiet environment; prompt sedation; hydration; anticonvulsant therapy, usually magnesium sulfate intramuscularly; and hypotensive drugs, if the hypertension is extreme. Blood samples are drawn for hematocrit (to be followed serially for hemoconcentration-dilution) and for routine studies, which include BUN, CBC, uric acid, total serum proteins, A/G ratio, blood electrolytes, and CO_2. Quantitative determinations of urinary albumin are performed every 24 hours. Quantitative cellular counts are made if the urinalysis on a single specimen is noted. The total volume of intravenous fluids is based on the carefully recorded urinary output but does not exceed 2.5 liters in 24 hours. No pelvic or rectal examinations are performed at this time. A careful fundoscopic examination is performed to evaluate the character of the optic discs and vessels and the retina.

Magnesium sulfate may be administered intramuscularly, 10 g. initially and 5 g. every 4 to 6 hours as long as the knee jerks are present, the respirations are 16 or more per minute and urinary output is 600 ml. (average 25 ml. per hour) daily. If convulsions seem imminent, 1.5 g. (15 ml. of 10 per cent) magnesium sulfate is given slowly intravenously, in addition to the initial intramuscular dose of 10 g. as described. Calcium for intravenous use (calcium chloride of calcium gluconate, 10 ml. of 10 per cent solution) is at bedside as an immediate antidote to magnesium. When hypertension is extreme and there is a grave risk on intracranial hemorrhage, an intravenous infusion containing 20 mg. hydralazine (Apresoline) and 5 mg.

cryptenamine (Unitensin) in 500 ml. of 5 per cent glucose in water is started at a rate of 20 drops per minute, with very frequent blood pressure checks and the rate of flow titrated to reduce the untreated levels by 25 per cent.

Morphine sulfate, 15 mg., may be given intramuscularly prior to any stimulation of the patient, and it is desirable to give a sedative prior to each injection of magnesium sulfate. A narcotic antagonist (nalorphine hydrochloride) should be available in case of overdose. A mouth gag and oxygen should also be at hand, and it is important to have a responsible attendant in constant attendance. Severe narcosis of the central nervous system interferes with evaluation of the patient, impairs respiration and reduces cerebral and renal blood flow and thus should be avoided.

Satisfactory response to these therapies does not alter the need to evacuate the uterus at the appropriate time after stabilization of the signs and symptoms of the toxemic process. At that time a pelvic examination is done, a sterile technique being used to determine the suitability of the obstetric situation for induction of labor. A difficult or delayed labor following induction should be sufficient indication to effect delivery by cesarean section. Fortunately, in most instances the uterine irritability encountered in such patients makes induction of labor a simple matter, usually terminating in delivery within 12 hours. Rupture of membranes alone or in conjunction with oxytocic stimulation is usually successful. If the cervix is long and tightly closed at the appropriate time for intervention, or if the patient's condition deteriorates despite several days of intensive therapy, cesarean section as the initial approach may be indicated.

The anesthetic choice is individualized, but a general balanced anesthetic with nitrous oxide, oxygen and a muscle relaxant offers a safe method. Conduction anesthetics are not preferred. In the uncontrolled patient who presents in advanced labor, inhalation or intravenous anesthesia may be required. By and large, there is little concern about inducing convulsions if 30 g. of magnesium sulfate has been administered before delivery at the therapeutic level of 7 mg. per 100 ml.

In the postpartal period, energetic therapy, including continuation of intramuscular magnesium sulfate administration and meticulous supervision, is continued until there is objective evidence of improvement and diuresis has occurred. Water and electrolyte replacement, including salt and potassium, may be required during the diuretic phase. When oliguria has been present or if shock has occurred and especially when abruptio placentae is a complication, mannitol can be used to promote diuresis. Sometimes this is achieved with hypertonic glucose solutions.

The prognosis for the mother in most cases of preeclampsia should be good; however, the perinatal mortality rates will be increased, perhaps to 5 to 6 per cent, primarily related to an incidence of prematurity of about 20 per cent.

Eclampsia. Convulsions or coma occurring in toxemia of pregnancy signifies eclampsia and represents a grave complication, since from 7 to 10 per cent may succumb to the disease. The incidence of eclampsia is probably 1 in every 1,000 to 1,500 deliveries. Roughly one half of the cases occur antepartally, while the remaining 50 per cent are equally divided between intrapartal and postpartal occurrences. All of these patients are critically ill, but those whose prognosis is gravest exhibit one or more of the following: numerous convulsions attended by prolonged coma; tachycardia, tachypnea, pulmonary edema and cyanosis, jaundice, oliguria or anuria, fever, extreme hypertension and neurologic signs indicative of central nervous system hemorrhage or hypoxia.

The immediate objective is to stabilize the process, control convulsions, promote diuresis, and to correct hemoconcentration, azotemia, metabolic acidosis, hypokalemia and hyperchloremia. Patients may benefit from digitalization, and oxygen is advisable under positive pressure if pulmonary edema is present. Initially, intravenous magnesium sulfate, 1.5 g., can be given along with intramuscular medication and administered subsequently in accordance with urinary output and the status of the reflexes. The details of management are much the same as those outlined for severe preeclampsia, except that the immediate use of intravenous thiopental, amobarbital or sodium phenobarbital may be required to help convulsions. Once convulsions are controlled, an effort is made to rely on magnesium therapy as the primary anticonvulsant therapy in preference to heavy sedation, because the latter interferes with evaluation of the patient's condition and aggravates cerebral anoxia. Infusions of hypotensive drug are given if blood pressure recordings are alarmingly high.

At this stage and for the ensuing day or two there is no need to be concerned about the patient's obstetric status. As long as either convulsions or coma persists, no thought should be given to delivery. The key features of control are stabilized blood pressure at lower levels, reduced albuminuria, normal respirations, adequate urinary output, clear sensorium, water and electrolyte balance, normal temperature, hyporeflexia or normal reflexes, diminished angiospasm in the eye grounds, normal pulse rate and absence of convulsions and coma for at least 24 hours. This postconvulsive and postcoma stage of the disease has been referred to as "intercurrent eclampsia," which implies that exacerbation can be anticipated if delivery is not effected.

When a judgment is made that the process has stabilized at an optimal level, the patient is evaluated to determine the least traumatic method of effecting delivery, the same as outlined for severe preeclampsia. Delivery alone is ultimately curative, but provoking delivery by any means before adequate stabilization has been achieved may lead to an aggravation of the patient's condition and maternal death.

Since eclampsia may occur postpartally as well as antepartally and intrapartally, appropriate regard for forewarning signs is mandatory. Following delivery of the eclamptic patient, magnesium sulfate, appropriate sedation and other supervisory and therapeutic measures are continued until evidence of the toxemic process dissipates and diuresis occurs, usually within several days of intensive care.

The overall maternal mortality rate is about 7 per cent, but the range is from about 3 to 35 per cent according to its severity. The prognosis appears to be worse among older patients, multiparas and those without significant edema. Persistent neurologic sequelae or permanent visual impairment is rare among the survivors. The reported incidence of recurrent eclampsia is not great, but from 25 to 30 per cent of the patients with pre-eclampsia have persistent hypertension or develop hypertension and associated phenomena in subsequent pregnancies.

Congestive heart failure, cerebral hemorrhage, peripheral circulatory collapse, complications of operative obstetrics, hemorrhage shock and afibrinogenemia, acute yellow atrophy, respiratory paralysis and bilateral pyelonephritis are the most common causes of death in eclampsia.

In eclampsia the prognosis for the fetus is likewise grave and a perinatal mortality rate of from 20 to 40 per cent can be expected depending upon the maternal condition and stage of pregnancy.

Chronic Hypertensive Vascular Disease. As the name indicates, this disease is a chronic disorder of the vascular system associated with high blood pressure. In other words, these patients have authenticated hypertension antedating the pregnancy or hypertension that is noted prior to the 24th gestational week. The kidneys may be affected, with the result the proteinuria may be present as well as diminution in the excretory power of the kidneys. A few patients have retinal hemorrhages and many will have minor changes. However, in the majority, an elevated arterial pressure is the only demonstrable finding. The patients usually are in the 30s or the late 20s; most are multiparas with a number of children, and the majority are obese. The course of pregnancy in these women often is troublesome, the blood pressure showing a tendency to higher and higher levels as they reach the last 3 months of pregnancy. The most common hazard faced by gravidas with chronic hypertensive vascular disease is the superimposition of pre-eclampsia, frequently as early as the 24th to the 28th week, which occurs in 25 per cent or more of cases (range 15 to 50 per cent depending upon the definition). Most patients do well in pregnancy and achieve a good outcome; however, fetal prognosis is poor in advanced cases. A falling or low estriol urinary secretion suggests advancing placental deterioration and portends poorly for the fetus. Termination of pregnancy as soon as the superimposed toxemic process is stabilized offers the best chance for fetal survival even though the fetus may be premature. Otherwise, quite apart from the maternal risks involved, further delay almost inevitably is associated with progressive fetal inanition, hypoxia and eventual death in utero. Placental abruption constitutes an additional risk. One can expect a perinatal mortality rate of up to 50 per cent in these patients.

Symptoms. Aside from the high blood pressure, the signs and symptoms of hypertensive vascular disease may be surprisingly few. Headache is rather common, but even this complaint may be absent. Examination of the retina very often shows a narrowing of the arterioles, indicative of the fact that there is a generalized sclerosis of the small arterioles throughout the body. However, in some, there may be a rapid appearance of retinal exudates and hemorrhages, nitrogenous retention, proteinuria, and edema.

Treatment. The decision as to the best way of managing a patient with hypertensive vascular disease will be made after taking into consideration a number of circumstances, such as the severity of the hypertensive process, the number of children in the family and the duration of the pregnancy when first seen. If the process is mild, the pregnancy may be allowed to continue with the patient under close observation for signs of impending trouble. Hypotensive drugs, particularly rauwolfia compounds, are helpful in controlling hypertension in some cases. Rest, sodium restriction and saluretics are necessary represent good therapy. Several hospitalizations for study and rest are advisable. Periodic tests of fetoplacental status are imperative. Should toxemia intervene, the process is controlled and delivery is indicated. In the absence of toxemia, early intervention, usually by induction of labor, is desirable at about the 37th or 38th week if significant hypertension is present. Even when the blood pressure has been successfully lowered, toxemia may supervene, or impaired uteroplacental blood flow may develop.

Although fetal monitoring involving stress tests is a valuable means of predicting the ability of a fetus to withstand the insults of labor, there remain many unanswered questions about validity. Fetal deaths have been reported within several days after a negative oxytocin challenge test. Although disturbances of fetal heart rate and pattern in response to the myometrial activity are definitely suspicious, a positive test is best predicated upon the presence of a persistent late deceleration from the previous baseline. The uteri of hypertensive patients are particularly sensitive to oxytocin and even test doses can be hazardous in some patients. Precise criteria for the oxytocin challenge test are not established universally, false negatives are well documented, and false positive tests are common (up to 50 per cent). In some instances there will be a fixed baseline tachycardia, irregularities or even at times an atypical variable deceleration. Loss of beat-to-beat variation and/or appearance of late decelerations represent a positive test, but it should always be repeated with the patient in a lateral recumbent position.

More recently, the nonstress test has been popularized as a somewhat safer procedure since the test is conducted in the same fashion with the same equipment as that used in the stress test but uterine contractions are neither desired not stimulated. The normal test is predicated upon the fact that the FHR accelerates in response to fetal movement and the beat-to-beat variation increases. An undulating FHR, with no beat-to-beat variability, very little fetal movement, and no accelerations with the occasional movements, are unfavorable factors associated with a perinatal mortality of 40 to 50 per cent.

If the process is very severe, especially with advanced degrees of cardiorenal insufficiency or fresh retinal hemorrhages, it may be necessary to interrupt the pregnancy in order to save the mother's life. In most cases in this group it is desirable to prevent further pregnancies by ligating the fallopian tubes or employing some method of contraception. Current therapeutic methods have improved the outlook for these patients during pregnancy, so that interruption of pregnancy is rarely contemplated in modern practice. However, many should have sterilization after the 6-week checkup.

Coincidental Complications of Pregnancy

Gravid women are naturally subject to all the diseases from which nonpregnant persons suffer. Most of these will not be aggravated by pregnancy, and the coincidental condition will not affect the normal course of gestation. The notable exceptions to this generalization are heart disease, diabetes mellitus, pyelonephritis, pneumonia, syphilis and rubella. Current opinion suggests that pregnancy exerts no deleterious effect on tuberculosis, and that therapeutic abortion is rarely indicated. As a rule, tuberculosis of the mother does not affect the infant.

Heart Disease. Heart disease, usually rheumatic, complicates pregnancy in about 1 per cent of gravidas and accounts for almost 10 per cent of all deaths from puerperal causes. Heart disease complicating pregnancy is generally regarded as the fourth most common cause of maternal death (after hemorrhage, toxemia and infection), although in certain teaching institutions it may rank first. In determining the prognosis of cardiac patients, emphasis should be given to the functional classification, the age of the patient, signs or history of heart failure, atrial fibrillation and complicating serious disease. Generally speaking, the prognosis is most serious in mitral stenosis, either alone or in association with insufficiency. Judging the severity of the heart condition by these several criteria, the unfavorable group of cases comprises about 20 per cent of the total, yet these women with poor prognostic signs account for about 85 per cent of the deaths attributable to heart disease. In addition to the deaths that bear a relationship to the functional classification, especially Classes III and IV of the New York Heart Association Classification, certain cardiovascular complications, such as vascular accidents, bacterial endocarditis and postpartal venoarterial shunts with vascular collapse, may take an additional toll. The principles of management are: adequate rest, reduced emotional strain, prevention or correction of anemia, proper diet to avoid excess weight and fluid retention, avoidance of infection, recognition of early signs of heart failure, allowing labor to ensue spontaneously, meticulous care in labor and allaying decompensation. Warning signs of early cardiac failure are decreased vital capacity, fatigue, orthopnea, resting tachypnea, rales at lung bases, and pulmonary congestion on a chest film. In the presence of heart failure, delivery by any known method carries with it a maternal mortality of more than 50 per cent. Should frank heart failure develop, digitalis and bed rest in the hospital are required throughout the remainder of the pregnancy. During pregnancy, cardiac failure constitutes a grave hazard since 15 per cent or more of patients die. It is probably wisest to hospitalize all patients with severity heart disease for rest throughout pregnancy in order to avoid overt cardiac decompensation. Mitral commissurotomy is not recommended during pregnancy except in rare circumstances, although it is too early to reach a final conclusion about the place of valvotomy in pregnancy since up to now fetal losses have occurred in about 33 per cent of the operated cases. Uneventful pregnancies have been reported following insertion of a pacemaker for complete heart block.

The presence of heart disease should be realized at the onset of pregnancy because gestational disturbances make the diagnosis difficult. Edema, fatigue, dyspnea, cardiac enlargement, left axis deviation and occasional T wave inversion on electrocardiogram, and apical or left sternal border systolic ejection-type murmurs are common in pregnancy and may falsely implicate a heart disease as the basis for these clinical manifestations. In pregnancy, it is best to rely on more reliable criteria established by Burwell and Metcalfe. These include diastolic or holosystolic murmurs, grade III or higher (thrill) systolic ejection murmurs, unequivocal cardiomegaly, arrhythmias, and definite electrocardiographic indications of myocardial damage.

The physiologic and medical circumstances of pregnancy, labor, and delivery are not favorable for the cardiac patient. Cardiac output rises 30 to 40 per cent (range 25 to 65 per cent) beginning at the 8th gestational week and peaks about the 30th gestational week before leveling off at this range. However, most decompensations occur after the 7th lunar month, and the cardiac workload steadily increases to term. Cardiac work is accentuated even more during labor and, following delivery, there are additional burdens imposed by the augmentation of the uteroplacental blood volume into the general circulation.

Of special concern are those patients who have had cardiac failure previously, because repeated cardiac decompensation in pregnancy is very likely. Another grave category is represented by women with congenital cyanotic heart disease. Here, not only are the perinatal risks great but the maternal mortality rate is also enhanced. In some instances, patients may be suitable surgical candidates even during pregnancy; however, in general, all women, particularly older women, classified as having class III and IV heart disease are extremely serious risks who should be considered for elective abortion prior to the 8th gestational week. Otherwise, hospitalization and bed rest through pregnancy is required along with the closest supervision. One of the most serious complications of cardiac disease in pregnancy is bacterial endocarditis. The streptococcus, (beta-hemolytic, Group A) is most often implicated, and penicillin is a major drug utilized in a prophylactic regime. Women who undergo complicated vaginal deliveries are highly vulnerable to bacterial endocarditis. Another likely candidate is the woman with a valve prosthesis; otherwise, the risks of pregnancy are generally low if the valve does not malfunction and there are no problems with heparin anticoagulation. In postsurgical patients, the prognosis depends upon any residual pulmonary hypertension or myocardial deterioration. Patients with the tetralogy of Fallot and Ebstein's anomaly fare reasonably well in pregnancy because there is no pulmonary hypertension. Successful pregnancy has followed a cardiac bypass operation.

Diabetes Mellitus. This is the most common and the most serious metabolic disease in pregnant women. The overall incidence of this maternal complication is about one per cent, although the incidence will be considerably higher in tertiary care centers (perhaps two to three per cent). The combination of diabetes and pregnancy occurs because the availability of insulin has created an improved life expectancy for women as well as a reasonable prospect for successful childbearing. Now, under optimal conditions, the maternal mortality is 0.5 per cent, although in the moderate to severe groups it may be much higher. In the absence of adequate prenatal care, the perinatal mortality will be 40 per cent, but it can be reduced to 10 per cent under more optimal conditions. The etiology of most of these deaths is unknown but it increases toward term and accentuates post term.

One of the stresses that can percipitate clinical diabetes in the prediabetic patient is pregnancy. Insulin demands are increased during the gestational state. The innate capacity for the pancreas to respond may be lacking, inability to metabolize or tolerate even normal amounts of glucose results. This creates a state of hyperglycemia along with glucosuria. Fasting plasma glucosa levels above 120 m g. per dl should be considered abnormal. Glycosuria should also be evaluated. A blood sugar test one hour after ingesting 50 g. glucose as a screening test for gestational diabetes is considered "positive" if the value is above 130 m g. per dl. First identification is usually based on the medical history, physical findings, gynecological background, past obstetrical performance, and laboratory data. Obviously, there are risk factors that make some individuals more vulnerable than others. A family history of diabetes in one close relative or two distant relatives should be taken into consideration. A gynecological history of wound healing problems, resistance to infection, recurrent urinary tract infections and refractory monilial vaginitis should be noteworthy. Obstetrically, an unexplained fetal death, neonatal respiratory death, child with anomalies, recurrent toxemia, fetal macrosomia, gestational obesity, diabetes in a prior pregnancy, polyhydramnios and other factors should be viewed with concern.

During pregnancy, a number of insulin antagonists are operative, including chorionic somatomammotropin, which induces lipolysis, increases free fatty acids, and inhibits the cellular uptake of glucose and gluconeogenesis. Normally, a pregnant woman can respond by increasing insulin synthesis and release. When an overt diabetic becomes pregnant, there is a glucose intolerance that may not be demonstrable until the last trimester. The placenta may contribute to the diabetic picture by producing insulinase. The resulting gestational diabetes can be diagnosed with an oral, 3 hour glucose tolerance test. For two or three days prior to the test, the patient should ingest a high carbohydrate diet. According to O'Sullivan's criteria, two of the four blood sugar levels should be elevated above the following baseline figures: Fasting of 90 mg. per dl.; one hour = 165 mg. per dl; two hours = 145 mg. per dl.; and 3 hours = 125 mg. per dl. If plasma sugar is determined, the values are approximately 15 per cent higher. If the fasting blood sugar is above 140 mg. per dl., the diagnosis is established and the GTT should not be performed because it could be dangerous. On the other hand, a negative study in early pregnancy in a high risk or suspect patient calls for a repeat GTT after the 28th week of gestation.

Once the diagnosis is established, the disease should be classified because this will bear on the pregnancy outcome and prospects for perinatal survival. For example, asymptomatic gestational diabetics almost always controllable by diet alone (Class A, Priscilla White Classification, 1949), is associated with the best survival rate, which is about 95 per cent. At the other end of the spectrum, patients with hypertension, proteinuria, and nephropathy have a survival rate of only 50 to 65 per cent. Generally, perinatal mortality rates are about 10 per cent for all cases throughout the United States.

Gestational diabetes occurs in about one in 110 to 120 prenatal registrants and frank diabetes occurs in about 1 in 300 deliveries. Among patients with gestational diabetes, approximately 25 to 30 per cent will progress to chemical diabetes mellitus within 5 years. In pregnancy, there may be a rapid onset of diabetic symptoms even among previously undiagnosed patients. Blood sugar should be relied upon in establishing the diagnosis because the lowered renal threshold for sugar in association with an increase in glomerular filtration rate may lead to glycosuria. After delivery, lactosuria is common. There is an augmented tendancy for acidosis in pregnancy and the presence of vomiting may create a confusing disturbance in the chemical balance. Insulin requirements are increased in more than two-thirds of patients, especially in the last two trimesters.

Maternal acidosis is probably the major factor in the markedly increased perinatal mortality. Other adverse factors are water imbalance, hypertensive disorders (up to 50 per cent), excessively sized fetus (somatic and splanchnic growth), and hydramnios (10 per cent). Monitoring the fetus should consider several adverse findings, signs that are indicative of a deteriorating fetal status include falling or a precipitous drop in urinary estriol excretion (levels falling well below 12 mg. per 24 hrs. or dropping 50 per cent below previous levels). The risk of fetal death rises substantially after the 36th week. Regardless of the initial classification according to White, Pedersen's bad signs in diabetic pregnancy include (1) pyelonephritis (premature labor), (2) ketoacidosis, (3) toxemia (25 per cent incidence creating a 25 per cent likelihood of fetal loss), and (4) "neglectors" who do not cooperate in the plan of clinical management.

The prime target in medical management is adequate blood sugar control to minimize fetal macrosomia and new born problems (potential for hypoxia, delayed pulmonary maturation, hypoglycemia, and hyperbilirubinemia). Thus, diet must be rigidly controlled and insulin requirements must be made precisely based on blood glucose levels. Ketoacidosis should be avoided meticulously by keeping fasting plasma glucose levels below 120 mg. per dl. and 2 hour post prandial levels below 135 mg. per dl. These two factors—hyperglycemia and ketoacidosis—are detrimental to fetal growth, development, maturation and survival. Oral hypoglycemics cannot be relied upon in achieving this level of control. Hospitalization is required initially to establish the workup necessary for classification and an individualized management plan. Insulin-dependent patients will require the most supervision. Hospitalization is required for any subsequent problem in managing the diabetes or in correcting an obstetrical complication. Most clinical diabetics should be admitted for evaluation in advance of a decision concerning the time and mode of delivery, usually at the 33rd to 34th week. Those with more severe diabetes should be admitted even earlier than one month in advance of a scheduled delivery date. Estriol excretion values are determined twice weekly or more and steps are taken to determine fetal maturity and the pattern of inutero growth; e.g., ultrasound for the biparietal diameter of the fetal head, L/S ratio in the amniotic fluid, cytohormonal studies, etc. The stress and nonstress tests are important in the final weeks in an effort to select the most appropriate time for delivery. Unfortunately, despite an L/S ratio of 2.0 or greater, about one-quarter of the infants of diabetic mothers will develop the respiratory distress syndrome neonatally. Because of fetal macrosomia, fragility, tendancy to be hypoxic, and compromised reserve, delivery by cesarean section should be used liberally. There is much more latitude in managing the gestational diabetic; however, in all cases the method of delivery is selected on the basis of the obstetrical situation and the anticipated ease of labor and delivery. Vaginal delivery can be achieved in 30 to 35 per cent of patients while maintaining optimal perinatal results. The optimal time for delivery of the average diabetic patient is 18 to 24 days before the expected date of confinement. The decision to deliver a patient prior to that time should be based on special indications such as the superimposition of toxemia, and clear evidence of fetal distress or chronic inutero growth retardation. Rarely, a very brittle diabetic will defy control and the intrauterine environment is so hostile that intervention must be considered.

Class A diabetics (those exhibiting only laboratory evidence of the metabolic disorders) subject their infants to the same hazards encountered in patients with the clinical disease, namely, respiratory distress syndrome, hypoxia, physiologic immaturity, macrosomia, risk of fetal death in utero and neonatal hypoglycemia. Thus, determination of glucose metabolism in suspect cases becomes an integral part of modern prenatal evaluation.

Abruptio Placentae

Placental abruption refers to obstetric bleeding from the premature separation of a normally implanted placenta. When the placental detachment occurs prior to the 20th gestational week, the mechanism may be similar but the process is referred to as an abortion. By definition, abruptio placenta is restricted to cases of placental attachment occurring after the period of fetal viability, e.g., the 20th gestational week. Mostly, this complication arises during the last trimester in about one per cent of patients. Bleeding from this cause should be distinguished from that of premature separation arising in an abnormally situated placenta, which characterizes placenta previa. Although these two conditions constitute the major causes of severe bleeding in the third trimester, there are many other nonplacental causes, including lower genital tract disease (such as infection, polyps, malignant lesions, etc.) or discharge of an endocervical mucus plug.

Although the precise etiology is unknown, placental abruption is found in association with maternal hypertension in about one-half of patients. The predisposing factors may be vascular disease, preeclampsia or chronic renal diseases. The previous occurrence of placental abruption is a risk factor. Others include a tumor or hyperirritable or overdistended uterus, or the sudden reduction of uterine volume as in delivery of one twin, or membrane rupture and escape of a large quantity of amniotic fluid (polyhydramnios). Other possible causes that have been cited include multiparity, trauma, malnutrition (including folic acid deficiency and low vitamin C levels), vena caval compression, short cord, and many others.

The clinical picture and amount of bleeding depends upon the size and location of the detached area and the number of uterine sinuses disrupted. When the abrupted portion of the placenta is centrally located while peripheral attachments remain intact, the bleeding is merely internal or "concealed." An extension of the hematoma to the placental edge where peripheral disruption occurs or an abruption arising at the periphery give rise to visible or "external" bleeding. Progression of the hematoma and disruption may cease when pressure is relieved by external bleeding or rupture into the amniotic cavity. However, the situation remains tenuous and bleeding may recur at any time, but particularly in response to the onset of uterine contractions. In the most severe cases there may be extensive hemorrhagic infiltration beneath the serosa of the uterus, the tubes and the adjacent ligaments and also between the uterine muscle bundles. The latter occurrence is known as the uteroplacental apoplexy of Couvelaire; the additional complication of uterine atony and further hemorrhage postpartally sometimes occurs.

The classic signs and symptoms of abruptio placenta are (1) intense abdominal pain; (2) vaginal bleeding; (3) a tetanically contracted myometrium; (4) absence of fetal heart sounds; and (5) symptoms of shock. Less than one-half of cases present so dramatically and, often, minor disruptions involving only one or two central cotyledons may go unrecognized until the placenta is inspected after its removal. Every effort must be made to establish the diagnosis as timely as possible without provoking additional bleeding. A gentle speculum examination, avoiding any direct cervical manipulation or deep vaginal intrusion, will be helpful in some cases to rule out lower genital tract pathology. In the latter and in most cases of placenta previa, the blood is bright, whereas in abruptio placenta the blood is usually dark or even clotted. Placental localization studies, particularly ultrasonography, can be helpful in determining the probable cause of bleeding in some doubtful cases, but such methods of study should be withheld in the presence of profuse vaginal bleeding or in managing women with a term or near term fetus. Delays caused by these examinations could be costly since the prognosis is associated with the timeliness of obstetrical intervention.

In the more severe grades of placental abruption associated with classic findings and shock, there may be disseminated intravascular coagulation. Fibrin obstruction occurring in periglomerular arterioles, hypotension, lack of adequate renal perfusion, and perhaps arteriolar spasm from the release of myoglobin from damaged tissues, may give rise to acute renal failure in the mostly severely abrupted cases. There may be an apparent level of hypovolemic shock out of proportion to the observed blood loss, since there may be considerable concealed hemorrhage associated with uterine enlargement, dysrhythmic myometrial contractility, and severe pain. A proper response to mannitol may be useful in distinguishing between a depressed urinary output from hypoperfusion (hypovolemia) and low output from renal failure.

A suspicion of placental abruption is an indication for blood to be drawn for a clot observation test and baseline coagulation studies. Defective clotting begins to occur when the concentration of plasma fibrinogen falls below 150 mg. per 100 ml. Fibrinogen replacement is of only temporary value since there is prompt conversion to fibrin as long as the disrupted placenta remains undelivered; there is also a risk of inducing hepatitis. The coagulopathy is satisfactorily treated only by adequate whole blood transfusion and prompt delivery. The urgency depends on the clinical situation involving the state of both the mother and fetus. There is no role for expectant management once the diagnosis of placental abruption has been made, even if the separation is presumably minor.

The hematologic problem in the severe cases involves a consumption coagulopathy characterized by a depression in platelet count and decline in circulating levels of fibrinogen, factors V, VIII, XIII, and to a lesser extent, prothrombin. Rarely, there may be primary activation of the fibrinolytic system resulting in the lysis of fibrinogen by fibrinolysins before fibrin can be formed. This possibility accentuates the consumption coagulopathy and exacerbates the hemorrhage. The suspicion of this complication calls for the determination of fibrinogen split products in the blood. If possible, fresh whole blood should be administered. Success in eliminating the underlying problem (which usually means delivery) is evidenced by a decline in the concentration of fibrin split products first and, subsequently, by a rise in plasma fibrinogen. Infusion of heparin may be useful in correcting blood coagulation induced by disseminated intravascular coagulation. If there is documentation of primary activation of the fibrinolytic system, epsilon aminocaproic acid therapy may be of value, since it inhibits the action of profibrinolysin activators. It should be noted that subsequent postpartal hemorrhage, even involving uteri of the Couvelaire variety, seldom necessitates hysterectomy because the myometrium can be made to contract sufficiently to close off bleeding sites in most instances.

Even in the mild cases of placental abruption concern for the fetus will justify cesarean section as the preferred method of delivery. If labor has already commenced, the membranes may be artificially ruptured to hasten its progress, and appropriate fetal monitoring can be instituted. There is greater flexibility in anticipating vaginal deliveries among multiparas than primigravidas; however, placental abruption has a tendency to speed parturition. Carefully administered oxytocin infusion is a highly successful means of inducing labor in low grade abruptions when obstetrical circumstances are favorable. However, prompt delivery by cesarean section may be the best approach regardless of fetal status, if profuse bleeding, shock, and worrisome clinical signs are endangering the mother.

The prognosis for the mother varies with the severity of the placental abruption, but overall the maternal death rate in the United States is one per cent or less. Among women surviving major shock, there may be postpartal necrosis with resultant destruction of the anterior lobe of the pituitary, which may be associated with a depression of gonadotropic, adrenal and thyroid functions, as well as the develoment of cachexia (Sheehan's Syndrome). The perinatal risks also vary with the degree and type of placental separation and the underlying maternal complications; e.g., hypertension, malnutrition, etc. In addition to the risks of hypoxia associated with maternal shock and placental disruption, the complications of premature birth impose additional grave hazards. Generally, the perinatal mortality rates are higher among black women than white women. Among those with partial placental separations, the rate is 15 to 30 per cent. The risk is much lower when only a marginal sinus ruptures. Contrariwise, in the presence of total placental abruption, perinatal mortality rates are about 80 per cent. Obviously, long term morbidities among survivors are likewise high.

Placenta Previa

Placenta previa is an important cause of antepartal bleeding, even though it is encountered in only about 1 in 200 deliveries. This condition has been referred to as premature separation of the abnormally implanted placenta. The cause is not known, but the abnormality of placentation occurs more often in multiparas. The types are designed on the basis of the relationship of the placenta to the internal cervical os as follows:

(1) Complete, total, or central placenta previa: the entire cervical os is covered by placental tissue at the time of the initial examination.
(2) Partial placenta previa: the internal os is only partially covered by placenta at the time of the initial examination. This relationship is not static, since the progress of labor with its retraction of the lower uterine segment can draw up the placenta as the cervix dilates. Thus, the entire os may be covered early in labor and may be only partially covered later on.
(3) Marginal placenta previa: the edge of the placenta extends to the margin of the internal os.

When the placenta lies well within the lower uterine segment but the edge does not reach to or encroach upon the internal os, the condition has been designated "low implantation." As apparent spontaneous conversion of a marginal placenta previa to a low implantation can occur when the placenta is drawn upwards in the development of the lower uterine segment during late pregnancy in response to "false labor pains."

The placental margin at or near the internal os is vulnerable and a cleavage plane occurs in the decidua spongiosa. When separation occurs, particularly in response to increasing myometrial activity, there may be external bleeding because muscular contractions in the lower uterine segment are poorer in quality than in the fundus and vessels are not shut off. The classic symptoms are recurrent episodes of bleeding, usually painless, particularly in the earlier stages of pregnancy. With uterine contractions, bleeding may be accentuated and there may be discomfort. The latter clinical condition may be quite similar to a partially separated placenta implanted normally in the fundus. Generally, the initial episode of bleeding ceases spontaneously or continues as only minimal drainage. The blood loss is ordinarily not life threatening to the mother unless and internal examination has been performed. However, recurrent episodes are the rule and the amount of blood loss is accentuated by contractions. In contrast with abruptio placenta, the bleeding is ordinarily entirely external and the degree of hypovolemia and anemia is proportional to observed blood loss. There should be no infiltrations of blood into the myometrium or other tissues and there is no tenderness or increase in the resting tone of the uterus.

Diagnosis. The most characteristic clinical presentation of painless, bright red vaginal bleeding calls for the presumptive diagnosis. Since abnormal presentations are found in one-quarter of the cases of placenta previa, the presence of a transverse lie or breech, particularly if the presenting part is riding high in the fundus, should provoke even more concern.

The definitive method of diagnosis is a vaginal examination consisting of careful inspection and digital exploration of the endocervical canal. This examination must be performed in context with some rigid safeguards and precise obstetrical indications, since manipulations may disrupt more placenta and create life-threatening hemorrhage. Thus, these potential risks can be tolerated only if the fetus is clearly viable or if delivery is required to stop heavy blood loss. An examination of this type can be undertaken only under sterile circumstances in the presence of a "double setup" capability which means that the operating room has been adequately prepared for immediate vaginal or abdominal delivery. There should be provisions for infusions, blood transfusions, oxygen, anesthesia, instruments, and the proper personnel to proceed with active intervention if necessary.

In the patient who does not require definitive diagnosis a plan of expectant management is indicated if it is necessary to postpone delivery until the fetus becomes mature. Preferably, the patient should remain at bed rest in the hospital under close observation with blood readily available. Sometimes, spontaneous heavy bleeding makes it necessary to abandon this conservative approach under emergency conditions. It is usually safe to conduct a careful speculum examination to inspect the lower generative tract for pathology. A noninvasive method of placental localization should be utilized to select those with lower uterine segment implantations consistent with placenta previa. Available techniques include soft tissue radiographs, radioisotopic technics, amniography, retrograde femoral arteriography, thermography and others; however, the preferred diagnostic method today is the sonographic examination. The technique is entirely safe and carries with it an accuracy of about 95 per cent. Unfortunately, the precise relationship of the lower placental margin to the internal cervical os cannot be determined; ultimately, the direct digital examination is required to establish the definitive diagnosis. Placental localization is not indicated if the clinical status requires active intervention with labor or heavy bleeding or the gestational age of the fetus is already around 36 weeks. If a conservative plan of management has been followed, it is terminated electively at about that stage and confirmation of fetal maturity can be determined by special tests, e.g., biparietal measurements by ultrasound studies, amniotic fluid studies (L/S ratio, etc.).

Active Treatment. Definitive treatment is indicated when labor ensues, when the amount of bleeding is hazardous to the life of the mother or when the fetus is approaching term size. A sterile vaginal examination, with the operating room set up for possible immediate surgery, is carried out to ascertain the diagnosis before definitive therapy is performed. It should be borne in mind that a wide variety of unrelated lower genital tract lesions, including carcinoma of the cervix, may be the cause of the vaginal bleeding.

The selection of definitive treatment in cases of placenta previa is based primarily on the status of the cervix, parity, degree of previa, presence or absence of labor and the amount of bleeding.

Pregnancy should be terminated at a time optimal for maximal perinatal salvage and protection of the mother against hemorrhage, trauma and unnecessary operations. Adequate blood replacement and combat of shock are basic considerations in any management. All patients with total placenta previa should be delivered by cesarean section, and most primigravidas who have even minor degrees of partial previa are better delivered by the abdominal route. Although there is somewhat more latitude in selecting a method of definitive management for multiparas who have partial placenta previa, patients in this category who are bleeding actively but who are not in labor and in whom the cervix is long and relatively closed, should be delivered by cesarean section. Multiparas with marginal previa, especially those with an open cervix or who are already in labor, are handled best by rupture of membranes in anticipation of vaginal delivery. Only rarely, when labor does not proceed normally or heavy vaginal bleeding continues, or the fetal presentation is abnormal, will it become necessary to resort to abdominal delivery.

It should be emphasized that a vaginal delivery might produce additional fetal hazards by compressing the placenta and creating partial obstruction of the fetal vessels. The additional hypoxia resulting from these vascular deficits could result in fetal death. However, a vaginal delivery, if it could be achieved safely, would be preferred in the presence of sepsis and/or a very immature or nonviable fetus. Occasionally, it might be appropriate to rupture membranes in a case of marginal or partial placenta previa and to apply scalp traction by placement of a Willett forceps. The effect of this procedure is to pull down the presenting part to tamponade the bleeding uterine sinuses. For the most part, such technique and use of the Voorhees bag and Braxton Hicks version to reduce maternal blood loss have no place in modern obstetrics.

Maternal risks involve primarily hemorrhage, shock and puerperal infection but the mortality rate in the United States is less than 0.25 per cent in modern hospitals. The perinatal risks are hypoxia, birth injury, and the consequences of premature birth, including respiratory distress syndrome and a slightly higher incidence of developmental defects. The perinatal mortality rate is in the range of 15 go 20 per cent.

Ectopic Pregnancy

Ectopic pregnancy means a gestation in which the fertilized ovum implants itself at some site other than the usual one in the endometrium. It includes: (1) pregnancy in any portion of the tube (tubal pregnancy), including its interstitial portion in the wall of the uterus (interstitial pregnancy); (2) pregnancy in a rudimentary uterine horn; (3) ovarian pregnancy; (4) abdominal pregnancy, either primary or secondary; and (5) cervical pregnancy. Ectopic pregnancies occur once in about 200 pregnancies in white women, but the incidence in nonwhite woman may be closer to 1 in 120 pregnancies. Tubal pregnancy is by far the most common form of ectopic gestation. The phenomena of implantation in tubal pregnancy are similar to those of normal uterine gestation when allowance is made for the striking deficiency of decidual response on the part of the tubal wall. The villi themselves have the same characteristics, although there is a high incidence of hydropic degeneration.

Ectopic pregnancy may be due to any condition that narrows the tube or brings about some constriction within it. Most common of these are developmental defects and inflammatory processes. These factors prevent or delay the passage of the fertilized egg into the uterine cavity, and when the burrowing apparatus of the ovum (trophoblast) develops, implantation occurs in the tube. Normally, the blastocyst has trophoblast development to achieve implantation at about 7 days following conception. Anything that delays transport through the tube for that period of time may cause a tubal implantation (e.g., diverticulum, peritubal adhesions, tumor distortions, prior tubal surgery, endosulpingitis, etc.). Factors increasing the receptiveness of the tubal mucosa to the fertilized egg (endometrium-like areas in the tube) also may rarely cause tubal implantation. It is important to note that tubal pregnancies occur among women using an intrauterine contraceptive device at a rate some 10 times higher than in normal women.

Tubal pregnancy may terminate in any one of the following ways: (1) internal rupture of the pseudocapsularis with resulting hemorrhage into the tube and from the fimbriated orifice; (2) tubal abortion, when the ovum may be expelled into the abdominal cavity; (3) tubal rupture, which is a frequent occurrence; (4) abdominal pregnancy secondary to tubal rupture; (5) broad ligament (intraligamentary) pregnancy secondary to tubal rupture; (6) spontaneous regression; (7) lithopedion formation or mummification; and (8) tubal hydatidiform mole of chorioepithelioma.

The symptoms of tubal rupture may be dramatic, resulting from the intraabdominal hemorrhage. Sudden lower abdominal pain, shock and collapse may be the outstanding symptoms. The symptoms of uninterrupted extrauterine pregnancy are usually so slight that a physician seldom is consulted before rupture, so that a diagnosis before rupture is rarely made. The presence of a unilateral tubal tumor in a patient with the symptoms of pregnancy suggests the diagnosis. An altered recent menstrual history is usual, but a history of amenorrhea is not obtained in one fourth or more of the cases. However, the incidence of vaginal spotting is about 75 per cent. If the fetus is dead before rupture, the continued uterine bleeding may be mistaken for an incomplete uterine abortion or menorrhagia. The pregnancy test is usually negative in the conventional tests. Characteristically, serum levels of human chorionic gonadotropin are lower with tubal pregnancy than with intrauterine pregnancy. However, with the advent of the radio ceptor assay for hCG and radio immuno assay for hCG subunit, it is possible to defect pregnancy at extremely low levels of trophoblast activity.

Diagnosis. The diagnosis of tubal rupture, on the other hand, is usually clear. The symptoms are sudden severe lower abdominal pain in a pregnant woman, who suddenly becomes faint and pale and may collapse, particularly if resistance is felt on either side of the uterus. There is often a history of "spotting." The pain need not be on the same side as the supposed mass. If the collapse becomes more profound, rupture has probably occurred. Certain of these cases may result in the subsequent formation of a pelvic hematocele. A bluish discoloration of the umbilicus indicates intraperitoneal hemorrhage but is rarely present (Cullen's sign). Tenderness on vaginal examination is exquisite; thus, an examination under suitable anesthesia is usually mandatory. In doubtful cases, the direct visualization of the pelvic pathology through the culdoscope is helpful in establishing the diagnosis. More recently, inspection of the pelvis through the laparoscope after intraabdominal instillation of CO_2 has proved to be more satisfactory. When the cul-de-sac bulges, needle aspiration or posterior culdotomy may be used to demonstrate free blood in the pelvis or to visualize the pelvic structures (culdescentesis). In about 20 per cent of cases, uterine currettings reveal decidua without villi; however this diagnostic approach in unrewarding in the great majority of cases since the decidua has been discharged inconspicuously in a piecemeal fashion over a time following the fall in endocrine support associated with placental deterioration. Rarely, by pelvic ultrasonography, tubal pregnancy can be established; but more frequently the absence of an intrauterine sac at the 5th to 6th gestational week makes a tubal pregnancy more likely.

Treatment. Laparotomy and blood transfusion are required. Blood for transfusion should be immediately available and may be lifesaving. Future childbearing potential is guarded. Attempts at tuboplasty are not desirable at this time, and in the presence of free blood the appendix should not be removed.

PATHOLOGY OF LABOR AND PUERPERIUM

Dystocia

Dystocia (difficult labor) may be defined as cessation of progress in parturition, and the causes fall into three main groups:

1. Subnormal or abnormal uterine forces that are not strong enough to overcome the natural resistance offered to the birth of the baby by the birth canal. Weakness of uterine action is called uterine inertia and is the most common cause of dystocia.
2. Faulty presentation or abnormal development of the fetus.
3. Abnormalities in the size or the character of the birth canal that form an obstacle to the descent of the fetus.

Dysfunctional Labor

The commonest cause of dysfunctional labor in healthy, well-nourished women is "abnormal uterine contractility." The dysfunction may take the form of "hypocontractility" in which uterine contractions occur less than twice per 10 minutes and average less than 25 mm. Hg. Progress in labor is arrested or retarded in terms of rate of cervical effacement and dilatation, and descent and rotation of the presenting part. Although abnormal cervical compliance (cervix remains firm and poorly effaced) has been implicated as the underlying cause in a small percentages of cases (approximately 3 per cent), this factor, too, is probably merely part of the dysfunctional pathophysiology. The investigation of patients with arrested labor must include evaluation for obstruction of the birth canal, fetal origin, placental origin, or, perhaps, poor patient effort, if the second stage of labor is adversely affected, which may be an effect of heavy analgesia. Dysfunctional labor may also present in the form of "hypercontractility" which is manifested by more than 5 contractions in 10 minutes with or without elevated resting pressures (normal range of 8 to 12 mm. Hg). This type of abnormal uterine behavior is seen in cases of placental abruption and in some preeclamptic parturients. There is a growing belief that the behavior of the uterine muscle is determined by the physiologic state of the population of myocytes participating in each contraction; and, when a sufficient number of these cells become excitable and develop depolarization rhythms, effective contractions are present at a mode repetition frequency of four per 10 minutes with a mean amplitude of 40 to 50 mm. Hg. The alternative hypothesis involving pacemaker activity and a spreading wave of contractility determined by well-defined organizational systems has been questioned recently, since there is no nervous system integration of activity and contractility seems to be the result of innate biochemical characteristics of the myocyte.

Uterine Hypocontractility

When uterine contractions are poor (uterine wall easily indented at the acme) from the very onset of labor, and there are cessation of cervical dilatation, descent and rotation of the fetal head for a period of hours in the first stage of labor after true labor has definitely been established, the condition is known as primary uterine inertia. The most common cause in modern obstetrics is the premature and the injudicious administration of analgesic drugs and conduction anesthesia. Emotional instability is a major contributing condition. It should be emphasized, however, that even minor degrees of pelvic contractions, slight fetal malposition such as mild extension of the head or posterior positions, uterine overdistention and pathologic conditions such as intramural myomas may give rise to serious inertia. There may be a significant and worrisome prolongation of the latent, acceleration or deceleration phases of labor that call for early recognition and prompt institution of therapy. No arbitrary time limits can be placed on these conditions; arrest of labor at any stage for a period sufficient to be recognized warrants a careful appraisal of the situation and search for possible causes. However, it is important to establish the fact that labor has truly begun. About one patient in 10 with presumed rest (morphine sulfate) and hydration will fail to develop uterine contractions after 4 to 6 hours, despite the fact they were presumed to be in a prolonged latent phase. They may be presumed not to have been in labor.

Biophysical intrapartal fetal monitoring, which will be discussed in more detail later, provides the opportunity of following fetal heart patterns and rates and to demonstrate the effects of uterine contractions upon cardiac behavior. Definite changes are observable in cases of established fetal hypoxia, which may call for prompt intervention to extricate the fetus from its hostile environment and resultant jeopardy. Assessment of fetal scalp blood pH as a means of identifying a hypoxic condition is a useful indicator in many instances or a means of corroborating other evidence of distress, particularly when the level is lower than 7.15. However, prognostic errors are not uncommon in terms of both false-positive and false-negative interpretations.

Uterine inertia of the second stage of labor is defined as cessation of rotation and descent of the fetal head over a 2-hour period after full cervical dilatation, and a uterine wall that is easily indented at the acme of each pain. This should not be confused with a prolonged second stage of labor, a condition in which the second stage exceeds 2 hours in length but does not imply a cessation of progress for 2 hours. The treatment is to give the patient more time. Repeated hot soapsuds enemas often are helpful. Supportive treatment, fluids and encouragement are important. Antibiotics should be administered, particularly if the membranes have been long or prematurely ruptured.

In *carefully selected cases,* Pitocin, administered intravenously in physiologic doses, will promote effective labor and delivery. Abnormal labors, caused by dysrhythmic uterine contractions, will not respond well to oxytocin but they may respond to rest and hydration. The transition may be due to coordinated subnormal contractions that will respond to oxytocin stimulation. Sometimes, however, discoordinated labors will respond to the administration of a conduction anesthetic.

A word of caution is needed, however, because uterine stimulation employed in cases of hypertonic or dyskinetic labor will seriously impair uteroplacental blood flow and embarrass the fetus. Moreover, the risk of uterine rupture is great unless the presenting part is engaged or near engagement, the pelvis is normal, the uterus is unscarred and normally developed, the patient's parity is low, the fetal presentation is normal, and the character of the labor is constantly monitored during administration. Oxytocin should be used only on strict indications. It should not be used in slow labors (not true inertia) or in normal labors for the sake of merely speeding parturition. Use of an oxytocin should be an indication for continuous fetal monitoring throughout the course of labor.

When the cervix is dilated 5 cm. or more and the bag of forewaters is present in front of the fetal head, artificial rupture of the membranes frequently will expedite labor. Postural therapy to effect pressure against the lower uterine segment often is helpful. Adequate hydration and the correction of acid-base imbalance are imperative. Any extension of either the first or the second stages of labor may result in increased perinatal mortality. Therefore, delay in any of the phases of cervical dilatation must be looked upon as a serious sign necessitating prompt attention, diagnosis of its etiology and a plan of action aimed toward proper and timely therapy and delivery as befits each individual case.

Secondary Uterine Inertia. In other cases, the pains are excellent in the initial hours of labor but then become weak, irregular and far apart. Often there is an associated quickening of the pulse rate. This condition is called secondary uterine inertia because it is secondary to exhaustion. This should be a rare occurrence

in modern obstetrics. The treatment should include rest and fluids. This usually is accomplished by giving morphine intramuscularly and 500 or 1,000 ml. of glucose solution (usually 5 per cent) intravenously. In these cases the uterus requires rest rather than stimulation. Also, it should be kept in mind that certain cases of dyskinetic labor—those characterized by painful, dysrhythmic and ineffectual contractions—are logically treated with rest rather than uterine stimulation. Moreover, it is imperative that all causes for dystocia other than uncomplicated uterine dysfunction be excluded, for many of these are best handled by prompt abdominal delivery. Long difficult exhausting labors should not be tolerated today in the interests of promoting optimal perinatal salvage.

Hypertonic Inertia. The occlusion of intramyometrial vessels supplying the placenta, which is a particularly prominent feature of precipitous and hypertonic labor, is a well-recognized cause of suppressed flow of blood through the intervillous space. Bradycardia or fetal hypoxia, or both, can be correlated with dysfunctional labor of this type, namely, short interval of contractions, high tonus, increased intensity, increased duration and dysrhythmic patterns. In a similar manner, the injudicious use of oxytocic stimulation, especially with sparteine sulfate administration, may induce dysrhythmic and hypertonic contraction patterns in the uterus, which greatly interfere with uteroplacental circulation. From whatever cause, this hypertonus prevents full reestablishment of placental circulation between uterine contractions. Fetal asphyxia persists and maintains abnormal stimulation of the vagus nerve, preventing the fetal heart rate from recovering the normal basal values; thus prolonged and profound bradycardia throughout the interval between contractions is probably the best criterion of fetal distress. If the hypertonic inertia persists, fetal death may occur. The patient may complain of considerable intermittent pain. The cervical dilatation remains stationary and, during a contraction, especially if there is a reversal of pressure gradient, the presenting part may actually rise slightly in the pelvis. The treatment is sedation and uterine rest, not stimulation, or abdominal intervention if there is evidence of obstructed labor or impending uterine rupture.

Precipitate Labor

Fetal welfare is compromised when the intensity of uterine contractions is increased, intervals are shortened and duration is increased. A combination of excessively forceful uterine contractions and minimal soft tissue resistance can give rise to precipitate labor, fetal anoxia and cerebral trauma, maternal lacerations and postpartal hemorrhage caused by uterine atony. Early recognition of the problem, timely preparation for delivery under controlled conditions and properly administered analgesia and/or anesthesia may minimize these risks.

Uterine Constriction Rings

In association with ineffectual uterine contractions, there may be annular, spastic muscular strictures that do not rise or change position as labor advances. Unlike the pathologic retraction ring of Bandle, they are not associated with obstructed labor and they cannot be palpated externally at the junction of the lower and upper uterine segments. The majority are palpable only on the uterine interior. Often, they arise from inappropriate manual or oxytocic stimulation. Relaxants including amyl nitrite, intravenous epinephrine or deep anesthesia may eliminate the localized myometrial spasms, but more often abdominal delivery is required.

Intrapartal Infection

Normally, there appear to be natural defenses in the mother that are effective in preventing intrapartal infections. Obviously, host resistance in general is affected by the overall health status; the cervical mucus plug, intact membranes and perhaps antibacterial activity in the amniotic fluid are also important factors. These defense mechanisms are lost when the membranes rupture. Within 24 hours the great majority of patients, perhaps 75 per cent, will have positive amniotic fluid cultures. The longer the duration of membrane rupture prior to delivery the higher the incidence of "chorioamnionitis," and, in some cases, a rapid invasion of gram-negative bacilli will produce septic shock. Thus, an accurate diagnosis of ruptured membranes is crucial. Usually, by observation or inspection or utilizing the nitrazine paper test (positive results due to alkaline amniotic fluid), fern test (amniotic fluid allowed to dry shows ferning, and cytologic examination (presence of vernix caseosa cells), the diagnosis can be established.

Once chorioamnionitis develops the fetus and the mother are at risk because fetal penumonia and/or septicemia may produce a perinatal death. Often, there is a dilemma because immaturity of the fetus at the time of membrane rupture may mean the chances of extrauterine survival would not be great. Unfortunately, prophylactic antibiotics do not protect the mother or the fetus. A delay of some 18 to 24 hours after rupture of the membranes tends to provoke fetal lung maturity and lessen the likelihood of the respiratory distress syndrome. Within 48 hours of administering betamethasone therapy to the mother, even greater lung maturation can be achieved in the fetus. If there is no evidence of infection in the mother and the gestation is less than 34 weeks duration, corticosteroid therapy and expectancy might be an appropriate management. About 80 per cent of these patients will go into labor spontaneously within 72 hours. Despite the risk of provoking a candida albicans infection in the infant, antibiotic coverage during labor may reduce the likelihood of puerperal morbidity. In an asymptomatic woman whose gestation is 34 weeks or more or with evidence of overt signs of infection at earlier stages, the presence of documented ruptured membranes calls for induction of labor or abdominal intervention, should this be contraindicated or unsuccessful within a latent period of some 12 hours.

Biophysical Intrapartal Fetal Monitoring

Continuous electronic monitoring of the fetus is a widely applied clinical means to detect fetal distress. When the amniotic membranes are intact, indirect techniques are used, but, with ruptured membranes, direct techniques utilizing electrodes attached directly to the fetal presenting part can be employed. Certainly, in major centers, all fetuses considered to be at risk are monitored in this manner during labor. In addition, such techniques employed prior to the spontaneous onset of labor can be studied under a Pitocin provocation circumstance to determine fetal response in relation to a short-term test labor. These responses may be helpful in deciding management; that is, a decision can be made with such objective evidence in hand whether acceptable risks are or are not present in relation to allowing normal labor to ensue.

The most significant variant in fetal heart rate is deceleration occurring late in the contracting phase of the uterus, usually caused by uteroplacental insufficiency. Poor perinatal outcome is associated with a fetal cardiac pattern of this type that persists and is uncorrected. Another significant pattern is variable deceleration, which is commonly causes by umbilical cord occlusion. Fetuses with ominous heart patterns in utero frequently develop the respiratory distress syndrome as newborn infants. Late deceleration, considered to be hypoxic bradycardia, is a cause of perinatal brain damage if left uncorrected. Lack of the normal baseline fetal heart rate variability is an ominous sign. The presence of such objective evidence of fetal distress in utero has been the basis for intapartal intervention on a timely basis. Modern salvage rates are predicated upon the use of such monitoring techniques in vulnerable patients whose fetuses are at risk.

Pelvic Contraction

The common types of pelvic contraction may be classified in four main groups: contraction of the inlet, contraction of the midpelvis, contraction of the outlet and combinations of inlet, midpelvic and outlet contraction. Inlet contraction is defined as diminution of the obstetric conjugate measurement (by roentgenogram) to 10.0 cm. or less of diminution of the diagonal conjugate measurement (clinical) to 11.5 cm. or less. The most common cause of inlet contraction is rickets. About two per cent of white women and about 15 per cent of Negro women have pelvic contraction of the inlet from this cause. When the interischial spinous diameter is 9.5 cm. or less (by roentgenogram), there is transverse contraction of the midpelvis. In outlet contraction the angle formed by the pubic rami is narrow, and the ischial tuberosities are close together; thus it resembles a male pelvis insofar as the outlet is concerned; often it is called a funnel pelvis. It is customary to make a diagnosis of outlet contraction whenever the intertuberous distance is 8 cm. or less (clinical) or 10 cm. or less by roentgenographic measurement. The sum of the interischial tuberous diameter (TI) and the posterior sagittal diameter of the outlet (PSO) should be 15.0 cm. or more by clinical measurement to be considered normal.

In addition to actual measurements, the pelvic architecture is important in determining pelvic capacity and compensatory space. This can be appreciated best with the aid of x-ray pelvimetry. It should be noted that the size of the pelvis is only one important factor in determining whether or not a given fetus can be delivered through a given pelvis. Other factors involved in the eventual outcome include size of the fetus, moldability of the fetal head, fetal position and presentation, rigidity of the maternal soft parts, the uterine powers and other clinical features. Therefore, x-ray pelvimetry cannot be a replacement for astute clinical evaluation of the factors of labor.

Pelvic Dystocia

The treatment of dystocia due to abnormal pelves varies with the degree of contraction, the size of the child and, in multiparas, the history of previous labors. Successful treatment depends on the ability to determine the extent of disproportion between the child and the pelvis. However, in general, a normally developed full-term child cannot be born spontaneously and alive when the true conjugate measure 8 cm. or less, and only rarely when it is below 8.5 cm. In the great majority of cases, a trial of labor is necessary before proper decision can be made concerning definitive management. However, in modern obstetrics, fetal monitoring is instituted and the decision for intervening at an optimal time is based more on the fetal status and clinical situation than any arbitrary set of pelvic measurements. Certainly, if the trial of labor is continued until there is a pathological retraction ring of Ban-

dle, indicative of an obstructed labor, the possibility of fetal jeopardy already exists.

Dystocia due to abnormalities in the fetus include: (1) excessive size, (2) monstrosities, (3) hydrocephalus, (4) multiple pregnancies and (5) transverse lie. In "shoulder presentations," external cephalic version can be carefully attempted before or early in labor, provided that the patient's parity is not great, the fetal membranes are intact and the presenting part is not markedly engaged. If this fails, as it often does, a careful examination should be made to rule out placenta previa (a very common cause of transverse lie) and contracted pelvis. Any primigravida at or near term whose fetus at the onset of labor is in transverse lie should be delivered abdominally if there is no tendency for spontaneous conversion. Any patient with a contracted pelvis, either primigravida or multipara, should be subjected to cesarean section. However, in multiparas with normal pelves, the treatment may be more elastic. Because of the extremely high perinatal mortality associated with premature rupture of the membranes and prolapse of the umbilical cord in this presentation, a multipara with a persistent transverse lie whose membranes rupture before near or full cervical dilatation is delivered best by cesarean section. If the membranes remain intact until late in labor, usually labor should be allowed to continue to full cervical dilatation, at which time version and extraction are performed, provided the infant is relatively small, the pelvis is known to be normal, and the mother's parity is not great. However, the grave risk of uterine rupture with these internal manipulations has made the procedure obsolete, except for small fetuses and second twins. Cesarean hysterectomy is preferable to a vaginal destructive procedure in neglected, infected cases of transverse position with fetal death in utero, especially if the fetus is of near-term size. Rarely, spontaneous evolution may occur—either by Douglas' or Denman's method—in which a small macerated fetus may be expelled spontaneously, or delivery may occur by a mechanism in which the fetus is doubled upon itself (*conduplicato corpore*).

Posterior Occipital Position

The majority of posterior positions are delivered ultimately in the anterior position. However, at the onset of labor, posterior position of the occiput is a common finding. Persistent occiput posterior includes those cases that do not deliver anteriorly (only about 5 per cent).

The diagnosis of right occipital posterior (ROP) position is made by:

1. The palpation of freely movable soft parts above and just to the left of the umbilicus

2. Maximum intensity of the heart sounds in the right flank; less frequently near the midline
3. Deflexion of the head in the inlet
4. The finding on rectal or vaginal examination that the sagittal suture occupies the right oblique diameter, the small fontanel being felt opposite the right sacroiliac synchondrosis and the large fontanel being directed toward the left iliopectineal eminence.

In ROP one of the following may occur:

1. Complete anterior rotation through 135 degrees to OA
2. Incomplete anterior rotation
3. Arrest in transverse position
4. No rotation—persistent ROP
5. Posterior rotation of occiput through 45 degrees (occipitosacral)

In the vast majority of ROP positions, anterior rotation takes place spontaneously if patience is exercised. In a very small minority (and only after the cervix is fully dilated) one of the following procedures may be necessary: (1) manual rotation of the head to OA, followed by application of forceps; (2) forceps rotation to OA followed by reapplication of forceps (Scanzoni maneuver); and (3) delivery with forceps as a posterior. If the fetal head is considerably molded or the pelvis is anthropoid or android in type or shows midpelvic contraction, delivery by forceps as an occiput posterior may prove to be the least traumatic to the mother and the fetus, but each case must be considered and treated individually.

Breech Presentation

Breech presentations are classified as follows:

1. *Complete,* when the feet and the legs are flexed on the thighs, and the thighs are flexed on the abdomen, so that the buttocks and the feet present.
2. *Incomplete,* when the foot or the knee, in any combination, presents through the cervix.
3. *Frank,* when the legs are extended and lie against the abdomen and the chest, and the buttocks present.

The diagnosis of breech presentation depends on palpating the hard ballotable head in the fundus with the irregular soft breech above the symphysis. Rectal or vaginal examination reveals the characteristic parts. The fetal heart sounds are heard through the back of the fetus at about the level of the umbilicus. The normal mechanism includes: (1) engagement and (2) descent, ordinarily in one of the oblique diameters.

Usually it is the anterior hip that first encounters the resistance of the pelvic floor, causing an internal rotation of 45 degrees that brings the anterior hip to the pubic arch. If the posterior hip descends first, internal rotation occurs through an arc of 135 degrees. Descent continues until the perineum is distended, when the posterior hip is delivered over the anterior margin of the perineum by lateral flexion of the body, followed by the spontaneous delivery of the legs and the feet. As the shoulders reach the perineum they undergo internal rotation to the anteroposterior diameter. The flexed head enters the pelvis in one of the oblique diameters and then rotates so that the posterior neck engages under the symphysis. The head is born in a position of flexion, with the chin, the mouth, the nose, the forehead, the bregma and the occiput appearing in succession over the perineum.

The relatively high perinatal mortality (approximately 15 per cent) of breech presentation is due mainly to the increased incidence of prematurity, complications of gestation and labor (especially inert labor) and fetal anomalies, the presentation itself being responsible for only about one third of the deaths, trauma and anoxia accounting for many of these. Prolapse of the umbilical cord is particular hazard of the complete and the incomplete varieties, the incidence being, respectively, about 12 and 22 times the usual incidence for vertex presentation.

In the latter weeks of pregnancy, substitution of a vertex presentation may be attempted by external version. This may be done even during the first stage of labor, provided that (1) the breech has not descended deeply into the pelvis, (2) the membranes are intact, and (3) the fetus is not of excessive size.

Breech deliveries may be of three types:

1. A spontaneous delivery is one in which the entire infant is expelled by natural forces.
2. A partial breech extraction is one in which the infant is extruded as far as the umbilicus by natural forces, but the remainder of the body is extracted by the attendant. This method of delivery is the one of choice whenever feasible.
3. A total breech extraction is one in which the entire body of the infant is extracted by the attendant. This method should be employed only when specific indications demand it.

The breech should be allowed to advance spontaneously until the umbilicus has been born. The completion of labor is facilitated if the arms remain crossed and the head is sharply flexed. This is best obtained by avoiding traction and by moderate downward pressure on the fundus as soon as the breech begins to emerge through the vulva.

When delivery by traction is necessary, the traction on the legs and the body should be downward until an axilla becomes visible, when the body is flexed upward, delivering the posterior shoulder over the perineum. By depressing the body of the fetus the anterior shoulder is brought to emerge beneath the pubic arch. The head usually occupies an oblique diameter with the chin posteriorly and is best delivered by Mauriceau's maneuver. The index finger of one hand is introduced into the mouth of the child and applied over the superior maxilla, while the body rests upon the palm of the hand. Two fingers of the other hand are then hooked over the neck and, grasping the shoulders, make downward traction until the occiput appears over the symphysis. The body is now extended upward, and the mouth, the brow, the nose and the occiput emerge successfully over the perineum. Piper forceps to the after-coming head are favored by many obstetricians.

The safe management of breech presentation, especially in the primigravida, necessitates an intimate knowledge of the maternal pelvis, usually obtainable only through x-ray pelvimetry. Cesarean section is a safer approach to breech delivery and yields better results than does a complicated and difficult extraction. If the fetus is large or there is any question whatever concerning pelvic adequacy, a cesarean section should be performed after labor is established.

Current management is predicated upon the findings that vaginal delivery is risky and that, in general, perinatal mortality and morbidity can be improved by utilizing abdominal delivery. The vulnerable groups include complete and incomplete (footling) breeches among whom the incidence of prolapsed cord may be 10 per cent, patients with premature labor or who have an in utero growth retardation problem (12 to 14 per cent), and primigravidas with average to large term-sized fetus. The trend now is to require specific indications and justification for vaginal delivery in breech presentations even among multiparas at term.

Face Presentation

Since face presentations result from extension of the fetal head, the characteristic sign is that the cephalic prominence is palpable on the same side as the back instead of on the side of the small parts as in vertex presentation. The heart sounds are heard on the side of the small parts and are louder than usual.

Delivery occurs by (1) descent, as in vertex presentation, with internal rotation and flexion, (2) extension and (3) external rotation.

Internal rotation brings the chin under the symphysis, the head being delivered by flexion, with the nose, the eyes, the brow, the bregma and the occiput appearing in succession over the anterior margin of the perineum. After the birth of the head the occiput sags backward and undergoes external rotation to the side toward which it was originally directed. The face must rotate, because delivery of a mature baby with the chin posterior is impossible. The initial position of the chin is posterior in about 30 per cent of these cases.

Anterior rotation usually occurs spontaneously, though very late. When this is not the case (about one instance in ten), conversion into a vertex presentation may be attempted, provided that the face is not deeply engaged, the pelvis is normal and the membranes are intact or recently ruptured. If the cervix is fully dilated and the fetus is less than average size, an internal podalic version may be attempted under such circumstances. However, in primigravidas in whom the chin remains posterior, cesarean section is preferable. Finally, if the baby is dead, craniotomy may be necessary. If the pelvis is normal and the chin anterior, spontaneous delivery or an easy forceps delivery should be anticipated, no treatment being necessary.

When a brow presentation is detected at the superior strait, it should be left alone until it promises to be persistent because the transient varieties will be born spontaneously as either a vertex or a face presentation. On the other hand, less than one half of the persistent cases—often attended by a true disproportion—can be expected to deliver uneventfully; thus, attempts at conversion or (usually) cesarean section are indicated on a basis similar to that outlined for face presentations.

Cesarean sections are advocated much more frequently in all cases of malposition and malpresentation of the fetus, and when labor becomes abnormal or fetal distress develops.

Birth Injury

Injury of the fetal brain may be the result of primary oxygen deficiency or of mechanical trauma. The former group includes any maternal, placental or cord condition that interferes with oxygenation of the fetus, while the latter group is made up of cases in which the fetus exhibits evidence of contusions, dural lacerations, hematomas, skull fractures or other forms of trauma.

The influence of hypoxia on the fetal brain is characterized by capillary congestion, endothelial injury and interstitial hemorrhage; involved vessels may rupture in response to less than ordinary stresses. A membrane that can withstand a certain strain when the force is applied gradually may rupture when the stress is applied suddenly. As long as the stress increases gradually and is directed toward the midline or is equally distributed to both sides of the head, there is little danger that the margin of either the falx cerebri or the tentorium will be disrupted. If the force is applied asymmetrically, one leaf of the tentorium will be relaxed, while the other is placed under excessive tension. If the force is sufficient, and especially if it is suddenly applied, the leaf under tension will rupture, often involving the great cerebral vein or one of the sinuses.

Prolapse of the Cord

Prolapse of the cord is most common in conditions that tend to interfere with engagement at the superior strait; hence, it is most common in transverse and foot presentations and less often found in frank breech. The cord may sometimes be seen or, provided that the fetus is alive, may be palpated as a cord with distinct pulsations. Hypotension in the fetus for any reason may cause the cord to become limp and possibly prolapse; hence, perinatal mortality rates of 30 per cent for all cases can be anticipated, since many of these infants are premature. Variable deceleration noted in the fetal heart pattern identified through biophysical intrapartal monitoring may help identify cord compression in occult prolapses.

If the cord prolapses after the cervix has become fully dilated, forceps are indicated when the head is deep in the pelvic canal. In breech presentation, a foot should be brought down and extraction completed.

If the cervix is only partially dilated, the patient should be placed immediately in the knee-chest position until preparations can be made for sterile vaginal manipulation. Then an attempt should be made to replace the cord, although the attempt is frequently unsuccessful. The chances for the child are poor unless cesarean section is performed, but this should not be attempted unless the fetal heart and the umbilical pulsations are strong after release of pressure from the cord. Oxygen should be administered to the mother. As a prophylaxis against this complication, it is advisable to make a sterile vaginal examination and to palpate for the cord when the diagnosis of abnormal presentation is first made. Close watch of the fetal heart in such cases is imperative.

Rupture of the Uterus

Rupture of the uterus occurs once in approximately every 2,000 cases and is a grave accident, carrying a composite maternal mortality of about 10 to 15 per cent and a perinatal mortality of about 50 to 75 per cent. There are two main types, spontaneous and traumatic, and each of these, in turn, may be classified according to whether it occurs in pregnancy or in labor. Ruptures that occur spontaneously may further be categorized into three groups: (1) those with a previous cesarean section scar; (2) those with previous operative scars; and (3) those with an intact uterus. The distinction is important because the maternal mortality rate for ruptures of intact uteri is between 20 and 40 per cent, while that associated with rupture of a cesarean section scar is only about 5 per cent. It is customary to distinguish between "complete" and "incomplete" rupture, according to whether the laceration communicates with the abdominal cavity or is separated from it by peritoneal covering (subperitoneal hematoma).

Causes. The spontaneous rupture of the uterus during labor is more common than traumatic rupture because of the modern trend away from difficult vaginal operations, especially the elimination of version and extraction as a frequent procedure. In the past, nearly one half of the traumatic ruptures resulted from this operation. Other cases resulted from a Braxton Hicks version, difficult or unsuccessful forceps breech extraction and the use of bags and bougies. The common antecedent factors in spontaneous rupture of the uterus are advanced maternal age and parity, contraction of the pelvis, a large fetus and such obvious dystocial factors as abnormal presentation and impacted pelvic tumors. Excessive stretching of the lower uterine segment with the development of a pathologic retraction ring plays an important predisposing role. Unfortunately, the injudicious use of Pitocin stimulation of the uterus remains a significant factor in uterine rupture. Other predisposing factors in the spontaneous rupture of the intact uterus are congenital defects of the uterus, adenomyosis and a history of previous curettage, manual removal of the placenta and postabortive or postpartum sepsis. However, with the increasing incidence of cesarean section, *rupture of the scar has become the most common cause of uterine rupture.* The risk of uterine rupture following a previous cesarean section is about 2 per cent. When the old scar merely disrupts and the myometrium is not freshly lacerated, the event is more properly referred to as a wound dehiscence than actual rupture, and the prognosis is much better. The overall incidence of uterine rupture is approximately the same following classic and low cervical operations; however, about one third of classic scars rupture in the later months of pregnancy and are apt to be complete and dramatic and to occur without warning, while the low cervical ruptures occur almost exclusively during labor and the signs and symptoms are insidious. A hematoma may develop within the broad ligament with few or no signs appearing until the patient begins to have pain and fever during the puerperium. When the bladder and the ureter are lacerated and the severed uterine artery has retracted far laterally into a hematoma, the definitive surgical procedure becomes exceedingly difficult and tedious.

Symptoms. Rupture occurring in the later months of pregnancy usually causes sudden, sharp abdominal pains followed by collapse, but in some cases the immediate symptoms are mild. If rupture occurs at the time of labor, the patient usually complains at the height of a uterine contraction of a sharp shooting pain in the lower abdomen, followed by sudden relief. There may be external hemorrhage, cessation of uterine contractions and sudden disappearance of the fetal heart beat. The lower uterine segment becomes more sensitive to pressure, the presenting part slips away from the inlet, and the firmly contracted uterus can be felt alongside the fetus. The symptoms of shock from hemorrhage are usually sudden and severe but may be delayed, especially if the rupture is in the lower uterine segment. Blood may appear in the urine.

If rupture occurs during delivery, extraction should not be attempted, but immediate laparotomy should be done. Hysterectomy is usually required, as is also blood transfusion.

Sound obstetric management will avoid uterine rupture in most cases. Although cases must be treated individually, the attitude generally held today is that in most instances, one cesarean section is enough to indicate this mode of delivery in following pregnancies. When the patient has had a previous normal vaginal delivery and all obstetric factors are favorable, or the patient appears in advanced labor, or the fetus is small, one can contemplate vaginal delivery under close observation in carefully selected cases. Some clinics report safe delivery by the vaginal route in up to 50 per cent of their cases.

Postpartal Hemorrhage

Serious bleeding following the birth of the child is usually due to (1) uterine atony, (2) placental retention or (3) deep tears of the birth canal. The most common of these is the first, which is responsible in over 90 per cent of these cases. Among the controllable causes of postpartal hemorrhage, the most common are: operative delivery, deep ether anesthesia, prolonged labor with maternal exhaustion and mismanagement of the third stage of labor. Postpartal hemorrhage should be anticipated and prepared for when any of these complications is present or when there has been overstretching of the uterus as in cases of an excessively large fetus, multiple gestation, hydramnios or uterine tumors. Postpartal hemorrhage is defined as bleeding from the birth canal in excess of 500 ml. during the first 24 hours after birth. Postpartal hemorrhage, as defined, is observed in about 10 per cent of all deliveries.

If hemorrhage after extrusion of the placenta is due to tears, it gives a steady flow of bright-red blood, beginning immediately after delivery. When due to retained placental tissue the blood escapes in gushes and frequently in large clots. In uterine atony there is a continuous flow, which may be very copious. If the bleeding commences immediately after delivery (third-stage bleeding), it is due to tears or to partial separation of the placenta. If the hemorrhage continues after the uterus has been emptied and is well contracted, tears should be looked for and sutured at once. On the other hand, if the uterus does not contract, the hemorrhage may be due to atony or the retention of a placental cotyledon, which will be shown by careful examination of the placenta. In the presence of marked bleeding before separation of the placenta has occurred, manual removal of the placenta should be carried out at once, certainly before appreciable blood loss has taken place. Also, if the placenta is retained for 10 or 15 minutes in the "absence" of bleeding, the placenta should be removed prophylactically. Recently there has been a trend toward even earlier manual removal if the placenta does not separate soon after delivery. In many clinics it is routine to explore the uterus after delivery of the placenta to assure complete evacuation as well as the intactness of the uterus. Certainly, it is advisable to explore the uterus if there is a question of incompleteness of placental removal, when bleeding continues after the placenta is expressed or following a difficult delivery when the uterine wall may have been injured.

Attempts to deliver the placenta by squeezing and kneading the uterus through the abdomen, as entailed in the original Credé procedure, are not only futile as a rule but also traumatize the myometrium and often aggravate the difficulties. When the placenta has been removed, and bleeding continues, 1 ml. vasopressin (Pitocin), followed by 0.2 mg ergonovine (Methergine), should be given intramuscularly or intravenously. If bleeding persists, bimanual compression and massage of the uterus are indicated. An oxytocin infusion may be helpful. If symptoms of shock appear, the usual treatment of adequate blood replacement is indicated. Uterine packing is losing favor as a means of controlling hemorrhage, except as a temporary procedure in rare instances when hysterectomy is contemplated.

Delivery by Forceps

Delivery by forceps is indicated in any condition that threatens the life of the mother or the child, where a reasonable prospect of being relieved by delivery without too much danger is offered. The most frequent indications in modern obstetrics are conditions in which it is desirable to spare the mother second-stage effort, in dysfunctional labor in the second stage and in certain situations of fetal distress. One of the most frequent indications is uterine dysfunction. In general, it is considered good practice, in the absence of disproportion, to apply forceps if advance is not made after 2 hours of satisfactory second-stage pains, or after 1 hour if the head is on the perineum, although each case must be individualized. When a large caput interferes with determination of station, a Thoms' lateral roentgenogram is desirable prior to attempted forceps delivery to avoid an ill-advised application of high forceps. It should be recognized that even in the second stage of labor, oxytocic stimulation, further delay or even abdominal intervention may be choices that are to be preferred to a difficult forceps delivery. The suggested time limits are appropriate points to evaluate the patient thoroughly but not necessarily to effect delivery in every case. The difficulty to be counteracted by the forceps operation and its inherent dangers to the mother and the fetus must be weighed against the hazards of allowing a protracted second stage with its significant fetal risks.

To forestall prolonged pressure of the fetal head against a more or less rigid perineum and to spare the mother the strain of the last few minutes of the second stage, the use of so-called elective low forceps has become popular in recent years, particularly in primigravidas.

The following conditions must be fulfilled before forceps are applied:

1. The child must present correctly, either a vertex or mentum anterior.
2. The cervix must be fully dilated.
3. Membranes must be ruptured.
4. There must be no marked disproportion between the head and the pelvis.
5. The head must have descended to the level of the ischial spines or below.
6. The bladder must be emptied by catheterization.

The most important function of forceps is traction, although they are frequently employed to rotate the fetal head. Forceps operations are classified according to the level of the fetal head at the time that the blades are applied:

1. *Low forceps*—the application of forceps when the head is visible, the skull is on the perineal floor, and the sagittal suture is in the anteroposterior diameter of the pelvis.
2. *Mid forceps*—the application of forceps before the criteria of low forceps (as stated above) have been met but after engagement has taken place, that is, after the plane of the greatest cephalic diameter (biparietal) has passed the inlet. Every effort must be made to avoid this type of poten-

tially hazardous vaginal delivery in the interests of perinatal welfare.
3. *High forceps*—the application of forceps before engagement has taken place. This variety of forceps delivery has no place in modern obstetrics.

For general use the ordinary Simpson forceps are very serviceable, but the particular forceps employed should be varied to suit the particular case. In certain mid-forceps extractions, axis traction is essential (Tarnier, Irving); and in certain cases of transverse arrest, the Kielland forceps have certain advantages. The Piper forceps generally are employed to deliver the after-coming head in breech deliveries. In modern obstetrics, most clinical situations requiring major forceps operations are best handled by cesarean section. Occasionally, there may be an indication for the use of a vacuum extractor as a substitute for forceps when pelvic space is limited.

Version

Version consists of turning the baby in the uterus from an undesirable into a desirable position. There are three types of version: external, internal and Braxton Hicks. According to whether the head or the breech is made the presenting part, the operation is spoken of as cephalic or podalic version, respectively.

External Version. This is an operation designed to change a breech or a transverse presentation into a vertex presentation by external manipulation of the fetus through the abdominal and the uterine walls. It is likely to be most successful when done about a month before full term; however, it often fails, either because it proves to be impossible to turn the fetus around or because the fetus returns to its original position within a few hours. Some obstetricians disapprove of it altogether because, in rare circumstances, the placenta is partially separated, the uterine integrity is jeopardized, or the cord is entangled or knotted. Also, in clinics where this procedure is carried out routinely when a case of breech presentation is discovered, the incidence of breech delivery is about the same as that noted in clinics where this procedure is not employed (about 3 per cent). It should never be done under anesthesia, since undue pressure can be exerted with the patient oblivious to pain. The chance of success is greatest if the presenting part is unengaged and the membranes are intact.

Internal Version. Sometimes called internal podalic version, internal version is an operation designed to change whatever presentation may exist into a breech presentation. With cervical dilatation complete, the whole hand of the operator is introduced high into the uterus, one or both feet grasped and pulled downward in the direction of the birth canal. With his other hand, the obstetrician may expedite the turning by pushing the head upward. When one hand manipulates through the abdominal wall, while two or more fingers of the other hand are introduced through the cervix, the procedure frequently is referred to as a *combined version.* The procedure usually is followed by breech extraction. Internal version finds its greatest usefulness in transverse lie and in cases of multiple pregnancy in which the birth of the second twin is retarded. However, the hazard of uterine rupture and the guarded fetal prognosis limit the usefulness of this procedure. Version and extraction always should be followed by internal exploration of the uterus to make certain that accidental rupture of the uterus has not occurred. In today's obstetrical practice, abdominal delivery is much the preferred method for transverse lie and, currently, even complicated in utero manipulations of a second turn are being discouraged. The use of Braxton Hicks version—compressing the lower uterine segment with the infant's buttocks in placenta previa or stretching the cervix with the infant's thigh so that labor may be initiated—has no place in modern therapy.

Cesarean Section

There are four main types of abdominal cesarean section: (1) classic, (2) low cervical, (3) extraperitoneal, and (4) cesarean hysterectomy. Low cervical is the type favored generally, although other types are preferred in special circumstances.

The one generally accepted indication for cesarean section is a serious disproportion between the size of the fetal head and the maternal pelvis. In certain cases of contracted pelvis, the operation may be indicated if the trial of labor is unsatisfactory. A history of previous difficult labors is significant. Aside from pelvic contraction and mechanical dystocia, the most common indication for cesarean section is fear that a previous cesarean section scar might rupture. In many clinics it is the most common indication. Other important indications for cesarean section, in descending order of importance, are: hemorrhagic complications (placenta previa, abruptio placentae); toxemias; intercurrent diseases (especially diabetes) and middle-aged primigravidas. There are other miscellaneous indications, such as carcinoma of the cervix, certain cases of uterine inertia and pregnancy following major vaginal repairs. Generally, perinatal risks are weighed very high and when the welfare of the fetus or mother is potentially compromised by waiting, or if fetal monitoring shows the potential of stress or actual stress in response to provoked or spontaneous myometrial activity, abdominal intervention may be desirable.

Except in the presence of an absolute pelvic indica-tion, abruptio placentae or central placenta previa, cesarean section should not be performed when the child is dead or in serious danger or the mother is in poor condition. Rarely, craniotomy may be necessary as in hydrocephaly presenting cephalically or by the breech. Cesarean section is usually contraindicated when the patient is grossly infected; if the operation is imperative, cesarean hysterectomy may be the treatment of choice. The maternal and the fetal morbidity and mortality are least if cesarean section is performed before the onset of labor; they increase progressively with the time the membranes have been ruptured and the duration of labor before the time of surgery. However, the modern chemotherapeutic agents have added a considerable margin of safety and flexibility to the use of cesarean section. Low cervical cesarean section, plus antibiotic therapy, has been used with good results in many mildly infected cases. In these circumstances some clinicians employ an extraperitoneal technique.

The more liberal use of cesarean section in recent years (range of 25 to 30 per cent) has unquestionably resulted in greater perinatal salvage, as in certain cases of transverse lie and mild abruptio placentae and in the management of middle-aged primigravidas. However, wider use of cesarean section should not be regarded as the ultimate solution for all antenatal problems, or even for the majority. Also, liberalizing surgical interventions will undoubtedly introduce certain new maternal risks. The perinatal loss in *elective* cesarean sections exceeds 1 per cent. Moreover, cesarean section is a frequent mode of delivery among premature infants dying of pulmonary problems during the neonatal period. Objective tests should be utilized to be assured of fetal lung maturity when intervening. It should be borne in mind, also, that if this mode of delivery is to yield satisfactory results, it must be selected as a proper and timely technique of definitive management, not as a last resort after all others fail or after the fetus has sustained irreversible brain injury.

Puerperal Infection

Puerperal infection, one of the three major causes of maternal death, is a postpartal wound infection of the parturient canal (usually of the endometrium) that may remain localized but often extends along lymphatic and vascular channels to produce systemic signs and symptoms. Puerperal infections are grouped under the general term *puerperal morbidity,* defined as a temperature of 100.4 F. (38.0 C.) occurring on any two of the first ten days postpartum, exclusive of the first 24 hours. In general, the most common cause of puerperal infection is the anaerobic streptococcus, but the hemolytic streptococcus is the most common cause of fulminating puerperal infection, as well as epidemics of the disease. Mixed infections are the rule and other organisms include various staphylococci, *Escherichia coli,* gonococci, *Proteus vulgans,* enterobacter, peppo-streptococcus, bacteroides, pneumococci, and clostridia. *Clostridium perfringens* is an uncommon cause of puerperal infection, but the dramatic course and the high mortality that usually attend such infections make this organism of signal interest. It is seen more commonly after criminal abortions than after deliveries near term. Gonorrheal puerperal endometritis, once considered the cause of 5 to 10 per cent of all fevers occurring in the puerperium, is rarely seen today, although an increase in venereal disease in recent years, coupled with the continuing problem of teen-age pregnancy, may well justify renewed concern about this infection. The overall incidence of puerperal infection is probably about 4 per cent of deliveries, although this figure may reach 25 per cent or more in patients delivered by cesarean section.

The most important predisposing causes of puerperal infection are hemorrhage and trauma at the time of labor. Pre-existing anemia, under nutrition and other debilitated states make puerperal infection more likely. Retention of placental tissue is a common predisposing factor to infection. However, the prime cause of puerperal infection is introduction of bacteria into the genital tracts by attendants, from the patients own skin, from the infected tissues of the patient or fellow patient, from instruments, bedding or other equipment.

It is desirable to regard puerperal infection as falling into two main groups:

1. Local processes (inflammatory lesions of perineum, vulva, vagina, cervix and endometrium). The most common local sources of infection are the episiotomy, and vulvar, perineal or vaginal lacerations.
2. Extensions of the original process (along the veins to produce thrombophlebitis and pyemia, through the lymph vessels to produce peritonitis and parametritis and along the surface of the endometrium and the endosalpinx to produce salpingitis).

The most common manifestation of puerperal infection is endometritis. Endometritis usually begins suddenly on the 3rd or the 4th day of the puerperium, with malaise, headache, chilliness or a definite chill and temperature of 103 F. or more that remains definitely elevated. The uterus is somewhat enlarged and tender to pressure. The lochial discharge may be increased and purulent and is often devoid of odor, particularly in virulent streptococcic cases.

If the infection is limited to the uterus, the patient slowly returns to normal. Rise in temperature indicates an extension, which may lead to abscess within the broad ligament, the posterior cul-de-sac or the anterior pelvis. The infection may extend through the uterine lymphatics to cause peritonitis, or pyemia may develop with typical spiking temperature, or rarely, septicemia with very rapid death. Thrombosis may arise in the pelvic veins and extend to the femoral, causing phlegmasia alba dolens (milk leg). The most common organisms causing the septic type are streptococci and staphylococci. Rarely, ovarian vein thrombosis may occur with its accompanying inflammation and give rise to protracted fever, pam and disability.

Another clinical variant is characterized by abundant, very foul-smelling and frequently frothy lochia. However, it should be remembered that *E. Coli* infections are odorless. There may be initial chill and high temperature, but the patient's condition does not appear so serious, and recovery is the rule. The most common causes are the colon bacillus, *Pseudomonas aeruginosa* and various anaerobes. Endotoxic shock following these infections carries a grave prognosis.

Prophylaxis. Most important are (1) maintenance of strict asepsis; (2) restriction of vaginal and rectal examinations; (3) omission of coitus and vaginal douches late in pregnancy; (4) immediate repair of lacerations; (5) puerperal examination of the genital canal in special circumstances only; (6) prevention of anemia; and (7) complete evacuation of placental tissue from the uterus at the time of delivery; (8) limiting long labors and traumatic deliveries; (9) supporting the patient's hydration; (10) proper bladder care; (11) proper postpartal perineal care; and (12) isolation of infected patients to protect others.

Since the advent of chemotherapy, adequate blood replacement, improved prenatal care and modern techniques of management, fulminating cases of puerperal infection are rarely encountered.

Treatment. The type, intensity and duration of specific therapy will depend upon the organism involved, drug sensitivities by in vitro tests, the extent of the infection, and the presence of complicating clinical conditions (e.g., septic shock; septicemia; thromboembolic disease, etc.). Appropriate cultures should be taken. The procedure of obtaining an intrauterine culture may, of itself, be beneficial because it promotes drainage. Ergot preparations may provoke uterine drainage. Collections of pus in the perineum, vagina or cul-de-sac will also require adequate drainage. Transfusions are needed to correct significant anemia. In the more serious cases, monitoring fluid administrations, electrolyte replacement, urinary output and fluid losses through a gastrointestinal tube (from ileum) will be necessary if the patient is to be supported properly. Clinical suspicion of lower limb and pelvic thrombophlebitis will call for diagnostic tests, e.g. Doppler ultrasonic flow detector, impedance phethysmography or, occasionally, the more accurate but invasive method of ascending contrast phlebography. The presence of thrombophlebitis requires bed rest, use of anticoagulants, and antibiotics. Initially, both heparin infusion and oral warfarin are administered; in 36 to 72 hours, when proper anticoagulation has been achieved with the oral medication, the heparin is discontinued. If there is femoral phlebitis accompanied by pain and fever, the involved extremity should be protected from external pressure and elevated until the acute process disappears. After that elastic support is needed often for many months to promote venous drainage.

When there is evidence of parametritis and pelvic cellulitis, it is desirable to perform frequent rectovaginal examinations to detect a cul-de-sac abscess because this must be drained to promote optimal recovery from the infection. Drainage and/or uterine debridement by curettage may be called for in endotoxic shock, which is treated according to the principles outlined for septic abortions. Otherwise, a curettage might be dangerous and generally it is best to avoid deep entry of disinfectant solutions or objects into the vagina. Manipulations should be avoided except for culture taking and checking on possible lacerations, hematomas, or collections of pus. Hematomas that are quite large, symptomatic, and continuing to expand should be incised and drained. There may be a combination of old blood and pus when the diagnosis is delayed a number of days. Occasionally, morbidity may be associated with a hematoma above the pelvic fascia, and the tumefaction is paravaginal or spread into the broad ligament. Retroperitoneal extensions may give rise to an inguinal ligament presentation or to rupture into the peritoneal cavity. Any suspicion of hematoma in the form of unexplained pelvic pain, fever, tachycardia, hypotension or anemia must be immediately investigated.

Puerperal infections may be delayed and/or refractory, characterized by persistent uterine red or purulent discharge (lochia). There may be continued bleeding with intermittent passage of old clots. There are usually pelvic complaints or backaches associated with subinvolution of the uterus and a low grade endometritis. The underlying cause may be retained placental fragments or, occasionally, an infected leiomyoma of the uterus.

Endometritis does not always respond sensitively to antibiotics, particularly if cervical drainage is poor. While waiting for the antibiotic sensitivity report, a drug may be chosen on the basis of a Gram-stained smear of the cervical discharge. Recent hospital antibiotic sensitivity patterns can be taken into account in the selection of a drug and it should be given in adequate doses intravenously. Mixed infections involving two or more organisms are common, and effective therapy may require a combination of drugs. Anaerobes frequently participate in mixed infections; their growth is promoted as secondary invaders into tissues that have become necrotic after initial infection by facultative pathogens. The appearance of anaerobic infections may be quite delayed after an apparent initial successful management.

The majority of offending organisms are sensitive to ampicillin or to a combination of ampicillin and gentamycin given intravenously. Most of the anaerobes are susceptible to ampicillin, penicillin and the cephalosporins. The presence of *Bacteroides fragilis* calls for the use of clindamycin or chloramphenicol. Massive doses of antibiotics (penicillin, ampicillin, or erythromycin) are used along with a hyperbaric oxygen chamber and subsequent surgical intervention in the presence of gas gangrene (clostridium perfringens) infection. The possibility of *Neisseria gonorrhoeae* infections in the vaginal tract should be considered in screening patients for pathogens. The uncomplicated case is treated with oral probenecid (ig) followed by intramuscular injections at two sites of aqueous procaine penicillin G (total of 4.8 million units).

STERILIZATION

A common method of terminating childbearing potential has become the surgical tubal ligation (Pomeroy or Irving technique) performed in the immediate postpartal period while the patient is still under anesthesia from her delivery. Very often a simple Pomeroy procedure can be performed through a small umbilical incision that scarcely interferes with the postpartal recovery or delays the patient's discharge date. Every attempt is being made today to simplify sterilization procedures. Male sterilization can now be achieved by simple vas deferens ligation performed on an ambulatory basis. Tubal electrocoagulation in the female via the laparoscope is almost as innocuous, despite certain serious potential hazards (hemorrhage, bowel injury, etc.), and the potential of hysteroscopic electrocoagulation of the proximal interstitial tube from within the uterine cavity is even less involved. Recently, laparoscopy by the "open" technique has been advocated to avoid the potential injures produced by the blind insertion of a sharp trocar. By the new technique, the small opening through the lower abdominal wall, including the parietal peritoneum, is made under direct vision before the sheath of the instrument is inserted and secured with sutures to prevent leakage of instilled carbon dioxide.

THE NEWBORN

Fetal Circulation

The fetal circulation carries nutritive material from the placenta through the umbilical vein, whose smaller branch unites with the portal vein and empties into the liver, and whose larger branch, the ductus venosus, empties directly into the vena cava. On entering the right atrium, most of the blood passes through the open foramen ovale into the left atrium and thus to the systemic circulation, returning to the placenta by the umbilical (hypogastric) arteries. Blood from the head region delivered via the superior vena cava is low in oxygen and tends to pass in a direct stream into the right ventricle. Since the lungs do not function, the greater part of the blood in the right ventricle passes directly from the pulmonary artery into the aorta through the ductus arteriosus and is mixed with blood of higher oxygen content pumped from the left side of the heart.

Arterial blood passing from the placenta to the fetus is only about 65 per cent saturated with oxygen. The maternal blood source in the intervillous space is mixed, thus reducing the effective saturation. In addition, oxygen diffuses slowly through a wet membrane. The oxygen supply under normal conditions is adequate for the fetal needs, since a number of adaptive mechanisms are operative, such as an increase in fetal red cell count and hemoglobin, differences in fetal hemoglobin as compared with the adult type that, in the plasma, result in a shift of the oxygen dissociation curve to the left, enabling an increased oxygen uptake at low gas tension, increased cardiac output several times that of the adult, and, finally, the mechanism allowing for anaerobic metabolism to help meet the fetal requirements. Therefore, the lactic acid content of fetal blood is only slightly greater than that of the mother. According to our present state of knowledge of the conditions under which anoxic survival is possible, the carbohydrate stores, particularly of the heart, may be of paramount importance. Oxygen tension in the fetal blood returning to the placenta may remain within the normal range for short periods despite considerable reductions in the oxygen level in the blood perfusing the uterus. In addition, the fetus has a number of autoregulatory, homeostatic mechanisms relating to placental blood flow, oxygen pressure gradients and control of transport of various substances that are sensitive to external or internal environmental changes.

In a variety of clinical situations, however, there may be serious disruptions of these defense mechanisms, and the fetus may exhibit obvious signs of distress. Impairment of placental exchange can occur (1) in the maternal circulation, (2) in the placental membrane, (3) in the fetal circulation, or (4) in combination, with several of these insults operative. Anoxia arising from any one of these conditions represents the principal basic cause of perinatal death in 25 per cent or more of cases.

The umbilical circulation ceases 5 to 15 minutes after birth, and blood from the right ventricle circulates through the lungs, causing mechanical closure of the foramen ovale. This is due to the increased volume of blood returning from the lungs as respirations are established and the diminished quantity of blood going to the inferior vena cava when the umbilical cord is ligated. The functionless umbilical vein becomes the ligamentum teres. The ductus venosus closes and forms the ligamentum venosum, and the obliterated umbilical arteries become the lateral umbilical ligaments. The ductus arteriosus closes as the lungs begin to function, becomes occluded and forms the ligamentum arteriosum. A large volume of blood is pumped by the right ventricle into the previously collapsed pulmonary arteries, thus reducing pressure within the lumen. Thus, within several days after birth, the adult type of circulation, in which the venous and the arterial systems are separate, develops; thereafter the blood is aerated in the lungs.

Care of the Newborn Child

Immediate care consists of clearing the nasopharynx, clamping and severing the umbilical cord and placing the infant in a heated crib or resuscitator unit, where further suction, oxygen administration, intubation or other care is given as required. The cord is ligated or clamped some 2 cm. from the abdomen, and an abdominal binder is applied. Chilling of the infant must be avoided. The infant is properly identified by beads or wrist band and foot prints. It is important to perform a thorough examination as soon as possible with special emphasis on the respirations, heart rate, muscle tone, reflexes and color, as recorded on the 1- and 5-minute Apgar scores. Generally, infants with scores of 6 or above do not require any special treatment. Search should be made for a single-umbilical artery because this is associated with anomalies in 15 to 20 per cent of cases. The incidence in singletons is about 1 per cent and up to 6 per cent in twins.

The eyes of the newborn should be treated routinely with one drop of one per cent silver nitrate solution. Previously, eyes were washed out afterward with a solution of sodium chloride. However, that practice may reduce the effectiveness of the medication. The alternative prophylactic use of penicillin drops is not recommended since the antibiotic can be sensitizing. While some ophthalmic ointments may be effective, others (Bacitracin) are not. And these do not represent the preferred method of treatment. All infants born to mothers with gonococcal infections should have cultures obtained (orogastric, rectal, blood) and should be treated if organisms are found.

Nursing may be started early in the postpartal period because of the stimulating effect even though only colostrum is present. The infant should nurse for 5 to 10 minutes at each breast during the hospital stay, usually at 4-hour intervals. The infant will usually lose about 5 to 8 per cent of the birth weight in the first few days.

In some clinics, a "birthing room" or rooming-in policy has been adopted, whereby the infant is kept in a crib at the mother's bedside rather than in the nursery. It stems from the modern trend to ambulate mothers early and to make all phases of childbearing as natural as possible. These natural practices are physiologic and promote a favorable "bonding" between the mother and her infant.

About one third of newborn infants will have mild icterus, usually between the 2nd and 5th days of life, probably caused by hepatic cell immaturity. The bilirubin is mostly free or unconjugated, and levels up to 4 to 5 mg. per 100 ml. of serum are not uncommon. Icterus is usually more severe and prolonged among prematures. Breast feeding aggravates the problem. Care should be taken to exclude the possibility of hemolytic disease and other pathologic causes of jaundice.

Apnea Neonatorum

If the newborn infant has not begun to breathe within 2 minutes after birth, the condition usually is referred to as apnea neonatorum. In the milder cases the color of the infant is livid, and the muscle tone good—*asphyxia livida*. In the severe cases the child is pale and limp—*asphyxia pallida*.

Failure of the baby to breathe at birth is usually due to one of three main causes, or to some combination of them: (1) anoxia, (2) cerebral injury, and (3) narcosis. Apnea resulting from narcosis is usually transient, rarely lasting more than 1 minute.

The clinical classification of infants with respiratory difficulties at birth is as follows:

1. *Primary apnea.* Infant does not breathe and has not breathed.
2. *Secondary apnea.* Infant breathes, gasps or cries initially and then ceases to breathe.
3. *Infant breathing but with poor air exchange.* The infant is cyanotic or has gasping, shallow or intermittent respirations with cyanosis or pallor.

Principles of Treatment. The best treatment of apnea neonatorum is its prevention by combating anoxia and trauma, avoiding excessive and ill-timed analgesia, and by avoiding multiple insults to the fetal respiratory center through a conservative atraumatic plan of management.

1. *Gentleness.* These infants are in a state of shock, and rough attempts to resuscitate them (vigorous spanking, shaking and plunging in ice) do more harm than good.
2. *Warmth.* Temperature and humidity must be maintained, since these babies are in a state of shock.
3. *Posture.* Slight Trendelenburg position is employed to favor gravity drainage of mucus.
4. *Establishment of an adequate airway.* The nasopharynx may be suctioned with bulb syringe and catheters. Gastric suction should be carried out on infants delivered by cesarean section and on the infants of diabetic mothers.
5. *Administration of oxygen.* If oxygen is delivered successfully to the infant's lungs, respirations will ensue in the great majority of cases. Positive pressure should be administered to infants with primary apnea, but it is contraindicated in secondary apnea until the obstruction has been relieved. In the latter cases, the trachea should be intubated under direct visualization, the laryngoscope being used. The secretions should be aspirated, and positive pressure oxygen administered through the tube. Since the amount of pressure cannot be controlled and an aftermath of infection is a potential risk, mouth-to-mouth insufflation is less desirable than administering oxygen under controlled pressure by means of resuscitator equipment. The amount of pressure required to expand the infant's lungs is best determined on an individualized basis by observing the movements of the chest and by listening to the entry of air into the lungs. Gas mixtures containing carbon dioxide and use of respiratory stimulants are not recommended.

6. *Drugs.* Nalline (0.2 mg.) can be given intravenously to the infant to combat the narcotic effects of morphine, Demerol or their derivatives. Antibiotics should be administered to minimize the danger of pneumonia. Increased tension of carbon dioxide and lowered pH should be corrected with bicarbonate administrations intravenously. Generally, it is the infant with an Apgar score of less than 6 at 5 minutes who develops metabolic acidosis and requires such special treatment. Infusions can be given through a catheterized umbilical vessel. The infusion of 10 per cent glucose intravenously should also be considered. An inaudible heart beat calls for intubation of the trachea, pulmonary inflation, external heart massage, and, possibly, an intracardiac injection of epinephrine.

7. *Postresuscitation.* After resuscitation the infant should be placed in an incubator with maintenance of body temperature, humidification and oxygen *not to exceed 40 per cent.*

Prematurity

From 7 to 10 per cent of babies are born a month or more prior to the expected date of confinement. Among the lower socioeconomic groups, the incidence may reach 14 per cent or more. Such infants usually weigh between 500 and 2,500 g. and are called premature. Their chance of survival is much less than that of mature infants and, as a consequence, premature infants account for more than half of all deaths in the first 30 days of life (neonatal period). Perinatal mortality rates vary between 15 and 20 per cent over all, but the smaller the infant the poorer the prognosis. The clinical cause of premature birth is apparent in slightly less than 40 per cent of cases. The causes most frequently responsible for the onset of premature labor are chronic hypertension, abruptio placentae, placenta previa, heart disease, toxemia, multiple gestation and congenital abnormalities of the fetus and, formerly, syphilis. Premature rupture of the membranes is the triggering factor provoking premature labor or active intervention in 20 to 30 per cent of the cases. Other known factors include incompatible blood groups, uterine pathology and anatomic defects, nutritional deficiency, endocrine dysfunction and placental steroid defects. Prematurity is often repeated in a subsequent pregnancy.

The best clinical weapon against the ill effects of premature birth is prevention. Often, the underlying etiology is obscure and cannot be addressed. Many patients will be in advanced labor by the time they are first seen. Efforts to halt established labor are usually unsuccessful if the cervix is fully effaced and dilated more than 3 cm. The membranes are already ruptured in a substantial minority of cases and in others the maternal complication is an overriding clinical issue. In these circumstances, an arrest of labor might be highly undesirable.

Bed rest itself may be a preventive because myometrial irritability may be reduced. In circumstances involving uterine overdistension, e.g., multiple gestation, polyhydramnios, uterine tumor, etc., bed rest may be an effective adjunct in delaying the onset of labor. The most commonly employed agent used in the past to diminish uterine contractions has been ethanol, since delays in delivery of 72 hours or more can be anticipated in more than three-quarters of the patients. Its action may be related to improved uterine blood flow and reduction in the release of oxytocin. The method is safe; however, the side effects of inebriation may be troublesome in managing the mother. Synthetic beta-adrenergic compounds (Terbutaline) and sympathomimetic amines capable of stimulating uterine beta-adrenergic receptors (Ritodrine hydrochloride) are capable of inhibiting myometrial activity in 80 to 90 per cent of patients. However, they have the disadvantage of producing both maternal and fetal tachycardia and hypotension in the mother. Isoxuprine hydrochloride is particularly troublesome with respect to these side effects. Recently, the inhibitory effects on uterine muscle contractility of magnesium sulfate have been recognized and utilized therapeutically in normotensive women experiencing threatening premature labor. The regime is identical to that utilized in treating women with preeclampsia and the same safeguards are required in terms of magnesium level control, urinary output, and periodic clinical assessments. Excessive serum levels can cause respiratory depression in the newborn since magnesium traverses the placenta.

Once premature labor is established, clinical management takes into account the particular vulnerabilities of the immature infant. Care must be exerted to avoid narcosis, hypoxia, and trauma. These insults are synergistic and must be given careful attention in programming management on an individualized basis. A generous episiotomy cut under a local or regional block might spare the fetal head and facilitate an easy spontaneous delivery. If there is a faulty labor, malpresentation, or reason to believe that more operative manipulations than desired would be necessary in achieving a vaginal delivery, abdominal intervention should be considered. A more liberal use of cesarean section even in the delivery of very small infants has been made possible by the great advances achieved in recent years in increasing the chances of neonatal survival. In today's intensive care nurseries, live-born infants with birth weights of only 750 to 1000 g. (25th to 27th gestational week) have about a one chance in three of surviving.

In considering low birth weight infants, it is very important to distinguish between those whose weight is commensurate with the gestational age and those whose birth weight is low for the stage of gestation. The latter are referred to as "small for gestational age" infants. By definition, their birth weight is below the tenth percentile for gestational age and they are said to have an in utero growth retardation. These make up about one-third of all low birth weight infants. They may be genetically small or defective or they may have suffered in utero malnutrition. Uteroplacental vascular damage, preeclampsia, chronic infections (syphilis, rubella, etc.), chronic hypoxia (hemoglobinopathies), heavy smoking, chronic alcoholism, drug addiction, severe diabetes, and other maternal illnesses may underly the fetal inanition and jeopardy. In some instances, there is a problem of postdatism beyond 42 gestational weeks. Serial ultrasonic cephalometry is useful but between 10 and 20 per cent of these fetuses are undergrown and have a reduced birth weight but skeletal proportions are normal. Cytohormonal assessments performed periodically after the 20th gestational week may identify fetuses at risk and stress tests may be used to determine those who may not be able to withstand the rigors of labor. Despite their vulnerabilities, these undergrown infants tend to have a more favorable neonatal prognosis than do infants of the same weight those whose weight is appropriate for gestational age. However, undergrown infants at birth are frequently hypoxic, hypoglycemic (two-thirds), and polycythemic because of hyperviscosity of the blood. Glucose infusion is ordinarily required and, in some, a phlebotomy followed by administration of plasma might be beneficial.

Among immature (premature) infants, a respiratory distress syndrome (Hyaline Membrane Disease) constitutes one of the gravest risks. This problem affects about 20 per cent of prematurely born infants but only one to two per cent of all live births. Premature infants do not produce adequate quantities of surfactant, which is a group of phospholipids, elaborated by type II alveolar cells. Surfactant, lecithin/sphingomyelin (L/S Ratio of 2:1), is produced in large quantities after the thirty-fourth or thirty-fifth week of gestation. After birth these phospholipids are surface active and they reduce the stickiness of the aveolar walls (diminish surface tension), increase compliance, and promote partial alveolar distention with residual air, even at the end of expiration. Without these properties, alveoli tend to collapse (atelectasis) and eosinophilic hyaline-like membranes develop on the surface of the alveoli and in the terminal bronchioles, presumably due to capillary plasma/fibrin transudation. Submembraneous epithelium becomes necrotic, vasoconstriction occurs, aeration is diminished, and hypoxia (acidosis) and systemic hypotension develop. This chain of events can lead to death in 4 to 72 hours. However, about three-quarters of these patients will survive with proper support.

It should be emphasized that the upper respiratory tract of all infants must be intubated and aspirated at birth to prevent the meconium aspiration syndrome, which is associated with mortality rates of up to 20 per cent. In this condition, there is mechanical obstruction, chemical irritation and inflammation, resulting in edema, hypoxia, atelectasis and possibly pneumothorax. An additional preventive is the need to empty the stomach to minimize the risks of regurgitation and meconium aspiration.

Another problem, which is largely preventable, that occurs in immature infants usually weighing less than 1,500 g. is the development of *retrolental fibroplasia* caused by exposure to high concentrations of oxygen. The prognosis is grave, most of the infants affected becoming partially or totally blind. However, since the condition is almost always caused by exposure of premature infants to high concentrations of ambient oxygen (about 40 per cent) over periods longer than 24 to 48 hours, certain prophylactic measures are preventive.

The incidence of cerebral palsy and mental retardation is also increased among premature infants. The mortality rate is higher during the first 2 years of life, and even after that time there is a higher incidence of disorders considered to be associated with birth injury.

A special comment is required concerning the documented ill effects of alcohol ingestion during pregnancy. The chronic alcoholic patient will have malnutrition in varying degrees, particularly when ingestion of alcohol negates the desire for food and an adequate diet is ignored. Alcohol traverses the placenta readily and newborn infants may suffer from withdrawal symptoms. Recently, the problem of maternal alcoholism has been shown to be of even greater concern since, in about one-quarter of the cases, there will be extremely serious effects upon fetal growth and development in utero. A so-called "fetal alcohol syndrome" has been described which is made up of several major defects, including growth retardation, microcephaly, and a variety of anomalies involving the face, eyes, heart, joints, and external genitalia.

The concept of dysmaturity tends to focus on small

for gestational age infants and those who are postmature, associated with an undergrown in utero compromised status. Dysmaturity can also characterize large for gestational age infants. There may be excessive weight because of severe water retention or hydrops, e.g., syphilis, erythroblastosis fetalis, maternal diabetes, or transposition of the aorta. A large for gestational age infant can be compromised by complications usually associated with immatures, e.g., increased prevalence of hyaline membrane disease among large infants born of diabetic mothers. Obviously, there are additional perinatal hazards of shoulder dystocia, birth trauma, operative obstetrics, hypoxia, and other problems.

HEMOLYTIC DISEASE OF THE NEWBORN (ERYTHROBLASTOSIS)

About one per cent of all newborn infants have hemolytic disease. Although a host of factors in the blood are immunologically and genetically important, there are at least nine red cell factors representing significant genetically independent antigen systems. These "families" include ABO, Rh, MNS, Kell, Duffy, Kidd, P, Lewis, Lutheran, but there is a growing list of others, mostly rare, which are unclassified. Practically all blood factors are inherited as mendelian dominants.

With the discovery of three specific anti-Rh sera, a constellation of eight Rh types, which fall into two groups of four each, was distinguished; the distinction is related to the presence or absence of the antigen D (Rh$_o$).

About 85 per cent of the population react positively with anti D (Rh$_o$) serum; roughly 15 per cent have a negative reaction. For each of the Rh antigens there is an allelomorphic Hr antigen (Fisher-Race designation). Rh antigens dominate over other blood group antigens in the causation of erythroblastosis fetalis. They are inherited independently of all other blood group antigens.

Approximately 13 per cent of all marriages in this country take place between an Rh-negative woman and an Rh-positive man. Isoimmunization occurs in about 7 per cent of all Rh-negative gravidas, and great majority becoming sensitized by the fourth pregnancy. A homozygous Rh-positive male will give rise to all Rh-positive fetuses; there is a chance of Rh-negativity in 50 per cent of the offspring of heterozygous Rh-positive males (the former exceed the latter by about three to one). The likelihood of sensitization depends also upon the quantity of fetal red cells reaching the mother's circulation, the relative antigenicity of the

Rh factor, variability of host responsiveness, and other factors. The various Rh factors, in diminishing degree of antigenicity, are: D (Rh$_o$); c (rh1); E (rh11); c (hr1); e (hr11); and d (hr$_o$).

Extravasation of fetal red cells into the maternal circulation is relatively rare; thus, isoimmunization in the first pregnancy is not a potential risk unless there has been a prior incompatible transfusion or an abortion. The moment of transfer of fetal red cells appears to be at the end of a pathologic pregnancy (placental abruption, previa, toxemia, etc.); during labor, especially with obstetric intervention; and at the time of actual delivery, particularly if there has been a cesarean section or manual removal of the placenta. Sensitization may follow operative termination of early pregnancy. Survival time of fetal red cells in the circulation of adults has been found to be an estimated 80 days. A fetomaternal transfusion of more than 50 cu. mm. has been found in at least one fifth of women at delivery. Apparently as little as 0.1 ml. Rh-positive blood can produce sensitization.

The clinical degree of anemia, hyperbilirubinemia and physical manifestations at birth is variable, and the prognosis varies accordingly. In the mildest form the fetus is only anemic without other stigmata and the outlook is excellent. A more serious stage is designated *icterus gravis*, in which there is jaundice which deepens progressively. Hepatosplenomegaly is present. Many will survive with optimal exchange transfusion. The most serious stage is hydrops fetalis, which rarely responds even to the most vigorous therapeutic regimen. In the more severe cases the placenta is also markedly edematous and boggy and exhibits large, grayish, friable cotyledons.

One of the postnatal phenomena of hemolytic disease is *kernicterus*, characterized by yellowish pigmentation of the basal nuclei, as well as other portions of the infant's brain. Approximately 6 per cent of those who survive the first week of life develop signs of central nervous system damage, particularly premature infants and those in whom high levels of hyperbilirubinemia were evident over a protracted period. This risk can be minimized with prompt exchange transfusion repeated as often as necessary to keep the plasma bilirubin considerably below 20 mg. per 100 ml. Likewise, improved, more refined management has succeeded in reducing the overall perinatal mortality rate to 15 to 20 per cent.

There are now four primary laboratory methods of following the progress of Rh-negative women during pregnancy:

1. Rh-antibody titers (albumin type)
2. Indirect Coombs titer—mix of the patient's se-

rum with Rh-positive cells and testing with anti-globulin.

3. The amount of pigment in the amniotic fluid–spectral absorption curve, in which the optical density is plotted on semi-log paper and the 450 mμ peak is measured on a line drawn from the peak to an intersection with a tangent connecting the beginning and ending curves of the rise (Liley technique). The degrees of fetal involvement (mild, moderate or severe) are represented by zones on the graph depicting the height of the peak of pigment in the amniotic fluid at different stages of fetal maturity.

4. Hormonal evaluations, rising hCG titers and falling urinary estrogen excretion

By first documenting sensitization, noting the trend of the titers, and then by performing serial hormonal tests as well as repeated examinations of the amniotic fluid, beginning as early as the 20th gestational week in patients with the poorest history and early prior fetal deaths, reasonably accurate estimates of the fetal condition can be obtained. Thus, management is based on objective tests as well as clinical notations regarding uterine growth and tone, presence or absence of hydramnios and evidence of maternal edema (mirror syndrome). Abdominal roentgenograms or pelvic sonography will help in estimating fetal size, skeletal normality and evidence of hydrops or hydramnios.

When the history, clinical and laboratory findings indicate severe fetal involvement (in the absence of hydrops or significant hydramnios) by the 26th to 32nd week of gestation, thereby forecasting certain death of the fetus prior to the 33rd to 34th week, an intrauterine fetal transfusion should be performed and repeated at biweekly intervals until there is sufficient fetal maturity to yield a reasonable chance of survival, usually about the 36th week. There is evidence that up to two-thirds or more of the transfused red cells are absorbed into the fetal circulation through the subdiaphragmatic lymphatics. Unfortunately, the fetal mortality rate with each in utero transfusion ranges between 5 and 20 per cent, depending upon the beginning status of the fetus. Amniotic fluid analyses are also important, when indicative of mild or no fetal involvement, in sparing the infant unnecessary premature delivery. Mildly affected fetuses occurring in sensitized mothers whose husbands are homozygous, even without a history of prior fetal erythroblastosis or perinatal loss, should be delivered a few weeks before term, usually in the 38th week. The choice of method of delivery in all cases, induction of labor or cesarean section, will depend upon the obstetric situation. However, it should be understood that these fetuses should not be subjected to any significant hypoxia or trauma since such insults increase their vulnerability to the deposition of bilirubin in the brain.

A small percentage of women who do not lack an Rh or an Hr antigen possessed by their husbands and show no evidence of immunization to these antigens have been reported as giving birth to infants suffering from hemolytic disease. Certain of these infants suffer from an ABO incompatibility, a situation in which the mother's blood contains anti-A or anti-B agglutinins incompatible with the fetal cells. Rh incompatibility and A-B hetero-specificity account for approximately 98 per cent of all cases of hemolytic disease. The principles of management are identical in the two conditions, particularly with reference to the behavior of hemoglobin and bilirubin. For simple transfusion or exchange transfusion, group O Rh-negative blood is used.

The patient with multiple losses who has 80 per cent or more chance of fetal death in any subsequent pregnancy, or one who has been subjected to intrauterine fetal transfusion, may desire tubal sterilization. A few may wish a pregnancy by an Rh-negative male donor.

One of the great advances in obstetrics, certainly in the management of Rh problems, has been the demonstration that high-potency, anti-D gamma globulin fraction administered to Rh-negative mothers shortly after delivery (within 72 hours) has been successful in preventing the development of sensitizing antibodies. An effective commercial preparation is available for such purposes, to be administered to Rh-negative unsensitized mothers following the birth of each Rh-positive infant. A standard dose of .300 μg. of Rh$_o$ (D) immune globulin has been prepared for routine use; this counteracts up to 15 ml. of packed fetal Rh$_o$ (D) erythrocytes. If clinical circumstances make it likely that the fetomaternal hemorrhage exceeds that volume, or the concentration of fetal erythrocytes in maternal blood are excessive as demonstrated by the Kleihauer-Betke acid elution test, additional immune globulin may be required. Hopefully the tragic prenatal losses and the tedious procedures of amniocenteses and intrauterine fetal transfusion will soon be relegated to the past.

Hyperbilirubinemia from Other Causes

It is important to recognize that hyperbilirubinemia of the newborn may arise from causes other than blood incompatibilities. All drugs administered to the mother should be evaluated for placental transmission, method of conjugation for excretion, hemolytic effect, ability to bind proteins and effect on hepatocellular function. Ideally, the treatment for hyperbilirubinemia, which is caused by excessive dosage of vitamin K, sulfonamides, other drugs, hypoxia, disordered carbohydrate metabolism or acidosis, is basically one of prevention, since the incidence of exchange transfusions to correct hemolytic diseases of this type seems to be increasing.

GYNECOLOGY

DISORDERS OF THE LOWER GENERATIVE TRACT

Leukorrhea

The literal meaning of the term leukorrhea is a white discharge. In practical usage it is applied to a wide range of vulvovaginal exudates that vary in color, consistency, odor, and cause. The proper environment for the vagina is maintained under the influence of estrogens and enough acidity to foster the growth of a normal bacterial flora. An acid pH of 3.5 to 4.0 is achieved in the presence of adequate lactobacilli (Döderlein's bacilli) and acidogenic corynebacteria. Endogenous estrogen causes proliferation of the stratified squamous epithelium of the vagina, which brings about a resistance to infection and trauma after puberty and during the premenopausal years. Normally, under estrogen stimulation, vaginal fluid contains a cellular debris resulting from a continuous process of desquamation. There may be an excess of mucus discharge in response to sexual excitement, increased estrogen stimulation, use of oral contraceptives, pregnancy, and pelvic congestion. There should be no real problem of soiling of underclothes or evidence of vulvovaginal irritation or offensive odor. Menstrual fluid reduces the acidity of the vagina. Estrogen depletion, caused by castration or aging, produces mucosal atrophy, reduction in cellular glycogen content, and decreased acidity of the vaginal fluid. The warm, moist condition of the vulva makes it vulnerable to irritation and infection when it is exposed to urinary and fecal soiling. Allergies, coitus, feminine hygiene practices, excessive douching, tight fitting, heat- and moisture-retaining pantyhose, abrasions (masturbation) and other practices, and potential insults may predispose to symptomatic leukorrhea by changing the vaginal flora. The overall physical and emotional health, nutritional and metabolic state, and general level of activity will affect the vagina. There may be specific causes of leukorrhea that arise in the cervix, endometrium and fallopian tubes and these discharges may adversely affect the vaginal flora and decrease the pH. Mucopurulent fluids, arising from infected endocervical mucosa, are alkaline and will change the bacterial flora by altering the vaginal pH. Anomalous development in the hind end may likewise disturb anatomy, function, and physiological processes in the vagina.

Vaginal infection is the most common cause of leukorrhea. Vulvar irritation resulting from contact with the vaginal discharge may give rise to the presenting complaint. There may be some pruritis, dyspareunia, and a sense of severe burning discomfort when the irritated areas on the vulva and perineum are exposed to urine. There may be mixed bacterial flora without predominant organisms, although one or more common pyogenic pathogens may be present in vaginal cultures. Nonspecific vulvovaginitis may be secondary to poor perineal hygiene, foreign bodies, mucosal atrophy, trauma, skin infections, intestinal parasites, or arise in association with a systemic illness. *Escherichia coli, Proteus sp., Enterobacter aerogenes, Klebsiella pneumoniae,* and other organisms common to the intestinal tract may be found in vaginal cultures. Occasionally, pinworms migrate into the vagina from the anus and deposit ova, which may lead to vulvovaginitis because of contamination with *Escherichia coli* and other intestinal bacteria. Sexual molestation involving the female child almost always causes injury to the immature vagina and such trauma may give rise to hematomas and infection. The thin vaginal mucosa is also susceptible to invasion by the gonococcus.

Many of the specific types of vulvovaginitis causing leukorrhea represent a wide variety of sexually transmitted infectious diseases. The offending organisms may be classified as bacteria, spirochetes, chlamydia, fungi, metazoans, mycoplasma, protozoans, and viruses. The most common symptom of vulvar disease is pruritis. Some of the more specific common entities associated with leukorrhea include:

Trichomoniasis. *Trichomonas vaginalis* vaginitis is a sexually transmitted disease caused by a unicellular protozoan flagellate that infests not only the vagina but also the lower urinary tract of both men and women. These organisms may occasionally be found in an asymptomatic female with normal vaginal acidity and bacterial flora. However, vulvovaginitis and urinary symptoms, when there is associated acute vulvitis, represent the typical clinical picture and the pH of the vagina usually exceeds 5.0. The characteristic leukorrhea is frothy, greenish, profuse and malodorous. The mucous membranes show generalized erythema and scattered small petechial hemorrhages. There may be vulvar edema and excoriations of the skin from scratching. The discharge may be blood tinged. The diagnosis is made by demonstrating the motile flagellates in a wet-mount preparation. These protozoa are smaller than a mature epithelial cell but usually larger than polymorphonuclear leukocytes. Although several antitrichomonal suppositories are available, the preferred method is the simultaneous treatment of both partners with metronidazole (Flagyl), one 250 mg. tablet orally three times daily for 7 days. In resistant cases and in the event of reinfections, oral courses may be repeated after 4 to 6 weeks. The couple should be warned about the possibility of intolerance to alcohol as an important side effect of metronidazole and this agent should be withheld during the first trimester of pregnancy and during lactation.

Candidiasis. *Candida albicans* vaginitis is a fungus infection arising from candidal organisms that may be normal inhabitants of both the vagina and the large bowel. There may be a disturbance of normal vaginal physiology that allows these ubiquitous organisms to overwhelm the normal bacterial flora. The pH may not be elevated. Large numbers of candida may be introduced during coitus or their growth may be promoted by metabolic disease (e.g., diabetes mellitus), pregnancy, or by certain drugs (e.g., antibiotics, corticosteroids, and oral contraceptives). Candidiasis is the most common cause of leukorrhea. The typical clinical picture is vulvar erythema, edema, maceration, and excoriation usually associated with the intense pruritis as evidenced by scratch marks on the skin. The characteristic discharge is a thick, tenacious, often cheesy-white (curdy) "thrush patch" or plaque overlying a red mucosal base that may bleed when scraped. Burning may be intense in the acute stage particularly following urination. Normally, there is no odor unless a secondary infection develops. The diagnosis is based upon the demonstration of filamentous forms (pseudohyphae) of the candida albicans organism in a wet slide preparation utilizing 10 to 20 per cent potassium hydroxide. Sabouraud's or Nickerson's medium can be used to grow the organism. The sexual partner should always be examined, particularly in refractory or recurrent cases, and there should be no coitus without the protection of a condum. There are several effective anti-candida preparations including Nystatin tablets (100,000 units) (one or two vaginal inserts twice daily for 14 days), Miconazole nitrate (Monistat) 2 per cent cream, one applicator full daily for one week, and a 0.25 to 1 per cent aqueous solution of Gentian violet. Nystatin-corticosteroid (Mycolog) cream can be used to eliminate vulvar pruritis and to treat the male partner.

Corynebacterium Vaginate Vaginitis. This type of vulvovaginitis is bacterial in etiology and the causative agent is a small, gram-negative bacillus. There may be a profuse purulent discharge with minimal vulvar irritation but there are no characteristic features. The vaginal pH is usually between 5.0 and 6.0. The offending organism can be demonstrated by Gram stain and culture. Epithelial cells containing many of the organisms within their cytoplasm appear to be stippled or dusted with tiny particles and these represent the so-called "clue" cells associated with this type of vaginal infection. Sulfonamide cream (Sultrin) applied twice daily for 2 weeks is usually effective but tablets containing oxytetracycline and polymyxin B, Furacin vaginal cream, or ampicillin may be used.

Atrophic Vulvovaginitis. In the absence of the stimulation of normal endogenous estrogen, the vaginal epithelium is quite thin and deficient in glycogen, and the bacterial flora becomes mixed in association with an abnormally high pH as the normal acidogenic flora is replaced. Multiplication of potentially pathogenic organisms, including many types of streptococci, coliform bacteria, and others, is encouraged. There may be pruritis, external burning discomfort, dyspareunia, and often an associated urgency-frequency syndrome caused by atrophic urethritis. The discharge is highly variable in amount, color and consistency but it may be thick and purulent or serosanguineous. The pH of the vaginal fluid is usually in the range of 5.5 to 7.0. Vaginal cytology on wet-mount preparations on stained smears shows a predominance of intermediate or parabasal cells. The treatment consists of nightly applications of topical estrogenic creams for about 10 days and, for maintenance of the vaginal mucosa, of periodic instillations twice weekly thereafter. A simple atrophic condition of the vulva must not be mistaken for a dystrophic lesion or perhaps an even more serious underlying condition, such as a malignancy, that has given rise to a bloody vaginal discharge.

Viral Vulvovaginitis. Vulvar infections caused by herpesvirus hominis type 2 are sexually transmitted and represent the most common viral disease of the lower genital tract. The typical clinical picture is one of extreme vulvar pain in association with vesiculation and skin maceration. The primary disability may be quite acute for 7 to 10 days before remission occurs; recurrences are common, although the symptoms may be less severe. There may be vaginal and cervical involvements without symptoms. When the infection is extensive, there may be excoriations and secondary abscess formation. Fever may develop and there may be enlarged inguinal lymph nodes. Burning may be present on voiding, or there may be urinary retention. If acute herpes genitalis occurs during late pregnancy, the potential for transmission of the virus to the infant during delivery is sufficiently serious to justify abdominal intervention, provided the membranes are intact or ruptured for less than 4 hours. There is no specific diagnostic procedure short of isolating the virus; however, this is rarely necessary. Histologically, epithelial cells may be swollen and bizarre nuclear changes may be present. There may be eosinophilic intranuclear inclusions (Lipschütz bodies) that are usually centrally located and surrounded by a pale halo. Treatment for these infections is nonspecific, supportive, and directed at relief of symptoms during the self-limiting acute phase. It is possible to confuse this type of vulvovaginitis with another self-limiting disease characterized by multiple gas-filled cystic structures involving the vagina and cervix. Vaginitis emphysematosa, which is the official designation, may be a manifestation of trichomoniasis; however, the lesions are often unattended by leukorrhea or irritation and no treatment is usually required. Another consideration has been circumstantial evidence and possibility that the herpes simplex virus is oncogenic and may be an etiologic agent in the development of cervical cancer.

Chlamydia Trachomatis.

These sexually transmitted infections may be manifested as cervicitis or acute salpingitis may be more common than those attributable to gonorrhea. In the male, these organisms may be a prominent cause of nongonococcal urethritis and acute epididymitis. Chlamydial and gonococcal infections may be acquired simultaneously. Both infections, which resemble each other, may cause a mucopurulent cervical exudate in association with erythema, congestion, and friability. A Gram stain shows polymorphonuclear leukocytes and mononuclear inflammatory cells but no gonococci. Subsequent cultures are likewise negative for *Neisseria gonorrhoeae* unless both organisms are present. More specific diagnostic methods consist of isolation of the organism, which requires sophisticated culture capabilities, or of demonstrating a rise in the microimmunofluorescent antibody titer. Chlamydial infections have a longer incubation period that *N. gonorrhoeae* and symptoms may not appear until several weeks after the latter was treated with antibiotics. Treatment with penicillin G, ampicillin, or spectinomycin may not eradicate the chlamydial organisms although these drugs are ordinarily effective against the gonococcus. Treatment of endocervical chlamydial infection is tetracycline hydrochloride (500 mg. twice daily for 14 days). Acute salpingitis requires larger doses for longer periods of time. The male sex partner must be examined for nongonococcal urethritis and treated accordingly.

Benign Ulcerative Lesions of the Vulva

Granulomatous lesions of the vulva are often sexually transmitted and are infectious, although they may be cancerous either as a primary lesion or coexisting with the infectious underlying process. Granulation tissue is simply a reaction to the infection, and the superimposition of nonspecific inflammation is almost inevitable. A variety of investigative tests and procedures are required to establish the proper diagnosis and to initiate the proper therapeutic plan. The various diseases of clinical significance may be outlined as follows:

Chanchroid. This lesion is an irregularly shaped shallow vulvar ulceration with a very short inoculation period of only about 3 or 5 days. An exudate aspirated from the buboes or pus obtained from the ulcer usually demonstrates *Hemophilus ducreyi*. Autoinoculation is common and the vesiculopustular ulceration is usually very painful. When there are lesions about the external urethral meatus, the resultant scarring may lead to stenosis. The ulcers may multiply or be confluent and spread toward the thighs; usually there will be a thick foul discharge, draining buboes and tender inguinal nodes. The *H. ducreyi* can usually be cultured on blood agar, and Gram stains of the material from open lesions or buboes with show gram-negative rods in strands. One can culture a biopsy specimen for the most accurate results. One or two weeks after an infection, Ducrey's intradermal skin test will become positive and will remain so for years. On culture there may be a mixed complex vaginal flora. These lesions usually heal quickly following sulfonamide therapy in usual doses for 7 to 10 days. Streptomycin may also be effective singly or combined with tetracyclines, but these drugs may mask the early signs of syphilis.

Granuloma Inguinale. This ulcerative granulomatous disease involving the vulva, perineum, and inguinal regions is sexually transmitted. The causative organism is *Calymmatobacterium granulomatis* and the incubation period is 8 to 12 weeks. Bacteria encapsulated in mononuclear leukocytes are known as Donovan bodies. Initially, there is a papule that ulcerates and satellite ulcers may coalesce to produce a large lesion. Inguinal swelling and abscess (bubo) formation are common features and ulcerative lesions may extend to involve the urethra and anal area. There may be vegetative lesions, ulcers, and introital cicatricial distortions leading to dyspareunia and pain on walking or sitting. The diagnosis is made on the basis of large mononuclear cells containing the Donovan bodies. Smear materials stained with Wright's Giemsa's or silver stain will demonstrate the cystic inclusions; in traditional hematoxylin and eosin preparations there will be small round or rod-shaped particles. The treatment of choice is tetracycline administered orally in doses of 500 mg. four times daily for 2 to 3 weeks. In about 10 per cent of the cases the disease will be recurrent.

Lymphogranuloma Venereum. This infectious

disease, caused by chlamydial, is transmitted by coitus and is characterized by a chronic process often occurring in an anemic person in poor health. The offending organism is a large virus of the psittacosis-trachoma group. The early clinical lesion is a painless erosion that proceeds to ulceration on the fourchette, urethral meatus, or medial surface of the labia. The ulcer itself may be irregular, shallow, poorly defined, and associated with lymphatic spread and finally a destructive phase which may lead to loss of urethra, vaginal narrowing and distortion, anorectal edema, ulceration and stricture, and systemic symptoms. The diagnosis is most reliably established by demonstrating a positive complement fixation test in a titer of 1:16 or more, or by obtaining a positive microimmunofluorescent test. Other suggestive features include vulvar elephantiasis (esthiomene), hypoproteinemia and reversal of the albumen/globulin ratio. The best treatment consists of tetracycline in daily doses of 2 g. for 2 to 4 weeks, depending on tolerance. Various local and surgical therapies may be required because of abscesses and strictures.

Vulvar Lesion of Syphilis. Two-thirds of the syphilitic lesions occur on the labia majora or minora and many are quite small and lie within the labial folds. The infecting organism known to be the treponema pallidum gives rise to single or multiple primary lesions at the portal of entry about 21 days (range 10 to 90 days) after exposure. The characteristic features are a firm painless ulcer with raised borders, lymphatic spread, inguinal adenitis, and discrete rubbery nodes. Treponemes will pass through intact mucous membranes or abraded skin. About 2 weeks to 6 months after disappearance of the primary lesion, a rash develops in the form of maculopapular, follicular, or pustular lesions. There may be latent syphilis, which becomes noncommunicable in 4 years or produces late destructive (tertiary) lesions in about one-third patients (fatal in one-fourth and nonclinical in one-fourth). The tertiary lesions are vascular and neurologic. A gravid female with latent syphilis may transmit the disease to her fetus. Primary lesions may be found in areas of the perineum, nose, breast, and mouth and moist papules in the anogenital area, the secondary lesions, take the form of raised white plaques covered with serous exudates and are known as condyloma lata. Serologic tests for syphilis are usually nonreactive when the primary chancre first appears but become positive one to four weeks later. In primary syphilis, dark-field microscopic findings are positive, while serologic tests are positive in only about one-quarter of the cases. Up to 10 per cent of false positive serologic tests for syphilis may be caused by collagen diseases, viral, protozoal, and other spirochetal infections. The standard treatment for primary and secondary syphilis is benzathine penicillin G, 2.4 million units intramuscularly (1.2 million units in each buttock), penicillin with aluminum monostearate in oil (PAM), 2.4 million units initially and 1.2 million units intramuscularly on two occasions at an interval of 3 days, or aqueous procaine penicillin G, 600,000 units intramuscularly daily for 8 days. Treatment of a patient with a positive spinal fluid examination indicating latent syphilis would call for benzathine penicillin G, 1.2 million units intramuscularly every week for 4 weeks.

Tuberculosis of the Vulva. The vulva may be infected by the excretion of tubercle bacilli from the genital tract, urine, stool, or infected sputum. Contact of the organism with damaged vulvar epithelium leads to ulceration. There may be a foul discharge and contact bleeding. Genitourinary tuberculosis in the sexual partner may rarely infect the female. Characteristic lesions include chronic ulcers with firm margins and irregular bases, granulation tissues at the fourchette, fistulous tracts to the rectum, and inguinal adenopathy. Diagnosis is suspected when biopsy and histologic examination show the typical tuberculous granuloma, consisting of epithelioid cells, Langerhans giant cells, and a collar of lymphocytes and plasma cells. Confirmation is achieved bacteriologically by smears, cultures, or animal innoculation. The standard treatment is multiple drug therapy consisting of streptomycin and Isoniazid according to standard therapeutic protocols.

Other Lesions. Other benign ulcerative lesions of the vulva consist of sclerosing lipogranuloma, hidradenitis suppurativa, diphtheric culvitis, noma (pudenti) vulvae, pyogenic granuloma, dexamethasone granuloma, and, of course, superficial desquamations associated with various dermatoses including acute monilial infections. In addition, there may be aphthous small yellowish painful ulcers, shallow ulcers associated with the *Bacillus crassus* (Lipschütz ulcer), and Behcet's syndrome, which is a conglomerate of eye and mouth lesions along with painful small ulcers in the labia, vestibule and vagina.

Lesions of the Vulva Involving Abnormal Pigmentation

The coloration of the vulva varies among individuals and racial groups; however, in general, the vulvar skin color depends not only upon pigment (melanin or blood) but also on vascularity of the dermis and thickness of the overlying epidermis. A dystrophic lesion may take on different appearances in the course of its evolution or maturation. There may be erythema early and a distinct white appearance later on when there is decreased vascularity (sclerosis and atrophy) or hyperkeratosis (vasculature is obscured by the thickened epidermis). White lesions may be associated with loss or absence of melanin, either diffusely (vitiligo) or focally (leukoderma). Inflammation, congestion, vasodilation and neovascularization may produce red lesions, particularly when there is superficial ulceration and the underlying vascular dermis becomes more apparent. Some specific vulvar lesions are typically velvety red (psoriasis and extramammary Paget's disease). Lesions that result in increased production or concentration of melanin or blood pigments will give rise to dark discolorations (bluish, purplish, brownish), e.g., melanosis, melanoma, pigmented nevus, etc.

Vulvar Dystrophies.   There is a spectrum of vulvar diseases that are associated with a variety of clinical terms, but these terms are being discarded in favor of a classification based on histologic features. When the vulvar epithelium is exposed to chronic irritations from long-standing infection, the clinical appearance in response to thickening and maceration may be localized or diffuse white raised lesions. These may extend to involve the perineum, perianal skin, and adjacent thighs. These conditions have been referred to as "lichen simplex chronicus," or neurodermatitis. This type of dystrophy is designated as "hyperplastic" because the principal histologic features are benign epithelial changes consisting of thickening, acanthosis, hyperkeratosis and inflammatory infiltration. In contrast, there may be pronounced atrophy in association with a profound reduction in endogenous estrogen or in conjunction with a systemic skin condition known as "Lichen sclerosus et atrophicus." Clinically, the vulvar skin becomes thin, inflamed, fragile, wrinkled, parchment thin, and contracted or stenotic. Histologically, the principal features are thin epithelium, homogenization, loss of rete, and inflammatory infiltration. There may be a combination of the two ("mixed" type) types of dystrophies. Intense pruritis may be associated with the several varieties of lesions along with dyspareunia and dysuria if there is an associated atrophic urethritis. Although symptomatic treatments encompassing topical applications of corticosteriod, testosterone, estrogenic, and possibly antibacterial creams may be effective, preliminary biopsies taken at multiple sites suggested by toluidine staining are imperative to exclude areas of dysplasia and carcinoma in situ that may merge with frank cancer. Malignant lesions may be found coexisting with atrophic and hyperplastic dystrophic conditions. A clear distinction between severe dysplasia and intraepithelial carcinoma may be difficult to derive.

Intraepidermal Carcinoma.   These focal or diffuse lesions often found in association with dystrophic and/or dysplastic lesions of the vulva, may be of the squamous (Bowenoid) or of the transitional or intermediary cell type. Either type may be at the periphery of an invasive lesion. Usually, the preinvasive lesion produces pruritis, burning, discomfort, dyspareunia, and sometimes dysuria. There may be considerable shrinkage of the introitus. One variant of the Bowenoid transformation is a lesion of definite intraepithelial malignancy that occurs only in the mucous membrane or at the mucocutaneous junction. This condition has been termed erythroplasia of Queyrat and has the capacity to terminate in frank squamous cell carcinoma and metastatic spread if left untreated. These lesions in their several forms are best treated with a total vulvectomy with resection lines wide enough to encompass the whole disease and provide at least a 1 cm. clear margin.

Extramammary Paget's Disease.   This uncommon vulvar disease derives its name from its histologic similarity to Paget's disease of the breast, although the two conditions are probably unrelated. In the breast there is an underlying primary mammary carcinoma, usually apocrine in type, which gives rise to an intraepidermal metastasis. Contrarily, the vulvar lesion arises in the epithelium and it may be either unifocal or multicentric. The epidermis should contain clusters of cuboidal cells that show very pale cytoplasm containing mucopolysaccharides (Paget's cells). This intraepithelial cancer usually presents as a sharply demarcated, slightly elevated, somewhat indurated, reddened lesion. There may be patchy excoriations and maceration and an appearance of eczema, or the disease may be somewhat similar to that of psoriasis. These lesions may be found in the vulva of women during the reproductive years or in the elderly at any age. The associated symptoms of pruritis, burning and tingling may have been present for many years before the nature of the condition was appreciated. If there is a malignant transformation, the progression will be downward from the epidermis along the several appendages or by lymphatic permeation. The primary lesion may represent one variant of an intradermal carcinoma and may coexist with other histological types. Total vulvectomy with adequate margins is adequate treatment unless the deep areas of the corium are involved and dictate an associated lymphadenectomy.

Melanotic Lesions.   The proportion of melanomas arising in the vulva is disproportionately high, and while these lesions are uncommon (one to three per cent of all malignant vulvar tumors), they tend to be highly aggressive. They may arise from pigmented nevi which must be removed by excisional biopsies to diagnose or exclude melanoma. Similarly, melanosis may undergo malignant transformation after a number of years. The typical lesion is brownish and the pigment is unequally distributed throughout ill-defined, irregular areas of spread. Treatment consists of adequate local excision. If malignant degeneration occurs, the surgical approach would be radical vulvectomy together with inguinal lymphadenectomy. In malignant melanoma, the overall prognosis for a 5 year survival is in the 35 to 40 per cent range but the prognostic variables depend on histologic picture, site of origin (worse with lesions near the vestibule), and size of lesion at the time of therapy.

Benign Vulvar Tumors

Condylomata Acuminata. Warty growths of viral etiology may be found over a large area involving the cervix, vagina, vulva, perineum and perianal tissues. They may appear as isolated predunculated lesions or as exuberant coalescing tumors. Usually, the base is not indurated or ulcerated but secondary infection is common. There may be a chronic discharge and irritation arising from an underlying venereal disease or pathologic lesion involving the genital tract, particularly in recurrent cases. Initial workup encompasses diagnostic steps to uncover one of these potential causative factors. Improved personal hygiene and a liberal use of sulfonamide cream may bring about rapid improvement. Discrete warty growths may be removed with applications of podophyllin or by surgical excision when the tumors are large. Histological evaluation of these lesions is routine, since one of the underlying problems or associated conditions may be early squamous cell carcinoma. Also, the Buschke-Lowenstein Tumor (verrucous carcinoma) has fungating, cauliflowerlike growth, it too may spread widely over a period of years, and it has a tendency to recur. There are histological features that distinguish this lesion, which can be treated by local excision except in the extensive stages. In the latter, electrocoagulation or topical 5-fluorouracil may be eradicative.

Molluscum Contagiosum. This condition is a proliferative virus-induced skin disease with a predilection for the vulva. The lesions are usually multiple, benign, tumors that vary in size from tiny growths up to about one centimeter. They are usually attached by a sessile base, although some are pedunculated. The tumors tend to be dome shaped and some may develop a central opening secondary to necrosis and infection. The epithelial cells degenerate because their cytoplasm succumbs to the formation of large inclusion "molluscum bodies" that contain the numerous elementary structures representing the virus. The disease is sexually transmitted and autoinoculation is common. The lesions may be treated individually by freezing, desiccation, or curettage and cauterization of the base.

Hidradenoma. These rare, small benign tumors

may be solid but the typical lesions are cystic and they present chiefly on the labia majora of Caucasian women as sharply circumscribed, movable, partially translucent (partly dark), elevated masses, rarely larger than 1.5 cm. They will make their appearance only after puberty when the apocrine glands from which these tumors arise become functional. The tumors are firmly attached to the overlying skin, which becomes thinned out or necrotic from the pressure. A central opening, or so-called umbilication, may show a protrusion of papillomatous, red, granular tissue. There may be associated infection, bleeding, and pain. Histologically, the highly papillary adenomatous proliferations may be mistaken for adenocarcinoma although the absence of anaplastic changes or stromal invasion should call attention to the benign nature of the tumor. These growths can be locally excised intact.

These cystic tumors may be grossly similar to others of epidermal or epidermal appendage origin, e.g., epidermal cysts (arising from buried squamous epithelium), Fox-Fordyce disease (formation of microcysts from the retention of sweat in the apocrine gland ducts), sebaceous cysts, or syringomata which arise in the eccrine sweat gland structures. These conditions may give rise to intense pruritis and some may need to be locally excised.

Cysts of Embryonic Origin. A benign cyst arising from vestigial remnants of the vaginal portion of the mesonephric (wolffian) ducts in the female is referred to as Gartner's duct cyst. A second variety may arise from vestiges of the paramesonephric (müllerian) duct system and these probably make up more than one half of all the simple vaginal cysts. These cystic tumors are far more commonly found in the vagina than in the vulva. The probable overall incidence is about one per cent and most are not clinically significant. Large cysts causing protrusion and mechanical symptoms can be excised, but care must be taken in the dissections to avoid injury to the ureter, bladder, urethra or rectum.

Bartholin's Duct Cyst. Obstruction of the Bartholin duct usually near its opening into the vestibule may give rise to cyst formation. A combination of congenital narrowing and inspissated mucus may be a much more common cause of obstruction than scarring secondary to primary bartholinitis from gonorrhea or other microbial organisms. Usually, the main duct is obstructed and the cyst is unilocular; however, multiloculations can occur if the deeper minor ducts or acini or the ductal system become occluded. Cysts enlarge in response to the secretions of sexual stimulation and the mass may be tender and cause pain. The cyst may become infected, and abscess formation will give rise to marked inflammation of the overlying skin and severe vulvar pain. In addition to the gonococcus, *Escherichia coli, Aerobacter aerogenes,* various types of streptococci and other organisms have been isolated. Large symptomatic cysts usually having diameters of greater than the average of 1 to 4 cm. or those associated with recurrent abscesses should be approached surgically. In most instances, simple marsupralization will suffice and the original opening into the cyst wall will shrink to a small permanent tract for the escape of secretions. The appearance of a tumor mass in the region of the Bartholin gland after the menopause, or development of an enlarging firm tumor, even if the tissues are inflamed, should arouse suspicion of a neoplasm.

Benign Solid Vulvar Tumors. In addition to a number of benign solid epidermal and epidermal appendage tumors, one can encounter many neoplasms of mesodermal origin. These include tumors arising from smooth muscle in the round ligament (leiomyomas), proliferations of fibroblasts (fibromas), combinations of fat cells and connective tissue (lipoma), neural sheath (neurofibromas or granular cell myoblastoma), blood vessels (hemangiomata), capillary hemangioma, possibly pyogenic granuloma, and hypertrophied lymphatic channels (lymphangioma). Generally, large tumors or those causing symptoms can be excised. Excision of the granular cell myoblastoma may be the most troublesome because the margins of the tumor are indistinct and there is poor encapsulation. Wide excision will be necessary and close subsequent followup to detect early recurrences in the area of the resection line. There may be a similar tumor in the lower respiratory tract which calls for evaluations of the chest as a routine. Cavernous hemangiomas are probably best treated expectantly unless there is ulceration, bleeding or extension into the underlying muscle.

One may encounter primary and secondary vulvovaginal endometriosis presenting as dark colored nodular lesions. The majority of lesions seem to occur in old scars from lacerations, episiotomies or colpoperineorrhaphies, or from extensions of pelvic endometriosis, usually through the posterior vaginal fornix. The cervix may be involved as isolated lesions or as a part of a much wider disease process. Histologically, endometrial stroma and glands are demonstrable. Lesions may be fulgurated or locally excised and it may be best to suppress subsequent menstruation until the operative sites have healed.

Another benign solid tumor is the urethral caruncle, which is caused by ectropion of the posterior urethral wall secondary to postmenopausal mucosal atrophy or possibly by chronic irritation and infection of the meatus. The tumors may be pedunculated but they are generally sessile and they rarely exceed one centi-

meter in diameter. The appearance may be red or fleshy and the tumor may be friable. Some lesions cause dysuria, pain, bleeding, dyspareunia and tenderness. Histologically, they may be papillomatous, angiomatous, or granulomatous. Symptoms may be relieved with topical estrogen, or symptomatic larger tumors may be removed by local caustics, fulguration, or surgery removal.

Invasive Vulvar Malignancies

Epidermoid Cancer. Squamous cell carcinomas make up about 85 to 90 per cent of vulvar malignancies and roughly 5 per cent of all malignant tumors of the female generative tract. These lesions occur in postmenopausal women (more than half being over age 60 years), usually after a long history of vulvar irriation, bleeding, venereal infections, discharges, granulomatous ulcerations, poor personal hygiene or preexisting dysplasia (one-third of the patients). There may be long physician and patient delays in appreciating the clinical significance of refractory pruritis and vulvar sores. About two-thirds of the tumors arise in the labia majora and minora, but the lesion may spread to involve the whole vulva, perineum, and anal margin. The gross lesions may be exophytic or infiltrating but the appearance does not seem to correlate either with the histologic grade of the tumors or presence of nodal metastases. The diagnosis is established by biopsy or excisional biopsy at a suitable local site.

The size of the local lesion at the time of therapy is a key prognostic variable. There will be lymph node involvement in more than half of the patients with local lesions over 3 cm. in diameter. Midline lesions involving the clitoris, urethra, or rectum are most often associated with metastases extending directly into the obturator and other deep pelvic nodes. Otherwise, the primary route of spread is by way of the superficial and deep inguinal, deep femoral and external iliac lymph nodes. Usually, if the Cloquet's node in the upper femoral canal is not involved, no higher glands will be involved. Contralateral spread may occur because there are rich intercommunicating lymphatics in the vulvar skin. In fact, the contralateral inguinal nodes may become involved first. The primary lesions may be localized, confluent, or multifocal, and the histologic appearance of the cancers may show a spectrum of types (Grades I, II and III) based on degree of differentiation, keratinization with distinct pearl formation and anaplasia. Stromal tissues with invasion may show a variable degree of inflammatory cell differentiation. The degree of dedifferentiation has prognostic significance in small lesions, but overall the gross size of the tumor at therapy is the more sensitive factor. Young women tend to experience lesions on the fourchette most commonly, while, in the elderly, midline lesions notably in the region of the clitoris are more common. Lesions that extend into the vagina are less favorable varieties, and when tumors involve the vulva bilaterally, nodular metastases are more frequent.

The optimal therapy is surgical and the principle is to excise the lesion widely to encompass the entire tumor together with regional lymphatic tissues. The commonest type of treatment failure is a local recurrence resulting from inadequate removal of tissue and lack of a wide margin of cancer-free tissue on the specimen. The usual procedure is the en bloc radical vulvectomy and bilateral lymphadenectomy devised by Way and others. Frozen section examination of the glands of Cloquet will determine the need to proceed to lymphadenectomy in the deep pelvis, in addition to the groin dissections involving both nodes and skin that are called for in the standard procedure. Radiation therapy and chemotherapy have limited place in the management of vulvar cancers, and seldom could a case be made for palliative surgery. Optimal treatment results in a 5 year survival rate of about 65 per cent; however, if nodes are not involved, the expectation for survival rises to about 90 per cent.

Basal Cell Carcinoma of the Vulva. These slow growing, locally infiltrating lesions are derived from primordial basal cells in the epidermis or hair follicles and account for about two to three per cent of vulvar cancers. Their site of origin is normally in the skin of the labia majora and they may be described as papillomatous, somewhat pigmented, or maculopapular eruptions. Since as many as one in five lesions give rise to a local recurrence, an adequate resection is the key to proper management. Distant metastases are not expected unless the tumor is of the basal-squamous cell type. The latter are more aggressive and have sufficient potential for metastatic spread to justify radical surgical therapy.

Other Malignant Lesions. Other malignant vulvar lesions include melanoma (2 per cent of vulvar cancers), cloacogenic carcinoma (arising from epithelial rests or remnants of the urogenital sinus or cloaca), mesonephric carcinoma (arising from the remnants of the wolffian or gartnerian ducts), sarcoma, hemangioendothelioma, lymphosarcoma, and various metastatic tumors (vaginal, cervical, endometrial, ovarian, trophoblastic, rectal, or urinary tract origins). Bronchogenic carcinomas, as well as other primary types, may spread to the vulva, and there can be leukemic infiltrations.

Carcinoma of Bartholin's gland deserves special attention because the diagnosis may be long delayed. The symptoms associated with carcinoma are the same as those noted in the much more common acute inflammatory conditions. Ultimately, there is degeneration of overlying tissues and an irregular ulcer or sinus tract may be formed. Carcinomas arising from the duct of the gland are squamous cell in type and the histological appearance is not different from the other epidermoid vulvar lesions. Tumors arising in the gland may be adenocarcinoma (most frequent variety), adenoacanthoma, or adenoid cystic in type. These tumors account for about five per cent of vulvar cancers. The prognosis is generally poor and the presence of a malignant lesion of this type calls for radical vulvectomy, and partial vaginectomy as required, along with bilateral lymphadenectomy.

Cancer of the Vagina

Primary carcinomas of the vagina are largely epidermoid (roughly 75 per cent) and the peak age of women with the disease is between age 60 and 70. Altogether, these lesions make up only one to two per cent of gynecological malignancies. An invasive tumor may be preceded by an in situ lesion for up to a decade or more. Early lesions high in the vaginal fornices may be inconspicuous, although cytology may be positive for malignant cells. The tumors may progress as ulcerative lesions or they may become exophytic. There may be direct spread into the bladder or rectum while proximal lesions tend to produce nodal metastases similar to those in the cervix (deep pelvis) and distal vaginal tumors spread like vulvar lesions into the lymphatic tissues of the groin. The likelihood of lymph spread and the prognosis are determined largely by the size of the primary lesion. Bleeding or foul discharge from ulceration are prominent early symptoms and there is usually no associated pain. The treatment may be surgery or radiation therapy. The prognosis depends upon the stage of the disease when treated (70 to 75 per cent 5 year survival for Stage I, 25 to 30 per cent for stage III).

Primary malignancies of the vagina may also take the form of adenocarcinomas, melanomas, and sarcomas. Young women, between the ages of 14 and 23, may have an increased incidence of clear cell adenocarcinoma of the vagina associated with intrauterine exposure to diethylstilbesterol (DES) administered to the mother usually prior to the 17th gestational week. The prospect for this occurrence is fortunately quite low, probably 0.8 cases per 1000 exposed individuals. A benign vaginal condition associated with DES exposure known as "adenosis" is much more common (32 per cent of cases or higher) but none has yet been observed to progress to adenocarcinoma. In addition, the squamous metaplasia that occurs in maturing lesions of adenosis has not been seen to develop into a squamous cancer. Thus, the current attitude towards the management of vaginal adenosis is conservative and quite optimistic.

Distant spread is rare and late in epidermoid vaginal cancers, while pulmonary and liver metastases with melanomas and sarcomas are more common, usually disseminating by the blood stream. Embryonal rhabdomyosarcomas occur in young girls while leiomyosarcomas and reticulum cell sarcomas are seen in the adult female.

Secondary vaginal malignancies are quite common and there may be extensions or metastatic spread from vulvar, cervical, endometrial, trophoblast, tubal, or ovarian cancer. A malignant lesion in the Bartholin gland, urethra, bladder, kidney, or rectum may extend into the vagina, but cancer from more distant sites is rare. Cases of adenocarcinoma have been reported to arise from mesonephric duct remnants, ectopic cervical glands, and vaginal endometriosis.

DISORDERS OF THE CERVIX

Benign Disorders

Acute, subacute and chronic forms of cervicitis probably represent the most common gynecologic disorders, and the cervix may participate in a variety of the infectious processes involving the vulva and vagina that have already been discussed. In addition to parasitic, bacterial, viral and other pathologic agents, the underlying causes may be anal-vaginal contamination (poor hygiene), hypoestrogenic state, hypovitaminosis, pressure necrosis (pessaries), foreign bodies, obstetric lacerations, or iatrogenic factors relating to perforations and other injuries associated with instrumental procedures. Symptoms may include purulent discharge, bleeding, irritation, dyspareunia, lower abdominal discomfort, secondary urethritis (if there is an associated vulvovaginitis), infertility (hostile environment for sperm, incompetency of the cervix, etc.) or even carcinoma, possibly related to granulomatous and herpes simplex type 2 viral infections. The cervix may appear acutely inflamed with erythema and edema or, in cases of chronic infection, it may have a denuded, red, granular (eroded) appearance at the mucosquamous junction. In long-standing infections, the cervix may be hypertrophied and elongated. There may be positive laboratory studies for specific pathogens that call for a particular type of therapy. In addition to local or systemic antibiotic and other medical treatments, severe chronic cervicitis may require surgical intervention in the form of electrocauterization (incision and coagulation), cryosurgery (tissue destruction by freezing), endocervical curettage (after polypectomy), or partial trachelectomy (conization or excision

of specific lesions). The preliminary diagnostic procedures must be adequate to exclude specific granulomatous infections before embarking upon these procedures (e.g., tuberculosis, tertiary syphilis, granuloma inguinale, etc.) in addition to carcinoma. There may also be virulent pathogens residing in polyps, and a simple local excision may be associated with rapid spread to the internal genitalia. Adequate broad-spectrum antibiotics are required at the first suspicion of extension of local infection. Rarely, lymphogranuloma venereum, chancroid chlamydial infections, fungi or parasites give rise to prominent cervical lesions that present as papillary tumefactions, fistulous tracts, and/or ulcerations.

Occasionally, mesonephric (wolffian) duct remnants lying deep in the stroma of the cervix will become cystic. Ectopic endometrium can also involve the cervix by implantation during surgery or possibly delivery or by direct extension of pelvic endometriosis through the culdesac. A papilloma arising on the portio vaginalis should be excised and carefully examined histologically because a small percentage will be anaplastic. Cervical leiomyomata are capable of becoming highly symptomatic, particularly if they are large, and may give rise to dyspareunia, bladder or rectal complaints, ureteral obstruction, or hematometra (pyometra) secondary to obstruction of the endocervical canal. Most cervical tumors of this type are associated with leiomyomas of the uterine fundus and can be treated surgically in context with the overall problem.

Gonorrhea

Although documented cases of nonvenereal transmission of gonorrhea are on record, the disease is contracted almost entirely by coitus and the major site of primary infection in the female is the cervix. There is about an 80 to 90 per cent risk of contracting the disease in the female following her exposure with an infected male, after an incubation period of probably about 2 weeks, although precise figures are unknown. Early symptoms may be quite subtle or absent although some will present with a purulent urethral discharge, urinary frequency or dysuria, unilateral swelling of a Bartholin gland, or, possibly, sore throat or rectal discomfort if there has been pharyngeal or anal exposures. Most affected women will be asymptomatic carriers; however, it is probable that about 10 to 15 percent of untreated women will develop pelvic infection. Presumably, when spread to the tubes and ovaries does occur, it is subsequent to the development of an endometritis often in association with the first menstrual period after contracting the disease. This extension may occur silently or it may provoke acute pelvic symptoms and a systemic reaction.

Diagnosis of gonorrhea is presumptive when gram-negative diplococcal organisms are demonstrated on Gram stain, typical growth is seen on Thayer-Martin media, and there is a positive oxidase reaction. Selective media are highly effective diagnostic procedures and sensitive serologic tests are available for detecting antibodies to *Neisseria gonorrhoeae* in special circumstances. A serologic test for syphilis should be obtained routinely since the two venereal diseases may coexist.

Treatment consists of aqueous procaine penicillin G, 4.8 million units intramuscularly in two injection sites, combined with 1 g. of probenecid by mouth. There are alternative management programs involving ampicillin, tetracycline, and spectinomycin. In the presence of upper tract involvements, a loading dose of oral ampicillin (3.5 gm.) has been recommended in addition to 1 g. of probenecid and 10 days of followup ampicillin (500 mg., four times daily). Alternative treatment programs are also offered if followup culture of specimens from the endocervix, urethra, rectum, or pharynx are positive 7 to 14 days after initial therapy. All contacts must be investigated and careful surveillance of the patient is required to prevent recurrences and subsequent infertility.

Cervical Intraepithelial Neoplasias and Microinvasive Lesions

Cervical "dysplasia" refers to a histologic condition in which there is cellular anaplasia, nuclear hyperchromatism, increased numbers of abnormal mitotic figures, and loss of polarity in the deeper layers, but only a part of the thickness of the squamous epithelium has been replaced by these abnormalities. These disturbances can be mild, moderate, or severe, depending upon the depth of the more superficial layers of cells still capable of maturation. In the severest form, only a few cell layers near the surface retain their normal status. This falls short of total loss of maturation from the base membrane to the surface that characterizes squamous cell carcinoma in situ. Although dysplastic lesions may regress, the more severe stages tend to progress more often and more rapidly than the minimal lesions. Exfoliated cells occurring in cervical-vaginal cytologic smears tend to show a degree of the same anaplasia, changes in the nuclear chromatin, as well as multinucleation and increased nuclear-cytoplasmic ratio. Usually, there is a fairly close correlation between the cytologic and histologic findings (better than 80 per cent). However, management and diagnostic investigations as well as treatment, are predicated upon the fact that a "dysplastic" smear does not rule out an in situ carcinoma, and an in situ lesion noted on biopsy does not necessarily exclude an early stromal invasion. Although most early lesions of the cervix arise in the region of the squamocolumnar junction and are confined to the distal 2 cm. of the endocervical canal, they can remain hidden from view. Thus, stages 0 (in situ lesion), Ia (microscopic invasion) and Ib occult clinical lesions may occur in grossly normal appearing cervices or actually these several types may coexist. One definition of microinvasion (stage Ia) is that the neoplastic epithelium invades the stroma in one or more places only to a depth of 3 mm. or less below the basement membrane. Thus, there may be the full spectrum in one cervix between the normal and the clearly malignant and in situ carcinoma can be found at the periphery of an invasive lesion.

The incidence of squamous cell carcinoma in situ of the cervix on initial population screening is probably about 7 per 1000, while it is estimated that about 2 per cent of women over age 40 will ultimately develop clinical cancer. The prevalence of cervical dysplasia is less than 4.0 per cent in nonpregnant women, probably 1.5 to 3.5 per cent. Cervical changes of the dysplastic type are much more common during pregnancy, but in the majority of patients the lesions regress postpartally. Although biological progressions from dysplasia to clinical cancer have been observed in a significant minority of cases, possibly one-third, many lesions may remain static for many years. However, overall, the suggestion of progression is underscored by noting that the average age of a patient with clinical cervical cancer is about 45, while the peak incidence for in situ cancers is age 35, and, dysplasias are usually noted in women from 25 to 35 years. The epidemiological variables related to causes and predisposing factors are not altogether clear; however, the most position correlation exists between cancer and coitus at an early age involving multiple experiences with different partners. Cervical cancer is virtually unknown among nuns. Thus, cancer screening should begin when the female becomes sexually active and attention should be paid to matters of personal hygiene since viral and chemical agents may be involved. Undoubtedly, hereditary immunity and cultural practices (circumcision, etc.) are also operative because the incidence of cervical cancer is very low in Jewish women. Prior cancer in another organ, multiparity, low socioeconomic status, herpes virus type 2 infections, and immunosuppressive therapy may be other factors.

A plan of management dictates that an abnormal cytologic examination in the presence of a normal appearing cervix requires colposcopic examination and target directed biopsies of any areas displaying atypism. Unstained areas representing immature cells not containing glycogen may be detected following painting of the cervix and proximal vagina with Schiller's (Lugol's) solution. These may be targets to focus upon in obtaining suitable biopsies. In general, disturbing features on colposcopy calling for histologic evaluation include white epithelium, mosaicism, or the course punctate pattern of the surface capillaries, and, particularly, bizarre capillary configurations (possibly indicative of stromal invasion). The entire limits of the transformation zone and margins of the lesion or lesions must be clearly visible, or a diagnostic cone biopsy is mandatory. This occurs in 10 to 15 per cent of premenopausal women and an even greater percentage of postmenopausal individuals. The same approach is indicated if there are significant discrepancies among the cytologic, colposcopic and histologic findings. Selection of a specific treatment is made on an individual basis. If abnormal cytology is found in association with infection in the cervix or vagina, eradication of the infectious process and further cytologic studies are indicated.

Mild to moderate dysplastic cervical lesions may be treated with cryosurgery, provided there are no extensions into the endocervical canal and adequate followup is assured. If a cone biopsy has been performed and all margins show only normal tissue, this should suffice as treatment, even for in situ carcinoma if the patient is young and is desirous of childbearing. An extrafascial total abdominal hysterectomy would represent a definitive treatment for an in situ cancer or certain stage Ia lesions. However, if there is microinvasion associated with deep cell nests, confluence of cell aggregates, or lymph or vascular involvements, it is best to consider the lesion an occult stage Ib (clinical type) and offer more radical treatment (see next section).

Clinical Cervical Malignancy

About 95 per cent of cervical malignancies are epidermoid (roughly 87 per cent) or the adenosquamous type (8 per cent), while the remaining 5 per cent present as adenocarcinomas, or very rarely as sarcomatous lesions. The usual histologic grading based on differentiation I to III is generally directly related to the biological potential. Undifferentiated tumors (grade III) tend to metastasize early. The adenocarcinomas are more difficult to classify in this manner. Most of these cancers arise from the glandular elements of the cervix although some may be derived from the mesonephric (wolffian) duct remnants.

Epidermoid lesions may be infiltrative or exophytic, and ulceration associated with abnormal bleeding (acyclic) and odorous discharge may be primary manifestations. There may be irregular indurated edges with central friable necrotic tissues that may give rise to frank bleeding. Histologically, the squamous lesions may be of the small cell type, large cell keratinizing type, or the large cell nonkeratinizing type. Extension

into the vaginal fornices will usually occur in untreated cases and, ultimately, there will be parametrial involvements (beginning with stage IIb) and metastases to the deep pelvic nodes in a progressive manner. These may be spread anteriorly to invade the mucosa of the bladder or rectum (stage IVa). Lateral spread may occur to the lateral pelvic wall (no cancer-free space, stage IIIb) which may be associated with hydronephrosis or nonfunctioning kidney. The extent of vaginal involvement also influences the stage, since disease that does not encroach upon the lower one-third is classified in stage II, while lesions that do become stage III. The clinical staging I–IV determines the likelihood of nodal metastases. Squamous cell carcinoma confined to the cervix from a clinical viewpoint (stage I) is associated with lymph node involvement in 15 per cent; and, in those patients with parametrial extensions, this incidence rises to 30 to 40 per cent for deep pelvic nodes and about 10 per cent for paraaortic nodes. The nodes in stages III and IV will be positive in 35 to 65 per cent. This relatively high percentage of pelvic extensions even with stages I and II demonstrates the fallibility of clinical staging technics, e.g., examination under anesthesia, cystoscopy, rectosigmoidoscopy, intravenous pyelogram, barium enema, chest roentgenogram, sonograms, lymphangiograms and chemical profiles for renal and liver functions. Recently, various radioscans have improved the likelihood of discovering parenchymal disease and positive nodes; however, the inherent errors in these clinical evaluations have led some to sponsor pretherapy staging operative procedures to obtain tissue samples for histologic study of pelvic and paraaortic nodes and the parametria.

In patients with stage Ib and IIa lesions (proximal vaginal but no parametrial disease). The 5 year survival rates for irradiation therapy and surgery are essentially the same under optimal standards of care. Since the ovaries can be preserved (rare site of metastases), surgery has some advantages if the young woman is reasonably thin and a good operative risk. The proper procedure would be a radical hysterectomy and bilateral deep pelvic lymphadenectomy. An adequate resection of parametrial and paracervical tissues requires dissection and displacement of the ureters bilaterally. Lesser degrees of surgery are adequate only for Stage Ia disease where the changes for the nodal disease are negligible. Even the high risk categories of microinvasion (occult Stage Ib) are probably best treated in a more radical manner since nodal involvements may occur in two per cent or more of the cases (possibly up to 15 per cent as the lesion expands to an overt clinical lesion). The presence of pelvic infection (chronic salpingitis, diverticulitis, ulcerative colitis, parametritis, etc.) or presence of tumor (large uterine leiomyomata or ovarian pathology) would tend to contraindicate irradiation therapy and favor the operative approach. The surgical approach has special appeal in all three trimesters of pregnancy, since the pregnancy will be eliminated along with early cancer (avoids additional potentially hazardous manipulations to evacuate the uterus either before or after irradiation therapy). Extensive pelvic and intraabdominal adhesions from prior surgery and disease states would likewise complicate radiation. The surgical approach may be used as a method of salvaging some patients with central pelvic recurrences following irradiation or surgery or those who may have been left with a cloaca from slough after radiotherapy (even without residual disease). In these cases, a pelvic exenteration is performed, which accomplishes removal of the bladder (with creation of urinary diversion), rectum (with sigmoid colostomy), vagina (residual cervix if present), remaining central parametrial and paravaginal tissues, lymph nodes (if appropriate) and even the vulvoperineal tissues as may be required. The direction and extent of tumor growth determines the nature of the operative procedure. There are major operative and postoperative complications in all cases of radical pelvic surgery. The mortality rate varies from about one per cent or less up to 2.5 per cent in the extended surgical approaches. An effort to preserve ureteral blood supply and prolonged catheterization of the urinary bladder should give rise to fistulas in only about three percent or less of patients. Vesicovaginal and rectovaginal fistulae should be even less common.

Except for the above considerations, radiation therapy is generally the best primary treatment for invasive carcinoma cervix, especially in stages IIb to IV. In planning therapeutic management, a critical concern must be given to the dose of radiation given to the organs adjacent to the cervix and vagina. Although the latter structures can tolerate doses up to 24,000 roentgens, serious damage can be created in the major blood vessels of the pelvis and the bowel at about 7000 to 9000 roentgens and in the bladder and terminal ureter at about 10,000 roentgens or higher. The delicate balance between cancericidal dose levels and the possibility for injury to important uninvolved tissues becomes clear when it is realized that a dose necessary to kill cervical carcinoma is in the range of 6000 to 7000 roentgens administered over a period of 4 to 5 weeks. Furthermore, the tumor dose will fall off rapidly and a central safe source of radium delivered by intrauterine tandem and lateral forniceal colpostats may need more therapy at the lateral pelvic wall. A standard technique is to use radium locally to deliver about 8000 roentgens to point A (2 cm. lateral to the central canal of the cervix and 2 cm. above the lateral fornix in the axis of the uterus). This is a trouble spot because it is the general point where the uterine artery crosses

the ureter. Excessive radiation must be avoided in this crucial area. Usually the dose needed is given in 144 hours broken into two sessions, 2 to 3 days each at a two week interval. The dosage may be reduced in older patients. In one month's time, a dose of 300 roentgens can be given to Point B (same level as Point A but 5 cm. lateral to the central canal of the cervix), which corresponds roughly to the pelvic wall where the major deep lymph nodes are present along the iliac vessels. External radiation generated by supervoltage equipment (60 CO, linear accelerator, betatron) can be delivered first (with or without central shielding of the pelvis) to be followed by one or two radium applications, depending upon the stage of disease and individual circumstances. The irradiation field can be extended as necessary (moving grid technique) in attempt to sterilize the paraaortic nodes.

Generally, chemotherapeutic agents have not been effective in the treatment of cervical carcinoma. A variety of protocols have been used, but the results have been discouraging. Recently, cis-platinum has been used to treat squamous lesions, but the drug is nephrotoxic to a worrisome degree. Overall palliative care and emotional support are extremely important features in managing incurable cases. Unfortunately, among patients with recurrences, the majority (probably 75 per cent) will have disease involving the lateral pelvic wall. Uremia resulting from bilateral ureteral obstruction is the commonest cause of death. In selected cases, urinary diversion or palliative colostomy may be rewarding adjuncts in providing chronic care.

The 5 year suvival rate for Stage I fall into the 85 to 90 per cent range for most major centers and there is about a 10 to 12 per cent salvage in the Stage IV cases. The moderate stages evidence 5 year survival rates of about 65 per cent for Stage II and 35 per cent in Stage III, although some individual institutions achieve higher salvages. The presence of positive nodes greatly reduces the chances of survival at all stages including Stage I (drop of 40 per cent or more).

Special comment about managing a patient with a bulky central lesion (barrel-shaped cervical carcinoma) is needed. The hypoxic deep stromal tumor cells are more resistant to ionizing irradiation and, since 5 year survivals in Stage I and II are reduced, followup extrafascial hysterectomy may be beneficial.

DISORDERS OF THE UTERINE CORPUS

Leiomyomata

These are the most common uterine tumors (20 to 30 percent of all women over age 30) and they develop from the immature mesenchymal cells or smooth muscle cells in the walls of myometrial arterioles. Occasionally, they arise in the cervix, round ligament, or broad ligament. The tumors contain connective tissues, but they are chiefly smooth muscle and are not derived from fibrous tissue sources. These tissues are estrogen dependent and the fibromuscular elements may be highly susceptible to estrogen stimulation. All of them decrease in size dramatically postmenopausally. Growth hormone may provoke their development (under estrogenic stimulation) and the associated erythrocytosis. They range in size from seedling tumors to masses of enormous size that fill the abdominal cavity. They may be discrete, but usually are multiple and each tumor tends to be demarcated from encompassing normal tissue and somewhat lighter in color. The varieties are submucous, intramural, subserous, and separate from the uterus and parasitic. The subserous varieties may lie within the broad ligament (intraligamentary) or come to rely on extrauterine blood supply from omental vessels. The pedicle under the latter circumstances may undergo atrophy and resorption and the tumor becomes parasitic. Unrelated to the clinical situation there may be a variety of degenerative changes, e.g., atrophic, cystic (liquefaction of marked hyalinization), calcific (precipitation of calcium carbonate and phosphate from circulatory obstruction), septic (subsequent to central necrosis), carneous (venous congestion, thrombosis, interstitial hemorrhage, aseptic degeneration, and infarction particularly during pregnancy), and myxomatous changes (fatty degeneration). Malignant change resulting in a leiomyosarcoma from abnormal generative processes of unknown type occur in less than 0.5 per cent of patients with leiomyoma.

Symptoms will depend not only upon the size of the tumor and nature of any degenerative changes but also upon its location, clinical state, and whether or not there is a pregnancy. Large tumors impacting on pelvic nerves may cause pressure and considerable pain radiating to the back and lower extremities. Abnormal uterine bleeding, usually in the form of hypermenorrhea, is a common manifestation and there may be a parasitizing effect on iron stores both from tumor growth and blood loss. A submucous tumor in particular may cause intermenstrual leukorrhea and bleeding in addition to hypermenorrhea and secondary dysmenorrhea may be a prominent complaint. With large tumors, there may be polycythemia (erythrocytosis) of unknown etiology, although it can be hypothesized that partial ureteral obstruction induces erythropoietin production. Hysterectomy usually reverses the hematological problem. Endometritis or carneous septic degeneration may incite a systemic reaction with leukocytosis and increased sedimentation rate. Significant uterine enlargements and distortions may make it difficult or impossible to cancer screen or adequately curette the uterus or to control bleeding mechanically and/or hormonally. Acute torsions of a pedunculated tumor may produce acute symptoms. The effects of pregnancy on the tumors and vice versa may be profound. The adverse effects on pregnancy may be early abortion, late abortion, abruptio placenta, placenta previa, premature birth and degenerative changes leading to tenderness pain and a systemic reaction. In addition, there may be malpresentation, uterine inertia, dystocia, retained placenta, and sepsis. Women with significant leiomyomata should probably be offered family planning methods other than oral contraceptives and postmenopausal women should be given supportive estrogens with great caution since these hormones promote tumor growth.

Rarely, treatment consists of emergency surgical intervention in the event of acute torsion of a pedunculated tumor or intestinal obstruction in association with the ensuring inflammatory process. Supportive measures may require blood transfusions and/or iron therapies to correct anemias. Occasionally, a submucous leiomyoma provokes severe uterine contractions, which deliver the body of the tumor into the vagina while the elongated pedicle is still attached in the endometrial cavity. There is almost always infection present. It is best to excise the bulbous tumor near the cervix and delay hysterectomy if it is indicated until 6 weeks later. For the most part, myomectomies are reserved for the minority of patients who wish to create or preserve a potential fertility. However, such procedures are likely to be associated with considerable blood loss (use a Bonny clamp or tourniquet in an effort to control bleeding) and postoperative sepsis, adhesions, tumor growth or intestinal obstruction are not uncommon sequelae. Obviously, recurrent curettages for refractory bleeding in association with large intramural tumors are not effective means of controlling excess blood loss. Cyclic hormones as a hemostatic approach is not rewarding and radiation therapy to shrink down the tumor has very little place in overall management. The definitive treatment is abdominal hysterectomy. It should be recognized that tumors rising out of the pelvis (larger than 12 week gestational size) deserve removal on the basis of their potential to cause symptoms, and a substantial minority will partially obstruct the ureter leading to a silent hydro-ureter and hydronephrosis.

Sarcoma

These mesenchymal tumors comprise less than 2 per cent of uterine malignancies. It is customary to identify a homologous type that is derived from mesenchymal cells normally present in the uterus and a heterologous tumor that may contain cartilage, bone, striated muscle, and fat. There are also mixed tumors involving both homologous and heterologous sarcomas in addition to the mixed mesodermal (müllerian) tumors, which contain both sarcomatous and carcinomatous elements, but none of the teratomatous features. Recently, it has been suggested that it may be best to discard the ambiguous terms carcinosarcoma, sarco botryoides and recurrent fibroids, and to restrict the classification to the more specific types known as leiomyosarcoma, endometrial stromal sarcoma, and rhabdomyosarcoma. If identification is impossible after appropriate diagnostic efforts, the tumor should be designated "unclassified." Another current attitude is the belief based on electron microscopic studies that leiomyosarcoma may be a distinct entity and that there is no malignant degeneration of a preexisting leiomyoma. The distinction between benign and malignant tumor is often difficult to make, although the number of mitoses per high-power field is a helpful histologic criterion. Those with few mitoses per high field are likely to be benign while those with 10 mitoses per 10 high-power microscopic (HPF) fields are likely to be malignant and metastasize. So-called recurrent fibroids are merely borderline or low grade leiomyosarcomas. Aggressive tumors may have more than 20 mitoses per 10 HPF.

Stromal endometrial tumors tend to bulge into the uterine cavity, produce necrosis and hemorrhage, and infiltrate the endometrium. Stromal myosis, which is the benign condition, occurs in the premenopause while the aggressive form known as stromal sarcoma is a postmenopausal occurrence. In most cases of sarcoma, the uterus is enlarged or there is a rapid enlargement within a preexisting uterine leiomyoma. Leukorrhea may be a presenting complaint, in contradistinction to abnormal uterine bleeding, and there may be pelvic discomfort. There may be progressive local extension. Epithelial components may be either squamous cell carcinoma or adenocarcinoma, or both, and heterologous elements include osteosarcoma with bone or osteoid formation, chondrosarcoma or rhabdomyosarcoma. The poorest prognosis is associated with unencapsulated tumors, frequent mitotic figures per high-power microscopic field, and cell types consisting of rhabdomyoblasts or osteoblasts. The grapelike, polypoid neoplasms noted in children (sarcoma botryoides) and the mixed müllerian tumors in adults are usually rhabdomyosarcomas. Interestingly, the metastatic lesions of sarcomas resemble adenocarcinoma in three-quarters of the cases.

The prognosis is poor and hematogenous and lymphatic spread continues in most cases despite therapy. The standard treatment is total abdominal hysterectomy and bilateral salpingo-oophorectomy. In the case of mixed tumors with endometrial stromal lesions preoperative irradiation has been reported to be of value but generally radiation therapy is not rewarding. Melphalan therapy may be of value as a palliative measure. Rarely, endometrial stromal sarcoma will be responsive to large doses of medroxy progesterone. Radical surgery is not indicated. The overall 5 year survival rate for uterine sarcoma is only 20 per cent or less.

Endometrial Carcinoma

Traditionally, the ratio of the incidence of cancer of the body of the uterus to that of the cervix is 1:2 or 1:3. However, a sharp increase in the frequency of endometrial carcinoma during the decade of the 1970's has changed this relationship; and now it may be the most common female pelvic malignancy. As a cause of gynecologic cancer death, it will continue to rank second to carcinoma of the cervix. It is worrisome that the incidence in premenopausal, as well as older women has increased and it is estimated that about 3 per cent of women in the adult reproductive age category will develop the endometrial lesion in their later years.

There appear to be precursors, predispositions, and various factors associated with the development of endometrial carcinoma. Large boned, heavy (obese), nulliparous women often suffering from diabetes mellitus and hypertension constitute a high risk group. In some there will have been evidence of long-standing anovulation, delayed or so-called bloody climacterium, and changes in the endometrium indicative of adenomatous hyperplasia or carcinoma in situ. Chronic estrogen exposure from endogenous or exogenous sources may predispose malignant transformations in the endometrium in susceptible women or those with a familial predisposition. Presumably, estrone represents the most potential carcinogenic threat and its major precursor is androstenedione, which is metabolized in peripheral fat in an augmented fashion among obese women and those with endometrial carcinoma. Presumably, chronic anovulation from any cause (polycystic ovary syndrome), estrogen-producing ovarian tumors, or prolonged estrogen intake represent risks even among relatively young women. Granulosa-theca cell tumors of the ovary are associated with endometrial cancer in as many as 20 per cent of the cases. In considering chronic estrogen usage, one cannot discount topical applications because the hormone is absorbed rapidly into the blood stream through the vaginal mucosa. The type of endometrium provoked by unopposed estrogen is also important because only about one per cent or less of patients with cystic glandular hyperplasia will develop endometrial carcinoma, while a progression to malignancy in atypical adenomatous hyperplasia is a common occurrence (possibly 45 per cent). The latter lesions often coexist and in some cases no clear distinction can be made on histologic grounds.

The key clinical feature is abnormal uterine bleeding, particularly of the acyclic intermenstrual or postmenopausal types, although hypermenorrheic patterns and other forms of refractory dysfunctional uterine bleeding may have preceded the malignant endometrial transformation by a decade or more. At least one-half of patients can be characterized by these presentations, both in terms of underlying etiology for the bleeding and predisposing menstrual disturbances. It is a wise policy to probe the endocervix (as in obtaining endocervical specimens for cytologic studies) in providing routine gynecological care particularly in women at risk for the development of adenocarcinoma. A cervical stenosis preventing the discharge of blood or pus (a vaginal discharge may also be a presenting complaint) can result in considerable delays in diagnosis. In these cases the initial symptoms of pain associated with the development of a hematometra or pyometra.

Endometrial lesions may be focal or diffuse. The types are usually adenocarcinoma, adenocanthoma (contain nests of benign squamous or metaplastic cells), or adenosquamous carcinoma which contains both malignant glandular and squamous cells (perhaps 25 per cent of the types in the United States). Adenocarcinoma often takes the form of a polyp but the transformation of a "benign endometrial polyp" into an adenocarcinoma while its pedicle remains free of malignant change is a rare occurrence. Likewise, an epidermoid carcinoma arising from the endometrium in squamous cell rests, metaplasia, or cell patches within atrophied uteri is extremely uncommon. Certain sarcomas may have their derivation in the endometrial stroma.

Most adenocarcinomas arising in the endometrium are fairly well differentiated, perhaps two-thirds are graded I or II, and this histologic grade together with or without presence of malignant squamous cells, depth of the uterine cavity, and depth of myometrial invasion are the key prognostic variables. Spread of cancer can occur by surface growth into the cervical canal (Stage II) and into the myometrium (often associated with a uterine cavity depth of more than 8.0 cm. which distinguishes Stage Ia from Stage Ib and represents a worsening of the prognosis). With increasing myometrial infiltrations, lymphatic and vascular spread, as well as direct penetrations of tumor through the serosa, become major threats. When the outer one-third of the myometrium is involved, there will be spread to the deep pelvic lymph nodes in about one-half of the cases and to the paraaortic nodes in a significant minority. There may be a spread to the vagina (into the urethra, bladder, or rectum) and into the parametrial tissues. Tumors confined to the pelvis are Stage III unless the bladder or rectum is directly infiltrated (Stage IV). Spread to the liver, bones, and lungs is not uncommon (also, Stage IV) which makes radio scans an important part of the metastatic survey.

Diagnostic procedures include in utero inspection (hysteroscopy), exfoliative cytology, or smears of endometrial cavity saline irrigation fluid (Gravlee Jet Washer), endometrial biopsy or suction curettage, radiographs of the endometrial cavity (hysterosalpingography) and other procedures. Vaginal cytology as a screening diagnostic tool is less reliable in fundal than cervical cancers. The definitive diagnostic method is a differential curettage whereby tissues are obtained from the uterus in two specimens from scrapings first within the endocervical canal followed by a scraping of the endometrium. An adenocarcinoma may arise as a primary lesion at either site and the biological potential and the approach to management may be quite different. Also, when an endometrial cancer spreads to the endocervix (Stage II), the lymphatic metastases become quite similar to those of primary cervical carcinoma (internal, external and common iliacs and obturators). Usually at the time of the fractional uterine curettage careful pelvic examination and inspection of the bladder (cystoscopy) and rectosigmoid colon (endoscopy) are done in an effort to "stage" the disease accurately. Proceeding to therapy on the basis of frozen section study of curetted tissues rather than awaiting reports on permanent sections can lead to clinical error. Sometimes, complications of the malignant disease will impose problems in following a standard management protocol. The metastatic survey may reveal large bowel obstruction (on barium enema), chest lesions (on pulmonary roentgenograms or laminograms), ureteral obstruction (on intravenous pyelogram), or the presenting problem may be salpingitis and/or pyometra. The latter would call for uterine drainage and appropriate antibiotics to clear the infection before the definitive curettage could be performed.

Definitive treatment should be an extrafascial total abdominal hysterectomy which encorporates a collar of proximal vagina and bilateral salpingo-oophorectomy. Among patients subjected to irradiation therapy alone, the commonest site of failure is local recurrence in the uterus itself. However, the common occurrence of vaginal spread after hysterectomy alone (10 to 15 per cent) and the probabilities of lymph node metastases even in presumed Stage I disease, make a combined irradiation and surgical approach the preferred therapeutic modality. Deep pelvic nodes and paraaortic nodes may be positive even in Stage Ia disease, roughly six and three per cent respectively; and, if, in addition, the cancer is highly undifferentiated, these nodal involvements may be present in about one-third of the cases. Thus, preoperative radium (platinum radium capsules) is usually offered to reduce the likelihood of vaginal vault recurrences (the lymphatic channels are sterilized and obliterated). Followup surgery can be performed within 48 hours of completion of therapy or after 6 weeks. Postoperative external irradiation (cobalt therapy) can be given to patients who are found to have positive nodes at the time of surgery or if pathologic study of the uterus reveals substantial myometrial extension. Radiation to the pelvis alone, or in combination with a paraaortic dose (5000 roentgens in 5 to 6 weeks), may be required. In the presence of Stage II disease, a radical hysterectomy together with bilateral pelvic lymphadenectomy is preferred over standard procedures if the patient is a reasonably good operative risk. Followup external irradiation to the paraaortic nodes can be administered. Occasionally, patients with Stage III Stage IV disease are candidates for an exenterative surgical approach. More commonly, patients with widespread disease are best managed with chemotherapy. Long-acting progesterone administered intramuscularly may be effective in bringing about tumor regression and remission (perhaps in up to one-half the patients with well-differentiated lesions involving the lungs). Various chemotherapeutic agents used to control metastatic disease have included 5-fluorouracil, cytoxan, chlorambucil, melphalan, megase, and others. However, the most promising single agent usually used in combination with some of the others is doxorubicin (Adriamycin) administered intravenously every 3 weeks contingent upon lack of toxicity (particularly myocardiopathy).

The overall 5 year survival rate varies with the stage. There should be roughly an 80 per cent salvage when only the endometrium or superficial myometrium are involved. When the uterus is atrophic and only the endometrium is involved, a "cure" can be expected in almost all cases even with surgery alone. When the endocervix or extensive myometrial involvements occur, the 5 year survival drops to 50 per cent or less even with extensive therapeutic approaches; and, in the presence of extrauterine disease, little more than 15 to 20 per cent of the patients will survive for that period of time.

Optimal gynecological care for all women calls for the identification of those at special risk. Good medical supervision assumes that states of chronic anovulation will be recognized and remedied and that the administration of estrogen will be reserved for special indications and not abused. Proper practices of cancer screening should be pursued in context with continuing health surveillance. In the presence of endometrial hyperplasia, estrogen should be opposed by prescribing oral progesterone on a cyclic basis. Progesterone reduces estrogen receptors in the endometrium and depresses the receptor-mediated stimulation of these tissues. Even some of the atypical or very early cancerous lesions have been revised by this medical approach.

Pelvic Infections

Pelvic infections involving the internal genitalia, peritoneum, and adjacent structures are common occurrences in gynecologic practice and their incidence is on the rise because of permissive sexual attitudes giving rise to more venereal diseases as well as to recurrent and super infections that increase the risk of extension to the pelvis. These infections may be obstetrical (postabortal, intrapartal, postoperative, postpartal), gynecological (IUD related, postoperative, foreign body, catheter related, etc.), or pelvic extensions of inflammatory processes originating outside the genital tract (appendicitis, diverticulitis, urinary fistula, etc., or blood-borne condition). There can be local cellulitis, wide spread peritonitis, abscess formation, pelvic thrombophlebitis, septicemia (septic emboli), thromboembolic phenomena, endotoxic shock, renal shutdown, and other formidable complications. Although the etiology is usually bacterial, pelvic infections may be viral, parasitic, fungal or mixed. Traditionally, so-called pelvic inflammatory disease was essentially synonymous with gonorrheal salpingo-oophoritis, and these infections were designated as initial attack or recurrent disease as well as acute, subacute or chronic in type. It is now known that more than one-half of these infections are mixed and the various organisms involved include aerobic cocci, coliforms, and anaerobic bacteria. The latter tend to dominate (anaerobic progression) when the pelvic infection progresses to abscess formation. These organisms, which reside in the normal vagina and endocervix, including even clostridia, bacteroides, anaerobic streptococci, and those indigenous to the gastrointestinal tract, tend to become virulent under these hypoxic environmental conditions. The eventual outcome may be a ligneous cellulitis, leakage or rupture of purulent contents into the peritoneal cavity, adherent tuboovarian inflammatory cyst, walled-off chronic abscess with recurrent flareups, distortions, adhesions, infertility and a variety of incapacitating symptoms. Occasionally, abscesses obstruct the ureter, give rise to marked ileus or bowel obstruction, or extend to give rise to perinephric, subdiaphragmatic or pleural pus collections.

A considerable amount of difficulty may be encountered in distinguishing gynecological etiologies from conditions arising in the gastrointestinal tract, appendix, gallbladder, pancreas, urinary tract, or elsewhere. Although anorexia, nausea and vomiting may occur with acute salpingo-oophoritis, these symptoms are more characteristic of appendicitis. Change in bowel habits, and especially presence of occult blood in the stool, favor diverticulitis over salpingitis or appendicitis. The sudden onset of pain is more typical of ruptured viscus (tubal pregnancy), or torsion of an adnexal mass. Back or flank pain of a colicky type along with chills and fever suggest ureteral calculus (or urinary infection) particularly if there is radiation into the groin, microscopic hematuria, or pyuria. There may be backache with acute pelvic inflammation, but usually it is sacral and the pain radiates down one or both legs, and the patient may complain of an associated deep pressure. There may be marked abdominal tenderness, intermittent pain, and distension, but unlike intestinal obstruction, the bowel sounds tend to be hypotonic rather than hypertonic. Also, in acute salpingitis, the tenderness on motion of the cervix is likely to be exquisite. There may be fullness in the cul-de-sac associated with the cloudy fluid of a peritoneal inflammatory reaction or beginning pelvic abscess. An adnexal mass may be present, which may appear to be unilateral on palpation even though the contralateral tube is acutely inflamed. Confusion with a degenerated leiomyoma or tort subserous tumor can be a problem, especially if the mass is on a pedicle and there are no other uterine irregularities. The pelvic infection may even arise from the endometrium as in IUD-related sepsis, and an enlarged, boggy, tender uterus may arouse the suspicion of infected abortion or even of malignancy. Acute pelvic symptoms associated with marked tenderness in the absence of much temperature elevation or leukocytosis tend to favor other conditions, notably ruptured ectopic pregnancy. However, it is disconcerting that recurrent pelvic infections may not give rise to systemic responses, and there can be chronic abscesses in the pelvis without elevated white blood count or sedementation rate. Acute cholecystitis is likely to produce epigastric pain, colic, anoxeria, nausea, vomiting, right upper quadrant tenderness, leukocytosis, and, sometimes, icterus (cholelithiasis). The presence of upper quadrant abdominal pain radiating into the back is suggestive of acute biliary colic. It should be noted that gonorrheal perihepatitis represented by adhesions between the liver and surrounding structures can mimic acute cholecystitis almost exactly (Curtis-Fitz-Hugh syndrome). Generally, it is helpful to observe that, for the most part, gonorrheal infections involving the pelvis are usually associated with mild clinical pictures in sharp contrast with invasion of the pelvis by virulent mixed infections or sepsis in context with an acute surgical disorder. Nevertheless, these clinical clues notwithstanding, specific radiographs, ultrasonograms, radioscans, culdocentesis, colpotomy, endoscopies, and other procedures and investigative methods, including exploratory operations, may be required before the diagnosis can be established in some cases.

In the event of a tuboovarian abscess which may follow an initial episode of acute salpingo-oophoritis, the gravest risk is leakage or sudden rupture. There may be the dramatic onset of tachycardia, tachypnea, oliguria, hypotension, disorientation, and sometimes hypothermia, indicative of septic shock. There will be four quadrant abdominal pain, tenderness and rebound in association with a bulging cul-de-sac (pelvic abscess) and gross pus on culdocentesis. Without intensive monitoring, adequate support measures and prompt surgical intervention, the mortality is very high.

Inflammatory masses in the pelvis that do not respond to medical therapy or decrease in size despite aggressive management may be leaking pus. Another possibility to be considered is pelvic "tuberculosis," particularly if ascites has developed. There may be a history of chronic pelvic disease and infertility; eosinophilia in the peripheral blood would be suggestive. Menstrual disorders are common, often including amenorrhea, because tuberculous endometritis occurs in a very high percentage of cases with pelvic involvement. Detection of acid-fast bacteria in a Ziehl-Neelsen stain and positive cultures on Lowenstein-Jensen medium are diagnostic, and these evaluative methods can be applied to endometrial tissues, menstrual discharges, cul-de-sac fluid or peritoneal biopsies. All serosal surfaces may show disseminated granulomatous disease. If the patient is mistakenly subjected to operative intervention before 12 to 18 months of appropriate medical therapy (combinations of isoniazid, aminosalicylic acid, streptomycin, ethambutol, or others), suspicion of the disease should be aroused by certain distinguishing features. These may include unusually dense adhesions and lack of any clear planes of cleavage in the dissections. The tubes may be dilatated segmentally, but the ostia remain open. Fistula formations are highly suspicious findings.

The possibility that a septic abortion underlies a pelvic infection when there is a recent history of menstrual disturbance (especially missed), crampy pain, bleeding, foul vaginal discharge or possible passage of tissue. A molar pregnancy may behave similarly. Occasionally, pelvic endometriosis associated with a chocolate cyst of the ovary, and an inflammatory reaction causing fibrosis, contractures, serosal adhesions and fixations, may be mistaken for chronic pelvic infection and result in inappropriate therapies. The primary focus of endometritis and source of spread resulting in serious pelvic infection, including tuboovarian abscess, may be an infected polyp, submucous leiomyoma, or intrauterine device. Sometimes, an IUD-related abscess is unilateral and restricted solely to the tube and/or ovary. Uterine perforation following biopsy, curettage, IUD insertion, etc. may underlie serious pelvic infection. Critical sequelae in all these conditions are pelvic thrombophlebitis and septic emboli. A septic clinical course associated with high fever that does not respond to aggressive medical therapy suggests these complications. In particular, a marked persistent tachycardia may be feature of pelvic thrombophlebitis, and the patient's clinical picture may not improve until heparin therapy is instituted. Pelvic veins become involved more often when anaerobic streptococci and bacteroides are the offending pathogenic organisms.

The principles of clinical management are based on the knowledge of likely causes of sepsis, ability to assess the clinical picture properly, to provide proper coverage of the major bacteria involved in aerobic/anaerobic polymicrobial infection, recognize associated complications (embolization, thrombophlebitis, foreign body, bowel injury, urinary leakage, etc.), and to intervene surgically when indicated (debridement, drainage of abscess, etc). The four main categories of bacterial organisms requiring antibiotic coverage are (1) the grampositive aerobes and anaerobes; (2) non-penicillin sensitive bacteroidaceae *(B. fragilis);* (3) Group D streptococci (enterococci); and (4) enterobacteriacae. For life-threatening pelvic infections, triple therapy consisting of penicillin, clindamycin and gentamycin should provide proper coverage for these organisms. In about one-third of the patients with gonorrheal salpingitis, there will be aerobic/anaerobic, polymicrobial organisms involved in the pelvic infection. Thus, in nonresponding or serious cases, this broader and intensified therapeutic coverage must be provided. An established lower genital tract gonorrheal infection is often associated with pelvic extension, as evidenced by the ability to culture organisms from a cul-de-sac aspirant (between one-half and two-thirds of the cases).

Generally, there is a favorable clinical outcome when acute salpingo-oophoritis is promptly and adequately treated in an appropriate manner. For some, however, there will be thickening and other tissue changes including hydrosalpinx or tuboovarian inflammatory cysts, which may give rise to acute or subacute flareups in addition to chronic pain recurrent tenderness, deep thrust dyspareunia, backache, rectal pain, menstrual disturbances and general fatigue. Symptomatic heat, repeat courses of appropriate antibiotic therapy, anal-

gesics, and careful followup will be adequate to control symptoms in some of these patients. Among those interested in childbearing, a form of tuboplasty may be indicated during a quiescent period under antibody coverage if there is tubal occlusion clearly demonstrated in the course of the infertility workup. If a large symptomatic adnexal mass persists, or if the patient remains symptomatic because of extensive chronic pelvic inflammatory disease, definitive pelvic extirpative surgery would be indicated, even among the relatively young. The most quiescent period possible must be selected for the pelvic "operation" to avoid considerable postoperative morbidity.

Endometriosis, Adenomyosis, and Dysmenorrhea

Endometriosis is a benign proliferative process consisting of functioning ectopic endometrium capable of invading and distorting normal tissues in the pelvis and elsewhere, or occasionally spreading by lymphatics to the umbilicus and deep pelvic nodes or by hematogenous dissemination to the pleura and other sites. Adenocarcinoma, particularly in the ovary, may rarely arise from these implants of endometrium residing outside the uterine fundus. Pelvic pain, dysmenorrhea, dyspareunia, low back ache, rectal discomfort, abnormal bleeding and infertility represent the principal clinical features of endometriosis, although many patients remain asymptomatic despite extensive pelvic disease. There appears to be no correlation between the severity of symptoms and the extent of pelvic involvement. Although the incidence of endometriosis is highest among caucasian women of high socioeconomic status, probably caused by delayed marriage and childbearing, the disease is common in women of all nationalities and can be found in teenagers as well as in women in their thirties and forties. The ability to observe the pelvis through the laparoscope in so many different clinical situations has brought us new insights about the true incidence of this disease.

It has been clearly documented that blood and detritus can flow retrograde through the fallopian tubes at the time of menses, and shedded viable endometrium will sometimes implant on the visceral peritoneum or serosal surfaces of pelvic organs. An inoculum of endometrium will implant more readily in some women than in others, but the length of exposure to such transplantations of viable tissues undoubtedly is a factor. This transplantation theory, proposed by Sampson in 1921, is made creditable by clear evidence of iatrogenically induced endometriosis at various operative sites following opening the uterine cavity and inadvertantly, contaminating the wounds with endometrial cells. In addition to the myometrium, there may be lesions in episiotomy wounds, abdominal incisions, or in scar tissues arising from lacerations in the vagina or cervix. However, not all sites of endometriosis can be explained on this basis. "Metaplasias of the coelomic epithelium," first proposed by Meyer and popularized by Novak, Meigs and others, or a similar "müllerian cell rest theory" advanced by Russell have been put forward to explain ectopic foci of endometriosis at distant sites or in the retroperitoneal areas of the pelvis. A continuation of these processes may account for the various types of ectopic sites and these may be spread by local propagation or through the lymph or vascular channels.

The ovary is the most common site of implantation, but other areas of involvement include the uterosacral ligaments and cul-de-sac peritoneum in the typical case. Other sites of predilection are the broad ligaments and posterior surface of the uterus, bladder peritoneum or that overlying the terminal ureters, and the serosa of the rectosigmoid colon. There is intraabdominal bleeding associated with functioning surface implants that gives rise to chemical peritonitis, fibrosis and adhesions. There may be pain of a crampy type associated with periodic intestinal distension, but also from the bleeding surrounding the deeply placed foci of endometriosis. The typical cul-de-sac lesions, including a fixed retroflexed uterus and adherent ovaries, give rise to dyspareunia, and when the rectovaginal septum is involved, painful defecation is a common complaint in addition to pain referred to the sacrum and coccyx. Serosal bowel lesions that create muscular involvements and contractures may be responsible for partial or total bowel obstruction. Rarely, the terminal ureter will be obstructed by extrinsic strictures. Mucosal involvements are very uncommon. Rectal or bladder bleeding may arise from extreme submucosal inflammation and congestion without invasion of the lining. Uncommon, however, are ectocervical surface lesions or erosion through the vaginal mucosa overlying an extensively diseased cul-de-sac. There may be contact bleeding and bleeding at the time of menses at these sites. Secondary dysmenorrhea is a classic presentation, but the cause is not clear since severe symptoms can occur in the absence of adenomyosis and the serum prostaglandin $F_2\alpha$ concentrations are not elevated above the norm. Similarly, menstrual disturbances, usually taking the pattern of polymenorrhea (short cycles) and hypermenorrhea (excessive flow), are common even in the absence of extensive bilateral ovarian disease. There may be associated constant premenstrual, menstrual and postmenstrual pain away from the midline in the region of the ovaries for periods up to one half the entire cycle, representing two weeks

or more of incapacitating complaints. The ovary is usually adherent and very tender to palpation at these times surrounding the menstrual period. It may or may not feel cystic. Sometimes, an endometrioma will rupture with very dramatic results characterized as an acute surgical abdominal emergency. For many, infertility will represent the most distressing problem. Among women who are infertile without apparent cause, laparoscopic investigation will reveal pelvic endometriosis often in association with perituboovarian adhesions in almost one-third of the cases. In a few women, the ovarian parenchyma will be destroyed by destructive endometriomas, or rarely the extent of tubal disease will obstruct the lumen; however, there is much more likely to be an egg "trapping" or "pickup" problem. The incidence of infertility tends to correspond to the extent of pelvic disease, but exceptions occur since a few implants here and there on peritoneal surfaces without adhesions can be associated with infertility, while a pregnancy may occur in some instances when the extent of disease makes the patient a pelvic cripple.

Endometrial implants classically appear as dark bluish or brownish-black cystic structures on the surface or imbedded in tissues where there is a rather characteristic surrounding zone of fibrosis and contracture in the form of a "puckering." Histological study of these lesions will show both endometrial glands and stroma, interstitial hemorrhage, fibrosis and inflammatory cells, including hemosiderin-laden macrophages, in the surrounding tissues. In longstanding cases or after the menopause these lesions may "burn out" and the glandular elements may disappear. In active disease, ectopic endometrium responds to cyclic ovarian steroid stimulation although it may go out of phase and become hyperplastic. Rarely, an adenocarcinoma may develop in a focal area of ectopic endometrium. In stromal endometriosis, the glandular elements are absent even with active proliferation of the stroma. A few cases of sarcomatous degeneration have been reported. These entities are poorly understood and the cause of stromal disease of this type is unknown. Presumably, tissues containing glandular elements can produce stroma while stromatous elements are incapable of forming glands.

In diagnosis, the occurrence of secondary dysmenorrhea in a nulligravidous woman in her 30s is endometriosis until proven otherwise. By the same token, asymptomatic endometriosis may come to light in the process of a routine pelvic examination, especially if there is a mass and tender nodules in the cul-de-sac. Occasionally, symptoms of cramps are attributed to endometriosis because of pelvic findings and the underlying cause is an endometrial polyp associated with anovulatory bleeding and hyperplasia. The ensemble of abnormal bleeding, nodular pelvic masses, and pain may be adenocarcinoma with pelvic metastases; and this type of differential diagnostic possibility must be considered and eliminated before resorting to medical therapies that would cost time. An accurate diagnosis must be established before a therapeutic plan is instituted. Pelvic and rectovaginal examination with a focus of attention on the cul-de-sac are imperative. Radiologic and sonographic studies will assist in confirming the presence of a pelvic mass, cystoscopy, intravenous pyelography, and rectosigmoidoscopy will be helpful in excluding damage to adjacent pelvic structures. Diagnostic laparoscopy can be used to take biopsies of suspicious lesions. Treatment should not be programmed without a specific diagnosis.

In managing a patient, the treatment plan will depend upon age of the patient, underlying cause of endometriosis, desire for childbearing, extent of pelvic disease, ovarian function, type of tubal involvement, general medical status, and emotional status. The range of clinical problems will vary enormously. On the one hand, there will be the 15 year old female with extensive endometriosis whose menses have been regurgitated into the pelvic cavity because there is distal vaginal agenesis coexisting with normal gonads and müllerian duct differentiation. On the other hand, there will be the highly symptomatic woman in her 40s who has no interest whatever in childbearing but wishes to be rid of pain. In context with these considerations, it is useful to attempt to stage the disease with respect to the nature and extent of the lesions. While there are several classifications available for review, the basic considerations revolve around patients who will or will not be expected to respond to conservative management, consisting of observation, and analgesics and endocrine therapy, in terms of both comfort and desire for childbearing. The second major consideration involves those individuals who fall into a more advanced group characterized by advanced disease, larger lesions, usually more symptoms, and need for more aggressive, often surgical, therapies if there is to be a realistic chance for childbearing.

In the palliation group, there are no endometrial implants as large as 5 mm. in diameter and there are no avascular adhesions, scarred fimbriae, adherent bowel, uterine fixation, or involvements of the bladder, appendix, lymph nodes, surgical wounds, vagina, or umbilicus. Only in these cases of mild and moderate degrees of disease should hormonal suppression be attempted, and even in these only temporary remission should be anticipated. Basically, modern approaches

to hormonal control of endometriosis have settled on three modalities:

1. Estrogen-progestogen (Ovral, Demulen, Norlestrin, etc.) consisting of combination-type oral contraceptive agents that contain the least amount of estrogen necessary to suppress ovulation and the amount of progestogen needed to induce a pseudodecidual reaction, necrosis and resorption in the ectopic endometrium.
2. Treatment with continuous low-dose oral androgens, which remain subvirilizing while they suppress growth of ectopic implants without preventing ovulatory menses.
3. Creation of a pseudomenopause by utilizing a weak impeded androgen, which acts as an antigonadotropin upon the hypothalamus and pituitary, as well as a direct androgen suppressor of the endometrium at the site of the estrogen receptors. Mild virilization may occur, which makes this type of therapy undesirable in hirsute women. The biggest problems at the present time are the great expense of the medication and side effects of edema, weight grain and menopausal symptoms. This hormonal therapy does provide a substitute for women who have not responded to creation of pseudo-pregnancy by the traditional approaches. If symptoms of thromboembolic disease appear, progestogen therapy should be discontinued.

If restoration of childbearing potential as well as relief of symptoms represent the primary therapeutic goals, surgical treatment promises the greater chances of success. Occasionally, certain limited fulgurations of implants and lysis of adhesions in the adnexa can be accomplished through the laparoscope, but conservative operations through a conventional laparotomy generally will be required. The objectives are to lyse adhesions involving the uterus, tubes, ovaries, cul-de-sac, and any bands between the bowel or bladder and the internal genitalia. All ectopic endometrial implants are excised or fulgurated. A meticulous reperitonealization is attempted, and the uterine fundus is suspended to mobilize the adnexal structures in an effort to prevent their adhering to the cul-de-sac peritoneum. If there is severe dysmenorrhea in association with minimal cul-de-sac disease, a presacral neurectomy may be effective in reducing pain. These conservative procedures are successful in restoring fertility in up to 80 per cent of carefully selected cases, but success rates in the 50 to 80 per cent range are acceptable. One disadvantage to this surgical approach is the high likelihood of persistent or recurrent disease that makes a second operation necessary (20 per cent of cases or more).

Extensive involvements of bladder or bowel may require surgical castration rather than resection of lesions from these important organs. Since endometriosis is estrogen dependent, this approach would be successful. Occasionally, endometriosis is so extensive even in a young woman that the risk of failure of the various conservative operative approaches would be prohibitive. Definitive surgery consisting of total abdominal hysterectomy and bilateral salpingo-oophorectomy is best for women with advanced disease or those who are highly symptomatic and have completed their family. Even in young women, this type of curative surgery may be required if there are refractory symptoms or evidence that lesions are obstructing the ureter or adversely affecting other important organs. There is little evidence that hormone therapy preoperatively will aid the dissections and postoperative administrations after conservative therapy may take away the most optimal time for conception to occur. One of the iatrogenic causes of symptomatic failure is the overly zealous treatment of menopausal symptoms with estrogen after definitive surgery, which keeps certain residual implants alive. Also, there may be tags of functional ovary left, and these pieces of tissue may produce enough estrogen to keep the ectopic endometrial implants alive. In these rare cases, the unfortunate necessity for a second attempt at ovarian extirpation may be needed, if hormonal suppression and conservative measures cannot control symptoms.

Adenomyosis

This condition consists of ectopic endometrial islands within the myometrial layer of the uterus that appear as discrete localized lesions (adenomyomas) without distinct capsules or more commonly as diffuse involvement extending into the muscle to variable degrees. The islands may or may not connect with the basal endometrium. There is usually hypertrophy and hyperplasia around the islands of ectopic endometrium, and this thickening causes a globular enlargement of the uterine fundus. Although this condition has been referred to as "endometriosis interna," it is probably misleading to link adenomyosis and "endometriosis externa" as if they were similar in origin or in patterns of symptoms. The etiology of adenomyosis is not known, but it appears to arise primarily in parous women over age 30, and usually becomes symptomatic in the fifth decade (about 70 per cent of the cases). It is a relatively common condition (20 per cent or more of hysterectomy specimens) and in some adenomyosis extends into the isthmic portion of the fallopian tube (so-called "salpingitis isthmica no-

dosa"). The latter form of the disease, which occurs in about one-fifth of the cases, is a rare cause of sterility because it is unusual for both tubes to become obstructed by these lesions. The ectopic endometrium in the myometrium is similar to the basalis layer, and the tissue probably does not bleed during menstruation, only about 15 to 20 per cent of patients will respond to progesterone therapy. Adenomyomas commonly coexist with uterine leiomyomas (more than one-half the cases) and less often are associated with pelvic endometriosis. The characteristic symptoms are hypermenorrhea and dysmenorrhea. There may be a sense of pelvic pressure in association with an enlarged, softened, tender uterus. Chronic anemia from excess menstrual flow occurs in some patients. Attempt to regulate the menses hormonally are generally unsuccessful. Uterine curettage is required to rule out other causes (submucous leiomyoma, endometrial polyp, adenocarcinoma, etc.), but cannot be expected to resolve the problem of hypermenorrhea. Hysterectomy establishes the diagnosis and represents the most satisfactory method of treatment.

Pelvic Congestion Syndrome

This entity, described by Taylor and often referred to as the Taylor's syndrome, tends to arise in patients of the hysterical personality type and is associated with a variety of symptoms mimicking adenomyosis and other organic conditions arising in the uterus and pelvis. As in adenomyosis, the uterus may be symmetrically enlarged, softened and tender and the associated symptoms may be menstrual disturbances, pelvic pressure, and dysmenorrhea. The presence of marked congestion, including a somewhat patulous cyanotic cervix along with marked tenderness and pain on palpation of the boggy uterus and supporting structures represent the classic features. There may be associated tissue edema and muscle spasms giving rise to lower abdominal pain, low backache, cramps, and dyspareunia on a cyclic, intermittent or nearly continuous basis. Premenstrual tension may be a significant part of the syndrome. Usually, the uterus is retroverted, and the pelvic veins are engorged and tortuous. The veins within the broad ligaments may take on the appearance of a container of worms. These patients who suffer from a major functional overlay do not respond to symptomatic therapies very well and the problem is not basically one to be approached surgically without considerable thought.

Primary Dysmenorrhea

Painful menstruation is the most common gynecological complaint and a leading cause of disability that causes absenteeism from school and the loss of many millions of working hours annually. There may be an organic basis (secondary dysmenorrhea), or incapacitating cramps may be idiopathic and not related to any identifiable gynecologic disorder (primary dysmenorrhea). Patients suffering severe menstrual cramps of the primary type tend to have a significant psychologic overlay, including recurring fear. Establishing rapport with the patient and gaining her confidence with simple psychotherapeutic methods represents an essential part of the management by creating faith in the therapeutic approaches. In addition to possible emotional factors, physiological disturbances in the form of strong, uncoordinated uterine contractions have been demonstrated in some patients. There is a likely connection between elevated uterine tone and higher levels of prostaglandin production by the endometrium. Levels are higher after ovulation during the secretory phase and highest during the menses. Prostaglandin levels are lower in the proliferative stage and lowest in atrophic endometrium and after oral contraceptive therapy. The latter approach constitutes a rational therapeutic approach and cyclic medications administered for 6 months will be successful in 90 per cent of cases. The use of prostaglandin inhibitors (indomethacin, maproxen, etc.) given 24 to 48 hours in advance of the anticipated onset of discomfort may be effective for the same reason. This type of therapy is a logical alternative to oral steroids when side effects arise and analgesics or hypnotics are poorly tolerated. Anticholinergic medications (isoxsuprine) given to relax the smooth muscle of the uterus may also be successful therapies. Rarely, refractory cases may require surgical attention. The sympathetic and parasympathetic autonomic nerve supply for the uterus is concentrated in the presacral nerve, uterosacral ligaments, and nerve endings and ganglia in the region of the internal cervical os. Thus, the surgical approaches have been to produce pressure necrosis of the sensory nerve endings in the endocervix (insertion of a stem pessary), transection of the uterosacral ligaments either vaginally or abdominally (Doyle procedure) or presacral neurectomy (Cotte operation); complete relief of pain can be expected in about one-half of these difficult cases.

Tumors of the Trophoblast

Hydatidiform mole (molar pregnancy) is a disorder of the chorion characterized by grapelike vesicular enlargements of the villi capable of filling the uterus and enlarging it to the size of a 6 to 7 month gestation. There may be genetic (racial) factors associated with its occurrence since the incidence may be high in some areas (Taiwan, 1 in 82 pregnancies), relatively uncommon in some (United States, 1 in 1500 to 2000 pregnan-

cies), and intermediate in others (Mexico, 1 in 200 pregnancies). Although the precise etiology is unknown, the molar tissue is of placental origin and it is assumed that the eventual tumor is a type of missed abortion following early death of the embryo. With early death of the embryo in the 3rd to 5th week, the disappearance of the fetal circulation results in accumulation of fluid in the villi, if the maternal circulation is intact. Excessive trophoblast proliferation occurs and the syncytiotrophoblast, which is the source of chorionic gonadotropin, will produce higher titers than in normal pregnancy, and this finding is diagnostic of the disease. The investment with syncytium is complete, and the cytotrophoblast becomes quite prominent and will persist even after the 4th to 5th month if the mole is not evacuated. There is a tendency for these molar pregnancies to develop in females at either end of the reproductive era, either under age 10 or above age 40. The malignant potential of these tumors will vary with the race. In the Orient, as many as 15 per cent of hydatidiform moles behave as a malignant condition, while in the US, only about 1 to 4 per cent become choriocarcinomas. A classification based on pathologic findings is unrewarding because the histologic pattern does not reflect the biological potential of the tissues. In about 15 per cent of the tumors, the histologic features will be those of a benign hydatidiform mole, but the trophoblast will be aggressive in its ability to erode into the surrounding tissues (invasive mole).

A strongly positive pregnancy test, even in high dilutions, is suggestive of mole or multiple pregnancy. The human chorionic gonadotropin (hCG) titer may exceed one million IU per 24 hours at a peak time of 60 to 70 days, when the normal pregnancy range is almost always 400,000 IU. The titer may remain persistently high or may even rise up to 120 days and beyond, when normally there is a gradual fall to much lower levels. In molar pregnancy, there is a type of thyroid-stimulating hormone (TSH) activity usually without clinical evidence of thyrotoxicosis associated with elevated T_4 levels.

Clinical signs and symptoms associated with molar pregnancy consist of excessive nausea and vomiting (roughly one-third of cases), uterus larger than one should expect by dates (about one-half), uterine bleeding or dark red or brownish vaginal discharge, usually by the 18th week (90 per cent or more), pain of uterine origin from overdistension (one-third of the cases), preeclampsia-eclampsia associated with hypertension, edema, and proteinuria (more than one-third of retained moles), absent fetal heart quickening or palpable fetal parts after the fifth month, and extrusion of vesicles. On examination there may be an unusual fullness, softness, and thinning of the lower uterine segment; in the adnexa, bilateral theca lutein cysts caused by the excessive hCG stimulation may be found in the ovaries (one-half the cases). Dramatic symptoms attend the serious complications of hemorrhage, intrauterine infection with the potential of septicemia, and the rare occurrence of spontaneous rupture of the uterus.

An x-ray examination of the abdomen will reveal no fetal skeleton, there will be no "R" wave demonstrable on fetal electrocardiographic tracings, and ultrasound techniques utilizing the Doppler principle will not yield a fetal pulse. The most satisfactory diagnostic method after the third month is the ultrasound B scan, which shows a "snowstorm pattern" of echoes or a mottling effect in the uterine cavity. Amniography is more difficult and hazardous but injection of hypaque will show a "honeycomb pattern" and no fetal parts.

The great majority of patients require no treatment other than evacuation of the molar tissue since routine followup care will show a rapid fall of the hCG until the highly sensitive radioimmunoassay of the serum beta subunit of hCG is negative (roughly 80 per cent of cases). The risk of recurrent mole in a subsequent pregnancy is less than 2.0 per cent.

Certain diagnostic evaluations are required to rule out metastases in anticipation of determining the type of management. In addition to hCG titers, roentgenograms of the chest (tomograms as necessary), intravenous pyelogram, liver, spleen, brain scans, electroencephalogram, and possibly CT scans and arteriograms would represent an appropriate workup.

In the absence of labor, uterine evacuation by suction curettage followed by sharp curettage under the protection of oxytocin infusion is the proper approach for most patients. Attempts to rely upon prostaglandins to stimulate labor have not been rewarding. Hysterotomy, which was the traditional means of evacuating large uteri, is rarely necessary today. When the molar pregnancy occurs in the older age group and/or there is no interest in further childbearing, women who are good operative risks are best treated by total abdominal hysterectomy. The hCG regression time is roughly cut in half over that of cases handled by curettage and there is a lowered incidence of residual disease.

Histologically, the typical tumor shows advanced hyperplasia or anaplasia of the trophoblast, edema of the stroma (hydropic degeneration), absence of fetal capillaries, and no evidence of an embryo, cord, or amniotic membrane. Genetic studies on the tissues determine the sex chromatin (Barr bodies are noted in 80 per cent of the stromal cells) and chromosomal defects. There is some evidence suggesting that moles that are androgenic in origin are more likely to be "complete" and have a greater malignant potential. Aneuploid chromosome constitutions are not uncommon in these tumors.

In the partial or "incomplete" mole, only a fraction of the chorion is involved and pregnancy may continue although premature birth of a dead fetus is a frequent clinical outcome. In binovular twins it is possible for a normal fetus and placenta to coexist with a complete mole.

Careful post-mole surveillance consists of weekly hCG titers (beta subunit) until three consecutive normal values are obtained. Pelvic examinations, including careful inspection of the vagina, should be conducted biweekly. Periodic chest roentgenograms are mandatory because metastatic spread involves the lungs most commonly (60 per cent). Metastases to the vagina are next most common (40 per cent). All other sites are involved in less than 20 per cent of cases, but the more important organs include brain, liver, and kidney. It is extremely important to eliminate pregnancy and the confusion it would cause by administering oral contraceptives for at least one year.

Utilizing the beta subunit method of determining the hCG regression time, one does not expect the hormone to disappear until about 90 days following mole evacuation by suction curettage. However, after hysterectomy with the mole in situ, that time period is reduced to less than 60 days. One would expect the hCG to fall progressively during that period after a rather precipitous initial fall. This pattern is more important than the actual regression time up to about 3 months. A plateau, or rising titer, serves as a basis for treatment. This occurs only in about 20 per cent of the cases. More than one normal test must be insisted upon because a negative report one week may be followed by a positive titer the next. Demonstration of a metastatic lesion at any time would of course indicate malignant trophoblast disease and call for primary therapy or change of drug.

Methotrexate is the standard drug used singly, but actinomycin-D is equally effective and perhaps somewhat less toxic. The internal between courses is usually about 3 weeks as dictated by toxicity, particularly bone marrow suppression, although a variety of allergic and gastrointestinal complaints may arise. Generally, prior to each course of chemotherapy, a complete blood count and platelet count is performed. Treatment is permissible when the hemoglobin is over 10 g. per dl., white count over 3500 per cu. mm., and platelet count over 100,000 per cu. mm. The serum glutamic-oxaloacetic transaminase (SGOT), BUN, and serum creatinine should not be rising. If response is not apparent or if toxicity arises to one drug, the other should be tried. It is customary to give two therapeutic courses after the hCG titers have been normal for 3 weeks. Hysterectomy might have be necessary when the uterine wall is perforated by an invasive mole or the patient is refractory to chemotherapy. Remission can be anticipated in a high percentage of patients with nonmetastatic disease. The highest risk patients include those with advanced duration of disease before therapy, exceptionally high titers of hCG if there is no apparent association with pregnancy (possible teratomatous origin) or follows a nonmolar pregnancy (60 per cent of cases). Choriocarcinoma in all cases or metastatic disease, particularly brain involvement. In these patients, as well as those who are nonresponsive to single-agent chemotherapy, multiple drugs must be given (methotrexate, Actinomycin-D, and cyclophosphamide, or others) as well as irradiation of the brain-metastatic sites. Even in these high risk categories, a favorable response can be achieved in about 75 per cent. The myometrium itself is a site of metastatic disease in about 10 per cent of patients, and its persistence in the absence of other lesions calls for hysterectomy. Usually surgical treatment is reserved for complications. Choriocarcinoma, which once was universally fatal, can now be controlled or even cured after appropriate therapy (perhaps 40 to 50 per cent), although toxic effects of the medications may be troublesome.

Malignancy of the Fallopian Tube

Malignancies of the oviducts (fallopian tubes) are overwhelmingly metastatic from other organs (about 90 per cent), but primary lesions may occur, usually as adenocarcinomas (95 per cent of the cases), even though they represent the rarest malignancies of the female genitalia. The predisposed woman is a nulligravida who is usually postmenopausal with a history of chronic salpingitis. The presence of an elongated, slightly tender mass in the adnexa usually unilateral, less than 10 cm in diameter, and associated with lower abdominal discomfort from tubal distension, colicky pain followed by a profuse watery, serosanguineous or yellowish discharge and reduction in the size of the mass (hydrops tubae profluens), is highly suggestive of a primary malignant tumor of the oviduct. The tube is usually distended by a papillary adenomatous malignant lesion which spreads by protruding through the fimbriated os and the lymphatic channels rather than invading through the myosalpinx. Ascites is not common and abdominal enlargement and intestinal obstruction occur late if at all. Postmenopausal bleeding is a common occurrence and tubal cancer should be suspected when endometrical curettings are benign and examination of the pelvis reveals a fusiform or sausage-shaped mass. Vaginal cytology, hysterosalpingography, and laparoscopy may lend credibility to the diagnosis of this rare pelvic condition. Characteristically, the diagnosis is delayed and not made preoperatively. A small malignant tumor found incidentally at the time of surgery for another condition might have a favorable prognosis. Otherwise, the outlook is grave despite total hysterectomy and bilateral salpingo-oophorectomy. Followup pelvic irradiation is recommended, but the 5 year salvage rate of less than 15 per cent points up the limited value of this modality or following a chemotherapeutic plan.

Other Conditions of the Oviducts and Parovarium

Rarely, there will be unilateral or bilateral absence of the fallopian tubes, unilateral duplication with a single cornual entrance, multiple open tubular structures with independent fimbriae, atresias, unconnected tubes, absent fimbrae, and other anomalies. Infertility is common, and tuboplastic efforts are usually not very successful. Related anomalies elsewhere in the müllerian duct (uterus) and urinary tract occur frequently.

Occasionally, there may be "ectopic ovarian accessory tissues" in the broad ligament near the cornu of the uterus or the normal ovary. They usually present as nodules of less than 1.0 cm. in diameter and they are predisposed to neoplastic transformation. Ovarian tissues may be found retroperitoneally near the kidney and in the groin in a hernia sac. Supernumerary ovaries should be removed when they are encountered.

Cysts may develop in the mesosalpinx from paramesonephric structures and come to lie between the tube and hilus of the ovary. Many of these are blind accessory lumens of the tube. The blind outer wolffian duct may become cystic and pedunculated (hydatid cyst of Morgagni). Rarely, they may produce acute symptoms by becoming necrotic or infected or by causing torsion of the tube and ovary. Benign, thin-walled, parovarian cysts may be single or multiple, and occasionally may become large enough to produce pressure symptoms or acute distress if infarction becomes a complication associated with torsion. The ureter may be displaced or buried in the posterior wall of the cyst, making surgical removal of the intraligamentary (retroperitoneal) mass a tedious exercise. Often, surgery is undertaken in the mistaken belief that an ovarian neoplasm is present. Symptomatic cysts should be removed but the majority are small, nonpalpable and not associated with pelvic complaints.

Ovarian Tumors

Benign tumors of the ovary may be cystic or solid. The cystic ones may be nonneoplastic (follicle, lutein, germinal inclusion and endometrial cysts) or neoplastic (cystadenoma, pseudomucinous or serous and benign cysticteratoma or dermoid). The solid ones are papilloma, fibroadenoma, fibroma, fibromyoma, angioma, lymphangioma, mesothelioma, chondroma and osteoma. Other solid tumors, probably benign, are Brenner tumors, adrenal tumors and hilus cell tumors. Malignant tumors of the ovary may also be solid or cystic. The cystic varieties are pseudomucinous and serous papillary cystadenocarcinomas and epidermoid carcinoma arising in dermoid cysts. Primary solid carcinomas of the ovary take the form of adenocarcinoma, papillary, medullary scirrhous, alveolar, plexiform, carcinoma simplex, mesonephroma and chorioepithelioma. A special group of embryonic or dysontogenetic tumors includes granulosa cell carcinoma, thecoma, luteoma, arrhenoblastoma and dysgerminoma. Other special malignant tumors are terotoma, sarcoma and melanoma. Metastatic carcinomas may be of the following types: adenocarcinoma, Krukenberg tumor from the gastrointestinal tract, epidermoid carcinoma and hypernephroma.

Cysts. Formation of cysts following atresia of a follicle is physiologic. Occasionally, one or more cysts may enlarge at the expense of the others forming a thin-walled mass up to about 5 cm. in size and filled with a clear transudate. Hemorrhage into the cavity of a cystic, atretic follicle is common (follicle hematoma). Follicle cysts are the most frequent ovarian cysts, but they are the least important clinically, although they may cause temporary menstrual irregularities and alterations of flow. Occasionally, rupture may cause acute pain or even peritoneal irritation.

Lutein cysts may take the form of granulosa lutein cysts (corpus luteum cysts) and theca lutein cysts (frequently associated with hydatidiform moles). The corpus albicans cyst is a variant or sequel of the corpus luteum cyst. Hematomas may develop in any of these structures. Corpus luteum hematomas, frequently associated with delayed menstruation, pain and palpable mass, are not infrequently confused with tubal pregnancy. Occasionally, their rupture gives rise to considerable hemoperitoneum and acute abdominal symptoms, requiring emergent operative intervention.

Neoplastic Cysts. The *pseudomucinous cystadenomas* are usually unilateral and grow very slowly, though they reach enormous dimensions. The histogenesis is thought to be from teratomatous elements within the ovary. They are multilocular and are lined with high cylindric epithelium that may be discolored by hemorrhage. They rarely become malignant or adhere to the intestines, being essentially benign and operable. Only about 10 per cent of these tumors are papillary. If the cyst content is spilled on the peritoneum, it sometimes forms implantation metastases that cause adhesions by their continued gelatinous secretion (pseudomyxoma peritonei). About 5 per cent of these tumors undergo malignant degeneration. The treatment is surgical removal of the tumor unilaterally (if the tumor is unilateral, free, nonpapillary and intact), or by total abdominal hysterectomy together with bilateral salpingo-oophorectomy in older women, or if there is a question of extension or bilateral involvement.

Serous cystadenomas, on the other hand, usually appear unilocular, though the larger ones are lobulated and multilocular. They arise from the germinal epithelium on the surface of the ovary. The cysts are lined with a low cylindric epithelium with papillary processes in both the inner lining of the cyst and the outer surface. The epithelium may show many of the characteristics of tubal epithelium. Psammoma bodies may be scattered throughout the stroma. They are filled with a clear, yellowish, serous fluid. Characteristically, these tumors grow in both ovaries, though not always simultaneously, and often spread between the leaves of the broad ligament. Those of the nonpapillomatous type usually are benign, but the papillary tumors have a tendency to malignant degeneration, as well as to form implantation papillomas on the peritoneum with prodigious ascites. When implants are present or there are papillary growths, a hysterectomy and bilateral salpingo-oophorectomy should be done; otherwise, a unilateral operation may suffice in young women, provided that the contralateral ovary is normal. To assure the latter, the contralateral ovary may be bisected and inspected.

Dermoid cysts, or *benign teratomas,* are also common tumors. Only about one per cent develop a malignant lesion arising in the squamous epithelium. The tumor is smooth coated and pearl gray and shows, on cut section, a semifluid sebaceous material; hair, teeth, bone and cartilage may be seen. Dermoid cysts are bilateral in nearly one fourth of the cases. There is a predominance of ectodermal elements, though mesodermal elements usually are also found, and occasionally even well-differentiated entodermal structures. Occasionally, thyroid tissue is present in the tumor in sufficient quantity to obscure or even exclude the presence of other elements. This tumor, the so-called struma ovarii, is usually a benign cystic variant, but in 5 to 10 per cent malignant changes are found.

Teratomas may also be malignant, the fetal elements being of undifferentiated type, usually representing all three germ layers, whereas the simple dermoid cyst has only two (ectoderm and mesoderm). The teratoma is basically a solid tumor, although it may have cystic elements, while the dermoid is the reverse. Solid teratomas constitute the very small percentage of ovarian teratomas that are not cystic, probably over 1 or 2 per cent. An extremely rare variant is the teratocarcinoma. Dermoid cysts are expanding lesions and destroy ovarian tissue by continued pressure. The cysts may be asymptomatic or, because of the long ovarian pedicle, may undergo torsion with acute symptoms or may undergo septic degeneration. Treatment is surgical, making every effort to leave intact all functioning ovarian tissue. The contralateral ovary should be bisected to exclude the possibility of leaving behind a small dermoid that could easily be enucleated. The malignant varieties are treated by total extirpation of the internal pelvic organs, but the prognosis is generally poor. The tumors do not ordinarily respond to radiation or cytotoxic drugs.

Torsion is one of the most important complications of ovarian tumors; it occurs in 10 to 20 per cent of all cases. The growth of an ovarian tumor causes it to ride out of the true pelvis, so that it may fall forward and rotate 90 degrees. Unequal growth in the cyst walls, trauma, intestinal peristalsis or pregnancy may increase the degree of torsion. Generally, torsion of 180 degrees produces symptoms, though the cyst may twist on its pedicle two or three or even five or six times. The torsion first causes venous blocking, the arterial circulation producing a rapid increase in size, and results in hemorrhage into the lumen and areas of infarction; the damage surface soon becomes adherent to the intestine and the omentum. If the torsion is acute, the symptoms are like those of acute peritonitis, with rigid, extremely sensitive abdomen and signs of shock. If there is no infection, the attack sometimes abates, but it generally recurs. Adhesions to the intestine may result in intestinal perforation, with peritonitis. If the tumor suppurates, it may rupture into the abdominal cavity. Uterine bleeding is common. If the patient seeks medical attention promptly, and the appropriate surgery is performed, the patient usually has an uneventful recovery; otherwise, suppuration, rupture and general peritonitis may ensue with dire results. At the time of surgery it is important to avoid undue manipulation and untwisting the pedicle to minimize the risk of embolization.

Carcinoma of the Ovary. This disease ranks next to uterine cancer in relative frequency insofar as the various forms of female reproductive organs are concerned. The cancer may be primary or secondary to a lesion in other organs. It may be solid or cystic, the latter being more common (serous cystadenocarcinoma is the most common lesion). The great majority arise in previously benign cystadenomas. Cancerous lesions are bilateral in about half of the cases. It is estimated that about 15 per cent of all ovarian tumors are malignant. The pathologic types have been outlined previously. From a histologic viewpoint the epithelial tumors are classifiable as serous, mucinous, endometrioid (similar to adenocarcinoma of the endometrium) mesonephroid lesions of the ovary (clear cell carcinoma), and tumors that cannot be assigned to one of the above categories. Ovarian carcinoma spreads frequently to the tubes and the uterus and onto the pelvic peritoneum. The lumbar lymphatic glands are frequently involved, and metastases occur by bloodstream to such distant organs as the lungs and the brain. Symptoms appear late and are of insidious onset. The presence of a mass or ascites may be the first indication of disease. Menstrual dysfunction and pelvic pressure or pain may occur but are often absent. Ascites is relatively common. Weakness, anemia, weight loss and gastrointestinal symptoms appear late.

The embryonic group of ovarian carcinomas may present special genital symptoms according to the type and the age of onset. The most common of this group is the feminizing mesenchymoma or estrogen-producing tumor (granulosa cell, thecoma or luteoma). The granulosa cell carcinoma is the most common variety, and it may arise at any time in life. Premenarcheal girls experience premature sex development and uterine bleeding and hypertrophy of the uterus and the endometrium. In older women, the hyperplasia may develop atypical features or carcinoma of the endometrium. The counterpart of this tumor is the masculinizing ovarian neoplasm, arrhenoblastoma. There is a progressive defeminization and then masculinization of the patient. Rarely, adrenal tumors of the ovary, hilus cell tumors and gynandroblastomas are responsible for masculinizing symptoms. As a rule, the secondary sex changes gradually reverse after the tumor is removed. Another rare embryonic tumor, the dysgerminoma, is sexually indifferent, although it frequently arises in patients with pseudohermaphroditic defects. About one-fourth of these embryonic tumors exhibit evidence of clinical malignancy. A conservative unilateral operation appears to be justified in young women in whom future pregnancies are important. However, some dysgerminomas are highly malignant and any suspicion of clinical malignancy (or positive evidence by frozen section) warrants a complete operation.

Prior to treatment, a malignant ovarian tumor must be staged and a systematic preoperative work-up, including diagnostic procedures and a metastatic survey, must be completed. In stage I growth is limited to the ovaries, as follows: substage Ia, one ovary involved without ascites; Ib, both ovaries involved without ascites; and Ic, one or both ovaries involved and presence of ascitic fluid containing malignant cells. In stage II there has been pelvic extension of the tumor: IIa, to internal pelvic organs only, or IIb, to other pelvic tissues. In stage III there is widespread intraperitoneal abdominal metastases, and in stage IV there is distant spread outside the peritoneal cavity.

The treatment and the prognosis for ovarian cancer will depend on the type of tumor, its histologic grade and degree of malignancy, the stage, presence of metastasis, the age, and general condition of the patient. The primary treatment is surgery, supplemented in selected cases by a follow-up course of cobalt radiation or chemotherapeutic agents or both. Recurrent ascites can frequently be controlled palliatively by the use of cobalt radiation and peritoneal cytotoxic drugs. Colloidal gold used for this purpose has limited value. Intraabdominal injections are followed by changes in the portion of the patient to permit maximum diffusion and time contact with the cytotoxic agent. If the capsule of the ovary is intact, cobalt radiation treatment is of little value. Even when the cancer has extended throughout the pelvis or to distant organs, it is advisable, whenever feasible, to excise the great bulk of the primary tumor and omentum because the procedure may result in good palliation or even temporary regression of implants at distant sites. Follow-up cobalt radiation to the pelvis and abdomen (moving strip) is worthwhile. Satisfactory palliation may also be achieved in certain patients with chemotherapeutic agents such as the alkylating agents (nitrogen mustards, chlorambucil, etc.).

Surgical treatment for ovarian carcinoma stage I, is a satisfactory approach but the 5 year survival is only about 65 per cent (range 50 to 80 per cent). Adding external irradiation does not result in any substantial improvement in that figure. These early cases often have paraaortic node metastasis (approximately one case in five). Therefore, pelvic irradiation alone would not be expected to improve salvage. The use of radioactive gold or chromic phosphate should probably be restricted to protective therapies in stage I disease when there is no gross intraabdominal spread, but the malignant tumor has ruptured or peritoneal washings are positive. The significantly improved salvage rates (90 to 95 per cent) seem to validate the value of this type of supportive therapy. Irradiation therapy in patients with spread to pelvic organs (stage II) seems to improve survival (30 to 70 per cent) but the problem of paraaortic and subdiaphragmatic spread restricts the value of this modality since the liver and kidneys can tolerate doses usually not considered to be cancericidal (about 2500 roentgens).

Unfortunately, ovarian malignancies are usually nonresectable when they are first recognized. They disseminate early and the extent of spread calls for reliance upon surgery to "debulk" the tumor to the smallest volume possible prior to appropriate chemo-

therapy. In contrast with the endometrium (under 9 per cent) and the cervix (about 12 to 13 per cent), there are distant lesions in ovarian carcinoma at the time of diagnosis in about two-thirds of the cases. Single agent therapy with melphalan or chlorambucil will offer a favorable tumor response for 12 to 18 months in two-thirds or more of the cases (except in poorly differentiated tumors). Cyclophosphamide and thiotepa have been effective as well in perhaps 50 to 60 per cent of the cases. Nonresponsive patients should be offered combination chemotherapy consisting of actinomycin-D, 5-fluorouracil, and cyclophosphamide, given in daily regimes for 5 days repeated every 4 weeks unless toxic effects justify delay or discontinuation. The possibility of cardiomyopathy leading to heart failure calls for a limit on the total dosage of doxorubicin (approximately 550 mg./m^2 body surface). Hexamethylmelamine and cis-platinum are drugs not yet fully evaluated for use in cases not responding to conventional therapies, and more clinical trials are needed.

Nearly all patients today receive surgical therapy to reduce the bulk of tumor to the smallest volume possible so that the maximum effectiveness of adjuvant chemotherapy can be realized. After about 12 courses of chemotherapy the patient can be evaluated for discontinuation of the drug or for possible modification if residual disease is present. Accordingly, a "second look" exploratory laparotomy may be useful to inspect, palpate and biopsy suspicious lesions and/or nodes in the pelvis and abdomen.

The management of advanced ovarian malignancy is very complicated. Bowel obstruction is a particular problem and the risk of fistula formation may call for a paliative a bypass procedure to accomplish an ileotransverse colon side-to-side anastamosis. Occasionally, diverting ileostomy or colostomy, nasogastric and enteric decompression, fluid administration, paracenteses, thoracocenteses, hyperalimentation and pam control may present complex management problems in addition to the requirement to provide the necessary emotional support.

The 5-year survival rate for all cases of ovarian cancer probably does not exceed 25 to 30 per cent. For this reason, the emphasis should be on a high index of suspicion, early diagnosis and prompt surgical intervention. Persistent masses of more than 5 or 6 cm. in size in the region of the ovary, particularly if there are solid components, should arouse the suspicion of malignancy until proved to be benign. Inspection of the pelvis via the laparoscope eliminate is helpful in establishing the diagnosis. In addition, cul-de-sac asperation and cell block studies, as well as a careful examination under anesthesia, may be required. All women over 30 years of age should have periodic pelvic examinations every 6 to 12 months and, at the same time, should have a cytologic examination of the vaginal posterior forniceal pool.

REMOTE EFFECTS OF THE INJURIES OF CHILDBIRTH AND GYNECOLOGIC THERAPY

Although insufficiency of the pelvic floor may arise from pelvic and vaginal surgery or on a congenital basis, the great majority of such defects result from the injuries of childbirth. These defects are accentuated in the postmenopausal era when poor estrogen support of the tissues gives rise to pelvic insufficiency of muscles and fascia. The specific defects may be classified on an anatomic basis as follows:

I. Injuries to the levator sling (disruption of endopelvic fascial layer in the rectovaginal septum)
   1. Rectocele (most common—bearingdown sensation, constipation—requires manual expression of fecal material in rectal pouch
   2. Enterocele—herniation of peritoneum between unterosacral ligaments into the rectovaginal septum
II. Injuries to the anterior vaginal wall (vesicovaginal septum is stretched or torn)
   1. Urethrocele—stress urinary incontinence and disappearance of the posterior angle between the posterior surface of the urethra and the bladder base
   2. Cystocele—protrusion of bladder downward into the vaginal canal; stasis and infection of urine, pressure symptoms
III. Injuries involving uterine support (injury or stretching of the cardinal ligaments)
   1. Descensus or prolapse of the uterus—pressure, decubitus ulcer of cervix with bleeding
      A. First degree—The cervix lies between the level of the ischial spines and the vaginal introitus.
      B. Second degree—The cervix protrudes through the introitus while the corpus remains in the vagina.
      C. Third degree—The cervix and the body of the uterus have passed through the introitus, and the vaginal canal is inverted.
   2. Retrodisplacement of the uterus—possibly backache, dyspareunia, rectal complaints, especially if fixed and enlarged
      A. Retroflexion—The body of the uterus lies posteriorly while the cervix retains its usual position in the vagina; the body is flexed posteriorly in the region of the isthmus.
      B. Retroverted—The fundus rotates posteriorly and the cervix anteriorly, maintaining a normal axis.
      C. Retrocession—The entire uterus has sagged backward into the posterior pelvis
IV. Genital fistulas (trauma of operations, pressure necrosis in prolonged labor, trauma in childbirth or extension of malignant disease)
   1. Urinary tract fistulas—vesicovaginal, vesicocervical or vesicouterine
      A. Vesicovaginal—most common type of fistula. They most often follow hysterectomy or extension of cancer from cervix and elsewhere. Injuries of childbirth are no longer a common cause. Frequently follows therapeutic radiation.
      B. Ureterovaginal—more frequent in recent years because of increased use of radical surgery
   2. Rectovaginal fistulas—rectal injury in childbirth, extension of cervical cancer, radiation necrosis
V. Injuries to the cervix uteri (lacerations, eversion, ectopion, erosion, chronic cervicitis, chronic discharge per vaginum; possible antecedent for cervical malignant disease)
VI. Injuries to pelvic joints
   1. Separation of the symphysis pubis—pain on locomotion
   2. Dislocation of coccyx—soreness and tenderness

The concept of the role of the levator muscles and the importance of providing a smaller aperture with an adequate obturator form the basis of modern vaginal surgery. It should be borne in mind that the great majority of multiparous women have some degree of relaxation of the pelvic floor; however, only a small percentage are symptomatic and require special gynecologic attention. Moreover, presenting symptoms must not be attributed to an obvious anatomic defect until other conditions have been excluded. For example, urinary incontinence, even in the presence of an obvious urethrocele, may be due to intrinsic or extrinsic bladder or pelvic conditions or even to a neurologic or emotional disturbance. Thus, a careful work-up is required, usually including cystoscopic, cystographic and cystometric studies, complete urinalysis and cultures or, occasionally, upper urinary tract studies.

In patients with stress incontinence, the vesical neck

assumes the most dependent portion of the bladder and becomes the point of maximal impact transmitted from the dome to the base. In the standing position the downward angulation of the proximal urethra in relation to the vertical is also increased beyond the usual 30 degrees or less if the defect is advanced (angle of inclination). Thus the proximal urethra is usually wide in diameter, funnel in shape and poorly contractile. When scarring is likewise present, there may be an additional loss of mobility, motility and elasticity, and loss of sphincteric action since the elevated intra urethral tone relative to the bladder is diminished. In the presence of bladder infection, there is an increase in detrusor irritability, and urge incontinence develops as well as stress incontinence.

It should be borne in mind that urgency and urge incontinence are symptomatic hallmarks of urinary tract infection, and associated factors are obstruction, neurologic disease, congenital malformations, tumors, polyps and drug therapy. Posturinary dribbling suggests expression of urine from a urethral diverticulum, although this symptom may also be a sign of urethral stricture. Weakness of detrusor action, or obstruction of the outflow of the urethra, or combinations of the two may be responsible for urinary retention and overdistention of the bladder, so-called overflow incontinence, which may be caused by a variety of abnormalities. Neurogenous chronic overdistention and retention must never be overlooked as classic causes of incontinence. Diabetic neuronitis is becoming a frequent and important cause of difficulty. Thus, it is apparent that in no other disorder of the genitourinary tract are the medical history and general as well as pelvic examination more important.

There is no single therapeutic approach to the management of patients with pelvic floor insufficiency. Some will respond to reassurance and perineal exercises. The use of a pessary for such conditions as retrodisplacement of the uterus, urinary incontinence and uterine prolapse must be considered palliative rather than a definitive plan of management except, perhaps, in elderly women who are not candidates for surgery. Most of the specific anatomic defects occur in combination, so that the surgeon usually has more than a single objective in reconstructing the pelvic floor. Moreover, the proper selection of surgical management in cases of pelvic insufficiency will depend on the age and the general condition of the patient, the desirability of preserving menstruation and childbearing function, the degree of descensus uteri, the condition of the uterus (including the cervix), the presence and the degree of cystocele and urethrocele, the presence and the degree of rectocele or enterocele, previous vaginal surgery and, above all, the presence and the duration of distressing symptoms. The symptoms do not always parallel the degree of pelvic relaxation.

Urinary loss that is potentially amenable to a successful reparative surgical effort must have strictly an anatomic basis. Urine is lost only in relation to stress or positional changes. Normal bladder function is present after involuntary losses. The patient is comfortable with voiding; there is no dribbling or bed wetting; the problem is gravitational, not associated with urgency and frequency. Most of all, the condition is a social problem about which the patient is concerned.

Checking the patient in the lithotomy and erect positions gives a fairly accurate comparison of the degree of severity of urinary incontinence. Elevation of the urethrovesical junction to a high retropubic position is a maneuver common to most of the tests devised to inhibit the loss of urine after water instillation, i.e., the Bonney test, two fingers; the Marchetti test, two Allis forceps applied to the vesical neck region of the vaginal mucosa in an area previously anesthetized; and the Read test, two rubber-covered clamps applied to the same region.

Determination of bladder capacity, caloric and tactile sensations, residual urine, cystometry and direct observation of the anatomy and the functional relationships through urethrocystoscopy and essential preoperative investigations. In studying the urethra and the urethrovesical relationships, the metallic bead chain permits accurate visualization of the essential structures and demonstration of their position, shape and mobility. The length of the urethra is measured with a special catheter, and the caliber measured with an olive-tipped bougie. In addition, x-ray cineurography is a helpful technique that makes it possible to study normal and abnormal structure and function of the bladder, the bladder neck and the urethra.

Sophisticated tests are now available for selecting patients who are surgical candidates and those who are best approached medically. It is essential to exclude neurological diseases and unstable bladder problems in identifying potentially correctable conditions. The appropriate workup includes tests associated with the cystometric examination. Important among these evaluations are the exteroceptive sensation tests demonstrating an intactness of touch and temperature perceptions as well as a rapid anal sphincter response to a pinprick of the bulbocavernosus muscle which indicates a proper functioning pudendal nerve parasympathetic motor pathway. Another evaluative technic is based on the fact that neurogenic bladders have a normal smooth muscle stretch reflex in response to instillation of 100 ml. of water at a flow rate of 60 ml. per minute (rise of 5 to 18 cm. of water). However, when urecholine is administered in small doses (2.5

mg., subcutaneously), bladder hypersensitivity at the neuromuscular junction and ganglionic synapse results in pressure responses of 15 cm. of water or more over control values. If there is a neurologic defect in all types of major disorders (e.g., cortico-regulatory tract, sensory limb of the lower reflex arc, motor limb of the segmental reflex arc), or any combination of the three, absence of sensation in the saddle area is noted in all neurogenic bladders except the uninhibited type (CNS damage). The neurogenic bladder may be the only sign of a neurologic deficit. Lesions above the micturitional reflex center at the sacral cord level of S_2, S_3 and S_4 gives rise to uninhibited neurogenic bladder (higher centers, multiple sclerosis, tumor, etc.), or reflex neurogenic bladder (upper motor neuron cord lesion associated with high cervical disease or syringomyelia). Lesions occurring below the micturitional reflex center may be motor paralytic (anterior horn cells; multiple sclerosis or Guillain-Barré syndrome); sensory neurogenic bladder (tabes dorsalis or diabetes mellitus); or autonomous neurogenic bladder (disc, tumor, meningomyelocele, trauma, etc.). Reflex neurogenic bladder and uninhibited neurogenic bladder have small bladder capacity and uninhibited contractions, whereas sacral lesions lead to a flaccid bladder and overflow incontinence.

Electromyography of the periurethral tissues shows that urinary continence is associated with surface continuity of the urinary tract, proper pressure gradient between the urethra and bladder favoring the former, and normal detrusor muscle activity. Motor unit firing increases progressively until bladder capacity is reached. When the normal patient either thinks of urination or actually performs the act, the motor impulses to the urogenital diaphragm abruptly stop. Normally, no uninhibited voiding contractions are noted in the bladder during filling in the cystometric evaluations or at capacity when the patient is in discomfort. There is no abnormal detrusor hyperactivity or involuntary contraction in response to coughing, heel bouncing, or percussing the bladder as it is filled. When these reactions are present, the bladder is usually unstable (dyssynergic) and the patient experiences a false type of stress urinary incontinence in which losses occur in response to detrusor contractions coming on after a slight delay following the stimulus (coughing, sneezing, laughing, changing positions, running, and walking). Once the urinary stream is provoked in relation to urgency and frequency, there may be an urgency incontinence that is not controllable by will. Classically, organically based stress urinary incontinence is associated with a measure of control in which the urinary stream can be stopped in the process of voiding. The patient with the unstable bladder loses urine in

large volumes, in contrast with small instantaneous leakages in immediate response to intraabdominal pressures in anatomically based problems. The unstable bladder is quiescent at night, but women losing urine on a gravitational basis will also not experience enuresis except possibly in changing positions in bed rather abruptly.

Carbon dioxide urethroscopy is quite important in assessing the sphincteric urethral segment, particularly in recurrent incontinent cases. Opening pressures of the sphincteric urethra may be low (25 to 50 cm. of water). Closures of the segment may be sluggish, asymmetric, and incomplete in the presence of marked periurethral scarring. These cases usually represent problems of loss of sphincteric urethra, which may give rise to considerable urinary incontinence, despite a retropubic anatomic position. Often, these patients will require a combined transvaginal and retropubic operative approach to break up the adhesive bands and to mobilize the vesical neck. It is important to individualize the workup and to select potential operative candidates very carefully.

It is estimated that about 10 per cent of patients with urinary incontinence have an unstable bladder; in about one-half of these, there will be an anatomic defect in addition. A bolus of urine sitting in a funneled dependent proximal urethra will often trigger detrusor hyperirritability and give rise to an urgency-frequency-urgency incontinence syndrome. These few patients represent exceptions to the rule that anatomically based urinary incontinence of the true stress type have a normal voiding pattern. Another exception is the patient who has a cystocele, urinary retention and infection in addition to a dependent vesical neck. Here, too, urgency, frequency, and even dysuria may be overriding symptoms.

Every effort should be exerted to make the initial surgical procedure the definitive one, for the likelihood of success is never again as good. It is unacceptable to insist on a single operative approach and to try to make every patient adapt to a stereotyped problem of management. The traditional failure rate of 15 to 20 per cent with the intitial operation emphasizes this lack of individualization of symptomatic cases.

Urinary stress incontinence usually can be corrected satisfactorily by plicating the pubovesicocervical fascia and the internal vesical sphincter (Kelly or Kennedy operation). If there is also relaxation of the vaginal and rectal walls, the procedure is ordinarily combined in one procedure as an anterior and posterior colporrhaphy. Likewise, the cervix may be amputated, and the cardinal ligaments plicated onto the anterior stump if the cervix is elongated (Manchester operation); however, this approach does not enjoy much favor as a procedure of choice in this country. When there is a significant degree of uterine prolapse, it is usually better to perform a vaginal hysterectomy. The Spalding-Richardson composite operation in which the cervical isthmus is spared and used in the reconstruction to gain better pelvic support is rarely used today. In certain elderly women, it is possible to do a simple colpocleisis (Le Fort operation) to correct uterine prolapse. When the patient's principal difficulty is descensus of the vesical neck and stress urinary incontinence, a retropubic urethral suspension (Marshall-Marchetti-Krantz operation) may be the approach. When the periurethral tissues (pubourethral ligaments) are sutured into the Cooper's ligament (Burch technique) there is a danger of overangulation of the urethrovesical angle and possibly of enterocele formation. The traditional Marshall-Marchetti-Krantz procedure calls for the suspensory sutures to be placed in the pubic periosteum. These tissues may be friable and highly vascular, tear out easily, or cause symptomatic periostitis. It is particularly advantageous when the adbomen needs to be entered for some benign pelvic condition. When a previous repair has failed, one may use a fascial sling to provide a suspensory support to the urethra, thereby producing the necessary acute angulation of the urethra at the vesical neck (Goebell-Stoeckel operation and its Aldridge and Studdiford modifications). After complete mobilization of the urethra and paraurethral tissues, monofilament, nonabsorbable sutures can be placed by a special instrument to suspend the urethrovesical junction retropubically by exposing the spaces of Retzius transvaginally (revised Pereyra procedure). The short, heavy-boned, obese woman or one whose condition is complicated by chronic coughing or sneezing may be handled best by a combined incontinence operation performed as the primary procedure. Likewise, it may often be the operation of choice in recurrent cases. This operation combines an anterior colporrhaphy with a suprapubic ventral urethrovesical suspension after complete mobilization of the urethrovesical segment. In addition, after all periurethral adhesions are lysed, the urethral fascia is pleated from above as well as below to eliminate funneling in the proximal portion and to lengthen the organ.

If the bladder descends appreciably below the lowest margin of the symphysis during the effort of straining (more than 4 cm.) or if there is considerable scarring and fixation of periurethral tissues, the retropubic ventral suspension operation must be combined with an anterior colporrhaphy if a high success rate is to be anticipated. To be successful, the urethra must be of normal tonicity, it must be well supported and yet be free to move and contract normally, and the proximal urethra must be located in front of the main target point in the transmission of the force in intraabdominal pressure from the dome to the base of the bladder where pressures as high as 75 mm. Hg or more may occur during times of abrupt stress.

In the last analysis, the best treatment is prophylaxis by providing good antepartal care (adequate nutrition), good intrapartal care (conservative obstetrics, prophylactic forceps and episiotomy) and good postpartal care (bladder care, prompt treatment of lacerations, infections, etc., and perineal exercises). Perineal exercises may be of value either as an effective means of correcting mild stress incontinence in patients with slight anatomic defects or as preoperative or postoperative supportive measures in surgical cases and after childbirth.

Urinary Tract Injuries

Urinary tract obstructions, fistulization and extravasations involving the urethra, bladder and/or ureter may be serious complications of gynecologic disease, childbirth and therapeutic intervention. There may be extensions of destructive granulomatous or cancerous lesions, irradiation damage, or direct tissue injuries sustained in the course of instrumentations and various operative procedures performed on genital tract organs in the immediate vicinity of urinary structures. Strangulations and tissue necrosis with slough following misplaced ligatures, acute angulations, and crushing injuries produce fistulae and extravasation of urine with tracts communicating between affected organs and structures. The direction of urine drainage may be external, intraperitoneal or retroperitoneal, depending upon the nature and site of injury. The various types of fistulae are designated on the basis of the affected organs between which there are communicating tracts, e.g., urethrovaginal; vesicovaginal, or ureterovaginal, occurring singly or in combination. Usually, gynecological surgery involving hysterectomy is the etiological factor in most fistulae found in the terminal ureters or bladder. Resection of a suburethral diverticulum, anterior colporrhaphy, and certain urologic procedures are more likely to give rise to urethrovaginal fistulae. The ureters may be damaged in the course of eradicating pelvic disease associated with massive adhesions (pelvic inflammatory disease or endometriosis), when the ureter is displaced (broad ligament cyst or leiomyoma), or by devascularizing it in the course of stripping it out of its bed in the process of pelvic lymphadenectomy and radical hysterectomy for malignant disease. Extensive bladder adhesions following prior low cervical cesarean sections can make mobilizations for a repeat cesarean birth or hysterectomy a risky undertaking. Postpartal urinary fistulae arise from prolonged labor resulting in ischemic necrosis from extreme continued pressure of the presenting part or, possibly, from a traumatic instrumentation. In modern obstetrics these causes are rare (less than 0.1 per cent of deliveries) although bladder injury in the course of repeat cesarian births remains a potential problem. Rarely, in the course of various pelvic operations there may be multiple injuries involving the bowel (uretero- or vesicoenteric or rectal fistula), uterus (uretero- or vesicouterine or cervical fistula), and free abdominal cavity (uretero- or vesicoperitoneal fistula).

The site or sites of damage, extent of injury, and the subsequent pattern of urinary drainage will determine the nature of symptoms and signs, therapeutic approach, and prognosis. The timing of the problem is also affected by the etiology, since unrecognized structural defects produced at operation may give rise to urinary leakage through the vagina, wound, or abdominal drain site almost immediately. Intraperitoneal leakage may produce acute peritonitis and ileus. Severe colicky flank pain referred into the groin, costovertebral angle (CVA), flank tenderness, and fever suggest ureteral injury with obstruction. When urinary leakage is delayed until 10 to 28 days postoperatively, progressive ischemic necrosis and tissue slough secondary to ligature or crushing injury are a likely possibility.

Proper management must be based on an appropriate urologic investigation to determine the extent, nature, and cause of the urinary injury. A bladder instillation of methylene blue coupled with intravenous phenosulfonphthalein (PSP) administration is a useful method of distinguishing between a vesicovaginal fistula (blue drainage) and a uterovaginal fistula (red drainage). Excretory urography, cystourethroscopy, retrograde pyelography when a ureteral catheter can be passed, and radioscans as necessary are important diagnostic methods. The possibility of multiple injuries must be considered which may call for uterine, bowel and other studies. Prompt diagnosis is required to prevent as array of potentially lethal complications including obstructive uropathy, hydronephrosis, perirenal or psoas abscess, peritonitis, thrombophlebitis, anuria and uremia.

Emergency treatments may consist of measures to combat shock, blood loss and dehydration, and to relieve acute urinary obstruction by an appropriate drainage method (catheter, gall-bladder, T tube in the ureter, nephrostomy, etc.). A vesicoperitoneal fistula with a deteriorating clinical situation necessitates an immediate laparotomy to stop the intraabdominal leakage. Otherwise, fistula repairs should be delayed until all the necrotic and inflamed tissues have resolved to create a clean epithelialized tract. This waiting period may require 4 to 6 months, although some time may be conserved by administering cortisone to accelerate the healing process. The great majority of the vesicovaginal fistulas can be successfully closed transvaginally by partial colpocleisis. Severe scarring, poor blood supply, and large defects may require using adjacent muscle tissues with their independent blood supply in the repair when the potential for healing is in doubt. A concomitant ureteral injury would require a combined abdominal-vaginal approach. Severely damaged or severed terminal ureters are best treated by excising the diseased segment and reimplanting the healthy proximal end into the bladder (ureteroneocystostomy). A splinting catheter can be used for 10 to 14 days.

The best treatment obviously is one of prevention. In the better medical centers in the United States, the incidence of urinary tract injuries on gynecological services should be less than 1.0 per cent following major gynecologic surgery. Modern technics to protect or augment ureteral blood supply in the course of radical hysterectomy and to suspend the ureter to remove it from a pool of extravasation have reduced fistulization from about 10 to 15 per cent down to less than 4.0 per cent in a number of studies. There should be no hesitancy to isolate or catheterize the ureters as a preliminary to difficult pelvic dissections, to inject dye into the bladder during or after the procedure before the abdomen is closed, or even to open the bladder to identify its margins in the "frozen" pelvis. If prevention of tissue injury is not possible, the best reparative results are at the time of damage in context with the initial operation. Subsequently, the decisive postoperative variable in success of repair is timing because no effort by any technic will be successful in diseased tissues. Rarely, small fistulae will heal in time and some will respond to local therapies. However, for the most part, the approach is surgical with anticipated successful results in the 90 per cent range for the initial effort.

GYNECOLOGIC ENDOCRINOPATHIES

Disorders of Menstruation

Irregular or excessive bleeding from the uterus is one of the most common symptoms that the gynecologist is called upon to treat. Abnormal bleeding may manifest itself by profuse, prolonged or too frequent periodic flow or by bleeding between periods. Menstrual disorders may be classified as follows (Fluhmann):

    I. Ovulatory cycles
        A. Disorders of incidence of menstruation
            1. Polymenorrhea—intervals are short.
            2. Oligomenorrhea—intervals are lengthened.

3. Amenorrhea
   a. Primary—Patient has never menstruated, and diagnosis is not made before age 18.
   b. Secondary—cessation of menses for 3 months or longer
   c. Physiologic—before puberty (or age 18), during pregnancy or lactation, after menopause
   d. Cryptomenorrhea—mechanical obstruction to the egress of uterine flow
   e. Uterine origin—good ovarian function but uterus does not respond
   f. Functional—general or local disturbance holds menses in abeyance.

B. Disorders in amount of menstrual flow
   1. Hypomenorrhea—scanty menstrual flow
   2. Hypermenorrhea—profuse or prolonged flow (menorrhagia); also, there may be a disturbance in the functioning of the corpus luteum with irregular shedding of the endometrium and prolonged flow.

C. Periodic intermenstrual bleeding—ovulatory bleeding

II. Anovulatory uterine bleeding
A. Anovulation (cyclic or irregular)—This is the most important single cause of abnormal bleeding in the absence of demonstrable pelvic lesions. Anovulatory periods are common at the time of puberty and during the climacterium, although they may occur from a variety of causes at any time during menstrual life. The atypical character of the uterine mucosa may be brought about by the prolonged action of moderate amounts of estrogen over a long time, or it may result from relatively short periods of hyperestrinism.

B. Hyperplasia of the endometrium (adenomatous pattern or Swiss-cheese type, typical or atypical)—In menopausal or postmenopausal women, atypical lesions may be noted that frequently predispose or coexist with adenocarcinoma.

C. Arrhythmic uterine bleeding (metrorrhagia)—The bleeding may be continuous (starting at the time of the expected menses), acyclic interval hemorrhage, intermenstrual spotting, bleeding after amenorrhea or atypical irregular hemorrhage. This bleeding may be due to a variety of local and systemic conditions, but, in all cases, cancer must be excluded. This type of abnormal bleeding occurs in more than one fourth of all nonpregnant women of childbearing age who seek treatment for a bleeding disorder. It is estimated that about 40 per cent of patients over 40 years of age have some uterine or pelvic pathology that may contribute to the symptom of abnormal uterine bleeding. The common causes of arrhythmic bleeding are carcinoma of the cervix, myoma uteri, endometrial hyperplasia, pelvic inflammatory disease, cervicitis, cervical or endometrial polyps, fundal cancer, systemic diseases and a small, miscellaneous groups of unknown etiology. Thus, a thorough uterine curettage is imperative in these cases to exclude cancer as a diagnostic consideration.

Since most abnormal bleeding is due to either organic causes or complications of pregnancy, these possibilities must be excluded. Many other cases are ascribable to psychogenic causes or no definite cause can be detected. Thus, it is a serious error to assume immediately that the cause is a disturbance of ovarian endocrine mechanisms without subjecting the patient to careful study. Moreover, an obvious ovarian dysfunction may be due to a primary defect or to some pathologic lesion, or it may be secondary to malfunction of other endocrine glands, notably the pituitary, the thyroid and the adrenals.

Menstruation: Regulation and Dysfunction

At the onset of puberty, the germ cell mass in the ovary has been reduced to about 300,000 units, which is a relatively small residuum from the 6 to 7 million endowment by the 20th week of fetal life and 1 to 2 million cortical germ cells at birth. The ovary is fully capable of an adult response before puberty, but these normal functions do not occur until there is a diminished sensitivity of the hypothalamic centers to a negative inhibitory feedback of gonadal steroids. When this sensitivity is gradually lost after about age eight, the gonadotrophin secretion increases, promoting estrogen production as the follicular units mature. The usual sequence of events are a growth spurt, breast development (thelarche), pubarche (sexual hair growth), and menarche which occurs between the ages of 10.5 and 15.5 years (mean of 12.6 years in the United States). The actual age is puberty and onset of menses are conditioned by genetic factors, socioeconomic conditions, nutrition, and general health. There will, therefore, be variation in the time and sequence of these events. In addition, there may be precocious pseudopuberty in a small number of cases caused by hormones arising from sources other than the normal gonads, e.g., hypothyroid disorder, adrenal adenoma, ovarian estrogen-producing tumor, choriocarcinoma (gonadotropin-producing lesions), or cerebral neoplasm, trauma, or infection. In the true form of puberty arising from estrogens elaborated by the ovaries, there is a sequence of progressive events characterized not only by formation and maintenance of secondary sexual characteristics, but also by biological events representing certain tissue changes in response to endogenous estrogen, e.g., cervical mucus, vaginal cornification, and proliferative endometrium. During the first year or 18 months after the menarche, uterine bleeding episodes are likely to be heavy and irregular since they represent merely the estrogen withdrawal responses of the endometrium. Finally, the definitive developmental response occurs; it is represented by the appearance of a positive feedback estrogenic mechanism on the hypothalamus. At this level of maturity in the hypothalamic-pituitary-gonadal axis, true menstrual function occurs by the creation of a cyclic LH surge and ovulation, which ends the so-called period of "adolescent sterility" and disordered bleeding pattern. Elaboration of progesterone resulting from ovulation and development of the corpus luteum has the effect of growth limitation on the endometrium. The corpus luteum has a normal life span of about 12 to 14 days, and during that time the structure secretes both estrogens and progesterone. In the absence of pregnancy, these hormones decline as the corpus luteum degenerates and menses follows as a consequence of universal, orderly and progressive events occurring in the endometrium. In response to rhythmic waves of vasoconstriction of increasing duration, there is widespread ischemia, disintegration and slough of the endometrium.

This recycling mechanism associated with normal menstrual physiology is dependent, therefore, upon the ability of gonadal steroids to evoke in the hypothalamus a negative feedback to promote gonadotropin (FSH/LH) secretion and a positive feedback to release LH-releasing factor (LHRH) to create the subsequent cyclic LH plus FSH peaks necessary for ovulation. The tonic LHRH center lies in the median eminence of the hypothalamus and the cyclic positive feedback hypothalamic center is located in the preoptic area. The ovaries must be responsive to the gonadotropins, and in turn the steroids elaborated must be able to affect the proper cyclic changes in the endometrium associated with preparation for egg implantation. Thus, any defect or disturbance of function arising in the hypothalamus, pituitary, ovaries, uterus, or extragonadal hormonal disorders involving the thyroid or adrenal glands, may lead to abnormal menses. The disordered pattern may vary from frequent heavy periods (polymenorrhea with hypermenorrhea) to infrequent light periods or absence of menses (oligomenorrhea with hypomenorrhea, or amenor-

rhea). These dysfunctions often associated with chronic anovulation are more prevalent at either end of the reproductive era, although they do occur at various times during adult menstrual life. In addition to the factors previously noted, a number of nonspecific causes may be found that include significant swings in weight, anemia, emotional stress, and the ill effects of certain drugs sometimes found in association with galactorrhea (tranquilizers, antidepressants, methyldopa, reserpine, and others).

In the face of a mature hypothalamic-pituitary-ovarian axis, chronic anovulation is often found in association with two major types of pathophysiologic disturbances, regardless of the specific underlying defect. On the one hand, the estradiol signal to the hypothalamus may be inadequate to evoke the LH surge through a positive feedback mechanism. On the other hand, estrogen levels may not fall sufficiently to achieve the proper FSH response for ovarian follicular stimulation. In context with these defects, postpubertal girls may remain anovulatory because of lack of a mature mechanism achieving ovulation through the positive feedback; and, in the premenopausal woman, the disturbance may have its genesis in the lack of ovarian follicles to secrete sufficient estrogen to provoke an LH surge. Impaired metabolism and clearance of estradiol (hepatic disease, hypothyroidism, etc.) may not permit the proper nadir in steroid levels to occur. There may be extragonadal peripheral conversion of C-19 precursors, such as androstenedione, which are capable of producing both estrone and testosterone. Obesity associated with a considerable amount of androstenedione conversion in adipose tissue or stress resulting in increased adrenal contribution of estrogenic precursor can sustain the blood level of estrogen at a time when decline is necessary for recyclicing and negative feedback on the FSH.

A state of chronic anovulation results in a tonic rather than a cyclic condition in which the constantly slightly elevated levels of estrogen bring about static, somewhat elevated LH and lowered FSH. The follicular apparatus in the ovary is stimulated continuously but not sufficiently to achieve the proper growth and maturation. Multiple follicle cysts at various stages of development and dense stromal tissues derived from atretic follicles tend to perpetuate the problem of chronic anovulation by producing androstenedion, which is continuously converted into estrone in the peripheral tissues. The resultant perpetuation of follicles in all stages of development and atresia, dense functional stroma and the grossly thickened tunica albuginea, represent the features of the classic polycystic ovaries. The pathophysiological features found in association with the chronic anovulation may be various patterns of abnormal menses ranging from irregular heavy periods in more than one-quarter and oligoamenorrhea in more than one-half of these patients. These patients are usually obese and more than two-thirds have some degree of hirsutism, although only one-third or less will be overly virilized. These basic problems of anovulatory dysfunction in association with abnormal bleeding, infertility and possibly hirsutism may arise from a variety of causes including gonadal as well as extragonadal but the common denominator is a steady state of asynchronous gonadotropin and estrogen production. This problem is quite different from hypergonadatropic hypogonadism (ovarian failure) or hypogonadotropic hypogonadism (central failure). Markedly high or significantly low serum gonadotropin levels and clinical or genetic stigmata characterize these latter conditions. For example, gonadal dysgenesis gives rise to high serum gonadotropin levels because of lack of follicular tissue on a genetic basis.

Chronic anovulation causes breakthrough bleeding from a faulty endometrium. Usually the endometrium is overgrown and the glandularity and vascularity outstrips the stromal support matrix. The fragile tissues break down in a random fashion and healing can only be temporary because the orderly physiologic process of rhythmical vasoconstriction and stasis does not occur. The bleeding may be acyclic, highly irregular and very heavy at times. There may be periods of amenorrhea followed by profuse bleeding and possibly cramps. In younger women, these disturbances arouse the suspicion of incomplete abortion, endometrial polyp, or submucous myoma. Chronic anovulation gives rise to endometrial hyperplasia and to adenocarcinoma even at an early age in the susceptible person who is subjected to long term unopposed estrogen stimulation. Adequate study of endometrial tissues is mandatory to exclude malignancy in such women above the age of 35.

Another pattern of menstrual disturbance associated with intermittent light bleeding of variable duration results from an unfavorably high ratio of progesterone to estrogen (progestin therapy or low dose estrogen therapy as in prolonged use of oral contraceptives). The lack of a proper tissue base for endometrial growth, structural support, stability, and healing calls for estrogens to promote hemostasis. Usually, high-dose estrogen therapy is so effective in correcting all types of dysfunctional bleeding that a failed response in 24 hours should arouse the suspicion of an underlying cause, e.g., polyp, placental fragments, blood dyscrasia, tumor, malignancy, etc. Administrations of estrogens in high doses should be considered as temporary therapy to be used only in the initial control of profuse bleeding. A critical issue in determining the approach pertains to the amount of endometrium present. In cases of longstanding bleeding there may be little endometrium and responses to progesterone or even progestin-estrogen combinations may not be effective in these exhausted tissues without proper preliminary estrogenic support. Similarly, a thorough curettage of the uterus will not solve the problem since it does nothing to correct the underlying pathophysiology unless there is organic disease. Moreover, one may produce synechiae (fibrous adhesions) in the uterus that could cause secondary amenorrhea (Asherman's syndrome).

Among the most important aspects of management is the patient's history. It is best to judge the normality or abnormality of the menstrual pattern based on the patient's own past menstrual history. A normal female can have normal ovulatory menses at intervals of several months; a change to monthly cycles might be an indication of chronic anovulation. The presence or absence of molimenal symptoms may be an indication of ovulation or its disappearance. An attempt is made to discern any clinical stigmata or genetic fault that would be associated with abnormal menses. Check for evidence of malnutrition, psychological stress, systemic illness, gynecological disease, or endocrinopathy. Sometimes, the symptoms are subtle and the menstrual disorder may be the first or possibly only manifestation of a serious medical problem. Investigation of the diet and documentation of shifts in weight are necessary. A check for galactorrhea is required, and a careful pelvic examination should exclude organic pathology of the internal genitalia, or complications of pregnancy. Routine laboratory studies should exclude anemia, blood dyscrasia, liver impairment, metabolic disorders, and renal dysfunction. Thyroid tests are often obtained, as are adrenal studies if there is hirsutism. If there is galactorrhea in association with anovulation and/or infertility, serum prolactin levels and polytomograms of the sella turcica should be obtained to rule out the presence of a pituitary adenoma.

Luteal phase defects with premenstrual spotting in association with deficient corpus luteum may require thyroid and adrenal studies (acquired adrenogenital syndrome). After complete assessment, including plasma testosterone, luteinizing hormone, prolactin levels and, possibly, morning and evening cortisol determinations, patients with hirsutism may be suppressed in the hope of establishing a satisfactory treatment. Elevated plasma testosterone levels may be suppressed with estrogen/progesterone-containing compounds; failing in this, a dexamethasone suppression test is helpful in assessing the suitability of corticosteroid therapy. Depending on these results, it may be possible to reduce the growth rate and apparent size of the hair. Antiandrogens that prevent androgens from expressing their activity on target sites hold promise for the future.

Nearly all women with hirsutism have increased testosterone production rates, elevated free testesterone levels and increased testosterone metabolic rates. Many hirsute women (about 30 per cent) have increased androgen production from both the ovary and the adrenal; in some, hypothyroidism is present and when that problem is corrected, an associated adrenal or ovarian disorder associated with anovulation is corrected. When dehydroepiandrosterone and its sulfated compound are prominent secretory products, adrenal tumors are likely. Extremely high testosterone levels in the serum (above 500 ng. per 100 ml.) and when androgen levels are fixed or unresponsive to suppression or stimulation testing, there is the probability of adrenal adenomas or carcinomas. Further studies are required. The same is true of hirsutism in the presence of an unilaterally enlarged ovary (granulosa cell tumor or ovarian thecoma), when signs and symptoms of Cushing's syndrome are present with an abnormally elevated plasma cortisol after attempted suppression with dexamethasone, or failure to suppress elevated plasma testosterone with progestin therapy for 6 months (ovarian tumor is a possibility). In the latter cases, a laparoscopy or pelvic sonogram might be helpful.

When the bleeding is heavy and the hemoglobin falls below 10 mg. per dl. and requires replacement of blood volume, hospitalization may be required to achieve initial hemostasis. Depending upon the circumstances, high-dose estrogen therapy utilizing conjugated estrogens in 20 mg. increments administered intravenously every four hours will usually cause heavy bleeding to subside within 12 hours. Oral high dose progestin-estrogen combination pills can also be used in less dramatic problem cases for periods of 1 week. Failure of cessation or abatement of heavy blood flow calls for uterine curettage, even in the teenager, to rule out the possibility of organic uterine disease. In older women, this procedure should precede hormone therapy in most cases to rule out malignancy as a prerequisite in the management. Underlying factors are studied and treated as necessary while cyclic hormone therapy is continued through 3 to 6 cycles. Establishing or reestablishing ovulatory menses is a goal only in the young and in those who are desirous of childbearing. Oral medroxyprogesterone administered in 10 mg. doses on a cyclic basis on days 15 or 20 to day 25 of the cycle will prevent hyperplasia in refractory anovulatory cases.

When there has been no sexual development by the age of 14 or an absence of menarche by age 18, puberty is delayed and there must be a search for possible genetic faults or a hypothalamic-pituitary-ovarian axis disorder. The appropriateness of height and bone age and use of Bayley-Pinnean tables to predict future adult height are proper evaluative methods. If there is short stature, there must be a check for the usual causes: malnutrition, chronic infectious disease, gonadal dysgenesis and panhypopituitarism. There may be a familial history of growth tardiness with eventual normal stature. The average growth in height after the menarche is about 2.5 inches. In some individuals exhibiting menstrual dysfunction, there may be disturbances in sexual behavior, social adjustment, marital relations, and family status, which may require psychiatric assistance.

Overall, about two-thirds of patients exhibiting dysfunctional uterine bleeding are either pubertal or premenopausal; about 30 per cent of the cases occur during the childbearing years. The problem occurs in approximately 15 per cent of females and accounts for a great majority of the justifications for uterine curettages, in addition to many hysterectomies. However, the latter must not be a means of eliminating refractory bleeding in the absence of pathology unless conservative medical measures have been exhausted. The potential problems of dysfunctional uterine bleeding can be both immediate (shock), remote (consequences of operative procedures, shock or blood transfusion) and potentially dangerous over time (carcinogenesis of long term unopposed estrogens either endogenous or offered exogenously on a chronic basis). The overall goals in specific therapies include (1) control of the present bleeding episode; (2) establishment of normal cyclic bleeding pattern in the future; (3) reestablishment of ovulatory cycles in the young if possible or indicated; and (4) establishment of cyclic progestational endometrium for women desirous of childbearing and of having that potential restored. Radiation has no place today in provoking ovulation and its use to stop ovulation by causing ovarian atrophy has no clear place in modern therapy. Polycystic ovaries ordinarily require no definitive therapy—wedge resection or attempt to provoke ovulation unless childbearing is a goal, although regularization of the bleeding pattern and opposing the estrogen are worthwhile objectives.

In patients with amenorrhea, if bleeding can be induced by an injection of 50 or 100 mg. of progesterone, one may generally assume that the amenorrhea is not due to any serious derangement of the pituitary, the ovary or the uterus. However, if bleeding does not occur, the cause may be any one of the three. In this instance, if bleeding occurs after estrogen withdrawal (following 21 days of therapy), the cause is due either to ovarian or to pituitary dysfunction, provided that the thyroid and the adrenal glands are normal. If bleeding does not occur, the factor is nonresponsiveness of the uterus and can be demonstrated by endometrial biopsy (tuberculosis or synechiae). Serum gonadotropins will usually distinguish the ovarian and the pituitary factors; a high titer indicates deficient ovarian function (agenesis, aplasia or hypofunction), while absence of or a low titer indicates pituitary hypofunction. These assumptions are based on the fact that all other systemic and local factors have been proved to be normal by previous work-up. For example, when amenorrhea is merely one manifestation of a problem of defeminization or masculinization, the problem is much more complex. The basic problem may be pituitary (basophilic adenoma, Cushing's syndrome), adrenal (cortical hyperplasia, adenoma or carcinoma) or ovarian (arrhenoblastoma, adrenal tumor of the ovary, gynandroblastoma, hilus cell tumor or the Stein-Leventhal syndrome). Obviously, a much more extensive work-up is required, including an ACTH or cortisone test, and others.

Infertility

Approximately 10 to 15 per cent of married couples of childbearing age in the United States have difficulty in achieving a pregnancy. Infertility is defined as failure to conceive after one year of regular coitus without contraception, in contrast with sterility, which is total inability to conceive. About 80 per cent of normal couples are capable of achieving pregnancy within one year; however, after another 6 months that percentage will rise only to about 85 to 90 per cent. Thus, it is generally advisable to investigate couples for infertility after one year of unprotected coitus if childbearing is their interest. A workup can be conducted sooner if clinical stigmata or symptoms raise other therapeutic objectives. Fecundability, which denotes the probability of conception, is maximal at about age 24 in both the male and the female. Among infertile couples, modern investigative capabilities make it possible to identify one or more potential causes in about 90 per cent of the cases. Appropriate therapy incorporating current modalities, both medical and surgical, will succeed in achieving pregnancy for only about one-half of these. Infertility can be attributed to a male factor either as the definitive cause or one of the contributing causes in about 40 per cent of cases. Both partners possess antifertility factors in almost one-third of the couples. A significant minority of patients will conceive without therapy at some time during the workup (perhaps 35 per cent), perhaps because of alleviation of anxiety and other emotional problems. By the same token, the tedious workup, including various tests and proce-

dures to obtain specimens and requirements for the couple to perform on schedule, may remove the favorable effects of spontaneity in lovemaking or even result in impotence in the male. It may be possible to evaluate the true motivation of the partners under these circumstances and to sort out the various fears, guilt, ambivalences and misinformation. Proper counseling and attention paid to these psychological aspects by attempting to establish and maintain a proper relationship between the husband and wife are central issues in the overall management plan. It is essential for the husband to be present at the initial interview and after he and his wife are studied separately and as a couple, he must be a party to the management planning sessions. In addition to emotionally based issues, prognostic variables affecting therapeutic success are age, frequency and technique of coital exposure, duration of infertility, number and type of antifertility factors, past reproductive performance in secondary infertility, quality of care, and patient compliance.

The cornerstone of the infertility workup initially is a careful history and thorough physical examination of both partners. Although the investigative process should follow an orderly pattern, focusing first on the potential of a male factor, these basic evaluations may give immediate insights into potential etiologies and focus upon certain targets in formulating a management plan for either partner. Routine laboratory screening may direct attention to problems affecting the workup, therapy and prognosis, e.g., anemia, diabetes, cervical neoplasia, urinary or prostatic infection, syphilis, gonorrhea and other conditions. More specialized tests, including those for specific endocrine disorders, need to be performed when clinically indicated. A check for subclinical hypothyroidism, which is a common endocrine-related antifertility factor, may be part of the routine investigation (measurement of serum TSH).

A management program of basic studies includes the following evaluative tests and procedures:

1. Evaluation of semen (usually two or more specimens). Determine the number, motility, and morphology of the spermatozoa. Sperm counts below 10 million/ml., total sperm counts below 25 million per ejaculate, and normal motile sperm of less than 12.5 million per ejaculate are frequent findings in infertile men. In addition, there may be enzymatic and certain chemical derangements, including serum fructose, which is normally produced in the seminal vesicles. If it is not found in the semen, there may be a congenital absence of the duct system. Presence of autoagglutinating antibodies in the semen may give rise to clumping

of the spermatozoa, while poor motility may be an indication of autoimmobilizing antibodies. The latter defect is a more serious prognostic factor. Abnormal sperm morphology with tapering forms predominating and greatly reduced sperm motility may be associated with varicocele.

2. Postcoital test: This test is performed on about the 12th to 14th day of the menstrual cycle, which is the time of peak spontaneous cervical mucus flow. Normally, there is a clear watery mucus with tenaciousness or stretchability (spinnbarkeit) in response to an estrogen level peak which promotes sperm penetration. A proper test reflects on sperm production and transport, coital technique, quality of the sperm and their motility and the cervical transport. The worrisome features include thick, opaque, nontenacious mucus (inadequate estrogen stimulation or defective cervical glands), presence of pus (cervicovaginal or seminalurinary infection), absence of sperm (azoospermia, failure of male transport mechanisms, or faulty coital technique), and poor sperm motility, (oligospermia, faulty mucus representing a physical barrier to penetration, or immunological incompatibilities). Absence of sperm is seen in retrograde ejaculation (check urine for spermatozoa).

3. Tests of tubal patency: Tubal transport function can be tested by uterotubal CO_2 insufflation (Rubin's test), hysterosalpingogram, dye instillation and determination of peritoneal spillage under direct laparoscopic view. The hysterosalpingogram has the advantage of demonstrating both tubal patency and uterotubal morphology (distortions of diseases, tumors or anomalous development). Unfortunately, misinterpretations may occur in a significant minority of cases. Follow-up pelvic sonography, curettage, or hysteroscopy may clarify some of the diagnostic problems relating primarily to the uterus. Antifertility factors involving congenital defects (septum), pathologic entities (submucous myoma), endometrial adhesions, infectious processes (tuberculous endometritis), old placental polyp, foreign body (unsuspected IUD) and other conditions may be disclosed in these investigations. Some times after a hysterosalpingogram, filmy adhesions about the tubes will become disrupted and normal mobility is restored.

4. Test for ovulation: The standard methods to test for ovulation include the basal body temperature (thermogenic effect of progestin produces a biphasic curve), serum concentrations of progesterone during the midluteal phase of the cycle (expen-

sive), and the endometrial biopsy taken on day 21 to 23 of the cycle (date the endometrium for appropriate secretory changes indicative of ovulation and progestational development). In the event of anovulation, adequate tissue studies of the endometrium will be required to check for hyperplasia and for evidence of malignancy in the older female. A uterine curettage may be needed. A careful pelvic examination for evidence of polycystic ovaries is indicated (sometimes), requiring sonography, examination under anesthesia, and/or diagnostic laparoscopy. Chronic anovulation calls for weight (diet) assessment and evaluation of potential emotional factors. The presence of hirsutism and virilism in particular would justify a more sophisticated workup (see the previous section). A unilateral ovarian enlargement likewise necessitates steps to rule out a functioning neoplasm. The response of an elevated 17-ketosteroid excretion level to dexamethasone suppression is helpful in distinguishing relevant entities. Suppression to a value consistent with normal ovarian function (2 mg. per 24°) is consistent with adrenal hyperplasia while lesser depressions (to 5 to 11 mg. per 24°) are more compatible with persistent anovulation. An increased urinary pregnanetriol level suggests 21- or 11-hydroxylase deficiency (acquired adrenogenital syndrome), particularly when 17-OH progesterone levels are elevated. Very high levels of 17-ketosteroid excretion (greater than 30 mg. per 24°), or of serum testosterone or androstenedione, suggest tumor in either the ovary or adrenal and these levels would not suppress appreciably. An elevated dehydroepiandrosterone or its sulfated compound (DHEA-S) is likewise suggestive evidence of adrenal tumor.

Polycystic ovaries may be associated with hypothyroidism (which should be checked for routinely, including tests for thyroid antibodies) but, also, in about 20 per cent of these cases, there is hyperprolactinemia. These elevated levels may interfere with LH release, or may possibly disrupt steroidogenesis at the gonadal tissue level; however, there seems to be little correlation between prolactin values and those of the adrogens and estradiol 17-a. Fear or anxiety and a host of drugs, including phenothiazine derivatives and oral contraceptives, sexual practices (suckling), and a variety of lesions involving the hypothalamus, thyroid, adrenal or pituitary glands may be at fault. Polytomograms of the sella turcica may detect some microadenomas of the pituitary, and these evaluations should be a standard part of the workup, particularly when galactorrhea is demonstrable. Bromocriptine is a synthetic ergot alkaloid which is a specific inhibitor of the release of prolactin, as well as TSH, capable of reducing elevated prolactin levels, suppressing galactorrhea, and of inducing ovulation.

5. Diagnostic laparoscopy: Inspection of the pelvis via the laparoscope adds a considerable dimension to the quality of the infertility workup. Detection of tubal and peritoneal adhesions that immobilize but do not obstruct can best be accomplished by endoscopy. The actual dynamics of the tubes subjected to transuterine dye injections can be appreciated, and the precise location and extent of adhesions or blockage can be determined in most instances. Often these subtle changes are not apparent on physical examination and there may be no history suggestive of prior pelvic disease. Adhesions associated with minimal endometriosis may be characterized in this way in many instances, locating to an unexpected "egg pickup" problem. Similarly, pelvic infection arising from an IUD, after abortion, following appendicitis or peritonitis of pneumococcal or fungal etiology, may result in "silent" adhesions.

Following these five major diagnostic approaches to infertility, the cause or causes of not conceiving are identifiable in 80 to 90 per cent of cases. In some, pregnancy will occur during the course of workup, perhaps even before a particular problem has been identified. However, in the others, no cause will be found on these basic investigations. A few more etiologic antifertility factors will be unearthed by very specialized tests. Among these cases of so-called "infertility of unknown etiology" or "normal infertile couple," cultures for particular organisms (*T. mycoplasma,* tubercle bacilli, fungi, etc.), refined assessments for immunologic incompatibilities, and chromosomal studies for pertinent genetic defects may pay dividends in some clinical situations. Sometimes, the multifactorial nature of the problem is not recognized until a more in depth study of the couple is made. This same type of restudy is required if treatment given to correct a particular problem such as anovulation fails after an adequate trial. A small percentage of patients with 45 X complements may have spontaneous menses, normal height and breast development. Those with a mosaic pattern of XX and XO gonadal dysgenesis with normal stature and appearance constitute an even greater likelihood of escaping detection. In about 5 to 10 per cent of couples with repetitive abortions, either the wife or the husband will have balanced translocation. Antenatal diagnosis for chromosomal disorders can be offered. About 5 to 10 per cent of fetal deaths involve an abnormal chromosomal complement although, that figure might be higher if macerated fetuses could be studied appropriately. Only about 0.5 per cent of liveborn infants have these defects.

In the workup, the more simple conditions with the best clinical prospects in the husband and the wife must not be overlooked through lack of an organized approach or preoccupation with the exotic. For example, plastic procedures on the penis, surgical correction of ductal obstruction, creation of artificial spermatoceles, and administrations of arginine, HMG, hCG, testosterone, and other approaches will yield some favorable results in selected cases. However, far better success can be achieved by eliminating faulty coital practices, detecting and treating hypothyroidism, eradicating a genital infection, and discovering and ligating a varicocele. Remeding adverse heat effects on the testicles, advising on rest, exercise, consumption of alcohol, tobacco, caffeine, drugs of various types, and offering emotional support may likewise contribute to the likelihood of success. These same principles pertain to the female partner.

Hormonal therapies may be effective modalities in correcting anovulation, corpus luteum insufficiency, thyroid dysfunctions, adrenogenital syndrome, adrenal hyperplasia, gonadotrophin deficiency, poor cervical mucus, and galactorrhea (hyperprolactinemia). In patients with polycystic ovaries with hirsutism, a trial on dexamethasone or estrogen/progesterone (oral contraceptives) will often determine the best hormonal treatment. A documented hypothyroidism might take first priority of attention because its correction often reestablishes ovulation despite apparent multiglandular defects. The mainstay in the induction of ovulation in the absence of thyroid deficiency, adrenal disorder and/or hyperprolactinemia (galactorrhea) is the use of clomiphene citrate. Candidates for this therapy must be estrogen sufficient and the hypothalamic-pituitary-ovarian axis and uterine integrity must be intact. If large polycystic ovaries are present, they may be hypersensitive to this therapy and the drug must be administered with care to avoid significant ovarian enlargement, abdominal distention, pain, nausea, vomiting, and many other side effects. When used in 5 day courses (usually days 5 to 10 of each cycle) and gradually increased in dosage at 50 mg. increments beginning at 50 mg. and stopping at a maximum of 200 mg., induction of ovulation can be expected in about 80 per cent of properly selected cases. That figure can be increased to about 90 per cent if refractory cases are offered human chorionic gonadotropin (hCG) to mimic an LH surge on about day 7 to 10 (10,000 IU per day). Under very special circumstances, a more complicated and potentially dangerous hormonal regime of human menopausal gonadotropin (hMG) and hCG may be required, but the risks of a hyperstimulation syndrome can be life threatening, and are prohibitive except in the hands of the expert. The discouraging feature is that while 90 per cent of women may ovulate, only about 50 per cent or less will conceive. Patients require reevaluation when they do not respond. Under clomiphene therapy, they may become somewhat hypoestrogenic, as evidenced by poor cervical mucus, which may require exogenous augmentation. Patients with low gonadotropins or hyperprolactinemia may not respond well to clomiphene. When ovaries are large, wedge resection may be the safer mode of therapy in an effort to avoid overstimulation. Also, patients who are refractory to hormonal therapies may respond to this surgical approach if the ovaries are not low normal or small in size. When immunologically based infertility is suspected, it may be possible to reduce the antibody titer by eliminating sperm contact through use of a condom for 3 to 6 months. Inadequate mucus creating a cervical sperm transport problem can sometimes be eliminated by administering preovulatory estrogen on about day 10 of the cycle. Progestogens (medroxy progesterone acetate, or dydrogesterone) or antigonadotropin (danazol) administrations may be administered to produce pseudopregnancy or pseudomenopause, respectively, in an effort to restore fertility in women with pelvic endometriosis. Subvirilizing oral androgens may be used for the same purpose. It is generally conceded by most that conservative surgical procedures may be more successful in restoring fertility than these hormonal approaches. Restoration of childbearing potential occurs in 50 to 80 per cent of cases, depending upon the individual circumstances, but one drawback is the risk of a second operation if there is progression of the disease.

There are surgical approaches to female infertility problems that can be directed to a number of problems relating to the uterus, e.g., hysteroplastic procedures (uterine unification and resection of septum), myomectomy, cervical circlage for incompetent cervix, etc. Tubal infertility, characterized by blockage and/or immobility, results from scarring secondary to infection or inflammatory responses to pathological conditions and peritoneal irritants (blood, etc.). There may be pelvic infections arising from or associated with uterine causes and in many of these the outlook is poor for restoring reproductive function, e.g., tuberculous endometritis and endosalpingitis, IUD-related pelvic

abscess, fungus infections of the pelvis, septic degeneration in submucus myomas, perforated uterus with abscess formation or pyometra, etc. Generally, endogenous infections of the tubes (gonorrhea) are less amenable to surgical correction than adhesions affecting the tube extrinsically, but the mucosa is normal. Evacuation of a conceptus implanted in the tube can sometimes be accomplished while the functional integrity of the organ is preserved, but this approach is restricted to highly selected cases. A subsequent pregnancy implanted in the affected tube is a considerable risk of conservative procedures.

A number of plastic procedures are now applicable to the problem of tubal infertility; and, recently, advances in microsurgical techniques have upgraded the chances of success even in cases requiring partial resections and reanastamosis. Salpingolysis, requiring only division of perituboovarian adhesions, carries the best results (50 to 80 per cent success rate). Fimbriolysis, salpingoplasty with or without a fimbrial prosthesis, midsegment reconstructions and uterotubal implantations are other feasible techniques in selected cases, but salvage are generally in the 20 to 40 per cent range. Tubal "reversal" (reversing a tubal sterilization) can be attempted, with the prospects for better results in ligations achieved by ligature and resection of small segment than by electrocautery, which may have inflicted extensive tubal drainage. A short residual tubal segment portends poorly for success, and inadvertently operating on a patient with residual salpingitis will doom any plastic attempt to failure.

Abnormal Sexual Development

Dysfunctional gynecological presentations are frequently associated with developmental sexual abnormalities that must be considered if a wide range of disorders of the female is to be managed safely and effectively. In practice, the question of chromosome abnormalities, intersex, and congenital anomalies of the female genital tract must be suspected in a host of abnormal presentations involving abnormal generative tract and reproductive functions. These considerations have been mentioned in other sections under discussions of menstrual dysfunctions, amenorrhea, ambiguous external genitalia, disturbed puberty, infertility, reproductive wastage, and several types of carcinogenesis. Abnormalities are generally identified with a frequency inversely related to the age of individuals. A relatively high incidence of chromosomal anomalies is found in early spontaneous abortuses (roughly 40 per cent). Defective developments in the ovary or testis may create morphological and functional disturbances manifested at any time during the embryonic (up to the 56th day), perinatal, or pubertal periods of life.

Particular maldevelopments may involve the gonads, müllerian ducts, genital tubercle, and urogenital sinus.

The Y chromosome appears to carry the testicular inductor in the human. Genetic or chromosomal sex is determined at the moment of fertilization, but the gonads remain in an indifferent stage until about the seventh embryonic week. At that time, histodifferentiation of the testes occurs at a rapid pace while differentiation in the female requires a little longer. The male set is stimulated preferentially while the female set undergoes atrophy if the testis-inducing Y chromosome is present. The X chromosome does not possess a counterpart gene to the Y chromosome. There must be two X chromosomes for the ovary to differentiate, since gonadal dysgenesis occurs if the second X is either missing or defective. Thus, if the testicular inductor is absent, the indifferent gonad develops as an ovary. Originally, germ cells of the 45XO karyotype contain the same number of germ cells as the normal 46XX type, but at some point, by unknown mechanisms, chromosomal sex material is lost. When the inductor is present, the testis is developed in its definitive form by the 10th to 11th week of intrauterine life. Hilar structures and the great proliferation of Leydig cells (distinctive interstitial cells) reach a peak at about 19 weeks. Seminiferous tubules without lumina are apparent, and their growth results in coiling and crowding prior to the lumina formation and the appearance of spermatogonia and sertoli cells. In gonads destined to be ovaries, one of the distinguishing features at about the 7 week stage is the presence of masses of ovogonia. Ultimately, deeper ones become surrounded by somatic (granulosa) cells of the primitive follicles. These structures are very prominent by the 17th gestational week.

The uterus and vagina slowly arise as distinctly identifiable structures during the 4th and 5th months of fetal life. The uterus, including the cervix and upper four-fifths of the vagina, are müllerian duct-derived. The lower one-fifth of the vagina is derived from a cord of epithelium that arises from the urogenital sinus and grows upward to displace at least in part the müllerian epithelium craniad and establishes the anlage of the future hollow tube. Canalization proceeds from the caudal region in the craniad direction and the fornices develop clefts to complete the definitive vaginal form. When sinus proliferation does not take place or grows to a certain point and atrophies, vaginal agenesis may occur. In the absence of a vaginal mass, the hymen is not formed. Also, incomplete fusion of the distal portions of the müllerian ducts results in various forms of partial or total duplication of the uterus and proximal vagina. In addition to septation of the upper vagina and incomplete fusion of the sinovaginal bulbs (arrests in development occurring between the eighth and twelfth week of fetal life), there may be transverse bars, adenosis, and various anatomic and histologic abnormalities occurring at the vault. The vagina is the last genital organ to be completed embryologically and masculinizing effects occurring relatively late may adversely affect its development.

Diethylstilbestrol (DES) exposure in utero in the first trimester creates morphologic and anomalous changes in both the cervix and vagina in a majority of young females, and very rarely there will be clear cell adenocarcinomatous development. There may be cervical and vaginal structural defects in the female as well as abnormal morphological genital defects in the male as a result of DES exposure, and there may be attendant problems relating to reproductive success. Transverse vaginal septae and bands of tissue in the upper segment may give rise to dyspareunia, while various deformities of the cervix may predispose to its incompetency in pregnancy. Cervical ectropion (erosion and eversion) and morphologic defects and vaginal adenosis and structural anomalies have been reported in a majority (up to 60 to 90 per cent in some reports) of DES-exposed offspring during the age period 14 to 24.

Anomalies are multiple in roughly one in four defective fetuses, and maldevelopments in the generative system are often coincident with those of the urinary organs. Development of the external organs of the genital system is so intimately interrelated that isolated anomalies are rare. In addition to sympodia, which represents an absence of the entire hind end of the body, other defects include agenesis of the perineum and phallus, exstrophy of the cloaca or of the bladder, imperforate anus, rectoperineal or rectovaginal fistulae, rectal agenesis, posterior displacement of the urogenital sinus, duplication of the external genitalia, and other anorectal and perineal anomalies.

Anomalies of the external genitalia in association with a positive buccal smear are usually associated with female pseudohermaptroditism. The classic underlying condition is congenital hyperplasia of the adrenal gland, but other causes may be female fetuses subjected in utero to maternal progestin or androgen therapy or, possibly, to an androgen secreting gonadal tumor. Despite the illusion of the urethra opening into the vagina or the vagina into the urethra, these structures are intact and open separately into a common passage consisting of a persistent urogenital sinus. The vaginal and urethral openings present well within the common passageway and there is one external opening located at the base of the phallus. The uterus and tubes are not affected. This problem is easily corrected surgically by resecting the urogenital membrane, providing access to the vaginal introitus and exposing the external urethral meatus. If ovarian suppression and virilization are present, these should be eliminated during adolescence by utilizing corticosteroid administrations. In most untreated patients, ovarian function does not occur and primoidial follicles diminish in number. Usually, premature closure of epiphyses of the long bones results in short adult stature. Hypospadius, varying failure of the labioscrotal folds, cleft in the scrotum resembling a vagina, urogenital opening or separate urethral and vaginal openings are reminiscent of the congenital adrenal hyperplasia syndrome in females.

The complete form of testicular feminization is associated with no androgen response. Only in the incomplete form is there a problem of sex assignment because usually there is normal external female development and these patients naturally are reared in that sex. In the case of partial response to androgens, there may be ambiguous genitalia. However, there is no müllerian development and in these circumstances, the vagina is short and ends in a blind pouch. These genetic males are phenotypic females with normal secondary sex characteristics except for sparse genital and axillary hair. Inguinal hernias are present in more than one-half of the patients, and often the gonads are found in the inguinal canal. The gonads have a malignant potential, justifying castration and estrogen hormone replacement. The clinical situation is confused by a number of incompletely masculinized male pseudohermaphrodites. The presence of a normal vagina, uterus, and tubes differentiates the Swyer syndrome. In the Reifenstein syndrome, there is a phallic enlargement at birth, along with a severe perineal hypospadius. After puberty, hypogonadism occurs with gynecomastia. The pseudovaginal periscrotal hypospadius condition is associated at birth with a normal steroid condition that rules out adrenal disorders.

Anorchia is similar to the Swyer syndrome, except that the affected individuals lack internal genitalia and a vagina. Patients with the uterine hernia syndrome are individuals who appear to be normally male, but a well-developed uterus and tubes may be found in an inguinal hernia sac.

It is apparent that confusion in the gender role with its attendant emotional stress is a common problem among children with contradictory sex structures. Reinforcement of the gender role in the selected sex of rearing, including the erotic component, which is independent of the gonadal and chromosomal sex, is essential in programming management. From a surgical viewpoint, the assignment of sex must depend upon the morphology of the phallus and whether or not a penis adequate for successful coitus can be constructed. The technical factors are all important. Construction of a satisfactory artificial cavity for coitus is the sim-

plest operative undertaking (transperineal rectovesical space dilations, McIndoe procedure with creation of rectovesical artificial space and split-thickness skin graft over a mold, or musculovascular transplant). Construction of an artificial penis with both erectile and erotic capacities has not been achieved to this same level of success.

In assessing the newborn, it is of interest to note that the number of cells with nuclear sex chromatin in normal female neonates will be falsely low in the first two days of life. A karyotype determination of the chromosomal sex is needed if the Barr body count is inconsistent with the appearance of the external genitalia. 17-ketosteroid and pregnanetriol excretion levels may be needed to distinguish between congenital adrenal hyperplasia (associated with elevated levels) and other types of hermaphroditism. By the same token, labial adhesions may resemble labioscrotal fusion. The preferred treatment is simple application of estrogen cream. If some type of operative separation is performed, the results will be painful inflammation and recurrence of adhesions. Occasionally, hypertrophy of the labia resulting in a distorted gross appearance is associated with excessive masturbation and deep seated psychological disturbances.

In male hermaphroditism, laparotomy may be required both for diagnosis and therapy. Disadvantageous sex structures should be removed. When these individuals are reared as females, testes should always be removed at puberty, regardless of hormone production, because a variety of tumors including malignant ones may develop in these abnormal gonads.

Family Planning

In global terms, there may be socioeconomic indications for birth control to cope with increasing population, excess pollution, and an inevitable decline in natural resources and quality of life. Contraception may be mandatory on medical grounds to safeguard a particular individual whose life would be put in jeopardy by a pregnancy. There may be eugenic indications for birth control that benefit both the individual and society by discouraging conception or interrupting a pregnancy that perpetuates a harmful genetic trait or gives rise to a hopelessly deformed offspring. Effective contraception has been sponsored to reduce adolescent and out-of-wedlock pregnancy, unwanted pregnancies among married couples, and in an effort to avoid the disastrous consequences of illegal abortion. In many instances, the quality of married life and the ability to realize goals for the family are predicated upon the ability to control the reproductive process. Traditionally, the folk and conventional practices of family planning have not been successful. These have included coitus interruptus, rhythm method, prolongation of lactation, and postcoital douches of various types. The barrier contraceptives consisting of the condom and diaphragm are much more reliable contraceptive methods, and they are of course medically safe, but mechanical and technical problems reduce their effectiveness. Nonetheless, the failure rate overall is low (2 or 3 pregnancies per 100 women per year of exposure with the vaginal (cervical diaphragm), if prescribed and used properly, and probably this record can be improved by using spericidal preparations for lubrication. The more modern methods consist of oral contraceptives, repeated injections of progestational steroids, intrauterine devices both, medicated and nonmedicated, surgical sterilization of the female transabdominally by laparotomy or laparoscopy, and male sterilization. In addition, there may be induced abortions by suction or surgical curettage, intraamniotic instillation of an oxytocic agent, (midtrimester), use of abortifacients (prostaglandin F_2 and $F_2\alpha$ administered orally or by intraamniotic injection) or, rarely, hysterotomy. Suction curettage within 2 weeks after a missed menstrual period may be instituted under the designation of "menstrual regulation" to prevent unwanted pregnancies before the fact of gestation is established.

Oral Contraceptives. Oral contraceptives used to inhibit ovulation contain a combination of synthetic estrogen, usually in the form of ethinyl estradiol (0.02 to 0.05 mg.) or mestranol (0.075 to 0.8 mg.) and progestin, usually Norethindione (0.3 to 5.0 mg.), dl-Norgestrel (0.3–0.5 mg.), Norethynodrel (2.5 to 5.0 mg.) or Ethynodiol diacetate (1.0 mg.). Under this therapy there is no rise of FSH or follicle growth in the first half of the menstrual cycle, and at midcycle there is no LH surge or ovulation. The course is a 21 day hormonal regime whereby one pill is taken daily during days 5 to 25 of the cycle and the patient bleeds by withdrawal 3 to 5 days later to commence the new cycle. The on-and-off intervals, which must be remembered, can be avoided since packets are now available that provide hormonally inert pills for the last 7 to 8 days when steroids are not being offered to the patient.

Except for sterilization, oral contraceptives are the most effective method for preventing pregnancy (less than 0.1 pregnancy per 100 woman-years). However, these steroids provoke a variety of systemic effects, the 1-year continuation rate is probably only about 70 per cent, and included among these significant side effects are alterations in hepatic function tests, hematologic and coagulation tests, thyroid evaluations, glucose tolerance tests (15 to 40 per cent) serum folate values, metyrapone test and others. Side effects may be gastrointestinal symptoms, breast discomfort, fluid retention and weight gain, megaloblastic anemia (diminished absorption of folate polyglutamates), pyridoxine deficiency, depression (sometimes reversible with vitamin B_6), and rarely, chloasma (2 to 5 per cent of cases). The most worrisome potential effects of pill usage is the increased risk of thromboembolic disease, thrombotic stroke, and myocardial infarction (among smokers). The likelihood of these serious complications is much more common among women with hypertension, advancing age, type II hyperlipoproteinemia, obesity, previous toxemia of pregnancy, diabetes mellitus, varicose veins, chronic disease and immobilization. There appears to be an increased risk of postsurgery thromboembolic complications, gallbladder disease, and benign hepatomas. Some patients will become hypertensive for the first time while taking oral contraceptives, presumably because of alteration of the renin-angiotensin mechanism. Long-standing chronic anovulation is a factor in the etiology of endometrial carcinoma, and prolonged pill usage may be implicated in some cases. There may be a steepening of the corneal curvature (lowered tolerance to contact lenses), allergic reactions, augmented vaginal (cervical) secretions, and other conditions. Obviously, patients must be selected and supervised in a most meticulous fashion if oral contraceptives are to be prescribed. Absolute contraindications would be thromboembolic, cerebral, or coronary artery disease, suspected carcinoma of the breast, known or suspected estrogen dependent neoplasia, undiagnosed abnormal genital bleeding, or known or suspected pregnancy. Visual loss, severe headache, icterus or pruritis, choletheasis, development of hypertension, and significant breakthrough bleeding are causes for alarm. Patients who have experienced oligoamenorrhea are not suitable candidates for oral contraceptives, since postpill amenorrhea may be a problem. Normally, fertility following pill usage is not a worrisome feature, since 95 per cent of the patients who are destined to ovulate will do so by the third cycle.

The "mini-pill," or nonstop progestin (Norgestrel, 0.35 mg. daily) is an effective oral contraceptive despite the fact that a high percentage of the menstrual cycles are ovulatory. The chief advantage of this approach is elimination of estrogen, its side effects, and the problems inherent in ovulatory withdrawal bleeding. Overall, the pregnancy rate ranges between 2 and 7 per 100 woman years; and, whereas the precise mechanism of action is unknown, out-of-phase endometrial activity and hostile cervical mucus have been suggested as antifertility factors.

Diethylstilbesterol, ethinyl estradiol, conjugated equine estrogens, or other estrogenic substances given alone, progestins administered alone, or in combination with estrogens have been used as postcoital, or "morning-after," pills with varying degrees of success. The effectiveness of a high dose of estrogen is based on its ability to suppress ovulation when ingested 2 to 6 days in advance of the event, or by accelerating transport of the fertilized ovum through the tube to reach the endometrium before it is properly prepared for implantation. The failure rate ranges up to nearly 2.5 per cent in some reports and there may be significant side effects of estrogen usage in these high doses. Recently, ethinyl estradiol and dl-norgestrel in substantial doses have been used in combination to achieve a very low failure rate. Contraceptive effectiveness is also very high when hormone injections are given to prevent ovulation by suppressing the pituitary and eliminating the midcycle surges of luteinizing hormone. For this purpose, a popular choice is medroxy progesterone acetate (Depo-Provera) administered intramuscularly in 150 mg. doses every 90 days.

Intrauterine Contraceptive Devices. Insertion of intrauterine devices to prevent conception is safe, effective, and inexpensive. Long-term protection is afforded without any attentiveness on the part of the patient that medications require. The preferred types are classified as "open" devices, which have no circumscribed aperture larger than 5 mm. Should uterine perforation occur and the device come to lie in the abdominal cavity, a bow or "closed" ring type might be receptive to omentum or bowel, leading to strangulation. The traditional intrauterine contraceptive devices have been nonmedicated, but more recently the device has been used as a vehicle for an active agent capable of enhancing local effects on the uterus. Copper is widely used for this purpose, and this metal as well as zinc evoke a profound leukocytic infiltration in the uterus that renders the endometrial environment unsuitable for implantation of the blastocyst. This inflammatory response is not dependent upon microbial invasion and the normal course is for the uterine cavity to be sterile within a few weeks after the device is inserted. Nonetheless, IUDs do not prevent bacterial invasion, and salpingitis or pelvic abscess can occur in wearers. Devices with complex multifilament tails tend to be potentially the most dangerous because bacteria can ascend from the vagina between individual fibers through a "wicking" action. For this reason, such devices should be replaced with those with monofilament tails. Even with the latter device, the risk of acute pelvic inflammatory disease is significantly higher in IUD users than in the women who are not. The most vulnerable women are nulligravidas of a lowly socioeconomic status; there is also the added risk of ectopic pregnancy among long-term users.

The most serious complication associated with the insertion of an IUD is perforation of the cervix or uterine fundus. An open, nonmedicated IUD is much less likely to evoke a prominent tissue reaction in the peritoneal cavity than the copper device. It is important to remove the latter type as soon as possible to avoid fixation by adhesions. The significant side effects are cramping pain, uterine bleeding, early infection (first few weeks after insertion), or expulsion. If pregnancy occurs with the IUD in situ, the risk of abortion spontaneously is roughly 50 per cent. If the IUD is not removable by simple traction on the tail, the device is best left in place if continuation of pregnancy is desired. There is no indication that even the medicated devices will increase the risk of fetal anomalies.

Overall the pregnancy rate per 100 woman-years is in the range of 2.7 (0.4 to 5.8) and the 1-year continuation rate is about 70 per cent (50 to 92 per cent). Another form of the medicated intrauterine device is the Progestasert, which contains a mechanism to slowly release progesterone into the uterine cavity. Its use has been questioned recently, because it appears that an accidental pregnancy occurring with this form of IUD in place is much more likely to be ectopic than with copper-bearing or nonmedicated devices.

Sterilization. Surgical sterilization is a definitive method of contraception which is legal in all states in the US. Tubal closure represents the most consistently effective permanent method of controlling childbearing, and, of course, the problem of continuation is avoided. Transabdominal operative technics include conventional laparotomy procedures or mini laparotomy, which can be performed in the immediate puerperium or in an interim period at any phase of the menstrual cycle. The sterilization can be performed concomitantly with an induced abortion. The classic technics of tubal occlusion include the various types of tubal transection, ligation, and retroperitonealization of stumps, e.g., Pomeroy, Madlener, and Irving technics. More recently, sterilization via the laparoscope on an ambulatory basis has become very popular, and by means of that endoscopic transabdominal approach it is possible to fulgurate (coagulate) the tubes with or without division or excision, and to clip or band them. The latter methods have the theoretical advantage of reversibility. In each one of the operative techniques, accidental pregnancy is likely to be tubal. Coagulation of the tubes only, without division or excision or application of tantalum hemoclips, is associated with higher failure rates. Overall, the pregnancy rate per 100 woman-years is in the 0.04 to 0.08 range, which is a slight improvement over the antifertility effectiveness of the combined type of oral contraceptives. Partial vasectomy is the most effective male contraceptic technique. Generally, intravas occlusive devices for controlled infertility potential in the male have not yet been adequately developed and tested.

Abortion. In some countries, voluntary abortion has become the principal method of controlling the size of the family. In the US, there is one legal abortion for every four live births, about 10 per cent of the teenage population become pregnant each year, and a significant number of abortions occurs in the very young who are not prepared for childbirth and child rearing. The duration of pregnancy at the time of anticipated interruption determines the preferred method. Termination of pregnancy at the 12th gestational week or less is most efficiently achieved by suction curettage with negative pressures ranging to about 30 to 50 cm. H_2O. Maternal mortality rates are exceedingly low (2 per 100,000 patients or less) and the morbidity associated with infection, bleeding and perforation of the uterus should be 5 per cent or less. Midtrimester abortions can be accomplished by instilling 200 ml. of 20 per cent saline solution into the uterine cavity (80 to 90 per cent success rate within 48 hours), but side effects, complications, and emotional stress factors are very common. The use of oxytocin for induction of labor is unreliable and the latent period and interval to abortion can be quite long. Prostaglandin therapy may be highly efficient in inducing labor, and vaginal suppositories introduced at the time of the expected menstruation can bring on a period and evacuate an early conceptus. Hysterotomy or hysterectomy should be considered only in context with the presence of coexisting pelvic disease. Overall, complications associated with midtrimester abortions (approaching 20 per cent after intraamniotic instillations) are so prevalent that the primary emphasis in family planning must be upon contraceptive methods or early interruption if accidental pregnancy occurs.

Climacterium, Menopause, and Postmenopausal Syndrome

The term menopause refers simply to the permanent cessation of menstruation. The physiological termination of menses which results from a progressive decline in ovarian function over a period of years usually occurs at age 52 in the US. The atresia of germ cells, which has now depleted functional follicular units, has far exceeded those used up in ovulation, which account for only 450 or less, but the process is not understood. Occasionally, premature ovarian failure occurs which results in premature menopause without discernible causes (approximately one menstruating woman in 20). Rarely, debilitating systemic illnesses, psychiatric disability, pelvic irradiation, and ovarian ischemia from pelvic surgery may cause early gonadal insufficiency.

An abrupt bilateral oophorectomy may produce more severe acute symptoms than the more gradual physiological process. There may be significant pathophysiologic changes resulting in autonomic nervous system instability, vasomotor changes, emotional upsets, and certain objective changes characterized by inovulation of the reproductive tract, urinary system, mammary ducts and body hair, as well as increased bone resorption. At this stage of life, there is a slight increase in the development of hyperthyroidism and maturity-onset diabetes mellitus. Preceding the actual menopause there may be polymenorrhea, hypermenorrhea, prolonged menstrual flow and perhaps metrorrhagia suggestive of uterine malignancy after a chronic period of anovulation. Symptoms may be emotional instability, atrophic urethrocystitis (urgency, frequency, dysuria, urgency incontinence, pyuria, occasional hematuria, and possible meatal pouting and caruncle formation), and atrophic vulvovaginitis and cervicitis. There may be diurnal hot flashes (flushes) and night sweats. The skin may lose its elasticity and turgor, breast size may regress, bone resorption (symptomatic osteoporosis) occurs in about one-quarter of postmenopausal women, and there may be symptoms and signs of atherosclerosis (more severe in women who were castrated before age 40). More than 50 symptoms have been attributed to the changes of the postmenopausal state, although a cause-and-effect relationship is doubtful for most. Laboratory data tend to support the level of estrogenic deprivation. The vaginal cytologic smear may show a lowering of the cornification counts, although this measure is crude and it is now clear that many postmenopausal women derive significant plasma levels of estrogen from extragonadal sources. The most significant postmenopausal endocrine alteration is the great increase in the secretion of pituitary gonadotropins involving both FSH and LH production (FSH increased three-fold over the increase in LH). Although sporadic gasps of menstrual function may occur before the final episode, the endometrium should be atrophic and clearly benign. Roentgograms of the lungs, bones, and blood vessels show only the changes ordinarily associated with the normal aging process. A variety of clinical conditions may mimic all of the signs and symptoms noted, which calls for appropriate evaluation of signs and symptoms as well as potential laboratory studies to sort out the proper diagnosis from among a host of masquerading diseases. Nothing can be done to stall a physiological menopause, although there is discretion in creating an artificial termination of menses in context with pathological entities of the internal genitalia. Probably, the potential consequences of artificial menopause can be justified in women who must be subjected to hysterectomy at age 40 or over.

At that stage of life, the elective removal of ovaries to prevent ovarian cancer, which will be a risk of increasing proportions throughout life is probably justified.

Although vulnerable women cannot be identified with precision, there is the likelihood that endometrial cancer can be triggered by prolonged estrogen therapy. Mitigating influences may be low doses, cyclic administrations, opposing the estrogen with progesterone therapies in each cycle, and emotional support to reduce the need for support. The experience of withdrawal blood loss after progesterone therapy suggests that there is estrogen overdosage, which is an indication to stop exogenous sources and to perform a uterine curettage to rule out an organic basis if bleeding continues. On the other hand, progestins may relieve vasomotor symptoms in a patient whose uterus is not primed with estrogen to the level of provoking withdrawal bleeding when these hormones are administered. Current studies tend to show that a close relationship exists between the occurrence of pulsatile LH release and objective (cutaneous temperature) plus subjective (experience of hot flashes and flushes) evidences of menopausal symptoms. Catecholamines may be involved in central thermoregulatory function and the therapy probably should be more specific than simple estrogen replacement, although the objectives in management seem to be rather broad. An estrogen-androgen therapy has been recommended to minimize the potential ill effects of the estrogenic administration as a sole therapeutic modality, but methyltestosterone does not add to the therapeutic efficacy against postmenopausal osteoporosis. Similarly, progestational therapies, while relieving some symptoms, will not replace entirely the estrogen deprivation in the minority who may not have endogenous sources in adequate amounts from extragonadal sources. The majority of patients will not need exogenous steroid therapy; but, in the small minority who do, estrogen therapy in modest doses for prescribed periods can be given without a documented increased risk of hypertension, atherosclerosis or heart, renal and cerebral disease.

QUESTIONS IN OBSTETRICS AND GYNECOLOGY

What are the principal objectives of obstetric care?

What is the definition of maternal death?

What are the principal causes of maternal mortality?

What has been the trend in maternal mortality rates in the United States over the last five decades?

What factors are responsible for these trends?

What are the direct causes of maternal death? indirect causes?

What are the principal causes of perinatal mortality and morbidity?

What are the recent trends in perinatal mortality in the United States?

What is the proportion of fetal deaths among perinatal deaths? What factors influence the risk of a fetal death?

Describe the true pelvis.

How is the true obstetric conjugate estimated?

Classify pelves according to type and describe the morphologic features of each.

Draw a sagittal section through the female pelvis, showing the vagina and the uterus and their relationship to the bladder and rectum.

Describe the relationship of the peritoneum to the uterus.

What is the main support structure for the uterus?

Describe the uterine ligaments.

What is the uterine blood supply?

Describe the fallopian tubes grossly and histologically.

Diagram a graafian follicle, indicating its principal parts.

Discuss the relation of the corpus luteum to the graafian follicle.

Describe the life cycle of the corpus luteum.

Describe the menstrual cycle and discuss the physiology of its production.

What is the relation of the hypothalamic-pituitary-ovarian axis to menstruation?

Where is the ovum fertilized?

Describe the retrogressive changes in the corpus luteum if pregnancy does not ensue.

What is meant by maturation of the ovum?

Describe some of the essential structures within the mature ovum and in its surroundings.

Describe the process of implantation.

What are the phases of the menstrual cycle?

Discuss the endocrine support of normal menses.

What are the vascular phenomena involved in the menstrual cycle?

What are some of the key histological characteristics of the endometrium in the menstrual cycle?

Describe the nuclear events in oogenesis and spermatogenesis.

What is the characteristic chromosomal pattern of cells in the human?

Describe the process of implantation.

What is the chorion? amnion? decidua? trophoblast? What are Langhans' cells? syncytial cells?

How is the embryo nourished before implantation? after implantation?

How does one classify the human placenta?

List the ancillary organs of the developing conceptus.

What triggers the endometrial decidual response after conception?

Discuss the maturation of the placenta from a vascular and functional viewpoint.

Describe the hemodynamics and metabolic exchange capabilities within the intervillous space.

What are the transport mechanisms within the placenta?

Outline proper prenatal care.

Give the positive signs, the probable signs and the presumptive signs of pregnancy.

What are the common laboratory tests that are employed to establish the diagnosis of pregnancy? What is the hormonal basis for these tests? Which one is highly sensitive and specific?

Discuss diet in pregnancy and effect of maternal nutrition upon fetal growth and development.

Discuss the current laboratory capabilities for estimating fetal status, welfare and maturity; indications?

What is a stress test? A non-stress test?

Describe the diagnosis of fetal presentation.

What are the stages of normal labor? What is the so-called fourth stage?

Describe the mechanism of normal labor.

How is placenta normally delivered?

Describe episiotomy. What is the purpose of this procedure?

Describe the care of the lacerated perineum.

What are the principal techniques used in obstetric analgesia and anesthesia?

Discuss the purpose of systemic analgesia. Outline a plan of management.

What factors influence the choice of technique?

Describe the postpartal care of the mother.

Discuss common methods of family planning.

Define abortion; premature birth.

Define habitual abortion.

What constitutes good preventive medicine in obstetrics as it applies to the problem of repeated abortion?

What are the principal causes of spontaneous abortion?

Give the prophylaxis of abortion; give the signs, the symptoms and the treatment of threatened abortion.

What clinical factors are known to influence the outcome in patients who are threatening to abort? What are the hazards of missed abortion?

What is the role of amniocentesis? of pelvic sonography?

Classify the toxemias of pregnancy. What are the early warning signs? Discuss the etiology.

Discuss the principles of management of pre-eclampsia; of eclampsia.

What are the special problems of chronic hypertensive vascular disease complicating pregnancy?

Discuss the significant factors that determine the prognosis for patients with heart disease during pregnancy. Outline the principles of management.

How does pregnancy influence the clinical course of diabetes? What are the principal obstetric problems of the diabetic patient?

What are the principal causes of antepartum hemorrhage? How are they treated?

What are the clinical signs and symptoms of severe abruptio placentae? What factors determine fetal prognosis? What are the principal hazards to the mother? Outline a plan of management in cases of abruptio placentae.

Which factors favor the occurrence of placenta previa? Describe 3 types. How is it diagnosed and treated?

Discuss the diagnosis of extrauterine pregnancy. Specify types. Give the diagnosis and the treatment.

What are the major types of dystocia? Classify the types of uterine inertia. Discuss its management.

What are the current brophysical intrapartal fetal monitoring capabilities? What are the indications for their use?

Outline the various worrisome fetal heart rate patterns that reflect fetal insult or jeopardy. What are the underlying causes?

Which factors must be considered in determining whether or not a given fetus will negotiate a given pelvis?

Define the common types of pelvic contraction.

What are the special problems of a shoulder presentation? Outline a plan of management.

Give the diagnosis and the delivery of R.O.P.

Discuss the diagnosis, the mechanism and the delivery of breech presentation. What are the principal fetal hazards? When should one perform a total breech extraction?

What is the current role of cesarean birth?

How is face presentation diagnosed and delivered? Discuss the clinical outcome of brow presentations.

Give the treatment for prolapse of the cord.

Give the etiology, the diagnosis and the treatment of rupture of the uterus. What are the important predisposing factors in spontaneous uterine rupture? When should one contemplate a vaginal delivery in a patient who has had a previous cesarean section?

What are the principal causes of postpartum hemorrhage? How is it treated? What are the indications for manual removal of the placenta?

What are the indications for the application of forceps? Which conditions must be fulfilled before forceps are applied? How are forceps operations classified?

What is the clinical attitude toward external version? internal version?

What are the indications for cesarean section? contraindications? types? When is a cesarean section indicated primarily for fetal indications?

What operative methods are available for female sterilization?

Into which main groups do puerperal infections fall? Discuss the prophylaxis and the treatment of puerperal infection. Define puerperal morbidity.

What are the common organisms involved? What are some of the late sequelae of puerperal infection?

Describe the fetal circulation. What are the maternal-fetal oxygen relationships? What are the compensatory mechanisms of the fetus to help meet its oxygen needs? Describe the changes in the infant's circulation after birth.

Describe the care of the newborn child.

What are the causes of apnea neonatorum? What are its signs and treatment? What constitutes good prophylaxis?

Discuss the special problems of prematurity. What are the principal causes of premature labor? What are the principal hazards to the infant?

How is premature labor best managed? What drugs are most effective in forestalling or arresting premature labor?

What are the clinical forms of hemolytic disease of the newborn? Discuss each type. What are the pathologic findings? Outline the objective of management of isoimmunized women. Upon what evaluation is the timing for induction of labor based?

Discuss the immunologic basis for this disease. What is the significance of antibody determinations? Discuss the significance of kernicterus.

How does one estimate the severity of the fetal hemolytic process? What therapeutic capabilities are available? What method of prophylaxis is currently available? What is the basis for the approach?

Discuss ABO incompatibility.

What are the special characteristics of gonococcal infections? What are the principal types of acute lower tract infections? Outline the symptoms, the diagnosis and the treatment.

Discuss the clinical varieties, the diagnosis and the treatment of acute upper tract gonorrheal infections.

What are the principal types of salpingitis? Discuss the differential diagnosis.

What are the pathologic varieties of chronic upper tract infections? Discuss the role of surgery in the management of such cases.

What are the immediate hazards of acute pelvic inflammation? Subsequent remote hazards?

How do gonococcal and streptococcal pelvic infections differ? Mixed infections?

Discuss the common tuberculous lesions of the pelvis. Outline the clinical symptomatology and the diagnosis. Give the appropriate plan of management.

Classify and discuss the etiology of the ulcerative lesions of the vulva.

What are the vulvar dystrophies? What are their significance?

Describe the common varieties of vaginitis, the predisposing clinical factors, the characteristic physical findings, the diagnostic procedures and the treatment.

What are the principal benign tumors of the vulva?

Describe the urethral caruncle. What are the histologic types?

What are the clinical characteristics of squamous cell cancer of the vulva?

Give the etiology, the symptoms, the types, the diagnosis and the treatment of uterine myomas. How do they influence pregnancy? Discuss the histogenesis of uterine sarcoma.

What are the diagnosis and the treatment of cervical polyps? Discuss the differential diagnosis.

Discuss the importance of detection of cancer in the cervix. Outline technique of detection and of diagnosis. What are the principal attributes of cytologic method? When is colposcopy indicated?

What risk does in utero exposure to maternal diethylstilbestrol impose upon young adult women?

Discuss carcinoma in situ, its histologic features, significance and treatment.

When should the cervix be sharply conized?

Describe the gross appearance of clinical cancers of the cervix. What are the principal symptoms?

What are the histologic types of cancer of the cervix? How does the lesion spread?

List and define the clinical stages of cancer of the cervix. What constitutes an adequate work-up for these patients?

What are the objectives of radiation therapy? Describe the methods of achieving these objectives? What is a cancer-lethal dose at point B, and why is this an important consideration?

Outline the role of surgery in the management of cancer of the cervix. What is considered to be an acceptable 5-year survival rate for the various clinical stages?

What palliative measures are available in uterine cancer management? cervix? endometrium?

What are the expectations of chemotherapy in these lesions?

What clinical conditions are associated with a higher incidence of cancer of the endometrium?

Describe the histologic and the clinical types of adenocarcinoma. What are the common symptoms? What diagnostic procedures are indicated? How does the fundal cancer spread? Discuss management and prognosis.

What agents are useful for endometrial cancer?

Define and discuss the significance of endometriosis. Discuss the etiology and the predisposing factors. What are the common sites of involvement? Discuss the characteristic symptoms and the physical findings. Discuss the differential diagnosis. What is the fundamental fact upon which treatment is based? Outline a plan of management for these cases. What is adenomyosis, its symptoms, and management?

How are infertile patients with pelvic endometriosis treated?

What is the derivation of hydatidiform moles? Describe the histologic characteristics. Discuss the clinical and the diagnostic features. Discuss the role of hormone studies. What is the differential diagnosis? What is the risk of malignant degeneration? How helpful is pelvic sonography? at what stage of pregnancy?

What are the special hazards of chorioadenoma destruens? What are the clinical and the pathologic features of choriocarcinoma?

Classify ovarian tumors according to type. What are the functional cysts of the ovary?

Discuss the benign neoplastic cysts of the ovary, their derivation, histologic features and clinical significance.

Distinguish between teratomas and dermoid cysts of the ovary. What are common complications arising in the dermoid cysts?

How does one stage the disease in malignant ovarian tumor?

What are the outstanding clinical characteristics of malignant ovarian tumors? What are the most common types? Discuss treatment and prognosis.

Classify the embryonic group of ovarian carcinoma, the clinical features according to type and the age of patient, and the malignant potentialities.

In what way is the surgical attitude with respect to management of ovarian cancer rather unusual?

What clinical and histologic variables influence outcome in the treatment of ovarian cancer? What is the role of chemotherapy? What are the most effective agents?

Classify the remote injuries of childbirth according to anatomic defects. What is the most common genital tract fistula?

Define the retrodisplacements of the uterus. Define the various degrees of uterine prolapse.

What are the causes of genital tract fistulas?

What general principle forms the basis of modern vaginal surgery?

Discuss the usual clinical and laboratory work-up of patients whose chief complaint is urinary incontinence. What is the differential diagnosis? What are the modern testing capabilities? What are the clinical features of an unstable bladder?

The proper selection of surgical management of pelvic insufficiency is dependent on what factors?

What is the principle objective in restoring normal urethral and vesical neck anatomy? What are the surgical approaches?

Discuss the principal prophylactic measures that tend to maintain pelvic sufficiency.

Classify according to type the common disorders of menstruation. Give a definition of each specific type.

What is the most important single cause of abnormal bleeding in the absence of demonstrable pelvic lesions? Discuss the etiology of this condition, its histologic features and its significance according to the age of the patient.

What are the common causes of acyclic bleeding and the relative frequency of such bleeding? Discuss the diagnostic work-up and the significance of this condition.

Discuss the differential diagnosis and work-up of patients with abnormal uterine bleeding due to anovulation. What are the principal goals in management? Outline the principles of hormone therapy in these patients. What are the hazards of chronic anovulation?

What are the causes of amenorrhea? Work-up? What is the significance of galactorrhea? What special evaluative methods are used? How does one check on the various hypothalamic-pituitary-ovarian axis defects?

What attitude should one have about treating patients with postmenopausal complaints?

Discuss the differential diagnosis in female patients with defeminizing or masculinizing signs and symptoms. What work-up is recommended to distinguish the conditions?

Discuss the principal clinical features, the etiology, the diagnostic work-up and the treatment of patients with polycystic ovaries. Describe the pathologic findings in the ovaries. What are the clinical results of surgical management? the results of hormone management? What endocrinopathies may underly the polycystic ovarian condition?

Define the term infertility. What are the incidence and the significance of this problem? What are the important causative factors in the male? in the female? Discuss a systematic program of investigation for these patients. Outline the general and the specific principles of management. What results can be expected?

How does one establish the presence of a tubal factor responsible for infertility?

Discuss abnormal sexual development by cause. What treatments are appropriate for abnormal sexual development?

What is the chromosomal defect in gonadal dysgenesis? How can an affected fetus be determined in utero?

What are the most effective methods of contraception? Indications for each? Side effects, hazards, contraindications? Level of effectiveness?

MULTIPLE CHOICE QUESTIONS

Indicate the best response. Answers are at the end of this chapter.

1. When should a female patient have her first complete pelvic examination?
   (a) As a newborn
   (b) As a child
   (c) When she begins to have sexual experiences regardless of age
   (d) At the time of menarche
   (e) At age 18

2. Puberty is the attainment of reproductive powers and may not be completed in all respects until about age 16 in females. Which is the last of the sophisticated developments in this progression of changes?
   (a) Menarche
   (b) Pubarche
   (c) Growth spurt
   (d) Hypothalamic cyclic center (positive feedback estrogen mechanism)
   (e) Thelarche

3. Which one of the following potential causes of maternal death is always classified as a "Direct Maternal Death?"
   (a) Heart disease
   (b) Infection
   (c) Embolization (thrombotic)
   (d) Hemorrhage
   (e) Toxemias (preeclampsia)

4. Puerperal infections are generally caused by which type of organisms?
   (a) Beta-hemolytic streptococci
   (b) *Staphylococcus aureus*
   (c) Anaerobic organisms
   (d) *Bacteroides fragilis*
   (e) Clostridia

5. A fetal death occurring between the 20th and 28th gestational week when the birth weight is between 500 and 999 grams is classified as:
   (a) intermediate fetal death
   (b) abortion

(c) late fetal death
(d) immature fetal death
(e) perinatal death

6. The commonest classification of fetal mortality by cause of death is:
   (a) erythroblastosis
   (b) placental or umbilical causes
   (c) congenital anomalies
   (d) maternal medical causes
   (e) no known cause

7. Which of the following is a positive sign of pregnancy?
   (a) Positive pregnancy test (sensitive radioimmunoassay method)
   (b) Outlining the fetus (Leopold's maneuvers)
   (c) Perception of fetal movements by the examiner
   (d) Ballottement
   (e) Intermittent uterine contractions (Braxton Hicks sign)

8. Which one of the following causes of abortion is most clearly associated with losses in the second trimester?
   (a) Abnormal chromosomes
   (b) Anomalous or pathologic uterus
   (c) Localized anomaly of embryo
   (d) Abnormal placentation/defective trophoblast
   (e) None of the above

9. The patient was in her 10th gestational week and she began to complain of crampy pain, gush of clear fluid followed by minimal vaginal bleeding. On examination, her uterus was compatible with dates with respect to size and the cervix was dilated to about 1 to 2 cm. size. What type of abortion listed below is the most likely diagnosis?
   (a) Inevitable abortion
   (b) Threatened abortion
   (c) Incomplete abortion
   (d) Missed abortion
   (e) Hydatidiform mole

10. Which one of the following entries is more effective in distinguishing between a missed abortion and hydatidiform mole?
    (a) Disappearing symptoms and signs of pregnancy
    (b) Dark brown turbid vaginal drainage
    (c) Presence of comsumption coagulopathy
    (d) Presence of cystic ovaries
    (e) Ultrasonic snowstorm pattern in the uterus

11. Which one of the following entries is best in identifying a high risk case of trophoblast dis-

ease that may require more aggressive initial therapy?

(a) Duration of disease prior to onset of chemotherapy of more than 4 months

(b) Initial hCG titers over 100,000

(c) Cerebral metastases

(d) Hepatic metastases

(e) All of the above

12. Three weeks postpartally following a normal term delivery, the patient developed persistent vaginal bleeding, uterine and subinvolution and bilateral cystic ovaries. The most likely diagnosis is:

(a) hydatidiform mole

(b) choriocarcinoma

(c) retained placental fragments

(d) pelvic inflamatory disease

(e) pelvic hematoma

13. Which one of the following types of ectopic pregnancy is more often associated with delayed rupture and marked hemorrhage?

(a) Ovarian implantation

(b) Interstitial tubal implantation

(c) Isthmic tubal implantation

(d) Ampullary tubal implantation

(e) Infundibular tubal implantation

14. A multipara stated that in the first trimester of pregnancy she experienced sudden pain and sensation of syncope which subsided but subsequently in the second and third trimesters, she has been experiencing gastrointestinal symptoms, painful fetal movements and now at term, attacks of false labor without bleeding. A probable diagnosis is:

(a) abdominal pregnancy

(b) abruptio placenta with concealed hemorrhage

(c) placenta previa

(d) silent uterine rupture with contained bivad ligament hematoma

(e) multiple gestation with impaired circulation in one twin

15. In which one of the following obstetrical situations would you least likely associate with the complication of consumption coagulopathy?

(a) Abruptio placenta

(b) Rupture of the uterus

(c) Placenta previa

(d) Amniotic fluid embolus

(e) Missed abortion

16. If a laboring patient you have been examining and following suddenly ruptures her membrane and develops minimal vaginal bleeding and fetal distress in the absence of increased pain or uterine tone, hypotension, tachycardia, oliguria or other local or systemic sign or symptom, which of the following underlying clinical conditions would you suspect?

(a) Ruptured umbilical cord vessel

(b) Cervical laceration

(c) Marginal abruptio placenta

(d) Silent uterine rupture

(e) Change of low implantation to placenta previa when cervix dilates

17. Based on your clinical impression from question 16, which one of the following methods of investigation would provide the best means of establishing the diagnosis?

(a) Pelvic sonogram (Placental localization)

(b) Check urine for blood indicative of bladder trauma

(c) Speculum examination of the lower generative tract

(d) Kleinhaur smear

(e) "Double set-up" examination

18. Abruptio placenta is a complication of one or more obstetrical conditions listed below. Which entry below is most likely response?

(a) Chronic hypertension

(b) Diabetes mellitus class D

(c) Chronic nephritis

(d) Preeclampsia/Aclampsia

(e) All of the above

19. There are clinical distinctions to be made between abruptio placenta and placenta previa. Which one of the following entries is the most accurate response?

(a) Placenta previa is always associated with painless vaginal bleeding, while in abruptio placenta the painful nature of the clinical picture is dominant.

(b) In abruptio placenta the uterus remains tetanically contracted, while in placenta previa it is flaccid.

(c) Initial bleeding in placenta previa is usually life threatening, while it is more likely minimal or even concealed in abruptio placenta.

(d) The absence of fetal distress tends to rule out placenta previa.

(e) Almost one third of the cases of abruptio placenta are first diagnosed "postpartally" when the placenta is available for inspection.

20. The least likely cause of postpartal hemorrhage is which one of the following potential etiologies?

(a) Uterine atony

(b) Laceration and/or hematoma; ruptured varix

(c) Retained placenta and/or membranes

(d) Ruptured uterus prolapsed uterus; or inversion of uterus

(e) Blood dyscrasia

21. Clinical signs and symptoms during labor characterized by cessation of uterine contractions, fetal distress with rapid disappearance of fetal heart sounds, regression of a previously engaged presenting part, hypovolemic shock and external or concealed hemorrhage, suggest which one of the following complications?

(a) Ruptured uterus

(b) Abruptio placenta

(c) Abdominal pregnancy (or intraligamentary)

(d) Heterotopic pregnancy (in utero gestation in addition to an ectopic gestation)

(e) Placenta accreta (or placenta with rupture through the wall by the myometrial trophoblast)

22. A primigravidous patient with hypertensive disease of pregnancy as well as edema and proteinuria seemed to be developing toxemia at the 18th gestational week. The uterus was soft and compatible with dates and there was no bleeding. There has been no prior evidence of hypertension or nephritis. What is the most likely diagnosis?

(a) Essential hypertension aggravated by pregnancy

(b) Multiple pregnancy

(c) Renal hypertension provoked by maternal physiological changes affecting the kidneys

(d) Hydatidiform mole

(e) Pheochromocytoma collagen disease (lupus erythematosus, nephrotic syndrome or other condition referred to as "pseudo-preeclampsia"

23. A 20-year-old primigravida had a normal pregnancy until the 37th gestational week when she developed a rise in the systolic blood pressure of 40 and a rise in diastolic pressure of 20. The other findings were hyperreflexia, proteinuria of 3 g. per 24 hr., urinary output of 100 ml. per 24 hr. and mild edema of the face and hands. There was no tachycardia, fever, pulmonary edema, anasarca, epigastric pain, CNS irritation or cloudy sensorum. Her past medical history was totally unremarkable. Apparently, the fetal growth and development was normal and the uterus was compatible with dates and there was no evidence of fetal dis-

tress. Which one of the following therapeutic approaches is the best?

(a) Force fluids to flush the kidneys but restrict the salt intake substantially

(b) Administer diuretics to correct edema and minimize risks of pulmonary edema

(c) Administer Digoxin to minimize the risks of congestive heart failure (Along with prescribed rest regime)

(d) Administer apresoline (hydralazine) to minimize the risks of intracranial hemorrhage

(e) Admit the patient immediately to the hospital for evaluation *without any* ambulatory treatments

24. The patient under discussion in question 23 was given intravenous fluids and magnesium sulfate intramuscularly. Which one of the following findings reflects most acutely upon the dose level and timing of $MgSO_4$ administrations?

(a) Lowered blood pressure in the first 30 minutes after administration

(b) Decreased variability of the fetal heart on the heart rate monitor

(c) Reduction in urinary output to 500 ml. per 24 hr.

(d) Increase in proteinuria to 4 g. per 24 hr.

(e) Absent knee jerks

25. The physiological action of hydralazine is best represented by which one of the following responses?

(a) All of the actions below

(b) Reflex tachycardia

(c) Increases renal flow

(d) Increases cardiac output

(e) Smooth muscle relaxant

26. Which one of the following statements about twins is correct?

(a) Monozygotic twinning is a recessive autosomal trait inherited from the female descendants of mothers of twins

(b) Monochorionic placentas are *always* monozygotic

(c) Divisions occurring in a single ovum before the differentiation of the trophoblast at day 5 or before result in single placentas with one chorionic

(d) Monochorionic placenta with vascular communications of the artery-to-artery or vein-to-vein are the most serious fetal risks

(e) The so-called fetus acardiacus is a fetal teratomatous tumor arising in the gonad which resembles a parasitic second twin

27. Which one of the following categories of multiple pregnancy constitutes the gravest hazard to the fetuses?
    (a) Monochorion diamniotic placenta
    (b) Dichorionic-diamniotic placenta
    (c) Dichorionic fused placenta
    (d) Velamentous insertion of the cord
    (e) Monoamniotic monochorionic placenta

28. Which one of the following entries pertaining to the progress of labor and eventual outcome represents the best response to the question of which major factor(s) is or are involved?
    (a) The passage
    (b) The powers
    (c) The passenger
    (d) The placenta
    (e) All of the above

29. Most pelves are morphologically of the:
    (a) gynecoid type
    (b) android type
    (c) anthropoid type
    (d) platepelloid type
    (e) mixed type

30. Initiation of labor may involve:
    (a) Myometrial stretch reflex increasing fetal cortisone
    (b) augmented estradiol and estrone
    (c) increase in Prostaglandin production and release of oxytocin
    (d) free calcium activates ATP-ase which acts on ATP to activate the contractile protein
    (e) all of the above

31. What is the most common dysfunction leading to abnormal progress in labor?
    (a) Soft tissue dystocia
    (b) Hypotonic labor
    (c) Dystonic labor
    (d) Hypertonic labor
    (e) None of the above

32. Oxytocin stimulation of dysfunctional labor has its greatest usefulness in certain types of clinical symptoms. Which one of the following entries is the best response relative to indication for this approach to management?
    (a) Hypertonic labor
    (b) Dystonic labor
    (c) Reverse peristalsis
    (d) Segmental tetanic contracture
    (e) None of the above

33. Which one of the following mechanisms of normal labor in vertex presentation is an abnormal occurrence before the fetal head reaches the perineum?
    (a) Engagement
    (b) Extension
    (c) Descent
    (d) Internal rotation
    (e) Flexion

34. The patient has a septic abortion associated with anaerobic organisms with a gram negative bacteremia. She was treated wtih ampicillin and chloramphenicol. After 3 days of some clinical improvement, she began to experience fatigue, pallor and tachycardia and when blood counts were evaluated she had a pancytopenia. There was an alarmingly low red count of 1 million/ul red blood cells and these were slightly macrocytic, the icteric index was low. A bone marrow study revealed normal hemosiderin on stained smear but the marrow was fatty with few red cells, white cells or magakaryocytes. The likely diagnosis is:
    (a) iron deficiency anemia
    (b) folic acid deficiency anemia
    (c) pernicious anemia
    (d) aplastic anemia
    (e) drug-induced anemia

35. An 18-year-old female with primary amenorrhea had normally developed secondary sex characteristics. On workup she failed to have withdrawal bleeding after the progestational challenge or cyclic conjugated estrogen-progesterone administrations. Workup revealed a normal 46XX karyotype. An intravenous pyelogram revealed an anomalous urinary tract on the left. On pelvic examination, a morphological defect was discovered. What do you suspect it is (indicate one of the following conditions)?
    (a) Testicular feminization
    (b) Asherman's syndrome
    (c) Müllerian agenesis
    (d) Transcerse vaginal septum
    (e) None of the above

36. A 30-year-old patient with secondary amenorrhea, galactorrhea and hyperprolactaemia is likely to have which one of the following disorders?
    (a) Hypothalamic amenorrhea
    (b) Disorder of the pituitary gland (adenoma)
    (c) Ovarian disorder (ovarian steroid defect)
    (d) Breast disorder (response to chronic suckling)
    (e) Disorder of genetic constitution with uterine or lower generative tract defect

37. Which one of the following statements is the best response concerning testosterone production in the normal female?

(a) Testosterone in the circulation arises from direct ovarian secretion.

(b) Testosterone in the circulation arises from direct secretion from the adrenal gland.

(c) Testosterone in the circulation arises from peripheral conversion, mainly from the reduction of androstenedione.

(d) A major fraction of secreted ovarian androgens is synthesized in the stroma.

(e) All of the above are correct.

38. Which one of the following statements is the best response concerning conditions associated with a steady state of estrogen stimulation that leads to irregular endometrial shedding characteristic dysfunctional uterine bleeding?

(a) Continously proliferating endometrium may outgrow its blood supply.

(b) The persistence of acid mucopolysaccharides causes a loss of nutrients by preventing depolymerization and diffusion of these substances.

(c) Asynchronous development of the glands, stroma, and blood vessels.

(d) Overdevelopment of Golgi-lysosomal complex capable of releasing excessive amounts of hydrolytic enzymes.

(e) All of the above are correct.

39. A 25-year-old patient developed dysuria, frequency, urgency, chills, fever, malaise, lower abdominal pain, yellow vaginal discharge and marked pelvic tenderness. Which one of the following simple investigative procedures is most likely to establish the diagnosis?

(a) Gram stain of cervical smear

(b) Wet preparation of vaginal discharge

(c) Nickerson's medium culture of vaginal discharge

(d) Papanicolaou smear

(e) Urine culture

40. Which one of the following causes of vaginitis is the best response to the clinical problem of vaginal burning, pruritis and dyspareunia in association with a thin, often watery, bubbly, frothy white to yellowish vaginal discharge, erythematous mucosa, petechial hemorrhages and "strawberry" spots?

(a) Trichomonas vaginalis

(b) Monilial vaginitis

(c) Atrophic vaginitis

(d) Nonspecific vaginitis

(e) Early cervical carcinoma

41. Which one of the following is the best response to the question of theories of etiology and mechanism of dissemination in pelvic endometriosis?

(a) Tubal reflux (Sampson Theory)

(b) Coelomic metaplasia

(c) Vascular dissemination

(d) Lymphatic dissemination

(e) All of the above

42. The patient is a 35-year-old who has aborted twice at the 18th gestational week and she has complained of severe dysmenorrhea, hypermenorrhea, some increased vaginal discharge and spotting intermenstrually. On pelvic examination the uterus was slightly irregular, firm and enlarged to an 8 week gestational size. The impression is that she has a leiomyomatous uterus. What type of uterine tumor is associated with these types of clinical presentations?

(a) Submucous leiomyoma

(b) Intramural leiomyoma

(c) Subserosal leiomyoma

(d) Intraligamentary leiomyoma or (parasitic)

(e) None of the above

43. What are the basic infertility screening procedures? Which entry below represents the best answer?

(a) Semen analysis

(b) Evaluation of ovulatory function

(c) Tubal patency tests

(d) The postcoital examination

(e) All of the above

44. The important causes of female infertility include the following factors:

(a) tubes and peritoneum

(b) the ovaries

(c) the cervix

(d) the uterine fundus

(e) all of the above in descending order of relative importance

45. If the basic tests in the infertility workup are uninformative, which one of the following special investigations is likely to be most rewarding?

(a) Tests for sperm allergy

(b) Skull roentgenogram for sella turcica

(c) Buccal smear (chromisomal analysis

(d) Laparoscopy

(e) Hysteroscopy

46. Which one of the five leading reversible methods of contraception is the most effective?

(a) Oral contraceptives (the pill)

(b) Barrier contraception with jelly

(c) The intrauterine device (IUD)

(d) Condom and foam

(e) Post ovulatory rhythm

47. Which one of the complications is least likely to be associated with the use of the IUD?
    (a) Breakthrough vaginal bleeding
    (b) Hypermenorrhea
    (c) Dysmenorrhea
    (d) Endometrial cancer
    (e) Pelvic infection

48. Which one of the following entries is the best response to the question of positive colposcopic findings in the cervix?
    (a) White epithelium
    (b) Punctation
    (c) Mosaic structure
    (d) Abnormal vessels
    (e) All of the above

49. A high risk microinvasive cervical lesion requiring special surgical attention involves which one(s) of the following histopathologic features? Mark the entity which represents the best response.
    (a) Microinvasive lesion of more than 3 to 5 ml. in depth
    (b) Deep cell nests
    (c) Confluence of nests of cells
    (d) Lymphatic or vascular involvements
    (e) All of the above findings

50. A 52-year-old woman who had never been able to conceive presented with anorexia, weight loss, nausea, abdominal discomfort, bloating, fullness and increasing tightness of the clothes. She was one year postmenopausal and there had been no vaginal bleeding. She had a positive family history of gynaecologic cancer. On pelvic examination, it was possible to feel a pelvic mass. The suspicion of a malignancy should focus upon which one of the following sites?
    (a) Ovary
    (b) Tube
    (c) Endometrium
    (d) Cervix or vagina
    (e) Nongynecologic organ

Based on your knowledge that a certain pattern of urine loss often characterizes a particular type of underlying defect or disorder, please match the following items (51-53) and (54-56) by writing the appropriate letter (a, b, or c).

51. Genito-urinary fistula   (a) slightly delayed loss after coughing
52. Neurogenic bladder   (b) continuous urine loss
53. Detrusor dyssynergia   (c) precipitous voiding

54. Irritable bladder   (a) without voiding action losses with increased abdominal pressure
55. Urethral deformity   (b) dribbling upon standing after emptying the bladder
56. Stress incontinence   (c) loss with urge

Recognizing that flexible clinical policies and some degree of controversy exist about the selection of proper definitive procedures in the management of early cervical neoplasia, please choose your preference of therapeutic modality listed in the right column (a-e) for each of the cervical lesions indicated in the left column.

57. Mild to moderate dysplasia   (a) radical hysterectomy with pelvic lymphadenectomy
58. Severe dysplasia   (b) extrafascial hysterectomy with or without excision of vaginal cuff
59. Carcinoma in situ   (c) intrafascial hysterectomy without excision of vaginal cuff
60. Microinvasion, less than 3mm, nonconfluent; absence of lymphatic or vascular channel invasion.   (d) cold knife conization and curettage
61. Microinvasion, 3 to 5mm, confluent; vascular and lymphatic invasion.   (e) cryosurgery (double freeze technic).

Please assign to each statement below, the proper letter based on the following key: (Pertains only to questions 62 and 63).
    (a) if only 1, 2 and 3 entries are best answers.
    (b) if only 1 and 3 are best answers.
    (c) if only 2 and 4 are best answers.
    (d) if only 4 is the best answer.
    (e) if some other combination is best.

The patient began to exhibit mild uterine irritability in the 35th gestational week despite a rigid best regime and a slight increase in her blood pressure occurred. Prompt hospitalization reversed these changes but monitoring tests were intensified. At the 36th week one or more of the following reports were worrisome.

62. (1) The urinary estriol level had fallen slightly below the 10th percentile of control normal values in our laboratory (also more than two standard deviations below the mean for normals)

(2) Serial ultrasonic cephalometry showed a fetal growth rate below the 10th percentile for the first time

(3) Amniocentesis yielded clear amniotic fluid, an L/S ratio of 2.2 and a creatinine concentration of 2.0 mg. per 100ml.

(4) The serum HPL levels of the mother had fallen to a level below 4 mcg./ml.

63. (1) The superimposition of preeclampsia is the most common hazard of hypertensive disease.

(2) Preeclampsia superimposed on chronic hypertensive disease manifests itself by a subtle rise in blood pressure, and the appearance of edema or substantial proteinuria is relatively uncommon.

(3) When preeclampsia develops in association with hypertension, it is likely to be earlier than in normal pregnancy.

(4) Control of blood pressure by antihypertensive drugs has been highly effective in reducing the incidence of preeclampsia and in reducing perinatal mortality.

64. The overwhelming majority of pelvic infections are produced by endogenous organisms. Which one of the following organisms is considered an "endogenous" type?
    (a) *N.* gonorrhoea.
    (b) Group A beta-hemolytic streptococcus.
    (c) *Myco* tuberculosis
    (d) *Staph. aureus*
    (e) Klebsiella

65. Which of the following anaerobic bacteria is the most likely species to be encountered clinically when serious pelvic infections develop?
    (a) Fusobacteria (gram-negative bacillus)
    (b) Clostridia (gram-positive bacillus)
    (c) Peptostreptococci (gram-positive coccus)
    (d) Actinomyces (gram-positive bacillus)
    (e) Bacteroides fragilis (gram-negative bacillus)

Please attempt to match the rather classic clinical lesions on the left with the corresponding venereal diseases.

66. Destructive vulvar ulceration, nodal masses and procto-colitis | (a) Granuloma inguinale

67. Nontender, raised, firm, indurated papules with a raised border. | (b) Chancroid

68. Tender, irregular, serpiginous ulcerations, soft erythe-matous grayish or yellowish necrotic exudate | (c) Primary syphilis (chancre)

69. Autoinoculation, beefy, granulations keloidlike depigmented scars, superficial ulcerations. | (d) Lymphogranuloma venereum

70. Multiple and flesh-colored pinkish papillary, or sessile growths on mucous membranes or perineum. | (e) Condylomata acuminata

The presence of suspicion of one veneral disease requires multiple tests to exclude others. Please match the relatively standard tests itemized on the left with the appropriate letter.

71. Diploid human fibroblast culture; cytologic changes in Pap smear | (a) Lymphogranuloma venereum

72. Culture purulent discharge (cervix) on modified Thayer-Martin medium agar; culture anus. | (b) Herpes virus 2

73. Gram stain, material at base of ulcer (Giemsa stain) to detect *H. ducreyi* bacillus | (c) Gonorrhea

74. Biopsy granulation tissue (Wright and Giemsa stains) to detect Donovan bodies. | (d) Chancroid

75. Positive chamydial complement fixation test; Frei test | (e) Granuloma inguinale

Please associate the following veneral diseases with their recommended treatment. Discount the fact that resistant organisms may be present and that alternative therapy may be required.

76. Gonorrheal cervicitis | (a) Tetracycline

77. Primary syphilis | (b) Sulfasoxazole

78. Lymphogranuloma venereum | (c) Aqueous procaine penicillin

79. Chancroid | (d) Tetracycline and gentamicin

80. Granuloma ingui-   (e) Benzathine penicillin
    nale   G

81. Which one of the following antepartal methods of assessing fetal jeopardy is most valuable in programming clinical management in patients with RH incompatibility?
    (a) Obstetrical history
    (b) Determination of maternal antibody titers
    (c) Spectrophotometric screening of amniotic fluid
    (d) Chemical assay amniotic fluid bilirubin
    (e) RH genotype test to determine zygosity of the father

Specific anatomic and functional changes occur at the several phases of the menstrual cycle in synchronized events involving glandular, vascular, and stromal components of the endometrium. Please match the following:

82. Shallow endome-   (a) Endometrial break-
    trium with desqua-   down
    mation and collapse
    of the supporting
    matrix representing
    a transitional state
    bridging exfoliative
    and growth stages.

83. Saw-tooth glands;   (b) Preparation for im-
    vacuoles, stromal   plantation
    edema; coiled spiral
    vessels; tortuous dis-
    tended gland lu-
    mina.

84. Shrinkage of en-   (c) Proliferative phase
    dometrial height; di-
    minished blood flow
    and venous drain-
    age; vasodilation,
    rhythmic vasocon-
    striction and relax-
    ation of spiral arte-
    rioles; ischemia;
    white cell migration;
    interstitial red cells,
    tissue disorganiza-
    tion

85. Continuous epithe-   (d) Menstrual Endome-
    lial lining; un-   trium
    branched spiral
    vessels; peripheral
    extension of gland
    epithelium pseudo-
    stratification, mi-

toses; loose, syncytial-like stroma; increasing endometrial height

86. Engorged subep-   (e) Secretory Phase.
    ithelial capillaries &
    spiral vessels; large,
    polyhedral stromal
    cells in superficial
    endometrium; lace-
    like edematous
    stroma; coiled spiral
    vessels; exhausted,
    dilated glandular
    ribbons of stratum
    spongiosum com-
    pressed gland necks.

87. Among DES—exposed young females with gross structural changes in the vagina and/or cervix which one of the following abnormalities is most likely to interfere with thorough evaluation and ultimately require surgical attention because of associated symptoms or worrisome epithelial changes, and potential of subsequent reproductive losses?
    (a) Transverse ridges, complete or incomplete bands of tissue in the proximal part of the vagina
    (b) Peaked, roughened anterior cervical lip (cock comb shape)
    (c) Cervical collar or hood
    (d) Hypoplastic cervix or eccentrically located cervical OS
    (e) Pseudopolyps of the cervix

88. Which one of the following genital organs originates from the involvement of two distinct embryologic structures?
    (a) Ovaries)
    (b) Tubes
    (c) Uterus
    (d) Vagina
    (e) External genitalia

Among apparently well women who suffer from abnormal or absent menstrual function disturbances within the hypothalamic, pituitary, ovarian axis may be classified broadly according to three major faults. Please match the resultant clinical expressions with the appropriate defect noted in Questions 89, 90, and 91.

89. ovarian failure   (a) hypogonadotropic
                           hypogonadism
90. central failure   (b) asynchronous gona-

dotropin & estrogen production.

91. anovulatory dys-
function

    (c) hypergonadotropic, hypogonadism

92. Among the various presenting symptoms of patients with ovarian malignancy, which one of the following manifestations is the most common?
    (a) Abnormal vaginal bleeding
    (b) Gastrointestinal symptoms
    (c) Abdominal distention and/or discomfort
    (d) Weight loss
    (e) Urinary complaints (pressure frequency)

93. Which one of the following surgical procedures designed to restore reproductive function in the presence of tubal and pelvic peritoneal disease enjoys the overall greater chance of success?
    (a) Salpingolysis
    (b) Fibrioplasty
    (c) Partial resection and reanastomosis
    (d) Tubal implantation
    (e) Tubal bypass (Estes procedure and replacement operations)

94. Which one of the following chemotherapeutic agents has documented activity and enjoys considerable popularity as the traditional drug of choice as initial adjuvant therapy in ovarian malignancy?
    (a) cyclophosphamide
    (b) actinomycin-D
    (c) methotrexate
    (d) adriamycin
    (e) melphalan

95. Roughly what percentage of patients with metastatic epithelial ovarian cancer will be benefited by treatment with an alkylating agent?
    (a) less than 10 per cent
    (b) 25 to 49 per cent
    (c) 50 to 74 per cent
    (d) 75 to 89 per cent
    (e) more than 90 per cent

96. The best prognosis in endometrial adenocarcinoma occurs in Stage I.a. Which ones of the following features are characteristic of the early lesion?
    (a) if only 1, 2, and 3 entries are best answers
    (b) if only 1 and 3 are best answers
    (c) if only 2 and 4 are best answers
    (d) if only 4 is the best answer
    (e) if some other combination is best
    (1) The disease is confined to the corpus of the uterus
    (2) The uterus sounds to less than 8.0cm

(3) The histological appearance is that of a well differentiated tumor
(4) Encocervical curetings are positive for tumor but not the ectocervix

97. Endometrial cancer is now considered to be the most common female pelvic malignancy with respect to the presence of associated conditions and epidemiologic variables. Which one(s) of the following entries and possible etiologic factors have been identified.
    NOTE: Please use the same key presented in Question 96.
    (1) Longstanding endogenous or exogenous estrogen exposure, particularly estrone.
    (2) Obesity and increased tissue conversion of androstenedione to estrone.
    (3) Diabetes mellitus and/or hypertension.
    (4) Endometrial polyps, adenomyosis and/or leiomyomata.

98. Which one of the following vulvar diseases is *not* one of the circumscribed or diffuse "white lesions"?
    (a) Hypertrophic dystrophy (lichen simplex chronicus or neurodermatitis)
    (b) Atrophic dystrophies (Lichen sclerosus et atrophicus)
    (c) Mixed vulvar dystrophies
    (d) Intraepithelial cancer
    (e) Extra mammay Paget's disease

99. In considering the hormonal interrelationships in lactation, which one of the following agent is primarily involved in milk ejection rather than breast preparation, initiation of lactation or maintenance of lactation
    (a) Drop in serum estrogen and prozesterone
    (b) Oxytocin
    (c) Prolactin
    (d) Placental lactogen
    (e) Thyroxin

100. Certain anatomic considerations of the cervix must be taken into account in obtaining materials for diagnostic study. Which one of the following statements is *least* likely to be correct?
    (a) The early lesions of the cervix are usually associated with the squamocolumnar junction.
    (b) The portio vaginalis which, is most visible and easiest to biopsy, is not the area of greatest interest in diagnosing early carcinoma.
    (c) As metaplasia develops in columnar epithelium, tongues of stratified squamous eipthelium may extend from the endocervical canal onto the portio vaginalis.

(d) The squamocolumnar junction is always within the distal two centimeters of the endo-cervical canal.

(e) Surgical biopsies taken properly should attempt to include intact and adequate epithelium from the endocervical canal in the specimen.

ANSWERS TO MULTIPLE CHOICE QUESTIONS

1. (c)	26. (b)	51. (b)	76. (c)
2. (d)	27. (e)	52. (c)	77. (e)
3. (e)	28. (e)	53. (a)	78. (a)
4. (c)	29. (e)	54. (c)	79. (b)
5. (a)	30. (e)	55. (b)	80. (d)
6. (e)	31. (b)	56. (a)	81. (c)
7. (c)	32. (e)	57. (e)	82. (d)
8. (b)	33. (b)	58. (c)	83. (e)
9. (a)	34. (d)	59. (b)	84. (a)
10. (e)	35. (c)	60. (b)	85. (c)
11. (e)	36. (b)	61. (a)	86. (b)
12. (b)	37. (e)	62. (e)	87. (a)
13. (b)	38. (e)	63. (b)	88. (d)
14. (a)	39. (a)	64. (e)	89. (c)
15. (c)	40. (a)	65. (e)	90. (a)
16. (a)	41. (e)	66. (d)	91. (b)
17. (d)	42. (a)	67. (c)	92. (c)
18. (e)	43. (e)	68. (b)	93. (a)
19. (e)	44. (e)	69. (a)	94. (e)
20. (e)	45. (d)	70. (e)	95. (c)
21. (a)	46. (a)	71. (b)	96. (a)
22. (d)	47. (d)	72. (c)	97. (a)
23. (e)	48. (e)	73. (d)	98. (e)
24. (e)	49. (e)	74. (e)	99. (b)
25. (a)	50. (a)	75. (a)	100. (d)

11

Pediatrics

PAUL R. PATTERSON, M.D.

Professor of Pediatrics, Albany Medical College of Union University

Pediatrics begins in utero! In fact, the problems of infancy and childhood may even begin before conception takes place. Nutritional deprivation, socioeconomic status, physical illness and genetic abnormalities in either parent have a predispositional effect upon the growing fetus. Even the mother's emotional attitude toward the unborn child may indirectly influence that infant's subsequent growth and development. Malnutrition, excessive cigarette smoking, drug addiction, moderate alcohol use, and coitus in the last trimester as an example may result in small fetal size or an increased incidence of minor birth defects or in prematurity or neonatal infection of the infant.

Fetal growth, likewise, may be influenced by primiparity, small heart volume, living at high altitude, chronic or preeclamptic hypertensive disease and other maternal diseases of sufficient duration and severity. As examples, mothers of White's class A–C may have large-for-dates babies, whereas mothers of classes D, E, F, and H have small-for-dates babies. Severe diabetes in the mother may result in fetal growth retardation although babies born to prediabetic mothers or fathers may be larger than normal.

It is recommended that infants weighing less than 2500 g. (5½ lb.) should be called *infants of low birth weight* instead of being given the customary label of premature. It may be difficult to distinguish an infant *small for gestational age* (SGA) secondary to genetic or hereditary causes as well as the environmental variety such as those caused by placental insufficiency (pseudopremature) from an infant born after a short gestation (true premature). An infant may have been born of a mother with placental insufficiency resulting from a variety of pathologic states of the placenta and, even though full term, may be underweight. The infant may go beyond term and be labeled postmature and still weigh less than a normal term infant.

Severe maternal illness caused by infectious agents such as mumps, influenza, measles, pneumonia, typhoid and paratyphoid fever may cause prematurity. Infections occurring late in gestation such as hepatitis, herpes simplex, syphilis, cytomegalic inclusion disease, rubella, Coxsackie B virus, smallpox, chickenpox, rubeola, and herpes virus type II are more likely to cause illness in the infant following birth. The only known infectious agents that unequivocally cause teratologic effects on the human fetus are the rubella, cytomegalic viruses and toxoplasmosis.

Radiation given for therapeutic reasons to the pelvic area of the mother may cause defects in 50 to 75 per cent of those children born alive. Microcephaly and mental retardation are increased significantly in pregnancy exposed between the seventh and fifteenth weeks of gestation. Subsequent growth retardation may be observed as well. Increased radiation does cause genetic mutation, but the long-term effects of background radiation on future generations cannot be predicted.

Chemicals and drugs administered to the mother may not only interfere with the subsequent resuscitation of the newborn but may produce congenital malformations. Permanent structural changes are the conspicuous effect of gonadal hormones, and fetal female masculinization may follow the use of steroid sex hormones (estrogen, testosterone, progesterone or their analogues) in certain pregnant women if administered during the first trimester. Administration of these hormones later during the pregnancy may lead to enlargement of the clitoris in female infants. Tetracyclines may interfere with the skeletal growth in addition to the staining of deciduous teeth and hyperplasia of the enamel as the result of transplacental acquisition by the fetus. While novobiocin and chloramphenicol have been observed to have adverse effects on the premature and newborn infant, no effect on the fetus has been noted. Sulfanilamides resemble aspirin in that they have a propensity for dissociating bilirubin from its protective binding to albumin. This freed bilirubin may diffuse into the central nervous system, exerting permanent damaging effects, as one may observe in the immediate postnatal period when there is a critical relationship between bilirubin production and the metabolism of bilirubin by the liver.

In the treatment of maternal thyroid difficulties, the use of radioactive iodine may lead to congenital malformations of the fetus in addition to destructive effects on the fetal thyroid. Congenital goiters may occur in the offspring of mothers who have received thiouracil derivatives inasmuch as the drug may inhibit thyroxine synthesis by the independently functioning thyroid of the fetus. Goiters may also develop in infants of asthmatic mothers treated with iodine-containing preparations.

Reserpine administered within 2 days prior to delivery has led to a recognizable syndrome in the infant characterized by lethargy, anorexia, respiratory depression and a nasal discharge, which subsides spontaneously within the first week. If symptoms persist choanal atresia needs to be ruled out by passing a catheter into both nares and down into the pharynx.

Paraldehyde administration to mothers has been associated with drowsiness in the newborn for as long as 5 to 6 days following birth. As would be expected, almost any hypnotic sedative will have some depressive effect on the newborn. The short-acting barbiturates are the drugs of choice if they are required. However, it is important to bear in mind that the inadequate excretory and metabolic mechanisms in the fetus may result in increased barbiturate concentrations that may then subsequently cause anesthesia of the infant who may succumb to depression of the respiratory center.

Unusual drug addiction, such as to morphine, may cause withdrawal symptoms in the newborn characterized by a high-pitched cry, irritability and convulsions several days after birth. Addicted mothers being treated with methadone may give birth to infants with new and delayed withdrawal symptoms that may become manifest several days or weeks after delivery. These infants may even be at greater risk than those of heroin-addicted mothers. LSD has been implicated as causing chromosomal abnormalities and may ultimately join other drugs such as thalidomide as being teratogenic.

The true incidence of malformations is difficult to ascertain, because we recognize that it is possible to have molecular malformation, chromosomal malformation, cellular malformation, anatomic malformation and even functional malformation or anomalies such as abnormal intelligence and behavior patterns developing at a later age. It is known, however, that certain chromosome abnormalities are found most frequently in the products of miscarriages in the first trimester. At the very least, the overall incidence of morphologic malformations in fetal deaths is about 9 per cent as contrasted with 15 per cent in deaths occurring within the first 28 days. However, careful examination of these products of conception would probably double these figures. A single umbilical cord artery is associated with an increased incidence of defects in the newborn. Diabetic mothers have five times the incidence of a single umbilical artery.

The United States ranks fifteenth among the nations of the world in the rate of survival in the perinatal period. In addition to the factors mentioned as causing increased mortality, one must consider the possibility that with improved obstetric care, infants are being born that did not survive in utero in years gone by.

Briefly, taking direct blood samples from the fetus to determine fetal blood pH as well as carbon dioxide and oxygen tension has helped to recognize fetal hypoxia. Amniocentesis, exchange transfusions in utero and many other dramatic obstetric procedures are being developed to treat the pediatric patient in utero.

At the time of delivery, one should be mindful that if the "bag of waters" has been ruptured for more than 24 hours there is the possibility that the fetus may have become infected with *Streptococcus faecalis, Escherichia coli, Aerobacter aerogenes,* wide group of beta streptococci, *Listeria monocytogenes* . . . and other paracolon bacteria. Chorioamnionitis occurs in about 10 per cent of all deliveries but may result from this premature rupture along with prolonged labor. Three methods may be utilized to determine inflammation of the fetal adnexa and thus direct attention to the infant as being a possible greater risk from neonatal infection.

a. The umbilical cord may be examined in frozen section to determine if there is infiltration of the vein wall by polymorphonuclear leukocytes. In fact, there may be migration of these leukocytes into the Wharton's jelly and subsequent inflammatory cells surrounding all three vessels of the cord.

b. A section of the amnion may be examined for the presence of leukocytes in the subamniotic tissue.

c. More frequently now the gastric aspirate or smears of the contents of the ear canal are being examined for increased WBC and organisms. The presence of organisms will tell that the body is colonized, but not infected.

Certain congenital defects may be predicted by the finding of a single umbilical artery. The incidence of not readily apparent defects may be as high as 15 to 20 per cent.

Severe oligohydramnios is indicated by the presence of numerous grayish yellow plaques on the fetal surface of the placenta as a result of the deposition of vernix on the surface of the amnion. This is associated with a high incidence of severe urinary tract anomalies and hypoplasia of the lungs in the newborn.

Polyhydramnios is associated with high G-I obstruction.

OBSERVATION AND CARE OF THE NEWBORN

After careful 9 months' observation of the mother, it behooves the physician to devote from 1 to 10 minutes in observing the newborn baby. To assist in this evaluation, the Apgar scoring system has been devised and recorded as the 1 minute and 5 minute Apgar. Table 11-1 depicts the five signs—heart rate, respiratory effort, muscle tone, reflex irritability and color—that are evaluated and given a rating of 0, 1 or 2. The scores are totaled and recorded. A score of 10 is optimal, and scores of 3 and below represent infants in very poor condition. It is a mistake to withhold resuscitation until the score is determined, especially in those infants suffering from unusual asphyxia due to prolapse of the cord, large breech presentation or impacted shoulders or those who have been found by intrapartum sampling of fetal scalp blood to be suffering from

acidosis. The pH of the infant's blood can drop from 7.4 to 6.9 in less than 5 minutes! The score at 1 minute does not reflect oxygenation but is rather a reflection of the acid-base status. In infants whose condition has produced concern, blood samples should be drawn from the umbilical artery rather than the vein to judge the condition of the infant, inasmuch as the umbilical vein reflects the placental exchange and not the status of the infant's arterial blood.

Most newborn infants weigh 2.7 to 4.1 kg. (6 to 9 lb.), the average weight being 3.4 kg. (7.5 lb.). The first newborn is often lighter than subsequent infants. There is usually initial loss during the first 3 or 4 days of life of approximately 10 per cent of the birth weight, which is regained by the seventh or eighth day.

The average length of the newborn is 50 cm. The average circumference of the head is 35 cm. This enlarges to 40 cm. at 4 months of age. These represent important measurements to be borne in mind in observing the early development of an abnormally enlarging head as in hydrocephaly or, conversely, of an abnormally small head as in primary microcephaly or craniosynostosis.

With one in every 60 infants born succumbing within the first 3 days of life and one in 40 dying within the first month of life, one should not take the examination of the newborn as an unimportant procedure. Inasmuch as more lives are lost in the first month of life than in the following 40 years of life, it is essential that there shall not only be a general knowledge of the obvious physical defects and abnormalities that may be present but also keen awareness of the normal physiology of the newborn as it differs from that of older children and adults.

At birth the infant is generally covered with vernix caseosa, a cheesy white substance. There may be edema of the scalp as a result of the passage through the birth canal with or without overriding of the bones of the skull. There may be reddened areas over the head where forceps have been placed. The natural folding of the infant reflects its position in utero. Sometimes we find that minor and occasionally major orthopedic abnormalities may be reflected by the intrauterine posture of the growing fetus.

Normal anatomic and physiologic variations may be observed that include telangiectases at the base of the nose and back of the head ("stork bites"); mongolian spot, which is a purplish discoloration at the base of the spine; phimosis; and little white epithelial pearls in the oral mucosa. The external auditory canal is short and the drum lies obliquely across the canal. The liver and spleen are commonly felt just below the costal margin, and the kidneys are often palpable. (An unusu-

TABLE 11–1. Apgar Scoring System

	Sign	0	Score 1	2
A	Appearance (color)	Blue; pale	Body pink; extremities blue	Completely pink
P	Pulse (heart rate)	Absent	Below 100	Over 100
G	Grimace (reflex irritability response to stimulation of sole of foot by glancing slap)	No response	Grimace	Cry
A	Activity (muscle tone)	Limp	Some flexion of extremities	Active motion
R	Respiration (respiratory effort)	Absent	Slow; irregular	Good strong cry

ally enlarged kidney at this age is more likely due to hydronephrosis than to Wilms' tumor at a later age.)

The establishment of a patent airway and adequate respiratory activity is the most important need of the newborn. The average respirations are 30 to 40 per minute. The infant will easily cry, sneeze, cough, yawn and stretch.

Heart rate ranges from 120 to 160 a minute. The heart appears larger in comparison to the size of the chest than is to be expected in the standard for older children. Murmurs heard in the first day of life may be less ominous than those heard at 1 to 2 weeks of age. Ninety per cent of these latter will subsequently represent congenital heart disease. Such loud murmurs as the machinery murmur of patent ductus arteriosus may not be heard at this time, however.

Normal reflexes such as rooting, which represents searching for the nipple, sucking, gagging and swallowing are present.

The newborn is relatively well supplied with body water and may easily go without feeding for several days if necessary. Sterile water should be utilized for the first feeding in case there is an abnormality of the esophagus or the trachea. Rectal temperature should be taken immediately to ascertain the patency of the anus.

The stools will be passed within 24 hours and will be black, representing meconium. The meconium stools may become greenish yellow to brown and be called transitional stools after oral feedings have begun. Intestinal stenosis and atresia and meconium ileus secondary to cystic fibrosis may permit a small passage of stools early, but the subsequent enlargement of the abdomen may suggest that these causes of intestinal obstruction are present. However, it is not unusual for a normal infant to have six to seven stools after the second day of life.

Epidemics of diarrhea occur from time to time in nurseries for newborn infants. Such outbreaks, called epidemic diarrhea of the newborn, are characterized by rapid spread through the nursery. The incubation period is usually short, in some outbreaks only a matter of a few hours, diarrhea being the first symptom. Resulting dehydration may end in death. In the majority of epidemics studied, the causative agent has been thought to be transferred from infant to infant for the most part by hands, linens or equipment as a result of error in nursery technique. Careful studies have revealed that various enteropathogenic strains of *Escherichia coli,* especially *E. coli* 055:B5, 011:B4 and 0127:B8, have been encountered more frequently than any other serogroups. Certain strains of staphylococcus and viruses such as ECHO virus 18 have likewise been isolated. Treatment consists of prompt isolation of the known cases with closure of the nursery from which the infant was transferred, institution of appropriate antibiotic therapy, but most of all, institution of prompt hydrating measures to correct the dehydration and acidosis before death results. In most neonatal bacterial infection, gentamycin and ampicillin in combination are the antibiotic of choice. Chloramphenicol may prove lethal to the neonate, and especially to premature infants, by producing the gray syndrome, which may progress to vascular collapse 6 to 48 hours after the onset of toxic signs. Sulfanilamides may cause kernicterus in premature infants. Streptomycin may cause deafness.

Ampicillin and gentamycin or kanamycin may be used as prophylactic antibiotic therapy when the amniotic fluid is obviously infected. Neonates should get a complete septic workup before initiation of therapy unless positive cultures have been obtained or there is evidence of clinical deterioration in the infant's status.

Antibiotic therapy is no longer recommended when meconium-stained skin or cord is noted, which may suggest possible aspiration of amniotic fluid, unless positive cultures have been obtained. Antibiotics are started on babies whose mothers have evidence of infection, an elevation of temperature, increase WBC with a shift to the left on differential peripheral blood count, positive smears in mothers who have a history of premature rupture of the membranes, and in those mothers who received antibiotics prior to delivery. The infants may not be symptomatic.

LOW BIRTH WEIGHT SYNDROME (PREMATURITY)

Low birth weight syndrome (prematurity), anoxia, birth injury and malformation are the four leading causes of perinatal mortality. The term perinatal mortality is applied to deaths of fetuses and infants weighing 1000 g. or over that occur between 28 weeks of gestational life and 28 days of neonatal life.

Because of the immaturity of the various systems of the body, the low birth weight infant is susceptible to pneumonia, septicemia, anoxia, cerebral injuries with hemorrhage and the idiopathic respiratory distress syndrome (hyaline membrane disease). The causes of respiratory distress and respiratory failure in newborn infants are listed in Table 11-2.

Idiopathic respiratory distress syndrome is by far the most common cause of death among true premature infants but is likewise seen in infants born of diabetic mothers following cesarean sections (where it may approach 50 per cent) and rarely in full-term infants.

In this condition, hyaline membranes are formed, lining the air spaces of the lungs. These are believed to be caused by an effusion from the pulmonary circulation with conversion of fibrinogen to fibrin (which probably has been increased by the thromboplastic activity of the aspirated amniotic fluid) and finally the absorption of the fluid leaving the fibrin deposit lining the pulmonary alveoli. However, it is thought by some that there may be absence of or alteration in the pulmonary surfactant, a phospholipid lining the alveoli, which has been implicated, but this theory is gradually losing disfavor as the pathophysiologic cause.

A third and alternative hypothesis is that the primary lesion is pulmonary hypoperfusion rather than the deficiency of surfactant. Intrauterine asphyxia produces increased vascular resistance (such as hypoxia produces in later childhood). This may cause shunting of almost all the cardiac output away from the lungs. The resulting ischemia of the lungs would cause damage to the alveolar lining cells that produce the surfactant and would explain the loss of surfactant and the resulting effusion. It is stated that when fibrinogen is changed to fibrin both peptide A and peptide B are produced. It is the peptide B that will potentiate the vasoconstriction in the lung.

Caution is given to resist administration of high levels of oxygen (over 40 per cent) inasmuch as retrolental fibroplasia may occur in the eyes, producing partial or complete blindness. Oxygen toxicity may result in pulmonary changes, with fibrosis eventually resulting.

Successful therapy may consist only of the use of oxygen, sodium bicarbonate to correct acidosis and assisted respiratory therapy. There is much debate as to what the treatment should be. Nevertheless, one

TABLE 11–2. Respiratory Distress and Failure in Newborn Infants

Type	Manifestations	Examples
Central nervous system failure	Apnea Slow irregular, gasping respiratory efforts	1. Narcosis 2. Prenatal or perinatal anoxia 3. Intracranial hemorrhage or trauma 4. CNS anomalies
Peripheral respiratory difficulty	Rapid respiratory rate Increasing respiratory rate Chest lag Intercostal retraction Subcostal retraction Xiphoid retraction Chin tug Expiratory grunt Frothing at lips	1. Primary atelectasis 2. Congestive pulmonary failure 3. Idiopathic respiratory distress (hyaline membrane syndrome) 4. Aspiration of amniotic fluid containing formed elements 5. Pneumonia 6. Diaphragmatic hernia 7. Lung cysts 8. Lobar emphysema 9. Pneumothorax 10. Aspiration of food or mucus

From: Nelson, W. E., et al: Textbook of Pediatrics. ed. 11. Philadelphia, Saunders, 1979.

should avoid cooling the delivery room and should maintain infants in a neutral thermal environment following prompt ventilatory resuscitation and use intravenous fluid and glucose with monitoring of the arterial oxygen and pH as appropriate correction is instituted for acidosis.

Do not hesitate to examine roentgenographically the lungs of all infants with respiratory difficulties, searching for pneumonia, pneumothorax, pulmonary hemorrhage and pulmonary dysmaturity.

Choking following the first feeding should always be considered to result from a tracheoesophageal fistula.

Cyanosis associated with heart murmur usually means some form of heart disease. However, cyanotic heart disease is not always accompanied by a murmur. Moreover, cyanosis of the hands and feet occurs very commonly in normal infants and may be caused by hypoglycemia, methemoglobinemia and the high hematocrit syndrome as well as by pulmonary difficulties. If one stimulates the infant to cry, a lessening of the cyanosis suggests pulmonary disease since the cry makes the infant breathe more deeply and this improves oxygenation of the blood. If cyanosis deepens, it is probably due to heart disease. Another important sign of heart disease is the change in intensity of the heart sounds. They are almost always loud and snapping in heart disease and in rare instances may be the only clinical sign of abnormality. The following list of congenital malformations is given in the order of frequency established in the first few days or weeks of life:

Complete transposition of the great vessels
Hypoplastic left heart syndrome
Tetralogy of Fallot
Multiple major cardiac defects
Coarctation of the aorta and venticular septal defect
Pulmonary atresia
Single ventricle
Pulmonary stenosis
Tricuspid atresia
Various other anomalies of lesser frequency.

Differential Diagnosis of RDS in the Newborn

A. Medical
  1. Respiratory
      Transient tachypnea
      Meconium inspiration
      Pneumonia—congenital or acquired
      Pneumothorax—pneumomediastinum
      Pleural effusion—hemothorax—chylothorax
      Pulmonary hypoplasia
      Pulmonary hemorrhage
  2. Cardiac
      Congenital heart defect
      Congestive heart failure
      Persistent fetal circulation
  3. Central Nervous System
      Intracranial hemorrhage
      Cerebral edema
      Withdrawal from addictive drugs
      Spinal cord injury
  4. Neuromuscular
      Diaphragmatic paralysis due to phrenic nerve injury
      Werdnig-Hoffman disease
      Myasthenia gravis
      Congenital muscular dystrophy
  5. Hematologic
      Acute blood loss
      Hyperviscosity syndrome
  6. Miscellaneous
      Hypoglycemia
      Hypermagnesemia
      Glycogen storage disease (types 0,11)
      Disorders of amino acid metabolism
      Thoracic dystrophy (Jeune's syndrome)

B. Surgical
  1. Choanal atresia—bilateral
  2. Goiter
  3. Vascular rings
  4. Tracheoesophageal fistula
  5. Diaphragmatic hernia
  6. Hernia pneumothorax
  7. Bronchogenic cyst
  8. Cystic adenoid malformation

JAUNDICE IN THE NEWBORN

While the causes of jaundice in the older child are due to the many etiologic factors seen in the adult, there are unique causative difficulties that produce jaundice within the first few days of life.

The following are the more common causes of jaundice or icterus in the newborn:

1. Physiologic jaundice
2. Hemolytic disease of the newborn: erythroblastosis fetalis (Rh and other secondary blood group incompatibilities) and ABO blood group incompatibilities
3. Deficiency of glucuronyl transferase resulting from:
  a. immaturity

b. genetic factors
c. hypoxia
d. excess pregnanediol in breast milk
e. sepsis
f. dehydration
g. disturbances of carbohydrate metabolism (e.g., galactosemia)
h. certain drugs
i. cretinism
j. occasionally Down's syndrome
4. Intrauterine infections
   a. cytomegalic inclusion body disease (CID)
   b. toxoplasmosis
   c. herpes
   d. rubella
   e. giant cell hepatitis
   f. infectious and possibly homologous serum hepatitis
5. Syphilis
6. Erythrocyte enzyme deficiencies: glucose-6-phosphate dehydrogenase, pyruvate kinase
7. Inspissated bile syndrome
8. Biliary atresia

The definition of physiologic jaundice can be met by the following criteria:

A. Term infant
   1. Jaundice visibly detectable at 36 hours of life
   2. Bilirubin peak level of 12 mg per 100 ml. or less on day 3 or 4
   3. Jaundice not visible after seven days
   4. No pathological process identified
B. Premature infant
   1. Jaundice visibly detectable at 36 hours of life
   2. Peak bilirubin level of 15 or less achieved on day 5 or 6
   3. Jaundice not visible after 14 days
   4. No pathological process identified

The following are factors that contribute to physiologic jaundice:

A. Decreased hepatocellular uptake of bilirubin
B. Decreased activity of the enzyme uridine diphospho glucuronyl transferase
C. Increased blood volume of the neonate
D. Decreased life span of the fetal red cell
E. Increased hemoglobin concentration in the neonatal period
F. Increased enterohepatic circulation
   1. Decreased intestinal motility
   2. Absence of normal intestinal flora
G. Increased early labeled peak production
   1. Caloric deprivation
   2. Oxytocin induction

The most significant form of jaundice requiring clinical judgment and treatment is that due to erythroblastosis. This entity causing hemolytic disease of the newborn results in the destruction of the fetal red cells as a result of antibodies produced by the mother. These develop as a response to fetal blood antigens that are absent in the mother's own cells. The Rh or D factor is the most common cause of severe disease while the ABO incompatibilities are more common but generally are much milder. The D-negative or Rh-negative mother may become sensitized in her first pregnancy with a D-positive fetus or by a transfusion of D-positive blood. The greater the number of pregnancies, the greater the risk of hemolytic disease. However, the first child usually escapes the hemolytic crisis unless an instrumental abortion has been performed on the mother previously or unless she has received a blood transfusion of D-positive blood. Approximately 10 per cent of marriages have the D incompatibility. However, a relatively low incidence of hemolytic disease (one in 150 pregnancies) results in any serious difficulty. Other factors such as Kell, Duffy, c, C or E may produce hemolysis and require treatment.

As a result of the hemolysis, hyperbilirubinemia occurs in the newborn usually within twenty-four to forty-eight hours, and may cause the development of kernicterus and resulting cerebral palsy. Exchange transfusions have been utilized when the bilirubin has risen to 10 mg. per 100 ml. in the first 24 hours, 15 mgm in 36 hours or 20 mg. per 100 ml. thereafter. Whereas nonerythroblastic hyperbilirubinemic infants do not seem to have quite the same risk of brain damage from kernicterus, nevertheless, premature babies who have an indirect bilirubin of 15 mg. per 100 ml. or more or full term infants who have 20 mg. per 100 ml. elevation may require a replacement transfusion. These figures do not apply to infants who are septic, acidotic or hypothermic, since kernicterus has been observed at much lower figures.

After complete evaluation of the cause and severity of the hyperbilirubinemic state has been made, exposing the eye-covered infant to 75 to 100 hours of blue-spectrum light definitely decreases the level of serum bilirubin and thereby reduces the number of babies requiring exchange transfusions. However, repeated determinations of hemoglobin and hematocrit are necessary during this treatment. Ultraviolet radiation after an exchange transfusion will likewise reduce the need to repeat the procedure.

The indications for exchange transfusion are as follows:

1. An alert is provided when the titer of anti-Rh antibody in the mother's blood is rising and in

the unusual situation in which the amniotic fluid has been examined for bilirubin pigments and intraperitoneal fetal transfusion has been performed or indicated.

2. A positive direct Coombs' test may not be an indication per se, inasmuch as 50 per cent of the erythroblastotic infants will have mild disease and a positive Coombs' test.

3. Cord blood hemoglobin less than 10 g. per 100 ml. or when the cord plasms bilirubin is greater than 4 mg. per 100 ml. This is an indication that an exchange transfusion should be done immediately. In the premature, if transfusion is needed, the cord bilirubin is over 3 mg. per 100 ml.

4. If the serum bilirubin rises at a rate of 0.75 to 1.0 mg. per hour after birth, this is almost presumptive evidence an exchange transfusion will be required.

5. If the cord hemoglobin is greater than 10 g. per 100 ml. and the cord plasma bilirubin is less than 4 mg. per 100 ml. the immediate replacement transfusion is not necessary; however, the infant's bilirubin and hemoglobin levels at 8 to 12 hour intervals should be observed, and the following values of bilirubin indicated at these times will be an indication:

8 to 10 mg. per 100 ml.	8 hr.
10 to 12 mg. per 100 ml.	16 hr.
12 to 15 mg. per 100 m.	24 hr.
18 to 20 mg. per 100 ml.	40 hr.
20 mg. per 100 ml.	at any given time

6. Observable edema, petechiae, paleness, hepatomegaly and splenomegaly are indications for exchange transfusions at any time.

7. Repeated exchange transfusions are indicated by any of the previous indications or if there is persistent heme pigment discoloration of the baby's serum. Of course, the heart failure should be treated first and a partial exchange transfusion performed with packed red blood cells.

8. Salt-poor albumin has been utilized in the hyperbilirubinemic baby when anemia and heart failure are not problems. The albumin serves to bind indirect bilirubin and thus moves the bilirubin from tissue spaces into the bloodstream. A micromethod for measuring reserve albumin-binding capacity has some indication of being promising in the treatment of these jaundiced babies.

The prevention of erythroblastosis fetalis by preventing Rh immunization in pregnancy can now be accomplished by giving potent anti-Rh antibodies to the Rh-negative mother within 36 hours after delivery of her *first* born Rh-positive infant.

INFANT FEEDING

The feeding of the infant under 6 months of age is no longer the problem that existed before the present methods of sterilization, commericaly prepared formulas and the addition of solid foods at a much earlier date.

The feeding of the premature infant calls for special individualized decisions, but in most nurseries, a low-fat high-protein formula containing 20 to 24 calories per ounce is preferred for infants weighing less than 3 pounds.

One should bear in mind in providing the necessary calories from carbohydrate, fat and protein that extra calories must always be provided for the element of growth and maturity of the infant. Undoubtedly in low income groups, the breast-fed infant has a much better chance for survival. A nursing mother should have adequate fluid, ranging from 2 to 3 quarts a day, and calcium in the amount of 1 to 2 g. a day, and she should have a diet relatively high in protein. Medications that the mother ingests that may be excreted in the breast milk include atropine, sulfanilamides, laxatives, barbiturates, iodides, aspirin, quinine, nicotine and caffeine.

For both breast and bottle-fed babies, the relatively self-demanding feeding schedule is recommended. Most infants adjust themselves to a 3 hour schedule for the first few weeks of life and then progress to a 4 hour schedule, and sleep through the night within 6 weeks time.

An infant receiving a protein-deficient formula or breast milk from a mother suffering from malnutrition may develop symptoms of kwashiorkor, i.e., growth retardation, edema, frequent infections, apathy, and some abnormal pigmentation of the hair and skin.

Formula Writing

Use of evaporated milk is probably the easiest method of preparing a formula. The amount to be used can be calculated as follows: 1 ounce of evaporated milk per pound of body weight of the infant, 2½ ounces total fluid per pound of body weight to provide the necessary total daily fluid requirements, carbohydrate in the form of sugar or Karo syrups to provide the remaining calories.

It is always expected that the milk in the formula is written for what the child should weigh at that age or for the anticipated progress in weight of the child. As an example, an 8 pound infant would be given 9 ounces of evaporated milk and 20 ounces of water. However, 4 ounces of the water may be given throughout the day, and the formula is concentrated more by using only 16 ounces of water. The extra carbohydrate may be made up by giving approximately 1½ tablespoons of cane sugar.

In actual practice, a formula consisting of 10 ounces of evaporated milk and 17 ounces of water with 1 ounce of added carbohydrates is used for the first few weeks of life with a gradual increase of evaporated milk until a half and half proportion with water is utilized. The added carbohydrates are generally omitted after 2 or 3 months of life when the half and half proportions are used.

When homogenized milk is used, such a routine formula, containing 21 ounces of whole milk and 7 ounces of water with an additional 1 ounce of sugar, is utilized in the same way. Whole milk is then offered by 3 months of age. It is recommended that multivitamins or vitamins A, D and C be administered once a day to all children under 5 years of age throughout the year.

There are many commercial formulas available and fortunately some specifically for children who may be allergic to regular cow's milk. The commercial hypoallergenic formulas made from soybean are undoubtedly the most popular.

Solids can be started by 3 months of age in the average child, beginning with cereals and fruits with gradual addition of vegetables and meat until the child is on a three-meal-a-day schedule.

GROWTH AND DEVELOPMENT

Nature's preparation of the infant for childhood, adolescence and adult life is to have him go through distinct stages of behavioral, physiologic and physical changes. In fact, one of the most important means of recognizing disease and abnormality developing in childhood is to know thoroughly what is normal for growth, development and behavior at any age.

Factors, both external, as from the environment, and internal, from the child, influence these changes. No longer are the terms underweight and overweight used as liberally as in the past. Charts have been prepared, called percentile charts, that represent lines of progress in which most children develop in both weight and height. The percentile is based on comparing any child with his position in comparison with 100 children. If a child is in the 25th percentile, this means that 75 children weigh more, or are taller, than this individual child. As he develops over the months and years, it will be found that he remains in the same curve that is calibrated upward. A drop below his percentile generally indicates some disease or environmental influence that has impaired his growth and development.

The normal infant after birth gains approximately 1 ounce a day during the first 5 or 6 months of age. This results in the doubling of the birth weight by 4 and at the most 5 months. From 6 to 12 months of age, the weight gain is approximately 3 to 4 ounces each week, and the birth weight is tripled by 1 year. After the first year, weight gain is relatively steady and averages 4 to 6 pounds a year. At about 2½ years of age, the birth weight is quadrupled. The following formulas may be useful in giving the average weights:

3 to 12 months of age weight in pounds
= age in months + 11
2 to 12 years of age weight in pounds
= age in years × 5 + 18

Height progresses less rapidly than weight. The average newborn measures about 20 inches in length and increases about 10 inches during the first year. A rough formula for a child between 2 and 12 years of age is as follows:

Height in inches = ages in years × 2 + 32

A frequent question asked by parents is "How many teeth should my child have?" Since the first tooth is cut at around 7 months of age, one can use the formula:

Age in months − 6 = number of teeth the infant
should have

In appraising actual hormonal development of the child, we determine what is called the bone age, inasmuch as different ossification centers of bones are formed at different ages. There are five ossification centers present in 90 per cent of newborn infants.

1. Calcaneus
2. Cuboid
3. Talus
4. Distal end of the femur
5. Proximal end of the tibia

The first ossification centers to appear after birth are those of the capitate and hamate bones in the wrist. Up to 6 years of age, an x-ray film of the wrist, with the aid of the following formula, will assist in determination of normal bone age:

Ages in years + 1 = number of ossification centers
in the wrist

In addition to the growth of the body as determined by weight, height and bone age, certain physiologic and enzymatic changes that may take place within the infant are responsible for many disturbances of metabolism characteristically found in children, some of which are outgrown; others are permanent. In fact, there are probably more than 100 so-called experiments of nature, inborn errors of metabolism, that may occur in childhood. The one most frequently tested for at birth is phenylketonuria, in an attempt to establish an early diagnosis and so prevent PKU-induced mental retardation. The phenylalanine level in the blood is determined in the newborn nursery; the hoped-for finding is in the normal range of below 5 to 6 mg. per 100 ml.

Congenital absence of the thyroid or an insufficiency of thyroid function may produce severe hypothyroidism or the severe state called cretinism in the first few months of life. Hypothyroid children may manifest all the different degrees of true cretinism, ranging from dry yellowish skin with porcine or pig-like face to slow motor development, leading subsequently to mental retardation. Constipation in association with umbilical hernia is sometimes called the classical sign of the hypothyroid infant. Diagnosis by clinical inspection and the determination of PBI or a T_3 and T_4 test will provide the basis for treatment with thyroid hormone.

To remember the letters LAMPS, which illuminate the growth of a child, is to remember to appraise the Language, Adaptive behavior, Motor development, and Personal-Social response of the growing child as a means of appraising his development, which is sometimes expressed as the developmental quotient or D.Q., which is not equivalent to I. Q.!! While texts are available to show the normal developmental quotient throughout childhood, it is most important to recognize neurologic, endocrinologic and metabolic diseases in the first 2 years of life. Awareness of normal development will greatly assist in diagnosis. The following chart depicts development of the first 24 months of life.

DEVELOPMENTAL MILESTONES

1 month	Cries; focuses eyes in line of vision; hold head up when prone; fists clench; body responds to head positioning reflexly
2 months	Follows moving objects; holds chest up when prone; hands left open; smiles and responds to people
3 months	Coos; hands held open; will open mouth on feeding; has good head control
4 months	Coos; chuckles and babbles; grasps rattle; puts hands in mouth; will look at own hands in front of face; laughs aloud
5 months	Will turn in response to sounds; rolls from back to stomach (rolls over)
6 months	Will respond differently to strangers than the household; puts feet in mouth when lying on back; reaches for objects given to him; bangs spoon on table; picks up small block with hands, not fingers; sits alone leaning forward on hands
8 months	Sits alone; picks up small objects by bringing the thumb and index fingers together (this is called prehensile ability); transfers objects from one hand to the other and looks for objects
10 months	Pulls self to standing position; will respond to own name by turning head; brings blocks together, will cruise around furniture while standing; crawls; points with index finger; plays peek-a-boo; will wave bye-bye
12 months	Walks with holding of hand; stands alone; will respond to criticism such as "no-no"; drops objects into a cup; will give toys back to you when requested; may say "da-da," "ma-ma," or "bye-bye"
15 months	Definitely walks alone; may say four or five words; will indicate wants; will use jargon with babbling sounding like words; may name objects that are familiar; crawls up stairs
18 months	Able to point to nose, eyes, hair; says "hello" and words equivalent to thank you; will sit down by himself and may be able to feed self; is able to run
24 months	Can run without stumbling; can go up and down stairs alone, may use three-word sentences; will refer to himself by his own name; will use pronouns and verbs in sentences; will use toilet during waking hours and may verbalize toilet needs. Toilet training easier in girls than boys; speech occurs earlier in girls than in boys.

In summary, the infant improves in his motor behavior from what is called cephalad to caudad progression. In other words, he lifts his head and then his motor ability goes downward over his body so that he can use his feet and walk as maturation of the nervous system occurs.

PREVENTIVE PEDIATRICS

Of the greatest importance in pediatric training is not only the early recognition of abnormalities but the provision of conditions conducive to optimum health during the developmental years preparatory for adulthood. In addition to recognition of diseases unique for childhood, every child is deserving of the immunization procedures available now to prevent diseases that in the past took thousands of lives. The following schedule of immunizations may change from year to year as rubella and mumps vaccine become as universally available as the measles vaccine is at the present time.

Immunization Procedures

Pediatrics is rightfully concerned as much with the prevention of illness as with the cure of disease. Vaccines are now available that prevent many of the infectious diseases that in the past claimed the lives of numerous children, so that these diseases are becoming more and more uncommon.

Table 11-3 is the immunization schedule currently recommended for United States infants by the American Academy of Pediatrics. Revisions are, of course, made from year to year as new information and new vaccines become available.

For clean, minor wounds, a booster dose of tetanus toxoid is not needed by a fully immunized child at the time of injury unless more than 10 years have elapsed since the last dose. For contaminated wounds, a booster dose should be given if more than 5 years have elapsed since the last dose.

Smallpox vaccination is no longer recommended on a routine basis. It is contraindicated in any child with skin eruptions or eczema or who has siblings with these problems and in children who are receiving immunosuppressive drugs.

In special situation, globulin or special immune serum globulins can also be used to provide passive immunity.

Pneumococcal vaccines are recommended for high risk groups such as children with sickle cell anemia and asplenic patients from any cause.

Haemophilus influenzae type b and meningoccal serogroups A and C polysaccharide vaccines have been shown to be quite effective in stimulating protective antibodies in older children and adults, but appear to be ineffective in younger infants below 15 months. They are not recommended for contacts of sporadic cases since their effectiveness depends on development of an immunological response over a period of several days. The majority of secondary cases, on the other hand, occur within 48 to 72 hours of an index case. Thus, these vaccines should be reserved for outbreaks of meningococcal disease.

Secondary cases of meningococcal meningitis can be prevented by prophylactic administration of an anti-

TABLE 11-3. Schedule for Active Immunization of Normal Infants and Children in the United States

2 months	DTP[1]	TOPV[2]
4 months	DTP	TOPV
6 months	DTP	TOPV
1 year	Measles[3]	Tuberculin Test[4]
1 to 12 years	Rubella[3]	Mumps[3]
1½ years	DTP	TOPV
4 to 6 years	DTP	TOPV
14 to 16 years	Td[5]	and thereafter every 10 years

[1] DTP—diphtheria and tetanus toxoids combined with pertussis vaccine.

[2] TOPV—trivalent oral polio virus vaccine. The above recommendation is suitable for breast-fed as well as bottle-fed infants although the passive immunity provided by breast milk may somewhat decrease the development of active immunity by the infant.

[3] May be given at 1 year as measles-rubella or measles-mumps-rubella combined vaccines. Rubella vaccine is recommended for preschool children not so much to protect them as to protect their unimmunized mothers who may become pregnant. All susceptible girls should definitely receive the vaccine prior to puberty. Both boys and girls, if susceptible, should receive mumps vaccine prior to puberty as the disease is much less mild in adults.

[4] The tuberculin test should be done prior to giving measles vaccine as viral infections may sometimes temporarily convert a positive TB skin test to negative and may exacerbate the disease if present. The frequency with which the tuberculin test should then be repeated depends on the risk of exposure of the child.

[5] Td—combined tetanus and diphtheria toxoids (adult type) for those over 6 years of age in contrast to diphtheria and tetanus (DT) containing a larger amount of diphtheria antigen.

Vaccine containing pertussis antigen should not be given past age 6.

microbial agent to close contacts of patients. Rifampin, in dosage of 10 mg. per kg. per day, should be used to provide chemoprophylaxis against meningococci.

Reimmunization of the high school age group against measles should be considered because 85 per cent of all reported cases are now occurring in this group.

Immune Defense and Immune Deficiency

A newborn infant comes into the world with a fairly well developed capacity for immune response, but with little preformed immunity. Initially, he does have IgG antibodies transferred across the placenta from his mother, at levels even higher than her own, but these disappear by 4 to 5 months, normally to be replaced by his own endogenous production. If he is breast fed, he also gets the benefit of immunoglobulins (largely IgA) in his mother's milk, which gives him additional protection from infection via the gastrointestinal route. IgM and IgA do not cross the placenta, and while the infant is capable of producing these immunoglobulins if stimulated, they are generally present in quite low levels in the healthy baby. IgM antibody is thought to have particular protection against gram-negative bacteria, which may partly explain why the newborn is especially susceptible to these organisms. IgM is also the first type of antibody formed as infection occurs, so that IgM levels can be used as an index of prenatal or perinatal infection.

All of these immunoglobulins increase as the child grows older and is exposed to an increased variety of antigens, with IgM, IgG and IgA reaching full development in that order. A fourth immunoglobulin, IgE, is thought to be a reaginic antibody of allergy and is often increased in allergic states; elevation of serum IgE is not essential for a diagnosis of allergy, however. A fifth immunoglobulin, IgD, has also been discovered, but its function is still unclear.

If these immunoglobulins, particularly IgG and IgM, are deficient, or if antibodies of IgG and/or IgM class cannot be formed, the child will begin to develop numerous bacterial infections (pneumonia, otitis media, meningitis, etc.) as his mother's prenatally transferred immunoglobulin wears off. These children will have less difficulty with viral illness, but may die of severe hepatitis or poliomyelitis to which they are very susceptible. This disease may occur sporadically or as an X-linked inherited disease (Burton type agammaglobulinemia). Most of these children can be markedly improved with repeated injections of gamma globulin (which contains only IgG), while some require periodic plasma infusions. Isolated IgA deficiency is quite common and generally requires no treatment. These children may be asymptomatic or may have problems with allergies, arthritis, malabsorption, and may have severe anaphylaxis after transfusion of blood containing IgA.

Immunoglobulins are made by plasma cells, which are in turn derived from lymphocytes, but most of the lymphocytes seen in the peripheral blood are not of this kind, but rather function more directly to protect the body against viruses, fungi, tubercle bacilli and tumors (with the assistance from other immune mechanisms, of course). They are also primarily responsible for the rejection of organ transplants. These lymphocytes not only have to be present in adequate numbers but must have been exposed to a functional thymus in order to perform properly. Hence they are called T cells, in contrast to the immunoglobulin-producing lymphocytes which are known as B cells, in allusion to their supposed site of origin in the bone marrow and to their similarity to the bursal-dependent cells of the chicken. As in the immunoglobulin system, the protection provided by T cells is directed against specific targets and is not fully developed until the antigenic stimulus has been encountered.

A fairly pure T cell deficiency is seen when the thymus is lacking, as in the Di George syndrome. As this is due to an embryologic maldevelopment of the third and fourth pharyngeal pouches, defects in the parathyroid are often present concomitantly, and such infants may present with resistent hypocalcemia rather than infection. Their immunologic defect is now treatable by grafts of fetal thymus.

Both the T and B cell systems are deficient in severe combined immunodeficiency disease (formerly called Swiss type agammaglobulinemia). This is thought to be due to absence or deficiency of a common lymphocyte stem cell. One form has recently been shown to be due to a missing enzyme. This disease may be transmitted either by autosomal recessive or by X-linked inheritance. As of now, treatment is possible only by marrow transplantation. As might be anticipated, untreated infants do not survive more than a few years or so in a normal environment.

Numerous other syndromes also affecting both of these systems but producing only partial deficiency are known, including most commonly, the **Wiskott-Aldrich syndrome** in which the classic triad of frequent infections, eczema and thrombocytopenia is found, and ataxia telangiectasiae in which there are skin and conjunctival telangiectasiae and progressive neurologic decline as well as immune deficiency. Treatment by bone marrow transplantation has produced cures.

The two systems just described, though vitally important, are not, however, the body's only means of active defense. Granulocytes and other phagocytic cells, in contrast to the lymphocytes of either type, do not appear to need to be "introduced" to their target before they can function but are able to act rapidly, giving first aid until the other immune systems have time to become operational. The risk of overwhelming bacterial sepsis in severe granulocytopenia of any cause is well known. The spleen also is an integral part of this system, and its removal, or absence, particularly in a young child, places the child at risk of overwhelming sepsis, particularly if he is exposed to a pathogen to which he does not have previously developed antibody. This is particularly dangerous in those children whose underlying disease already places them at risk of infection, such as children with the Wiskott-Aldrich syndrome or children with malignant disease who are taking immunosuppressive drugs.

It is possible, of course, for granulocytes to be present but unable to function properly, as is best known to occur in chronic granulomatosis, in which bacteria of some types are phagocytosed but cannot be killed. These children, generally boys, develop granulomas in much the same way as tuberculosis patients do. These patients' granulocytes cannot kill any organism except streptococci and pneumococci, which are catalase negative and bring their own H_2O_2 along, and, hence, destroy themselves inside the powerless polymorphonucleur leucocytes. Prophylactic use of sulfisoxazole has been of some help in managing these children. Multiple additional defects of phagocytosis are also known but are of greater rarity.

Assisting the above systems is complement, a cascade of nine serum proteins that aids in the lysis of bacteria and other particulate antigens targeted by antibodies, as well as functioning in the clotting system. Deficiencies of complement components have been reported for each of the nine major complements, deficiency of C'_5 (Leiner's disease) being the most well known. However, the aggregate total of complement deficiencies equals the frequency of cystic fibrosis.

Of course, when one is confronted with a child with persistent or recurrent pulmonary infections, intrinsic immune deficiency is only one of the things to be considered in the differential diagnosis. Diseases such as cystic fibrosis and neurologic or anatomic problems leading to recurrent aspiration can present similarly. Infections may also persist if the causative organism was not properly identified and the infection was therefore not adequately treated even in a patient with a perfectly normal immunologic system.

DISEASES OF ORGAN SYSTEMS

Subsequent to the newborn period and the first year of life, diseases occurring in later childhood and in adulthood are somewhat similar, and in general the discussion of those diseases in other chapters are applicable. However, there are many diseases characteristic of childhood that are too numerous to review, and the reader should refer to standard textbooks of pediatrics. There are, however, a number of entities that occur uniquely in childhood that are of sufficient frequency to be highlighted in the following system disease summaries.

Pituitary

Arising from the craniopharyngeal duct and lying usually above the sella turcica, may be found craniopharyngiomas, which clinically present symptoms usually before 15 years of age. These are manifested by diplopia and variable neurologic signs, but especially papilledema. Radiologically, calcification is noted in the suprasellar area with destruction of the clinoid processes and a resulting flat sella turcica.

Since craniopharyngiomas are resistant to radiation, surgical removal of the tumor, followed by substitution therapy with pitressin as well as thyroid and adrenal hormones, is the only treatment. While these tumors may cause obesity, 99 per cent of obesity in childhood results from overeating, with a frequent family history of obesity. Breasts may be enlarged in the male chiefly because of an increase in fatty tissue, and the genitals may look small because they are hidden by the pubic fat pad. If there has been a history of obesity in the preadolescent period and in early childhood, obesity may persist to some degree throughout adolescence.

Cachexia and wasting of the body resembling anorexia nervosa occurring before puberty is almost always of hypothalamic or diencephalic origin. After puberty, especially in girls, the psychologic basis for marked wasting and lack of appetite is due to severe emotional changes secondary to crash dieting undertaken to prevent or overcome obesity.

Laurence-Moon-Biedl syndrome is a rare autosomal recessive trait characterized by obesity, hypogonadism, mental retardation, retinitis pigmentosa, syndactyly or polydactyly. Various degrees or incomplete forms may be present. There is no treatment.

Albright-McCune syndrome is characterized by unilateral cafe-au-lait spots (resembling tanned discoloration occurring with neurofibromatosis), sexual precocity with monoostotic or polyostotic fibrous dysplasia. It occurs most commonly in females and is due to congenital anomaly of the hypothalamus.

Diabetes insipidus may occur without symptoms, or obesity may be its only manifestation. In some cases there may be distinct signs of deficiency of the anterior pituitary hormones giving rise to hypopituitary dwarfism and sexual infantilism. Occasionally there may be disturbances of temperature regulation with prolonged somnolence.

Diabetes insipidus–suggesting lesions of the pituitary hypothalamic axis occur with Hand-Schüller-Christian disease or result from a neoplasm arising from the third ventricle. Diabetes insipidus may occur transiently following a severe head injury or infection such as meningitis or encephalitis. (The nephogenic type is due to failure of the renal tubules to respond to the normally secreted antidiuretic hormone and occurs as a sex-linked dominant genetic disease that may be associated with mental retardation.) The third type of diabetes insipidus is idiopathic, with no etiologic factor known at the present time.

The symptoms may resemble those of diabetes mellitus inasmuch as there may be polyuria with bed wetting, associated with polydipsia, fever, irritability, fatigue and sleep disturbances. Small infants may have severe dehydration with actual circulatory collapse resembling shock.

In true diabetes insipidus (in contradistinction to psychogenic polydipsia, salt-losing adrenogenital syndromes and diabetes mellitus) there is a definite increase in the 24 hour urine volume (6 to 12.1) with specific gravity of 1.001 to 1.006, accompanied by increased serum levels of sodium. The Hicky-Hare test consists of giving a 2.5 per cent solution of sodium chloride (hypertonic saline) intravenously. In children with psychogenic polydipsia, and also of normal children, there is a marked reduction in urine volume. There is no response in patients with true diabetes insipidus of the nephrogenic type.

The pitressin test consists of giving 0.1 unit of aqueous pitressin intravenously. In the patient with true diabetes insipidus, there is prompt reduction in urinary volume and increase in specific gravity within 30 minutes. Patients with the nephrogenic type do not respond.

Dwarfism. A child has been arbitrarily considered a dwarf if he is at least 5 cm. shorter than 90 per cent of the children of the same chronologic age. Dwarfism is erroneously thought to be caused chiefly by a pituitary deficiency, but the following represent some of the more frequent causes of stunting of growth in infancy and childhood:

1. Endocrine disorders such as hypopituitarism, hypothyroidism, ovarian agenesis (Turner's syndrome), or premature sexual precocity with early closing of the epiphyses
2. Chronic malnutrition such as may occur with starvation, cystic fibrosis or the celiac syndrome
3. Chronic renal disease such as congenital hydronephrosis or base-losing nephritis
4. Metabolic disorders such as glycogen storage disease, Hurler's-Hunter's disease, galactosemia, or idiopathic infantile hypercalcemia
5. Congenital heart disease or chronic anemia with chronic hypoxia
6. Skeletal disorder, osteogenesis imperfecta, achondrodystrophy, rickets and various diseases of the spine
7. Central nervous system disturbances associated with severe mental retardation or brain damage
8. Most common is a familial cause when members of the family are short, a condition sometimes referred to as primordial dwarfism; or a delay in puberty so that those children who have not reached the normal height for their age

Thyroid

Hypothyroidism is far more frequent in childhood than hyperthyroidism and undoubtedly is the most frequent endocrine disorder observed in children. It can be readily diagnosed by the experienced clinician when it occurs in infancy as congenital cretinism, but the diagnosis is more difficult in older children when it develops as the so-called acquired hypothyroidism.

Congenital hypothyroidism may be caused by defective hormonogenesis or an inborn enzymatic defect, or it may be secondary to maternal ingestion of goitrogens or lack of maternal dietary iodine.

A second type is due to agenesis or true dysgenesis of the thyroid gland and is frequently referred to as athyrotic cretinism. More recently it has been demonstrated that some of these cases may be due to maternal autoimmunization.

Acquired hypothyroidism may be idiopathic or may possibly be due to autoimmunization. In the presence of panhypopituitarism, thyroid-stimulating hormone deficiency may be the cause. Other causes of acquired hypothyroidism are the same as those found in the adult, e.g., following thyroiditis or thyroidectomy.

The clinical features of cretinism may not be apparent until 2 or 3 months after birth because of the mother's thyroid hormone still circulating within the infant's body. The physical findings are those of a sluggish-appearing infant with coarse hair that may grow downward onto the forehead, which can be wrinkled quite readily by placing one's hand on the scalp and pushing downward toward the eyes; stunted growth with shortening of the extremities; skin that is dry and cool and may be yellowish; a protuberant abdomen with an umbilical hernia because of poor muscle tone; and constipation. Retarded growth may not be so severe in early infancy but occurs in later childhood. Mental retardation may not result if the thyroid deficiency begins after 5 or 6 years of age although the child is very sluggish. The laboratory findings are the same as those in an adult hypothyroid patient. Treatment is essentially the same except that triiodothyronine is not recommended for use in cretins.

Adrenal Glands

Acute adrenal insufficiency in children is much more common than the chronic form seen in adults. It is mentioned inasmuch as many clinicians are not aware that it may occur in infancy and early childhood during the course of an overwhelming infection or severe septicemia. Its occurrence secondary to adrenal hemorrhage in the newborn infant is quite well known. It may also result from the presence of congenital hypoplastic adrenal glands or the congenital adrenogenital syndrome.

Adrenogenital Syndrome. This syndrome may be of the autosomal recessive type, which is strongly familial and is frequently referred to as the congenital type due to bilateral hyperplasia of the adrenal cortex. Adrenal tumor may produce the same symptomatology. Congenital adrenogenital syndrome is due to one of several enzymatic defects in the biosynthesis of hydrocortisone associated with excessive accumulation of various precursors, many of which are androgenic and may result in virilism. It has been shown that the pituitary secretes large amounts of ACTH in an attempt to supply the physiologic requirements of hydrocortisone in a compensatory fashion. This stimulation brings about the adrenal hyperplasia but likewise may increase the production of the androgens and other steroids. The most common cause of virilizing adrenal hyperplasia is a C-21 hydroxylase defect. A salt-losing defect may be associated with the disturbance in aldosterone biosynthesis and occurs in one third of this group as a salt-losing syndrome associated with vascular collapse and early death unless treated with the hydrocortisone and mineralocorticoids.

Females with this disorder are frequently diagnosed as pseudohermaphrodites, inasmuch as abnormalities of the external genitalia are quite apparent at birth, with an extremely enlarged clitoris, the presence of a urogenital sinus and possibly even labioscrotal fusion, although the internal genitalia may be perfectly normal. There is accelerated growth of the bony structures, with actual early epiphyseal fusion, precocious appearance of sexual hair and masculine muscular development with small breasts or absence of breast development and a deep voice. Untreated patients do not develop normal menstruation. They may likewise fail to thrive, exhibit marked dehydration and die in acute adrenal crisis owing to the salt-losing characteristics.

It should be mentioned that a woman treated with progesterone, adrenocortical steroids or testosterone during pregnancy may give birth to a female infant with an enlarged clitoris. These girls continue to grow normally.

In the male, the adrenogenital syndrome is sometimes referred to as macrogenitosomia praecox, inasmuch as the penis is exceptionally large and there may be frequent erections. The testes, however, remain of normal prepubertal size. There may be precocious development of secondary sex characteristics such as a deep voice and abundant sexual hair as well as acne. Accelerated growth also occurs, as in the female, and the salt-losing symptomatology is present.

In these infants the first symptom may be projectile vomiting and dehydration, and the erroneous diagnosis of pyloric stenosis may be made. For this reason, any child suspected of having pyloric stenosis should have a careful examination of the genitals.

The laboratory findings in both boys and girls are important. If there is any difficulty in determining the sex of the female, and this determination is always recommended, a buccal smear should be obtained to determine the Barr body count. This would determine the genetic sex. The urinary 17-ketosteroids are increased, there is no response to the ACTH stimulation test, and there is increased urinary pregnanediol in the congenital adrenogenital syndrome and, characteristically, increased dehydroepiandrosterone in adrenal tumors.

In the salt-losing type, there is a decrease in serum sodium and chloride and in plasma CO_2 content. The serum potassium level is generally elevated. There is a therapeutic test to separate adrenal tumors from simple hyperplasia by the use of cortisone. Cortisone is given intramuscularly in a dose of 20 to 100 mg. daily for 10 days in order to suppress the pituitary ACTH. At the end of this period, the urinary 17-ketosteroids are decreased if the adrenogenital syndrome is secondary to congenital hyperplasia. No response will be found in the case of adrenal tumors. In the latter, surgical removal is the only treatment, especially if the adrenocortical tumor produces virilism.

The treatment for congenital adrenal hyperplasia is the use of cortisone, indefinitely for females and until puberty for males. The doses are kept minimal to suppress the oversecretion of the ACTH as followed by the decreased urinary secretion of 17-ketosteroids. In the salt-losing type, 9-alpha-fluorocortisol is administered daily along with salt.

Pancreas

Hypoglycemia. The newborn infant appears to be able to function perfectly normally with blood sugar levels of 40 or 50 mg. per 100 ml. If the infant is a full-sized, normal infant the symptoms of hypoglycemia manifest themselves if the glucose is under 30 mg. per 100 ml. in the first 3 days of life. The low birth weight infant may not manifest any symptoms at this time unless the glucose level is under 25 mg. per 100 ml. These symptoms may be manifested as apathy, with difficulty in feeding and tremors that may go into convulsions. Interestingly enough, the symptoms may resemble those of the respiratory distress syndrome. Treatment consists of intravenous use of glucose and saline, and, if no response is elicited, the giving of hydrocortisone at 12 hour intervals may be necessary. Treatment should be continued until the blood glucose remains normal for 48 hours and all feedings are being received satisfactorily.

In the older infant and the child, the symptoms of increased perspiration, irritability, vomiting, tremors, excessive hunger, pallor and behavior disorders may be the clinical manifestations of hypoglycemia. Convulsions and death may occur in certain cases.

Hypoglycemia in the older child may be due to hypersensitivity to the amino acid, leucine. The condition may manifest itself by hypoglycemia following increased protein intake. When no cause can be found, the hypoglycemia may be classified as idiopathic or functional. Hypoglycemia associated with glycogen storage disease may result from the deficiency of glucose-6-phosphatase. Other causes are present in older children and adults, particularly hyperinsulinism, glucagon deficiency, Addison's disease, pituitary insufficiency, liver failure, insulin shock and defective intestinal absorption as in the chronic diarrhea of celiac disease. Rarely, in those children sensitive to fructose, hypoglycemia may follow a large ingestion of fructose.

Diabetes Mellitus. Juvenile diabetes mellitus in general can be assumed to resemble the adult type, but there are sufficient differences to warrant a brief discussion of the subject. Diabetes beginning before 15 years of age occurs in approximately 6 per cent of all diabetics but presents such a disproportionate degree of problems and complications that the diabetes is referred to as the juvenile type. The mean age of onset is 8 years, with no differences based on sex.

The following information serves to contrast the juvenile-onset diabetes with the adult type.

Whereas diabetes usually develops insidiously in adults, the onset in children may be extremely abrupt, with the development of coma and severe acidosis in a matter of days or even hours. In fact, cases have been known in which urine was checked for glucose on one day and found to be normal, but 3 days later was found to be 4+ when the child was admitted to the hospital in diabetic coma. Usually, however, the prodromal symptoms may manifest themselves as enuresis, nausea, vomiting, fatigue, dehydration and abdominal pain. A change in personality with weight loss in spite of excessive food intake may be noted. The sudden consumption of many bottles of soft drinks is a common symptom.

There is a marked variation in insulin response with swings from hypoglycemia to hyperglycemia in the first year of treatment. Sometimes within two or three months following the initiation of insulin therapy there may be a temporary remission of the diabetic state. Oral hypoglycemic agents are usually not effective except with the early stages of diabetes, and should not be utilized. Activity and exercise have a much greater lowering effect on the blood glucose than in adults.

Pathologically, early in the disease hypertrophy and hyperplasia of the islet cells are characteristic, and the plasma insulin reaches above-normal levels. But atrophy of the cells soon follows, with full-blown diabetes appearing in 4 to 6 years. Unfortunately, severe renal and ocular complications develop as time goes on, and by 20 years following the onset rapid physical deterioration of the patient has taken place and death results.

It is important to mention here that occasionally the development of an entity called pseudodiabetes may be noted in the newborn. This condition is characterized by hyperglycemia and glycosuria, which respond to 1 unit or less of insulin, and ultimately disappears completely. In cases of this kind the physician has to be certain that the child is not overtreated with insulin, for the result could be the development of hypoglycemia with subsequent brain damage.

Hemopoietic System

The average blood cell values determined during infancy and childhood vary with the age. In fact, normal values occurring in the first few days and weeks of life might well represent disease if they occurred in the older child.

At birth, the erythrocyte count may average between 4 and 5.5 million per cu. mm., rise on the second day to between 4.5 and 6.5 million, only to fall by the third month to between 3.4 and 4.8 million. Hemoglobin at birth may range from 16 to 20 g. per 100 ml., increase at 2 days to between 18 and 22 g. per 100 ml., only to fall to between 10 and 11 g. per 100 ml. at 3 months of age. As one would expect, a few nucleated red cells are a normal finding at birth and during the first few days of life.

For the first few days of life, the total white blood count may range from 14,000 to 24,000 per cu. mm., suggesting an infection but representing a perfectly normal finding. The lymphocytic per cent may rise to as high as 68 by 3 months of age and persist to nearly 1 year of age, giving the appearance of lymphocytosis but being normal.

Because of this marked physiologic variation in the erythrocyte and hemoglobin levels during the first year of life, one must not hasten to make the diagnosis of anemia. In fact, the so-called physiologic anemia that occurs around 3 months of age is a normal phenomenon and not a true anemia.

Anemia due to Iron Deficiency. This occurs mostly in infants between the ages of 8 and 24 months. Iron deficiency is the most common cause of anemia at this age. When this anemia occurs before 8 months of age, it may mean that it was present from birth as a result of severe iron deficiency in the mother or as the result of severe blood loss in the infant during the neonatal period. It may also result from prematurity or the fact that there were multiple births.

Excessive milk drinking without adequate supplemental foods may result quite frequently in iron deficiency, which may even be accompanied by subtle gastrointestinal bleeding.

For these iron deficiency anemias the prophylactic administration of iron can routinely be employed during the first months of life. The daily dose is calculated on the basis of 8 mg. elemental iron per kg. body weight daily. There is a hazard in administering blood transfusions to infants, as is done in adults, because of the danger of overloading the already disturbed homeostatic mechanisms of the infant's body. Therefore, even in severe iron deficiency anemia, blood transfusions can usually be avoided, thus avoiding the hazards associated with blood transfusion.

Sickle Cell Anemia. A hereditary form of hemolytic disease occurring almost exclusively in Negroes, sickle cell anemia is due to the presence in the red cells of sickle hemoglobin, which represents the gene for the homozygous state. Its incidence in newborn American blacks is approximately 0.2 per cent.

The disease is marked by anemia associated with episodes of pain and fever and occasionally by aplastic crises and other varieties of clinical manifestations. The sickle-shaped red blood cell gives the disease its name.

The bulk of the hemoglobin is of the *S* variety (60 to 100 per cent). The remainder consists of fetal *F* hemoglobin (usually 2 to 24 per cent). Normal *A* hemoglobin is absent.

The disease is usually recognized during the preschool period. In half of the patients, symptoms are present by 2 years of age, although clinical symptoms are rare in the first 6 months of life.

The newly perfected accurate test for sickle cell disease, using microcolumn chromatography or acid agar gel electrophoresis, can now be performed on cord blood at birth.

The anemia is chronic, normochromic and normocytic. Sickle-shaped cells are noted on blood smears in numbers varying from 0.5 to 25 per cent along with many distorted cells.

One of the standard deoxygenation techniques shows sickling to be complete and rapid in all red cells in patients with sickle cell anemia, in contrast to the slow development in the red cells of those with the sickle cell trait.

The *sickle cell trait* represents the heterozygous state (hemoglobins A and S) and occurs in 7 to 9 per cent of American blacks. Thus, of those showing sickling about one in 50 of those shows sickle cell anemia.

The amount of sickle cell hemoglobin in the blood of persons with the trait as determined by electrophoresis varies from 34 to 45 per cent of the total hemoglobin. The remainder is adult hemoglobin. Hemoglobin F is not found in the trait after infancy.

Persons with the trait are not anemic, show no physical abnormalities and are usually asymptomatic. However, just as in sickle cell anemia, splenic infarction, resulting from vascular occulsion by sickled cells, may occur at moderate and high altitudes during flight. Badly administered anesthesia or severe pneumonia

may cause a condition of deoxygenation in a "sickling crisis" of the type that occurs, quite frequently with sickle cell anemia.

While the presence of the sickle cell trait is relatively benign, the prognosis for sickle cell anemia is not favorable, with a fatal outcome occurring in many patients in childhood and early adult life.

The outlook for the patient with the variants (e.g., thalassemia and sickle cell trait) of sickle cell disease is more favorable than for the patient with homozygous sickle cell anemia.

Megaloblastic Anemia. Megaloblastic anemia is not as frequent in infancy and childhood as it was previously when goat's milk was utilized in infant's feeding and when severe malnutrition secondary to chronic diarrhea was more prevalent. However, it still occurs in children who have a congenital defect of absorption of either folic acid or vitamin B_{12} or those children who have inadequate intestinal absorption such as might occur following ileal resection of the bowel. Patients with kwashiorkor and juvenile addisonian (pernicious) anemia have a deficiency of the intrinsic factor. This type of anemia occurs most frequently in infancy between the ages of 2 and 20 months. Most cases are due to deficiency of folic acid secondary to frequent diarrhea occuring with the celiac syndrome.

The distinction between folic acid and vitamin B_{12} deficiency cannot be made by inspection of the peripheral blood or bone marrow. Determination of folic acid levels in the blood is the most reliable method of differentiation. Measuring the urinary formiminoglutamic acid (FIGLU) is another method used to recognize the folic acid deficiency since it will be increased in the presence of folate deficiency. The treatment for folic acid deficiency is accomplished with the utilization of 5 to 10 mg. folic acid daily for at least 2 weeks. Vitamin B_{12} deficiency is treated by the use of several daily intramuscular injections of 25 to 100 μg. Thereafter, the patient is maintained by a monthly intramuscular dose of 50 to 100 μg. In juvenile pernicious anemia, maintenance therapy of course is essential.

Chronic Hereditary Anemia. The principal chronic hereditary anemias such as thalassemia major, sickle cell anemia and congenital hemolytic jaundice may occur in infants and children. However, the discussion under general hematology is applicable to children.

Disorders of Leukocytes. Leukemoid reactions in the peripheral blood occur quite commonly in children and present an appearance resembling leukemia because of the presence of a high total count and the immaturity of some of the cells. In many diseases occurring in the pediatric age group, such as whooping cough, meningococcemia, infectious lymphocytosis and occasionally in severe bacteremia or in erythroblastosis, the blood picture may resemble that of leukemia. A bone marrow examination will usually exclude leukemia.

Leukemia. While cancer, including leukemia, is the chief medical cause of death in children (after poisons and accidents) one-third of the malignant diseases in children under 16 years of age are due to leukemia of the acute leukemic type. The type of chronic lymphatic leukemia that occurs in adults is practically unknown in childhood.

About 80 per cent of acute leukemia in childhood is lymphoblastic. With modern therapy utilizing various chemotherapeutic agents and central nervous system prophylaxis, more than 50% of these children will survive without relapse for at least 5 years, and most of them are considered cured.

Purpura. Nonthrombocytopenic purpura resulting from increased capillary permeability and called anaphylactoid purpura (Henoch-Schönlein purpura) is a common form of purpura in children, usually between the ages of 2 and 4 years and occurring mainly in the fall and spring. The child may present with a red macular eruption that becomes purpuric in appearance and is associated frequently with abdominal pain, arthralgia, and edema of hands and feet. Occasionally the abdominal pain is so severe that surgical intervention is decided upon, the assumption being made that a more serious condition is present.

Fortunately the disease is usually benign, lasting approximately 4 weeks, sometimes with recurrences. Attacks resembling acute glomerulonephritis with hematuria may occur. In these cases, prognosis must be more guarded inasmuch as the condition may progress to chronic glomerulonephritis.

Idiopathic thrombocytopenic purpura may occur in childhood as in adult life, following viral illnesses. About 90 per cent of children with idiopathic thrombocytopenic purpura will have a remission within weeks or months. Splenectomy may be required when the disease is severe, and has continued for 6 to 12 months or more. Splenectomized children are in danger of overwhelming and sometimes fatal infections due to pneumococci, meningococci, and H. influenzae, and should be protected by prophylactic antibiotics and pneumococcal vaccine.

Central Nervous System

The greatest incidence of central nervous system disorders in childhood is reflected in the occurrence of mental retardation, cerebral palsy and convulsions secondary to either metabolic or structural defects. Over 100 inborn errors of metabolism, primarily involving amino acids, have been identified, any of which may contribute to the dysfunctioning of the brain. In addition, genetic and chromosomal disorders may effect the metabolism of the central nervous system. Finally, there may be inadequate brain development as a result of antenatal factors or disturbances produced by hypoxia and brain injury, either at birth or subsequently. Sequelae from meningitis and encephalitis secondary to either viral or bacterial infections have also continued to contribute to permanent neurologic changes. Evidence of disturbances such as learning disabilities, symptoms of minimal brain damage and cerebral dysfunctioning syndromes are being discovered more and more frequently among school children, in some cases up to 10 or 15 per cent of the school population.

Meningitis. Even the diagnosis of meningitis may be difficult in the first year of life, inasmuch as the infant may not manifest the classical signs of stiff neck with Kernig and Brudzinski signs. The small infant before the anterior fontanelle is closed may manifest symptoms of irritability and fever with bulging of the fontanelle and either excessive crying or listlessness.

In the newborn period, meningitis, may occur secondary to gram-negative microorganisms such as *Escherichia coli*. In later infancy influenza meningitis is most frequent, especially between the ages of 6 and 12 months. It rarely occurs in later childhood. However, pneumococcal meningitis is a frequent type, occurring in infants and younger children and may follow otitis media or pneumonia. Meningococcal meningitis occurs throughout childhood, as may tuberculous meningitis.

While all meningitides may have any number of the frequently presenting features such as the bulging fontanelle, opisthotonos, neck rigidity, vomiting, headache, fever, twitching, convulsions, hyperactive reflexes, positive Kernig and Brudzinski signs and rash, the differential diagnosis can be made with certainty only by spinal fluid examination. Therapy past the newborn period may still consist of the use of chloromycetin and ampicillin until the specific microorganism is recognized. Recently the treatment with a single broad-spectrum antibiotic, ampicillin, is gaining favor. Tuberculous meningitis, as might be expected, is treated specifically as an acid-fast infection.

Convulsions. Since tremors, twitching and massive motor seizures occur quite frequently in infancy and childhood secondary to a rapid rise in temperature, the seriousness of this clinical phenomenon is often overlooked by equating a convulsion in a child with a headache in an adult. Any child who has a convulsion should be considered to have an infection or an irritation of the central nervous system, either primary or secondary, such as might occur during the course of a communicable disease.

Convulsions are sometimes classified as symptomatic

convulsive disorders when studies by electroencephalography exclude the idiopathic or genetic type. The cause of seizures can be grouped to some degree according to the age of the child:

From birth to 6 months of age:

1. Brain injuries
2. Developmental defects of the central nervous system
3. Bacterial and viral meningitis
4. Hypoglycemia
5. Rarely hypocalcemia

1. Febrile convulsions secondary to infections such as roseola infantum, gastroenteritis or bronchial pneumonia
2. Bacterial and viral infections of the brain
3. Secondary to birth injuries or anomalies of the brain

From 2 to 6 years of age:

1. Infections of the central nervous system
2. Residual of birth injuries and anomalies
3. Onset of idiopathic or genetic epilepsy
4. Manifestation of degenerative diseases of the central nervous system
5. Brain tumors

From 6 to 15 years of age:

1. Genetic idiopathic type of epilepsy
2. Brain anomalies as at 2 to 6 years of age
3. Brain tumors
4. Infections of the central nervous system
5. Degenerative diseases

The major motor seizures and petit mal seizures are not unlike those seen in older individuals. They generally occur most frequently between the ages of 4 and 8 years. A more specific type of seizure for childhood occurs between 1 and 12 months of age in a brain-damaged child. This type produces a jackknifing of the body sometimes referred to as salaam seizures. The majority of these children remain mentally retarded.

Another type of seizure that is beginning to be recognized more often is the so-called temporal lobe seizure, which may manifest itself as a behavior disorder, in some cases specifically associated with smacking the lips and grasping movements of the hands and a dazed countenance.

Cerebral Palsy. Contrary to common belief, cerebral palsy is not necessarily the result of a birth injury but may be secondary to any malformation, injury or infection of the central nervous system before birth, at birth or in later childhood. Four types are described: ataxic, rigid, athetoid and spastic. Gross tremors may occur in isolation or in conjunction with the developing spastic type. Hypotonia, nearly leading to atonia, may well be present also.

Hydrocephalus resulting from excessive accumulation of cerebral spinal fluid is of two types, obstructive and communicating. In both types the head may appear to enlarge suddenly, and at 4 months of age the normal head circumference of 40 cm. may be greatly exceeded. In the communicating type, the block is in the subarachnoid space. This prevents the cerebrospinal fluid from reaching the arachnoid villi but permits the ventricles to communicate with the spinal subarachnoid space. In the obstructive type, the block is within the ventricular system itself.

Respiratory System

Congenital defects involving the airway passages may be responsible for deaths in the newborn period if these conditions are not recognized. They may vary from choanal atresia with complete obstruction of the nasal passage to the various forms of tracheoesophageal fistulas. It is for these reasons that it is advised that a small catheter be passed through the nose of every newborn child to confirm the patency of the airway. Its passage into the stomach and not into the trachea or bronchus may assist in excluding a congenital fistula. It is likewise recommended that plain water be utilized for the first feeding to be certain that milk is not passed into the tracheobronchial tree.

While infections of the respiratory system, both acute and chronic, occur in childhood as they do in adults, there are many specific entities that are more common for the pediatric age group. In the process of developing immunity, there are undoubtedly myriad viruses to which the young child is exposed so that coryza and bronchitis are not uncommon. Then too, both hypogammaglobulinemia and agammaglobulinemia may occur in children of this age group, and if these conditions are not discovered early, they may result in the death of the child from infection.

The tonsils and adenoids are normally enlarged between 3 and 5 years of age and are mistakenly diagnosed as being diseased with the result that tonsillectomies and adenoidectomies are needlessly performed. Nearly 500 deaths a year may occur following these procedures. The indications for this operation may need to be individualized, but the most frequent indications are repeated otitis media, severe nasal obstruction with chronic adenoiditis and repeated attacks of tonsillitis, especially when airway obstruction results. Performing tonsillectomy and adenoidectomy, incidentally, does not eliminate sore throats.

Stridor, noisy breathing in a small child, may result from the enlarged tonsils and adenoids. It may also result from infantile tetany, croup, edema of the larynx, bronchiolitis, foreign body, epiglottic edema as in *Haemophilus influenzae* infection or congenital laryngeal stridor.

Congenital stridor is a crowing inspiration in the newborn infant that may persist up to 2 years of age and is caused by a flabby epiglottis. No treatment is required. However, retropharyngeal abscess, which occurs most commonly in infancy, must be excluded by direct examination and palpation of the posterior pharyngeal wall.

Bronchiolitis, sometimes erroneously called asthmatic bronchiolitis, is a much more severe infection. It may be caused by specific viruses or by bacteria. The viruses most frequently implicated are the influenza A, parainfluenza, respiratory syncytial, ECHO 11 and the adeno-viruses. *H. influenzae* is the most frequent bacterial incitant. These same microorganisms may also cause acute infectious laryngitis.

Acute infectious laryngitis, sometimes known as laryngotracheitis, laryngotracheo-bronchitis or descending croup, is an acute infection of the larynx, the trachea and both large and small bronchi. The condition may manifest itself first as hoarseness, but as the disease progresses downward, it becomes much more serious and may even prove to be fatal in some cases. Bacterial cultures should always be taken to be certain that *Corynebacterium diphtheriae* and other microorganisms such as beta hemolytic streptococcus, staphylococcus and *H. influenzae* have been excluded. Treatment should consist of specific antibiotics such as ampicillin and cold humidification and oxygen as required. This is one condition in which tracheotomy should always be considered a possibility, especially when edema of the epiglottis is present. The rule of thumb often given as an indication for tracheotomy is "that time when one wonders whether one should perform the procedure."

While infants and children may develop the same types of viral and bacterial pneumonias as adults, chemical pneumonia, frequently referred to as lipoid pneumonia, is found not uncommonly in children as a result of mineral oil or other petroleum products being placed in the child's nose or mouth. Oily nose drops or sprays should never be given to infants and children, and water-soluble vitamins should always be utilized in young infants. Indeed, it is worth mentioning here that chemical pneumonitis or pneumonia sometimes may result from the ingestion of kerosene by the small child. X-ray examination of the chest in lipoid pneumonia discloses a butterfly-like distribution of the shadows spreading out from the hilum.

A warning should be given here that a foreign body must always be excluded in every child who presents with evidence of any respiratory difficulty.

Bronchiectasis, was in the past considered to result most frequently from the aspiration of some type of organic foreign body like a peanut or to follow tonsillectomy. The most frequent causes of bronchiectasis at present are cystic fibrosis of the pancreas with its pulmonary complications and chronic bronchitis secondary to asthma or bacterial infection. In this light, one can be suspicious of either of these entities when polyps are noticed in the nose and a chronic cough is present. A sweat test for cystic fibrosis should be performed on every child with a history of frequent or chronic cough, pneumonia, wheezing, bronchiectasis or asthma. A value of sweat sodium chloride over 60 mEq. per liter is diagnostic.

Cardiovascular System

Heart. With the marked reduction in the incidence of acute rheumatic fever, congenital heart disease, both cyanotic and acyanotic, is now the main cardiac difficulty seen in infancy and childhood. These conditions are alluded to in the section on medicine, but the reader is referred to a standard text for systematized clarification of the cyanotic and acyanotic types and the frequency with which they occur.

It is estimated that about 8 of every 1,000 infants born have congenital heart disease. The order of frequency of the different causes of acyanotic heart disease may vary from institution to institution, but in our experience the order is as follows: ventricular septal defect, patent ductus arteriosus, atrial septal defect, isolated pulmonary stenosis, aortic and subaortic stenosis, coarctation of the aorta, primary endocardial fibroelastosis, idiopathic dilatation of the pulmonary artery, vascular rings, anomalous left coronary artery, glycogen storage disease and aortic pulmonary window.

Cyanosis may occur in congenital heart disease and the order of frequency of the causes is as follows: tetralogy of Fallot, transposition of the great vessels, pulmonary stenosis with either atrial or ventricular septal defects, Eisenmenger's complex, tricuspid atresia, persistent truncus arteriosus, levocardia and anomalous drainage of all pulmonary veins. Visible cyanosis is present if a right-to-left shunt is sufficient to cause a concentration of 5 g. of reduced hemoglobin per 100 ml. of capillary blood.

No longer can a congenital heart lesion be diagnosed

with dogmatic assurance by auscultation alone since we now know that 50 per cent of all children have a functional, nonpathologic murmur that disappears with time. Reliance must therefore be placed on the skilled services of a pediatric cardiologist who in turn will use x-ray examinations, electrocardiography and cardiac catheterization with gas studies to arrive at the proper diagnosis.

Functional murmurs are always short in duration and are midsystolic in time and are never diastolic. They generally are soft, low pitched, usually heard best at the left base of the heart along the upper left sternal border and occasionally to the right of the apex. A second type is the loud, low-pitched murmur that is heard best to the right of the apex and may be transmitted to the left of the sternum.

Rheumatic fever is discussed in detail elsewhere, but the chorea that so characteristically accompanies rheumatic fever in childhood is rarely seen in adults with rheumatic fever. It occurs most often in females, usually from 5 to 16 years of age. These children may appear to be little more than emotional problems with easy laughing and crying. They may become moody, irritable and restless and sometimes almost maniacal. The purposeless, incoordinated movements characteristic of chorea may result in scolding by the parents, which only aggravates the condition. The fact that 75 per cent of children with chorea have other rheumatic fever manifestations should help to recognize the symptoms of this condition.

Paroxysmal tachycardia may actually begin in utero and has sometimes been recognized by the obstetrician, or it may develop in the newborn or result from rheumatic fever or digitalis overdosage. The attacks are characterized by a rapid pulse, exceeding 250 beats a minute, with pallor and an appearance suggesting vascular collapse. Cardiac failure may actually occur in children under 18 months of age and if not recognized in time may result in death. Various means such as pressure on the eyeballs or the carotid sinus have been employed to stop the paroxysm, but digitalis is usually effective. In children under 18 months of age, digitalis should be continued for at least 6 months to a year because of the high rate of recurrence.

Hypertension. Blood pressure normally increases in children from infancy through adolescence, although blood pressure levels in children correlate better with height and weight than with age. It is unclear what level of pressure can be considered distinctly abnormal at any given age or size. Less than 1 per cent of children and 15 per cent of adolescents may have some elevated blood pressure. The underlying cause for elevated pressure may be found in children under 10 years of age or in adolescents with diastolic pressures over 110 mm.Hg. In black adolescents of either sex and white adolescent boys, a diastolic blood pressure less than 100 mm.Hg probably is due to essential hypertension. White adolescent girls with even mild to moderate hypertension usually have some underlying lesion. It behooves the physician to identify the potentially curable forms of hypertension in children as well as to recognize its presence as a signal of conditions that may give transient or intermittent hypertension. The clinical signs elicited in hypertensive children depend heavily upon the underlying cause of the entity, and most children present with few symptoms. It is only when the diastolic blood pressure has been sustained at a high level, such as over 120 mm.Hg, for a relatively prolonged time in diseases associated with chronic hypertension that the elevation of the pressure itself produces little or any clinical evidence. As in adults, the heart and kidneys in children become the target organs for damage from sustained systemic hypertension. Low-salt diet and the customary antihypertensive agents need to be utilized in those children who have sustained elevation of blood pressure.

Gastrointestinal Tract

The gastrointestinal tract is the first organ system of the newborn infant to share the contributions of its mother and society. In fact, one of the initial tensions that the newborn experiences is that of hunger with relief derived from feeding and having the nipple placed within its mouth. This developing personality quickly learns that, in a tension-producing environment, reaching for one's hand or thumb and duplicating the sucking experience of feeding may release other induced tensions. It is this necessity to feed that brings mother and child together, and it is no surprise that love and eating soon become synonymous. An overloving mother may overfeed the infant, who soon becomes fat and overweight. On the other hand, a rejected infant may reach for oral satisfaction or may refuse entirely to feed and become withdrawn and underweight, the so-called love-starved personality. In later childhood, the term psychogenic obesity is applied to that form of obesity that appears in the child who finds solace and comfort in overeating. The primary instinct to such to release tension may possibly be an underlying need in those individuals who in later life find release of tension in sucking on a pipe, cigar or cigarette.

Vomiting or diarrhea in infancy and early childhood is an extremely common symptom, not only of an intestinal tract disturbance but sometimes of disturbances in other organ systems, for conditions such as otitis media, tonsillitis and renal infection may lead to these symptoms. However, cases of previously labeled parenteral diarrhea may really represent a gastrointestinal response to a generalized infection that may have manifested itself locally in some other organ or organs of the body.

Vomiting occurring in patients in the newborn nursery, provided the formula offered the child was designed for this age and degree of immaturity, almost always suggests an abnormality of the gastrointestinal tract. The congenital defects that may cause vomiting under these conditions, with or without abdominal distention, may be any one of a number of congenital defects of the intestine. Intestinal stenosis or atresia, duodenal bands, annular pancreas, volvulus and meconium ileus secondary to pancreatic insufficiency of cystic fibrosis need always to be considered.

Black meconium is usually passed within the first 12 hours of life, and if there has been any delay beyond this time, especially if associated with vomiting, any one of these conditions should be considered. As one would suspect, obstruction lower down in the intestine would delay the onset of vomiting while an obstruction in the upper tract would precipitate vomiting almost immediately after the first feeding.

One should be warned that the passing of meconium does not exclude the possibility of complete intestinal obstruction. If microscopic examination of the meconium discloses the absence of lanugo hair and squamous cells this would tend to confirm the diagnosis of intestinal atresia.

X-ray examination should be made with the infant in an upright position in order to demonstrate air and fluid levels in the dilated intestinal loops. Barium swallow is usually unnecessary. In fact, air can be inserted by way of a decompression tube in order to assist in the visualization of the intestine. A barium enema, however, may be necessary if air has passed further down into the intestinal tract so that one cannot distinguish the small intestine from the colon. If intestinal obstruction has been excluded, other causes for the vomiting, such as sepsis, brain injury and other parenteral causes, may need to be excluded.

In cases of this kind, time is essential, and no delay should be considered, since prompt surgical intervention is essential when obstruction is present. However, N-acetylcysteine or pancreatic enzymes sometimes may be instilled through a nasal decompression tube in cases of meconium ileus in an effort to soften the inspissated meconium characteristic of the cystic fibrosis picture.

Vomiting in an otherwise healthy-appearing infant may result from an intolerance to the formula that is being administered. The formula may be either too rich or actually allergenic to the child. If the vomiting persists throughout the first 3 to 4 weeks of life, other congenital defects may be the underlying cause, such as spasm of the lower end of the esophagus or the opposite, excessive relaxation, called chalasia, which permits the stomach contents to pour back into the esophagus when the infant is lying flat. Obviously, the treatment is to premit the infant to be propped up after each feeding and to carry out this procedure for a number of weeks.

A partial duodenal or small intestinal obstruction may now become apparent. The duodenal obstruction characteristically gives the "double-bubble" sign on x-ray examination, which is the phenomenon of seeing two dilated segments of intestine in the upper abdomen, with the dilated proximal duodenum being on the right and the stomach on the left.

Allergic reactions to feedings of cow's milk and orange juice may produce spasm of the pylorus with vomiting, which may actually be projectile in character.

Pyloric stenosis is a not uncommon diagnosis made in the first-born male who gradually develops vomiting that turns eventually into projectile vomiting. In these cases, the patient may retain the previous feeding within the stomach for 4 to 6 hours. This condition occurs in approximately a 4 to 1 ratio in favor of the first-born males, and occasionally there is a family history of its occurrence in aunts and uncles during their infancy. The vomiting may persist to such an extent that electrolyte disturbances result, with associated listlessness and obvious dehydration, or the child may develop alkalosis due to loss of hydrochloric acid. On palpation, one can often detect a smooth pyloric tumor 2 to 4 cm. in size in the region of the right costal margin along the border of the right rectus muscle after the child has been fed. Fluoroscopy, using contrast material, may reveal the narrow pyloric canal, sometimes referred to as the "string sign," along with the delayed emptying time of the stomach.

Surgery is required to split the hypertrophied muscle of the pylorus. The operation is known as the Fredet-Ramstedt pyloromyotomy. There should be complete correction of the dehydration and electrolyte disturbances before surgery is attempted.

Projectile vomiting may also occur not infrequently in childhood secondary to gastritis, infections or generalized disease. Renal acidosis, adrenogenital syndrome and brain tumor will also cause this annoying symptom.

Intussusception, in which one portion of the intestine invaginates or telescopes into an adjacent portion, is not uncommon in infants and children. Three quarters of the cases occur within the first year of life, and as is characteristic of most childhood diseases, they occur more commonly in males. The most common type begins at the ileocecal valve and characteristically produces the classical symptom of extremely severe spasmodic pain, which causes the infant suddenly to cry out. In fact, the infant may throw up its arms and flex it legs, at the same time emitting an excruciating cry. A period may follow when the child lies quiet, exhausted and pale. Vomiting is more characteristic than diarrhea, inasmuch as occasionally the patient may have missed one or two customary bowel movements.

Since adenovirus infection has been implicated as a causative factor in many cases of intussusception in children, attention has been drawn to the comcomitant occurrence of gastroenteritis and upper respiratory infections. However, purgation from severe catharsis or chronic diarrhea may also be the etiologic factor in some children. In older children, polyps or duplication of the intestine may serve as the precipitating anatomic cause of intussusception.

Intussusception is the disturbance that is associated with the well-known "currant jelly" stools that appear a few hours after the onset of symptoms. This type of stool is really bloody mucus that can be detected by rectal examination. Palpation of the abdomen may reveal the tender, sausage-shaped mass usually found in the right upper quadrant of the abdomen.

When intussusception has been diagnosed early, surgery can often be avoided by the reduction of the invagination by the use of a barium emena under carefully controlled pressure. Indeed, many of these children with intussusception recover spontaneously without surgical reduction. However, surgery must always be considered in order to make sure that strangulation and gangrene of the intestine do not develop.

Acute gastroenteritis with severe diarrhea and dehydration was at one time the most frequent cause of death in children. With the improvement of sanitation in both the environment and feedings, the mortality rate from this condition has been reduced markedly. An example of the seriousness of infections of this type occurs with epidemic diarrhea of the newborn, a condition that begins with a contagious infection in the nursery.

The essential treatment is based on recognition of the need to provide electrolytes and suitable fluids by the intravenous route in any infant or child who has become dehydrated as a result of vomiting or of "stooling" for many hours without adequate fluid intake. Fortunately, the majority of the cases are due to virus infection, although shigella, salmonella and staphylococcus infections occasionally still may play a role. During an epidemic of infectious hepatitis within a neighborhood or institution, many of the children will exhibit an apparent attack of acute gastroenteritis without evidence of jaundice. Indeed, only about 1 of 20 children who are infected with the infectious hepatitis virus will become icteric. Finally, 100 per cent of patients under 2 years of age with acute appendicitis will suffer rupture of the appendix but will manifest only symptoms of diarrhea and vomiting. Therefore, it is essential that the physician always keep in mind that the symptoms of gastroenteritis may result from parenteral infections as well as specific involvement of the gastrointestinal tract.

Abdominal pain in children is not uncommon and may result from dietary indiscretions, for example, the well-known "after eating green apples" syndrome, as well as simple fatigue or nervousness. Colic, a form of paroxysmal abdominal pain occurring in the first year of life, has a variety of causes, among which are underfeeding, apprehensive parents, swallowing of air or flood intolerance.

In later childhood, acute mesenteric adenitis causes abdominal pain from enlargement and inflammation of the lymph nodes within the abdomen. Pyelonephritis or infections of the genitourinary system with congenital renal defects may be a cause of acute or chronic abdominal pain.

Acute appendicitis is the most common condition requiring abdominal surgery in childhood. After the first 18 to 24 months of life, the symptomatology and complaints of appendicitis are not unlike those in adults. Typically, the onset is sudden, with generalized abdominal pain that, within 12 to 24 hours, becomes localized in the right lower quadrant. Nausea and vomiting, associated most frequently with constipation, follow. Fever, an increased white cell count and direct and rebound tenderness are present as well. However, in children, other apparently unrelated conditions such as pneumonia, rheumatic fever and the acute onset of diabetes must always be excluded before operation is decided upon. Every child with acute abdominal symptoms should have a chest film made to exclude the diagnosis of pneumonia.

Constipation in children is one of the conditions mothers most frequently find disturbing, for it often causes needless concern and great anxiety to a tense parent. If the constipation has persisted since the first few days of life and is characterized by days without a movement followed by the passage of a large voluminous stool, the diagnosis of rectosigmoid spasm or Hirschsprung's disease (congenital megacolon) is the diagnosis to be considered. This form of constipation occurs more often in males, as distinguished from functional constipation, which predominates in females. In early infancy the condition may actually resemble intestinal obstruction with vomiting, abdominal distention, hyperperistalsis and listlessness. Occasionally, by-pass diarrhea may result, causing leaking from the rectum with soiling of the clothes. Such a condition may be misdiagnosed as chronic diarrhea instead of constipation.

In general, rectal examination will differentiate this type of constipation from functional, sometimes erroneously called psychogenic, megacolon. On rectal examination, no feces can be felt within the rectum, while in functional constipation the rectum is usually paked with fecal material. Rectal biopsy will reveal the absence of ganglion cells in the colonic wall, since this entity is the result of a congenital defect of the parasympathetic ganglion cells of Auerbach's plexus. Skilled barium enema administration without overfilling the colon can often disclose the diagnosis as well. The treatment of choice is the Swenson operation, which consists of removing the contracted portion of the rectosigmoid colon and pulling the remaining colon down and fastening it to the rectal area once again.

Chronic diarrhea in infants and children is extremely frequent, with many causes known and unknown. Celiac syndrome is the term sometimes applied to all the conditions that produce malabsorption and frequent bowel movements from any number of causes. However, as more medical information is gained concerning the etiology of these conditions, specific identification of the causes of some forms is being made, and these are no longer included in this blanket terminology. Cystic fibrosis of the pancreas and gluten-gliadin enteropathy are examples. The listing of the many causes of this syndrome is beyond the scope of this review other than to mention milk and food allergy, the deficiency of sugar-splitting enzymes such as occurs with disaccharidase deficiencies of the mucosa and the defective absorption of monosaccharides. Disturbances causing malabsorption of different sugars are sometimes grouped together and called carbohydrate malabsorption syndromes. The ingestion of an offending sugar results in persistent diarrhea with the characteristic stool of low pH containing unabsorbed sugar.

Chronic infection of the intestinal tract or the genitourinary system is not infrequently the cause of chronic diarrhea, as are abnormal reactions to oral antibiotics and other medications.

Celiac disease caused by the intolerance of the child to the gluten present in the cereals rye, wheat and oats can be most dramatically treated by maintaining the child on a diet in which these offending cereals are eliminated. The patient will need to remain on this diet throughout childhood and into adulthood to some degree. If the removal of the offending cereals is followed by relatively prompt reduction of the number of stools, followed by a gain in weight, this result is almost diagnostic of this form of celiac disease. Further confirmation can be made by obtaining an intestinal biopsy through a duodenal biopsy tube, for histologic examination will reveal the characteristic blunting, clubbing and fusion of the villi of the small intestine.

Cystic fibrosis of the pancreas, sometimes shortened to CF, originally was thought to be a severe form of celiac disease, causing eventual death of the child before the adolescent period, in which the final diagnosis was made only at autopsy. By use of the iontophoresis sweat test—a method of collection and subsequent measurement of the sodium and chloride in the sweat (under normal 60 mEg. per liter for both sodium and chloride)—the condition may now be diagnosed even before the symptoms of pancreatic insufficiency, so characteristic of this disease, manifest themselves. This test has revealed many variations of this disease, not only in symptomatology but also in the degree of involvement. In many children the symptoms are primarily pulmonary, with chronic cough and frequent bouts of pneumonia, while in others the predominant symptoms are those of frequent foul-smelling bowel movements resulting from pancreatic insufficiency.

Cystic fibrosis is characterized by the secretion in the bronchi of viscid, gluey mucus that obstructs the pulmonary passages, resulting in the lack of aeration of different segments in the lungs, together with secondary infections caused by *Staphylococcus aureus* and eventually *Pseudomonas aeruginosa*. The child may have all the symptoms of asthma and whooping cough and other chronic pulmonary diseases before the persistence of symptoms stimulates the need to have a sweat test performed.

The symptoms relative to the gastrointestinal tract are undoubtedly related to the lack of pancreatic enzymes secondary to the destruction of the pancreas and the loss of acini. Prolapse of the rectum occurs quite frequently in these patients before replacement therapy of pancreatin (powered hog pancreas) is begun.

Cirrhosis of the liver with varices of the esophagus, as well as a form of diabetes characterized by the lack of acetone in the urine, may develop as the child survives into the adolescent period.

Before the present-day intensive therapy regimen had been developed, 50 per cent of these children succumbed to the disease by 4 or 5 years of age, and only 2 per cent ever reached the adolescent period. Now by the administration of anatomically oriented bronchial drainage by clapping and percussing the chest several times a day in order to remove the mucus, along with the daily use of antibiotics both oral and aerosol, 60 per cent of these children are now able to survive at least into the adolescent period.

Since the incidence of this disease is 1 in every 1,500 births, it has been estimated that for every cystic fibrosis child discovered there are three cases that remain undiagnosed. One should always perform sweat tests on the siblings in the family when one C F child is discovered. It is now recognized that in the milder forms of the disease, symptoms do not begin until much later in childhood.

A warning should be given that no screening test should be utilized for this disease. Only the iontophoresis sweat test should be performed; it should be performed two or more times to confirm or exclude the diagnosis.

The chronic diarrhea or loose stools can be treated by administration of pancreatic enzymes, with or without bile salts, with meals.

Chronic ulcerative colitis and regional enteritis; in children these diseases may have the same symptoms as those in the adult. However, the surgical resection of the diseased colon is indicated much more frequently than in the adult, usually with complete recession of all symptoms. A warning is given—ulcerative colitis in childhood should not be treated as a specific psychiatric disease!

Genitourinary System

As in all organ system difficulties in the pediatric age group, congenital defects should always be considered as a possible etiologic factor in any type of symptomatology manifested relative to that system. Congenital defects of the genitourinary system are usually confined to the internal organs, with the exception of hypospadias and aberration of the external genitalia secondary to hormonal or chromosomal defects or to both. Congenital hydronephrosis and hydroureter frequently are associated with congenital abnormalities of the lower gastrointestinal tract as in megacolon, or they may occur independently. One may even discover this condition by suspicion in the process of investigating fever of unknown origin, symptoms relative to the gastrointestinal tract or a failure to gain. Intravenous pyelography is almost always indicated in any child who has had at least two attacks of pyelonephritis.

Pyelonephritis is an extremely common disease of the diaper age and older children and occurs more frequently in the female than in the male. Increased numbers of white blood cells may not be found in any single urine specimen, so that repeated examinations of the urine are required. More specifically, both qualitative and quantitative urine cultures are recommended in the case of any child suspected of having an infection of the genitourinary system. In addition to an intravenous pyelogram a retrograde pyelogram and a voiding cystogram may be required to exclude both ureter and bladder abnormalities, such as posturethral "valves" in the male.

Acute glomerulonephritis in childhood does not have the same seriousness as when it occurs in adults, although 2 to 5 per cent of patients may go on to develop subacute and chronic glomerulonephritis and eventually die. Complete clinical healing results in 8 to 16 weeks in the majority of cases.

Acute glomerulonephritis is probably due to hypersensitivity to the beta-hemolytic streptococci, especially of group A, type 12 or 5. The first manifestation of the disease may be the passing of dark urine (hematuria) or periorbital edema on awakening in the morning. The evaluation of the kidney condition and subsequent therapy are carried out as in adults. It has been recommended, however, that penicillin be utilized only to eradicate the primary streptococcal infection and that the child no longer be prescribed constant bed rest and prophylactic penicillin therapy as in the past. The sedimentation rate is always elevated, along with an abnormal 12 hour Addis count. These two tests may remain abnormal for months in the presence of clinical healing.

A warning should be given regarding apparent hematuria in childhood. In the newborn period, for example, uric acid may give the appearance of hematuria. Also, the children readily pass red urine following the eating of red beets or rhubarb or after the administration of laxatives containing phenolphthalein or cascara.

Childhood nephrosis is a type of nephrosis that appears to occur as a specific entity in the early pediatric age group, although many characteristics of the disease are not unlike those in adults in whom there is an association of glomerular involvement as well. This disease in children is sometimes referred to as pure or lipoid nephrosis after the exclusion of the nephrotic syndrome, which is secondary to chronic glomerulonephritis and other disease conditions. Childhood nephrosis is probably caused by an antigen-antibody reaction for which no specific identifying test has been developed.

The disease occurs most frequently within the first 5 years of life and is less common in older children. The most frequent age is 2 years. The condition develops slowly and may first manifest itself as massive edema of the face or body, which goes on to the development of pitting edema and ascites.

There is copious albumin in the urine with associated

hypoproteinemia. Levels of alpha$_1$ and beta globulins are usually normal, but alpha$_2$ is characteristically increased as in the serum cholesterol. Serum complement is generally depressed in most cases. Occasionally renal biopsy by way of a percutaneous needle may be required to differentiate this type of nephrosis from other chronic renal diseases that present the same clinical picture.

This is a disease characterized by its chronic course with remissions and exacerbations, unless immunosuppressive therapy, primarily with adrenal steroids, is initiated. In the past, two-thirds of these children died within a 5-year period. Now, however, after a 21 day period of daily cortical steroid therapy, followed by the use of either cortical steroids every other day or steroids for 3 days on and then 4 days off, the mortality has been reduced to about 10 to 15 per cent.

Albuminuria secondary to lordotic positioning of a child's back should be mentioned as a unique entity, sometimes referred to as orthostatic albuminuria of childhood, a condition that corrects itself as the child matures and reduces the lordosis. This form of albuminuria disappears when the child is kept in bed but returns upon ambulation. However, studies have disclosed that many of these children will eventually have evidence of chronic renal disease. For this reason, all patients with albuminuria should have a complete evaluation of the genitourinary system.

GENETICS

Undoubtedly, no other branch of medicine in recent years has grown from the theoretical to the practical as rapidly as the field of genetics. While most students in the past were content to be aware that chromosomes and their genes were the carriers of genetic information, these have now become laboratory identifiable entities in human cells. Deoxyribonucleic acid (DNA), considered to be the genetic material, is localized in the chromosomes and is relatively constant from one generation to the next. The genes are located at specific sites or loci in any given chromosome and are linearly arranged along the chromosomes. A set of two morphologically similar chromosomes is called a diploid chromosome with one set from the mother and one from the father at the time of fertilization. This means that the chromosomes are the link between one generation and the next.

Forty-six is considered the diploid number of chromosomes, which represents 21 homologous pairs and 2 sex chromosomes labeled X and Y. The homologous pairs of autosomes are numbered 1 to 22 and divided into seven groups labeled A to G. Even within these groups, individual chromosomes can sometimes be identified by their features and by the relative rates of replication. The X and Y chromosomes can be identified by their morphologic structure as well. Females have two X chromosomes while the male has a single X and Y chromosome.

Numerous clinical entities can now be identified by performing both chromosomal counts and analyses. The reader is referred to standard texts on genetics.

A number of diseases, inheritance of which has been assigned to the X chromosome, represents the largest group that has been associated with a single chromosome in any mammal. There are more than 60 X-linked conditions known at the present time. Examples of X linkage are represented by hemophilia A, total color blindness, agammaglobulinemia, nephrogenic diabetes insipidus, congenital cataract, hyperparathyroidism and hydrocephalus due to congenital stenosis of the sylvian aqueduct.

There may likewise be clinical abnormalities resulting from the number of X and Y chromosomes. This may range from the occurrence of extra chromosomes, such as an XXY that results in Klinefelter's syndrome, which may manifest itself as infertility with small testes, to a mentally retarded male with gynecomastia, small testes and infertility. The female with Turner's syndrome may have 44 autosomes and only 1 X chromosome, in contrast to the double X in the normal female. Chromosomal counts of cells from tissue culture then would usually reveal 44 chromosomes, although mosaicism is occasionally encountered. Girls with Turner's syndrome tend to be dwarfed and fail to develop secondary sex characteristics except pubic hair. Also present may be webbing of the neck, coarctation of the aorta, widely spaced nipples and ovarian agenesis. A type called the Bonnevie-Ullrich syndrome may have lymphedema of the extremities. In fact, edema of the hands and feet in the newborn is quite characteristic of Turner's syndrome.

Since there are many possible combinations of the abnormalities of the sex chromosomes and at the same time there are clinical entities that might be associated with sex chromosome abnormalities, it is more feasible to obtain a buccal smear and stain for the chromatin-positive mass, which is referred to as sex chromatin or Barr body, that is seen normally in 20 to 60 per cent of the epithelial cell nuclei in normal women. Women are referred to as being chromatin positive while men, in whom the sex chromatin is absent are called chromatin negative. This analysis of buccal cells serves as an excellent screening procedure for recessive X-linked conditions and may also prove helpful in cases of indefinite external genitalia occurring in either boys or girls.

Some indications for chromosome studies include:

1. Confirmation of suspected chromosomal syndromes (e.g. Down's, Turner's, etc.)
2. Infants of parents who are translocation carriers
3. Multiple congenital anomalies of unknown etiology
4. Mental retardation
5. Parents of children with mental retardation and multiple congenital anomalies of unknown etiology
6. Ambiguous external genitalia
7. Girls with inguinal mass or peripheral lymphedema
8. Cryptorchidism
9. Poor reproductive fitness—sterility, abortion, prenatal mortality
10. Abnormal Barr body count or one not consistent with the phenotypic sex

The indications for chromosomal analysis may be based on the abnormalities of sex differentiation or specific clinical entities identified as having chromosomal abnormalities such as the trisomy entities, trisomy 18 syndrome and trisomy 21, and Down's syndrome, known more commonly as mongolism. As examples, chromosome studies should be made in boys who demonstrate chromatin-positive material in their buccal smears and, conversely, in girls who demonstrate chromatin-negative smears, as well as in boys and girls who have a very low sex chromatin count or multiple chromatin masses or Barr bodies and in boys who may have marked hypogonadism in the presence of a normal buccal smear.

In essence, the main reason for making chromosomal studies would be to establish the diagnosis of any obscure clinical entity as well as to identify individuals in whom there may be an increased incidence of affected offspring as a result of chromosomal or genetic abnormalities. One must remember, however, that there are many genetic disorders, birth defects and somatic malformations that are not identifiable by chromosomal studies. Likewise there are many clinical conditions that could be confused with those due to genetic abnormalities that are actually secondary to viral infections during pregnancy, such as mental retardation, cataracts, and congenital defects of the heart secondary to rubella infection during the first trimester of pregnancy in an epidemic year of rubella. Parenthetically, all children, especially girls, should be immunized with the new rubella vaccine to prevent rubella encephalitis later in childhood and rubella infection during pregnancy.

METABOLISM

In recent years, the description of many diseases has become biochemical rather than clinical with the result that a considerable number of biochemical aberrations have been discovered long before any manifest clinical disease has been recognized.

Inborn errors of metabolism, or what are called philosophically "experiments of nature," were recognized 20 years ago as comprising only phenylketonuria, tyrosinosis, cystinuria, cystinosis, alkaptonuria and albinism. Today, it is estimated that there are over 100 biochemical aberrations that are either clinically recognizable or undoubtedly will be in the future.

The clinical manifestations of inborn errors of amino acid metabolism comprise the majority of these aberrations. Some have absolutely no effect on the patient's normal life span or activity, while others, if not recognized promptly and treated in time, result in gross mental retardation and even early death. Phenylketonuria, or as it is commonly known, PKU, is a well-known example of those cases that must be recognized and treated early, for it results in mental retardation of the infant if not diagnosed immediately after birth by measuring the phenylalanine of the infant's blood and then placing the child on a low phenylalanine diet.

Characteristically, inborn errors of metabolism occur more frequently among close relatives and are common in the offspring of consanguineous marriages. It is sometimes stated that they represent a characteristic type of pedigree even to the pattern of the appearance of symptoms, which manifest themselves sometime after birth, following a very short time in which the patient is symptom free. This interval depends on the accumulation and toxicity of certain metabolic products. However, in most instances, the inborn errors can be discovered within the first month of life.

While there is no specificity in the symptomatology of the inborn errors of amino acid metabolism, there may be suggestive clinical clues such as the knowledge that 50 per cent of these errors are associated with a moderate to severe degree of mental retardation, although there is no special characteristic of this retardation to point to a specific inborn error. This is why the early biochemical detection of the error, before brain damage has been produced, is the goal for the future. This is the basis for the many screening procedures that are being studied at the present time.

The term aminoacidopathies is sometimes applied to the various disturbances affecting different amino acids, their pathways and the specific involvement of a single enzyme. When excessive amounts of a substance are present in the urine the suffix "uria" is added, such as homocystinuria, which produces a Marfanlike syndrome with osteoporosis, fractures, arachnodactyly, subluxation of lenses, mental retardation, pectus excavatum and other clinical characteristics. In this condition, there are increased plasma and cerebrospinal fluid levels of methionine and homocystine, resulting in copious amounts of homocystine being excreted in the urine, which in turn gives a positive cyanide-nitroprusside test.

When the suffix "emia" is added it implies an increased blood level and the excessive urinary output of the substance results from this increased level. However, it is to be noted that the patient may excrete certain amino acids or byproducts in the urine and yet the blood level of the product is either normal or only slightly increased. In most inborn errors the plasma values are usually normal or close to normal. As a general rule, one can remember that the plasma levels for most amino acids are in the range of approximately 1 to 2 mg. per 100 ml.

Among the other biochemical studies that may be useful is the checking of the patient's biochemical fluids for the presence of the metabolites of the amino acid's subsidiary pathway. This is generally done by giving the patient a tolerance or loading test by oral administration of 100 to 200 mg. of the specific amino acid per kilogram of body weight. The plasma level of the substance following administration of the load and the percentage of the dose recovered in the 24 hour urine are then determined. Occasionally the same studies are carried out on the parents or siblings.

Phenylketonuira has been recognized clinically and diagnosed biochemically before clinical manifestations of the disease frequently enough to deserve specific discussion. Many states have a law requiring that the phenylalanine level in the infant's blood be determined at about the third day of life. Values above 6 mg. per 100 ml. plasma are highly suggestive of this disorder. However, the diagnosis needs to be confirmed by repeated quantitative determinations of the plasma phenylalanine value.

In typical PKU, the plasma phenylalanine values rise quite rapidly during the first 10 days of life, reaching levels of about 30 mg. per 100 ml. It is at this time that phenylpyruvic acid and orthohydroxyphenylacetic acid appear in the urine.

The infant may exhibit nonspecific symptoms such as irritability, vomiting, infantile eczema or may even show low weight gain. The evidence of mental retardation may not appear for several months. However, if they are not placed on a low phenylalanine diet, 90 per cent of these individuals become mentally retarded. They may exhibit irritability, with or without convulsions.

In addition to the disorders of carbohydrate metabolism resulting in the malabsorption syndrome discussed under the gastrointestinal system, there are other hereditary carbohydrate abnormalities. Some are perfectly benign, such as essential pentosuria, which is characterized by the excretion of pentose L-xylulose in the urine. It occurs predominantly in those of Jewish extraction and is inherited by an autosomal recessive gene. This disorder must not be confused with diabetes.

Essential fructosuria is characterized by excretion of fructose in the urine of perfectly asymptomatic children. It likewise is due to an autosomal recessive gene.

Hereditary fructose intolerance, however, is a serious disease characterized by hypoglycemia, irritability, seizures, vomiting, wasting, hepatomegaly, and aminoaciduria. When fructose is eliminated from the diet, the symptoms and abnormal findings disappear. An intravenous fructose tolerance test using 3 g. per sq. m. will establish the diagnosis. There is a marked decrease in blood glucose and inorganic phosphorus during the test procedure. This disease is thought to be due to an autosomal recessive gene.

Galactosemia is a much more well known condition occurring in infancy. It is due to deficiency in the liver of the enzyme galactose monophosphate uridyltransferase, which converts galactose monophosphate to glucose monophosphate.

Galactosuria, aminoaciduria and **albuminuria** may be detected in those children who develop vomiting and diarrhea and enlargement of the liver within the first week or two after the introduction of milk containing galactose. Quite frequently the child will present a problem in differentiating the cause of jaundice. Eventually, cirrhosis may develop. Characteristically, brain damage and mental retardation eventually result. The mental retardation can be prevented if the diagnosis is recognized immediately, although frequently all other symptoms except this complication can be reversed when galactose is removed from the diet by providing milk-substitute formulas made of amino acids or soybean milk and containing no galactose.

The galactose tolerance test, unlike the fructose tolerance test mentioned above, may produce a dangerously low blood sugar level that can result in death, and hence it should never be performed. The erythrocytes are analyzed for their content of galactose monophosphate uridyltransferase. The finding of reducing substances in the urine by tests such as Benedict's—but not by specific glucose-detecting reagents—is suggestive of galactose and may serve as a screening test, provided the infant is receiving galactose in his diet, e.g., cow's milk.

Usually in the process of differentiating the causes of hypoglycemia or enlargement of the liver in children the clinician considers the glycogen storage diseases as contributing to hepatomegaly, growth retardation and periods of acidosis. In these diseases, there is defective mobilization of deposits of glycogen from the liver, heart, skeletal muscles and kidneys. Presently it has been established that there are six types of these diseases, classified as Cori type 1 to Cori type 6, each being based on a corresponding or specific enzymatic defect. As an example, Cori type 1 is sometimes referred to as Von Gierke's disease, in which there is enlargement of the liver at birth (often resulting in tremors of seizures) associated with marked hypoglycemia. This form is specifically diagnosed by demonstrating that the liver contains a high glycogen content and absence of glucose-6-phosphatase. It is thought to represent inheritance probably by an autosomal recessive gene.

In contrast, Cori type 6 is due to an enzymatic defect in the liver glycogen phosphorylase and is probably inherited by an autosomal dominant gene. While the symptomatology may resemble somewhat that of Cori type 1, it is more readily diagnosed by measuring the leukocyte phosphorylase, which is low, in addition to the hepatic phosphorylase. The prognosis is good in contrast to the poor prognosis in type 1. However, if an infant with type 1 survives to at least 5 years of age, he may be able to live a perfectly normal life from then on.

NEOPLASMS OF INFANCY AND CHILDHOOD

Malignant disease is the chief medical cause of death following poisoning and accidents in the 1- to 14-year age group. Leukemia, lymphomas, and other neoplasms of the hemopoietic system account for over 50 per cent of all malignant tumors of childhood. Tumors of the central nervous system rank second at 23 per cent, followed by those of the kidney and adrenal region at 6 per cent and those of the bone at 4 per cent. Carcinoma is relatively rare in childhood in contradistinction to adults.

Birthmarks, classified as hemangiomas and nevi of the skin, are the most common tumors seen and normally require no therapy as the years progress. The lesions most frequently disappear without surgical or radiation therapy.

Neoplasms may occur in the fetus or during the newborn period or at any time thereafter; in fact, solid tumors occur in the highest incidence during the first year of life and again between 6 and 9 years.

Acute stem cell leukemia, which comprises 80 per cent of all leukemias in childhood, accounts for approximately one-third of deaths from malignant disease in children under 16 years of age. Death usually results within 8 months without therapy, but survivals of 5 years or longer and cures occur with the use of steroids 6-mercaptopurine, cyclophosphamide, amethopterin or other antineoplastics such as vincristine.

The peak incidence of leukemia in children is between the ages of 2 and 4 with a second peak in the adolescent period between 15 and 19 years. The cause of leukemia is still obscure, although viral etiology is constantly suggested. There is an unusually high incidence of leukemia in patients with Down's syndrome, without explanation.

The symptoms are generally those of pallor with easy bruising, nose bleeds, petechiae and increased numbers of infections, either of the respiratory tract or elsewhere in the body. Sometimes a manifestation may be limited to joint or leg pain suggesting acute rheumatic fever. It is generally recommended that any child under 5 years of age who has symptoms of rheumatoid arthritis or rheumatic fever should have a bone marrow examination to exclude the diagnosis of leukemia.

Tumors of the central nervous system are common. In two thirds of the cases they are infratentorial in location, with symptoms referable to the cerebellum, namely, ataxia, incoordinate movements of the arms and legs and projectile or nonprojectile vomiting, as well as papilledema. Vomiting may be unrelated to meals and may occur upon arising in the morning. It is sometimes erroneously considered to be due to anxiety about attending school. Interestingly enough, headaches occur relatively infrequently in younger children. Specific symptomatology varies with actual location of the tumor.

Astrocytomas of the cerebellum are the most frequent type of brain tumor in children and account for 25 per cent of intracranial tumors. They occur generally between 6 and 9 years of age. They grow slowly and may manifest their presence by unilateral ataxia accompanied by the tilting of the head to the side of the tumor. Surgical removal is the treatment of choice, but since the tumors are radiosensitive, children should receive radiation therapy after surgery even though this treatment provides only a fair prognosis.

Medullablastomas account for 20 per cent of intracranial tumors and tend to be located in the posterior vermis. They are usually rapid growing and tend to occur more often in boys from 5 to 6 years of age.

The prognosis is very poor in spite of surgical removal followed by radiation.

Gliomas of the brain stem constitute 15 per cent of cerebral tumors and quite frequently are confused with encephalitis. Those generally located in the fourth ventricle are ependymomas and constitute about 10 per cent of brain tumors in children.

Supratentorial tumors include those of the hypothalamus and the optic chiasm, such as the craniopharyngioma discussed previously. The symptomatology depends largely upon whether the hypothalamus or the optic chiasm is involved. There may be polyuria, polydipsia, excessive appetite, atrophy of the genitals, irregular defects in the temporal portions of the visual fields and excessive sleepiness.

Those tumors in the region of the pineal body may produce sexual precocity, predominantly in males, and if the midbrain is involved there may be difficulty in upward gaze and loss of the pupillary reflex.

Palpable masses in the abdomen of infants and children are always considered to represent the possibility of malignant disease until proven otherwise. While neuroblastoma is frequently stated to be the most frequent abdominal tumor in children, Wilms' tumor is probably the most commonly palpable tumor in the abdomen. In the newborn period, polycystic kidneys, congenital hydronephrosis, omental or mesenteric cysts, as well as reduplication of the intestine may be the chief cause of a palpable mass.

Neuroblastoma originates from the neuroblasts making up the adrenal medulla or any of the sympathetic ganglia along the posterior wall of the abdomen or thorax. While the palpation of an abdominal mass may be the presenting feature, quite commonly the presence of unilateral exophthalmos with hemorrhage about the eye may be the first symptom. Enlargement of the liver or abdominal pain from metastases is not an uncommon complaint. Neuroblastoma may cause joint and leg pains, suggesting rheumatoid arthritis or rheumatic fever. The diagnosis is frequently made by simple observation of the patient or more definitively by the biopsy of a peripheral lymph node, the study of bone marrow aspirate, or by x-ray revelation of the presence of a retroperitoneal mass in the abdomen. Laboratory determination of catecholamines or other breakdown products in the urine has been of value in many cases. In most hospitals, vanilmandelic acid (VMA) and homovanillic acid (HVA) tests have been the most reliable.

Treatment consists of surgery, radiation and chemotherapy in combination. The most effective drugs are the alkylating agent cyclophosphamide and the alkaloid vincristine sulfate.

Wilms' tumor, sometimes called nephroblastoma, is the most common malignant tumor of the kidney in childhood and occurs most frequently during the first 3 years of life. It is usually unilateral but may be bilateral in 5 or 10 per cent of the cases. It occurs most often between the first and fifth year of life, although it has been diagnosed at birth. Occasionally it may make its appearance during late childhood and is generally discovered by the mother who, in the process of bathing the child, notices a large mass in the abdomen.

As soon as attention has been drawn to the abdominal mass, an intravenous pyelogram obtained in an attempt to isolate the tumor to the one kidney and to help differentiate the growth from neuroblastoma or a neoplasm of the adrenal.

Surgery, x-ray therapy and chemotherapy, with actinomycin D or vincristine sulfate or the combination of these two, is the recommended therapy. Prognosis has greatly improved; recovery may result in over 50 per cent.

With few exceptions, "rates of curing" rather than simple "survival rates" can be determined for malignant neoplasms in infants and children. If recurrence or metastasis has not taken place following removal of the tumor after a period equivalent to the age of the child at the time of removal plus 9 months, the probability of the tumor's recurring subsequently is very slight. This is called Collin's law.

The reticuloendothelioses form a group of relatively rare diseases whose causes are still unknown but which are characterized by proliforation of the cells of the reticuloendothelial system at one or more different sites in the body, such as lymph nodes, liver, lungs, spleen, skin and bone marrow.

Histiocytosis X is a term that lumps together the three diseases that are thought to be variants of the same pathologic process and are known as Letterer-Siwe disease, Hand-Schüller-Christian disease and eosinophilic granuloma. While these conditions are not tumors in the strict sense of the word, they are included here because of their invasiveness and the diffuseness of involvement of organs resulting in death of the children. There is a diffuse, generalized invasion of affected organs with histiocytes and occasional eosinophils. The infant may manifest eczema over the face and behind the ears, have chronic otitis media, exhibit small yellowish xanthomatous and purpuric skin lesions, develop enlargement of the spleen and liver and suffer from anemia. There may be both skeletal and lung infiltrations as seen on x-ray examination. The prognosis is very poor, and the course is rapid even though adrenal cortical steroids in large doses may help to maintain it for long periods. This is particularly characteristic of Letterer-Siwe disease, which progresses more rapidly than Hand-Schüller-Christian disease. The latter is a more benign form of reticuloendotheliosis occurring usually in older children and young adults. It may be characterized by punched-out lesions in the skull with bilateral exophthalmos and diabetes insipidus and may run its course for many years with occasional spontaneous remissions.

Eosinophilic granuloma is the most benign member of this group. The lesions are generally limited to the skeleton and are either solitary or develop as so-called eosinophilic granulomas of one bone or several bones. They appear cystic on x-ray examination.

Another group of lesions sometimes resembling tumors are the familial lipoidoses such as Gaucher's disease, Niemann-Pick disease and xanthoma tuberosum. Because of their rarity they will not be described here, and the reader is referred to standard texts of pediatrics for their description and therapy.

MENTAL RETARDATION

Approximately six million retarded individuals are living in the United States at the present time. Approximately three per cent of all children born annually in this country are retarded.

Mental retardation refers to below average general intellectual functioning that originates during the developmental period and is associated with impairment in adaptive behavior. Most significantly, and contrary to general belief, the largest group of retarded children, representing 2.6 of the annual birth rate, will with care and training be able to develop selfsufficiency to the point of being labeled "mildly retarded."

Retardation has been classified etiologically into four groups. The first results from antenatal conditions that are initiated before birth and includes all the familial and hereditary types as well as what are sometimes called the congenital types. The second type, called prenatal retardation, is due to factors occurring in pregnancy. The third type is called perinatal retardation and is due to birth injuries and hypoxia. The fourth type is called postnatal retardation and is due to infections, trauma and intoxication. Over 200 causes of retardation have been identified up to the present time. However, one third of all cases of retardation in children cannot be given a definite etiologic classification.

With increased interest in economic-social factors, undoubtedly there will be a reduction in actual retardation and pseudoretardation resulting from a socially deprived environment in the early years of life. The more widespread use of vaccines and improved obstetric care will also assist in reducing still further the number of retarded individuals.

Every retarded child should be intensively investi-

gated from the neurologic approach and the chromosomal approach, as well as from an environmental one. Deafness may sometimes give a false impression of retardation and should always be excluded.

Any condition that affects the central nervous system in infants and children appears also to affect emotionally the entire family. It is therefore the duty of every physician to provide emotional support and erase any feelings of guilt on the part of the parents. Whereas in the past physicians readily recommended that most retarded children be institutionalized, this is no longer true. The pendulum has now swung to the opposite pole, namely, to keeping the children at home within a relatively normal environment with acceptance by both the family and the community. However, there are children who may be hyperactive and destructive, who suffer from excessive numbers of convulsive seizures, and who may disrupt the entire home life of the normal children. These should be institutionalized. Down's syndrome or mongolism undoubtedly is one of the most commonly identified of those conditions. Chromosomal studies in these cases most often reveal trisomy 21, and as a result these studies not only lead to an accurate diagnosis but may well offer a dependable prediction to the parents as to the possibility that subsequent children may be born with this entity. Down's syndrome occurs more frequently in children of a middle-aged mother and may sometimes occur after the birth of several perfectly normal children.

These children have in common a characteristic facies, which makes them look alike whether they are born to different families or not. Because of the peculiar maldevelopment of the skull, the head is small and flat in the anterior-posterior diameter with a broad face and high cheek bones. The nose is small because of hypoplasia of the nasal and facial bones. The eyes are wide apart and slant upward and outward with narrow palpebral fissures and prominent epicanthal folds. The ears may be malformed, the lips thick and the tongue large and protruding.

There is a characteristic short fifth finger that is curved inward with the middle and distal phalanges often appearing rudimentary on x-ray examination. There are widely spaced first and second digits of the short stubby hands and feet with abnormal palmar and plantar prints. There is one major simian line or crease.

Hypotonia of the muscles with hypermobility of the joints is characteristic, and in a considerable number of cases congenital cardiac abnormalities such as interatrial septal defects may be present. These children are very susceptible to infections.

Skill and warm understanding are required by the physician in informing the parents of his impression of retardation, and his advice as to the care, treatment and the ultimate disposition of the child should be given as gently as possible.

EMOTIONAL GROWTH

The newborn infant, like all animals, requires warmth, cuddling and loving fondling from its mother and the environment in addition to provision of all physical needs. Some mothers are much more maternal than others and are not pressured to accept their child as a duty thrust upon them. One of the main advantages of breast feeding is that it brings the infant in loving contact with its mother, and the mother in turn responds to the infant's need for food and love.

Undoubtedly, the relationship any child has with its parents, and more specifically with its mother during the formative years, molds and shapes the total personality as evidenced in later childhood and adult life. A child who feels rejected by its parents will frequently become withdrawn and insecure and somewhat nonsocial as time goes by.

There are those psychiatrists who firmly believe that one's entire personality is molded and formed in the first 4 to 5 years of life. Indeed, many physicians place on the mother the blame for all the maladjustment problems of childhood and adolescence. Fortunately, however, many others recognize the fact that the growing child really does develop aspects of his own personality that are quite independent of what he has learned from his mother. In fact, there are certain children, such as the autistic child who from early infancy appears to withdraw from his environment, who in fact appear to require no cuddling or loving. It is understandable in such cases that the mother may in turn respond with negative feelings to a child who appears not to require her love.

Schizophrenia in childhood has become more and more to be recognized as a subtle metabolic central nervous system disorder that may either increase vulnerability to environmental influences or may interfere with the adaptive behavior of the child.

Neurologic dysfunctioning resulting from minimal brain damage may produce a hyperkinetic hyperimpulsive child who finds it difficult to control his activity and impulses and emotional behavior. A child of this kind could upset the entire environment to such an extent that the physician may carelessly see only the secondary effects in the parents and place the blame on them. One of these types of disorders apparently involves the temporal lobe, which has begun to manifest evidence of being an emotional controlling center of the brain that is relatively unresponsive to therapy.

No child in any family is raised in the same environment as its siblings and hence will have a personality that is different from theirs as a result of both hereditary and subtle developmental influences. It is not uncommon to find that the first child receives ten times the scoldings and spankings that the subsequent child or children receive merely because the parents, though they may have raised dogs or cats or pigs, have never raised a child before and under the pressure of our society wish to raise a perfect specimen for the admiration of relatives and neighbors.

It is quite frequent to find the second child of the family tending to be jealous, resenting the privileges that the first child appears to receive because of his age.

In any large family, the parents will note that they may have one child whom they could practically hit on the head every day with a skillet, and such violent action would not affect his personality in the least. On the other hand, another child may be so sensitive that the very sternness of a parent's glance may cause the child to cry. Rivalry and jealousy are perfectly normal between siblings of the same sex and the opposite sex.

Pediatricians generally believe that the entire personality of maleness and femaleness is not entirely learned but that much is instinctual. However, a basic part of sex education of children is to teach them the comfortableness of being a member of their own sex. In other words a young girl learns the joy of being a girl and the desire of becoming a woman. Contrariwise, the young boy is taught the advantage of identifying with his father or the male world and of experiencing his role in relationship to the female.

It is not unusual to note early signs of homosexuality in young boys when they appear to want to dress in girls' clothes or mimic mother's behavior, or both. With the development of a matriarchal society, it has been suggested that the young boy may be handicapped in accepting his mother as his identifying object instead of his father, who in general is so preoccupied with the business world during the week and with golf on the weekends.

It is advised that children never be compared with each other, ridiculed or punished by emotional rejection by the parents, who may temporarily withdraw their love in order to make the child regret his behavior. It apparently has been demonstrated that the ultimate adjustment of most children does not depend on whether they receive frequent spankings or not. Some parents react to abnormal behavior by administering corporal punishment to children, while others remain extremely calm and accept the immature behavior as part of the process of growing up. In general, it can be said that most children are good most of the time except when they are hungry or tired, do not feel well or are just bored.

It is a rule of the thumb that most children will mature with a satisfactory personality provided they have received adequate love, recognition, security, a sense of independence and at the same time have the feeling of belonging to the family or group.

With the pressure for success in school, we find many children emotionally handicapped by pressures outside of the home that may lead to feelings of inferiority and subsequent withdrawal. In fact, specific learning disabilities affect 10 to 15 per cent of the school population as demonstrated by the number of children who have difficulty in reading. Prior to fourth grade the ratio of boys to girls having reading difficulties is 4 to 1; after fourth grade the ratio rises to approximately 20 to 1. Careful neurologic and hormonal studies have demonstrated that those boys are neurologically handicapped, although their emotional behavior might suggest maladjustment as the etiologic factor.

Every child should be made aware of the fact that he is recognized for his abilities and his abilities alone. He is not required to overachieve or to live up to any expectation or desire of his parents. With the coming of adolescence, the young body is going through changes both hormonally and emotionally that are so rapid as to interfere with his normal feeling of happiness. Strong emotions, including a strong sex drive, may become manifest. Indeed, Kinsey demonstrated that the peak of the sex drive in the male is at 15 and 16 years of age.

It is quite normal for girls between 11 and 16 years of age to talk quite nastily to their mothers and to experience of periods of moodiness, loneliness and withdrawal. Boys may become more sullen or aggressive and concerned about their sexual drive and the need to masturbate. It is now considered by most religious authorities that masturbation is not a sin and is a normal phenomenon of adolescent growth, representing the discovery of one's self before being able to reach out to touch and to desire someone outside of one's own body. The normal crushes and gang activities of the adolescent are not abnormal homosexual experiences but represent the gradual emotional maturation that takes place at this time of life.

It is said that every adolescent goes through a "normal schizophrenic" period and that while he may accept life as a serious problem he quickly forgets the emotional turmoil he suffered when he has passed through the difficult years of rebellion, loneliness and variations in mood. A sense of humor on the part of the parents during these trying times can be most helpful. The role of the mother is to provide succor, love and the physical needs of the child, and the role of the father is to provide security, calmness and a sense of humor in the home.

Every parent should eventually learn that one does not completely mold children; one only sits back and watches them unfold. Many problems of life have resulted from the parents' mistaken belief that it is their role to shape and guide their child's destiny and life. Guidance can be provided without at the same time controlling all feelings and emotions of the developing child and adolescent. It is normal for the child to want to continue to mature and gradually to remove himself from the need of counsel and guidance from his parents. Moreover, the wise parents will recognize this normal rebellion and accept it without the child's needing to overreact and to project his hostility against the environment or the "establishment" as represented by parental authority.

With the pressures of society and confusion of parents as to their role, we find that today many of the young are using alcohol and drugs such as marijuana to a greater degree than ever before. Some of them use these "escape products" only occasionally for a trial, while others soon become addicted, using drugs as a means of escaping from the anxieties they feel. Schizophrenic psychotic behavior may manifest itself in adolescence. Often these individuals instead of withdrawing may become misfit heroes of their class, as one occasionally sees on the college campuses.

Many families that have been in the turmoils of emotional upheaval have been restored to calmness by the judicious talking out of their problems as a group either within the family home or in the physician's office.

QUESTIONS IN PEDIATRICS

REVIEW QUESTIONS

Write a formula for a 1-month-old infant who weighs 6 pounds 14 ounces and weighed 7 pounds at birth.

List 10 causes of the respiratory distress syndrome of the newborn.

What is the approximate weight and length of a normal 4-month-old child?

List the developmental milestones, month by month, for the first 12 months of life.

Outline the immunization schedule for the normal child.

List the cause or causes of dwarfism involving every body system.

What is the symptomatology of the adrenogenital syndrome in males? In females?

Name six causes of stridor in a 14-month-old child.

What are the signs and symptoms of intussusception?

List six congenital causes of acyanotic heart disease and six of cyanotic heart disease.

What are some of the causes of acute abdominal pain in children?

How is functional constipation differentiated from rectosigmoid spasm or Hirschsprung's disease?

List the signs and symptoms of cystic fibrosis.

List the causes of celiac syndrome.

Discuss childhood nephrosis in regard to age at onset, symptoms, treatment and prognosis.

What is the importance of a Barr body count?

What are inborn errors of metabolism? Give one example.

Discuss the diagnosis and treatment of Wilms' tumor.

What is histiocytosis X?

How many causes of mental retardation may be identified?

What is Down's syndrome?

Read the following case histories carefully and do not quickly jump to conclusions. Answer in five words or less and give only one diagnosis unless you are requested to give more. Make your diagnoses specific, not vague, e.g., "The diagnosis is patent ductus arteriosus," not "The diagnosis is some sort of congenital heart lesion."

A 4-hour-old infant is seen convulsing. What is the most likely cause?

A mother states that both she and her husband have been strongly allergic since childhood. She wants to know whether you would prefer that she (a) breast feed the new baby, (b) feed the baby goat's milk, (c) feed the baby boiled milk, (d) use a milk substitute, (e) not worry. Which would you advise her to do? First? Second?

In a hospital nursery eight cases of watery, loose, explosive stools develop within 1 week. What is the diagnosis?

A 5-month-old girl has been constipated since birth. She goes 3 and 4 days without a bowel movement. Physical examination is normal except for an umbilical hernia. Formula changes have been of no avail. What are the probable diagnoses?

A 4-year-old blond girl is brought in to you because of red scaly eczematoid eruption in the popliteal and antecubital areas. This has been present for "months." What has caused the eruption?

A 1-day-old baby has been unable to retain any feeding but vomits bile-stained material. What are the possible diagnoses?

A 3-month-old child who was started on "junior" vegetables last week has been passing lumps of carrots in her stools. What is the treatment?

A month-old baby, according to the mother, has sneezed "considerably" since birth. Since both parents have hay fever, does this represent a possible allergy?

A 3-month-old infant, previously well, is found dead in the crib. What is the probable cause?

A father calls you hysterically and says their 4-month-old baby had suddenly "turned bluish color" and "looks like he is dying." What three possibilities do you think of?

A mother states that her 1-week-old baby is passing green stools. What could cause this?

A 24-hour-old infant of a diabetic mother has been "twitching his legs and arms" for the past 6 hours. Oral and intravenous glucose has not relieved the symptoms. What are the probable diagnoses?

A 1-day-old infant becomes cyanotic at each feeding. What is the most likely diagnosis?

A 3-year-old boy who has always received vitamins has a history of recurring abdominal pain "since birth." He is below the third percentile for both weight and height. Albumin in the urine has consistently been 1 to 2+ for at least 2 years. It is noted that he has a prominent forehead and flaring of the wrists. What is a possible diagnosis?

A 5-year-old kindergarten pupil has had a cold for 6 days with coryza and cough and for the past 4 days has been running a temperature up to 105.6° F., in spite of having had penicillin for 5 days. What is a probable diagnosis?

A 5-year-old boy swallowed a nickel 1 hour ago. What should be done?

A 10-year-old boy with a "negative allergic history" states that he sneezed every morning for years and has a cold that lasts all winter long. Doctor A says he needs his adenoids removed, Doctor B says he has a deviated septum, Doctor C says he is allergic to feathers or house dust, Doctor D says he has agammaglobulinemia. Which physican do you support?

A 2-day-old infant has been taking his feeding, but his abdomen is becoming distended. He has passed meconium, which has a negative Farber test. What is the probable diagnosis?

A mother who states that she herself has always bled easily and has prolonged menstrual periods calls to tell you her 5-year-old daughter has developed "bruise marks throughout her body" since breakfast 2 hours ago. What diagnosis do you consider first?

A 5-month-old child with a head circumference of 42 cm. has been previously well until he began convulsing 4 hours ago. The junior medical student listed the following to be ruled out: (a) microcephaly, (b) hydrocephaly, (c) dolichocephaly, (d) infection, (e) tetany. What is the most likely diagnosis?

What are the common causes of "colic" in a 3-month-old baby?

A 3-month-old infant who weighs 8 pounds 2 ounces is receiving a formula of 8 ounces of evaporated milk,

14 ounces of water and 5 tablespoons of Dextri-Maltose. Is this adequate?

The mother of a 9-month-old baby complains that the child passes mucus frequently in its stool. What could cause this?

A 9-year-old girl is seen with a 7 hour history of vomiting, temperature of 102° F. and unlocalized abdominal pain. She has a cold and has had one loose stool. What are the possibilities?

A newborn baby is passing black tarry stools. What is the most likely diagnosis?

An interpreter informs you that this young mother and her 2½-year-old son arrived in the United States from India yesterday. Today, the child was found to have small red spots, blotches and little blisters over his chest and back. Temperature is 101° F., and the boy has vomited once. What is the probable diagnosis?

A 10-month-old white male was seen in your office because of pallor and poor appetite. He was born after an 8 month gestation. Birth weight was 5 pounds 1 ounce. The mother vomited one or two times daily during pregnancy. The baby has always taken solids poorly. He had diarrhea 2 weeks ago. His weight gain has been satisfactory. Examination discloses a well-developed and well-nourished pale infant. He has "small" cervical, axilliary and inguinal glands. The liver and spleen are not enlarged. The hemoglobin is 6.5 gm., RBC 4.11 million. Smear shows hypochromia, anisocytosis and poikilocytosis. What is the probable diagnosis? What is the treatment, if any?

A 2-day-old infant has a poor rooting and sucking reflex and thus takes its feedings poorly. What are the possible causes?

A 7-year-old girl was "feverish" for the past 2 days. For the past 12 hours she has not urinated and has complained of pain in her back. The mother states that she has been constipated for 3 days and is "slightly feverish" now. When you see her she is sitting up in bed with both her arms propped behind her on the bed. Her neck is obviously not rigid, but her back appears stiff. What is the probable diagnosis?

A 2-month-old bottle-fed baby has been spitting up some of his milk, sometimes in projectile fashion. He apparently has some abdominal distress after feeding, which is relieved by the passing of "gas." Symptoms began 5 days ago when (a) his paternal grandmother came to live with the family, (b) he started on orange juice, and (c) vitamins were started. Which of the three would you recommend be removed?

MULTIPLE CHOICE QUESTIONS

Select the correct answer or answers for the following statements. Answers are at the end of this chapter.

1. Prophylactic antibiotic therapy is indicated in the newborn:
   (a) to prevent pneumonia during winter
   (b) when the mother's membranes were ruptured more than 24 hours and labor was extremely prolonged and difficult
   (c) when the birth weight is less than 4 pounds
   (d) when the amniotic fluid is infected
2. Successful therapy of hyaline membrane disease entails:
   (a) reducing the metabolic rate
   (b) administering high levels of oxygen
   (c) correcting acidosis
   (d) monitoring the infant's arterial pH and O_2
3. Icterus of the newborn may be caused by:
   (a) infectious hepatitis
   (b) sulfanilamides
   (c) ABO blood group incompatibilities
   (d) gallstones
4. Indications for an exchange transfusion in the newborn are:
   (a) physiologic jaundice
   (b) a positive Coombs' test
   (c) a cord blood hemoglobin of less than 10 g. per 100 ml.
   (d) bilirubin of 14 mg. per 100 ml. at 16 hours of age
5. Diabetes insipidus in children may result from:
   (a) a sex-linked dominant genetic disease of the kidneys
   (b) Hand-Schüller-Christian disease
   (c) head injuries
   (d) hyperinsulinemia
6. The adrenogenital syndrome in early childhood:
   (a) occurs only in males
   (b) may result from an autosomal recessive familial abnormality
   (c) can be caused by an adrenal tumor
7. Hypoglycemia in children may result from:
   (a) glucose-6-phosphatase deficiency
   (b) hypersensitivity to an amino acid, leucine
   (c) adrenal insufficiency
   (d) islet cell insufficiency
8. Juvenile diabetes is characterized by:
   (a) insidious onset
   (b) absence of acetone
   (c) easy treatment with oral hypoglycemic agents
   (d) easy regulation
9. Anaphylactoid purpura:
   (a) is the same entity as idiopathic thrombocytopenic purpura
   (b) is the same entity as Henoch-Schönlein purpura

(c) is the same entity as black measles

(d) may cause acute abdominal pain

10. Meningitis in children is most frequently caused by the following microorganisms:
    (a) *Staphylococcus aureus*
    (b) *Haemophilus influenzae*
    (c) *Escherichia coli*
    (d) Pneumococcus
    (e) Meningococcus

11. The most likely cause of convulsions in a newborn infant is:
    (a) brain tumor
    (b) birth injury
    (c) congenital or developmental brain defects
    (d) hypoglycemia
    (e) infection

12. Bronchiolitis:
    (a) is the same as asthma
    (b) may be caused by the respiratory syncytial virus and influenzal viruses
    (c) is a mild benign disorder
    (d) may be caused by *Haemophilus influenzae*

13. Congenital cyanotic heart disease:
    (a) can be caused by tetralogy of Fallot
    (b) is associated with functional murmurs
    (c) can be diagnosed specifically by electrocardiography
    (d) is best studied by cardiac catheterization

14. Vomiting that occurs in infants in the newborn nursery may be caused by:
    (a) intestinal volvulus
    (b) intestinal atresia
    (c) meconium ileus
    (d) improper formula
    (e) nervousness

15. Double-bubble sign on x-ray film:
    (a) occurs with pyloric stenosis
    (b) is found in duodenal obstruction
    (c) results from faulty feeding
    (d) is found in meconium ileus

16. Children under five years of age with joint pain may have:
    (a) growing pains
    (b) leukemia
    (c) neuroblastoma
    (d) rheumatoid arthritis

17. Coombs' test should be done on cord blood from:
    (a) placenta side
    (b) infant's side
    (c) after exchange transfusion
    (d) before exchange transfusion

18. Sickling of red blood cells occurs in:
    (a) eight per cent of blacks
    (b) megaloblastic anemia
    (c) only in sickle cell anemia, not sickle cell trait
    (d) thalassemia and sickle cell trait occurring together

19. Children with diabetes mellitus
    (a) usually have an abrupt onset compared to adult onset
    (b) should not be treated with oral hypoglycemic agents
    (c) need not be concerned about developing renal and eye complications at any time
    (d) have marked variations in insulin response

20. An infant with an enlarged clitoris may have been born to a mother who received:
    (a) progesterone
    (b) adrenocortical steroids
    (c) testosterone
    (d) stilbesterol

21. Hypothyroidism in children:
    (a) can be chemically detected at birth
    (b) results from agenesis or dysgenesis of the thyroid
    (c) results from maternal autoimmunization
    (d) results from lack of maternal dietary iodine

22. A child with diabetes insipidus may have:
    (a) a third ventricle tumor
    (b) ingested excessive salt
    (c) mental retardation and renal dysfunction
    (d) a high urinary specific gravity

23. Anorexia nervosa:
    (a) occurs twice as frequently in obese boys
    (b) of the psychogenic origin should not be diagnosed in prepuberty children
    (c) can be treated with pituitary hormones
    (d) follows crash dieting

24. An infant with frequent lung infections may have:
    (a) cystic fibrosis
    (b) milk allergy
    (c) deficiency of a blood complement
    (d) gastric reflux

25. Immunodeficiency may be:
    (a) inherited
    (b) limited to IgA
    (c) caused by B cell deficiency
    (d) always treatable with gammaglobulin

26. Household contacts of a patient with meningococcal meningitis:
    (a) should receive penicillin
    (b) should receive meningococcus vaccine
    (c) rifampin in a dose of 1 mg. per kg per day
    (d) be watched for symptoms, and then treated to avoid adverse drug reactions

27. A six-month-old child should:
    (a) sit alone with support
    (b) have four teeth
    (c) laugh
    (d) wave "bye, bye"
28. The growing child:
    (a) at four years of age may weigh 40 pounds and measure 40 inches in height
    (b) double its birth weight by three months
    (c) may weigh 68 pounds at 10 years of age
    (d) at four months of age have a head circumference of 40 cm.
29. Physiological jaundice:
    (a) lasts longer in the premature
    (b) can cause clay-colored stools
    (c) result from decreased activity of uridine diphospho glucuronyl
    (d) can cause kernicterus
30. Cyanosis of the hands and feet in newborn infants:
    (a) may be normal
    (b) be caused by hypoglycemia
    (c) can indicate congenital heart disease
    (d) can be caused by the high hematocrit of the newborn

TRUE OR FALSE QUESTIONS

1. Cataracts of infancy may be caused by galactosemia.
2. Choanal atresia should be suspected in an infant with feeding difficulties.
3. Epidemic diarrhea of the newborn may be caused by strains of pathogenic *Escherichia coli*.
4. Accidents are the leading cause of death of children over 1 year of age.
5. One of every 60 babies born in the United States dies by the third day of life.
6. Anal atresia is frequently associated with congenital renal abnormalities, and an IVP is recommended.
7. A child with morning vomiting may have a subtentorial brain tumor.
8. Enuresis beginning in a 6-year-old girl may be due to organic causes.
9. A child with hyperimpulsivity may be misconstrued as hyperkinetic, but both conditions may result from minimal brain damage.

10. Milk allergy may produce symptoms of pyloric stenosis.
11. The adrenogenital syndrome occurs in both boys and girls and may cause vomiting and death.
12. Two or more attacks of pyuria in a child warrant a urological workup.
13. A sweat chloride of 85 mEq. per liter is compatible with the diagnosis of cystic fibrosis of the pancreas.
14. Glycogen storage disease is associated with either hepatomegaly or cardiomegaly and frequently with ketonuria.
15. Influenza meningitis occurs most frequently in infants under 1 year of age.
16. The most likely cause of a palpable abdominal mass in the newborn is a congenital renal defect such as polycystic or hydronephrotic kidney, but in a 3-year-old it is Wilms' tumor.
17. The Coombs test is negative in ABO incompatibility.
18. An asymptomatic 2-year-old with a positive tuberculin test should receive INH therapy.
19. A formula of evaporated milk, 13 ounces; water, 18 ounces; cane sugar, 2 tablespoons, will supply all nutritional needs of a normal 2-month-old infant except for vitamins.
20. So-called physiologic jaundice tends to be more severe and prolonged in the premature than in the full-term infant.
21. A rigid neck does not frequently occur in meningitis that develops in a child under 6 months of age.

ANSWERS TO MULTIPLE CHOICE QUESTIONS

Multiple choice questions:

1. b, d	**9.** b, d	**17.** b, d	**24.** a, c, d
2. c, d	**10.** b, c, d, e	**18.** a, d	**25.** a, b, c
3. a, c	**11.** b, c, d, e	**19.** a, b, d	**26.** c
4. c, d	**12.** b, d	**20.** a, b, c	**27.** a, c
5. a, b, c	**13.** a, d	**21.** a, b, c, d	**28.** a, c, d
6. b, c	**14.** a, b, c, d	**22.** a, c	**29.** a
7. a, b, c	**15.** b	**23.** b, d	**30.** a, b, c, d
8. none	**16.** b, c, d		

True or false questions:

1 to **21.** All are *true!*

12

Public Health and Community Medicine

CHARLES M. WYLIE, M.D., DR. P.H.

Professor of Public Health Administration, Department of Health
Planning and Administration, University of Michigan School of Public
Health

A major concern of most practicing physicians continues to be that of doing their best for individual patients. A new concern now rises—how each may have the greatest impact on community health; it reinforces the view that something more than the individual physician–patient contact is needed to help those sections of society with the greatest problems of disease. It is to this new concern that this chapter will direct full attention.

A difficult question, the answers to which are basic to all that this chapter contains, is: When do health problems become public health problems? The most usual answer is that health problems become public health problems when they cannot be solved by individual effort. This answer is dissatisfying, because personal values and political beliefs dominate our efforts to follow this rule-of-thumb. Have coronary artery disease and lung cancer become public health problems because their incidence is high? Do patients become public health problems when their personal habits reduce their expectation of life? Do physicians become public

health problems if they do not apply new techniques that will significantly improve the health of their patients? The health sciences give no uniform answer to these question; the answers relate as much to our beliefs and attitudes as they do to an organized body of knowledge.

Public health activities used to be limited to sanitary measures taken to control nuisances and environmental health hazards; such conditions were not subject to abatement through individual effort alone or were amenable to less expensive control by group effort. However, as techniques emerged from microbiology and immunology, the concept of preventing infectious disease in the individual benefited from such efforts. Public health in the early 20th century thus integrated sanitary science and medical science.

Public health efforts went further, however; it became clear that the incidence of illness was excessively high in low socioeconomic groups of the population. The gap has widened in recent decades, for example, between white and black death rates at each age, and it seems likely that this change was not biologically inevitable. It thus became acceptable for government funds to support personal health services to lower income groups and the elderly, through Medicaid and Medicare respectively. The relative shortage of health personnel, the gradual disappearance of the family physician, the slow application of new medical knowledge, the rising cost of hospital care and the increasing proportion of illness that is long term and disabling, all became concerns of American society and further broadened the outlook of public health.

Thus has evolved *community medicine*—the overlap between public health and medicine. Community medicine is concerned with the medical needs of all residents in the community, not only those who currently seek care. Community medicine is also interested in the future development of comprehensive health services at reasonable cost for all population groups, an ideal situation that is growing slowly in the United States in the 1980s.

What Is Health?

In most fields of activity, our morale and job satisfaction improve when we clearly define our goals. For centuries, however, we have had great difficulty in developing a clear picture, and good working definition, of health. A somewhat idealized definition, given in the Constitution of the World Health Organization (WHO) in 1948, has been widely used: "Health is a state of complete physical, mental, and social well-being, and not merely the absence of disease or infirmity."

Many respected persons, including examiners in public health, may still accept this statement as a feasible if somewhat distant goal; others regard this goal as unrealistic, for society continues to change its expectations as health conditions and knowledge improve. The WHO definition is open ended, setting a goal that slips over the horizon each time we move in its direction. Nor does the statement help greatly in separating healthy patients or communities from unhealthy ones. It requires that we exclude disease or infirmity; more difficult and perhaps impossible is the second step, to show that "complete physical, mental and social well-being" is present.

We may reach good definitions only by trying out and improving on a series of bad ones. A second group of definitions, widely held by the ancient Greeks, have again come to the fore in the 1980s. They relate health to an ability to resist threats of disease, and picture a positive interaction between the individual or community and the environment. One such example says that "Health is the perfect continuing adjustment of

an organism to its environment." From this definition we deduce that disease occurs when man and the environment are poorly balanced.

Society tends to associate disease with conditions of the body that shorten the duration of life or that cause unusual symptoms or signs, discomfort, disability or death. We are more certain that conditions are diseases when they can be recognized, labeled, and understood by physicians. When medical intervention helps these conditions, their classification as diseases seems no longer in doubt.

We thus realize that our concept of disease is closely related to what physicians do in society and to the degree of advancement of medical practice. Physicians are helped to determine the presence or absence of disease by means of laboratory tests and other measuring devices. With few exceptions, each new device tends to encourage the medical profession to classify an increasing proportion of the population as diseased.

In practice most physicians regard health as being the absence of disease. In their written descriptions, they often summarize a system in terms of abnormalities detected or absent. This may well be the most practical, although oversimplified, view to hold in the coming years.

The value of health lies in the worthwhile activities and goals that are made possible by the possession of it. People strive for food, shelter, sexual expression, and perhaps for some apparent luxuries in life, before striving for complete health. Health professionals must accept philosophically, at least for a time, this system of priorities. Government inevitably plays a large part in public health, because many activities can be carried out only by group or community action. Some individual liberty is surrendered in return for increased opportunity and security, but some parts of American society and some health professionals may not always be convinced that this exchange is good.

HEALTH STATISTICS

To some extent, definition is a first step in measurement; it sets clear limits that should tell us whether we fall between or outside the limits. Measurement goes further to indicate more precisely that part of a scale upon which we fall. Most devices that we use to measure the public health are part of the field of health statistics.

Since the population is the base for most health statistics, complete enumeration of the population is important. In the first year of each decade, such as in 1980, the United States Census Bureau conducts a national census to provide this information. For most purposes, the estimates made for intermediate years are sufficiently reliable.

Population trends in the United States differ from those in the developing countries. In many developing countries birth rates have not fallen far enough to compensate for a more rapid fall in death rates. These countries are rapidly adopting the lifesaving techniques that the more advanced countries took decades to acquire. Somewhat slowly, family planning activities are being included in the health programs for these countries. No form of life can continue to multiply without eventually coming to terms with its environment. Thus the rate of human population growth must inevitably slow down and level off; the major unknowns are when, at what levels, and with what cost to the public health this will occur.

In contrast to population figures, which form the denominators of most health statistics, vital facts such as births and deaths form the numerators. Registration of births and deaths is required throughout the United States and is a function of the departments of health of the various states. The attending physician is responsible for filing birth certificates with the local registrar. The funeral director is responsible for filing death and stillbirth certificates.

In the death certificate, emphasis is placed on the underlying cause of death as determined by the certifying physician. Because many older patients die with multiple diseases, the way in which physicians select the underlying cause of death has an important effect on time trends in death rates. There is good evidence that some changes in death rates in recent decades relate more to changes in diagnostic habits of physicians than to true changes in incidence of diseases.

The cause of death should be reported in accordance with the nomenclature developed by the International Statistical Classification of Diseases, Injuries and Causes of Death, which is distributed by the World Health Organization. The ninth revision of this publication, first used in the United States for 1978 death statistics, will produce some artificial changes in death rates between 1977 and 1978. Such changes in classification of causes of death must be taken into account when interpreting the significance of death rates. In addition to providing important data on health problems, the death certificate is needed legally for the settlement of estates and insurance claims.

The mortality statistics compiled from the death registrations are usually expressed as rates:

1. **The crude death rate** is formed by the number of deaths in the calendar year per 1,000 population at the middle of the year. After having fallen rapidly between 1930 and 1950, the crude death rate for the United States changed little in the 1950s and 1960s, and fell again in the 1970s (Fig. 12-1). This rate hides the fact that the falling death rates in each age group are partly hidden by the rising number of persons in the older population, among whom death rates are high. Crude death rates fall more swiftly in the developing countries, however, where older age groups form a smaller proportion of the total population. In

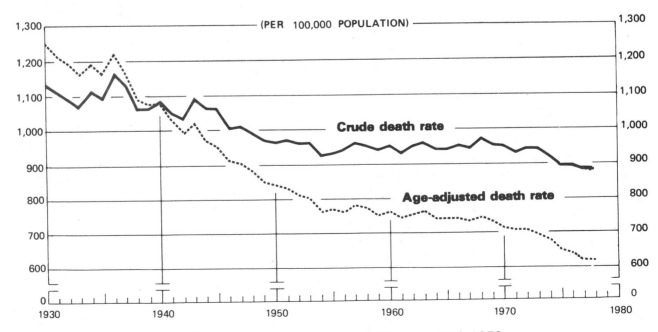

Fig. 12-1. Crude and age-adjusted death rates, 1930–1978.

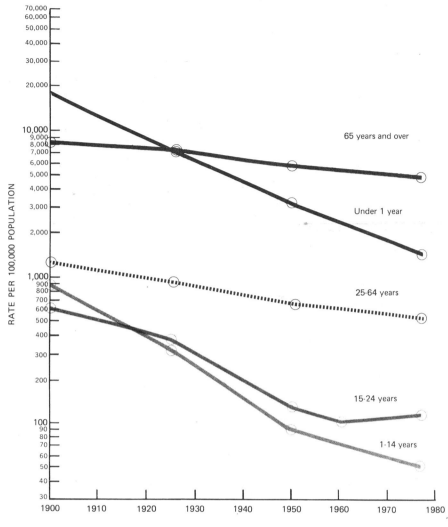

RATE PER 100,000 POPULATION

65 years and over

Under 1 year

25-64 years

15-24 years

1-14 years

NOTE: 1977 data are provisional, data for all other years are final. Selected years are 1900, 1925, 1950, 1960 (for age group 15-24 years only), and 1977.

SOURCE: National Center for Health Statistics, Division of Vital Statistics.

Fig. 12-2. Death rates by age: United States, selected years 1900–1977. Note: 1977 data are provisional; data for all other years are final. Selected years are 1900, 1925, 1950, 1960 (for age group 15–24 years only), and 1977. (National Center for Health Statistics, Division of Vital Statistics)

the United States, death rates also fall more steeply when adjusted for the increasing age.

2. **Specific death rates** are calculated for certain groups because the crude death rate is much affected by age, sex, race, marital and socioeconomic changes in the population being studied. One example is the age-specific death rate, formed by the number of deaths in a specific age group in a given year per 1,000 population at that specified age. Figure 12-2 shows time trends in age-specific death rates in the United States. At every age, these rates have fallen since 1900. Since 1960, however, rising death rates for accidents, suicides and homicide have caused the 16 to 24 age-specific death rate to increase through 1979.

At almost every age, mortality in women is now lower than in men; this is not the case in the developing countries, where complications of childbirth occuring under adverse conditions raise the mortality rates of women in the reproductive ages. Age-specific death rates have fallen more for women than men in the United States, and more for whites than for blacks. Socioeconomic factors and perhaps inferior health care of blacks are believed to be partly responsible for this latter difference.

Specific death rates are also developed for sex, race, marital status and other factors. At each age, for example, death rates among the married are lower than among the unmarried; this finding is partly explained by the likelihood that persons who marry are already more healthy than those who do not, but other factors may play a part. A disease-specific death rate is the number of

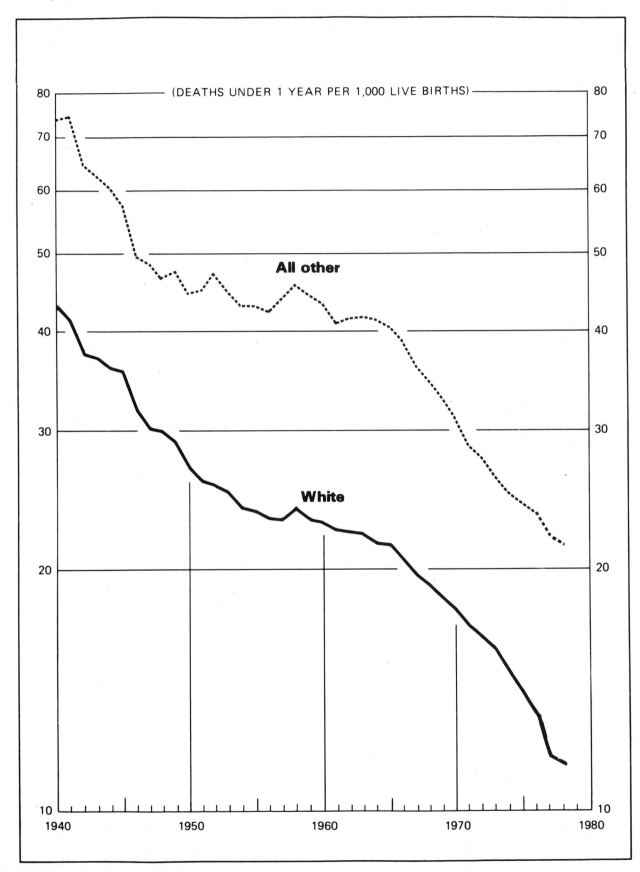

Fig. 12-3. Infant mortality rates by race: United States, 1940–1978.

deaths from the specific disease in a given year per 100,000 population for the same year. Specific rates for tuberculosis and other infectious diseases have been useful reflectors of changes in the health status of population groups.

3. **The infant mortality rate** is the number of deaths under 1 year of age in a given year per 1,000 live births in the same year. This rate was once regarded as a good (and perhaps the best) measure of the effectiveness of public health programs, which caused the rates to fall rapidly. It was sensitive to many changes in society, including improvements in health care. In the developed countries in recent years, however, further public health and medical efforts had less impact on infant mortality rates in the 1950s and early 1960s. They began falling again in the late 1960s, and this fall has continued in the 1970s with rates for blacks consistently higher than rates for whites (Fig. 12-3). Figure 12-4 shows that low birth weight has been associated with many infant deaths in recent years, both in whites and blacks.

It seems likely that reductions in infant mortality exaggerated the effectiveness of environmental health, communicable disease, and maternal and child health programs in former years, and now reflects less well our efforts to treat patients with chronic disease, the mental illnesses, and other problems of the older population. Infant mortality rates are lower in many developed countries than they are in the United States, and it seems clear that some differences are real, not caused artifically by the way in which data are reported. Infant mortality rates continue to fall rapidly in many developing countries. The debate over the value of infant mortality rates in assessing the health of populations has been strong in the United States. We may expect both the advocates and opponents of infant mortality rates, including some with vested interests, to continue the debate in coming years.

4. **The maternal mortality rate** is formed by the number of deaths from puerperal causes in a given year per 1,000 live births in the same year. Like the infant mortality rate, this rate is falling more slowly than before in the United States and is considerably higher for nonwhites than for whites.

The leading causes of death have changed markedly since 1900. At the turn of the century, the picture was dominated by such infections as tuberculosis and influenza and pneumonia (Fig. 12-5). In 1977 noninfectious long-term illness dominated the picture, with cardiovascular disease and cancer being the important causes of death. From the viewpoint of those who set priorities for disease control programs for society, however, the average age of death and the likelihood of success in disease prevention are among other factors that must be considered. Communities pay less attention to problems of cerebrovascular disease, for example, because this group of diseases mainly affects persons at an advanced age.

Another commonly used measure of health is the expectation of life at a given age. Although the *average expectation of life* is sometimes advocated as a "positive" measure of health—the higher the figure, the better the health—it is basically determined by the death rates of the population involved. The lower the subsequent death rates, the higher will be the expecta-

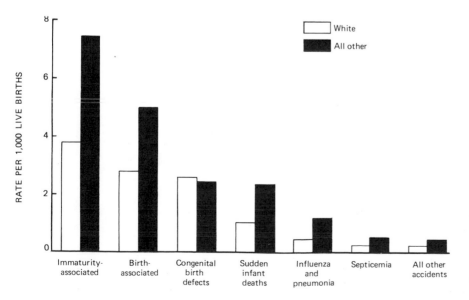

Fig. 12-4. Major causes of infant mortality: United States, 1976. (Based on data from the National Center for Health Statistics, Division of Vital Statistics)

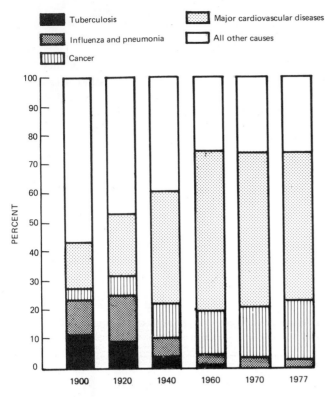

Fig. 12-5. Deaths for selected causes as a percent of all deaths: United States, selected years, 1900–1977. Note: 1977 data are provisional; data for all other years are final. (National Center for Health Statistics, Division of Vital Statistics)

tion of life. The case is weak, therefore, to suggest that the expectation of life measures something different from the force of mortality. Figure 12-6 shows that life expectancy at birth has slowly risen in recent decades and is consistently higher for women than men, between whom the gap has widened.

Morbidity Reporting

Reportable diseases are those that by law must be reported to health authorities. The list varies from state to state, and from time to time, according to the importance attributed to the given disease. Such reporting is rarely complete and gives a distorted picture of the frequency of disease in communities. Moreover, the incidence of many disease groups, such as the mental illnesses and the arthritides, is poorly reflected in death rates. Attempts to require the reporting of noninfectious disease have had limited success, with cancer registries being the most common example of this activity.

The United States National Health Survey is trying to correct these deficiencies through use of interviews of a nationwide sample of households, and other surveys, including medical examinations, to provide clinical information that is not obtainable from household interviews. This survey now provides good information on many nonfatal conditions, such as the frequency of acute conditions in the United States population (Fig. 12-7). This figure shows that the seasonal fluctuation in all acute conditions is produced partly by the swings in acute respiratory disease. Figure 12-8 shows that acute conditions fall with increasing age, and are more frequent in females than males at every age. In

Fig. 12-6. Life expectancy by sex: 1930–1978.

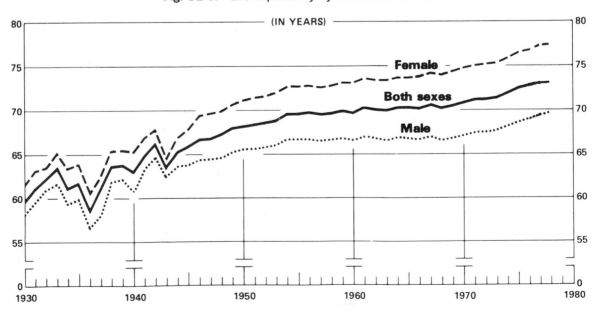

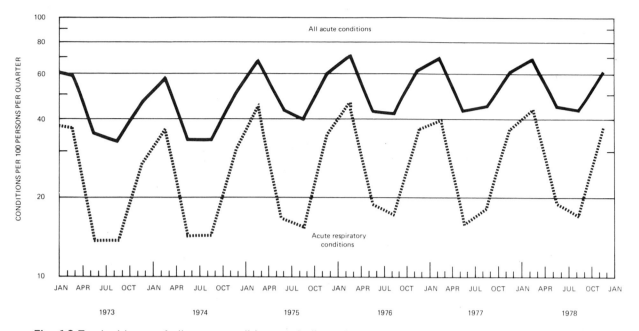

Fig. 12-7. Incidence of all acute conditions and all respiratory conditions per 100 persons per quarter.

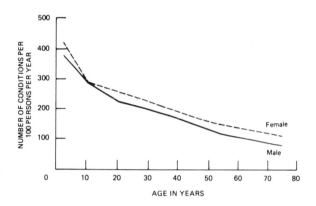

Fig. 12-8. Incidence of acute conditions per 100 persons per year by sex and age: United States, July 1976–June 1977.

addition to the reporting of disease and death, other methods are available to measure the health of individuals and population groups. They include (1) questions about early or mild symptoms of physical, mental or social malaise; (2) routinely testing the asymptomatic person for abnormal changes in blood pressure, weight, hemoglobin and other parameters; (3) measuring the performance of specific tasks; (4) recording over certain periods the frequency of absence from work due to illness; (5) observing behavior in controlled social settings; (6) routinely collecting hospital discharge data.

Statistical Methods and Reasoning

In the use of statistical methods to answer important questions, the critical first step in a study is a clear statement of the problem. This determines the kind of data to be collected and the manner in which it is to be done.

Samples may then be selected in several ways. Once collected, the data must be organized or tabulated systematically to show clearly the interrelationships and the variations in the phenomena that are being studied. Tables must be organized so as to be understood without referring to the text. Data can be presented in graphic form to emphasize salient points that large tables may hide.

The next step in analysis involves comparison of one set of data with another. Rates, ratios, averages and measures of variation are aids in analysis of data. There are statistical procedures for adjusting data so that they can be compared and interpreted more readily. Thus, death rates can be adjusted for differences in the age distribution of the populations being compared.

Two indices are often used to describe the frequency of disease in the population. The first is the incidence rate, which is the number of new cases of the disease occurring annually per 100,000 population; it is often adjusted for the age, race and sex distribution of the specified population, so that figures from relatively young and relatively old groups may be compared as in Figure 12-8. The second is the prevalence ratio, which is the number of cases of the disease per 100,000 population present at one moment in time. These figures again are often made specific for age, sex and race. The longer the duration of illness, the greater the number of cases there are in the population at any one moment. Thus, a high prevalence ratio may reflect a high incidence rate, a long duration of illness, or both.

Inasmuch as the results of many studies form the basis for generalization, one must consider the reliability of the data for this purpose. This requires knowledge of how samples vary when taken from the same population. There are several ways of measuring sampling variation. The standard deviation is suitable, for example, when the experimental and control groups are each divided into two classes only, such as "living" and "dead". When each group has more than two classes, the chi-square test is useful. Both methods help the investigator to confirm or deny the hypothesis that the differences between the experimental and the control groups may be caused by chance. This procedure is usually described as testing the null hypothesis.

Record linkage involves the collation of several items of information about the same person. For example, hospital and public health records may eventually be linked with data from physicians' offices so that complete health records covering an individual's lifetime may be compiled. If this is to be successful, each individual must be reliably and unambiguously identified on each record. Thus, record linkage depends on the availability of an identifying system that can be handled by computers. A possible system would assign a unique number, such as the Social Security number, to each individual at birth. For effective use the individual himself must know the number. Such developments raise serious misgivings about privacy and confidentiality; nevertheless, record linkage has great potential value for improving health care and for long-term studies of the natural history of disease.

EPIDEMIOLOGY

Many fields of science play a role in public health and community medicine. Perhaps foremost is the field of epidemiology, which is both an organized body of knowledge and a group of techniques used to produce that knowledge. The knowledge describes the distribution of a disease or a physiological condition in human populations, and identifies the factors that influence that distribution. Epidemiologic techniques advance and strengthen that knowledge.

Epidemiologic studies inevitably involve both the sick and healthy populations. When cases cannot be related to the population from which they come, it is less possible to perform a study that is acceptable to other epidemiologists. In helping determine etiology of disease, epidemiologic studies join with data from clinical and laboratory research; the former involve population-based studies, while the latter focus on individual humans and animals. In addition to determining cause, epidemiological studies have a second purpose of developing and evaluating the effectiveness of preventive, treatment and control measures used to alleviate disease in human populations.

Epidemiologic Reasoning. The process of epidemiologic reasoning has two principal stages. The first is to show that there is a statistical association between a characteristic of human groups, usually called an independent variable, and the frequency of disease or a physiological condition, usually called the dependent variable. The second stage is to develop a biologic or other explanation for the statistical association which has been found. At times the association between the population characteristic and the frequency of disease is not cause-and-effect. Another independent variable related to the first characteristic may be the determinant of disease. Epidemiologic studies face the problem of separating spurious from cause-and-effect relationships; only through understanding the latter can disease be controlled and prevented.

The Population. The population that interests epidemiologists is not necessarily the same as the populations that appeal to politicians or demographers. The useful group for epidemiologic studies is the *population at risk,* the population that creates the cases of the disease being studied. The frequency of accidents in hospital must be related to the hospitalized population in which these accidents occur; the nonhospitalized population is not exposed to the risk of having an accident in the hospital. The frequency of autopsies must relate to all deaths, not to the living population that undergoes no risk of being autopsied. Thus the population at risk has some basic characteristic that produces the event being studied. That characteristic should enable the population to be defined, counted, and sampled when necessary. The characteristic may be demographic, occupational, geographic or health related in nature.

The Case. How repeatable is the decision that an individual in the population is a "case," an example of the dependent variable being studied? That decision is more difficult now than in the past, when it was reasonable to assume the existence of two classes, the sick and the well, the affected and unaffected, the malignant and the benign. Advances of knowledge increasingly suggest that a continuum exists, such as from benign, premalignant dysplasia, carcinoma in situ, early asymptomatic cancer leading eventually to the patient dying of advanced cancer. Among the rare exceptions to the usual continuum is the genetic disease with high penetrance, such as achondroplasia.

Each epidemiologic study is expected to explain how the status of being a "case" is determined. One procedure is a statistical guideline, that populations which are beyond two standard deviations from the mean enter the abnormal classification. The procedure may be clinical, which usually requires the case to have an abnormal test result and also to have symptoms. The decision may be based on prognosis, cases being those persons whose risk of dying is significantly raised. Finally an arbitrary or operational decision may be made, based on the ability to treat or alleviate a condition. Each of these decisions has strengths and defects, but investigators are expected to explain clearly how the decisions are made. The procedures used to define a case should have two desirable characteristics:

1. *Validity,* or accuracy, producing a result close to the state being measured. Using the pulse rate to measure the frequency of ventricular beats is invalid in cases of atrial fibrillation. Using a urine sugar test to determine the population frequency of diabetes mellitus also is invalid, missing a large proportion of early cases.
2. *Reliability,* or repeatability, with repeat measurements of the same entity closely matching each other. For example, the rise in human weight between morning and evening causes weight to be an unreliable measure of the amount of adipose tissue. This does not prevent obesity control procedures that include the administration of diuretics.

Observations performed in real life may be distant from these requirements. To a limited extent, the same person may emerge from the offices of different physicians after being given different diagnoses and treatment advice. Some errors of clinical observation are random, fluctuating around the true value; in that situation, the average of many observations may give a valid result. Some errors may be biased in one direction, which does not produce a valid result through more numerous observations. Some alleged errors, such as the possibility that male physicians may make biased judgments of female patients, have been poorly studied. Other alleged errors among consumers, such as the subjective judgment of quality of care, may produce swings in the risk of malpractice suits.

The review of patient records also involves many random and biased errors. A large group of community agencies that arise from medical societies, the Professional Standards Review Organizations (PSROs), work extensively in this area. The epidemiologic stricture to "have dirty hands, but a clean mind" leads to the hope that PSROs understand the weaknesses of hospital data, but interpret and act on them with insight and intellectual rigor.

Epidemiologic Concepts. Some basic epidemiologic concepts originate from the field of infectious disease. They suggest that the frequency of much disease may be explained on the basis of a host (the susceptible person) interacting with an agent (factor causing disease) and with the environment (including its psychosocial, biological and other aspects). Also coming from the infectious disease field is the concept of an incubation period, the time between exposure to a possible etiologic agent and the onset of disease. A final concept is that of herd immunity; this emphasizes the finding that populations will no longer spread infectious disease even before they are fully immunized against the condition. For example, in a population which has 70 per cent of persons immune to an infection, the person-to-person spread may never become established since the infectious agent reaches many individuals who do not transmit the disease. That proportion which produces herd immunity varies with the infectivity of the agent, and with the size and social behavior of the community. The phenomenon of herd immunity makes it unnecessary to have 100 per cent participation in some immunization programs, although it is common to aim at as close to that level as possible. Epidemiologic concepts and methods can be applied to accidents, poisonings, measurements, attitudes, and, indeed, to any observable characterisic of people. Epidemiologic studies involve all cases with a given characteristic or disease in a defined population and usually collect information about unaffected as well as affected persons. Such studies often develop rates (or ratios) in which the numerator represents those with the characteristic under study and the denominator represents the total population.

Often the first clues to the etiology or the mode of transmission of disease come from field observations and lead to confirmatory observations in the clinic and the laboratory. For example, a number of carcinogenic substances, such as chromates, uranium-bearing ores and cigarette smoke, have been identified by observation of the excessive frequency of cancer among those exposed to the agent. Sometimes the situation is reversed, and the field study confirms or changes the conclusions of clinical or laboratory studies.

Epidemiologic methods may be classified broadly as:

1. Experimental
2. Observational
   a. Controlled
   b. Uncontrolled

In the experimental method a hypothesis is tested by prospective studies which follow two comparable groups of people. During the study the environment is changed for, or treatment is offered to, one group, while no change is made for the second group, which serves as a control. Whenever possible, the study should be double blind, with neither observer nor subject knowing to which group the subject belongs.

More common than studies that use the experimental method are observational studies, conducted in situations in which nature has changed the environment or altered the treatment. Sometimes the investigator can study two populations that are similar except for the factor under study; this is the controlled observational procedure, or case-control study. In uncontrolled observational studies, there are no explicit controls. Instead, the investigator must compare the attributes of the cases with those of random samples of the population from which they were drawn. In general, conclusions based on uncontrolled observation are least certain, and those based on an experimental study are most certain.

One dramatic use of epidemiologic methods is the determination of the cause of a food poisoning epidemic. There are two ways to present the evidence that relates food to illness. In one, the history of the consumption of specific foods is obtained from persons who ate the suspected meal, a group of those with symptoms and a group of the unaffected. The frequency of consumption of each food by members of the first group is contrasted with the corresponding frequency in the second group. In the second method, all the available foods are identified, and then two attack rates for each food are derived: One rate represents the frequency of illness among persons who ate the food; the other, among those who did not eat it.

A common mistake is the restriction of such investigations to ill persons only. We then measure merely the popularity of each food. For a number of reasons, the food that caused the epidemic rarely is listed as having been eaten by all affected persons, and another more popular food may be blamed wrongly. It is the size of the difference between figures for affected and unaffected persons that gives the most reliable lead to the casual agent.

HEALTH SERVICES ADMINISTRATION

Health services administration is an activity that involves the application of all available knowledge toward the prevention of disease, the prolongation of life and the promotion of physical and mental efficiency. The nature of public health programs has changed markedly over the years. The earliest efforts were to prevent the introduction and the spread of infection by quarantine of infected communities and isolation of infectious cases. As knowledge concerning

infectious disease increased, the control of public water supplies, milk, and many other foods was found to be necessary. Control of the disposal of human, household and industrial wastes also was found to improve the health of the people, as were improvements in housing.

In some parts of the world, government became involved in control or eradication of disease carriers, such as certain species of insects. Particularly in the United States and Western Europe, social reforms have taken place in which public health was an important issue. Governments have become greatly interested in maternal and child welfare, in aid to the physically handicapped and in special disease problems such as tuberculosis, venereal disease, cancer, cardiovascular disease and mental illness. Indeed, rehabilitation, the early detection of chronic illness and the assurance of continuity of medical care are becoming symbols of modern public health. The rising cost and better distribution and financing of personal health services has also become a leading concern of the United States government in the 1980s.

Whereas previously the emphasis of public health administration was on the establishment of basic public health services, there is now equal emphasis on the better use of existing services and the development and evaluation of new programs. In theory, new developments in public health are intended to reduce the need for individual action (such as regular visits to the dentist) or to motivate larger numbers of individuals to participate in voluntary programs. These developments have changed materially the character of the organization within government for the protection of the public health. The impersonal mass approach through environmental controls is being complemented by the financing of personal health services and by controlling the rising cost of health care.

Federal Health Services in the United States

The political structure and beliefs of the United States have guided the historical development of its public health services. A national government formed by a federation of the member states possesses only those powers delegated to it by the sovereign states. The provision in Article I of the Constitution of the United States for the interest of the federal government in the general welfare gave some authority for the development of national health services. The Constitution also delegated power to the federal government specifically for interstate and foreign quarantine.

In 1980 Congress created the Department of Health and Human Services (HHS), embracing federal agencies involved in health. It is the successor to the Depart-

TABLE 12-1. Federal Government Health Budgets (in millions)

(1) Fiscal Year	(2) Medicaid and Predecessors	(3) Medicare	(4) Dept. of Defense	(5) Veterans Services	(6) Indian Health Services	(7) Federal Civilian Employees Health Insurance	(8) Other Health Services	(9) Research	(10) Medical Facilities Construction*	(11) Total	(12) % of Total Federal Budget
1960	$ 200	N.A.	$ 880	$ 879	N.A.	—	$ 798	$ 448	$ 295	$ 3,500	3.8%
1965	555	N.A.	937	1,115	$ 71	$ 149**	843	1,040	450	5,160	4.4
1966	766	$ 65†	1,107	1,161	75	165**	869	1,315	405	5,928	4.4
1967	1,205	3,395	1,432	1,252	83	202**	1,524	1,364	344	10,801	6.8
1968	1,834	5,347	1,648	1,343	94	223	1,714	1,547	382	14,132	7.9
1969	2,298	6,598	1,750	1,431	107	230	2,132	1,528	482	16,556	8.9
1971	3,374	7,875	1,957	1,874	143	350	2,499	1,565	541	20,178	9.5
1973	4,997	9,479	2,468	2,587	198	561	3,253	2,002	485	26,030	10.6
1975	7,056	14,781	3,085	3,287	283	1,029	4,190	2,453	626	36,790	11.3
1977	9,714	21,391	3,815	4,708	395	1,654	3,712	3,147	1,100	49,636	12.4

N.A.—Not Available.

* Except Veterans Administration, Department of Defense and Indian Health Services facilities construction.

** Fiscal year estimates based on calendar year data provided by U.S Office of Personnel Management.

† July to December.

NOTE: Data include administrative expenses.

SOURCES: U.S. Office of Management & Budget, *Special Analyses. Budget of the United States Government,* various years; Social Security Administration, "Social Welfare Expenditures," *Social Security Bulletin,* various years; U.S. Department of Health, Education and Welfare, Indian Health Service; U.S. Civil Service Commission.

ment of Health, Education and Welfare. Many health activities remain in other departments of the national government, however. Examples are the extensive health efforts of the Veterans' Administration, the armed forces, the Occupational Safety and Health Administration (OSHA), and the Environmental Protection Agency (EPA).

The United States Public Health Service. The Public Health Service is one principal federal agency concerned with public health. Originally formed to provide health care to sailors in the merchant marine, its functions now include interstate and international quarantine, research and demonstration programs, advice on technical matters, and the loan of personnel to other agencies with health services. A significant impact on health services is made through financial support to state and local health agencies for the expansion and improvement of their programs, and to area Health Systems Agencies (HSAs) responsible for health planning and certificate of need programs. Federal legislation requires HSAs to support or disapprove any request for new equipment or other resources that cost more than a certain amount, such as $150,000 in 1980. If appropriate, state government then issues a certificate of need to the agency, usually a hospital, that desires to make the new investment.

Since the Public Health Service and other federal health agencies undergo frequent reorganization, most descriptions are obsolete before they appear in print. Interested students may obtain details of the current organization by writing to the US Public Health Service in Washington, D.C.

Health Care Financing Administration. Established in 1977, the Health Care Financing Administration is the federal agency responsible for Medicaid and Medicare, both launched in 1966. It also guides the activities of Professional Standards Review Organizations (PSROs), which monitor length of stay and quality of hospital care through peer review efforts. Medicaid and Medicare now form about two-thirds of the total federal budget on health (Table 12-1).

The State and Local Health Organizations. The state government is the sovereign power in the United States. The national and local governments, in theory, possess only those powers delegated to them by the states. In practice, however, financial strength has given the federal government more influence in the development of state and local health programs than might otherwise have occurred.

Health laws differ greatly among the 50 states. Some have extensive, detailed health legislation; in others, only broad principles are laid down, and special laws are enacted as urgent needs are recognized. All states make some provision for a board of health or a comparable body with advisory and legislative functions. Complementary in function are the state health planning and development agencies, which are organized to given consumers a majority voice in the future development of health services in the states. Federal funds finance the state and area HSAs that plan for the future needs of smaller geographic areas.

In most states, the state health officer is appointed by the governor with the advice of the state board of health. The state health officer's qualifications, duties and compensation are usually specified by law. In the early years of the state health departments, control of communicable disease was the first objective, followed by environmental sanitation, dealing with water supply and the safe disposal of wastes. In recent years a number of states have created environmental protection agencies which have taken over most environmental services.

Other responsibilities of state health departments are maternal and child health services, the recording of health statistics, medical and hospital care for special groups and certain rehabilitation services. Most state health departments have a division of local health services to provide grants-in-aid to local communities, and to advise local health departments. Most local health services are maintained by cities or counties, while the state delegates authority and often provides funds to the local community for developing the program. Local health departments give direct services, such as water purification and the supervision of sewage disposal, and a wide range of clinical services. Sparsely populated areas have only limited public health services, and in three states the state health department directly provides local health services.

Voluntary Health Agencies. A voluntary health agency is formed by a group, the members of which wish to pursue a common interest; membership is voluntary, and the agency is independent of the state. Although the United States is reputed to be a nation of joiners, probably less than 20 per cent of its population participate actively in its 100,000 voluntary health agencies. Such associations have become more common as society has grown more complex and techniques more numerous. In situations of rapid social change, voluntary associations are considered to be important as a means of achieving new goals, raising new funds or providing new labor.

The ideal voluntary health agency is more sensitive than government to the changing needs of society; many agencies have begun health services that were later assumed by government. However, at a time when many voluntary agencies have become stable and con-

servative, government agencies and funding have, in contrast, become more innovative in recent years. Thus, the rationale for voluntary health agencies has become less definite, while public resistance has risen against giving funds for health activities over and above the high taxes paid to government. It is now accepted policy to have voluntary associations carry out public functions, such as payment for medical and hospital care and professional licensure; thus some voluntary agencies receive increasing support from government funds.

Voluntary health agencies take many forms. First comes the large group which focuses on specific disease (e.g., the American Cancer Society) or organs (e.g., American Heart Association), or on specific populations or techniques (e.g., planned parenthood); these agencies concentrate more on health education and less on service. More service oriented are such agencies as hospitals, group practice clinics and health maintenance organizations (HMOs), and visiting nurse associations. Health maintenance organizations are medical groups that contract with an enrolled population to provide complete health services, preventive and curative, inpatient and outpatient, in return for an annual payment per enrollee. A third group includes the funding associations, such as the Rockefeller or Kellogg Foundations or the United Fund, which distribute funds to hospitals and physicians, also fall in this category. Planning and coordinating associations, such as community councils, form a fourth group of voluntary agencies; although funded by government, HSAs must originate from a voluntary group. A fifth, and influential, group is composed of the professional associations, such as the American Medical Association, concerned with setting standards for, and licensing, the profession, public and professional education and legislation related to the beliefs and activities of the profession; state and local medical societies guide the PSROs, even though federal funds support these agencies which monitor hospital care. Last, but not least, may be included some academic institutions that are concerned with research and teaching of health professionals.

Voluntary health associations help stimulate social change and mediate between population groups and government. They help communities set priorities in health and influence the decisions of local government. They create interest and consensus among their members but also induce stresses between one organization and another. If this conflict results in improved health services for a reasonable expenditure of funds, the end results will help American society. At present, however, our verdict on voluntarism has to be based on intuition and personal opinion rather than on scientific findings.

PRIORITIES FOR PREVENTION

Prevention and treatment cannot be mutually exclusive or one-shot affairs, although health services tend to approach them in that fashion. In the 1980s, part of the effort to control rising costs of treatment involves a rising intensity of preventive services. In contrast to the brief preventive measures of immunizations, much prevention in the future will be long term, continuous, and aimed at improving the individual's knowledge of disease and of health-related behavior patterns. The following sections cover some high priority areas of prevention in the coming years.

Hypertension

Hypertension is a potent risk factor for coronary heart disease and stroke, and contributes to deaths from heart and renal failure. In 1980 about 15 per cent of the population had definite high blood pressure, most with mild hypertension for which intervention seems warranted. High prevalence groups in the US include the black population and the elderly; with the latter, uncertainty exists about the benefit of early detection and treatment of isolated systolic hypertension.

Although elevated blood pressures can be lowered, the cause of most hypertension is not known. Despite this uncertainty, we have many reasons to raise public awareness that increased physical activity and avoidance of obesity are important. The public should also learn that a daily intake of over 5 g. of total sodium chloride may contribute to some hypertension.

Industry should be encouraged to promote the prevention and treatment of high blood pressure among its employees. Both among individuals and groups, blood pressure reduction and weight control could be encouraged by lowering the cost of life insurance premiums to those taking preventive measures. It is unfortunate that many health professionals pay insufficient attention to the failure to follow a lifetime of treatment for elevated blood pressures. The need for more extensive early detection efforts and for stronger attention to noncompliance with treatment raises the possibility that allied health professionals could be permitted legally to practice in these areas.

Since the etiology of hypertension is multifactorial, new knowledge may not eliminate it soon as a public health problem. Thus the basic components of successful control will continue to be earlier detection, better diagnostic evaluations, and more systematic treatment and followup.

Family Planning

Every population contains groups that do not contribute to the economy of the country—the young, elderly, sick and disabled and the unemployed. The dependent part of the population consumes goods and services formed by the producers. When mortality falls more rapidly than reproduction, the dependent population forms an expanding part of the total population. Education, urbanization, mechanization and industrialization have to advance speedily to raise the productivity of the contributors. Without population control, these social changes must advance more rapidly than is feasible in many developing countries.

Family planning is based on the voluntary decisions and actions of individuals who wish to reduce unintended fertility or to correct infertility. It may or may not be compatible with national population policy, but enables individuals to decide for themselves about reproduction.

Compared with other ages, pregnancies among teenagers are more likely to be unintended and unwanted. Such pregnancies are associated with markedly increased risks of maternal morbidity and mortality, with high rates of serious neurological impairment in infants, and with an increased proportion of low birth weight infants. Moreover, unwanted pregnancies impose psychological and social costs that may be lifelong.

Childbearing among unmarried American women is increasing. Low income women and black women have high rates of unintended pregnancy. Moreover, the risk of maternal death associated with temporary methods of contraception, sterilization, and legal abortion is less than the risk of death from childbearing. A small number of preventable deaths, associated with family planning, are caused by (a) oral contraceptive use in cigarette smokers, (b) oral contraceptives with unnecessarily high estrogen dosage, (c) legal abortions performed after the first trimester, and (d) illegal abortion.

It seems essential to strengthen educational measures for both health professionals and consumers. Teenage girls particularly should learn more about nonprescription contraceptives, including how they work, their relative effectiveness, how to use them effectively, and their availability and cost. Individuals who work in health care settings that serve adolescents should be encouraged to upgrade their counseling skills. Finally, we should improve access to and the acceptability of contraceptive services, including voluntary sterilization.

Maternal and Child Health

The maternal and child health activities of a community to provide complete and continuous health supervision of a child from conception to adulthood. Because problems and health needs change throughout this pe-

TABLE 12-2. Preventive Services for the Pregnant Woman and Fetus

	Services	Initial Visit[1]	Subsequent Visits[2]
History	General medical	•	
	Family and genetic	•	
	Previous pregnancies	•	
	Current pregnancy	•	•
Physical Examination	General	•	
	Blood pressure	•	•
	Height and weight	•	•
	Fetal development		•
Laboratory Examinations	VDRL	•	
	Papanicolau smear	•	
	Hemoglobin/hematocrit	•	
	Urinalysis for sugar and protein	•	•
	Rh determination	•	
	Bloodgroup determination	•	
	Rubella HAI titre	•	
	Amniocentesis (for women over 35)[3]		
Counseling with Referrals as Necessary and Desired	Nutrition during pregnancy	•	•
	Nutrition of infant, including breast-feeding	•	•
	Cigarette smoking	•	•
	Use of alcohol, other drugs during pregnancy	•	•
	Sexual intercourse during pregnancy	•	•
	Signs of abnormal pregnancy	•	•
	Labor and delivery (including where mother plans to deliver)	•	•
	Physical activity and exercise	•	•
	Provisions for care of infant	•	•
	In response to parental concerns	•	•

Labor and Delivery[4]

Post-partum Visit (including family planning counseling and referral, if desired)

[1] Initial visit should occur early in the first trimester.

[2] Subsequent visits should occur once a month through the 28th week of pregnancy; twice a month from the 29th through the 36th week; and once a week thereafter.

[3] If desired, amniocentesis should be performed at about the 16th week for women who are over 35 or who have specific genetic indications.

[4] Although not a "preventive" service, labor and delivery should be included in a package of pregnancy-related services.

riod, the program usually is divided into certain segments: maternal supervision and care, including the antenatal, the delivery and the postpartum periods; infant hygiene; preschool hygiene and school hygiene.

This important activity depends partly on other health programs for its success. Obviously, without basic sanitation programs in milk and water supply control, the maternal and child health activities would lose much of their effectiveness. The maternal and child health program makes use of the laboratory services, communicable disease control and mental hygiene programs, which are of vital interest to it.

Mortality and morbidity rates range markedly between different population groups. Maternal mortality among blacks is about three times that for whites. Infant mortality in blacks is about twice that of whites (Fig. 12-3). Comparing different geographic regions, the state with the highest infant mortality rate has about twice the incidence of the lowest.

The greatest single problem associated with infant mortality is low birth weight (Fig. 12-4). In turn, low birth weight babies are more common in young and elderly mothers, those of minority status, high parity, low socioeconomic status, poor nutrition, smoking, alcohol abuse, drug consumption, or with lack of prenatal care. High quality prenatal care can decrease the risk of low birth weight as well as of other complications in the newborn and their mothers. The preventive

TABLE 12-3. Preventive Services for the Normal Infant

	Services	Birth Visit	Second Visit[1]	Subsequent Visits[2]
History and Physical Examination	Length and weight	•	•	•
	Head circumference	•		
	Urine stream	•		
	Check to congenital abnormalities	•		•
	Developmental assessment			•
Procedures	PKU screening test		•	
	Thyroxin T4		•	
	Vitamin K		•	
	Silver nitrate prophylaxis	•		
Immunizations	Diphtheria			•
	Pertussis			•
	Tetanus			•
	Measles[3]			
	Mumps[3]			
	Rubella[3]			
	Poliomyelitis			•
Parental Counseling, with Referrals as Necessary and Desired	Infant nutrition and feeding practices (especially breastfeeding)		•	•
	Parenting		•	•
	Infant hygiene		•	•
	Accidental injury prevention (including use of automobile restraints)		•	•
	Family planning and referral for services		•	•
	Child care arrangements		•	•
	Medical care arrangements		•	•
	Parental smoking, use of alcohol, and drugs		•	•
	Parental nutrition, physical activity and exercise		•	•
	In response to parental concerns		•	•

[1] Second visit should occur within 10 days or before leaving the hospital.
[2] Four health visits the rest of first year or enough to provide immunizations.
[3] Measles, mumps, and rubella immunizations occur at 15 months.

services recommended in prenatal care are summarized in Table 12-2; those advised for the normal infant care shown in Table 12-3.

Health education programs in schools and communities should emphasize lifestyles and risk factors that impair maternal and child health. Society must try more seriously to improve the distribution of professionals and paraprofessionals who deliver perinatal and infant care. Such personnel and their services should be regionalized so that most women and newborns receive care appropriate to their needs. Direct federal financing of local health departments may be needed to expand maternal and child health services to reach neglected populations. Curtailment of smoking, alcohol consumption, exposure to toxic substances, and improved nutrition are all important preventive measures (Fig. 12-4).

Surveillance and Control of Infectious Diseases

Methods used for the control of communicable disease have changed markedly in recent years. The changes have resulted from better knowledge of the sources and the modes of transmission of disease and from improved methods of treatment. Early programs of communicable disease control relied on isolation and quarantine. However, the discovery that many infectious diseases result from contact with healthy carriers of the organism has greatly reduced confidence in such methods.

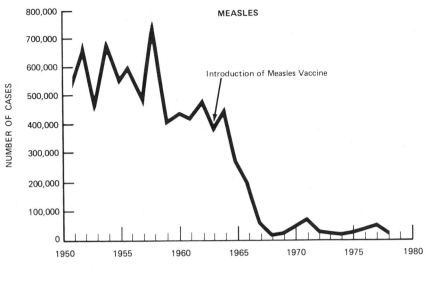

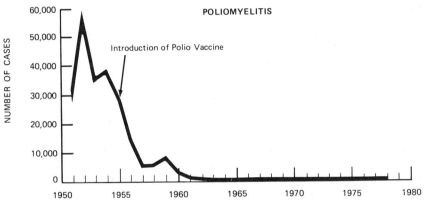

Fig. 12-9.   Reported cases of measles and poliomyelitis: United States, 1951–1978. Note: Polio incidence dropped below 1000 cases annually in 1962: 1978 data for measles and poliomyelitis are preliminary. (Based on data from the Center for Disease Control)

The way deaths are now classified tends to underestimate the importance of infectious diseases. Because only one category, influenza and pneumonia, is ranked among the top ten causes of death, we tend to forget the likelihood that all infectious diseases probably cause about 300,000 annual deaths, slightly less than those caused by all cancers. Infectious diseases are the most common reason for acute care visits to physicians offices and for absences from work and school. Moreover, nosocomial infections, acquired in patient care institutions, affect over 2 million persons each year in the United States.

In controlling the infectious diseases, we need to improve surveillance measures so that data are collected speedily and accurately. The current reporting of these diseases, while legally required, covers only a fraction of all cases. Data from the National Health Interview Survey give a more complete picture for the total US, although they cannot be subdivided into precise diagnoses and figures for small geographic areas. Consumers must better understand and practice basic hygienic measures, such as handwashing and proper handling of food. Public and professional education must improve the individual awareness of the need to obtain immunizations, and of the infectious disease consequences of substance abuse, including cigarette smoking. Improved water treatment, food processing, food service and waste disposal are all technologic measures needed to improve the environment of large populations.

Immunization

Figure 12-9 shows that the wide use of immunizing agents has dramatically lowered the incidence of measles and poliomyelitis, diphtheria, mumps, pertussis, rubella, and tetanus have also been much reduced, while smallpox was classified in 1980 as eradicated. With the exception of smallpox, however, the causal agents have not been eradicated. Cessation of immunization, for example, would lead to the recurrence of annual epidemics of measles causing hundreds of deaths in the US. During periodic pandemics, thousands of the chronically ill and elderly in the US may die prematurely as a result of influenza.

While preventable infections become scarce the rare adverse effects of immunization have become increasingly visible and publicized. Lawsuits for compensation of those injured by immunization have hampered these preventive services. Thus, we need an effective maintenance system for delivering routine immunization services. Making immunizations available without financial barriers in all health care settings would seem to be a rational arrangement. Such economic measures could include reimbursement for immunizations under Medicare and Medicaid, and providing immunizing agents free to all health care providers so long as they do not charge for them. Obviously, this is also a social, political, and economic problem in addition to one of public health concern.

Education and information measures tend to be more acceptable and less controversial than legislative and regulatory steps. Thus, we continue to debate how strongly we should enforce existing school immunization requirements, whether we should require immunization as a condition of employment in health care institutions, and whether we should require rubella immunization in family planning clinics and in the postpartum settings. Controversial as they may be, such legislative steps sometimes make the crucial difference between partial and full immunization of high risk groups.

Sexually Transmitted Diseases

Sexually transmitted diseases (STDs) are grouped separately from other infections because they spread from person to person during sexual contact. They cause much human suffering and use hundreds of millions of dollars for resources used in their control and cure. Women and children bear an inordinate share of STD complications: pelvic inflammatory disease, sterility, ectopic pregnancy, infant pneumonia, fetal and infant deaths, and mental retardation. STDs also disproportionately affect the poor. We thus need good financial support and adequate specialized clinics and programs to control and prevent these diseases.

Effective and more sustained health education programs must aim at high risk groups. Patient education should be improved, partly through the use of peers who can be as effective in education and counselling as are physicians. We must screen to detect early selected STD. Personnel from local health departments should be encouraged to trace and treat the contacts of patients, an effort too complex to be done well by private practitioners. Finally, properly used condoms are the best known measure during sexual activity to avoid acquiring or transmitting many of the STDs.

Occupational Safety and Health

Industrial hygiene is concerned with all factors that influence the health and the productivity of working people. Industrial health physicians are particularly concerned with occupational diseases, i.e., those that arise out of employment, either in the course of employment or subsequently. Such diseases may result from the physical state of the environment or from mechanical factors, or they may be caused by chemical or infectious agents. There are no reliable statistics on the incidence of occupational diseases. However, dermatitides usually are the diseases reported most frequently; diseases caused by chemical agents and by repeated motion and pressure are less common but usually more serious.

Occupational exposure to chemical or physical hazards may produce lung disease, cancers, sensory loss, degenerative changes in a number of organ systems, birth defects, and genetic changes. Some agents also increase the frequency of stillbirths, spontaneous abortions, reduced fertility, and sterility. While the reduction of occupational injuries has progressed in recent decades, many work accidents still occur that are potentially preventable (Fig. 12-10).

In addition to educational efforts to improve the knowledge and awareness of workers, service measures are needed to strengthen occupational health programs. Government agencies may have to give consultative help to small businesses. More physicians should become better trained in the diagnosis and treatment of occupational illness and injuries; in the absence of that change, large industries may have to develop a personal health service delivery system within each industry.

Within the federal government, the National Institute of Occupational Safety and Health (NIOSH) performs research and recommends standards for toxic substances used in industry; implementing that information, the Occupational Safety and Health Administration (OSHA) promulgates the standards and inspects industries to ensure compliance. In the 1980s, it seems necessary for OSHA to streamline its efforts, eliminating many details that weaken occupational safety and health programs. In addition, it may be necessary for NIOSH, located in the Center for Disease Control in 1980, to become an independent institute in the Public Health Service and to be given the more

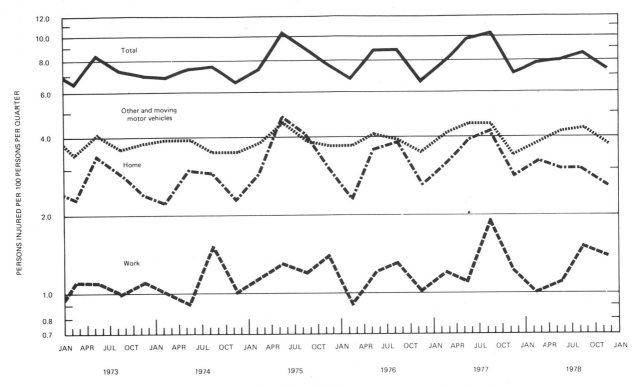

Fig. 12-10. Persons injured per 100 persons per quarter, by class of accident.

abundant resources needed to strengthen its efforts. State and local systems for recognizing and preventing occupational health and safety hazards must also be developed and improved.

Surveillance and Control of Toxic Agents in the Environment

Though we understand poorly the mechanisms by which certain toxic agents produce disease, recent experience confirms that serious health hazards exist in the environment. New evidence comes often showing previously unsuspected associations between specific environmental agents and diseases. The detection of specific causes is complicated because: (a) many agents may contribute to the same disease; (b) there may be long latent periods between exposure and disease onset; and (c) data are sometimes absent or inappropriately presented to reveal the possible association.

The speed of industrial change confuses the scene. Over 13,000 substances now in commercial use have been identified as toxic, with more introduced each year. Perhaps half of the current U.S. population dose of ionizing radiation comes from man-made sources and thus is potentially reducible.

Government control measures seem essential to reduce exposure to hazardous agents. Physicians must become more sensitive to and educated about the diag-nosis and reporting of environmental and occupational diseases. Government must also help develop the control technology and process redesign when industry cannot do the job. The regulatory agencies, EPA and OSHA, need to hire well-trained professionals to enforce the many laws which control hazardous substances in the environment. Moreover, we may have to withhold from commerce new chemicals until industry can show the safety of their uses and disposal. The permissible exposure levels must reflect real-life multiple exposures, the history of previous exposure, individual susceptibilities and the changing effects with increasing age.

Pharmaceutical and biological hazards also deserve full attention. We have yet to resolve the conflicting social goals of increased consumption and adequate health protection in the US. Because the balance is complex, we cannot depend on mechanical decision rules using simple cost-benefit analysis.

Accident Prevention and Injury Control

In the United States, accidents rank fourth as a cause of death, and they are the leading cause of death of persons between 1 and 43 years of age. Motor vehicle accidents cause about half of all accidental deaths. Approximately one-fourth of all accidental deaths occur at home.

Many accidents do not result in death, however, and the incidence of these nonfatal accidents is shown in Figure 12-10. These data come from the continuing National Health Survey mentioned earlier. Inasmuch as most accidents have multiple causes, research is difficult in this field. Personal and social maladjustment is found more commonly among accident repeaters than among accident-free groups. The likelihood of motor vehicle accidents increases steadily with increasing blood alcohol levels of vehicle operators. Such "host factors" are important in determining the incidence of accidents.

The characteristics of the "agent" of the accident are also important. A control lever that is difficult to reach and operate, or the obstruction of vision, even temporarily, may contribute directly to an accident. It is believed that the forces involved in many automobile accidents are within the body's physiologic limits of survival; fatal consequences can be prevented if the momentum of the body is properly checked and the forces are dissipated. Seat belts and passive restraints are used increasingly to achieve this aim.

About half of all accidental deaths in infants used to be classified as suffocation; an unrecognized overwhelming infection now is believed to have occurred in many such cases. Poisonings cause a relatively small proportion of all accidental deaths in children and have been combatted through educational programs and poison control centers. Aspirin ingestion has been the most common cause of poisoning.

Unintended events that injure human beings are partially preventable events, despite our tendency to describe them as accidents and to view them as beyond our control. When we take a less fatalistic view of these events, we may prevent a major proportion of these injuries and deaths.

Gunshot wounds are second only to motor vehicle crashes in causing death from trauma. However, about 93 per cent of the gunshot wounds are classified as homicides or suicides, producing death rates that are particularly high in black males. Falls, drowning and burn injuries are also important causes of death and morbidity. Particularly common in children and the elderly, burns are significantly related to alcohol consumption and cigarette smoking in the elderly.

Safety education programs help create the climate for change, but so far have not been convincingly shown to reduce injury rates. Injury prevention has been most effectively influenced by technological changes, such as improved automobile design, many changes in industry, and such passive measures as window guards for apartment buildings. Psychologically unappealing but also effective have been regulatory measures, such as building codes, fire codes, reduced highway speed limits, and the reduced availability of handguns through licensing. Still to be tested but with a strong potential for improved prevention is the use of economic incentives, such as low insurance rates for documented safe drivers, and higher taxes and life insurance rates with cigarette and smoking and alcohol consumption. Thus the field of injury control involves a complex variety of measures, which can be expedited if physicians use their social consciences as well as their therapeutic techniques.

Fluoridation

Fluoridation is the adjustment of the fluoride content of drinking water, which is deficient in naturally occurring fluoride, to the optimum level for dental health. This measure prevents dental caries and reduces the dental treatment bills of children.

Dental caries is a disease problem of massive proportions, affecting 98 per cent of the US population. Low income children have much more untreated decayed teeth than high income children. Fluoridated water supplies serve about 60 per cent of the US population. However, extension to the remaining population faces a number of barriers: (a) Community inaction. Many communities make no effort to fluoridate. They may not know its effectiveness and safety, and may be reluctant to confront the opponents of fluoridation. (b) Financial inability. Usually local funds are needed to pay the costs of fluoridation. In recent years, it has become increasingly difficult for communities to find this money, despite the fact that fluoridation is the cheapest way to control dental caries. (c) Improper supervision. Many fluoridated water supplies are maintained below the recommended optimum level.

Thus, we need to improve the quality of surveillance, testing, monitoring, and other engineering procedures. Federal funds also seem necessary to support the expansion of community and school water fluoridation. It would be rational to reduce premiums for dental insurance for families with children who live in fluoridated communities. In the United States the optimum fluoride level is between 0.7 and 1.2 parts per million.

Smoking

Cigarette smoking causes much unnecessary and preventable illness and death. It is a causal factor for the following conditions: coronary heart (Fig. 12-11) and peripheral artery disease; cancers of the lung, larynx, mouth and esophagus; chronic bronchitis and emphysema; and allergic conditions. It is associated with retarded fetal and childhood growth, decreased resistance to many infections, and greater use of health care. It acts synergistically with oral contraceptives

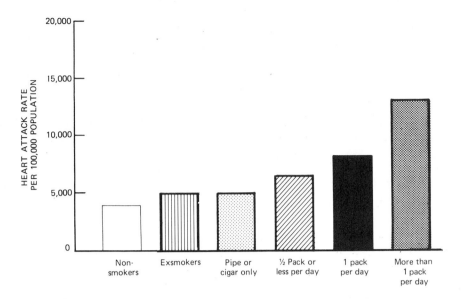

Fig. 12-11. Age-adjusted rates of first heart attack by smoking status for white males ages 30–59 years: United States. Note: age-adjusted to the United States white male population, 1960. Data based on the pooled results of five longitudinal investigations conducted in the 1950s and 1960s. Rates based on ten-year followup. (National Cooperative Pooling Project, National Heart, Lung, and Blood Institute, 1970)

to enhance the probability of coronary and other thromboembolic disease.

Involuntary or passive inhalation of cigarette smoke has measurable adverse effects. Smoking also contributes to death and injury from fires and burns. Finally, it is well established that after ten years of smoking cessation, the risk of smoking-related conditions and overall mortality approaches that of nonsmokers.

Education, information, fiscal, and regulatory measures are key strategies in a national smoking prevention program. Education measures focus on the specific health consequences, on self-initiated cessation, on less hazardous ways of smoking, on immediate benefits of cessation, and on the effects of passive smoking. Specific educational campaigns aim at high risk groups, such as pregnant women. Programs focused on the psychosocial factors influencing the initiation of smoking in youth usually include the immediate physical, cosmetic and esthetic consequences of smoking.

Technologic measures include the development of less hazardous cigarettes, while cautioning consumers that even the lowest-yield cigarettes present health hazards much greater than those affecting nonsmokers. Legislative and regulatory measures involve banning TV and radio advertising, health warnings in advertising, and the provision of nonsmoking areas in public places. Finally, economic measures include increased excise taxes on cigarettes, approving personal income tax deductions for the cost of participating in smoking cessation programs, and bonuses to employees who quit or do not smoke.

The cessation of smoking is most common among the educated, but may spread into other socioeconomic groups with appropriately vigorous techniques. Counselling on smoking by physicians and other health professions must reinforce the community efforts; positive lifestyle promotion programs should incorporate smoking education as an intrinsic and important effort. Probably we shall also find that the availability and use of smoking cessation service programs will steadily increase to support the counseling activities of physicians.

Alcohol and Drug Abuse

Alcohol and other drug problems have pervasive effects: biological, psychological, and social consequences for the abuser; psychological and social effects on family members and others; increased risk of injury and death to self, family members, and others, particularly by accidents, fires, and violence; and socioeconomic consequences for society. Thus prevention and control efforts need considerable resources and vigorous implementation.

Excessive alcohol consumption directly raises death rates from injuries, cirrhosis, alcoholism, or alcoholic psychosis, in addition to birth defects in infants suffering from fetal alcohol syndrome. In the US, most users of "other drugs" are marijuana users, more commonly adolescents. More serious, but less common and apparently declining in the US, are heroin-related medical problems. Deaths from barbiturates have also markedly fallen.

Regulatory measures have been the nation's primary tool to prevent and control drug abuse during most of the 20th century; the value and limitations of current prohibitions are much debated. The falling trends for heroin and barbiturate use suggest that regulatory approaches have had some impact. Regulation of alcoholic beverages has not traditionally been focused on public health considerations. Probably the availability of alcohol affects the level and type of alcohol problems; availability has been linked fairly conclusively

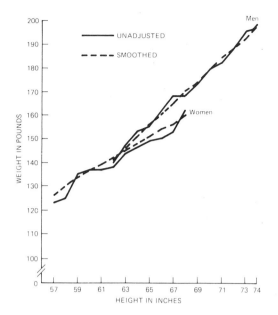

Fig. 12-12. Unadjusted mean weights and smoothed mean weights (estimated from the regression equations) of men and women aged 18–74 years, by height: United States, 1971–1974.

to the relative price of alcohol, and less conclusively to such factors as the legal purchase age, limiting the hours of sale, and limiting the number of retail outlets.

Special education and information programs can target high risk populations. A broad range of treatment services need to be developed in the general health care settings, with the acceptance that alcohol and drug abuse are disease problems, not only social or behavioral abnormalities. Some damage caused by these conditions may be alleviated by accident prevention efforts, free taxi service for intoxicated persons, and by other technological measures. Finally, the trend seems likely to continue toward less punitive administration of the criminal law in cases involving arrests for personal possession of all drugs.

Nutrition

Inappropriate food consumption practices, especially when combined with other risk factors, contribute to the incidence of major chronic disease problems in the United States. Changes in diet may help both in prevention and treatment.

Figure 12-12 shows that, at heights above 63 inches, average weights for men are greater at each height than average weights for women. The greater muscle mass in men causes much of this difference between the sexes.

Obesity may increase the risk for cardiovascular disease, hypertension, gallbladder disease, diabetes melli-

tus, and the osteoarthroses. High sucrose consumption is associated directly with increased dental caries. High sodium intake appears to associate with at least some cases of essential hypertension. Excess saturated fat seems to raise coronary heart disease, while excess total fat associates epidemiologically with some cancers. Inadequate nutrition is associated with poor pregnancy outcome, and iron and folic acid deficiency is still common in pregnant women.

Prenatal and perinatal care should include good nutritional advice. General education in nutrition needs strengthening in school, work and health care settings. Breakfast and lunch programs are useful services for school children and elderly populations. Livestock practices that produce leaner meat, a step that reduces intake of saturated fat, should be encouraged. Fortifying bread and developing new products that are lower in fat, saturated fat, cholesterol, and sodium are useful technologic measures. Other useful improvements include better food labeling and decreasing local sales taxes on foods that should be increased in the diet. It seems likely that health professionals will play a larger role in the provision of nutrition information in the coming years, and will themselves need a stronger scientific body of knowledge to convey to their patients.

Physical Fitness and Exercise

More than half of all American adults do not engage in regular physical activity (Fig. 12-13). Their inactivity is associated with an increased risk of developing obesity and coronary heart disease. Moreover, appropriate physical activity helps in treating obesity, coronary heart disease, diabetes mellitus, musculoskeletal problems, and depression/anxiety; nevertheless, such physical activity is not routinely prescribed for these conditions. Recently there has been a large reduction in school physical education programs.

The case seems strong that increased physical activity will improve the public's health. It seems likely, however, that an individual, personal commitment to improve physical fitness is needed to spur exercise activities. The groups that show disproportionately low participation in exercise include females (Fig. 12-14), the elderly, inner city and rural residents, and those from low socioeconomic groups.

Improved public education about exercise must be backed by increased availability of programs in school and in the workplace, developing bicycle and walking paths, and reducing health and life insurance premiums for those who are physically active. Employers and communities should provide more programs of appropriate physical activity, and make the public aware of using these resources. Physicians should also pro-

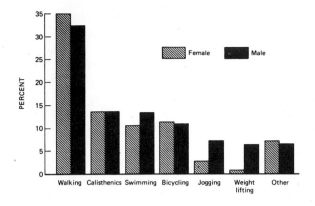

Fig. 12-13. Percent of persons 20 years of age and over who reported regular exercising, by type of exercise and sex: United States, 1975.

mote the wider imvolvement of their patients in exercise programs.

Stress Control

The term stress usually refers to those pressures, tensions, behaviors, or environmental influences which, unless suitably managed, lead to strain; the latter may manifest as fatigue, headache, absenteeism, illness, accident proneness, or other signs. Strain represents a harmful response, determined by a unique set of factors that determine the individual's response to a given stress. The same individual's perception of a stress will change with time and other circumstances.

Comprehensive programs which help individuals manage stress are held to be of high priority. However, it is essential to provide health professionals with ethically credible information; in the many areas where the answers are not known, we must formulate clearly the questions to be answered and support the research which will give the answers.

In the 1980s, the scientific base for stress management is limited. Simplistic ideas have led to techniques which may be harmful or may impede successful long-

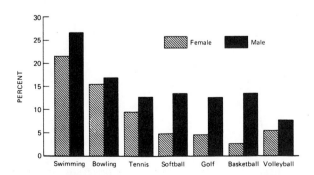

Fig. 12-14. Percent of persons 20 years of age and over who participated in seven specified sports, by sex.

term management. Overoptimistic claims or widespread premature application without pilot testing and evaluation can lead to failure and disillusionment.

Health Behavior

If we understand current health behavior, we may become more effective in persuading people to improve this behavior. One might expect that the use of health services depends on the frequency of disease or discomfort suffered by individuals or groups. This expectation proves to be partly false however. For the many preventable or treatable conditions that are more common in lower income groups, persons at greatest risk use health care and take preventive measures less often than those at lower risk.

When compared with higher income groups, the poor have higher infant mortality rates, a higher incidence of infectious disease, and a higher prevalence of untreated dental disease. However, almost all surveys show lower utilization rates by the poor of preventive and ambulatory health care. Within the poverty group, blacks usually show lower utilization rates than whites of comparable income.

Hospital admission rates are high, both for the poor and nonpoor, but the former have longer durations of stay. Such findings suggest that the poor delay longer before seeking care, and when admitted they have developed more serious illness. This interpretation is confirmed by the finding that, for almost every diagnostic group, death is a more frequent outcome among the lower income patients admitted to hospital.

How can these situations be explained? The vast literature on health services utilization describes possible approaches:

1. The *economic approach* studies the impact of financial barriers on seeking health care. The arrival of Medicare in 1966 raised hospital discharge rates for those 65 years and over and temporarily increased length of stay. In contrast, for those under 65 years, hospital discharge rates fell while little change occurred in length of stay. Such financial barriers are important, and should be reduced; but even when eliminated, wide variations still occur among income and ethnic groups. The factor of education is believed to perpetuate the lower use rates among the poor, even in countries with a national health service.

2. The *sociodemographic approach* analyzes utilization rates for various easy-to-identify groups. Such studies show that utilization tends to be higher for women than men of the same age, income and education. The problem with this approach is that it offers no explanation of the

reason that differences exist, nor does it explain the wide variations that occur within similar groups.

3. The *geographic approach* studies the association between geographic proximity of services to clients and utilization rates. The existing studies suggest that geographic convenience has slight or moderate importance.

4. The *social-cultural approach* studies cultural values, norms, beliefs and life styles. This approach focuses, for example, on the differences between "middle-classness," which is deemed to show the desired or ideal norms, and working or "lower-classness." The so-called culture of poverty is believed partly responsible for the low utilization rates of health care among low-income groups.

5. The *organization approach* emphasizes elements of the health delivery system that foster or impede utilization. Some studies suggest that large organizations, in order to survive financially, may neglect clients in greatest need of health care but with least ability to pay for it. Other critics say that the delivery system is so arranged as to maximize the convenience of health care providers, with less attention given to the needs of consumers. Further aspects of health services organization will be reviewed later in this chapter.

6. The *social-psychologic approach* emphasizes motivation, individual perceptions and learning. Using this approach, one group of investigators suggests that a number of conditions seem important in seeking and following professional health advice: (a) The individual must believe that he is suffering from an illness or that he is liable to develop an illness of serious consequence. (b) He must believe that the illness can be prevented, controlled or cured. (c) He must be sufficiently "future oriented" to justify taking immediate action to ward off health threats that are far in the future. (d) His social group—family, friends, peers—must approve of his use of the professional health care system. (e) He must be willing to overcome whatever obstacles exist to obtaining health care. (f) He must be willing to follow professional advice.

This list of conditions, which is likely to change in the coming years as further research is carried out, exemplify the many factors that health educators must consider as they try to improve health behavior. Clearly the conveying of information about health and disease is not sufficient to correct the absence of some of the above requirements. However, as we develop more effective ways to create these essential conditions,

so will we become more effective in improving health behavior.

ECONOMIC ASPECTS OF HEALTH CARE

Health care differs from other goods and services in a number of ways. The first difference is that it produces "external benefits"; thus health care includes many procedures that benefit society as well as the individual who receives the service. A second difference is that health care, besides being a "consumption commodity," something that we use up and spend money on, is partly an "investment good"; dollars spent on it now may raise future productivity and return the same dollars with interest. A third difference is its "collective nature"; when it is used by one person, there is no decrease in its availability to others. When one person consumes fluoridated water, for example, an abundance remains to give the benefits of fluoridation to other drinkers. The large dollar investment needed—such as for water and sewer systems, or for the buildings and personnel to provide hospital or nursing home care—also applies to health services.

The amount in dollars that individuals are willing to pay for preventive measures tends to be below its true value to society, for the individual does not care to pay for the additional benefits to society or for intangible benefits that are somewhat far off in the future. When the income of the average American family doubles, its demand for preventive care more than doubles, while that for curative care rises less. Low-income families give priority to paying for treatment when ill, and regard more as a luxury the preventive measures that are also indicated. Thus the argument is strong that government funds should support health services, and should be particularly funneled into preventive health services. The controversy over the appropriate area for government funds is in the support of curative health care. Science does not guide the development of a consensus on this point, and future decisions will be made on a political basis.

In recent years the costs of medical care have risen more steeply than other costs in the United States, particularly in the field of hospital care (Fig. 12-5). The main reasons for the rise in hospital costs have been:

1. Hospitals, which previously required many employees to work long hours at low wages, have been closing the gap in wages and working conditions between themselves and other industries.

2. Many scientific advances have increased the complexity of hospital care. Rarely does an improve-

ment replace a step that was more expensive; most often the innovation forms an extra step to improve the quality of care.

3. Hospitals make intensive use of personal services and less of mass production technology; they have not raised their productivity as fast as the economy at large.

4. The cost of educational and training programs has now risen much above the value of the benefits obtained. It is often suggested that government should do more to finance the training of nurses, interns and residents.

An increasing amount of money spent on health services comes from health insurance plans, sometimes described as third-party payments. Persons with hospital insurance have higher rates of hospital use than those without insurance. However, there is evidence to suggest that those without insurance have greater, rather than less, need for hospitalization. The government-financed Medicare program helped reduce this problem for those aged 65 years or older. The debate on nationwide compulsory health insurance focuses on the need for better coverage of other groups as well.

When third-party payments cover a service, rising prices cause less individual protest and less change in use. Thus, the price of a health service does not relate so inversely to its consumption as does price in other fields. Other rationing devices tend to develop when the price mechanism is not effective. Waiting lists for services develop, and registration at outpatient clinics may become unpleasant, partly to discourage a rapid return of patients. These deterrents have a different impact on different groups; price deters high-income patients less than low-income ones; long waiting times deter the unemployed less than those eager to return to the job they hold. Thus there is no universally fair way of rationing services that are scarce, which in theory almost all personal health services are.

Health Care Facilities

The system of health care facilities can be pictured as forming a bridge that carries the individual seeking service to the health worker who provides that service. The system also provides the necessary equipment and technology to make the service as effective and as efficient as possible.

There never will be a single, "best" system of health care. The way in which personal health services and facilities are organized depends mainly on factors outside the control of health professionals. The most prominent characteristics of the existing system of health care facilities are its complexity, and the difficulty it has in responding to the increasing demands of an affluent society.

Although there is no ideal pattern of organization, the goals to be aimed at are clearer. The health care facilities should be so organized that they produce health services that are:

1. Readily accessible, with no socioeconomic or geographic barriers to important populations groups.
2. Adequate in quantity, doing most of each necessary job.
3. Comprehensive, covering the range of needed services, and facilitating continuity of care.
4. Effective, reaching their stated goals, which will rise as techniques improve.
5. Efficient, reaching their goals with a reasonable degree of economy.
6. Of good quality, satisfying the consumer, as well as the producer, of health services.

What steps should be taken toward meeting these goals? Only partial and political answers to this question exist; the complex solutions will depend largely upon the judgment of those who have power to decide about community health problems. The current diversity of ownership and facilities makes it difficult for HSAs to plan for improved accessibility to health services. Fragmentation of care is common; continuity of care now depends upon the individual patient being able to find his way to the appropriate points of the health care system at the right time. We particularly need to integrate into the system those facilities that provide long-term care, rehabilitation and mental health services. To facilitate this integration, the HSAs and the developing Health Maintenance Organizations (HMOs) may help.

We also need to develop further the alternatives to institutional care. Many patients now admitted to institutions may be cared for in the future by home care programs, geriatric day centers, foster family programs and outpatient clinics. The current restrictions of health insurance programs and government funding slow the development of these alternatives.

Health Care Personnel

The physician, who will continue to dominate among providers of health care, is the major topic of discussion in this section. The classic ideal of an authoritarian but understanding physician who provides complete medical care to several generations of the family may never have been so common as hearsay suggests. Whether common or not in the past, this relationship cannot be successfully maintained in the face of changing patient demands and the wide expansion of medical knowledge.

Much of the medical profession's strength is based on the legally supported monopoly concerning practice. This monopoly operates through a system of licensing, which gives physicians the privilege to hospitalize patients and the right to prescribe drugs and order laboratory tests that are otherwise virtually inaccessible to the layman. The economic and political autonomy of physicians varies from country to country and may vary in the United States at different times. More constant is their scientific autonomy, because even the most socialized countries leave the profession fairly free to develop its special area of knowledge and to determine what practices are scientifically acceptable. Similarly, the medical profession has almost everywhere remained free to control the technical instruction of medical students.

Medical Training

Just as much as other professionals, physicians consider medical education to be the major single factor determining performance. Part of the content of medical education indoctrinates the student in the existing values and beliefs of the profession; it also provides the knowledge that allows the physician to deal with patients without undue anxiety and helps him cope with basic uncertainty in clinical practice.

Like students in other fields, medical students view their educational experience differently from their instructors. However, most students adopt two dominant values of the faculty, which they use to guide their learning experience and select their careers. These values are *medical responsibility* and *clinical experience*.

The traditional value of medical responsibility is that the physician holds the life of a patient in his hands and must take the blame for bad results. This value is stressed by many lectures about the way in which mistakes of omission or comission endanger the patient's life. It is stressed further by the hierarchy of hospital physicians—only the physicians of high status in teaching hospitals carry out the most dangerous procedures.

Clinical experience refers to direct contact with patients and their diseases. Experience is valued as superior to abstract textbook knowledge and even to general, scientifically verified knowledge. On ward rounds or at roundtable discussions, argument from experience seems unanswerable except by the same type of argument from someone with greater experience.

These values guide the student in selecting from the enormous mass of facts presented to him the information he is really to learn. They lead him to discount basic science and to focus on practical information not found in books. He seeks tasks in which medical responsibility is apparent, and avoids those that involve no risk or danger. His choice of career also hinges on how much he is exposed to the possibility of killing or disabling patients when he makes a mistake. Specialities such as dermatology, allergy, physical medicine, those that involve chronic illness, public health or pathology are unpopular.

Professional Control

Like those in most professions, physicians control their own performance in private practice. In isolated, solo practice, the burden of control rests solely on the physician's motivation, capacity and conscience. In urban areas, even solo practitioners usually belong to a "colleague network"; by referring patients to each other, practitioners can observe some of one another's performance; and by being economically and technically interdependent, physicians can influence one another.

Group practices and HMOs increase the opportunity for physicians to observe and influence one another's performance. In this increasingly common situation, physicians from two or more specialities collaborate and pool their earnings, which are divided among them according to some prearranged plan. Most groups function on a fee-for-service basis, but a few operate a health insurance program in which patients receive all the services they need for a fixed annual fee. Convenience for the physicians and improved accessibility of care for their patients are the basic motivating factors in the information of group practices; the physicians' improved ability to monitor each other's performance is a secondary benefit to both patient and doctor, rarely stated openly as an objective of group practice. Perhaps crucial in prevention of most strict control of the quality of medical care is the ideology of independence and autonomy held by physicians throughout the world.

Formal and Informal Organization

The national, state and local medical associations make up the formal organization of physicians. These associations do only part of the job of ensuring high quality care by setting minimum standards and the basic core of training required for licensing, by publishing new knowledge, and by educating the practitioners.

At least equally important is the informal structure of the profession. As mentioned above, most physicians in urban areas join a network of colleagues which is likely to be fairly homogeneous within itself. The networks probably interact little with each other, and their standards and practices differ from one another. One basic control mechanism is the "boycott"—practitioners refuse to refer patients to those of whom they disapprove. This device may or may not change the physician's performance; sometimes it merely pushes him outside a network of high standards into the company of those with lower standards.

Individual Physician Behavior

Once physicians were seen as powerful, wise and charismatic, possessing knowledge about human beings denied to other mortals. Recent decades have seen a reaction against this view, for social, administrative and therapeutic reasons, in favor of seeing him as one of many professionals providing health care in society. Acceptance of the newer view is patchy among physicians but more widespread among consumers in the United States.

The physician's behavior will reflect his adaptation to the medical role as he sees it. For example, the physician may prefer to treat critically ill patients, when he can rely mainly on his knowledge and technical skills, and ignore the patient as a person. In a crisis situation the physician is active and the patient passive. In an acute but less desperate situation, the physician guides while the patient cooperates, with the latter knowing what goes on and exercising some judgment. The third relationship is that of mutual participation, where the physician helps the patient to help himself, particularly useful in chronic disease and disability. This last role is closest to the newer view of physicians, particularly since medical knowledge and technical skills of other health professionals who can also help the chronic disease patient. The treatment of both chronically ill and elderly patients, therefore, tends not to appeal to many physicians since it reinforces the reaction against the physician-on-a-pedestal.

The strain of the physician role may be greater than that of other professionals. One reason may be that the physician cannot adapt by behaving regressively such as by screaming that he cannot cope with the demands placed upon him. Recourse then to alcohol or drugs, hostility to patients or family or forms of professional suicide may represent attempts to resolve the conflict at a level short of real suicide.

Other Health Personnel

A continuing national problem is the shortage of health personnel of all kinds and the more effective use of currently available personnel. Progress in the manpower field will partly depend on breaking the task of health care into its component parts according to the skills needed to do each part. The health care system is now trying to introduce greater degrees of personnel flexibility so that paramedical personnel can be trained and legally permitted to do some jobs normally done by physicians and nurses.

The most rapid rise in numbers, now and in the future, is likely to occur in the relatively new groups of personnel with shorter training. A new and mixed group of "physician extenders" is now being trained and studied, with such names as physician assistants and nurse practitioners. Also being trained in much larger numbers are the assistants and aides to various health professions. The lack of theoretical training results in their having a persistent low capacity to make even minor decisions about therapy and a continuing high need for supervision. These nonprofessionals will provide increasingly more direct patient care in institutions, while the professionals must inevitably spend more time on supervision. Such changes have already affected the nursing profession and may increasingly affect physicians in the coming decades.

QUESTIONS IN PUBLIC HEALTH AND COMMUNITY MEDICINE

REVIEW QUESTIONS

When do health problems become public health problems? Discuss the value and limitations of your answer.

How can health be simply explained, in terms of what it is and what it does? Discuss the good and bad points of the WHO definition, and give an alternative description which more closely approaches our real life activities.

What factors affect time trends in the crude death rates of the United States? If crude death rates are slowly rising while age-specific rates are falling slowly in a given developed country, what is the most likely explanation for this contrast?

What are the differences between incidence and prevalence, and how do they relate to each other?

What is record linkage, and what are its advantages and disadvantages? If more widely used in the coming years, how will it improve our understanding of the public's health?

Can infant mortality rates remain level in a country that is truly improving its health services? Justify your answer.

Discuss one well-established method of reducing the incidence and prevalence of a major chronic disease in the United States.

From the economic viewpoint, how does health care differ from other goods and services appearing in the marketplace?

Review the current status and possible future changes that may occur in the medical profession in the United States.

How do governmental health agencies differ from voluntary health agencies?

Suggest ten different areas that deserve high priority in prevention in the coming years. Review in detail the procedures which would be part of the preventive effort in one high priority area.

Should family planning and population control services be subsidized by government in a developed country? Justify your answer.

MULTIPLE CHOICE QUESTIONS

Choose the best answer for each question. Answers are at the end of this chapter.

1. The group of "physician extenders," now being trained and studied in the United States, includes such personnel as:
   (a) nurse practitioners
   (b) licensed practical nurses
   (c) occupational therapists
   (d) physical therapy assistants
2. A questionnaire mailed to 1,000 adult women asked about the presence or absence of joint stiffness. 500 women returned the questionnaire, and 100 stated that they had stiff joints. The appropriate rate for the prevalence of stiff joints would be:
   (a) 100/1000, provided the questionnaires are correctly answered
   (b) 100/500, provided the nonrespondents are similar to the respondents
   (c) 500/1000, provided women with stiff joints are likely not to reply
   (d) none of the above alternatives
3. Epidemiologic studies of hepatitis have been more productive than of diabetes mellitus in orienting prevention programs because:
   (a) the causes of hepatitis are more easily controlled by antibiotics than the causes of diabetes
   (b) hepatitis is more accurately diagnosed than diabetes
   (c) it is easier to classify hepatitis cases by the causal agents than it is to classify diabetes cases
   (d) hepatitis has more risk factors associated with it than does diabetes
4. Japanese migrants to Hawaii develop more cancer of the colon than Japanese who live in Japan. This difference is best explained by:

   (a) migrants from a country may differ from these remaining in the country
   (b) Hawaii may have environmental carcinogens which are absent from Japan
   (c) Japanese in Hawaii may eat different foods from Japanese in Japan
   (d) all of the above factors may play a part
5. In recent decades, the U.S. public has come to believe that health care is a human right. The response of government to this demand has been mainly at the federal level primarily because:
   (a) state and local governments have no authority to respond
   (b) many state governors disagree with the "human right" view
   (c) local government officials neither have the training, nor the experience to respond
   (d) federal government officials are more sensitive to public demands
   (e) financial resources are most abundant at the federal level
6. When a measurement, such as blood pressure level, leads to a diagnosis of disease or no disease, the cutoff point between the two groups may be defined:
   (a) by statistical means, such as two standard deviations from the age-specific average
   (b) by clinical means, such as the level at which symptoms and complications become more frequent
   (c) by prognosis, such as an elevated risk of future disease
   (d) by any of the above means, depending on the purpose of the cutoff point
7. A small study attempted to guide health planners as to whether death certificates for esophageal cancer form a useful guide to the frequency of that disease. Its findings were:

diagnosed before death	74
confirmed at autopsy	53
not confirmed at autopsy	21
first diagnosed at autopsy	22

   Please check whether each of the following statements is correct or wrong:

	Correct	*Wrong*
(a) 22/74 of individual cases were missed before death.		
(b) The false positive diagnoses before death about balance the false negatives.		
(c) Autopsies are essential to obtain the approximate population frequency.		

8. The average expectation of life at birth
   (a) rises with improvements in health
   (b) falls as death rates increase
   (c) is higher for United States females than males
   (d) has all of the above characteristics

9. The legal requirement that physicians report selected diseases
   (a) has succeeded particularly for mental illnesses
   (b) gives an incomplete picture of disease incidence
   (c) has been used mainly for noninfectious conditions
   (d) has slowed the control of infectious disease

10. Epidemiologic studies of disease usually involve
    (a) both the sick and healthy populations
    (b) discarding the clinical knowledge of disease
    (c) emphasizing the cases of advanced disease
    (d) relating local cases to the national population

11. The frequency of much infectious disease can best be explained by
    (a) host factors
    (b) characteristics of the infectious agent
    (c) environmental factors
    (d) interaction of all of the above

12. An epidemiologic study is "double blind" when
    (a) the subjects know that they belong to the control group
    (b) the investigators do not understand the pathology of the condition
    (c) neither observer nor subject knows to which group the subject belongs
    (d) all of the above conditions are met

13. In an epidemic of food poisoning, the contaminated food must
    (a) be eaten by all cases
    (b) have been avoided by all who remained well
    (c) be consumed by most cases and by few of the well
    (d) be characterized by none of the above

14. In the United States, the Public Health Service is
    (a) a federal agency with many public health functions
    (b) the agency using about two-thirds of the federal health budget
    (c) the guide for the activities of PSROs
    (d) a federal agency responsible for Medicare and Medicaid

15. The prevention and better control of hypertension involves
    (a) obesity control and reduced salt intake
    (b) a lifetime of antihypertensive treatment in established cases
    (c) more extensive screening for elevated blood pressure in employees
    (d) all of the above steps

16. Maternal and child health activities usually include
    (a) use of Medicare funds for immunizations
    (b) the supervision and care of mothers and children
    (c) the early detection and treatment of atherosclerosis
    (d) all of the above measures

17. The delivery of routine immunizations could be widened by
    (a) eliminating charges for these procedures
    (b) funding preventive measures through government subsidies
    (c) offering vaccines free to physicians who do not charge their patients for immunizations
    (d) all of the above steps

18. Identifying the environmental causes of disease is complicated because
    (a) the period may be short between exposure and disease onset
    (b) clear data are usually available, but overlooked, that reveal the association
    (c) many agents may contribute to the same disease
    (d) all of the above reasons play a part

19. About 40 per cent of the United States population drink water that is deficient in fluoride. Extending fluoridation to this remaining population faces the barriers of
    (a) a continued deep concern about dental caries
    (b) community reluctance to confront the opponents of fluoridation
    (c) weak scientific knowledge about the safety of fluoride
    (d) inadequate documentation that fluoride reduces caries

20. The Health Care Financing Administration is
    (a) a voluntary agency that funds health care
    (b) a philanthropic association, such as the Rockefeller Foundation
    (c) a professional association that guides health administrators
    (d) a federal agency responsible for Medicare and Medicaid

ANSWERS TO MULTIPLE CHOICE QUESTIONS

1. (a)
2. (b)

3. (c)
4. (d)

5. (e)
6. (d)

7. (a) wrong
(b) correct
(c) wrong

8. (d)
9. (b)
10. (a)
11. (d)

12. (c)
13. (c)
14. (a)

15. (d)
16. (b)
17. (d)

18. (c)
19. (b)
20. (c)

13

Psychiatry

Gordon H. Deckert, M.D.

Professor and Head, Department of Psychiatry
and Behavioral Sciences,
University of Oklahoma at Oklahoma City—
Health Sciences Center

Ronald S. Krug, PH.D.

Professor and Director of Undergraduate Education, Department of
Psychiatry and Behavioral Sciences, University of Oklahoma at
Oklahoma City—Health Sciences Center

Psychiatry is a science and a medical specialty. As a science, it seeks to understand disorders of the psyche (mind). The term "mind" is part of a psychological language reference system, along with such concepts as personality, anxiety, ego, neurosis, etc. The organ of the mind is the brain. The term "brain" is part of a physiological language reference system, along with such concepts as neurotransmitters, the limbic system, higher cortical functions, etc. Psychiatry employs both language systems. As a medical specialist, a psychiatrist seeks to study, diagnose, treat and prevent mental, emotional, behavioral, and psychophysiological disorders, and adverse psychological responses to illness. While those five areas of major concern overlap, most students of the field distinguish between them.

A given person, his mind, emotions, behavior, and soma (body) are influenced by many factors—so many that it becomes difficult to define the limits of psychiatry. There are various language models for describing human behavior, multiple theories to facilitate understanding, and even a variety of medical nomenclatures. No wonder the student may find all this perplexing. Nonetheless, despite these difficulties and differences, there is considerable agreement as to the major clinical entities and their management.

Mental illness is ubiquitous. The Institute of Medicine of the National Academy of Sciences, summarzing recent epidemiological studies, states that approximately 25 to 30 per cent of visits to ambulatory care medical facilities are attributed directly to mental illness. The majority of these visits relate to the manifestations of anxiety and depression. At any one time, as many patients with mental illnesses occupy hospital beds as do all other patients combined, even though the number of patients resident in state and country mental hospitals has decreased over the last several decades. Rates of admission and discharge have, however, increased at mental hospitals. In the United States, approximately one in ten individuals will be hospitalized in a psychiatric hospital for mental illness. Many others are admitted to general hospitals. One person in every three or four will seek specific medical assistance for a mental disorder. Increasing numbers of patients are being seen in community mental health centers and hospital emergency rooms. These figures and statements do not even include patients with psychosomatic illnesses, or those who present with psychological response to disease. Virtually *every* disease has accompanying psychological consequences. No wonder, then, that studies indicate that 75 to 90 per cent of all patients present with psychological factors playing some role in their discomfort. Add to this the increasingly recognized problem of compliance, that is, the relatively low percentage of patients who follow their prescribed medical regimen. Consider the mounting interest in prevention. One can understand those who predict a resurgence of interest in psychiatry over the next several decades. Undergraduate and graduate medical curricula have placed increasing emphasis on behavioral sciences, psychiatry, psychological medicine and behavioral medicine. This, in turn, is reflected nationally on certification, licensure and speciality examinations.

Practicing physicians frequently work with patients who *somatize,* that is, focus on their body, tend to ignore or deny psychological dimensions to their illness and resist efforts at psychological intervention. Less well recognized is another group of patients who *psychologize,* that is, who tend to ignore their body or the possibility of illness in their body and resist appropriate medical intervention. The physician by education, training and role is potentially in a unique position to help both groups of patients. Ideally, a physician has a biological and a psychological perspective and the capability to understand, manage and treat "disease."

Psychiatry in the United States is undergoing a major change in its diagnostic nomenclature. The *Diagnostic and Statistical Manual of Mental Disorders of the American Psychiatric Association* (DSM-III) will be officially in use by the time this chapter is published. Therefore, the language and outline of DSM-III will be followed in this section. Where necessary, comparable terms from DSM-I and DSM-II will be placed in parentheses so the student can correlate this material with the various headings used by most psychiatric texts now in print.

HISTORY

Man is curious about himself. He has always attempted to explain his behavior, including that behavior called mental illness. He has had a tendency to ascribe the phenomena of mental illness to supernatural causes, especially to possession by some outside influence. Nonetheless, many early Greek physicians, including Hippocrates, taught that mental illness resulted from natural causes, and both Hippocrates and his near contemporary in India, Susruta, held a rather sophisticated view of psychosomatic processes. After the death of the Roman physician, Galen, in 200 A.D., a gradual return of primitive attitudes in the West culminated in demonology and the persecution and execution of so-called witches. This practice was much more pervasive in parts of Europe than is generally recognized. In the late 15th and early 16th centuries, conservative estimates put the figure of executions to approximately 100,000 in Germany and a similar number in France. *Malleus Maleficarum* (The Witch's Hammer) published by two Dominicans, Sprenger and Kramer, has had a profound influence on Western medicine. Medicine's separation of mind from body during this time was perhaps inevitable given the theology of the day. Thomas Aquinas spoke for his culture when he argued that the soul could not be sick. During this era, advances in medical psychology were found primarily in the Moslem world, especially among Arab physicians.

The first effective answer to demonology was *De Praestigiis Daemonum,* by Johann Weyer (1515–1588), often called "the father of psychiatry." Two centuries later in 1792, Philippe Pinel struck the chains from the mental patients in the Bicetré in France. His contemporary, Benjamin Rush, a physician and a signer of the Declaration of Independence, was considered the father of American psychiatry because of his efforts for the mentally ill in Philadelphia.

During the 19th century, French and German psychiatrists, especially Emil Kraepelin (1855–1926), applied descriptive and statistical methods to clinical studies and elaborated a classification of personality disorders and mental illness. This classification influences ours today. Later, Eugene Bleuler revised the Kraepelinian concept of dementia praecox and introduced the term "schizophrenia."

Paralleling the development of descriptive psychiatry was an increasing understanding of psychological mechanisms. Many scholars trace a sequence of ideas from Paracelsus (1493–1541) to Franz Anton Mesmer (1733–1815) to James Braid (1795–1860), who coined the term "hypnosis," and Jean Martin Charcot (1825–

1893) among others to the first giant in dynamic psychiatry, Sigmund Freud (1856–1939). His concepts of the unconscious, the ego, id and super ego, defense mechanisms, and neurotic conflict have become an integral part of psychiatric thought. Some of these terms are now used on an everyday basis by the public as well. His emphasis on early life experiences as a determinant of later behavior was one stimulus among many for the increasing interest in psychological growth and development. Piaget's study of the development of the intellect is one example. Modification of Freudian psychoanalytic theory to include broader sociological and cultural influences is perhaps most prominently evident in the work of Erik Erikson.

More recently, a series of discoveries involving the brain, its neurophysiology and neurochemistry have brought biology into modern psychiatry, along with descriptive (phenomenological), psychological, sociological and cultural approaches. Today when examining a given patient, the physician must be capable of thinking and working within this multiple framework of understanding human behavior, whether the behavior in question is molecular or molar.

EVALUATION

CONCEPTS

When evaluating patients, certain critical concepts are essential to facilitate a complete diagnosis and a positive therapeutic outcome.

Unified Concept of Mind, Brain and Body

Modern clinicians in their thinking and in their approach to patients avoid the historical mind/brain/body trichotomy still inherent in our language system. They function from the thesis of empirical parallelism. With any human event, there is the component that is *experienced,* for example, any phenomenal event of seeing, hearing, thinking, wishing, etc. This *subjective* experience can be communicated to another with words. The other component of the event is that *observed* by those others outside the event. When these observations are consensually validated, we tend to call the evidence *objective.* An example is a neurophysiological or neurochemical response in the brain. By the parallelism thesis, these two components are not separate events, nor does one cause the other. A given thought does not cause a given neurophysiological response, nor does the neurophysiological event cause the thought. There is instead a single unitary event. In parallel, empirically, what I experience, you observe; what you experience, I observe.

This concept when applied to the clinical setting has very practical consequences. For example, we will recognize that what the patient experiences is not necessarily what we see. What we see, the patient may not experience. The question of whether the patient's problem is a physical illness or an emotional illness is seen as an increasingly useless and potentially destructive dichotomous question. Only patients can experience their distress or declare their dis-ease. It is not the physician's task to decide whether someone is sick. The physician's task is to help the patient understand the disease process, and given that understanding, to help the patient with appropriate intervention. The mind/brain/body trichotomy can no longer be supported by the weight of scientific evidence. Physics has understood this for several decades. It is puzzling that biology and medicine have lagged so far behind. To hold to this view, as unfortunately many physicians still do, is to risk inefficiency, ineffectiveness and even harm to the patient.

The Concept of Multiple Etiology

Any event (or constellation of events) labeled disease is multiply determined. More often than not in medical practice it is no longer useful to assume that for a given effect there is a given cause. Rather, we deal with multiple causality, multiple factors, multiple determinants in any disease process. Hence, multiple interventions at multiple levels are usually required.

The Concepts of Individual versus Stimulus-response Specificity

These concepts originate in physiology. *Individual response specificity* states that before one can predict the response of a given human to a given stimulus, one must first understand, the individual. Or, given a particular response, one can postdict the events leading to that response only by knowing the individual organism. Only in the individual is there a specific response to a specific stimulus. More often than not, this applies to the practice of medicine with most patients most of the time. The *stimulus-response specific assumption* states that a lawful, predictable relationship exists between the stimulus and the response. One can predict, therefore, the response by simply knowing the stimulus or postdict the stimulus by knowing the response. Knowledge about a particular, unique individual is not required. A light falling on the eye will constrict the pupil. This model is very efficient and powerful when applicable. It has been and continues to be a valuable model in the development of scientific medicine. However, many physicians attempt to use this model, often unknowingly, when it simply does not apply. Understanding and distinguishing between these two models and knowing when one is more applicable than another is critical to the day by day, even moment by moment, practice of medicine. When employed appropriately, these two complimentary concepts shape the priorities of the doctor/patient interaction and enhance accuracy of evaluation and effectiveness of intervention.

Purpose

Although seemingly almost self evident, it is useful nonetheless to keep in mind the various purposes of the interviewing-evaluating process. These may be outlined as follows:

1. to give patients the opportunity to express and share their distress
2. to observe and to elicit data
3. to establish rapport, an effective working relationship
4. to develop understanding of the disease in question
5. to exchange information with the patient
6. to develop a working contract, an intervention strategy and to effect implementation of that strategy.

PROCESS

A prerequisite for an effective evaluation process is an understanding of the doctor/patient relationship and a skill in developing that relationship. Another is in knowing how to utilize certain communication styles when interviewing. Finally, a fairly thorough knowledge of the phenomenology of mental processes is required. Given all the above, the interaction with a patient may proceed.

Interviewing Priorities

Usually the encounter begins with the patient and the physician confronting each other visually. Very early in the encounter, often with a glance, the physician determines whether or not there is an immediate medical emergency, e.g., cardiac standstill. Next, observing the patient's behavior the clinician makes a fairly early and accurate judgment as to whether the patient is oriented. Evidence for the possibility of an organic mental disorder should have a major influence on the remaining interaction. Also relatively early in the interview, a skilled clinician can usually determine whether or not there may be a profound thought disorder by carefully listening to the patient's speech. In the overwhelming number of instances, there is no immediate medical emergency, the patient is oriented and does not demonstrate a thought disorder of psy-

chotic proportions. In short, the physician has another "brain" with which to work. Then should come the question, "What is it that I would like to know next?" From the principle of individual response specificity, comes the answer, "I would like to know something fairly reliable about this particular individual." The royal road to understanding a given individual at a given moment is to conduct an inventory of that individual's primary emotions.

Identifying the Primary Emotions and Obtaining Congruence

Let's take a specific example. A male family physician in an office setting introduces himself to his next patient and notes that she is in no acute medical distress and seems oriented. She appears to be in her mid-30s, is neatly and well dressed, is sitting on the edge of her chair with one foot ahead of the other and greets him with wide open eyes. She licks her lips and says at the height of inspiration, "I'm certainly glad to see you." Many physicians in this situation would then say something like, "Thank you. Well, what brings you to see me?" But a more efficient and a more effective response is something of the order, "Yes, you look anxious." With this the patient responds, "Frankly, Doctor, I'm more than anxious. I'm scared to death. A week ago, while riding my horse, I hit my head on the limb of a tree. I felt a little dazed but not anything else and I went on with the ride, but several days later I started having headaches unlike any kind of headaches I've ever had in my life and I'm worried that maybe I have a subdural hematoma like my younger sister had after an automobile accident."

This patient looks anxious or fearful. The physician wonders if she feels anxious. He structures his response accordingly. Indeed, through her words, it is clear; she feels anxious and fearful. In short, the objective and subjective evidence, the behavioral and the verbal evidence, are *congruent*. Psychologically healthy individuals in trusting situations "look how they feel and feel how they look." Also when patients are congruent, they characteristically have a very good idea why they are feeling the way they are feeling. If this information is not volunteered, the physician can ask and the answer usually can be taken at face value. This particular patient volunteers this information in a direct and succinct manner.

The first step, then, in an interview process, is to ask oneself questions about the patient's primary emotion: Do I hear words indicating that the patient is aware of this emotion? Do I see evidence which portrays this emotion? In short, is the patient congruent? If the patient presents objective evidence, for example, of anger, one must attempt to determine whether the patient is aware of feeling angry. If the patient states that he or she is feeling a particular way in the absence of objective evidence for that particular emotional state, the effective interviewer notes that discrepancy and often draws the attention of that incongruity to the patient. Patients with neurotic conflict tend to be incongruent in one fashion or another. The patient's words and behaviors often suggest the particular defense mechanisms whereby they either hide their feelings from others or hide their feelings from themselves. Such patients usually are not completely aware of the factors that precipitate the feeling as experienced or portrayed. However, this was not the case with our example.

Establishing Consensus Regarding the Stress

Once congruence is established, the patient and the physician usually can come to an agreement as to what may account for the distress fairly quickly. However, with many patients this can be difficult. They have been trained or have trained themselves not to show their distress or even to be aware of it. Usually, this is accomplished through the elaboration of a neurotic personality. Accompanying this structure is usually a lack of accurate awareness of the constellations of events, past and present, leading to the disease in question. In contrast, this patient, a genial character (psychologically healthy, nonneurotic), looks anxious, feels anxious and knows why he or she is anxious and is ready to work toward a solution with the physician. The physician's response might be, "Your anxiety is understandable. From what you have told me so far, a subdural hematoma, while possible, is unlikely." Consensus is established. When effective physician interviewers are studied, they then tend to verbally summarize their understanding of the patient's visit before proceeding to the next step.

Making a Contract

At this point in the process, effective physicians usually obtain the patient's chief expectation. In our example, the physician might say, "I take it you're here to get to the bottom of these different kind of headaches you're having." The patient nods and says, "Yes, indeed!" What follows is an explicitly stated understanding of how the two of them will work together to solve the problem, what length of time will be required for more detailed history taking, physical examination, the possibility of laboratory studies, etc. Through an exchange of information, a decision is made as to the nature of the problem. This allows the final step in the process of a therapeutic interaction.

Developing a Strategy for Intervention and Implementation

The physician's particular knowledge of disease processes will be very helpful to the patient at this point. The patient's special knowledge of himself or herself, in turn, can be very helpful to the physician, as together they develop a strategy of intervention and create a specific plan for implementation. Each, then, proceeds to fill their particular role in that plan.

National competency examinations are paying increased attention to the measurement of interpersonal skills. By attending to the five process steps outlined above, a candidate may answer a whole series of questions on such examinations. (See the examples at end of chapter.) But more importantly, patient outcome research increasingly points to this particular sequence as enhancing therapeutic outcome. Training and practice are required for any physician to become an accurate diagnostician and an effective therapist especially when working with those many patients that resist the process.

STRUCTURE

In the context of the doctor/patient interaction and during the process of effective interviewing as outlined above, the clinician keeps in mind an historical outline. During and after the interview, the physician organizes this history into a particular format. In the practice of psychiatry and behavioral medicine, the structural outline of a usual medical history is perfectly appropriate and will not be detailed here. The chief complaint or the presenting complaint is significant and usually easily obtained, but again, for effective interviewers, it is not their first concern. In the preceeding example, if the physician's first response or inquiry was toward the chief complaint, the patient would undoubtedly have presented her headaches. Typically what would follow would be a whole series of questions and answers regarding the specific nature of the headaches. By paying attention first to the patient's emotional state, the patient volunteered very salient information, after which there can be the necessary medical interrogative interview and in *less* time and with a *better* outcome. In addition to the presenting complaint, information is gathered regarding the history of the presenting illness and the past personal and family medical history.

Especially when psychological factors seem particulary significant to the patient's problem or to the doctor/patient interaction, it is frequently very helpful, even necessary, to obtain a more detailed personal, familial and social history. Special attention should be paid to growth and development issues, the history of present and past family relationships, an education and work history and a history of leisure activities. Patients' descriptions of themselves as persons and patients' descriptions of their significant others as personalities are often of special value.

Also in the context of the interview process and while obtaining a history, a mental status examination is conducted. This is sometimes called the psychological examination. (See Behavioral Sciences, Chapter 14.)

Some aspect of a physical examination is required for evaluation purposes in most, but not all instances in a medical setting. Indeed on many occasions a rather thorough physical examination is very much in order even if the patient presents primarily with what seems like an emotional or mental problem. This is particularly true if one suspects an organic mental disorder or a psychosomatic illness. Also in some patients, certain illnesses mimic conversion hysteria, just as conversion hysteria often mimics certain medical problems.

EVALUATION BEYOND HISTORY, MENTAL STATUS AND PHYSICAL EXAMINATION

Involvement of Family, Friends and Other Health Professionals

Perhaps next in significance to the evaluation of the patient is interviewing one or more members of the patient's family and/or friends. Their view of the problem can be extraordinarily valuable; their involvement with strategies for intervention may be crucial. This is especially true for children. A review of the patient's past medical records is also too frequently overlooked as is direct contact with other health professionals with whom the patient has worked.

Psychological Tests

In some instances, formal psychological testing is helpful. (See Behavioral Sciences, Chapter 14.)

Laboratory Tests

When certain nosolotical entities are suspected, specific roentgenographic and/or laboratory tests are often indicated. These are covered under the various diagnostic headings in the clinical chapters.

Electroencephalographic Examination

The electroencephalogram (EEG) is a recording of the electrical activity of the brain. Leads are attached to the scalp, and the brain waves are recorded by pens on paper that moves at the rate of 3 cm. per second. The paper is commonly divided into 1 sec. and 0.2 sec. divisions for ease in determining the frequency of the waves. The amplitude of normal brain activity

is from 20 to 70 microvolts, which usually results, depending upon calibration, in pen deflections of 6 to 7 millimeters for every 50 microvolts.

Brain waves vary from 1 to 50 cycles per second. The most conspicuous activity is *alpha,* 8 through 13 cycles per second, especially seen in recordings from the occipital region. This rhythm tends to disappear when the eyes are opened, or when the subject is tense, engaged in mental activity or experiencing considerable anxiety. In the normal waking population, *theta* activity is also seen, ranging from 4 to 7 cycles per second. *Delta* activity refers to waves under 4 cycles per second. Delta activity is very unusual in a normal waking person. When seen it suggests sleep, delirium or diffuse brain damage. When slow wave activity seems to be localized over one area of the brain, it may suggest a space-occupying lesion. Fast activity beyond 13 cycles per second is called *beta* activity. Sudden bursts of high voltage disordered activity different from background rhythm of paroxysmal nature are frequently seen in patients with epilepsy. Random activity from recordings over the temporal lobe is reported with increased frequency in patients with temporal lobe epilepsy, but many patients without any pathology whatsoever also show occasional spiking in these areas. Some patients with temporal lobe epilepsy have normal EEGs. A characteristic pattern is often seen with petit mal epilspsy, that is, a pattern of 3 cycles per second spike and wave activity (spike and dome pattern).

It is often stated that the EEG is not of particular value in psychiatry. While this may be true generally with the traditional recording techniques, sophisticated measurements involving computer analysis are making it clear that certain psychiatric illnesses are accompanied by dysrhythmias of one kind or another. Most of this work is still experimental and does not as yet have wide diagnostic or therapeutic application.

NOSOLOGY

DISORDERS USUALLY FIRST EVIDENT IN INFANCY, CHILDHOOD OR ADOLESCENCE

Mental Retardation

Mental retardation is defined as lower than average general intelligence with resulting deficits or impairments in adaptive behavior. The four sub-types—mild, moderate, severe and profound—have prognostic implications. Milder cases often are not diagnosed until scholastic difficulty is noted in grade school. They may attain a sixth grade performance level. The moderate group is also educable, perhaps to the fourth grade level. The severe are trainable to some degree. The profound require custodial care.

About three per cent of the population of the United States is mentally retarded. The term *primary* designates those instances where no specific etiology can be identified or reasonably postulated. This constitutes the largest group, approximately 30 per cent of the patient population. They usually have no other symptoms. There may be family history. All others are referred to as *secondary*. Perinatal infections, especially viral, and early childhood encephalitides cause about 20 per cent of cases. Prematurity and birth trauma may account for another 20 per cent. Causes may be categorized under *prenatal* factors, e.g., phenylketonuria, Gaucher's disease, cretinism, Hurler's syndrome (gargoylism), Down's syndrome (mongolism). About 10 per cent of retardates suffer from mongolism. *Perinatal* factors are a second category, e.g., prematurity, birth injury, kernicterus. Examples of *postnatal* factors include viral meningoencephalitis, lead poisoning and malnutrition. Sociocultural factors may play a role. Emotional problems and environmental deprivation may result in a picture sometimes called pseudomental retardation, a particularly important diagnosis to make. Prevention of retardation should be a special concern of all health professions. Treatment should focus on etiological factors whenever possible. In the main, treatment means bringing appropriate support to the family and to the child with particular attention to special classes in school or appropriate institutional or custodial care to those instances of profound retardation.

Attention Deficit Disorder with or without Hyperactivity (Hyperkinetic Reaction)

This syndrome is characterized by inattention, e.g., having difficulty concentrating on school work, and impulsivity and, sometimes, hyperactivity. Onset is before age seven. The diagnosis should not be made unless symptoms have been present for at least 6 months. Parents report excessive activity and short attention span. Similar reports come from teachers. Present thinking about etiology points to central nervous system maturational factors interacting with environmental stresses. Treatment is directed toward parental counseling, education, environmental manipulation and usually medication with methylphenindate or pemoline.

Conduct Disorders

This diagnosis may be made in patients under eighteen when there is repetitive and persistent pattern of conduct for at least six months in which the basic rights of others are either ignored or violated. The behaviors may be *aggressive,* e.g., physical violence against property or persons, theft, or *nonaggressive,* e.g., a recurring and chronic tendency to violate rules, or lying. Another important distinction is whether the disorder is of the *undersocialized* or *socialized* variety. Techniques of intervention tend to be different. The undersocialized group fails to establish normal bonds of affection with others. In the socialized variety, there is evidence of emotional bonding or attachment to others, frequently to peers, often with considerable loyalty to the peer group (this variety previously was called group delinquent reaction). This disorder commonly is found in the slums of our large cities where security and self esteem are found in antisocial acts supported by peers. Etiology relates primarily to faulty parental attitudes, poor child rearing practices, emotional conflicts and a variety of sociocultural factors. Intervention follows accordingly.

Anxiety Disorders of Childhood and Adolescence

The *separation anxiety disorder* is characterized by manifestations of excessive anxiety clearly relating to separation from a significant person to whom the child feels attached. Symptoms should be present for at least two weeks before this diagnosis is made.

The *avoidant disorder* (withdrawal reaction) of childhood or adolescence is characterized by persistent shrinking from contact with strangers, often to the degree that social functioning with peers may not occur. Usually there are satisfying relationships with family members. For diagnosis, symptoms should persist for six months.

The *overanxious disorder* involves symptoms of anxiety for at least six months. There is a generalized and persistent worry regarding future events or past behaviors or competence and generalized tension and self-consciousness. If the symptoms are present for a relatively short period of time and relate to a specific stress, the diagnosis of an adjustment reaction is usually more appropriate. Here, the symptoms persist and tend to be symptomatic of an underlying neurotic disorder. Various psychological and counseling techniques are indicated. Antianxiety medication generally should be avoided except in special cases and for brief periods of time.

Eating Disorders

Pica refers to the eating of nonnutritive substances repeatedly for at least one month.

Bulimia refers to recurrent episodes of binge eating of large quantities of food, often with termination by self-induced vomiting, repeated attempts to lose weight by severely restrictive diets, marked weight fluctuation, awareness that the eating pattern is abnormal and a fear of being unable to stop, together with depression and self-deprecatory thoughts. This group is to be distinguished from those with anorexia nervosa.

Anorexia nervosa, more common in adolescent girls than boys, presents with all of the physiological findings of what is essentially self-induced starvation. The syndrome is not related to a known physical illness. The diagnosis should be considered when there is weight loss of at least 20 per cent of the original body weight, a refusal to maintain body weight over a minimum normal for the age and height, and when there is an intense fear of becoming obese and/or a disturbance of body image. These patients may report feeling fat when objectively they are almost emaciated. Many feel quite energetic and may even engage in body building exercises. Without effective intervention, there is significant mortality to this syndrome. Hospitalization may be necessary as a life-saving procedure. Intervention is often complicated because there is a tendency on the part of the patient and the family to deny the presence of serious psychological difficulties. With therapy severe conflicts regarding dependency and sexuality usually become apparent.

Stereotyped Movement Disorders

Tics are to be distinguished from choreiform, dystonic and athetoid movements. They are characterized as recurrent, involuntary, repetitive, purposeless movements. The patient is able to suppress the movement voluntarily for minutes to hours. A tic disorder may be subclassified either as *transient,* i.e., at least a month but no more than a year, or *chronic.* The syndrome is usually thought to be psychogenic in origin, and hence counseling and psychotherapy are indicated.

A separate syndrome, relatively rare, is *Tourette's disorder.* The tics involve multiple muscle groups. There are frequently vocal tics as well, sometimes with compulsive and stereotyped coprolalia. Here also the movements may be suppressed for minutes to hours and symptoms vary in intensity over weeks to months. The criteria for diagnosis include the presence of symptoms for more than a year. Organic pathology of the central nervous system has consistently been suspected as playing a role in this disorder. To date, there is no reliable effective treatment, although recently haloperidol has been reported to be helpful in some cases.

Other Disorders with Physical Manifestations

Stuttering is a syndrome for which there is considerable controversy regarding etiology and treatment. However, in some cases psychological factors clearly play a role and psychological intervention is effective. In others such is not the case.

Functional enuresis and *functional encopresis* are not due to a physical disorder by definition. They are manifested by the repeated, involuntary voiding of urine by day or night or the voluntary or involuntary passage of feces. One or both may be present. There should be a history of at least one event per month in children over age four or five for this diagnosis. Eighty to ninety per cent of children are dry, that is, not enuretic by age four and one-half. By age 18 the percentage of enuretics in the general population drops to about 2 per cent. With enuresis there is a growing opinion that causation in many cases may relate more to maturational or developmental factors than to classic psychodynamic considerations. Encopresis is much less common and is more frequent in boys than girls. When these symptoms appear transiently in essentially healthy young children in response to a specific stressful life event, the diagnosis of an adjustment reaction is more appropriate.

Sleepwalking and *sleep terrors* occur during non-REM periods of sleep, in contrast to nightmares. Nightmares have psychological significance but sleep terrors relate more to maturational lags in CNS development than to psychodynamic factors, and reassurance and counseling to parents is in order.

Pervasive Developmental Disorders

The child with *infantile autism* seems within his own world and out of reach. He lacks responsiveness to other people. There is a gross deficit in language development. Responses to environment are bizarre. Onset is before age three. There is considerable controversy about etiology but a recent emphasis is on biological factors rather than environmental or psychological factors. Normal siblings are common. Patterns of interaction seen between parents and such children probably relate more to the parents' reaction to the frustration of dealing with such a child and should ordinarily be viewed in that context rather than seeing the interaction as pathogenic for the syndrome.

Childhood onset pervasive development disorder is the current term for a group of patients whom earlier would have been called childhood schizophrenia. However, there is an absence of delusions, hallucinations of marked loosening of association. What is seen is marked impairment in social relationships with lack of appropriate affective responsivity and often sudden episodes of excessive and unexplained anxiety, inappropriate affect, marked resistance to change in the environment, various oddities of motor movement and speech, hyper- or hyposensitivity to stimuli, and selfmutiliation. Both of these diagnostic categories are relatively uncommon.

Specific Development Disorders

These disorders are to be distinguished from inadequate schooling, impaired vision or hearing, mental retardation or infantile autism. The deficit may relate specifically to *arithmetic* or to *spoken language*. With language the problem may be primarily expressive or receptive or relating to articulation. Another category are those with a deficit related to the *written or printed language*. This is often called dyslexia. It tends to occur in children who have average or better than average intellectual endowment and achievement in non-language-related subjects. There are few if any positive signs on classical neurological examination, and these are of the so-called "soft" variety. The diagnosis may be suspected by teachers. It should also be considered by physicians in children who may present with a variety of psychophysiological, behavioral and emotional symptoms but symptoms that develop secondary to the stress of attempting to cope with what has heretofore been an unrecognized problem by peers, parents, and teachers. Learning disorders are quite common. What happens to these children depends upon the support they get from their family, the kind of remedial help they receive from their school plus their own capacity to learn coping techniques to compensate for the specific deficit.

Other Issues Relating to Children

Most children and adolescents that present to health professionals with psychological problems do *not* fall into one of the above categories. First, there are *age-appropriate behaviors* that are of concern to parents for whom educational techniques and reassurance are indicated. Examples include the expected stranger anxiety of 8 months, the oppositional behaviors of the 18 to 36-month-old toddler, the transient phobias of the 4 or 5-year-old and the insecurity and identity issues of early adolescence.

Second, many responses in children are most appropriately diagnosed as *adjustment disorders* in response to such environmental stresses as illness, hospitalization, surgery, divorce of parents, birth of siblings, loss of a playmate, difficulty in school, etc. These symptoms tend to be transient, especially when given support in a system by concerned others. The symptoms may be regressive to earlier behaviors such as thumb-sucking or wetting the bed. Or, depending upon the age, the symptoms may be manifested as a conduct disturbance of one kind or another or that group of symptoms which have been called neurotic traits.

Persistent neurotic behaviors with evidence for psychopathology in children and/or adolescents should be diagnosed as one of the *neurotic disorders* to be outlined and described later in this chapter. *Schizophrenia* essentially indistinguishable from that seen in young adulthood in onset can also develop in late childhood and early adolescence. Finally, diagnostically, many symptoms presented by children fall into the *psychophysiological disorder* category now categorized in DSM-III under *psychological factors affecting physical condition.*

Other issues of considerable concern to child psychiatry are such psychological problems as maternal deprivation, child abuse, the cultural aspects of delinquent behavior and substance abuse in children and adolescents. (See Behavioral Sciences, Chapter 14.)

ORGANIC MENTAL DISORDERS

Organic Brain Syndromes

A group of brain syndromes of organic etiology or presumed organic etiology are fairly well defined and recognizable. Each has multiple possible etiologies. These syndromes will be described first. We will then discuss more specific disorders linked to more specific etiologies.

Delirium. Delirium develops over a relatively short period of time, usually hours or days, and tends to fluctuate over the course of the day. Symptoms include clouding of consciousness, disorientation, memory impairment, frequent perceptual disturbances such as illusions or hallucinations, speech which may be incoherent, a disturbed sleep-wakefulness cycle and either increased or decreased psychomotor activity. With this syndrome, as with all those that follow, from history, physical examination or laboratory tests, there is reason to believe that a specific organic factor may be etiologically related to the disturbance. Delirium is to be differentiated from acute schizophrenic illness. In general, acute visual hallucinations should suggest a delirium. Auditory hallucinations are more characteristic of schizophrenia. The type of thinking disorder typical of schizophrenia tends to be absent with organic delirium. Clouding of consciousness, typical of delirium, is absent in schizophrenia.

Dementia. With dementia, in contrast to delirium, there is not a clouding of consciousness, and symptoms usually develop over a longer period of time. There is evidence for loss of intellectual ability, memory difficulties (especially for recent memory), impairment of abstract thinking with substitution of concrete thinking and impairment of judgment. Emotional lability is common. Other disturbances of higher cortical function such as aphasia, apraxia, agnosia may be present.

Often a personality change that tends to be an accentuation of premorbid personality traits is noted. Especially in elderly individuals, severe depression may be confused with dementia and vice versa. It is critical that this differential is made, since depression with treatment tends to have a better prognosis.

Amnestic Syndrome. With the amnestic syndrome, there is both short term memory impairment and long term memory impairment but in the absence of clouding of consciousness, as in delirium, and in the absence of general loss of major intellectual functions, as in dementia.

Organic Delusional Syndrome. In the absence of clouding of consciousness and loss of intellectual abilities and prominent hallucinations, delusions are the prominent clinical feature.

Organic Hallucinosis. Persistent or recurring hallucinations are the predominant feature.

Organic Affective Syndrome. Most prominent here is a mood disturbance, either of the manic variety or of the major depressive variety.

Organic Personality Syndrome. This syndrome is characterized by a marked change in behavior or personality. Here, as with the organic hallucinosis and affective syndromes, there is absence of clouding of consciousness, as in delirium, and absence of significant loss of intellectual abilities, as in dementia.

Intoxication. This term is used when a substance-specific syndrome develops following the recent ingestion of that substance. Maladaptive behaviors such as disorientation, impaired judgment and belligerence result from the impact of the substance on the central nervous system. Intoxication has many features comparable to delirium.

Withdrawal. This refers to the development of a substance-specific syndrome following the cessation of that substance or reduction of intake of that substance when previously used by the individual to induce a state of intoxication. Clinical features are similar to delirium or to other of the various organic syndromes.

Disorders

Alzheimer's Disease, Pick's Disease (Senile Dementia, Presenile Dementia). While this disease may begin at any age, it usually develops insidiously later in life. The final features are usually that of dementia but the disorder may begin as an amnestic syndrome. The dementia may be accompanied by delirium, delusions and/or depression. Some authors estimate that from 5 to 15 per cent of persons over 65 living outside of hospitals have a mild dementia and of these about 50 per cent have dementia of this category. Throughout the world this disorder results in one of our most significant medical and sociological

problems. The precise etiology is unknown. There may be a hereditary factor. Current research suggests other exciting possibilities, but none of the hypotheses generated to date are confirmed. Early in the illness, the patient may be aware of losing previous capacity and may react to this loss with grief or depression. However, later in the course of the illness, patients often show little indication of being aware of their problem.

Multi-infarct Dementia. Most of the statements made above apply to this category of dementia as well. The syndrome is secondary to multiple infarcts. Diagnosis is made by history and course and later by pathological findings. Arteriosclerotic dementia is a diagnosis that is being used less and less as evidence increases that these so-called cases, when closely examined, tend to be either Alzheimer's disease or multi-infarct dementia.

Disorders Induced by Alcohol. Alcohol can produce the whole spectrum of organic brain syndromes described above. In addition to the very common *alcohol intoxication,* there is also *alcohol idiosyncratic intoxication,* in which there is a marked behavioral change with behavior atypical of the person when not drinking but behavior secondary to an ingestion of an amount of alcohol insufficient to induce intoxication in most individuals. The *alcohol withdrawal syndrome* (delirium tremens) is well known and may or may not be accompanied by delirium. The syndrome develops within one week of withdrawal and is characterized by a course tremor of hands or tongue, frequently nausea and vomiting, weakness, anxiety, depressed mood or irritability, orthostatic hypotension and various signs of autonomic hyperactivity. While withdrawal may be limited to these symptoms, a delirium may be superimposed as may seizures. This illness without vigorous medical treatment has significant mortality. *Alcohol hallucinosis* may be confused with an acute schizophrenic illness. On withdrawal from alcohol, usually within 48 hours, there are vivid hallucinations, predominately auditory. In contrast to delirium tremens, there is no clouding of consciousness. The *alcohol amnestic disorder* (blackouts) is a pathognomonic indicator of alcohol dependency. Prolonged, heavy ingestion of alcohol may also result in *dementia.*

Disorders Induced by Other CNS-Active Agents. *Barbiturates* may result in intoxication and withdrawal syndromes with or without delirium. The same can be said of almost any similarly acting *sedative* including the *benzodiazepines. Opioid intoxication* is usually accompanied with pupillary constriction and a change in mood, that is, euphoria, dysphoria, or apathy. *Opioid withdrawal* is characterized by pupillary dilation, lacrimation, rhinorrhea, piloerection, sweating, diarrhea, yawning, mild hypertension, tachycardia, insomnia, and fever. *Cocaine intoxication,* in addition to physical symptoms and signs of hyperactivity of the autonomic nervous system, often includes symptoms of psychomotor agitation or elation with elements of grandiosity or hypervigilance. *Amphetamines* or similarly acting sympathomimetic agents can result in intoxication, delirium and withdrawal. The intoxication is similar to that of cocaine. The delirium and especially the accompanying delusional disorder may be very similar to an acute schizophrenic illness with rapidly developing persecutory delusions as a prominent feature. Withdrawal is characterized by depressed mood, disturbed sleep and increased dreaming. *Phencyclidine* or similarly acting agents may result in intoxication and/or delirium. The *hallucinogens* may produce an hallucinosis or a delusional disorder or an affective disorder. Perceptual changes are characteristic of the hallucinosis with synesthesias, hallucinations, illusions, depersonalization or merely the report of subjective intensification of perceptions, all occurring in a state of full wakefulness and alertness. Again, physiological symptoms and signs, mainly of hyperactivity within the autonomic nervous system, frequently accompany this disorder. *Cannabis intoxication* is characterized by tachycardia, euphoria or apathy, a sensation of slowed time and a subjective intensification of perceptions. Physical symptoms and signs often include increased appetite, dry mouth and conjunctival injection. Cannabis can also result in a delusional disorder but one that does not persist beyond six hours following cessation of its use. Many other substances can produce intoxication and withdrawal including *caffeine* and *tobacco* in sufficient doses.

Disorders Secondary to Other Etiologies. In addition to multi-infarct dementia and arteriosclerotic dementia, *circulatory disturbances* can result in a variety of organic brain syndromes. Acute *cerebral infarction* may include a deliriumlike syndrome in addition to focal signs. Bilateral lesions of the hippocampus may result in an amnestic syndrome. Any *hypoxic state,* whatever the etiology, can accentuate delirium or superimpose upon dementia an increased confusionlike state. Of particular interest are the confusional states following *cardiac surgery.*

In the category of *metabolic and endocrine disorders,* delirium is a feature of *hepatic, uremic and hypoglycemic encephalopathies* as is *diabetic ketoacidosis.* Symptoms of anxiety and emotional instability, even delirium, may accompany *acute intermittent porphyria.* Endocrine disorders, whether involving the thyroid, the parathyroid or the adrenal gland can be accompanied by changes in personality, impairment of mental functions and memory. *Myxedema* may mimic depression and/or early dementia.

Huntington's chorea, although relatively rare, is a hereditary disorder characterized by choreiform movements and dementia that begins in adult life.

Normal pressure hydrocephalus may be characterized by a progressive dementia. These patients have enlarged ventricles but normal cerebrospinal fluid pressure. There may be associated gait disturbances.

Brain trauma can present acutely as a delirium and over time a Korsakoff-like syndrome showing elements of amnesia and confabulation. Delayed sequelae, depending upon the nature of the trauma, and whether the trauma is repetitive, can result in the whole spectrum of brain syndromes.

Infections of the CNS or systemic infections frequently include features of delirium. If the CNS infection is more chronic, a dementia can result, the classic example being the general paralysis of the insane secondary to syphilis (dementia paralytica).

Organic brain disorders may be associated with *intracranial neoplasia.*

Certain organic brain disorders may be associated with *epilepsy.* Following a grand mal seizure, the patient's confused state has features of delirium. Temporal lobe seizures may be difficult to differentiate from dissociative reactions. Some epileptics between seizures may show brief, inter-seizure psychotic episodes. The majority of these occur in cases of psychomotor epilepsy.

Treatment

Treatment of the organic brain syndromes should focus on the underlying etiology. The more specific medical treatments will not be reviewed here. But beyond this, certain guidelines regarding general management can be made.

With delirium in particular, general medical support measures are indicated—fluids, electrolyte balance, nutrition, etc. Sedatives and all other nonvital drugs should be discontinued. Precautions against suicide should be considered. Human contacts with others, especially friends, should be encouraged. Friends and personnel can be extremely helpful in providing reassuring, orienting verbal input. When the patient is awake the light should be on in the room. Avoid mechanical restraints if at all possible. Urge the patient to accept their hallucinations as bad dreams. If medication becomes necessary to manage agitated or aggressive destructive behavior, avoid barbituates and consider haloperidol 5 to 10 mg. orally or intravenously or chlorpromazine beginning 10 mg. orally three times a day, gradually increasing the dose, being attentive to the possible development of hypotension. Chlordiazepoxide is often helpful with alcohol withdrawal syndromes.

With the dementias, in addition to instituting a specific treatment aimed at a known etiology, general treatment should be focused on consulting with the patient's family, providing a protected physical and social environment, maintaining activity and avoiding social isolation, physical isolation or immobilization. Appropriate supportive psychotherapeutic and environmental maneuvers can sometimes result in dramatic improvement. Again, depression can be superimposed on a dementia or be confused with it. Any medical illness can intensify the symptoms of dementia. Some patients with "dementia" improve dramatically when unnecessary medications are withdrawn or inappropriately high doses of medication are reduced.

SUBSTANCE ABUSE

The definitions of substance abuse and substance dependence are discussed in Chapter 14, Behavioral Sciences.

Clinically, indicators of alcoholism (alcohol dependence) include a steady increase in alcohol intake and/or drinking "sprees," solitary drinking, early morning drinking and occurrence of blackouts. Operationally, an individual may be considered an alcoholic if he continues to drink despite the fact that his drinking is clearly causing physical illness or repeated difficulty for him with his employer, his family or the police. Multiple therapeutic approaches are utilized including alcohol treatment programs in hospital and community settings, psychotherapeutic intervention in selected patients, the use of conditioned reflex treatment involving disulfiram (Antabuse), Alcoholics Anonymous and other group therapies or support systems. Initially, denial is a major mechanism seen in most alcoholics. Many are experts in self destruction and are skilled in manipulating their environment to provide a continuing source of alcohol. Many physicians have severe countertransference problems with these patients. Nonetheless, if the illness is viewed as a chronic one and intervention is persistent, the prognosis for many can be quite good.

The abuse and dependence on different drugs varies from time to time and from country to country. Many addicts state they take drugs to experience euphoria or to feel "normal" or to overcome states of depression. Narcotic addicts have a wide range of personality characteristics, but many are described as immature, impulsive and emotionally unstable. Treatment programs, as with alcohol treatment programs, are multifaceted. Addicts Annonymous is modelled after Alcoholics Anonymous. Substitute programs in which, for example, methadone is substituted for heroin, are widely used but still seen by many as experimental and subject to increasing criticism in recent years. In the clinical setting, nalorphine (Nalline), an antagonist, may be used to test for evidence of readdiction. A current trend for individuals who abuse drugs is involvement with more than one agent.

SCHIZOPHRENIC DISORDERS

Schizophrenia is one of the psychoses. A salient feature is a defect in reality testing which may be manifest in the schizophrenics' relationship to self, to the objects in the world or to others. Bleuler distinguished between primary and secondary symptoms. The primary or fundamental symptoms include disturbances in associations (e.g., loosening, blocking, neologisms), disturbances in affect (disharmony or incongruity between ideas and emotion), ambivalence (multiple and contradictory feelings of extreme degree), and autism (preoccupation with self). Secondary or accessory symptoms include hallucinations, delusions, and bizarre behavior.

Modern criteria emphasize the thought disorder. The disorder may be so profound that speech is incoherent. Examination more commonly reveals tangentiality, loosening of association, or poverty of content of speech. A mixture of autistic and concrete thinking is common. This may be accompanied by blunted or inappropriate affect. Disorganized behavior is common. Delusions are bizarre in content. They may be somatic, grandiose, religious, nihilistic or persecutory. Hallucinations, especially auditory hallucinations, may be evident. When one or more sets of these symptoms are accompanied by deterioration of previous level of functioning, whether relating to taking care of self, relating to significant others or to educational activities or work, and when these signs have been present for at least six months, the diagnosis is warranted. Differential diagnoses include the organic mental disorders and manic-depressive illness. The full-blown illness may be preceded by a prodromal phase with symptoms which include social isolation or withdrawal, impairment in role functioning, peculiar behavior, impairment in personal hygiene, affect disturbances, thought disturbances manifested by vague, digressive, circumstantial or metaphysical speech, bizarre ideation or magical thinking and unusual perceptual experiences which may not be diagnosable as clear hallucinations. Similar symptoms are seen in remission with or without treatment.

The currently recognized subtypes are as follows:

Disorganized Type (Hebephrenia)

In addition to the clinical picture outlined above, this relatively uncommon type shows blunted, inappropriate and especially silly affect. Systemized delusions are characteristically absent and speech is frequently incoherent. Prognosis tends to be poor.

Catatonic Type

Here the schizophrenia is dominated by any of the following: catatonic stupor, catatonic negativism, catatonic rigidity and/or posturing and catatonic excitement. Onset is often acute. Introjection is a common defense mechanism. Prognosis is relatively good.

Paranoid Type

This is the most common of the differentiated schizophrenias and is dominated by persecutory or grandiose delusions and/or hallucinations with persecutory or grandiose content. Projection is a prominent defense mechanism.

Undifferentiated Type

This category is utilized when the criteria for schizophrenia are met, but when one of the above three differentiations is not in evidence.

Residual Type

This diagnosis is utilized when there has been the history of at least one previous episode of frank schizophrenia but on the present occasion, the clinical picture does not present prominent psychotic symptoms although there is continuing evidence of illness.

Schizophrenia constitutes the largest group of severe behavioral disorders in our culture. Circa 1 to 3 per cent of the population are affected. It is seen most commonly in lower socioeconomic groups, especially in areas of high mobility and social disorganization. One explanation for the prevalence in these groups is the "downward drift" hypothesis, which essentially states that schizophrenic patients move toward such a lower socioeconomic categorization. Onset is usually in persons between 20 and 40 years of age although onset may be earlier. It is unusual for a first episode to appear after age 45. Longterm studies suggest that there is not a separate category of childhood schizophrenia and that schizophrenia in childhood or adolescence simply represents the earlier appearance of schizophrenic illness.

The etiology of schizophrenia is unknown. As discussed in the Behavioral Sciences chapter, there is evidence for both a genetic component and a biochemical component. Psychodynamic formulations are many but currently focus on a disturbance of ego with an inability to differentiate between self and object and unusual sensitivity to sensory input. Psychoanalytic theory views the logic of schizophrenia as *primary process* thinking and sees similarity to the associative patterns present in dreams and in fantasies especially those of imaginative children.

Two broad categories of schizophrenia have been proposed: *process* schizophrenia, a variety in which the illness begins at a younger age and progresses slowly, seemingly inevitably toward a final state of deterioration, and *reactive* schizophrenia which begins temporally in relationship to a traumatic event and is often of acute onset. The latter seemingly has a better prognosis. In fact, if a patient is hospitalized for less than three months with the first illness, the remission rate is at least 75 per cent. If the patient has been hospitalized for over two years, the remission rate is approximately 1 to 2 per cent.

Treatment is empirical. Hospitalization during the acute illness is often required. Although difficult to obtain, the development of a trusting doctor/patient relationship which can be maintained over time seems particularly important where the physician, so to speak, becomes an auxiliary reality tester for the patient and helps the patient in a growing-up process. The absence of a familial and/or community support system seems to trigger exacerbation of illness and rehospitalization. Today, every schizophrenic patient should also be given an adequate trial of pharmacological treatment, usually one of the phenothiazines.

OTHER PSYCHOTIC DISORDERS

Some patients who are psychotic do not present with the full picture of schizophrenia, but show persistent persecutory delusions or delusions of jealousy with emotion and behavior appropriate to the content of these delusions but without prominent hallucinations. There is no evidence of organic mental disorder nor are the criteria for the manic-depressive syndrome present. If the illness is of at least one week's duration, the diagnosis *paranoid disorder* is made. If such symptoms become chronic and stable for at least six months' duration, the diagnosis *paranoia* is most appropriate. The latter is relatively rare.

The diagnosis *schizophreniform disorder* according to modern evidence and thought is the appropriate appellation for patients who present with the symptoms of schizophrenia but in whom the illness, while lasting more than two weeks, has been present less than six months. Since many patients with such an acute illness recover without recurrence, labelling such individuals as schizophrenics is inappropriate. Frequently this disorder is in reaction to an acutely stressful life event. Patients with a borderline personality seem particularly subject to such responses.

Some patients seem to have a mixture of schizophrenia and a major affective disorder with symptoms such that neither diagnosis can clearly be made. For some clinicians, the diagnosis *schizoaffective disorder* is utilized. There is controversy as to whether such a category is warranted or not.

AFFECTIVE DISORDERS

The principle and characteristic feature of the affective disorders is a disturbance of mood, especially depression, but mania or hypomania, anxiety and anger may be present as well. These patients may be psychotic.

Major Affective Disorders

A *manic episode* is characterized by a distinct period of an elevated or expansive or irritable mood. Duration is at least of one week. In addition to the mood disturbance, there are frequently several or more of the following: increase in activity or physical restlessness, increased talkativeness, flight of ideas or at least the subjective experience that thoughts are racing, inflated self esteem to the point of grandiosity, seemingly decreased need for sleep, distractability, and an excessive involvement in activities which have a high potential for painful consequences, such as buying sprees, sexual indiscretions, etc. In some patients, this may be accompanied with psychotic features, i.e., impairment in reality testing with delusions, hallucinations or bizarre behavior. Many patients with a manic episode do not present with psychotic features.

A *major depressive episode* is characterized by dysphoric mood and/or anhedonia (loss of interest or pleasure in usual activities and pasttimes). The patient may describe the mood as depressed, sad, down in the dumps, irritable. A sense of helplessness and hopelessness is very common as is guilt and such accompanying emotional states as anxiety and anger. These symptoms should be present nearly every day for a period of at least two weeks. They are accompanied by several of the following: poor appetite and significant weight loss or, in some patients, increased appetite with significant weight gain; insomnia or, in some patients, hypersomnia; psychomotor agitation or retardation; loss of interest in usual activities and/or decrease in sexual drive; loss of energy, a sense of fatigue; feelings of worthlessness, self reproach with excessive or inappropriate guilt; complaints of diminished ability to think or concentrate; recurring thoughts of death or suicidal ideation or a history of a suicide attempt. There may be psychotic features with delusions and hallucinations. When the subjective experience of depression is particularly severe, when the depression is particularly worse in the morning and often accompanied by early morning awakenings as well as psychomotor retardation or agitation and significant anorexia or weight loss, and profound guilt, the term "melancholia" is often used.

Bipolar Disorder (Manic-depressive Illness). Patients in this category over time show features cyclically of both manic episodes and depressed episodes. In some individuals, depressive episodes predominate and in others manic episodes predominate. In a smaller percentage, the episodes are intermixed, rapidly alternating every few days.

Major Depression (Unipolar, Endogenous). Patients with this type of affective disorder meet the requirements of a major depressive episode as described above but have never had a manic episode.

Over one-half of patients with bipolar disorders become ill prior to age 30. Unipolar onsets reach their peak in the 40s. Bipolar disorders are equally predominant in men and women. Manic episodes typically begin more suddenly than depressive episodes and may last from a few days to months but tend to be briefer in duration than depressive episodes. In some patients, perhaps 20 per cent, the course seems chronic. Epidemiological evidence suggests that circa 20 per cent of females and 10 per cent of males will have a depressive episode sometime in life with hospitalization required in about 6 per cent of females and 3 per cent of males.

The precise etiology of this disease is unknown. There is good evidence that the illness is familial and for some there is a genetic component, especially those with bipolar illness. There is also evidence of a disturbance in the neurotransmitter systems.

Depending upon the severity of the illness, treatment may involve electroshock therapy (ECT), drug therapy, and/or psychotherapy. Electroshock is particularly efficacious in a high percentage of patients with depression. Most clinicians utilize electroshock therapy after an unsuccessful trial of drug intervention. Phenothiazines, especially haloperidol, may be initially useful in manic states. Lithium, however, is the treatment of choice in bipolar disease, especially to effect prevention of manic episodes. Lithium may also be useful in the treatment of some patients with recurring unipolar depression. However, a full trial of a antidepressive tricyclic drug is the treatment of choice for major depression. Psychotherapy is *extremely* difficult and is usually disappointing if there is the expectation of significant improvement in mood or energy level. However, studies do show that patients can show significant improvement in self esteem and in their interpersonal relationships. Also the relationship established with the physician facilitates psychopharmacological intervention.

Other Affective Disorders

Cyclothymic Disorder (Cyclothymic Personality).

Some patients present with a history of numerous periods in which some symptoms characteristic of both depressive and manic syndromes are present but not of such severity to meet the criteria of either a major depressive or manic episode. These episodes are also separated by periods of normal mood which may last for months at a time. While some patients may proceed over time to frank bipolar illness, many do not and these tend to be viewed as individuals who have developed this personality disorder in response to psychological factors.

Dysthymic Disorders (Depressive Neurosis).

Current criteria for this diagnosis require at least a 2 year history of symptoms characteristic of a depressive syndrome most of the time but not of such severity to meet the criteria for a major depressive episode. There may be periods of normal mood lasting for a few days to a few weeks. There are clearly no psychotic features. This diagnostic entity is more common than bipolar disease in primary care settings. While some patients benefit from antidepressant medication, many do not. In fact, some seem even worse. Psychotherapy is the usual mode of treatment. In recent years, careful studies evaluating the effectiveness of psychotherapy show distinct benefit compared to control groups, and in some studies psychotherapy alone shows better outcome than psychotherapy plus antidepressant medication. Psychotherapy seems particularly helpful when the depression has been triggered by an identifiable life stress. The term *reactive depression* is often used in this instance. A careful study of these patients often suggests a vulnerability to certain kinds of stress, especially loss, through earlier life events and the elaboration of a particular character structure. Introversion is a common defense mechanism. Some patients' complaints especially in primary care settings, are primarily somatic. If treatment is focused only on the somatic complaints, improvement at best is only transitory. The underlying depression must be recognized and treated. Some clinicians see these patients as suffering from a *depressive equivalent.*

Many, maybe most, patients in ambulatory primary care settings whose complaints suggest depression do *not* represent patients who fall into *any* of the above diagnostic categories. Recall that modern criteria for the diagnosis of depressive neurosis requires a two year history. Further, depression as described above is a clinical entity and is *not* synonymous to a grief reaction. Many patients who speak of themselves as depressed have experienced losses and are responding appropriately with grief. We are speaking here of *uncomplicated bereavement.* Therapy facilitating the grief work is the physician's major responsibiiity with these many patients. Others are responding to an identifiable stressor, often a loss, in a maladaptive way, and the diagnosis *adjustment disorder with depressed mood* is appropriate. Here again, psychotherapeutic intervention is indicated and rarely psychopharmacological intervention. Finally, a number of physical conditions may be accompanied by depression, including carcinoma of the lung, carcinoma of the head of the pancreas, myxedema, etc. Certain drugs can precipitate a depressive syndrome, e.g., reserpine and many antihypertensive medications. The appropriate diagnosis in these instances is an *organic affective disorder,* and such patients should be treated accordingly. The point has already been made but deserves reemphasis. In older individuals depression may mimic or accompany dementia.

All in all, depression is one of the most common complaints bringing patients to physicians. Some studies indicate that it is *the* most common complaint. Other studies suggest anxiety, and still others, depending on the season, list upper respiratory complaints. A final reminder—depression should alert the physician to evaluate the risk for suicide.

ANXIETY DISORDERS

This nosological category and several that follow represent disturbances or disorders that have been called the *psychoneuroses.* The psychoneuroses do not show gross disturbances of reality testing nor severely antisocial behavior and in the main are determined mostly by environmental factors. The factors in part are in the present, those precipitating stresses which immediately precede an exacerbation of psychoneurotic symptoms. These factors also relate to the past when environmental influences acting on the infant and/or the child produced a defect in personality development, leaving the person vulnerable to the later elaboration in adult life of neurotic patterns of response. To a degree, the childhood experience for all of us becomes the paradigm for all those that follow.

Key to understanding psychoneurosis is the concept of conflict, conflict which may be partially conscious but which is predominately unconscious. An individual must be carefully evaluated to determine what in fact represents a significant conflict and beyond that, a conflict related to a neurotic disorder. Conflict tends to develop around the issues of dependency, aggression or sexuality or some mixture thereof. Subjective and objective evidence for emotions during the evaluation frequently suggests the nature of the conflict, especially those emotions experienced or displayed when discussing significant present situations reminiscent of past events and those linked to the exacerbation of neurotic symptomatology.

Phobic Disorders (Phobic Neurosis)

With phobic disorders, repression followed by isolation and displacement are characteristic defense mechanisms. In some patients, the neurotic response evolves from those conflict issues typical of a child from age three through age six. Premorbidly an avoidant or compulsive personality is common.

Agoraphobia. These patients have a marked fear of and thus avoid being in public places from which there may be no immediate escape. They usually restrict their normal activities to the point that avoidance behavior dominates their life. To venture forth is to experience overwhelming incapacitating anxiety. One group of patients have a history of severe panic attacks while another group do not. In the group with panic attacks especially, the panic attacks often occur without evidence of there being a particular understandable situational stress related to a particular underlying conflict. The individual's response to these panic attacks is to become increasingly phobic. Management of the panic attacks with imipramine together with appropriately structured psychotherapy may be the treatment of choice for this particular group.

Social Phobia. These patients experience a persistent, irrational fear of and a desire to avoid a situation in which they are exposed to possible scrutiny by others. The patient recognizes that the fear is excessive or unreasonable but feels powerless to effect change.

Simple Phobia. Here the irrational fear is of an object or a situation other than being away from home (agoraphobia) or anxiety regarding social situations (social phobia). Fear of animals, heights, close spaces, are examples. Again, the patient recognizes that the fear is excessive or unreasonable. Therapy may include dynamic psychotherapy, the technique of reciprocal inhibition, or behavioral therapy employing some schedule for desensitization.

Anxiety States (Anxiety Neurosis)

Panic Disorder. With this disorder the patient presents with a history of distinct panic attacks which occur in the absence of a life-threatening situation or marked physical exertion. The patient describes subjective awareness of anxiety, apprehension or fear and usually reports several or more physical symptoms which are in the category of the typical psychophysiological manifestations of anxiety such as dyspnea, palpitations, sweating, trembling, etc.

Generalized Anxiety Disorder. This disorder is characterized by the manifestations of anxiety either consistently present or frequently recurring. The patient may report a subjective awareness of this anxiety using such expressions as fear, afraid, apprehension, worry, etc.; or describe feeling constantly on the alert, dreading some unknown and unidentified danger or tragedy; or report various of the psychophysiological manifestations of anxiety, e.g., sweating, feeling cold, clammy hands, lightheadedness, etc. or some combination of the various groups of symptoms. Patients who report the physiological manifestations of anxiety may deny feeling apprehensive, anxious or fearful. Other patients who describe overwhelming fear and anxiety may not in fact look fearful or anxious to the physician. Psychotherapeutic intervention will be different for the different subgroups described. However, even when the patient feels anxious and reports the symptoms of anxiety and appears anxious to the physician, the patient rarely understands the basis for the anxiety or if he does link it to a particular situation or event, the linkage does not make sense to him. Anxiety is an extraordinarily common complaint of patients in primary care ambulatory settings. This disorder is to be distinguished from normal fear of real life-threatening situations or from an adjustment reaction manifested by anxiety. Some illnesses mimic this disorder, e.g., hyperthyroidism, mitral valve prolapse syndrome, pheochromocytoma; however, the description of the symptoms by these patients are qualitatively different, e.g., they describe their symptoms as feeling *as if* they were afraid. Repression and denial are common defense mechanisms. The neurotic personality structure (often a histrionic personality) and the neurotic symptoms frequently date to those conflicts and issues typical of children ages four through seven. Psychopharmacological agents if used should be used judiciously and then for only brief periods. Some form of psychotherapy ordinarily is the treatment of choice.

Obsessive Compulsive Disorder (Obsessive Compulsive Neurosis). Obsessions and/or compulsions become a significant source of distress to the individual to a degree that they interfere with social or role functioning. These patients are particularly distressed in knowing their symptoms are irrational. Reaction formation, undoing, and overintellectualization are typical defense mechanisms. The promorbid personality is often a compulsive personality which in many patients dates to particular responses to conflicts and issues of childhood typical of ages one and one-half to 3. Frequently the patient presents behaviorally as a clean, neat, overly polite individual who speaks in a rather controlled and guarded fashion. While subjective awareness of anxiety and sadness may be present, there is typically an absence of evidence for anger. In fact, many patients either take pride in the infrequency of their experiencing anger or express considerable fear of it. Psychotherapy is the treatment of choice, but the course may be quite long and difficult.

Post-traumatic Stress Disorder

This recently recognized syndrome seems to merit a separate diagnostic category. In response to a specific recognizable stressor that would tend to evoke symptoms of distress in almost anyone, these patients, however, *continue* to reexperience the trauma. This is manifest through either recurring dreams, or intrusive recollections of the event, or subjective sensations that the event is occurring again, triggered in association to some environmental or thought stimulus reminiscent of the trauma. Examples of typical stressors include accidents, surgery, deaths, etc. In addition, these patients report a numbing of responsiveness to the external world manifest by marked diminished interest in previously significant activities and subjective feelings of detachment or estrangement from significant others. In addition, there are frequently exaggerated startle responses, sleep disturbances, guilt about surviving when others have not, trouble concentrating, avoidance behavior toward activities that might trigger recollection of the event, and intensification of symptoms by exposure to events that symbolize the traumatic occurrence. Some form of psychotherapy is the preferred treatment. Prognosis is usually good.

SOMATOFORM DISORDERS

Somatization Disorder (Briquet's Syndrome)

This syndrome is characterized by multiple somatic complaints not adequately explained by physical disorder, injury or side effects of medication or drugs. These patients typically report that they have been sickly all their life or a good part of their life. Complaints include symptoms that might fall into the conversion or pseudoneurological category (e.g., loss of voice, double vision, muscle weakness, difficulty urinating), gastrointestinal symptoms (e.g., abdominal pain, nausea, bloating, etc.), female reproductive symptoms (e.g., painful menstruation, menstrual irregularity, severe vomiting through pregnancy), psychosexual symptoms (e.g., pain during intercourse, sexual indifference, lack of pleasure during intercourse), pain (e.g., in back, joints, extremities), and cardiopulmonary symptoms (e.g., shortness of breath, palpitations, dizziness). Current diagnostic criteria require at least a dozen of such symptoms and a history of several years duration beginning before age 30. There may be a genetic disposition to this disorder. There is often a family history

of a similar syndrome, especially in female relatives, or antisocial behavior, especially in male relatives, or alcoholism. A history of multiple trials of medications without significant change in symptomatology is common. Pharmacotherapy seems to have little value. These patients are very resistant to treatment and psychotherapeutic intervention is difficult.

Conversion Disorder (Hysterical Neurosis, Conversion Type)

This disorder is characterized by an involuntary psychogenic loss or disorder of function often suggesting a physical illness. Symptoms typically are limited to impairment of motor or sensory functions (e.g., blindness, paresthesia, paralysis), but also may involve the autonomic system to a lesser degree. Symptoms characteristically begin and end suddenly. Often symbolic of an underlying conflict, the symptoms solve, so to speak, the underlying dilemma. In psychodynamic terms, this is called the *primary gain*. A *secondary gain* is often superimposed, such as avoiding some unpleasant activity, obtaining additional attention from significant others, avoiding responsibility, etc. Many patients give the impression of being naive, behave in a seductive fashion toward the examiner, may seem strangely indifferent or aloof to their symptomatology *(la belle indifference)* and yet under certain circumstances demonstrate poor emotional control. These patients are frequently misdiagnosed as malingerers by the general medical profession. Repression, denial and dissociation are common defense mechanisms. It is not unusual for a patient to have few if any memories prior to age six. A premorbid histrionic character is common, frequently with an underlying sexual conflict reminiscent of the Oedipal conflict of ages four through seven. Psychotherapeutic intervention may be dramatically successful especially early in the course of the illness. Hypnotherapy may be especially helpful in some patients. If symptoms have been present for months or years, therapy becomes difficult.

Psychogenic Pain Disorder

Here the predominant feature is severe, prolonged pain, often inconsistent with the anatomic distribution of the nervous system, in the absence of organic pathology or when there is organic pathology the pain is grossly in excess of what would be expected from findings. Psychological factors are judged to be etiologically involved in the genesis of the pain. Some clinicians would see this syndrome as being a variation of a conversion disorder. Except for the symptom presentation, many of the statements made above would apply to this category as well.

Some of these patients develop a *chronic benign pain*

syndrome (a term used by many authors). Patients with chronic depression constitute another major group. Many utilize multiple medications in large doses. Some in fact are addicted. An intensive multidisciplinary treatment approach is required with individual, group and family therapy and a conservative approach toward pharmacotherapy. This syndrome is attracting increasing attention for many reasons one of which is that a high percentage of resources from the health arena is devoted to this group of patients.

Hypochondriasis (Hyponchondriacal Neurosis)

The predominant disturbance here is an unrealistic interpretation of physical signs or sensations as abnormal leading the patient to a preoccupation with the fear of having or the belief in having a serious disease, a disease which tends in their view to go unrecognized by family and physicians. The malady causes considerable social and occupational impairment, tends to persist despite medical reassurance that no such disease exists, and often becomes the central theme around which the family is organized. In this manner control and attention are obtained simultaneously. Patients, therefore, tend to have serious conflicts in the area of dependency and aggression. Considerable psychotherapeutic skill is needed in working with this group of patients.

DISSOCIATIVE DISORDERS (HYSTERICAL NEUROSIS, DISSOCIATIVE TYPE)

Subgroups in this category include *psychogenic amnesia, psychogenic fugue, multiple personality* and *depersonalization disorder* (depersonalization neurosis). All are predominately psychogenic in origin. Amnesia refers to the sudden inability to recall important personal information that is too extensive to be explained by forgetfulness. A fugue is characterized by the assumption of a new identity by the patient, often traveling away from home or usual place of work with inability to recall the past. During a fugue a patient may not seem to behave unusually or abnormally to the casual observer. Multiple personality is defined as the existence within a given individual of two or more distinct personalities, each of which predominates at a particular time. Many statements made about patient characteristics, etiology and treatment under the conversion disorder apply to this group as well. Patients with multiple personality usually have a very complex personality structure and considerable psychotherapeutic skill is required for a successful outcome.

Patients with a depersonalization disorder respond to neurotic conflicts in such a manner that they experience parts of their bodies as not belonging to them or greatly expanded or changed in size or shape, or they may experience themselves as unreal, phony, in a fog, etc. The experience is often transient and in response to a meaningful life event but usually not recognized as such by the patient. When severe, patients may seem psychotic. Symptoms of derealization may or may not accompany the depersonalization, i.e., the sensation or feeling that the surround is strange or unreal.

PSYCHOSEXUAL DISORDERS

Current nosology categorizes psychosexual disorders into the *gender identity disorders,* including *transsexualism* and *gender identity disorder of childhood;* the *paraphilias,* including *fetishism, tranvestism, zoöphilia, pedophilia, exhibitionism, voyeurism, sexual masochism, sexual sadism;* and the *psychosexual dysfunctions. Ego-dystonic homosexuality* is also considered a psychosexual disorder. Ego dystonia refers to the fact that the individual is uncomfortable with and does not want a particular set of symptoms. In this instance, the patient wishes not to be a homosexual in terms of fantasy, sexual arousal or overt behavior. Behaviors that are ego syntonic do not cause subjective distress.

Of the above, the psychosexual dysfunctions are by far the most commonly seen in medical practice. Categories include *inhibited sexual desire.* Here, the patient reports a persistent and pervasive inhibition of sexual interest. Often the patient does not experience this as a source of personal distress; the report of distress comes from the partner. Next is *inhibited sexual excitement.* Here, the patient reports sexual interest, but for males there is partial or complete failure to attain or maintain erection throughout the sexual act and for females the partial or complete failure to attain or maintain the lubrication and swelling response of sexual excitement throughout the act. *Inhibited female orgasm* relates to a recurring and persistent pattern of delay or absence of orgasm, although there has been normal sexual excitement. *Inhibited male orgasm* is similarly defined. *Premature ejaculation* refers to ejaculation occuring before the individual wishes it because of an inability to bring reasonable voluntary control of ejaculation to the sexual act. Obviously the term "reasonable control" requires clinical judgment. This diagnosis is probably made too frequently by both physicians and their patients. A patient may insist that he is a premature ejaculator, yet upon careful inquiry the length of time or the number of sexual thrusts during intercourse is at or above average. *Functional dyspareunia* refers to pain during intercourse of psychogenic origin. This diagnosis also is made too frequently. Discomfort may occur because the penis is inserted before the female has reached the plateau phase; communication between partners solves this problem. Foreplay may take place with the patient exclusively on her back and introital lubrication does not take place given the slant of the vagina. In some women, with deep penetration, penile thrusting impinges on the cervix, causing pain; here a change in position of intercourse effects a solution. For all these circumstances, educational counseling is indicated. Major psychogenic factors may not be playing a role. *Functional vaginismus* refers to voluntary spasm of the musculature of the outer one-third of the vagina hindering or preventing insertion. In some patients, this is essentially a conversion reaction. In others it has become a learned response. Psychotherapy is probably the treatment of choice for the former group, behavior therapy for the latter group.

All of the diagnostic categories under psychosexual dysfunction are disturbances not caused exclusively by organic factors. In fact psychogenic factors predominate. Anxiety regarding the sexual act and/or hostility between partners is the typical psychodynamic picture. Commonly symptoms may be present with one partner but not another. Or historically symptoms may not be present before marriage but may appear after marriage. The reverse is just as frequent. In some instances an unresolved Oedipal problem plays a dynamic role. In others, the symptoms seem to result from early life messages that the individual was not to assume an adult sexual role or that the sexual act in some fashion was ugly or dirty. When evaluating these patients, especially patients where functional dyspareunia and inhibited orgasm are suspected, a careful medical workup including history and laboratory tests is indicated, since a number of medical conditions may first be manifest with one of these problems as the primary symptom. Penile erection studies in sleep laboratores are increasingly being utilized in this regard since full erections take place during REM sleep, and if demonstrated with such a study, erectile difficulties are most likely psychogenic in origin.

ADJUSTMENT DISORDER (TRANSIENT SITUATIONAL REACTIONS)

This diagnosis should be used frequently, especially in primary care settings. These patients present with mental, emotional or behavioral symptoms in response to a given life event, but the criteria of the diagnostic categories outlined above are not met. However, there is evidence of a maladaptive reaction to an identifiable social stressor within three months of the onset of the stressor. The maladaptive nature of the reaction is indicated by impairment in social or occupational function or by symptoms that seem in excess of a normal or an expected response to such a stressor. With this diagnosis it is assumed that the symptoms would remit should the stressor cease or a new level of adaptation achieved should the stressor persist.

Depending upon the predominant manifestation, the diagnosis of adjustment disorder is modified by one of the following self-explanatory phrases: with anxious mood, with depressed mood, with mixed emotional features, with disturbance of conduct, with mixed disturbance of emotions and conduct, with work or academic inhibition, with withdrawal, and finally with atypical features.

Most patients with adjustment disorders can be helped with supportive or educational psychotherapy and/or counseling. In general, pharmacotherapy is not indicated nor is referral for intensive psychotherapy. If a new level of adaptation does not occur or if symptoms persist or become worse, then the diagnosis adjustment disorder no longer applies, the diagnosis should be changed to one of the categories outlined above, and treatment strategies developed accordingly.

PSYCHOLOGICAL FACTORS AFFECTING PHYSICAL CONDITION (PSYCHOPHYSIOLOGICAL DISORDERS)

Psychologically meaningful environmental stimuli may be temporally related to the initiation or exacerbation of physical conditions, conditions which either have a demonstrable organic pathology or a known pathophysiological process. An example of the latter would be tension headaches and of the former, ulcerative colitis. A great number of patients fall into this category. The pathophysiology of such illness is increasingly well known and will not be reviewed in detail here. Psychologically significant events or trains of events often linked to situations or events reminiscent of childhood or adolescence are interpreted in the cortex. Then, with involvement of the limbic system, the hypothalamic/pituitary/adrenal axis or the hypothalamic/autonomic nervous system axis triggers pathophysiologic responses or accentuates existing pathology. Many patients have difficulty in understanding how psychological or social factors can contribute to their illness. A trusting relationship with their physician is of prime importance as skill in communicating this understanding. Even then patients frequently do not recognize their conflict areas or area of stress. In fact in many instances it is difficult for the clinician to determine these as well. A careful psychosocial history relative to the onset of the illness and/or the exacerbation or remissions in the illness may be clues in this regard, as may the patient's utilization of "body language," that is, such figures of speech as "pain in the neck," "he makes me sick to my stomach," "it just breaks my heart," etc. Therapeutic intervention often requires the cooperation of a number of medical specialties. In addition to traditional medical management, the use of psychotropic medication, behavioral modifying techniques and psychotherapy may be utilized as well. The following represents a brief outline of the organ systems to which disorders of this category may apply.

Skin Disorders

Psychological factors are prominent in patients with dermatitis factitia, trichotillomania, pruritus and neurodermatitis and may be significant with alopecia, urticaria, rosacea, psoriasis, herpes and hyperhidrosis, as well as others.

Musculoskeletal Disorders

Musculoskeletal tension headache is one of the most common symptoms of mankind. Similarly, pain involving skeletal musculature elsewhere whether in the chest or in the back or in the extremities can result from similar underlying psychophysiological mechanisms. Immunological abnormalities seem significant in *rheumatoid arthritis,* but it should be remembered that stress reactions acting through the hypothalamus can affect immune mechanisms. The common observation that some patients with rheumatoid arthritis have exacerbations of symptoms under emotional stress should not be ignored.

Respiratory Disorders

The *hyperventilation syndrome* is the most common syndrome in this category. Frequently it is a manifestation of underlying anxiety. However, depressed patients may hyperventilate, and hyperventilation may be a learned response without there necessarily being an underlying psychodynamic conflict of major significance. Psychological factors also seem to play a role in some patients with bronchial asthma and some patients with vasomotor rhinitis.

Cardiovascular Disorders

Some patients with an underlying anxiety syndrome or acute sensitivity to body sensations may become aware of their cardiac function and become alarmed at what is essentially normal tachycardia. Emotional factors may play a role in certain cardiac arrhythmias. The precise relationship between anxiety syndromes and the mitral valve prolapse syndrome requires further study. Certain categories of patients with hyper-

tension, when studied psychiatrically, present evidence for a psychological component in their etiology. Difficulty in handling hostile feelings, difficulty in being assertive and the presence of obsessive-compulsive traits are not uncommon. Recently, the so-called "type A personality" has been reported as being particularly prone to angina and/or coronary artery disease. This personality is characterized by an excessive competitive drive, a chronic sense of time urgency, a tendency to overcommit to a series of responsibilities, achievement orientation and an immersion in self-imposed deadlines. Emotional factors play a role in vasodepressor syncope. In fact there is evidence that emotional factors in some instances may precipitate sudden death in certain patients.

Gastrointestinal Disorders

In addition to anorexia nervosa and bulimia, already described, here would also be included cardiospasm, nervous vomiting, diarrhea and constipation. Psychogenic factors play a role in ulcerative colitis in certain patients. In patients with peptic ulcer, most psychiatric investigations have reported a basic conflict between passivity and aggressiveness. Reaction formation is a common defense mechanism. Clinical investigations have estimated that circa 80 per cent of the gastric hyperactivity and hyperacidity is related to life situations.

Genitourinary Disorders

In addition to the various sexual dysfunctions already reviewed, psychological factors can play a role in a wide variety of disturbances of genital and urinary functions. In certain individuals life conflict influences menstrual disorders, abortion, leukorrhea, urinary frequency, urgency and retention and prostatitis. Perhaps most dramatic is the amenorrhea of false pregnancy (pseudocyesis) in which there are other signs of pregnancy including breast changes, weight gain and abdominal distention. This syndrome is almost entirely psychogenic in origin.

Endocrine Disorders

Obesity has been defined as an increase in adipose tissue of 15 per cent or more above the norm for a given height and age. Psychological responses to obesity are nearly universal, and in a great majority of patients, psychological factors play a role in etiology. Group therapy seems particularly helpful in the treatment of obesity. Therapy limited to reducing diets and drugs frequently fails or if successful, tends in the overwhelming number of instances, to be followed by weight gain once again. The course of diabetes mellitus, hyperthyroidism and myxedema is affected by psychological factors, and some investigators attribute such factors to playing a role in disease onset.

In contrast to the somatoform and dissociative disorders where the symptom is frequently symbolic of the conflict, this is not the case in this group of disorders. In general, the effort to identify a specific constellation of psychological conflicts and relate them to specific psychophysiological disorders has not been successful. If there is a personality type prone to psychosomatic disease, it would be the compulsive personality. However, all individuals seem more vulnerable to stress in one organ system than another. Genetic predisposition and early developmental factors probably play a more significant role in organ selection than pesonality type or the category of conflict. With these patients in particular, the conceptual principle of individual response specificity is particular significant. What life situations and life events represent a psychological stress to a specific patient or which longterm psychological conflicts in fact are significant to a psychophysiologic process must be determined on an individual basis. The process of evaluation outlined earlier is helpful in this regard.

PERSONALITY DISORDERS

Each of us has certain characteristic attitudes and reaction patterns in our relationship to the world, to others and to ourselves that make us a unique individual. For each of us the development of this character structure has a history. It beings in our early years and is elaborated over time. In general, there is very little evidence that our various personality patterns have prominent genetic determinants. Much more prominent etiologically are all those events and situations of life to which a person reponds over time with learned, acquired response patterns. Early mother/child interactions, familial example, discipline and teaching from significant others, peer relationships, unique personal experiences, cultural shaping, all contribute to our personality. When these ways of behaving become exaggerated, when behavior to some degree becomes stereotyped regardless of the external reality, the individual then may be said to suffer from a character or personality disorder.

Usually the individual experiences little sense of distress with his personality. More often others find them disturbing, or the individual is distressed by the consequences of his character structure, often without awareness of how his character determined the very consequence he or she finds dis-easing. Each personality pattern disorder to some degree predicts that person's response to stress. A wise physician includes in his thinking the personality diagnosis of his patient. The management of appendicitis in a paranoid character is quite different than the management of appendicitis in a hysterical character. A paranoid character in delirium tends to behave differently from an hysterical character. The adjustment reactions of each to an identical stressful life event will be different. Therapeutic intervention, therefore, in each instance is different.

In reviewing the following personality disorders the reader would do well to ask for each a series of questions. If this personality disorder decompensated, would there be a tendency for the emergence of a particular mental disorder? If there was superimposed a delirium or a dementia, what would be the manifestations? If this kind of individual would develop an anxiety disorder, what kind of stress, what kind of conflict would be most likely, and how would this affect management and treatment? How would this category of personality tend to respond to pregnancy, bronchoscopy, herniorrhaphy, diabetes mellitus, on intensive care unit, renal dialysis, paraplegia, loss of a job, malignancy in a young son, infidelity, divorce, death of spouse, my characteristic way of opening an interview, my particular style of asking questions and giving suggestions? The list is endless.

Any nosology of personality disorders would be somewhat arbitrary. Many individuals show features of more than one category. Even within categories the principle of individual response specificity still holds. Nonetheless, even when the personality pattern of a given patient does not warrant the label of a disorder, a physician limits his therapeutic potential if he fails habitually to diagnose the personality of his patients.

The following group of disorders tends to show greater psychopathology than those that follow, utilize more primitive defense mechanisms and with decompensation under stress move toward more serious categories of mental illness.

Schizotypal Personality Disorder

While not meeting the criteria for schizophrenia, this personality type, as the name implies, has certain features of that illness. There tends to be magical thinking, ideas of reference, recurrent illusions, depersonalization not associated with manifest anxiety, and paranoid ideation. There is usually evidence for social isolation and undue social anxiety or hypersensitivity to real or imagined criticism. Their speech is often odd, vague, circumstantial, metaphorical, but without loosening of association or incoherence. There is inadequate rapport in face to face interaction with others.

These individuals seem to have introjected a semi-crazy world.

Paranoid Personality Disorder

Individuals of this type show a propensity for using projection as a defense mechanism. They demonstrate pervasive, unwarranted suspiciousness and mistrust of people. Hence, they are hypervigilent, expect trickery, are guarded or secretive, question the loyalty of others, tend to avoid accepting blame even when blame is warranted, look for hidden motives in the behavior of others and often show unusual jealousy. In addition, they are often hypersensitive, tending to take offense quickly. They show restricted affectivity, appearing to be cold or unemotional, often taking pride in being, in their view, objective or rational. They often lack a sense of humor, and frequently there is an absence of soft, tender, sentimental feelings. In short, these individuals have been taught to distrust the world.

Schizoid Personality Disorder

This type of personality is characterized by emotional coldness or aloofness, or absence of tender feelings toward others, relative indifference to praise or criticism or to the feelings of others. They tend to have very few if any close friends but may be very attached to animals. They may have outstanding academic records, having spent hours alone in studying. As adolescents they tend to be seen as shy, withdrawn, alone. They give the appearance of being quiet loners. In contrast to the schizotypal personality disorders, there are, however, no major eccentricities in speech, behavior or thought. In short, these individuals have been taught to expect hurt from the world but defend themselves by becoming indifferent to it.

Antisocial Personality Disorder

Several of the following features are found in the history of these patients with onset before age 15: truancy, expulsion or suspension from school, behavioral delinquency, running away from home, persistent lying, casual sexual intercourse, repeated drunkenness or substance abuse, thefts or vandalism, poor school performance, chronic violation of rules at home and/or initiation of fights. After age 18, there are manifestations of the disorder as follows: an inability to sustain consistent work behavior, an inability to function in a consistent way as a responsible parent, failure to accept social norms with respect to lawful behavior, an inability to maintain enduring attachments to a sexual partner, irritability and aggressiveness as indicated by repeated physical fights or assaults which may include spouse or child beating, failure to honor financial obligations with repeated defaulting on debts, failure to provide child support, failure to plan ahead, impulsively traveling from place to place without a clear goal in mind, disregard for the truth as indicated by lying, using aliases, "conning" others and recklessness. Current diagnostic criteria require that such a behavioral pattern be present for at least five years without any intervening period in which the syndrome is absent. These individuals constitute a major social problem, consuming a considerable percent of the manpower and fiscal resources of law enforcement, social service and health agencies. To date, this disorder stands alone in this category in there being relatively convincing data suggesting a genetic factor in etiology. Early psychological factors also play a major role. Particularly striking is the finding of a parental disciplinary pattern which is demanding, inflexible and punitive one moment and permissive and nonpunitive the next. In short, these individuals behave as if they have failed to incorporate any set of value systems; hence, they are often described as without conscience.

The following group of disorders tend to show less psychopathology than those above but more than those that follow.

Borderline Personality Disorder

These individuals show many of the following characteristics. First, there tends to be impulsivity in areas that are potentially self damaging, for example, spending, sex, gambling, shoplifting, overeating or physically self damaging acts such as recurring accidents, self mutilation or suicide attempts. Second, there tends to be a pattern of unstable and/or intense personal relationships. Third, there is often inappropriate intense anger or a lack of control of the expression of anger. Identity disturbances are commonly manifest by uncertainty over such issues as choice of friends, values, loyalties, or career. There is considerable difficulty, in short, with self image. Next, there is frequently affective instability with marked shifts from normal mood to depression or irritability, usually lasting several hours but rarely for more than a few days with then a return to normal mood. They tend to be intolerant of being alone and experience chronic feelings of emptiness and/or boredom. For periods of time they seem to block out incoming stimuli, but on other occasions seem exquisitely sensitive to it. Certain of these individuals under stress develop "micropsychotic" episodes. During such episodes the diagnosis of schizophreniform reaction may be appropriate. Many physicians find these patients particularly difficult to understand or treat. They seem neither psychotic nor neurotic, simultaneously both, but also normal from moment to moment. Although there is no evidence to date for a genetic determinant for this disorder, the possibility of CNS dysfunction secondary to maturational lag or early developmental trauma is frequently raised by clinical investigators.

Narcissistic Personality Disorder

Narcissists seem to possess a grandiose sense of self importance or uniqueness and often are preoccupied with fantasies of unlimited success, power, brilliance, or beauty. There may be a quality of exibitionism, that is, requiring attention. They may show cool indifference or marked feelings of rage, shame or humiliation in response to criticism by others. Interpersonally, they tend to operate from the posture of entitlement, that is, the expectation of special favors from others without assuming reciprocity. There tends to be, therefore, interpersonal exploitiveness. They lack empathy and tend to relate to others alternating between the extremes of overidealization and devaluation. Having never received or having received without the expectation of reciprocity, psychologically they seem like little babies who simply expect the world to revolve about them; they would be quick to take umbrage with this description.

Dependent Personality Disorder

These individuals lack self confidence and see themselves as helpless and/or stupid. They tend to subordinate their own needs to those of persons on whom they depend. Their passivity allows others to assume responsibility for major areas of their life because of their inability to function independentally. Because they seem so obedient and compliant, they are sometimes viewed by physicians as being "good" patients. Nonetheless, there is a tendency, in order to maintain their dependency, for them to stay "sick" in one fashion or another. They can feel literally devastated with the loss of those upon whom they depend, parent, spouse, employer, son or daughter. They have been taught that they cannot or should not function in the world as independent beings.

This last group of disorders with decompensation tend to move toward less serious categories of mental illness than those that precede it. It should be understood that this is a general statement and not applicable in all instances. Further, the hierarchy is ordered with the assumption that serious refers to the more psychotic end of the spectrum of mental illness and the less serious move toward the neurotic. There would be those clinicians who would argue, quite appropriately, that this does not necessarily indicate less psychopathology.

Passive-aggressive Personality Disorder

These individuals express their hostility in an indirect fashion, hence, they resist demands for performance in occupational or social settings through procrastination, dawdling, stubbornness, intentional inefficiency, or forgetfulness. A longstanding history of educational, social or occupational ineffectiveness and inefficiency is common. These behaviors presist even under circumstances in which more self-assertive behavior would be possible and effective. These individuals tend to evoke frustration, impatience, anger and eventually rejection from others including, of course, physicians.

Compulsive Personality Disorder

These individuals tend to be preoccupied with details, rules, order, organization, schedules and lists. They often give themselves or are given the appellation of "perfectionist." The perfectionism is one that attends to details and fails to grasp the larger picture. The compulsive frequently is unduly conventional or formal, has restricted ability to express warm and tender emotions, is unaware of feelings of anger even though the anger may be communicated to others nonverbally, or, if aware of anger, places premium on control of expression and may be devoted almost excessively to work or studies to the exclusion of pleasure or interpersonal relationships. They tend to insist that others submit to their particular ways of doing things and seemingly are unaware of the feelings elicited in others by this behavior. Nonetheless, quite often they are indecisive, i.e., decision making is postponed or avoided or protracted from inordinate fear of making a mistake. In response they adopt rules, principles and belief systems that they automatically impose on themselves or on others in an arbitrary, unthinking fashion even when the situation does not particularly warrant that approach or response. They lack flexibility. Intellectualization, rationalization, compartmentalization and reaction formation are typical defense mechanisms. In short, these individuals psychologically seem fixated on that stage of life where great emphasis is placed on "doing things right" or risk punishment, shame, withdrawal of love or rejection.

Avoidant Personality Disorder

This pattern of personality is characterized by hypersensitivity to rejection, an unwillingness to enter into relationships unless given strong guarantees of uncritical acceptance, social withdrawal, a desire for affection and usually extremely low self esteem. Outwardly they may behave in a manner similar to the schizoid, but these individuals are not indifferent to the world they are afraid of the world's shame and ridicule.

Histrionic Personality (Hysterical Personality)

These persons demonstrate behavior that is overly dramatic, reactive and intensely expressed. This may be manifest by some of the following characteristics: self dramatization with exaggerated expression of emotions, drawing of attention to self, a craving for activity and excitement, overreation to minor events including irrational angry outbursts or tantrums. In addition, there are disturbances in interpersonal relationships. Often they are perceived by others as shallow and lacking in genuineness even if superficially charming, or as egocentric, self indulgent, vain and demanding, or sometimes dependent and helpless, seeking constant reassurance. They demonstrate considerable denial and repression and at an unconscious level often sexualize their relationships with others, yet find sexual experience incomplete or unrewarding or unsatisfying. These individuals psychologically seem stuck, fixated in the role of staying little boys or little girls.

One characteristic of normal, nonneurotic individuals is a personality structure that is not stuck or fixated into a particular pattern; hence, they demonstrate flexibility and adaptability. These individuals, sometimes called *genital characters,* may show features of any or all of the above personality disorders. But, none of the above patterns predominate or endure when such behavior becomes maladaptive to a given situation. There are those who would insist that no one is normal, that everybody is neurotic or has some kind of neurotic personality disorder. However, this is simply not true. From studies from a variety of sources one can estimate that circa 20 to 30 per cent of the population are genital characters. The concept of integration of certain features within a personality is useful when working with patients who are genital characters. It is useful to think in such terms as a genital character with integrated compulsive features or a genital character with integrated histrionic features, etc.

CONDITIONS NOT ATTRIBUTABLE TO A MENTAL DISORDER BUT A FOCUS OF ATTENTION OR TREATMENT

All individuals over a lifetime regardless of diagnosis are confronted with particular problems of one kind or another and frequently turn to their physicians for assistance. When the problem is not due to a mental disorder, when it is not a feature of one of the diagnostic categories described above, this problem should be recognized without attaching a diagnosis of mental disorder. In DSM-III, common examples of such problems which may be a focus of attention or treatment are *borderline intellectual functioning, adult antisocial behavior* (for example, manifest in some professional thieves, dealers of illegal substances, etc.), *academic problems, occupational problems, uncomplicated bereavement* (especially common in the practice of medicine), *noncompliance with medical treatment, phase of life problem, marital problems, parent-child problems* and *other interpersonal problems.*

PREVENTION

From within the health professions and from without, the growing emphasis on prevention derives from multiple factors: the realization that in some domains of medicine there seems to be almost no limit to the possible growth of treatment programs, the dramatically rising costs of medical care and a genuine interest in the prevention of disability and suffering. We will consider here the prevention of smoking, obesity, alcohol abuse and the prevention of behavioral and emotional disorders in children. There is considerable evidence to suggest that successful techniques for prevention in these areas would have considerable impact on the incidence of a whole variety of diseases.

Abstinence can be achieved among heroin addicts, alcohol abusers and smokers. This has been demonstrated. For those who successfully maintain their abstinence decreased incidence of certain illnesses has been documented. However, the relapse rates for these three addictions follow essentially a similar curve. After achieving abstinence, at 3 months only 40 per cent remain abstainers and after 12 months the figure falls to approximately 20 per cent. A similar pattern holds for obesity. Programs for prevention too often are judged only in terms of immediate rates.

For example, initial reports on the utilization of behavior therapy compared to conventional programs for weight reduction were impressive with behavior therapy programs outperforming the other approaches by impressive margins. However, more recently, with longrange studies, the overly optimistic expectations in this field have turned to disillusionment and pessimism at least for some. Obesity after all is a lifestyle disorder. To effect the maintenance of weight reduction requires a lifestyle change. Some programs devoted to prevention have failed to confront the complexity of the problem and the repeatedly demonstrated difficulty in effecting major and enduring change in human behavior.

Another example is smoking. When smoking behavior is analyzed, it would appear that the main purpose in smoking technique is to get nicotine into the blood and particularly into the brain as quickly as possible. The various models of addiction are discussed in the behavioral sciences chapter. Here we are considering the prevention of smoking in the first place. The usual attempts at primary prevention tend to be educational programs. There is evidence that there has been a decrease of smoking of tobacco in the United States. This has been attributed to a large-scale national education effort. However, if one considers the increasing incidence of marijuana smoking in segments of population, it is highly questionable whether there has in fact been an overall decreased incidence of smoking *per se*. The proportion of persons 18 to 25 years old who have used marijuana has increased from 4 to 68 per cent since 1962. The incidence of tobacco smoking has increased among adolescents in recent years in spite of this educational effort.

The primary prevention of alcohol abuse poses similar problems. Alcohol education programs have been developed in schools. From studies of these programs students do make significant gains in their knowledge of alcohol, but changes in attitude and behavior do not necessarily follow. Actually, broader sociological techniques may be more effective. For example, it is fairly clear from a variety of studies that those states that have lowered the legal drinking age have seen an increase in traffic accidents and fatalities and an increase in the number of young drinkers in treatment for alcoholism. Some studies suggest that the number of alcohol distribution outlets can be correlated to rates of consumption and of alcoholism.

Other techniques for prevention have been developed to involve the popualtion at risk more directly. An example is an instrument that asks the individual to characterize their lifestyle. Then utilizing that data they determine the liklihood of their succumbing to various diseases, given that lifestyle. Whether this approach effects change remains to be researched. The effect of a book on self health care distributed to 460 families in a prepaid health plan was recently reported. At 6 and 12 month study periods, there was *no* significant effect on the number of physician visits made, even though it was determined that half of the families read most of the book and a third used it specifically for a particular medical problem. All in all in these areas it is clear that prevention on a large scale is a complex problem. Some have concluded that there has been more rhetoric regarding prevention than programs which have been demonstrated to work. Others point to studies showing some success and argue that this is too pessimistic a view.

Various studies suggest that children born into a wanted and nurturant environment tend to receive good parenting and tend to develop fewer behavioral and emotional problems in childhood. By inference this group may show a lower incidence of mental illness as adults. But to actually effect an increase in the likelihood of children being born into such settings is difficult. In fact the number of unwanted pregnancies, especially among teenagers, has increased as has the number of teenagers keeping their babies. Sex education and abortion issues tend to generate very strong opinions. Current trends in the United States do *not* suggest a decrease in the number of unwanted children born into our population. Programs more narrowly focused, however, show promise. Involving parents in the process of preparing their children for surgery is one example.

Some observers have suggested rather caustically that society will know when the medical profession takes prevention seriously when we see effective stress reduction programs in medical schools and in health science centers for the health professionals and the staff who work in such centers.

TREATMENT

The Physical Therapies

The most common of the physical therapies is electroconvulsive therapy or electroshock therapy (EST, ECT). Although many theories have been postulated, the mode of action of this treatment is not certain. Empirically, there is no question that treatment will produce remission in a high percentage of patients with severe depression. Major depression is almost a universally accepted indication for electroshock therapy, especially when the depression has not responded to psychotherapy and/or pharmacotherapy. On some occasions, patients with manic episodes also are treated with this modality. Patients with schizophrenia or with severe psychoneurosis are also sometimes treated in this manner, but indications here are controversial.

After appropriate patient preparation, treatment is instituted by applying an alternating current at a frequency of 60 cycles per second with voltage varying between 70 to 150 volts for a 0.1 to 1 second duration through electrodes placed bitemporally. Considerable variations of technique have been introduced, including electrode placement at other sites, changes in the way the current is administered or in the properties of the current and utilization of unidirectional currents and unilateral treatments. The advantages of the various methods are still primarily a matter of opinion; however, seizures, confusion and memory loss are not necessarily required for therapeutic success. Treatments are typically given three times a week up to 8 to 14 in a series, although the number may be as few as 3 or 4 or as high as 15 to 20. The most common complication is an induced organic brain disorder with blurring of memory. This clears spontaneously. The death rate is usually given at about .08 per cent. With modern techniques, the procedure has become exceedingly safe. There is certainly much less risk to the patient than the risk of suicide with unrelenting depression. Fractures and dislocations, especially compression fractures of the spine, have been considerably reduced with the use of muscle relaxants and/or subconvulsive therapy. Personnel must be prepared to deal with an occasional respiratory arrest or cardiac arrest. Some clinicians routinely use atropine prophylactically. EEG changes occur almost universally with slowing in all leads, becoming maximal after 10 to 12 treatments and disappearing in most cases within a few weeks. There would seem to be very few if any absolute contraindications, but special consideration should be given to patients who are pregnant, have bone and joint disease, an aortic aneurysm, coronary artery disease or a brain tumor.

Other techniques for inducing convulsions are now primarily of historical interest although some are still used today but with decreasing frequency. These include the use of an inhalant, hexafluorodiethyl ether (Indokolon) and insulin to induce severe hypoglycemic states.

Electrosleep has been investigated by Russian scientists for many years and has attracted the interest of certain American investigators more recently. Continuous sleep therapy for periods up to 2 weeks and even to 2 months induced and maintained by pharmacological agents is still widely used in Russia but rarely in North America. Carbon dioxide inhalation therapy for the treatment of neurosis with the inhalations being utilized to induce narcosis also is rarely used today. With the widespread use of tranquilizing medications, psychosurgery is also now mainly of historical interest. Its most frequent application is in cases of intractable pain. Depth electrode stimulation techniques are still primarily research techniques.

Pharmacotherapy

While the treatment of the mentally ill by means of drugs is not new, there has certainly been a renewed interest, even excitement, regarding drug therapy in the last several decades. The era of psychopharmacology came into being with the synthesis of chlorpromazine by Laborit in 1951. Psychopharmacotherapy aims at achieving better control of psychological symptoms. They do not cure patients in the usual sense of the word. When prescribing medication, it must be prescribed on an individual basis with thorough knowledge of the patient's condition, a knowledge of the patient's reaction to the drug in question and with a clear view of the therapeutic goal in mind. There are many drugs used in the practice of psychological medicine. What follows is a brief and cursory review.

Antipsychotic Agents (Major Tranquilizers, Neuroleptics, Ataractics). Like the barbiturates, these agents have a quieting or calming effect, but unlike the older hypnotic agents, this occurs without producing marked drawsiness. Subcortical sites of action are more prominent than cortical effects. In general these drugs cause accumulation of the O-methylated metabolites of dopamine and noradrenalin within the brain, suggesting that they block these brain receptor sites. Highest concentrations of these receptors are in the hypothalamus, the basal ganglia, the thalamus, the hippocampus and in the septum. In addition to an antipsychotic effect, these drugs have an antiemetic effect, can result in extrapyramidal symptoms such as pseudo-Parkinsonism, akathisia (motor restlessness), dyskinesia and torsion spasms. Some of these effects may be controlled by synthetic anticholinergic agents (e.g., methanesulfonate, Cogentin; trihexyphenidyl, Artane). Of particular concern is tardive dyskinesia which has a chronic course and usually appears after prolonged administration of such agents with the symptoms often exaggerated when the drug is withdrawn. The dyskinesia is characterized by Parkinson-type activity of a choreiform character especially involving the tongue and the mouth. Other adverse side effects include gynecomastia, heat intolerance (especially chlorpromazine), pigmentation of the exposed areas of the skin, retinal pigmentation (especially thioridizine), jaundice of the cholestatic type on occasion, and less commonly dermatitis and various blood dyscrasias. These drugs enhance the effects of central depressants such as barbiturates. This class of drugs is most useful with schizophrenic disorders. They also are utilized to help control the agitated or the hyperactive states of mania and the organic brain disorders. In some patients in particular, they have a marked lessening effect on the intensity of delusions and hallucinations. The accompanying table provides examples of the various categories of antipsychotic agents with the generic name followed by the trade name and in parentheses the daily dose range.

Antianxiety Agents (Anxiolytics, Minor Tranquilizers). These drugs are used primarily to control the tension and anxiety seen in patients with neuroses and in patients with depression accompanied by agita-

TABLE 14-1. Effects of Antianxiety Agents

Class	Generic Name	Brand Name	Daily Dosage
Antipsychotic Agents			
Phenothiazines			
Aliphatic	Chlorpromazine	Thorazine	50–1000 mg.
Piperidine	Thioridazine	Mellaril	50–800 mg.
Piperazine	Fluphenazine	Prolixin	1–20 mg.
Thioxenthines	Thiothixene	Navane	5–60 mg.
Butryophenone	Haloperidol	Haldol	1–100 mg.
Dibenzoxazepine	Doxapin	Loxitane	20–250 mg.
Antianxiety Agents			
Benzodiazepines			
	Chlordiazepoxide	Librium	15–100 mg.
	Diazepam	Valium	4–40 mg.
	Oxazepam	Serax	30–120 mg.
Antihistamines			
	Hydroxyzine	Atarax	50–400 mg.
Carbonates			
	Meprobamate	Equanil	200–1200 mg.
Antimanic Agents			
	Lithium Carbonate	Eskalith	1200–1800 mg.
Antidepressants			
Tricyclics	Imipramine	Tofranil	75–300 mg.
	Nortriptyline	Aventyl	75–150 mg.
	Desimipramine	Norpramine	75–200 mg.
	Amitriptyline	Elavil	75–300 mg.
	Doxepin	Sinequan	75–300 mg.
Monomine Oxidase Inhibitors			
	Phenelzine sulfate	Nardil	60–90 mg.
	Tranylcypromine	Parnate	10–30 mg.

tion. They have essentially replaced the barbiturates and sedatives in this regard. They have become the most commonly prescribed group of medications in the United States in all categories, psychiatric or otherwise, and are subject to considerable abuse. They are frequently used in suicide attempts and can become psychologically addicting. It is increasingly evident that considerable caution should be utilized in prescribing these medications espeically for more than short periods of time. Perhaps the most serious side effect is that longterm use tends to support the patients' tendency to avoid facing their psychological problems and effecting more appropriate solutions. The drugs produce mild sedation without major impairment of psychomotor performance. Physiologic relaxation is another effect. Drowsiness is perhaps the most common side effect. Patients should be warned about any activity involving skilled motor coordination, for example, driving a car. These drugs have synergistic effects with alcohol and other sedatives, and patients should be forewarned. Other effects include dizziness, headache, dry mouth and on occasion paradoxical hyperactive and/or rage reactions. Less common are hematological, allergic, renal and hepatic reactions. Table 14-1 gives common examples of these agents.

Sedatives and Hypnotics

These drugs are utilized less and less in the practice of psychological medicine, but still are employed for nighttime insomnia and severe daytime anxiety. The antianxiety agents or even certain of the phenothiazines are probably better drugs of choice for severe daytime anxiety. After two to three days, the nighttime sedative effect begins to abate. In sleep laboratories, sedatives can be shown almost universally to have a disrupting effect on the sleep cycle. Earlier reports suggested there might be one exception to the latter statement, namely, flurazepam (Dalmane), but more recent studies raise questions regarding its disruption of the sleep cycle as well. As an adjunct to certain phases of psychotherapy, shortacting barbiturates are used to induce a state of light narcosis (narcotherapy).

Central Nervous System Stimulants

There are perhaps only two indications for utilization of this class of drugs in the modern practice of psychological medicine. One is in the management of hyperkinetic children where methylphenidate (Ritalin) and pemoline (Cylert) are widely used. Methylphenidate and other amphetamines are also useful in the treatment of narcolepsy.

Antimanic Agents

Lithium carbonate is considered to be the only specific antimanic drug for use in bipolar depression. Since it requires 7 to 10 days to achieve a threshold level in body tissues, acute episodes are usually managed initially with antipsychotic agents (e.g., Haldol) until the lithium can begin to take effect. Longterm maintenance on lithium of patients with manic attacks is reported to prevent the recurrence of such attacks in 50 to 80 per cent of patients. There is controversy as to whether lithium is effective in preventing recurring episodes of depression. Utilization of lithium requires the monitoring of blood levels. A therapeutic serum level of .5 to 1.5 mEq/liter is usually in the therapeutic range. Since lithium competes with the sodium ion, it is not surprising that lithium is contraindicated in patients with renal, hepatic or heart disease. With longterm administration, asymptomatic thyroid enlargement can occur. The range between a therapeutic level and toxicity is relatively narrow. Most common effects are polyuria, polydipsia, and a fine hand tremor. These tend to be transient in most patients. As more toxic levels are reached, there is progressively the appearance of nausea and diarrhea, malaise, vomiting, muscle weakness, ataxia, abdominal pain, slurred speech, nystagmus, vesiculations, choreoathetoid movements, convulsions, circulatory failure, stupor, coma and death. Extreme toxic effects have been reported at levels above 2.5 mEq/liter.

Antidepressants

As a group, these medications elevate mood, enhance mental alertness, improve sleep and appetite patterns, increase physical acitivity, reduce morbid preoccupations and lower the risk of suicide in patients with depression. Tricyclics act by inhibiting the reuptake of norepinephrine and serotonin by the neuronal terminals. Monomine oxidase inhibitors block intracellular metabolism of biogenic amines resulting in an increased amine concentration at the terminals. Imipramine, nortryptyline and desipramine seem to have more effect on norepinephrine systems whereas amitriptyline and doxepin have a greater impact on serotonin. Patients who may not respond to one class of tricyclics may respond to another. All these compounds require one to three weeks before there is symptomatic response.

Tricyclics can aggravate the symptoms of schizophrenia and may convert depression into mania. Side effects include dry mouth, constipation, hyperhidrosis, and blurred vision. Weight gain has also been reported; less frequently, tachycardia, anorexia, increased ocular tension, urniary retention and orthostatic hypertension. Monomine oxidase inhibitors are less effective than tricyclics and are usually utilized only after failure with tricyclics or ECT. Careful monitoring is needed because adverse reactions can be serious. These drugs should not be administered to patients taking other sympathomimetic compounds, often present in cold remedies, decongestants, etc. Foods with high tyramine content should be avoided since hypertensive crisis may be precipitated. Subarachnoid hemorrhage has been reported. Other adverse reactions include orthostatic hypotension, dizziness, headache, cardiac arrhythmias, fatigue, dryness of mouth, blurred vision and constipation.

At the present time, there is probably a tendency to *overprescribe* all these classes of pharmacotherapeutic agents, especially the antianxiety drugs and the antidepressants. Normal fear responses and normal grief reactions do *not* require medication. Oft times these medications make such individuals feel even worse. A second trend, however, is seen as well. Once a given psychoactive agent is indicated, there is a tendency to *underdose* the patient. Doses should be gradually increased and given for a sufficient length of time so that the patient truly has been given an adequate trial before the drug is discontinued.

Psychotherapy

Interviews are conducted for many purposes—research, education, selling merchandise, moral persuasion, among others. Even when the interaction is intended to be therapeutic, such may not be the case. A good doctor/patient relationship sets the stage, but whether an interview or a series of interviews has a therapeutic outcome depends on many other factors. Outcome depends upon the motivations of both parties, the capacities of both participants, the nature of the communication process, the experiences facilitated by the encounter, the resulting inner permission given by the patient to himself to experiment with new patterns of action, the practice opportunities within the context of the interview to effect change, and the balance between resistance and assistance for change in the patient's environs.

Psychotherapy Effects Change

Psychotherapy, if effective, facilitates change, a giving up or a modification of maladaptive responses and the acquisition of more adaptive behaviors. Without change at some level—biochemical, intrapsychic, behavioral, interpersonal—the patient stays sick. He holds to a response pattern; he maintains a character structure vulnerable to illness. Although therapists may utilize different theoretical frameworks for understanding human behavior, may belong to different schools of therapeutic intervention and have different styles in their work, they are similar in their effort to facilitate change.

The process of psychotherapy can be described. As is the case with acquiring any new skill, whether walking or talking for a child or farming or performing a surgical operation for an adult, the first step is increased *awareness*. Without awareness for the possibility of change, without awareness of possible options, without awareness of some of the determinants in these options, choices remain elusive. The effective therapist facilitates increased awareness often in the face of resistance of unconscious if not conscious opposition from the patient. The evaluation process described earlier in this chapter not only sharpens diagnostic accuracy and enhances interviewing efficiency, but encourages increased awareness as well.

From this awareness evolves *understanding*. It is not enough for the child to be aware of the possibility of walking. To walk there must also be understanding of that process, whether acquired by imitation or formal study. As therapy proceeds, awareness fosters fuller and more complete understanding of the maladaptive process in question. Ultimately more significant than the physician's understanding is the patient's understanding.

From this understanding, a range of possible alternatives comes into view, and after due consideration, *decision*. To continue our analogy, awareness of the possibility of walking, understanding the process of walking, does not make a walker. Insight in and of itself is not enough. To walk requires the decision to walk. To effect change requires a decision as to the what, the how and the when of change.

Acquiring and integrating a new behavior requires *practice*. The effective therapist encourages and supports such practice, again often in the face of resistance. Any new behavior is unskilled, awkward and doesn't feel natural. The new behavior also opposes, so to speak, the dynamics in the neurotic solution to the conflict. Beyond this, change when manifest may be resisted by the patient's surround. For example, a male patient with a dependent personality recovering from depression may experience resistance from his wife and children as he moves behaviorally toward more independence.

Finally, with sufficient practice, the circle is complete. The new behavior now integrated feels natural. The new behavior allows a new level of awareness.

Having learned to walk, no longer having to pay attention to the walking *per se,* the child becomes aware of a whole new world. Many patients avoid change because, to oversimplify, they wait for the feeling to change first. They say, for example, "When I no longer feel so terrified, then I'll be able to get on the elevator." Change in feeling comes after practice, not before. Others avoid change because they obsess, waiting for the "right" decision, the "perfect" solution, the "answer" which has no consequences other than the relief of symptoms.

The emphasis may be different between therapies. Traditional psychoanalysis emphasizes awareness and understanding and tends to assume that the patient will work through the decision/practice part of the change cycle. With appropriately selected patients, this can occur. Certain behavior therapies tend to ignore awareness and understanding, focus on a particular decision often prescribed, and detail a schedule for practice. Again, with appropriate selection, there can be good outcome. Most psychoanalysts and behavior therapists would object to this somewhat sterotyped description and appropriately so. Neither completely ignores the principles of the other. The principle of individual response specificity would suggest that some patients would be more likely to benefit from one method than the other and vice versa. Studies of therapeutic efficacy are beginning to demonstrate the validity of this statement.

Characteristics of Effective Physicians

The following represents a summary of the characteristics of effective physicians based upon outcome studies, that is, given a group of physicians whose patients have an effective outcome by some measure, what are their characteristics compared to those physicians whose patients by the same measure do not have a comparable outcome. Interestingly, the results of these studies suggest comparable characteristics, whether the study relates to pediatricians and the rates of recurring otitis media in their patients, family physicians and maintenance of weight reduction by their patients, surgeons and morbidity rates following gallbladder surgery, psychiatrists and rates of rehospitalization of schizophrenic patients, therapists and measured improvement in their depressed patients with cognitive psychotherapy, etc.

First, it is interesting to notice what is not significantly different between the two groups of physicians in a given study. There do not seem to be significant differences in any cognitive measurement, e.g., I.Q., grades in medical school, or performance on national testing examinations. Apparently the system that selects individuals into medicine and the system that educates them accomplishes the cognitive mission. Physicians learn what they need to know. At least in these studies there appears to be no significant differences between the two groups in this domain. However, there are differences in other dimensions.

First, the good physician is appropriately nurturant, that is, appropriately supportive. Some physicians tend to be "too nurturant," taking a stance which might be characterized in the following message to their patient: "I care about you. You simply should trust me and place yourself in my hands. Don't worry. I know what is in your best interest." Others tend to be "insufficiently nurturant." Their message may be characterized in this manner: "I know what to do. I intend to do it. You follow my instructions. If you don't get better, it's essentially your fault." Patronizing communication is characteristic of the first example, whereas blaming communication is characteristic of the second. Neither is appropriately nurturant in most instances.

From the data, even more powerful in the statistical sense than the above, is the second characteristic. A good physician is extraordinarily skilled in providing a cognitive model so that the patient understands their disease process. This is not surprising when considered. The patient who understands their hypertension is more likely to follow the antihypertensive regimen than one that does not, especially through periods when there may be no symptoms and in fact even side effects from the medication. With psychotherapy, despite what adamant adherents to given schools of psychotherapy may proclaim, a given theroetical model cannot be shown from data to be consistently more powerful than another. A therapist who uses transactional analysis does not necessarily have better outcome than one who uses the model of Freudian psychoanalysis or another who employs a model from learning theory. The nihilist may jump to the conclusion that it is not necessary to have a model at all. But this is not the case either. Apparently what these good therapists have in common is some model of understanding, a model they understand very well and are able to employ, and especially a model they can communicate to their patients.

Finally, what seems to emerge from the evidence is the following characteristic. The good physician is very skilled in involving the patient in the problem solving. This is in striking contrast to the sick role as defined by Western culture which tends to exempt the patient from being responsible for his illness and which simply expects the patient to comply with the recommendations of the health expert. It is also in striking contrast to the all too frequently observed process of the physician making his diagnosis after evaluation and simply prescribing a therapeutic regimen.

Involving certain patients in the problem solving process requires considerable skill.

Types of Psychotherapy

Before reviewing the various types of psychotherapy, it should be noted that in the last decade studies of therapeutic outcome are demonstrating the significant effect of appropriately conducted psychotherapy. The studies involve control groups, counterbalanced design, reliable measurements, careful statistical analysis, the usual requirements in scientific medicine. Of course, clinical experience has for years suggested such an effect. This kind of research is just beginning. Much remains to be done. The results of such studies seem to show a greater effect than therapeutic nihilists might have anticipated but less effect than therapeutic enthusiasts would have predicted.

Hypnotherapy. Historically, hypnosis was one of the earliest psychotherapies. It was utilized initially to effect suggestion during the hypnotic state or to accomplish psychological catharsis and abreaction. The technique also can facilitate dynamic understanding of the pathological process. In the modern era, it is probably used most successfully for control of pain and for early intervention into conversion or dissociative disorders. The technique tends to foster dependent attitudes in some patients. For others it savors of magic. To others it seems to threaten their need for control. Of course, all effective therapies have potential adverse side effects.

Relaxation Therapy and Biofeedback. The teaching of relaxation techniques also has a long history. A more sophisticated version utilizes biofeedback techniques, although the effect of biofeedback is probably not related simply to skeletal muscle relaxation in all instances. There are reports of therapeutic effect in many kinds of patients, but most consistently in patients with generalized anxiety and accompanied by generalized muscular tension and in patients with specific psychophysiologic syndromes, in particular, tension headache, and certain varieties of hypertension.

Individual Psychotherapies. *Psychoanalysis* or psychoanalytic oriented therapy makes considerable use of the technique of *free association* which encourages the patient to put into words whatever comes to his mind without censuring. At first, this is difficult for most patients to do. However, over time this technique carries the possibility of fostering more complete understanding of the pathological process.

Related to psychoanalysis is a variety of *dynamic psychotherapies*. Here also, there is considerable emphasis on increasing awareness and developing understanding. As is the case with psychoanalysis, *transference* may be fostered and utilized through *inter-*

pretation to bring greater understanding to the pathological process. Transference refers to the unconscious tendency of the patient to respond to the therapist as if he or she were someone else, a significant other in the patient's present or the patient's past. The concept of *fixation* is also characteristic of many of these therapies, namely, that maladaptive behavior patterns are old patterns which persist from specific points in time of psychological development and revolve around certain issues. Returning to those situations and events in the patient's past history, reexamining them, reinterpreting them, identifying their role in the present is a process effecting change.

Supportive psychotherapy emphasizes the development of a more effective support system for the patient in his family setting or work setting. It also seeks to discover the more healthy behaviors in the patient and encourages their elaboration. Uncovering the past, making the unconscious conscious, is not emphasized, even avoided. There is, of course, a supportive element to all effective therapies.

Educational psychotherapy is a term given to that intervention which focuses primarily on educational techniques. There is also an element of education in all therapies.

Behavior therapy using the principles of learning theory also has many variations but focuses specifically in some fashion on a program of practice of behaviors to help the patient extinguish old inadequate responses and/or learn new, more adaptive ones. Some forms of behavior therapy may be particularly helpful to patients who have phobias or in patients who clearly need to alter specific destructive habit patterns, e.g., overeating, smoking, etc.

Group Psychotherapy.   The group psychotherapies are as varied as the individual therapies. They share in common patients working together in the context of a group. Some therapists employ a psychoanalytic theoretical background with an emphasis on developing an understanding of each member of the group and/or an understanding of the group process as a whole. Others may be more active and experiential, for example, those who utilize psychodrama. Conjoint marital therapy, that is, working with both husband and wife, might be viewed as the smallest group possible. Family therapy focuses on therapy with the whole family. Particular indications for these techniques may be in those situations where pathological interactions occurring between the dyad or between members of the family perpetuate pathological processes. Group psychotherapy has an advantage in that it provides the patient with a particular opportunity to practice such new behaviors as more openly sharing feelings, responding to angry confrontations, etc. in a safe and supportive setting and with individuals who are not part of the patient's family or work group.

Self-help Groups.   These groups can be extraordinarily helpful in some situations in fostering therapeutic outcome. Perhaps the best known is Alcoholics Anonymous. It is effective in helping a significant percentage of alcoholics maintain abstinence. Other groups have been modeled after Alcoholics Anonymous including, such groups as Addicts Anonymous and Weight Watchers. There are self-help groups made up of individuals who have recovered from severe mental illness, groups who share in common a particular kind of chronic disease or have undergone similar surgery, e.g., colostomy, mastectomy, or share in common the death of a child or the loss of a marital partner. Finally, given the primary intent of this chapter, indeed the intent of this book, it might be useful in closing that self-help groups have been formed by individuals who share in common the anticipated taking of national certifying or competency examinations.

MULTIPLE CHOICE QUESTIONS

Choose the *best* answer in the following multiple choice questions. This does *not* mean, necessarily, that there is only one right and four wrong answers.

1. Identify the most accurate statement:
   (a) Rates of admissions and discharges of patients to and from state mental hospitals are decreasing.
   (b) Circa one in three or four persons during a lifetime will be hospitalized in a psychiatric hospital for mental illness.
   (c) The most common diagnosis for patients with mental illness seen in ambulatory care medical settings is alcoholism.
   (d) Twenty-five to 30 per cent of all visits to ambulatory care medical care settings in the United States are related directly to mental illness.
   (e) The number of patients resident in county and state mental hospitals over the past decade has increased.
2. A surgical resident making early morning rounds of patients scheduled for elective surgery during that day makes one of the following opening statements to each patient as he enters. Which statement most clearly suggests the concept of stimulus–response specificity?
   (a) "Good morning. How was your night?"
   (b) "I know you are a little anxious about the surgery. Would you like to talk about it?"

(c) "Well, how are you feeling this morning?"

(d) "Anything you would like to ask me this morning?"

(e) "Well, we're all set for your surgery. Are you?"

3. During the first moments of an initial visit to a family physician, a man about 24 licks his lips and with tremulous voice states, "Well, Doctor, it's good to meet you. I suppose you are interested in why I'm here?" The physician nods and the patient continues, "Well, there is no problem really. I'm just here for a regular checkup." Choose the best response.

(a) "You are obviously anxious. What's bothering you?"

(b) "Is there anything in particular you would like me to check?"

(c) "Any particular reason you decided to have a checkup right now?"

(d) "I am wondering if you are feeling a little uneasy."

(e) "So there is nothing in particular and you're just here for a regular checkup. Right?"

4. An experienced pediatrician has completed his initial evaluation of a 9-year-old boy brought to his office by his mother. He has interviewed the mother. Given the evidence from history and physical, he strongly suspects an attention deficit disorder with hyperactivity. Which of the following is most likely to be helpful to the physician for diagnosis and management of this patient?

(a) Consultation with the patient's teacher

(b) Referral to a clinical psychologist for psychologic tests

(c) Referral to a neurologist for a detailed neurologic examination

(d) Electroencephalographic examination

(e) A blood chemistry battery (especially to rule out hyperthyroidism)

5. While reviewing an electroencephalographic tracing from an adult patient with a long history of epilepsy, a physician notes considerable delta activity. Which is most likely? The patient

(a) has diffuse brain damage.

(b) is entering a toxic delirium.

(c) fell asleep during the tracing.

(d) may have a space-occupying lesion.

(e) has the petit mal variety of epilepsy.

6. Which of the following accounts for the fewest number of cases of mental retardation in the United States?

(a) Perinatal infections and early childhood encephalitides

(b) Prematurity and birth trauma

(c) Primary mental retardation

(d) Down's syndrome

(e) Phenylketonuria, Gaucher's disease, cretinism, Hurler's syndrome and kernicterus

7. Patients with anorexia nervosa

(a) more commonly are adolescent boys than adolescent girls.

(b) rarely die from this disorder.

(c) frequently report feeling fat when objectively emaciated.

(d) complain bitterly of nausea.

(e) commonly report symptoms of hypersomnalence and lethargy.

8. Of the following childhood disorders, psychogenesis is clearly most prominent in

(a) the hyperkinetic reaction.

(b) a conduct disorder, aggressive socialized type.

(c) Tourette's disorder.

(d) infantile autism.

(e) the avoidant disorder (withdrawal reaction).

9. A psychiatric house officer is seeing a 30-year-old man in the emergency room. He has been hospitalized previously for a schizophrenic disorder, paranoid type. On this occasion he presents all of the following symptoms. Which is most suggestive of a delirium (acute brain syndrome)?

(a) Visual hallucinations

(b) Speech bordering on incoherence

(c) Persecutory delusions

(d) Concrete thinking

(e) Clouding of consciousness and disorientation

10. In contrast to the alcohol withdrawal syndrome with delirium, alcohol hallucinosis is characterized by

(a) clouding of consciousness.

(b) visual hallucinations.

(c) the comparative absence of physiological withdrawal symptoms.

(d) a disturbed sleep/wakefulness cycle.

(e) autistic thinking.

11. For persons over 65 living outside of hospitals, the most common of the dementias is

(a) Alzheimer's disease.

(b) multiple infarct dementia.

(c) arteriosclerotic dementia.

(d) normal pressure hydrocephalus.

(e) uremic encephalopathy.

12. All of the following substances produce a withdrawal syndrome *except*

(a) barbiturates.

(b) opioids.

(c) cocaine.

(d) caffeine.

(e) tobacco.

13. The intoxication most likely confused with an acute schizophrenic disorder is that produced by
    (a) barbiturates.
    (b) cocaine.
    (c) amphetamines.
    (d) alcohol.
    (e) lysergic acid diethylmide.

14. The possibility of suicide must be considered in all of the following. In which is it *least* likely?
    (a) Dementia with a depression
    (b) Alcoholism
    (c) Delirium (acute brain syndrome)
    (d) Schizophreniform disorder
    (e) Bipolar disorder, mixed type

15. Identify the most accurate statement regarding schizophrenic disorders.
    (a) An example of a primary symptom (Bleuler) is a persecutory delusion.
    (b) Process schizophrenia has a better diagnosis than reactive schizophrenia.
    (c) Hebephrenia is more common than catatonia.
    (d) Schizophrenia affects about 2 per cent of the population.
    (e) Schizophrenia with a chronic course shows deterioration toward dementia.

16. A genetic component probably plays a role in the genesis of all of the following mental disorders. However, the evidence is *least* compelling in
    (a) schizophrenia.
    (b) manic depressive illness.
    (c) Alzheimer's disease.
    (d) Huntington's chorea.
    (e) antisocial personality disorder.

17. Compared to the unipolar disorders, bipolar disorders
    (a) are less likely to respond to lithium during the acute phase.
    (b) are less likely to benefit prophylactically from lithium treatment.
    (c) have an older age of onset.
    (d) are more common in women than in men.
    (e) may have an acute episode precipitated by imipramine (Tofranil).

18. In primary care ambulatory settings, patients frequently have as their presenting complaint "depression." In such instances the most common diagnosis is

(a) manic depressive illness (bipolar disorder).

(b) major depression with melancholia.

(c) dysthymic disorder (depressive neurosis).

(d) adjustment disorder with depressed mood.

(e) uncomplicated grief in response to loss.

19. Imipramine is most likely indicated in patients with
    (a) agoraphobia with panic attacks.
    (b) social phobias.
    (c) generalized anxiety disorders.
    (d) obsessive-compulsive disorders.
    (e) post-traumatic stress disorders.

20. A patient with a major depression with psychotic features is hospitalized. He is given a trial of imipramine (Tofranil) but is unresponsive. A decision is made to attempt a different drug. Which of the following would probably be the drug of choice?
    (a) Nortriptyline (Aventyl)
    (b) Desipramine (Norpramin)
    (c) Amitriptyline (Elavil)
    (d) Phenelzine sulfate (Nardil)
    (e) Lithium carbonate (Eskalith)

21. A 32-year-old man reports difficulty maintaining erections during intercourse with his wife. This has developed gradually over the past 3 years since his marriage at 29. He had experienced no such difficulty prior to marriage. He reports noting full morning erections with wakening. He has had a sexual experience on a recent business trip and noted no difficulty with erection on that occasion. He says he is embarrassed in having this difficulty, and he frequently looks embarrassed as he gives his history. He volunteers no other symptoms of significance. Given the above, the most appropriate tentative diagnosis would be
    (a) psychosexual dysfunction, inhibited sexual excitement.
    (b) psychosexual dysfunction, inhibited male orgasm.
    (c) latent ego-dystonic homosexuality.
    (d) adjustment disorder with anxious mood.
    (e) adjustment disorder with depressed mood.

22. In which of the following are psychological factors probably *least* significant etiologically?
    (a) Dermatitis factitia
    (b) Urticaria
    (c) Rosacea
    (d) Hyperhidrosis
    (e) Acne

23. In which of the following are psychological factors *most* significant etiologically?
    (a) Dermatitis factitia

(b) Urticaria

(c) Rosacea

(d) Hyperhidrosis

(e) Pemphigus

24. Which of the following personality disorders is probably *most* prone to psychophysiological disorders?

(a) Compulsive personality disorder

(b) Dependent personality disorder

(c) Histrionic personality disorder

(d) Narcissistic personality disorder

(e) Passive aggressive personality disorder

25. Identify the most accurate statement.

(a) After 1-year follow-up, heroin addicts who have achieved abstinence are more likely to return to use of heroin than tobacco addicts are likely to return to smoking.

(b) Patients with obesity who successfully lose a significant amount of weight through behavior therapy techniques tend to maintain the weight loss over the next 2 years.

(c) In the United States, in response to a national education program, there has been a decreased incidence in smoking.

(d) Alcohol-abuse educational programs have resulted in a decreased intake of alcohol among high-school students.

(e) Distribution of self-care health books to families in prepaid health plans to date have not shown significant decreases in number of physician office visits.

26. All of the following statements about electro-shock therapy are correct *except*

(a) The most commonly accepted indication is major depression.

(b) Risk of mortality in patients with depression is considerably less than the risk of mortality in such patients who are untreated.

(c) The most common complication is an organic brain disorder.

(d) The muscle relaxants have decreased the incidence of compression fractures of the spine.

(e) The therapy is absolutely contraindicated in patients with aortic aneurysms or coronary artery disease.

27. Based on patient-outcome studies, therapists with good outcome compared to therapists with poorer outcome are more likely to demonstrate

(a) utilization of the psychoanalytic model of therapy compared to the transactional analysis model of therapy.

(b) a higher performance on the Boards of Psychiatry and Neurology.

(c) a tendency to use patronizing communication.

(d) skill in involving the patient in the problem-solving process.

(e) a tendency to use psychopharmacological agents less frequently.

28. Which of the following therapies emphasize increasing awareness and understanding the *least?*

(a) Behavior therapy

(b) Psychoanalysis

(c) Dynamic psychotherapy

(d) Educational psychotherapy

(e) Hypnotherapy

29. Transference refers to

(a) the unconscious tendency of the patient to respond to a situation in the present as if in some measure it were a situation from the past.

(b) the unconscious tendency of the patient to respond to the physician as if he or she were someone else.

(c) the unconscious tendency of the physician to respond to the patient as if he or she were someone else.

(d) the conscious tendency of the patient to displace feelings felt toward others toward the physician.

(e) the conscious tendency of the physician to displace feelings felt toward others toward the patient.

30. Careful evaluation of a man who complained of feeling discouraged about his marriage indicated that the problem in the main seemed to relate to pathological communication patterns between husband and wife. This suggests referral for evaluation for which of the following?

(a) Psychoanalytically oriented psychotherapy for the patient

(b) Group therapy for the couple

(c) Group therapy for the patient

(d) Conjoint marital therapy

(e) Educational psychotherapy for the couple

Questions 31 to 33 and 34 to 36 are sets.

31. A medical resident enters an emergency room to see a patient. The patient, a man about 43, is sitting on the examining table. His shoulders are slumped. His head and eyes are downcast. His eyes are red. He looks up slowly and after a deep sigh says at the end of inspiration, "I am sorry to bother you, Doctor, but I have to talk to someone. I have been so discouraged again and so depressed lately that I've been afraid I might try to kill myself." At this point, there is

(a) verbal and behavioral evidence for anxiety.
(b) verbal and behavioral evidence for sadness.
(c) verbal and behavioral evidence for anger.
(d) only behavioral evidence for anxiety.
(e) only behavioral evidence for sadness.

32. Given the above, choose the most effective immediate response on the part of the physician.
    (a) "Don't worry, you're not bothering me."
    (b) "Have you ever tried to kill yourself before?"
    (c) "What is it exactly you are afraid might happen?"
    (d) "You look and feel depressed. Do you have any idea what has you so discouraged?"
    (e) Would you like to talk to a psychiatrist?"

33. Given the available evidence, which of the following is the most likely diagnosis?
    (a) Uncomplicated bereavement
    (b) Organic affective syndrome
    (c) Schizoaffective disorder
    (d) Dysthymic disorder (depressive neurosis)
    (e) Major depressive disorder

34. A well-dressed woman in her early thirties consults a pediatrician for the first time. While fidgeting with her hands she states, "I want to talk to you about my 7-year-old daughter. She has me worried. She hasn't done anything like this since she was two or three. Last week she wet the bed on two nights. I have been reading, and frankly I'm afraid of what this might mean." The patient pauses and looks at the pediatrician with wide open eyes. Noting the behavioral and verbal evidence for emotion, the pediatrician responds, "Yes, I can see that you are
    (a) concerned. What in particular about this has you worried?"
    (b) concerned. I doubt that this is anything very serious."
    (c) concerned. Has your daughter complained of burning when she goes to the bathroom?"
    (d) concerned. This sometimes is a reflection of tension in the home."
    (e) concerned. Symptoms like this can be alarming."

35. After the above, the physician learns that the daughter has had no urinary tract complaints, has been previously healthy, has been doing well in school, enjoys playing with several playmates, has a younger sister age 5 and recently was very excited about the pending arrival of another sister. She seemed disappointed one week ago when her mother returned home from the hospital with a baby boy. Given this information, which of the following is the most likely diagnosis?
    (a) Adjustment disorder
    (b) Functional enuresis
    (c) Occult cystitis
    (d) Conduct disorder
    (e) Age-appropriate behavior

36. Assume that the diagnosis above is supported during the initial visit with additional evidence following evaluation of the mother and the daughter. Which of the following would then be most appropriate therapeutically?
    (a) Referral of mother for psychological evaluation and possible individual psychotherapy
    (b) Referral of child for psychological evaluation and possible individual psychotherapy
    (c) Referral of child to urologist for further diagnostic evaluation
    (d) Referral of child for psychological evaluation and behavior therapy
    (e) Educational psychotherapy by pediatrician

For the following matching questions, an answer may be used *once, more than once* or *not at all*.

(37–41) Match the following common side effects with the appropriate agent.
    (a) Polyuria, fine hand tremor
    (b) Dry mouth, hyperhidrosis
    (c) Dry mouth, akathisia
    (d) Drowsiness, especially subject to psychological addiction
    (e) Hypertensive crisis with ingestion of foods with high tyramine content

37. Phenelzine sulfate (Nardil)
38. Imipramine (Tofranil)
39. Lithium carbonate (Eskalith)
40. Diazepam (Valium)
41. Chlorpromazine (Thorazine)

(42–46) For each of the following, assume the presence of the given illness and *match* with the psychiatric disorder *most likely* to be missed as a superimposed disease thereby.
    (a) Major depression
    (b) Schizophrenia, paranoid type
    (c) Generalized anxiety disorder (anxiety neurosis)
    (d) Conversion disorder (hysterical neurosis, conversion type)
    (e) Dissociative disorder (hysterical neurosis, dissociative type)

42. Multiple sclerosis
43. Mitral valve prolapse syndrome
44. Temporal lobe epilepsy
45. Hypothyroidism
46. Phencyclidine abuse

For the following matching questions a given answer should be used *once* and *once only*.

(47–51) Link the following diagnosis with the defense mechanisms characteristic of each.
- (a) Displacement
- (b) Projection
- (c) Reaction formation
- (d) Conversion
- (e) Introversion

47. Schizophrenic disorder, paranoid type
48. Phobic disorder
49. Obsessive compulsive disorder
50. Psychogenic pain disorder
51. Major depression with melancholia

(52–56) *Match the following:*

52. Eugene Bleuler   (a) Father of Psychiatry
53. James Braid   (b) Introduced the term schizophrenia
54. Sigmund Freud   (c) Coined the term hypnosis
55. Johann Weyer   (d) Elaborated the concept of defense mechanisms
56. Erik Erikson   (e) Emphasized cultural influences in human behavior

(57–61) In an ambulatory setting, a physician asks a 25-year-old man, "What brings you to see me?" The patient responds with a series of statements. *Match* each with the following.
- (a) Neologism
- (b) Logical thinking
- (c) Autistic thinking
- (d) Concrete thinking
- (e) Clang association

57. "A Ford."
58. "A fine, flashy ford, my lord."
59. "You'd understand if your stomach made as much gas as mine did."
60. "I am an outstanding gasogenic member of *Homo sapiens.*"
61. "That sounds crazy, doesn't it?"

(62–66) Consider five patients, each with a different personality disorder. Assume that each decompensates with what for each is the severe stress of a recent death of a parent. Considering the structure of the personality, *match* with the following responses.
- (a) Schizophreniform disorder
- (b) Major depression with psychotic features
- (c) Panic disorder
- (d) Psychophysiological disorder, neck/shoulder/arm syndrome
- (e) None of the above

62. Borderline personality disorder
63. Dependent personality disorder
64. Compulsive personality disorder
65. Histrionic personality disorder
66. Genital character

(67–72) Assume that each of the following patients as adults have the following diagnoses. Match with the most likely diagnosis of a childhood disorder made when the patient was a child.
- (a) Sleep terrors
- (b) Overanxious disorder
- (c) Stereotyped movement disorder—tics
- (d) Avoidant disorder
- (e) Conduct disorder, aggressive undersocialized type

67. Antisocial personality disorder
68. Phobic disorder—social phobia type
69. Anxiety neurosis (generalized anxiety disorder)
70. Conversion disorder (hysterical neurosis)
71. Genital character

(72–76) During a formal mental status examination, a physician asks a series of patients, "What does the following proverb mean to you? 'The grass is always greener on the other side of the street.'" Consider the responses. Although a single response to a proverb is not conclusive, given the following choices, *match* with the *most likely* diagnosis.

- (a) Schizophrenia, indifferentiated
- (b) Bipolar disorder, manic phase
- (c) Primary degnerative dementia, senile onset
- (d) Dysthymic disorder (depressive neurosis)
- (e) Bipolar disorder, depressed phase

72. "That means when you look across the street, the grass looks greener."
73. "Well, Doc, sometimes that's true. If you know where to look, you can make a mint, and I'm on my way to a fortune. If you put some of your money in with me, I'll make you a millionaire."
74. "I don't know."
75. "Green is not my color."
76. "That's the story of my life. No matter what I've done, on my side of the street, so to speak, it seems like there's been nothin' but bad luck. Of course, it's all my fault, I realize."

(77–96) Consider the following five patients, all being seen for the first time by a family physician. In each instance, the physician makes the observations noted. The patient is making his opening statement.

Mrs. Alport, age 42. Average weight. Neat but old-fashioned dress. Sitting comfortably with hands in lap.

She speaks with a hint of whine in her voice. "Well, Doctor, I hardly know where to begin. I don't think I've had a well day in my life since I was in high school. I guess the worst are these excrutiating headaches. Half the time I can't even fix meals, but my husband and children try to take care of me. It's all very upsetting. They do the best they can, but I get annoyed and irritable sometimes because I don't think they realize how much I suffer! But then I have these dizzy spells and bowel trouble. Unless I'm very careful with what I eat I get sick to my stomach and my periods have never been right."

Mr. Brazil, age 19. Dressed in red sport shirt and white slacks. Sitting with right leg crossed over left. He speaks with considerable inflection. "Well, there's *nothing* serious. I don't know why my parents are so *concerned.* I have this little headache." (Patient smiles.) "It's right here most of the time." (He gestures dramatically with his right hand to an area circa 5 to 6 cm. in diameter over his right ear.) "As you can see, I don't like to touch it because it is sensitive and shoots pains. Sometimes, it's kinda numb, though."

Mr. Cooper, age 54. Dressed in a conservative, expensive suit. Sitting with his right hand in a fist resting on arm of chair. Eyebrows are knit. Forehead is in a scowl. He speaks in a quiet and controlled manner. "I'll be brief. For 4½ years, almost on a daily basis, mainly at work—I'm Vice President of First National Bank, in charge of the loan division—beginning at noon, becoming severe in the late afternoon, I develop rather painful bilateral frontal headaches. I'll be frank with you. You are the third physician with whom I have consulted. I have not been satisfied with my experience in seeking relief from this malady to date." (With the last statement, he points his finger toward the physician.)

Mrs. Duncan, age 37. Dressed in skirt and blouse. Hands fidget somewhat. Patient looks at physician with wide open eyes, "Doctor, I'm frightened. For the last two weeks, I have been waking up early in the morning with a kind of a dull, throbbing headache mainly over my right eye. I've had headaches before but nothing like these, and this morning while reading the newspaper I happened to shut one eye and I noticed that the print was blurred, especially with my left eye closed."

Mr. Eagleton, age 41. Sitting in a rumpled sport coat. Hair uncombed. Head and eyes downcast, looking toward the floor. He speaks quietly and with little inflection. "Well, Doctor, I need help, but I don't think anybody can help me. I know I have to do it myself, but I can't seem to pull myself together since I got laid off at work, almost a year ago now. My wife is very understanding. I don't deserve her. She'd be better off without me. I just sit home and hardly don't want to get up. To be honest, I'm just awfully discouraged. I feel awful, just awful. I don't know what's going to become of me."

(77–81) Match the following. A given answer may be used *once, more than once* or *not at all.*
   (a) Evidence for anxiety
   (b) Evidence for anger
   (c) Evidence for sadness
   (d) Evidence for disgust
   (e) Little evidence for any of the above, either objective or subjective

77. Mrs. Alport
78. Mr. Brazil
79. Mr. Cooper
80. Mrs. Duncan
81. Mr. Eagleton

(82–86) Given the following, choose the most likely diagnosis. Here an answer should be used *once and once only.*
   (a) Major depression
   (b) Meningioma
   (c) Conversion disorder
   (d) Somatization disorder (Briquet's syndrome)
   (e) Musculotension headache

82. Mrs. Alport
83. Mr. Brazil
84. Mr. Cooper
85. Mrs. Duncan
86. Mr. Eagleton

(87–91) Given the following, choose the most likely character structure. Here also an answer should be used *once and once only.*
   (a) Narcissistic character
   (b) Compulsive character
   (c) Histrionic character
   (d) Dependent character
   (e) Genital character

87. Mrs. Alport
88. Mr. Brazil
89. Mr. Cooper
90. Mrs. Duncan
91. Mr. Eagleton

(92–96) Recall that objective evidence refers to behavioral data and subjective evidence to verbal data. Identify the physician's most appropriate move in the interview given the above. Again, an answer should be used *once and once only.*
   (a) Noting neither objective nor subjective evidence for a distressing emotion when one would be expected, physician inquires

how the patient is feeling about his or her symptom.

(b) Noting congruence of objective and subjective evidence, the physician acknowledges the emotion and formulates a question attempting to identify the category of stress.

(c) Noting subjective evidence for an emotion but without objective evidence, physician inquires whether the patient is feeling that way right now, intending to then confront the patient with the absence of objective evidence.

(d) Noting objective evidence but an absence of subjective evidence, physician inquires how the patient is feeling about the symptom and the situation just expressed.

(e) Noting congruence between objective and subjective evidence and sensing already a consensus regarding the stress, the physician inquires what in *particular* the patient is distressed about.

92. Mrs. Alport
93. Mr. Brazil
94. Mr. Cooper
95. Mrs. Duncan
96. Mr. Eagleton

ANSWERS TO MULTIPLE CHOICE QUESTIONS

1. (d)	**25.** (e)	**49.** (c)	**73.** (b)
2. (b)	**26.** (e)	**50.** (d)	**74.** (e)
3. (d)	**27.** (d)	**51.** (e)	**75.** (a)
4. (a)	**28.** (a)	**52.** (b)	**76.** (d)
5. (c)	**29.** (b)	**53.** (c)	**77.** (b)
6. (e)	**30.** (d)	**54.** (d)	**78.** (e)
7. (c)	**31.** (b)	**55.** (a)	**79.** (b)
8. (e)	**32.** (d)	**56.** (e)	**80.** (a)
9. (e)	**33.** (e)	**57.** (d)	**81.** (c)
10. (c)	**34.** (a)	**58.** (e)	**82.** (d)
11. (a)	**35.** (a)	**59.** (c)	**83.** (c)
12. (c)	**36.** (e)	**60.** (a)	**84.** (e)
13. (c)	**37.** (e)	**61.** (b)	**85.** (b)
14. (d)	**38.** (b)	**62.** (a)	**86.** (a)
15. (d)	**39.** (a)	**63.** (b)	**87.** (a)
16. (e)	**40.** (d)	**64.** (d)	**88.** (c)
17. (e)	**41.** (c)	**65.** (c)	**89.** (b)
18. (e)	**42.** (d)	**66.** (e)	**90.** (e)
19. (a)	**43.** (c)	**67.** (e)	**91.** (d)
20. (c)	**44.** (e)	**68.** (d)	**92.** (c)
21. (a)	**45.** (a)	**69.** (b)	**93.** (a)
22. (e)	**46.** (b)	**70.** (c)	**94.** (d)
23. (a)	**47.** (b)	**71.** (a)	**95.** (e)
24. (a)	**48.** (a)	**72.** (c)	**96.** (b)

14

Behavioral Sciences

Ronald S. Krug, PH.D.

Professor and Director of Undergraduate Education, Department of
Psychiatry and Behavioral Sciences, University of Oklahoma at
Oklahoma City—Health Sciences Center

Gordon H. Deckert, M.D.

Professor and Head, Department of Psychiatry and Behavioral
Sciences, University of Oklahoma at Oklahoma City—
Health Sciences Center

Behavioral Sciences Defined

Behavioral sciences is literally defined as the science
of behavior. Because it is not defined as the "art" of
behavior, this topic appropriately belongs in the basic
science section of medical education preparatory to
the study of the clinical art of medicine.

As a science it shares with other sciences the generation of hypothesis about its content arena and method-
ology for testing those hypotheses. This is termed the
scientific method, which is a self-correcting style of
thinking and inquiry. That is, from curiosity about
and observation of the world a general theory of how
an event occurs is formulated. Hypotheses are then
generated to test aspects of the theory; and, through
appropriate controlled research design the hypotheses
are tested for their reliability and validity. Results of
the hypothesis testing (be they directly applicable to
basic theory or of more hueristic value) are used to

refine the theory with the ultimate goal of replacing
theoretical formulation with established fact.

The "behavioral" portion of behavioral sciences is
not as readily defined due to national influence from
the "behaviorism" school, which posited "if you can't
see it or measure it, it doesn't exist." Fortunately, this
extreme stance has been tempered. Psychomotor (or
sensorimotor) actions are, in fact, a part of what is
labeled; however, there are other behaviors. The basic
parameters of mental functioning, particularly as they
contribute to the practice of medicine, are legitimate
concerns for scientific study: e.g., thought processes,
thought content, subjective emotional state, personal
perceptual phenomena, etc. The "static" personality
structure of individuals (their *traits*) as well as adaptation to fluctuating internal and external *states* (the *dynamic* aspects of human behavior) are also valid foci
of scientific investigation. Included in the definition

of the science of behavior are those phenomena that are expressions of the "collective man" (society, culture, subculture, mores, etc.).

Behavioral sciences in medical education is an aggregate body of knowledge which has been argued and refined. The most common concensus of content is referenced in the publications of the Association of Behavioral Sciences in Medical Education (ABSAME) and the varied constituency of the Behavioral Sciences committees of the National Board of Medical Examiners. Both of these organizations have representation from throughout the United States and each operates from the studied and organized conglomerate of data supplied by it's nonstatic membership. The academic discipline sources of the data are varied. From the basic sciences of biochemistry, genetics, pharmacology and physiology come a series of data loosely termed behavioral biology—the relationship between more molecular events and human behavior. From the social sciences of anthropology and sociology come concerns of cultural, group and system influences; and, from, psychology comes the information of abnormal behavior, assessment of behavior, developmental processes, personality, psycholinquistics and psychophysiology.

The behavioral sciences are a group of data that have wide application to all of the subdivisions of medicine. Sabshin indicated that ". . . Patients with psychiatric problems constitute a major portion of the work load of those . . . in general medical practice . . ." and ". . . more patients with mental illness are treated by health professionals than by mental health professionals. . . ." Rakel reported psychofamilial patient problems as the third most common patient problem seen in a family physicians office. Large scale studies have cross-validated the finding that 59 to 60 per cent of randomly sampled adults report psychophysiologic symptomotology. With these and other validating data it is clear that it is necessary to rely upon Behavioral Sciences to accomplish theraputic goals. It would be erroneous and perhaps dangerous to misconstrue behavioral sciences as the introduction to psychiatry. Certainly it would be an injustice to both these areas of medicine, which have common and unique content, as do behavioral sciences and all clinical medical specialties.

Integration of Behavioral Sciences and Psychiatry

We have noted that behavioral sciences is not the introduction to psychiatry; however, there are two practical ties between these fields of study and practice. The first is academic history. For the most part, behavioral sciences was introduced through the departments of psychiatry in medical schools in the United

States. The second is an apparent content tie. Within behavioral sciences is a subsection of "abnormal behavior." Obviously, the diagnosis, intervention and followup of many of these conditions is within the purvue of psychiatry, not behavioral sciences. It should be remembered that the predisposers, precipitators and maintainers of "abnormal behavior" may be orthogonal phenomena that are totally independent and call for different approach strategies. For example, a person may be genetically predisposed to alcoholism; however, that individual may only begin to drink because of the death of an offspring; and, continues to drink because of biochemical addiction to the drug. The genetic predisposition would have required genetic counseling; the precipitating stress would have required grief and bereavement work that provided more available and attractive alternatives than alcohol; and, the biochemical addiction would demand medical detoxification from this class of depressant compounds. Some of these activities are the legitimate domain of some behavioral scientists and all are in the purvue of the practicing physician regardless of medical specialty. It is only through applied research that the issues and answers surrounding predisposers, precipitators and maintainers can be addressed.

PHENOMENOLOGY OF MENTAL PROCESSES

The mental processes are those functions that constitute the concept of "mind"; that is, the dimensions of behavior to which physicians attend as they evaluate the total person. These are the arbitrarily assigned basic elements of mental functioning upon which all other more complex forms of human behavior are constructed. It is assumed that many of these processes are unique to man and not shared with subhuman forms. By assumption these elements are processes and not static events. They wax and wane, and are in dynamic interchange with the person's internal and external environment.

Basic Concepts

Motivation. Motivation is a concept that represents the energy which moves a person to actively satisfy physical, psychological and social needs. It is *drives* or tension states created by "survival" needs as well as *impulses,* which are unexpected urges over which the individual has little or no control. Other terms from various theories are libido and will. It is a common assumption that all primary needs are basically physiologic in origin and that through man's symbolic and communication ability psychological or social needs (secondary needs) develop.

Fig. 14-1.

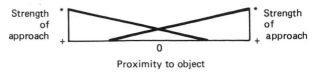

Fig. 14-2.

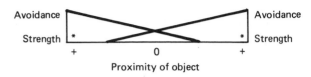

Fig. 14-3.

Gradient. Gradient refers to the slope of a line on a graph which depicts a relationship between two elements. For example, in Figure 14-1, as one progresses on the X axis, the value of Y increases. For example, if a patient is unmedicated and X represents the distance from the surgical suite, and Y represents anxiety levels, the gradient would state that the closer the surgical suite the more anxious the patient.

Stress. Stress is that concept which involves an internal homeostatic state which persons attempt to maintain. If the homeostatic balance is disrupted, the individual is understood to be stressed. Cannon characterized the attempt to correct this lack of homeostasis as the "fight or flight" syndrome demonstrable by: increased blood sugar, dilated pupils, increased blood pressure and increased muscle tone to prepare the person for battle or rapid retreat. Selye posited *the general adaptation syndrome* which ultimately implicated activation of the entire endocrine system in response to psychosocial stress. Arthur said, "Constant activation of the endocrine system can lead to adrenal exhaustion and deleterious bodily effects elsewhere from secondary processes such as elevated blood sugar." Selye's work is perhaps most applicable in those conditions where the stress emanates from an internal condition of the person from which it is not possible for the person to "fly" or which the individual cannot "fight." The three conditions which seem to be most important in internal psychologically based stress are: loss of significant objects (e.g., a body part, loved one, occupation); injury or threat of injury (e.g., surgery, illness, terminal disease); and frustration (e.g., rejected lover, crowded living space, sitting in a waiting room). These three will be elucidated below.

Conflict. Conflict is present when two or more drives arise simultaneously, e.g., to study for specialty board exams or to attend a desirable social event; or, when two or more incompatible responses (including feelings) are aroused simultaneously, e.g., love and hate toward one's parents. By definition, conflict is within the individual. Basically conflict can be classified into three types: approach-approach, avoidance-avoidance and approach-avoidance. Figure 14-2 displays the schema for approach-approach conflicts. The conflict is maximal where the two gradients cross, e.g., taking a vacation in Tahiti or Hawaii. Once the individual has moved past the conflict point on either gradient,

no consequent difficulty arises because the level of the nonchosen gradient decreases as the individual approaches the chosen object.

Figure 14-3 displays the schema for avoidance-avoidance conflict. Again, conflict is maximal where the gradients intersect, e.g., "stop smoking or get lung cancer." However, in avoidance-avoidance conflict, once the individual makes a decision and moves towards one object, the avoidance gradient increases and pushes the individual into conflict again.

Figure 14-4 demonstrates approach-avoidance conflicts. Here the same object has both approach (gradient a) and avoidance (gradient b) attributes. The person begins the approach gradient *before* encountering the avoidance gradient, e.g., marriage; and again, the conflict is maximal where the two gradients cross. If the individual proceeds on the approach gradient, the avoidance increases, and if the person retreats, the approach becomes more attractive once again. The resolution is to either increase the positive value or decrease the negative value of the object so the gradients never cross.

Organic-Functional. Organic-functional is a distinction that refers to the etiology of a given human condition which is usually "pathologic." Basically, organic means the etiology is known and usually, in pathologic states, is on the basis of one or more of the following conditions which affect the central nervous system (CNS) either directly or indirectly: metabolic, inflamatory, traumatic, toxic, infectious, neoplastic, cardio-vascular, or degenerative. Behaviors that are organic in etiology can present to the physican as any of the syndromes discussed in the chapter on psychiatry. However, organic brain syndromes are usually distinguishable by a disordered sensorium or unique types of perceptual experiences discussed below under the heading Mental Status Exam. The term functional implies that at the present time there is no known

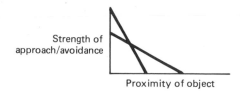

Fig. 14-4.

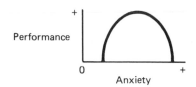

Fig. 14-5.

organic condition that is responsible for the observed behavior pattern. Functional etiology does not imply malingering, lying, etc. Functional pain, while sometimes inappropriately dismissed as "all in the head" does not make the experience of the pain any less for the patient who has it. Functional etiology also implies a psychological base to the behavior pattern observed by the physician.

Acute-Chronic. The acute-chronic dimension used in behavioral sciences, and specifically the psychiatric conditions of behavior, is applied differently than in medicine as a whole. In psychiatry and behavioral sciences acute infers that the condition is reversible and chronic means that it is not reversible. In certain situations multiple acute episodes (e.g., acute alcoholic intoxication) can produce a chronic-organic condition (e.g., Korsakoff's psychosis).

"The Mind"

Emotions. For this discussion, emotions and affect will be considered synonymous. Emotions accompany the alteration of the homeostatic state of the human organism. The alterations may be small and often ignored by the person, or large and overwhelming. The accompanying emotion can covary accordingly. Both large and small alterations and the emotional concomitants are important because small unnoticed changes can accumulate into a large overwhelming situation. Emotions can be judged positive (e.g., happy) or negative (e.g., sad); however, because people usually do not seek help from the physician when they are "happy," the following discussion will focus on the more disruptive emotions of anxiety-fear, anger-hostility and sadness.

Anxiety-fear is the typical emotional response to some type of real or imagined injury or threat of injury. However, a distinction between fear and anxiety can be made. Fear as an emotion is related to a real thing that the frightened person recognizes, usually understands, and against which the person can make protective behavioral responses. Anxiety as an emotion is best understood as fear of something that the anxious person cannot identify. The symptoms of anxiety are experienced subjectively but not linked to an object in the anxious person's awareness. The event responsible for the anxiety is said to be repressed. It is not that the anxious person will not tell the physician the source of experience anxiety, but rather that he cannot because he has no awareness of the threatening object.

The subjective evidence of anxiety (what the patient reports) includes statements like "I'm nervous," "I have butterflies in my stomach," "My knees are shakey," etc. The objective evidence (what the physican sees) includes: excessive perspiration, fine motor tremor, speaking at the height of inspiration, head pulled back (as if avoiding a blow to the face), eyes open wide so sclera is visible above and below the iris, eyebrows elevated leading to a wrinkled brow, frequent and rapid changes in body posture, fidgeting of the hands and feet; and, if the patient is sitting, the feet and lower legs positioned with one in front of the other as if to enable a fast getaway.

The physiologic correlates of anxiety include an epinephrine-like response and suggest gross overactivity of the sympathic nervous system. These include excessive perspiration, skeletal muscle tension (resulting in tension headaches, constriction of the back of the neck and/or chest, quivering voice, low back pain); cardiovascular irritability (e.g., transient systolic hypertension, premature contractions, tachycardia, hypotension); genitourinary dysfunction (e.g., urinary frequency, dysuria, erectile dysfunction in men and decreased vaginal lubrication in women); functional gastrointestinal disorders (e.g., abdominal pain, anorexia, nausea, diarrhea and constipation); and respiratory difficulties. The extreme instance of the latter is known as the *hyperventilation syndrome,* which includes: dyspnea; dizziness; paresthesias of the fingers, toes and perioral area; and, in extreme cases, carpopedal spasm. Generally, hyperventilating patients subjectively report that they are oxygen deficient, but in fact their O_2 blood level is above normal.

Besides anxiety's role as either etiologic or at least an accompaniment of pathologic behavior syndromes, there is a clear relationship between anxiety and performance, as expressed in Figure 14-5. To a certain degree anxiety can enhance performance by making the person alert, activated and motivated. However, too much anxiety effects a decrease in performance.

The most common situations that provoke anxiety are: *anticipatory anxiety* where individuals frighten themselves with the unknown in advance of a given event (e.g., stage fright); *castration anxiety* which originated from psychoanalytic theory, meaning the anxiety/fear associated with the son's fear that the father will cut off his penis for "loving" the mother. Today the concept has been expanded to any situation where the person encounters threat from an authority figure such as a supervisor; *separation anxiety,* which is experienced when one is separated from another person who is needed (e.g., the first day of school, frequently for both the child and the parents); *stranger anxiety,* which is a normal development event occurring in an infant between six and twelve months when the infant is confronted with anyone who is "nonmother." This is frequently distressing (anxiety provoking) for the nonmother figure—usually father; however, separation anxiety simply indicates that the child has begun to discriminate between objects.

These specific examples demonstrate the signal-alerting quality of anxiety/fear. The anxiety/fear signals the individual that danger is present. It is frequently difficult for a person to "unlearn" anxiety/fear attached to a specific event that is no longer dangerous because the symptoms are so uncomfortable that the frightened/anxious person automatically avoids the source of the distress whenever the alerting signals are perceived.

Anger as an emotional response usually has frustration as its stimulus. Frustration occurs when motivated behavior (goal directed) is either blocked or there is a threat to obtaining the goal. The goal may be a real or symbolic object that will satisfy a given primary or secondary need, e.g., pulling into a parking space and someone else blocks the entry. The aim of the resultant anger is to remove the blocking agent and allow the accomplishment of the drive. Anger is termed a drive discharge emotion in that the emotion appropriately directed, allows for satisfaction of the frustrated drive/need state.

Anger is also related to hostility. The major distinction between anger and hostility is that anger is relatively short-lived if the frustrating stimulus is removed. Some authors suggest anger should not last longer than 20 minutes. Also, anger is not necessarily destructive, but more aggressive in nature. *Hostility,* however, is an emotional condition that pervades the person's entire behavioral repertoire, is present over extended periods of time (e.g., years) and is physically or psychosocially destructive in outcome. Hostility may or may not be related to a specific frustrating stimulus or condition.

Subjective reports from the angry patient include statements like "I'm mad," "I'm angry" and "I'm pissed off." Objective signs the physician can observe include narrowed eyelids, eyebrows "knitted," flared nares, clenched teeth (protruding masseter muscles), lips thin and tightly pursed, head and neck jutted forward, protruding and throbbing temporal and neck blood vessels, rigid back, arms crossed tightly across the chest and feet planted flatly and firmly on the floor.

The psychophysiologic concommitants of anger are epinephrine (and possibly norepinephrine) in nature. These include increased heart rate and blood pressure, dilated pupils, increased muscle tension, increased energy, constriction of peripheral vessels and increased metabolic rate.

Through primate studies the diencephalic-limbic system has been implicated in anger. Rage reactions have been observed after intercollicular section, nocioceptive stimulation in the posterior and lateral portions of the hypothalamus as well as other areas of the limbic system. Also, there appear to be modifying influences from the forebrain and rostral thalamic muclei. The "forced activity" observed in the temporal lobe epileptic; and, the absence of fear and aggression responses as well as the hypersexuality of the Kluver-Bucy Syndrome associated with bilateral lesions of the amygdala, must be considered here.

Sadness as an emotional response usually has loss of a significant object as the etiologic event. The lost object may be a person, job, health, youth or anything to which the individual is strongly attached. The subjective evidence for sadness is the patient's report that "I feel down," "I feel blue," "I am sad," etc. The objective evidence the physician can observe includes: flacid faces, downcast gaze, sighing respirations, speaking at the end of expiration, head tilted down, shoulders slumped, decreased associative arm movement in walking, hands held loosely in the lap, legs crossed at the ankles and general decreased amounts of body movements.

Sadness as an accompaniment of the mourning process is expected and must be distinguished from the depressive syndrome. Mourning should be completed 6 to 12 months after loss. If mourning extends into the second year, the physician should know that the patient is no longer mourning, but is depressed and should be treated accordingly.

There are two important variations of sadness. First, *guilt* which can be conceptualized as a mixture of sadness plus anger turned back upon the self. The individual angrily blames the self for some event. For example, a mother whose child is born retarded may be sad over the "loss" of a "normal" child and, in addition, may inappropriately assume the responsibility for the retardation with a statement such as, "If only *I* had (not) done_____." *Shame,* on the other hand, can be conceptualized as sadness in the face of external environment disapproval. For example, with the same mother noted above, the immediate family might say "If only *you* had (not) done_____."

There are essentially five major descriptions that characterize emotions. First, they are bipolar in nature: anxious-calm; angry/hostile-warm (similar to hate-love continuum); and sad-happy. Next, an emotion can be ambivalent in that an individual simultaneously experiences both ends of the bipolar continuum towards the same object. This is similar to the approach-avoidance conflict noted above, e.g., loving and hating an individual at the same time. Third is the ability to *express* emotions. Some persons have decreased or constricted expression, some have increased expression and some demonstrate no emotional response. This absence of emotional expression is termed "flat affect." Fourth is the *appropriateness* of an expressed emotion relative to the content to which it is attached. It is generally appropriate to cry at the loss of a loved one, but not to laugh. Last is the rapidity of emotional change. All persons experience fluctuations in their emotional state; however, some individuals' emotions change markedly quite frequently (e.g., every 30 seconds). This is termed *lability* of affect.

Thought. Thinking is "mental" manipulation of symbolic processes usually for creative and/or problem solving purposes. Since thoughts are intangible, thinking can only be judged objectively by verbal, written or other products. For discussion purposes, thought will be divided into two separate portions: the process and the content.

This first major division, *process* describes *HOW* a person thinks. There is a given *production rate,* which may be inferred from the rapidity with which a person speaks, but geographic and cultural variations may be misleading. It is clearer to conceptualize production rate of thoughts as a person walking. *Accelerated thought process* is similar to a person descending a steep hill and about to lose balance. That person takes short rapid steps to prevent stumbling. The physician may try to intervene, but the person cannot help but continue rapidly down the hill. *Retarded thought process* is similar to a person ascending a steep hill. The progress is slow and labored; and, regardless of the physicians' attempt to assist, the person maintains a slow pace. *Blocking* is exemplified by the person who, while walking, encounters sudden darkness in which the appropriate direction cannot be ascertained. This individual is confused, doesn't understand why the darkness occurred and can't extract himself from the darkness. Accelerated and retarded production rates generally accompany major affectives disorders and certain organic conditions. Blocking is usually psychologically determined, precipitated by content issues

that are conflicted and are the most common in major thought disorders.

When examining *how* a person thinks, besides rate is the continuity with which thoughts are connected. Most formal thought process is characterized by Aristotelian logic; i.e., $A \rightarrow B \rightarrow C \rightarrow D \ldots Z$. The term *looseness of association* refers to thought process that is non-Aristotelian, where associations between thoughts are formed on unique bases that have very loose connections. Sometimes this is called "predicate logic" (e.g., von Damerus's Principle), i.e., "The Virgin Mary was a woman, I am a woman, I am the Virgin Mary." In other forms the association between thoughts is on the basis of sounds and are called "clang associations," e.g., bang, rang, dang, sang, . . . clang. Another disorder of continuity is *circumstantial thinking* in which the person produces *every* detail surrounding a given event. For example, when asked, "what did you do this morning?" the person might respond: "I heard the alarm, opened my left eye, then my right eye, opened my mouth, yawned, stretched my right arm, then my left, . . . (3 hours later) and then stood up at the side of the bed." These persons will eventually arrive at the end goal; however, the physician hardly has time to wait. *Tangential thinking* is that process characterized by the person slightly missing the goal aimed for, e.g., "are you a good tennis player?" answer "I like to play tennis." While the questioner has some data relative to the inquiry, an "on-target" response was not made. The thought process known as *perseveration* is when persons repeat the same response regardless of the context of the question. For instance, Q: "How old are you?" A: "30." Q: "How many children do you have?" A: "30." Q: How tall are you?" A: "30."

The second major division, thought content, is concerned with the message or meaning of the thoughts themselves. The first consideration is *the relationship of thoughts to external reality,* and must be examined from three viewpoints: (1) sense of reality, e.g., knowing that the four-legged object on which one is sitting is a chair; (2) testing reality, e.g., validation with someone else or through functional experimentation that the object is, indeed a chair; and (3) adapting to reality e.g., using the chair to sit comfortably at a table to eat when the table is too high or low without it. The most significant aspect of relationship to reality is whether the individual is either realistic or *autistic* in thought content. Autistic means that the individual has a private understanding of the world or external events which is not shared by others, e.g., Einstein's theory of relativity when initially posited. If the autistic thinking becomes fixed in the face of contrary, overwhelming evidence and takes on a maladaptive and/

or malevalent quality the thought content is called delusional. *Delusions* are defined as false-fixed belief systems. Autistic thinking is characteristic of major thought disorders like schizophrenia.

The second aspect of thought content to be considered is the relative level of abstraction that an individual can attain. For example, upon request, can the individual abstract the common essence from examples of a general category (an organge and banana are both fruit) and distill a general principle from a concrete example (e.g., "a stitch in time saves nine" = prevention is cost effective). If abstractability is impaired, the person can only identify superficial concrete qualities of diverse objects of a general class (e.g., an orange and banana both have peelings) or can only repeat the example or give a literal interpretation of the example (e.g., "sew a tear when it starts and it won't take as many stitches to fix"). While poor abstractability is found in functional organic thought disorders, it is also indicative of mental retardation.

The next characteristic of thought content is if the individual can develop *insight*. Can the person interdigitate relations between events in a cause-effect manner; or, can the individual recognize stress events or internal conflicts and their subsequent emotional effects. Related to insight is *judgement*. Given insight, how does the person relate in social situations, generally exercise control over life, and judge the consequences of given situations and adjust to them.

The last significant element of thought content is the relative obsessional nature. That is, whether the same thought content characteristically intrudes uncontrollably into the persons' awareness; or whether characteristic thoughts are varied and rich in content.

Orientation. Orientation is knowing who, when and where one is at the present time. There are four dimensions of orientation that are considered: person, place, time and situation.

Orientation to person means does the individual know who (s)he is, (Name, birthdate, identity of parts of the body or that the body belongs to that person). The phenomenon of *depersonalization* is a disorientation to person in which the body as a whole or parts of it seem dissociated away from the "mind," e.g., the "mind" drifts from the body and observes events from the corner of the room. Two other disruptions in orientation to person are: anosognosia, not knowing that one is ill; and autotopagnosia, not being able to correctly locate one's own body parts.

Orientation to place means can the individual locate himself geographically and spatially? If orientation to place is disrupted, the most common forms are: *derealization,* a sensation of distortion of spatial relations

and unreality; *deja vu,* a feeling when in a strange environment that "I've been here before"; and *jamais vu,* the reverse of deja vu where the individual is in a familiar environment and suddenly feels "where am I?"

Orientation to time is the individual's ability to know present position in linear time: e.g., day or night, morning or evening, day of the week, month and year. The latter is emphasized because of the common assumption that if a person knows the date and month, that person automatically knows the year. This is frequently untrue particularly, in the various forms of organic brain syndromes.

Orientation to situation is a synthesis of the above three. That is, to repeat the definition of orientation: does this person know who (s)he is, where (s)he is, when it is and what the present contextual situation is that relates these three together?

Consciousness. Within behavioral sciences, the concept of conscious-unconscious mental processes has three distinct definitions. First, consciousness is used to refer to the relative level of physiologic arousal. Second, it can mean that the person is physiologically alert, but there is a psychodynamic condition present that may grossly affect mental processes. Third, it is used to define whether a piece of data is in a person's awareness at the present time, with the assumption that the individual's physiological arousal level is normal and alert.

The first point (relative physiologic arousal) is referable to the level of activation of the central nervous system (CNS) and the associated constant, nonfluctuating nature of consciousness. This aroused condition of the organism is intimately tied to the integrity and functioning of the reticular activating system (RAS). Apparently the RAS is also central to the behavioral alerting-orienting response which is the primary determinant of *attention*. If the RAS is functioning in an activating manner, it is transmitting signals to other portions of the brain and the person is alert and attending to (orienting to) incoming stimuli. However, if the RAS is compromised in function the individual experiences conditions ranging from mental confusion through clouding of consciousness, to stupor (the individual's senses are dulled and the person is capable of very little environmental interchange), and finally coma where there is no awareness of the environmental surroudings. These alterations in physiologic alertness are common sequelae of CNS dysfunction and particularly traumatic head injury. In addition to the characteristic level of consciousness, fluctuating levels of consciousness (or attention) frequently accompany pathologic CNS conditions as well as psychologically based disease. Organic conditions should be suspected if the person is well-rested and attempting to focus attention or *concentrate*.

The second definition of consciousness implys that the person is physiologically alert; however, some *psychologically based conflict* has precipitated a condition in which the person seemingly functions in a "normal" manner but is unaware of massive amounts of personal experience. The most common of these conditions are: *fugue* states characterized by the assumption of a totally "new life" without being aware of a different earlier life. Upon recovery of the earlier memory, the "fugue" life is forgotten; *dream or twilight states* in which the physiologically alert person seems to focus all attention on an inner or far off event. During the condition the person is relatively immobile and markedly unresponsive to environmental stimuli. Amnesia for the event is expected; *sonambulism* or sleep walking is the third major type of psychologically based alteration in consciousness. It is similar to a short-lived fugue state, except that it begins while the person is asleep. Again, upon awakening the individual has no recollection of the events that transpired during the sleepwalking episode.

The third definition of consciousness derives from psychoanalytic theory and refers to whether given material is in the awareness of the person. Freud spoke of three levels: first, *conscious* material which is in full awareness; second, *preconscious* material which is not in awareness but can be readily recalled at will, e.g., one's own telephone number; third, *unconscious* material which is not in awareness and cannot be brought into awareness without special techniques like hypnosis or free association.

Sensation. Sensation is defined as the experience that results from stimulation of sensory nerve endings of any of the five senses: sight, sound, touch, smell/taste, and kenesthesia.

Primary sensation, because of its "unknown" quality tends to provoke anxiety. This "unknown" disrupts the homeostatic condition of the person which the person attempts to correct through understanding or *perception* discussed below. Toxic conditions (e.g., various drugs) and other neuropathologic conditions, such as irritating lesions of the visual cortex or migraine headache can produce sensory pheonmena. It is emphasized that primary sensations without environmental stimuli (e.g., visual scotoma and "sparklers", tinnitus, foul odors, etc.) usually imply organic conditions. The primary sensory pathways, their projection sites in the brain and behavioral correlates will be included in the discussion of the physiologic contributions to the determinants of behavior.

Psychogenically based disorders of sensation are best represented by the phenomenon of chronic, psychogenic pain. This condition is discussed in the chapter on psychiatry.

Perception. The understanding of sensory stimuli referred to above is the operational definition of perception. As stimuli enter the brain in addition to the specific sensory nerve tracts that pass to the sensory cortical areas, there are collateral sensory imputs to the reticular formation which apparantly activates the RAS. This activation results in attention to the stimulus and is called an orienting response. With attention and concentration on the nature of stimuli and past experience or frames of reference, the person "understands" or perceives the stimuli. For example, one is awakened in the night by a noise. Until the etiology of the noise is perceived, arousal (orienting response) and/or anxiety remain at high levels. With perception, anxiety may change to fear or disappear depending upon the etiologic event. The arousal (orienting response or attention) may turn to concerted effort to deal with the perceived stimulus. Sometimes for either organic or functional reasons, misperceptions of environmental stimuli occur. A drape blown by a draft is perceived as someone entering a window or the shadow of a leaf on a wall at night is perceived as a tarantula spider. These are *illusions,* defined as misinterpretations or misperceptions of real environmental events.

However, exteroceptive stimuli are not always necessary for perception to occur such as imagination or dreaming. On occasion internal stimuli like thoughts can become so intense that they are projected as perceptions onto the external world in the form of *hallucinations.* That is, the person perceives an imaginary or interoceptive event as an exteroceptive reality. While hallucinations are usually considered "pathologic" (auditory being more functionally based; and, visual, tactile, olfactory/taste and kinesthetic more organic) there are two forms of hallucinations that seem to be unrelated to significant pathologic conditions. In stages of sleep when control over "conscious" processes is marginal, hallucinations (particularly auditory types) are frequently reported. If a hallucination occurs as one enters sleep it is called a *hypnogogic* hallucination; and, if it occurs as one is gaining wakefulness it is called a *hypnopompic* hallucination.

Memory and Forgetting. Memory (mnesis) is the ability upon demand to bring into awareness past events and experiences. It is customary to divide the concept of memory into three arbitrary types. *Immediate memory or recall* is the ability to reproduce data to which one has just been exposed. For example, finding a telephone number in a telephone book and having the number available for a few seconds; or, the repetition of a serial set of numbers. This ability is apparently limited to seven "bits" or "chunks" of data. *Recent, or short-term memory* is the ability to remember information after at least a ten minute interval between exposure to and recollection of the data; e.g., recollection of three independent items presented by an interviewer at the beginning of an interview, recent notable news events within the last week, etc. *Remote, or long-term memory* refers to the availability of information learned by the individual a considerable time before; e.g., personal activities on the day Pearl Harbor was bombed (verified by reliable sources).

Research has established that both neuroanatomical sites and neurochemical substances are important in the mnestic process. Apparently the mesencephalic reticular system is important early in the memory process, and activation of the thalamic reticular system with attendent inhibition of the mesencephalic reticular system is crucial later in the memory process. RNA and protein synthesis is important in the formation and storage of particularly long term data. The hippocampus appears to be particularly central to the transfer of information from short term to long term memory. Special states of memory include: *hypermnesia,* or unusual memory for detail of a specific or selected situation; *iconic* memory, or the brief detailed retention of visual stimuli; *eidetic,* or "photographic" memory, which is the unusual ability to glance at an object like a book page, look away and recite it without error as if reading the page.

Forgetting (amnesia) is the *nonrecollection* of material to which one has been previously exposed. It is assumed that the forgetting of material has either a "dynamic" or functional base (the information is "blocked" from awareness by psychological processes) or is organic in nature. The most common types of amnesia are: *Patchy, or lacunar amnesia:* the person has intact memory around a given amnesic "hole." For example, the grandparents who can remember all grandchildren's names and birthdates except the one who's mother died at its birth. *Anterograde amnesia:* the person forgets all information following a given significant life event, e.g., memory loss for 24 hours after being raped. *Retrograde amnesia:* the loss of memory for events preceding a significant life event, e.g., 24 hours prior to being knocked unconscious from an automobile accident. *Paramnesia* (retrospective falsification): the distortion of remembered data. The person who experiences this is firmly convinced of the valadity of the recollection. One specific instance of this phenomenon is called *confabulation,* characteristic of the organically based Korsakoff's Psychosis. In con-

fabulation the individual weaves data from the here and now into the recalled experience. Sometimes the interwoven data is suggested by the physician as a way to test for confabulation.

In general, a memory defect is considered to be of psychogenic origin if the individual has no disturbed level of consciousness and there is no intellectual impairment. Organically based memory disorders have the following associations. Bilateral lesions of the hippocampus and/or mammilary bodies produce profound deficits particularly in short term memory. Long-term memory is usually unaffected by organic conditions unless accompanied by psychosis. If organic memory loss occurs, recovery is typically *gradual* and from the extremes to the precipitating event, e.g.,

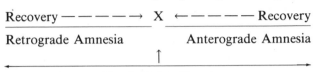

By implication, if recovery of lost memory is abrupt, a psychogenic etiology is implied.

Intelligence. The concept of intelligence is defined as "the aggregate or global capacity of the individual to act purposely, to think rationally and to deal effectively with his environment."

Intelligence is usually subdivided into two types: verbal and performance. These can be related to CNS lateralization of higher mental or cognitive processes in the brain with verbal abilities under executive control of the left hemisphere and visual-spatial skills associated with the right hemisphere functioning for most people, regardless of hand dominence.

A central issue in the discussion of intelligence involves the "nature-nurture" controversy or whether intelligence is determined by heredity or environment. Evidence in favor of the nature position includes: twin studies have consistently shown that there is an IQ concordance rate between monozygotic twins that is higher than the rate for dyzogotic twins which, in turn, is higher than that of natural siblings; an adopted child's IQ correlates higher with that of biological parents than with the IQ of adoptive parents.

For the nurture postion, the favorable evidence is: social, cultural and interpersonal deprivation is correlated with low IQ scores; rural, isolated and mistreated children have lower IQ scores than matched urban, stimulated and well treated peers; minority children taught in inferior school systems who are moved to enriched schools have positive correlations between IQ scores and length of time in the enriched school system.

The Intelligence Quoteint (IQ) is a mathematical expression of the relation between mental ability and age. It will be discussed in detail below under psychological assessment; however, dependent upon the particular IQ test administered, an average IQ is 100 with 10 to 15 points of variation on either side.

The distribution of intelligence is assumed to follow a normal or "bell shaped" curve; however, due to early trauma, infections, poor maternal prenatal health care, etc., there is a higher than expected number of persons with lower intelligence in the universe. Generally intelligence scores are grossly classified as below normal, normal and above normal.

In the below-normal range are those persons diagnosed as primary mentally retarded. Primary mental retardation is a syndrome defined by low intelligence, poor social adaptation and developmental problems. This definition excludes those persons whose intellectual ability is compromised by brain dysfunction and related disorders. These are classified as having secondary mental retardation. The IQ distribution and functional classification according to the Diagnostic and Statistical Manual of Mental Disorders II (American Psychiatric Association, 1968) is:

IQ 20: Profound mental retardation
IQ 21–35: Severe mental retardation
IQ 36–51: Moderate mental retardation
IQ 52–67: Mild mental retardation
IQ 68–85: Borderline mental retardation

Another classification that is sometimes more useful is based on prognosis in self care. This divides retarded individual into:

IQ 30: *Custodial.* These persons cannot distinguish between safety and danger and therefore must live in a protected custodial environment.
IQ 30–50: *Trainable.* Persons classified here can distinguish safety between danger; however, they cannot learn the essentials of symbolic communication (reading, writing and arithmetic).
IQ 50–70: *Educable:* These individuals can learn the basics of symbolic communication but, encounter difficulty in abstract thinking and complex judgement.

Normal intelligence then is bordered by IQ scores between 90 and 109. The greatest majority of persons fall within this range of IQ scores.

The above-average intelligence person has an IQ score greater than 109. The classification according to Wechsler is:

110–119: Bright normal
120–129: Superior
130 and above: Very superior

In addition to intelligence, there are persons with outstanding unique abilities. On the low IQ end of

this continuum people are sometimes born with IQs in the range of "retarded", but show dramatic excellence for some singular talent. These individuals are called *idiot savants.* Some have spectacular achievement in arithmetic calculation, playing musical instruments by imitation, and calander calculation in the remote past and future. On the high end of the continuum are persons with IQs in the range of genius but who have singular outstanding deficits. For example, Albert Einstein for all practical purposes had an IQ which was so high as to be untestable. However, at age 15 his grades in history, geography and language were poor and he left school with no diploma.

These aspects of the mind comprise what can be conceptualized as the phenomenology of mental process. The focus has been on delineating mental activity, which constitutes the basis of an individual's interface with the external environment. These parameters are conceptualized as biological "givens" which must function in a "normal" manner for the individual to be maximally adaptive in the world.

Frequently the physician must determine if a given individual's "mind" is functioning correctly. To do this in a valid manner, the physician must use a given procedure which is standard and reflects the important dimensions of mental processes. This procedure is called the *Mental Status Examination.* Various authors arrange the content somewhat differently; however, the following outline is presented because of meaningful diagnostic implications which can be drawn from dysfunction reflected in the various groupings.

1. Sensorium
   Consciousness: level and stability
   Orientation: four spheres
   Memory: immediate, recent and remote
   Attention and concentration.

   The first letters of these variables spell the *mnemonic* (memory aid) COMA which is particularly meaningful since dysfunction in any of these four areas should alert the physician to a possible organic condition.
2. Thought Process
   Production rate
   Continuity

   Dysfunctions of thought process have implications for the major psychotic-proportion affective and thought disorders, as well as organic brain syndrome.
3. Thought Content
   Relationship to reality: (autism and/or delusions)
   Concept formation: Relative abstractability
   Intelligence
   Insight and judgement

Characteristic topics

These parameters are disrupted mostly in the major thought disorders, but also in affective psychotic conditions and organic brain syndromes.

4. Perceptions

Hallucinations

Illusions

Dysfunction in perception should always alert the physician to possible organic substrates.

5. Emotional Regulation

Subjective and objective evidence for emotional states and relative congruence

Ambivalence

Appropriateness to thought content

Disruptions here can accompany any major psychotic condition, but especially thought disorders.

6. Relevant Somatic Functioning

Sleep

Appetite

Weight

Sexual functioning

These are vegetative behaviors which, when dysfunctional in a syndrome complex usually accompany affective disorders and suggest immediate and vigorous intervention is necessary.

DETERMINANTS OF BEHAVIOR

The preceding section addressed mental process of behavior. This section summarizes how behavior is influenced, beginning with genetic events, proceeding through biochemical influences, psychophysiologic parameters, learning and growth and development, to sociocultural considerations and psychosocial issues in current American society.

Genetic Influences on Human Behavior

Genetic factors are responsible for unique human conditions. Basic genetic concepts are:

Genes: the elemental unit of heredity composed of a biochemical substance called deoxyribonucleic acid (DNA) which provides hereditary information and controls.

Chromosomes: the 23 pairs of "strands of genes" that are present in virtually all cells of the body. The exception are sex cells, which are unpaired and have only 23 chromosomes.

Genotype: the genetic makeup of the person.

Pheontype: the expression of the genotype. Sometimes unless special conditions are present, the genotype may not be observable or manifested as a phenotype.

X Chromosome: "Female" chromosome (XX). The X chromosome can be provided by either the male or the female.

Y Chromosome: "Male" chromosome (XY). The Y chromosome can only be provided by the male.

Karyotype: the chromosome composition of the somatic or body cells.

Mutations: alterations in the chemical composition of genes so new cells produce substances different from those produced by the cells that preceded the mutation. Some are "spontaneous" (meaning unknown etiology), which are rare: and some are due to exposure to x-rays, chemical actions, etc.

Centromere: the palely staining primary constriction on each chromosome which divides the chromosome into two arm lengths.

Sex chromatin, or Barr body: a chromatin mass present in the somatic nuclei of normal females during interphase. Normal males have no Barr bodies. These are thought to be inactivated by X chromosomes. The number of Barr bodies is always one less than the number of X chromosomes.

Autosome: the 22 homologous pairs of *nonsex* chromosomes formed at the union of the sperm and the egg. Because each complement of chromosomes from each parent is a chance assortment of half of each parents' chromosomes, every human is a unique genetic entity. This also leads to an equal or random distribution of an autosomal trait between sexes.

Sex-linked: the gene responsible for a trait is located on an X or Y sex chromosome. This results in an unequal distribution of the given trait between the sexes.

Homozygus: both corresponding genes of a sperm-egg chromosome pair carry a given trait.

Heterozygus: only one gene of a sperm-egg chromosome pair carries a given trait.

Dominant single gene inheritance: when the genetic effect (phenotypic expression) requires only one gene of a sperm-egg chromosome pair to carry a trait.

Recessive single gene inheritance: when the genetic effect (phenotypic expression) requires both genes of the sperm-egg chromosome pair to carry a trait.

Chromosomal Disorders in Man. Those behavioral disorders that have been established to be genetic in etiology can be divided into four major subgroups.
Sex chromosome disorders:

1. *Turner's Syndrome* occurs in one per 3000 to 5000 girls and is characterized by underdeveloped external female genitalia, a small uterus, short stature, webbed neck and usually a lack of ovaries. Often these girls show intellectual impairment but not usually severe mental retardation.

The karotype of these women shows 45 chromosomes with a sex chromosome constitution of XO and there is no Barr body observed. Presumably this is due to nondisjunction of an X chromosome of one parent during gametogenesis.

2. *Klinefelter's Syndrome* is an anomaly of males and is characterized by external male genitalia with small atrophic testes. These men are usually sterile, often have gynecocomastia, sparse body hair, long legs and an increased excretion of gonadotrophin. It has a rate of one per 340 to 500 male births. Mental retardation is usually present but not invariably. The etiology also is presumed to be nondisjunction of an X chromosome, leading to a karotype of 47 chromosomes with an XXY sex chromsome constitution. There is a Barr body present, which is unusual for males.

3. *XYY Karotype* has led to a great deal of controversy because of a suggested link between this karotype and criminality. These men ("supermales") have been characterized as tall, displaying poor impulse control, having disrupted interpersonal contacts and a greater than average sexual drive. If they have criminal histories, the criminality tends toward crimes of violence. The XYY karotype has been demonstrated to have a higher prevalence rate in incarcerated men. Further research, however, has also demonstrated a higher frequency of the karotype among nonincarcerated males.

4. XXX KAROTYPES are females ("superfemales") who are sexually infantile, sterile and amenorrheic. These women have two Barr bodys.

Inborn errors of metabolism:

1. *Phenylketonuria (PKU)* results from insufficient amounts or absence of the enzyme phenylalanine hydroxylase, which oxidizes phenylalanine to tyrosine. As a consequence, phenylalanine is metabolized by alternate pathways and either the excessive unmetabolized phenylalanine or the alternative metabolites alter brain metabolism. The disease can be diagnosed in the infant by detection of phenylpyruvic acid in the urine. Through dietary control (low phenylalanine content), mental retardation can be prevented. Most states in the United States require urine testing of newborns for PKU (Guthrie Test). The incidence is about 1 per 16,000. If untreated, mental retardation appears at about 6 months; the ultimate result is severe retardation. This is an autosomal recessive transmission and persons who are carriers have no clinical manifestations. However, carriers can be detected by their inability to metabolize rapidly test loads of phenylalanine.

2. *Tay-Sachs* disease is a disorder caused by a specific enzymatic deficiency. It has an autosomal recessive transmission, most prevalent in (but not confined to) the Ashkanazi Jewish group from eastern Europe. The disease is characterized by progressive mental deterioration, loss of visual function, cerebromacular degeneration and accumulation of lipid substances throughout the central nervous system. The usual onset is 4 to 8 months with death by 3 years. The infants become hypotonic, display slow developmental progression, and are weak and apathetic. They become spastic with primitive postural reflexes, frequently have convulsions and display progressive mental and physical deterioration. A cherry-red spot in the macula lutea of each retina can be discerned upon examination.

Genetically Transmitted Blood Disorders:

1. *Sickle cell anemia* is a disease confined mostly to blacks whose ancestors originated in the central-costal zones of Africa. The red blood cells have a sickle shape, which apparently promotes a tendency to "clumping" resulting in chronic lifelong illness or death, resulting from a homozygous abnormal hemoglobin (SS). Persons who are sickle cell carriers are much more resistant to malaria than non carriers. In the United States, about .25 per cent of blacks have the disease and about 9 per cent are carriers. The carriers, who have only one abnormal hemoglobin gene (AS) are very susceptible to the hypoxia of high altitudes, indicating that the gene has some partial effect on the hemoglobin molecule. It apparently is an autosomal recessive disorder displaying decreasing prevalence rates as malaria is brought under control.

2. *Hemophilia* is a recessive sex-linked genetic disorder. The responsible recessive gene is on the X chromosome. The disorder occurs almost exclusively in males, but is transmitted from generation to generation by a heterozygus female who carries the responsible gene. The father cannot pass the disease to his son, since the father only contributes a Y chromosome to his son.

Translocation/nondisjunction errors:

1. *Down syndrome ("mongolism")* is characterized by a prominence of the median folds of the eyelids, short stature, stubby hands and feet, and peculiarity of palm prints. Other congenital malformations, (e.g., cardiovascular) may be present.

Mental retardation is present. This condition *represents the single most definable clinical entity causing severe mental retardation.* There are two causes of Down syndrome, which are phenotypically identical. The first type, (trisomy 21) has chromosome 21 represented three times instead of two. This produces a karotype with 47 chromosomes. Apparently this is due to nondisjunction of chromosome 21. The second type apparently is due to translocation of chromosomes 21 and 15. There are 46 chromosomes: the two 21s are normal; one of the 15s is normal; and there is one large unpaired chromosome that is interpreted as a fusion of 15 and 21. While there is no absolute reason why these alterations occur, it is known that they have a higher prevalence in offspring of older mothers; and, there is some relationship to the mother's having been exposed to x-rays within the recent past.

The Inheritability of emotional disorders:

1. *Schizophrenia,* as with intelligence noted above, has a concordance rate between family members that varies with the degree of genetic similarity. Kallman's work demonstrated that monozygotic twins raised together have a concordance rate of 86 per cent and monozygotic raised apart have a somewhat lower concordance rate; however, monozygotics reared apart have a higher rate than fraternals reared together (15 per cent). Other studies suggest concordance figures for monozygotic that range from 50 per cent to 88 per cent. Children of schizophrenic mothers who were raised away from the mother since day three were studied and found to experience significantly more difficulty on a number of relevant variables than did the controls (e.g., total years incarcerated in mental institution was 112 for children of schizophrenics versus 15 for children of nonschizophrenics). Lastly, the degree of relationship to a schizophrenic has an expectancy rate for becoming schizophrenic as follows:

general population	.85 per cent
half sibs	7–8 per cent
full sibs	5–15 per cent
parents	5–10 per cent
children of one index case	8–16 per cent
children of two index cases	53–68 per cent

2. *Manic depressive illness* appears to be the major affective disorder that has a possible hereditary component. Some authors have suggested a 100 per cent concordance rate in monozygotic twins; and postulate evidence for a X-linked, dominant

mode of transmission. Reported expectancy rates are:

half sibs	16.7 per cent
parents of an index case	23.4 per cent
siblings	22.7 per cent
fraternal twins	25.5 per cent
monozygotic twins	100 per cent

3. *Other behavioral complexes* for which there has been some minimal support for a genetic base include:
   various neurotic symptom complexes
   homosexuality
   criminality (discussed under XYY genotypes)
   alcoholism
   In each of these, other factors seem more important than the suggested genetic substrate.

Biochemical Determinants of Behavior

Neurotransmitters are biochemical substances that facilitate transmission of nerve impulses from one neuron across the synapse to the next neuron; or, from neuron to muscle fibers at the myoneural junction. Apparently, they are released from the presynaptic neuron into the synaptic cleft where they are attached to receptors at the postsynaptic site. They may be eliminated from the body through metabolism or they may be taken up by the presynaptic neuron. Their action is very short and different specific types of neurotransmitters are stored in different neurons in different parts of the nervous system. The receptors of neural tissues have a high degree of specificity for specific neurotransmitters. Acetylocholine is the principle chemical mediator at the myoneural junction of skeletal muscles and at the preganglionic synapses of autonomic ganglia. There is also evidence for its role as a central neurotransmitter also. The best recognized neurotransmitters of the CNS are epinephrine, norepinephrine (NE), dopamine (DA), serotonin (5-HT), angiotensin II, and endorphins. The catecholamines are formed by the breakdown of phenylalanine to tyrosine, tyrosine to DOPA, DOPA to dopamine and dopamine to norepinephrine and epinephrine. Other likely central neurotransmitters include histamines and gamma-aminobutyric acid (GABA).

Catecholamines. There is evidence that the catecholamines NE and DA may be important in the pathogenesis of the depressive syndrome. This evidence is based first on the observation that rauwolfia drugs (whose action reduces catecholamines) produce depression in some patients. Second, the mode of action of drugs that are most effective in the clinical management of depression all increase the available NE (and 5-HT) at the receptor sites. More recent evidence suggests that certain depressions may be associated with low NE synthesis and release, and others with low 5-HT. Research on urine surveilance for decreased metabolites of NE and 5-HT to detect altered levels of these neurotransmitters in depressive syndrome persons is ongoing at this time. Additional evidence documents a significantly higher activity level of cathecoholo-methyl transference (COMT) in psychotically depressed versus normal persons. COMT is responsible for the first step in breaking down neurotransmitter substance.

There is strong evidence that the antipsychotic or neuroleptic compounds have antidopamineric effects, but also, all antidopaminergic agents apparently possess antipsychotic activity. This, of course, has led to the "dopamine hypothesis of schizophrenia" which suggests schizophrenics have increased amounts of dopamine at the nerve terminals, increased sensitivity of dopamine receptors, or reduced dopamine antagonists. However, to date no definitive answers have been established.

Indolamines. The suspected role of 5-HT in affective disorders has been noted above. 5-HT has also been postulated to be etiologic of schizophrenia because the hallucinogenic drugs (e.g., LSD) that at first were thought to be "psychotomimetic" (psychosis mimiking) contain an indol nucleus similar to the indolamines. 5-HT's role in the major thought disorders is unclear at this time.

Endorphins. One of the most dramatic developments in the biochemical determinants of behavior has been the documentation of naturally occurring morphinelike peptides in the human body. Three terms have been established: endorphin (used in the generic sense to refer to any morphine-like peptide); beta-endorphin (refers to long pituitary peptides); and encephalin (means the small brain peptides).

The encephalins are present in the brain, spinal cord and intrinsic nerve network of the intestines. They are found in the nerve terminals of short neurons in the manner of other neurotransmitters, and therefore can be released to act on opiate-like receptors located in other nerve cells. Encephalin-containing neurons are clustered along pain pathways where the release of encephalin apparently can inhibit pain messages. Encephalin-containing cells occur in other regions of the CNS that are involved in motor function, mood control, emotions, hormone release, memory storage, etc. These encephalins are destroyed extremely rapidly in brain tissue.

The beta-endorphins are found in high concentration in the pituitary gland, in cells that also contain ACTH (the pituitary hormone released by stress). Beta-endorphin is very stable, with long-lasting effects. There appears to be a system of neurons in the brain (a single cluster in the hypothalamus that send out long processes throughout the brain) that are involved with the beta-endorphin/ACTH substances. These neurons contain no encephalins. Thus, there are two separate neuronal systems in the brain containing morphinelike peptides.

Functionally, it may be that these substances are released as a result of artifical pain used to induce analgesia (e.g., electrical stimulation of the floor of the fourth ventricle and acupuncture). A narcotic antagonist (e.g., naloxone) does block the analgesic effect of either of those two procedures. Because of the close relationship between beta-endorphin and ACTH one could reasonably conclude that the endorphins play a role in the body's reaction to stress.

A number of hypotheses have arisen regarding endorphin dysfunction and behavioral abnormalities. The following have been demonstrated: (1) The endorphins have been demonstrated to inhibit nerve activity and diminish the release of other neurotransmitters like NE and DA. The relationship between endorphins, dopamine and schizophrenia is being addressed at this time. (2) Narcotic antagonist administration to some schizophrenic patients has improved the patients' status under some conditions. The implication then is that excessive endorphin activity might play a role in some major thought disorders. (3) Narcotic antagonist administration to manic-depressive patients had demonstrated some improvement of the manic phase of the illness. (4) A single case study of congenital insensitivity to pain, using a doubly-blind administration of narcotic antagonist versus saline, produced recovery of sensitivity to pain with the narcotic antagonist.

Current *speculation* regarding narcotic addiction involvement with the endorphin system involves the hypothesis that constant external supply of morphine substances suppresses the natural production of endorphins. Withdrawal, then, would be defined as an endorphin deficiency that takes an extended period of time to return to normal functioning level. This would in part account for the long-lasting depression and protracted abstinence syndrome. A second hypothesis concerns congenital endorphin deficiency. Since congenital endorphin excess can be postulated from the case study of insensitivity to pain noted above, it is logical the converse can occur. Such a finding would assist in understanding how some persons can use narcotic substances without becoming addicted; and others report addiction like "craving" behavior from first exposure to narcotic substances.

Physiologic Determinants of Behavior

Limbic System. The limbic system is made up of the phylogenetically older cortex and its associated structures; the hippocampus, fornix, mammillary bodies, anterior thalamic nuclei, cingulate gyrus, septal nuclei and amygdala. This system is arranged into circuits and influences behavioral expression regulated by the hypothalamus. Activities of the limbic system include modulation and coordination of the central processes of emotional elaboration, motivation, establishment of conditioned reflexes and memory storage. The major behavioral correlates of limbic system dysfunction are:

Bilateral lesions of the hippocampus produce profound deficits of short term memory storage.

Patients with irrepressible rage reactions demonstrate spiking on EEG tracings originating from the intraamygdala.

The Kluver-Bucy syndrome of submissive behavior, hypersexuality, visual agnosia and oral exploration of objects (first noted in vicious monkeys after removal of the temporal lobes, uncus, amygdala, hippocampus and the tail of the caudate) has been demonstrated in humans with lesions to the amygdala.

Electrical stimulation of the septal region produces intense pleasurable responses and pain/seizure blockade.

Electrical discharges from the uncus (uncinate fits) are correlated with: olfactory hallucinations of foul odors (feces, burning rubber); anxiety-fear ("empty feeling in the stomach"); jamais vu and/or deja vu.

Reticular Activating System. The reticular activating system (RAS) and its thalamic projections is one of the phylogenetically oldest parts of the brain involved with determining behavior. As noted in the section on consciousness, the RAS is intimately involved in attention. All sensory and motor impulses pass through the RAS as they enter and exit the brain. Functionally the RAS can: through diffuse activation, "prime" the entire brain to process stimuli; facilitate or inhibit sensory and/or motor stimuli; "filter" incoming information; and, facilitate the active process of sleep through inhibition of the midbrain reticular system.

Based on evidence that all antipsychotic preparations have their effect in the RAS and limbic system some theorists have postulated RAS dysfunction in the schizophrenias. In this framework schizophrenia would be seen as the behavioral expression of improper filtration of environmental stimuli. The resultant stimulus influx overwhelms the schizophrenia's cortical function, reflected in the schizophrenic's inability to appropriately cope with the world.

Sensory Deprivation. Sensory deprivation is a physiologic condition presumably tied to activity of the RAS. Sensory deprivation in the laboratory is attained through constant control of visual, auditory, olfactory, kinesthetic, thermal, tactile and gustatory stimuli. When environmental sensory stimuli are decreased and/or removed, apparently the RAS can no longer maintain a homeostatic balance between internal and external reality. In perceptual terms all external frames of reference to interpret cues are absent. The major correlates of sensory deprivation are: profound anxiety; depression and/or hostility (irritability); auditory, visual and tactile hallucinations; depressed level of consciousness and alertness; and extreme stimulus hunger. The basic similarity between monotonous night driving, isolation for "brainwashing" or suggestability effects (stimulus hunger), and sensory deprivation is apparent.

Sleep. Sleep behavior is an active physiologic process. Apparently structures in the lower pons and medulla are responsible for initiating and/or maintaining sleep through synchronization of cerebral cortical rhythms. Presumably these mechanisms act through inhibition of the midbrain reticular system. Sleep is divided into stages reflected by EEG activity.

Stage 1: the EEG is characterized by low voltage-mixed frequency, but most predominate in theta activity (5 to 7 per second). This is the same wave form demonstrated by experienced meditators.

Stage 2: the EEG shows waxing and waning bursts of regular waves called sleep spindles. Sleep spindles are 12 to 14 per second and each spindle lasts 1 to 2 seconds. These are present against a background of low voltage irregular rhythms.

Stage 3: high voltage slow EEG activity is observed.

Stage 4: continuous high voltage slow EEG activity at about 1/second is seen. Night terrors in children apparently are due to arousal from this stage directly into half wakefulness.

Rapid eye movement (REM): the background EEG is indistinguishable from Stage 1, except that bursts of rapid eye movement are recorded. Accompaniments of REM sleep are: Vivid visual dreams approximating hallucinations are reported. Nonvisual dreams (like thoughts running through the mind) occur in other sleep stages; penile tumescence in males from infancy through elderly; Torso EMG disappears and muscles are in a state of total relaxation except for some twitches of fingers, toes and limbs; Sedative-hypnotic medications reduce REM, and withdrawal of these medications results in REM rebound; In the autonomic nervous system (ANS) all measures are at their highest and lowest producing the greatest variability: REM deprivation is correlated with subsequent neural hyperexcitability and decreased electroconvulsive seizure threshold.

Apparently REM sleep interrupts non-REM sleep on an average of every 90 minutes, with the amount of REM sleep increasing during the total sleep period. Over a lifetime, progressively less REM (and less sleep overall) is needed. During a single normal sleep period individuals proceed regularly through consecutive stages of sleep, with few or no full awake episodes during the period. Also with increased age the trend is towards lighter sleep patterns and, therefore, more awakenings are to be expected. CNS depressant drugs like alcohol produce similar effects.

Disorders of sleep other than those noted above include *narcolepsy*, which is characterized by four symptoms: excessive daytime sleepiness; cataplexy, a sudden loss of muscle control and tone, precipitated by strong emotion or excitement; sleep paralysis; and hypnagogic hallucinations. There is evidence for a recessive genetic component in the dysfunction. *Sleep apnea syndromes*, or sleep-induced respiratory impairment, which are characterized by three types: those associated with REM and NREM (type A); those associated with NREM only (type B); and those associated with REM and the transitions from wakefulness to stage 1, and transition to REM (type C). *Drug dependency insomnia*, which results from chronic habitual use of hypnotics and tranquilizers. *Nocturnal myoclonus* sometimes occurring with the "restless leg syndrome." *Circadian rhythm disturbance*, or "jet-lag" occurs due to dissonance between the internal body clock and external time zone. In *phase lag syndrome* the individual has difficulty falling asleep and in *phase lead syndrome* the patient falls asleep and awakens too early. *Pseudoinsomnia*, in which the patient sleeps six or more hours but believes (perhaps dreams) he is not sleeping.

Circadian Rhythms. Circadian rhythms are those cyclic physiologic activities of the body which may have significant influence on behavior. The different rhythms have regulators of two origins. The first are endogenous regulators that arise from within the person. With total isolation from atmospheric and/or other relevant influences, these will continue in a more or less regular fashion. The second are exogenous regulators that originate outside the person. The major exogenous regulators that have been studied to date are the 24 hour light-dark cycle (the disruption of which is responsible for "jet-lag"); chemicals like alcohol, amphetamines and other drugs that can produce

a new pattern to the circadian rhythms; and, stress (emotional/physical) that can disrupt the normative rhythm.

The major circadian rhythms are: sleep-wakefulness period of the 24 hour day, menstrual cycle in women, adrenal steroid secretion, liver enzymes for metabolism, REM-NONREM variations in sleep, body temperature, heart rate, blood pressure, and cell reproduction and sensitivity. The latter rhythm has clinical significance for conventional radiation therapy, in that radiation of some tumors may kill more cancerous cells in the morning than at other times.

Neuroanatomical Sites. Neuroanatomical sites are in executive control of much of human behavior. The left cerebral hemisphere is responsible for verbal abilities (with the exception of a very few right hemisphere dominant persons). Prerolandic areas are correlated with the motor act of speech. Dysfunction here results in motor/Broca's or expressive *aphasia* (synonymous terms). A person with such an aphasia usually is able to understand symbolic communication, but may have difficulty expressing themselves freely in good grammatical form. Postrolandic areas (temporal and parietal) appear to be in executive control of the comprehension of symbolic communication. Lesions here produce sensory/Wernike's/or receptive *aphasia*.

The right cerebral hemisphere in postrolandic areas are correlated with visual-spatial aspects of behavior. Lesions here produce spatial dysfunctions (e.g., inability to follow a blueprint or road map) and construction dyspraxias (the inability to motorically reproduce a visual stimulus). Sensorimotor abilities tend to be under control of the contralateral sensory/motor gyri of the cortex. Audition is primarily contralateral in executive control; although there is an 80 to 20 per cent split of fibers from the choclea to the temporal lobes, with the 20 per cent being represented on the ipsilateral cortex.

Vision is somewhat more complex. *Visual fields* are divided into quadrants. The right half of each *RETINA* (and therefore the left visual field) is represented on the right occipital cortex; and conversely the left half of each retina (the right visual field) is represented on the left occipital cortex. Fibers from the upper quadrants sweep through the temporal lobes and fibers from the lower quadrants course through the parietal region. When corresponding fields in each eye are defective, it is called a homonymus hemianopsia if both upper and lower quadrants are defective. A homonymus hemianopsia implies either occipital lobe dysfunction *or* temporal AND parietal dysfunction in the brain hemisphere *contralateral to the field defect*. Upper-outer field cuts imply temporal lobe dysfunction of the *contralateral* hemisphere. Lower-outer field cuts imply a *contralateral* parietal dysfunction. Bitemporal field cuts imply dysfunction at the optic chiasm (usually tumors of the pituitary gland). Single eye impairment suggests dysfunction anterior to the optic chiasm. Stereognosis is the ability to perceive spatial configuration of objects from tactile sense along. This is characteristically under executive control of the contralateral post rolandic area. Dysfunction in this ability is astereognosis.

Acquisition of Behavior (Learning)

Genetic, biochemical and physiologic determinants of behavior address "inborn" or "natural" events over which the individual has little control. The following discusses behaviors that are either acquired or strongly influenced by "learning."

Learning is defined as the relatively permanent change in a behavioral tendency that occurs as a result of reinforced practice. This definition involves a number of assumptions. First, "change" infers that one can learn *to do* or learn *not to do*. Second, "behavioral tendency" implies that learning is inferred from behavior. Third, practice accompanied by reinforcement is the "cause" of acquisition and maintenance of a change in behavioral tendency.

Reinforcement has the central role in all acquisition of behavior. Reinforcement is a "payoff" and is commonly conceptualized as positive (the person given something which strengthens the response tendency like food, money, etc.) or negative (the person has something withdrawn which strengthens the response tendency (e.g., pain or other discomfort is removed). In addition to the positive or negative dimension of reinforcement is the schedule of reinforcement i.e., the person is placed on either an absolute reinforcement schedule: *always reinforce* every time the behavior occurs, or *never reinforce* when the behavior occurs; usually the latter will extinguish a given behavior, but periodically the extinguished behavior will reoccur "just to see if maybe it will work this time." This is called *spontaneous recovery* or a *partial reinforcement* schedule. Partial reinforcement schedules produce the most stable behavior patterns which are resistant to extinction. The major ones can be diagrammed as follows:

	Fixed	Variable
Interval		
Ratio		

Fixed-interval means reinforcement is available only after a given consistent period of time has elapsed. This produces "bursts" of behavior immediately prior to the time reinforcement is available, e.g., "cramming" for scheduled exams. This yields the fewest responses per unit of time and the least consistent rate of response (4th place).

Variable-interval means reinforcement again is available after a period of time; however, the time period changes e.g., an instructor gives random "pop quizzes." This improves response and consistency rates to 3rd place.

Fixed-ratio improves response and consistency rates to 2nd place. In this mode reward is available after a given constant amount of responding, e.g., being reimbursed $5.00 per 100 stitches sewn.

Variable-ratio schedules produce the highest response and consistency rates. Again, reinforcement is available after the person produces a given number of responses; however, the response rate for "payoff" varies; e.g. playing a slot machine. This partial reinforcement schedule produces high rates of behavior because the person *knows* it's a variable-ratio reward system; therefore, the more responses the sooner the reinforcement will appear. And, maybe the ratio will be smaller "next time."

In addition to the positive or negative dimension and the schedules of reinforcement, two general types of reinforcement have been demonstrated. Primary reinforcements are those that address some type of primary need the organism has, e.g., food, sleep, water, etc. Secondary reinforcers are *learned,* such as money, a smile, verbal approach, job promotion, etc.

As a general rule, the acquisition of behavior is maximal if practice is *distributed* over a series of trials rather than the same number of responses massed into fewer numbers of episodes.

Different types of learning are discussed below. These are ordered in terms of increasing complexity as well as chronological appearance.

1. *Instincts.* Instincts are defined as inborn predispositions to behave in a specific manner when appropriate stimulation is experienced. Today most writers refer to instincts as "primary drives" or "primary needs." While inborn and, therefore, not generally learned, their expression in humans is strongly modified by the milieu. Those instincts central to psychodynamic theories are sexuality, aggression, dependence and death. Other writers include curiosity, nutrition, oxygen and other vegetative functions. Whether called instincts, primary drives or needs, these motivations presumably originate from genetic-biochemical-

physiologic substrates; therefore, while they can be modified in expression (and actually, in some instances, suppressed for extended periods of time) they will recur given appropriate stimulation of the sources or circadian fluctuation.

2. *Imprinting.* Imprinting was considered by Konrad Lorenz to be an innate mechanism, released by a set of stimuli at a critical time in neonates in which the role of reward was minimal which precipitated attachment to a significant parenting person. Lorenz adequately demonstrated the phenomenon in ducks and geese as they "imprinted" him as their "mother." Subsequent theoreticians have linked imprinting in lower animals to "bonding" in human infants. While the analogy is tempting, the reality has not been established.

3. *Classical Conditioning.* Classical conditioning is that form of learning popularized by Pavlov, which is described as stimulus substitution. In classical conditioning, an event that does not produce a given effect is presented immediately prior to an event that will produce the given effect. With multiple paired repetitions, the initial event will produce the given event. That is, the first stimulus (event) has been substituted for the second. A clarifying example is the child who is only brought to the physician for immunizations. The child walks in the door, sees the doctor, is stuck with a needle and begins to cry. With repetition the child begins to cry when the doctor is first encountered. In classical conditioning terms the needle stick is the "unconditioned stimulus (UCS)" that produces the cry, or "unconditioned response (UCR)." The physician is the "conditioned stimulus (CS)" and the cry on seeing the physician is the "conditioned response (CR)." The conditioning is *the new bond* between the physician and the cry. Sometimes not only the physician but the waiting room, the nurse, the word "doctor," the front door of the office and all things associated with the needle stick begin to elicit the same conditioned response of crying. This is called *stimulus generalization* or *stimulus gradient* and is probably the responsible factor for the observation that hypertensive patients produce more hypertensive readings in the physician's office than in their home environment.

Classical conditioning has been demonstrated in all animal life forms from unicellular animals through man (both pre- and post-natal). Classical conditioning is associated with sympathetic and parasympathetic responses of the ANS and therefore is not normally under much cognitive control. There is an optimal time interval of 0.5 seconds separation between the CS and the UCS for the stimulus substitution to occur. Also, the UCS must occur regularly for the behavior to remain stable. If it does not, then *extinction* (weakening, and eventually disappearance of the CR) occurs. If the child does *not* experience the prick of the needle each time the physician is seen, soon the child will no longer cry when the physician enters the room. Heart rate, galvanic skin response, insulin shock and immune reaction are a few of the ANS responses which have been classically conditioned to neutral stimuli like a word or picture.

Classical conditioning is thought to be the basic process by which certain early fears and emotional responses are acquired. Many authors feel the foundations of "psychosomatic" illnesses are laid down in the infant by this process. Presently there is some evidence that the "placebo reaction" maybe a classically conditioned endorphin response.

4. *Operant Conditioning.* Operant (or instrumental) conditioning has had its impact through the scientific, theoretical and philosophical work of B. F. Skinner. Operant conditioning is the production of a given response through environmental reinforcement. The child stops crying and the physician gives the child a piece of candy, or, the medical student diligently studies and receives an "F." Later the same student doesn't study and receives an "A." The student learns to *discriminate* which responses the environment will differentially reinforce and thereafter does not study.

Operant conditioning is the general case of learning and affects all behavior including activity of the ANS system. Biofeedback is a direct outgrowth of operant conditioning. In biofeedback, a person receives positive secondary reinforcement (a light or buzzer is activated for increasing periods of time, a smile or approval from the experimentor, etc.) for controlling a body function (be the function under ANS control or not). The body function that is trained to appear is one that is incompatible with distress. For example, tension headache sufferers are trained to decrease frontalis muscle EMG. Biofeedback has been applied experimentally to a wide variety of medical problems including migraine and tension headaches, hypertension and peripheral circulatory disorders. The technique, however, is still controversial as a therapeutic modality.

In direct opposition to classical conditioning where the UCS (the reinforcement) must always be present to insure stable response patterns, in operant conditioning the reinforcement is present 100 per cent of the time *only* during the response acquisition phase. After acquisition, a schedule of partial reinforcement is instituted to maintain a stable response pattern. For example, parents who want to guarantee that children are disruptive should inconsistently provide approval of the behavior either through interparental inconsistency or only sometimes disapproving it. This partial reinforcement produces behaviors that are resistent to extinction.

Skinner views future social survival as based on rigorously planned environmental reinforcements which will yield adaptive, stable and socially compatible behavior patterns.

A variant of operant conditioning that has been useful in developing certain complex behaviors is *shaping*. In this procedure, successive approximations of a complete behavior are developed through 100 per cent reinforcement, stabilized with partial reinforcement, and then a more complex form is developed, stabilized, etc. For example, an elective mute child first would have sounds developed through 100 per cent reinforcement and stabilized by partial reinforcement; then syllables; then words; then phrases; then sentences; etc. Shaping can also be used to decrease given unwanted behaviors like toewalking; e.g., the child first is reinforced for partial toewalking, then for partial sole walking, then for flat foot walking.

5. *Cognitive Learning*. Cognitive, as opposed to conditioned, learning emphasizes the role of understanding. It assumes the individual is fully aware and attention is focused. Data acquired by classical and operant conditioning may be employed to acquire material through this process.

Piaget and associates have contributed most to elucidating cognitive learning. Piaget emphasized that the cognitive apparatus to understand the world changes dramatically as the human being matures; and the child is *not* a miniature adult. Rather the child at different ages and stages has different capacities to comprehend. The child is moved into more mature ways of understanding through the *equilibration* process defined by two parts. First, *assimilation* means that the child, through *active* interchange with the environment, incorporates data from the external world. The child assimilates data until the extant mental structure can't manage the mass of assimilated data. At this point the second part, *accomodation*, takes place and the mental apparatus changes

to the next more complex structure of cognitive processing and understanding. With this new structure the child assimilates more data until forced to accomodate the mass of assimilated data through a new more complex stage of cognitive structure.

In addition to the equilibration process, Piaget posited that physical maturation, active experience with environment, and social transmission of information were the essential elements for changing cognitive structure. Depreviation of any or all of these was believed to result in less than maximal cognitive functioning.

Piaget posited four stages of cognitive development.

(a) Sensorimotor stage. During this stage (birth to roughly 18 months) the infant employs senses and motor activity to interface with the environment. The focus is coordination of senses and motoric acts. Pure sensations are relied upon, therefore the infant operates on the principle of "out of sight out of mind" (which explains why "peek-a-boo" can be a never ending source of distraction and pleasure for the infant). During this stage the infant moves beyond its body to interaction with the world. Continued practice produces more systematic and well-organized interaction. This sensorimotor period ends with the infant having an active interest in new behaviors and novel events. The infant has shifted from reflex activity to intentional means-ends action sequences, with independent motor systems purposely coordinated.

(b) Preoperational stage. In this stage (roughly 18 months to 7 years) the child relies specifically on perception and "intuition" in thought processes to comprehend the world. However, the conservation of identity of objects is not possible yet. For example, if one of two same sized pieces of clay is elongated it is reported to be "more" or "bigger," etc. than the one that was not altered. The child at this stage can only center cognitive processes on one dimension at a time.

(c) Concrete operations stage. At this time (roughly 7 to 11–13 years) the child begins to abstract commonalities from tangible objects. When the child can see, touch or gain images from objects, similarities between them can be extracted. This child can add and substract elements to or from each other and yet conserve the essence of separate elements. Totally abstract discussions are not possible yet and "reversibility" in thought processes is difficult.

(d) Formal operations stage. This last stage, beginning at about 11 to 13 years, is characterized by the ability to indulge in abstract, conceptual thinking where tangible objects are not necessary for the conceptualization to occur. This individual can think in terms of relations and reversibility. Reflective-conceptual cognitive reasoning and understanding is a reliable process at this stage.

Social Learning. Social learning theories focus on reciprocal interpersonal relations and those behaviors acquired as a result of modeling. The learner observes another person perform an act and models behavior after the observed person. The observer learns without the reinforcement necessary for conditioning type learning. Indeed *vicarious reinforcement* as well as vicarious *extinction* has been observed in children. If a child sees another rewarded for a behavior, the observing child will produce the same behavior and visa versa with vicarious extinction. It is assumed that the intergrated, conforming, social behavior which children acquire is based on observation of either peers being reinforced for producing a behavior or through imitation of parental behavior. The most current controversial issues in social learning are those that involve the influence of media on childrens' behaviors, (most specifically sexuality, aggression and violence observed on television) and peer influence in substance abuse.

While reinforcement (especially primary reinforcement) does not play a truly central role in social learning theories, it is important. Models may provide behavioral roles for others to follow; however, if primary or secondary reinforcement of the newly acquired modeled behavior does not occur, it will soon extinguish.

Growth and Development

In addition to biochemical, physiologic, genetic and learned influences on behavior there is impact from the natural unfolding growth and development process. This process will be presented in two parts: the theories and the phenomenal observations.

Theories. Psychoanalytic theory, associated most with Sigmund Freud and his cohorts, focuses on the *intra*psychic aspects of the mind and psychosexual development. Psychoanalytic theory evolved from observations of emotional pathology and, therefore, extrapolates normal function from pathological condition. Central to psychoanalytic theory is the concept of "libido," defined as "psychic" energy (motivation), and presumed to emanate from tissue metabolism. During "psychosexual" development, this psychic energy, or libido, is invested (concentrated or "collected") in different somatic areas at different stages of maturation. There are five stages:

1. *The oral stage:* (approximately birth to 18 months) during which the child's major source of interest and gratification is the mouth which serves as the major mechanism for exploration of the environment. "Oral receptivity (sucking)" is characteristic of the early portion and "oral aggression (biting)" of the latter portion of this stage. The central psychological "personality" issues involved are trusting others, the relative safety of the world and dependency needs.

2. *The anal stage:* (approximately 18 months to 3 years) in which the anus is the major repository of libidinal energy and the primary source of gratification or pleasure. Personality issues of learning to control (excretory functions), attitudes about authority's rules, saving and spending are considered to eminate from this stage.

3. *The phallic/urethal stage:* (about 3 years to 6–7 years) when libidinal energy is invested in the sexual organs. Activity is concentrated in extension to others and awareness of sex differences. It is at this stage that the Oedipal/Electra complex develops and is (hopefully) resolved.

    Oedipal/Electra complex is a *normal* phase through which all persons develop. It encompasses the child's developing a "love" attachment to the parent of the opposite sex, and a simultaneous desire to "get rid of" the parent of the same sex so the son-mother or daughter-father love can be consumated. Characteristic of this phase is the child's saying to the loved parent, "I want to marry you when I grow up." Successful resolution of this conflict is through the child realizing the same-sexed parent is more powerful; therefore, attempts to "get rid of" that parent may backfire and precipitate dire consequences including for the boy removal of the penis (castration anxiety). To resolve this, the child identifies with the same sexed parent, gives up the opposite sexed parent as a primary love object and says "when I grow up I want to be like my (daddy/mommy) and marry a (woman/man) *like* you."

4. *The latency stage:* (approximately 7 to 12 years) is a period during which libidinal energy is not concentrated in any specific body zone. It is chacterized by same-sex peer relations and avoidance of opposite sex interactions; although, girls seem to be more interested in relations with boys than are boys to girls. Socalization, acquisition of social customs and companionship are major issues.

5. *The genital stage:* (about 12 years to adult) is described by fully integrated, aware activities which involve persons of the opposite sex and include romantic love. Independence from parents, establishment of sexual identification, selecting a spouse and vocational goals should be established during the early portion of this stage.

Throughout this maturational process, difficulty can be encountered through two separate mechanisms. First, *fixation* can occur at a particular stage of development and no progress is made toward increasingly adaptive or mature levels of functioning. Second, normal progression through various stages occurs but during periods of stress, *regression* to an earlier stage of maturity can be observed. This is particularly true if a significant trauma occurred at an earlier stage producing a "weakness" there. In this case normal development may continue but later under stress that is either literally or symbolically similar to the original trauma, the individual regresses to the stage at which the original trauma occurred. Because the original trauma was repressed (forgotten), the individual experiences the anxiety/fear from the original threat without cognitive awareness of the frightening stimulus.

The concepts of conscious, preconscious, and unconscious (as nonphysiologic referents) stem from psychoanalytic theory. *Conscious* means material that is in present awareness of the person (e.g., what is being read at this time). *Preconscious* refers to material not presently in awareness but which can readily be brought to awareness (e.g., one's personal phone number). *Unconscious* refers to material which is not in the person's awareness and cannot be brought into awareness without special techniques like hypnosis or selected psychotropic medication.

In addition to stages of development and levels of consciousness, Freud also posited the pleasure principle, meaning that people seek pleasure and avoid pain. The pleasure principle, modified by experience, is the reality principle which allows for the delayed gratification of needs until an appropriate time.

Freud divided intrapsychic life ("mind") or personality into three conceptual subdivisions: the *ego, super-ego,* and *id.* The ego is that portion which interfaces internal needs with the external reality. It has the most conscious awareness and operates predominantly by the reality principle. The functions that are characteristically assigned to the *ego* are:

1. *Reality:* the relationship to, testing and sense of whether one is operating in the real world or in delusion.
2. *Object relations:* whether one can establish and maintain long term close interpersonal relations with at least one other person.
3. *Autonomous Functioning:* the ability to care for oneself and meet the ordinary demands of living. This includes those "conflict free" such as memory, mobility, vocabulary, etc.
4. *Defensive:* protection of the ego from being overwhelmed by demands from the other sectors of

"the mind." A partial list of ego defensive mechanisms is presented below.

5. *Synthetic:* the ability to integrate data about the self and portions of behavior into a meaningful integrated whole, e.g. "I am a physician."
6. *Identity:* usually refers to sexual identity (maleness/femaleness) or a sense of "who am I?"
7. *Thinking:* those elements discussed above under the process of thought. A helpful mnemonic (memory aid) for ego functions in ROADSIT—comprised of the first letters of each word.

The *id* is the repository of basically unconscious instinctual drives (needs) and impulses. It operates on the pleasure principle and therefore constantly seeks gratification of needs which is unrealistic.

The *super-ego* is the "conscience" or value system that was acquired at a very young age from parenting figures, through introjection and identification. Because it is acquired at an early age in its pure form, it is usually irrational, punative and rigidly understood as a child might. Its function is control of instinctional needs (id), "thou shalt not!"

The unconscious instincts of the id constantly seek gratification and are controlled by ego reality functioning and superego restrictiveness. In order for the ego to function in reality and not be overwhelmed by demands from the id protective mental devices develop called *ego defense mechanisms.* These allow at least partial gratification of instinctual needs. All people have defense mechanisms, but some are more healthy than others. The major ego defense mechanisms are:

1. *Repression: involuntary* exclusion of material (particularly conflictual data) from conscious awareness. Repression is considered to be the basic defense mechanism, operating in conjunction with one or more of the following.
2. *Suppression:* the *intentional* exclusion of material from consciousness.
3. *Introjection:* the total assimilation of the values, attitudes, and prejudices from parenting figures into one's own ego and most specifically the super-ego.
4. *Identification:* while similar to introjection, is less total or complete. It is modeling oneself after another significant other. It can also be the conforming to the values and attitudes of a group.
5. *Displacement:* when the object that will satisfy an instinctual need is changed. For example, a resident physician on the house staff may strike his spouse instead of the attending physician at whom the resident feels rage.
6. *Projection:* the attribution of one's own impulse

and/or thoughts (particularly if they are unacceptable) to another person. This is the mechanism underlying scapegoating, the central core of prejudice.

7. *Reaction formation:* turning an impulse, feeling or thought into its opposite (e.g., persons who cannot accept their own sexual impulses may work as a censor of pornographic movies, thereby, partially gratifying their sexual needs).

8. *Sublimation:* turning "unacceptable" impulses, thoughts, or feelings into socially acceptable ones (e.g., an individual may have murderous rage as a characteristic feeling state, but become a butcher). Sublimation is one of the healthiest defense mechanisms because of constructive end products and elements of conscious decision making involved.

9. *Compensation:* when one encounters failure or frustration in one activity or arena, (s)he overemphasizes another (e.g., an uncoordinated child may overstress intellectual pursuits).

10. *Denial:* the failure to recognize or be aware of obvious and logical consequences of a thought, act, or situation. (e.g, the student who blatantly cheats on an exam while a proctor is observing the student.) This is a rather primative defense mechanism and is almost always pathological in the adult.

11. *Conversion:* the somatic representation of conflicted impulses, feelings, or thoughts. The representation is in body functions under executive control of sensory nerves or voluntary nervous system. Usually, there is secondary gain from a conversion reaction so the symptom is a symbol of the conflict. (e.g., the student fearful of failing an exam may experience paralysis of the dominant hand.) This defense mechanism is the only one which is *always* pathologic because it doesn't facilitate free functions of the individual.

12. *Somatization:* in contrast to conversion, this is the physical expression of conflicts through body parts under executive control of the ANS, both the sympathetic and parasympathetic branches. (e.g., peptic ulcer).

13. *Regression:* the return to an earlier level of maturation or personality development. As noted above, this usually occurs under periods of stress and can be expected to appear in two specific situations: first at the birth of a sibling an older sib may begin to behave below their achieved maturation level; second, patients admitted to hospital characteristically become whining, demanding, dependent, etc. This is a *normal* expected event in illness.

14. *Dissociation:* this is the responsible defense mechanism in "multiple personalities." A group of thoughts, feelings, actions, etc. is split off from the main portion of consciousness, i.e., they are compartmentalized. One personality is "good," the other is "bad."

15. *Rationalization:* offering a socially acceptable and more or less logical reason for an act usually produced by unconscious or nonverbalized impulses e.g., "I was drunk, therefore, I sexually approached my attendings' spouse." The person misleads self as well as others.

Since psychoanalytic theory eminated from observations of and attempts to intervene in pathology some concepts unique to management of patients are important. *Transference* refers to that situation where the patient begins to inappropriately project thoughts, feelings and impulses onto the health care provider which derive from unconscious internal states of the patient. Presumably these are from unmet needs the patient is experiencing. Frequently attendant to transference is the behavior complex called "acting out." Instead of dealing maturely with the transference the patient behaviorally expresses (displaces) the impulses outside of treatment setting. In *countertransference* the health care provider projects personal unmet needs, feelings, and impulses from unconscious processes onto the patient. Frequently there also is "acting out" by the professional with the patient, which ends in a malpractice suit or divorce.

The *psychosocial model* is also psychoanalytic but emphasizes the person in interface with the environment. Eric Erikson postulated eight stages in the psychosocial development of man. Each stage has a "task" for resolution before the next stage can be entered successfully. Defective resolution of a stage forms an inadequate foundation upon which subsequent stages are constructed. The stages and tasks follow:

1. *Trust versus mistrust* (ages 0 to 18 months). To know and feel that the world is intrinsically safe and trustful, the developing infant must have basic needs met appropriately, e.g., the hungary infant must be able to trust that when it cries, it will be fed. There must be continuity between the infant's action and the world's reaction.

2. *Autonomy versus shame and doubt* (18 months to 3 years). In this stage the young child must attain confidence in its ability to operate in the world autonomous of parents or significant others. It must not end this period doubting "it can stand on its own two feet" or ashamed of attempts to differentiate from significant parenting others. Issues of self-control (including bodily functions)

are primary at this stage exemplified by toilet training and the automatic "no" of the "terrible twos."

3. *Initiative versus guilt* (4 to 6 years). Here the child must achieve the ability to initiate independent activities in the world, and effectively carry these iniatives to fruition without others overwhelming the plans. Disproportionate fear (inadequate resolution of the Oedipal/Electra complex) and super-ego anger can combine to form guilt as an inadequate resolution of this stage.

4. *Industry versus inferiority* (6 to 13 years). Industry refers to the child's accomplishments of goals without parental support. The child attends school with peers who are relative equals in ability to produce. If the child, in interaction with these peers without the support of the parenting persons, does not successfully compete, then a sense of inferiority develops which can color the remaining stages of development. This frequently produces in children the overwhelming impression of having nothing to offer others.

5. *Identity versus role confusion* (13 to 18 years). During this phase the young adult experiences extremely rapid physical/endocrine changes and is simultaneously impacted by numerous new environmental influences. The major task is to maintain a sense of personal identity, which includes the establishment of a solid sexual role. The adequate resolution must be "I know me and I can make it as an adult." If in the face of these extreme pressures, the young adult can't establish a sense of "who I am," then adult role confusion develops.

6. *Intimacy versus isolation* (18 to 25 years). With foregoing stages resolved, the adult has the task of developing an intimate, trusting and committed relationship with at least one other person. If by the end of this stage individuals have not established that intimate relationship, a pervasive state of singular isolation is experienced in which persons feel they can neither share their life with nor gain support from others.

7. *Generativity versus stagnation* (25 to 40 years). Generativity refers to both establishment of offspring and the guidance of those children's development; and, entering into an occupational arena where accomplishment and continued growth is feasible. Without developing children as personal extensions of self or opportunities for occupational advancement, individuals find no meaning in life and becomes stagnant. By the end of this stage individuals must take active personal responsibility for themselves. That is, if at age 40 the person still attributes all responsibility for present conditions to parents and early childhood experiences, serious difficulty in adaptation usually occurs.

8. *Integrity versus despair* (40+). During this time persons develop emotional integration, examine their lives and begin to evaluate the status. Hopefully, the individual looks at the past, present, and future and perceives a continuity of which that person is proud. If this examination results in unrectifiable disapproval, despair is the consequence.

In summation, these theories (psychoanalytic and psychosocial) and the concepts that Piaget noted should not be regarded in adversary positions. All three examine different, but complimentary, dimensions of human development. Freud's theory focuses on psychodynamic/psychosexual internal processes, Erikson examines interpersonal or psychosocial issues; and Piaget attends to development of the cognitive mind.

The Life Cycle of Growth and Development. From *conception to birth* a number of variables impact the fetus. Maternal emotional stimuli are reported to result in high levels of ACTH and epinephrine substances in the fetal bloodstream, irritability of the fetus as well as cholic conditions have been observed. Maternal attitudes towards the pregnancy, as well as the number of siblings, predict post partum child rearing practices (Warmth-Coldness: Permissive-Restrictive).

An area of recent concern is maternal psychoactive drug dependence during pregnancy. A *general withdrawal syndrome* in neonates born to mothers who consistently use psychoactive drugs during pregnancy has been documented and a rating scale of severity established. This syndrome can be fatal to neonates if not appropriately managed, with fatality apparently due to pervasive CNS hyperactivity resulting in dehydration and consequent seizure activity. Long-term effects of the general withdrawal syndrome have not been established. Also, the *fetal alcohol syndrome* (FAS) has recently resurfaced as a primary concern. The syndrome has been associated with heavy maternal alcohol consumption during pregnancy. In severe cases the syndrome can include microcephaly, mental retardation, various system abnormalities and stigmata suggestive of Down's Syndrome. To date, an exclusive causal relationship between alcohol and/or its metabolites alone and the described syndrome has not been definitely established, suggesting it may be the result of interaction between alcohol and other idiosyncratic factors.

The utilization of CNS depressant medications and anesthesias to assist the *birth* process is being scrutinized. The most common include inhalation anesthetics, barbituarates, meperidine, "major tranquilizers," and local anesthetics. Most of these drugs may affect the maternal physiology and labor by changing the intrauterine environment; the newborn directly by altering activation of functions that have been dormant; or the neonates' behavior by altering EEG activity level and its behavioral correlates.

Due to these medication issues and suggested "dehumanization" of hospital births, natural or prepared childbirth is being reexamined. Lamaze and Dick-Reed have been major proponents of unmedicated labor and birth, with the father present and providing a support system for the delivering mother. At birth, neonatal function can be assessed by using the Apgar rating system. Assessment is done at one minute and 5 minutes using 5 indicators: heart rate, respiratory effort, muscle tone, reflex irritability and color tone. Each indicator is rated on a three point scale: 0 = no function; 1 = function present, but poor; 2 = function perfect. The 5 minute score in combination with birth weight has the best predictability with the following correlates: 0 to 3 = likely death; 4 to 6 serious subsequent problems; 7 to 9 = later attentional defects and possible learning disability; 10 = perfect functioning (See Chapter 11, Pediatrics).

The major abilities with which the neonates can interact with the world are reflexes. The main primative reflexes are:

1. *Babinski:* when scratched on the lateral aspect of the sole of the foot, heel to toes, the infant responds with dorsiflexion of the big toe and fanning of the others. This response continues from birth to between 12 and 18 months when it disappears in normal children.
2. *Moro:* any sudden movement of the infant's head and neck stimulates a rapid abduction, extension and supination of the arms with opening of the hands. The fingers of the hands adopt a distinctive "C" formation of the thumb and index finger and other digits of the hand are extended. In normal infants the reflex persists until 4 to 6 months of age. The reflex is absent in newborns with diffuse central nervous system depression and other brain stem disorders. Its persistence beyond 4 to 6 months has been associated with mental retardation and brain damage.
3. *Eye blink:* tactile stimulation of eyelashes, tapping the bridge of the nose; a bright light or loud noise provokes the blink response.
4. *Grasp:* palmar pressure causes a grasp response in infants from one to 5 to 6 months of age. A similar response of plantar flexion can be elicited up to 9 to 12 months by pressing an object on the sole of the foot behind the toes.
5. *Crossed extensor:* if the leg of a supine infant is extended by pressure exerted on the knee and the sole of the extended foot stimulated with a sharp object, the result is extension and slight abduction of the unstimulated limb. This reflex normally disappears by 2 months.
6. *Deep tendon reflexes:* the response of striated muscles to sudden stretching is termed a deep tendon reflex. Those characteristically tested in infants are: jaw jerk (C5); biceps (C5-6); radical-periosteal (C5-6); triceps (C6-8); knee (L2-4); and ankle (S1-2).
7. *Suck:* stimulation of the perioral and oral area results in orientation to the stimulus and sucking behavior of the mouth if the stimulus is encountered.

Normative *motor control* in the infant is always individually different and no developing infant is "normal" at all milestones of development. The following are presented as general guides:

1 month: Can lift head briefly
2 months: Can raise chest for brief periods
3 months: Makes stepping motions; can lift the head and hold it above the body plane; and retain a hold on objects.
4 months: Can sit on a lap, look around and display some lumbar back curvature. The hands can be grasped together, played with, and a unilateral open handed approach to objects can be observed.
5 months: Can sit alone briefly and grasp objects in a one hand directional motion.
6 months: Can do knee push or swimmer movements and can get up on hands.
7 months: Can roll over unassisted.
8 months: Can stand with help.
9 months: Can sit alone unassisted and make some progress on the stomach.
10 months: Can scoot backwards and is able to crawl.
11 months: Can stand holding on to furniture. Can grasp an object in each hand and bring them together; and can use the thumb and opposing forefinger to pick up small objects.
12 months: At the end of the 1st year can pull to a stand, walk when led, take and release small objects and place them in containers.
15 months: Can stand and walk alone.
18 months: Can walk forward and backwards, throw a ball, feed itself and use a cup.
24 months: Can hold a pencil and draw with it.

Social behavior development in the infant is characterized by milestones of appearance of selected behaviors. Appropriate *social smiling* appears at about two months. *Stranger anxiety* (a fear response to "non-mother" persons) normally appears between 6 to 12 months (note: this indicates the capability of Piagetian object constancy has developed). During infancy play activity is singular and concentrated in sensorimotor exercise. This moves the infant from reflexive-respondent behavior into controlled-purposive externally directed activity.

Verbalizations by the end of the first two years have reached an average frequency of 200 words. The acquisition of language is from early reflexive laughing and crying to self motivated babbling which appears at about 6 to 8 months. Words as meaningful symbols first appear at about 12 months; however, a range of 1 to 3 years is normal.

Toilet training is not feasible until sphinter control has developed at between 1.5 and 2.5 years. This is contrary to data that many American parents "toilet train" their children between 9 and 14 months. Essentially, if a child is "toilet trained" prior to 18 months, it is the "mothering person" who has been trained to observe when elimination is imminant and consequently rushes the child to the "potty". In the later stages of infancy the *"terrible twos"* appear in which the child responds with *"No!"* to any request. This behavior is the reflection of the infants initial attempts to establish autonomy and reflects entrance into Erikson's second stage.

During the latter stages of infancy and extending into the first preschool year, the gender identity is established. Dependent upon how parents and significant others interact with the child, he or she establishes the basic feeling of being male or female. This feeling is learned and set by age 3 years.

Major problem areas with infants include maternal deprivation which may precipitate the infants withdrawal from all social interaction. If no mothering substitute is provided the infant can enter an extremely withdrawn condition known as *marasmus* and die. Institutionally raised children display milder but similar withdrawn characteristics; and, while they may not die, their ability to form close interpersonal relations in later life is seriously compromised, they are unresponsive, and demonstrate retardation in cognitive, language and motor development. In addition to maternal deprivation, highly nervous mothers have a higher prevalence rate of infants who demonstrate behavioral dysfunctions, such as sleep disorders, irritability, hyperactivity, feeding disorders and prematurity.

During the *preschool age* (2 to 5 years) psychomotor maturation involves gross and fine motor skills development and handedness is typically established.

Parental childrearing attributes seem to be most in-fluential here. The Warmth-Cold and Restrictive-Permissive dimensions in parental childrearing practices are correlated with characteristic behavior patterns in children. This relationship is characterized in the following figure:

WARMTH, AFFECTION, LOVE	
Creative	Obedient
Spontaneous	Other Centered
Independent	Self Controlled
PERMISSIVE	RESTRICTIVE
Belligerent	Dependent
Rebellious	Not a "free thinker"
Selfish	
COLD (HOSTILE)	

Play activities progress to "parallel play" in which two children are in close physical proximity; however, each is playing alone with its own toys and games. The only reliable interaction is one child taking a toy from the other, precipitating a relatively violent interchange.

During preschool years the child is extremely egocentric with all understanding of events in the external world being referred to the self for causal relations; e.g., "the sun came up because it's time for me to get up." Serious problems often arise from this egocentricity. If parents argue and/or divorce during this stage, the child may assume personal responsibility for that event; e.g., "my daddy left because he doesn't like me."

In these first 5 years, *language* has fully developed and that progression is presented here as a cohesive whole process. The structure of language is roughly divided into phonemes, morphemes, syntax and semantics. A *phoneme* is the smallest possible unit of language identifiable as a discrete sound, e.g., in the word "pot," the p (written |p|) is a phoneme; and, the "k" sound of both words "cow" and "keep" is the same phoneme (|K|) even though the two words are spelled differently. A *morpheme* is comprised of several phonemes and is the smallest linguistic unit that can have independent meaning. The word "apples" has two morphemes: (1) "apple," and (2) the "s" which makes it plural. *Syntax* is the rules by which people speak and understand a language. Syntax or grammar rules specify how morphemes are connected to produce meaningful units like phrases and sentences. *Semantics* is the inherent meaning (frequently involving emotional attachment) which is assigned to a particular piece of syntax. It is in this portion of language that major communication difficulty arises between persons, particularly if they are from different backgrounds. For example, the meaning of the word *white* is different depending upon one's skin color (e.g., black, red, white or yellow), occupation (artist versus bleach manufacturer), etc.

Acquisition of language is interpersonal and represents an interplay between developmental process and the milieu within which a child is raised. Developmentally, prior to age six months infants produce random sounds which are used in every known language. These sounds are identical regardless of the infant's nationality, and are probably due to neuromuscular development of the throat and mouth. Apparently during the 6th to 12th month, when selfmotivated babbling appears, selective reinforcement by significant others shapes the infants babbling into characteristic national language. The first words to appear are nouns, next are verbs, third are adjectives, and finally pronouns. Between ages 1 and 2 years the phrases and sentences are simple and may be only one word, e.g., "water." Between 18 months and 2 years, the utterances become longer, with brief phrases and rudimentary sentences being assembled. By age 5 adult syntax (including past tenses, plurals and active as well as passive sentences) is established. Severly retarded persons are very slow to develop speech; however for the normal and higher intellect persons, there is not correlation between the rapidity with which children talk and intelligence.

Issues in language development as influences on behavior include most specifically minority-majority issues. The majority of social institutions in America are white, Anglo-Saxon, and Protestant (WASP). Children who are not from a WASP background have been raised in a cultural milieu which may have different syntax than WASP, and/or may assign a semantic meaning to the WASP syntax which is at variance with WASP language. The result is that a minority child entering a majority school must become semantically bilingual and live in two different semantic worlds (the one of school and the one of home) in order to progress in WASP educational structure. Majority instructors frequently do not recognize this variance; therefore, when using a specific WASP word or phrase in the presence of a minority student, two things may occur: the student translates the word to and from minority semantics which gives the appearance of the student being slow; and/or the student may display a different emotional reaction to the word than the instructor expects, and therefore seem "strange" or "crazy."

By the time the child has reached *school age* (6 to 12 years) psychomotor development is complete and play activities have developed to a phase of cooperative interactional activity. In Erikson's framework, industry and adequacy in peer relations are of foremost importance. The beginning school years are when the child leaves the primary influence of parents and enters the control sphere of other adults (teachers) and peers. Typically, there is eager anticipation towards school

entry which lasts for the first two years. The relationship which children develop with teachers can be predicted by the child's relation to parents, i.e., there is generalization between parents and teachers. Physical handicaps, eye-hand motor coordination difficulties, learning disabilities, perceptual problems, hyperactivity, etc., can become barriers to adequate school performance which in turn will impact the child's feeling of adequacy. Research suggests that males, children from lower classes and children from minority groups (particularly if they also form a minority in the school) have a more difficult time adjusting to the WASP school situation characteristic of American public education.

During this stage, increased sexual exploration of self (masturbatory activity) and others is normal. Because this age group is also characterized by same-sex interpersonal relations, same-sex sexual activity is also normally expected.

Sex role differences which began to appear in the previous stage are further defined and refined. Children learn at this time to regulate and sometimes to totally inhibit natural emotions. For instance, male children are taught not to cry ("big boys don't cry") i.e., not to demonstrate sad feelings; however, they are groomed to display aggressive, angry, hostile emotions. Conversely, female children learn that crying is perfectly permissible but "nice girls never say 'damn'." As a consequence of this sex role training, males often display anger when in fact they are sad, and females often cry when angry. Fortunately, several of the issues described above relating to language development, physical handicaps, physical orientation and sex role differences are being perceived by educators and are being corrected.

Child abuse sometimes occurs during infancy, preschool and subsequent school age phases. Child abuse encompasses neglect, active physical trauma, and sexual abuse. Each state in the United States has laws against child abuse, which both require physicians to report suspected child abuse, and protect the physician from retaliatory acts. According to the National Center on Child Abuse and Neglect and other researchers, characteristics of the parent reported for abuse of their children include: the parents themselves were abused children; the parent seldom looks at or touches the child; the family is isolated (unlisted phone number, no social club memberships, cannot be located, seem to trust no one, do not participate in school activities or events); the parents expect or demand behavior beyond the child's years or abilities; they don't care for the physical hygiene of the child; the parents over- or underreact to the child's condition; they appear to be misusing alcohol or other drugs; and they are over-critical of the child. These parents perceive the child's expression of needs as being purposeful acts of frustration and irritation to the parent; e.g., a hungry child cries at night and the parents say "that child won't let me sleep." They are reluctant to give information about the child's injury or condition and are either unable to explain injuries or offer illogical and/or contradictory information. They appear to lack control or at least they fear losing control.

Characteristics of the abused or neglected child include obvious welts or skin injuries; clothes inappropriate for the weather; severely abnormal eating habits (e.g., eating from garbage pails and drinking from toilet bowls) and begging or stealing food; and, exhibiting extremes of behavior from aggression to extreme passivity/withdrawal. While these children appear overly mature, they also seem unduly afraid of parents. They generally cause trouble with peers, are wary of any physical contact, and are apprehensive around other children who are crying. They frequently engage in vandalism, sexual misconduct, use alcohol, and use drugs. Often these children need glasses or other medical attention, show severely retarded physical growth, and are often tired and without energy.

The onset of *adolescence* (12 to 17 years) this period is introduced by the onset of puberty: menstruation for females and seminal emissions for males. At puberty there is a physical growth spurt accompanied by radical endocrine shifts that control the onset of secondary sex characteristics (distribution of body fat, pubic hair, voice changes, facial hair in males, etc.). This endocrine shift also provides the overwhelming sexual drive observed in this phase. Females have an earlier onset of puberty than males; and there is evidence that onset of menses is occurring at younger ages with the average age at 12.5 years and the range of 10.5 to 15 years. Sperm production in males begins at about 14.5 years with a range of 12.5 to 16.5 years. Both masturbatory and interpersonal sexual activity heightens during this phase. Each year in America there are approximately 30,000 pregnancies to females under the age of 15 years old, and 1,000,000 to females between 15 to 19 years old. As a result, teenage marriages frequently occur, fifty per cent of which are because of pregnancy. While some of these are extremely stable and endure, one third end in divorce within four years.

During adolesence, a major achievement is for the young person to separate from the dependent role with parents. Cognitively, adolescents can meaningfully ask the question, "why are things like they are," but, because they have not fully developed delay of gratification, they want changes in perceived inequities *now!* In this constellation, the adolescent is faced with the necessity of separating from the parents, requiring affectional and emotional support needs, being associated with peers who share the perceived inequities and can supply the support system. This configuration in combination with the adolescent's perception of personal invulnerability contributes to: high levels of illicit substance abuse; accidents being the leading cause of death among white teenagers (National Center for Health Statistics, 1977); suicide being the third leading cause of death (National Center for Health Statistics, 1977); crimes of violence peaking in incidence at the 15-year-old age range; and, homicide being the leading cause of death of black youth.

Throughout the above stages, moral development has also been maturing along with other psychosexual, psychosocial and cognitive abilities. Dependent upon social model transmission, cognitive ability development and other issues, by the end of adolesence and entering into young adulthood, the individual should have reached a high level of moral sophistication. As with all developmental phases, persons may become fixated at one level or regress under special conditions of internal or external stress. Kohlberg provided the following framework for understanding moral development:

Stage 1: Punishment and obedience orientation. The physical consequences determine "goodness' or "badness." "It was bad because I got punished."

Stage 2: Instrumental relativist position. An action is right because it satisfies my needs.

Stage 3: Interpersonal concordance. Good behavior is that which pleases or helps others and is approved by them.

Stage 4: Orientation to authority. Respect for law, authority and order for its own sake.

Stage 5: Social contract orientation. Laws are agreements or contracts; and the contracts are what make right and wrong. Contracts are changable.

Stage 6: Universal ethical principal orientation. Universal principals of justice prevail, e.g., taking another's life is wrong.

In Erikson's framework, the major tasks during the *young adult* period (18 to 35 or 40 years) are developing an intimate relation and establishing oneself in an occupational position. An intimate relationship in the United States usually implies love and, according to Maslow, this is either "B" love or "D" love. "B" love is that which is based on each individual feeling personally secure, a full "genital" character in psychodynamic framework. These persons like themselves, feel complete individually and have an appreciation of "being." From this security and well being, two persons choose each other to share their life and create children from the union. Within this nuclear family there is a maximum of respect for individuality with no ulterior motive to change the other person. Children in these families are guided through warmth and permissiveness towards self-discovery and maximizing individual potential. "D" love is deficient love. In this framework each person comes to the relationship out of perceived personal deficit and selects the other to fill the missing characteristic in the self. Such marriages frequently have an ulterior motive to alter the other person after the marriage is established. Children in these nuclear families are acquired to fulfill needs the parents have, (e.g., to be an "average" family, to hold the marriage together, so the mother has "something to do," etc.). Such arrangements dynamics predispose a nuclear family to later difficulties when the marriage partners can't or won't meet each other's needs and/or the children leave the home.

The resolution to the second part of this Eriksonian phase, occupational choice, and particularly professional choice, is frequently based on irrational decisions. Early childhood or adolescent experiences often shape a premature decision which is retained as an irrevocable law. Sometimes persons enter a particular field due to familial or other social pressures ("all the women in this family have always been nurses") and maintain in their training "until. . . .". Unfortunately "until" never comes and these persons frequently shift jobs at middle age. Terkel described four aspects of work. It influences the conception a person has about self and the surrounding world. It is used as a social locator. It can provide a source of power and autonomy. It can be a source of major frustration and devaluation. In the United States there is a work ethic that values and promotes productivity. While this orientation provides solid base to the economy, it creates considerable difficulty for youth who can't produce and the elderly who are forced into idleness at retirement age, particularly with regard to the first three of Terkel's items. Since socioeconomic status is based on income, education and occupation, the young and old clearly fit a nonvalued lower socioeconomic status "label."

A major complicating factor which develops for young adults is forced incompatibility between marriage partners in Erikson's psychosocial context. Because extended family structure in the United States is no longer the rule, each new nuclear family must quickly establish its own independent existence. This forces the husband to be preoccupied with work (generativity) leaving the wife to raise the children and be the major source of warmth and intimacy. By the later part of this stage, the husband frequently has established himself occupationally and wants to return to

the family for the intimacy he has foregone while "becoming a success." However, the wife has "run out" of intimacy and wants to begin her generativity. This decrease in extended family dependence and psychosocial incompatibility is probably responsible for the observed increase in American divorce rates (40 per cent in 1977 and the rate is increasing at about 5 per cent per year). About 1.5 million families in the United States have a separated or divorced person as head of the family; and, those families involve 2,365,000 children, 90 per cent of whom live with their mothers. This condition, coupled with data presented earlier regarding sex role acquisition, egocentricity of youth, etc., provides a situation in which youth can become confused in identity, assume responsibility for the divorce of parents and, in frustration, act out maladaptively. Whether the increase in the number of wives entering into the work-force over the past decade will alter these astounding data remains to be seen.

As individuals enter the *middle years* (40 to 60 or 65) regardless of their previous occupational role (housewife or financial provider), they encounter the "career clock" phenomenon. They critically review accomplishments to date, reexamine the reasons for entering the role and evaluate whether things should remain as they are. Frequently the occupational, marital, social and a geographic status changes at this point because of no wish to carry through previous decisions that are inappropriate at this time. Others evaluate their present situations, find them unacceptable yet do nothing to alter them, resulting in a subsequent life of desparation. Others evaluate, are happy with their present state and continue with an integrity between previous, present and anticipated future life style. During this time, sex role stereotypes are better modulated, prejudices are relaxed and overall tension levels reduced. Consistently, this age range is reported as the most gratifying for the majority of persons.

On the negative side, women who have overinvested in their children sometimes develop the "empty nest syndrome" and frequently experience a rather severe depressive episode when the last child is gone. Men at 45 to 54 years old are at the peak of their earning power and careers; consequently stress syndromes (e.g., gastrointestinal distress, myocardial infarctions, hypertension) may become manifest. Divorce also may occur due to waiting "until the children are grown" or to both persons being required to deal with each other rather than through the children.

The technocracy in the United States has provided a socioeconomic climate which has drawn attention to the *elderly* of America. In this focus on the elderly, a number of myths have been generated. The most popular are:

1. The elderly live alone in nursing homes. The reality is that 5 per cent of elderly live in residential institutions; 60 per cent own their own homes; and, between 65 and 80 per cent live with someone else.

2. The elderly are asexual. Realistically, 70 per cent of elderly males and 20 per cent of females report active sexuality. The disparity between males and females probably reflects the fact that males marry younger females and have a shorter life expectancy; therefore, more females are left without a sexual partner in later life.

3. The elderly are senile. While senility does have some correlation with plaque formation in the CNS, the major determinant of senility is social isolation, forced inactivity and lack of insignificant interpersonal involvement. One needs only consider Albert Einstein to realize age *per se* has little to do with senility.

The realistic issues with which the elderly are confronted are multiple.

1. *Mental Processes:* as persons age, two significant changes occur. First, reaction time slows. As a consequence, because quick sensorimotor reactions are the basis for performance items on most intelligence tests, there is an apparent but illusionary decrease in IQ as persons age. Second, new or recent memory seems to be attenuated while remote memory is unimpaired. This results in older persons "boring" younger adults with repetition of remote data. However, young children are fascinated with these recollections as they are with the retelling of fairy tales. While these acquisitional problems are relative and not absolute, (older persons can and do learn) it does take longer for them to acquire new data.

2. *Fixed income:* 15 per cent of American elderly are living on poverty level, fixed incomes which makes them most vulnerable to fluctuations in national economics.

3. *Chronic health conditions:* 85 per cent of the elderly have at least one chronic health problem: twice as many are likely to be hospitalized; medicare meets about 50 per cent of total health care costs; 14 per cent need assistance in their homes; 50 per cent of the blind are 50 years old or older; 25 per cent of all prescribed drugs are consumed by the elderly; and, 15 per cent of the elderly make serious errors in the consumption of prescribed medication, mainly due to the recent memory problems (forgetting if and when they took medications).

4. *Nutrition:* nutritional deficiencies affect about 10 per cent of the elderly due to fixed income and rising food costs; if they live alone, they loose interest in preparing food and eating; compromised access to food based on transportation problems listed next.

5. *Transportation:* the breakdown of extended families has led to the elderly being excluded from regular travel previously provided by their children. Health problems may limit the ability for the elderly to drive; and, inadequate or expensive public transportation further limits mobility.

6. *Inactivity:* enforced idleness due to mandatory retirement with financial penalities for earning extra money; lack of mobility; and, decreased social contacts as friends and relatives of the same age die. The people who successfully age are those who actively planned for retirement, continue activities of the middle years, maintain an active social involvement and provide themselves with continued growth experiences. The best predictor of successful aging is a good IQ, higher education, and how active and intergrated the individual was prior to onset of the rapid aging process.

Interpersonal and Small Group Determinants of Behavior

Group Dynamics. When an individual interfaces with one or more person(s), the needs of the single individual are placed in a context of the needs of the other(s). Usually in such a setting no single individual's needs are completely met. Group size dictates some basic influences on human behavior. Two interacting people (a dyad) have an opportunity to devlop intimacy and resolve differences when lack of concensus develops. Three people (a triad) are involved in a more complex issue in that relations must be maintained at less than an intimate or dyadic level to avoid exclusion of one person. If dyadic intimacy does develop between persons in groups larger than two, priorities must be clearly established; e.g., children in a family must understand they cannot destroy the marital bond and be the primary intimate object for one of two parents. Likewise, parents must align solidly together for the child to mature appropriately. Triads always have the potential to move into the "drama triangle" where the roles of persecutor, victim and rescuer are stable; but persons in the triangle assume different roles at different times. When more than three people interact members tend to subdivide and form relations to at least one other person in the group which are affiliative (attraction) and differentiating (repulsion). The affiliations and differentiations occur along multiple dimensions (sex, age, race, ethnicity, occupation, socioeconomic status, etc.) as well as various combinations. These dimensions of affiliation and differentiation within a group frequently get superimposed upon the nature of the group.

The nature of the group is defined as whether the group has an end product, task or goal (task oriented group), or whether it assembles to support a given identity (sentient group) with no task or goal product expected.

Related to these affiliation-differentiation and task-sentient dimensions is the focus of the group, i.e, does the group focus on the *content-decision* issue of a topic (which is more characteristic of task groups) or does the group focus on the *process* of how things are occuring? Typically these content-process issues are always ongoing but difficult to attend to simultaneously. A neurosurgical team doing surgery is a *task group* focused on content decision outcome issues. The outcome may be less acceptable if all team members are in the *process* of undercutting the other members' effectiveness. That same team later in an informal setting discussing the outcome of the surgery, "rehashing" how well everyone performed and sharing personal feelings with each other, transforms to a sentient group which is process oriented and no tangible product is expected.

Leadership. Leadership is tied to the nature, focus and needs of the group. Leaders are typically polemically divided into authoritarian or democratic styles. Democratic leaders provide a setting in which group members are true contributors to decision making. Their groups perform consistently, display high morale and produce when the leader is absent. They perceive themselves as an integral part of a whole. Authoritarian leaders have groups which have sporadic high performance when the leader is present, but when absent production diminishes noticeably. Typically, in a group that is product oriented but led by an authoritarian person who makes all meaningful decisions, the group concerns itself with irrelevant process issues or incidental content items. This group is not productive either in a task oriented or a sentient support sense.

Group needs and the consequent expectation by the group of the leader interact with the relative maturity of the group. Rioch has defined these issues in Table 14-1. Leaders who attempt to fulfill the fantasy demands of an immature group or who approach leadership from the fantasy/immature posture generally fail and the group either ostrasizes the leader or deteriorates in functioning.

Destructive Issues. Other destructive variables to internal group structure are competition and aggression. Both of these variables not only interfere with group performance but in some instances also dissolve the extant group. The group, however, can extrude the offending member(s), close the group to the extruded person(s) and gain solidarity by closed rank resistance to attempts from the extruded person(s) to

TABLE 14-1. Group Expectations

Group need	Group Expectations of Leader	
	Fantasy-Immature	Mature
Dependency	Omnipotence	Dependable
Fight-Flight	Unbeatable	Courageous
Pairing/		
Affiliation	"Marvelous unborn"	Creative

either rejoin or further destroy the group structure.

Group as a System. A basic assumption underlying large and small groups is that a group is a relatively rigid closed system that is tightly interdependent. Any alteration in the system (a person entering, exiting or changing) requires compensatory alteration in another person in the system to maintain stability.

Families can be viewed as such systems in which there are extremely stable roles that are resistant to change; however, the individual who fills a role can be variable; e.g., the mothering role can be assumed by any family member. This role stability and resistance to change exists regardless of the relative functional adaptability or health of the family. Attempts to enter or alter the structure are either resisted or the system structure of the family group must change.

Family systems characterized by inclusion factors have changed considerably in the recent past. A *nuclear family* is a unit of procreation (mother, father and children). *Extended families* are those in which there is inclusion of more than one unit of procreation; e.g., grandparents, parents, grandchildren, great grandchildren, aunts and uncles. As a general rule, in America today most families are nuclear with only loose ties to other familial procreative units. This weakening of bonds in extended family units has serious implications for a support system for orphaned, single, older or new family members. Previously, new marriages in an extended family could rely on that system to provide support while the new family stabalized. Now new marriages must establish a stable nuclear family in an extremely short period of time.

Assessment of Behavior

Observation of specific aspects of human behavior has been standardized into formal and consistent samples called psychological tests. Because these are standard observations, normative data has been collected about performance of people. Consequently, any one person's performance can be compared to the norms and statements about that person's relative standing on a particular variable can be made. Normative data comprising the sample against which an individual's score is compared can be collected by selecting people *randomly* (everyone in a given population has an equal opportunity to be selected for the sample) or through stratification of the sample. That is, the sample is constituted to reflect relevant variables in the over all population, at the rate the variables occur in the overall population (e.g., including the per cent of Eskimos in the sample which reflects the rate of Eskimos in the population). The major types of psychological tests are described below. While some are administered in a group fashion, individualized assessment is always more valid.

Developmental Scales. These are standard observations of the psychomotor/social development of infants and children. For example, the Denver Developmental Scale is applicable from birth to six years old, and provides data on gross developmental progress in personal-social, fine motor, language and gross motor areas. The Vineland Social Maturity Scale is a standard interview (usually with the parent) about a child's socialization level that can be applied from birth to maturity.

Intelligence Tests. These are psychological tests that presumably reflect the concept of intelligence presented earlier. An intelligence quotient (IQ) is derived by one of two methods. The first is the mental age concept where a mental age (MA) score is derived from a standard test. That MA is divided by the person's chronological age (CA) and multiplied by 100 to yield the IQ. The formula is $MA/CA \times 100 = IQ$. The Stanford-Binet Intelligence Test is an example of this process.

The second method of IQ derivation, called the deviation IQ, is exemplified by the Wechsler scales (Wechsler Adult Intelligence Scale) for those 16 years old and older and the Wechsler Intelligence Scale for Children for those under 16. The IQ is derived from age subgroup norm tables and therefore age-related factors that might contaminate scores are controlled. The Wechsler tests provide a verbal IQ (VIQ), a performance IQ (PIQ), and a full scale (FSIQ). The separate verbal scales that are combined to obtain the VIQ are information (general fund of knowledge); comprehension (social judgement); arithmetic (mathematical ability); similarities (ability to abstract commonalities from objects of a class); digit span (rote recall forward and backward); and, vocabulary (general vocabulary level). The timed performance scales that are combined to obtain the PIQ are digit symbol (a coding task); picture completion (visual recognition of incomplete data); block design (psychomotor reproduction of progressively more complex visual geometric designs); picture arrangement (visual appreciation of non-verbal social judgement situations); and object assembly (recognition of a gestalt from diverse parts of an object). The Verbal and Performance scales are combined through norm tables to prove the FSIQ. IQ tests tend to be highly correlated with adequate education. Also the norms on IQ tests tend to be nonhandicapped "WASP" biased; therefore, one must carefully interpret test results if the person examined is non-"WASP", poorly educated or has a physical or mental handicap.

Achievement Tests. These are norm-based assessments which usually have been established on stratified representative national samples. They purport to reflect the amount an individual has "learned" or accomplished. The National Board of Medical Examiners tests are examples, as is the Wide Range Achievement Test (WRAT). The WRAT has subdivisions of reading, spelling and arithmetic with national norms applied from preschool through high school years.

Aptitude Scales. Ability or aptitude tests are those attempts to assess "native" endowment in areas like creativity, musical and artistic aptitude, and psychomotor coordination and speed.

Interest Tests. Scales like the Strong Vocational Interest Inventory were empirically derived by administering many diverse items to persons who were successful and satisfied in different occupations. Those items to which persons in a given vocation responded uniquely were combined into a scale. Persons who answer items in a similar manner are presumed to be good candidates for that vocation. In such empirical derivation, it is not necessary that item content have "face validity" (make sense).

Personality Scales. These tests presume to assess dimensions of stable intra and interpersonal interaction patterns. They are typically subdivided into objective (empirical) versus subjective (projective) tests:

1. The Minnesota Multiphase Personality Inventory (MMPI) is the best known *objective* test. It is objective in that it was derived from empirical analysis and not theory. The MMPI has hundreds of true-false psychiatric symptom-related questions which are scored on ten clinical scales and three validity scales. It is not a true personality inventory because the clinical scales presumably reflect the relative absence or presence of psychopathology but not underlying personality dimensions.

2. The Meyers-Briggs Inventory is an *objective* personality scale based on Jungian theory. The major dimensions reflected by this test are:
   Extroversion-Introversion
   Sensation-Intuition
   Feeling-Thinking

These, in combination, yield 8 "types", which are personality descriptions, not degrees of psychopathology as with the MMPI. Norms are available for an individual's "type" as well as "type" compatibility in some special professions.

The projective or subjective personality tests are those derived from personality theories and based on the projective hypothesis. The *projective hypothesis* states that given an ambiguous stimulus, people will structure the ambiguity according to their own needs and personality. The clinician analylizes responses to the ambiguous stimuli and infers internal needs and underlying dynamics. The major projective tests are the Rorschach ("ink blot" test), which is associated more with unconscious intrapersonal dynamics; and the Thematic Appreception Test (TAT), which consists of ambiguous pictures of different persons and objects in vague settings about which the person creates a story. Again, the examiner infers from the stories the underlying personality needs. The TAT reflects more interpersonal dynamics although some intrapersonal data can be obtained. There is a Children's Appreception Test (CAT) similar to the TAT which involves animals instead of humans in the poorly structured pictures. Other projective tests are the Draw-A-Person (DAP) and the Sentence Completion Test (e.g., Right now I feel —————).

Neuropsychological Tests. These are psychological instruments sensitive to cerebral (most specifically cortical) dysfunction. The Bender-Gestalt (a test of graphic reproduction of nine rather simple geometric designs) has been used for this purpose. The Halstead-Reitan battery (combination of many different tests) has a long research and clinical history of proven utility in reflecting specific brain-behavior relationships. The Luria scales currently show promise in this regard. With biomedical advances (e.g., CAT scans), the utility of these as primary differential diagnostic tools has decreased; however, they are helpful as noninvasive techniques for documenting relative progression of dysfunction and/or relative recovery of function after cerebral insult. They are particularly meaningful in those situations where structural lesions are not present and other biomedical procedures cannot detect disease progression, e.g., posttraumatic syndrome and it's legal sequelae.

PSYCHOSOCIAL ISSUES IN HEALTH CARE DELIVERY

The following section addresses generic topics that have surfaced as major areas of concern in delivery of health care. They represent the interface between internal psychological/biological processes and social efforts to exert control of them. For clarity, they have been divided into those issues associated with the patient versus those associated with the health care delivery system. However, in reality the issues are present

for both the patient and the physician at all times in an interactive process.

Issues Associated With The Patient
Sociocultural Influences. The sociocultural milieu in which the patient is immersed defines for the patient what behavior is "normal", allowed or sanctioned against, how expression of allowed behavior is permitted and how the patient can attend to illness. The cultural subgroup to which the patient belongs establishes the rewards, and through application of those rewards controls behavior. While the term *minority* means a group which has less representation in the United States population, in the past it has been used to connote a value judgement of "weak" and "inferior" or "bad". It has been most specifically applied to ethnic subgroups and has provided the basis for prejudice and negative discrimination. In health care delivery this has resulted in at least two classes of health care delivery: that applied to the majority (which tends to be private fee for service or private health insurance); or that delivered through a public health service model which is government subsidized and usually not considered to be as adequate or "caring" about the patient.

Attitudes, beliefs, prejudice and values are at the core of the psychosocial issues in health care delivery.

Beliefs are the cognitive information an individual has about an object. The belief may or may not be based in fact; and varies in strength from an opinion (a lightly held belief) to a strong belief for which a person may die; e.g., "woman and children first."

Attitudes are the evaluative (good-bad) *and* affective aspects of responses toward a given object or situation. There are two basic components to an attitude: first, a belief portion and second, an affective part; e.g., not only must a physician believe that the medical profession is worthwhile but also that physician must enjoy a positive feeling from the practice of medicine.

Prejudice is an attitude that is harmful and based upon the distortion of some small element of truth; and usually is directed towards a subgroup of people. The distortion involves overgeneralization, oversimplification, alteration of reality and employs the phenomenon of *scapegoating*. In scapegoating, the defense mechanism of projection is used to project onto the victim qualities about which prejudiced persons are unconsciously ashamed or afraid in themselves. The case against the scapegoat must be justified by some vices that are attributed (correctly or incorrectly) to the scapegoat; the scapegoat must be weak enough not to retaliate effectively but strong enough not to be easily victimized; and the scapegoat must be easily accessible and identifiable.

Typically, prejudice begins to appear at about the

preschool age and apparently is conveyed by the parenting persons in the child's life. While influenced by cultural norms and the significant group to which the person belongs, prejudices also vary with socioeconomic status, education and religious affiliation. Persons who are strongly prejudiced tend to have aggressive, authoritarian personalities which do not allow them to consider alternative views of the scapegoated object.

The alteration of prejudice (and other attitudes) is a complex process which involves variations on the basic theme of extended exposure to the prejudiced object over time. This allows the distorted facts to be recognized as such and negative affects to extinguish and be replaced with affiliative bonds. Other factors in prejudicial attitude change include: the creditability and prestige of the source; the source must display disinterest in changing the attitudes (e.g., "overheard" conversations); the source apparently argues a position against their own self-interest; arousal of emotions (except fear, which leads to further avoidance of the object); and, moderately held prejudices are easier to change than are extreme ones.

Values are the personal guide an individual develops that give direction to life. They help the person relate to the world and take decisive personal action. Values are usually developed later in life as the result of rational-conscious considerations of various alternatives, and usually have three aspects: choosing them consciously, prizing or feeling good about them and acting on them.

Human behavior is significantly affected by the *roles people play* under given conditions.

Scapegoating was explained earlier; however, it has been reported that persons who are subjected to scapegoating for protracted periods of time take on the attributes of the scapegoating role.

People from different professional, socio-economic, sexual and ethnic backgrounds display *illness* differently. For example, health professionals frequently won't recognize illness in themselves because of the "omnipotent" role forced on them by the culture. There is no more confining prison than being incarcerated on a pedestal. Women tend to seek more health care than men, even when the effects of pregnancy are controlled. Lower socioeconomic persons do not seek as much preventive care as do the middle and upper classes. Consequently, hospital stays for lower class persons tend to be longer because illness progresses further in its course before care is sought. Basically, lower socioeconomic status persons define illness when, in the course of dysfunction, there is impairment of earning power.

Ethnicity helps shape how individuals display their

TABLE 14-2. Sexual Stages

Stage	Female	Male
Excitement	Vaginal ballooning	
	Vaginal lubrication	Penile erection
	Nipple erection	Nipple erection
	Clitoral erection	
Plateau	Clitoral retraction	Testes increase in size
	Further vaginal ballooning	Additional penile engorgement HR, BP, Resp. increase
Orgasm	Vagina and uterus contract at about ¾ sec. intervals for 3–15 contractions.	Ejaculation of seminal fluid: Marked penile and prostrate contraction at .8 sec. for 3–4 major contractions. HR, BP, Resp. may increase further
Resolution	All changes return to unstimulated state within 30 minutes	All changes return to unstimulated state within 30 minutes.

illness. Cultures which encourage open display of emotions, e.g., Italians, will be volatile in expression, while less emotionally apparent cultures, e.g., Chinese, will endure in quiet reservation. Ethnicity also determines what health care person is sought—medicine man, priest, chiropractor, physician, midwife, etc.

The psychosocial environment provides at least four additional considerations. Hollingshead and Redlick demonstrated that some types of mental illness are more likely to receive medical treatment at earlier stages among the rich as compared to the poor; and, in cities compared with rural areas. There is a correlation between low socioeconomic status and severe symptom impairment, particularly schizophrenia. There does *not* seem to be a relationship between rural versus urban setting with regard to overall rates of mental disturbance. Rates for all functional psychosis tend to be higher in rural settings; and rates for neuroses and personality disorders appear higher for urban areas.

Holmes and Rahe established a strong relationship between life change events and illness. Their Social Readjustment Scale has proven effective in predicting relative mental and physical illness from cumulative social events such as divorce, Christmas holidays, etc.

Human Sexuality.   Reviewing developmental data presented above, the gender refers to sexual anatomy. The gender identity refers to the sexual role the child

TABLE 14-3. Sex and the Elderly

Stage	Female	Male
Excitement	Decreased vaso-congestion Delayed vaginal lubrication	Decreased vasocongestion Increased time to erect
Plateau	Vaginal expansion is reduced	Increased duration of erection and activity without orgasm Full erection not until entering orgasmic phase
Orgasm	Contractile phase reduced in duration	Slower ejaculatory experience with decreased contractions Prostatic contractions are absent
Resolution	Very rapid return to unstimulated state	Very rapid detumnescence of the penis

TABLE 14-4. Sexual Dysfunction

Stage	Female	Male
Excitement	General sexual dysfunction ("frigidity") Vaginismus (strong vaginal contractions) Dyspareunia (painful intercourse)—usually organic base	Erectile dysfunction ("impotence") Dyspareunia (painful intercourse)—usually organic base
Orgasm	Inorgasmia (usually due to low trust level of partner)	Inorgasmia (performance anxiety) Premature ejaculation (inadequate learning or control).

feels it belongs in—either that of a man or woman. Sex role identification means how the child through modeling (social learning), is taught to act, whether masculine or feminine. These three can be independent of each other.

Sexual behavior which is considered normal includes sexual excitement from birth until death; masturbation from early adolescence until death; same sex exploration from late childhood/early adolescence until opposite sex attachments occur in the late teens or early twenties; and opposite sex attachments in middle to late teens until death.

Masters and Johnson pioneered modern medicine's objective knowledge about adult human sexuality. Their work separates the human sexual response cycle into four phases. Table 14-2 summarizes their data, the work of Sherfey and Sadock and Sadock.

In addition to these states, a refractory period after orgasm occurs for males during which time he cannot erect or have additional orgasms. Females can be multiorgasmic. Recent data suggested some females may also have ejaculate at orgasm.

The normal effects of aging on the human sexual response are shown in Table 14-3. In the man over 60 years old, it has been observed that the refractory period is quite extended (to perhaps days) before the male can erect again.

The human sexual response cycle is biologically stable and apparently correlated with normal biochemical/physiological functioning. Dysfunction can occur at any or all of the stages of the cycle for both males and females. These dysfunctions are noted in Table 14-4. Generally, the etiology of these dysfunctions can

be traced to inadequate education and social programming, getting out of the "here and now pleasure" and anxiously going into remembered past or projected future, assuming a critical spectator role during sexual activity. It should also be noted that a number of primary physiologic illnesses (e.g., diabetes mellitus), aging and drug use (prescription and otherwise) can produce identical sexual dysfunctions.

The utilization of behavioral modification techniques, resolution of physical abnormalities and counseling towards improved communication between sexual partners (oriented to trust and taking personal responsibility for one's own pleasure) has resulted in high rates of resolution of these dysfunctions.

Besides the predominant heterosexual pattern there are *different sexual preferences* which form large subgroups within the population. While there is some minimal evidence that some of these preferences occur on a genetic basis, most are viewed as being the result of early learning experiences based in either the gender identity formation prior to age 3 or role identification issues later in childhood.

Kinsey reported that four per cent of adult white males live an exclusive *homosexual* existence, and about ten per cent are "more or less" exclusively homosexual for at least 3 years between the ages of 16 and 65. 48 per cent of adolscents report same sex genital play.

According to Kinsey, there are a third to a quarter as many female *(lesbians)* as male homosexuals. Apparently the discrepancy is correlated with relative definitions and differentially allowed or accepted behaviors between males and females in American society.

Transvestism is defined as intermittant but regular

dressing in clothes of the opposite sex, which the practicing transvestite finds sexually pleasurable. This syndrome in the United States is confined to males, since females are allowed to crossdress with no social proscriptions.

In these three conditions, the gender identity is consistent with the gender or biologic sex, and the major etiologic issue would seem to be one of gender identification.

Transexuality is apparently due to gender identity inversion (the gender identity is opposite of the biologic sex). Since first memories, these persons *feel* as if they are the opposite sexed person trapped in the body of the biologic sex of birth. They crossdress frequently from early childhood but it is not for sexual pleasure but role fulfillment. They usually are married with a family and, in middle years (30 to 50), seek surgical intervention to align the external genitalia with internal feelings.

Other sexual variances include Organic Based differences, such as Turner's syndrome and Klinefelter's Syndrome.

Functionally Based differences include *Pedophelia,* which is defined as sexual interest in young children. This syndrome is predominately heterosexual (95 per cent) and is illegal in all states. *Voyeurism* is sexual gratification from watching sexual acts or looking at sexual organs. This is believed to be confined to males; however, differential allowed (prosecuted) behavior between males and females must be considered. *Exhibitionism* is the compulsive need to expose one's genitals, usually only prosecuted in males as with the above syndromes. The act of exposure does not provide release of sexual tension, but the reaction from the female to the exposure does. Exacerbation of these syndromes apparently occurs when the male is faced with defeat, ego deflation or other threat to adult functioning. Theoretically these alternatives are taken because approaching a mature female in a situation where rejection is possible is too threatening.

While *incest* is a universal sexual taboo, high prevalence rates in some subgroups of the population are reported. Incest is defined as sexual activity between members of a family. Father (or step-father) and daughter is most common by report, although mother-son and sibling (heterosexual and homosexual) are not infrequent patterns. Typically parent-child incest is correlated with a family constellation in which the same sex parent as the child involved is an extremely poor and incompetent marriage partner who (at least passively) encourages and condones the relationship because it relieves that parent of unwanted and overwhelming responsibilities. Alcohol consumption is frequently involved in incest. While general statistics

imply this is a phenomenon of lower socioeconomic status persons, clinical experience suggests a differential legal prosecution and detection rate among the social classes.

Death and Dying

Death and the process of dying in the United States has become a hospital-focused issue, since today few Americans die in their homes. Elizabeth Kubler-Ross pioneered the therapeutic work in death and dying. Since that time, the process stages identified by her (listed below) have been recognized to accompany any serious health loss of which the patient is informed. That is, if the patient is informed of a serious, though not fatal illness, these stages can be observed; and, until the patient works through the stages, compliance with proper medical regimene is not good.

The Adult. The stages of dealing with death in an adult are:

Denial: The patient firmly insists there is a diagnostic error. Frequently, requests for independent validation are made or the patient disappears from the physician's practice.

Anger: In this phase the patient moves out of the denial stage and enters a phase of angrily asking the question "why me?"

Bargaining: As the anger is dissipated, the patient attempts to strike compromises with the physician, self or a diety. These frequently take the form of "If I can live until *(given time or event),* then I won't ask for more," or "I'll do *(usually a sacrifice)."* Temporary remissions during this phase frequently are interpreted by the patient as fulfillment of the bargain. These should be anticipated by medical personnel and carefully discussed with the patient to prevent over interpretation.

Sadness or depression: During this stage, the patient becomes fully cognizant of the terminal nature of the condition and emotionally experiences the finality of the diagnosis. The anger and bargaining of previous stages is replaced with appropriate sadness which accompanies any significant loss.

Acceptance: This is not a euphoric happiness but rather a condition in which the patient resolutely gives up the sadness and depression, puts their life in order and make plans to live out the remainder of their life with the given situation.

While these stages are listed as discrete entities, in reality they are fluid, and overlap each other. The individual moves in and out of a given stage in a progression-regression pattern; however, there is usually predominance of one stage over the others. The issue for the physician is *how* to tell the patient of a serious condition, not *whether* to tell the patient. Collusion between health care personnel and relatives not to inform the patient are ill advised. It should be the patient's choice not to hear (denial), not the physician's preference to withhold the information. Dying patients have also pointed up the serious error of the physician announcing to the patient what stage they are in as a way of circumventing dealing with the patient as a dying person. For example, "Oh, you're in the stage of anger, you'll be out of it soon and start bargaining with me."

The Child. The dying child poses special management issues. Because the child is in preoperational or concrete-operations stage, the full cognitive understanding of imminent death is not a true reality. The child comprehends it as going to sleep and from which the child believes (s)he will awaken. Willis reported that dying children do not fear death but rather they are most disturbed by separation from parents and mutilation that will make them different.

Management Issues. Commonly, physicians and other health care providers have avoided dealing with the dying patient by giving the patient no entree for discussion (busily making rounds and moving in and out of the patient's room quickly); geographically isolating the patient in a single room at the end of the hall and/or keeping the room door closed; making a contract with significant others not to inform the patient of the nature of the condition; extending unrealistic hope ("we're expecting a breakthrough any day") or automatically saying "you're going to be just fine"; and, maintaining a clouded sensorium in the patient through medication.

These realities, coupled with the American penchant for keeping dying relatives isolated in social institutions, has led to the "hospice" movement, where persons with terminal illnesses are assisted in their dying process by allowing the patient to be afraid and discuss the fear; providing physical contact in a warm, supportive atmosphere; allowing the patient to talk and cry about the loss; managing temporary remissions to not build unrealistic hope; providing as much dignity in the health care as is feasible; and using medications that provide pain relief without clouding the sensorium (e.g., Brompton's mixture, a combination of narcotics and stimulants).

Grief and Bereavement

The persons remaining after the loss of a loved one (and some authors report after the loss of a body part like a limb, breast, testicle, etc.) undergo predictable reactions. The grief and bereavement process reflects significant loss; therefore, it is related to the emotion sadness. The expression of these reactions is culturally determined and varies by ethnic subgroup. It is ex-

pected that the normal process of mourning should be completed within 6 to 12 months after loss. The grieving/mourning is a process not a condition; and, as such, changes with time like a contusion that is in the process of resolution.

The Adult. The stages of the grief process for adults are:

Acute disbelief or phase of protest: This may last for minutes, hours or days during which the individual is not fully aware the object is gone. It is a state of mental "shock" during which the person may intellectually know the loss has occurred, but not affectively experience it. Anger is often projected towards the physician, relatives and friends because these support people allowed the loved one to die or will not help the grieving person recover the loved one.

Grief work or phase of disorganization: In this second phase the grieving person develops an emotional sense of loss. The world is experienced as empty, meaningless and barren. The grieving person tends to withdraw from social contacts and isolates him/herself. Initially, mental activity is almost exclusively involved with memories of the lost object. Frequently, the mourner will report feeling the "presence" of the individual in the room or close by. As this stage continues, the mental preoccupation with the dead one and the withdrawal/isolation noted in the early part of this phase diminishes.

Resolution or phase of reorganization: Through the first two phases the mourner emerges with an acceptance that the loss is real. They have formed a new relationship with the loss object in terms of realistic memories, not vows to preserve the world, literally and figuratively, as it was the day the loss occurred. This phase signals that the grieving individual is ready to return to the world and form relations without experiencing guilt over fantasized unfaithfullness or what might have been.

Age-Related Grieving. Humans react differently to the death of another depending upon their age and ability to comprehend the loss. The conditions listed below are not rare or abnormal accompaniments of mourning.

Infants may withdraw from social contact, refuse to eat, and die if a mother figure is lost and not replaced. This condition, known as marasmus was discussed previously. *Children* will frequently react with hyperactivity and assume a jocular attitude. *Adolescents and young adults* may develop dissocial behavior including hypersexuality, delinquent activity and significant substance abuse. *Adults to elderly* often develop psychosomatic illnesses or an exacerbation of a previous pathologic condition; and, are highly vulnerable to physical disease. Again, substance abuse is a potential problem. *Elderly,* like infants, frequently withdraw from social contact and often die within the one year of mourning unless support system steps are taken to involve them in a life process.

Normal Variants. *Anticipatory grief* sometimes accompanies the death of someone who has had protracted illness. The grieving person has worked through the loss prior to the actual death and frequently at the time of demise is ready to begin establishing new relationships (guilt free) immediately. The major problems observed from this pattern are that the person may feel guilty because they are relieved at the death, and they are not reacting as others expect. *Delayed grief* is the maintaining of the affectless shock from stage I until a protracted period of time after the death. Often delayed grief is triggered by accidentally finding a possession of the dead person. It is as if the possession or event has "slipped through" a defense mechanism and triggered the grief.

Anniversary reactions are exacerbations of the pain, sadness and loss triggered by birthdays, wedding anniversarys or death anniversary of the dead person. Usually these decrease in intensity with years; however, when they serve as a trigger for a delayed grief reaction, the initial grieving may be of equal or more intensity than would have been expected with an immediate grief reaction.

Delayed grief reactions frequently appear in the person who was strong for the other grieving persons, made all funeral arrangements and postponed the mourning. Similarly persons who have been separated from a parent at a young age and subsequently learn of that parent's death may experience a variant of a delayed grief reaction. They mourned the loss with the original separation and with the final one they experience the old grief and also the anger that the parent died before a reuniting and resolution of desertion issues were managed. These delayed grief reactions can precipitate profound acute clinical depression with impulsive suicidal acts.

Abnormal Grief Patterns. Abnormal variants of the grief process are usually of two types. First the individual may become fixated in one of the age related reaction patterns noted above and not move beyond it. For example, an adolescent may react to the loss of a sibling, friend or parent with substance (drug) abuse. The substance abuse becomes a defense against addressing the loss. Consequently when the loss begins to surface (or the patient develops tolerance to the drug or begins to withdraw from it) drug use is increased to manage the uncomfortable feelings. Obviously, physicians who chronically medicate grieving patients are preventing the patient from appropriately working through the grief and sometimes create iatro-genic addiction. Second, the adult patient may become fixated in the second stage of the grief process and not move into resolution. If grieving extends more than 12 months, the patient should be assumed to be clinically depressed and be treated appropriately.

Substance Abuse

Substance or drug abuse involves use of psychoactive chemicals taken for nonmedical reasons in a nonprescriptive pattern which are harmful to the person or society. Basically these are alcohol, narcotics, sedative-hypnotics, psychedelics and stimulants. Definitions for substance abuse are not clear because substance abuse is socially defined and subject to social subgroup variation regarding "normal" or "deviant."

Alcoholism. This is best defined as that pattern of alcohol consumption which results in dysfunction in one or more of five areas: marital, social, legal, occupational or physical, and the person cannot stop drinking (the individual has *lost control* of consumption). Problem drinking is defined as problems in any or all of the same 5 areas; but when the person is confronted with these as a result of alcohol consumption, the person can alter the drinking pattern so it no longer creates the problem.

Addiction. Addiction is defined as the nonprescription use of a drug harmful to society and/or self which has the following properties:

Tolerance: increasing amounts of the drug are needed over time to achieve the same experience effect. This is a cellular, biochemical event.
Dependence: Abrupt cessation of use of the drug precipitates a recognizable withdrawal syndrome. Again this is a biochemical-physiologic condition.
Habituation: the drug is taken for the psychological effects and/or it may be taken out of "habit."

Prevalence. Prevalence data for substances of abuse vary with time and the substance in question. However, the figures of 9 to 10 per cent of *adult* Americans having alcoholism or problem drinking and 300,000 narcotics addicts seem to be stable consensual estimates of these problems. Statistics on prevalence of other drugs of abuse, particularly marijuana, indicate increases in use; however, whether this is a higher rate of actual use versus report of use is not clear at this time. What is true is that substance abuse is a significant health care problem and is extending to younger populations as well as all socioeconomic and ethnic groups.

Etiology. The etiologic theories of substance abuse (particularly alcoholism) fall into three major categories:

1. Physiologic and Biologic Models
   (a) Genetotropic issues include research on inherited metabolic defects which result in the need for greater than average consumption of some food stuffs such as alcohol.
   (b) Endocrine research data emphasize a defect which leads to episodic hypoglycemia. This produces emotional symptoms that stimulate drug taking to balance the system.
   (c) Normalizing effect of drugs. Multiple studies have demonstrated physiologic, biochemical and neurophysiologic differences between substance abusers and non-substances abusers which disappear *after* acute drug ingestion. Unfortunately, no presubstance abuse measures have been available on the subjects therefore it is not possible to know if observed differences are drug induced.
   (d) Genetic marker variables (inherited color blindness), genetic mice strains which drink alcoholically, and concordance rates between adopted children and biologic alcoholic parents all suggest a genetic component to substance abuse *for some persons.*
2. Psychological Models
   (a) The psychodynamic model focuses on unconscious conflicts and low self esteem as stress variables. The reinforcer of substance abuse is the stress reduction induced by the drug consumption.
   (b) Personality trait models have identified low stress tolerance, dependence, decreased self image, insecurity, impulsiveness and tolerance for deviant behaviors as traits associated with substance abuse.

   Both the psychodynamic and personality trait models have only identified their core findings in persons who are substance dependent. They have neither examined the dependent persons prior to the substance dependence nor presented data on the number of persons who possess the traits and are not substance dependent.
   (c) Behavioral learning models explain drug ingestion as a learned response which decreases felt stress. As a result of the chemical's properties and reported use, the body becomes physiologically dependent leading to continued drug use to avoid withdrawal.
3. Sociocultural Models
   (a) Cultural and socialization issues focus on cultural norms being established which promote substance abuse.
   (b) The cultural stress factors model relates substance abuse to the degree of stress and inner tension produced by the culture. It also explores the cultural drinking attitudes and the alternatives for stress management provided by the culture.
   (c) Familial pattern research is focused on role modeling with social learning providing the basis for the substance abuse.
   (d) Environmental instabilities and crises produce changes in individual life situations or social roles which precipitate instability, confusion and stress. In this model drugs are taken as a mechanism to decrease these conditions.

Drug Effects and Treatment. The effects of various psychoactive substances of abuse, their toxicology and some aspects of treatment are presented in Table 14-5. Different levels of drug toxicity involving different chemicals of abuse are frequently misdiagnosed as functional emotional disturbances. Most notably psychedelics and stimulants have produced conditions similar to acute manic or paranoid schizophrenic reactions; and phencyclidine (PCP) can present as a dissociated, catatonic (agitated or depressed) schizophrenic reaction. These toxic conditions can be complicated by unusually long abstinence syndromes from some drugs (sometimes weeks) presumably on the basis of the lipaphilic binding properties. Failure to obtain toxicologic studies on patients with distorted behavior patterns can result in improper medical regimens that exacerbate and/or prolong the episode rather than assist in its resolution. Sometimes inappropriate management due to inadequate diagnostic studies can be fatal.

Violence

Violence may be a special case of uncontrolled aggression or a separate entity that has independent etiologies. While aggression can be directed towards a single person, groups of people or an inanimate object, violence usually denotes interpersonal acts. For both aggression and violence, it is important to distinguish the intentionality of the act. That is, while war and crime are aggressive and violent acts, they are usually not premediated to do harm to an individual person.

In the United States, reported juvenile crime has increased 245 per cent over the last 13 years and one out of every nine youths below the age of 18 will be arrested and go through the court system. Data reported in 1977 regarding violence and school age children suggests the following involving teachers and peers: 100 murders, 12,000 armed robberies, 9,000 rapes, 204,000 aggravated assaults and 270,000 school burglaries. Most school violence is predictable and occurs during school hours, at midweek, in February,

TABLE 14-5. Drug Effects

Physiologic Aspects	Alcohol	Narcotics	Sedative Hypnotics	Psychedelics	Phencyclidine	Stimulants	Marijuana
Tolerance	X	X	X	X	X	X	X
Dependence	X	X	X		?	X	X
Habituation	X	X	X	X	X	X	X
Fatal in:							
a. Overdose	X	X	X	?	X	?	
b. Withdrawal from addiction	X		X		?		
Discomfort on withdrawal from addiction	X	X	X		?	X	?
Psychological Effects							
Pain blockade	X	X	X	X	X	X	?
Euphoria	X	X	X	X	X	X	X
Energy level							
increase	?			?	?	X	
Decrease	X	X	X	?	X		X
Anxiety							
decrease	X	X	X		X		X
Perceptual changes (e.g., hallucinogens)				X	X	X	X
Psychomotor impairment	X	X	X		X		X
Time sense changes	X	X	X	?	?	X	X
Toxicologic test available	X	X	X		X	X	
Treatment							
Titrated withdrawal recommended	X	?	X				
Chemical blockade available	X	X					
Antagonist available		X					

Adapted from the National Institute on Drug Abuse Medical Monograph Series (1976).

between classes, and to a victim who is a 7th grade male minority (minority in the school) who has been victimized before. The offender is usually the same age and sex and known to the victim.

Toch reported that adult acts of violence fall into the following categories: Preservation of self image (41 per cent): promoting (28 per cent), defending (13 per cent); pressure removing (12 per cent); as a tool (26 per cent): exploitation (10 per cent), bullying (6 per cent), self defense (6 per cent), self indulgence (6 per cent); norm enforcing (4 per cent); cathartic (3 per cent).

Specific data on the predictability of adult violence is not as clear as for youth. The major correlates are that most murders are a family affair in the heat of a quarrel; there is a strong correlation between alcohol consumption and violence/aggression (50 per cent of all arrests; 24 per cent of violent deaths; 50 to 64 per cent of all homicides—killer or victim; 34 per cent of all forcible rapes; and 41 per cent of all assaults); and, repressive social conditions precipitate outbursts of violence.

Four special forms of violence are frequently seen by the physician: chemically induced (most frequently alcohol, amphetamines or phencyclidine); child abuse (discussed above); spouse beating; and rape (⅓ occur in the victim's home; and most are executed by someone known to the victim, particularly if the victim is younger).

Recommendations for control of aggression (and perhaps violence) include: eliminate sources of frustration, don't reinforce aggressive behavior, reinforce nonaggressive behavior, eliminate associated objects (e.g., toy guns), provide alternatives to violence, react to aggression with nonaggression, and decrease the use of physical punishment.

Suicide

If aggression can't be directed appropriately, displaced or scapegoated, it may be turned upon the self and suicide occurs. Four different definitations or descriptions can be applied: anyone who takes their own life; taking one's own life where a given set of circumstances (physical health; environmental conditions, etc.) are so hopeless that a person actively "gives up"; taking one's own life where unexpressed hostility towards others is involved (e.g., "I'll show you, you son-of-a-bitch, you'll miss me when I'm gone"). Menninger wrote about this angry self-destruction as simultaneously containing the wish to kill, the wish to be killed, and the wish to die; and taking one's own life as an accompaniment of a serious depressive syndrome.

The latter three definitions all incorporate the feeling of hopelessness for change ("things will never get any better and I don't want to continue like this"). Hopelessness and loss of future orientation are the best predictors of active suicidal intent.

Statistically, approximately 26,000 persons in America are reported to commit suicide each year and about 10 times that number attempt it. The National Center for Health Statistics (1975) reported that in adolescents and college students (age 15 to 24) suicide is the third leading cause of death, homicide is second and accidents are first. It is likely that many accidents (particularly single person auto deaths) are truly suicides. Overall, suicide is one of the 10 leading causes of death in America.

The demographics correlated with successful suicides are (those with an asterisk are most significant): *previous attempts, *more males than females are successful (more females attempt it), *single, widowed or divorced, *living alone, *over 45 years old, *white, *unemployed, *a suicide note, *poor health, *early stages of recovery from depression (energy and concentration levels have improved to where the individual can make plans and carry them through), eight out of ten have given a warning, hits all social classes (relative standing is difficult to ascertain due to differential recording), 25 to 36 per cent are alcohol related, and it increases in incidence after a national crisis.

It is commonly reported that physicians have a higher rate of suicide than the general population; however, if socioeconomic status is controlled, their rate is not significantly different.

Since suicidal persons are only actively suicidal for a short period of time, appropriate management of the suicidal person should entail close supervision. Preferably this is done by a close support system (family or friends) on an ambulatory basis (admission to a mental hospital presupposes subsequent release and the rate for suicidal persons discharged from mental hospitals is 34 times that of the general population). However, if no adequate ambulatory support system is available, hospitalization is indicated.

Psychosocial Issues Associated with the Health Care Delivery System

The "Doctor-Patient" Relationship. A major factor in the care of patients is the rapport that develops between the physician and the patient. Rapport is not simply or necessarily that "I like you," it is the understanding each has of the other; *and* the cooperative effort to cure or control the patient's condition. That is, both the patient and the physician must be involved in the treatment process and the patient must actively attempt to "get well." This is best accomplished by the physician talking *with* the patient, not at them.

The verbal and non-verbal messages that physicians convey must be congruent and of a particular nature. The physician must be a warm, "nurturant parent." That does not necessarily mean totally permissive or all-giving. It does mean caring enough to sometimes set very specific boundaries ("I won't let you kill yourself") and being honest ("your test results and examination suggest you have a malignancy"). The physician must maintain a mature adult reality with all patients. The physician must have an active inventive mind to bring new solutions to patients problems; e.g.,

M.D.: Has the Valium worked?
PT: Yes.
M.D.: Good, now we can discontinue it. Or, in the opposite case:
PT: No.
M.D.: Well, we'll discontinue it and try for a better solution.

There are three major interviewing styles which will predictably produce different outcomes with patients. None are correct or incorrect; however, each can be used differentially for specific purposes.

Laundry List: the physician asks a series of preprogrammed, structured questions, which effectively communicates to the patient "I will tell you when to talk and what to talk about." This interview style is probably the *least* efficient in gathering data meaningful to the care of patients and certainly does the least to promote effective doctor-patient rapport. It is useful to structure persons with thought disorders or affective disorders (particularly mania) and to intervene in obsessive compulsive verbal detail. That is, it can assist some patients by structuring their internal state and maintaining effective communication patterns.

Associative: in this style, the physician listens to and observes the patient. Any communication from the physician is associated to what the patient is presenting. The physician inserts minimal structure into the interview. This is considered the most efficient method of relevant data collection first because more pertinent information is elicited than by laundry list interviewing; and second, the best rapport is developed. Obviously, those conditions listed above for which a laundry list interview is indicated are those for which the associative interview is contraindicated.

Open-ended: this format is not truely appropriate for general medical interviewing since it tends to focus on process rather than content issues. In true open-ended interviewing, whatever the patient wishes to verbalize is the topic at hand and no focus is necessary. This is useful in certain psychotherapeutic encounters, but not the greater majority of medical practice.

Some specific concepts for interviewing:

1. Support: any response (verbal or nonverbal) that demonstrates interest in, concern for or understanding of the patient.
2. Reassurance: a physician's response that helps the patient feel good about her/himself. These include feelings of merit and self-assurance.
3. Empathy: a response that informs the patient that the doctor recognizes the feeling a patient has; and, there is no judgement or criticism of that feeling (even though the doctor may feel that it is wrong).
4. Confrontation: a physician's response that points out to the patient the patient's feeling or behavior. Confrontation need not be a hostile or accusatory action.
5. Reflection: a response that echos or mirrors a portion of what a patient has just said. Generally this is intended to allow patients to become aware of what they have verbalized.
6. Interpretation: a confrontation from the physician based on inference rather than an observation; e.g., "given those frustrating events, I assume you became angry."
7. Silence: a physician can provide different types of verbal silence; interested silence, disinterested silence and withdrawn silence. However, silence is a very effective communication device.
8. Summation: a physician's response that reviews information given by the patient.

Legal and Ethical Considerations

The major controversial ethical considerations today, as in the past, are those associated with life and death.

Birth Control. A central issue is the physician's legal right to disseminate information and/or contraceptive devices to persons below the age of majority. While such information is available to adults in each state in the United States, some states maintain laws prohibiting the physician's dissemination of information to minors without parental consent.

Abortion. The arguments are multifaceted but include these major points: public financing of abortion for indigent persons; the general ethics of performing elective abortions; whether a wife, without consent of her husband, should be able to receive an abortion; the physical or mental health conditions under which abortions should be available.

The Patients' Right to Die. These are important issues: first, if the patient is of sound mind, is in severe discomfort and/or has a condition which, without medical support, will be fatal and the patient does not want the medical support; should it be withdrawn, particularly if the legal next of kin opposes the removal of life support system? Second, if the patient only has vital signs, there is clear indication that cortical death has transpired and auxiliary life support systems are presumably maintaining basic physiologic functioning, by whose authority can the life support systems be withdrawn?

The Patients' Right to Live. While this is beginning to be a focal issue, as medical economics tighten it will become more critical. It encompasses the reality that as medical science advances expensive technologies are developed. The available public health care dollar may not be able to subsidize these services for all persons who cannot personally afford them; and if private third-party health insurance carriers attempt to provide them, premium payments for all persons will increase sharply. However, if a mechanism is not provided for the less affluent, then "rich people" and "poor people" health care delivery will demonstrate more disparity than presently exists.

Parental Refusal of Child Medical Care. This life and death issue involves the emergent medical care of children whose parents reject medical intervention on religious or personal grounds. The basic legal maneuver to circumvent this difficulty has been to have the child declared a ward of the court and treatment effected. The aim is to provide care until the child is of legal and mental age to personally decide about medical intervention.

Legal Aspects. The issues that form a present major focus are those that surround informed consent and the committed "mentally ill" person.

1. *Informed consent* involves the patient knowing what a particular treatment regimen involves, including what specifically is being prescribed (medicine, surgery, etc.), what the probable outcomes are and what side effects are known to occur. The latter is particularly relevant both with

antipsychotic medications and their association with tardive dyskinesia, as well as the utilization of addictive drugs. If a patient is not physically or mentally able to comprehend the information, it is generally permissable to administer the least traumatic effective treatment, if that treatment is responsible medical practice. As soon as the patient is able to comprehend the management the patient must be fully informed. A better option (if available) is to discuss management with responsible family and follow their wishes. In either case, documentation with time and date is essential.

2. *Committed mentally ill.* Committed mentally ill adults legally are entitled to the following:

they must have treatment available

they can refuse treatment

they can require a jury trial to determine "sanity"

they retain their competence for conducting business transactions, marriage, divorce, voting, driving, etc.

the words "sanity" and "competence" are legal, not psychiatric terms. They refer to prediction of dangerousness, and all medical-psychological studies show that health care professionals cannot realiably and validly predict dangerousness.

the committed *only* lose the civil liberty to come and go

emergency detention can be effected by a physician and/or a law enforcement person for 48 hours pending a hearing

a physician can *detain* only, a judge can commit. With children, special rules exist:

physicians cannot detain. Besides parents, only juvenile courts have authority over children.

children can be committed only if: they are in imminent danger to self and/or others; they are unable to care for themselves in daily needs; the parents have absolutely no control over the child and the child is a danger (e.g., fire setter).

RESEARCH METHODOLOGIES FOR THE STUDY OF HUMAN BEHAVIOR

Statistical Distributions

In research, a statement of significant difference is made based on statistical probabilities. The statement, "the results are significant at the .05 level" means that by chance alone the results are expected 5 times out of 100. The often quoted statement should be remem-

bered, "statistics are like a light pole—they can be used for support as does the drunk or to illuminate a given area as does the sober person."

Normal Distribution. The "normal distribution" is the "bell shaped" curve, which has been used to describe human traits. The curve is presented below. The percentage figures given in this diagram reflect the proportion of events that fall within a given standard deviation of the curve. Abnormality is defined as the amount of deviation from the mean or statistical average, not by social agreement.

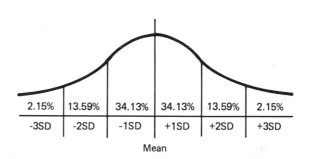

| 2.15% | 13.59% | 34.13% | 34.13% | 13.59% | 2.15% |
| -3SD | -2SD | -1SD | +1SD | +2SD | +3SD |

Mean

Irregular Distributions. Other distributions that do not have a "bell-shape" or normal curve are:

Bimodal

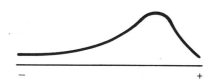

Skewed-negative

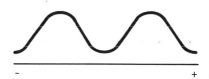

Skewed-positive

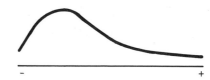

Skewed distributions are named in terms of their "tail."

Distribution Statistics. There are various statistics that describe the distribution of events (scores). The major ones are:

Measures of Central Tendency

1. *Mean* ($\overline{X}$) is the arithmetic average of all individual scores.
2. *Mode* is the most frequent score.
3. *Median* is the point above and below which 50 per cent of scores occur.

For normal distributions, these are all the same point.

Measures of Variation

1. *Standard Deviation (SD)* is the mathmatical expression of the variability of all scores around the mean. Usually plus and minus 1 SD is considered to be "normal variation"; e.g., if the $\overline{X}$ IQ score is 100 and the SD is 10, then "normal" scores would be 90 through 110.
2. *Variance* is the standard deviation squared.
3. *Range* is the highest and lowest scores of a distribution.

Research Concepts

Control Groups.   Control groups are the core of experimental designs. These are groups which are as identical as possible to the experimental group upon which experimentation is done; and, which hopefully only differ in the experimental treatment being applied. There are two major types of control groups.

No treatment control groups are used for example with pathologic groups where a disease exists. In this design, this control group doesn't get an investigational treatment. After treatment is applied to the experimental group, both groups are examined for improvement in disease course. Use of such a design helps examine treatment efficacy relative to spontaneous remission rates.

Same subject control groups are those where measurement on the criterion of change is taken before a treatment is applied, and again after the treatment. Scores are examined for significance of change. This design helps control extraneous factors which might arise from using a matched control design of totally independent persons.

Independent and Dependent Variables.   Independent variables are those which are manipulated; e.g., a given medication. Dependent variables are those which reflect the effects of the independent variable; e.g., decrease in a febrile condition after a certain medicine is administered.

Validity.   Validity refers to the true accuracy of the observed experimental effect. Using the above illustration, if the febrile condition decreased was it the effect of the medication or the differential time of day the temperature reading was taken? Generally, cross validation of an experimenter's results by independent researchers is required before a given conclusion is acceped as valid.

Reliability.   Reliability means with what regularity can the experimental effect be reproduced? Using the example from above, does the medication reduce the febrile condition 100 per cent of the time it is administered or 50 per cent of the time?

Epidemiologic Concepts.   Special statistics related to rates of occurence of a phenomenon in a given population or sample from the entire population are important in behavioral sciences. There are four major epidemiologic statistics. *Incidence* is the rate of *new* cases of a phenomenon in a given group of persons. *Prevalence* is the rate of *all* cases of a phenomenon in a group. *Morbidity* is the ratio of the number of ill persons to the total population of a community. *Mortality* is the death rate in a given population.

Research Designs

The manner in which data is collected on a given research topic constitutes the research design.

Longitudinal.   Longitudinal studies are those which track the same group of subjects (S s) over an extended time period. Periodic observations are made and changes in the group over time are tested for significance of change or are related through correlational statistics. This design can incorporate no treatment or same subject control groups and is employed when unpredictible extra-personal events like a world war may confound results.

A special form of longitudinal study is the treatment *followup design;* e.g., after patients have received a given treatment does the treatment last or is it a temporary phenomenon? This is a particularly relevant research question when the treatment is expensive in physicians' time, financial cost and/or social-personal consequences.

Cross Sectional.   Cross-sectional designs examine different groups at various levels of a given variable *all at the same time* and compare the different groups for a given effect; e.g., groups at ages 10, 20, 30, 40, 50, 60, and 70 are administered IQ tests (all on one day) and results compared to evaluate the hypothesis that IQ decreases with age. This design does not control for the extrapersonal events (such as living through a world war) which are controlled through the longitudinal design. This design is most applicable when one wishes to examine the effects of a given treatment on various levels of a variable; e.g., the response of different aged carcinomas to a given chemotheraputic regimen.

Double Blind. Double-blind designs are those in which neither the subject *(S)* nor the experimenter *(E)* knows if the treatment an *S* is receiving is true treatment or a "placebo." This design is useful to control the subjective bias of both the *S* and *E* which frequently, without awareness, enters the outcome of research.

Cross-Over. Cross-over designs are a combination of no treatment and same subject control groups in which to prove the efficiency of a given treatment, midpoint through the experiment, the experimental group is subjected to the events applied to the control group and vice versa. If the experimental treatment is effective the respective positions of the two groups relative to the dependent variable will shift. Or if treatment is permanent, the control group should approximate the experimental group. This is a powerful design and not only assures treatment effect, but also addresses the ethical issue of withholding a treatment for a group of persons (e.g., patients with carcinoma not receiving a given type chemotherapy).

Research Statistics

Research statistics in Behavioral Sciences essentially test how similar or how different groups of *S*s are.

Measure of Difference. Central to probability statistics based on the normal curve is testing if an observation is significant or if it is a common "chance" variation within the normal range.

Distribution data characterized by a mean and standard deviation can be tested to see if two groups (e.g., experimental and control) differ significantly on the dependent variable. This is done with the "*t*" test. This statistic compares the difference between the means of two samples using the standard deviations of each sample to "pace off" the distance between the two means. If the distributions don't overlap a great deal it is concluded the two groups are "significantly different." The size of the "*t*" value is determined by reference tables based on sample size and level of significance. The larger the sample and the lower the significance one is willing to accept the smaller the "*t*" and vice versa.

The "*F*" statistic is similar to "*t*" except the "*F*" statistic can compare more than two means at a time (e.g., different doses of a medication or the effects of different medications, time of day administered, and different doses of each on the dependent variable). The "*F*" statistic can reflect whether each of the independent variables is associated with the change in the dependent variable or whether it is the interaction between given variables that is significant.

Measures of Relationships. Besides the statistics of central tendency and variation used to test differences between groups and generally describe how a group of people present, there are also statistics of relationship between conditions.

The basic relationship statistic is the correlation coeffecient *(r)*. This statistic tells how two variables relate to or co-vary with each other. The *r* which is positive means as one variable increases so does the other; the *r* which is negative means as one variable increases the other decreases. The value of *r* can only range from 0.00 to 1.00; the higher the value the stronger the relation. Therefore *r* values can vary from -1.00 to $+1.00$. An $r = -.85$ expresses a stronger relation than an $r = +.75$. Correlational statistics can *NEVER* be interpreted as cause-effect. There are three possible interpretations to all correlational data. If the *r* is between variables a and b permissible interpretations are: a leads to b; b leads to a; or a and b are related through a third variable, c. Correlations can be tested for significance of the size of the correlation; i.e., significantly different from $r = 0$. One can also establish correlations among multiple variables. Multivariate analyses (e.g., factor analysis) are examples of this approach.

MULTIPLE CHOICE QUESTIONS

1. The latency phase of psychoanalytic theory occurs at the same time as which of Erikson's stages?
   (a) Trust vs mistrust
   (b) Identity vs role confusion
   (c) Industry vs inferiority
   (d) Autonomy vs shame & doubt
   (e) Initiative vs guilt

2. A 32-year-old housewife from an upper middle class background is married to an affluent junior executive who must travel a great deal. She does not work but pours herself into volunteer organizations, bridge club, working at the local orphanage, and visiting sick people in hospitals. In a social gathering she rather pointedly occupies the center of attention and generally gives the impression of "anything you can do, I can do better." She is also deathly afraid of riding on elevators. At which stage of Erikson's tasks of development is this woman fixated?
   (a) Initiative vs guilt
   (b) Industry vs inferiority
   (c) Identity vs role confusion
   (d) Intimacy vs isolation
   (e) Generativity vs stagnation

3. Which of the following defense mechanisms would you naturally expect to occur as a psycho-

logical concomitant of physical illness, where the person is placed in a hospital?

(a) Symbolization
(b) Regression
(c) Isolation
(d) Compensation
(e) Introjection

4. According to the *Diagnostic and Statistical Manual of Mental Disorders,* Edition II, (DSM-II), an IQ of 65 classifies a person as:

(a) borderline mental retardation
(b) mild mental retardation
(c) moderate mental retardation
(d) severe mental retardation
(e) pround mental retardation

5. Which of the following is *not* expected after one hour of sensory deprivation?

(a) Anxiety
(b) Depression
(c) Hostility
(d) Fugue
(e) Hallucinations

6. A 14-year-old male is brought into your office by his mother. They have had an argument over the length of his hair. The boy reacts to you in a hostile, argumentative fashion even though you have reasonably long hair, a beard, and have not provoked the reaction from the young man. You would say that the phenomenon which is occurring is:

(a) countertransference
(b) transference
(c) acting-out
(d) regression
(e) synthesis

7. With regard to children who have debilitating and terminal illness, their greatest fear is:

(a) pain
(b) death
(c) separation from parents
(d) what will become of their pets
(e) being anesthetized

8. In the prediction statistic, the correlation, the value which would have the most predictive power would be:

(a) +.95
(b) −.35
(c) 0
(d) −1.0
(e) +.65

9. Which of the following defense mechanisms is always pathological?

(a) Rationalization
(b) Isolation

(c) Denial
(d) Disassociation
(e) Conversion

10. In a crisis management of persons who abuse drugs, there are certain drugs of abuse from which persons often die if they are abruptly withdrawn from the substance. Which of the following preparations constitutes a danger of death from abrupt withdrawal?

(a) Stimulants
(b) Sedative hypnotics
(c) Psychedelics
(d) Opiates
(e) Volatiles

11. In the grieving and mourning process we know that at different ages the mourning can take different forms. Which of the following is an *INCORRECT* statement?

(a) The infant might protest, deny, and detach itself away.
(b) A child in the latency stage would probably be jocular and perhaps hypomanic.
(c) A child in the adolescent stage might turn to antisocial acting out.
(d) Middle-age persons quite frequently turn to hypochondriacal symptoms.
(e) Elderly persons typically are relieved and feel somewhat released.

12. The Thematic Apperception Test (TAT) is an example of what type of psychological test?

(a) Intelligence
(b) Achievement
(c) Ability
(d) Interest
(e) Personality

13. In speaking of orientation, four spheres are usually examined. All of the following are included *except:*

(a) relationship of self to a place in time
(b) awareness of self as a person
(c) knowledge of geographic location
(d) awareness of internal affective state
(e) knowledge of present position in time

14. In terms of etiology, anxiety is usually viewed as repressed or forgotten:

(a) fear
(b) guilt
(c) sorrow
(d) grief
(e) anger

15. All of the following are true statements about the memory process *except:*

(a) Long-term memory is rarely defective in organicity unless accompanied by psychosis.

(b) If memory loss occurs, recovery is typically from the extremes of loss to the precipitating event.

(c) Memory is particularly disrupted with bilateral lesions of the hippocampus and/or mammilary bodies.

(d) In general, memory defect is psychogenic if there is no disturbance of consciousness and no intellectual impairment.

(e) If there is short-term memory loss and motivation and attention is good, it is suggestive of psychogenic involvement.

16. In Freudian theory, a child who has begun to be strongly attached to the parent of the opposite sex and display some "fear" of the parent of the same sex would be in which stage of psychosexual development?
(a) Oral
(b) Latent
(c) Anal
(d) Phallic/urethral
(e) Genital

17. All of the following are considered to be functions of the ego *except:*
(a) personal values
(b) defense mechanisms
(c) object relations
(d) reality testing
(e) thought processes

18. In Erikson's theory of psychological tasks, which of the following is *not* a correct task?
(a) Integrity vs despair
(b) Industry vs inferiority
(c) Intimacy vs isolation
(d) Generativity vs stagnation
(e) Identity vs shame and doubt

19. The patient states: "I feel uptight about my new job." This is an example of:
(a) objective evidence of anxiety
(b) subjective evidence of anxiety
(c) inappropriate affect
(d) repression of affect
(e) a drive discharge emotion

20. All of the following are examples of psychophysiologic responses to anxiety *except:*
(a) excessive perspiration
(b) tension headaches, constriction in the chest, backache

(c) aphasia, apraxia, and a right homoymus hemianopsia
(d) dyspnea, dizziness, and paresthesias
(e) transient systolic hypertension, premature contractions and tachycardia

21. A student did poorly on an examination which was given in a specific room. The student is afraid he will fail the course. On the next occasion he walks into the room he experiences fear. This is an example of:
(a) classical conditioning learning
(b) social learning
(c) cognitive learning
(d) inhibition learning
(e) fixed schedule learning

22. In learning theory, grades in an academic course would be an example of:
(a) acquisition
(b) generalization
(c) primary reinforcers
(d) secondary reinforcers
(e) ratio reinforcement

23. All of the statements below regarding adolescence (age 13 to 18) are true *except:*
(a) in Erikson's framework the basic task to be resolved is to develop affiliation with others.
(b) 50 per cent of teenage marriages occur because of pregnancy
(c) One-third of teenage marriages end in divorce within 4 years
(d) are in Piaget's stage of formal operations
(e) must maintain a sense of identity in the face of rapid changes

ANSWERS TO MULTIPLE CHOICE QUESTIONS

1. (c)	7. (c)	13. (d)	19. (b)
2. (a)	8. (d)	14. (a)	20. (c)
3. (b)	9. (e)	15. (e)	21. (a)
4. (b)	10. (b)	16. (d)	22. (d)
5. (d)	11. (e)	17. (a)	23. (a)
6. (b)	12. (e)	18. (e)	

Index